MEDICAL ASSISTING CLINICAL SKILLS CD QUICK LOCATOR

This is your link to *Delmar's Medical Assisting Clinical Skills* CD-ROM, which is found on the inside back cover of this book.

Text Chapter	Skills and Their Location on the CD-ROM	Text Chapter	Skills and Their Location on the CD-ROM
9	CPR	21	Cold Treatment
9	Heimlich	21	ROM Exercises
9	Accidental Poisoning	21	Assisting with Crutches
10	Handwashing	21	Elastic Bandaging
10	Gloves and Gowns	21	Splint
10	Removing Items	21	Arm Sling
10	Sterile Gloves	21	Casting
12	Taking a Temperature	21	Cast Care
12	Taking a Pulse	24	Oral Meds
12	Counting Respirations	24	Ear Meds
12	Taking a Blood Pressure	24	Eye Meds
12	Weighing	24	Skin/Topical Meds
18	Clean Catch Urine	24	Nasal Meds
18	Testing Urine	24	Rectal Meds
18	Collecting Nose, Throat, Sputum Specimens	24	Nebulized Meds
18	Testing for Occult Blood	24	Intradermal Injection
18	Skin Puncture	24	Subcutaneous Injection
18	Blood Glucose	24	Intramuscular Injection
18	Oxygen Therapy	24	Z-Track Injection
18	Peak Expiratory Flow	24	Vial
19	Sterile Gloves	24	Ampule
19	Handwashing	24	Mixing Meds
19	Gloves and Gowns	25	EKG
19	Removing Items	28	Venipuncture
19	Wound Specimen	30	Clean Catch Urine
19	Bandaging	30	Testing Urine
19	Dry Dressing	31	Wound Specimen
19	Sutures/Staples	32	Collecting Nose, Throat, Sputum Specimen
21	Safe Lifting	32	Occult Blood
21	Safe Falling	32	Skin Puncture
21	Moist Heat	32	Blood Glucose
21	Dry Heat	32	Wound Specimen

DELMAR'S CLINICAL MEDICAL ASSISTING

Delmar's **CLINICAL**

MEDICAL ASSISTING

2nd Edition

Wilburta Q. Lindh

Marilyn S. Pooler

Carol D. Tamparo

Joanne U. Cerrato

DELMAR

THOMSON LEARNING ™

Australia   Canada   Mexico   Singapore   Spain   United Kingdom   United States

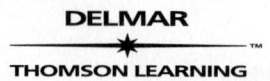

DELMAR

THOMSON LEARNING

Delmar's Clinical Medical Assisting, 2nd Edition
by Wilburta Q. Lindh, Marilyn S. Pooler, Carol D. Tamparo, and Joanne U. Cerrato

Health Care Publishing Director:
William Brottmiller

Executive Marketing Manager:
Dawn F. Gerrain

Production Coordinator:
John Mickelbank

Acquisitions Editor:
Rhonda Dearborn

Executive Editor:
Cathy L. Esperti

Art/Design Coordinator:
Mary Colleen Liburdi

Senior Developmental Editor:
Elisabeth F. Williams

Project Editor:
David Buddle

Cover Design:
The Drawing Board

Editorial Assistant:
Jill Korznat

Technology Manager:
Laurie Davis

Technology Assistant:
Sherry McGaughan

For permission to use material from this text or product, contact us by
Tel   800-730-2214
Fax 800-730-2215
www.thomsonrights.com

Library of Congress Cataloging-in-Publication Data

Delmar's clinical medical assisting / Wilburta Q. Lindh . . . [et al.].—2nd ed.
      p. cm.
   Includes bibliographical references and index.
   ISBN 0-7668-2426-8
   1. Physicians' assistants.   2. Clinical competence.
   I. Title: Clinical medical assisting.   II. Lindh, Wilburta Q.
R697.P45 D45 2001
610.73'7—dc21

                                          2001047099

NOTICE TO THE READER

Publisher does not warrant or guarantee any of the products described herein or perform any independent analysis in connection with any of the product information contained herein. Publisher does not assume, and expressly disclaims, any obligation to obtain and include information other than that provided to it by the manufacturer.

The reader is expressly warned to consider and adopt all safety precautions that might be indicated by the activities herein and to avoid all potential hazards. By following the instructions contained herein, the reader willingly assumes all risks in connection with such instructions.

The publisher makes no representation or warranties of any kind, including but not limited to, the warranties of fitness for particular purpose or merchantability, nor are any such representations implied with respect to the material set forth herein, and the publisher takes no responsibility with respect to such material. The publisher shall not be liable for any special, consequential, or exemplary damages resulting, in whole or part, from the readers' use of, or reliance upon, this material.

CONTENTS

Managing Authors   xiii

Acknowledgments   xiv

Reviewers   xv

Contributors   xvi

List of Procedures   xvii

Preface   xix

How to Use This Book   xxii

How to Use the Medical
Assisting Clinical Skills CD-ROM   xxiv

SECTION I: GENERAL PROCEDURES   1

Unit 1:   Introduction to Medical
           Assisting and Health
           Professions   2

Chapter 1: Medical Assisting as a
            Profession   3

Personal Attributes of the
Professional 4
Empathy 5
Attitude 5
Dependability 5
Initiative 5
Flexibility 5
Desire to Learn 6
Physical Attributes 6
Ability to Communicate 7
Ethical Behavior 7
Historical Perspective of
Medical Assisting 7
American Association of
Medical Assistants 8
Accreditation 8
Certification 8
Continuing Education 9
Registered Medical Assistant . . 9

Education of the Professional
Medical Assistant 9
Preparation for Externship . . . 10
Career Opportunities 11
Regulation of Health Care
Providers 11
Scope of Practice 11

Chapter 2: Health Care Settings and
            the Health Care Team   15

Ambulatory Health Care
Settings 16
Individual and Group Medical
Practices 16
Urgent Care Centers 17
Managed Care Operations . . . 17
The Impact of Managed Care
in the Health Care Setting . . 18
The Health Care Team 18
The Role of the Medical
Assistant 18
Health Care Professionals and
Their Roles 19
Allied and Other Health
Professionals and Their Roles . . 21
The Role of Integrative or
Alternative Health Care
Therapies 24
The Value of the Medical
Assistant to the Health Care
Team 25

Chapter 3: History of Medicine   29

Cultural Heritage in
Medicine 30
Medical Specialists 30
Medical Education 31
Attitudes toward Illness 31
Medical Treatments 32
Significant Contributions to
Medicine 33
New Frontiers in Medicine . . 34

⊙ For practice activities, this icon
tells you when to turn to *Delmar's
Medical Assisting Clinical Skills*
CD-ROM in the back of the book.

v

Unit 2:   The Therapeutic Approach   36

Chapter 4:   Therapeutic Communication Skills   37
Importance of Communication 39
Cultural Influence on Therapeutic Communication 39
Biases and Prejudices 40
The Communication Cycle . . 40
The Sender 40
The Message 40
The Receiver 41
Feedback 41
Listening Skills 41
Verbal Communication 41
The Five Cs of Communication 41
Nonverbal Communication . 42
Facial Expression 43
Territoriality 43
Posture 43
Position 44
Gestures and Mannerisms 44
Touch 44
Congruency in Communication 44
Perception 45
Maslow's Hierarchy of Needs . 45
Technology and Communication 45
Roadblocks to Therapeutic Communication 45
Defense Mechanisms 46
Introjection 46
Denial 46
Compensation 46
Regression 46
Repression 46
Sublimation 46
Projection 46
Displacement 46
Rationalization 47
Interview Techniques 47
Telephone Techniques 47

Chapter 5:   Coping Skills for the Medical Assistant   51
What Is Stress? 52
Adaptation to Stress 52
Coping with Stress 53
What Is Burnout? 54
Burnout in the Workplace . . . 54
What to Do If You Are Burned Out 55
Preventing Burnout 55
Goal Setting as a Stress Reliever 55

Chapter 6:   The Therapeutic Approach to the Patient with Life-Threatening Illness   59
Life-Threatening Illness 60
Cultural Perspective on Life-Threatening Illness 60
Choices in Life-Threatening Illness 61
The Range of Psychological Suffering 62
The Therapeutic Response to the Patient with AIDS 62
The Challenge for the Medical Assistant 63

Unit 3:   Responsible Medical Practice   66

Chapter 7:   Legal Considerations   67
Civil and Criminal Law 69
Medical Practice Acts and the Medical Assistant's Role 69
Patient Rights 69
The Physician, the Medical Assistant, and the Law 69
Contracts 69
Termination of Contracts 71
Standard of Care and the 4 Ds of Negligence 72
Torts 72
Battery 73
Defamation of Character 74
Invasion of Privacy 74
Medical Records 74
Informed Consent 74
Implied Consent 75
Consent and Legal Incompetence 75
Subpoenas 75
Confidentiality 76
Statute of Limitations 76
Public Duties 76
Drug Screening 76
AIDS 77
Abuse 77
Good Samaritan Law 77
Physician's Directives 78
Americans with Disabilities Act (ADA) 78

Chapter 8:   Ethical Considerations   83
Ethics Defined 84
Bioethics Defined 85
Keys to the AAMA Code of Ethics 86
AMA Ethical Guidelines . . . 87
Advertising 87
Media Relations 87
Confidentiality 87
Medical Records 88
Professional Fees and Charges 88
Professional Rights and Responsibilities 88
Abuse 88
Bioethical Dilemmas 89
Allocation of Scarce Medical Resources 89
Abortion and Fetal Tissue Research 89
Genetic Engineering/ Manipulation 90
Artificial Insemination/ Surrogacy 90
Dying and Death 90
HIV and AIDS 90

Chapter 9:   Emergency Procedures and First Aid   93
⊚ **CPR**
⊚ **Heimlich**
⊚ **Accidental Poisoning**
Recognizing an Emergency . . 95
Responding to an Emergency . 95
Primary Survey 96
Using the 911 or Emergency Medical Services System 97
Good Samaritan Laws 97
Blood, Body Fluids, and Disease Transmission 97
Preparing for an Emergency . 97
The Medical Crash Tray or Cart 98
Common Emergencies 99
Shock 99
Wounds 100
Burns 101
Musculoskeletal Injuries 105
Heat- and Cold-Related Illnesses 107
Poisoning 107
Sudden Illness 108
Cerebral Vascular Accident (CVA) 110
Heart Attack 110
Procedures for Breathing Emergencies and Cardiac Arrest 111
Heimlich Maneuver (Abdominal Thrust) 111
Rescue Breathing 112
Cardiopulmonary Resuscitation (CPR) 112

SECTION II: CLINICAL PROCEDURES   129

Unit 4:   Integrated Clinical Procedures   130

Chapter 10:   Infection Control, Medical Asepsis, and Sterilization   131
⊚ **Handwashing**
⊚ **Gloves and Gowns**
⊚ **Removing Items**
⊚ **Sterile Gloves**
Impact of Infectious Diseases 133
The Process of Infection . . 134
Chain of Infection 134

Infectious Agents 134
Reservoir 137
Portal of Exit 137
Means of Transmission 137
Portal of Entry 137
Susceptible Host 137
The Body's Defense
Mechanisms for Fighting
Infection and Disease 138
Inflammatory Response 138
The Immune System and
Immunity 138
Stages of Infectious
Diseases 140
Incubation Stage 140
Prodromal Stage 140
Acute Stage 140
Declining Stage 140
Convalescent Stage 140
Disease Transmission 140
Acquired Immunodeficiency
Syndrome and Hepatitis B . . 140
AIDS 142
Acute Viral Hepatitis
Diseases 142
Transmission of HIV and
HBV 142
Principles of Infection
Control 142
The Centers for Disease Con-
trol and Prevention, and Its Role
in Infection Control 142
Universal Precautions 145
Standard Precautions 146
Transmission-Based
Precautions 146
Blood and Body Fluids 146
Personal Protective
Equipment 150
Needlestick 150
Disposal of Infectious Waste . . 150
Occupational Safety and
Health Administration
(OSHA) Regulations 150
The Bloodborne Pathogen
Standard 151
OSHA Regulations and
Students 159
Avoiding Exposure to
Bloodborne Pathogens 162
Medical Asepsis 163
Handwashing 163
Sanitization 163
Disinfection 164
Surgical Asepsis and
Sterilization 165
Gas Sterilization 165
Dry Heat Sterilization 165
Chemical Sterilization 165
Steam Sterilization
(Autoclave) 166

**Chapter 11: Taking a Medical History,
the Patient's Chart,
and Methods of
Documentation   183**

The Function of the Medical
History 185
The Cross-Cultural Model . . 185
Patient Information
Forms 185
Administrative or
Demographic Data Forms . . . 185
Medical Forms 186
Computerized Health
History 189
The First Office Contact . . 189
Telephone Contact. 189
Personal Visit 189
Emergency Visit 189
Completing the Medical
History Forms 189
Interacting with the Patient. . 189
Displaying Cultural
Awareness 190
Handling a Difficult Patient . . 191
Dealing with Sensitive
Topics 191
Parts of the Medical
History 192
Chief Complaint 192
Present Illness 192
Past Medical History 192
Family History 193
Social History 193
Review of Systems 194
The Patient's Record and
Its Importance 195
Contents of Medical Records 195
Methods of Charting/
Documentation 195
Source-Oriented Medical
Records 195
Problem-Oriented Medical
Records 196
Computer-Modified Records . . 196
SOAP Method of
Charting 198
Abbreviations Used in
Charting 198
Correcting an Error 198
Chart Organization 199

**Chapter 12: Vital Signs and
Measurements   205**

◉ **Taking a Temperature**
◉ **Taking a Pulse**
◉ **Counting Respirations**
◉ **Taking a Blood Pressure**
◉ **Weighing**
The Importance of
Accuracy 207
Temperature 207
Terms Used to Describe Body
Temperature 208
Types of Thermometers 208
Recording Temperature 210
Measuring Temperature 210
Cleaning and Storage of
Thermometers 211
Pulse 212

Pulse Sites 212
Measuring a Pulse 213
Normal Pulse Rates 213
Pulse Abnormalities 213
Recording Pulse Rates 213
Respiration 213
Respiration Rate 214
Abnormalities 214
Blood Pressure 215
Equipment for Measuring
Blood Pressure 215
Measuring Blood Pressure . . . 216
Recording Blood Pressure
Measurement 217
Normal Blood Pressure
Readings 217
Blood Pressure
Abnormalities 217
Height and Weight 218
Height 218
Weight 219
Significance of Weight 219
Measuring Chest
Circumference 219

**Chapter 13: The Physical
Examination   235**

Methods of Examination . . 236
Observation or Inspection . . . 236
Palpation 237
Percussion 237
Auscultation 238
Mensuration 238
Manipulation 238
Positioning and Draping . . . 239
Examination Positions 239
Equipment and Supplies for
the Physical Examination . . 241
Basic Components of a
Routine Physical
Examination 242
Patient Appearance 242
Gait 242
Stature 242
Posture 242
Body Movements 242
Speech 243
Breath Odors 243
Nutrition 243
Skin and Appendages 243
The Physical Examination
Sequence 243

**Unit 5:   Assisting with Specialty
Examinations and
Procedures   256**

**Chapter 14: Obstetrics and
Gynecology   257**

Obstetrics 259
Initial Prenatal Visit 259
Subsequent or Return
Prenatal Visits 262
Complications of Pregnancy . 262

Parturition 264
Postpartum Period 264
Gynecology 265
The Gynecological
Examination 265
Gynecological Diseases and
Conditions 269
Other Diagnostic Tests Used
to Detect Female Reproductive
System Diseases 270

Chapter 15: Pediatrics   281
What Is Pediatrics? 282
Preparation of Vaccines for
Administration 284
Recommended Vaccination
Schedule 284
Growth Patterns 285
Developmental Patterns 285
Measuring the Infant or
Child 285
Height and Weight
Measurements 285
Height and Weight
Measuring Devices 289
Measuring Head
Circumference 289
Measuring Chest
Circumference 290
Pediatric Vital Signs 290
Temperature 290
Pulse 291
Respirations 291
Blood Pressure 292
Collecting a Urine
Specimen from an Infant . . 292
Screening Infants for
Hearing Impairment 292
Screening Infant and Child
Visual Acuity 292
Common Disorders and
Diseases 293
Otitis Media 293
The Common Cold 294
Tonsillitis 294
Pediculosis 294
Asthma 294
Child Abuse 294

**Chapter 16: Male Reproductive
System   303**
Testicular Examination . . . 304
Disorders of the Male
Reproductive System 306
Benign Prostatic Hypertrophy 306
Prostatitis 306
Prostate Cancer 306
Testicular Cancer 307
Sexually Transmitted
Diseases 307
Assisting with the Male
Reproductive Examination . 308
Diagnostic Tests and
Procedures 308
Vasectomy 308
Semen Analysis 308

Chapter 17: Gerontology   311
Societal Bias 312
Facts about Aging 313
Physiological Changes 313
Senses 313
Integumentary System 314
Nervous System 314
Musculoskeletal System 314
Respiratory System 314
Cardiovascular System 314
Gastrointestinal System 315
Urinary System 315
Reproductive System 315
Prevention of
Complications 315
Psychological Changes 316
The Medical Assistant and
the Geriatric Patient 316
Memory-Impaired Older
Adults 316
Visually Impaired Older
Adults 317
Elder Abuse 318

**Chapter 18: Examinations and
Procedures of Body
Systems   321**
◉ **Clean Catch Urine**
◉ **Testing Urine**
◉ **Collecting Nose, Throat,
Sputum Specimens**
◉ **Testing for Occult Blood**
◉ **Skin Puncture**
◉ **Blood Glucose**
◉ **Oxygen Therapy**
◉ **Peak Expiratory Flow**
Urinary System 323
Signs and Symptoms of
Urinary Conditions and
Disorders 323
Diagnostic Tests 323
Urinary Catheterization 326
Digestive System 328
Signs and Symptoms of
Digestive Conditions and
Disorders 330
Diagnostic Tests 331
Fecal Occult Blood Test 334
Sensory System 335
The Eye 335
The Ear 340
Respiratory System 343
Spirometry 343
Musculoskeletal System . . . 344
Fractures, Casting, and Cast
Removal 346
Cast Care Guidelines 347
Neurological System 347
Components of a
Neurological Screening 349
Circulatory System 350
Blood and Lymph System . . 351
Integumentary System 352
Allergy Skin Testing 354

**Unit 6:   Advanced Techniques
and Procedures   382**

**Chapter 19: Assisting with Minor
Surgery   383**
◉ **Sterile Gloves**
◉ **Handwashing**
◉ **Gloves and Gowns**
◉ **Removing Items**
◉ **Wound Specimen**
◉ **Bandaging**
◉ **Dry Dressing**
◉ **Sutures/Staples**
Surgical Asepsis 385
Handwashing for Surgical
Asepsis 385
Sterile Principles 385
Common Surgical Procedures
Performed in Physicians'
Offices and Clinics 386
Alternative Surgical
Methods 387
Electrosurgery 387
Cautery 387
Cryosurgery 388
Laser Surgery 388
Suture Materials and
Supplies 388
Suture/Ligature 388
Suture Needles 389
Instruments 389
Structural Features 389
Categories and Uses 389
Care of Instruments 398
Chemical "Cold"
Sterilization 399
Supplies and Equipment . . . 399
Sponges and Wicks 399
Solutions/Creams/
Ointments 400
Dressings and Bandages 400
Anesthetics 403
Patient Care and
Preparation 404
Patient Preparation and
Education 404
Informed Consent 404
Medical Assisting
Considerations 404
Postoperative Instructions . . . 404
Wounds, Wound Care, and
the Healing Process 404
Basic Surgery Setup 406
Basic Rules and Concepts
for Setup of Surgical Trays . . . 406
Minor Surgery Process 406
Preparation for Minor
Surgery 406
Using Dry Sterile Transfer
Forceps 408

Chapter 20: Diagnostic Imaging   431
X-ray Machine 432
Radiation Safety 432
Contrast Media 433
Patient Preparation 433

Positioning the Patient 435
Fluoroscopy 436
Diagnostic Imaging 436
Ultrasonography 436
Positron Emission
Tomography (PET) 437
Computerized Tomography
(CT) 437
Magnetic Resonance
Imaging (MRI) 438
Flat Plates 438
Filing Films and Reports 439
Radiation Therapy 439
Nuclear Medicine 440

**Chapter 21: Rehabilitation and
Therapeutic Modalities   443**
◉ **Safe Lifting**
◉ **Safe Falling**
◉ **Moist Heat**
◉ **Dry Heat**
◉ **Cold Treatment**
◉ **ROM Exercises**
◉ **Assisting with Crutches**
◉ **Elastic Bandaging**
◉ **Splint**
◉ **Arm Sling**
◉ **Casting**
◉ **Cast Care**
The Role of the Medical
Assistant in Rehabilitation . 445
Principles of Body
Mechanics 445
Posture 445
Using the Body Safely and
Effectively 446
Lifting Techniques 448
Transferring Patients 448
Assisting Patients to
Ambulate 449
Assistive Devices 449
Walkers 449
Crutches 450
Canes 453
Wheelchairs 454
Therapeutic Exercises 455
Range of Motion 455
Muscle Testing 455
Types of Therapeutic
Exercise 456
Electromyography 456
Electrostimulation of
Muscle 456
Range of Motion Exercises . . 456
Therapeutic Modalities . . . 457
Heat and Cold 457
Moist and Dry Heat
Modalities 458
Moist and Dry Cold
Modalities 460
Deep Tissue Modalities 460

**Chapter 22: Nutrition in Health
and Disease   475**

Nutrition and Digestion . . . 476
Types of Nutrients 476
Energy Nutrients 477
Other Nutrients 480
Reading Food Labels 485
Items on the Nutrition
Label 486
Comparing Labels 486
Nutrition at Various Stages
of Life 486
Pregnancy and Lactation . . . 486
Infancy 488
Adolescence 488
Elderly 488
Therapeutic Diets 488
Weight Control 488
Diabetes Mellitus 489
Cardiovascular Disease 489
Cancer 490
Diet and Culture 491

Chapter 23: Basic Pharmacology   497

Medical Uses of Drugs 499
Drug Names 499
History and Sources of
Drugs 499
Plant Sources 499
Animal Sources 499
Mineral Sources 499
Synthetic Drugs 500
Genetically Engineered
Pharmaceuticals 500
Drug Regulations and Legal
Classifications of Drugs . . . 500
Controlled Substance Act
of 1970 500
Prescription Drugs 502
Nonprescription Drugs 503
Proper Disposal of Drugs . . . 503
Administer, Prescribe,
Dispense 504
Drug References and
Standards 505
How to Use the PDR 505
Other Reference Sources . . . 506
Classification of Drugs 506
Principle Actions of Drugs . 506
Factors that Affect Drug
Action 506
Undesirable Actions of
Drugs 508
Drug Routes 508
Forms of Drugs 509
Liquid Preparations 509
Solid and Semisolid
Preparations 509
Other Drug Delivery
Systems 509
Storage and Handling of
Medications 510
Emergency Drugs and
Supplies 510
Drug Abuse 511
Effects of Drug Abuse 511

**Chapter 24: Calculation of Medication
Dosage and Medication
Administration   515**
◉ **Oral Meds**
◉ **Ear Meds**
◉ **Eye Meds**
◉ **Skin/Topical Meds**
◉ **Nasal Meds**
◉ **Rectal Meds**
◉ **Nebulized Meds**
◉ **Intradermal Injection**
◉ **Subcutaneous Injection**
◉ **Intramuscular Injection**
◉ **Z-Track Injection**
◉ **Vial**
◉ **Ampule**
◉ **Mixing Meds**
Legal and Ethical
Implications of Medication
Administration 517
Ethical Considerations 517
The Medication Order 517
The Prescription 517
Drug Dosage 518
Age 518
Weight 518
Gender 519
Other Factors 519
The Medication Label 519
Calculation of Drug
Dosages 520
Understanding Ratio 520
Understanding Proportion . . 521
Weights and Measures 521
Medications Measured in
Units 524
How to Calculate Unit
Dosages 524
Insulin 525
Diabetes 525
Calculating Adult
Dosages 526
Calculating Children's
Dosages 527
Body Surface Area 528
Kilogram of Body Weight . . . 529
Administration of
Medications 529
The "Six Rights" of Proper
Drug Administration 530
Medication Error 532
Patient Assessment 532
Administration of Oral
Medications 533
Equipment and Supplies for
Oral Medications 533
Administration of Parenteral
Medications 533
Hazards Associated with
Parenteral Medications 534
Reasons for Parenteral Route
Selection 534

Parenteral Equipment and
Supplies 534
Site Selection and Injection
Angle 539
Marking the Correct Site for
Intramuscular Injection 539
Basic Guidelines for
Administration of
Injections 542
Z-Track Method of
Intramuscular Injection . . . 544
Administration of
Allergenic Extracts 544
Inhalation Methods of
Medication Administration . 545
Implications for Patient
Care 545
Administration of Oxygen . . 545

Chapter 25: Electrocardiography   565

◉ EKG
Anatomy of the Heart 567
Electrical Conduction
System of the Heart 568
The Cardiac Cycle and
the ECG Cycle 569
Calculation of Heart Rate
on ECG Graph Paper 569
Types of Electrocardio-
graphs 570
Single-Channel ECG 570
Multichannel ECG 571
Automatic ECG Machines . . 572
ECG Telephone
Transmissions 572
Facsimile Electrocardiograph 572
Interpretive Electro-
cardiograph 572
ECG Equipment 572
Electrocardiograph Paper . . . 572
Electrolyte 572
Sensors or Electrodes 573
Care of Equipment 574
Lead Coding 574
The Electrocardiograph
and Lead Placement 574
Standard Limb or Bipolar
Leads 575
Augmented Leads 576
Chest Leads or Precordial
Leads 576
Standardization of the
Electrocardiograph 576
Standard Resting
Electrocardiography 576
Mounting the ECG
Tracing 577
Interference or Artifacts . . 577
Somatic Tremor Artifacts . . . 578
Alternating Current (AC)
Interference 578
Wandering Baseline
Artifacts 579
Interrupted Baseline
Artifacts 579
Cardiac Conditions and
Diseases 579

Myocardial Infarctions
(Heart Attacks) 579
Cardiac Arrhythmias 579
Atrial Arrhythmias 580
Ventricular Arrhythmias 580
Defibrillation 582
Other Cardiac Diagnostic
Tests 582
Holt Monitor (Portable Ambu-
latory Electrocardiograph) . . 582
Treadmill Stress Test or
Exercise Tolerance ECG 584
Echocardiography 585

Unit 7:   Laboratory
Procedures   595

Chapter 26: Safety and Regulatory
Guidelines in the
Medical Laboratory   597

Clinical Laboratory
Improvement Amendments
of 1988 (CLIA '88) 598
The Intention of CLIA '88 . . 599
General Program
Description 600
Categories of Testing 600
Contents of the Law 601
CLIA '88 Regulation for
Quality Control in Automated
Hematology 605
Aftermath of CLIA '88 605
Impact of CLIA on Medical
Assistants 605
Where to Find More
Information Regarding
CLIA '88 606
Occupational Safety and
Health Administration
(OSHA) Regulations 606
The Standard for Occupational
Exposure to Hazardous
Chemicals in the Laboratory . 606
Chemical Hygiene Plan 606
OSHA Regulations and
Students 612
Avoiding Exposure to
Chemicals 612
Cumulative Trauma
Disorders 613

Chapter 27: Introduction to the
Medical Laboratory   615

The Laboratory 616
Purposes of Laboratory
Testing 617
Types of Laboratories 618
Laboratory Personnel 618
Laboratory Departments 619
Quality Controls/Assurances
in the Laboratory 623
Control Tests 623
Proficiency Testing 623
Preventative Maintenance . . 623
Instrument Validations 624

The Medical Assistant's
Role 624
Laboratory Requisitions
and Reports 624
Specimen Collection 626
Proper Procurement, Storage,
and Handling 626
Processing and Sending
Specimens to a Laboratory . . 627
Microscopes 628
Types of Microscopes 629
How to Use a Microscope . . . 629
How to Care for a Microscope 630

Chapter 28: Phlebotomy: Venipuncture
and Capillary Puncture   635

◉ Venipuncture
Why Collect Blood? 636
The Medical Assistant's
Role in Phlebotomy 637
Anatomy and Physiology of
the Circulatory System . . . 637
Collection of Blood Samples . . 638
Venipuncture Equipment . . 640
Syringes and Needles 640
Safety Needle 640
Evacuated Tube System 641
Anticoagulants 642
Tourniquets 642
Specimen Collection Trays . . 644
Venipuncture Technique . . 644
Approaching the Patient 645
Preparing Supplies and
Greeting the Patient 645
Patient and Specimen
Identification 645
Positioning the Patient 646
Selecting the Appropriate
Venipuncture Site 646
Performing a Safe
Venipuncture 647
Syringe Specimen
Collection 648
Evacuated Tube Specimen
Collection 649
Butterfly Collection System . 650
Patient Reactions 650
The Unsuccessful
Venipuncture 650
Criteria for Rejection of a
Specimen 651
Factors Affecting Laboratory
Values 651
Capillary Puncture 652
Composition of Capillary
Blood 652
Capillary Puncture Sites 652
Preparing the Capillary
Puncture Site 653
Performing the Puncture 653
Collecting the Blood Sample 653
Order of Draw 654

Chapter 29: Hematology   665
Hematological Tests 667

Hemoglobin and Hematocrit
Determinations 668
White and Red Blood Cell
Counts 671
White Blood Cell
Differential 675
Examination of a Blood
Smear 677
Erythrocyte Indices 679
Using Erythrocyte Indices to
Diagnose 679
Erythrocyte Sedimentation
Rates (ESR) 679
Wintrobe Method 680
Westergren Method 680
Using the ESR to Diagnose . . 681
Automated Hematology
Instrumentation and
Quality Control 681
Hematology Instruments
That Require Sample
Dilutions 682
Hematology Instruments
That Do Not Require
Sample Dilutions 682

Chapter 30: Urinalysis **697**
◉ **Clean Catch Urine**
◉ **Testing Urine**
Urine Formation 698
Filtration 698
Reabsorption 699
Secretion 699
Urine Composition 699
Safety 700
Quality Control 700
CLIA '88 700
Urine Containers 701
Urine Collection 701
Urine Specimen Types 701
Collection Methods 702
Examination of Urine 703
Physical Examination of
Urine 703
Chemical Examination of
Urine 705
Microscopic Examination of
Urine Sediment 708

Chapter 31: Basic Microbiology **721**
◉ **Wound Specimen**
The Medical Assistant's
Role in the Microbiology
Laboratory 723
Microbiology 723
Classification 723
Nomenclature 724
Cell Structure 724
Equipment 725
Autoclave 725
Microscope 725
Safety Hood 725
Incubator 726
Anaerobic Equipment 726
Inoculating Equipment 726
Incinerator 727
Media 727

Refrigerator 727
Safety When Handling
Microbiology Specimens . . . 727
Personal Protective
Equipment 727
Work Area 728
Specimen Handling 728
Disposal of Waste and Spills . 728
Quality Control 728
Collection Procedures 729
Specific Collection
Requirements 732
Microscopic Examination
of Bacteria 734
Bacterial Shapes 734
Dyes (Stains) 735
Simple Stain 735
Differential Stain 735
Acid-Fast Stain 736
Special Techniques 737
Potassium Hydroxide (KOH)
Preparation 737
Culture Media 738
Media Classification 739
Microbiology Culture 740
Inoculating the Media 740
Other Types of Streaking . . . 740
Primary Culture 741
Subculture 741
Biochemical Tests 742
Direct Tests 742
Biochemical Tube Testing . . 743
Identification Systems 744
Streptococcus Screening
(Rapid Strep Testing) 744
Packaged Systems 745
Semiautomated and
Automated Instruments 746
Sensitivity Testing 746
Parasitology 747
Examination Methods 747
Specimen Collection 747
Common Parasites 748
Mycology 749

**Chapter 32: Specialty Laboratory
Tests** **759**
◉ **Collecting Nose, Throat,
Sputum Specimen**
◉ **Occult Blood**
◉ **Skin Puncture**
◉ **Blood Glucose**
◉ **Wound Specimen**
Pregnancy Tests 761
Commercial/Home
Pregnancy Tests 761
Testing Methods 761
Slide Test or Agglutination
Inhibition Test 761
Enzyme Immunoassay (EIA)
Test 762
Infectious Mononucleosis . . 762
Transmission of EBV 763
Symptoms of Mononucleosis . 763
Treatment of Mononucleosis . 763
Diagnosis of Infectious
Mononucleosis 763

Slide Test for Infectious
Mononucleosis 764
Blood Typing: ABO Blood
Groups and Rh Factor 765
ABO Blood Typing 765
Rh Blood Typing 766
Semen Analysis 766
Semen Composition 767
Altering Factors in Semen
Analysis 767
Phenylketonuria (PKU)
Test 767
Blood Testing for PKU 768
Urine Testing for PKU 768
Tuberculosis: Mycobacterium
and TB Testing 768
Cause of Tuberculosis 769
Resistance in Mycobacteria . . 769
Transmission of Infectious
Tuberculosis 769
Diagnosis of Tuberculosis . . . 769
Screening for Tuberculosis:
Skin Testing 769
The Mantoux Test 769
Blood Glucose 770
Fasting Blood Glucose 770
Two-Hour Postprandial
Blood Glucose 771
Glucose Tolerance Test 771
Automated Methods of
Glucose Analysis 771
Testing Profiles 772
Glycosylated Hemoglobin . . . 773
Cholesterol 773
The Chemistry of
Cholesterol 773
Functions of Cholesterol 774
Lipoproteins and Cholesterol
Transport 774
Triglycerides 774
Blood Urea Nitrogen
(BUN) Test 775

SECTION III:
PROFESSIONAL
PROCEDURES   787

**Unit 8: Office and
Human Resource
Management** **788**

**Chapter 33: The Medical Assistant as
Office Manager** **789**
The Medical Assistant as
Manager 791
Qualities of a Manager 791
Management Styles 792
People-oriented Personality . . 792
Things-oriented Personality . . 792
Idea-oriented Personality . . . 792
Other Management Styles . . 792
Changing Styles for the
Twenty-first Century 793

The Importance of
Teamwork 793
Getting the Team Started ...794
Using a Team to Solve a
Problem 794
Planning and Implementing
a Solution 794
Recognition 794
Supervising Personnel 794
Staff Meetings 795
Supporting Staff Members ...796
Travel Arrangements 796
Itinerary 796
Supervising Student
Practicums 797
Time Management 798
Procedures Manual 798
Organization of the
Procedures Manual 798
Updating and Reviewing
the Procedures Manual 799
Marketing Functions 799
Seminars 799
Brochures 800
Newsletters 801
Press Releases 801
Special Events 801
Record and Financial
Management 801
Payroll Processing 803
Facility and Equipment
Management 804
Inventories 804
Equipment and Supplies
Maintenance 805
Risk Management 805
Liability Coverage and
Bonding 805

**Chapter 34: The Medical Assistant
as Human Resources
Manager   813**

Tasks Performed by the
Human Resources
Manager 814
The Office Policy Manual . 815
Recruiting and Hiring
Office Personnel 815
Job Descriptions 815
Recruiting 816
Preparing to Interview
Applicants 816
The Interview 817
Selecting the Finalists 818
Orienting and Training
New Personnel 819
Evaluating Employees and
Planning Salary Review ...819
Performance Evaluation 819
Salary Review 822
Dismissing Employees 822
Involuntary Dismissal 823
Voluntary Dismissal 823
Exit Interview 823
Maintaining Personnel
Records 824

Complying with Personnel
Laws 824
Special Policy
Considerations 824
Temporary Employees 824
Smoking Policy 826
Discrimination 826
Employees with Chemical
Dependencies or Emotional
Problems 826
Providing/Planning
Employee Training and
Education 826
Conflict Resolution 827

**Unit 9:   Entry into the
Profession   832**

**Chapter 35: Preparing for Medical
Assisting Credentials   833**

Purpose of Certification ...834
Preparing for the
Examination 834
Registered Medical
Assistant (RMA) 835
Examination Format and
Content 835
Application Process 836
Application Completion
and Test Administration
Scheduling 836
Certified Medical Assistant
(CMA) 836
Examination Format and
Content 836
Application Process 837
Eligibility Categories and
Requirements 837
Grounds for Denial of
Eligibillity 837
How to Recertify 838

Chapter 36: Employment Strategies   843
Resume Writing
Developing a Strategy 844
Self-Assessment 844
Job Analysis and
Research 844
Budgetary Needs
Analysis 846
Resume Preparation 847
Resume Specifications 847
Clear and Concise
Resumes 847
Accomplishments 847
References 848
Accuracy 848
Resume Styles 848
Vital Resume Information ...852
Application/Cover
Letters 852
Completing the Application
Form 852
The Look of Success 854

Personal and Professional
Poise 854
The Interview Process 855
Preparing for the Interview ..855
The Actual Interview 855
Closing the Interview 856
Interview Follow-Up 856
Follow-Up Letter 856
Follow Up by Telephone 857

**Appendix A Common Medical
Abbreviations and
Symbols   861**
**Appendix B Top 200 Drugs by Retail
Sales in 2000   867**
**Appendix C Medical Assistant Role
Delineation Chart 871**
**Appendix D Answers to Case Study
Reviews   873**
Glossary of Terms   889
Index   907

MANAGING AUTHORS

Wilburta (Billie) **Q. Lindh**, CMA, holds professor emeritus status at Highline Community College, Des Moines, Washington, and currently serves as program director and consultant to the Medical Assistant Program. She is a member of the SeaTac Chapter of the American Association of Medical Assistants (AAMA) and has lectured at AAMA seminars on the importance of communication. Lindh is co-author of *Therapeutic Communications for Allied Health Professions* published by Delmar. She has also co-authored *The Radiology Word Book* and *The Ophthalmology Word Book*, texts frequently used by transcriptionists. Lindh also authored the medical assistant chapter for *Guide to Careers in the Health Professions*.

Marilyn S. Pooler, RN, CMA-C, MEd, is a professor in the Medical Assisting Department at Springfield Technical Community College, Springfield, Massachusetts. Pooler has taught at Springfield for 24 years and previously served as chair of the Medical Assisting Department. She has served on the certifying board of the AAMA task force for test construction and is a member of the executive board of the New England Association of Allied Health Educators. She also is a site surveyor for AAMA, reviewing medical assisting programs at schools and colleges seeking accreditation.

Carol D. Tamparo, CMA-A, PhD, is Dean of Business and Allied Health at Lake Washington Technical College in Kirkland, Washington. Tamparo, who taught at Highline Community College in Des Moines, Washington, for 23 years, is a member of the SeaTac Chapter of the AAMA. Tamparo, a speaker at numerous AAMA seminars and educational conferences, is recognized as an expert on medical law, ethics, and bioethics. She is the co-author of *Diseases of the Human Body*; *Medical Law, Ethics, and Bioethics for Ambulatory Care*; and *Therapeutic Communications for Allied Health Professions*.

ACKNOWLEDGMENTS

The managing authors personally acknowledge the following people:

To my husband, who continually supports and assists in so many ways, thank you. To my family for support and encouragement, and to Laura, who provided expertise for some chapters, thank you. To the students, graduates, and fellow colleagues who challenge me to stay current with skills and up-to-date with technology, thank you.

Billie Q. Lindh

Thanks to my friends who were very supportive of my efforts, and a special thanks to my husband, Jud, for his patience and understanding during this endeavor.

Marilyn S. Pooler

To all my students in health care programs who keep me current, to my school administrators and family members who have been supportive of this project, and to the health care providers who patiently and lovingly cared for my mother in an assisted living Alzheimer's unit until her death in April 2001, my thanks and deepest regard and respect.

Carol D. Tamparo

A sincere thank you to Joanne Cerrato, former co-author, for her many invaluable contributions to the formation of the first edition of this text.

A special thank you to William Patten, MHS, MT (ASCP), for editing Unit 7, Laboratory Procedures. Bill is a laboratory supervisor at the Baystate Medical Center in Springfield, Massachusetts. He is a certified medical technologist and has a master's degree with a concentration in allied health education. He has 25 years of experience in the laboratory field. His responsibilities have included program director of a Committee on Allied Health Education and Accreditation (CAHEA)-approved medical technology program, Director of Education for the Department of Pathology at Baystate Medical Center, and, most recently, Service Coordinator for the Baystate Reference Laboratories. He is also a faculty member at a number of area academic institutions. He has taught phlebotomy, clinical chemistry, and other laboratory science courses during the past 10 years. He is a member of the American Society of Clinical Pathologists and has served as a site surveyor in the inspection process for the National Accrediting Agency for Clinical Laboratory Science (NAACLS) and the College of American Pathology (CAP).

REVIEWERS

Kaye Acton
Director of Medical Assisting
    Program
Alamance Community College
Graham, NC

Magdalena Andrasevits, NRCMA
Medical Assistant Program Director
Sanford-Brown College
North Kansas City, MO

Joseph DeSapio, RMA
Director of Facility and Library
    Resources
Medical Assisting Instructor
Ultrasound Diagnostic School
New York, NY

Eleanor K. Flores, RN, BSN, MEd
Briarwood College
Southington, CT

Tova Green
IVTC Fort Wayne
Fort Wayne, IN

Karen Jackson, NR-CMA
Medical Program Chair
Education America, Dallas Campus
Garland, TX

Barbara G. Kalfin, BS, AAS,
    CMA-C
Medical Assisting Extern Coordinator
Instructor, Medical Assisting Program
City College
Ft. Lauderdale, FL

Theresa Offenberger, PhD
Professor of Medical Assisting
Cuyahoga Community College
Cleveland, OH

Agnes Pucillo, LPN
Medical Assisting Program Director
Ultrasound Diagnostic School
Iselin, NJ

Patricia Schrull, RN, MBA, MEd,
    CMA
Program Director, Medical Assisting
    Program
Lorain County Community College
Elyria, OH

Janet Sesser, BS Ed. Admin., RMA,
    CMA
Corporate Director of Education,
    Allied Health
High-Tech Institute, Inc.
Phoenix, AZ

Kimberly A. Shinall, RN
President and CEO
KAS Enterprises
Virginia Beach, VA

Lois M. Smith, RN, CMA
Arapahoe Community College
Golden, CO

Susan Sniffin
Suffolk Community College
Great Neck, NY

Alisa M. Tetlow, RMA
Medical Assistant Program Director
Ultrasound Diagnostic School
Philadelphia, PA

Nina Thierer
Tidewater Technical Institute
Virginia Beach, VA

Fred Valdes, MD
Medical Department Chairman
City College
Ft. Lauderdale, FL

Sujana Wardell, RMA, RPT (AMT),
    AS
Program Director for Clinical and
    Administrative Medical Assisting
San Joaquin Valley College, Visalia
    Campus
Visalia, CA

Sally Wooten
Whitman Education Group
Miami, FL

Terri Wyman, CMA
Director of Health Information
    Specialties
Ultrasound Diagnostic School
Springfield, MA

CONTRIBUTORS

Julie B. Brown, RNC, MSN, CMA
Chapter 10: *Infection Control, Medical Asepsis, and Sterilization*

Barbara Dahl, CMA
Chapter 10: *Infection Control, Medical Asepsis, and Sterilization,* Chapter 19: *Assisting with Minor Surgery,* and Chapter 27: *Introduction to the Medical Laboratory*

Bonnie Lou Deister, MS, BSN, RN, CMA-C
Chapter 33: *The Medical Assistant as Office Manager* and Chapter 34: *The Medical Assistant as Human Resources Manager*

Walter R. English, MA, MT
Chapter 30: *Urinalysis*

Lynn B. Hoeltke, MBA, MT (ASCP), PBT, DLM
Chapter 28: *Phlebotomy: Venipuncture and Capillary Puncture*

Diane Klieger, RN, MBA, CMA
Chapter 18: *Examinations and Procedures of Body Systems* and Chapter 25: *Electrocardiography*

Sharon Paff, AS, RMA (AMT)
Chapter 12: *Vital Signs and Measurements,* Chapter 13: *The Physical Examination,* and Chapter 18: *Examinations and Procedures of Body Systems*

Tom Palko, MEd, MCS, MT (ASCP)
Chapter 29: *Hematology*

Theresa Perry, MS, BS, CMA
Chapter 22: *Nutrition in Health and Disease*

Jane Rice, RN, CMA-C
Chapter 23: *Basic Pharmacology* and Chapter 24: *Calculation of Medication Dosage and Medication Administration*

Lisa Shimeld, MS
Chapter 32: *Specialty Laboratory Tests*

Sylvia Taylor, BS, CMA
Chapter 2: *Health Care Settings and the Health Care Team*

Virginia Lawless Thompson
Chapter 9: *Emergency Procedures and First Aid*

Ginny Torres, CMA
Chapter 11: *Taking a Medical History, the Patient's Chart, and Methods of Documentation*

Adrianne C. Williams
Chapter 21: *Rehabilitation and Therapeutic Modalities*

LIST OF PROCEDURES

9-1   Control of Bleeding
9-2   Applying an Arm Splint
9-3   Heimlich Maneuver for a Conscious Adult
9-4   Heimlich Maneuver for an Unconscious Adult or Child
9-5   Heimlich Maneuver for a Conscious Child
9-6   Back Blows and Chest Thrusts for a Conscious Infant Who Is Choking
9-7   Back Blows and Chest Thrusts for an Unconscious Infant
9-8   Rescue Breathing for Adults
9-9   Rescue Breathing for Children
9-10 Rescue Breathing for Infants
9-11 CPR for Adults
9-12 CPR for Children
9-13 CPR for Infants
10-1 Medical Asepsis Handwash
10-2 Sanitization of Instruments
10-3 Removing Contaminated Gloves
10-4 Chemical Disinfection of Instruments
10-5 Wrapping Instruments for Sterilization in Autoclave
10-6 Steam Sterilization of Instruments (Autoclave)
11-1 Taking a Medical History
12-1 Measuring an Oral Temperature Using a Mercury Thermometer
12-2 Measuring an Oral Temperature Using a Disposable Oral Strip Thermometer
12-3 Measuring an Oral Temperature Using a Digital Thermometer
12-4 Measuring an Aural Temperature Using a Tympanic Thermometer
12-5 Measuring a Rectal Temperature Using a Mercury Thermometer
12-6 Measuring a Rectal Temperature Using a Digital Thermometer
12-7 Measuring an Axillary Temperature
12-8 Measuring a Radial Pulse
12-9 Taking an Apical Pulse
12-10 Measuring the Respiration Rate
12-11 Measuring a Blood Pressure
12-12 Measuring Height
12-13 Measuring Adult Weight
13-1 Positioning Patient in the Supine Position
13-2 Positioning Patient in the Dorsal Recumbent Position
13-3 Positioning Patient in the Lithotomy Position
13-4 Positioning Patient in the Fowler's Position
13-5 Positioning Patient in the Knee-Chest Position
13-6 Positioning Patient in the Prone Position
13-7 Positioning Patient in the Sims' Position
13-8 Positioning Patient in the Trendelenburg Position
13-9 Assisting with a Complete Physical Examination
14-1 Assisting with Routine Prenatal Visits
14-2 Instructing Patient in Breast Self-Examination
14-3 Assisting with Gynecologic or Pelvic Examination and a Papanicolaou (Pap) Test
15-1 Measuring the Infant: Weight, Height, Head, and Chest Circumference
15-2 Taking an Infant's Rectal Temperature with a Mercury or Digital Thermometer
15-3 Taking an Apical Pulse on an Infant
15-4 Measuring Infant's Respiration Rate
15-5 Obtaining a Urine Specimen from an Infant or Young Child
16-1 Instructing Patient in Testicular Self-Examination
18-1 Performing a Urine Drug Screening
18-2 Performing a Urinary Catheterization on a Female Patient
18-3 Performing a Urinary Catheterization of a Male Patient
18-4 Assisting with Proctosigmoidoscopy
18-5 Fecal Occult Blood Test

18-6   Performing Visual Acuity Testing Using a Snellen Chart
18-7   Measuring Near Visual Acuity
18-8   Performing Color Vision Test Using the Ishihara Plates
18-9   Performing Eye Instillation
18-10   Performing Eye Patch Dressing Application
18-11   Performing Eye Irrigation
18-12   Assisting with Audiometry
18-13   Performing Ear Irrigation
18-14   Performing Ear Instillation
18-15   Assisting with Nasal Examination
18-16   Performing Nasal Irrigation
18-17   Performing Nasal Instillation
18-18   Obtaining a Sputum Specimen
18-19   Administer Oxygen by Nasal Cannula for Minor Respiratory Distress
18-20   Instructing Patient in Use of Metered Dose Nebulizer
18-21   Spirometry Testing
18-22   Assisting with Plaster-of-Paris Cast Application
18-23   Assisting with Cast Removal
18-24   Assisting the Physician During a Lumbar Puncture
18-25   Assisting the Physician with a Neurological Screening Examination
19-1   Applying Sterile Gloves
19-2   Assisting with Minor Surgery
19-3   Suturing of Laceration or Incision Repair
19-4   Dressing Change
19-5   Suture Removal
19-6   Application of Sterile Adhesive Skin Closure Strips
19-7   Sebaceous Cyst Excision
19-8   Incision and Drainage of Localized Infections
19-9   Aspiration of Joint Fluid
19-10   Hemorrhoid Thrombectomy
19-11   Chemical "Cold" Sterilization
19-12   Preparation of Patient Skin for Minor Surgery
19-13   Setting Up and Covering a Sterile Field
19-14   Opening Sterile Packages of Instruments and Supplies and Applying Them to a Sterile Field
19-15   Pouring a Sterile Solution into a Cup on a Sterile Field
21-1   Transferring Patient from Wheelchair to Examination Table

21-2   Transferring Patient from Examination Table to Wheelchair
21-3   Assisting the Patient to Stand and Walk
21-4   Care of the Falling Patient
21-5   Assisting a Patient to Ambulate with a Walker
21-6   Teaching the Patient to Ambulate with Axillary Crutches
21-7   Assisting a Patient to Ambulate with a Cane
21-8   Range of Motion Exercises, Upper Body
21-9   Range of Motion Exercises, Lower Body
24-1   Administration of Oral Medications
24-2   Administration of Subcutaneous, Intramuscular, and Intradermal Injections
24-3   Withdrawing (Aspirating) Medication from a Vial
24-4   Withdrawing (Aspirating) Medication from an Ampule
24-5   Administering a Subcutaneous Injection
24-6   Administering an Intramuscular Injection
24-7   Administering an Intradermal Injection
24-8   Reconstituting a Powder Medication for Administration
24-9   Z-Track Intramuscular Injection Technique
25-1   Perform Twelve-Lead Electrocardiogram, Single-Channel
25-2   Perform Twelve-Lead Electrocardiogram, Three Channel
25-3   Perform Holter Monitor Application
27-1   Using the Microscope
28-1   Finding a Vein in the Upper Arm
28-2   Venipuncture by Syringe Procedure
28-3   Venipuncture by Evacuated Tube System
28-4   Venipuncture by Butterfly Needle System
28-5   Capillary Puncture by Fingerstick
29-1   Hemoglobin Determination (Manual Method Using a Spectrophotometer)
29-2   Hemoglobin Determination (Hemoglobin Analyzer)
29-3   Microhematocrit
29-4   White Blood Cell Count (Unopette® Method)

29-5   Red Blood Cell Count (Unopette® Method)
29-6   Preparation of a Differential Blood Smear Slide
29-7   Staining a Differential Blood Smear Slide
29-8   Differential Leukocyte Count
29-9   Erythrocyte Sedimentation Rate
30-1   Assessing Urine Volume
30-2   Observing Urine Color
30-3   Observing Urine Clarity
30-4   Using the Refractometer to Measure Specific Gravity
30-5   Performing a Urinalysis Chemical Examination
30-6   Testing for Sugar in the Urine
30-7   Microscopic Examination of Urine Sediment
30-8   Performing a Urinalysis
31-1   Procedure for Obtaining a Throat Culture
31-2   Preparing a Bacteriological Smear
31-3   Gram Stain
31-4   Ziehl-Neelsen Stain
31-5   Wet Mount and Hanging Drop Preparations
31-6   Specimen Inoculation and Dilution Streaking
31-7   Broth Tube Inoculation
31-8   Deep Inoculation/Slant
32-1   Pregnancy Tests
32-2   Slide Test for Infectious Mononucleosis
32-3   Analyzing Semen
32-4   Obtaining Blood Specimen for Phenylketonuria (PKU) Test
32-5   Obtaining Urine Specimen for Phenylketonuria (PKU) Test
32-6   Mantoux Test
32-7   Measurement of Blood Glucose Using an Automated Analyzer
32-8   Cholesterol Testing
33-1   Preparing a Meeting Agenda
33-2   Making Travel Arrangements
33-3   Making Travel Arrangements Via Internet
33-4   Supervising a Student Practicum
34-5   Developing and Maintaining a Procedures Manual
34-1   Develop and Maintain a Policy Manual
34-2   Preparing a Job Description
34-3   Interviewing
34-4   Orient and Train Personnel

PREFACE

The world of health care has changed rapidly over the past few years, and as we travel through the 21st century, health care professionals will encounter more challenges than ever before. As medical assistants you will be called on to do more and respond to an increasing number of clinical responsibilities, especially in this age of managed care. Now is the time to equip yourself with the skills you will need to excel in the field. Now is the time to maximize your potential, expand your base of knowledge, and dedicate yourself to becoming the best multifaceted, multiskilled medical assistant that you can be.

The new edition of *Delmar's Clinical Medical Assisting* will guide you on this journey. This text is part of a dynamic learning system that also includes a skills CD-ROM and a workbook. Together, these learning tools conform to the standard and advanced areas of competence defined by AAMA's Role Delineation Study and AMT's Registered Medical Assistant Competency Inventory. They emphasize the importance of interpersonal communications in the medical environment. They explore changes in the health care setting including the development of standard precautions and the implications of managed care. This powerful learning system gives you an intimate look at the challenges you'll face and the opportunities you'll find as a medical assistant.

Unlike many texts, *Delmar's Clinical Medical Assisting*, 2nd edition, was written not just by one or two individuals but by many talented authors—experts who give you a sound and thorough understanding of the fundamentals. The text then moves beyond theory and develops all concepts in a real-life situation. What is it like to be working in the field? What are the problems you may encounter?

You'll discover common challenges faced by medical assistants through realistic scenarios woven into the chapter introductions. Case studies depict the ambulatory care setting where you, as a medical assistant, may very well be employed. Patient teaching tips provide practical advice. Proper documentation is emphasized.

How the Text Is Organized

Delmar's Clinical Medical Assisting, 2nd edition, presents a logical, in-depth review of all clinical competencies required of today's multiskilled medical assistants—*in full color!*

- **Section I, General Procedures (Chapters 1 through 9)**, provides the groundwork for understanding the role and responsibilities of the medical assistant. Topics include the medical assisting profession, the health care team, history of medicine, therapeutic communications, coping skills for the medical assistant, legal and ethical issues, and emergency procedures and first aid.

- **Section II, Clinical Procedures (Chapters 10 through 32)**, gives you a thorough understanding of all clinical, diagnostic, and laboratory procedures important to today's ambulatory care settings. Topics include medical asepsis, medical history, vital signs and measurements, physical examination, obstetrics and gynecology, pediatrics, male reproductive system, gerontology, body systems, assisting with minor surgery, diagnostic imaging, rehabilitation medicine, nutrition, pharmacology, medication calculations, EKG, safety guidelines, venipuncture, hematology, urinalysis, microbiology, and specialty tests.

- **Section III, Professional Procedures (Chapters 33 through 36)**, examines the role of the medical assistant as office and human resources manager and provides tools and techniques to use when preparing for externship, medical assisting credentials, and employment.

- **Appendices** include (A) Common Medical Abbreviations and Symbols, (B) Top 200 Drugs by Retail Sales in 2000, (C) Medical Assistant Role Delineation Chart, and (D) Answers to Case Study Reviews.

- **Glossary of Terms** includes definitions of all key terms, with related chapter numbers indicated.

- **The Medical Assisting Clinical Skills CD** is found on the inside back cover of this book. This interactive software challenges you to apply content, think critically, develop competency in skills, and improve your knowledge base.

How Each Chapter Is Organized

All chapters include similar features and presentation and function as building blocks to a comprehensive medical assisting education. However, each chapter is also a self-contained module and can be studied in any order or independently of other chapters in the text.

Features include:

- A listing of *key terms*
- *Role delineation components*, both standard and advanced

- An *outline of the chapter*
- *Objectives*
- An *introduction* with a real-life scenario
- *Graphic icons, tables, and figures*
- *Full-color illustrations and photographs*
- *Procedures* with step-by-step instructions
- *Patient teaching tips*
- *Spotlight on AAMA Essentials through CAAHEP* boxes
- *Case studies with review questions*
- *Summary*
- *Review questions*
- *Web Activities*
- *Bibliography* for further study

To receive the full value of *Delmar's Clinical Medical Assisting*, 2nd edition, it is important to understand the structure of the text and each chapter. Review the following information, plus "How to Use This Book" and "How to Use the Medical Assisting Clinical Skills CD-ROM." Together, these materials will make your medical assisting education comprehensive and meaningful, providing you with the skills and understanding to enable you to practice your profession with confidence and competence.

EXTENSIVE TEACHING/LEARNING PACKAGE

The complete supplements package helps instructors efficiently manage time and resources and helps students develop the necessary skills and competencies required by the demanding profession of medical assisting.

Instructor's Manual

Order #0-7668-2427-6
This compact resource is designed as a quick reference tool for classroom activity and instruction. Chapters include:

- Proficiency assessments
- Answers to text review questions
- Answers to text critical thinking questions
- Answers to workbook exercises
- Answers to workbook case studies

Student Workbook

Order #0-7668-2428-4

The workbook helps you learn and reinforce the essential competencies needed to become a successful, multiskilled medical assistant. Each chapter includes:

- Vocabulary builder exercises
- Learning review
- Investigation activity
- Case study
- Skills assessment checklist

Instructor's Resource Kit (Comprehensive)

Order #0-7668-2419-5

This dynamic resource is a must-have for all instructors. This comprehensive three-ring binder includes:

Instructor's Guide. Complete with teaching strategies and learning concepts, this print and electronic resource offers:

- Teaching/learning concepts
- Objectives and evaluation
- Instructional strategies
- Lesson plans
- Classroom activities

Computerized and Printed Testbank. Both electronic and printed testbanks are included, containing approximately 1,200 multiple choice questions.

PowerPoint Slides. The CD included in the *Instructor's Resource Kit* contains over 250 PowerPoint slides, making a backdrop with impact for your classroom presentations.

Medical Assisting CD-ROM. This is an innovative, comprehensive multimedia learning reference tool to enhance classroom presentations and increase student learning.

HOW TO USE THIS BOOK

Delmar's *Clinical Medical Assisting, 2nd edition,* contains many features that make it an easy-to-use learning system. They include:

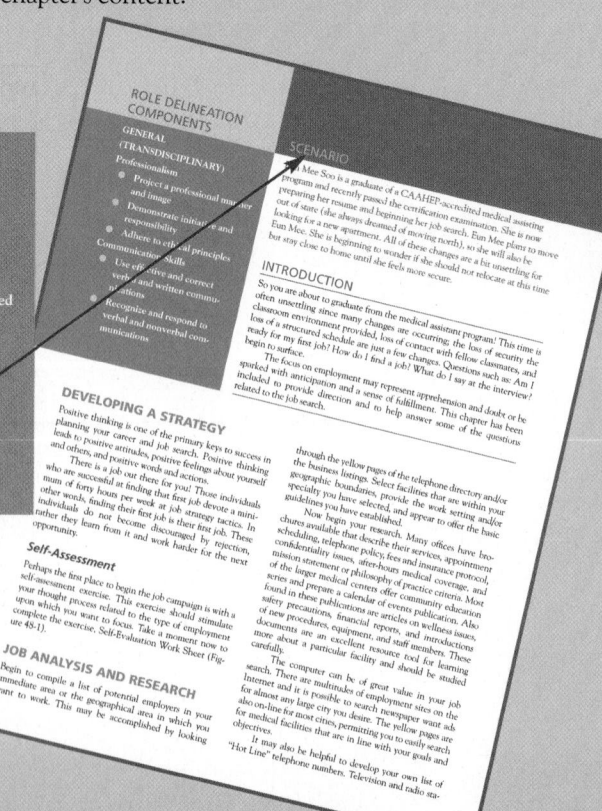

1 Key Terms

All key terms are listed at the beginning of each chapter. Within the text, the term is always boldfaced at its first occurrence for easy identification. Turn to the glossary for definitions of all key terms.

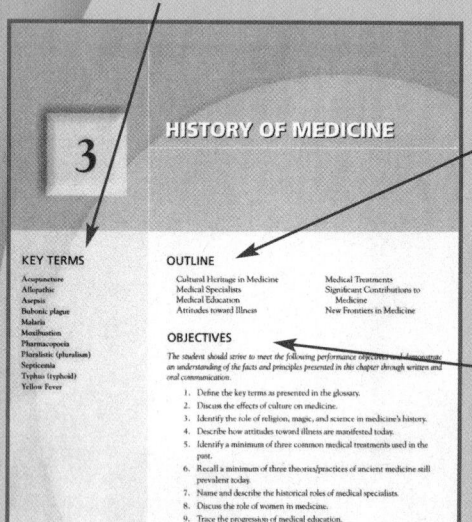

HISTORY OF MEDICINE

3

KEY TERMS
Acupuncture
Allopathic
Asepsis
Bubonic plague
Malaria
Moxibustion
Pharmacopoeia
Pluralistic (pluralism)
Septicemia
Typhus (typhoid)
Yellow Fever

OUTLINE
Cultural Heritage in Medicine   Medical Treatments
Medical Specialists   Significant Contributions to
Medical Education   Medicine
Attitudes toward Illness   New Frontiers in Medicine

OBJECTIVES
The student should strive to meet the following performance objectives and demonstrate an understanding of the facts and principles presented in this chapter through written and oral communication.

1. Define the key terms as presented in the glossary.
2. Discuss the effects of culture on medicine.
3. Identify the role of religion, magic, and science in medicine's history.
4. Describe how attitudes toward illness are manifested today.
5. Identify a minimum of three common medical treatments used in the past.
6. Recall a minimum of three theories/practices of ancient medicine still prevalent today.
7. Name and describe the historical roles of medical specialists.
8. Discuss the role of women in medicine.
9. Trace the progression of medical education.
10. Name at least five significant contributions to medicine.
11. Identify a minimum of three recent developments in medicine.

2 Chapter Outline

At the beginning of each chapter, you'll find an outline of all major headings. Review these headings of topic areas before you study the chapter. They are a road map to your understanding.

3 Objectives

Performance objectives test your knowledge of the key facts presented in the chapter. Use these objectives, together with review questions, to test your understanding of the chapter's content.

ROLE DELINEATION COMPONENTS

GENERAL (TRANSDISCIPLINARY)

Professionalism
● Project a professional manner and image

Legal Concepts
● Maintain and dispose of regulated substances in compliance with government guidelines
● Comply with established risk management and safety procedures

Operational Functions
● Evaluate and recommend equipment and supplies

4 Role Delineation Components

This opening list in each chapter keeps the focus on the medical assistant's actual job functions as defined by the accrediting bodies.

5 Real-Life Scenarios

The introductions to most chapters include an overview of the material *and* a real-life scenario based on two distinct ambulatory care settings and their physicians, medical assistants, and patients. Through these scenarios you'll come to understand some of the stimulating challenges faced by medical assistants and gain insight into how these challenges are overcome.

6 Patient Teaching Tips

This feature helps all current and future medical assistants anticipate patient concerns and provides sound suggestions for effective patient communication.

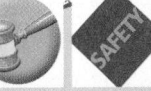

Patient Teaching Tip

Encourage patients to think of themselves as members of the health care team for they can provide information about their medical history. Use good communication skills to encourage the patient to describe symptoms and provide other information that is useful in diagnosis and treatment.

7 Icons

Graphic icons pinpoint information that relates to legal, safety, computer, managed care, and global or cultural issues.

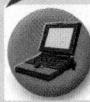 

8 Procedures

Step-by-step procedures are now conveniently grouped together at the end of each chapter. They give detailed information on all important administrative, clinical, and general competencies as defined by AAMA and AMT.

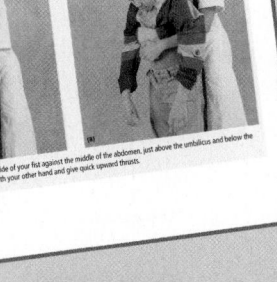

Procedure 9-5 — Heimlich Maneuver for a Conscious Child

STANDARD PRECAUTIONS:

PURPOSE:
To open up a blocked airway

EQUIPMENT/SUPPLIES:
None needed

PROCEDURE STEPS:
1. Place the thumb side of your fist against the middle of the child's abdomen, just above the

umbilicus and below the xiphoid process (Figure 9-21A).
2. Grasp your fist with your other hand. Give quick upward thrusts (Figure 9-21B). Repeat the procedure until the object is expelled or until the patient loses consciousness (see Heimlich maneuver for unconscious child, Procedure 9-4).
3. Wash hands.
4. Document the procedure.

Figure 9-21 (A) Place the thumb side of your fist against the middle of the abdomen, just above the umbilicus and below the xiphoid process. (B) Grasp your fist with your other hand and give quick upward thrusts.

9 Spotlight on AAMA Essentials through CAAHEP

These psychology tips help you focus on the CAAHEP-mandated understandings required of medical assistants.

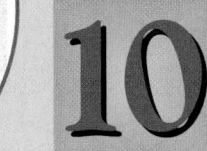

SPOTLIGHT ON AAMA ESSENTIALS THROUGH CAAHEP

- Recognizing a patient's cultural background is part of caring for the patient as a whole person.
- Human kindness often eliminates fear of the unknown.
- A positive attitude helps to lessen a negative feeling.

10 Web Activities

This new feature at the end of each chapter gives you practice navigating the Internet by suggesting online activities to help you begin to use those sites.

11 Case Studies

The case studies with accompanying review questions encourage a problem/solution approach. Use the case studies to put your knowledge into practice and arrive at a deeper understanding of the profession. Answers to the case studies are included as an appendix of the text.

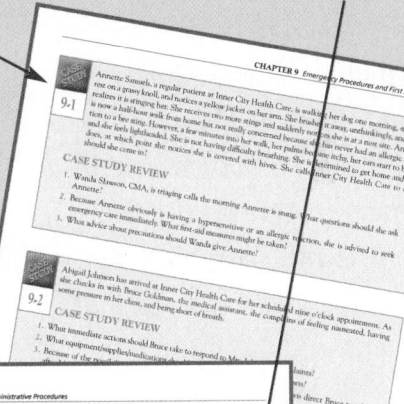

12

Review Questions

Test your comprehension of the chapter with structured multiple choice questions and open-ended critical thinking questions that require you to combine an understanding of chapter material with your personal insight and judgment.

13 Clinical Skills CD Quick Locator

This invaluable tool located in the table of contents tells you when to turn to your skills CD-ROM for practice activities that will strengthen your understanding of the chapter you are reading.

HOW TO USE THE MEDICAL ASSISTING CLINICAL SKILLS CD

The Skills CD is designed to accompany **Delmar's Clinical Medical Assisting, 2nd edition,** so you can review and reinforce the important concepts you are learning in the textbook. By using this CD, you'll challenge yourself and make your study of medical assisting concepts more effective and fun.

The Clinical Skills CD-ROM is designed to be easy to use. It includes basic clinical skills used in medical assisting, a glossary of words used in the office, important infection control information, a help feature, and a tutorial that will assist you in using the CD-ROM.

If you need to go back to the previous screen, just hit the **Previous** button.

The **Next** button takes you to the next step in the procedure.

The skills menu lists each of the clinical skills contained on the CD-ROM. Click on the button of the skill you wish to study.

As you choose each skill, a menu will appear listing each of the sections included with the skill. By clicking on the buttons, you will navigate through the skill.

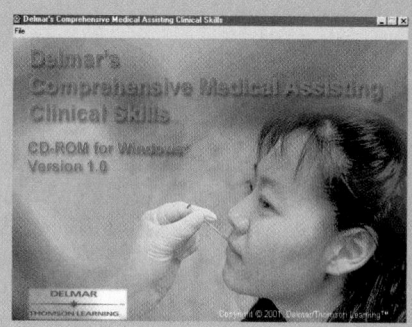

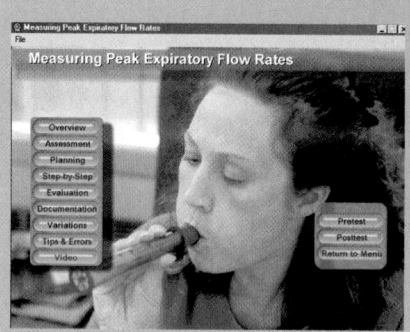

A glossary of terms is included to help you with your medical terminology. To find a term, just scroll down or use the buttons to advance you to the place in the alphabet where the word is found.

Clicking on the skills menu will take you to the main menu of skills you will be reviewing.

At any time you may return to this menu by clicking on the **Main Menu** button.

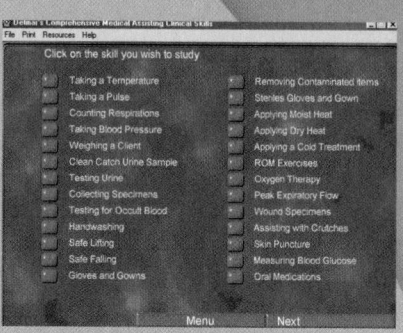

Each skill includes a pretest and a post-test section so you may enhance your learning by checking your knowledge before and after viewing the skill.

Each question on the pretest and post-test gives you a chance to answer correctly. You will be asked if that is the answer you want to go with, and you are able to change your answer. The correct answer will be displayed and your score will be tallied as you advance through the questions.

At the end, your final score with your percent rate for passing will be given. You are able to reset the questions and try again by simply clicking on the **Reset** button.

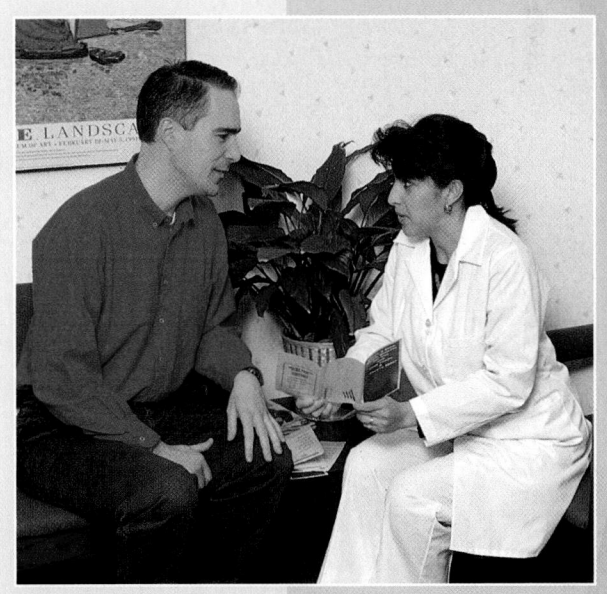

GENERAL
PROCEDURES

INTRODUCTION TO MEDICAL ASSISTING AND HEALTH PROFESSIONS

1

MEDICAL ASSISTING AS A PROFESSION

KEY TERMS

Accreditation
Ambulatory Care Setting
Attribute
Baccalaureate
Certification
Certified Medical Assistant (CMA)
Competency
Compliance
Credentialed
Disposition
Empathy
Externship
Facilitate
Improvise
Integrate
Internship
License
Licensure
Litigious
Practicum
Proprietary
Registered Medical Assistant (RMA)

OUTLINE

**Personal Attributes
of the Professional**
Empathy
Attitude
Dependability
Initiative
Flexibility
Desire to Learn
Physical Attributes
Ability to Communicate
Ethical Behavior
**Historical Perspective
of Medical Assisting**

**American Association of
Medical Assistants**
Accreditation
Certification
Continuing Education
Registered Medical Assistant
**Education of the Professional
Medical Assistant**
Preparation for Externship
Career Opportunities
**Regulation of Health Care
Providers**
Scope of Practice

OBJECTIVES

The student should strive to meet the following performance objectives and demonstrate an understanding of the facts and principles presented in this chapter through written and oral communication.

1. Define the key terms as presented in the glossary.
2. Identify and discuss nine personal attributes that are important for a professional medical assistant to possess.
3. Discuss the history of medical assisting.
4. Describe the American Association of Medical Assistants and list its three major functions.
5. Explain accreditation, certification, and continuing education as they pertain to the professional medical assistant.
6. Identify the importance of the accreditation process to an educational institution.
7. Recall two methods to obtain recertification.
8. List five means of obtaining continuing education units.   *(continues)*

3

OBJECTIVES (*continued*)

9. Describe the certifying agency that certifies medical assistants as registered medical assistants (RMA).
10. Describe the externship experience.
11. Recall two criteria for the selection of externship sites.
12. List three benefits of externship to student and site.
13. Describe the profession of medical assisting and analyze its career opportunities in relationship to your interests.
14. Differentiate among certification, licensure, and registration.
15. State the importance of understanding the scope of practice for the medical assistant.

ROLE DELINEATION COMPONENTS

GENERAL (TRANSDISCIPLINARY)

Professionalism

- **Project a professional manner and image**
- **Adhere to ethical principles**
- **Demonstrate initiative and responsibility**
- **Work as a team member**
- **Adapt to change**
- **Promote the CMA credential**
- **Enhance skills through continuing education**

Legal Concepts

- **Maintain confidentiality**
- **Practice within the scope of education, training, and personal capabilities**

INTRODUCTION

Historically, medical science has been fascinating to most people. Perhaps you have been drawn to medical assisting because you too are intrigued by medicine and want to learn about advances in health care and want to become involved in providing care to patients. More than likely you have a desire to help others.

Medical assistants have always played an integral role in physicians' offices and ambulatory care settings such as clinics and urgent care facilities, where health care services are offered on an outpatient basis. And now more than ever, because of the explosion of knowledge and high technology in medicine, medical assistants are involved in an ever-widening scope of clinical and administrative duties. With the medical assistant's expanded role has come the responsibility to become a well-educated and highly competent professional dedicated to providing the highest quality of health care.

Consumers of health care have become increasingly aware, primarily through the media, of the availability of the latest advances, techniques, and discoveries in medicine. They realize that they have a right for health care to be provided to them by educated, skilled, and competent professionals.

As you study to become a medical assistant, it is important for you to understand what a professional is. According to *Merriam-Webster's Collegiate Dictionary*, 10th edition, it is "one who has acquired a specialized body of knowledge, skills, and attitudes."

You will learn to integrate, or unify, your desire and need to help others with the knowledge, skills, and attitudes you acquire through your studies. By blending all of these, you will be able to provide patients with the best health care possible and learn what it means to be a professional medical assistant.

PERSONAL ATTRIBUTES OF THE PROFESSIONAL

There are certain characteristics or personal qualities that medical assistants should strive to cultivate. These are the attributes that identify a true professional; when caring for patients these qualities should come from the heart. They will enable the patient to trust you, the caregiver.

Empathy

To have **empathy** means to consider the patient's welfare and to be kind. It means stepping into the patient's place, discovering what the patient is experiencing, and then recognizing and identifying with those feelings.

Medical assistants should treat patients as they themselves would want to be treated. A visit to the doctor is often a time of fear and anxiety. Apprehension can be allayed tremendously when patients realize that their caregiver understands their feelings and desires to make their lives more pleasant and comfortable. See Figure 1-1.

It is important to realize that patients' health problems can have a profound effect on the caregiver. By maintaining a balanced outlook, medical assistants can safeguard themselves from becoming too emotionally involved with patient problems. Empathy is extremely important in the health care profession; however, emotionalism can cloud one's judgment.

Attitude

A friendly, warm **disposition** and a sense of humor will help patients feel more at ease. A sincere affection for people can be conveyed by actions that **facilitate** open and honest communication. Your attitude should radiate genuine interest.

On occasion, difficult patients can test the tolerance level of the most experienced medical assistant because they seem never to be content with the care or services received. But no matter what the circumstances, patients should never be treated with disinterest or in an unfriendly manner. The medical assistant should always be pleasant and courteous.

When giving care to patients, do so unrestricted by your concerns about their attitudes, disease, race, religion, economic status, or sexual orientation.

As a member of the health care delivery team, the medical assistant needs to be cooperative and supportive of all other members, working with the team in an honest, open manner while keeping in mind the patient's right to privacy and confidentiality.

Dependability

When providing for a patient's well-being, it is important to focus attention on activities in the office or clinic environment that will demonstrate being well-organized, accurate, and responsive to the patient's needs.

Being dependable means that employer and coworkers rely on the medical assistant to be respectful of them, of patients, and of equipment and materials. Other members of the health care team will expect duties and responsibilities to be carried out responsibly. A depend-

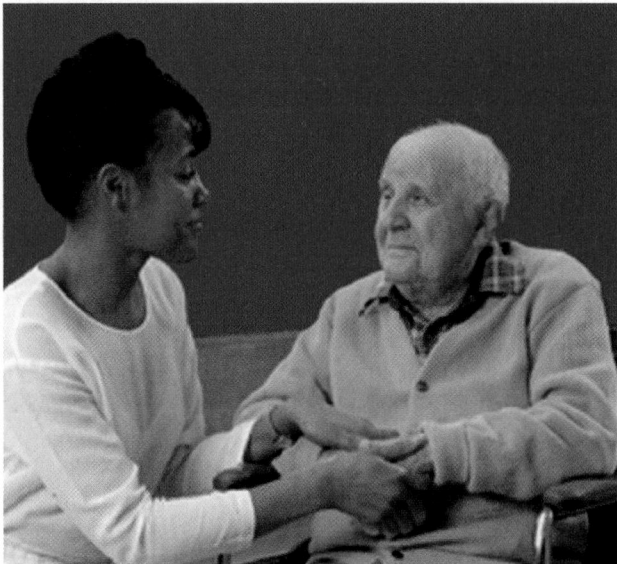

Figure 1-1 The medical assistant should have a friendly disposition and communicate empathy for the patient.

able person interacts with coworkers in a supportive manner, is punctual, and limits absences from work.

Initiative

The willingness and ability to work independently shows initiative. A person with initiative is observant, notices work that needs to be done, and then takes action to complete those tasks without being told to do them. Employer and coworkers must be able to count on one another to anticipate patients' needs and be attentive to work that needs to be accomplished. The successful medical assistant will be ready to pitch in and recognize when others need assistance.

By asking appropriate questions and seeking information that will improve performance, medical assistants will demonstrate that they have the foresight and the "get up and go" needed to complete the numerous and varied tasks of the ambulatory care environment.

Flexibility

The ability to be adaptable is a trait that serves all professionals well. When caring for ill people, unexpected situations arise daily and medical assistants must be able to respond to a variety of situations (many of them emergencies and unanticipated) without losing a sense of equilibrium. Finding solutions to problems and developing alternative action plans demonstrates flexibility. To **improvise,** or solve problems that arise either routinely or spontaneously, is a characteristic worth nurturing.

Desire to Learn

A willingness to continually learn and grow is the mark of a true professional. With the growing technology in medicine, there is an ongoing necessity for constant learning. Medical assistants must be dedicated to high standards of performance, which can be accomplished by showing a desire to acquire information and by constantly updating their knowledge and skills. Keeping abreast of the latest diseases, treatments, procedures, and techniques can be achieved in a variety of ways, such as college courses, seminars, workshops, reading, and simply by being observant. The sharper the power of observation, the more the medical assistant will learn from physician, employer, and coworkers.

Physical Attributes

Appearance is important in patients' perceptions of the delivery of their care. Imparting the look of a professional requires an appearance that is clean and fresh and wholesome; in general, an appearance that reflects good health habits (Figure 1-2). Good personal hygiene practices, weight control, healthy-looking skin, hair, teeth, and nails all contribute to a professional appearance. Rest, good nutrition, regular exercise, and recreation all promote good health.

Female medical assistants should wear appropriate light daytime makeup. For the safety of both the profes-sional and the patient, no necklaces or dangling earrings should be worn. The only jewelry worn should be single earposts or wedding rings. Hair should be neat and off the collar. Wear only clear, unchipped nail polish over short, manicured nails. Male medical assistants should be clean-shaven and have short hair. The only jewelry should be a wedding ring. Colognes, perfumes, and aftershave should not be worn at work. Tattoos should not be visible.

Patient care can place physical demands upon medical assistants. Lifting and moving patients is often required and the use of correct body mechanics will help minimize injuries to the back. While every reasonable accommodation is made for physically challenged medical assistants, to be mobile without assistance is important because medical assistants move about throughout the day while performing tasks and procedures. It is frequently necessary to bend, stoop, kneel, and crouch, especially when filing and retrieving patients' records, and for other tasks as well. Most procedures require that medical assistants have the ability to hear and see well for the accurate completion of tasks (Figure 1-3). Listening to blood pressures, taking a medical history, observing patients, performing phlebotomy, and identifying microorganisms under a microscope are some of the routine tasks and procedures performed daily in a medical facility.

Manual dexterity is also needed for manipulating certain instruments and for entering data using a computer.

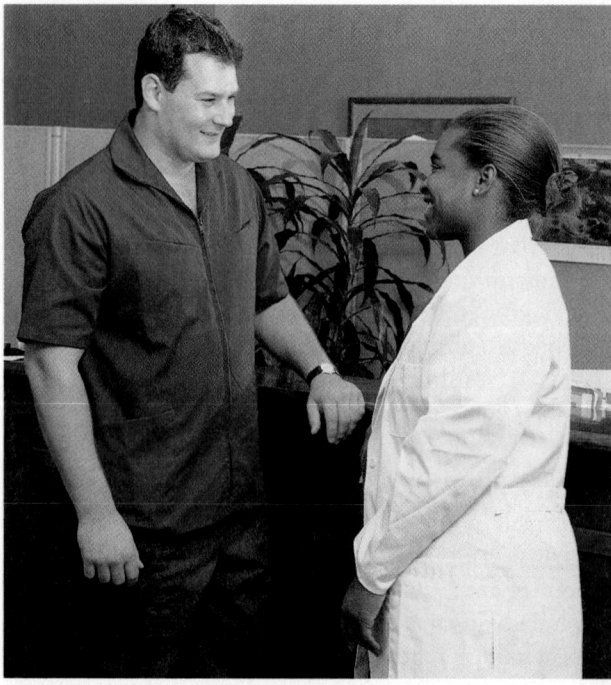

Figure 1-2 A professional, neat appearance makes patients feel at ease with their health care provider.

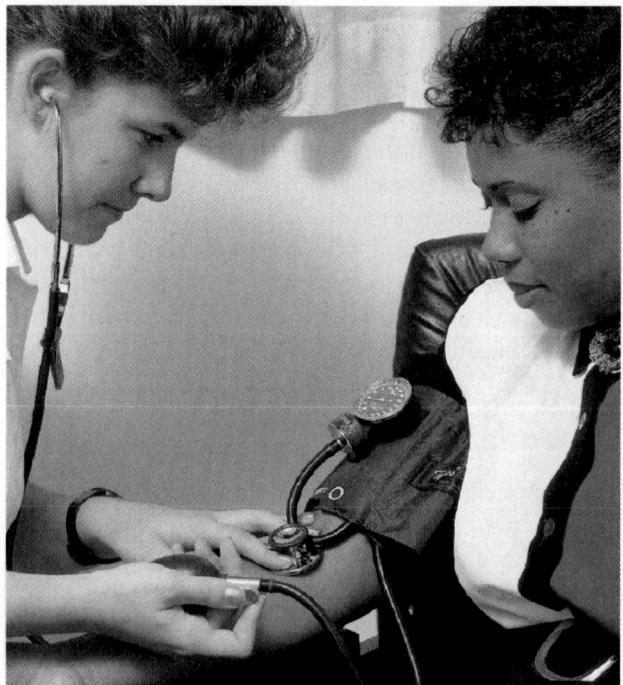

Figure 1-3 Measuring blood pressure is a task that requires the medical assistant to see and hear well.

Ability to Communicate

It is important that medical assistants learn to develop the ability to communicate well verbally and nonverbally with patients, staff, and other professionals.

Compliance with the physician's treatment plan is important for a positive outcome of patients' illnesses (Figure 1-4). Also, patients will feel more comfortable and less threatened in a medical office or ambulatory center that encourages staff to keep them informed.

Ethical Behavior

No discussion about personal attributes is complete without the mention of ethics. Ethics is a system of values each individual has that determines perceptions of right and wrong. Our life experiences mold this set of values, which is considered a personal code of ethics.

Medical ethics govern medical conduct or that behavior practiced as health care providers. These ethics involve relationships with patients, their families, fellow professionals, and society in general. Good ethical behavior will have a positive impact on the profession of medical assisting and on the medical community as well. By adhering to the medical assistants' Code of Ethics, we endeavor to elevate the profession to a position of dignity and respect. (A more in-depth discussion of this Code of Ethics can be found in Chapter 8.)

The personal qualities of empathy, healthy attitude, dependability, initiative, flexibility, the desire to learn, a wholesome physical presence, the ability to communicate well, and ethical behavior are some of the characteristics that any professional possesses and that medical assistants should strive to develop. When entering into the profession of medical assisting, it is important to learn more about these and other qualities and to begin to cultivate and refine them.

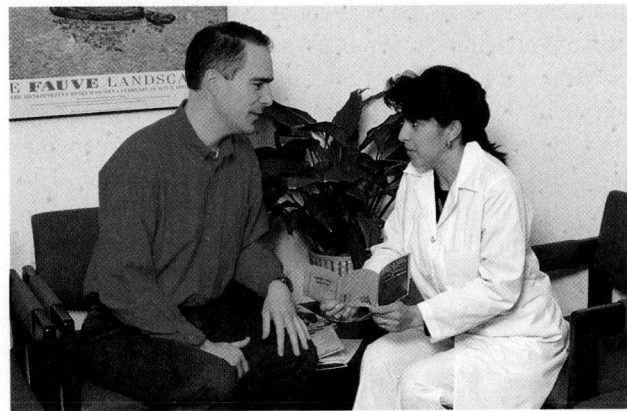

Figure 1-4 Patient education requires skill in communicating instructions to patients in language appropriate to their needs.

SPOTLIGHT ON AAMA ESSENTIALS THROUGH CAAHEP

- It is your attributes that enable others to trust you as their caregiver.
- A true professional behaves in an ethical manner.
- Continuing education should be an ongoing and life-enhancing experience.

HISTORICAL PERSPECTIVE OF MEDICAL ASSISTING

Historically, when physicians began their practices, it was common for them to hire individuals and train them on the job. Physicians originally hired nurses, but eventually they came to realize that nurses could not perform the variety of duties that are required in medical offices and ambulatory care centers. The nurse's role was limited to assisting the physician with clinical procedures, whereas the medical assistant's role was and is much broader and includes a large number of activities, procedures, and responsibilities, both administrative and clinical.

Today, with a much more informed patient comes the need for educated and credentialed medical assistants. Additionally, in today's litigious atmosphere, which makes health care providers vulnerable to malpractice suits, most employers recognize the importance of employing medical assistants who are professionally prepared through formal education. Employers want knowledgeable and dependable medical assistants so that physicians can focus their time and attention on the medical decisions, treatments, and techniques for which they have been educated and licensed. This leaves in the hands of the medical assistant, assisting the physician and the operation and management of the practice.

It was in 1978 that the profession of medical assisting was formally recognized by the United States Department of Education. Twenty-four years prior to this official recognition of the profession, a group of medical assistants gathered to establish a professional organization. With support, encouragement, and guidance from the American Medical Association (AMA), the American Association of Medical Assistants (AAMA) was founded in 1956 (Figure 1-5). The first president of the organization was Maxine Williams.

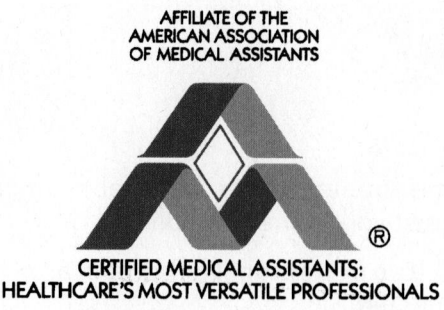

AFFILIATE OF THE
AMERICAN ASSOCIATION
OF MEDICAL ASSISTANTS

®

CERTIFIED MEDICAL ASSISTANTS:
HEALTHCARE'S MOST VERSATILE PROFESSIONALS

Figure 1-5 Logo of the American Association of Medical Assistants, a professional organization founded in 1956. (Courtesy of the AAMA)

In 1991, the AAMA's board of trustees approved the present definition of medical assisting:

> Medical Assisting is an allied health profession whose practitioners function as members of the health care delivery team and perform administrative and clinical procedures.

AMERICAN ASSOCIATION OF MEDICAL ASSISTANTS

The American Association of Medical Assistants has three major purposes:

1. Accreditation
2. Certification
3. Continuing education

Accreditation and certification standards were developed by the AMA and the AAMA through the Commission on Accreditation of Allied Health Education Programs (CAAHEP) for schools wishing assurance that their medical assistant programs are of the highest quality and satisfy CAAHEP criteria.

Accreditation

The AAMA works jointly with the AMA to define the essential components and appropriate standards of quality that educational institutions offer in their medical assistant curriculum. The United States Department of Education has approved the AAMA and AMA as an **accreditation,** or approving, body for educational programs for medical assistants. A medical assisting program that is accredited meets the standards as outlined in the *Standards and Guidelines for an Accredited Education Program for the Medical Assistant. Standards* are the minimum standards of quality used in accrediting programs that prepare individuals to enter the medical assisting profession. On-site review teams evaluate the program's **compliance** with, or adherence to, the standards. All aspects of programs seeking accreditation status undergo scrutiny to ascertain the program's quality and to ensure continued compliance with the standards.

Certification

As the profession grew and developed, some states came to require special licensure or certification to perform certain tasks, and in other states health professionals were challenged by the skill and broad spectrum of the medical assistant's ability. To defend medical assistants whose right to practice clinical procedures was being challenged, the AAMA responded at their 1995 convention with the following policy, which became effective February 1, 1998:

> that any candidate for the AAMA Certification Examination be a graduate of a CAAHEP-accredited medical assisting program. This requirement would become effective February 1, 1998. Anticipated benefits of the recommendation are to: (1) safeguard the quality of care to the consumer; (2) ensure the CMA's role in the rapidly evolving health care delivery system; and (3) continue to promote the identity and stature of the profession.

For a three-year trial period beginning in March 1998, graduates of medical assisting programs accredited by the Accrediting Bureau of Health Education Schools (ABHES) with 12 months of full-time health work experience or 24 months of part-time health work experience were eligible to take the AAMA certification examination.

Certification is voluntary, not mandatory, for medical assistants to practice, although the AAMA strongly urges those eligible to take the national certification examination. The exam measures professional **competency** at job entry level. Successful completion of the examination earns the individual the status of being certified and of being known as a **certified medical assistant (CMA).** The initials follow the individual's name. Conferring of the CMA status is referred to as being **credentialed** (Figure 1-6). It signifies recognition of competency by having attained a certain level of knowledge and skill.

In some areas of the United States, employers hire only certified medical assistants. The examination is offered twice yearly simultaneously at more than 200 test sites across the United States.

Recertification of the credential must be undertaken within five years from the date of certification in order to maintain current status as a CMA. Two routes are available to recertify. One is by accumulating approved continuing education hours, the other is by taking the certification examination again.

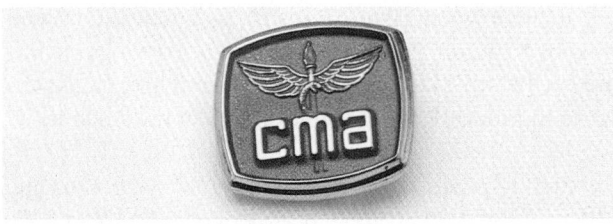

Figure 1-6 CMA pin awarded by the American Association of Medical Assistants upon successful completion of the national certification examination.

The status of a medical assistant's credentials (whether current or not current) is a public record available at the AAMA executive office, 20 N. Wacker Dr., Suite 1575, Chicago, IL 60606-2963. The AAMA Board of Trustees approved a policy change at the association's 1999 annual convention in Nashville. Effective January 1, 2003, all certified medical assistants who are employed or seeking employment *must* have current status as a CMA in order to use the credential. The mandatory current status for use of the CMA designation protects patients, employers, and the medical assistant's right to practice. Certification and recertification attest to the medical assistant's desire for professional development.

At one time, the credentials CMA-A (Certified Medical Assistant, Administrative); CMA-C (Certified Medical Assistant, Clinical); CMA-AC (Certified Medical Assistant, Administrative and Clinical); and CMA-Ped (Certified Medical Assistant, Pediatrics) were awarded to candidates who successfully passed specialty examinations in addition to the basic CMA examination.

While these specialty examinations have been phased out for newly graduated medical assistants, current medical assistants who have already earned these specialty credentials can maintain them and continue to be recertified through the Continuing Education Unit method.

Continuing Education

The AAMA vigorously encourages continuing education for all medical assistants. This can be accomplished through various means such as educational meetings, seminars, workshops, conventions, and the "Quest for Excellence," AAMA's series of home study courses for continuing education credit.

Membership in the AAMA is tri-level: local, state, and national. Educational meetings are held regularly at local and state meetings and conventions. The annual AAMA national convention provides an excellent forum for attaining knowledge through its educational offerings and for networking with other medical assistants.

Continuing an education is a lifelong process and serves as testimony to a commitment to professionalism.

REGISTERED MEDICAL ASSISTANT

The American Medical Technologists (AMT) is a national agency that certifies several different health professionals including medical assistants. In 1972, the AMT began offering and administering a national certification examination to medical assistants. The AMT offers a computerized examination year-round to qualified candidates. Upon successful completion of the examination, medical assistants receive a certificate designating them as **registered medical assistants (RMA).**

The association is similar to the AAMA. It has its own committees, conventions, bylaws, state chapters, officers, registrations, and revalidation examinations.

RMAs have been active in legislation to protect medical assistants, assuring improvement in medical assistant education, and providing for continuing education opportunities.

The RMA certification examination is given yearly in June and November at schools that have been accredited by the Accrediting Bureau of Health Education Schools (ABHES). To sit for the examination, applicants must have graduated from a medical assisting program accredited by ABHES or must meet certain experience requirements. AMT continuing education programs for renewal of the RMA credential also are available. The credential is awarded through the AMT (Figure 1-7). For more information, call 1-800-275-1268 or write to AMT, 710 Higgins Rd., Park Ridge, IL 60068.

EDUCATION OF THE PROFESSIONAL MEDICAL ASSISTANT

Formal education of medical assistants takes place in community and junior colleges as well as in **proprietary** schools. The AAMA has established educational requirements for program directors to follow for their programs to be considered accredited. These requirements were previously known as the DACUM Competencies. In 1997, in coordination with the National Board of Medical Examiners, educators, and practicing CMAs, the AAMA developed the Medical Assistant Role Delineation Chart, which is the occupational analysis of the medical assisting profession, and is included as an appendix of this

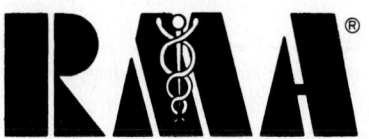

Figure 1-7 Logo of Registered Medical Assistant. Courtesy of American Medical Technologists.

text. In addition, the entry-level competencies that must be mastered by students in academic programs and the *Standards* (formerly *"Essentials"*) *and Guidelines for an Accredited Education Program for Medical Assistants* will be revised to reflect the findings of the Role Delineation Study.

Educational institutions seeking accreditation for a medical assisting program must develop the curricula to these *Standards and Guidelines* to ensure the highest quality medical assistant education and employment preparedness.

While not a complete list, some of the administrative, general (transdisciplinary), and clinical courses include those shown in Table 1-1.

Another aspect of an educational medical assisting program is the externship, a period of time when students participate in a practicum. This provides an excellent opportunity to apply theory to practice.

Preparation for Externship

Externship, practicum, and internship are all terms used to define the transition period between the classroom and actual employment. An externship is planned and supervised by a coordinator from the medical assisting program and the health care facility that agrees to become a partner in the education and employability of the student.

Externship Sites. Sites for externship are chosen carefully to ensure that a variety of experiences is available for the student. The sites should provide the student with adequate administrative, clinical, and general experiences. The staff at the various sites must be willing to make a commitment to the medical assistant's education by spending appropriate time observing and instructing the student.

Benefits of Externship. The externship experience is mutually beneficial to the student and staff at the health care facility that is providing the educational experiences.

Some of the benefits to the student are the opportunity to:

- Apply classroom knowledge and skill in a real-world medical setting

- Recognize improvement in performance and knowledge

- Understand that there may be more than one acceptable method of performance

- Begin to establish a network of support through colleagues

Some of the benefits to the externship site are:

- Greater alertness of staff because of their educational responsibilities to the student

- Opportunity for staff to observe students who will soon be seeking employment

- Possibility that staff will learn more about the profession of medical assisting

Educational institutions that confer associate or baccalaureate degrees require general education courses for graduation in addition to the administration and clinical courses.

There are four-year institutions of higher learning that offer a baccalaureate degree to medical assistants who have graduated with an associate's degree from a community or junior college. The graduate is accepted as a third-year student and can obtain a baccalaureate degree in such areas as health care management or health care facility administrator.

Because there is a demand for medical assistant educators, some medical assistants take education courses to become allied health educators.

TABLE 1-1   TYPICAL ADMINISTRATIVE, GENERAL, AND CLINICAL COURSES IN AN ACCREDITED MEDICAL ASSISTING PROGRAM
Administrative Courses
Computer Applications
Manual Recording of Patients' Data
Scheduling Appointments
Maintaining Medical Records
Word Processing/Typewriting/Keyboarding
Billing/Collections/Managing Patients' Accounts
Coding/Insurance Claims
Telephone Triage
Personnel Management
General Courses
Anatomy and Physiology
Medical Terminology
Diseases
Patient Education
Medical Law and Ethics
Clinical Courses
Pharmacology/Administration of Medications
Assisting Techniques/Physical Examination
Assisting with Minor Surgery
Basic Laboratory Procedures/Routine Blood and Urine Testing
Cardiopulmonary Resuscitation

CAREER OPPORTUNITIES

Medical assistants have been described as health care's most versatile, multifaceted professionals. The fact that medical assistants possess a broad scope of knowledge and skills makes them ideal professionals for any ambulatory care setting. Indeed, owing to such versatility, medical assistants find employment in a variety of settings: offices, clinics, hospitals, medical laboratories, insurance companies, government agencies, pharmaceutical companies, and educational institutions. Although the range of employment opportunities continues to grow, in the past decade, about four out of five medical assistants were employed in physicians' offices and clinics. About one in five worked in offices of other health care practitioners, such as chiropractors, optometrists, and podiatrists. The outlook for employment for medical assistants is very promising. According to the AAMA, there are presently 1.3 million medical assistants in the work force. The United States Department of Labor Bureau of Statistics listed medical assisting as one of the fastest growing allied health professions for the years 1998–2008.

Increased employment opportunities for medical assistants result from the increased medical needs of an aging population, growth in the number of health care practitioners and their desire to hire the most qualified person for the task, increased diagnostic testing, greater volume and complexity of paperwork and computer information, managed care's emphasis on ambulatory care, and the insurance-mandated shorter stay of patients in hospitals.

REGULATION OF HEALTH CARE PROVIDERS

One way health care providers can be regulated is through the process of credentialing. Credentialing recognizes health care providers who are professionally and technically competent. Recognition comes from professional associations, certifying agencies, and the state or federal government. Regulation ensures:

- Competence of health care providers
- A minimum standard of knowledge, training, and skill
- The limiting of the performance of certain procedures to a specific occupation

Licensure, certification, and registration are three kinds of regulations/credentialing. See Table 1-2.

Scope of Practice

Medical assisting is not licensed as a profession; however, some states require that medical assistants be graduates of an accredited medical assisting program in order to work as medical assistants.

Two examples of licensed professions are medicine and nursing. A **license** regulates the activities of these professions by enacting laws that specify educational requirements and by defining the scope of practice. A license is conferred upon an individual who successfully completes specialized educational requirements and successfully passes an examination administered by the state in which the individual resides. The state grants a license to that individual to practice medicine or nursing. Licensure forbids anyone who is not licensed from performing activities that are designated by that particular license. For example, the law states that the physician's license allows diagnosing and prescribing treatment. If someone were to diagnose or prescribe without a license, that individual would be committing an illegal act and would be practicing medicine without a license, which is considered a felony.

There are state laws that govern the practice of medicine and nursing (medical practice acts, nursing practice acts), and many states have acts that give physicians the right to delegate certain clinical procedures to

TABLE 1-2	COMPARISON OF REQUIREMENTS FOR CERTIFICATION, LICENSURE, AND REGISTRATION		
	Certification	**Licensure**	**Registration**
Practice Requirement	Voluntary	Mandatory	Voluntary
Conferred by	Nongovernmental agency or professional association	Legislated by each state	Professional association
	If qualified and meets requirements	If qualified and meets requirements	Listed on an official roster
	Must pass examination	Must pass state examination	Passing examination not always required
How restrictive	Used by most professional associations	Most restrictive	Least restrictive

qualified allied health professionals. Because medical assistants are not required to be licensed, they are allowed to perform clinical procedures only under the supervision of the physician or other licensed health care professional who is granted the right and who delegates the specific clinical procedures to them.

In some states, including California, Washington, and others, unlicensed health care providers are required to have authorization from the state to perform allergy testing, venipuncture, and to give injections. A registration fee and mandatory training are required. In such circumstances, medical assistants or other health care providers would be breaking the law if they performed these procedures without registration and training.

In some states, authorization is required for unlicensed health care providers to expose patients to X rays.

Medical assistants do not perform procedures for which they have not been educated and trained. The AAMA's Role Delineation Chart in the appendices is an excellent reference source that identifies which clinical, administrative, and general (transdisciplinary) procedures medical assistants are educated to perform. However, due to the variability of state statutes, the medical assistant would be wise to check with the executive director of the AAMA if there is doubt regarding the legality of performing certain clinical procedures.

SUMMARY

Progress has been made in the advancement of the profession of medical assisting since the first group of medical assistants gathered to become organized and formed the American Association of Medical Assistants. For example, the number of certified medical assistants has exceeded 70,000 and continues to grow since certification began in 1963. The total number of medical assistants in the work force is 1.3 million and employment opportunities continue to grow. Educational requirements have become increasingly important. The AAMA continues to promote standards of excellence for its members, encouraging continuing education and awarding continuing education credits to members of AAMA via various means.

All of these factors are evidence of a strong professional perspective and should offer encouragement and support to any student or graduate of medical assisting.

Becoming a professional is a gradual process and cannot be learned in its entirety from a textbook. The challenge of becoming a professional medical assistant will require open-mindedness and a desire for continued learning and education, certification, and recertification of the CMA credential, and professional involvement through organizational participation.

As the scope of work done by medical assistants broadens and medical assistants seek and require formal education, the professional medical assistant will gain additional respect and be in even greater demand. Medical assistants must continuously pursue excellence, which is the hallmark of all professional behavior.

REVIEW QUESTIONS

Multiple Choice

1. Medical assisting has been recognized by the United States Department of Education as a profession since what year?
   a. 1956
   b. 1964
   c. 1978
   d. 1995
2. The AAMA was established as a professional organization in what year?
   a. 1945
   b. 1956
   c. 1962
   d. 1967

3. The "Quest for Excellence" is:
   a. a professional publication for medical assistants
   b. a code of professional behavior for medical assistants
   c. otherwise known as ethical behavior
   d. the AAMA's series of home study courses
4. The designation Registered Medical Assistant is awarded by:
   a. American Association of Medical Assistants (AAMA)
   b. Accrediting Bureau of Health Education Schools (ABHES)
   c. American Medical Association (AMA)
   d. American Medical Technologists (AMT)

5. Increased employment opportunities for medical assistants result from:
   a. decreases in diagnostic testing
   b. computers decreasing volume of paperwork
   c. managed care's emphasis on ambulatory care
   d. longer hospital stays for patients

Critical Thinking

1. For each personal attribute used in your textbook to describe a professional, identify individuals from your family, friends, church, or community who possess one or more of these traits.
2. Patients and physicians desire professional medical assistants who have had the benefit of a formal education to care and work for them. Discuss the impact of this education on patients and employers. Why is it important to both groups?
3. Discuss the importance of certification and recertification.
4. Differentiate among certification, licensure, and registration.
5. Describe externship and its benefits.

WEB ACTIVITIES

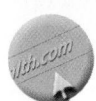

1. Visit the National Accrediting Agency for Clinical Laboratory Sciences (NAACLS) web site at http://www.naacls.org
   • What allied health professions other than medical technologist and clinical laboratory scientist are accredited by NAACLS?

• Does NAACLS have a code of ethics for the medical assistant?
2. Visit the American Association of Medical Assistants web site at http://www.amaa-ntl.org
   • What allied health profession does the AAMA accredit?
   • What resources are available on the web for medical assistants interested in continuing education?
3. Visit the American Medical Technologists web site at http://www.amtl.com

REFERENCES/BIBLIOGRAPHY

Balasa, D. (2000). Securing the future for medical assistants to practice. *Professional medical assistant*, January/February 2000, 6–7.

Keir, L., Wise, B. A., & Krebs, C. (1998). *Medical assisting: Administrative and clinical competencies* (4th ed.). Albany, NY: Delmar.

Kinn, M. E., & Woods, M. A. (1999). *The medical assistant: Administrative and clinical* (8th ed.). Philadelphia: W. B. Saunders.

Merriam-Webster (1998). *Merriam-Webster's collegiate dictionary* (10th ed.). Springfield, MA: Author.

Prickett-Ramutkowski, B., Barrie, A., Keller, C., Dazarow, L., & Abe, C. (1999). *Medical assistant: A patient-centered approach to administrative and clinical competencies* (1st ed.). Princeton, NJ: Glencoe/McGraw Hill.

2

HEALTH CARE SETTINGS AND THE HEALTH CARE TEAM

KEY TERMS

Acupuncture
Allied Health Professionals
Ambulatory Care Setting
Fringe Benefit
Health Maintenance Organization (HMO)
Holistic
Independent Physician Association (IPA)
Integrative Medicine
Managed Care
Managed Care Operation
Managed Competition
Partnership
Preferred Provider Organization (PPO)
Sole Proprietorship
Triage

OUTLINE

Ambulatory Health Care Settings
   Individual and Group Medical Practices
   Urgent Care Centers
   Managed Care Operations
The Impact of Managed Care in the Health Care Setting

The Health Care Team
   The Role of the Medical Assistant
   Health Care Professionals and Their Roles
   Allied and Other Health Professionals and Their Roles
   The Role of Integrative or Alternative Health Care Therapies
   The Value of the Medical Assistant to the Health Care Team

OBJECTIVES

The student should strive to meet the following performance objectives and demonstrate an understanding of the facts and principles presented in this chapter through written and oral communication.

1. Define the key terms as presented in the glossary.
2. Analyze the benefits and limitations of working in the different health care settings.
3. Assess the role and impact of managed care in the health care environment.
4. Identify and describe the three primary medical management models.
5. Describe the function of the health care team.
6. Discuss the role of the medical assistant in the health care team.
7. List and describe a minimum of twelve physician specialists.
8. List and describe a minimum of five nonphysician health care specialists.
9. List and describe a minimum of twelve allied health professionals.
10. Compare and contrast the types of nurses.
11. Critique alternative therapies and discuss their role in today's health care setting.

GENERAL
(TRANSDISCIPLINARY)

Professionalism

- Project a professional manner and image
- Adhere to ethical principles
- Demonstrate initiative and responsibility
- Work as a team member
- Promote the CMA credential

Communication Skills

- Serve as liaison

Legal Concepts

- Practice within the scope of education, training, and personal capabilities

INTRODUCTION

There are few professions in our society as rich and complex as the health care profession. In recent years, especially, the health care environment has been very much in flux as the profession seeks ways to provide quality care while containing costs. This effort to curtail costs has resulted in the rise of what is known as managed care, which, in turn, has spawned a number of medical models such as health maintenance organizations (HMOs) and preferred provider organizations (PPOs), two well-known managed care entities.

Many other types of physician networks and alliances are also being established as providers merge in order to give patients the best of care while controlling their costs. Ambulatory care settings, where services are provided on an outpatient basis, have become increasingly pivotal to consumer health care as insurers direct dollars away from hospitals and toward outpatient care.

Just as the medical setting continues to evolve to meet new societal needs, health care technology is ever-changing. Health care is a dynamic, stimulating industry that requires the medical assistant and other professionals to constantly develop new skills if they are to contribute to the team effort. The range of skills within the health care team is astonishing, and includes physicians, or medical doctors, in more than 25 specialties, more than 20 kinds of allied health professionals, and an increasing number of nontraditional alternative practitioners.

AMBULATORY HEALTH CARE SETTINGS

While medical assistants may work in a number of different environments, including laboratories or hospitals, most are employed in an **ambulatory care setting** such as a medical office (either a solo-physician or group practice), an urgent or primary care center, or a managed care organization such as an HMO.

Often, the medical assistant will choose to work in one setting rather than another based on interests, personality, and work preferences. For instance, the individual practice may provide medical assistants with the opportunity to use their full array of skills, while in urgent care centers, the work of the medical assistant may be more specialized in nature.

Medical assistants should also be aware of the three major forms of medical practice management and how they affect salary, benefits, and liability issues (Figure 2-1).

Individual and Group Medical Practices

For years, the most common form of medical office was the individual physician or group practice. Although this model now competes with a variety of other models such as urgent care centers and HMOs, many medical assistants will still find the individual or group practice a challenging place of employment.

Individual Practices. In the individual practice, also called the solo practice, one primary physician sees and treats all patients. While this type of arrangement is limited in the number of people it can serve, many patients feel secure in this kind of health care setting for they come to know and trust their doctor. Because they always see the same doctor, they feel their health care is being managed in a personal way. The solo-physician practice, however, can be an expensive arrangement, because one doctor must undertake the costs of office space, equipment, and personnel.

Group Practices. In today's managed care environment, group practices are attractive arrangements where two or more physicians can share the high costs of space, equipment, and personnel. The advantages of a group practice are not solely economic, however; physicians learn from and consult one another, while patients receive the benefit of this exchange of information and knowledge. Often, a group practice may have more than one office and some employees may be asked to travel between sites to cut overhead. Group practices may also be formed to offer specialized care, such as oncology or women's health care.

In most smaller group practices, patients may

FORMS OF MEDICAL PRACTICE MANAGEMENT

Medical assistants employed in ambulatory care settings or medical offices and clinics are likely to see three major forms of medical practice management. They are sole proprietorships, partnerships, and corporations.

Whatever form of management is chosen by physicians, they are responsible for the employees that serve with them. (Refer to the discussion of *respondeat superior* in Chapter 7.) Physician-employers and their medical assistants must have the kind of healthy working relationship where mutual trust and respect are apparent. The physician must understand the skill level of the medical assistant, and the medical assistant must feel secure enough to ask any questions necessary or admit any errors. Critical errors are often made when this trust does not exist between employer and employee. This causes a breakdown in the delivery of the best health care for patients.

Sole Proprietorships

In the past, many physicians preferred a solo practice. A solo practice entitles the physician or sole proprietor to hold exclusive right to all aspects of the medical practice or sole proprietorship, including profits and debts. If the business fails, the sole proprietor's personal property may also be attached.

A sole proprietorship may employ other physicians to participate in the practice. The employed physician(s) would be entitled to any employee fringe benefits such as health insurance and paid vacation, but the solo practitioner is not so entitled.

It is predicted that the business of practicing medicine may become more generalized and government regulated. Trends indicate more group practices and managed care facilities may gain dominance over the sole proprietorship

form of management for physicians. The accelerating cost of maintaining an office has become more prohibitive for a physician in a sole proprietorship, especially the new-graduate physician.

Partnerships

When two or more physicians join together under a legal agreement to share in the total business operations of the practice, a partnership is formed. Several physicians who share a facility and practice medicine are often referred to as a group. Partners share expenses, income, debt, equipment, records, and personnel according to a predetermined agreement. Partners are liable for only their own actions, but may be liable for the whole amount of the partnership debts.

Corporations

Physicians may form a corporation, usually referred to as a professional service corporation. The physician shareholders are considered employees of the corporation. A corporation allows income and tax advantages to all employees. A variety of fringe benefits can be offered to the employees, which may include pension, profit-sharing plans, medical expense reimbursement, and life, health, and disability insurance. These benefits are separate from salary. Another advantage is that professional employees of a corporation are liable only for their own acts, and personal property cannot be attached in litigation. A sole proprietor may incorporate if the practice is large enough.

The health maintenance organization (HMO) is one type of corporation in which physicians often practice. Basically, physicians are employees of the HMO and are paid by various methods; physicians in the HMO usually serve as the primary care physician (PCP). In this situation, a referral from the PCP may be necessary before a patient can see a specialist or allied health professional.

Figure 2-1   Different forms of medical practice models and how they may affect the medical assistant.

request that they see the same physician for all appointments, although sometimes patients are assigned to the next available doctor. For emergencies, group practices have the staff and flexibility to ensure that there is always a doctor on call.

Urgent Care Centers

Urgent care centers are usually private, for-profit centers that provide services for primary care, routine injuries and illnesses, and minor surgery. Sometimes lab services and a radiology department are located on the premises. Physicians and other health care professionals in the center are often salaried employees, not owners who share in the profits, and often are associated with other medical facilities.

The pace in most urgent care centers is brisk and typically a number of doctors are working at one time. Patients may be requested to make appointments, but in some centers drop-ins are accepted, especially for emergencies.

Because these centers can see a higher volume of patients, usually for a lower cost than the traditional solo-physician or small group practice, some experts predict that ambulatory care settings will continue to grow as private practices decrease in number.

Managed Care Operations

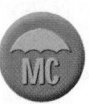 Health maintenance organizations, or HMOs, are probably the most familiar managed care operation. Originally, HMOs were

designed to provide a full range of health care services under one roof. More recently, the HMO without walls has become established, which is typically a network of participating physicians within a defined geographic area.

Originally, the HMO with walls was conceived to provide patients with comprehensive health care services at one facility. Today, as managed care and managed competition sweep the health care industry, other arrangements include the **preferred provider organization (PPO)**, where physicians network to offer discounts to employers and other purchasers of health insurance, and the **independent physician association (IPA)**, whose members agree to treat patients for an agreed-upon fee.

THE IMPACT OF MANAGED CARE IN THE HEALTH CARE SETTING

The emergence of **managed care** in today's society provides new administrative and clinical challenges to members of the health care team as they struggle to provide the best health care while working within limitations often imposed by insurance carriers. Virtually all health care settings, whether they are individual practices or urgent care centers, are experiencing the impact of managed care and **managed competition,** where physicians network and compete to serve patients better and more cost-efficiently.

Under managed care, critics charge, health care dollars have grown scarce, physicians must strive to provide the same quality for reduced reimbursement, preapprovals must be obtained for many services, and some services may be denied because they are not considered cost-effective.

Clinically, managed care may set limits on services or length of services. Second opinions are encouraged and sometimes required. In some systems, the patient selects a primary care physician, who is considered the gatekeeper and who must provide a referral for specialist care. Critics of managed care point out that restricting or denying services may lead to an increase in professional liability.

Administratively, paperwork and documentation have become increasingly important to assure proper reimbursement. While it is the patient's responsibility to understand the conditions of the insurance policy, these are often difficult to understand or interpret. The medical office or center must be fully aware of when a preapproval or treatment plan is required, when a second opinion is necessary for reimbursement, and of other clauses and restrictions that affect care and reimbursement for care.

At the same time, while managed care is challenging even the most resilient of providers, the very real need to keep costs down has also generated considerable creativity and energy among the health care profession as

SPOTLIGHT ON AAMA ESSENTIALS THROUGH CAAHEP

- Working as a team member and adapting to change makes a professional medical assistant stand out from others.
- Communication makes the difference between competency and negligence.
- Compassion and a caring attitude provide a positive experience for patients even when they are too ill to express their feelings.

physicians seek to use technology more efficiently, as they collaborate on new, cost-effective delivery methods, and as everyone involved in health care—insurers, providers, and patients—works together to contain costs by emphasizing prevention and lifestyle changes.

THE HEALTH CARE TEAM

In every kind of health care setting, the team concept is critical to the quality of patient care. A primary care physician is most likely the main source of health care for patients. From time to time, however, a specialist will be sought or recommended. A number of different allied health professionals, including the medical assistant, will supply additional health care as ordered by the physician. Increasingly, patients are looking outside traditional medicine for portions of their health care. While alternative care may not be covered by medical insurance, traditional and nontraditional health care practices are nonetheless blending in many areas. For example, **acupuncture** is becoming recognized as effective in the treatment of chronic pain. In whatever manner health care is sought, all members of this health care team must communicate, sometimes in person and sometimes just through the medical history and record, with one another to assure quality patient care.

The Role of the Medical Assistant

In the ambulatory care setting, a critical **allied health professional** is the medical assistant. The medical assistant, performing both administrative and clinical tasks under the direction of the physician, is an important link between patient and physician. The medical assistant serves in many capacities—receptionist, secretary, transcriptionist, bookkeeper, insurance coder and biller, patient educator, and clinical assistant. The latter requires the medical assistant to be able to administer injections and perform venipuncture, prepare patients for examinations, assist the physician with examinations and special procedures, and perform electrocardiography and various laboratory tests. Medical assistants triage and assess patient needs when scheduling appointments and tests. However, while medical assistants have a broad range of responsibilities, it is critical that they perform only within the scope of their training and personal capabilities and always function within ethical and legal boundaries and state statutes.

Because medical assistants are often the patient's first contact with the facility and its physicians, a positive attitude is important. They must be excellent communicators, both verbally and nonverbally, and project a professional image of themselves and their physician-employer. Medical assistants who believe in their work, who are proud of their career, and who convey compassion and caring provide a positive experience for patients who may be ill or in a great deal of discomfort.

Health Care Professionals and Their Roles

The public is often confused by the title *doctor*. The term implies an earned academic degree of the highest level in a particular area of study. Physicians have earned the MD or Doctor of Medicine degree. A doctorate in medicine and/or a license to practice allows a person to diagnose and treat medical conditions. The doctor of medicine candidate will attend four years of medical school after receiving a baccalaureate degree. An internship of one to two years follows in a hospital or major medical center. If a physician chooses to specialize, as many do, a residency

Patient Teaching Tip

Encourage patients to think of themselves as members of the health care team for they can provide invaluable information about their medical history. Use good communication skills to encourage patients to describe symptoms, identify their medications, and provide other information that is useful in diagnosis and treatment.

of two to five years in that specialty is required. In the medical field, the abbreviation *Dr.* is used and the title *doctor* is addressed to the person qualified by education, training, and licensure to practice medicine.

Other medical degrees include the Doctor of Osteopathy (DO), Doctor of Dentistry (DDS), Doctor of Optometry (OD), Doctor of Podiatric Medicine (DPM), Doctor of Chiropracty (DC), and Doctor of Naturopathy (ND). This group of doctors completes a different training regimen than that required for the Doctor of Medicine. The training is highly specialized and very specific but still grants the title of doctor upon completion, and when licensed, allows these health care professionals to diagnose and treat medical conditions.

In other nonmedical disciplines, the persons who have achieved a doctorate conferred by a college or university include the Doctor of Education (EdD) and the Doctor of Philosophy (PhD). Both the EdD and PhD have several areas of specialty.

Table 2-1 gives a selected listing of medical and surgical specialties, while Table 2-2 lists other health care specialists.

TABLE 2-1 SELECTED MEDICAL AND SURGICAL SPECIALTIES			
American Board of Medical Specialties	**General Certificates**	**Subspecialty Certificates**	
Allergy & Immunology	Allergy & Immunology	Clinical & Laboratory Immunology	
Anesthesiology	Anesthesiology	Critical Care Medicine	Pain Management
Colon & Rectal Surgery	Colon & Rectal Surgery		
Dermatology	Dermatology	Clinical & Laboratory Dermatological Immunology	Dermatopathology Pediatric Dermatology
Emergency Medicine	Emergency Medicine	Medical Toxicology Pediatric Emergency Medicine	Sports Medicine Undersea & Hyperbaric Medicine
Family Practice	Family Practice	Geriatric Medicine	Sports Medicine

(continues)

TABLE 2-1 *(continued)*

American Board of Medical Specialties	General Certificates	Subspecialty Certificates	
Internal Medicine	Internal Medicine	Adolescent Medicine Cardiovascular Disease Clinical Cardiac Electrophysiology Clinical & Laboratory Immunology Critical Care Medicine Endocrinology, Diabetes & Metabolism Gastroenterology	Geriatric Medicine Hematology Infectious Disease Interventional Cardiology Medical Oncology Nephrology Pulmonary Disease Rheumatology Sports Medicine
Medical Genetics	Clinical Biochemical Genetics Clinical Cytogenetics Clinical Genetics (MD) Clinical Molecular Genetics Ph.D. Medical Genetics	Molecular Genetic Pathology	
Neurological Surgery	Neurological Surgery		
Nuclear Medicine	Nuclear Medicine		
Obstetrics & Gynecology	Obstetrics & Gynecology	Critical Care Medicine Gynecologic Oncology	Maternal & Fetal Medicine Reproductive Endocrinology
Ophthalmology	Ophthalmology		
Orthopaedic Surgery	Orthopaedic Surgery	Hand Surgery	
Otolaryngology	Otolaryngology	Otology/Neurotology Pediatric Otolaryngology	Plastic Surgery within the Head and Neck
Pathology	Anatomic Pathology & Clinical Pathology Anatomic Pathology Clinical Pathology	Blood Banking/Transfusion Medicine Chemical Pathology Cytopathology Dermatopathology Forensic Pathology	Hematology Immunopathology Medical Microbiology Molecular Genetic Pathology Neuropathology Pediatric Pathology
Pediatrics	Pediatrics	Adolescent Medicine Clinical & Laboratory Immunology Development-Behavioral Peds Medical Toxicology Neonatal-Perinatal Medicine Neurodevelopmental Disabilities Pediatric Cardiology Pediatric Critical Care Medicine Pediatric Emergency Medicine Pediatric Endocrinology	Pediatric Gastroenterology Pediatric Hematology- Oncology Pediatric Infectious Diseases Pediatric Nephrology Pediatric Pulmonology Pediatric Rheumatology Sports Medicine

Physical Medicine
  & Rehabilitation
	Physical Medicine
	  & Rehabilitation
		Pain Management
		Spinal Cord Injury Medicine
			Pediatric Rehabilitation
			Medicine

Plastic Surgery	Plastic Surgery	Surgery of the Hand Plastic Surgery within the Head and Neck	
Preventive Medicine	Aerospace Medicine Occupational Medicine Public Health & General Preventive Medicine	Medical Toxicology Undersea & Hyperbaric Medicine Undersea Medicine	

Psychiatry & Neurology	Psychiatry
	Neurology
	Neurology with Special
	  Qualifications in Child
	  Neurology
		Addiction Psychiatry
		Child & Adolescent Psychiatry
		Clinical Neurophysiology
			Forensic Psychiatry
			Geriatric Psychiatry
			Neurodevelopmental
			  Disabilities
			Pain Management

Radiology	Diagnostic Radiology Radiation Oncology Radiological Physics	Neuroradiology Nuclear Radiology Pediatric Radiology	Vascular & Interventional Radiology
Surgery	Surgery	Pediatric Surgery Surgery of the Hand	Surgical Critical Care Vascular Surgery
Thoracic Surgery	Thoracic Surgery		
Urology	Urology		

Copyright 2000 American Board of Medical Specialties

TABLE 2-2 OTHER HEALTH CARE SPECIALISTS

Title	Degree	Function
Chiropractic Medicine	Chiropractors are licensed in their field of practice. They hold a degree of DC, or Doctor of Chiropractic.	Manipulative treatment of disorders originating from misalignment of the spinal vertebrae
Dentistry	Dentists are licensed in their field of practice, which can range from general to highly specialized. They hold the degree of DDS, or Doctor of Dental Surgery.	Diagnosing and treating diseases and disorders of the teeth and gums
Optometry	Optometrists are licensed in their field of practice. They hold the degree of OD, or Doctor of Optometry.	Measuring the accuracy of vision to determine if corrective lenses are needed
Osteopathy	Osteopaths are physicians who hold the title DO or Doctor of Osteopathy.	A therapeutic system that restores or preserves health through manipulation of the skeleton and muscles. Osteopaths also rely upon physical, medicinal, and surgical methods
Podiatry	Podiatrists are licensed in their field of practice. They hold the degree of DPM, or Doctor of Podiatric Medicine.	Diagnosing and treating diseases and disorders of the feet
Psychology	Psychologists are licensed in their field of practice. They hold the degree of PhD, or Doctor of Philosophy. (Some hold only a master's degree, or MA, and are not permitted to use the title *doctor*.)	Evaluating and treating emotional problems. These professionals give counseling to individuals, families, and groups

Allied and Other Health Professionals and Their Roles

In the health care team, allied health professionals bring specific educational backgrounds and a broad array of skills to the medical environment. Medical assistants are considered allied health professionals. Table 2-3 lists some of the allied health professionals recognized by the Commission on Accreditation of Allied Health Education Programs (CAAHEP) and other national accrediting bodies.

TABLE 2-3 ALLIED HEALTH PROFESSIONS

Occupation	Abbreviations	Job Description
Anesthesiologist Assistant	AA	Performs preoperative tasks, performs airway management and drug administration for induction and maintenance of anesthesia during surgery under direction of a licensed and qualified anesthesiologist
Athletic Trainer	AT	Provides a variety of services including injury prevention, recognition, immediate care, treatment, and rehabilitation after athletic trauma
Cardiovascular Technologist	CVT	Performs diagnostic exams under the direction of a physician in (1) invasive cardiology, (2) noninvasive cardiology, and (3) noninvasive peripheral vascular study
Clinical Laboratory Scientist	CLS	Develops data on the blood, tissues, and fluids of the human body by using a variety of precision instruments
Clinical Laboratory Technician *Associate Degree*	CLT	Performs all routine tests in a medical lab and is able to discriminate and recognize factors that directly affect procedures and results. Works under direction of pathologist, physician, medical technologist, or scientist
Clinical Laboratory Technician *Certificate*	CLT	Performs many routine uncomplicated procedures in medical lab where discrimination is clear and errors are few and easily corrected. Works under direction of pathologist, physician, medical technologist, or scientist
Cytotechnologist	CT	Works with pathologists to detect changes in body cells that may be important in early diagnosis of cancer or other diseases primarily through microscopic analysis

(continues)

TABLE 2-3 *(continued)*

Occupation	Abbreviations	Job Description
Diagnostic Medical Sonographer	DMS	Provides patient services using medical ultrasound under the supervision of a physician
Electroneurodiagnostic Technologist	EEG-T	Possesses the knowledge, attributes, and skills to obtain interpretable recordings of a patient's nervous system functions
Emergency Medical Technician—Paramedic	EMT-P	Recognizes, assesses, and manages medical emergencies of acutely ill or injured patients in prehospital care settings, working under the direction of a physician (often through radio communication)
Health Information Administrator	RRA	Manages health information systems consistent with the medical, administrative, ethical, and legal requirements of the health care delivery system
Health Information Technician	ART	Possesses the technical knowledge and skills necessary to process, maintain, compile, and report patient data
Medical Assistant	MA, CMA, RMA	Functions under the supervision of licensed medical professionals and is competent in both administrative/office and clinical/lab procedures
Medical Illustrator	MI	Creates visual material designed to facilitate the recording and dissemination of medical, biological, and related knowledge through communication media
Nuclear Medicine Technologist	NMT	Assists the nuclear medicine physician to make diagnostic evaluations of the anatomic or physiologic conditions of the body and to provide therapy with unsealed radioactive sources
Occupational Therapist	OT	Educates and trains individuals in the application of purposeful, goal-oriented activity in the evaluation, diagnosis, and/or treatment of loss of the ability to cope with the tasks of living and impairment due to physical injury, illness, or emotional disorder, congenital or developmental disability, or the aging process
Occupational Therapy Assistant	OTA	Directs an individual's participation in selected tasks to restore, reinforce, and enhance performance; facilitates learning of those skills and functions essential for adaptation and productivity; diminishes or corrects pathology; and promotes and maintains health (under the direction of an occupational therapist)
Ophthalmic Medical Technician or Technologist	OMT	Assists ophthalmologists to carry out diagnostic and therapeutic procedures
Orthotist/Prosthetist	OP	Orthotists design and fit devices to provide care to patients who have disabling conditions of the limbs and spine; prosthetists design and fit devices for patients who have partial or total absence of a limb
Perfusionist	PERF	Operates extracorporeal circulation equipment during any medical situation where it is necessary to support or temporarily replace the patient's circulation or respiratory functions
Physician Assistant (includes Surgeon's Assistant)	PA	Practices medicine under the direction and responsible supervision of a doctor of medicine or osteopathy; performs diagnostic, therapeutic, preventive, and health maintenance services in any setting in which the physician renders care
Radiation Therapist	RADT	Administers radiation therapy services to patients under the supervision of radiation oncologists
Radiographer	RT(R)	Provides patient services using imaging modalities, as directed by physicians qualified to order and/or perform radiologic procedures
Respiratory Therapist	RRT	Applies scientific knowledge and theory to practical clinical problems of respiratory care
Respiratory Therapy Technician	CRTT	Administers general respiratory care
Surgical Technologist	ST	Works as integral member of the surgical team, which includes surgeons, anesthesiologists, registered nurses, and other surgical personnel delivering patient care and assuming appropriate responsibilities before, during, and after surgery

Adapted from Health Professions Directory, 2000–2001, 28th ed. © American Medical Association, Chicago, IL

As a medical assistant, you may not work directly with all the identified allied health care professionals, but you are likely to have contact with many of them by telephone and written or electronic communication. Knowledge of the roles these health professionals play enables you to interact more intelligently with all members of the health care team.

In addition to the professionals listed in Table 2-3, you may encounter some or all of the following health care professionals in daily patient care.

Health Unit Coordinator (HUC).

Health unit coordinators (HUC) perform nonclinical patient care tasks for the nursing unit of a hospital. This profession requires a self-motivated, mature individual who can handle the stress and hectic pace of coordinating personnel and their duties at the nurses' station. Also called unit secretary, administrative specialist, ward clerk, or ward secretary, a health unit coordinator receives on-the-job training with an emphasis on administrative office skills.

Medical Laboratory Technologist (MLT).

Medical laboratory technologists physically and chemically analyze, as well as culture, urine, blood, and other body fluids and tissues. They work closely with physician specialists such as oncologists, pathologists, and hematologists. Knowledge of specimen collection, anatomy and physiology, biochemistry, laboratory equipment, asepsis, and quality control is essential. The American Society of Clinical Pathology (ASCP) is a professional organization that oversees credentialing and education in the medical laboratory professions. See Figure 2-2.

Nurses.

The nursing profession is not listed in Table 2-3 because CAAHEP is not responsible for nurses' training

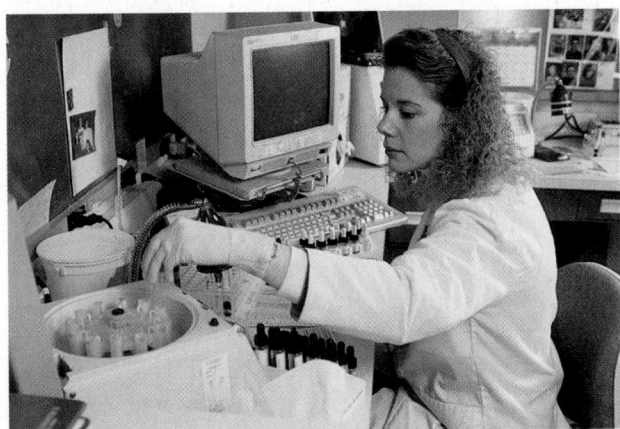

Figure 2-2 Medical technologists perform blood analyses and analyze and culture other body fluids as well. (Photo by Marcia Butterfield, courtesy of W. A. Foote Memorial Hospital, Jackson, MI)

and accreditation. Nurses are licensed by the state in which they practice. Although nurses' education and training are oriented to bedside care, some are employed in medical offices as clinical assistants, especially in offices where surgery is performed. Nurses play a number of roles on the health care team.

Registered Nurse (RN). In the United States, RNs are professionals who have completed at a minimum, a two-year course of study at a state-approved school of nursing and passed the National Council Licensure Examination (NCLEX-RN). They are licensed only by the state to practice. Employment settings most often include hospitals, convalescent homes, clinics, and home health care.

Licensed Practical Nurse (LPN). An LPN is a professional trained in basic nursing techniques and direct patient care. LPNs practice under the direct supervision of a registered nurse or physician and are employed in similar settings to RNs. Training includes completion of a state-approved program in practical nursing and successful completion of a national licensure examination.

Nurse Practitioner (NP). A nurse practitioner is a registered nurse who, by advanced education (usually a master's degree) and clinical experience in a branch of nursing, has acquired expert knowledge in a specific medical specialty. Nurse practitioners are employed by physicians in private practice or in clinics, and sometimes practice independently, especially in rural areas.

Registered Dietitian (RD).

Registered dietitians have specialized training in the nutritional care of groups and individuals and have successfully completed an examination of the Commission on Dietetic Registration. Dietitians assist patients in regulating their diets. Although they are typically employed in hospitals and clinics, they can also be found working with the public in personal nutritional counseling. Education includes a baccalaureate degree with a major in dietetics, food and nutrition, or food service systems management plus completion of an approved internship. See Chapter 22, Nutrition in Health and Disease, for more information.

Pharmacist (RPh).

Pharmacists are licensed by each state to prepare and dispense all types of medications as well as medical supplies related to medication administration. They may practice in hospitals, medical centers, and pharmacies. The minimum training for a pharmacist is a five-year baccalaureate degree; some pharmacists pursue a Doctor of Pharmacy degree (Pharm D), offered by major universities in the United States. Pharmacy technicians assist the pharmacist with preparation and administration

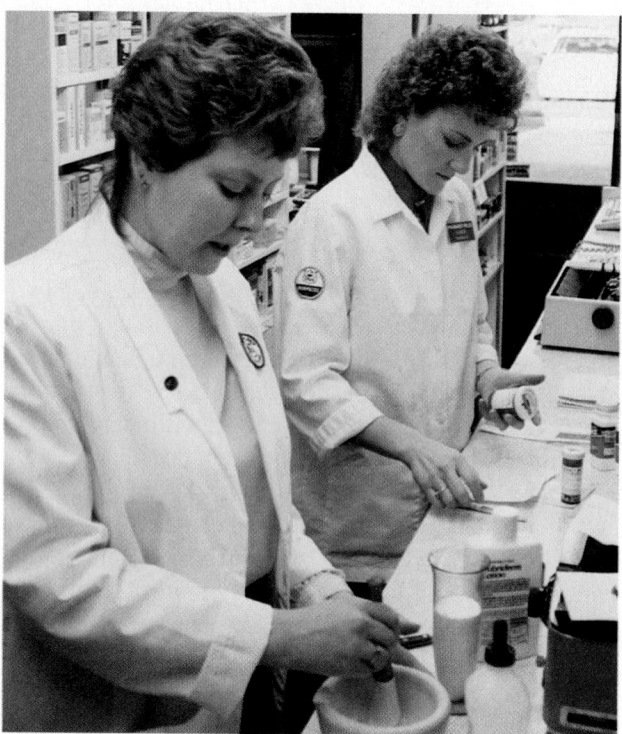

Figure 2-3   Pharmacy technicians prepare medications to be dispensed. (Courtesy of the Michigan Pharmacists Association and the Michigan Society of Pharmacy Technicians)

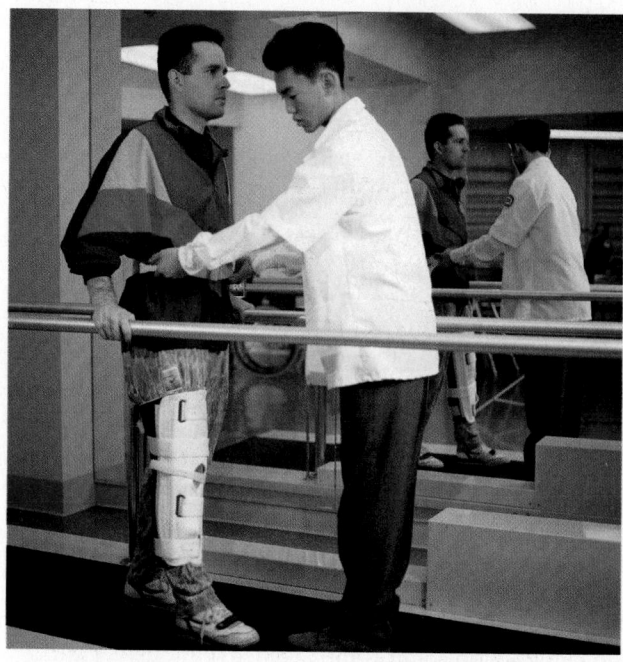

Figure 2-4   Physical therapists work with disabled and physically challenged individuals and with patients who require physical rehabilitation.

of medications, as well as perform receptionist and billing duties. Professional certification of pharmacy technicians varies from state to state and is administered by state pharmacy associations. See Figure 2-3.

Phlebotomist (LPT). Phlebotomists are trained in the art of drawing blood for diagnostic laboratory testing. Phlebotomists are also referred to as lab liaison technicians. Phlebotomists may be nationally certified and are employed in medical clinics, hospitals, and laboratories. Training consists of one to two semesters in a community college program or on-the-job training.

Physical Therapist (PT). Physical therapists are licensed professionals who assist in the examination, testing, and treatment of physically disabled or challenged people. They also assist in physical rehabilitation of patients following an accident, injury, or serious illness using special exercises, application of heat or cold, *ultrasound* therapy and other techniques. Educational requirements for a physical therapist are a minimum of a four-year baccalaureate degree (bachelor of science) or a special certificate course after obtaining the bachelor of science in a related field. Physical therapists must also successfully complete a state licensure examination. See Figure 2-4.

Physical Therapy Assistant (PTA). Physical therapy assistants are trained to use and apply physical therapy procedures such as exercise and physical agents under the supervision of a physical therapist. The physical therapy assistant is a graduate of an accredited associate of science degree program and must pass a licensure or registry examination in selected states.

The Role of Integrative or Alternative Health Care Therapies

Increasingly, integrative medicine or alternative forms of health care are being perceived as complements to traditional health care. As mentioned earlier, some nontraditional approaches, such as acupuncture, have been very successful in pain management or in reducing stress-related illnesses. For example, a patient being treated with medication for high blood pressure may also try to manage the hypertension with diet, exercise, and relaxation techniques. Sometimes this is considered a holistic approach to patient care, which takes into account the whole person.

While there is often controversy and confusion about the role of many alternative approaches, medical assistants should nonetheless be aware of the philosophy and intent of nontraditional therapies. Table 2-4 reviews some of the more common approaches.

TABLE 2-4   SELECTED EXAMPLES OF ALTERNATIVE APPROACHES TO HEALTH CARE

Type of Approach	Description of Approach
Acupuncture	A piercing of the skin by long needles into any of 365 points along twelve meridians that transverse the body. Each point is related to a particular organ. Acupuncture is often successful in managing pain and has been successfully used to treat drug dependency.
Biofeedback	A relaxation technique that uses monitoring devices to gain information about certain automatic body responses such as heart rate or blood pressure in order to help the patient gain some voluntary control over that function. Biofeedback is often used to treat hypertension and migraine headaches.
Holism	An approach that treats the whole body, mind, and spirit. A holistic practitioner considers the needs of the patient in all areas, including physical, emotional, social, spiritual, and economic.
Homeopathy	A method of treating disease by administering very dilute doses of remedies that are typically made from natural substances. In more massive doses, these remedies would produce symptoms of the disease being treated. This is in contrast to traditional allopathic medicine, which typically treats disease with remedies that produce effects different from those caused by the disease itself.
Hypnotherapy	An approach that encourages patients to enter a trance-like state in which they are more open to suggestion. The hypnotherapist makes verbal suggestions in the attempt to bring some desired behavior change.
Naturopathy	Naturopaths are licensed in their field of practice and hold the degree of ND, Doctor of Naturopathy. Naturopaths diagnose and treat patients using the relationship between mind/body/spirit and nature.
Therapeutic Touch	Therapeutic touch uses the hands to facilitate healing and to restore wholeness, harmony, and well-being to the patient. Often practiced by nurses, therapeutic touch is considered a modern interpretation of ancient healing practices. It is thought to be effective for producing relaxation, reducing pain, and promoting wound healing.

The Value of the Medical Assistant to the Health Care Team

With their broad range of competencies in both administrative and clinical areas, medical assistants are increasingly valued as health care team members. Medical assistants are the great communicators, serving as liaison between physician and hospital staff and between physician and any number of allied and other health professionals. Because they are the first providers to see or speak with patients, they undertake responsibility for directing, informing, and guiding patient care while establishing a professional and caring tone for the entire health care team. The value of a competent, professional, caring medical assistant is immeasurable in today's fast-paced and challenging health care environment.

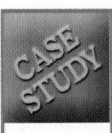

The number of sole proprietors is declining in this country.

CASE STUDY REVIEW

2.1

1. Identify at least five reasons for this decline.
2. Describe the impact, if any, this decline has on quality health care.

SUMMARY

The health care environment is a dynamic profession and one that changes rapidly in response to new technology and societal needs. In an effort to reduce the cost of health care, managed care has had and will continue to have a profound impact on all health care settings. A strong health care team is critical in the health care setting, as primary care physicians, specialists of all disciplines, and allied and other health professionals collaborate on the best way to provide patient care. Increasingly, selected alternative treatments may begin to complement traditional health care solutions. In almost any health care environment, but especially the ambulatory care setting, the medical assistant is a vital link in the team and is responsible for a range of responsibilities, both clinical and administrative.

REVIEW QUESTIONS

Multiple Choice

1. Medical assistants are employed for the most part in:
   a. hospitals
   b. nursing facilities
   c. ambulatory care settings
   d. insurance companies
2. A health maintenance organization is one kind of:
   a. managed care operation
   b. individual practice
   c. sole proprietorship
   d. hospital
3. With its emphasis on controlling costs, managed care is likely to affect:
   a. only hospitals
   b. all health care settings
   c. only physicians in private practice
   d. only patients
4. The health care team:
   a. should exclude the patient from being part of the team
   b. is only important in the hospital setting
   c. is made up of physicians and nurses
   d. is made up of physicians, nurses, allied and other health care professionals, patients, and sometimes a practitioner of nontraditional medicine
5. Integrative or alternative health care approaches:
   a. are increasingly accepted as complementary to traditional health care
   b. are always covered by insurance
   c. are not safe to practice
   d. are not important to understand
6. A medical assistant permitted by law to draw blood for diagnostic laboratory testing performs a procedure similar to those performed by a:
   a. health unit coordinator
   b. radiation therapist
   c. phlebotomist
   d. cytotechnologist
7. The distinct difference between the PA and the MA is that the PA:
   a. draws blood and gives injections
   b. practices medicine
   c. performs diagnostic services
   d. both b and c
8. Physicians just establishing their practice often seek to work with another physician in the same field. When expenses and profits are shared, this form of management is called a/an:
   a. HMO
   b. corporation
   c. sole proprietorship
   d. group or partnership
9. Managed care may be identified as care that:
   a. offers unlimited services
   b. forbids second opinions
   c. establishes a primary care physician as gate-keeper
   d. offers protection to physicians against liability
10. An alternative approach to medicine that treats patients using the relationship between mind/body/spirit/and nature is:
    a. homeopathy
    b. holism
    c. acupuncture
    d. naturopathy

Critical Thinking

1. Evaluate the different health care settings and discuss the pros and cons of working in each setting.
2. From a patient point of view, which health care setting do you think offers more benefits? Why?
3. Review the three forms of medical management models. Which is probably the most advantageous from the physician's point of view? From the medical assistant's point of view?
4. Discuss the purpose of managed care. What impact is it having on health care?
5. What kinds of professionals make up the health care team?
6. Discuss the role of the medical assistant in the health care team. What qualities does the medical assistant need to possess?
7. If you were attending a family reunion and overheard a discussion about the title *doctor*, how would you clarify the situation? What are some examples of individuals who might be referred to as a doctor?
8. What organization recognizes allied health professionals?
9. Recall a few types of allied health professionals and, working in small groups, have each student create a scenario in which the medical assistant needs to coordinate with two or three allied professionals.
10. What role might alternative therapies play in the health care setting? Describe a few different alternative approaches and their philosophies.

WEB ACTIVITIES

 Visit http://www.abms.org for the most current list of the American Board of Specialties. What does board certified mean? Who credentials a specialist? How is this different from the certification or registration of medical assistants?

REFERENCES/BIBLIOGRAPHY

American Board of Medical Specialties (1997). *The official ABMS directory of board certified medical specialists* (26th ed.). Evanston, IL: author.

Burton Goldberg Group (1995). *Alternative medicine*. Fife, WA: Future Medicine Publishing.

Health professions directory (27th ed.). (1999–2000). Chicago: American Medical Association.

Humphrey, D. D. (1996). *Contemporary medical office procedures* (2nd ed.). Albany, NY: Delmar.

Mosby's medical, nursing and allied health dictionary (5th ed.). (1998). St. Louis: Mosby-Year Book, Inc.

Smith, G. L., Davis, P. E., & Dennerll, J. T. (1999). *Medical terminology: A programmed systems approach* (8th ed.). Albany, NY: Delmar.

Stanfield, P. S. (1995). *Introduction to the health professions* (2nd ed.). Sudbury, MA: Jones & Bartlett Publishers.

Taber's cyclopedic medical dictionary (18th ed.) (1997). Philadelphia: F. A. Davis.

Warden, C. D. (1986). *Health care in the 1980s from a consumer's perspective*. Unpublished doctoral dissertation, Union Graduate School, Seattle, WA.

Weil, A. (1995). *Spontaneous healing*. New York: Alfred A. Knopf.

HISTORY OF MEDICINE

3

KEY TERMS

Acupuncture
Allopathic
Asepsis
Bubonic Plague
Malaria
Moxibustion
Pharmacopoeia
Pluralistic (Pluralism)
Septicemia
Typhus (Typhoid)
Yellow Fever

OUTLINE

Cultural Heritage in Medicine
Medical Specialists
Medical Education
Attitudes toward Illness

Medical Treatments
Significant Contributions to
  Medicine
New Frontiers in Medicine

OBJECTIVES

The student should strive to meet the following performance objectives and demonstrate an understanding of the facts and principles presented in this chapter through written and oral communication.

1. Define the key terms as presented in the glossary.
2. Discuss the effects of culture on medicine.
3. Identify the role of religion, magic, and science in medicine's history.
4. Describe how attitudes toward illness are manifested today.
5. Identify a minimum of three common medical treatments used in the past.
6. Recall a minimum of three theories/practices of ancient medicine still prevalent today.
7. Name and describe the historical roles of medical specialists.
8. Discuss the role of women in medicine.
9. Trace the progression of medical education.
10. Name at least five significant contributions to medicine.
11. Identify a minimum of three recent developments in medicine.

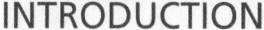

INTRODUCTION

A historical overview of medicine must do more than identify a series of contributions by physicians. It must remind us that more than one discipline and more than one philosophy have contributed to medicine. This is perhaps more true now than ever as our world becomes smaller and our society becomes increasingly **pluralistic,** ethnically, culturally, and religiously.

CULTURAL HERITAGE IN MEDICINE

Today's health professional will give care to individuals of varied cultures who hold differing philosophical beliefs toward medicine. The informed and caring health professional will recognize that a person's culture and ethnic heritage play an enormous role in any kind of health care. For example, if the cultural experience leans toward a more natural, nonmedical form of health care, treating the patient with prescription drugs will necessitate an explanation and rationale for the use of medications. Otherwise, the patient may refuse to take all or part of the medications, thus hindering recovery. It would be better to seek a treatment for the patient that embraces both the health care professional's desire to heal and the individual's wish to respect cultural tradition.

In every society, medicine has been an important element for its people. From the earliest time, culture was an important influence on medicine, and modern day medicine is in many ways a reflection of this diverse and rich heritage.

It is certain that religion, magic, and science all played a vital part in the history of medicine. Religion was important because it was perceived that certain gods were to be called upon for a cure through ceremonies, prayers, and sacrifices. Magic was practiced because it was such an important part of many societies and was seen as an essential ingredient to chase away evil spirits. The importance of science was demonstrated in the use of plants and minerals for medicinal purposes. The use of plants and minerals is found throughout medicine's history. Unearthed clay tablets reveal hundreds of plants, minerals, and animal substances used for medicinal purposes in ancient Mesopotamia and Babylon. The Chinese **pharmacopoeia** was rich in the use of herbs.

Skeletal remains of prehistoric cultures show advanced stages of arthritis, a nearly toothless jaw and only a 20- to 40-year lifespan for humans. Skull bones reveal round holes (trephination) believed to be necessary to release the evil spirits thought to be causing a person's ill-

ness. Mesopotamian cultures believed that illness was a punishment by the gods for violation of a moral code. Ancient Egyptians believed the body was a system of channels for air, tears, blood, urine, sperm, and feces. All the channels were thought to come together in the rectum, and were believed to become easily clogged. Thus, emetics, enemas, and purges of the anus were common treatments. In ancient India, plastic surgery was practiced. Punishment for adultery was cutting off the nose, therefore allowing physicians many opportunities to practice and refine the art of nose reconstruction.

The ancient Chinese examined and carefully monitored the pulse in each wrist. It was believed that the pulse had hundreds of characteristics important in medical treatment. There were five methods of treatment to bring a person back to the right track. They were:

1. Cure the spirit.
2. Nourish the body.
3. Give medications.
4. Treat the whole body.
5. Use acupuncture and moxibustion.

Acupuncture is the piercing of the skin by long needles into any of 365 points along twelve meridians that transverse the body and transmit an active life force called "ch'i" (pronounced chee). Each of these spots is related to a particular organ. **Moxibustion** requires the use of a powdered plant substance that is made into a small mound on the person's skin and then burned, usually raising a blister.

Even today's **allopathic,** or traditional, physicians would agree that the first four methods of treatment from Chinese culture are excellent guidelines for health care. There is an increasing awareness, also, that acupuncture has a valid place in allopathic medicine, especially for the control of pain.

MEDICAL SPECIALISTS

Medicine's history gives early evidence of many "specialists" in the healing arts. They were known by various names—witch doctors, medicine men and women, shamans or healing priests, and physicians. These healers were more than ancestors of the modern physician, however, for they performed many functions that involved the welfare of the entire community or village. By today's standards, they were considered to be equivalent to spiritual advisers, social workers, counselors, and teachers.

While women were accepted as healers in primitive societies, later cultures reduced their status to that of being allowed to care only for women and to assist in childbirth. In any culture that granted women only secondary status, women are also considered unqualified to become physicians. In Chinese culture, the first reference to a female physician mentioned by name is in documents from the Han dynasty (206 B.C.–A.D. 220). In Muslim society, the reluctance of Arabic physicians to violate social taboo and touch the genitals of female strangers further encouraged relegating the practice of obstetrics and gynecology to midwives.

Women were not accepted as medical doctors in Western culture until the nineteenth and twentieth centuries. Italy granted women the status earlier than other cultures. In America, the first female physician was Elizabeth Blackwell, who was awarded her degree in 1849. While she was snubbed by the public, she soon earned the respect of her colleagues. When she refused to be absent from class when the male reproductive system was discussed, her fellow male students supported her actions.

From the earliest times, it appears that some payment was expected for medical services rendered. In many instances, the payment was dependent upon the status of the physician as well as the patient. At the same time, some cultures punished a physician who was not successful in treatment by forcing that physician to treat only those too poor to pay.

MEDICAL EDUCATION

During the rise of Christianity, emphasis was placed on the soul rather than the body; therefore, early Christian monks held great control over medicine. This is evidenced by St. Benedict of Nursia (480–554) who forbade the study of medicine. The care of the sick was encouraged, but only through prayer and divine intervention. Thus, Christ's healing mission was institutionalized in a fashion that was to control medical care almost completely for the next 500 years, until the seventh century.

At that time, however, the religion of Islam moved to preserve the classical learning that had been achieved in medicine, and practitioners were not only able to return to the same methods as those practiced by earlier Greeks and Romans, but medical study was now encouraged.

Medical education in established universities began in the ninth century. These universities included Salerno in southern Italy, the University of Montpelier in southern France, and the University of Paris. By the time the Renaissance was at its height in the midfifteenth century, the physician had become licensed, was receiving great status, and was attending the ill in a velvet bonnet and fur-trimmed cloak.

Art and science were more closely related during the Renaissance than at any other period of time. Michelangelo (1475–1564) spent years on careful human dissection and this anatomical detail is evident in his paintings in the Sistine Chapel in the Vatican in Rome. Leonardo da Vinci (1452–1519) made anatomical preparations from which he produced drawings representing the skeletal, muscular, nervous, and vascular systems. His accurate sketch of the spinal vertebrae went undiscovered for more than 100 years.

ATTITUDES TOWARD ILLNESS

Various attitudes prevailed toward the ill person. A sick person might be excused from daily activity, but was likely to be shunned if the disease was believed to be a punishment by the gods for mortal sin. This forced isolation may well have been beneficial to the community. In contrast, touching by Jesus was an important component of healing, as was the faith of the individual involved. The New Testament parable of the Good Samaritan helped establish a nexus between the early church and a concern for the sick. It was felt that though the body might be wasted and foul with disease, the purity of the soul guaranteed life everlasting. This was unlike the pagan religions that tended to abandon individuals thought to be ill because they were in disfavor with the gods.

 Native Americans had various feelings about illness. The ill were treated with kindness among the Navaho and Cherokee, and some who recovered from serious illness were considered to have extraordinary powers. However, if a tribe was faced with famine, suicide by the aged and infirm was considered a highest form of bravery. The Eskimos put their elderly unprotected onto ice floes. Neither the Romans nor the Greeks treated the hopelessly ill or deformed, and unwanted infants were disposed of quickly or left to die.

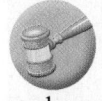 Some of these attitudes are seen even today. The Western medical community and the consumers it serves are heatedly debating the right to choose life or death and the ethics and legality of physician-assisted suicide, which is acceptable in many other cultures. Even with our vast knowledge of medicine and the disease process, many individuals are still very fearful of any illness they do not understand or that they perceive as threatening their health—AIDS is a good example. This fear is often accompanied by public ill treatment of the individuals suffering from certain diseases. For example,

Cuba quarantines everyone who tests positive for the human immunodeficiency virus (HIV), even if they show no signs of illness.

MEDICAL TREATMENTS

The writings of ancient Egypt reveal that when a woman suspected she was pregnant, she urinated over a mixture of wheat and barley seeds combined with dates and sand. If any of the grains sprouted, she was surely pregnant. If the wheat grew, she would have a boy. If the barley grew, it would be a girl. Urine is still used in modern tests to determine pregnancy.

Early medical treatments were often crude. For a sore throat, a physician might mix barley water, vinegar, and mulberry syrup for a gargle. Someone suffering with rheumatism might be given a prescription of chopped mice, lynx claws, and elk hooves. Rhubarb, senna, bitter apple, turpentine, camphor, and mercury were among the physicians' staples. Some physicians washed the instru-

ments used in treating the ill; others scoffed at such a practice. **Malaria,** diphtheria, tuberculosis, **typhoid,** and dysentery were commonplace. Leprosy was prevalent and venereal diseases were rife. Smallpox was frequent in villages; sometimes the sufferer would be placed in a meat pickling vat and fumigated. The death toll from such diseases was particularly high among children. Finally in the eighteenth century, Edward Jenner made a great contribution to the prevention of disease by discovering a method of vaccination against smallpox.

Medicine progressed rapidly during the nineteenth century. Two very important discoveries occurred: anesthesia to alleviate pain during surgery and the realization that some bacteria cause disease. Once it had been proven that certain bacteria were causes of diseases and were transmissible agents responsible for contagion, greater care was taken to prevent that transmission. **Asepsis** became important to reduce the risk of infection. The Hungarian physician and obstetrician Ignaz Phillipp Semmeweis (1818–1865) was able to prove that physicians who came from an autopsy directly to the care of postpartum women, without scrubbing their hands and washing instruments, carried infection with them that often caused puerperal fever (**septicemia** following childbirth) and death to the new mothers.

The names of Louis Pasteur (1822–1895), Joseph Lister (1827–1912), and Robert Koch (1843–1910) are familiar to all bacteriologists. Louis Pasteur has sometimes been referred to as the father of preventive medicine as the result of his work in recognizing the relationship between bacteria and infectious disease (Figure 3-1). Joseph Lister revolutionized surgery because of his belief in Pasteur's theory of using carbolic acid as an antiseptic spray. He insisted that all instruments and physicians' hands be washed with the solution (Figure 3-2). Robert Koch used the culture-plate method for isolating bacteria

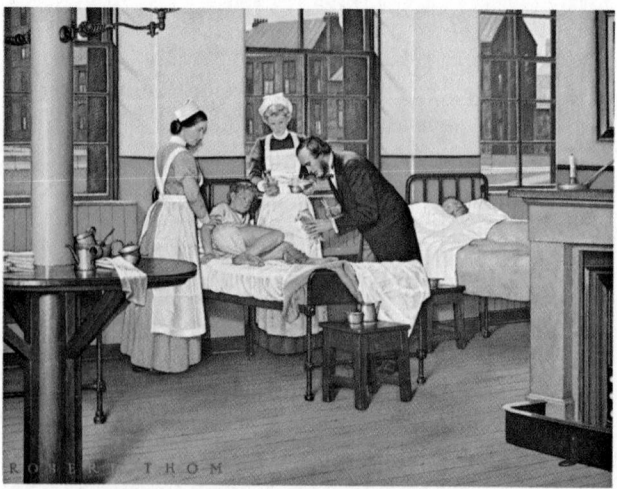

Figure 3-1   Louis Pasteur, the father of preventive medicine. (Courtesy Parke-Davis & Company, © 1957).

Figure 3-2   Joseph Lister revolutionized surgery by introducing antisepsis. (Courtesy Parke-Davis & Company, © 1957)

and demonstrated how cholera was transmitted by food and water. His discovery changed the way health departments cared for persons with infectious disease.

Fortunately, early in the twentieth century, society was finally liberated from many of the infectious and epidemic diseases that had scourged the human race for millennia. Smallpox vaccinations became common and causes of **yellow fever, typhus,** and **bubonic plague** were determined. Life expectancy increased. Tuberculosis became less frequent. In 1922, Frederick G. Banting and a medical student, Charles Best, were able to isolate and inject insulin into a fourteen-year-old boy who was dying of diabetes. Two weeks later, the boy was alive and alert. By 1923, insulin was available for general sale in pharmacies throughout the world. Antibiotics were discovered and the Salk and Sabin vaccines were found for poliomyelitis.

Yet, as we enter the twenty-first century, we are quite aware of the limitations of modern medicine. The rise of AIDS is a reminder that plagues are still possible. In developing countries torn with war and strife, cholera causes the deaths of thousands simply because there is no proper sanitation. In the microbial world, there are new, drug-resistant strains of malaria, tuberculosis, and other diseases that are not responding to known treatments. The challenge of medicine is as strong today as it was 100 years ago.

SIGNIFICANT CONTRIBUTIONS TO MEDICINE

Hippocrates (c. 460–c. 377 B.C.) is the physician most recall from the Greek culture (Figure 3-3). It is not known

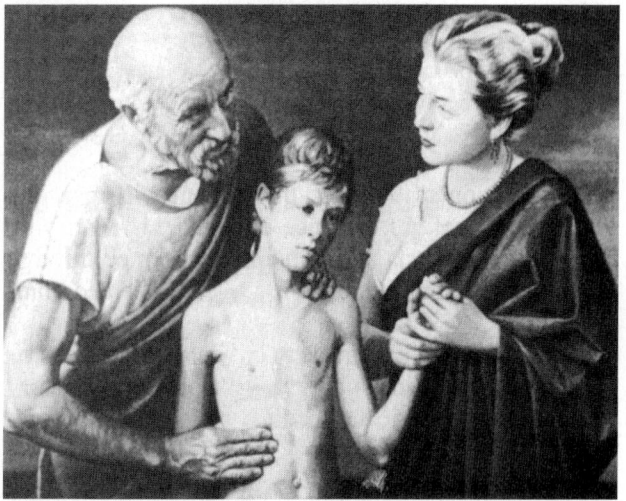

Figure 3-3 Hippocrates examining a child.

why his name surfaces above all other Greek physicians, for some were surely just as prominent. His writings, however, have contributed much to today's medical culture. Hippocrates is remembered by many for his well-known Hippocratic Oath, which established guidelines for a physician's practice of medicine. While few physicians swear to this oath today when they embark on their medical career, it is still recognized for its validity and wisdom. There are various translations of the Hippocratic Oath, although all communicate the same fundamental message.

It would be impossible to identify all the other individuals who made significant contributions to medicine in this text. There are several of note, however, who are mentioned in Table 3-1.

TABLE 3-1 INDIVIDUALS OF NOTE IN THE HISTORY OF MEDICINE	
Moses c. 1205 B.C.	Advocate of health rules in Hebrew religion
Hippocrates c. 460–c. 377 B.C.	Greek physician; "father of medicine"
Andreas Vesalius A.D. 1514–1564	Brussels physician; wrote first anatomical studies
Anton van Leeuwenhoek 1632–1723	Dutch lens grinder; discovered lens magnification
John Hunter 1728–1793	Founder of scientific surgery
Edward Jenner 1749–1823	Developed smallpox vaccine
Rene Laennec 1781–1826	Invented the stethoscope
W. T. G. Morton 1819–1868	Massachusetts physician; introduced ether as anesthetic
Florence Nightingale 1820–1910	Founder of modern nursing
Elizabeth Blackwell 1821–1910	First female physician in America
Clara Barton 1821–1912	Started American Red Cross in 1881
Louis Pasteur 1822–1895	"Father of bacteriology"
Joseph Lister 1827–1912	Laid the groundwork on asepsis
Elizabeth G. Anderson 1836–1917	First female physician in Britain
Robert Koch 1843–1910	Bacteriologist; developed culture-plate method
Wilhelm Roentgen 1845–1923	Discovered X rays (roentgenograms)
Sir Alexander Fleming 1881–1955	Discovered penicillin in 1928

THE OATH OF HIPPOCRATES

I swear by Apollo Physician and Aesculapius and Hygeia and Panacea and all the gods and goddesses, making them my witnesses, that I will fulfill according to my ability and judgment this oath and this covenant:

To hold him who has taught me this art as equal to my parents and to live my life in partnership with him, and if he is in need of money to give him a share of mine, and to regard his offspring as equal to my brothers in male lineage and to teach them this art—if they desire to learn it—without fee and covenant; to give a share of precepts and oral instruction and all the other learning to my sons and to the sons of him who has instructed me and to pupils who have signed the covenant and have taken an oath according to the medical law, but to no one else.

I will apply dietetic measures for the benefit of the sick according to my ability and judgment; I will keep them from harm and injustice.

I will neither give a deadly drug to anybody if asked for it nor will I make a suggestion to this effect. Similarly, I will not give to a woman an abortive remedy. In purity and holiness I will guard my life and my art.

I will not use the knife, not even on sufferers from stone, but will withdraw in favor of such men as are engaged in this work.

Whatever houses I may visit, I will come for the benefit of the sick, remaining free of all intentional injustice, of all mischief, and in particular of sexual relations with both female and male persons, be they free or slaves.

NEW FRONTIERS IN MEDICINE

There has been phenomenal growth in medicine in the past two decades. Only a few advances are mentioned here. Much better imaging leading to much better diagnosis is now available. Where exploratory surgery might have been performed in the past to determine a diagnosis, noninvasive ultrasound, CT scans, and MRIs assist in diagnosis now. People who have worn glasses or contact lenses for many years are turning to eye laser surgery and implantable lenses.

Recently surgeons performed the first successful human larynx transplant. Consider the implications of an AIDS saliva test that creates a needle-free way to test for HIV. Needleless injections are now possible. There is a flu prevention inhaler and an osteoporosis pill.

Experimentation with aromatherapy reveals that some aromas actually improve brain function. Research has shown that individuals suffering from dementia often respond favorably to the odor of freshly roasted coffee and bread baking. Inhaling the scents of green apple, banana, and peppermint stimulates positive feelings. It is thought that with aromatherapy we will soon accelerate learning and speed up rehabilitation for people who have had a stroke.

Who can possibly predict what the future will bring in medicine?

SUMMARY

Medicine's history leaves us with a rich heritage and a sound basis for the future of health care. Medical history continues to be in the making today. For example, research in gene manipulation has the potential benefit of being able to reverse the progression of many debilitating diseases. One day we will look upon medical discoveries of this decade and be impressed by how much further medicine has advanced.

REVIEW QUESTIONS

Multiple Choice

1. A pharmacopoeia is:
   a. a book describing drugs and their preparation
   b. an ancient religious rite used in medicine
   c. a source of magic
   d. used only by twentieth-century physicians

2. In later cultures, women were typically allowed to use their health care skills to:
   a. cure everyone in society
   b. care only for women and to assist in childbirth
   c. become physicians
   d. care only for the elderly

3. An accurate sketch of the spinal vertebrae was created during the Renaissance by:
   a. Leonardo da Vinci
   b. Michelangelo
   c. early Christian monks
   d. Louis Pasteur
4. Hippocrates is considered by many to be:
   a. the founder of scientific surgery
   b. the inventor of the smallpox vaccine
   c. the father of medicine
   d. the father of preventive medicine
5. The first woman physician in the United States was:
   a. Florence Nightingale
   b. Clara Barton
   c. Elizabeth Anderson
   d. Elizabeth Blackwell

Critical Thinking

1. With a group of peers, identify the effects of culture on today's medicine.
2. How does the role of a medical specialist today compare to the role of a medical specialist in the past? Consider both similarities and dissimilarities.
3. You are a male physician on call in your hospital's emergency room when a woman, five months pregnant, is brought in. She is hemorrhaging. Her husband shuns you and demands a female physician. You quickly realize this couple is Muslim. Role play this scenario with a classmate. How can you solve the dilemma? Consider the possibility that your only female physician is out of the country on vacation.
4. You are the medical assistant. Your physician has just prescribed analgesics for a young Oriental woman suffering from migraine headaches. You overhear the young woman arguing with her mother who thinks that she should see a Chinese acupuncturist. What, if anything, would you do?
5. Discuss with a peer the role of women in medicine today. What difficulties, if any, might a female physician face today? Compare today's difficulties to those of female health care practitioners 100 years ago.
6. Write a one-page report on one significant person who contributed greatly to medicine.

WEB ACTIVITIES

The World Wide Web is an ideal place to seek evidence of new and emerging technologies in medicine. One such avenue is "Medical Breakthroughs" reported by Ivanhoe Broadcast News, Inc. Identify at least two or three recent discoveries you find particularly interesting from your research on the Web.

REFERENCES/BIBLIOGRAPHY

Keir, L., Wise, B. A., & Krebs, C. (1998). *Medical assisting: Administrative and clinical competencies* (4th ed.). Albany, NY: Delmar.

Kinn, M. E., & Woods, M. A. (1999). *The medical assistant: Administrative and clinical* (8th ed.). Philadelphia: W. B. Saunders.

Lewis, M. A., & Tamparo, C. D. (1998). *Medical law, ethics, and bioethics for ambulatory care* (4th ed.). Philadelphia: F. A. Davis.

Lyons, A. S., & Petrucelli, J. R., II (1978). *Medicine: An illustrated history.* New York: Harry N. Abrams, Inc.

Taber's cyclopedic medical dictionary (18th ed.) (1997). Philadelphia: F. A. Davis.

Warden, C. D. (1986). *Health care in the 1980s from a consumer's perspective.* Unpublished doctoral dissertation, Union Graduate School, Seattle, WA.

Unit

2

THE THERAPEUTIC APPROACH

Chapter 4

THERAPEUTIC COMMUNICATION SKILLS

KEY TERMS

Active Listening
Bias
Body Language
Buffer Words
Closed Questions
Clustering
Communication Cycle
Compensation
Congruency
Decode
Defense Mechanism
Denial
Displacement
Encoding
Facial Expressions
Feedback
Gestures/Mannerisms
Hierarchy of Needs
Indirect Statements
Interview Techniques
Introjection
Kinesics
Masking
Modes of Communication
Open-Ended Questions
Perception
Position
Posture
Prejudice
Projection
Rationalization
Regression
Repression

(continues)

OUTLINE

Importance of Communication
Cultural Influence on Therapeutic Communication
Biases and Prejudices
The Communication Cycle
  The Sender
  The Message
  The Receiver
  Feedback
Listening Skills
Verbal Communication
  The Five Cs of Communication
Nonverbal Communication
  Facial Expression
  Territoriality
  Posture
  Position
  Gestures and Mannerisms
  Touch

Congruency in Communication
  Perception
  Maslow's Hierarchy of Needs
Technology and Communication
Roadblocks to Therapeutic Communication
Defense Mechanisms
  Introjection
  Denial
  Compensation
  Regression
  Repression
  Sublimation
  Projection
  Displacement
  Rationalization
Interview Techniques
Telephone Techniques

OBJECTIVES

The student should strive to meet the following performance objectives and demonstrate an understanding of the facts and principles presented in this chapter through written and oral communication.

1. Define the key terms as presented in the glossary.
2. Identify the importance of communication.
3. Recall at least four influences on therapeutic communication related to culture, and describe four common biases/prejudices in today's society.
4. List and define the four basic elements of the communication cycle.
5. Identify the four modes or channels of communication most pertinent in our everyday exchange.

(continues)

KEY TERMS (*continued*)

Roadblocks
Sublimation
Territoriality
The Message
The Receiver
The Sender
Therapeutic Communication
Touch

OBJECTIVES (*continued*)

6. Discuss the importance of active listening in therapeutic communication.
7. Differentiate the terms verbal and nonverbal communication.
8. Analyze the five Cs of communication, and describe their effectiveness in the communication cycle.
9. Demonstrate the following body language or nonverbal communication behaviors: facial expressions, territoriality, position, posture, gestures/mannerisms, touch.
10. Identify and explain congruency in communication.
11. Discuss the use of Maslow's hierarchy of needs in therapeutic communication.
12. Discuss communication modification for electronically transmitted messages.
13. Recall eight significant roadblocks to therapeutic communication.
14. List and describe seven common defense mechanisms.
15. Discuss the possible impact on therapeutic communication that the unequal relationship between physician and patient might have.
16. Compare/contrast closed questions, open-ended questions, and indirect statements.
17. List four tools or considerations when communicating on the telephone.
18. Demonstrate the correct way to speak into the mouthpiece of a telephone by answering an incoming call and closing a telephone conversation.

ROLE DELINEATION COMPONENTS

GENERAL (TRANSDISCIPLINARY)

Communication Skills

- **Treat all patients with compassion and empathy**
- **Recognize and respect cultural diversity**
- **Adapt communications to individual's ability to understand**
- **Use effective and correct verbal and written communications**
- **Use medical terminology appropriately**
- **Use professional telephone technique**

(continues)

SCENARIO

In the two-doctor office of Doctors Lewis and King, four medical assistants constantly interact with patients, allaying their concerns, scheduling their appointments, instructing them on medications, and helping them understand their insurance coverage. On any given day, office manager Marilyn Johnson, CMA, is greeting patients warmly as they arrive for their appointments. Some patients, like Anna and Joseph Ortiz, are new to the practice. Marilyn's warm manner puts them at ease. Other patients, like Martin Gordon, who has prostate cancer, may be depressed and anxious. Marilyn tries to create an environment where they feel free to share their concerns and anxieties.

While Marilyn is busy with patients, administrative medical assistant Ellen Armstrong is on the telephone, scheduling appointments, answering patient questions, and making decisions about what calls need priority attention. Ellen projects a warm, courteous presence over the telephone; she maintains her composure, even when faced with difficult calls and tries always to ask the right questions of callers in a nonthreatening manner.

- Recognize and respond to verbal and nonverbal communications
- Receive, organize, prioritize, and transmit information
- Serve as a liaison
- Promote the practice through positive public relations

INTRODUCTION

Of all the tasks and skills required of the medical assistant in the ambulatory care setting, none is quite so important as communication. Communication is the very foundation for every action taken by health care professionals in the care of their patients. Because medical assistants are often the liaison between patient and physician, it is critical to be aware of all the complexities of the communication process.

Every day, Marilyn and Ellen and the two clinical medical assistants at the offices of Doctors Lewis and King face many communication challenges. This chapter will describe effective communication principles, apply those principles to face-to-face communication as well as telephone communication, and describe the basic roadblocks to communication. The key word to all communication in the medical setting is *therapeutic*. In all conversation with patients, the more therapeutic the conversation, the more satisfied the patient will be with the care provided.

IMPORTANCE OF COMMUNICATION

Communication in the health setting is the foundation for all patient care and is of the utmost importance. The majority of this communication in the ambulatory care setting will be therapeutic—it will utilize specific and well-defined professional skills. Patients' satisfaction with their medical care is as much related to the effectiveness of the communication between themselves and their chosen health care provider as it is to the actual care itself.

A patient choosing a physician wants a clear understanding of the physician's professional and technical skills as well as the physician's ability to communicate. The patient may question family members and friends regarding their personal physician's professional manner and communication skills. Questions often asked include: "Will your doctor talk with me so that I understand what is being said?" "Will your doctor listen to what I have to say?" "Can I talk to your doctor honestly and openly?"

When communication is therapeutic, patients feel validated and respected. Therapeutic communication skills create a feeling of comfort for patients even when difficult or unpleasant information must be exchanged.

CULTURAL INFLUENCE ON THERAPEUTIC COMMUNICATION

For true therapeutic communication to take place, the influence of culture must be considered. Cultural influences include one's ethnic heritage, geographic location and background, genetics, age, gender, economics, educational experiences, life experiences, and value systems.

Any or all of these influences may exhibit themselves when health care is sought by patients. A patient's ethnic heritage may indicate a slant toward the Eastern influence in medicine as opposed to the traditional Western style more commonly taught and practiced in the United States today. Geographic location and background may reveal that a person is more comfortable with a family physician in a very small clinic than one in a large metropolitan multispecialty practice.

Age and gender are factors with a strong influence on communication. How and when do you communicate with a young child? What do you communicate to that child? How do you impress upon an elderly gentleman who has taken little medications throughout his lifetime that he now must take his pill every day? In a culture where the husband is the authority, how does the doctor discuss with the female patient the inadvisability of another pregnancy at this time?

Language barriers will prevent therapeutic communication if great care is not taken. If an interpreter is necessary, it is important to remember to speak directly to the patient, not the interpreter. If English is the second language or a heavy accent is involved, speaking clearly and slowly (not loudly) can greatly enhance communication. It must always be emphasized, however, that the lack of clear and understandable language does *not* imply lack of intelligence.

The influence of economics may reveal a discomfort if the office staff and patients have a different perception about how billing is managed and when and how payment is expected. A discussion of billing and payment procedures at the first office visit or before a major procedure will be beneficial to all concerned parties.

Educational and life experiences will, in part, determine how patients react to their care. Patients with family members being treated for a chronic illness will have more knowledge and understanding of that illness in their own lives. Individuals who have already suffered a great deal of loss and grief in their lives may handle the information of a life-threatening illness more easily than someone who has experienced little grief.

BIASES AND PREJUDICES

Personal preferences, biases, and prejudices will enter into many physician-patient relationships. Such biases affect the types of communication possible. When individuals are not aware of their biases or prejudices, hostile attitudes may prevail.

For therapeutic communication to take place, biases must be examined, a person's comfort level with each bias determined, and measures taken to ensure that a hostile attitude is not present. **Bias** is defined as a slant toward a particular belief. **Prejudice** is defined as an opinion or judgment that is formed before all the facts are known; prejudice is a preconceived and unfavorable concept. Common biases and prejudices in today's society include:

1. A preference for Western style medicine
2. Choosing physicians according to gender
3. Prejudice related to a person's sexual preference
4. Discrimination based on race or religion
5. Hostile attitudes toward people with different value systems than one's own
6. A belief that people who cannot afford health care should receive less care than someone who can pay for full services

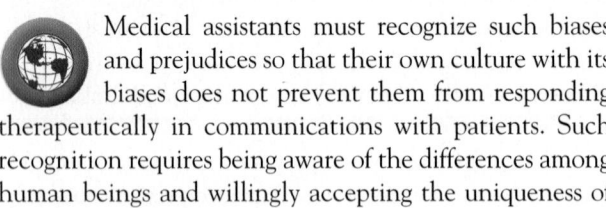 Medical assistants must recognize such biases and prejudices so that their own culture with its biases does not prevent them from responding therapeutically in communications with patients. Such recognition requires being aware of the differences among human beings and willingly accepting the uniqueness of each person.

THE COMMUNICATION CYCLE

All communication, whether social or therapeutic, involves two or more individuals participating in an exchange of information. The **communication cycle** involves sending and receiving messages even when unconsciously aware of them.

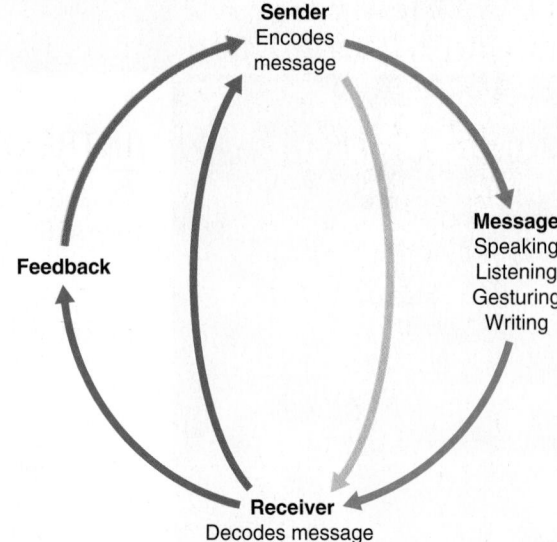

Figure 4-1 The communication cycle and channels of communication.

Four basic elements are included in the communication cycle. They are (1) the sender, (2) the message and a channel or mode of communication, (3) the receiver, and (4) feedback (Figure 4-1).

The Sender

The sender begins the communication cycle by **encoding** or creating the message to be sent. This is an important step, and much care should be taken in formulating the message. Before creating the message, the sender must observe the receiver to determine the complexity of the words to be used within the message, the receiver's ability to interpret the message, and the best channel by which to send the message.

The Message

The message is the content being communicated. The message must be understood clearly by the receiver. Various levels of complexity in communication are used depending upon the ability of the receiver to recognize and understand the words contained within the message. Children do not have the vocabulary base nor the cognitive skills to communicate and understand the same as adults. The health of the receiver also must be considered. A patient who is stressed or in pain may find it difficult to concentrate on the message. If the patient is of a different nationality and/or culture from the sender, verbal communication may require special skill. When visual or hearing acuity is impaired, another challenge must be surmounted.

The four **modes of communication**, also called channels of communication, most pertinent in our everyday exchange include (1) speaking, (2) listening, (3) gestures or body language, and (4) writing. These modes or channels are affected by our physical and mental development, our culture, education and life experiences, our impressions from models and mentors, and in general by how we feel and accept ourselves as individuals. Each mode or channel of communication has its appropriateness and must be considered when formulating the message.

The Receiver

The receiver is the recipient of the sender's message. The receiver must decode, or interpret, the meaning of the message. The primary sensory skill used in verbal communication is listening. It is hard work to concentrate and listen. When decoding the message, the receiver must be aware that not only the spoken words, but the tone and pitch of the voice and the speed at which the words are spoken carry meaning and must be evaluated.

Feedback

Feedback takes place after the receiver has decoded the message sent by the sender. Feedback is the receiver's way of ensuring that the message that is understood is the same as the message that was sent. Feedback also provides an opportunity for the receiver to clarify any misunderstanding regarding the original message and to ask for additional information.

LISTENING SKILLS

A vital part of feedback in the communication cycle is listening. A good listener is alert to all aspects of the communication cycle—the verbal and nonverbal message as well as verification of the message through appropriate feedback.

Active listening is one method used in therapeutic communication. In this technique, the received message is sent back to the sender, worded a little differently, for verification from the sender.

Sender: "How can I possibly pay this fee when I have no insurance?"

Receiver: "You're worried about paying your bill?"

The preceding example illustrates how the receiver is able to validate the sender's concerns at the same time the message is checked for accuracy. The door is then left open for a therapeutic response such as:

Sender: "Our bookkeeper will be glad to work out a payment plan with you that will fit your resources."

VERBAL COMMUNICATION

Verbal communication takes place when the message is spoken. However, one must keep in mind the fact that unless the words have meaning, and unless the sender and the receiver apply the same meaning to the spoken words, verbal communication may be misunderstood. If, for example, you overhear a conversation in a language foreign to you, you are indeed a witness to verbal communication, but you may not understand the message. To have any meaning, the spoken word must be understood by all parties of the communication (Tamparo & Lindh, 2000).

The Five Cs of Communication

In their book *Professional Development*, Mary Wilkes and C. Bruce Crosswait (1991) identified the five Cs of Communication in business. They are (1) complete, (2) clear, (3) concise, (4) courteous, and (5) cohesive. These five Cs apply equally well in health care professions.

Complete. The message must be complete, with all the necessary information given. The medical assistant cannot expect the patient to be compliant if all the instructions are not given and understood.

Clear. The information given in the message must also be clear. The use of eye contact enhances clarity. Health care professionals must be able to articulate by using good diction and by enunciating each word distinctly. The patient must be allowed time to process the message and verify its meaning. The message must also be heard to promote understanding.

Concise. A concise message is one that does not include any unnecessary information. It should be brief and to the point (Figure 4-2). Patients must not be overloaded with technical terms that may not be understood or that tend to distract them by diverting their attention away from the balance of the message.

Patient Teaching Tip

When patients speak a different language or when English is their second language, you may need to urge them to communicate nonverbally; you can encourage them to do so by using appropriate, nonthreatening gestures. Sometimes, it may be important to communicate verbally with a family member to gain specific information. Be sure not to violate any confidentiality of the patient, however.

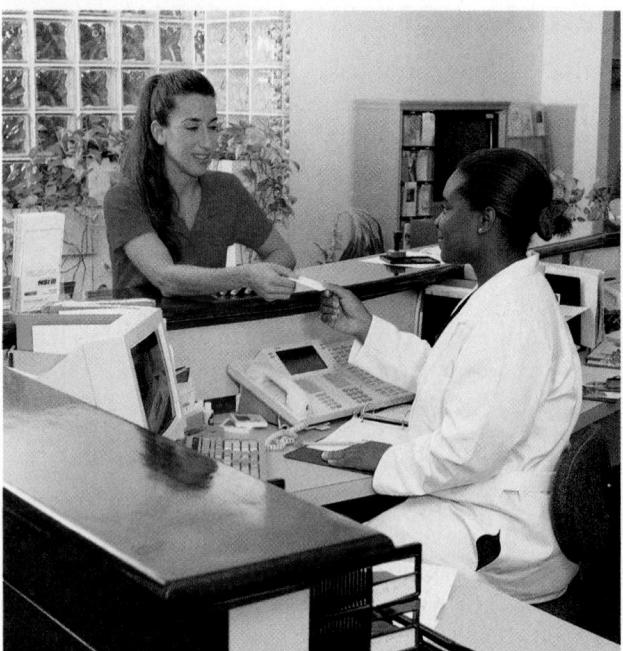

Figure 4-2 To say to the patient after greeting her by name, "I've completed an appointment card to remind you of your next appointment, Tuesday at 2:00 P.M." is an example of a concise message, brief and to the point.

Courteous. Courtesy is important in all aspects of communication. It only takes a moment to acknowledge a patient with a smile or by name. Knocking on the exam room door before entering validates the patient's right to privacy and builds self-esteem.

When a patient must be placed on hold on the telephone, thank the patient for waiting. Try not to keep the patient waiting too long if you must find information.

Remember to be courteous to colleagues in the office. Good working relationships and professionalism are always enhanced by simple courtesy.

Cohesive. A cohesive message is organized and logical in its progression. The cohesive message does not ramble and does not jump from one subject to another. The

Patient Teaching Tip

Sensitive medical assistants will encourage patients to verbalize their concerns. The ability to ask questions in a nonprobing way and to elicit patient response is an important function in any ambulatory care setting, for it is critical to know a patient's history, current medications, and other relevant data.

patient should be able to follow the message easily. The medical assistant should always allow time to summarize detailed messages and utilize responding skills to verify that the patient fully understands the message.

When communicating within the health professions, keep in mind the following:

1. Good communication skills are necessary in establishing rapport with patients.
2. Patients feel respected and validated when called by their full name, such as Mary O'Keefe or Mrs. O'Keefe.
3. Patients should be encouraged to verbalize their feelings.
4. Give technical information to patients in a manner that they can understand.
5. Allow patients to make practical application to their personal health needs.

NONVERBAL COMMUNICATION

Verbal communication alone is not always adequate in conveying the message being sent. In most instances, more than one mode or channel of communication is employed. Nonverbal communication, often referred to as **body language,** includes the unconscious body movements, gestures, and facial expressions that accompany speech. The study of body language is known as **kinesics** (Figure 4-3).

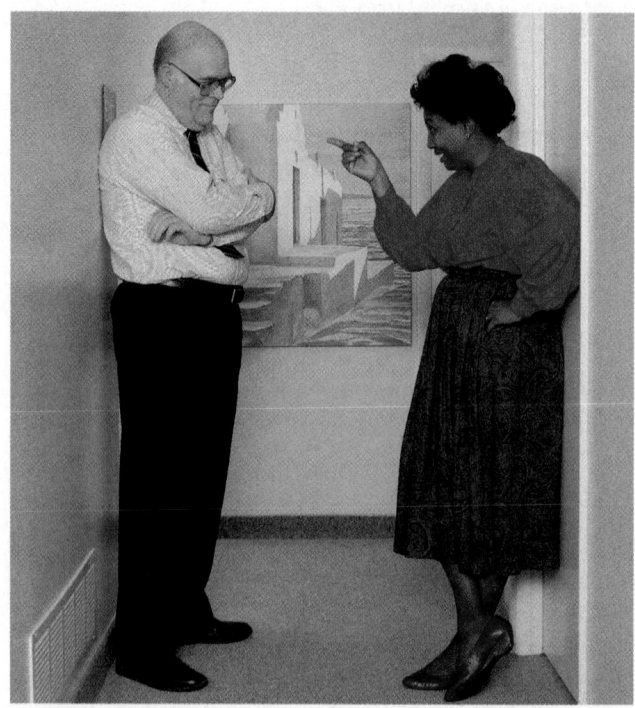

Figure 4-3 Body language can communicate more than spoken words.

Nonverbal communication is the language we learn first. It is learned seemingly automatically when infants learn to return a smile or respond to touches on the cheek. Much of our body language is a learned behavior and is greatly influenced by the primary caregivers and the culture in which we are raised.

Feelings and emotions are communicated most often through nonverbal means. The body expresses its true repressed feelings using body language. Most of the negative messages we communicate are also expressed nonverbally and usually are unintentional. Experts tell us that 70 percent of communication is nonverbal. The tone of voice communicates 23 percent of the message—only 7 percent of the message is actually communicated by the spoken word (Wilkes & Crosswait, 1991).

Facial Expression

Facial expression is considered one of the most important and observed nonverbal communicators. Each facet or aspect of the anatomy of the face sends a nonverbal message.

Often expressions of joy and happiness or sorrow and grief are reflected through the eyes. The anatomy of the eyes does not change, but the movements of the structures surrounding the eyes enhance or magnify the message being communicated.

Children are told it is not polite to stare at people. It is acceptable to stare at animals in the zoo or art objects in the museum, but not at humans. Staring is dehumanizing and is often interpreted as an invasion of privacy.

The medical assistant must learn not to stare when patients present with ailments that make them "look" different. Patients such as these are individuals who have needs and who perhaps feel pain, discomfort, and have decreased self-esteem and value. These feelings will only be amplified if the medical assistant and other health professionals are unable to "see" them as humans. A lack of eye contact may also be viewed as avoidance or disinterest in being involved.

The movements of the eyebrow indicate many nonverbal cues as well. Surprise, puzzlement, worry, amusement, and questioning are often nonverbal messages reflected by the position of the eyebrow. Wrinkling of the forehead sends similar messages.

Cultural influences affect customs and different forms of facial expressions. In many Latin and Asian countries, it is unacceptable to look adults in the eye so people from these cultures often stare at the floor. This expression may be misinterpreted and misunderstood. Many persons of Eastern cultures communicate nonverbally differently from persons of Western cultures. These differences also may lead to confusion and misunderstanding.

Territoriality

Territoriality is the distance at which we feel comfortable with others while communicating. In the classroom, for example, students claim their territory the first day of class. The area is well-defined by using books and papers or by placing the arm, hand, or chair on boundary lines. When another invades the territory, a shift in body position or the use of eye contact sends the message "This is my area." Individuals may feel threatened when others invade their personal space without permission. Some examples of comfortable personal space follow:

- Intimate
  touching to 6 inches
- Personal
  1½ to 4 feet
- Social
  4 to 12 feet
- Public
  12 to 15 feet

As with facial expressions, territoriality or personal space will be handled differently by various cultures. For example, there is no word for privacy in the Japanese language. Population numbers require crowding together publicly as well as privately. Public crowding is often viewed as a sign of warmth and pleasant intimacy in Japan. In the private home, several generations may live together; however, each considers this space to be his own and resents intrusion into it.

 Arabs like to touch their companions, to feel and to smell them. To deny a friend your breath is to be ashamed. When two Arabs talk to each other, they look each other in the eyes with great intensity.

The medical assistant may perform many invasive tasks during the course of an office visit. Examples include taking vital signs or giving injections, both of which require touching the patient. It is beneficial to explain procedures that invade another's space before beginning the procedure so that it will not be perceived as threatening. This helps to empower the patient by involving the patient in the decision-making process and builds a sense of trust in the medical assistant.

Posture

Like territoriality, **posture** is important to allied health care professionals. Posture relates to the position of the body or parts of the body. It is the manner in which we carry ourselves, or pose in situations. We tend to tighten up in threatening or unknown situations and relax in nonthreatening environments. Those who study kinesics feel a posture involves at least half the body and that the position can last for nearly five minutes.

When the patient is seated with the arms and legs crossed, the message of closure or being opinionated may be relayed. On the other hand, sitting in a chair relaxed with the hands clasped behind the head indicates an attitude of being open to suggestions. Slumped shoulders may signal depression, discouragement, or in some cases even pain.

Position

Position, the physical stance of two individuals while communicating, is a key factor to consider while communicating with the patient. Most physician-patient relationships utilize the face-to-face communication arrangement. When speaking with a patient, the physician or medical assistant will want to maintain a close but comfortable position enabling observation of all cues being sent, both verbal and nonverbal (Figure 4-4).

Standing over a patient can convey a message of superiority, and too much distance between the two parties may be interpreted as avoidance or being exclusive. Generally, leaning toward the patient expresses warmth, caring, interest, acceptance, and trust. Moving away from the patient may be interpreted as dislike, disinterest, boredom, indifference, suspicion, or impatience.

Whenever possible, it is best to have a chair in the examination room and to have the patient seated comfortably there to begin the communication cycle. The medical assistant or physician can sit on a stool that can easily be moved toward the patient. This arrangement aids the patient in feeling valued, listened to, and cared for as a fellow human being.

Gestures and Mannerisms

Most of us use gestures and mannerisms when we "talk" with our hands. This form of body language may be useful in enhancing the spoken word by emphasizing ideas, thus creating and holding the attention of others.

Touch

Touch is a powerful tool that communicates what cannot be expressed in words. Its appropriateness in the patient/ health professional relationship has well-defined boundaries and requires the use of good judgment on the part of the professional. Infants who are not touched, cuddled, and loved do not grow and develop as those who receive these reassuring gestures. The touch that communicates caring, sincerity, understanding, and reassurance is usually welcomed and considered to be a therapeutic response. Most patients will understand and accept the touching behavior as it relates to the medical setting; however, we

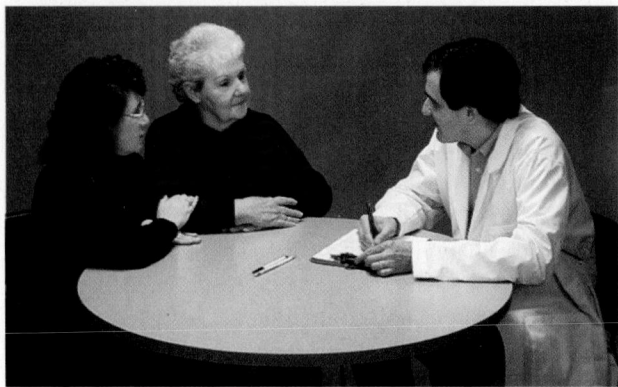

Figure 4-4   Positive posture and position encourage therapeutic communication.

must remember that not all patients are comfortable with touch. Whenever the patient is not comfortable with touch, ask permission and create as safe and reassuring an environment as possible.

CONGRUENCY IN COMMUNICATION

There are some keys to successful communication to employ for communication to be effective. There must be congruency between the verbal and nonverbal communication. The two messages must agree; you cannot shake your head NO while saying YES verbally. This response sends a mixed message, and in most cases, the nonverbal messages will be accepted as the intended message.

It is also important to remember that most nonverbal messages are sent in groups of various forms of body language. The grouping of nonverbal messages into statements or conclusions is known as clustering. Masking involves an attempt to conceal or repress the true feeling

---

SPOTLIGHT ON AAMA ESSENTIALS THROUGH CAAHEP

- Respect your patient's cultural diversity, and adapt your skills to meeting the patient's needs.

- Remember that body language can often convey feelings not otherwise expressed through verbal communication.

- Consider that a patient may use defense mechanisms to mask true feelings.

or message. The perceptive professional will be aware of all these messages.

Perception

Perception as it relates to communication is the conscious awareness of one's own feelings and the feelings of others (Fast, 1970). To be most useful and therapeutic as health professionals, we must first explore our own feelings and appreciate and accept ourselves.

Learning to use perception involves the ability to sense another's attitudes, moods, and feelings. It takes practice and experience to develop and use this skill effectively. Being attentive to other professionals and observing their use of perception will yield insight into its usefulness and provide an example to emulate. A word of caution—the use of perception may easily be misinterpreted, especially when going with your feeling or assessment of what is happening regarding the patient. Always follow perceived assessments with verbal validation before assuming your perception of the circumstance is correct.

Nonverbal communication is easily misinterpreted. Careful observation for congruency between verbal and nonverbal communication, and clustering nonverbal cues being sent into nonverbal statements will strengthen the ability to interpret the message accurately.

Maslow's Hierarchy of Needs

Abraham Maslow is considered the founder of humanistic psychology and is most well known for his hierarchy of needs (Figure 4-5) (Miliken, 1998).

If you can understand this hierarchy, you can assess a patient's needs. If the most basic of needs are not met, it is highly unlikely that a patient can be successful with any

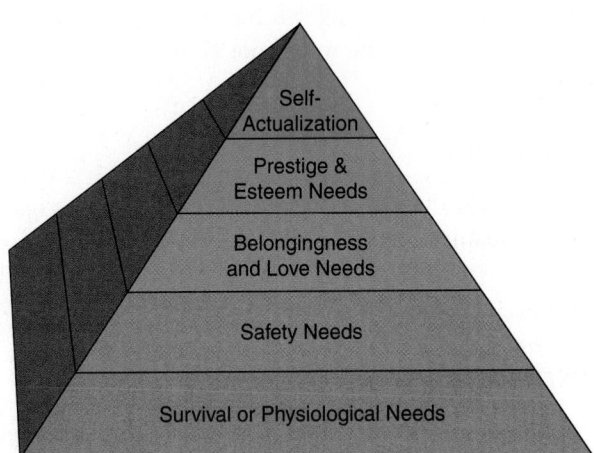

Figure 4-5 Maslow's hierarchy of needs.

treatment protocol. Keeping this hierarchy in mind will help facilitate therapeutic communication.

TECHNOLOGY AND COMMUNICATION

Face-to-face communication is the mode of choice in most physician offices today. However, technological devices are becoming more and more accepted as a means of communication. Technology-mediated communication and a greater reliance on cyberspace technology will greatly affect communication in the twenty-first century. Examples of new technologies in medical offices include fax machines, telecommunication conferences, e-mail, and laptop computers linked to a network of computers that communicate with satellite offices in another part of the community or even in another country.

Do these new communication methods change the communication cycle? There is still a message, a sender, a receiver, and feedback. What changes is the way in which the message is encoded and decoded. The content of the message will be examined for credibility rather than one's dress, eye contact, facial expression, vocal inflection, and posture. Technology does not convey emotions nearly as well as face-to-face or even telephone conversations. Another factor to consider is that your composed message may not look like what your reader sees. The software and hardware that you use for composing, sending, sorting, downloading, and reading may be completely different from what your recipient uses. Modifications to the format may change the intended emphasis or meaning of the message.

There are several advantages for the use of e-mail rather than postal mail (commonly referred to as "snail mail"). E-mail is less expensive and faster than mailing a letter. Because the turnaround time can be so fast, e-mail is more conversational than traditional paper-based media. An e-mail transmission is less intrusive than a telephone call and less bother than a fax. When one uses e-mail transmissions, differences in location and time zone are less of a problem.

ROADBLOCKS TO THERAPEUTIC COMMUNICATION

Being sensitive to patients' unique personalities and needs will enable the health care professional to avoid roadblocks to communication (Table 4-1).

It must be the concern of each health care professional to facilitate communication by encouraging and enabling patients to express themselves honestly without

TABLE 4-1 ROADBLOCKS TO COMMUNICATION	
Roadblock	**Example**
Reassuring clichés	"Don't worry, Mr. McKay, about not having a job; you'll find another one really soon."
Moralizing/lecturing	"If you were smart, Mrs. Johnson, you'd lose fifty pounds and you wouldn't have such a problem with your diabetes and hypertension."
Requiring explanations	"Why would you not want to have chemotherapy, Mr. Gordon? Seeing your wife die of cancer should surely make you want to seek treatment."
Ridiculing/shaming	"Ha, ha, Mr. Gordon! It's not *prostrate*—it's prostate cancer."
Defending/contradicting	"Mr. Marshal, I assure you the physician is *very busy*. He will not see you until he has finished with his other patients."
Shifting subjects	"Yes, Mrs. Jover, your work is very interesting, but I must ask you to sign this permission form to test for HIV."
Criticizing	"Mrs. O'Keefe, why in the world would you stay with an abusive husband?"
Threatening	"There is no way you will get rid of this cough if you do not stop smoking, Mr. Fowler."

fear. Roadblocks close communication and prevent quality care of the total person.

DEFENSE MECHANISMS

Defense mechanisms are used often by individuals and may further block the communication cycle. The use of defense mechanisms may be the result of individuals feeling threatened, ashamed, or guilty. In this situation, patients tend to respond defensively to protect themselves. Defense mechanisms are used unconsciously by all individuals at one time or another. They allow individuals to gain composure and/or control in a situation. They can become harmful when they prevent patients from seeing problems through to a satisfactory solution. Recognizing common defense mechanisms enables individuals to communicate effectively.

Introjection

Introjection is the identification with another person or with some object. The patient assumes the supposed feelings and/or characteristics of the other personality or object.

Denial

Denial (rejection of or refusal to acknowledge information) is often found in the health care setting. When patient Abigail Johnson does not comply with her diet, she is denying the consequences that might occur as a result.

Compensation

Compensation is the overemphasizing of characteristics to make up for a real or imagined failure or handicap.

Regression

Regression is moving back to a former stage to escape conflict or fear. When three-year-old Chris is faced with another baby in the family, he may feel left out, unwanted, and demand to be nursed or to have a bottle like the baby.

Repression

Repression is temporary amnesia—being unable to cope with the overwhelming situation by temporarily forgetting. When Mary O'Keefe confronts her husband about his hostile attitude, he is likely to deny her allegation because he has repressed his frustration and anger at not having a satisfactory job.

Sublimation

Sublimation is an example of redirecting a socially unacceptable impulse into one that is socially acceptable. If John O'Keefe could release his anger and frustration by playing handball, he would not be so hostile in other settings.

Projection

Projection is the act of placing one's own feelings upon another. Juanita Hansen, who is suspected of child abuse, accuses the medical assistant of being unduly rough with her son.

Displacement

Displacement occurs when individuals displace their negative feelings onto something or someone with no significance to the situation. Cele Little is agitated when Dr. Woo tells her that her hearing is seriously impaired and suggests going to an audiologist for a hearing aid. She yells at her sister, Dottie, about being so clumsy and falling and injuring her back.

Rationalization

Rationalization is the act of justification, usually illogically, that one uses to keep from facing the truth of the situation. Leo McKay rationalizes that his stomach pains are the result of his lousy cooking and have nothing to do with the stress he may be feeling as the result of being laid off his job.

Recognizing defense mechanisms and understanding how best to communicate to get beyond the defense mechanisms to the truth is an art. It takes practice and patience. Medical assistants must be observant, always looking for the nonverbal cues while listening closely to the verbal message. Being present in the moment and giving each patient your full attention will enable you to communicate therapeutically.

INTERVIEW TECHNIQUES

All health professionals must be adept at **interview techniques**—knowing how to encourage the best communication between themselves and the patient. It is important to remember that an unequal relationship exists between the health professional and the patient. The health professional, whether it be the physician or the medical assistant, is in the power position and has a great deal of control over the patient. Therefore, it is important to equalize the relationship as much as possible. That is the reason why some professionals use the term *client* rather than *patient*.

Early in the interview, the patient must feel comfortable enough to risk being honest with the health professional. The health professional must build an atmosphere of trust by showing concern for the patient. A gentle touch and a warm, caring facial expression may be all that is necessary. Always be honest and genuine in your responses to patients. Be sympathetic and empathic and create an environment that is free of hypocrisy.

When the medical assistant is interviewing the patient for the chief complaint, it is important to listen with a "third" ear. Listen to what the patient is not saying but is apt to exhibit through nonverbal communication.

You might choose to share your observation of the nonverbal message with the patient, thus encouraging the patient to verbalize more freely. When feelings are shared, validate and acknowledge those feelings through such statements as "I understand your distress." You can verify the communication by reflecting or paraphrasing what the patient has said.

You will be asking **closed questions** during the interview. Closed questions can be answered with a simple yes or no.

> "Are you still taking your medication?"
> "Are you in pain now?"

You will also use **open-ended questions** with the patient. These questions encourage therapeutic communication because the patient is required to verbalize more.

> "What kind of help will you have at home during your recovery?"
> "How are you coming along on this diet?

Indirect statements will also prove helpful in facilitating therapeutic communication. An indirect statement will elicit a response from a patient without the patient feeling questioned.

> "Tell me what you've been doing since you retired."
> "I'd like to know more about your exercise program."

TELEPHONE TECHNIQUES

It has often been said that the telephone is the lifeline of the physician's office. Communication over the telephone requires understanding on the part of each communicator (Figure 4-6).

Each medium uses the proper tools to get the job done. Speaking on the telephone is much like a conversation

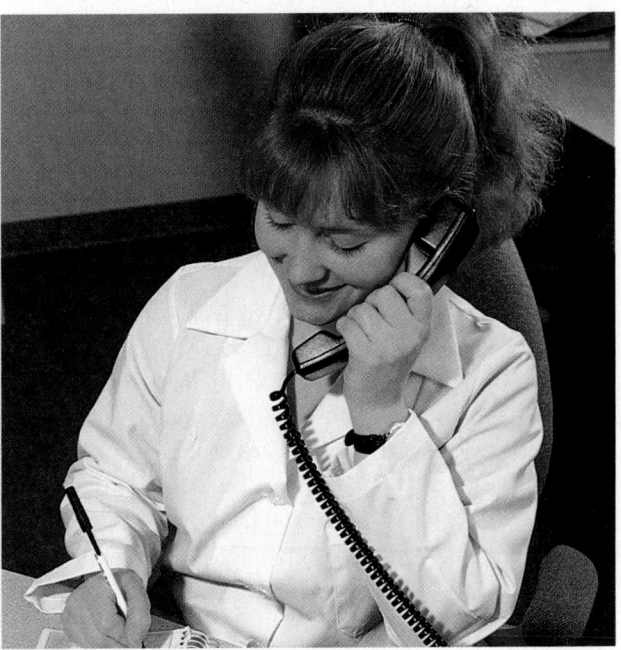

Figure 4-6 When communicating over the telephone, listen with full attention to make certain the message sent and received is correct.

between two blindfolded individuals. The facial expressions cannot be seen, there is no eye contact, and there is no visual feedback. The listener will interpret mood by the tone and pacing of voice and the words spoken. When speaking on the telephone, quick conclusions are drawn. Often, we jump to conclusions, and the communication is misinterpreted.

The old, cold, aloof, formal business greeting comes across like frostbite in the medical office setting. It sounds curt, bored, and uncaring. Think of welcoming a new acquaintance into your home, then practice the same characteristics when speaking on the telephone. Speaking clearly, use words that will be easily understood, and ask questions to verify that the patient has understood the message being conveyed.

Concentrate on enunciating and being understood. If you hear, "What? I didn't understand you. I can't hear you," slow down and speak a little louder with distinct enunciation directly into the mouthpiece. The mouthpiece should be held one to two inches away from the mouth. Project your voice at the mouthpiece and then project another foot further. Your voice is the delivery system for your words and thoughts. Speak with confidence and conviction.

Have you ever called an office and had the firm name clipped off? The name of the office is important. To avoid clipping off the office name, practice using buffer words. **Buffer words** are expendable; if you clip them off, at least the office name remains intact. Use buffer words before the office name and before you identify yourself. "Good morning, this is Inner City Health Care. This is Walter, how may I help you?" *Good morning* and *this is* are buffer words.

All the techniques for effective face-to-face communication must be more intentionally observed when the communication is over the telephone because you cannot see the person with whom you are speaking. You must listen with full attention to make certain that the message sent and received is correct.

To close a telephone conversation to schedule an appointment, for example, consider the following:

1. Use the patient's name if it can be done without announcing the name to persons in the reception area.
2. Confirm the date and time of the appointment.
3. Identify the physician if there is more than one physician in the office.
4. Give any specific instructions that may be necessary.
5. Say goodbye.

SUMMARY

Throughout this text you are reminded of the importance of effective communication techniques. Good communication takes practice. Use the techniques identified in this chapter with your family and with your peers. Watch for roadblocks, be aware of defense mechanisms, and remember the five Cs of communication.

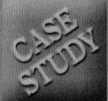

CASE STUDY 4.1

It is a typically active day at the offices of Doctors Lewis and King. Despite the three emergencies in early afternoon and the full schedule of patients, everything is running smoothly with Dr. Lewis and the entire staff responding quickly but thoroughly to patient concerns.

At 4:00 P.M. another emergency patient arrives; at the same time Jim Marshal, an architect in a downtown firm, comes in early for a routine appointment and demands to be seen immediately. Jim, a regular patient, has a history of being difficult and impatient; being a bit arrogant, he tends to put his needs first. However, Dr. Lewis is occupied with another patient. It is critical to treat the patient with the emergency as soon as possible, and Jim is half an hour early.

Joe Guerrero, CMA, the office's administrative and clinical medical assistant, calmly asks Mr. Marshal to please wait until his scheduled appointment time. When he threatens to leave, Joe explains to Mr. Marshal that there are two patients ahead of him but that the doctor will see him at his scheduled appointment time.

continues

CASE STUDY REVIEW

1. What communication roadblocks did medical assistant Joe Guerrero avoid in reacting to Jim Marshal's demands to see the doctor?

2. With another student, role-play the scenario, with one student taking the role of patient and one student the role of the medical assistant. Identify roadblocks to communication imposed by the patient. How is the medical assistant using the five Cs of communication to deal with the situation?

3. Do you think the medical assistant reacted appropriately? What else could he have done? What should he *not* do in this situation?

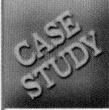

4-2

You have learned in this chapter that communication has not been successful until the cycle is complete. Consider the following scenario:

An 82-year-old woman with moderate dementia and a hearing impairment is brought to the surgeon's office for a follow-up appointment after hip replacement surgery. The woman's daughter accompanies her. The goal of the appointment is to make certain the hip is healing nicely and to discuss precautions before the patient returns to her assisted-living apartment. Almost immediately the conversation is directed toward the daughter because it is so much easier to explain to her what should be done.

CASE STUDY REVIEW

1. What might the staff do to help the patient understand the following?
   - Use the walker consistently.
   - Shoes must be leather tennis shoe type or uniform style; consider Velcro closure as opposed to laces that have to be tied.
   - Do not wear pantyhose.
   - You will not be able to walk your dog on a leash.

2. Should the patient be left out of the conversation? Should the daughter be included?

3. In cases such as these, is something other than verbal communication indicated?

REVIEW QUESTIONS

Multiple Choice

1. Culture influences which of the following?
   a. biases and prejudices
   b. ethnic heritage, age, and gender
   c. educational and life experiences and value systems
   d. b and c only

2. In the cycle of communication, encoding means:
   a. deciphering a message
   b. creating the message to be sent
   c. sending the message
   d. receiving the message

3. Body language:
   a. is used to express feelings and emotions
   b. is not as important as verbal communication
   c. only makes up 7 percent of the message
   d. is only used in Eastern cultures

4. A comfortable social space is defined as:
   a. touching to 6 inches
   b. 1½ feet to 4 feet
   c. 12 to 15 feet
   d. 4 to 12 feet

5. A reassuring cliché is:
   a. a way of calming down a patient
   b. a means of rationalizing a decision
   c. a roadblock to communication
   d. always useful in daily communications

6. Redirecting a socially unacceptable impulse into one that is socially acceptable is an example of which of these defense mechanisms?
   a. sublimation
   b. rationalization
   c. projection
   d. displacement

7. When using an open-ended question with a patient, we expect:
   a. a yes or no answer
   b. them to tell us the truth
   c. a response that permits the patient to elaborate
   d. only the right answers
8. Buffer words:
   a. help us get through the day
   b. are meant to soothe a patient's feelings
   c. are expendable words used in answering a telephone call
   d. are important in face-to-face communication

Critical Thinking

1. The 15-year-old girl awaiting a sports physical exam complains that she is overweight and has pimples. What is your therapeutic response?
2. Bill, who is 28 years old, comes for his annual checkup. When reviewing his social data sheet, you discover he is now living in an apartment and has a new phone number. He mumbles to you that his wife left him and won't let him see the kids. What is your verbal therapeutic response?
3. You try to be gentle and gracious with Edith. She is very fragile and difficult to please. While positioning her for an X-ray, she sneers and says, "You are about the roughest person who ever cared for me." What is your therapeutic response?
4. When you report to Herb that his cholesterol is quite high and that the doctor wants to discuss medication and diet, he responds, "That is impossible; you must have made some mistake." What is your therapeutic response?
5. Lenore uses a wheelchair for mobility. When you offer to help her, she says, "Buzz off! I can do this myself." What is your therapeutic response?
6. Leo, age 62, comments on his being laid off, "I simply don't know what I will do with all the extra time on my hands." What is your therapeutic response?
7. Martin says to you, "I wish it would just end," as you schedule him for another series of chemotherapy treatments. What is your therapeutic response?

8. Your physician/employer is leaving for hospital rounds. He must tell the Ward family that their father will never recover. If he does not die within the next thirty-six hours, the physician recommends disconnecting the ventilator. Your physician is close to this family; he has given them care for many years. What is your therapeutic response?

WEB ACTIVITIES

Select three cultures of particular interest to you personally and search the World Wide Web for information regarding these cultures and communication traditions. How might this new information be applied to the physician whose clientele is primarily made up of these cultures? How might this new knowledge benefit a medical assistant employed in this type of setting?

REFERENCES/BIBLIOGRAPHY

Blair, G. M. (January 23, 2000). *Conversation as communication* [On-line]. Available: http://www.ee.ed.ac.uk/~gerard/Management/art7.html

Fast, J. (1970). *Body language*. New York: M. Evans and Company.

Kinn, M. E., & Woods, M. A. (1998). *The medical assistant: Administrative and clinical* (8th ed.). Philadelphia: W. B. Saunders.

Miliken, M. E. (1998). *Understanding human behavior: A guide for health care providers*. Albany, NY: Delmar.

Purtillo, R. (1990). *Health professional/patient interaction*. Philadelphia: W. B. Saunders.

Sherwood, K. D. (January 25, 1999). *A beginner's guide to effective email* [On-line]. Available: http://www.webfoot.com/advice/email.top.html

Taber's cyclopedic medical dictionary. (18th ed.). (1997). Philadelphia: F. A. Davis.

Tamparo, C. D., & Lindh, W. Q. (2000). *Therapeutic communications for health professions*. Albany, NY: Delmar.

Wilkes, M., & Crosswait, C. B. (1991). *Professional development: The dynamics of success*. San Diego: Harcourt Brace Jovanovich.

5

COPING SKILLS FOR THE MEDICAL ASSISTANT

KEY TERMS

Burnout
Goal
Inner-Directed People
Long-Range Goals
Outer-Directed People
Parasympathetic Nervous System
Self-Actualization
Short-Range Goals
Stress
Stressors
Sympathetic Nervous System

OUTLINE

What Is Stress?
    Adaptation to Stress
    Coping with Stress
What Is Burnout?
    Burnout in the Workplace
    What to Do If You Are Burned Out
    Preventing Burnout
Goal Setting as a Stress Reliever

OBJECTIVES

The student should strive to meet the following performance objectives and demonstrate an understanding of the facts and principles presented in this chapter through written and oral communication.

1. Define the key terms as presented in the glossary.
2. Differentiate between stress and stressors.
3. Describe Hans Selye's GAS theory.
4. Identify seven approaches to coping with stressors in the ambulatory care setting.
5. Identify three characteristics associated with burnout in the workplace.
6. Identify seven signs or symptoms of burnout.
7. List five aspects of personality that promote burnout.
8. List a minimum of five ways to reduce the risk of burnout.
9. List five considerations when setting a goal.
10. Differentiate between long-range and short-range goals.

**GENERAL
(TRANSDISCIPLINARY)**

Professionalism

- Project a professional manner and image
- Demonstrate initiative and responsibility
- Work as a team member
- Prioritize and perform multiple tasks
- Adapt to change

At the office of Doctors Lewis and King, there are four full-time medical assistants who collaborate to make the office run smoothly, both administratively and clinically. One day a month, though, office manager Marilyn Johnson, CMA, is out of town, leaving Ellen Armstrong, the administrative medical assistant, in charge of a busy reception area and an ever-ringing telephone.

On these days, Ellen is particularly careful to organize her work so that things run as they should. She organizes some work the night before, she sets priorities so she is confident that the critical work will get done, and she tries to maintain her calm by taking a short break every couple of hours to review new needs that have come up during the day. While Ellen can't anticipate every emergency, she does try to influence the situation rather than let events control her.

INTRODUCTION

Even in the most well-managed ambulatory care setting, medical assistants and other health providers are likely to feel the effects of stress from time to time. They may be overworked on certain days; they may face difficult patient situations; they may find that the administrative and paperwork load is getting ahead of them.

This chapter helps today's busy, multifaceted medical assistant pinpoint the symptoms of stress and provides ideas for coping with stress as it occurs. The better equipped the medical assistant is to confront and solve the sources of stress, the less likely stressors will become so overwhelming as to lead to burnout on the job. Goal setting, recognizing one's limitations and potentials, setting priorities, and keeping a balanced perspective can work together to reduce stress and enable the medical assistant to take pleasure in working with patients and colleagues.

WHAT IS STRESS?

The body's response to change is termed **stress**. Stress is the "wear and tear" our bodies experience as we continually adjust to a changing environment. Stress has physical and emotional effects on the body, which create either eustress-positive feelings, or distress-negative feelings. Feeling positive leads to a sense of well being, increased motivation, and awareness of new opportunities and perspectives. Positive stress adds anticipation and excitement to life and is enhancing to our lives. Some stress is beneficial and helps us focus on details, achieve difficult goals, and perform at our best.

Negative feelings, or distress, may result in boredom, frustration, rejection, distrust, anger, and depression. Physical symptoms of distress may include cigarette smoking, obesity, and lack of exercise. It has been estimated that 50 percent of all diseases in the United States have a stress-related origin. Included in these diseases are hypertension, migraine headaches, ulcers, anxiety, allergies and asthma, and some types of cancer and cardiovascular disease (Tecco, 1999).

The demands to change that cause stress are called **stressors.** Stressors cause the body to go into arousal or alarm and may be anything from fear, worry, threat, or even challenging events. When we experience any type of stress that exceeds what our body can comfortably handle, we are more susceptible to depression and anxiousness. If we become very stressed, the ability to think clearly and objectively may be impaired.

Adaptation to Stress

Hans Selye's General Adaptation Syndrome (GAS) theory proposes that adaptation to stress occurs in four stages, which he defines as alarm, fight-or-flight, exhaustion, and return-to-normal (Figure 5-1).

Alarm. Awareness of perceived stress is recognized by the body during the alarm stage. Pain is a part of this system as it tells us when body tissue is being damaged. A therapeutic response in the ambulatory care setting is to recognize the fact that pain does produce a stress response. The medical assistant who falls behind during the daily rush of scheduling may also experience a slight rise in blood pressure caused by the alarm stage of stress.

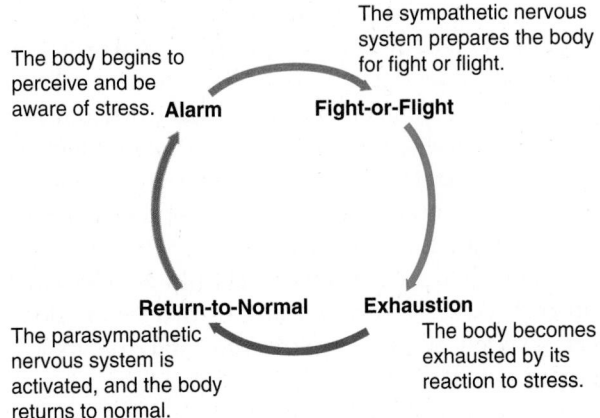

The body begins to perceive and be aware of stress. **Alarm**

The sympathetic nervous system prepares the body for fight or flight.

Fight-or-Flight

Return-to-Normal

The parasympathetic nervous system is activated, and the body returns to normal.

Exhaustion

The body becomes exhausted by its reaction to stress.

Figure 5-1 Hans Selye's General Adaptation Syndrome (GAS) theory proposes that four stages are involved in adapting to stress.

Fight-or-Flight. The sympathetic nervous system prepares the body for fight-or-flight. The eyes dilate and the mouth becomes dry. The heart rate is increased, as is the pulse and respirations. Blood vessels in the skin constrict, and blood vessels in the heart and brain dilate. There is decreased motility in the gastrointestinal and genitourinary tracts. All these changes prepare the body for whatever action may need to be taken.

Exhaustion. The body can only stay in the fight-or-flight state for a limited time. If you have ever stretched a rubber band to the maximum and held it there for a period of time, eventually you tired of holding it and released the rubber band. If you were to examine the rubber band after its release, you would find that it has lost some of its elasticity, which can never be regained. The same principle applies to the blood vessels throughout the body. After repeated periods of dilation and relaxation, they become weakened. If you have ever overstretched a rubber band, you know it snaps in two. Blood vessels may burst when they are dilated to an extreme or have developed weakened areas.

Return-to-Normal. During the return-to-normal stage, the parasympathetic nervous system is activated, and the body returns to normal. The eyes constrict, salivary glands begin to function, and heart rate, pulse, and respirations decrease. Blood vessels dilate in the skin and constrict in the heart and brain. The gastrointestinal and genitourinary tracts begin to function again (Tamparo & Lindh, 2000).

Each stage in Selye's GAS theory is a mechanism to help protect the body and prepare it to escape from danger. When demands are placed on the body, stress occurs. The way a person reacts to those demands determines the level of stress and whether health is threatened or harmed.

Stress is often considered harmful to health. In reality, stress is essential to one's well-being. The body continually goes through change in the course of a twenty-four-hour period. For example, a quick response while driving to work may be necessary to avoid a collision with another vehicle. During your working hours the telephone rings, the exam rooms are full, and the physician is called to the hospital on an emergency. Immediately the body's stress mode is activated. A moderate to high level of stress for short periods of time enables you to make quick judgments and decisions, to be organized and efficient, and to accomplish tasks within minimal time limits.

When too much stress is experienced or if the stress lasts for a long period of time, it begins to affect the body in a negative way. Often one of the first signs of stress may be a headache caused by an increase in blood pressure. Feeling tired even after plenty of rest may be another signal of stress. If these conditions continue, other vital organs, such as the heart and lungs, for example, may also be affected negatively. Cardiac or respiratory arrest, transient ischemic attack, or fainting may be experienced.

For the medical assistant, new technology, a demanding work load, responding to the needs of people who are ill or hurting, patient diversity, and the continuing need for creative problem solving are examples of the stressors encountered daily in ambulatory care settings.

Coping with Stress

The following suggestions may be helpful in coping with stressors in the work environment.

1. Plan ahead
   - Review the schedule for the next day, and pull charts before leaving the office for the day.
   - Keep an accurate inventory of supplies; order before the last items are used.
   - Read journals and keep current with new technology.
   - Participate in continuing education activities.
2. Arrive early
   - Review the patient charts for the day; notice any special problems or needs.
   - Be sure that each exam room is well-equipped and ready for patients.
3. Personal assessment
   - Get plenty of rest.
   - Exercise and eat balanced meals.
   - Dress appropriately. Clothing or shoes that are too tight cause stress.

4. Laugh
   - Learn to laugh at life's little problems.
   - Laugh at yourself.
   - Establish an appropriate level of humor with other members of the staff.
5. Music, color, light
   - Soft background music has been proven to soothe and promote relaxation.
   - Use color and light to create a calm atmosphere.
6. Breaks
   - Build morning and afternoon breaks into the schedule, even if only five or ten minutes.
   - Close the office during the lunch hour, and if possible, leave the facility.
7. Work smarter, not harder
   - Employ time management techniques for reducing stress by completing one task before moving on to another.
   - Prioritize tasks; when possible do the most difficult task early in the day.
   - Do not procrastinate.
   - Be motivated.
   - Be a team member as well as working well independently.
   - Plan your work, then work your plan.

Incorporating these suggestions for coping with and relieving stress will help you operate efficiently and effectively in the ambulatory care setting. You may begin to experience what Abraham Maslow termed **self-actualization.** During self-actualization, you develop your full potential and experience fulfillment and job satisfaction. See Table 5-1 for some suggestions for relieving tension and stress during your daily work routine.

WHAT IS BURNOUT?

According to New York psychologist Herbert J. Freudenberger, PhD, who coined the term, **burnout** is a state of fatigue or frustration brought about by a devotion to a cause, a way of life, or a relationship that failed to produce the expected reward (Gehmeyer, 2000). Burnout exhausts one's physical and mental resources, and leaves one feeling angry, helpless, and trapped. The military term for burnout is "battle fatigue." As a medical assistant you are a member of the health care team that battles disease and the ravages of disease on a daily basis.

Burnout does not occur suddenly as does stress. Rather, burnout is a gradual process that occurs slowly over a period of time. Typical signs and symptoms of burnout include:

- Emotional and physical exhaustion
- Anger
- Self-criticism
- Irritability
- Hair-trigger display of emotions
- Impatience
- Negativism
- A sense of being constantly under attack
- Inability to keep even daily frustrations in perspective

Burnout in the Workplace

Burnout happens to people who previously were enthusiastic and bursting with energy and new ideas when first hired on the job or beginning a new experience. When individuals with a high need to achieve do not reach their goals, they are apt to feel angry and frustrated. Failing to recognize these signs as symptoms of burnout, they may throw themselves even more fully into work-related goals. Unless there is some type of revitalization outside of the workplace, burnout occurs.

Three characteristics associated with burnout in the workplace include:

- Role Conflict: When employees have conflicting responsibilities, they feel pulled in many directions. The perfectionist tries to do everything equally well without setting priorities. Fatigue and exhaustion associated with burnout begin to set in after a period of time.

- Role Ambiguity: The employee does not know what is expected and how to accomplish it because there may not be a role model to follow or ask, or established guidelines to follow.

- Role Overload: If the employee cannot say no and continues to accept more responsibility than they can handle, burnout is sure to set in (Gehmeyer, 2000).

TABLE 5-1 TECHNIQUES FOR REDUCING STRESS AT WORK
• Stretch or change positions.
• Slowly roll your head from side to side and forward and back.
• Slowly rotate your shoulders forward and backward several times.
• Turn away from the computer or close your eyes for several seconds.
• Walk around and deliver charts or lab specimens, and so on.
• Stand or sit tall and take a few deep breaths.
• Meditate for 30 seconds.
• Know your limits and be aware of your body's needs.

What to Do If You Are Burned Out

When you recognize the signs and symptoms of burnout, it is time to do some self-analysis by asking yourself some hard questions. Recall and analyze when you began feeling so tired and unable to relax and enjoy your work. Have you always been a perfectionist? Have you always had a higher need than most of your peers to do a job well? Are you irritable toward coworkers or patients? At what point did you lose your sense of humor? Do you always see work as a chore? Are you so intensely striving to achieve your goals that if you do not succeed you consider yourself a failure? Are you physically and emotionally exhausted?

The next step is to make some changes.

- Make a list of negative words or phrases that you most often use. Now replace the negatives with more neutral words or phrases.

- Create some job diversity for yourself. Drive to work via a different route; enter the building through a different door; change your work routine slightly; change your start time.

- Become creative. Redecorate your area.

- Establish some long- and short-term realistic goals and write them down.

- Take care of yourself; change your eating habits; exercise more; get more sleep.

- Renew friendships; go to lunch with coworkers; laugh with them.

- Implement time management techniques.

- Delegate responsibility to others who are capable.

Table 5-2 will help you assess your risk for burnout.

Preventing Burnout

The best way to treat burnout on the job is to prevent it. This can be accomplished by leaving work-related issues at the office when leaving for the day. Other things you can do to reduce the risk of burnout include:

- Maintain a positive self-esteem and self-image
- Have regular physical examinations
- Take a vacation
- Give up unrealistic goals and expectations
- Develop interests outside of your profession
- Separate work from the rest of your life
- Develop time management techniques
- Develop clear and complete job descriptions for each position in the office

GOAL SETTING AS A STRESS RELIEVER

Do you direct your life or do you allow others to influence and make decisions for you? **Outer-directed people** let events, other people, or environmental factors dictate their behavior. By contrast, **inner-directed people** decide for themselves what they want to do with their lives. Laurence Peter, author of *The Peter Principle*, stated, "If you don't know where you are going, you will end up somewhere else" (Wilkes & Crosswait, 1991).

Discoveries prove that goal-oriented employees are more effective and assertive than colleagues with no goals or future objectives. Recognizing the value of goal planning, many employers arrange planning sessions and/or

---

TABLE 5-2   ASSESS YOUR RISK FOR BURNOUT

This simple test, developed by the Center for Professional Well-Being, can help you determine your predisposition to distress in your life. The more questions with a "yes" response, the greater your risk for burnout.

	Yes	No
1. Are you highly achievement-oriented?	☐	☐
2. Do you tend to withdraw from offers of support?	☐	☐
3. Do you have difficulty delegating responsibilities to others, including patients?	☐	☐
4. Do you prefer to work alone?	☐	☐
5. Do you avoid discussing problems with others?	☐	☐
6. Do you externalize blame?	☐	☐
7. Are your work relationships asymmetrical; that is, are you always giving?	☐	☐
8. Is your personal identity bound up with your work role or professional identity?	☐	☐
9. Do you often overload yourself and have a difficult time saying no?	☐	☐
10. Is there a lack of opportunities for positive and timely feedback outside of your professional or work role?	☐	☐
11. Do you abide by the laws "don't talk, don't trust, don't feel?"	☐	☐

Musick, J. L. (1997). *How Close Are You to Burnout?* American Academy of Family Physicians. [On-line]. Available: http://www.aafp.org/fpm/970400fm/lead.html

SPOTLIGHT ON AAMA ESSENTIALS THROUGH CAAHEP

- Planning ahead will help the medical assistant deal with stressful situations encountered daily in the ambulatory care setting.

- Maintaining a positive self-esteem and self-image and being able to separate work from the rest of one's life, will help the medical assistant prevent burnout.

- Setting goals and promoting a sense of pride in one's work are two ways the medical assistant can help reduce the stress on the job and cope better with the daily ups and downs of a busy medical practice.

seminars to encourage goal setting as a practical application for coping with stress and/or burnout and to develop career objectives. If this does not happen in your work environment, seek your own seminars for goal setting. Such an activity not only "centers" you in your current employment but helps you clearly picture your future plans and hopes.

What is a goal? The dictionary definition of a goal according to *Merriam-Webster's Collegiate Dictionary* is, "the result or achievement toward which effort is directed." To reach a desired goal, a person must implement planning along with a sincere desire to work hard. Skill in goal setting allows the medical assistant to clarify what must be accomplished and to develop a strategic plan to successfully achieve the goal.

A goal must be specific, challenging, realistic, attainable, and measurable. Specific goals are focused and have very precise boundaries. A goal that is challenging creates enthusiasm and interest in achievement. Realistic goals are practical or beneficial for the present and for future self-actualization. An attainable goal refers to the fact that the goal is possible to fulfill. Measurable goals achieve some form of progress or success. By reflecting on the process, one is encouraged to establish additional goals.

Long-range goals are achievements that may take three to five years to accomplish. Long-range goals give direction and definition to our lives and serve to keep us "on track" so to speak. Much discipline, perseverance, determination, and hard work will be expended in accomplishing long-range goals. Some adjustment and readjust-

ment to your goals may be necessary, however. The rewards of goal achievement include satisfaction, pride, a sense of accomplishment, and a job well done.

Short-range goals take apart long-range goals and reassembles the required activities into smaller, more manageable time segments. The time segments may be daily, weekly, monthly, quarterly, or yearly periods.

As a graduate and new employee, one of your long-range goals might be to become the office manager in the ambulatory care setting in which you are currently employed. You may wish to attain this goal within the next three to five years; by breaking it into three longer range goals and a series of short-range goals, you will be able to measure progress and feel a sense of accomplishment. Examples of long- and short-range goals might include:

Long-range goal 1:

To become proficient in all back-office clinical skills during the first year of employment.

Short-range goals necessary to achieve this:

- Practice accuracy and proficiency when performing tasks and skills.

- Practice efficiency by planning ahead for the equipment and supplies needed for each task performed.

- Evaluate your progress on a regular basis, and identify areas that need improvement.

Long-range goal 2:

To add front-office administrative tasks and skills to your routine during the second year of employment.

Short-range goals necessary to achieve this:

- Practice accuracy and proficiency when performing all front-office tasks and skills.

- Practice efficiency by planning ahead for the equipment and supplies needed for each task performed.

- Evaluate your progress on a regular basis, and identify areas that need improvement.

Long-range goal 3:

To begin to focus on office management during the third year of employment.

Short-range goals necessary to achieve this:

- Develop a procedures manual for all back- and front-office tasks and skills.

- Enroll in office management classes.

- Focus on team-building skills.

By year four, you will be ready to move into the office manager position.

Long-range and short-range goals work together to help make changes in our lives. Goals keep life interesting and give us something for which to strive. We can all reach goals successfully with some planning, hard work, discipline, and dedication.

SUMMARY

Stress is very much a part of the medical profession. Each individual working in a medical career experiences consecutive days of demanding, emotionally and physically draining interactions with patients and staff members. This highly technical and ever-changing career requires its professionals to maintain a high level of skill and training and to be familiar with the newest technology.

Goal setting is one approach to reducing stress and burnout and promoting a sense of pride in the workplace, self-actualization, and possible employment promotion. Both long-range and short-range goal planning work together to help make changes in our lives.

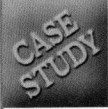

Ellen Armstrong, CMA, is an administrative medical assistant with Doctors Lewis and King. This is her first job. She is just two years out of school, and she is trying to learn everything she can to achieve her long-range goal of becoming office manager at this or some other ambulatory care setting.

Ellen has a great deal in her favor, for she is good with patients, both face-to-face and over the telephone. She is not daunted by the complexity of administrative work her job requires. Ellen knows she has a great deal yet to learn and, although she is a bit intimidated by her, Ellen looks to Marilyn Johnson, CMA, the office manager, for guidance and advice.

CASE STUDY REVIEW

1. How would you advise Ellen to go about achieving her long-term goal of office manager?
2. What are some of the short-term goals Ellen should set? Why are short-term goals important to her success?
3. Besides learning on the job, what else can Ellen do to achieve her goal?

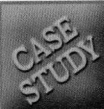

Ellen Armstrong, CMA, has been employed for five years as an administrative medical assistant with Doctors Lewis and King. Ellen is a perfectionist and has pushed herself to achieve many of her short- and long-term goals. The office staff has become aware of the fact that Ellen does not have a sense of humor lately. She seems frustrated and irritable, and is becoming critical of herself and others. Ellen has felt physically and emotionally exhausted, yet she continues to focus on her high standard of job performance; however, work is becoming a chore. At the end of the day if everything has not been completed to her satisfaction, she feels like a failure.

CASE STUDY REVIEW

1. Do you feel Ellen is stressed or experiencing burnout? What do you base your conclusions upon?
2. What might Ellen do to differentiate these two conditions?
3. What changes might Ellen implement to resolve this problem?

REVIEW QUESTIONS

Multiple Choice

1. Which answer is *not* true about stress?
   a. It does not occur suddenly.
   b. It has physical and emotional effects on the body.
   c. It may be positive or negative on its affects on the body.
   d. It is the body's response to change.
2. Hans Selye's GAS theory proposes that adaptation to stress occurs in how many stages?
   a. 2 stages
   b. 3 stages
   c. 4 stages
   d. 5 stages
3. Which is *not* a stage in the General Adaptation Syndrome?
   a. fight-or-flight
   b. exhaustion
   c. burnout
   d. alarm
4. Burnout occurs often if:
   a. a person is aged
   b. the individual works as a health care professional
   c. an individual has certain personality traits
   d. the individual isn't interested in the job
5. Signs and symptoms of burnout include all of the following *except:*
   a. emotional and physical exhaustion
   b. hair-trigger display of emotion
   c. feelings of accomplishment and pride in work
   d. irritability and impatience
6. Working smarter, not harder includes:
   a. taking a sick day now and then, even if you're not sick
   b. prioritizing your tasks and employing time-management techniques
   c. giving as much work to others as possible
   d. making sure others are not taking advantage of you
7. Self-actualization is a term used by:
   a. Laurence Peter
   b. Abraham Maslow
   c. Hans Selye
   d. Harry Levinson
8. Long-range goals are easy to achieve if:
   a. they are not too challenging
   b. they are divided into a series of short-range goals
   c. they don't involve too much hard work
   d. you never change or adjust them

Critical Thinking

1. Discuss a minimum of five methods of dealing positively with stress.
2. Through self-analysis, determine whether you are an outer-directed person or an inner-directed person and what impact this trait may have upon your medical assisting career.
3. List two long-range goals you personally would like to attain within the next five years. Now determine the short-range goals necessary to achieve your long-range goals.
4. Discuss the causes and manifestations of burnout.
5. Discuss the causes of burnout in the workplace and ways in which it may be decreased.

WEB ACTIVITIES

 Search the World Wide Web for additional information on burnout in the workplace. Compile your information into a report for your instructor. Be sure to include a bibliography identifying your web sources.

REFERENCES/BIBLIOGRAPHY

Cooper, J. R. (1993). *The medical reporter: Beware of professional burnout* [On-line]. Available: http://none.coolware.com/health/medical_reporter/burnout.html

drkoop.com. (1998–2000). Wellness: Mental health, stress, ways stress affects individuals. [On-line]. Available: http://www.drkoop.com/wellness/mental_health/stress/page_337_765.asp

Gehmeyr, A. (June 14, 2000). *Burnout* [On-line]. Available: http://155.187.10.12/fun/burnout.html

Gehmeyr, A. (1993). *Prescription for burnout* [On-line]. Available: http://155.187.10.12/fun/burnout.html

Keir, L., Wise, B. A., & Krebs, C. (1998). *Medical assisting: Administrative and clinical competencies* (4th ed.). Albany, NY: Delmar.

Merriam-Webster's collegiate dictionary (10th ed.). (1994). Springfield, MA: Merriam-Webster.

Musick, J. L. (1997). *American Academy of Family Physicians: How close are you to burnout?* [On-line]. Available: http://www.aafp.org/fpm/970400fm/lead.html

Stress management. (2000). [On-line]. Available: http://www.ivf.com/stress.html

Tamparo, C. D., & Lindh, W. Q. (2000). *Therapeutic communications for allied health professions.* Albany, NY: Delmar.

Tecco, A. (1999). *Stress management* [On-line]. Available: http://www.drkoop.com/wellness/prevcenter/stress/stress.asp

Vikesland, G. (1999). *How to prevent burnout and ridding yourself of burnout* [On-line]. Available: http://www.employer-employee.com/Burnout.html

Wilkes, M., & Crosswait, C. B. (1991). *Professional development: The dynamics of success.* San Diego: Harcourt Brace Jovanovich.

THE THERAPEUTIC APPROACH TO THE PATIENT WITH LIFE-THREATENING ILLNESS

KEY TERMS

Acquired Immunodeficiency Syndrome (AIDS)

Culture

Dementia

Durable Power of Attorney for Health Care

Human Immunodeficiency Virus (HIV)

Libido

Living Will

Physician Directive

Psychomotor Retardation

OUTLINE

Life-Threatening Illness
   Cultural Perspective on Life-
   Threatening Illness
**Choices in Life-Threatening
Illness**
**The Range of Psychological
Suffering**

**The Therapeutic Response to the
   Patient with AIDS**
**The Challenge for the Medical
   Assistant**

OBJECTIVES

The student should strive to meet the following performance objectives and demonstrate an understanding of the facts and principles presented in this chapter through written and oral communication.

1. Define the key terms as presented in the glossary.
2. Describe possible patient perspectives when facing a life-threatening illness.
3. Define "life-threatening" illness.
4. Discuss cultural manifestations of life-threatening illness.
5. Identify the strongest cultural influence in the life of a patient.
6. List at least four choices to be made when facing a life-threatening illness.
7. Briefly describe the use of living wills and physician directives.
8. Discuss the range of psychological suffering that accompanies life-threatening illnesses.
9. Discuss additional concerns/fears when the life-threatening illness is AIDS.
10. Recall a number of challenges faced by the medical assistant when caring for people with life-threatening illnesses.

**GENERAL
(TRANSDISCIPLINARY)**

Communication Skills

- **Treat all patients with compassion and empathy**

Legal Concepts

- **Maintain confidentiality**

Instruction

- **Instruct individuals according to their needs**

- **Teach methods of health promotion and disease prevention**

- **Locate community resources and disseminate information**

You have seen the medical reports and have agonized with your physician who must tell Suzanne Markis when she comes in today that she has inoperable pancreatic cancer. When she arrives, you treat her as you normally would, making certain she suspects nothing from you. When she emerges from the physician's room, you make certain to meet her, take her arm, and ask if you can call someone for her. You do not present her with a bill or make another appointment at this time. You recognize that anything you say will probably not be remembered, so you focus entirely upon this patient and her immediate needs. In a day or two, as instructed by your physician employer, you will make a phone call to set an appointment for Suzanne and any family members she might want present to visit with your physician so any questions might be answered for them.

INTRODUCTION

Everything learned in Chapter 4 regarding therapeutic communications is heightened and considered more difficult when the patient has a life-threatening illness. If you were told today that your life would probably be shortened because of a serious illness, your perspective would change completely. What was important yesterday may mean little or nothing now. Something that meant nothing to you yesterday suddenly takes on great importance to you now. It is essential for the medical assistant to remember this difference in perspective and what is likely to be important to patients with a life-threatening illness.

It also must be remembered that no two individuals respond to a life-threatening illness in the same way. Some respond with denial and act as if the information had never been shared with them. Others alter their lives radically and drastically change their priorities. Still others quietly continue their lives changing very little outwardly but recognize that their choices may now be limited (Figure 6-1).

LIFE-THREATENING ILLNESS

A life-threatening illness is not easily defined. Some will use the word *terminal*; others refuse to use that word because they believe it removes any hope from the situation. Also, what is life-threatening for one individual may not be for another. For our purposes, life threatening is used to imply a life that in all probability will be shortened because of a serious or debilitating illness or disease. It may be defined as death that is imminent; it may be defined in terms of a serious illness that one will battle for many years but will ultimately shorten his/her life.

Cultural Perspective on Life-Threatening Illness

Strong cultural manifestations will be seen in the treatment of a life-threatening illness and for anyone facing death. Culture is defined as how we live our lives, how we think, how we speak, and how we behave.

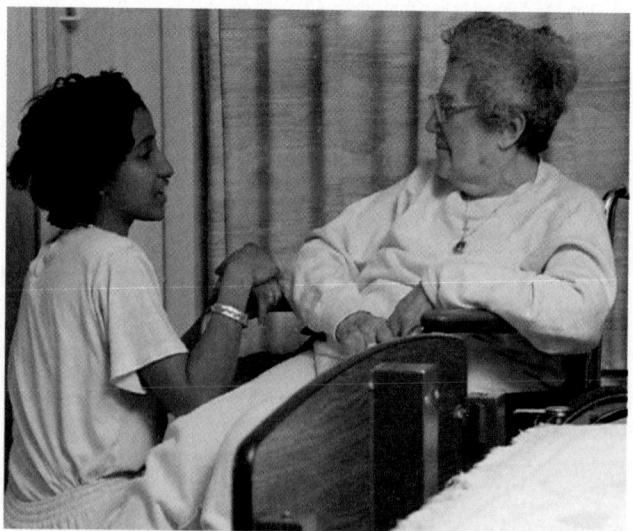

Figure 6-1 Establishing a caring and trusting relationship will help the patient come to terms with a life-threatening illness.

SPOTLIGHT ON AAMA ESSENTIALS THROUGH CAAHEP

- Taking care of a patient with a life-threatening illness should not constitute a fear of caring for that patient.

- Patients with life-threatening illnesses need not only skillful medical care but compassionate, sensitive treatment.

- Interacting with the seriously ill patient should include care that is appropriate to the patient's developmental age and cultural preferences.

Some cultures prefer that the life-threatening illness not be shared with the patient in the beginning, but with the family who helps to prepare the patient for the inevitable. A few cultures generally do not seek care for an illness until it is quite advanced; this practice can make pain management and treatment more difficult or impossible in some cases. Some cultures surround the person who is ill with great attention, never leaving the person alone. Other cultures view the illness as something that must be removed from the body, perhaps even believing that the individual has been visited upon with this illness due to some past sin or transgression.

In the same manner, pain is viewed. Some cultures believe it is to be endured quietly without complaint; others believe there is to be no pain and family members will go to great lengths to have health care providers relieve the pain. When questioning a patient about the pain level, it must be within a cultural perspective. For example, cultures with an Asian influence are more likely to describe pain in general terms related to the imbalance of the body than in terms of "piercing, intermittent, or throbbing" or on a scale of 1 to 10.

It must also be remembered that the strongest influence in managing any life-threatening illness in the life of the patient is *not* the health care team; it is the family and those closest to the patient. Therefore, great care must be taken to determine and understand the patient's cultural perspective as much as possible, and the patient must be given great respect. Many times the cultural influence may contradict the standard of care preferred by the health care provider. It is better to understand the culture and work within it than to deny it and continually work against the patient's belief system and influence of family.

CHOICES IN LIFE-THREATENING ILLNESS

Many choices are available to a patient with a life-threatening illness, and many decisions are to be made. The urgency of the decisions will depend in part upon possible life expectancy. Sometimes these decisions may seem contrary to recommended medical intervention.

Patients have the right to choose or to refuse treatment in most cases. Some rush into a treatment protocol only to discover later that their choices have brought them pain, disability, and expense far beyond what originally was assumed. While it is the health care professional's goal to heal, if healing is not likely or possible, patients ought not to be "urged" into treatment protocols that are likely to be contrary to their personal wishes for the sake of treatment only.

While health care professionals are less comfortable with death than they are with saving life, there are some issues appropriate to discuss with patients especially when facing life-threatening illness. Those issues include the following:

1. **Living will** or **physician directive** documents may be used in making end-of-life decisions.
2. **Durable power of attorney for health care** allows another to make decisions for the patient when the patient is no longer able to do so.
3. Discussions of pain management and treatment may or may not be a part of a living will document but should be discussed at some point with the patient and/or patient's family.
4. Alternative methods of treatment should be discussed as well as the outcome if no treatment is sought.
5. Finances are to be considered. What will insurance cover (if there is insurance)? Who makes the decisions if managed care is an issue? What family resources can or will be used?
6. Emotional needs of the patient and family members are important. From where does the patient's primary support come? Friends, clergy, other?

It is not the responsibility of the health care professionals treating the individual with life-threatening illness to provide all these services, but a health care professional who raises these issues for patients and families to deal with is more closely in tune with a patient's power in the illness.

While some states were slow to recognize living wills, there is a piece of legislation that is available to all. The federal government passed the

Patient Self-Determination Act in 1991 giving all patients receiving care in institutions receiving payments from medicare and medicaid written information about their right to accept or refuse medical or surgical treatment. The act also requires that patients be given information about their options to create living wills and to appoint someone to act on their behalf in making health care decisions (durable power of attorney for health care). When facing a life-threatening illness, it can be very helpful to have some decisions made about what should be done and who can make decisions if the patient becomes unable to do so.

Any documents of this nature the patient has should be copied in the medical chart that goes with the patient when hospitalized. At any time the patient makes a change in such a document, the old document is to be replaced with the new one.

The time when such documents are formulated can be the time for physicians to discuss with patients their right to decisions regarding pain management and treatment alternatives. Patients often fear pain and loss of independence more than anything when facing a life-threatening illness. It is better to have those discussions early in treatment than later when the patient may not be so clear on options. Sometimes treatment alternatives the patient may consider are not within the realm of recognized medical acceptability, but it is better to have that discussion than to ignore the possibility. Remember the earlier statement indicating that the family and friends bring more influence to bear than does the health care professional. If the physician and patient are seen as partners in the patient's care, then the patient may not be so fearful in discussing any nonmedically accepted protocol being considered.

Finances are no one's favorite subjects, especially physicians. However, such a discussion is important. Often patients fear not being able to meet their financial obligations as much as they fear the illness. What methods of payment are there? What does insurance cover? How far will insurance go? What restrictions does any managed care agency hold in a particular illness? Can the medical insurance be cancelled when the patient is no longer able to work or when a life-threatening illness is diagnosed?

Emotional support is vital when dealing with a life-threatening illness. Health care professionals will want to determine where that support comes from for the patient. Should a support group be suggested for the patient and family members? For some patients and families, an individual giving spiritual guidance is seen as a member of the family and a member of the health care team. For others, no spiritual influence is recognized or sought.

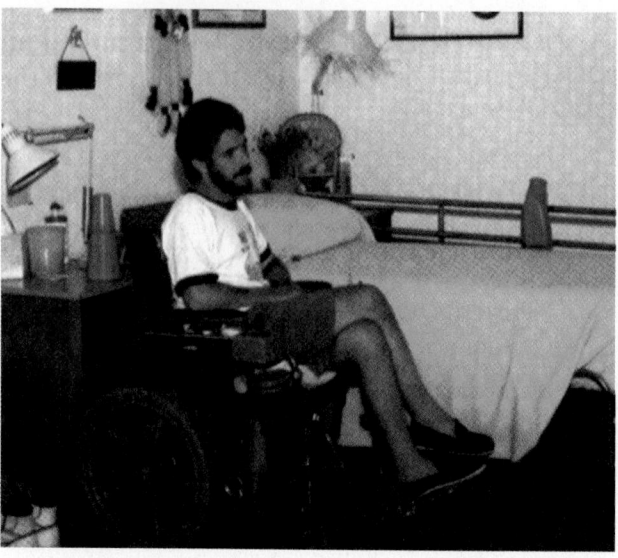

Figure 6-2   Patients living with a serious illness may experience a wide range of emotions.

THE RANGE OF PSYCHOLOGICAL SUFFERING

The range of suffering associated with a life-threatening illness is extensive. Patients feel extreme distress. Anxiety and depression are common. At the time of diagnosis, patients' responses may include denial, numbness, and inability to face the facts. Sadness, hopelessness, helplessness, and withdrawal often are exhibited (Figure 6-2).

The range of psychological suffering leads to physical symptoms, such as tension, tachycardia, agitation, insomnia, anorexia, and panic attacks. The physician may be so intent on treating the physical ramifications of the illness that the psychological suffering is mostly ignored.

THE THERAPEUTIC RESPONSE TO THE PATIENT WITH AIDS

It is not the intention of this chapter to specifically identify the many life-threatening illnesses and their particular needs. However, a few comments about patients testing positive for **human immunodeficiency virus (HIV)** and suffering from **aquired immunodeficiency syndrome (AIDS)** are important.

The discovery of infection with HIV is extremely stressful and is typically accompanied by the fear of developing AIDS. Patients are often preoccupied with illness and the fear of getting other life-threatening diseases. Patients are angry at the disease, at the discrimination that often accompanies it, at the prospect of a lonely, painful death, at the lack of effective treatment, at medical staff, and at themselves.

In many cases, guilt develops about past behavior and lifestyles, or about the possibility of having transmitted the disease to others. When the disease has been contracted through contaminated blood or blood products or by individuals who felt they were protected or safe from the disease, the anger may turn to rage.

Some patients contemplate suicide. Because social and physical assistance are needed, a strong network of friends and family is particularly important. In the case of homosexuals and those addicted to intravenous drugs, however, there are a large number who are estranged from their family's support system. People with AIDS may feel added strain if this is the first knowledge their families have of any high-risk behaviors associated with the transmission of the disease.

Patients with AIDS are apt to suffer central nervous system involvement. Forgetfulness and poor concentration may be followed by **psychomotor retardation** (the slowing of physical and mental responses), decreased alertness, apathy, withdrawal, diminished interest in

work, and loss of **libido** (sexual drive). Some patients later experience confusion, progressive impairment, and profound **dementia** (progressive impairment of intellectual function).

THE CHALLENGE FOR THE MEDICAL ASSISTANT

As a medical assistant, you face the challenge of caring for people with a life-threatening illness; you must comfort those who face great suffering and death. You will become a source of information for patients and their support members. You must be particularly sensitive and respectful toward individuals who may be viewed as social pariahs. You will have to examine your own beliefs, lifestyle, and biases. You must be comfortable treating all patients, no matter what the illness is or how it was contracted.

As well as assisting your physician or employer in providing the best possible medical care, many nonmedical forms of assistance may be required by patients suffering from a life-threatening illness. You may need to make referrals to community-based agencies or service groups. Health departments, social workers, trained hospice volunteers, and AIDS volunteers may also be helpful to you, your patients, and their families.

The best therapeutic response to the patient with a life-threatening illness will build upon the person's own coping abilities, capitalize on strengths, maintain hope, and show continued human care and concern. Patients may want up-to-date information on their disease, its causes, modes of transmission, treatments available, and sources of care and social support. Be prepared to recommend support groups where patients can discuss their feelings and express their concerns. Treat patients with concern and compassion and assure them everything will be done to provide continuity of care and relief from distress. Patients may be encouraged to call upon clergy for spiritual support.

For example, at Inner City Health Care, Dr. Ray Reynolds is known for his compassion and great warmth toward people. On difficult days at the center, this attitude holds him in good stead. Sometimes, he tends to take on the more challenging cases: patients with life-threatening diseases, often young people with AIDS who should be in the prime of their lives.

Clinical medical assistant Wanda Slawson always tries to learn from Dr. Reynolds' example. While she is quieter and not as outgoing as Dr. Reynolds, Wanda always tries to be both courteous and comforting to patients, especially those who are anxious. She makes it a point always to help patients discover a new way to cope with debilitating diseases.

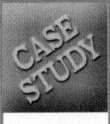

CASE STUDY 6-1

The extended family of Wong Lee is concerned about his illness and his care. Chronic obstructive pulmonary disease (COPD) has ravaged his body. He is on oxygen all the time now. He wants to remain at home to die; his family wants that, too. Yet you are uncertain of how much information to give to members of this expanded family when they call. You wish to protect Mr. Lee's confidentiality.

CASE STUDY REVIEW

1. Are the questions the extended family members raise intended to harm or help Mr. Lee?
2. Is there a durable power of attorney for health care in place?
3. What, if any, of this concern is related to the culture?
4. What can you and your physician-employer suggest to be of help to everyone involved?

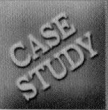

CASE STUDY 6-2

Inner City Health Care, a multi-doctor urgent care center in a large city, has a large roster of patients, some of whom have AIDS. While clinical medical assistant Bruce Goldman tries not to be, sometimes he is wary of patients who he thinks might be homosexual. When patient Bill Swartz was seen for a change in a mole on his calf, Bruce did his best to interact in a professional manner even though he suspected Bill was homosexual. After this patient exchange, medical assistant Bruce Goldman decided it was time to deal with his prejudices against homosexuals and his fear of AIDS and all AIDS patients.

CASE STUDY REVIEW

1. While medical assistant Bruce Goldman may not admit it, he is threatened by AIDS. What should he know about AIDS transmission that may reduce his fears?

2. In the future, Bruce would like to be more open and supportive when he is dealing with an AIDS patient. What are some of the things he can do to help patients?

3. What are some things Bruce can do to reduce wariness regarding patients he feels might be homosexuals?

SUMMARY

Medical assistants must be aware that when caring for people with a life-threatening illness, having even the slightest fear of death can undermine the ability to respond professionally, with empathy and support. If you feel yourself losing the ability to be helpful, it is time to briefly step aside. This does not mean withdrawal from your position or refusal to care for your patients. It means that you do whatever is necessary so that your perspective is not lost. It may mean taking a day off from work to "fill up your soul" and to give your psyche a rest. If the ambulatory care setting has an abundance of patients with life-threatening illnesses, it may require that you spend some time in a support group of your own so that you are better able to cope. Never be afraid to feel sad or weep with your patients. It is better to sense their pain and, at times, feel the pain with them, than it is to be so clinically objective you miss their true needs.

REVIEW QUESTIONS

Multiple Choice

1. When a practice treats patients with AIDS, it is important for medical assistants to:
   a. warn other patients about the dangers of transmission
   b. segregate AIDS patient reception areas from other patient areas
   c. be supportive and free of prejudice
   d. deny any information to patients regarding the seriousness of the illness

2. The Patient Self-Determination Act:
   a. allows a patient to have a choice of physicians
   b. ensures a patient's right to accept or refuse treatment
   c. gives patients the right to formulate advance directives

   d. all of the above
   e. only b and c

3. The strongest influence in a patient with a life-threatening illness is:
   a. the physician
   b. the hospital
   c. the family
   d. the patient

4. Life-threatening illness is defined as:
   a. a life shortened due to serious illness or disease
   b. death that is imminent
   c. serious illness to battle for many years but may shorten life
   d. all of the above

5. Culture may be defined as:
   a. how we live our lives
   b. how we think

c. how we speak and behave
d. all of the above

6. Therapeutic communication with a patient with a life-threatening illness:
   a. is no different than communicating with any patient
   b. is heightened and considered more difficult
   c. is left to nonmedical support staff
   d. comes naturally and requires no special skill

7. Cultural influence may in part determine:
   a. when/how to involve family members
   b. whether spiritual support is sought
   c. how the illness and pain associated with it is managed
   d. all of the above

8. Durable power of attorney for health care:
   a. enables someone other than the patient to make only health care decisions
   b. enables someone other than the patient to make any decisions for the patient
   c. makes certain that patients' financial responsibilities are met
   d. makes certain a patient's wishes are followed
   e. only a and d

9. Additional problems people with AIDS may encounter are:
   a. loss of family and friends for support
   b. being treated as social pariahs in some settings
   c. that living wills are not recognized
   d. only a and b

10. Effective pain management may depend upon:
    a. patient's needs
    b. family wishes
    c. cultural systems
    d. all of the above
    e. only a and c

Critical Thinking

1. Research other sections in this text that discuss end-of-life legal documents. Describe additional information that you find.

2. Discuss with a friend what cultural influences might affect each of you if you were facing a life-threatening illness. What choices would each of you make?

3. In a paragraph seen only by yourself, describe your greatest fears in caring for patients with AIDS.

4. List common psychological reactions people might have from learning they have a life-threatening illness.

5. Research other sections in this text that discuss AIDS. What additional information do you find beneficial?

6. What steps would you personally take to make certain you do not burn out from caring for persons with a life-threatening illness?

7. List the advantages/disadvantages of the physician directives available.

8. Discuss with a nurse or a nursing student in your school how health care professionals deal with the psychological suffering in persons with a life-threatening illness.

9. Discuss with a classmate your concerns in dealing with patients with a life-threatening illness. Would you choose to work where you seldom lost a patient to a life-threatening illness? If so, what are the reasons?

10. Research the agencies available in your community that can provide support for people and family members facing life-threatening illness.

REFERENCES/BIBLIOGRAPHY

Lewis, M., & Tamparo, C. (1998). *Medical law, ethics, and bioethics for ambulatory care*. Philadelphia: F. A. Davis Company.

Purnell, L., & Paulanka, B. (1998). *Transcultural health care: A culturally competent approach*. Philadelphia: F. A. Davis Company.

Tamparo, C., & Lindh, W. (2000). *Therapeutic communications for health professionals*. Albany, NY: Delmar.

Unit

3

RESPONSIBLE MEDICAL PRACTICE

Chapter

7

LEGAL CONSIDERATIONS

KEY TERMS

Agent
Civil Law
Criminal Law
Defendant
Doctrine
Durable Power of Attorney
Emancipated Minor
Expert Witness
Expressed Contract
Implied Consent
Implied Contract
Incompetence
Informed Consent
Libel
Litigation
Malpractice
Mandate
Minor
Negligence
Noncompliant
Plaintiff
Risk Management
Slander
Statute
Subpoena
Tort

OUTLINE

Civil and Criminal Law
Medical Practice Acts and the Medical Assistant's Role
  Patient Rights
The Physician, the Medical Assistant, and the Law
Contracts
  Termination of Contracts
Standard of Care and the 4 Ds of Negligence
Torts
  Battery
  Defamation of Character
  Invasion of Privacy

Medical Records
  Informed Consent
  Implied Consent
  Consent and Legal Incompetence
  Subpoenas
  Confidentiality
  Statute of Limitations
Public Duties
  Drug Screening
  AIDS
  Abuse
Good Samaritan Law
Physician's Directives
Americans with Disabilities Act (ADA)

OBJECTIVES

The student should strive to meet the following performance objectives and demonstrate an understanding of the facts and principles presented in this chapter through written and oral communication.

1. Define the key terms as presented in the glossary.
2. Compare/contrast civil and criminal law.
3. Define the medical assistant's role in legal issues.
4. Describe the use of contracts in the ambulatory care setting.
5. Discuss the standard of care for health care professionals.
6. Explain the 4 Ds of negligence.
7. Define and give examples of torts.
8. Explain the necessity of informed consent.
9. Describe how to handle subpoenas.
10. Recall the special consideration for patients related to the issues of confidentiality, the statute of limitations, public duties, and AIDS.   *(continues)*

OBJECTIVES (*continued*)

11. Describe procedures to follow in documenting and reporting abuse.
12. Discuss Good Samaritan Laws, physician's directives, and the Americans with Disabilities Act.

ROLE DELINEATION COMPONENTS

GENERAL (TRANSDISCIPLINARY)

Legal Concepts

- Prepare and maintain medical records
- Document accurately
- Use appropriate guidelines when releasing information
- Follow employer's established policies dealing with the health care contract
- Follow federal, state and local legal guidelines
- Maintain awareness of federal and state health care legislation and regulations
- Comply with risk management and safety procedures

SCENARIO

At the ambulatory care center of Doctors Lewis and King, a two-doctor family physician office, Dr. Lewis and Dr. King are especially careful about establishing stringent risk management procedures to protect patients from harm and the practice from potential liability.

Dr. King has worked with office manager Marilyn Johnson, CMA, to assemble a policy and procedures manual outlining everything from how telephone calls are answered to how patient medical records are documented and stored. Marilyn, in turn, seeks the input of the other administrative and clinical medical assistants as she frequently updates the manual. To ensure that they are providing the best care for patients while protecting themselves, four times a year the entire staff meets to review office policies, changing them as necessary or incorporating new procedures to meet new situations or legal mandates.

INTRODUCTION

The law as it relates to health care has grown increasingly complex in the past decade. The agendas of federal and state governments include an investigation of quality health care, a desire to control health care costs (while hoping to assure equitable access to health care), and an interest in protecting the patient. A full discussion of health law requires several volumes; therefore, only the laws designated to protect the patient will be identified in this chapter, and emphasis will be placed on the ambulatory care setting.

Being aware of the law and its implications and establishing sound practices and procedures will both safeguard patient rights and protect the health care professional.

CIVIL AND CRIMINAL LAW

The most frequent law exercised in the ambulatory care setting is **civil law**, or law as it is related to individuals. Restitution awarded when a civil wrong is committed is usually monetary in nature. **Criminal law** addresses wrongs committed against the welfare and safety of society as a whole; punishment is usually imprisonment or a fine.

If a charge is brought against a physician as the **defendant** in a civil case, the goal is to reimburse the **plaintiff**, the person bringing charges (usually a patient), with a monetary amount for suffering, pain, and any loss of wages. For example, a physician who has caused harm to a patient in the course of treatment may be sued in a civil case by the patient for the recovery of time lost from work as well as the pain and suffering that was the result of treatment.

In a criminal case, charges are brought against the defendant by the state with the intent of preventing any further harm to society. For example, a physician practicing medicine without a proper license may be subject to disciplinary action from a professional association and criminal action by the courts.

MEDICAL PRACTICE ACTS AND THE MEDICAL ASSISTANT'S ROLE

Each state has medical practice acts that regulate the practice of medicine with the intent of protecting its citizens from harm. These **statutes**, or laws, govern licensure, standards of care, professional liability and negligence, confidentiality, and torts. Some states also regulate personnel who may be employed in the ambulatory care setting. For example, some states require that medical assistants be licensed or certified to be able to perform any invasive procedures. Other states require additional training in radiology for the medical assistant to be able to take X rays. Further, some states are so strict in their regulations that medical assistants perform mostly clerical functions. Certainly, medical assistants desiring to utilize their skills must be aware of state regulations and always perform only within the scope of those regulations.

Patient Rights

The Patient's Bill of Rights was developed by the American Hospital Association in 1973 and revised in 1992 to establish more effective patient care and greater satisfaction for patient, physician, and hospital (Figure 7-1). While this Bill of Rights was written with the hospital patient in mind, patients in ambulatory care settings should be accorded the same rights. Although no list of rights can guarantee the kind of treatment patients have a right to expect, medical assistants should make every effort to conduct activities with the concern of the patient in mind.

THE PHYSICIAN, THE MEDICAL ASSISTANT, AND THE LAW

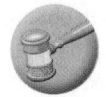

There are a number of ways in which the law governs physicians and their employees. Some of these issues are particularly pertinent to the ambulatory care setting and the medical assistants who work in these health care environments.

CONTRACTS

A contract is a binding agreement between two or more persons. A physician has a legal obligation, or duty, to care for a patient under the principles of contract law. The agreement must be between competent persons to do or not to do something lawful in exchange for a payment.

A contract exists when the patient arrives for treatment and the physician accepts the patient by providing treatment. An example of a valid contract occurs when a patient calls the office or clinic to make an appointment for an annual physical examination. Assuming both physician and patient are competent and that the physician performs the lawful act of the physical examination and the patient pays a fee, all aspects of the contract exist.

There are two types of contracts, expressed and implied. An **expressed contract** can be written or verbal and will specifically describe what each party in the contract will do. A written contract requires that all necessary aspects of the agreement be in writing. An **implied contract** is indicated by actions rather than by words. The majority of physician-patient contracts are implied contracts. It is not required that the contract be written to be enforceable as long as all points of the contract exist. An implied contract can exist either by the circumstances of the situation or by the law. When a patient complains of a sore throat and the physician does a throat culture to diagnose and treat the ailment, an implied contract exists by the circumstances. An implied contract by law exists when a patient goes into anaphylactic shock and the physician administers epinephrine to counteract shock symptoms. The law says that the physician did what the patient would have requested had there been an expressed contract.

For a contract to be valid and binding, the parties who enter into it must be competent; therefore, the mentally incompetent, the legally insane, persons under heavy drug or alcohol influences, infants, and some minors cannot enter into a binding contract.

A PATIENT'S BILL OF RIGHTS

First adopted by the American Hospital Association in 1973.

This revision approved by the AHA Board of Trustees on October 21, 1992.

1. The patient has the right to considerate and respectful care.

2. The patient has the right to and is encouraged to obtain from physicians and other direct caregivers relevant, current, and understandable information concerning diagnosis, treatment, and prognosis.

   Except in emergencies when the patient lacks decision-making capacity and the need for treatment is urgent, the patient is entitled to the opportunity to discuss and request information related to the specific procedures and/or treatments, the risks involved, the possible length of recuperation, and the medically reasonable alternatives and their accompanying risks and benefits.

   Patients have the right to know the identity of physicians, nurses, and others involved in their care, as well as when those involved are students, residents, or other trainees. The patient also has the right to know the immediate and long-term financial implications of treatment choices, insofar as they are known.

3. The patient has the right to make decisions about the plan of care prior to and during the course of treatment and to refuse a recommended treatment or plan of care to the extent permitted by law and hospital policy and to be informed of the medical consequences of this action. In case of such refusal, the patient is entitled to other appropriate care and services that the hospital provides or transfer to another hospital. The hospital should notify patients of any policy that might affect patient choice within the institution.

4. The patient has the right to have an advance directive (such as a living will, health care proxy, or durable power of attorney for health care) concerning treatment or designating a surrogate decision maker with the expectation that the hospital will honor the intent of that directive to the extent permitted by law and hospital policy.

   Health care institutions must advise patients of their rights under state law and hospital policy to make informed medical choices, ask if the patient has an advance directive, and include that information in patient records. The patient has the right to timely information about hospital policy that may limit its ability to implement fully a legally valid advance directive.

5. The patient has the right to every consideration of privacy. Case discussion, consultation, examination, and treatment should be conducted so as to protect each patient's privacy.

6. The patient has the right to expect that all communications and records pertaining to his/her care will be treated as confidential by the hospital, except in cases such as suspected abuse and public health hazards when reporting is permitted or required by law. The patient has the right to expect that the hospital will emphasize the confidentiality of this information when it releases it to any other parties entitled to review information in these records.

7. The patient has the right to review the records pertaining to his/her medical care and to have the information explained or interpreted as necessary, except when restricted by law.

8. The patient has the right to expect that, within its capacity and policies, a hospital will make reasonable response to the request of a patient for appropriate and medically indicated care and services. The hospital must provide evaluation, service, and/or referral as indicated by the urgency of the case. When medically appropriate and legally permissible, or when a patient has so requested, a patient may be transferred to another facility. The institution to which the patient is to be transferred must first have accepted the patient for transfer. The patient must also have the benefit of complete information and explanation concerning the need for, risks, benefits, and alternatives to such a transfer.

9. The patient has the right to ask and be informed of the existence of business relationships among the hospital, educational institutions, other health care providers, or payers that may influence the patient's treatment and care.

10. The patient has the right to consent to or decline to participate in proposed research studies or human experimentation affecting care and treatment or requiring direct patient involvement, and to have those studies fully explained prior to consent. A patient who declines to participate in research or experimentation is entitled to the most effective care that the hospital can otherwise provide.

11. The patient has the right to expect reasonable continuity of care when appropriate and to be informed by physicians and other caregivers of available and realistic patient care options when hospital care is no longer appropriate.

12. The patient has the right to be informed of hospital policies and practices that relate to patient care, treatment, and responsibilities. The patient has the right to be informed of available resources for resolving disputes, grievances, and conflicts, such as ethics committees, patient representatives, or other mechanisms available in the institution. The patient has the right to be informed of the hospital's charges for services and available payment methods.

Figure 7-1   A Patient's Bill of Rights. (Reprinted with permission of the American Hospital Association)

Medical assistants are considered **agents** of the physicians they serve and as such must be cautious that their actions and words may become binding on their physicians. For example, to say that the doctor can cure the patient may cause serious legal problems when in fact a cure may not be possible.

Termination of Contracts

A broken contract or breach of contract occurs when one of the parties does not meet contractual obligations. A physician is legally bound to treat a patient until:

- The patient discharges the physician
- The physician formally withdraws from patient care
- The patient no longer needs treatment and is formally discharged by the physician

Patient Discharges Physician. When the patient discharges the physician, the physician should send a letter to the patient to confirm and document the termination of the contract. The notice should be sent by certified mail with return receipt requested. Keep a copy of the letter in the patient's record (Figure 7-2).

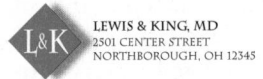

LEWIS & KING, MD
2501 CENTER STREET
NORTHBOROUGH, OH 12345

January 6, 20--

CERTIFIED MAIL

Jim Marshal
76 Georgia Avenue
Millerton, TX 43912

Dear Mr. Marshal:

This will confirm our telephone conversation today in which you discharged me as your attending physician in your present illness. In my opinion your condition requires continued medical supervision by a physician. If you have not already done so, I suggest that you employ another physician without delay.

You may be assured that after receiving a written request from you, I will furnish the physician of your choice with information regarding the diagnosis and treatment which you have received from me.

Very truly yours,

Winston Lewis

Winston Lewis, MD
WL:ea

Figure 7-2 Letter confirming physician's discharge by the patient.

Physician Formally Withdraws from the Case. To avoid any charges of abandonment, the physician should formally withdraw from the case as, for example, when the patient becomes **noncompliant** or the physician feels the patient can no longer be served. Again, notice should be sent to the patient by certified mail with return receipt requested and a copy of the notice should be filed in the patient's record (Figures 7-3 and 7-4).

Inner City Health Care
222 S. First Avenue
Carlton, MI 11666

May 9, 20--

CERTIFIED MAIL

Lenny Taylor
260 Second Street
Carlton, MI 11666

Dear Mr. Taylor:

You will recall that we discussed our physician-patient relationship in my office on May 6, 20--.

Your son, George Taylor, and Bruce Goldman, my medical assistant were also present. As you know, the primary difficulty has been your failure to cooperate with the medical plan for your care.

While it is unfortunate that our relationship has reached this stage, I will no longer be able to serve as your physician. I will be available to you on an emergency basis only until June 10, 20--. Meanwhile, you should immediately call or write the Medical Society, 123 Omega Drive, Carlton, MI 11666, Tel. 123-456-7899 and obtain a list of gerontologists. Any delay could jeopardize your health, so please act quickly.

Your physical (and/or mental) problems include: hypertensive heart disease, decreased kidney function, and arteriosclerosis. You could have additional medical problems that may also require professional care. Once you have found a new physician have him or her call my office. I will be happy to discuss your case with the physician assuming your care, and will transfer a written summary of your case to them upon the receipt of a written request from you to do so.

Thank you for your anticipated cooperation and courtesy.

Very truly yours,

James Whitney

James Whitney, MD
JW:kr

Figure 7-3 Letter reiterating "for the record" the physician's decision to withdraw from the case discussed during meeting with patient.

Inner City Health Care
222 S. First Avenue
Carlton, MI 11666

December 5, 20--

CERTIFIED MAIL

Rhoda Au
41 Academy Road
Carlton, MI 11666

Dear Ms. Au:

I find it necessary to inform you that I am withdrawing further professional medical service to you because of your persistent refusal to follow my medical advice and treatment.

Since your condition requires medical attention, I suggest that you place yourself under the care of another physician without delay. If you so desire, I shall be available to attend you for a reasonable time after you have received this letter, but in no event later than January 7, 20--. This should give you sufficient time to select a physician from the many competent practitioners in this area.

You may be assured that, upon receiving your written request, I will make available to the physician of your choice your case history and information regarding the diagnosis and treatment which you have received from me.

Very truly yours,

Mark Woo

Mark Woo, MD
MW:kr

Figure 7-4   Letter notifying patient of physician's withdrawal as attending physician.

The Patient No Longer Needs Treatment.
Unless a formal discharge or withdrawal has occurred, a physician is obligated to care for a patient until the patient's condition no longer requires treatment.

STANDARD OF CARE AND THE 4 DS OF NEGLIGENCE

Physicians, medical assistants, and all health care providers have the responsibility and duty to perform within their scope of training and to always do what any reasonable and prudent health care professional in the same specialty or general field of practice would do. That is what is expected of every physician when a contact is made by a patient. Failure to do what any reasonable and prudent health care professional would do in the same set of circumstances can be seen as a breach of the standard of care.

Negligence is defined as the failure to exercise the standard of care that a reasonable person would exercise in similar circumstances. Negligence occurs when someone suffers injury because of another's failure to live up to a required duty of care. This is a primary cause of malpractice suits. **Malpractice** is professional negligence. The four elements of negligence, sometimes called the 4 Ds, are:

1. Duty: duty of care
2. Derelict: breach of the duty of care
3. Direct cause: a legally recognizable injury occurs as a result of the breach of duty of care
4. Damage: wrongful activity must have caused the injury or harm that occurred

If an individual has knowledge, skill, or intelligence superior to that of a layperson, that individual's conduct must be consistent with that status. Medical assistants are held to a high standard of care by virtue of their skills, knowledge, and intelligence. As professionals, medical assistants are required to have a standard minimum level of special knowledge and ability. This is what is known as duty of care.

Physicians and members of their staff may be called to testify in court to the standard of care. In such a case, they are usually considered **expert witnesses**. An expert witness is one who has knowledge and experience enough in a field to be able to testify to what is the reasonable and expected standard of care. Expert witnesses are expected to tell what they know to be fact and are best counseled to use lay terms rather than complicated medical language. The goal is for jurors and judges to understand the nature of any medical information shared. Visual aids, charts, and computer simulations are often used to illustrate or clarify testimony given by expert witnesses.

TORTS

A **tort** is a wrongful act that results in injury to one person by another. Medical assistants may commit a tort that may result in **litigation**. If it can be proven that the injury resulted from the medical assistant (or other health care professional) not meeting the standard of care governing their respective professions, then litigation is a possibility. If, however, the medical assistant (or other health care professional) commits a wrongful act but the patient suffers no injury or harm, then no tort exists. If, for example, the medical assistant changes a wound dressing, breaks sterile technique, and the patient suffers a severely infected wound, the medical assistant has committed a tort and can be held liable, and legal action can be taken. On the other hand, if the medical assistant changes a wound dressing, breaks sterile technique, and the patient's wound does not become infected, no harm has been suffered, and a tort does not exist. If a medical assistant fails to report to the physician a negative result on a blood test that causes the physician to fail to make an early diagnosis of a disease, the assistant's omission of an act has caused a breach in the standard of care.

There are two major classifications of torts, intentional and negligent. Intentional torts are deliberate acts of violation of another's rights. Negligent torts are not deliberate and are the result of omission and commission of an act. Malpractice is the unintentional tort of professional negligence; that is, a professional either failed to act in a reasonable and prudent manner and caused harm to the patient or did what a reasonable and prudent person would not have done and caused harm to a patient.

There are two Latin terms that can be used to describe aspects of negligence. These are known as **doctrines**. *Res ipsa loquitur*, or "the thing speaks for itself," is the term used in cases that involve situations such as a nick made in the bladder when the surgeon is performing a hysterectomy. The negligence is obvious. The other doctrine, *respondeat superior*, "let the master answer," expresses that physicians are responsible for their employees' actions. If a medical assistant violates the standard of care, therein lies the basis for a suit of medical malpractice. For example, the medical assistant used the incorrect solution to clean the patient's wound and the patient sustained injuries to the wound. The physician-employer can be sued under the doctrine of *respondeat superior* because the physician-employer is responsible for the acts of employees committed in the scope of their employment. The medical assistant also can be sued because individuals are responsible for their own actions.

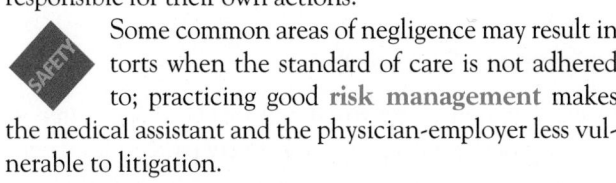 Some common areas of negligence may result in torts when the standard of care is not adhered to; practicing good **risk management** makes the medical assistant and the physician-employer less vulnerable to litigation.

- Protect patients from falling from an examination table, wheelchair, or stretcher.

- Check for faulty electrocautery. Have repair done by qualified technicians.

- Check patient identification by correctly identifying patient before performing a procedure or administering a medication.

- Never leave a patient unattended. If you must leave, pass the responsibility for the patient's care on to another individual.

- Be particularly watchful with patients who have special needs such as the elderly, pediatric patients, and those with physical and emotional disabilities.

SPOTLIGHT ON AAMA ESSENTIALS THROUGH CAAHEP

- Looking at a neighbor's medical record out of curiosity, and not as part of your responsibility as a medical assistant, is not against the law, but it is unethical.

- Practicing good risk management, such as protecting patients from falling, checking identification, and never leaving a patient unattended, makes the medical assistant less vulnerable to litigation.

- A healthy relationship between the medical assistant and the patient, as well as respect for one another's rights, lowers the potential for the likelihood of a lawsuit.

- Properly label and identify all specimens. Handle specimens properly.

- Make certain the patient has signed a consent for surgery and other care.

- Follow all policies and procedures established by your employer.

- Do not misrepresent your qualifications.

- Document fully only facts and do not alter medical records.

- Admit any error that may have occurred.

Some specific examples of common torts that can occur in the office or clinic are battery, defamation of character, and invasion of privacy.

Battery

The basis of the tort of battery is unprivileged touching of one person by another. A patient must consent to being touched. When a procedure is to be performed on a patient, the patient must give consent in full knowledge of all the facts. It does not matter whether the procedure that constitutes the battery improves the patient's health. Patients have the right to withdraw consent at any time.

One example of battery is when a medical assistant insists on giving the patient an injection the physician ordered for the patient even though the patient refuses the injection. Another example can be seen when a physician performs additional surgery beyond the original procedure (the surgeon performed a hysterectomy for which consent was given, but is liable for battery for removing an abdominal nevus from the patient's abdomen without consent). It does not matter that the physician does not charge for the additional procedure. It also does not matter if the patient would have given consent if asked in advance.

Defamation of Character

The tort of defamation of character consists of injury to another person's reputation, name, or character through spoken or written words for which damages can be recovered. Two kinds of defamation are libel and slander. Libel is false and malicious writing about another such as in published materials, pictures, and media. An example can be seen when the medical assistant writes in the patient's record, "Mr. O'Keefe's wife appears to be the cause of his ulcer." A copy of Mr. O'Keefe's records were later sent to a new physician who reviewed the record and saw the remarks quoted by the medical assistant.

Slander is false and malicious spoken words. Slander can be seen in the following comment directed by a patient toward the physician, "Dr. Woo is incompetent. He should have his license revoked." The statement is overheard by the office receptionist and other patients waiting in the reception area.

In order for a tort of defamation of character (either libel or slander) to exist, a third party must see or hear the words and understand their meaning.

Invasion of Privacy

Invasion of privacy is another kind of tort. It includes unauthorized publicity of patient information, medical records being released without the patient's knowledge and permission, and patients receiving unwanted publicity and exposure to public view. For example, if a minor unmarried girl has been examined for possible pregnancy, and the medical assistant telephones the laboratory report to the girl's home and inadvertently gives the results to someone other than the patient, her privacy has been invaded. A second situation exists when persons other than those providing care and performing examinations and procedures (essential or nonessential personnel) are allowed to be present without the patient's consent. Yet another example of the patient's right to privacy being violated is when the patient is asked to walk from the examination room across the hall to a treatment room while wearing only a patient gown in full view of other patients and personnel.

Medical assistants and other health care professionals should:

- Close a door, pull a curtain, or provide a screen when looking at, handling, or examining the patient's body
- Expose only body parts necessary for treatment (drape the patient's body, exposing only that part which is being treated)
- Discuss patients with no one except those individuals involved in the patient's care and then discuss only those aspects that relate to the needs of the patient for care

It is not an invasion of privacy to disclose information required by a court order (subpoena) or by statute to protect the public health and welfare, as in the reporting of violent crime.

MEDICAL RECORDS

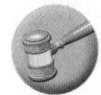

A major responsibility of the physician and the medical assistant is to maintain an accurate and up-to-date record of the patient's care. Whatever style of record is used, the credibility of the medical record will be a key factor in any litigation.

All matters related to a patient's care must be charted, and these charts must be an accurate reflection of actual care rendered and charges made. An act not recorded is generally considered an act not done. Charts that are incomplete or illegible are not easily defensible. Necessary corrections should be made by drawing one line through the error and placing the correction above it with the person's initials and date. All entries should be properly signed and dated, also. Consistency in the medical records becomes a powerful defense for the physician.

Informed Consent

Documentation of informed consent becomes an important part of the medical records. Every patient has a right to know and understand any procedure to be performed. The patient is to be told in language easily understood:

1. The nature of any procedure and how it is to be performed
2. Any possible risks involved as well as expected outcomes of the procedure
3. Any other methods of treatment and those risks
4. Risks if no treatment is given

It is the responsibility of the health care provider to make certain the patient understands. If an interpreter is necessary, the physician must procure one.

Often, consent forms will be signed if there is to be a surgical or invasive procedure performed (Figure 7-5). The medical assistant may be asked to witness the patient's

---

CONSENT FOR TREATMENT

Date _____ Time _____

 I authorize the performance of the following procedure(s) _____ on _____ (name of patient) _____ to be performed by _____ (name of physician) _____, MD.

 The following have been explained to _____ by Dr. _____ (name physician) _____.

 Nature of the procedure _____ (describe procedure) _____.

 For the purpose of _____ _____.

 The possible alternative methods of treatment are _____.

 The possible consequences of the procedure are _____.

 The risks involve the possibility of _____ _____.

 The possible complications of this procedure are _____.

 I have been advised of the serious nature of this procedure and have been further advised that if I desire a more detailed explanation of any of the foregoing or further information about the possible risks or complications, it will be given to me.

 I do not request a more detailed listing and explanation of the above information.

 Signed _____
 (Patient/Parent/Guardian)
Witnessed by: _____

Figure 7-5 Model formal consent for treatment form.

signature and may be expected to follow through on any of the physician's instructions or explanations but is not expected to explain the procedure to the patient. The signed consent form is kept in the medical chart and a copy is also given to the patient.

Implied Consent

Two circumstances related to consent are worth mentioning at this point. **Implied consent** occurs when there is a life-threatening emergency or the patient is unconscious or unable to respond. The physician, by law, is allowed to give treatment without a signed consent. Implied consent

occurs in more subtle ways, also. The patient who rolls up a shirt sleeve for the medical assistant to take a blood pressure reading is implying consent to the procedure by the action taken.

Consent and Legal Incompetence

Consent for treatment is not valid if the patient is legally incompetent to give consent. Legal **incompetence** means that a patient is found by a court to be insane, inadequate, or to not be an adult. In such instances, consent must be obtained from a parent, a legal guardian, or the court on behalf of the patient. Consent for treatment may be given only by the natural parent or legal guardian as determined by the court for a **minor** child, typically defined as one under eighteen years of age or the age of majority. An **emancipated minor** is one considered by the courts to be an adult. Emancipated minors may be defined as persons living on their own, who are self-supporting, who may be married, or who are in the military. They can legally give consent for treatment.

 Consent problems may arise when providing care to minors. Consent for medical care such as treatment of sexually transmitted diseases, pregnancy, alcohol or drug abuse, abortion, or birth control pose special problems. Some states allow minors to give their consent in these special situations.

 Questions of ability to give consent related to minors and emancipated minors often must be determined on a case-by-case basis because state statutes vary. Placing a telephone call to the state attorney general's office can help clarify issues, questions, and concerns that involve consent and treatment of minors.

Subpoenas

The medical records may be subpoenaed and/or the physician and health care provider (*subpoena duces tecum*) may be subpoenaed to testify in court. The subpoena is a court order naming a specific date, time, and reason to appear. The staff in the ambulatory care setting usually will have ample time to make certain the record is current and complete prior to its inclusion in court. Out of courtesy, the physician will notify patients whose records have been subpoenaed. If, for any reason, the patient does not want the record released, the physician must call for legal advice on how to respond to the subpoena.

 Certain records, because of their sensitive nature, may require more than a subpoena to be released. These include records related to sexually transmitted diseases, including AIDS and HIV testing, mental health records, substance abuse records, and sexual assault records. For the courts to have access to these records, a court order is required in some states.

Confidentiality

The care taken with subpoenas and court orders for certain information is to assure patients of confidentiality. The information in the medical record, including the information a patient shared with the physician and medical assistant, is private.

No patient information can be given to another (another physician, patient's attorney, insurance company, federal or state agency) without the expressed written consent of the patient. Care must be exercised at all times to ensure that the patient's right to confidentiality is not breached. For example, information given to unauthorized personnel associated with the physician's or clinic's practice in regard to the patient's condition or financial status regarding payment of bills violates the patient's right to confidentiality. Likewise, when discussing issues over the telephone that can be overheard—such as the patient's account being turned over to a collection agency—the patient's right to confidentiality has been violated.

There are certain disclosures of information about a patient's conditions and suspected illnesses that are required by law. Legally required disclosures are necessary when the public needs to know certain information for its safety and welfare. The disclosures supersede the patient's right to privacy and confidentiality. See "Public Duties" in this chapter.

Statute of Limitations

No discussion of medical records is complete without a brief statement regarding the statute of limitations which will, in part, determine how long medical records are kept. Generally speaking, all records should be retained until after the statute has run, usually three to six years. Statutes of limitations most commonly begin at the time a negligent act was committed, when the act was discovered, or when the care of the patient and the patient-physician relationship ended. It is easy to understand why many physicians choose to keep their records indefinitely.

State and federal statutes set maximum time periods during which certain actions can be brought or rights enforced; there is a time limit for individuals to initiate legal action. The statute of limitations varies from one jurisdiction to another and a lawsuit may not be brought after the statute of limitations has run. For example, in the Commonwealth of Massachusetts, the statute of limitations for an act of medical malpractice committed on an adult is three years. If harm to a patient resulted from a medical assistant administering the wrong dose of medication to a patient in Massachusetts, a lawsuit must be brought within three years from the time the medication error was made, with the three years commencing at the time the negligent act was committed.

PUBLIC DUTIES

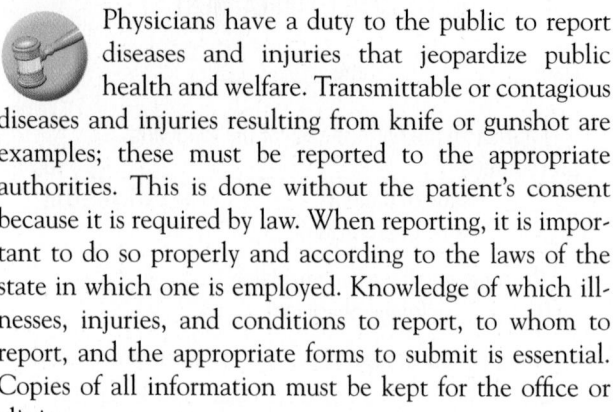 Physicians have a duty to the public to report diseases and injuries that jeopardize public health and welfare. Transmittable or contagious diseases and injuries resulting from knife or gunshot are examples; these must be reported to the appropriate authorities. This is done without the patient's consent because it is required by law. When reporting, it is important to do so properly and according to the laws of the state in which one is employed. Knowledge of which illnesses, injuries, and conditions to report, to whom to report, and the appropriate forms to submit is essential. Copies of all information must be kept for the office or clinic.

Other generally required reportables include: births, deaths, childhood immunizations, rape, and abuse toward a child, elder, or domestic partner.

Some states have laws specific to the release of information relative to mental or psychological treatment, human immunodeficiency virus testing, acquired immunodeficiency syndrome diagnosis and treatment, sexually transmitted diseases, and chemical substance abuse.

Local or state health departments can provide lists of diseases and injuries to report and will also provide the appropriate forms.

Drug Screening

States vary in the laws they have regarding the abuse of alcohol and other drugs. In general, employers are allowed to screen an employee for chemical substances if they believe the employee's work performance is being affected by the abuse.

Great controversy surrounds preemployment and random screening for drugs in the workplace. Some states allow widespread random testing of employees. It is important that the worker's right to privacy not be violated. A tort of defamation of character could be claimed against an employer if the results of the testing become known to others.

Get the patient's written consent when asked to collect a specimen for drug screening. Be certain the laboratory that performs the screening is qualified to perform the test. The possibility of liability is great if the ambulatory care setting does not have specific policies and procedures to employ in regard to specimen collection and testing. It should be carefully documented on the patient's record which medical personnel are responsible for the specimen from the time it was collected until the results are known.

The release of patients' records that pertain to chemical substance abuse is protected by federal laws under the Federal Drug Abuse Prevention, Treatment, and Rehabilitation Act. The law prohibits disclosure of information that identifies the patient as a chemical substance abuser. Also, information about the patient's treatment cannot be divulged without the patient's written consent. The records can, however, be released by order of a subpoena to another health care professional during an emergency situation or if the records are to be used for research and program evaluation.

AIDS

The Americans with Disabilities Act of 1990 (ADA) offers protection to persons with AIDS or diseases associated with AIDS. Controversy surrounds the mandatory testing for human immunodeficiency virus (HIV) in medical assistants and other health care professionals and the release of the results to patients who say they have the right to know the HIV status of their caregivers. Health care professionals insist on their right to privacy.

Patients also insist on their privacy. A written informed consent form specific to HIV testing is signed by the patient prior to testing. Laws regarding HIV and AIDS vary from state to state. The best approach regarding release of information regarding the HIV status of a patient is never to disclose this or any confidential patient information.

Abuse

Child abuse, elder abuse, and domestic violence are becoming more common in our society and as a result, patients suffering such abuse may be seen in the ambulatory care setting. In all cases of abuse, medical records hold valuable information if a court procedure ensues. Careful documentation is critical. State laws are fairly specific in mandates to report child abuse, but laws related to elder abuse and domestic violence are not so detailed. In any case, the rights of the victim must be protected.

Child Abuse. The law **mandates**, or requires, that physicians and health care professionals, teachers, social workers, and certain others who suspect child abuse report the incident to the proper authorities. Confidentiality in the physician-patient relationship does not exist when parents abuse children. If a person has a reason to suspect abuse and reports the abuse to the police and in the case of child abuse to the child protective agency, this individual is protected against liability as a result of making the report. Failure to report could result in criminal or civil penalties. Usually, the Child Protective Unit of the State Department of Social Services is called in to investigate suspected cases of child abuse. Some injuries that are commonly seen in child abuse are bruises, welts, burns, fractures, and head injuries.

If a suspicion of abuse exists, the physician and health care professional should:

- Treat the child's injuries
- Send the child to the hospital for further treatment when necessary
- Inform parents of the diagnosis and that it will be reported to the police and social services agency
- Notify the child protective agency (keep phone number posted)
- Document all information
- Provide court testimony if requested

Elder Abuse. Elder abuse may consist of neglect, physical abuse, punishment, physical restraint, or abandonment. Examples are seen when elders are overmedicated or undermedicated, physically restrained, intimidated by shouting or profanity, sexually abused, neglected or abandoned, or in any other way have their rights and dignity violated. The person reporting the abuse is generally a health care professional, and the reporting agency is most likely one of a social service or welfare nature.

Domestic Violence. Incidents of spousal abuse have escalated since the 1970s. The battered women's syndrome is recognized as a significant problem. The violence of it is a criminal act and failure to report it may be considered a misdemeanor in some states. Victims of domestic violence should be treated as soon as possible after the assault so as to preserve evidence for legal purposes. Community agencies such as rape hot lines are available and the physician may refer the patient for additional services.

GOOD SAMARITAN LAW

Most states have laws regarding the rendering of first aid by health care professionals at the scene of an accident or sudden injury. Good Samaritan laws, although not always clearly written, encourage physicians and health care professionals to provide medical care within the scope of their training without fear of being sued for negligence. In an emergency situation, medical assistants cannot be held liable should an injury result from some form of first aid rendered or from first aid they omitted to render as long as they acted in a reasonable way within the scope of their knowledge. Medical assistants and other health care professionals with skills in cardiopulmonary resuscitation (CPR) who are present when CPR is needed must perform the procedure on the victim or otherwise could be declared negligent. Emergencies that arise in the ambulatory care setting generally are not covered by Good Samaritan laws.

PHYSICIAN'S DIRECTIVES

Medical assistants in the ambulatory care setting will be asked to attach physicians' directives or living wills to patients' charts (Figure 7-6). These directives are legal documents in which patients indicate their wishes in the case of a life-threatening illness or serious injury. Such documents should always accompany the patients to the hospital for any treatment or care. They may be updated from time to time, and the patient can ask to rescind such a document at any time. Medical assistants must remember that these documents reflect the choices of their patients and are to be respected as such.

Another document often seen in the ambulatory care setting is the **durable power of attorney** for health care or Designation of Health Care Surrogate (Figure 7-7). These documents allow a patient to name another person who is appointed as the official spokesperson for the patient should the patient be unable to speak for herself. The documents may allow another person to manage finances and personal matters or just to make medical decisions. These documents should be recognized and honored.

Every state has different versions of the Living Will and Designation of Health Care Surrogate forms as well as requirements for filling them out. To assure the correct language is used, these forms should be prepared either by an attorney familiar with your state requirements, or by contacting Partnership for Caring, 1035 30th Street NW, Washington, DC 20007, 800-989-9455.

AMERICANS WITH DISABILITIES ACT (ADA)

The federal government established new laws in 1990 to protect physically challenged persons. Barrier-free accommodations are required in public and commercial facilities. The ADA law applies to businesses with at least fifteen employees, but some states have more stringent laws.

Figure 7-6   Living will declaration. Choice In Dying makes available legally recognized document forms to residents of states that have enacted right-to-die laws. For people in states that have not enacted right-to-die laws, Choice In Dying provides statutory advance directives for each state free of charge, as well as other materials and services relating to end-of-life medical care. (Reprinted by permission of Choice in Dying, 200 Varick Street, New York, NY 10014, 212-366-5540)

FLORIDA LIVING WILL

INSTRUCTIONS

PRINT THE DATE

PRINT YOUR NAME

Declaration made this _____ day of _____, _____,
(day)   (month)   (year)
I, _____, willfully
and voluntarily make known my desire that my dying not be artificially
prolonged under the circumstances set forth below, and I do hereby
declare that:

PLEASE INITIAL EACH THAT APPLIES

If at any time I am incapacitated and
_____ I have a terminal condition, or
_____ I have an end-stage condition, or
_____ I am in a persistent vegetative state

and if my attending or treating physician and another consulting
physician have determined that there is no reasonable medical
probability of my recovery from such condition, I direct that life-
prolonging procedures be withheld or withdrawn when the application of
such procedures would serve only to prolong artificially the process of
dying, and that I be permitted to die naturally with only the
administration of medication or the performance of any medical
procedure deemed necessary to provide me with comfort care or to
alleviate pain.

It is my intention that this declaration be honored by my family and
physician as the final expression of my legal right to refuse medical or
surgical treatment and to accept the consequences for such refusal.

In the event that I have been determined to be unable to provide express
and informed consent regarding the withholding, withdrawal, or
continuation of life-prolonging procedures, I wish to designate, as my
surrogate to carry out the provisions of this declaration:

PRINT THE NAME, HOME ADDRESS AND TELEPHONE NUMBER OF YOUR SURROGATE

Name: _____
Address: _____
_____ Zip Code: _____
Phone: _____

© 2000
PARTNERSHIP FOR CARING, INC.

FLORIDA LIVING WILL — PAGE 2 OF 2

I wish to designate the following person as my alternate surrogate, to
carry out the provisions of this declaration should my surrogate be
unwilling or unable to act on my behalf:

PRINT NAME, HOME ADDRESS AND TELEPHONE NUMBER OF YOUR ALTERNATE SURROGATE

Name: _____
Address: _____
_____ Zip Code: _____
Phone: _____

ADD PERSONAL INSTRUCTIONS (IF ANY)

Additional instructions (optional):

I understand the full import of this declaration, and I am emotionally
and mentally competent to make this declaration.

SIGN THE DOCUMENT

Signed: _____

WITNESSING PROCEDURE

Witness 1:
    Signed: _____
    Address: _____

TWO WITNESSES MUST SIGN AND PRINT THEIR ADDRESSES

Witness 2:
    Signed: _____
    Address: _____

© 2000
PARTNERSHIP FOR CARING, INC.

Courtesy of **Partnership for Caring, Inc.**   6/00
1035 30th Street, NW Washington, DC 20007 800-989-9455

Figure 7-7 Health care surrogate form. (Reprinted by permission of Choice in Dying, 200 Varick Street, New York, NY 10014, 212-366-5540)

The ADA allows preemployment physical examinations only after an individual has been offered employment. Medical records of these persons are kept confidential and separate and accessible only to persons who must know what restrictions the patient may bring to a job. Job qualifications and the specific standards for employment must be the same for all applicants. Disabled persons cannot be screened using different standards for employment.

Former drug users and those who are being rehabilitated also are covered by the ADA and cannot be denied employment because of their past history of drug use.

Employers are required to post notices regarding employee and applicant rights and obligations.

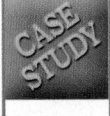

CASE STUDY 7-1

Three weeks ago, Dr. King treated a new patient, Boris Bolski, for lower back pain, which the patient felt was the result of consistent heavy lifting at his job. Medical assistant Joe Guerrero assisted Dr. King during the examination and, today, both Joe and Dr. King were served with subpoenas by Mr. Bolski's attorney. Mr. Bolski is alleging that unsafe conditions at his workplace caused severe strain on his back and he is suing his employer for damages. Dr. King and Joe Guerrero were called as expert witnesses to a civil hearing; Joe, especially, is a bit nervous about this, as he has never been on the witness stand in court and is not sure what is expected of him.

CASE STUDY REVIEW

1. How will Mr. Bolski's medical record help Joe answer questions at the hearing?

2. What information should Joe gather in order to be prepared to testify?

3. As an expert witness, what is Joe expected to communicate to the judge in this case?

SUMMARY

Changing societal values have contributed to an explosion of lawsuits in medical practice. Patients are more aware than ever of their rights, especially those of confidentiality and the right to privacy, consent, and records ownership. They readily seek redress when they perceive their rights to be violated.

A healthy relationship between physicians and patients and between medical assistants and patients, as well as respect for the patient's rights, lowers the likelihood of a lawsuit.

Knowledge of the laws that regulate medical and business practices in your state is necessary in order to be in compliance. Sources of information regarding state and federal laws can be obtained from the state medical society, the physician's liability insurance company, the state medical assistant society, the state attorney general's office, or the public library.

REVIEW QUESTIONS

Multiple Choice

1. The type of contract that most often exists between physician and patient is:
   a. expressed
   b. implied
   c. privileged
   d. civil
2. Which of the following claims of negligence would fit into the category of *res ipsa loquitur*?
   a. improper use of X-ray equipment
   b. failure to use X-ray equipment
   c. incorrect administration of anesthesia
   d. discovery of a surgical instrument inside the patient's body
3. Slander is defamation through:
   a. spoken statements that damage an individual's reputation
   b. written statements that damage a person's reputation
   c. written falsehoods about an individual
   d. a, b, and c
4. Occasionally, a physician will be sued for the negligence of a partner or employee, even though the physician is not guilty of any negligent act. This is done on the basis of the doctrine of:
   a. *res ipsa loquitur*
   b. *respondeat superior*
   c. proximate cause
   d. contract law
5. The standard of care expected of a physician is held by the courts to mean:
   a. on a par with all other physicians engaged in the same medical specialty anywhere
   b. reasonable, attentive, diligent care comparable to other physicians of the same specialty in the same or similar community

   c. the best possible under the circumstances
   d. the same as the national norm
6. Physician's directives:
   a. allow patients to direct how their billing is to be handled
   b. are designed to encourage physicians to render first aid in an emergency
   c. direct physicians based on a patient's wishes in life-threatening circumstances
   d. are not considered legal documents
7. A subpoena:
   a. is a court order requesting data and/or an appearance in court
   b. is sufficient to enforce a release of any type medical record or information
   c. may be ignored without consequences
   d. allows the person being served to select a specific date or time to appear
8. The 4 Ds of negligence are:
   a. duty, danger, damage, and disaster
   b. derelict, direct cause, damage, and danger
   c. danger, direct cause, damage, disaster
   d. duty, derelict, direct cause, damage
9. Emancipated minors:
   a. are considered adults and can consent to treatment
   b. live on their own and are self-supporting
   c. may be married or serve in the military
   d. all of the above
   e. only b and c
10. Torts:
    a. include battery, defamation of character, invasion of privacy
    b. are always intentional in nature
    c. do not require that harm has occurred
    d. do not include malpractice

Critical Thinking

1. Chris is a six-year-old girl whom Dr. King has seen for a broken leg. Chris' parents fail to follow Dr. King's treatment plan for Chris. What, if any, action can Dr. King take? What is the legal term for this situation?

2. Audrey, the medical assistant at Lewis & King MD, has accidentally used an incorrect solution to irrigate a patient's eyes. The patient suffers injuries to both eyes. Can Audrey's error be considered malpractice? Explain your reason.

3. Explain the standard of care as it applies to medical assistants. Give an example.

4. Jaime arrived in the clinic having sustained a serious laceration at his construction site. Dr. Woo ordered Demerol R 100 mg. 1.m - stat which Wanda, the medical assistant, administers. Dr. Woo determines surgery is required. Should a consent form be prepared? If so, by whom, and what should be included?

5. Give two examples of routine office or clinic procedures that might constitute violation of the patient's right to privacy.

6. Discuss the federal law regarding HIV testing, AIDS, and drug screening.

7. What are public duties? Discuss the physician's and medical assistant's obligations in regard to public duties.

8. What is the Good Samaritan Law? What must a medical assistant and any other health care professional remember when giving first aid at the scene of an accident?

9. Describe three types of abuse. Tell what your role and responsibilities are as a medical assistant when Juanita brings her son Henry into the clinic. Henry appears to have bruises on his face and chest.

10. Lenore McDonnell, who uses a wheelchair, has applied for employment in a large bookstore in town. She has not yet been offered the job. She has an appointment today for a preemployment physical examination and tells Audrey, the medical assistant, that the bookstore wants a copy of the results of Dr. Lewis' findings. Discuss the situation in light of the Americans with Disabilities Act.

WEB ACTIVITIES

Research the World Wide Web for the statute of limitations related to claims injuries. What is the time span in your state?

REFERENCES/BIBLIOGRAPHY

Cowdrey, M., & Drew, M. (1995). *Basic law for the allied health professions* (2nd ed.). Sudbury, MA: Jones and Bartlett.

Flight, M. (1998). *Law, liability, and ethics for medical office professionals* (3rd ed.). Albany, NY: Delmar.

Lewis, M. A., & Tamparo, C. D. (1998). *Medical law, ethics, and bioethics for ambulatory care* (4th ed.). Philadelphia: F. A. Davis Company.

McWay, D. A. (1997). *Legal aspects of health information management*. Albany, NY: Delmar.

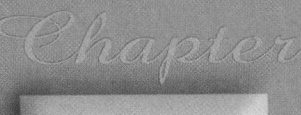
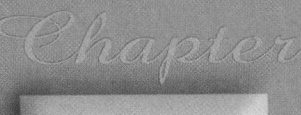

ETHICAL CONSIDERATIONS

KEY TERMS

Bioethics
Ethics
Genetic Engineering
Surrogate

OUTLINE

Ethics Defined
Bioethics Defined
Keys to the AAMA Code of Ethics
AMA Ethical Guidelines
  Advertising
  Media Relations
  Confidentiality
  Medical Records
  Professional Fees and Charges
  Professional Rights and Responsi-
    bilities
  Abuse

Bioethical Dilemmas
  Allocation of Scarce Medical
    Resources
  Abortion and Fetal Tissue
    Research
  Genetic Engineering/Manipula-
    tion
  Artificial Insemination/Surrogacy
  Dying and Death
  HIV and AIDS

OBJECTIVES

The student should strive to meet the following performance objectives and demonstrate an understanding of the facts and principles presented in this chapter through written and oral communication.

1. Define the key terms as presented in the glossary.

2. Identify the two prominent Codes of Ethics.

3. Compare/contrast the AAMA and the AMA Codes of Ethics.

4. Recall the five principles of the AAMA Code of Medical Ethics.

5. Relate the five principles of the AAMA code to patient care in the ambulatory care setting.

6. Recall the seven principles or standards of conduct adopted by the AMA.

7. Discuss the guidelines identified in at least six ethical issues presented by the *Current Opinions of the Council on Ethical and Judicial Affairs of the AMA.*

8. Restate the dilemmas encountered by the following bioethical issues: (a) allocation of scarce medical resources; (b) abortion and fetal tissue research; (c) genetic engineering/manipulation; (d) artificial insemination/surrogacy; (e) dying and death.

**GENERAL
(TRANSDISCIPLINARY)**

Professionalism

- ● **Adhere to ethical principles**
- ● **Promote the CMA credential**

Legal Concepts

- ● **Maintain confidentiality**
- ● **Prepare and maintain medical records**
- ● **Use appropriate guidelines when releasing information**

On occasion, ethical dilemmas occur because patients are unsure of the role of the medical assistant. For example, the medical assistants of Inner City Health Care are truly multidisciplinary and have a range of administrative and clinical skills. However, patients sometimes think of them as nurses who have an entirely different set of skills. While most of the medical assistants gently correct patients and make it a point to practice only within their area of expertise, occasionally newer members of the medical assistant staff may feel more "important" when patients regard them as nurses or physicians' assistants.

A few weeks ago, medical assistant Liz Corbin, who is in her early twenties, was taken aback when Walter Seals, the office manager, spoke up about Liz's tendency to let patients assume she was a nurse. While Liz never deliberately intended to mislead patients, she never corrected them about their misconceptions. Walter pointed out that to present a good example of the medical assisting profession, Liz should gently but firmly help patients understand that she was a medical assistant with a specific range of skills that complemented, but did not substitute for, nursing skills.

INTRODUCTION

It is impossible in today's world to function as a medical assistant without an awareness of the impact of ethics and bioethics on health care. Just as an understanding of the law and working within the law is vital information for the medical assistant, it is equally important to understand ethics and bioethics.

From the previous chapter, you have come to realize that there are many circumstances and situations that occur in health care that are guided and directed by state and federal laws. You, personally, are expected to be above reproach in all your actions in this regard. You must also work with your employer and other members of the health care team to assure that each member of the staff functions within the law—protecting both patients and providers.

Ethics plays a huge role in such an endeavor. To function ethically demands that you never function outside the law. Ethics, however, demands something more—ethics calls for honesty, trustworthiness, integrity, confidentiality, and fairness. To function ethically, you must know yourself well and understand weaknesses and any vulnerabilities that might prevent you from acting ethically.

The scenario described above is just one situation in which medical assistants may need to reflect on their actions and be sure that they are acting ethically and within the range of their skills. Medical assistants also need to recognize the warning signs that they, or some other staff member, may be about to breach a code of ethics. Often, this kind of breach occurs when one has, or seeks to have, too much power; when one attempts to take too much authority; and when one has too little knowledge and experience. When a breach seems about to occur, the individuals involved should be encouraged to step back and review their actions and the likely consequences of those actions.

ETHICS DEFINED

Traditionally, **ethics** has been defined in terms of what is right or wrong. For health care professionals, ethics is often defined by a code or creed as seen in the Code of Ethics from the American Association of Medical Assistants (AAMA) or the Principles of Medical Ethics from the American Medical Association (AMA). While these codes, and many others like them, are essential and very helpful, they lose their vitality unless they are understood by individuals who possess a personal and sound moral code or set of values.

Unlike the law, which seldom changes unless challenged and examined in the courts, codes of ethics constantly change and evolve just as personal values and morals change and evolve. Every time values are challenged and examined, a medical assistant's personal ethical codes become stronger, the understanding of others' perceptions becomes clearer, and professionalism is enhanced.

BIOETHICS DEFINED

Bioethics brings the entire focus of ethics into the field of health care and into those ethical issues dealing with life. Never before in the history of medical care has bioethics been such a topic of concern. In the past, most bioethical decisions were made by physicians and esteemed members of the medical and/or legal profession. However, advancing technology giving patients and consumers numerous choices regarding their health care causes each one of us to take an active role in bioethics.

Medical assistants will encounter ethical and bioethical issues across the lifespan. In Figure 8-1, a few issues are identified for contemplation and discussion. Issues of bioethics common to every medical office are the allocation of scarce medical resources, abortion and fetal tissue research, genetic engineering or manipulation, and the many choices surrounding life, dying, and death.

For medical assistants to fully comprehend a discussion of ethics and bioethics, they must be familiar with the Code of Ethics of AAMA (Figure 8-2) and the AMA's Principles of Medical Ethics (Figure 8-3).

A FEW ISSUES FOR CONTEMPLATION AND DISCUSSION

Infants

- In premature, deformed, or severely disabled infants, ethical issues include the decision to provide or withhold treatment. Health care professionals and parents are not always in agreement. Central to this issue, also, is the expense involved in certain treatments and deciding who pays the cost of treatment.
- Vulnerability of infants can lead to issues of negligence, abuse, or rejection. Parents are also vulnerable because they may be unable to cope with the needs of the entire family.

Children

- Children who are ill-fed, housed, educated, and clothed exhibit great needs for preventive, curative, and rehabilitative health care.
- Minors with sexually transmitted diseases can seek treatment without the parents' knowledge. Treatment also must be offered without parental consent to pregnant, infected, or addicted minors.
- Child abuse presents an ethical dilemma, especially when a child confides physical, sexual, or emotional abuse to a health care worker but does not want the information divulged. Health care professionals, as mandated reporters, must report suspected child abuse. Will the child/patient view this as a violation of confidence or suffer dire consequences as a result of the reported abuse?

Adolescents

- Adolescents as young as 13 to 18 years old may seek abortion without parental knowledge or consent. Is this a violation of parents' right to medical information regarding their children? Or should the adolescent, fearful of parental reaction, have the right to decide?
- The adolescent's growing autonomy, need for independence, changing values, and desire for peer acceptance lead to a number of ethical issues that may involve the health care environment. These include the adolescent's decision to be sexually active, to use birth control, to protect against sexually transmitted diseases, and to use drugs and/or alcohol.

Adults

- Many low-income women do not have sufficient access to prenatal care, which has proven to be a cost-saving medical measure that is critical to the health of both mother and infant.
- As employers seek to reduce the cost of health insurance benefit programs, many individuals and families are finding themselves shifted from one insurance program to another, leaving them with little or no continuity of care. Also, in some managed care programs, adults may receive medical services from a number of health care professionals with whom they have no opportunity to establish an ongoing physician-patient relationship.
- Even with a physician's directive or a living will, a dying patient's wishes may not be followed. Technological advances in medicine have created a situation where patients may not be able to exercise a choice in the death issue.

Senior Adults

- Dementia is a common problem that is physically and financially exhausting for the caregiver, who is usually a spouse or adult child. How do caregivers cope with their own needs and the needs of dependent adults? Often, the elderly may reject nursing home placement, and there may be limited funds for such long-term care.
- Elderly patients have the right to maintain dignity and privacy, but their dependency on others may deprive them of these basic rights.
- Physician-assisted suicide for terminally ill patients is a prominent issue in our society, especially when elderly patients sense a total loss of dignity.

Figure 8-1 Ethical issues across the lifespan. (Compiled by Carol Tamparo, CMA-A, PhD, and Marilyn Pooler, RN, CMA-C, MEd)

AAMA CODE OF ETHICS

The Code of Ethics of AAMA shall set forth principles of ethical and moral conduct as they relate to the medical profession and the particular practice of medical assisting.

Members of AAMA dedicated to the conscientious pursuit of their profession, and thus desiring to merit the high regard of the entire medical profession and the respect of the general public which they serve, do pledge themselves to strive always to:

A. render service with full respect for the dignity of humanity;
B. respect confidential information obtained through employment unless legally authorized or required by responsible performance of duty to divulge such information;
C. uphold the honor and high principles of the profession and accept its disciplines;
D. seek to continually improve the knowledge and skills of medical assistants for the benefit of patients and professional colleagues;
E. participate in additional service activities aimed toward improving the health and well-being of the community.

CREED

I believe in the principles and purposes of the Profession of Medical Assisting.
I endeavor to be more effective.
I aspire to render greater service.
I protect the confidence entrusted to me.
I am dedicated to the care and well-being of all people.
I am loyal to my employer.
I am true to the ethics of my profession.
I am strengthened by compassion, courage, and faith.

Figure 8-2   AAMA Code of Ethics and Creed. (Copyright by the American Association of Medical Assistants, Inc. Revised October, 1996)

KEYS TO THE AAMA CODE OF ETHICS

Medical assistants should consider the more salient points in the AAMA code of ethics and ask themselves the following questions:

A. *Render service with full respect for the dignity of humanity.*

- Will I respect every patient even if I do not approve of his or her morals or choices in health care?
- Will I honor each patient's request for information and explain unfamiliar procedures?

PRINCIPLES OF MEDICAL ETHICS: AMERICAN MEDICAL ASSOCIATION

Preamble

The medical profession has long subscribed to a body of ethical statements developed primarily for the benefit of the patient. As a member of this profession, a physician must recognize responsibility not only to patients, but also to society, to other health professionals, and to self. The following Principles adopted by the American Medical Association are not laws, but standards of conduct which define the essentials of honorable behavior for the physician.

I. A physician shall be dedicated to providing competent medical service with compassion and respect for human dignity.
II. A physician shall deal honestly with patients and colleagues, and strive to expose those physicians deficient in character or competence, or who engage in fraud or deception.
III. A physician shall respect the law and also recognize a responsibility to seek changes in those requirements which are contrary to the best interests of the patient.
IV. A physician shall respect the rights of patients, of colleagues, and of other health professionals, and shall safeguard patient confidences within the constraints of the law.
V. A physician shall continue to study, apply, and advance scientific knowledge, make relevant information available to patients, colleagues, and the public, obtain consultation, and use the talents of other health professionals when indicated.
VI. A physician shall, in the provision of appropriate patient care, except in emergencies, be free to choose whom to serve, with whom to associate, and the environment in which to provide medical services.
VII. A physician shall recognize a responsibility to participate in activities contributing to an improved community.

Figure 8-3   American Medical Association Principles of Medical Ethics. (Source: Code of Medical Ethics Current Opinions with Annotations, 2000–2001 Edition, American Medical Association, Copyright 2000)

- Will I give my full attention to acknowledging the needs of every patient?
- Will I be able to accept the indigent, the physically and mentally challenged, the infirm, the physically disfigured, and the persons I simply do not like as equal and valid human beings with an equal right to service?

B. *Respect confidential information obtained through employment unless legally authorized or required by responsible performance of duty to divulge such information.*

- Will I refrain from needless comments to a colleague regarding a patient's problem?
- Will I refrain from discussing my day's encounters with patients with my family and friends?
- Will I always protect a patient's chart and everything in it from unnecessary observation?
- Will I keep patients' names and the circumstances that bring them to my place of employment confidential?

C. *Uphold the honor and high principles of the profession and accept its disciplines.*

- Am I proud of serving as a medical assistant?
- Will I always perform within the scope of my profession, never exceeding the responsibility entrusted to me?
- Will I encourage others to enter the profession and always speak honorably of medical assistants?

D. *Seek to continually improve the knowledge and skills of medical assistants for the benefit of patients and professional colleagues.*

- Will I always be willing to learn new skills, to update my skills, and seek improved methods for assisting the physician in the care of patients?
- Will I keep my certification current and valid?
- Can I always remember that I am a member of a group of broad-based health care professionals and that my goal is to complement rather than to compete with that team?

E. *Participate in additional service activities aimed toward improving the health and well-being of the community.*

- Will I be able to serve in the community where I reside and work to further quality health care?
- Will I promote preventive medicine?
- Will I practice good health care management for myself, being a model for others to follow?

AMA ETHICAL GUIDELINES

The American Medical Association and its nine-member Judicial Council publish a guide for ethical behavior for physicians that is beneficial to medical assistants who act in concert with their physician/employer. The guidelines are based on the Code of Medical Ethics in the publication *Current Opinions of the Council on Ethical and Judicial Affairs of the American Medical Association, 2000.* Information shared here is not meant to be exhaustive; however, physicians and their employees will find it helpful to con-

sider information on the following topics, which was summarized from this publication. The complete guide can be purchased from the AMA in Chicago, IL.

Advertising

Physicians and professional people have traditionally not advertised; however, it is not illegal or unethical to do so if claims made are truthful and not misleading. Advertisements may include credentials of physicians and a description of the practice, kinds of services rendered, and how fees are determined. Managed care agencies may advertise their services and the names of participating physicians. Testimonials from patients are best avoided. Indeed, most physicians discover that word-of-mouth advertisement from patients is the best source of advertisement for their practice.

Media Relations

Physicians and all of their employees are not allowed to discuss a patient's medical condition with any member of the media without the patient's expressed approval. This does not apply to information that is considered "public domain," which includes births, deaths, accidents, and police records. While more hospitals than ambulatory care settings will be involved in media relations, the following is an example of information that is considered public domain and does not require the patient's consent.

"Jaime Carrera, a local construction worker, suffered a severe laceration to the head as a result of an accident at the construction site. He remains hospitalized in good condition."

Confidentiality

 Physicians must not reveal confidential information about patients without their consent unless they are otherwise required to do so by law. Confidentiality must be protected so that patients will feel comfortable and safe in revealing information about themselves that may be important to their health care. The following list contains examples of the kinds of reports that allow or require health professionals to report a confidence.

- A patient threatens another person and there is reason to believe that the threat may be carried out.

- Certain injuries and illnesses *must* be reported. They include injuries such as knife and gunshot wounds, wounds that may be from suspected child abuse, and communicable diseases such as influenza, AIDS, and sexually transmitted diseases.

- Information that may have been subpoenaed for testimony in a court of law.

When in doubt, it is always recommended that a physician have the patient's permission to reveal any confidential information.

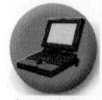 Extra caution must be taken to protect the confidentiality of any patient's data that is kept on a computer database. As few people as possible should have access to the computer data, and only authorized individuals should be permitted to add or alter data. Adequate security precautions must be utilized to protect information stored on a computer.

Medical Records

The medical chart and the information in it are the property of the physician and the patient. No information should be revealed without the patient's consent unless required by law. The record is confidential. Physicians should not refuse to provide a copy of the record to another physician treating the patient so long as proper authorization has been received from the patient. Also, physicians should provide a copy of the record or summary of its contents if a patient requests it. A record cannot be withheld because of an unpaid bill.

Upon a physician's retirement or death, or when a practice is sold, patients should be notified and given ample time to have their records transferred to another physician of their choice.

Professional Fees and Charges

Illegal or excessive fees should not be charged. Fees should be based on those customary to the locale and should reflect the difficulty of services and the quality of performance rendered. Fee splitting (a physician splits the fee with another physician for services rendered with or without the patient's knowledge) in any form is unethical. Physicians may charge for missed appointments (if patients have first been notified of the practice) and may charge for multiple or very complex insurance forms. Physicians and their employees must be diligent to assure that only the services actually rendered are charged or indicated on the insurance claim. Only what is documented in the patient's chart is to be billed.

Professional Rights and Responsibilities

 Physicians may choose whom to serve, but may not refuse a patient on the basis of race, color, religion, national origin, or any other illegal discrimination. It is unethical for physicians to deny treatment to HIV-infected individuals on that basis alone if they are qualified to treat the patient's condition. Once a physician takes a case, the patient cannot be neglected nor refused treatment unless official notice is given from the physician to withdraw from the case.

Patients have the right to know their diagnoses, the nature and purpose of their treatment, and to have enough information to be able to make an informed choice about their treatment protocol. Physicians should inform families of a patient's death and not delegate that responsibility to others.

Physicians should expose incompetent, corrupt, dishonest, and unethical conduct by other physicians to the disciplinary board. It is unethical for any physician to treat patients while under the influence of alcohol, controlled substances, or any other chemical that impairs the physician's ability.

Physicians who know they are HIV positive should refrain from any activity that would risk the transmission of the virus to others.

Any activity that might be regarded as a "conflict of interest"(for example, a physician holding stock in a pharmaceutical company and prescribing medications only from that company) should be avoided. Financial interests are not to influence physicians in prescribing medications, devices, or appliances.

Abuse

 It is the responsibility of physicians and their employees to report all cases of suspected child abuse, to protect and care for the abused, and to treat the abuser (if known) as a victim also. This is not an

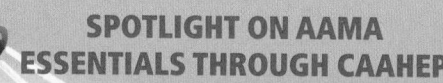

SPOTLIGHT ON AAMA ESSENTIALS THROUGH CAAHEP

● Medical ethics involves providing patients of all socioeconomic backgrounds with quality care.

● Professional and empathetic medical assistants never judge patients whose belief systems differ from their own.

● If a medical assistant suspects that an HIV-seropositive patient is infecting an unsuspecting person, he or she should make every attempt to protect the individual at risk and to encourage the infected person to cease endangering other people.

easy task. Abuse is not easy to witness. While there are very specific laws regarding suspected child abuse, and in most states medical assistants are mandated to report abuse, the laws are vague or nonexistent in elderly and spousal abuse. However, whatever form the abuse takes, it is best to treat all forms of abuse in the same manner by providing a safe environment for those abused and seeking treatment for the abuser and the abused.

BIOETHICAL DILEMMAS

Guidelines for bioethical issues are even harder to define than are guidelines for ethics, because each of the bioethical issues calls upon us to make decisions that directly affect a person's life. In some instances, the bioethical issue requires a choice about who lives and requires a definition of the quality of life. Such dilemmas are difficult, if not impossible, to approach from a neutral point of view even though medical assistants should strive not to impose their own moral values upon patients or coworkers.

Allocation of Scarce Medical Resources

The issue faced daily by health care workers is the allocation of scarce medical resources. Even with the government's attempts at health care reform, medical resources still will not be available to everyone. When the receptionist determines who receives the only available appointment in a day, when patients are turned away because they have no insurance or financial resources to pay for services, when Medicare/Medicaid patients are denied services because of low return from state and federal insurance programs, scarce medical resources are being denied.

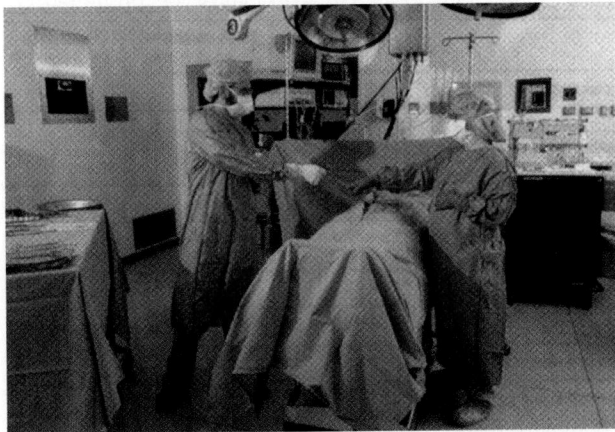

Figure 8-4   Scarce medical resources may limit surgery options for patients whose conditions are not immediately life threatening; some patients may lack insurance and not be able to afford necessary surgical procedures. (Photo courtesy of the U.S. Army)

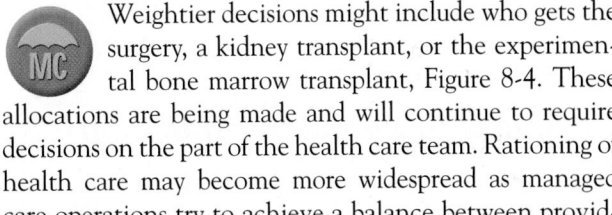 Weightier decisions might include who gets the surgery, a kidney transplant, or the experimental bone marrow transplant, Figure 8-4. These allocations are being made and will continue to require decisions on the part of the health care team. Rationing of health care may become more widespread as managed care operations try to achieve a balance between providing access to care while still curtailing costs.

Decisions made by Congress, health systems agencies, and insurance companies are termed macroallocation of scarce medical resources. Decisions made individually by physicians and members of the health care team at the local level are termed microallocation of scarce resources. No matter what the level, physicians and medical assistants will be involved.

Abortion and Fetal Tissue Research

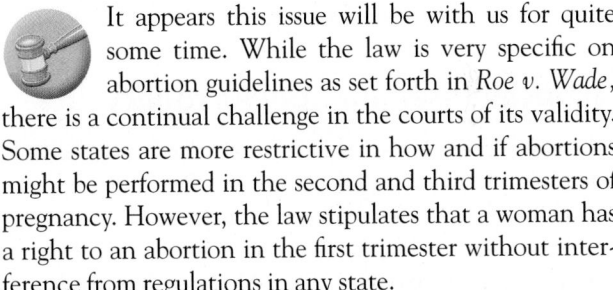 It appears this issue will be with us for quite some time. While the law is very specific on abortion guidelines as set forth in *Roe v. Wade*, there is a continual challenge in the courts of its validity. Some states are more restrictive in how and if abortions might be performed in the second and third trimesters of pregnancy. However, the law stipulates that a woman has a right to an abortion in the first trimester without interference from regulations in any state.

A physician must decide whether to perform abortions and under what circumstances (within the legal parameters). A physician cannot be forced to perform abortions, nor can any employee be forced to participate or assist the physician to perform an abortion. Employees not wishing to participate in abortions are advised to seek employment where they are not performed.

There are many unanswered ethical questions related to abortion that make it difficult for health care professionals. Should abortion be considered a form of birth control? If not, should birth control be readily available to all who seek it regardless of age? Is it ethical to deny a woman on welfare an abortion while providing one to the woman who either has money for the procedure or whose insurance pays for it? And, of course, the major unanswered question that must be determined by every physician is: when does life begin?

The abortion issue raises another bioethical issue—fetal tissue research and transplantation. Research has shown that transplanted tissue from aborted fetuses can be instrumental in benefiting individuals with serious, life-threatening diseases. This issue is political as well as bioethical, and it changes with each major political shift in our government. If fetal tissue research is allowed, the primary ethical concern is that that fact not be used to encourage women to have abortions; rather, the tissue would be available only after a decision had already been made regarding abortion.

Genetic Engineering/Manipulation

So much is possible today in the area of **genetic engineering** and more is being discovered daily. Through genetic engineering, we have the potential of identifying genes that predispose individuals to certain illnesses and diseases and manipulating or altering those genes to prevent or lessen the disease or illness. Who among us would not want to be free of certain illnesses? But at what cost? How far do we go in genetic engineering? Would we prefer a society where everyone is healthy and beautiful? If it is determined that a fetus suffers from a serious defect, should abortion be encouraged? If we manipulate the genes prior to implantation, are we playing god? If fertilization takes place *in vitro*, is discarding defective embryos a reasonable and presumed choice?

Artificial Insemination/Surrogacy

For many individuals, artificial insemination is the only means by which they can conceive. Physicians can be called upon to perform artificial insemination for couples, single women, or lesbians who want a child. If artificial insemination is practiced, the AMA recommends the signed consent of each party involved. It is also recommended that physicians practicing AID (Artificial Insemination by Donor), not continually use the same donors for semen, and that meticulous screening be performed prior to the insemination.

Surrogacy is another bioethical issue. Men have been used as **surrogates,** or substitutes, for decades with the practice of artificial insemination, but society has a more difficult time with surrogate mothers than artificial insemination with male donors. Under what circumstances should a surrogate mother be considered? How should the rights of each individual in the exchange be protected? For many of these issues, there is little or no protection or guidance under the law; therefore, physicians and their employees must make decisions on the basis of their own belief systems. The AMA is not supportive of surrogacy as a viable route to parenthood.

Dying and Death

Patients are making more choices regarding their death. We all have the right to direct health care professionals regarding our death in the case of a life-threatening illness. Through a living will or a physician's directive, we can mandate that life support systems be removed. Sometimes, patients make these decisions before physicians are ready to remove the life support. Other times, physicians can determine when a case is hopeless far quicker than the patient or the patient's family. What should be done then? When a physician is committed to sustaining life, it is very difficult to make decisions to terminate life. In 1994, Oregon voters passed a physician-assisted suicide law. Other states are considering similar laws.

In 1990, Congress passed a bill called the Patient Self-Determination Act, which encourages patients to make living wills and advance directives before life-sustaining measures become necessary. Nearly all states have legislation regarding advance directives.

Choices available to patients who are dying always cause us to ask ourselves what is "quality of life"? While the answer to that question is different for everyone, it is a question often in conflict with today's medical technology that can, in many instances, keep a patient alive much longer than the patient might prefer. The benefits of advanced technology will continue to be weighed against what many consider the right to die with dignity and a minimum of medical intervention.

HIV and AIDS

The general public's fear of AIDS has caused some serious bioethical issues. Patients who may suspect they have come into contact with HIV or AIDS should be tested for the virus. Their confidentiality must be protected as much as possible since persons with AIDS often face loss of employment, medical insurance, and even loss of family and friends. It is unethical to deny treatment to HIV-infected individuals because they test positive for HIV.

While persons with AIDS must be protected, so must the public. Therefore, if physicians suspect that an HIV-seropositive patient is infecting an unsuspecting individual, every attempt should be made to protect the individual at risk. Health professionals must first encourage the infected person to cease endangering any person. Second, if the patient refuses to notify the person at risk or wishes the physician to notify the person, the physician can contact authorities. Many states and cities have Partner Notification Programs that will anonymously notify the patient at risk, keeping the source confidential. The Program informs them that it has been brought to their attention that they are a "person at risk" and provides them with free testing. Third, the physician can notify the person at risk.

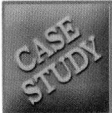

At the end of a busy afternoon, Juanita Hansen, a single mother in her twenties, brings in her son Henry after he fell down a flight of steps. He is badly bruised and crying and also seems to be somewhat fearful of his mother. Medical assistant Liz Corbin recognizes Henry, for his mother brought him in the week before when he fell off his bike. At that time, Liz had assisted Dr. Esposito in examining Henry and both were concerned about the possibility of child abuse, for Henry had been in before for various "accidents." Today, when Liz assists Dr. Esposito once again to examine Henry, it becomes clear that Henry is probably the victim of abuse.

CASE STUDY REVIEW

1. Because Liz and Dr. Esposito strongly suspect that Henry is being repeatedly abused, what are they obligated to do?

2. How can Liz best help Henry to cope with his situation?

3. How can Liz attempt to help Henry's mother come to terms with the fact that she is physically abusing her son?

SUMMARY

As medical technology continues to advance, a greater need for ethical guidelines will be necessary. Physicians and health care professionals at all levels must stay abreast of the issues and carefully consider all aspects prior to any decision making.

Medical assistants must, however, keep the following legal and ethical guidelines in mind: (1) always practice within the law; (2) preserve the patient's confidentiality; (3) maintain meticulous records; (4) obtain informed, written consent; (5) do not judge patients whose belief system differs from yours.

REVIEW QUESTIONS

Multiple Choice

1. Typically, ethics has been defined in terms of:
   a. what is right and wrong
   b. whether an action is legal
   c. the expedient thing to do
   d. professionalism in the workplace

2. Bioethics has to do with:
   a. biological reproduction
   b. the act of artificial insemination
   c. genetic engineering
   d. ethical issues that deal with life and health care

3. The Code of Ethics of AAMA:
   a. is concerned with principles of ethical and moral conduct
   b. defines the duties the medical assistant can perform
   c. is intended for physicians only
   d. applies only to patient rights

4. When a physician or medical assistant suspects child abuse, she should:
   a. give the parent a warning
   b. report it to the proper authorities
   c. not impose her values on the parents
   d. give the child some hints on how to protect against abuse

5. When a patient has HIV:
   a. it is ethical for the physician not to provide treatment
   b. it is unethical for the physician not to provide treatment
   c. other patients should be warned of the possibility of infection
   d. all friends and family members of the patient should be notified

6. A copy of a medical record may be granted to:
   a. a physician the patient is being referred to
   b. a physician's attorney when subpoenaed or released by patient

c. the patient
d. all of the above
e. only a and b

7. A patient's living will or physician's directive:
   a. is a legal document to be kept in the chart
   b. can be changed at any time by the patient
   c. should accompany the patient to the hospital
   d. all of the above
   e. only a and c

8. Your physician employer is considering changing the practice's announcement in the yellow pages of the phone book. Which of the following is not recommended?
   a. Name and specialty of practice
   b. Names and credentials/specialties of participating physicians
   c. Patient testimonials
   d. Managed care participation

9. Which of the following is true?
   a. A physician can choose whom to serve.
   b. A physician may charge for completing multiple and complex insurance claims.
   c. Physicians and their employees cannot be forced to perform abortions.
   d. All of the above
   e. None of the above

10. You are most likely to make ethical decisions correctly when:
    a. you have a clear picture of the situation
    b. you leave emotion out of the decision as much as possible
    c. you understand your weaknesses and vulnerabilities
    d. honesty and integrity are hallmarks of your entire life
    e. all of the above

Critical Thinking

1. In your own words, define ethics and bioethics.
2. List the similarities of and the differences between the AAMA Code of Ethics and the AMA Principles of Medical Ethics.
3. The physician observes another physician put a patient at risk while under the influence of alcohol and does nothing about it. What would constitute ethical behavior?

4. A physician attends a medical seminar related to medical practice every month and charges the seminar fee to the business. Would you consider this ethical or unethical? Why?
5. A physician refuses to accept any more Medicaid patients for medical care. Is this the physician's right? Is it ethical?
6. A medical assistant whispers to the receptionist, "There goes the guy with AIDS." How should the receptionist view this behavior?
7. The services reported on the insurance claim are more complex than those actually rendered. Is this ethical or unethical? State your reasons.
8. The physician refuses to perform a legal abortion. Do you consider this an ethical issue? Why?
9. A physician performs artificial insemination for a lesbian couple; however, the medical assistant refuses to participate or assist the physician. What are the ramifications of the medical assistant's behavior? Do you believe the medical assistant has a right to refuse?
10. Referring to Figure 8-1, select an ethical issue with which you may have had some personal experience. Now, form a small group, with each student leading a discussion on a different issue.

WEB ACTIVITIES

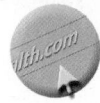 Using the World Wide Web, research particular guidelines to be used for artificial insemination either by donor or by husband. Look under the Current Opinions of the Council on Ethical and Judicial Affairs.

- What are the guidelines for medical records? Why?
- Why is frozen sperm recommended?

REFERENCES/BIBLIOGRAPHY

American Medical Association. (2000). Code of medical ethics. *Current opinions of the council on ethical and judicial affairs, 2000.* Chicago: Author.

Flight, M. (1998). *Law, liability, and ethics for medical office personnel* (3rd ed.). Albany, NY: Delmar.

Lewis, M. A., & Tamparo, C. D., (1998). *Medical law, ethics, and bioethics for ambulatory care* (4th ed.). Philadelphia: F. A. Davis Co.

9

EMERGENCY PROCEDURES AND FIRST AID

KEY TERMS

Cardiopulmonary Resuscitation (CPR)
Crash Tray or Cart
Crepitation
Emergency Medical Services (EMS)
First Aid
Fracture
Heimlich Maneuver
Hypothermia
Lackluster
Occlusion
Rescue Breathing
Shock
Splint
Sprain
Standard Precautions
Strain
Syncope
Triage
Universal Emergency Medical
    Identification Symbol
Wound

OUTLINE

Recognizing an Emergency
  Responding to an Emergency
  Primary Survey
  Using the 911 or Emergency
    Medical Services System
  Good Samaritan Laws
  Blood, Body Fluids, and Disease
    Transmission
Preparing for an Emergency
  The Medical Crash Tray or Cart
Common Emergencies
  Shock
  Wounds
  Burns

Musculoskeletal Injuries
Heat- and Cold-Related Illnesses
Poisoning
Sudden Illness
Cerebral Vascular Accident
  (CVA)
Heart Attack
**Procedures for Breathing Emer-
gencies and Cardiac Arrest**
  Heimlich Maneuver (Abdominal
    Thrust)
  Rescue Breathing
  Cardiopulmonary Resuscitation
    (CPR)

OBJECTIVES

The student should strive to meet the following performance objectives and demonstrate an understanding of the facts and principles presented in this chapter through written and oral communication.

1. Define the key terms as presented in the glossary.
2. Learn to recognize, prepare for, and respond to emergencies in the ambulatory care setting.
3. Understand the legal and disease transmission considerations in emergency caregiving.
4. Perform the primary assessment in emergency situations.
5. Identify and care for different types of wounds.
6. Understand the basics of bandage application.
7. Discriminate among first-, second-, and third-degree burns.
8. Assess injuries to muscles, bones, and joints.
9. Describe heat- and cold-related illnesses.

(continues)

10. Describe how poisons may enter the body.
11. Recall the eight types of shock.
12. Define a cerebral vascular accident.
13. Describe the signs and symptoms of a heart attack.
14. Demonstrate proficiency in Heimlich maneuver, rescue breathing, and cardiopulmonary resuscitation (CPR).

ROLE DELINEATION COMPONENTS

CLINICAL
Patient Care
- **Adhere to established triage procedures**
- **Recognize and respond to emergencies**
- **Obtain patient history and vital signs**
- **Prepare and maintain examination and treatment areas**
- **Prepare patient for examination, procedures, and treatment**

GENERAL (Transdisciplinary)
Instruction
- **Instruct individuals according to their needs**

SCENARIO

Inner City Health Care, which is located in Carlton, Michigan, has its share of cold, snowy winters and when the temperature drops near freezing, that snow sometimes turns to ice. Last night, as Clinical Medical Assistant Wanda Slawson, CMA, was leaving for the evening, she noticed a woman from an adjacent office slip and fall in the parking lot. Wanda immediately went over to the woman to lend assistance and saw that, in falling, the woman had cut the palm of her hand. Apparently, she had tried to break her fall with her hand only to sustain a large wound that was now bleeding moderately. Fortunately, Wanda knew that one of the physicians was still in the office and she led the woman back to the building, reassuring her all the way. Once in the office, Wanda assisted Susan Rice, the physician, to examine the wound. After determining that sutures were not needed, Dr. Rice and Wanda cleansed the wound, applied a dry, sterile dressing, and covered it with an elastic bandage. The patient was instructed to call her physician first thing in the morning.

INTRODUCTION

While the ambulatory care setting is primarily designed to see patients under nonemergency conditions, occasionally the physician will need to administer emergency care and the medical assistant will be called upon to assist the physician in this care. For the medical assistant who may need to triage or assess the patient's condition, the first and most critical step in responding to an emergency is developing the skill to recognize when emergency measures should be taken.

While some emergencies can be treated in the office, others cannot and the medical assistant must know when to call for outside help. If the emergency occurs in the ambulatory care setting, the physician usually provides immediate care. It is possible, however, that the medical assistant may be the first emergency caregiver should the physician be out of the office. The medical assistant also may be called upon to provide care in an emergency outside of the office environment.

This chapter will acquaint the medical assistant with types of emergency situations that may occur either inside or outside of the office. However, this chapter is merely an introduction to emergency topics and does not substitute for first aid and cardiopulmonary (CPR) instruction taught either through the college curriculum or through the American Red Cross or the American Heart Association. These hands-on classes are vital teaching tools and all medical assistants should take them on a regular basis in order to continually update their skills.

RECOGNIZING AN EMERGENCY

An emergency is considered any instance in which an individual becomes suddenly ill and requires immediate attention. Some common signs that an individual has an emergency include unusual noises, such as yelling, moaning, or crying. A person may appear to be behaving strangely when choking or if having difficulty breathing. To recognize when an emergency exists, it is important to have sharp senses of hearing, sight, and smell and be acutely sensitive to any unusual behaviors.

In the ambulatory care setting, medical assistants will encounter a range of emergency situations requiring first aid techniques. **First aid** is designed to render immediate and temporary emergency care to persons injured or otherwise disabled prior to the arrival of a physician or transport to a hospital or other health care agency.

Emergency situations can include:

- Wounds
- Bleeding
- Burns
- Shock
- Fractures
- Poisoning
- Sudden illnesses such as fainting
- Illnesses related to heat and cold
- Heart attack
- Choking and breathing crises

Some of these will be life-threatening; all will require immediate care. In either case, it is critical to remain calm, to follow the emergency policies and procedures established by the ambulatory care setting, and to be well-versed in first-aid and cardiopulmonary resuscitation techniques.

Responding to an Emergency

Once it has been determined that an emergency exists, it is essential to act quickly. Before making any decisions about how to proceed, it is necessary to assess the nature of the situation. Does it include respiratory or circulatory failure, severe bleeding, burns, poisoning, or severe allergic reaction?

Sometimes, it is possible that more than one type of care must be administered. In this case, it is necessary to **triage** the situation, which is a method of prioritizing treatment. When an individual suffers more than one illness or injury, care must be given according to the severity of the situation. When two or more patients present with emergencies simultaneously, triage also determines which patient is treated first. The main principle of triage states that absence of breath and severe bleeding are immediate life threats. See Table 9-1 for the common ordering of triage situations.

To identify the nature of the emergency and respond effectively, it is critical that the patient be assessed. If the patient is conscious, ask for personal identification and identification of next of kin. Try to obtain information about symptoms being experienced in order to identify the problem. Always check for a **universal emergency medical identification symbol** (Figure 9-1) and accompanying identification card, which will describe any serious or life-threatening health problems of the patient. Quickly observe the patient's general appearance, including skin color and size and dilation of pupils. Check pulse.

TABLE 9-1	EXAMPLES OF TRIAGE SITUATIONS	
First Priority	**Next Priority**	**Least Priority**
Airway and breathing problems	Second-degree burns not on the neck and face	Fractures
Cardiac arrest	Major or multiple fractures	Minor injuries
Severe bleeding that is uncontrolled	Back injuries	Sprains
Head injuries	Severe eye injuries	
Poisoning		
Open chest or abdominal wounds		
Shock		
Second- and third-degree burns		

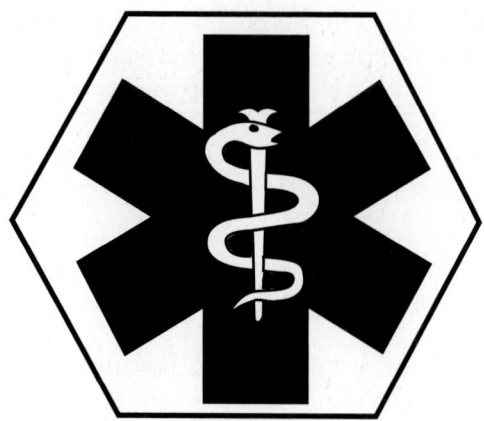

Figure 9-1   The universal emergency medical identification symbol.

Primary Survey

If the patient is unresponsive, it is critical to assess the ABCs, which include:

- Airway (A)
- Breathing (B)
- Circulation (C)

To assess whether the unresponsive patient is breathing and to determine if there is an open airway, place your face close to the patient's face and look, listen, and feel.

Look at the patient's chest and notice whether the chest rises and falls with breathing. Listen for air entering and leaving the nose and mouth and feel for moving air.

If the individual is not breathing, first open the airway by either tilting the head and lifting the chin (Figure 9-2A); or by the jaw-thrust maneuver, which involves placing both thumbs on the patient's cheekbones and index and middle fingers on both sides of the lower jaw (Figure 9-2B). **CAUTION:** Do not attempt to tilt the head and lift the chin when the patient has a head, neck, or spinal cord injury.

If the patient still does not breathe after the airway has been opened, rescue breathing must be performed, which is covered later in this chapter.

To assess circulation, check for the presence of a pulse at the carotid artery on the side of the neck below the ear. If no pulse is present, the patient may be in cardiac arrest and must be given cardiopulmonary resuscitation. CPR techniques are covered in detail later in this chapter.

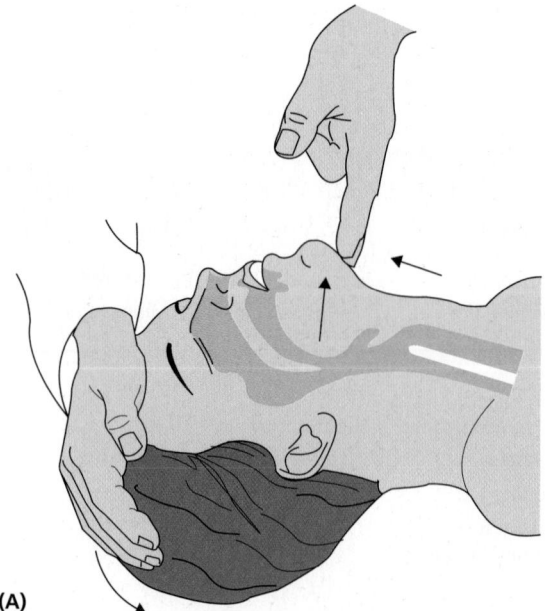

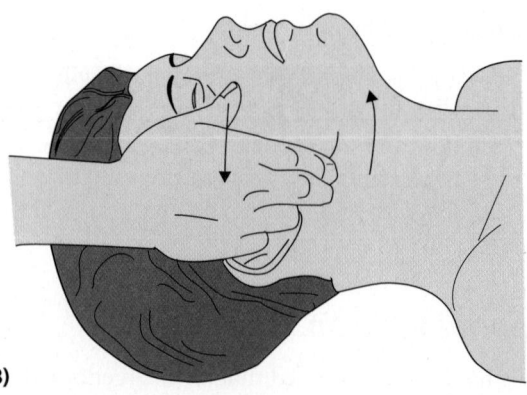

(A)   (B)

Figure 9-2   If the individual is not breathing, first open the airway: (A) By tilting the head and lifting the chin or (B) By the jaw-thrust maneuver, which involves placing both thumbs on the patient's cheekbones and index and middle fingers on both sides of the lower jaw.

Using the 911 or Emergency Medical Services System

The **Emergency Medical Services (EMS)** system is a local network of police, fire, and medical personnel who are trained to respond to emergency situations. Other community experts and volunteers also act as resources in an EMS system. In many communities, the network is activated by calling 911. Even when preliminary emergency care is provided by the ambulatory care physician, the patient may still need to be transported or may require follow-up care. It is also possible that the physician may not be equipped to deliver the type of emergency care required, in which case one person should call for EMS help while another stays with the patient until help arrives. Never leave a seriously ill or unconscious patient unattended.

Good Samaritan Laws

When delivering or assisting in delivering emergency care, the medical assistant may be concerned about professional liability. Most states have enacted Good Samaritan laws, which provide some degree of protection to the health care professional who offers first aid.

Most Good Samaritan laws provide some legal protection to those who provide emergency care to ill or injured persons. However, when medical assistants or any other individuals give care during an emergency, they must act as reasonable and prudent individuals and provide care only within the scope of their abilities. Remember that a primary principle of first aid is to prevent further injury.

While Good Samaritan laws give some measure of protection against being sued for giving emergency aid, they generally protect *off-duty* health care professionals. Also, conditions of the law vary from state to state. As part of establishing emergency care guidelines, every ambulatory care setting should understand the explicit and implicit intent of the Good Samaritan Law in its state. See Chapter 7 for more information on legal guidelines.

Blood, Body Fluids, and Disease Transmission

When providing emergency care, medical assistants should always protect themselves and the patient from infectious disease transmission. Serious infectious diseases, such as hepatitis B (HBV) and HIV, which causes AIDS, can be transmitted through blood and body fluids (see Chapter 10 for detailed information).

By establishing and following strict guidelines, the risk of contacting or transmitting an infectious disease while providing emergency care is greatly reduced.

- Always wash hands thoroughly before (if possible) and after every procedure.
- Use protective clothing and other protective equipment during the procedure.
- During the procedure, avoid contact with blood and body fluids, if possible.
- Do not touch nose, mouth, or eyes with gloved hands.
- Carefully handle and safely dispose of soiled gloves and other objects.

Refer to Chapter 10 for more information on standard precautions. **Standard precautions** were issued by the Centers for Disease Control and Prevention (CDC) in 1996 and combine many of the basic principles of universal precautions with techniques known as body substance isolation. These augmented 1996 guidelines represent the standard in infection control and are intended to protect both patients and health care professionals.

PREPARING FOR AN EMERGENCY

Emergencies are unexpected but can and should be anticipated and prepared for in the ambulatory care setting. Being properly prepared assures that the office has the materials and resources needed to respond to emergencies.

An in-office handbook of policies and procedures should be developed and should be familiar to all staff. Telephone numbers for the local emergency medical services (often this is 911) and the poison control center should be posted and kept in an established place so that there is no delay in calling for outside assistance. Materials and supplies should be maintained in proper inventory. All personnel should be trained in the basics of first aid and CPR, so that every staff member can respond to or

---

**SPOTLIGHT ON AAMA
ESSENTIALS THROUGH CAAHEP**

- Treat all patients with compassion and empathy.
- Identifying a patient's cultural needs during an emergency may help to save his or her life.
- Listening to how a patient "feels" is just as important as how the patient appears.

assist the physician in providing care. Proper documentation should be completed after any emergency situation. The office environment itself should be a safe one and as accident-proof as possible. Wipe up spills to avoid falls on a slippery floor, keep corridors clutter-free, and keep medications out of sight. These basic risk management techniques will help medical personnel focus on giving emergency care and also protect the facility from any possible litigation.

The Medical Crash Tray or Cart

Every health care facility should have a **crash tray or cart**, with a carefully controlled inventory of supplies and equipment (Figure 9-3). These first-aid supplies should be kept in an accessible place, and the inventory should be routinely monitored to assure that all supplies are replaced and that all medications are up to date and have not reached their expiration date.

A smaller practice may require only a portable tray for emergency and first-aid supplies; larger urgent care centers may respond more frequently to emergencies and thus may need a cart that can hold a large inventory and variety of supplies. Whether a tray or cart is used, supplies should be customized to the facility and the type of emergencies frequently encountered. Remember that only physicians can order medications or treatment.

Following is a brief list of some common supplies found on most trays and/or carts. Also see Chapter 23 for more information on supplies and medications.

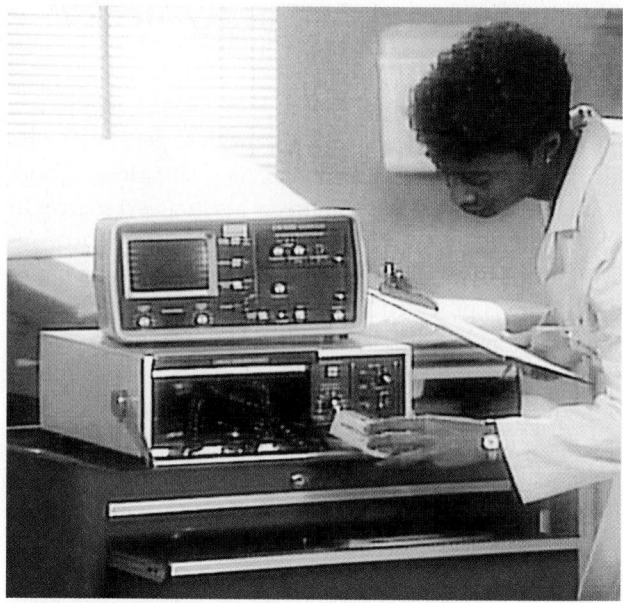

Figure 9-3 Medical crash cart.

General supplies:

- Adhesive and hypoallergenic tape
- Alcohol wipes
- Bandage scissors
- Bandage material
- Blood pressure cuff (standard, pediatric, large)
- Constriction band
- Defibrillator
- Gloves
- Hot/cold packs
- IV tubing
- Needles and syringes for injection
- Orange juice for diabetics (refrigerated)
- Penlight (with extra batteries)
- Personal protective equipment
- Spirits of ammonia
- Sterile dressings
- Stethoscope

Emergency medications:

- Activated charcoal
- Aramine
- Aspirin
- Atropine
- Dextrose
- Diphenhydramine
- Epinephrine
- Glucagon
- Insulin
- Lidocaine
- Nitroglycerin tablets
- Phenobarbital and diazepam (controlled substances; must be kept in a locked cabinet)
- Sodium bicarbonate
- Spirits of ammonia
- Sterile water
- Syrup of ipecac
- Verapamil
- Xylocaine and marcaine

Respiratory supplies:

- Airways of all sizes for nasal and oral use
- Ambu bag™
- Bulb syringe for suction
- Oxygen mask
- Oxygen tank

This list represents just some of the supplies to be found on a well-stocked crash cart or tray. The type and list of supplies should always be overseen by facility physicians and tailored to the emergency demands of the practice. The medical assistant should be familiar with the equipment and medication on the crash cart or tray. Practice "drills" simulating various emergency situations are helpful for preparing staff members for actual emergencies.

COMMON EMERGENCIES

Included in this discussion are shock, wounds, burns, musculoskeletal injuries, heat- and cold-related illnesses, poisoning, sudden illness, cerebral vascular accident, and heart attack.

Shock

When a severe injury occurs, shock is likely to develop. Shock is basically a condition in which the circulatory system is not providing enough blood to all parts of the body, causing the body's organs to fail to function properly.

Shock is always life threatening, and EMS should be activated. The body's attempt to compensate for a massive injury or illness, especially those involving severe bleed-ing, often leads to other problems. During shock several things occur.

- The heart becomes unable to pump blood properly.
- Consequently, the body does not get enough oxygen, which is carried by the blood.
- The body tries to compensate by sending blood to critical organs and reducing the flow of blood to arms, legs, and skin.

Signs and Symptoms of Shock. Learn to recognize the signs and symptoms of shock.

- Patient may be restless or feel irritable.
- Weakness, dizziness, thirst, or nausea may occur.
- Breathing may be shallow and rapid.
- Skin is cool, clammy, and pale.
- Pulse is weak and rapid.
- Blood pressure is low.
- Area around the lips, eyes, and fingernails may turn blue from lack of oxygen.
- The patient may be confused and/or become suddenly unconscious.
- Dilated pupils and lackluster eyes are notable.

Types of Shock. There are eight major types of shock, including respiratory, neurogenic, cardiogenic, hemorrhagic, anaphylactic, metabolic, psychogenic, and septic. See Table 9-2 for a description of each.

TABLE 9-2 EIGHT TYPES OF SHOCK WITH DESCRIPTIONS	
Type of Shock	**Description**
Respiratory	Trauma to the respiratory tract (trachea, lungs) which causes a reduction of oxygen and carbon dioxide exchange. Body cells cannot receive enough oxygen.
Neurogenic	Injury or trauma to the nervous system (spinal cord, brain). Nerve impulse to blood vessels impaired. Blood vessels remain dilated and blood pressure drops.
Cardiogenic	Myocardial infarction with damage to heart muscle; heart unable to pump effectively. Inadequate cardiac output. Body cells not receiving enough oxygen.
Hemorrhagic	Severe bleeding or loss of body fluid from trauma, surgery, or dehydration from severe nausea and vomiting. Blood pressure drops, thus blood flow is reduced to cells, tissues, and organs.
Anaphylactic	Results from reaction to substance to which patient is hypersensitive or allergic (allergen extracts, bee sting, medication, food). Outpouring of histamine results in dilation of blood vessels throughout the body, blood pressure drops and blood flow is reduced to cells, tissue, and organs.
Metabolic	Body's homeostasis impaired; acid-base balance disturbed (diabetic coma or insulin shock); body fluids unbalanced.
Psychogenic	Due to overwhelming emotional factors; i.e., fear, anger, grief. Sudden dilation of blood vessels, results in fainting because of lack of blood supply to the brain. In most cases, may not be life-threatening unless it leads to physical trauma as a result of a fall.
Septic	An acute infection, usually systemic, that overwhelms the body (toxic shock syndrome). Poisonous substances accumulate in bloodstream and blood pressure drops impairing blood flow to cells, tissues, and organs.

Treatment for Shock. A person suffering from shock needs immediate medical attention. Call for outside emergency help first, then care for the patient until help arrives. **CAUTION:** Shock requires immediate medical help. Shock is progressive and if not treated immediately, most types are life threatening. Once shock reaches a certain point, it is irreversible.

To care for a patient in shock, follow these procedures.

- Lie the patient down. This minimizes pain and decreases stress on the body.

- Loosen clothing.

- Check for an open airway.

- Control any external bleeding.

- Help the patient maintain normal body temperature. A blanket over and under the patient can help avoid chilling. Do not overheat.

- Reassure the patient.

- Elevate the legs about 12 inches, unless you suspect spinal injuries or broken bones involving the hips or legs.

- Do not give the patient anything to eat or drink.

- Ascertain that outside help has been called and stay with the patient until help arrives.

Wounds

Typically, **wounds** are classified as open wounds or closed wounds. In the closed wound, there is no break in the skin; a bruise, contusion, and hematoma are common closed wounds. An open wound represents a break in the skin and can be classified as an abrasion, avulsion, incision, laceration, or puncture wound.

Closed Wounds. Most closed wounds do not present an emergency situation. If there is pain and swelling, the application of a cold compress can be effective. Protect the patient's skin by placing a cloth beneath the source of cold; apply the compress for 20 minutes, then remove for 20 minutes; continue for 24 hours. Then apply heat 20 minutes on and 20 minutes off for the next 24 hours. A common procedure for treating closed wounds is to RICE it:

- *Rest*

- *Ice*

- *Compression*

- *Elevation*

Some closed wounds, such as hematomas, can be very dangerous and may cause internal bleeding. If the patient is in severe pain and was subject to an injury caused by high impact, call for help and keep the patient comfortable until the help arrives. Watch for symptoms of shock and monitor vital signs.

Open Wounds. Open wounds can be minor tears in the skin or more serious breaks, but all open wounds represent an opportunity for microorganisms to gain entry and cause an infection. Some major open wounds may involve heavy bleeding, which will need to be controlled, probably by suturing. A tetanus injection is indicated for an open wound if the patient has not had a booster in the past seven to ten years. See Chapter 10 for immunization information.

There are five common types of open wounds.

1. *Abrasions* are a superficial scraping of the epidermis. Because nerve endings are involved, they can be painful. However, they are not usually serious, unless they cover a large area of the body. Administer first aid by cleaning the area carefully with soap and water, apply an antiseptic ointment if prescribed by a physician, and cover with a dressing.

2. In an *avulsion*, the skin is torn off and bleeding is profuse. Avulsion wounds often occur at exposed parts: fingers, toes, ear. First, control bleeding (Procedure 9-1) if necessary. Then clean the wound. If there is a skin flap, reposition it. Apply a dressing, then bandage as necessary. Note that pieces of the body may be torn away. If possible, save the body part, keep moist, and transport with the patient.

3. *Incisions* are wounds that result from a sharp object, such as a knife or piece of glass. Incisions may need sutures. The wound must be cleaned with soap and water and a dressing applied.

4. *Lacerations* tear the body tissue and can be difficult to clean, so care must be taken to avoid infection. If there is not severe bleeding, which in itself is a cleansing mechanism, these wounds may need to be soaked to remove debris. If there is severe bleeding, it must be controlled immediately (Procedure 9-1). Lacerations with severe bleeding are likely to need suturing.

5. *Punctures* pierce and penetrate the skin and may be deep wounds while appearing insignificant. Usually, external bleeding is minimal, but the patient should be assessed for internal bleeding. Because a puncture wound is deep, the risk of infection is great and the patient should be advised to watch for signals of infection, such as pain, swelling, redness, throbbing, and warmth.

Use of Tourniquets in Emergency Care. In the past, tourniquets were regularly used in the field to control hemorrhaging from an extremity when all other attempts to control bleeding were unsuccessful. However, because tourniquet application was meant to completely stop blood flow, many times this complete lack of blood flow resulted in the death of the arm or leg. Often, the affected extremity needed to be amputated.

To remedy this situation, a "constriction band" was substituted for the tourniquet and is now widely used. The constriction band is made of a material similar to that used in the tourniquet. When the band is applied to an extremity to control bleeding, it is applied tightly enough to stem the rapid loss of blood but loosely enough to allow a small amount of blood to continue to flow. A pulse should be felt distally to the constriction band. The use of the constriction band applied in this manner allows a blood supply to the remainder of the extremity unlike the tourniquet, which cuts off all blood flow.

For information on wounds and minor surgery, see Chapter 19.

Dressings and Bandages. When a patient presents with an open wound, after treatment it is critical to dress and bandage it properly to curtail infection. This covering of the wound is accomplished by a series of dressings and bandages.

Typically, dressings are sterile pads placed directly on the wound; they often have nonstick, sterile surfaces, but they are absorbent and will soak up blood and protect the wound from microorganisms. They are often made of a gauze-type material.

Bandages, which are nonsterile, are placed over the dressing. They hold the dressing in place and are made to conform to the area to be covered. Sometimes, as in a Band-Aid, the dressing and bandage are combined. Roller bandages, such as those made of elastic, can be placed over a dressing and used to control bleeding or swelling.

Kling gauze, a type of gauze that stretches and clings as it is applied, and roller bandages, long strips of soft material wound on itself, are other types of bandage materials.

Bandages and their applications can take many shapes and forms, depending on the type of injury and the injury site. In all cases, a bandage must be secure, but not constricting. Avoid too tight or too loose a wrap.

- Spiral bandages are useful for injuries to the arms or legs (Figure 9-4).

- A figure-eight bandage will hold the dressing in place on a wound on the hand or wrist, knee, or ankle (Figure 9-5).

- Fingers, toes, arms, and legs can also be bandaged using a tubular gauze bandage (Figures 9-6, 9-7, and 9-8). Using a cylindrical applicator, a quantity of gauze is stretched over the wound site.

- Commercial arm slings are used to support injured or fractured arms (Figure 9-9). To apply, support the injured arm above and below the injury site while applying the sling.

Burns

Most burns are commonly caused by heat, chemicals, explosions, and electricity. Critical burns can be life threatening, requiring immediate medical care. According to the American Red Cross, critical burns:

- Involve breathing difficulty

- Cover more than one body part

- Involve the head, neck, hands, feet, or genitals

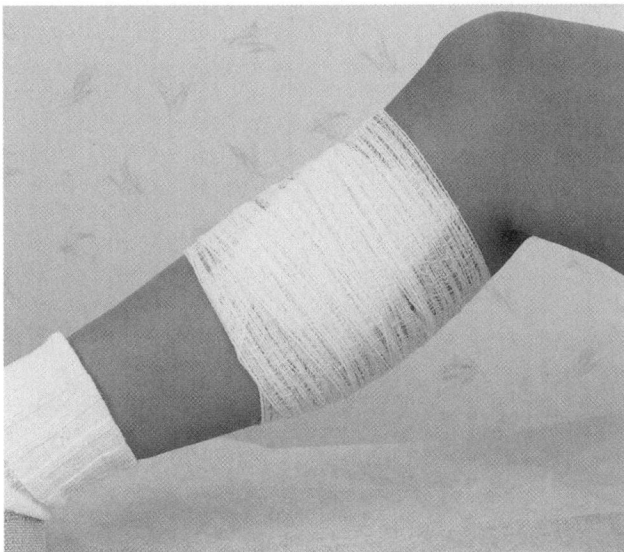

Figure 9-4   The spiral bandage is an option for arm and leg injuries.

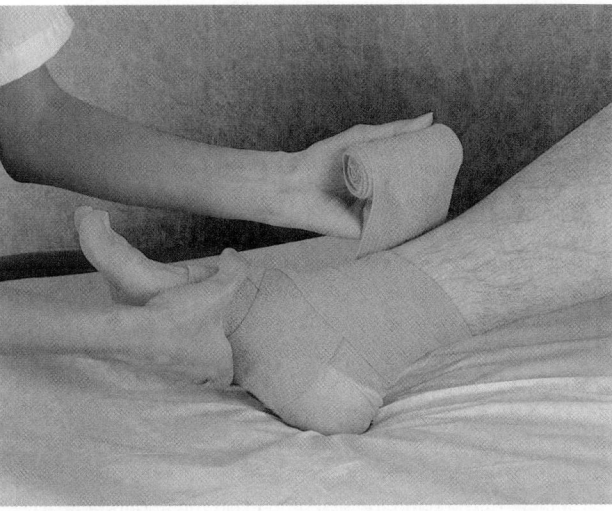

Figure 9-5   An elastic figure-eight bandage holds dressings in place or can be used for immobilization as with an ankle sprain.

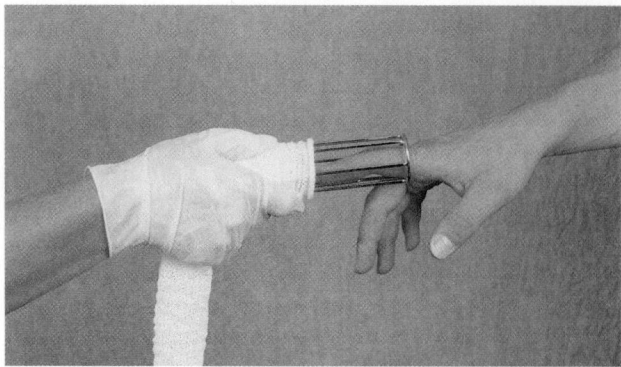

Figure 9-6   There are several types and sizes of tubular gauze applicators, including plastic, solid metal, and metal cage applicators; the metal cage is shown here. All applicators use a seamless elastic gauze bandage (also available in various sizes) that slides over the applicator. The applicator with the gauze then fits over the appendage to be wrapped.

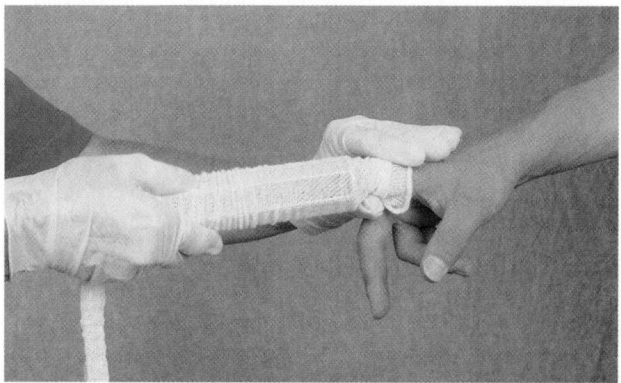

Figure 9-7   The gauze bandage is stretched over the appendage by pulling the applicator away from the base of the appendage. At the same time, the bandage should be held in place at the appendage base with the other hand.

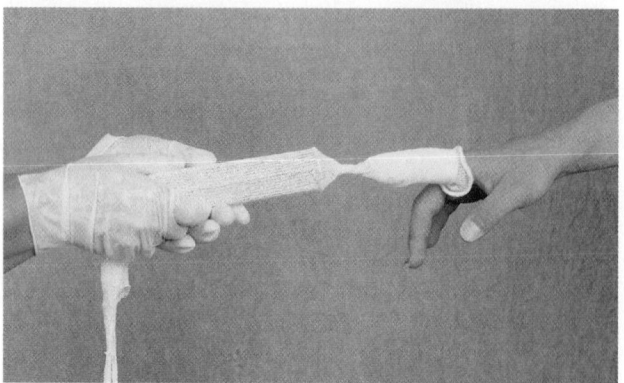

Figure 9-8   Once the applicator has been pulled off the finger, a layer of the bandage will remain on the appendage. To apply another layer, the applicator is again fitted over the finger and a new layer is applied in the same manner as before.

● are any burns to a child or elderly person (other than minor burns)

To distinguish critical from minor burns, it is important to understand the degrees of burns and what they mean.

First-, Second-, and Third-Degree Burns. First-degree burns are superficial burns that involve only the top layer of skin. The skin appears red, feels dry, is warm to the touch, and is painful. First-degree burns usually heal in a week or so with no permanent scarring (Figure 9-10).

In a second-degree burn, the skin is red and blisters are present. The healing process is slower—usually a month—and some scarring may occur. Second-degree burns affect the top layers of the skin, are very painful, and

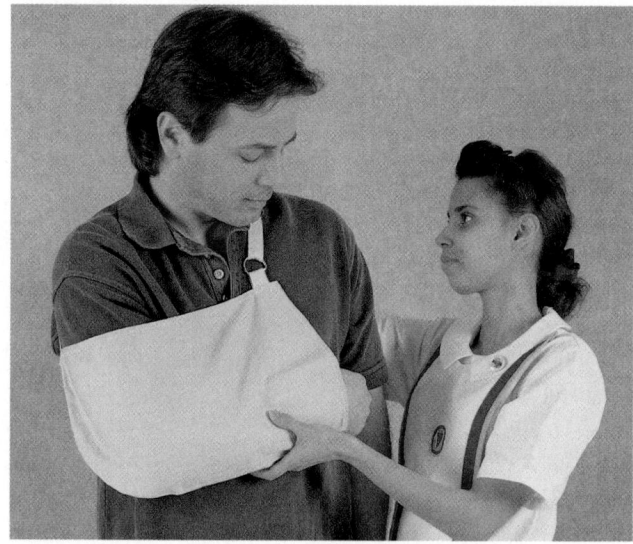

Figure 9-9   A commercial sling is used to support injured or fractured arms.

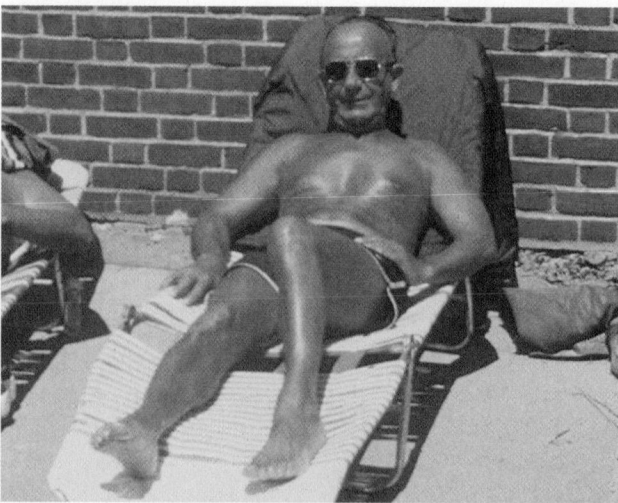

Figure 9-10   First-degree burns involve the top layer of skin.
(Courtesy of the Phoenix Society of Burn Survivors, Inc.)

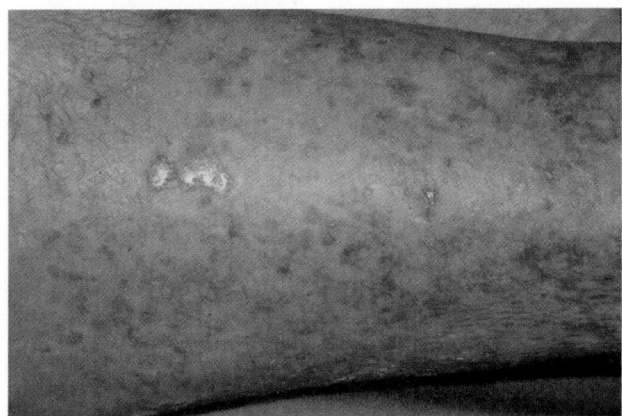

Figure 9-11 Second-degree burns affect the top layers of skin. The healing process is slower and scarring may occur. (Courtesy of the Phoenix Society of Burn Survivors, Inc.)

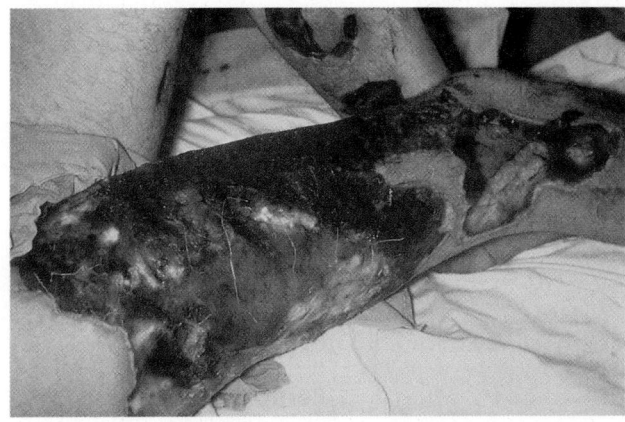

Figure 9-12 Third-degree burns are the most serious, affecting or destroying all layers of skin plus the fat, muscle, bones, and nerves. (Courtesy of the Phoenix Society of Burn Survivors, Inc.)

may take three to four weeks to heal. Some scarring may occur (Figure 9-11).

Third-degree burns are the most serious, affecting or destroying all layers of skin, plus the fat, muscles, bones, and nerves under the skin. These burns look charred or brown. There may be great pain or, if nerve endings are destroyed, the burn may be painless. Victims of third-degree burns must receive immediate medical attention both for the burn and for shock. Of serious concern with a third-degree burn, is the likelihood of infection and the amount of scarring that can result in loss of body function. Skin grafts may be necessary (Figure 9-12).

Figure 9-13 shows the relative penetration level of each degree of burn into the skin and underlying structures.

General Guidelines for Caring for Burns. Treatment for burns depends on the type of agent causing the burn. General treatment strategies for any degree of burn include the following:

- Cool the burn with large amounts of cool normal saline.
- Cover the burn with a sterile dressing if one is available and burn is minor. Otherwise, cover the burn with a sheet or other smooth textured cloth for a burn over a large area of the body.
- Be sure the patient is protected from being either chilled or overheated.

However, it is important to follow these guidelines:

- Do not apply ice or ice water to a burn.
- Do not touch a burn, except with a clean sterile dressing.
- Do not clean a severe burn, break blisters, or use any kind of ointment.
- Do not remove pieces of clothing that may be sticking to the burn.

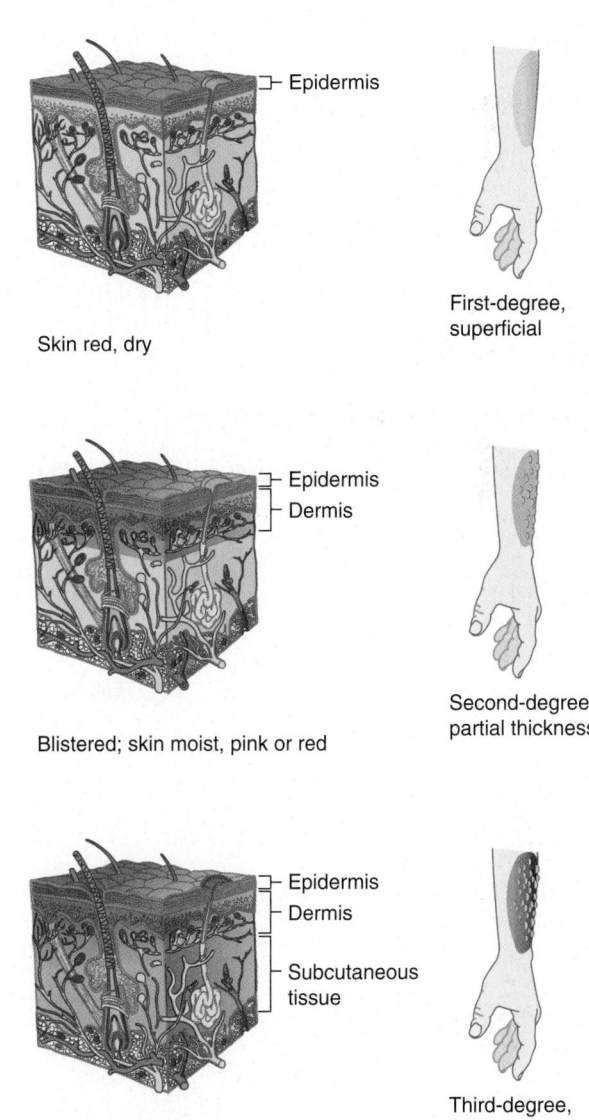

Figure 9-13 Classification of burn injuries.

First Aid for Burns. First aid for burns is outlined in Table 9-3.

Types of Burns. Most burns are caused by heat; however, burns can also be caused by chemicals, electricity, and solar radiation.

Chemical Burns. These can occur in the workplace or even in the home with "ordinary" household chemicals. In order to stop the burning process, the chemical must be removed from the skin. Have someone call an ambulance while you flush the skin or eyes with cool water. Remove any clothing contaminated by the chemicals unless they

---

TABLE 9-3   FIRST AID FOR BURNS

First-Degree Burn Response Guide

Questions	Responses	Action to Take	Rationale
Is skin reddened without blisters?	YES ⇨	Submerge in cool normal saline ⇨ 2–5 minutes.	Stops burning process.
NO ⇩			
Does area involve: • hands? • feet? • genitals? • face?	YES ⇨	Patient to come to office. ⇨	These are potential danger areas and require evaluation by the physician.
NO ⇩			
Is patient: • elderly? • very young?	YES ⇨	Patient to come to office. ⇨	These groups are very susceptible to burn complications.
NO ⇩			
Consult physician.			Physician has final decision whether patient is seen.

Second-Degree Burn Response Guide

Questions	Responses	Action to Take	Rationale
Is skin reddened with blisters or splitting of the skin?	YES ⇨	Submerge in cool normal saline ⇨ 10–15 minutes if skin is intact. Use compresses if skin is broken. Do not break blisters. Do not use anesthetic creams or sprays.	Stops burning process. If blisters are broken, can allow infection in burn. Creams or spray may slow healing process and increase severity of a burn.
NO ⇩			
Does area involve: • hands? • feet? • genitals? • face?	YES ⇨	Patient to come to office. ⇨	These are potentially dangerous areas and require medical attention.
NO ⇩			
Is the area involved larger than a child's hand?	YES ⇨	Patient to come to office. ⇨	Burns of this size are very susceptible to complications.
NO ⇩			
Is patient experiencing trouble breathing?	YES ⇨	Patient should go to emergency ⇨ room.	There may be swelling of the airways because of heat.
NO ⇩			
Consult physician.			Physician has final decision whether patient is seen.

(continues)

TABLE 9-3 *(continued)*

Third-Degree Burn Response Guide

Questions	Responses	Action to Take	Rationale
Is skin gray, black, or charred appearing? Can muscle, fat, or bone be seen in wound?	YES ⇨	Call EMS immediately. Do not ⇨ apply cold; do not remove burnt clothing from burn area.	Life-threatening emergency that requires prompt attention.
NO ⇩			
Is patient experiencing: • pallor? • loss of consciousness? • shivering?	YES ⇨	Patient in shock: ⇨ • maintain body temp. • elevate feet if appropriate. • monitor breathing. • call EMS.	Need to control shock due to loss of fluid.
NO ⇩			
Consult physician.			Physician has final decision whether patient is seen.

adhere to the skin. If clothing clings to the skin, it can be cut with scissors. Do not attempt to pull clothing away from burned area.

Electrical Burns. Electrical burns can be caused by power lines, lightning, or faulty electrical equipment in the home or workplace. **It is important to remember never to go near a patient injured by electricity until you are sure the power has been shut off because you could be injured.** If there is a downed line, call the power company and emergency medical services (EMS).

A victim of an electricity burn may be suffering from two burns: one where the power entered the body, and one where it exited. Often, the burns themselves may be minor. Of more serious consequence are the possibilities of shock, breathing difficulties, and other injuries. CPR is often needed here.

Solar Radiation. Most "sunburns," while not advisable nor good for the skin, present minor burns. If the patient has a severe burn, however, he should see a physician who will cover the burn area to reduce infection and protect the patient against chill.

Musculoskeletal Injuries

Most injuries to muscles, bones, and joints are not life threatening, but they are painful and, if not properly treated, can be disabling. Some injuries, such as those to the spinal cord, can be quite serious and can result in paralysis. These injuries are not typically seen in the ambulatory care setting.

Types of Injuries. A sprain is an injury to a joint, often an ankle, knee, or wrist, that involves a tearing of the ligaments. Most sprains are minor and heal quickly; others are more severe, include swelling, and may not heal properly if the patient continues to put stress on the sprained joint. Signs of a sprain are rapid swelling, discoloration at the site, and limited function. Many times it is difficult to determine whether the patient has sustained a sprain or a fracture because the degree of pain may not be a true indicator of the patient's injury. As with most closed wounds, treating the injury with the RICE method is beneficial.

A strain results from the overuse or stretching of a muscle or group of muscles, as with improper lifting or

---

Patient Teaching Tip

Some burns can be prevented. Advise patients who insist on sunbathing to protect themselves against harmful rays by using a sunscreen and avoiding the sun between 10 A.M. and 2 P.M.

Patient Teaching Tip

Advise patients not to run should their clothing catch on fire. They should fall to the ground or wrap themselves in a blanket or rug and roll on the ground to extinguish the flames.

moving heavy objects. Applications of ice and heat (as described for treatment of sprains), as well as rest, are indicated for treatment of strains.

Dislocations are painful and involve the separation of a bone from its normal position. These usually occur from the kind of wrenching motion that might result from a fall, automobile accident, or sports injury.

Fractures involve a break in a bone and can be caused by a fall, by a blow, from bone disease, or from sports injuries. There are several types of fractures, but all are classified as either open fractures or closed fractures. An open fracture involves an open wound and is characterized by a protruding bone. In a closed fracture, the skin is not broken. Signs and symptoms that occur with a fracture may include swelling, discoloration, pain, deformity, and immobility of the body part. It is not unusual for patients to tell you that they heard the bone break or that they sensed a grating feeling. **Crepitation** is the term that describes the grating sensation experienced when bone fragments rub together. Fractures are further defined as follows:

- Incomplete or greenstick: fracture in which the bone has cracked but the break is not all the way through. Frequently seen in children.

- Simple: complete bone break in which there is no involvement with the skin surface.

- Compound: fracture in which the bone protrudes though the skin surface, creating the possibility of infection.

- Impacted: fracture in which the broken ends are jammed into each other.

- Comminuted: more than one fracture line and several bone fragments are present.

- Spiral: fracture that occurs with a severe twisting action, causing the break to wind around the bone.

- Depressed: fracture that occurs with severe head injuries in which a broken piece of skull is driven inward.

- Colles: fracture often caused by falling on an outstretched hand. Involves the distal end of the radius and results in displacement, causing a bulge at the wrist.

See Figure 9-14 for examples of these fractures.

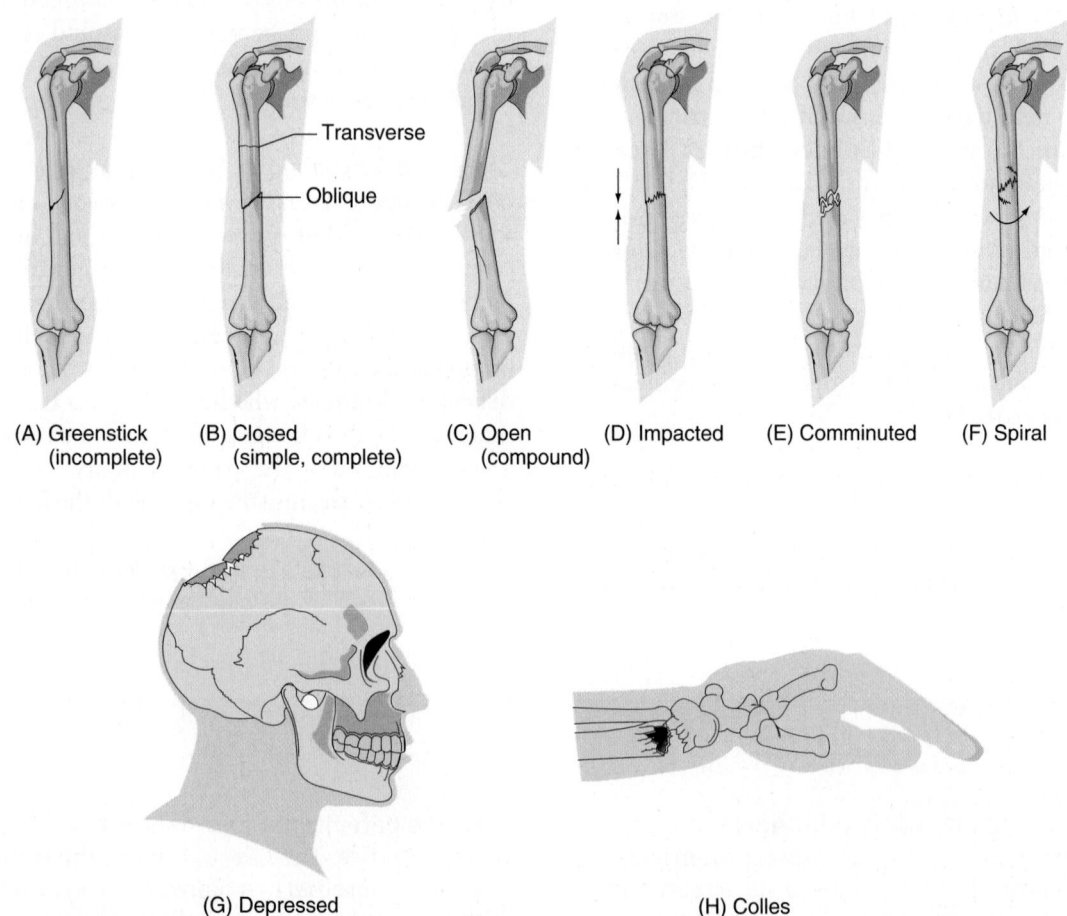

(A) Greenstick (incomplete)   (B) Closed (simple, complete)   (C) Open (compound)   (D) Impacted   (E) Comminuted   (F) Spiral

— Transverse
— Oblique

(G) Depressed   (H) Colles

Figure 9-14   Types of fractures.

Assessing Injuries to Muscles, Bones, and Joints. Sometimes it is difficult to determine the extent of an injury, especially in closed fractures. There are some assessment techniques to call upon, however, to gauge the seriousness of an injury.

- Note the extent of bruising and swelling.

- Pain is a signal of injury.

- There may be noticeable deformity to the bone or joint.

- Use of the injured area is limited.

- Talk to the patient: what was the cause of the injury? What was the sound or sensation at the time of injury?

Caring for Muscle, Bone, and Joint Injuries. Most injuries to muscles, bones, and joints are treated in a similar way; all require rest, elevation of the injured part, immobilization, and the application of ice to the injury.

After calling for outside care (always check for life-threatening symptoms, such as breathing difficulties, bleeding, or head, neck, or back injuries), it is important to immobilize the injured area if the patient must be moved. EMS personnel employ a variety of **splints** to immobilize bones and joints. See Procedure 9-2 for splinting an arm in the ambulatory care setting.

Heat- and Cold-Related Illnesses

The condition of patients who have been subject to extreme heat and cold can deteriorate very rapidly and either a heat- or cold-related illness can result in death. Individuals especially vulnerable to extreme exposures include the very young and very old; individuals who must work out of doors; and people who may suffer from poor circulation.

Heat-Related Illnesses. Illnesses related to heat, in increasing degree of severity, include heat cramps, heat exhaustion, and heat stroke. Heat cramps, the least serious, involve cramping in the legs and abdomen due to excessive body exposure or exercise in hot weather. Heat cramps should be considered a signal to stop, slow down, rest in a cool place, and drink plenty of water. Salt tablets should not be taken. The individual should lightly stretch the muscles. Heat cramps can progress to heat exhaustion or heat stroke, both more serious conditions.

Heat exhaustion, often experienced by people who work or exercise in extreme heat, is a more serious reaction and is signaled by exhaustion, cold and clammy skin, profuse sweating, headache, and general weakness. The individual should come out of the heat immediately, apply cool, wet towels, and slowly drink cool water. The physician will advise the patient not to resume activity in the heat.

Heat stroke is the least common, but the most dangerous of heat-related illnesses and requires immediate medical attention. Heat stroke is characterized by red, dry, hot skin, an abnormal, weak pulse, and breathing that is shallow and fast. In heat stroke, the body systems are extremely taxed. EMS should be alerted; until they arrive, stay with the patient, watch for breathing problems, and attempt to lower body temperature by applying cool, wet towels or sheets.

Cold-Related Illnesses. Exposure to extreme cold for prolonged periods can lead to frostbite or hypothermia.

Frostbite, which typically affects the extremities such as fingers, toes, ears, and nose, involves the freezing of exposed body parts. Symptoms include skin that becomes off-color, that is cold, or that takes on a waxy appearance. Severity can range from the superficial (frostnip) to more penetrating stages, which may require amputation.

Individuals with frostbite need immediate medical attention. To care for frostbitten extremities, warm the area of injury by wrapping clothing or blankets around the affected body part. Be careful in handling the frozen part. It is best to have the patient transported as soon as possible to emergency care. This type of facility is better able to properly rewarm the frozen part, preventing further tissue damage.

Hypothermia is a serious illness in which the body temperature falls to a perilously low level. It can result in death if the individual does not receive care and if the progression of hypothermia is not reversed. Hypothermia occurs when a person falls through the ice or is exposed to cold temperatures, for example, after getting lost in the woods while hiking. Symptoms include shivering, cold skin, and confusion.

After checking for breathing problems and alerting EMS, care for the patient. Make the individual comfortable, provide a source of warmth, such as a blanket, and *gradually* warm the body. If clothing is wet or cold, remove and put on dry clothing. In extreme cases, it may be necessary to provide rescue breathing, which is covered later in this chapter.

Poisoning

Poisons can enter the body in four ways:

- *Ingestion.* Ingested poisons enter the body by swallowing. Swallowed poisons may include medications, plant material, household chemicals, contaminated foods, and drugs.

- *Inhalation.* Poisons are inhaled into the body in poorly ventilated areas where cleaning fluids, paints and chemical cleaners, or carbon monoxide may be present.

- *Absorption.* Poisons absorbed through the skin include plant materials such as poison oak or ivy, lawn care products such as chemical pesticides, and other chemical powders or liquids.

- *Injection.* Drug abuse is the most common cause of injected poisons. The stingers of insects inject poisons into the body and can be extremely dangerous and lead to anaphylactic shock in allergic individuals.

Whenever a patient calls regarding poisoning or there is a suspicion of poisoning, call the local poison control center or the local emergency number and ask for advice. Telephone numbers of the poison control center should be posted in a familiar and accessible place.

The treatment for poisoning will vary according to the source of the poisoning and must be tailored to the specific incident. The physician will have advised staff regarding specific poisoning antidotes. Generally, do not give the patient anything to eat or drink; try to determine what poison the patient was exposed to and, if ingested, how much was taken; if the patient vomits, save some of the vomitus for analysis.

If prescribed by a physician, two medications used to treat poisoning include syrup of ipecac, which can induce vomiting, and activated charcoal, which is used to absorb certain swallowed poisons.

Insect Stings. The medical assistant in the ambulatory care setting is likely to receive a number of calls every summer from patients who have been stung by insects, typically yellow jackets, hornets, honeybees, or wasps. In the nonallergic patient, the sting is likely to result in localized swelling and tenderness and slight redness. The physician will recommend that these localized symptoms be managed with a topical cream and oral antihistamines. Swelling can be significant and cause for serious concern if the sting occurred in a vulnerable area of the body such as the mouth or tongue. Swelling in these locations can be

Patient Teaching Tip

Remind patients who are parents of young children to remove any potential sources of poisoning from their homes or to keep them in locked cabinets. Also advise them to include the nearby poison control center in their list of emergency phone numbers. They should also keep syrup of ipecac and activated charcoal on hand.

Patient Teaching Tip

Advise all patients with known allergic reactions to be particularly careful when working or playing outdoors. Insects are not usually aggressive until their nests are approached; however, often these nests are not easy to detect and an individual may approach one without being aware of its presence. Patients with allergies to insects should always wear shoes out-of-doors, wear light-colored clothing, preferably with long sleeves and pant legs, look before taking a sip from a beverage when outdoors, and inspect lawn areas, shrubbery, and building walls periodically for evidence of stinging insect nests.

frightening and dangerous because it can impair breathing. An antihistamine, administered as soon as possible after the sting, may help to curtail symptoms somewhat. Treatment for insect stings in nonallergic individuals consists of removing the stinger by scraping it off with the edge of something rigid such as a credit card or your fingernail. Tweezers can cause more venom to be dispersed into the patient's body tissues so should not be used. Wash the area with soap and water, apply a cold pack to the site, and watch for an anaphylactic reaction.

The individual who experiences an allergic reaction or hypersensitivity to a sting needs to be seen immediately, for in severe cases a sting may induce an anaphylactic reaction which can lead to death. If allergic, individuals who have been stung are likely to experience symptoms within a half-hour after the incident. Symptoms are generalized throughout the body and may include hives, itching, lightheadedness, and may progress to difficulty breathing, faintness, and eventual loss of consciousness.

For individuals with known allergic reactions, the physician will prescribe epinephrine, which patients should carry with them and self-inject should they not be able to get immediate emergency care. The patient should then seek immediate emergency treatment. For individuals who present at the ambulatory care setting with an apparent allergic reaction to a sting, the physician will prescribe epinephrine. Attempt to allay patient apprehension and monitor vital signs while waiting for EMS personnel to arrive.

Sudden Illness

Sudden illness is, by definition, an unexpected occurrence. While the cause of the illness may be inexplicable, it is important to respond sensibly and responsibly within the parameters of knowledge and resources.

Sudden illnesses include, but are not limited to, fainting, seizures, diabetic reaction, and hemorrhage.

Fainting. Also known as syncope, fainting involves a loss of consciousness, caused by an insufficient supply of blood to the brain. Loss of consciousness may simply be the result of a fainting episode or it may indicate a more serious medical problem such as diabetic coma or shock. A fall during a fainting incident may result in bodily harm.

If a patient in the office or clinic "feels faint," indicated by lightheadedness, weakness, nausea, or unsteadiness, have the individual lie down or sit down with head level with the knees. This may prevent a fainting spell. As a part of office policy, aromatic spirits of ammonia may be administered to revive the patient who faints. **CAUTION:** Hold the crushed ampule of ammonia at least six inches away from the patient's nose and eyes. Move it back and forth since the fumes are very irritating to eyes and mucous membranes.

If a patient faints, gradually lower the patient to a flat surface, loosen any tight clothing, and check breathing and for any life-threatening emergencies. Elevate the legs if there is no back or head injury. If vomiting occurs, place the patient on the side. While fainting is typically not serious in itself, 911 or EMS may need to be called since the problem may be indicative of a more complex medical condition.

Seizures. Seizures or convulsions occur when normal brain functioning is disrupted, which can occur for a variety of reasons including fever, disease such as diabetes, infection, or injury to the brain. Epilepsy is a common cause of convulsions. Involuntary spasms or contractions of muscles characterize seizures.

To the onlooker, seizures look frightening and painful, which may lead inexperienced individuals to try to stop the seizure when they see it occurring in another individual. A patient suffering from a seizure should never be restrained; simply care for the victim of a seizure with compassion and medical understanding. The goal is to protect the patient from self-injury during the episode. Also, do not force anything between the patient's clenched teeth—individuals experiencing seizures cannot "swallow" their tongues.

Most patients will recover from a seizure in a few minutes. During the seizure, protect the patient from injury, cushion the patient's head, and roll the patient to the side if any fluid is in the mouth. After the seizure subsides, calm and comfort the patient.

If a patient is known to regularly have seizures, and the patient's seizure subsides in a matter of minutes, EMS personnel do not need to be summoned. Repeated seizures during the same time frame, however, dictate a call to emergency services, as does any seizure if the patient is diabetic, pregnant, injured, or does not regain consciousness after the incident.

Diabetes. Diabetes is defined by the American Diabetes Society as the "inability of the body to properly convert sugar from food into energy."

Under normal functioning, the body produces a hormone called insulin, which transports sugars into body cells. In some cases, the body does not produce insulin or does not produce enough insulin; this results in diabetes.

Diabetes occurs in two major types:

- Type I, or insulin-dependent diabetes.

- Type II, or noninsulin-dependent diabetes, which usually occurs in adults. In Type II, the body produces insulin in insufficient quantities.

Complications from diabetes, which you may encounter in a medical office or clinic setting, include diabetic coma (acidosis) and insulin shock or reaction. The physician will prescribe either insulin or glucose prior to the patient being transported to the hospital. Both are serious emergencies that require immediate EMS assistance. See Table 9-4 for common causes and symptoms of diabetic coma or insulin shock.

Hemorrhage. The different sources of bleeding determine the seriousness of hemorrhage, or bleeding.

External Bleeding. External bleeding includes capillary, venous, and arterial bleeding. Capillary bleeding, often from cuts and scratches, usually clots without first-aid measures. Bleeding from a vein, which is characterized by dark red blood that flows steadily, needs to be controlled quickly (see Procedure 9-1) to avoid excessive blood loss. Bleeding from an artery produces bright red bleeding that spurts from the wound; this is the most serious type of bleeding and occurs when an artery is punctured or severed. Like venous bleeding, arterial bleeding requires immediate emergency care, for serious loss of blood and profound irreversible shock can quickly ensue.

Epistaxis, or nosebleed, may be the result of breathing dry air for a long period of time; may result from injury or blowing the nose too hard; may be caused by high altitudes; may be caused by hypertension (high blood pressure); or may result from overuse of medications such as aspirin and anticoagulants.

To control nosebleeds, seat the patient, elevate the patient's head, and pinch the nostrils for at least ten minutes. Assist the patient to sit with head tilted forward so blood running down the back of the throat will not be aspirated. If bleeding cannot be controlled, the physician may request that you activate EMS.

TABLE 9-4   CAUSES AND SYMPTOMS OF DIABETIC COMA AND INSULIN SHOCK

Diabetic Coma or Acidosis		Insulin Shock or Reaction	
Causes	Too little insulin, too much to eat, infections, fever, emotional stress	Causes	Too much insulin or oral hypoglycemic drug, too little to eat, an unusual amount of exercise
Symptoms	Skin: Dry and flushed	Symptoms	Skin: Moist and pale
	Behavior: Drowsy		Behavior: Often excited
	Mouth: Dry		Mouth: Drooling
	Thirst: Intense		Thirst: Absent
	Hunger: Absent		Hunger: Present
	Vomiting: Common		Vomiting: Usually absent
	Respiration: Exaggerated, air hungry		Respiration: Normal or shallow
	Breath: Fruity odor of acetone		Breath: Usually normal
	Pulse: Weak and rapid		Pulse: Full and pounding (gives patient feeling of heart pounding)
	Vision: Dim		Vision: Diplopia (double)
	Blood glucose over 200 mg/100 ml		Blood glucose low (40–70 mg/100 ml)
First aid	Keep patient warm	First aid	If conscious, give patient sugar or any food containing sugar (fruit juice, candy, crackers, etc.)
	Obtain medical help immediately		Obtain medical help immediately

Internal Bleeding. Internal bleeding may be minor or serious depending on the cause of the injury. A contusion, or bruise, will result in minor internal bleeding. A sharp blow may induce severe internal bleeding.

Because there is no visible blood flow, it is important to recognize other symptoms of internal bleeding. Symptoms are similar to those of shock and include a rapid, weak pulse, shallow breathing, cold, clammy skin, dilated pupils, dizziness, faintness, thirst, restlessness, and a feeling of anxiety. There may be pain, tenderness, or swelling at the injury site. The abdomen may be board-like.

If internal bleeding is suspected, ask another staff member to call EMS; until they arrive, stay with the patient and take measures to prevent shock. Monitor vital signs.

Cerebral Vascular Accident (CVA)

The common term for a cerebral vascular accident (CVA) is stroke. A stroke is the result of a ruptured blood vessel in the brain; it can also be caused by the occlusion of a blood vessel or by a clot. Both these situations can result in blood spilling over brain cells and depriving them of oxygen, causing them to die. Symptoms of a stroke

include numbness in face, arm, leg on one side of the body, loss of vision, severe headache, mental confusion, slurred speech, nausea, vomiting, and difficulty in breathing and swallowing. Paralysis may be present. If a patient is suspected of having a stroke, call EMS, loosen tight clothing, lie the patient down and keep her comfortable. Position the patient's head to facilitate flow of secretion from the mouth to avoid choking and maintain an open airway. Do not give anything by mouth and monitor vital signs. Immediate emergency care is critical for all individuals experiencing strokes. If the stroke is caused by a clot that blocks blood flow, a recently released drug may be able to protect the individual from permanent injury. Rapid transport to the hospital is important for treatment to be instituted as soon as possible. Treatment with the clot-dissolving drug must be given within three hours of onset of symptoms.

Heart Attack

Heart attack, also known as myocardial infarction, is usually caused by blockage of one or more of the coronary arteries. Symptoms include tightness of the chest, pain radiating down one or both arms, or pain radiating into the left shoulder and jaw. Other signs include rapid and weak pulse, excessive perspiration, agitation, nausea, and cold, clammy skin.

If you suspect the patient is experiencing a heart attack, contact EMS immediately, loosen tight clothing, and keep the patient comfortable. Prepare to give oxygen and other medications such as aspirin as directed by the physician. Monitor vital signs. If the patient suffers an

Patient Teaching Tip

Advise the patient not to blow the nose for several hours following an epistaxis.

episode of cardiac fibrillation, cardioversion or defibrillation may be necessary. See Chapter 18. Prepare to begin CPR if necessary.

PROCEDURES FOR BREATHING EMERGENCIES AND CARDIAC ARREST

Breathing or respiratory emergencies occur for a variety of reasons, including choking, shock, allergies, and other illnesses or injuries such as drowning and electrical shock. When an individual stops breathing, artificial breathing must be given quickly, for without a constant supply of oxygen, brain damage or death will occur.

When the breathing problem is accompanied by cardiac arrest, the rescue breathing must be accompanied by chest compressions. This is known as **cardiopulmonary resuscitation (CPR)**. Cardiac emergencies may occur in the medical office due to the large number of patients who have heart disease.

The procedures that follow will help you respond to breathing emergencies in your clinic or office until EMS arrives. The techniques vary for conscious and unconscious individuals, and for adults, children, and infants. These procedures are for review purposes only; it is essential that every medical assistant take first aid and CPR courses and frequent refresher courses.

Heimlich Maneuver (Abdominal Thrust)

A common cause of breathing difficulty results from choking. If an individual signals distress from choking, assist the patient in coughing up the object (Figures 9-15 and 9-16). If the patient cannot cough up the object, and the breathing airway is becoming completely blocked, act immediately. It is apparent that the airway is becoming blocked when the patient cannot cough or speak and the patient uses the universal sign for choking.

Have someone call an ambulance while you perform abdominal thrusts, known as the **Heimlich maneuver**. Patients can be taught to give themselves abdominal thrusts if they are alone and choking (Figure 9-17).

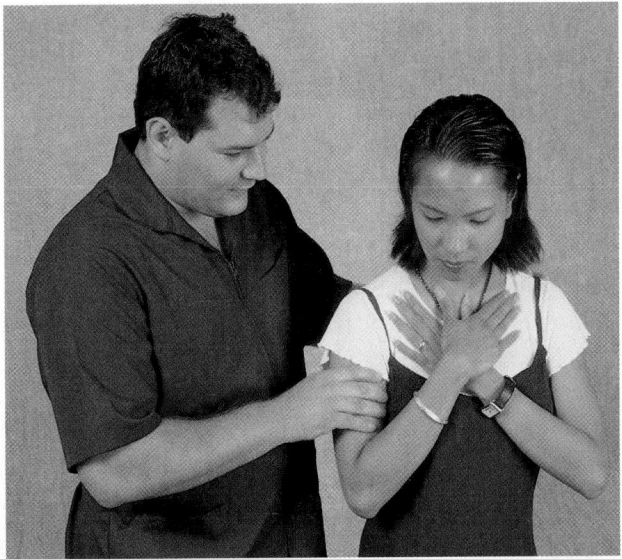

Figure 9-16 Assist the patient in coughing up an object by encouraging continuous coughing.

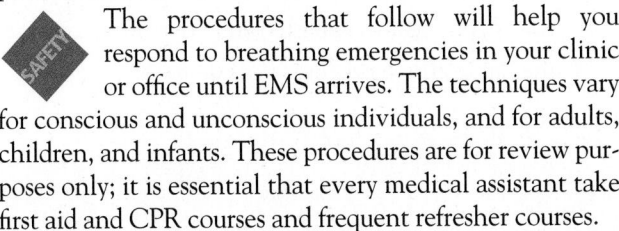

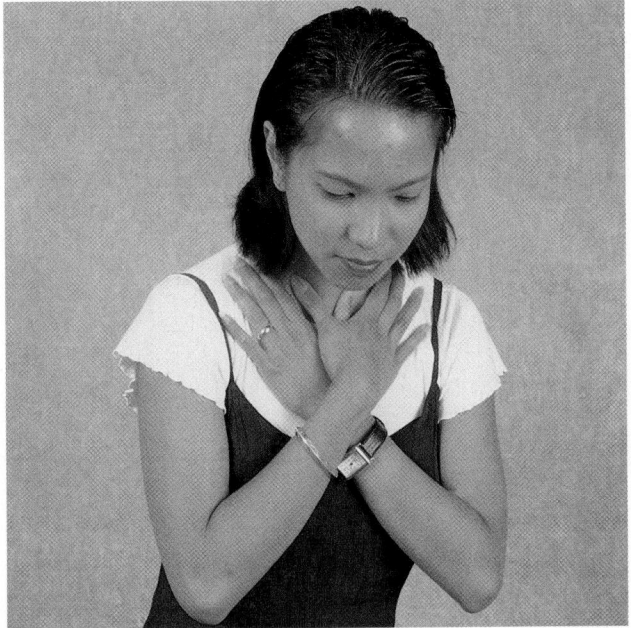

Figure 9-15 Universal sign for choking.

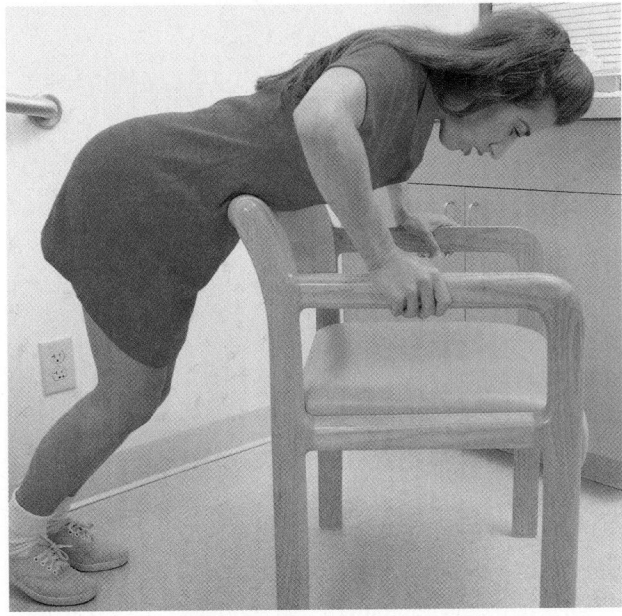

Figure 9-17 If alone, individuals can self-administer the Heimlich maneuver by using the back of a chair or similar hard object.

Patient Teaching Tip

Teach patients to perform the abdominal thrust when they are alone and choking. To perform the Heimlich maneuver when alone, use the fist or thrust against a chair back or any other hard object of adequate height that reaches just below the navel. See Figure 9-17.

Procedures 9-3, 9-4, 9-5, 9-6, and 9-7 describe how to perform the Heimlich maneuver for adults, children, and infants; these reflect the American Red Cross updates effective July 2001.

Rescue Breathing

Individuals in respiratory arrest require immediate emergency care. **Rescue breathing**, previously called mouth-to-mouth resuscitation, provides oxygen to the patient until emergency personnel arrive.

When performing rescue breathing procedures in the ambulatory care setting, it is recommended that resuscitation mouthpieces be used and that direct mouth-to-mouth (i.e., with no personal protective equipment) resuscitation never be used.

Procedures for rescue breathing differ for adults, children, and infants. See Procedures 9-8, 9-9, and 9-10.

Cardiopulmonary Resuscitation (CPR)

The combination of rescue breathing and chest compressions is known as CPR, which stands for cardiopulmonary resuscitation. Alone, CPR cannot save an individual from cardiac arrest—it represents preliminary care until advanced medical help is available to the heart attack victim. See proceedures 9-11, 9-12, and 9-13.

When performing CPR, the rule is that you do not stop until

- another trained person can take over
- EMS arrives and takes over care of the patient
- you are physically exhausted and not able to continue
- the environment becomes unsafe for any reason

Procedure 9-1   Control of Bleeding

STANDARD PRECAUTIONS:

PURPOSE:
To control bleeding caused by an open wound.

EQUIPMENT/SUPPLIES:
Sterile dressings
Sterile gloves
Mask and eye protection
Gown
Biohazard waste container

PROCEDURE STEPS:
1. Wash hands.
2. Put on gloves.
3. Apply eye and mask protection and gown if splashing is likely to occur.
4. Assemble equipment and supplies.
5. Apply dressing and press firmly (Figure 9-18A).
6. Apply pressure bandage over the dressing.

7. If bleeding continues, elevate arm above heart level (Figure 9-18B).
8. If bleeding still continues, press adjacent artery against bone (Figure 9-18C). Notify the physician if bleeding cannot be controlled.

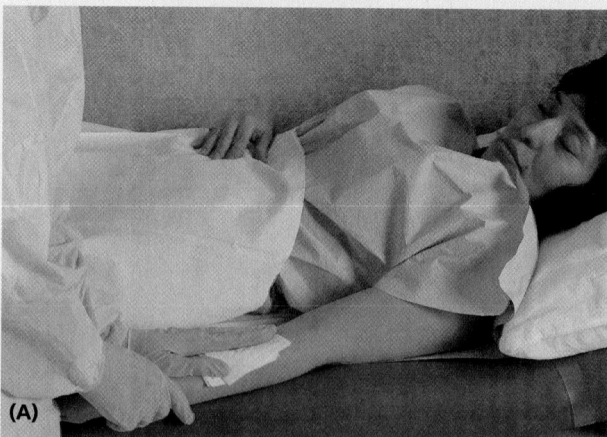
(A)

Figure 9-18   (A) Apply dressing and press firmly.

(continues)

Procedure 9-1 (continued)

9. Dispose of waste in biohazard container.
10. Remove gloves, dispose of in biohazard container.
11. Wash hands.
12. Document procedure.

CAUTION: If bleeding is not controlled, the patient may go into hemorrhagic shock. Be prepared to call EMS immediately.

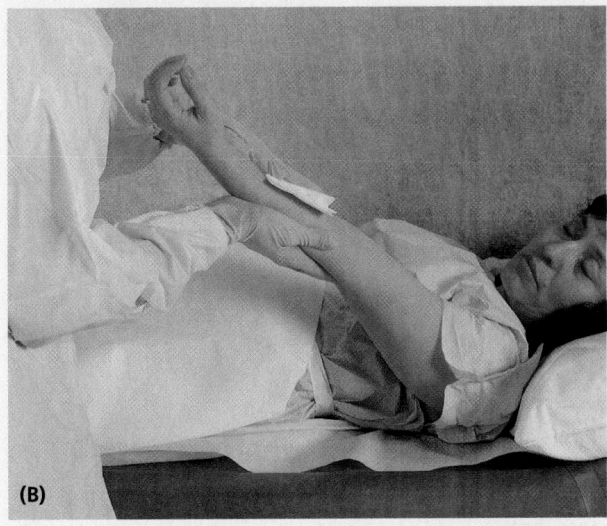
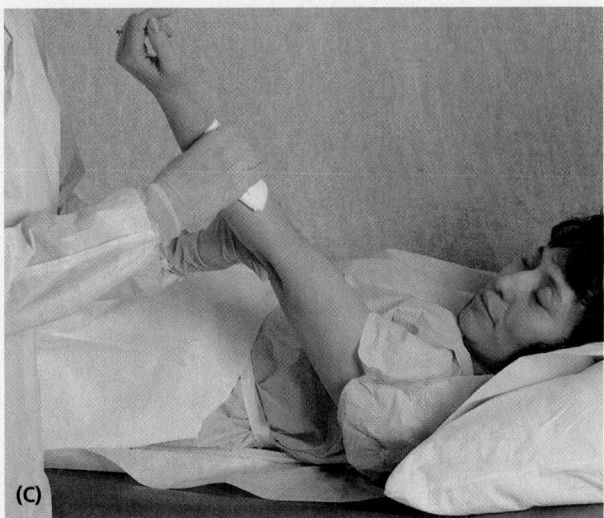

Figure 9-18   (B) Elevate arm above heart level. (C) Press artery against bone.

Procedure 9-2 Applying an Arm Splint

STANDARD PRECAUTIONS:

PURPOSE:

To immobilize the area above and below the injured part of the arm in order to reduce pain and prevent further injury.

EQUIPMENT/SUPPLIES:

Thin piece of rigid board; cardboard can be used if necessary
Gauze roller bandage

PROCEDURE STEPS:

1. Place the padded splint under the injured area.
2. Hold the splint in place with gauze roller bandage.
3. After splinting, check circulation (note color and temperature of skin, check pulse) to ascertain that the splint is not too tightly applied.
4. A sling can now be applied to keep the arm elevated, which increases comfort and reduces swelling.
5. Wash hands.
6. Document the procedure.

Procedure 9-3 Heimlich Maneuver for a Conscious Adult

STANDARD PRECAUTIONS:

PURPOSE:
To open up a blocked airway.

EQUIPMENT/SUPPLIES:
None needed

PROCEDURE STEPS:
1. Place the thumb side of your fist against the middle of the abdomen, just above the umbilicus and below the xiphoid process.
2. Grasp your fist with your other hand and give quick upward thrusts (Figure 9-19).
3. Repeat the procedure until the patient coughs up the object. If the person becomes unconscious, perform abdominal thrusts for an unconscious individual (Procedure 9-4).
4. Wash hands.
5. Document the procedure.

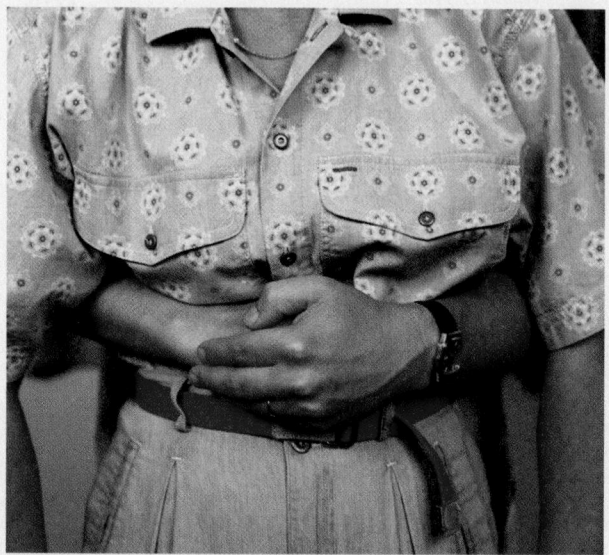

Figure 9-19   Grasp your fist with your other hand and give quick thrusts.

Procedure 9-4 Heimlich Maneuver for an Unconscious Adult or Child

STANDARD PRECAUTIONS:

  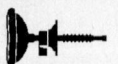

PURPOSE:
To open up a blocked airway.

EQUIPMENT/SUPPLIES:
Gloves
Resuscitation mouthpiece
Biohazard waste container

PROCEDURE STEPS:
1. Have someone call emergency services.
2. Put on gloves if available.

3. Lie person on back. Open victim's mouth and look for foreign object. Position resuscitation mouthpiece. Tilt back person's head (Figure 9-20A).
4. Give two breaths (Figure 9-20B).
5. If air will not go in, retilt head to try to give two breaths again. If air will not go in, give 15 chest compressions.
6. Find hand position on breast bone 2 inches above xiphoid and compress 2 inches deep. (For child, give 5 compressions, 1½ inches deep.)
7. Lift the jaw, look for object, and sweep it out of the mouth with finger, if seen (Figure 9-20C).
8. Tilt back the head, lift the chin, and give breaths again slowly. Continue giving breaths and com-

(continues)

Procedure 9-4 *(continued)*

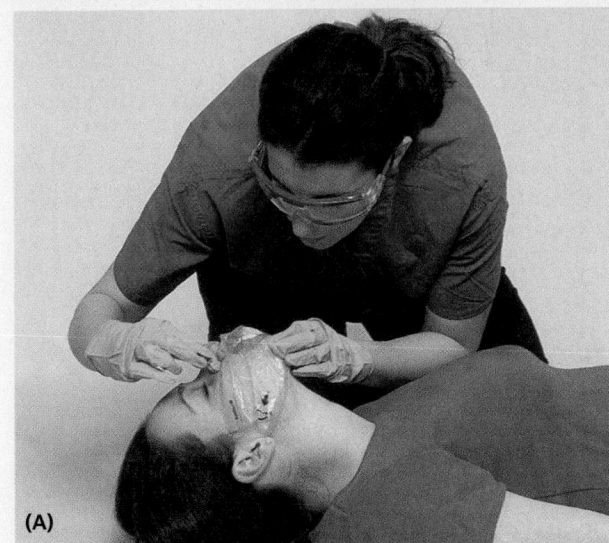

(A)

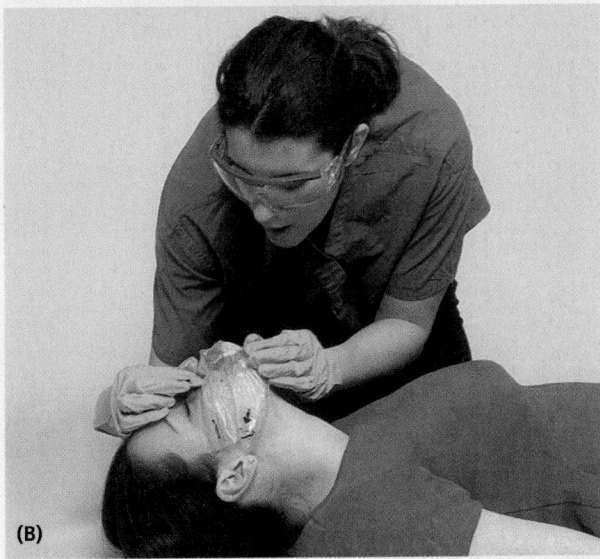

(B)

pressions, looking for object and sweeping it out if seen. Continue breathing until breaths go in. If the airway is cleared and victim does not begin to breathe on his own, prepare to perform CPR (Procedure 9-11).

9. Dispose of waste in biohazard container.
10. Remove gloves, dispose of in biohazard container, and wash hands.
11. Monitor vital signs.
12. Document the procedure.

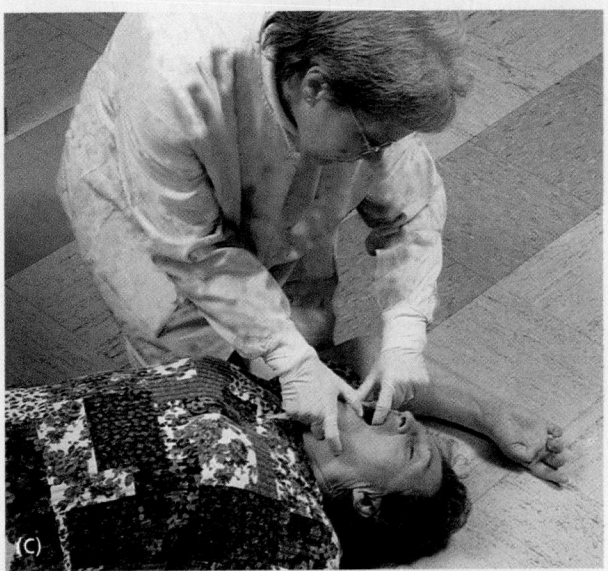

(C)

Figure 9-20   (A) Tilt back head. (B) Give breaths. (C) Lift jaw and sweep out mouth.

Procedure 9-5   Heimlich Maneuver for a Conscious Child

STANDARD PRECAUTIONS:

PURPOSE:
To open up a blocked airway.

EQUIPMENT/SUPPLIES:
None needed

PROCEDURE STEPS:
1. Place the thumb side of your fist against the middle of the child's abdomen, just above the umbilicus and below the xiphoid process (Figure 9-21A).
2. Grasp your fist with your other hand. Give quick upward thrusts (Figure 9-21B). Repeat the procedure until the object is expelled or until the patient loses consciousness (see Heimlich maneuver for unconscious child, Procedure 9-4).
3. Wash hands.
4. Document the procedure.

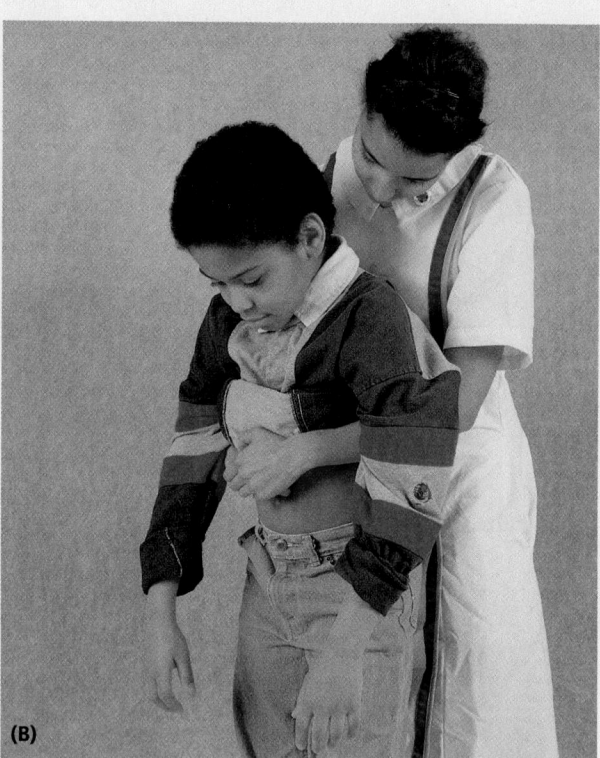

(A)   (B)

Figure 9-21   (A) Place the thumb side of your fist against the middle of the abdomen, just above the umbilicus and below the xiphoid process. (B) Grasp your fist with your other hand and give quick upward thrusts.

Procedure 9-6

Back Blows and Chest Thrusts for a Conscious Infant Who Is Choking

STANDARD PRECAUTIONS:

PURPOSE:
To open up a blocked airway and assist an infant unable to cough, cry, or breathe.

EQUIPMENT/SUPPLIES:
None needed

PROCEDURE STEPS:

1. With the infant face down on your forearm, give five back blows between the infant's shoulder blades with the heel of your hand (Figure 9-22A).

2. Position the infant face up on your forearm.
3. Give five chest compressions ½ to 1 inch deep, on about the center of the breastbone (Figure 9-22B).
4. Look in the infant's mouth for the object. Repeat the back blows and chest compressions and look for object until the infant begins to breathe on own. If the infant becomes unconscious, use back blow and chest compression techniques for unconscious infants (Procedure 9-7).
5. Wash hands.
6. Document the procedure.

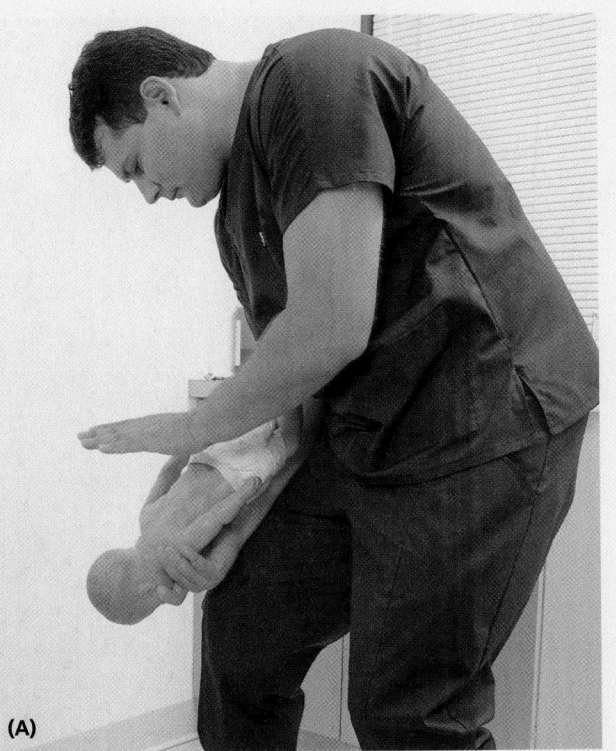

(A)

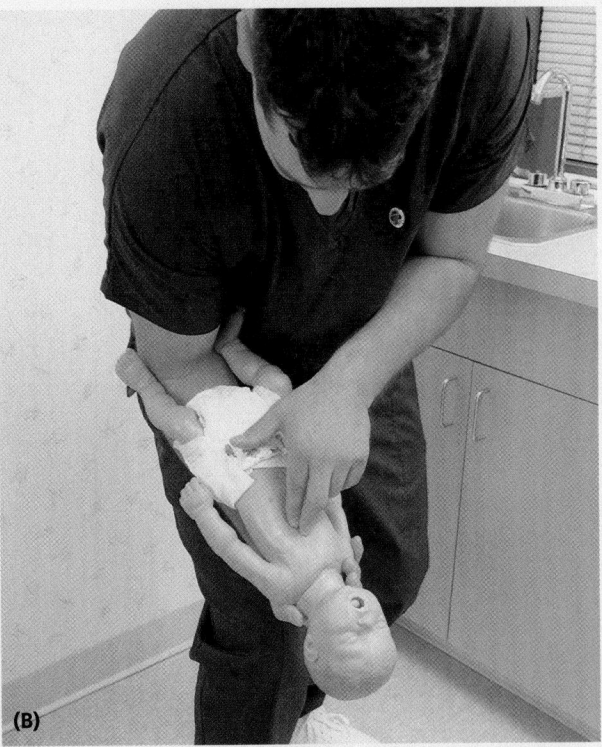

(B)

Figure 9-22   (A) With the infant face down on your forearm, give five back blows. (B) With the infant face up on your forearm, give five chest thrusts.

Procedure 9-7

Back Blows and Chest Thrusts for an Unconscious Infant

STANDARD PRECAUTIONS:

PURPOSE:
To open up a blocked airway.

EQUIPMENT/SUPPLIES:
Gloves
Resuscitation mouthpiece

PROCEDURE STEPS:
1. Have someone call emergency services.
2. Don gloves. Tap the infant gently to check for consciousness.
3. Gently tilt back the infant's head. Do not hyper-extend (Figure 9-23A).
4. Listen and watch for breathing.
5. Apply resuscitation mouthpiece. Give two breaths, covering infant's nose and mouth with your mouth (Figure 9-23B).
6. If air will not go in, retilt head, attempt to give breaths again.
7. If breaths still will not go in, give chest compressions ½ to 1 inch deep.
8. Lift jaw and tongue and check for object. If you see the object, sweep it out (Figure 9-23C).
9. Tilt back head and give one breath again.
10. Repeat breaths and chest compressions, and check for object until breaths go in. If the infant does not begin to breathe on his own, prepare to perform CPR.
11. Remove gloves. Wash hands.
12. Document the procedure.

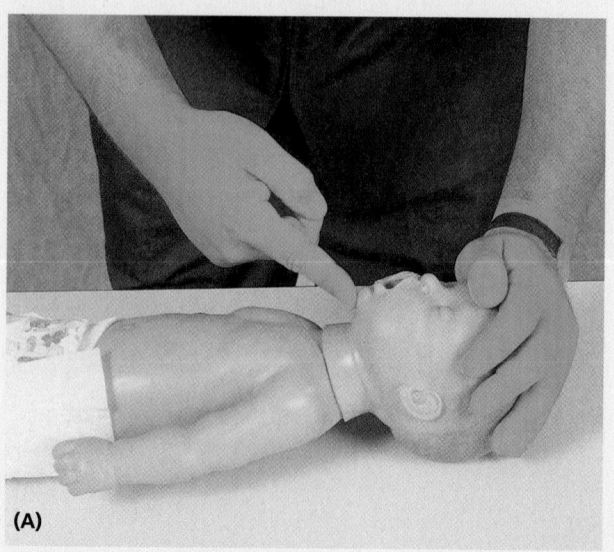

(A)

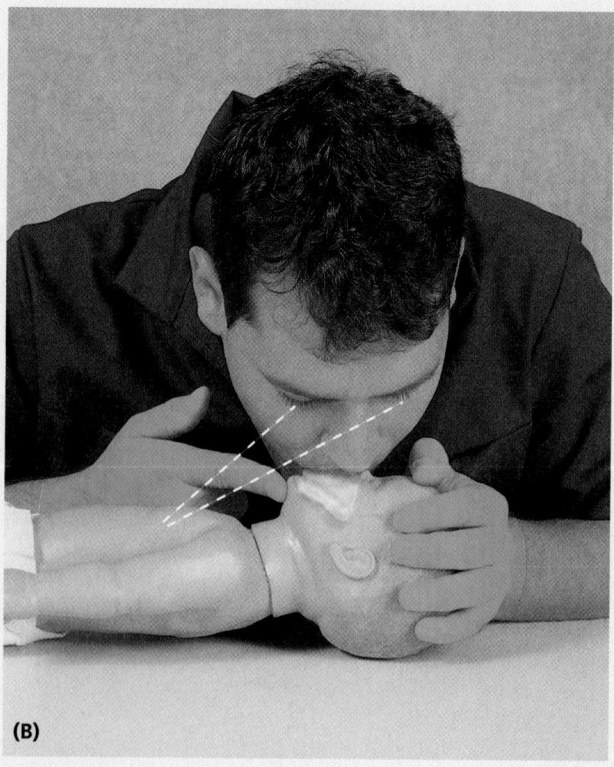

(B)

Figure 9-23   (A) Gently tilt back head. (B) Give two breaths, covering the infant's nose and mouth.   *(continues)*

Procedure

9-7 **(continued)**

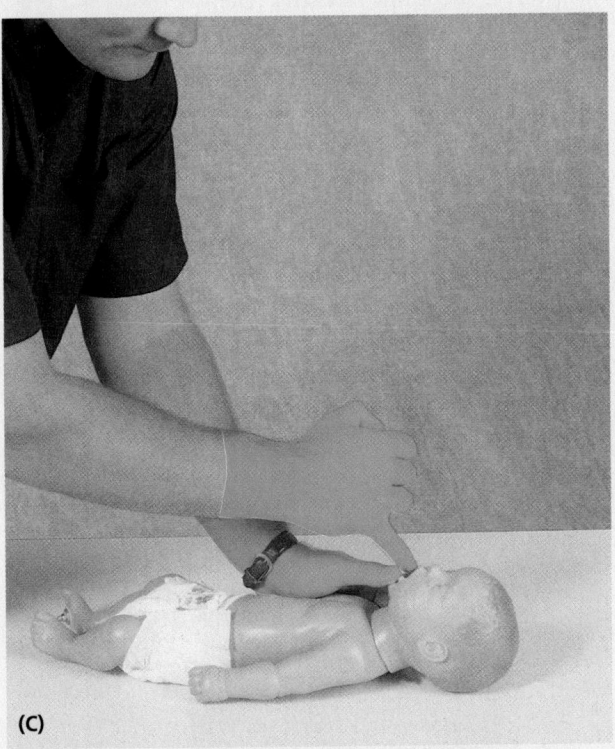

(C)

Figure 9-23 (C) Lift jaw and tongue. Check for object and, if seen, sweep out.

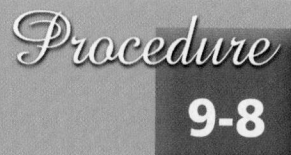

9-8   Rescue Breathing for Adults

STANDARD PRECAUTIONS:

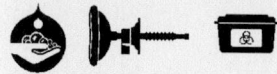

PURPOSE:
To respond to a breathing emergency.

EQUIPMENT/SUPPLIES:
Biohazard waste container
Resuscitation mouthpiece

PROCEDURE STEPS:

1. Have someone call emergency services.
2. Tilt back the head, lift the chin, position resuscitation mouthpiece, and pinch the nose closed (Figure 9-24A).
3. Give two slow breaths. Breathe into patient until the chest gently rises. Turn your face to the side and listen and watch for air to return.
4. Check for pulse on the carotid artery (Figure 9-24B).
5. If pulse is present, but the person is not breathing, give one slow breath every five seconds. Do this for one minute.
6. Recheck pulse and breathing every minute.
7. Continue rescue breathing as long as pulse is present and the person is not breathing. Continue until breathing is restored or another person takes over.
8. Dispose of waste in biohazard container.
9. Wash hands.
10. Document procedure.

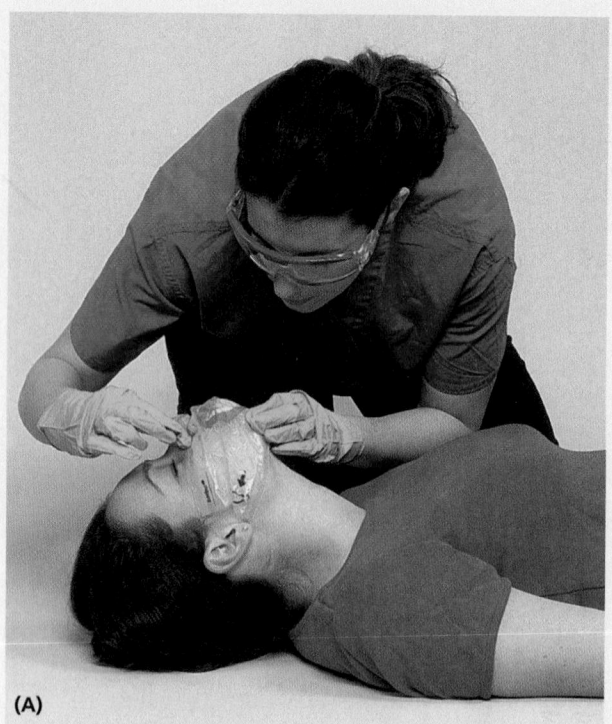

(A)

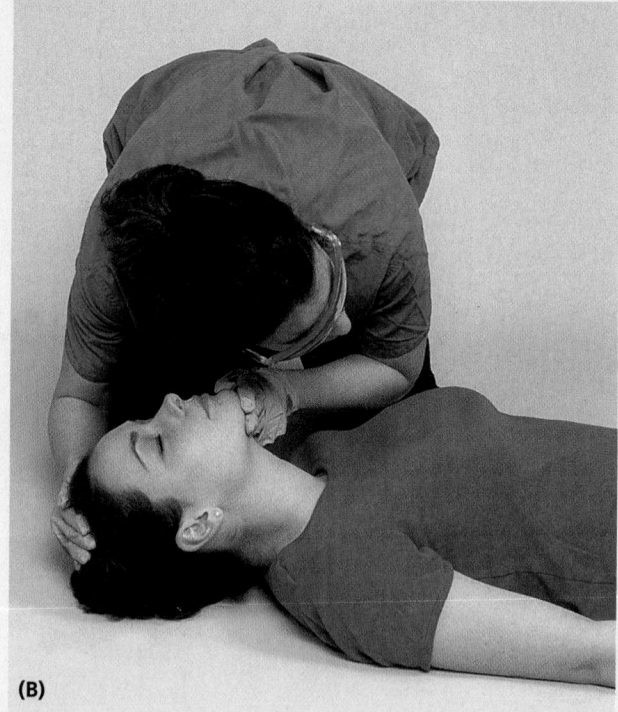

(B)

Figure 9-24   (A) Tilt back head, lift chin, position resuscitation mouthpiece, pinch nose closed, and give two short breaths. (B) Check for pulse at the carotid artery.

Procedure

9-9 Rescue Breathing for Children

STANDARD PRECAUTIONS:

PURPOSE:
To respond to a breathing emergency.

EQUIPMENT/SUPPLIES:
Gloves
Resuscitation mouthpiece

PROCEDURE STEPS:
1. Have someone call emergency services.
2. Don gloves.

3. Tilt back the head, lift the chin, position the resuscitation mouthpiece, pinch the nose closed, and give two short breaths (Figure 9-25A). If air does not go in, retilt head and breathe again.
4. Check for a pulse at the carotid artery (Figure 9-25B).
5. If pulse is present, but the child is not breathing, give one slow breath every three seconds. Do this for one minute.
6. Recheck pulse and breathing every minute.
7. Continue rescue breathing as long as pulse is present but the child is not breathing.
8. Remove gloves. Wash hands.
9. Document the procedure.

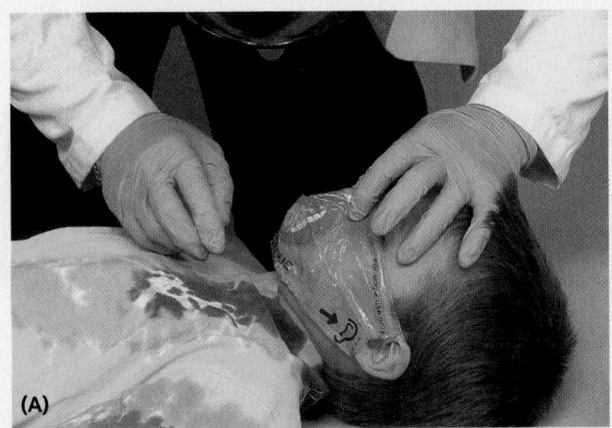

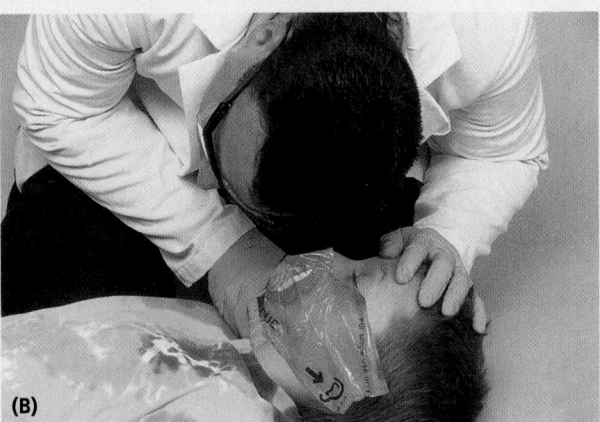

Figure 9-25 (A) Tilt back head, lift chin, position resuscitation mouthpiece, pinch nose closed, and give two short breaths. (B) Check for pulse at the carotid artery.

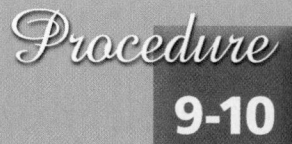

Procedure

9-10   Rescue Breathing for Infants

STANDARD PRECAUTIONS:

PURPOSE:
To respond to a breathing emergency.

EQUIPMENT/SUPPLIES:
Gloves
Resuscitation mouthpiece

PROCEDURE STEPS:
1. Have someone call emergency services.
2. Don gloves.
3. Tilt back the head (Figure 9-26A).

4. Position resuscitation mouthpiece. Seal your lips tightly around the infant's nose and mouth (Figure 9-26B).
5. Give two slow breaths. Breathe into the infant until the chest rises.
6. Check for a pulse at the brachial artery (Figure 9-26C).
7. If pulse is present, but infant is not breathing, give one slow breath every three seconds. Do this for one minute.
8. Recheck pulse and breathing every minute (Figure 9-26D).
9. Continue rescue breathing as long as pulse is present but the infant is not breathing.
10. Remove gloves. Wash hands.
11. Document the procedure.

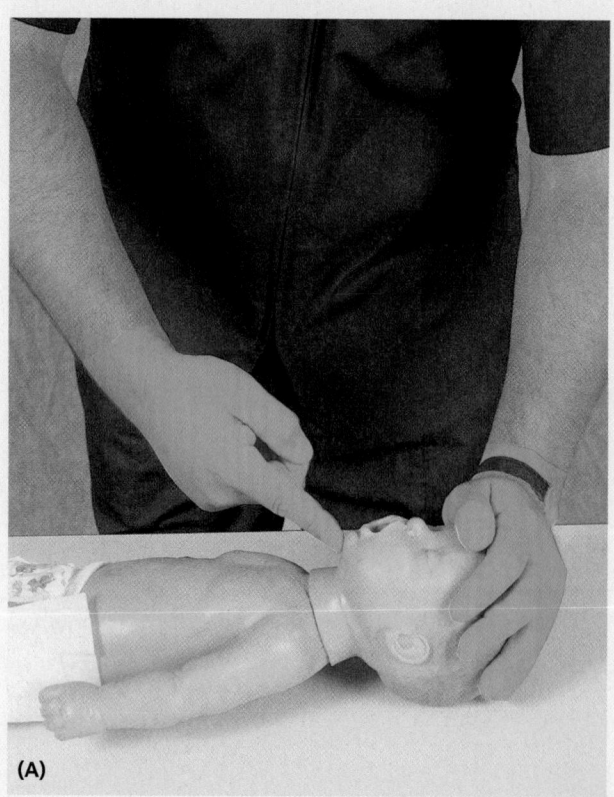

(A)

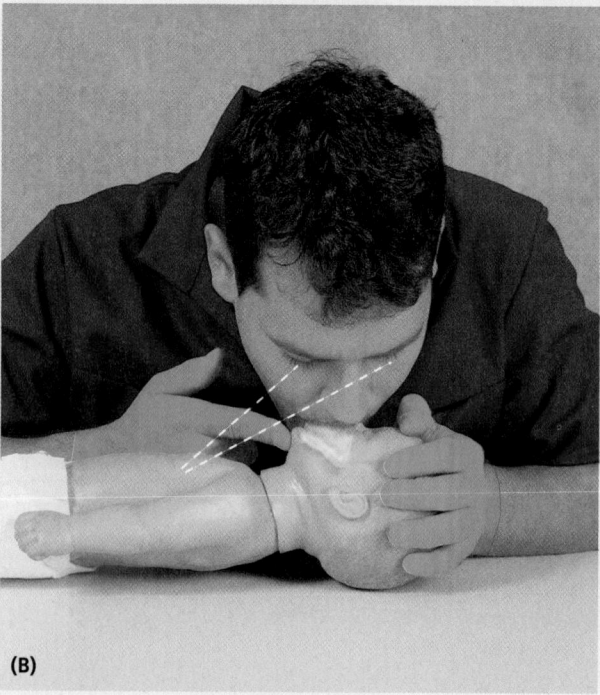

(B)

Figure 9-26   (A) Tilt back head. (B) Position resuscitation mouthpiece. Seal lips around nose and mouth, and give two slow breaths.

(continues)

Procedure
9-10 (*continued*)

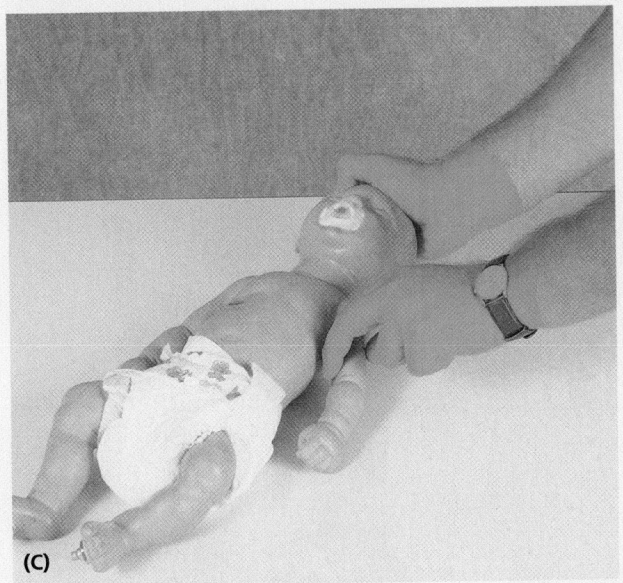
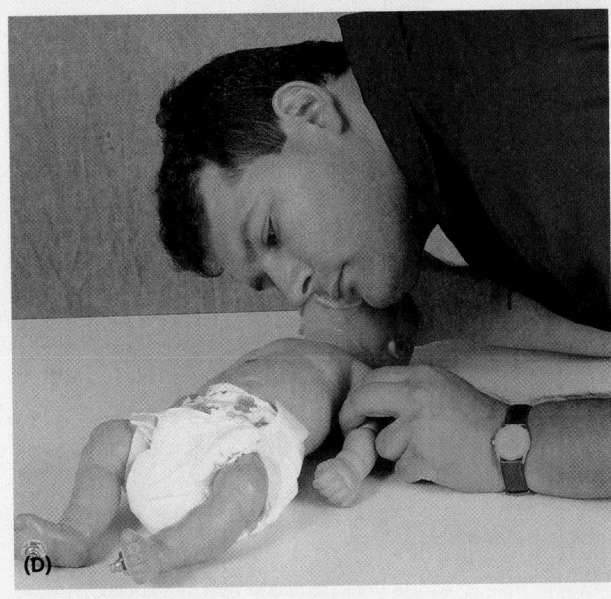

(C)   (D)

Figure 9-26   (C) Check for pulse at the brachial artery. (D) Recheck pulse and breathing every minute.

Procedure
9-11   **CPR for Adults**

STANDARD PRECAUTIONS:

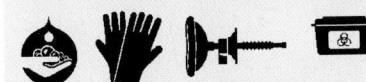

PURPOSE:
To respond to a breathing and cardiac arrest emergency.

EQUIPMENT/SUPPLIES:
Biohazard waste container
Resuscitation mouthpiece
Gloves

PROCEDURE STEPS:
Ask, "Are you OK?" If no response:
1. Have someone call emergency services.
2. Put on gloves if available.
3. Tilt back head and lift chin.

4. Look, listen, and feel for breathing for 10–15 seconds. If the patient is not breathing, keep the airway open, pinch the nose, position the mouthpiece, seal your mouth over the device, and give two breaths through the mouthpiece into the patient's lungs.
5. Check the pulse at the carotid artery for 10 to 15 seconds. If the patient has a pulse, continue rescue breathing. If the patient does not have a pulse, start chest compressions.
6. After locating the area on the abdomen 2 inches above the xiphoid (Figure 9-27A), position your shoulders over your hands and compress the chest about 2 inches fifteen times (Figure 9-27B).
7. Give two slow breaths, holding the nose (Figure 9-27C).

(*continues*)

Procedure 9-11 *(continued)*

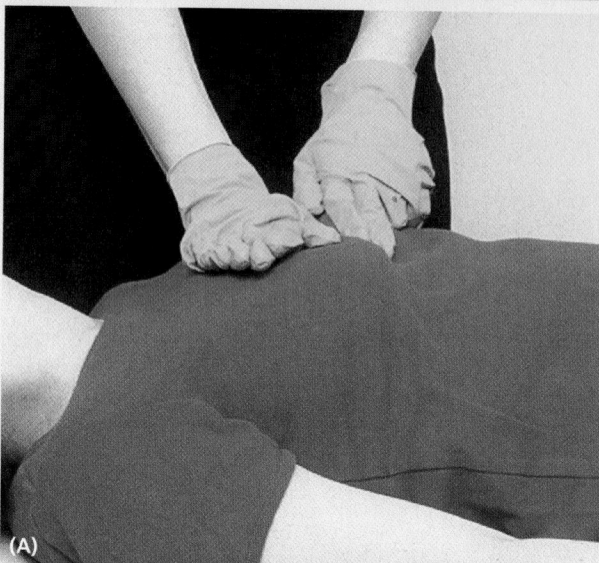

(A)

Figure 9-27   (A) Tilt back head and lift chin. Locate hand on the breastbone two inches above xiphoid process. (B) Position your shoulders over your hands and compress the chest fifteen times. (C) Give two slow breaths, holding nose.

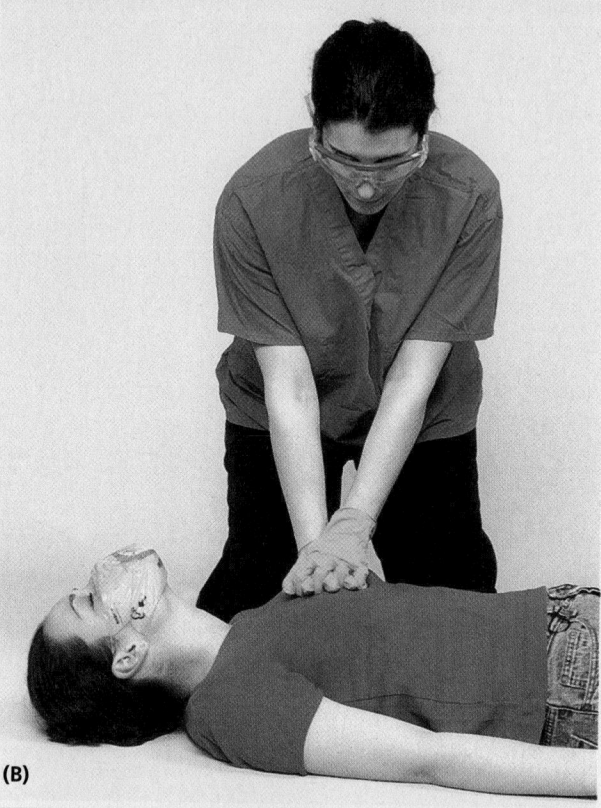

(B)

8. Do three more sets of fifteen compressions and two breaths.
9. Check the pulse and breathing for about 10–15 seconds.
10. If there is no pulse, continue sets of fifteen compressions and two breaths.
11. Dispose of waste in biohazard container.
12. Remove gloves, dispose of in biohazard container, and wash hands.
13. Document the procedure.

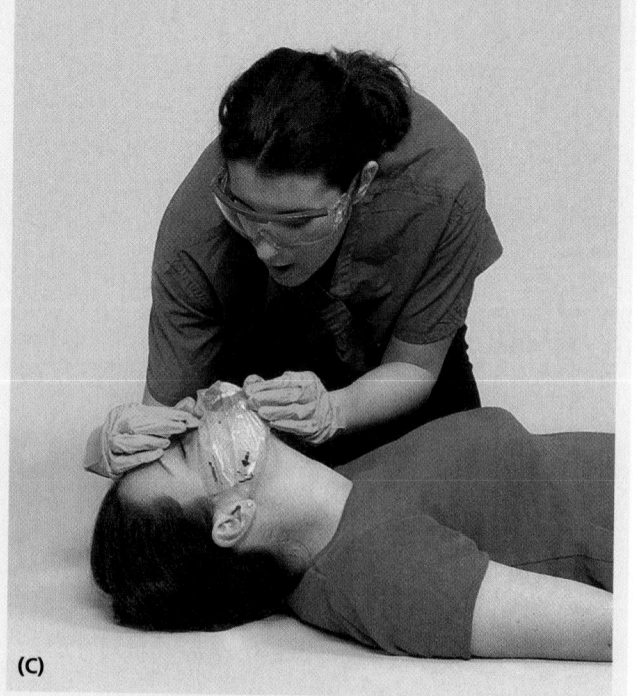

(C)

Procedure

9-12 CPR for Children

STANDARD PRECAUTIONS:

PURPOSE:
To respond to a cardiac arrest emergency.

EQUIPMENT/SUPPLIES:
Gloves
Resuscitation mouthpiece

PROCEDURE STEPS:
1. Put on gloves.
2. Tap child to check consciousness level. Activate EMS.
3. Tilt head, look, listen, and feel for breathing. If there is no breathing, give two slow breaths. Check carotid artery for pulse.
4. Locate one hand on the breastbone and one hand on the forehead to maintain an open airway. Use heel of hand only. Position your shoulders over the child's chest and compress the chest five times (Figure 9-28A).

5. Position resuscitation mouthpiece. Give one slow breath, while pinching the nose (Figure 9-28B).
6. Repeat cycles of five compressions and one breath for about 1 minute.
7. Check the pulse and breathing for about 5–10 seconds (Figure 9-28C).
8. If there is no pulse, continue sets of five compressions and one breath.
9. Recheck the pulse and breathing every few minutes.
10. Remove gloves. Wash hands.
11. Document the procedure.

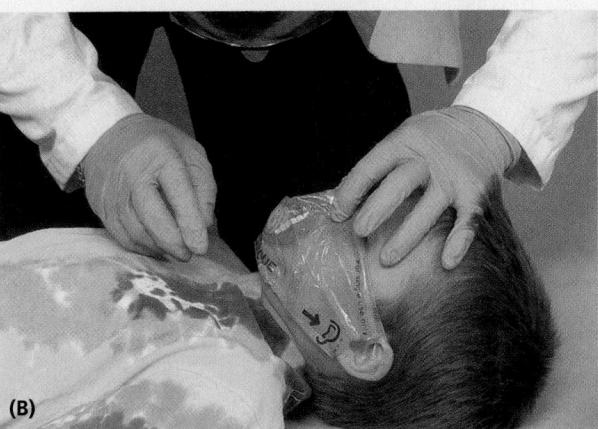

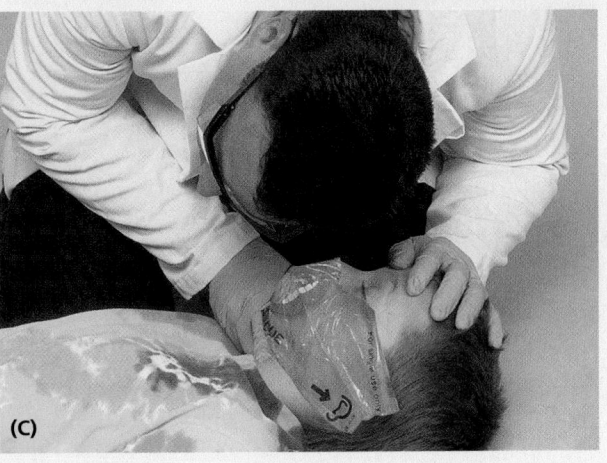

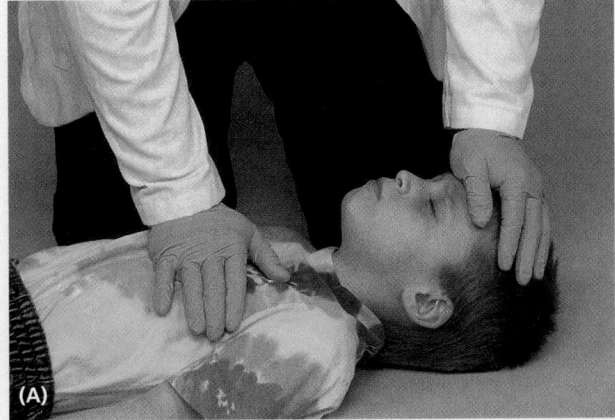

Figure 9-28 (A) Position your shoulders over the child's chest and compress the chest five times. (B) Give one slow breath, holding the nose. (C) Check pulse and breathing for 5 seconds.

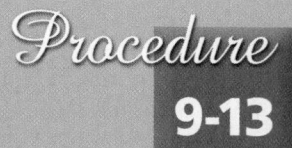

9-13   CPR for Infants

STANDARD PRECAUTIONS:

PURPOSE:
To respond to a cardiac arrest emergency.

EQUIPMENT/SUPPLIES:
Gloves
Resuscitation mouthpiece

PROCEDURE STEPS:
1. Don gloves.
2. Gently tap the infant to determine consciousness level. Activate EMS.
3. Tilt head. Look, listen, and feel for breathing. If there is no breathing, position resuscitation mouthpiece and give two slow breaths, covering mouth and nose. Check brachial artery for pulse for 5–10 seconds.
4. Find your finger position on the center of the sternum.
5. Compress the infant's chest five times about ½ inch to ¾ inch.
6. Give one slow breath (Figure 9-29A).
7. Repeat cycles of five compressions and one breath for 1 minute.
8. Recheck brachial pulse and breathing for about 5–10 seconds (Figure 9-29B).
9. If there is no pulse, continue cycles of five compressions and one breath.
10. Recheck the pulse and breathing every few minutes.
11. Remove gloves. Wash hands.
12. Document the procedure.

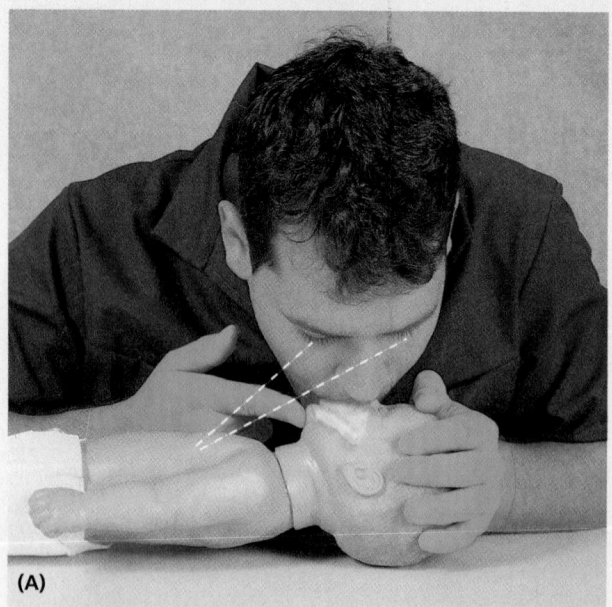

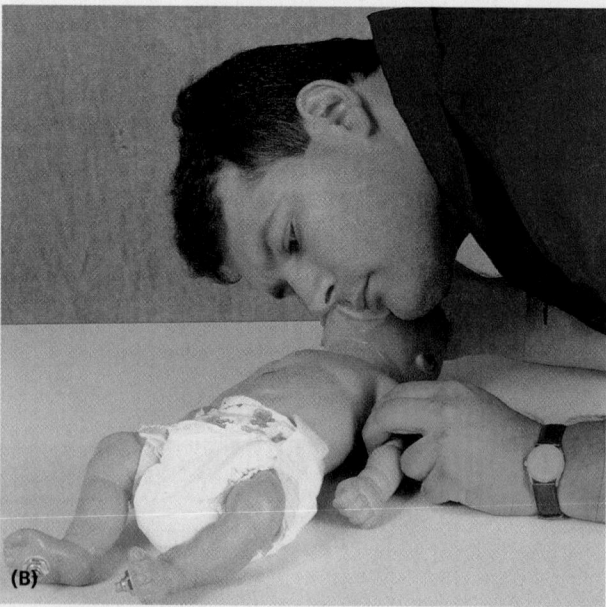

Figure 9-29   (A) Give one slow breath. (B) Recheck brachial pulse and breathing for 5–10 seconds.

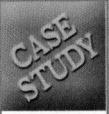

Annette Samuels, a regular patient at Inner City Health Care, is walking her dog one morning, stops to rest on a grassy knoll, and notices a yellow jacket on her arm. She brushes it away, unthinkingly, and then realizes it is stinging her. She receives two more stings and suddenly notices she is at a nest site. Annette is now a half-hour walk from home but not really concerned because she has never had an allergic reaction to a bee sting. However, a few minutes into her walk, her palms become itchy, her ears start to burn, and she feels lightheaded. She is not having difficulty breathing. She is determined to get home and she does, at which point she notices she is covered with hives. She calls Inner City Health Care to ask: should she come in?

CASE STUDY REVIEW

1. Wanda Slawson, CMA, is triaging calls the morning Annette is stung. What questions should she ask Annette?
2. Because Annette obviously is having a hypersensitive or an allergic reaction, she is advised to seek emergency care immediately. What first-aid measures might be taken?
3. What advice about precautions should Wanda give Annette?

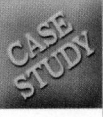

Abigail Johnson has arrived at Inner City Health Care for her scheduled nine o'clock appointment. As she checks in with Bruce Goldman, the medical assistant, she complains of feeling nauseated, having some pressure in her chest, and being short of breath.

CASE STUDY REVIEW

1. What immediate actions should Bruce take to respond to Mrs. Johnson's complaints?
2. What equipment/supplies/medications should be ready and available for Dr. Lewis?
3. Because of the possibility of myocardial infarction, what action would Dr. Lewis direct Bruce to take after Mrs. Johnson has been stabilized?
4. What patient education can Bruce employ in this situation?

SUMMARY

While many of the emergencies covered in this chapter may never be seen by the medical assistant in the ambulatory care setting, it is nonetheless important to develop a broad base of information about the various types of potential emergency situations. This knowledge gives the medical assistant the confidence and the preparation to manage the emergencies that do occur with speed, accuracy, and understanding until outside emergency help arrives. Staff will need to assess their response to emergencies on a continual basis. Was protocol followed? Were there difficulties in the delivery of care? Were staff and equipment pre-pared and ready to deal with these potentially life-threatening situations? Staff meetings should be held to discuss these and other questions that may have arisen and to allow staff the opportunity to talk about any fears or concerns they might have. It must be stressed that this chapter is at best an introduction to the topic of emergency procedures and first aid; it is highly recommended that all medical assistants in all ambulatory care settings, whether large or small, enroll in either a Red Cross or American Heart Association first aid and CPR program and take refresher courses at least every two years to update skills.

REVIEW QUESTIONS

Multiple Choice

1. Good Samaritan laws:
   a. are designed to protect the public
   b. only protect non-health-care professionals
   c. require that all individuals providing assistance act within the scope of their knowledge and training
   d. only protect health care professionals on the job

2. First-degree burns:
   a. are the most serious and penetrate all layers of skin
   b. affect only the top layer of skin
   c. often leave scar tissue
   d. usually take more than a month to heal

3. A fracture in which the bone protrudes through the skin is called:
   a. greenstick fracture
   b. compound fracture
   c. depressed fracture
   d. comminuted fracture

4. To control a nosebleed, it is important to:
   a. have the patient lie down
   b. tilt the patient's head back
   c. tilt the patient's head forward
   d. call 911 immediately

5. Another name for a heart attack is:
   a. cerebral vascular accident
   b. cardiac arrest
   c. angina pectoris
   d. myocardial infarction

Critical Thinking

1. Discuss the Good Samaritan law and define its purpose and the extent of its protection.
2. Recall what ABC stands for and describe actions that may need to be taken when doing a primary survey of a patient in distress.
3. Define the purpose of a crash cart or tray and compile a list of the major supplies and medications it should contain.
4. Describe shock and tell how and why it is important to prevent a patient from going into shock.
5. Recall three types of bandages and give examples of their use.
6. Describe the difference between first-, second-, and third-degree burns.
7. Recall and describe the four ways that poisons may enter the body.

8. What is hemorrhaging and what kinds of bleeding may the medical assistant encounter? What are the symptoms of each?
9. Explain when and why Heimlich maneuver, rescue breathing, and CPR techniques are performed.
10. What courses should every medical assistant take at least every two years and why?

WEB ACTIVITIES

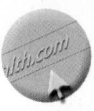

1. Search the web for sites and resources on the Emergency Medical Services (EMS) System. Are there any cities or towns within 100 miles of your place of residence that do not use the EMS System?
2. What sites can you recommend to patients and their families who are looking for first aid information about diabetes and heart attack?
3. What organizations could you use to search for information that deal with first aid for convulsions?
4. Search the web for information regarding first aid for insect stings.
5. What sites are available for information about poisonings?

REFERENCES/BIBLIOGRAPHY

American Red Cross. (1993). *Community first aid & safety.* St. Louis, MO: Mosby-Year Book, Inc.

Bonewit-West, K. (2000). *Clinical procedures for medical assistants* (5th ed.). Philadelphia: W. B. Saunders.

Frew, M. A., Frew, D., & Lane, K. (1995). *Comprehensive medical assisting, competencies for administrative and clinical practice* (3rd ed.). Philadelphia: F. A. Davis.

Keir, L., Wise, B. A., & Krebs, C. (1998). *Medical assisting: Administrative and clinical competencies* (4th ed.). Albany, NY: Delmar.

Kinn, M. E., & Woods, M. A. (1999). *The medical assistant: Administrative and clinical competencies* (8th ed.). Philadelphia: W. B. Saunders.

Prickett-Ramutkowski, B., Barrie A., Keller, C., Dazarow, L., Abel, C. (1999). *Medical assisting: A patient-centered approach to administrative and clinical competencies* (1st ed.). Princeton: Glencoe/McGraw Hill.

Taber's cyclopedic medical dictionary (18th ed.). (1997). Philadelphia: F. A. Davis.

Tuttle-Yoder, J., & Fraser-Nobbe, S. (1996). *STAT! Medical office emergency manual.* Albany, NY: Delmar.

II

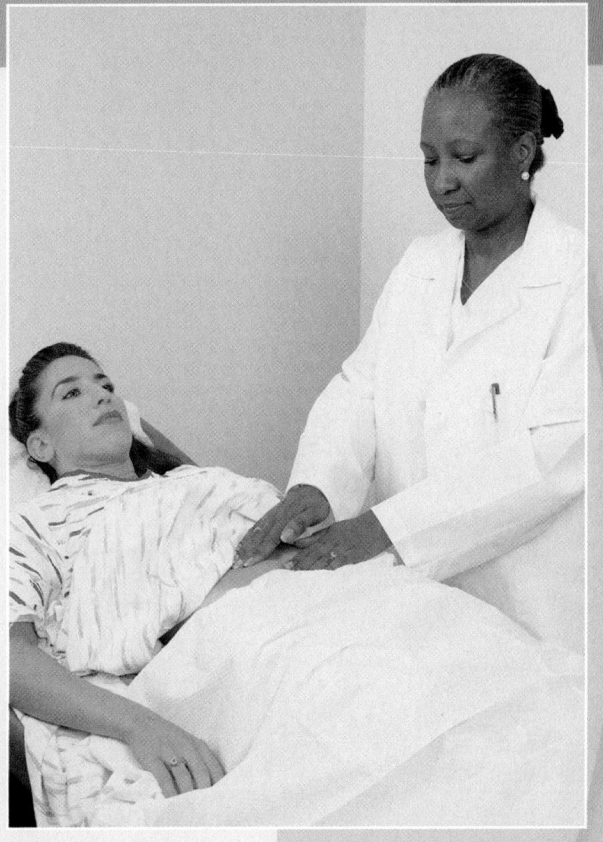

CLINICAL
PROCEDURES

Unit

4

INTEGRATED CLINICAL PROCEDURES

INFECTION CONTROL, MEDICAL ASEPSIS, AND STERILIZATION

KEY TERMS

Acquired Immunodeficiency
  Syndrome (AIDS)
Airborne Transmission
Amniocentesis
Amoebic Dysentery
Antibodies
Antigen
Aspirate
Barrier
Biohazard
Bloodborne
Bloodborne Pathogen
Body Substance Isolation
Carrier
Cell-Mediated Immunity
Communicable
Contact Transmission
Contaminate
Contracting
Declination Form
Dermatitis
Disinfection
Documentation
Droplet Transmission
Endoscopy
Engineering Controls
Epidemiology
Epistaxis
Excoriated
Excretion
Fomite
Human Immunodeficiency Virus
Humoral Immunity
Immune System

(continues)

OUTLINE

Impact of Infectious Diseases
The Process of Infection
Chain of Infection
  Infectious Agents
  Reservoir
  Portal of Exit
  Means of Transmission
  Portal of Entry
  Susceptible Host
**The Body's Defense Mechanisms
  for Fighting Infection and
  Disease**
  Inflammatory Response
  The Immune System and
    Immunity
Stages of Infectious Diseases
  Incubation Stage
  Prodromal Stage
  Acute Stage
  Declining Stage
  Convalescent Stage
Disease Transmission
**Acquired Immunodeficiency
  Syndrome and Hepatitis B**
  AIDS
  Acute Viral Hepatitis Diseases
  Transmission of HIV and HBV
Principles of Infection Control

**The Centers for Disease Control
  and Prevention, and Its Role in
  Infection Control**
  Universal Precautions
  Standard Precautions
  Transmission-Based Precautions
  Blood and Body Fluids
  Personal Protective Equipment
  Needlestick
  Disposal of Infectious Waste
  Educational Institutions and
    Standard Precautions
**Occupational Safety and Health
  Administration (OSHA)
  Regulations**
  The Bloodborne Pathogen
    Standard
OSHA Regulations and Students
  Avoiding Exposure to Bloodborne
    Pathogens
Medical Asepsis
  Handwashing
  Sanitization
  Disinfection
Surgical Asepsis and Sterilization
  Gas Sterilization
  Dry Heat Sterilization
  Chemical Sterilization
  Steam Sterilization (autoclave)

KEY TERMS
(continued)

Immunity
Immunoglobulins
Immunosuppressed
Incinerate
Infection Control
Infectious Agent
Infectious Waste
Inflammatory Response
Invasive Procedures
Isolation
Isolation Categories
Jaundice
Lesion
Leukorrhea
Lochia
Lumbar Puncture
Malaria
Medical Asepsis
Menses
Microorganisms
Morbidity
Mortality
Normal Flora
Palliative
Parenteral
Pathogen
Phlebotomy
Regulated Waste
Resistance
Sanitization
Scabies
Secretion
Sharps
Sodium Hypochlorite
Spill Kit
Sputum
Standard
Standard Precautions
Surgical Asepsis
Thermolabile
Thoracentesis
Transmission
Transmission-Based Precautions
Trichomoniasis
Universal Precautions
Vaccine
Vacutainer®
Vector
Virulence
Virulent
Work Practice Controls

OBJECTIVES

The student should strive to meet the following performance objectives and demonstrate an understanding of the facts and principles presented in this chapter through written and oral communication.

1. Define the key terms as presented in the glossary.
2. Define and state the critical importance of infection control in the ambulatory care setting.
3. Outline the six links in the chain of infection.
4. Define the five classifications of infectious microorganisms.
5. Recall and elaborate on the four phases the immune system uses to defend against infectious disease.
6. State the four stages of infectious diseases.
7. Recall at least five infectious diseases, their agents of transmission, and symptoms.
8. Compare the routes of transmission of AIDS and hepatitis and discuss the risk of infection from needlestick.
9. Explain why Universal Precautions were introduced in 1985.
10. Describe the purpose of Standard Precautions and give six examples of ways health care providers should practice Standard Precautions.
11. Differentiate among the three types of Transmission-Based Precautions, defining what they are and how they are applied.
12. List eight types of body fluids and give an example of each.
13. Describe personal protective equipment.
14. Recognize five situations in which exposure to a patient's blood can occur and discuss why Standard Precautions are important.
15. Describe disposal of infectious waste.
16. Discuss components of the bloodborne standard. Analyze what the law covers.
17. List human fluids that may contain HIV and HBV.
18. Define medical asepsis.
19. Define surgical asepsis.
20. Compare and contrast medical asepsis and surgical asepsis.
21. State four methods of sterilization.
22. List supplies and equipment necessary to achieve surgical asepsis when using an autoclave.
23. Explain competent wrapping and operation of the autoclave.
24. State storage measures and expiration periods for autoclaved materials.

ROLE DELINEATION
COMPONENTS

CLINICAL

Fundamental Principles

- Apply principles of aseptic technique and infection control
- Comply with quality assurance practices

GENERAL
(TRANSDISCIPLINARY)

Legal Concepts

- Comply with established risk management and safety procedures
- Follow federal, state, and local legal guidelines
- Maintain awareness of federal and state health care legislation and regulations

Instruction

- Teach methods of health promotion and disease prevention

SCENARIO

At Inner City Health Care, a multiphysician urgent care center, medical assistant Bruce Goldman, CMA, assumes responsibility for all infection control measures taken in the ambulatory care setting. In addition to his daily responsibilities related to medical and surgical asepsis, Bruce also makes it a point to stay current with infection control principles. Recently, he noticed that the Centers for Disease Control and Prevention (CDC) issued new guidelines, called Standard Precautions, that augment Universal Precautions. The CDC also issued another tier of precautions called Transmission-Based Precautions. When Bruce receives new information on any form of infection control, he makes it a point to become thoroughly familiar with the guidelines and to share his knowledge with other urgent care staff.

INTRODUCTION

Infectious diseases have plagued humans since the beginning of time. Recent scientific advances have changed our thoughts and behaviors regarding infectious disease. Advances such as antibiotic therapy and vaccination have significantly reduced risks of mortality from some previously fatal or debilitating infectious diseases. Infectious diseases that once were highly feared due to their likelihood of causing premature death are now preventable or treatable, causing us to forget the **virulence** and destructive potential of epidemics of infectious disease. The presence of AIDS as an incurable and fatal infectious disease has caused the world to realize the enduring impact of pathogens on the human race.

Although these medical advances have reduced the incidence of **mortality** and **morbidity** from infectious diseases, humans must never underesti-

mate the potential of resurgent infectious diseases. Tuberculosis has been the single leading cause of death in the history of mankind, yet was drastically reduced with the discovery of anti-tuberculosis drugs. Today, however, the tuberculosis organism may be found that has adapted to the drugs, thereby becoming resistant to our only line of defense. Medical assistants must pay close attention to the prevention of infectious diseases in the ambulatory care setting.

This chapter addresses the principles of the process of infection and control measures for use in ambulatory care settings. Since medical assistants deal directly with patients and other health care professionals, stringent adherence to the principles can greatly reduce **transmission,** or spread, of infectious disease. Continuous reliance on infection control measures ensures a clinical environment that is as safe as possible for employees, patients, and families. When infection control principles are not followed, infectious diseases may be transmitted to self, coworkers, or patients. The goals of infection control are to limit the presence of **infectious agents,** to create bar-

riers against transmission, and to decrease the risk to others of contracting infectious diseases. These goals can be achieved through medical asepsis and sterilization, by observation of all Standard Precautions and Transmission-Based Precautions set forth by the Centers for Disease Prevention and Control, and the Occupational Safety and Health Administration guidelines.

IMPACT OF INFECTIOUS DISEASES

Since the discovery of the germ theory by Louis Pasteur and Robert Koch in the nineteenth century, we have seen dramatic changes in global mortality and morbidity statistics from infectious diseases. Many scientists devoted their professional lives to the quest for the prevention and cure of infectious diseases, which were the main cause of death in earlier centuries. In developed countries, deaths from such diseases as tuberculosis, pneumonia, and smallpox have been significantly reduced due to pharmacologic agents such as antibiotics and vaccines. Antibiotic agents were widely introduced during World War II reducing deaths from traumatic wound infections. Edward Jenner is credited with the discovery of the first vaccine to protect against smallpox. Due to the vaccine, smallpox is considered to have been eradicated worldwide.

Epidemiology is the science that studies the history, cause, and patterns of infectious diseases. This field of medicine is credited to a Japanese bacteriologist in the late nineteenth century who correlated incidences of bubonic plague with rat infestation. Recent epidemiological studies have traced infectious diseases such as AIDS from the inception of the epidemic. The future of studies in infectious diseases will focus on increasing the pharmacological war against infectious diseases.

Reliance only on treatment of infectious disease does not address the crucial step in the spread of infectious diseases; that is, of prevention, or infection control. Emerging issues related to infectious diseases involve microorganisms that are resistant to present technology, bloodborne pathogen transmission, increased immunosuppressed populations, and global access to infection control and treatment. Developed countries become accustomed to anti-infectious medications, clean water, and laws that protect the public from infectious agents found in food and other consumables. These safety measures may not be present in other locations where political or economic factors limit access to infection control measures.

In the future, drug-resistant infectious diseases will place greater emphasis on prevention because there may never be a safe and universally effective drug for all infectious diseases.

Study of the history of infectious diseases allows us to realize the impact these diseases have on the lifestyles of people in various cultures. Infectious diseases such as AIDS and other sexually transmitted diseases have differing levels of social or cultural impact. Medical assistants should be aware of facts regarding the infectious process of specific diseases to reduce cultural isolation for the patient and to dispel myths regarding infectious diseases. Also see Chapter 6.

THE PROCESS OF INFECTION

Infectious diseases are caused by pathogenic microorganisms that are capable of causing disease. Microorganisms are microscopic living creatures capable of transmission and reproduction in specific circumstances. Pathogens are microorganisms that can cause infectious disease. Although all pathogens are capable of causing disease, not all microorganisms cause disease. Many microorganisms

are necessary for human, animal, and plant life survival. In the absence of microorganisms, life would not be possible. The term normal flora is used to recognize the beneficial role of microorganisms in certain parts of the body, in which microorganisms normally occupy space and use nutrients, thus retarding the potential of pathogenic growth in that specific body area. A fundamental concept in the study of infectious disease is that similar steps or phases occur in all infectious diseases; however, each specific microorganism causes unique characteristics and alterations in the process of infection. Medical assistants must apply the theoretical process of infectious disease growth and transmission in order to relate to specific pathogens. The goal is to reduce transmission and incidence of infectious diseases in patients, employees, and families.

CHAIN OF INFECTION

In order for infectious diseases to spread, several necessary steps must occur. These steps, or links, are known as the "chain of infection." Each link or step in the infectious process must occur for the spread of infection to take place. Infection control is based on the fact that the transmission of infectious diseases will be prevented when any of the levels in the chain are broken or interrupted (Figure 10-1). The steps are:

1. Infectious agent
2. Reservoir
3. Portal of exit
4. Means of transmission
5. Portal of entry
6. Susceptible host

Infectious Agents

Infectious agents are microorganisms that can be grouped into five classifications: viruses, bacteria, fungi, protozoa, and rickettsia. In order for an infection to occur, an infectious agent must be present. When infectious diseases are identified according to the specific disease-causing microorganism, the disease may be prevented with the use of anti-infective drugs or infection control practices. Each of the five classifications of infectious microorganisms will be explored.

Virus. Viruses are pathogens that require a living cell for reproduction and activity. These microorganisms are considered intracellular parasites, because they must live inside cells in order to multiply. They do so by altering particles of genetic material, such as DNA (deoxyribonucleic acid) or RNA (ribonucleic acid). Since viruses live

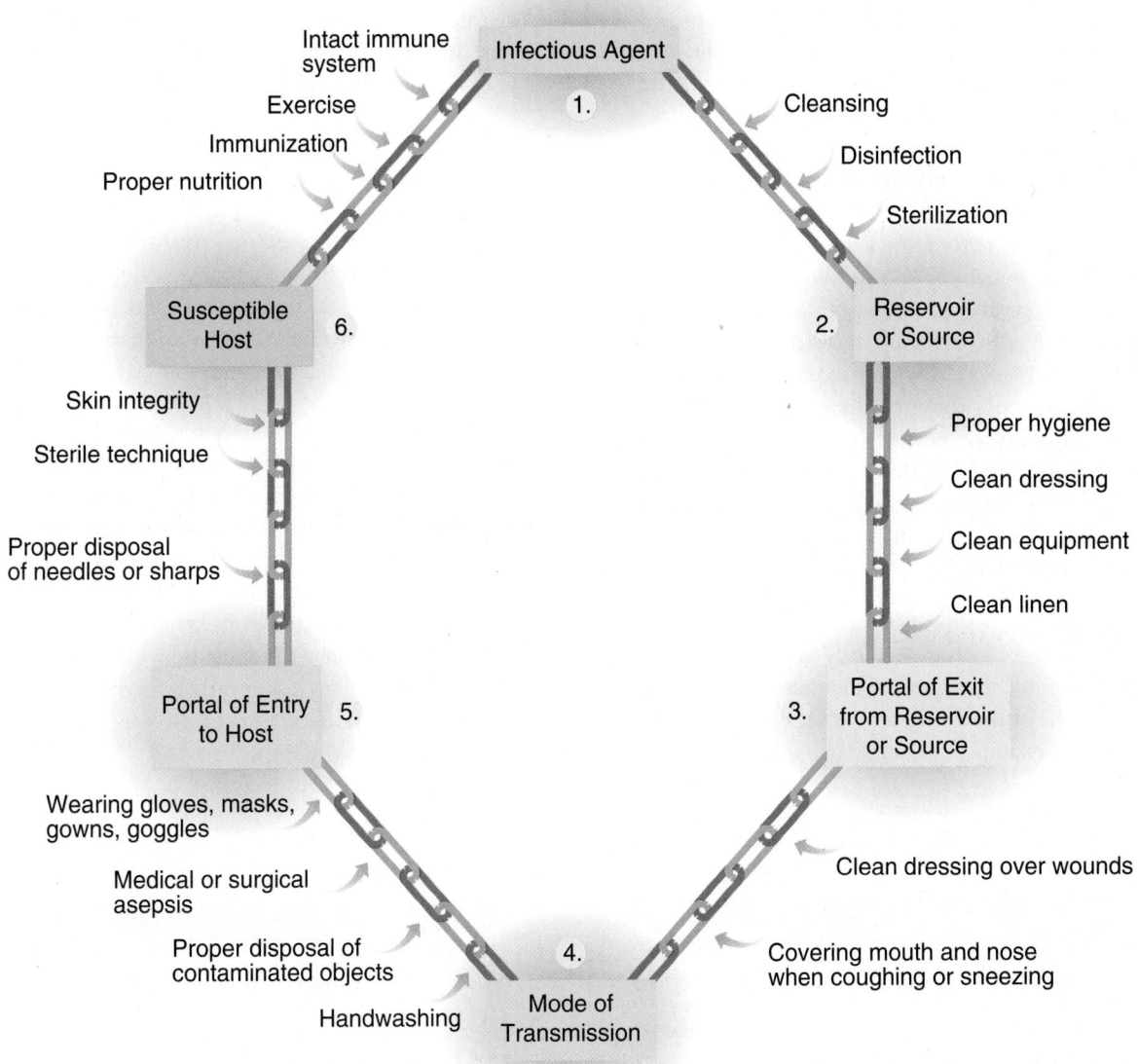

Figure 10-1 Health care worker's interventions used to break the chain of the infection transmission.

inside cells, they are protected against agents such as chemical disinfectants. Viruses are susceptible to heat. In order to survive, viruses have a notable characteristic of being able to change specific characteristics over time. For instance, viruses can adapt to their environment so they remain resistant to efforts to limit their growth. Viral infections have only a few pharmacological treatment agents, and usually these agents are **palliative** because they only relieve symptoms of the disease instead of curing the infection.

Bacteria. Bacteria are single-celled microorganisms that live in tissues rather than in body cells and are iden-

tified by characteristic shapes, or morphology. Bacteria may also be grouped according to ability to accept laboratory staining agents. Gram-negative bacteria stain visibly red under the microscope, whereas gram-positive bacteria stain purple. The bacteria that do not accept stain are considered spores, which are bacteria with a covering that protects them from many chemical disinfectants and higher levels of heat. The three classifications of bacteria are cocci (sphere or dot shaped); bacilli (rod shaped); and spirilla (spiral shaped). Bacteria are either pathogenic or nonpathogenic. Nonpathogenic bacteria normally reside on the skin of humans and in mucous membrane areas of the body. These are known as *normal flora.* The nonpathogenic bacteria use nutrients and occupy space, competing with the pathogenic bacteria. When nonpathogenic bacteria are reduced, the opportunity exists for pathogenic organisms to take over and cause infectious disease. A common cause of the reduction of nonpathogenic microorganisms is the use of anti-infectious drugs. Certain conditions favor bacterial growth and in fact are necessary for them to survive. They are darkness (promotes bacterial growth), oxygen (aerobic bacteria need oxygen to live, anaerobic bacteria live without oxygen), temperature (body temperature favors bacterial growth), and moisture (bacteria grow well in moist places). By depriving bacteria of their growth requirements they can be kept from causing an infection. This can be accomplished by providing light since certain bacteria will die in direct light or sunlight; providing or withholding oxygen according to the needs of the bacteria (aerobic or anaerobic); lowering temperatures to reduce bacterial growth; and keeping surfaces dry to inhibit bacterial growth. Examples of bacterial pathogens are listed in Table 10-1.

Fungi. Fungi are microorganisms that may be unicellular (single-cell) or multicellular (many cells). Mushrooms and molds are examples of fungi that are nonpathogenic. Pathogenic fungi cause athletes' foot, ringworm, and candida infections. Other pathogenic fungi include histoplasmosis and toxoplasmosis, which are fungal infections spread through the air from infected fowl and bird waste.

Parasites. Organisms that live in or on another organism are classified as parasites. They may be single-celled or multicelled. Examples include protozoa (single-cell microscopic organisms that cause **malaria, amoebic dysentery,** and **trichomoniasis**); metazoa (multicellular organisms that cause pinworms, hookworms, and tapeworms); and ectoparasites (multicellular organisms that live superficially on another host, such as lice and **scabies**).

Rickettsiae. Rickettsiae are intracellular parasites, similar to the virus. However, they are larger than viruses and can be seen under conventional microscopes following staining procedures. These microorganisms are susceptible to antibiotic therapy. Examples of rickettsiae infections include typhus (transmitted by the body louse); Lyme disease (transmitted by ticks); and Rocky Mountain Spotted Fever (transmitted by ticks). Characteristic of rickettsia infections is a skin rash caused by the rickettsia invading the small blood vessels. This appears on the skin as a small hemorrhagic rash.

TABLE 10-1   INFECTIOUS BACTERIAL DISEASES

Disease	Infectious Agent	Mode of Transmission
Botulism (food poisoning)	Clostridium botulinum	Ingestion
Chlamydia (sexually transmitted disease)	Chlamydia trachomatis	Sexual contact
Clostridial myonecrosis (Gas gangrene)	Species of gram-positive clostridia	Wound entry
Gonorrhea (sexually transmitted disease)	Neisseria gonorrhoeae	Sexual contact
Legionnaires' disease (pneumonia)	Legionella pneumophila	Inhalation
Meningococcal meningitis	N. Meningitidis, S. Pneumoniae, or H. Influenzae	Direct contact, inhalation
Nosocomial (hospital-acquired) infection	Gram-negative bacteria	Normal flora transmitted during illness/procedures; opportunistic pathogens transmit during debilitated condition
Pulmonary tuberculosis	Mycobacterium tuberculosis	Inhalation
Samonellosis (food poisoning)	Salmonella	Ingestion
Shigellosis (bacillary dysentery) (diarrhea)	Shigellae	Fecal-oral
Staphylococcal infection (abscesses, food poisoning, urinary tract infections)	Staphylococci	Direct contact, ingestion, inhalation, bloodborne, vectors (animals)
Streptococcal infection (strep throat, otitis media, pneumonia)	Hemolytic streptococci (usually beta-hemolytic group A)	Inhalation
Syphilis (sexually transmitted disease)	Treponema pallidum	Sexual contact
Tetanus (lockjaw)	Clostridium tetani	Wound entry
Typhoid fever (enteric fever)	Salmonella typhi	Fecal-oral

Reservoir

The second level in the chain of infection is the reservoir or location of the infectious agent. Reservoirs are people, equipment, supplies, water, food, and animals or insects (known as vectors). Methods of infection control in the reservoir level include handwashing, environmental hygiene, disinfection, sterilization, and maintenance of employee health standards, such as annual tuberculosis skin testing.

Portal of Exit

Although the infectious agent is housed or living in the reservoir, it must leave the reservoir to infect another person. The portal of exit is the method by which an infectious agent leaves the reservoir. Microorganisms may leave the human body with normally occurring body fluids, such as **excretions**, **secretions**, skin cells, respiratory droplets, blood, or any body fluid. The portal of exit may be continuous, such as with respiratory droplets, or dependent on the body fluid exiting the body under unusual circumstances, such as when blood leaves the body during a surgical procedure or phlebotomy.

 Standard Precautions and Transmission-Based Precautions are infection control methods based on the knowledge that exiting infectious diseases can be spread to others. These precautions attempt to control the spread of infectious diseases as infectious agents exit the reservoir.

Means of Transmission

The means of transmission are specific ways in which microorganisms travel from one place (reservoir) to another (susceptible host). Transmission depends on the characteristics of the microorganisms. Types of routes of transmission include:

- Direct contact (touching an infected person)
- Airborne transmission (inhaling the microorganism into the susceptible host's respiratory system)
- Bloodborne transmission (infected blood enters susceptible host)
- Ingestion (eating or drinking contaminated items)
- Indirect contact (microorganism on a fomite, a nonliving object such as a table or piece of equipment that can absorb and transmit infection)
- **Vector** (a carrier of disease, usually an insect)

Infection control measures in the ambulatory care area specifically address the transmission stage of the process of infection.

 Methods that reduce the transmission of pathogens include adherence to Standard and Transmission-Based Precautions, handwashing, sanitization, disinfection, and sterilization. Methods of infection control are used in food handling, water and sewage processing, and child care.

Portal of Entry

Following transmission, the infectious agent must enter another person, or a susceptible host. The portal of entry allows the agent access to the next person. Common entrance sites to the human body include broken skin, mucous membranes, and systems of the body exposed to the external environment, such as the respiratory, gastrointestinal, and reproductive systems. Breathing in airborne microorganisms allows infectious diseases to be spread to the lungs. Eating or drinking contaminated water is the cause of gastrointestinal infectious diseases. Sexually transmitted diseases spread through vaginal, oral, and anal intercourse. Care of patients with infectious diseases includes careful consideration of infection control to limit further spread of the microorganism. Methods such as sterile wound care, transmission-based precautions, and aseptic technique limit the transmission of infectious microorganisms. The portals of exit and entry need not be the same.

Susceptible Host

Finally, infectious microorganisms must enter another person who is susceptible. This means that the person is able to contract the pathogenic organism. The susceptible host is therefore not resistant or immune to the organism. Causes of susceptibility include the presence of other diseases, immunosuppression (weakened immune system), surgical procedures, trauma, or the absence of immunity to the specific microorganism. Susceptibility of a person depends on several factors, including:

1. Number and specific type of pathogen
2. Duration of exposure to the pathogen
3. General physical condition
4. Psychological health status
5. Occupation or lifestyle environment
6. Presence of underlying diseases or conditions
7. Youth or advanced age (young and old at greater risk)

The goal of infection control at this level of the chain of infection is to identify patients at risk for susceptibility, treat their underlying conditions if possible, and isolate them from those reservoirs that could be hazardous to the susceptible person.

THE BODY'S DEFENSE MECHANISMS FOR FIGHTING INFECTION AND DISEASE

There are two primary defense mechanisms that protect the body from infection and disease. One is known as inflammation or the inflammatory response, a non-specific immune response; the other is an individual's immune system or specific response.

Inflammatory Response

Inflammation is the body's natural way of responding when invaded by a pathogen or trauma. The body goes through a distinct process in an attempt to destroy and get rid of the pathogenic microorganisms and their by-products, and if this is not possible, to restrict the amount of damage done. The response is identical whether the agent is a pathogen, trauma, foreign body, or extremes in temperature. The cardinal signs of inflammation are redness, heat, swelling, and pain. Inflammation is a response to infection (invasion by a pathogen) and the two should not be confused. Inflammation can occur without infection, but infection cannot exist without inflammation.

These are the steps in the inflammatory process:

- Local dilation of blood vessels increases blood flow to injured (infected) area causing redness or heat

- Plasma moves into the tissue causing swelling and pain due to pressure on nerve ending

- White blood cells move into injured tissue to fight infection and phagocytes destroy invading pathogens

Following destruction of the pathogen, tissue repair can begin. If the inflammatory response is not effective, the specific immune response is necessary.

Indications that an inflammatory process is inadequate are (1) the accumulation of purulent matter in the area (due to destroyed pathogens, white blood cells, and body cells), (2) lymph node enlargement (swollen glands), and (3) septicemia may result because pathogens have spread to the blood stream.

Immediate antibiotic therapy is indicated in these circumstances due to the inadequacy of the inflammatory response.

The Immune System and Immunity

In order to fight infectious diseases, our bodies are equipped with several effective physical and chemical barriers such as the skin, mucous membranes, body excretions and secretions, and a complex, highly specific immune system. The immune system's purpose is to protect against pathogens and abnormal cell growth. The system is composed of various cells that collectively recognize, subdue, attack, and eliminate pathogens. The two types of immune responses include cell-mediated immunity and humoral immunity. Cell-mediated immunity is usually involved in attacks against viruses, fungi, organ transplants, or cancer cells. This type of immunity does not produce antibodies. Humoral immunity produces antibodies that are capable of killing microorganisms and of recognizing the pathogen in the future. Generally, both types of immune responses occur in four phases:

1. *Recognition of the invader.* The immune system is equipped with cells that identify agents, pathogens, and abnormal cell growth as foreign substances. Macrophages and helper T cells recognize foreign invaders, whether they are pathogens, cancer cells, or transplanted tissues.

2. *Growth of defenses, which allows for multiplication of helper T cells and B cells.* Following foreign substance recognition, the immune system alerts T cells and B cells to multiply and move to the site of the foreign substance. In cell-mediated immunity, activation of helper T cells means that the T cells are specifically oriented to a unique antigen, a substance such as bacteria the body recognizes as foreign. Activated T cells divide, forming memory T cells and killer T cells. In humoral immunity, activated B cells are antigen-specific and divide into memory B cells and plasma cells.

3. *Attack against the infection.* Cell-mediated immunity uses killer T cells and macrophages to phagocytize, or engulf and destroy the pathogens. Humoral plasma cells have the ability to produce specific antibodies that lock on to specific antigens, which prevents the disease-producing characteristics of the pathogen from forming. These antibodies are called immunoglobulins and they render the pathogen unable to reproduce or continue growth.

4. *Slowdown of the immune response following death of the infectious agent.* Following the death of the foreign substance, the immune response is halted. T cells and B cells return to normal levels, and in the case of humoral immunity, the presence of antibody production causes the immune system to resist the specific infectious pathogen in future contacts with the pathogen.

Susceptibility to some infectious diseases is closely linked to the person's unique resistance, or immunity. Immunity means the ability of the body to resist specific pathogens and their toxins. Resistance occurs following an exposure to a pathogen, which is the antigen-antibody reaction. This natural body defense to fight infectious disease occurs gradually and over time as pathogens and other foreign substances such as antigens enter the human body. When the antigen enters the body, the immune system recognizes the antigen as foreign and attempts to contain and subdue the foreign invader. Specific chemical antibodies to the antigen are produced by B cells, which attempt to prevent the antigen from further growth. Following the completion of the stages of that infectious disease, the body retains the ability to produce antibodies in response to that specific microorganism or antigen. Therefore, immunity can last for some length of time, possibly to provide lifetime protection against specific infectious microorganisms. Several forms of immunity can occur in response to specific antigens:

- Acquired active immunity results from contracting an infectious agent and experiencing either an acute or subclinical infectious disease

- Artificial active immunity is achieved following administration of vaccines

- Congenital passive immunity occurs when antibodies pass to a fetus from the mother providing short-term immunity for the newborn

- Passive immunity may be achieved through administration of ready-made antibodies, such as gamma globulin used to treat or prevent infectious diseases

The Body's Natural Barriers. The body has several natural barriers that serve to help inhibit infection. The greatest barrier is intact skin. Other barriers include mucous membranes that line body orifices, the gastrointestinal tract with hydrochloric acid that inhibits infection, cilia in the respiratory tract that filter out potential infectious agents, and the lymph and blood systems that fight pathogens through phagocytosis.

Immunization. Immunizing individuals against specific infectious diseases provides immunity with active or passive vaccines. Although most of severe childhood communicable diseases can be prevented, the U.S. Department of Health and Human Services has estimated that only about three-fourths of U.S. preschoolers under two years old are fully vaccinated according to recommended schedules (U.S. Department of Health and Human Services, 1999). Several factors influence vaccination rates, such as access to health care, cost of vaccinations, and irregularity or confusion in maintaining young children on the recommended schedule. Since most of the vaccinations are administered in ambulatory health care settings, medical assistants may have the

SPOTLIGHT ON AAMA ESSENTIALS THROUGH CAAHEP

- It's important for the medical assistant to develop an inner sense for the need to practice good aseptic procedures, since this is one of the very few tasks that directly affect the health of the patient, the physician, and the entire office staff.

- A medical assistant needs to be aware of the importance of taking time to discuss proper medical asepsis and handwashing techniques, as well as the relationship of infection control to good hygiene, so that the patient understands the necessity of following these procedures.

- All patients coming into your office should have absolute assurance that they are being taken care of in an aseptic atmosphere, under aseptic conditions, free of pathogens and disease-producing microorganisms.

responsibility to administer, document, and monitor immunizations.

Vaccines produce active or passive immunity by stimulating the immune system to recognize antigens without having to contract the infectious disease to provide natural immunity as described previously.

There are various classifications of vaccines, depending on the method of immune stimulation:

1. *Live attenuated (changed) pathogens.* These pathogens stimulate the body's own antibody production. However, the patient does not contract the infectious disease (or only a mild or subclinical case) since the pathogen has been altered in some mechanical or chemical means by the manufacturer. Examples of live attenuated pathogens include OPV (oral poliovirus vaccine), to protect from poliomyelitis.
2. *Pathogenic toxins.* Some pathogens produce toxins (poisonous substances) that can stimulate antibody production. Examples of toxin vaccines include tetanus and diphtheria.
3. *Killed pathogens.* Inactivated pathogens stimulate antibody production; however, several vaccines may be required to provide sustained protection. Examples include pertussis and rabies.

STAGES OF INFECTIOUS DISEASES

Depending on the specific pathogen causing an infectious disease, several stages occur from the time of exposure until full recovery and the absence of infection. These stages are often predictable and offer guidelines for patient education and treatment opportunities.

Incubation Stage

The incubation stage is the interval of time between exposure to a pathogenic microorganism and the first appearance of signs and symptoms of the disease. Some infectious diseases have very short incubation stages, whereas other infections have lengthy stages, lasting for years. If an exposure to an infectious agent occurs, the patient will manifest the disease if the patient's immune system cannot contain the agent or if therapeutic medications are available to prevent disease progression. Not all infectious agents are treatable or preventable.

Prodromal Stage

Prodromal means vague or undifferentiated from symptoms of other illnesses. The prodromal stage is characterized by common, general complaints of illness, such as malaise and fever. It is the interval between the earliest symptoms and the appearance of fever or rash that suggest an impending disease process is occurring.

Acute Stage

Disease processes reach their peak during the acute stage. Symptoms are fully developed and can often be differentiated from other specific symptoms. Treatment modalities are useful to reduce patient discomfort, reduce possibilities of debilitation and adverse effects, and to promote healing and recovery.

The inflammatory process is the body's natural defensive reaction to the invasion by a foreign substance such as a pathogen, and it is in this acute state that the response is evident.

Declining Stage

Patient symptoms begin to subside or wane during the declining stage. The infectious disease remains, however, though the patient will demonstrate improving levels of health.

Convalescent Stage

Recovery and recuperation from the effects of a specific infectious disease are called the convalescent stage. The patient regains strength and stamina, and the overall goal of this stage is that the patient is returned to the original state of health.

DISEASE TRANSMISSION

When providing patients with health care, medical assistants run the risk of contracting, or acquiring, an infection from pathogens that are causing patients' illnesses. Such pathogens are viruses, bacteria, fungi, and others that can be found in patients' blood and body fluids. In medical offices, ambulatory care centers, and hospitals, many ill patients are seen every day. Pathogens can be easily transmitted to another person if care is not taken to prevent such an occurrence.

Consistent use and adherence to infection control measures significantly reduce the risk of disease transmission. The CDC recommends that health care providers consider each patient to be potentially infectious for AIDS, hepatitis B, and other bloodborne pathogens and to routinely and conscientiously apply the techniques of Standard Precautions as a means of infection control.

Infectious diseases are caused by unique infectious agents, are characterized by various symptoms, are transmitted by differing means, and have unique treatments and prognoses. Medical assistants must recognize the unique characteristics of specific infectious diseases to prevent their transmission and treat patients suffering from these infections. Table 10-2 classifies common infectious diseases by critical components. When patients have contracted an infectious disease or are exposed to the risk of transmission, patient education plays an important role in infection control. Although a family member may have an infectious disease, proper training and education may protect other family members and close contacts.

Medical assistants also are responsible for when specific infectious diseases are encountered in the health care setting. With the increasing risk of drug-resistant pathogens, all health care professionals must habitually use infection control measures as well as oversee prudent treatment of patients with existing infectious diseases. For instance, tuberculosis was only recently the major cause of death, and the discovery of effective antituberculosis drugs slowed death rates dramatically. However, we are experiencing resurgent strains of the mycobacterium, which in some instances are resistant to drugs.

ACQUIRED IMMUNODEFICIENCY SYNDROME AND HEPATITIS B

A great deal of attention is focused on the human immunodeficiency virus (HIV) that causes AIDS, because there is yet no cure for the disease. With the focus on AIDS, other potentially life-threatening and fatal illnesses do not come to mind so quickly. Hepatitis B and other viral hepatitis diseases are examples of other diseases that place health care providers at great risk for serious illness or death. Acute viral hepatitis also deserves close attention.

TABLE 10-2   COMMON INFECTIOUS DISEASES

Disease	Agent	Transmission	Symptoms	Diagnosis	Treatment	Comments	Patient Education
AIDS (Acquired Immunodeficiency Syndrome)	Human Immunodeficiency Virus (HIV)	• Bloodborne • Sexual contact • Intrauterine • Lactation	Opportunistic infections, lymphadenopathy, fatigue, malaise, fever	CD4 level less than 200 cells/mm^3	Palliative care and treatment for opportunistic infections, antiviral drugs	WHO (World Health Organization) estimates 20–40 million people will be infected with HIV	1. Careful infection control to reduce contact with pathogens that cause opportunistic infections 2. Use of latex condoms in conjunction with effective spermicide 3. Support groups
Hepatitis B	Hepatitis B virus (HBV)	• Bloodborne • Sexual contact • Intrauterine	Fatigue, malaise, anorexia, headache, icterus, liver tenderness and enlargement, fever	Serum antibody tests; liver function studies elevated	Immunization of all those at risk of exposure, palliative therapy, monitor bilirubin levels, bedrest, frequent low-fat, high-carbohydrate diet	Mortality 1–10%	1. Follow-up required to monitor liver function studies 2. Close personal contacts of patient should receive HB vaccine or HBIG (HB immunoglobulin) 3. Teach infection control to patient to prevent spread to close contacts 4. Avoid alcohol, sedatives, or aspirin during acute phase
Tuberculosis (TB)	Mycobacterium tuberculosis bacillus	• Inhalation of contaminated airborne mucous droplets • Possibly ingestion	Productive cough, fatigue, fever, weight loss (elderly: behavior changes, anorexia, weight loss)	Sputum culture for M. tuberculosis, Mantoux skin test (PPD), chest X ray, pleural needle biopsy	Antituberculosis agents, airborne transmission-based precautions, until drug agents started, BCG vaccine for children at high risk (controversial)	Increase in incidence of TB, especially among persons with AIDS and the homeless; may be drug resistant; health care professionals should have annual skin testing	1. Encourage handwashing and proper sputum tissue disposal 2. Promote compliance with medications 3. Encourage close contacts to have skin tests 4. Well-balanced diet
Food poisoning and gastroenteritis	Bacteria or viruses (i.e., staphylococci, clostridium, botulinum, E. coli, shigella)	• Ingestion of contaminated food or water	Nausea, intestinal cramps, vomiting, diarrhea, dehydration, respiratory failure, death	Culture of emesis, feces, vomitus, or suspected food or water	Fluid balance restoration, medications, emergency treatment as required	Report outbreaks to local authorities	1. Teach proper food handling 2. Carefully washing hands prior to handling all food 3. Report to physician all signs of dehydration 4. Gastroenteritis usually communicable via feces for up to seven weeks following exposure
Influenza	Influenza viruses A, B, or C (various strains)	• Inhalation • Aerosolized • Mucous droplets	Acute upper/lower respiratory infection, severe cough, fever, malaise, sore throat, coryza	Tissue culture of nasal or pharyngeal secretions	Palliative therapy, active immunization (annual vaccine recommended for persons at risk [elderly, heart patients] for complications from infection)	Report cases to local health authority	1. Bed rest for two to three days after fever decline 2. Force fluids 3. Report signs of secondary infections
Chickenpox (Varicella)	Varicella-zoster virus	• Direct and indirect contact with respiratory droplets	Sudden onset fever, malaise, maculo-papular-vesicular skin rash	Vesicular fluid tissue culture during first three days after eruption; serology: increase antibodies two weeks after rash; lesion appearance characteristic of varicella	Acyclovir helpful to reduce severity of disease; zoster immune globulin (ZIG) for high-risk persons only within 96 hours of exposure; palliative therapy	Vaccine (varicella virus vaccine live) available in U.S. for children over 12 months of age	1. Communicable one to two days before rash until lesions crust 2. Avoid scratching lesions to prevent secondary infection and scarring

AIDS

Acquired immunodeficiency syndrome, or AIDS, is caused by a bloodborne virus, human immunodeficiency virus (HIV), and then ensuing infection directly affects the immune response. The HIV is responsible for T cell destruction; T cells are the white blood cells that provide immunity.

HIV is carried in semen, blood, and other body fluids, and the virus can penetrate mucous membranes. Once inside the body, the depletion of helper T cells leaves the patient vulnerable to a wide range of infections and malignancies. The infections that the patient contracts are devastating. There is no curative treatment for AIDS, but there are antiviral drugs such as AZT (azidothymidine), ZDV (zidovudine), Videx, and others that are used to halt cellular synthesis and incapacitate cell protein, which is important in the virus's reproduction.

Acute Viral Hepatitis Diseases

In any of the acute viral hepatitis diseases, the liver becomes inflamed and hepatic cells can be destroyed. Healthy persons can regenerate cells, but elderly patients cannot. There are several types of viral hepatitis, including hepatitis A (HAV); hepatitis B (HBV): hepatitis C (HCV); hepatitis D (HDV); and hepatitis E (HEV).

The hepatitis B virus (HBV) represents the greatest risk to health care providers. While a new type B vaccine that confers 96 percent immunity is available for high-risk groups, it is nonetheless critical to practice standard precautions to curtail the transmission of this very preventable disease.

Symptoms of Hepatitis B. Hepatitis B (HBV) is considered the greatest biohazard for health care providers. The American Medical Association has said that loss of health care workers to HBV overshadows the risk of AIDS and is almost entirely preventable.

Hepatitis B (HBV) is easier to contract than HIV. Symptoms of HBV include loss of appetite, fatigue, nausea, headache, fever and jaundice, a yellow discoloration of the skin. The liver function is impaired and, in severe cases, may even be lost. It is important to note that in some individuals HBV may be asymptomatic and can still damage the liver and possibly lead to cancer of the liver. Usually, once patients become infected, they remain so for life, and are capable of transmitting the virus to others.

Transmission of HIV and HBV

HIV and HBV are transmitted essentially through the same means. Contracting either disease requires direct contact with the virus living in infected blood and body fluids. The viruses are transmitted primarily through the following means:

- Sexual contact with an infected person (heterosexual, homosexual, or bisexual). The virus enters the bloodstream through small tears in the mucous membrane of the vagina, rectum, penis, or mouth

- Sharing needles for intravenous (IV) drug use with an infected person

- Using unsterilized tattoo and body piercing tools after their use on an infected person

- Receiving blood or blood products from an infected person. (All blood collected for transfusions is routinely checked for HIV and HBV; therefore, risk from this is now rare.)

- Intrauterine infection of the fetus by a pregnant infected woman

- Human bite

Despite the similarities between HIV and HBV, the risk of contracting HBV is far greater than contracting HIV. See Figure 10-2 and Table 10-3.

Medical assistants and all other health care providers must understand the importance of protecting themselves from the viruses that cause AIDS and hepatitis B and other pathogenic microorganisms as well. Through strict adherence to Standard Precautions and routine infectious disease control measures such as those found in medical asepsis, the risk of contracting an infectious disease is minimized.

PRINCIPLES OF INFECTION CONTROL

By understanding the dependent nature of the chain of infection which holds that each link in the process must occur for infectious disease to occur, medical assistants may apply principles of infection control to eliminate or reduce the transmission of infectious microorganisms in the ambulatory care setting. Conscious and continual reliance on infection control is a professional standard and protects employees, patients, and families from contracting infectious diseases. There are two general types of infection control: medical asepsis and surgical asepsis. Each is indicated in specific circumstances and each is achieved by the various techniques that are described in this chapter and Chapter 19. Stringent application of infection control measures should be the foundation of clinical care in the ambulatory care setting.

THE CENTERS FOR DISEASE CONTROL AND PREVENTION, AND ITS ROLE IN INFECTION CONTROL

The Centers for Disease Control and Prevention (CDC) is responsible for studying pathogens and diseases in an

BLOODBORNE FACTS

WHAT IS HBV?

Hepatitis B virus (HBV) is a potentially life-threatening blood-borne pathogen. Centers for Disease Control estimates there are approximately 280,000 HBV infections each year in the U.S.

Approximately 8,700 health care workers each year contract hepatitis B, and about 200 will die as a result. In addition, some who contract HBV will become carriers, passing the disease on to others. Carriers also face a significantly higher risk for other liver ailments which can be fatal, including cirrhosis of the liver and primary liver cancer.

HBV infection is transmitted through exposure to blood and other infectious body fluids and tissues. Anyone with occupational exposure to blood is at risk of contracting the infection.

Employers must provide engineering controls; workers must use work practices and protective clothing and equipment to prevent exposure to potentially infectious materials. However, the best defense against hepatitis B is vaccination.

WHO NEEDS VACCINATION?

The new OSHA standard covering bloodborne pathogens requires employers to offer the three-injection vaccination series free to all employees who are exposed to blood or other potentially infectious materials as part of their job duties. This includes health care workers, emergency responders, morticians, first-aid personnel, law enforcement officers, correctional facilities staff, launderers, as well as others.

The vaccination must be offered within 10 days of initial assignment to a job where exposure to blood or other potentially infectious materials can be "reasonably anticipated." The requirements for vaccinations of those already on the job took effect July 6, 1992.

WHAT DOES VACCINATION INVOLVE?

The hepatitis B vaccination is a noninfectious, yeast-based vaccine given in three injections in the arm. It is prepared from recombinant yeast cultures, rather than human blood or plasma. Thus, there is no risk of contamination from other bloodborne pathogens nor is there any chance of developing HBV from the vaccine.

The second injection should be given one month after the first, and the third injection six months after the initial dose. More than 90 percent of those vaccinated will develop immunity to the hepatitis B virus. To ensure immunity, it is important for individuals to receive all three injections. At

this point it is unclear how long the immunity lasts, so booster shots may be required at some point in the future.

The vaccine causes no harm to those who are already immune or to those who may be HBV carriers. Although employees may opt to have their blood tested for antibodies to determine need for the vaccine, employers may not make such screening a condition of receiving vaccination nor are employers required to provide prescreening.

Each employee should receive counseling from a health care professional when vaccination is offered. This discussion will help an employee determine whether inoculation is necessary.

WHAT IF I DECLINE VACCINATION?

Workers who decide to decline vaccination must complete a declination form. Employers must keep these forms on file so that they know the vaccination status of everyone who is exposed to blood. At any time after a worker initially declines to receive the vaccine, he or she may opt to take it.

WHAT IF I AM EXPOSED BUT HAVE NOT YET BEEN VACCINATED?

If a worker experiences an exposure incident, such as a needlestick or a blood splash in the eye, he or she must receive confidential medical evaluation from a licensed health care professional with appropriate follow-up. To the extent possible by law, the employer is to determine the source individual for HBV as well as human immunodeficiency virus (HIV) infectivity. The worker's blood will also be screened if he or she agrees.

The health care professional is to follow the guidelines of the U.S. Public Health Service in providing treatment. This would include hepatitis B vaccination. The health care professional must give a written opinion on whether or not vaccination is recommended and whether the employee received it. Only this information is reported to the employer. Employee medical records must remain confidential. HIV or HBV status must NOT be reported to the employer.

U.S. Department of Labor
Occupational Safety and Health Administration

Single copies of fact sheets are available from OSHA Publications, Room N3101, 200 Constitution Ave. N.W., Washington, D.C. 20210 and from OSHA regional offices.

Figure 10-2 *Bloodborne Facts,* published by the United States Department of Labor, Occupational Safety and Health Administration. This publication includes facts about hepatitis B virus, vaccination, declination, and steps to be taken by the employer should exposure to blood, body fluids, or OPIM occur.

TABLE 10-3   HEPATITIS VIRUSES A–E

	A	B	C	D	E
Etiologic Agent	Hepatitis A virus (HAV)	Hepatitis B virus (HBV)	Hepatitis C virus (HCV)	Hepatitis D virus (HDV)	Hepatitis E virus (HEV)
Transmission	Fecal-oral; contaminated water or food; person to person	Blood; sexual; perinatal; breast milk	Blood	Only persons with hepatitis B can get hepatitis D; blood and blood products; needlesticks; seldom sexual; rarely perinatal	Oral-fecal route; contaminated water; person-to-person uncommon
Risk Groups	Household/sexual contact with infected person; international travelers	Injection drug users; sexual/household contact with infected person; infants born to infected mothers; health care workers; multiple sex partners	Recipients of blood transfusions or organ transplants prior to 1992; people sharing needles; people exposed to blood and blood products	People sharing needles; health care workers	Travelers to countries where HEV is endemic
Incubation Period	15–50 days	45–160 days	14–180 days	15–60 days	15–60 days
Infectious Period	Usually less than 2 months	Before symptoms appear; lifetime if carrier	Before symptoms appear; lifetime if carrier	Not determined	Not determined
Diagnostic Tests	IgM anti-HAV	HBsAG	Anti-HCV; serum ALT increased 10x; HCVRNA	IgG anti-HDV	None available
Symptoms	Flu-like; jaundice; dark yellow urine; light-colored stools	Flu-like; may have jaundice; dark yellow urine; light-colored stools	Many have no symptoms; flu-like	Flu-like; may have jaundice; dark yellow urine; light-colored stools	Abdominal pain, anorexia; dark yellow urine; jaundice; fever
Prevention	Standard Precautions; enteric precautions; hepatitis A vaccine (entire series); immune globulin (for short term)	Standard Precautions; reduce risk behaviors; hepatitis B vaccine (entire series); immune globulin (for short term)	Standard Precautions; reduce risk behaviors; no vaccine	Standard Precautions; reduce risk behaviors; hepatitis B vaccine; if client already has hepatitis B, no prevention for hepatitis D	Standard Precautions; be sure water is safe when traveling; no vaccine
Treatment	Immune globulin within 2 weeks of exposure	Immune globulin (HBIg) Alpha interferon	Alpha interferon; ribavirin (Virazole)	Alpha interferon	None given
Prognosis	Rarely fatal; not a carrier	No cure; may become a carrier	85% or less have chronic infection; 70% develop chronic liver disease	Chronicity uncommon	No evidence of chronicity

(Courtesy Hepatitis Foundation International)

Data from: Centers for Disease Control and Prevention (CDC) (2000). Viral hepatitis. [On-line] Available: www.cdc.gov/ncidod/diseases/hepatitis; Lau, D. T., Kleiner, D. E., Park, Y., DiBisceglie, A. M., & Hoofnagle, J. H. (1999). Resolution of chronic delta hepatitis after 12 years of interferon alpha therapy. *Gastroenterology,* 117(5), 1229–33; National Institute of Diabetes and Digestive and Kidney Diseases (NIDDK) (1997). What I need to know about hepatitis A [On-line] Available: www.niddk.nih.gov/health/digest/pubs/hep/hepa/hepa.htm; NIDDK (1998). What I need to know about hepatitis B. [On-line] Available: www.niddk.nih.gov/health/digest/pubs/hep/hepb/hepb.htm; NIDDK (1999). What I meed to know about hepatitis C. [On-line] Available: www.niddk.nih.gov/health/digest/pubs/hep/hepc/hepc.htm; NIDDK (2000). Chronic hepatitis C: Current disease management. [On-line] Available: www.niddk.nih.gov/health/digest/pubs/chrnhepc/chrnhepc.htm; NIDDK (2000). The digestive diseases dictionary: E–K. [On-line] Available: www.niddk.nih.gov/health/digest/pubs/dddctnry/pages/e-k.htm.

effort to prevent their spread. A division of the United States Public Health Department, the CDC has issued a number of guidelines over the past twenty-five years that have enabled health care professionals to practice responsible infection control. As diseases evolve, and as new diseases are introduced into our society, the CDC revises and updates existing guidelines or issues new control measures to contain the spread of infection.

In 1970, the CDC developed a system of seven **isolation categories** for patients with known infectious diseases. This category system included strict **isolation**, respiratory isolation, protective isolation, enteric precautions, wound and skin precautions, discharge precautions, and blood precautions.

In 1985, the agency released a set of guidelines known as Universal Blood and Body Fluid Precautions, or simply **Universal Precautions**. These infection control practices were written in response to an increase in acquired immunodeficiency syndrome (AIDS) and hepatitis B, both bloodborne diseases, and to other infectious diseases as well.

Beginning in 1991, the CDC infection control guidelines were reviewed and subsequently revised. In 1996, a new set of guidelines was released. **Standard Precautions** reflect improved recommendations intended to protect all health care providers, patients, and their visitors from a wide range of **communicable** diseases. At the same time that the CDC issued the new Standard Precautions, they also released a second tier of precautions called **Transmission-Based Precautions**. These are intended to be used in addition to Standard Precautions when caring for patients with specific infectious diseases.

To understand the evolution and intent of these various CDC infection control guidelines, Universal Precautions, Standard Precautions, and Transmission-Based Precautions will be examined in more detail.

Universal Precautions

In an effort to curb the transmission of AIDS, hepatitis B, and other infectious diseases, in 1985 the CDC issued guidelines known as Universal Blood and Body Fluid Precautions or simply Universal Precautions. It is now known that consistent use and adherence to these guidelines greatly minimizes the risk of infectious disease transmission. At the recommendation of the CDC, health care providers were to consider every patient potentially infectious for AIDS, hepatitis B, and other bloodborne pathogens and to routinely and consistently use the techniques of Universal Precautions as a means of infection control.

While most of the basic tenets of Universal Precautions have now been incorporated into the new Standard Precautions, it is nonetheless important to know and understand the primary preventive measures of these 1985 recommendations.

Following is a summary of the CDC's Universal Precautions and guidelines for control of AIDS, hepatitis B, and other infectious diseases:

1. Consider all (patients') blood and body fluids to be contaminated.
2. Always wash hands before and after (patient) contact.
3. Always wash hands if contaminated with blood or body fluids.
4. Wear gloves when handling or touching blood, body fluids, body tissue, mucous membranes, nonintact skin, or contaminated equipment and supplies.
5. Wear gloves when performing venipuncture and other blood access treatments or procedures.
6. Change gloves after each patient contact.
7. Wash hands after glove removal. Gloves do not replace handwash technique.
8. Wear gloves, gown, mask, goggles/face shield if splashing of blood or body fluids can occur or if exposure to droplets of blood or body fluids is a possibility. Examples of this are wound care and **endoscopy**.
9. Use extreme caution when handling needles, scalpels, and other sharp instruments (**sharps**) during procedures and when handling them after procedures are completed. Dispose of sharps in an approved puncture-proof container that should be located as close as practical to the work area.
10. Use a mouthpiece if performing cardiopulmonary resuscitation. The risk of transmission of **human immunodeficiency virus (HIV)** through saliva is very low.
11. Clean blood and body fluid spills with agency disinfectant or a 10 percent solution of **sodium hypochlorite** (household bleach).
12. Report needlesticks, splashes, and contamination by wounds or body fluids. Follow up with employee health services, physician, and other appropriate personnel.
13. Health care workers with open **lesions** (injury or wound) or **dermatitis** (skin rash) should avoid direct contact with patients and their supplies and equipment until healed.
14. Laboratory specimens and their containers are modes of disease transmission and gloves should be worn during handling.
15. Pregnant health care providers should be especially careful to adhere to the guidelines so as to protect themselves and the unborn child.

Standard Precautions

The CDC spent several years researching, improving, and developing recommendations to protect health care providers, patients, and their visitors from infectious diseases. This intensive period of research resulted in Standard Precautions, a set of infection control guidelines that should now be utilized by all health care professionals for all patients.

Standard Precautions combine many of the basic principles of universal precautions with techniques known as **Body Substance Isolation (BSI)**, a system that maintains that personal protective equipment should be worn for contact with all body fluids whether or not blood is visible. Although BSI was developed not by a federal or state agency but by a private hospital, its techniques nonetheless have been adopted by many health care facilities.

The rationale behind developing the new Standard Precautions was that while Universal Precautions and Body Substance Isolation provide a good degree of protection, the CDC recognized that both could be improved upon. Advantages of the new Standard Precautions are that they include all of the major recommendations of Universal Precautions and Body Substance Isolation, while incorporating new information; they simplify medical terminology to be as user-friendly as possible; they use new terms to avoid confusion with existing infection control and isolation systems; and they are intended to protect all patients, all health care providers, and all visitors.

According to the CDC, Standard Precautions are "designed to reduce the risk of transmission of microorganisms from both recognized and unrecognized sources of infection in hospitals" (CDC, 1997). They apply to:

1. Blood
2. All body fluids, secretions, and excretions regardless of whether or not they contain visible blood
3. Nonintact skin
4. Mucous membranes

To be effective, Standard Precautions must be practiced conscientiously at all times. Although Standard Precautions were intended primarily for use in acute care facilities such as hospitals, they can and should be applied in other types of facilities including the ambulatory care settings where many medical assistants are likely to be employed.

Figure 10-3 provides a comprehensive review of the Standard Precautions.

Transmission-Based Precautions

When the CDC was in the process of developing a new guideline for isolation precautions in hospitals, the agency arrived at what it terms two tiers of precautions. The first

---

Latex Sensitivity

Health care providers should be aware that some people, including professionals and patients, can be allergic to latex products. Some personal protective equipment (PPE) is made from latex; medical and surgical products also are often made from this product.

The allergic reaction can be a localized one such as dermatitis or a more severe systemic reaction such as anaphylaxis (see Chapter 9), a form of shock marked by vascular collapse, respiratory failure, hypotension, arrhythmia, and laryngeal edema. Vinyl gloves can be worn in place of latex for hypersensitive individuals. Any person with an allergy to latex should wear a bracelet or other form of identification indicating this fact since, in any emergency, medical personnel wear latex gloves.

---

tier is called the Standard Precautions, discussed earlier in this chapter, designed for all patients regardless of their diagnosis or presumed infection status. The second tier of precautions is intended for patients diagnosed with or suspected of specific highly transmissible diseases. These are known as Transmission-Based Precautions.

Transmission-Based Precautions condense the seven existing categories of isolation precautions developed by the CDC in 1970 into three sets of precautions based on routes of infection. Released in 1996 to complement Standard Precautions, Transmission-Based Precautions reduce the risk of **airborne**, **droplet**, and **contact transmission** of pathogens and are always to be used *in addition to* Standard Precautions.

These airborne, contact, and droplet precautions also list specific syndromes that can appear in adult and pediatric patients who are highly suspicious for infection. They identify the appropriate Transmission-Based Precautions to be used until a diagnosis can be made. See Figures 10-4, 10-5, and 10-6 for specific information on these three Transmission-Based Precautions. Remember that these precautions are for specific categories of patients and are to be used in addition to Standard Precautions, which are used for all patients.

Blood and Body Fluids

In all infection control efforts, it is important to understand what is meant by blood and body fluids. Specifically, they are described as the blood, secretions, and excretions of a patient. Examples of blood and body fluids and some of the areas in which medical assistants may become exposed to them are:

STANDARD PRECAUTIONS
FOR INFECTION CONTROL

Wash Hands (Plain soap)
Wash after touching **blood, body fluids, secretions, excretions, and contaminated items.**
Wash immediately **after gloves are removed** and **between patient contacts.** Avoid transfer of microorganisms to other patients or environments.

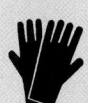

Wear Gloves
Wear when touching **blood, body fluids, secretions, excretions, and contaminated items.** Put on **clean** gloves just **before touching mucous membranes** and **nonintact skin.** Change gloves between tasks and procedures on the same patient after contact with material that may contain high concentrations of microorganisms. Remove gloves promptly after use, before touching noncontaminated items and environmental surfaces, and before going to another patient, and wash hands immediately to avoid transfer of microorganisms to other patients or environments.

Wear Mask and Eye Protection or Face Shield
Protect mucous membranes of the eyes, nose and mouth during procedures and patient-care activities that are likely to generate **splashes** or **sprays** of **blood, body fluids, secretions,** or **excretions.**

Wear Gown
Protect skin and prevent soiling of clothing during procedures that are likely to generate **splashes** or **sprays** of **blood, body fluids, secretions,** or **excretions.** Remove a soiled gown as promptly as possible and wash hands to avoid transfer of microorganisms to other patients or environments.

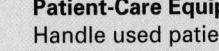

Patient-Care Equipment
Handle used patient-care equipment soiled with **blood, body fluids, secretions,** or **excretions** in a manner that prevents skin and mucous membrane exposures, contamination of clothing, and transfer of microorganisms to other patients and environments. Ensure that reusable equipment is not used for the care of another patient until it has been appropriately cleaned and reprocessed and single use items are properly discarded.

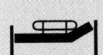

Environmental Control
Follow hospital procedures for routine care, cleaning, and disinfection of environmental surfaces, beds, bedrails, bedside equipment and other frequently touched surfaces.

Linen
Handle, transport, and process used linen soiled with **blood, body fluids, secretions,** or **excretions** in a manner that prevents exposures and contamination of clothing, and avoids transfer of microorganisms to other patients and environments.

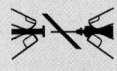

Occupational Health and Bloodborne Pathogens
Prevent injuries when using needles, scalpels, and other sharp instruments or devices; when handling sharp instruments after procedures; when cleaning used instruments; and when disposing of used needles.

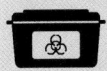

Never recap used needles using both hands or any other technique that involves directing the point of a needle towards any part of the body; rather, use either a one-handed "scoop" technique or a mechanical device designed for holding the needle sheath.

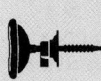

Do not remove used needles from disposable syringes by hand, and do not bend, break, or otherwise manipulate used needles by hand. Place used disposable syringes and needles, scalpels blades, and other sharp items in puncture-resistant sharps containers located as close as practical to the area in which the items were used, and place reusable syringes and needles in a puncture-resistant container for transport to the reprocessing area.

Use **resuscitation devices** as an alternative to mouth-to-mouth resuscitation.

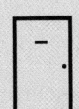

Patient Placement
Use a **private room** for a patient who contaminates the environment or who does not (or cannot be expected to) assist in maintaining appropriate hygiene or environmental control. Consult Infection Control if a private room is not available.

Figure 10-3   Standard Precautions for Infection Control issued by the CDC in 1997. (Courtesy Brevis Corp.)

AIRBORNE PRECAUTIONS
(in addition to Standard Precautions)

VISITORS: Report to nurse before entering.

Patient Placement
Use **private room** that has:
   Monitored negative air pressure,
   6 to 12 air changes per hour,
   Discharge of air outdoors or HEPA filtration if recirculated.
Keep room door closed and patient in room.

Respiratory Protection
Wear an **N95 respirator** when entering the room of a patient with known or suspected infectious pulmonary **tuberculosis.**
Susceptible persons should not enter the room of patients known or suspected to have **measles** (rubeola) or **varicella** (chickenpox) if other immune caregivers are available. If susceptible persons must enter, they should wear an **N95 respirator.** (Respirator or surgical mask not required if immune to measles and varicella.)

Patient Transport
Limit transport of patient from room to essential purposes only.
Use **surgical mask** on patient during transport.

Figure 10-4   Airborne Precautions, one category of Transmission-Based Precautions. (Courtesy of Brevis Corp.)

CONTACT PRECAUTIONS
(in addition to Standard Precautions)

VISITORS: Report to nurse before entering.

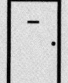

Patient Placement
Private room, if possible. Cohort if private room is not available.

Gloves
Wear gloves when entering patient room.
Change gloves after having contact with infective material that may contain high concentrations of microorganisms (**fecal** material and **wound drainage**).
Remove gloves before leaving patient room.

Wash
Wash hands with an **antimicrobial** agent immediately after glove removal. After glove removal and handwashing, ensure that hands do not touch potentially contaminated environmental surfaces or items in the patient's room to avoid transfer of microorganisms to other patients or environments.

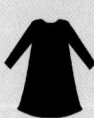

Gown
Wear gown when entering patient room if you anticipate that your clothing will have a substantial contact with the patient, environmental surfaces, or items in the patient's room, or if the patient is **incontinent,** or has **diarrhea,** an **ileostomy,** a **colostomy,** or **wound drainage** not contained by a dressing. **Remove** gown before leaving the patient's environment and ensure that clothing does not contact potentially contaminated environmental surfaces to avoid transfer of microorganisms to other patients or environments.

Patient Transport
Limit transport of patient to essential purposes only. During transport, ensure that precautions are maintained to minimize the risk of transmission of microorganisms to other patients and contamination of environmental surfaces and equipment.

Patient-Care Equipment
Dedicate the use of noncritical patient-care equipment to a single patient. If common equipment is used, clean and disinfect between patients.

Figure 10-5   Contact Precautions, one category of Transmission-Based Precautions. (Courtesy of Brevis Corp.)

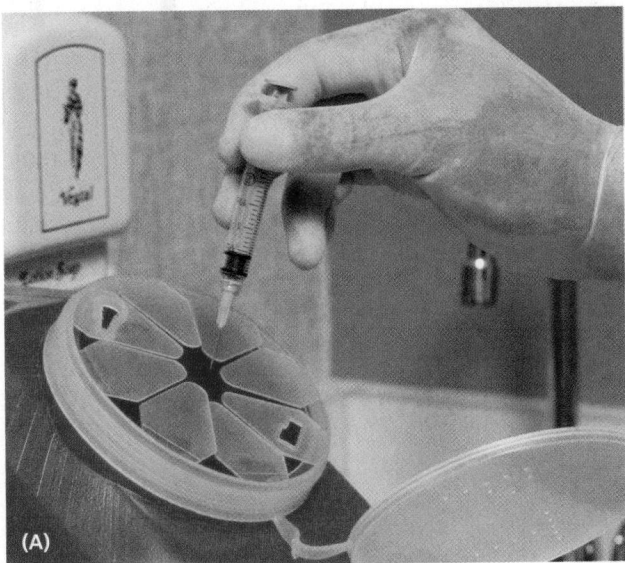

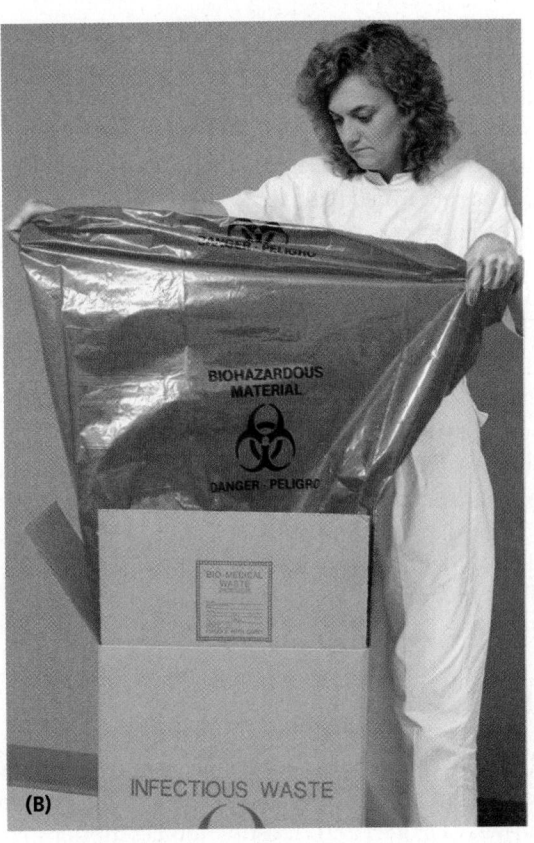

Figure 10-8 (A) Discard the entire disposable syringe with used needle intact in the biohazardous puncture-proof sharps container. (B) The medical assistant is placing a sturdy disposable plastic bag marked with the biohazardous waste symbol into a durable cardboard box for collection of infectious waste material. When full, these boxes are picked up by an agency for incineration or for autoclaving before disposal in a public landfill.

standards are rules established to measure quality, weight, extent, or value.

The Bloodborne Pathogen Standard

The Bloodborne Pathogen Standard became effective in March 1992. It came about principally in the hope of reducing the occupational-related cases of human immunodeficiency virus and hepatitis B infections among health care workers.

It covers all employees who can be "reasonably anticipated" to come into contact, as a result of performing their job duties, with blood and other potentially infectious materials (OPIM). It seeks to limit exposure to the pathogens. The law covers:

- Exposure determination
- Methods of control of exposure, especially Standard Precautions
- HBV vaccine
- Post-exposure follow-up
- Disposal of biohazardous waste
- Labeling
- Housekeeping and laundry functions
- Training for employee safety and documentation

Blood and Other Potentially Infectious Material (OPIM). Blood and OPIM are defined by the Centers for Disease Control and the Occupational Safety and Health Administration as the following human fluids:

- Blood and blood components
- Semen
- Vaginal secretions
- Cerebral spinal fluid
- Synovial fluid
- Pleural fluid
- Pericardial fluid
- Peritoneal fluid
- Body fluids visibly contaminated with blood
- Saliva in dental/oral procedures
- Unfixed human tissue (alive or dead); e.g., breast tissue from a frozen section biopsy
- Any tissue culture, cells, or fluid known to be HIV- or HBV-infected
- When the origin of a specimen is unknown, it must be handled as if it were infectious.

It is possible for medical assistants to come into contact with the majority of the fluids listed. Refer to "Blood and Body Fluids" earlier in this chapter.

Bloodborne Pathogens.

Disease-producing microorganisms are called pathogens; bloodborne refers to the manner in which the microorganisms can be transmitted—via blood or OPIM. Two pathogens of particular importance to health care providers are hepatitis B virus (HBV) and human immunodeficiency virus (HIV).

Hepatitis B causes diseases that directly affect the liver; the virus can be transmitted through blood from exposure to a contaminated needle. HIV is responsible for acquired immunodeficiency virus (AIDS), a fatal illness. HIV can be transmitted through blood from a contaminated needle and through direct contact with blood via broken skin. For a more in-depth discussion of both HBV and AIDS, refer to "Disease Transmission" earlier in this chapter.

Exposure Determination.

Exposure determination requires an employer to list all of the job classifications and employees in those job classifications that are exposed to blood and OPIM in the course of performing their jobs (Figure 10-9). Existing job descriptions can be used by the employer to identify the job categories that are considered high risk for exposure to blood and/or OPIM (Figure 10-10). It is important to note that exposure determination is made without regard to the use of PPE.

Plan to Control Exposure.

Every employer who has an employee(s) who is identified and determined to be at risk because of exposure potential must have a written exposure control plan (Figures 10-11 through 10-13). The plan must consist of methods of compliance for prevention of exposure, hepatitis B vaccination and post-exposure evaluation, communication of hazards to employee(s), documentation of the bloodborne standard, and a procedure for the determination of the events surrounding the exposure occurrence. The written plan must be employee accessible, updated regularly (at least annually), and modified when necessary and appropriate, especially to reflect changes in employee positions.

Methods of Compliance to Prevent Exposure.

There are seven major strategies mandated by OSHA for the prevention of exposure to bloodborne pathogens and OPIM.

1. *Standard Precautions*
   Adherence to the CDC's Standard Precautions is required; i.e., treating ALL bodily fluids and materials as if they are infectious. Handwashing is stressed and employers must provide handwashing facilities and must ascertain that employees use them frequently and especially following exposure to blood or OPIM.

2. *Engineering Controls and Work Practice Controls*
   Engineering controls and work practice controls consist of the physical equipment and mechanical

SAMPLE

Exposure Activity Form for Category 2 Employees.
Tasks Involving Occupation Exposure to Blood and Body Fluids

Employee at Risk and Job Title	Task Involving Risk and PPE	Risk Rating

Figure 10-9 Sample Exposure Activity Form for Category 2 Employees (no exposure to blood or body fluids), including tasks and risk rating. (Courtesy of POL Consultants)

SAMPLE

Exposure Classification Record of Employee

The following employee was classified according to work task exposure to certain body fluids as required by the current OSHA infection control standard on (Date) _____ as follows:

Employee Name: _____ SS# _____

_____ Category 1. "All procedures or other job related tasks that involve an inherent potential for mucous membrane or skin contact with blood, body fluids, or tissues, or a potential for spill or splashes of (blood or body fluids)."

_____ Category 2. Tasks in which "The normal work routine involves no exposure to blood, body fluids, or tissues, but exposure or potential exposure may be required as a condition of employment." For example, receptionists, accounting, or insurance staff or others who may, as a part of their duties, be asked to help in clean up, instrument recirculation, laboratory, or other similar procedures where exposure may result.

_____ Category 3. Tasks in which "The normal work routine involves no exposure to blood, body fluids, or tissues. Persons who perform these duties are not called upon as part of their employment to perform or assist in emergency medical care or first aid or to be potentially exposed in some other way."

Employer Signature _____

Because of a change of job assignment, the above employee was reclassified according to tasks exposure on (Date) _____ as follows:

_____Category 1
_____Category 2
_____Category 3

Employer's Signature _____

Because of a change of assignment, the above employee was reclassified according to task exposure on (Date) _____ as follows:

_____Category 1
_____Category 2
_____Category 3

Employer's Signature _____

NOTE: This record should be retained for length of employment plus thirty years.

OFFICE WORK PRACTICE EXPOSURE CONTROL PLAN

Effective Date: _____

Office of _____

As of the above date the office will follow the rules below to reduce exposure and contamination:

Observe Standard Precautions.

Wear gloves when drawing blood and performing procedures/tests.

Wash hands after removing gloves.

Change gloves frequently during the day and between patients.

Not answer phone or type while wearing gloves.

Not cap or break needles.

Dispose of all needles in sharps containers.

Not allow sharps containers to fill beyond ⅔ full.

Wear lab coats when performing tests.

Leave lab coats in laboratory/work area.

Dispose of all contaminated material in infectious waste container.

Disinfect the laboratory work surfaces frequently.

Disinfect the examining room surfaces, daily and as needed.

Sterilize nondisposable examination and testing equipment.

Monitor sterilization procedure.

Not eat or drink in work area.

Place gauze over tops of blood tubes when removing caps.

Clean up all specimen and chemical spills properly and immediately.

Label all chemicals according to OSHA regulations.

Label refrigerator that blood is stored in.

Centrifuges will have lids or specimens will be capped when spun.

Centrifuges will be disinfected regularly.

Hepatitis B vaccines will be offered to all employees.

Employees will take a safety training program.

Figure 10-10 Sample Exposure Classification Record of employee shows exposure categories into which employee's tasks fall. This record is kept for thirty years. (Courtesy of POL Consultants)

Figure 10-11 Office Work Practice Exposure Control Plan indicates a sample list of precautions to take to minimize employee risk exposure. (Courtesy of POL Consultants)

SAMPLE

Office Procedures Safety Form

PROCEDURE: _____

Type of hazard: _____

Person performing procedure: _____

Person assisting procedure: _____

Personal protective equipment used: _____

_____

Proper techniques for safety:

_____

_____

_____

What is done with used materials and soiled instruments?

_____

_____

_____

What chemical products are involved?

_____

_____

_____

What are the specific risks of procedure?

_____

_____

_____

Additional comments:

_____

_____

_____

_____

Prepared By: _____ Date: _____

Figure 10-12 Sample Office Procedures Safety Form lists procedures, type of hazard, employee performing procedure, employee assisting with procedure, and PPE. (Courtesy of POL Consultants)

SAMPLE

Safety/Work Practice Controls for Office Procedures

Each office has special safety procedures that are unique to that particular practice. These are also known as work practice controls. The fundamental work practice control is using Standard Precautions. Work practice controls reduce the likelihood of exposure to hazards. Many times the risks can be eliminated by changing the way a procedure is performed. Make copies of the PROCEDURES SAFETY FORM. Fill in the information for any procedure that involves exposure to potentially infectious body fluids. File these procedures in the office operation section of your manual. Do not limit this section to only body fluid exposures. General safety for other hazards such as chemicals and X-ray should be listed as well. Common examples are listed below. Check the ones you do and add to this list.

____ Patient exams	____ Arthroscopies
____ Aspirations	____ Vaginal exams
____ Inoculations	____ PAP smears/
____ Taking blood	IUDs
samples	____ OB care
____ Lab testing	____ Norplants
____ Lesion excisions	____ Vasectomies
____ Wound care	____ Biopsies
____ Dressing changes	____ Sigmoidoscopies
____ Colposcopies	____ _____
____ Surgical	____ _____
procedures	____ _____
____ X-rays	

Figure 10-13 Sample Safety/Work Practice Controls for Office Procedures lists procedures that involve exposure to blood, body fluids, and OPIM. (Courtesy of POL Consultants)

devices an employer provides in an attempt to safeguard and minimize employee exposure. A common example of an engineering control is sharps disposal containers (Figure 10-14). Others are mechanical pipettes, fume hoods, and splash guards. If and when occupational exposure continues after the engineering controls are in place, PPE must be used. Handwashing facilities or appropriate antiseptic hand cleanser (when handwashing facilities are unavailable) must be readily available. If antiseptic hand cleanser is used, hands must be washed with running water and soap as soon as possible. Employers must ascertain that employees wash their hands as soon as possible following the removal of gloves or other PPE, that employees wash hands and other skin surfaces with soap and water, flush eyes at the eyewash

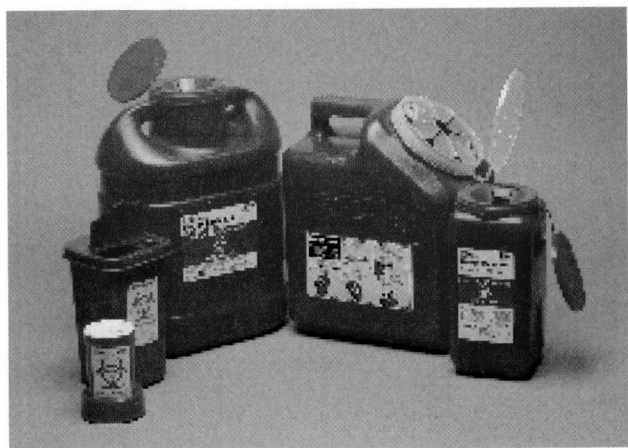

Figure 10-14 Various sizes of puncture-proof sharps containers. These and other biohazard waste containers are autoclaved when full and sent out to a biohazard agency for safe disposal.

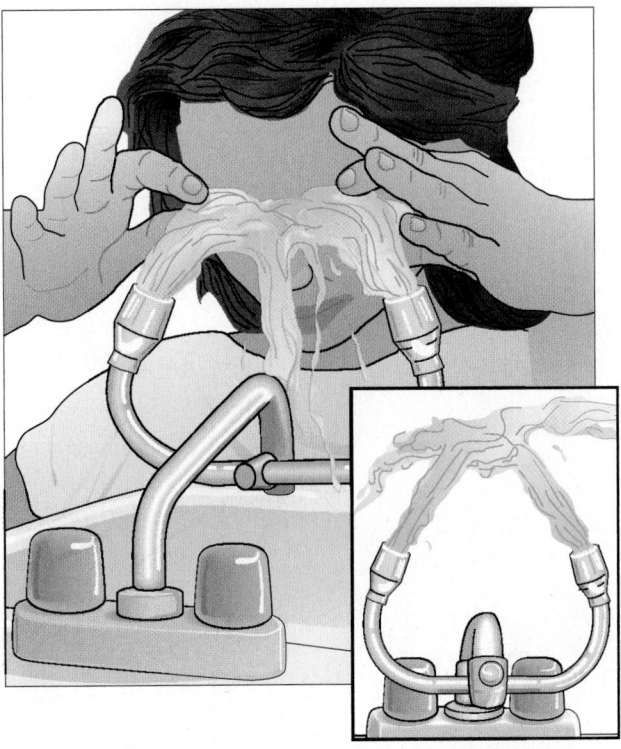

Figure 10-15 Emergency eyewash station: two streams of water wash both eyes simultaneously and continuously.

station, and flush mucous membranes with water as soon as possible following contact of these body parts with blood or OPIM (Figure 10-15).

Contaminated or used needles and other sharps must not be recapped, bent, nor removed unless required by a specific medical procedure. In such circumstances, a one-handed technique using a mechanical device must be used. (*In this instance, the needle has not been used on a patient.*) Contaminated sharps and needles must be placed immediately following use in a puncture-resistant container that is leak-proof and properly labeled with a biohazard label.

Eating, drinking, applying makeup, and so on are not allowed in areas when there is a possibility of exposure. Foods and drinks must be kept in a different refrigerator from one being used to store blood or OPIM.

Splashing, splattering, and spraying of blood or OPIM during procedures must be avoided if possible.

Mouth pipetting is not permissible.

Specimens must be put into containers that are labeled as biohazardous and the container must be leak-proof to prevent exposure during transport, handling, and collecting.

If equipment is contaminated with blood during its use, it must be decontaminated before it is serviced on-site or before it is sent out for service. It must also be labeled as biohazardous.

3. *Personal Protective Equipment (PPE)*
When workplace exposure still exists after using engineering and work practice controls, employers must provide PPE at no cost to the employee. PPE is used to place a barrier between the employee and

blood and/or OPIM that can contaminate skin, mucous membranes, or non-intact skin. PPE consists of such items as latex gloves, masks, goggles, face shields, gowns, laboratory coats, and plastic mouthpieces used during cardiopulmonary resuscitation (Figure 10-16). PPE provides protection only if it prevents blood or OPIM from permeating through it onto clothes, eyes, skin, mouth or other mucous membranes.

The employer must be certain that PPE is available and accessible and provide an alternative type of glove if an employee is allergic to those originally provided. Cleaning and laundering and disposal of PPE is the responsibility of the employer and the employee does not incur any expense for such.

All PPE must be removed before the employee leaves the work site and placed in an appropriate container that is supplied by the employer.

Gloves must be worn when there is a possibility of hand contact with blood or OPIM, with mucous membranes and nonintact skin, and when performing such procedures as phlebotomy. Disposable gloves cannot be decontaminated. They must be discarded into a biohazard container used for **regulated waste**.

Masks, face shields, and goggles must be worn if there is a possibility of splashing or splattering of

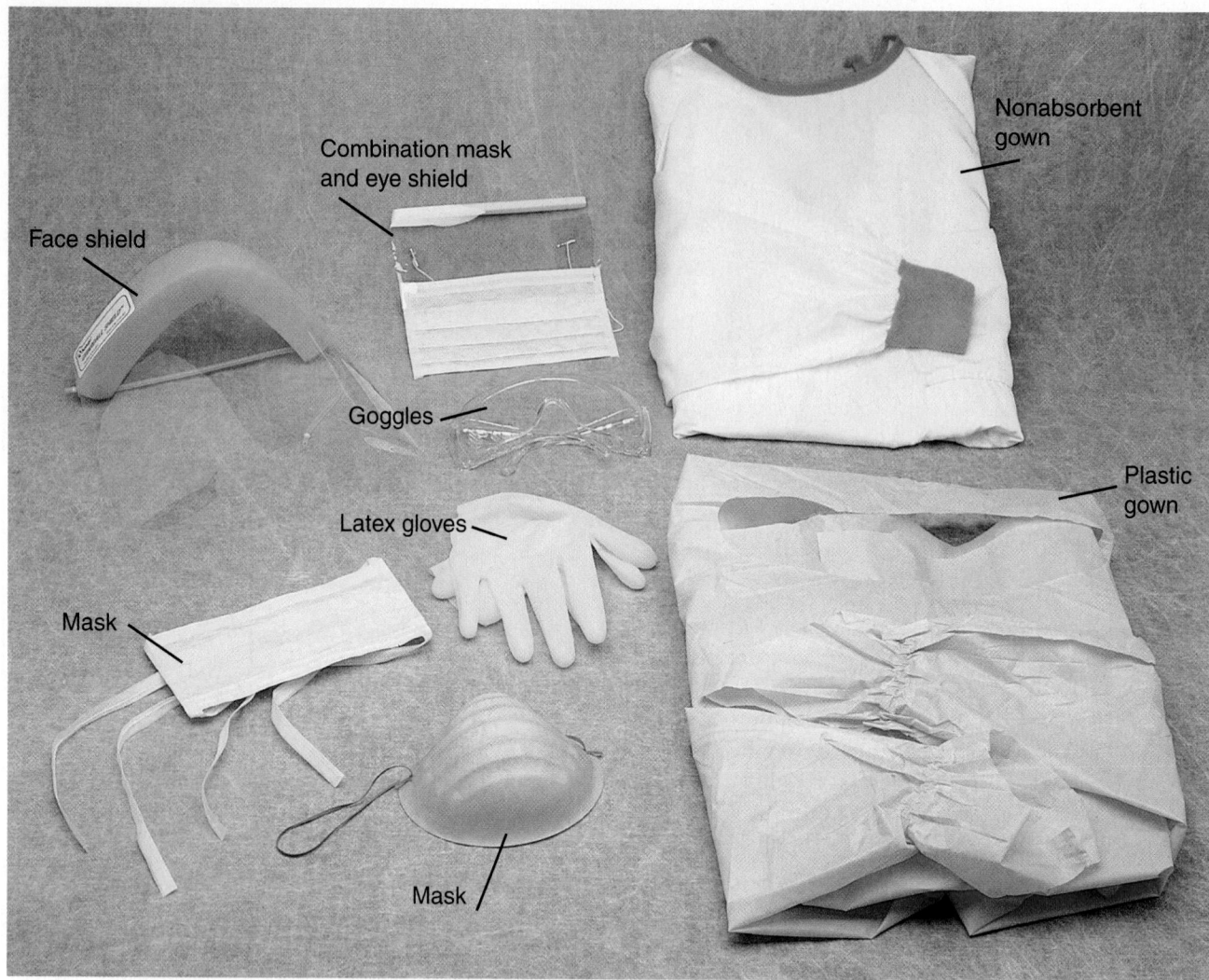

Figure 10-16   Personal protective equipment (PPE).

blood or OPIM. Gowns, laboratory coats, and other clothing must be worn to protect against exposure and must be left at the work site in an area set aside for their storage.

4. *Cleanliness of Work Areas*

The employer must maintain a work site that is clean and sanitary and have a written schedule for cleaning and decontaminating the work area after contact with blood and/or OPIM. Work surfaces that can become contaminated with blood or OPIM must be decontaminated after the work procedures are completed, after surfaces are contaminated, or at the end of the work shift. Some of the areas include counter tops, floors, examination tables, and wastepaper baskets.

When cleaning a work surface where there is the possibility of blood or OPIM present, latex gloves must be worn. A 10 percent solution of household bleach is used; alcohol is ineffective. Gloves should be worn when the spill is wiped with paper towels.

Both the towels and gloves are disposed of in a biohazard container and then the area is decontaminated (Figure 10-17).

Broken glass is placed in a sharps container after using cardboard or a dust pan and brush to remove it.

Laundry that is contaminated is handled with gloves and placed in a labeled container. If the laundry is damp or wet, gloves and other appropriate PPE must be worn and the damp/wet laundry must be placed in a plastic bag(s) to prevent blood or OPIM from leaking through it. PPE cannot be laundered at home (Figure 10-18).

Contaminated needles and other sharps must be disposed of into a puncture-resistant, leak-proof, and closable container immediately after use. The container must be labeled as biohazardous or orange-red in color and must be readily accessible to employees.

All other regulated waste must be placed into containers that are leak-proof and labeled as biohazardous or color coded orange-red.

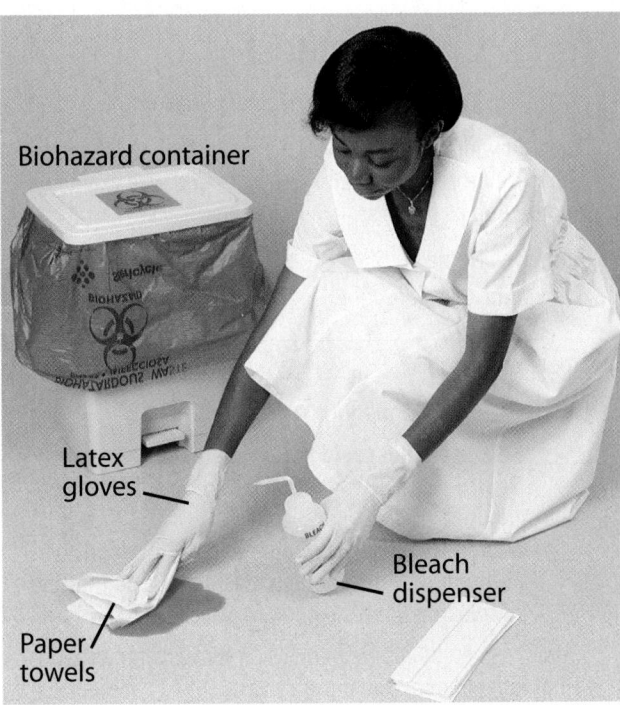

Figure 10-17 Medical assistant is wearing latex gloves to clean up a specimen spill. The biohazard waste bag is used to dispose of contaminated materials. The spill area is then cleaned with a 10 percent bleach solution.

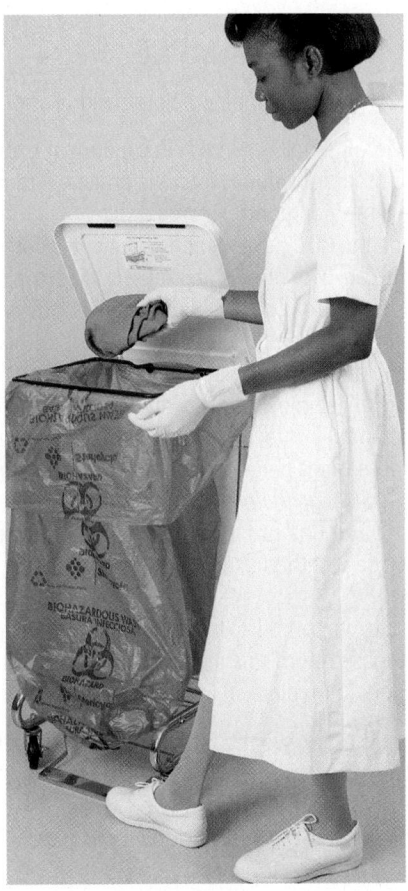

Figure 10-18 Medical assistant disposing of contaminated laundry in a covered laundry hamper containing a plastic biohazard bag.

5. *Hepatitis B Vaccine*

Hepatitis B vaccine must be made available free of charge to every employee, full-time, part-time, or temporary within ten days of work assignment (Figure 10-19). This refers to employees who have the potential for occupational exposure, and who can "reasonably" be expected to have skin, eye, mucous membrane, or **parenteral** contact with blood or OPIM. The vaccine is given in three doses over a six-month time period and is used to protect the employee from infection with the hepatitis B virus. It is an intramuscular injection with an approximate 96 percent rate of effectiveness.

An employee has the right to decline taking the vaccine, but must sign a **declination form**. There is the option to reconsider receiving the vaccine at a later time.

6. *Follow-Up After Exposure*

An accidental exposure is broadly defined as one in which blood, blood-contaminated body fluids, or body fluids or tissues to which Standard Precautions apply are introduced onto a mucous surface, onto nonintact skin, or to the conjunctiva via a needle-stick, skin cut, or direct splash. If an incident exposes an employee to any of these, the employer must make available a confidential medical evaluation in which is documented:

- The circumstances surrounding the event
- The route or routes of exposure
- The identification of the person who was the source of the exposure

The following procedure describes the steps to take following an exposure incident:

- Immediately wash exposed area with soap and warm water.
- If mouth area is exposed, rinse with water or mouthwash.
- If eyes are exposed, flush with large amounts of warm water.
- Report incident to a supervisor immediately for **documentation** (Figure 10-20).

Additionally, OSHA requires the following information:

- The exposed employee must be tested for HBV and HIV only if consent is given. An employee may refuse or may have blood drawn and stored for ninety days at which time the choice can be made whether to have the blood tested.

SAMPLE

Hepatitis B Employee Vaccination Form

MEMO: To all employees with occupational exposure to blood or other infectious materials on an average of one or more times per month.

OSHA and the CDC have identified the potential exposure of health care workers to hepatitis B virus (HBV) in the course of performing their duties in this office. For the protection of our employees, we are offering prescreening testing and the HBV vaccination with follow-up evaluation to all employees who are exposed to blood or other potentially infectious materials on an average of one or more times per month. *In accordance with recommended OSHA guidelines, this vaccine and testing will be offered at no cost to the employee.* You have the ability to decide whether or not you want the testing and/or vaccine.

At the bottom of this memo, you may indicate your choice. Please return this memo with your signature and date to your immediate supervisor.

[ ] I want to receive the prescreening (optional)
[ ] I want to receive the vaccine and follow-up evaluation testing
[ ] I *do not* want the vaccine and testing and have read the following statement:

I understand that due to my occupational exposure to blood or other potentially infectious materials I may be at risk of acquiring hepatitis B virus (HBV) infection. I have been given the opportunity to be vaccinated with hepatitis B vaccine at no charge to myself. However, I decline hepatitis B vaccination at this time. I understand that by declining this vaccine I continue to be at risk of acquiring hepatitis B, a serious disease. If in the future I continue to have occupational exposure to blood or other potentially infectious materials and I want to be vaccinated with hepatitis B vaccine, I can receive the vaccination series at no charge to me.

NAME _____   DATE _____

SIGNATURE _____   SS# _____

PRESCREENING DATE _____   RESULTS _____
DATE OF VACCINATIONS _____
DATE OF FOLLOW-UP EVALUATION _____
RESULTS _____
NOTES:

Figure 10-19   Sample Hepatitis B Employee Vaccination Form provides employee information regarding hepatitis B vaccine and space to sign indicating whether employee wants to receive the vaccine or whether employee declines vaccine. (Courtesy of POL Consultants)

SAMPLE

Post-Exposure Management Record

The following employee was the subject of an infectious exposure incident on (date) _____ and was examined and treated as follows:

Employee Name: _____ SS# _____
Type of Incident (describe) _____
_____

Route of Exposure: _____

Source Patient Information:

____ Source patient could not be identified.
____ Source patient was identified but refused to contribute blood.
____ Source patient was identified and blood was secured from such patient. Results of blood testing of source patient's blood are attached to this form.

Employee hereby grants permission for tests for antibodies of human immunodeficiency virus (HIV-1) and/or hepatitis B virus and acknowledges that the employee has been counseled concerning such tests.

Employee Signature _____ Date _____

The following test(s) were administered under supervision of a qualified physician:

____ Human Immunodeficiency Virus (HIV-1) Antibodies
____ Hepatitis B Virus Antibodies

Date(s) of Tests(s): _____ Results of Test(s)— See attached Physician's or Laboratory statement/report.

Employee hereby acknowledges that the employee was counseled and a written copy(ies) of the results of the above test(s) were furnished to such employee on (date): _____

Employee Signature _____ Date _____

____ Additional follow-up was performed as indicated by attached reports.

NOTE: This record should be retained for length of employment PLUS thirty years.

Figure 10-20   Sample Post-Exposure Management Record can be used to document employee exposure to blood, body fluids, or OPIM, tests performed on the employee by a qualified physician, and their results. (Courtesy of POL Consultants)

- The source individual's blood, if permission is granted, is tested for HBV and HIV, and the employee shall know the results (unless protected by the law).
- The employee is offered prophylaxis, gamma globulin, and/or HB vaccine following the exposure according to the current recommendation of the United States Public Health Service.
- The employee is counseled regarding precautions to take to avoid possible transmission and is provided information on potential illnesses for which to be alert.
- An OSHA 200 form must be filed.

7. *Medical Records*

Medical records of an employee who has suffered an occupational exposure must be kept for the length of employment plus thirty years and confidentiality must be guaranteed.

The following information is to be included in the employee's record: name and social security number, HB vaccination status with dates, results of any examinations or tests, a copy of the health care provider's written opinion, and a copy of the information that was provided to the health care provider.

The records must be available to the employee, to OSHA, and anyone with the written consent of the employee, but *not* the employer.

Hazard Communication for Blood. The employer is required to label containers of regulated waste, refrigerators, freezers, and other containers that are utilized to keep or transport blood or OPIM with warning labels that are orange or orange-red in color and have the biohazard symbol affixed to them. Red bags may be used in place of labels. The labeling serves to warn employees of the hazard possibility of container contents (Figure 10-21).

Information and Training for Employees. Employers must ascertain that employees take part in training sessions during working hours at no cost to employees. The initial session must be provided when occupational exposure may occur and annually thereafter. If employee tasks and job description change, training must take place at that time.

Training consists of:

- An explanation of the bloodborne standard
- The symptoms of the bloodborne disease
- An explanation of the modes of transmission
- An explanation of the exposure control plan
- Appropriate engineering and work practices
- PPE to utilize to limit exposure

BIOHAZARD LABELS

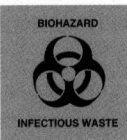

Containers that hold biohazardous materials must be properly labeled. Biohazardous materials include blood and body fluids as well as garments, gloves, masks, needles, gauze, wipes, aprons, and so on that may be contaminated with blood or other potential contaminated body fluids. Labels shall be used to identify the presence of an actual or potential biological hazard.

CONSIDERATIONS:

- Labels shall be fluorescent orange or orange-red, with lettering or symbols in a contrasting color.
- Labels should be affixed onto or as close as feasible to the container by adhesive, string, wire, or other method.
- Red bags or red containers may be substituted for labels.
- If blood or control serum is stored in a refrigerator, the refrigerator shall be marked with a biohazard label.
- If blood is stored in a refrigerator for transport or same-day shipment, it does not need to be labeled but should be put in containment bags.

Figure 10-21 Biohazard labels alert employees to biohazardous materials such as blood, body fluid, and OPIM.

- Information on the hepatitis B vaccine
- Procedures to follow should an exposure occur
- Information regarding post-exposure evaluation
- An explanation of the biohazard labels and color-coded containers

Documentation of training sessions must be available and kept for three years.

For an overview of the OSHA *Bloodborne Pathogen Standard*, see Figure 10-22.

OSHA REGULATIONS AND STUDENTS

With the passage of the OSHA law, all students with potential exposure to chemicals and bloodborne pathogens should follow all safety procedures as outlined by OSHA. Because students are not considered employees of a health care facility and are attending an educational institution, they do not fall under the OSHA guidelines. They should, however, take precautions to avoid contact with potentially infectious materials and toxic chemicals wherever learning is taking place.

Scope and Application

- The Standard applies to all occupational exposure to blood and other potentially infectious materials (OPIM), and includes part-time employees, designated first aiders, and mental health workers as well as exposed medical personnel.
- OPIM includes saliva in dental procedures, cerebrospinal fluid, unfixed tissue, semen, vaginal secretions, and body fluids visibly contaminated with blood.

Methods of Compliance

- General—standard precautions.
- Engineering and work practice controls.
- Personal protective equipment.
- Housekeeping.

Standard Precautions

- *All* human blood and OPIM are considered to be infectious.
- The *same* precautions must be taken with *all* blood and OPIM.

Engineering Controls

- Whenever feasible, engineering controls (devices that isolate or remove health hazards from the workplace) must be the primary method used to control exposure.
- Examples include needleless IVs, self-sheathing needles, sharps disposal containers, covered centrifuge buckets, aerosol-free tubes, and leak-proof containers.
- Engineering controls must be evaluated and documented on a regular basis.

Sharps Containers

- Readily accessible and as close as practical to work area.
- Puncture-resistant.
- Labeled or color-coded.
- Leak-proof.
- Closeable.
- *Routinely replaced* so there is no overflow.

Work Practice Controls

- Handwashing following glove removal.
- No recapping, breaking, or bending of needles.
- No eating, drinking, smoking, and so on in work area.
- No storage of food or drink where blood or OPIM are stored.
- Minimize splashing, splattering of blood, and OPIM.
- No mouth pipetting.
- Specimens must be transported in leak-proof, labeled containers. They must be placed in a secondary container if outside contamination of primary container occurs.

- Equipment must be decontaminated prior to servicing or shipping. Areas that cannot be decontaminated must be labeled.

Personal Protective Equipment (PPE)

- Includes eye protection, gloves, protective clothing, resuscitation equipment.
- Must be readily accessible and employers must require their use.
- Must be stored at work site.

Eye Protection

- Is required whenever there is potential for splashing, spraying, or splattering to the eyes or mucous membranes.
- If necessary, use eye protection in conjunction with a mask or use a chin-length face shield.
- Prescription glasses may be fitted with solid sideshields.
- Decontamination procedures must be developed.

Gloves

- Must be worn whenever hand contact with blood, OPIM, mucous membranes, nonintact skin, contaminated surfaces/items, or when performing vascular access procedures (phlebotomy).
- Type required—Vinyl or latex for general use.
    - Alternatives must be available if employee has allergic reactions (i.e., powderless).
    - Utility gloves for surface disinfection.
    - Puncture-resistant when handling sharps (i.e., Central Supply).

Protective Clothing

- Must be worn whenever splashing or splattering to skin or clothing may occur.
- Type required depends on exposure. Prevention of contamination of skin and clothes is the key.
- Examples —Low-level exposure lab coats.
    - Moderate-level exposure fluid-resistant gown.
    - High-level exposure fluid-proof apron, head and foot covering.
- *Note:* If PPE is considered protective clothing, then the *employer must* launder it.

Housekeeping

- There must be a written schedule for cleaning and disinfection.
- Contaminated equipment and surfaces must be cleaned as soon as feasible for obvious contamination or at end of work shift if no contamination has occurred.
- Protective coverings may be used over equipment.

(continues)

Figure 10-22   Overview of *The Bloodborne Pathogen Standard.* (Courtesy of the Occupational Safety and Health Administration, U.S. Department of Labor)

Regulated Waste Containers (non-sharp)

- Closeable.
- Leak-proof.
- Labeled or color-coded.
- Placed in secondary container if outside of container is contaminated.

Laundry

- Handled as little as possible.
- Bagged at location of use.
- Labeled or color-coded.
- Transported in bags that prevent soak-through or leakage.

Laundry Facility

- Two options:
  1. Standard precautions for all laundry (alternative color coding allowed if recognized).
  2. Precautions only for contaminated laundry (must be red bags or biohazard labels).
- Laundry personnel must use PPE and have a sharps container accessible.

Hepatitis B Vaccination

- Made available within ten days to all employees with occupational exposure.
- At no cost to employees.
- May be required for student to be admitted to college health program as well as for externship.
- Given in accordance with United States Public Health Service guidelines.
- Employee must first be evaluated by health care professional.
- Health care professional gives a written opinion.
- If the vaccine is refused, the employee signs a declination form.
- Vaccine must be available at a future date if initially refused.

Post-Exposure Follow-Up

- Document exposure incident.
- Identify source individual (if possible).
- Attempt to test source if consent obtained.
- Provide results to exposed employee.

Labels

- Biohazard symbol and word *Biohazard* must be visible.
- Fluorescent orange/orange-red with contrasting letters may also be used.
- Red bags/containers may be substituted for labels.

- Labels required on—Regulated waste.
  - —Refrigerators/freezers with blood of OPIM.
  - —Transport/storage containers.
  - —Contaminated equipment.

Information and Training

- Required for all employees with occupational exposure.
- Training required initially, annually, and if there are new procedures.
- Training material must be appropriate for literacy and education level of employee.
- Training must be interactive and allow for questions and answers.

Training Components

- Explanation of bloodborne standard.
- Epidemiology and symptoms of bloodborne disease.
- Modes of HIV/HBV transmission.
- Explanation of exposure control plan.
- Explanation of engineering, work practice controls.
- How to select the proper PPE.
- How to decontaminate equipment, surfaces, and so on.
- Information about hepatitis B vaccine.
- Post-exposure follow-up procedures.
- Label/color code system.

Medical Records

Records must be kept for each employee with occupational exposure and include:

- A copy of employee's vaccination status and date.
- A copy of post-exposure follow-up evaluation procedures.
- Health care professional's written opinions.
- Confidentiality must be maintained.
- Records must be maintained for thirty years plus the duration of employment.

Training Records

Records are kept for three years from date of training and include:

- Date of training.
- Summary of contents of training program.
- Name and qualifications of trainer.
- Name and job title of all persons attending.

Exposure Control Plan Components

- A written plan for each workplace with occupational exposure.

(continues)

Figure 10-22   *(continued)*

- Written policies/procedures for complying with the standard.
- A cohesive document or a guiding document referencing existing policies/procedures.

Exposure Control Plan

- A list of job classifications where occupational exposure control occurs (e.g., medical assistant, clinical laboratory scientist, dental hygienist).
- A list of tasks where exposure occurs (e.g., medical assistant who performs venipuncture).
- Methods/policies/procedures for compliance.
- Procedures for sharps disposal.
- Disinfection policies/procedures.
- Procedures for selection of PPE.
- Regulated waste disposal procedures.
- Laundry procedures.
- Hepatitis B vaccination procedures.
- Post-exposure follow-up procedures.
- Training procedures.
- Plan must be accessible to employees and be updated annually.

Employee Responsibilities

- Go through training and cooperate.
- Obey policies.
- Use universal precaution techniques.
- Use PPE.
- Use safe work practices.
- Use engineering controls.
- Report unsafe work conditions to employer.
- Maintain clean work areas.

Cooperation between employer and employees regarding *The Bloodborne Pathogen Standard* will facilitate understanding of the law, thereby benefiting all persons who are exposed to HIV, HBV, and OPIM by minimizing the risk of exposure to the pathogens.

Meeting the OSHA standard is not optional and failure to comply can result in a fine that may total $10,000 for each employee.

To obtain copies of *The Bloodborne Pathogen Standard*, contact OSHA at 800-321-6742 or www.osha.gov.

Figure 10-22 *(continued)*

Avoiding Exposure to Bloodborne Pathogens

Students can come into contact with blood and OPIM whenever in direct contact with patients or patients' specimens. The potential for exposure and contact increases whenever **invasive procedures** are being performed. Some examples of invasive procedures are:

- **Phlebotomy**, the process of withdrawing blood
- Administering an injection
- Performing or assisting with medical/surgical procedures such as suturing of wounds, removal of sutures, assisting with certain procedures such as Pap smears, arthroscopies, amniocentesis, thoracentesis, or lumbar puncture. Dressing changes, colposcopies, vaginal exams, obstetrical care, vasectomies, biopsies, and sigmoidoscopies are other examples in which students can contact blood and OPIM.

Students must be aware of and think about the procedures they are involved in and be certain that they use essential safety equipment (PPE) and procedures when necessary. Students should adhere to the same responsibilities that employees do.

PPE should be available in the student laboratory and used as necessary. Standard precautions must be strictly adhered to.

Gloves must be worn:
- During phlebotomy
- When giving injections
- When performing or assisting with invasive procedures
- When processing blood specimens

Eye protection with side projections must be worn:
- Whenever there is the potential for chemical exposure or the possibility of spray, splash, or splatter from blood or body fluids

Face shields or masks must be worn:
- When there is a chance of spray, splash, or splatter from blood or body fluids

Gowns or **aprons** must be worn:
- Where there exists any potential for exposure to contaminated materials

Lab coats must be worn and buttoned:
- When performing laboratory procedures

Students should always be on guard and make safety a priority by taking all precautions to avoid injuries. Some of the precautions are:

- No recapping of needles

- No bending or breaking needles

- Do not remove a needle from a syringe or a **Vacutainer®**

- Immediately dispose of needles and other sharps into a puncture-proof container

- No eating, drinking, smoking, or applying makeup in the area where there are patients or human specimens being handled and processed

- Never handle contaminated glass

- Clean spills with a device such as a shovel, cardboard, or paper towels, even if wearing gloves

- Know how to use a **spill kit**

- Know where the eyewash stations and showers are and know how to operate them

Students should decontaminate work areas with a 10 percent bleach solution and place contaminated waste into clearly marked biohazard containers. Some examples of contaminated waste items include disposable vaginal specula, patient swabs, gauze or dressing materials, and disposable suture removal kits, and any other equipment and supplies used during invasive procedures.

An exposure to blood or OPIM suffered by a student must be immediately reported to the instructor if the accident occurs at the college or to the supervisor of the clinical agency if the student is exposed during externship. OSHA procedures as outlined earlier in this chapter should be followed with the exception of the filing of the OSHA 200 form.

Many colleges require students studying the health professions to obtain the hepatitis B vaccine since it is approximately 96 percent effective against HBV. Because the vaccine is given in three doses over a period of six months, students should plan to have the injections in a timely fashion in order to be prepared for college laboratory courses and the externship period.

MEDICAL ASEPSIS

Medical asepsis is the destruction of pathogenic microorganisms after they leave the body. These techniques are used to decrease the risk of transmission to others. Objects should be medically aseptic if they are to be used in procedures that are on the external body or if they will enter a usually contaminated body part, such as the mouth. Medical asepsis also involves environmental hygiene measures such as equipment cleaning and disinfection procedures. Careful attention to methods of medical asepsis greatly reduces the presence of pathogens that could cause disease in others. Specific procedures to achieve medical asepsis include adherence to standard and transmission-based precautions. Standard Precautions and Transmission-Based Precautions are considered methods of medical asepsis. These precautions should be followed stringently to provide barriers between potentially infectious blood and body fluids and those people who may come into contact with the fluids. Use of PPE, disinfection and waste control are crucial steps in practicing these precautions. Handwashing, sanitization, and disinfection of instruments or equipment are also essential.

Handwashing

Handwashing is perhaps the most important aspect of all infectious control procedures. Proper handwashing reduces pathogens that could be transmitted by direct or indirect contact to others. Since handwashing is frequently required, the use of a mild antibacterial lotion is acceptable to reduce the possibility of skin breaks due to dryness.

Procedure 10-1 outlines the steps of a medical asepsis handwash.

Sanitization

Sanitization of instruments and equipment, another procedure used in medical asepis, is needed to rid contaminated reusable instruments and equipment of tissue, debris, blood, secretions, excretions, or other contaminates. **Sanitization** is physically cleaning and scrubbing to remove contaminated debris. Mild instrument detergent is used with a scrub brush on an instrument, paying careful attention to interior surfaces, hinges, crevices, and serrations. Disposable gloves should be worn by the medical assistant to protect from blood and body fluids. Use of a special detergent designed for a medical setting ensures that instruments will be more easily and thoroughly rinsed to protect them from corrosion. A critical component to promoting effective sanitization is to complete the procedure as soon as possible following contamination, so tissue or body fluids do not have the opportunity to dry on the instruments. Dried debris are more difficult to remove and may require much scrubbing. Instruments may be left to soak in disinfectant solution or water with a solvent if sanitization cannot be performed immediately following use.

To avoid the risk of punctures or cuts from sharp instruments during sanitization, heavy-duty gloves should be worn. Some facilities use an ultrasonic cleaner for sanitizing instruments prior to sterilizing them. Goggles are worn to protect eyes from splashing of contaminated debris during the scrubbing procedure. A plastic apron provides protection from splashing of clothing. (See Chapter 19.) Hot water may be used for rinsing in order to remove all residue and aid in the drying process. Drying thoroughly will prevent damage from rust or water spots.

Larger items such as instrument trays or Mayo stands, stools, chairs, examination tables, and lamps should also have a decontaminating sanitization process with thorough washing, rinsing, and drying.

See Procedure 10-2 for instrument sanitization and Procedure 10-3 for removing contaminated gloves. Gloves contaminated with biohazard substances should be removed carefully in order to contain the contamination. Procedure 10-3 describes how to remove contaminated gloves while preventing further exposure to biohazard substances.

Also see Latex Sensitivity on page 146 for a description of allergic reactions to latex products such as disposable gloves.

Disinfection

Disinfection, a third procedure used in medical asepsis practices, consists of various chemicals that can be used to destroy many pathogenic microorganisms but not necessarily their spores. Chemicals are used on inanimate objects. Because of their caustic nature, chemicals can irritate the skin and mucous membranes. Chemicals can be used to disinfect items or equipment made from materials that could be damaged by heat or that are too large to fit into an autoclave such as glass mercury thermometers, percussion hammers, examination tables, and Mayo stands. These and other items are used during *external* physical examination or procedures.

Boiling water (temperature 212°F) is considered a form of disinfection because it will kill some forms of microorganisms. It is important to note that this method *cannot* be used as a technique to sterilize goods because the temperature is not high enough to kill the hepatitis virus or microbial spores. Articles such as nasal and aural specula can be disinfected by vigorous boiling for at least fifteen minutes. The only reasonable use for boiling as a means of disinfection in today's medical setting is for items that:

1. Will *not* be used in invasive procedures
2. Will not be inserted into body orifices nor be used in a sterile procedure

Prior to either chemical disinfection or disinfection by boiling, articles must first be thoroughly sanitized. Of special note are stainless steel gynecological and proctologic examination instruments. These instruments are not sanitized with other instruments due to the risk of transmission of sexually transmitted diseases (STDs). They are sterilized in the autoclave following sanitization to eliminate transmission of microorganisms.

Fiberoptic endoscopes are sanitized and chemically sterilized. See chemical sterilization in this chapter. (See also Chapter 19.)

Chemical disinfectant solutions must be carefully prepared and used according to the manufacturer's instructions in order to ensure effective disinfectant properties. Medical offices should use the disinfectant solution that best meets the needs of the ambulatory care setting as to quantity of instruments to be disinfected, preparation requirements, storage needs, and handling procedures. When choosing a chemical disinfectant solution, pay close attention to the manufacturer's report of the chemical disinfectant properties of the product. Some solutions are effective against a wide spectrum of microorganisms, whereas other solutions may be selective for certain common microorganisms. If instructions for use are closely followed, the chemical disinfectant properties will be considered to have been met. Environmental hygiene procedures ensure disinfection of large pieces of equipment, furniture, and other fomites. Protocols for agency disinfection should address the frequency, solutions, and fomites (substances that absorb and transmit infectious material) for disinfection.

Procedure 10-4 outlines steps involved in chemical disinfection of instruments.

Some specific examples of appropriate use of medical asepsis include:

- Wash hands before and after handling equipment and supplies and before and after working with each patient even if gloves were worn.

- Handle all specimens as if they were contaminated.

- Use disposable equipment whenever possible and dispose of it properly in a biohazard waste container. All equipment is contaminated after patient use.

- Use personal protective equipment (PPE) as outlined in Standard Precautions and wash hands after removal of any PPE.

- Keep contaminated equipment and supplies away from clothing to prevent transmission of pathogens to self and others.

- Place dressing materials, gauze, cotton balls, and any other absorbable material that is damp or wet in a waterproof bag prior to disposal in the biohazard waste container.

- Any break in the medical assistant's skin should be covered with a sterile dressing.

- Items that fall to the floor are contaminated. Either discard or sanitize and disinfect or sterilize before using.

● If uncertain whether equipment or supplies are clean or sterile, clean or sterilize them before use.

For surfaces such as countertops, the least expensive and most readily available chemical is a 1:10 solution of ordinary household bleach (sodium hypochlorite). However, besides the obvious disadvantage of bleaching clothing, bleach is not easily rinsed and it is only effective if the solution is mixed fresh daily. Nevertheless, its effectiveness is so highly respected that many medical laboratories depend almost entirely on bleach to chemically kill pathogens on countertops.

In summary, medical asepsis includes procedures for which all medical assistants must be qualified and responsible to incorporate into daily work practices. The responsibility for maintaining medical asepsis is the combined goal of the office staff and physician.

Refer to information presented earlier in this chapter for information on environmental hygiene and daily work practices.

SURGICAL ASEPSIS AND STERILIZATION

Surgical asepsis means all microbial life, pathogens and nonpathogens, are destroyed before an invasive procedure is performed. Therefore, all equipment used is sterile. The terms *surgical asepsis* and *sterile technique* often are used interchangeably. (See Chapter 19.)

The main purpose of surgical asepsis is to prevent organisms from entering the patient's body during an invasive procedure. An invasive procedure is either creating or treating an opening in the skin such as a surgical incision, laceration, or an injection; or exposing a sterile inner surface to possible invasions of microorganisms such as when a urinary catheter is inserted through the urethra and into the urinary bladder.

Because the microorganisms are on virtually every surface such as the skin, instruments, surgical instrument trays, clothing, and even in the air, it is necessary to destroy as many of them as possible prior to doing any surgical (sterile) procedure. Any item that will come into contact with the sterile field (the area in which the sterile procedure will be performed or where sterile supplies will be maintained during the procedure) must be sterilized using physical or chemical agents. Once the surfaces are sterilized, every precaution must be taken to prevent contamination of the sterile areas either from a nonsterile surface or from airborne contamination. To **contaminate** is to make impure; e.g., by the introduction of microorganisms or infectious material.

● Before items can be sterilized, they must first be thoroughly sanitized. The contaminated instruments are taken to a work area designated for that purpose. See Procedure 10-5 regarding sanitation of instruments. Care must be taken to prevent contamination of self. Heavy-duty gloves, goggles, and a plastic apron are worn for protection. Always check instruments for their working condition. Check ratchets, serrations, alignment, and ensure that they open and close readily. Separate improperly working instruments. Instruments are now ready to be wrapped for sterilization.

Living tissue surfaces such as skin cannot be sterilized but can be rendered as free of pathogens as possible before the use of a sterile covering. One example of this concept is preparing the patient's skin with a surgical scrub solution prior to applying sterile drapes around the intended surgical site (see Chapter 19). Another example is the use of surgical handwashing technique prior to applying sterile gloves. The differences between handwashing for medical asepsis as discussed in this chapter (Procedure 10-1) and handwashing for surgical asepsis are addressed in Chapter 19.

There are four methods of sterilization:

1. Gas sterilization
2. Dry heat
3. Chemical sterilization
4. Steam sterilization (autoclave)

Gas Sterilization

Gas sterilization is accomplished in a gas oven large enough for wheelchairs and beds and takes hours for the extremely toxic gases to permeate and dissipate. These features make the gas oven very useful in a large hospital setting, but much too costly for the office.

Dry Heat Sterilization

Dry heat sterilization requires higher temperatures than steam sterilization and requires longer exposure times as well (at least one hour at 320°F). This method can be used for instruments that easily corrode such as sharp cutting instruments. Powders, oils, ointments, rubber goods, and plastic tubing may be sterilized using the dry heat method. Procedures for wrapping are the same as when wrapping for steam sterilization, see Procedures 10-5 and 10-6.

Chemical Sterilization

Chemical sterilization, or cold sterilization (see Chapter 19), uses the same chemical agents used to chemically disinfect instruments or fomites. However, the exposure time for sterilization is achieved through prolonged immersion. The handling of instruments following chemical sterilization differs from handling procedures for instruments that are steam sterilized.

Chemical sterilization (also see Chapter 19) is a very effective method used in many medical offices when the object being sterilized is too large or too heat sensitive for autoclaving (see following information on autoclaving). Fiber-optic endoscopes are one of the most common items sterilized with the use of chemicals. These items are delicate and unable to withstand the high heat of an autoclave. The necessary equipment for chemical sterilization is a container or basin of adequate size for the intended item (and should be maintained for that purpose only) with a well-fitting lid and the chemical of choice. Two of the most popular brands available through medical supply sources are Wavecide and Cidex. Both have advantages and disadvantages. Offices must make individual choices based on convenience, expense, and other personnel preferences.

The effectiveness of any of these products depends greatly on the strength of the solution. If the strength is a 1:1 ratio of water to chemical, effectiveness will be lost if the solution is not mixed according to that dilution. Any attempt to cut cost by mixing a weaker solution will greatly compromise the effectiveness. Sometimes solutions are weakened unintentionally by placing wet items into them, thereby adding more water than is intended. For this reason, wet items must be carefully dried prior to chemical sterilization. To avoid evaporation, which also interferes with the strength of the solution, a well-fitting lid is essential. The lid also lessens the chance of dust and airborne microbes from falling into the solution.

Another factor influencing the effectiveness of the sterilizing chemicals is exposure time. The manufacturer will provide specific time charts for each purpose. Manufacturer's directions will also include a time frame for replacing the solution. The ability of the solution to kill pathogens will be directly related to its freshness or shelf life. Regardless of the chemical used for sterilization, ventilation is very important.

 When using commercial chemicals, make certain the lid is placed on the soak basin at all times except when placing or removing items. Care must be taken to avoid contact with skin, eyes, and mucous membranes. Wear protective gloves, goggles, and apron if splashing is anticipated. The effects on skin can range from slight irritation to serious caustic burns. See Procedure 19-1 in Chapter 19.

Before any chemically sterilized items are used for patient contact, the chemicals must be thoroughly rinsed off using sterile transfer forceps to remove the item from the container. In order to maintain sterility, sterile water must be used for the rinsing process. Then dry with a sterile towel, and place onto a sterile field with new sterile transfer forceps.

Steam Sterilization (Autoclave)

Steam sterilization is the most widely used method of sterilization in the medical office. An autoclave, basically a pressure cooker, is used to achieve sterilization. The autoclave uses steam under pressure to obtain higher temperatures than can be achieved with boiling (Figure 10-23). Water reaches a maximum temperature of 212°F through boiling. When under pressure, water is converted to steam and is then able to reach a temperature of 250–254°F. Exposing items to this extremely high heat and at least 15 pounds of pressure for a specific amount of time assures that all microorganisms and their spores are eradicated. The autoclave is actually an inner sterilizing chamber surrounded by a metal jacket. This creates a middle steam chamber between the inner sterilizing chamber and the jacket. Inside the jacket is a reservoir for water. When water is poured into the reservoir, the autoclave door closed and secured, and the autoclave turned on, several processes occur. The water in the reservoir heats until vapor is produced. The vapor enters the middle steam chamber inside the jacket. The air in the steam chamber is pushed out and replaced with steam. Since the air has been pushed out, the pressure increases. The increase of pressure causes the steam to then enter the inner sterilizing chamber (this is where the surgical instruments are placed) which pushes out the air. With the air being displaced with steam, the pressure increases in the inner chamber. The steam under pressure is able to reach a much higher temperature than boiling water. When the steam is able to reach all surfaces of the items placed in the autoclave and exposure is maintained for adequate amounts of time, sterility of those items is assured.

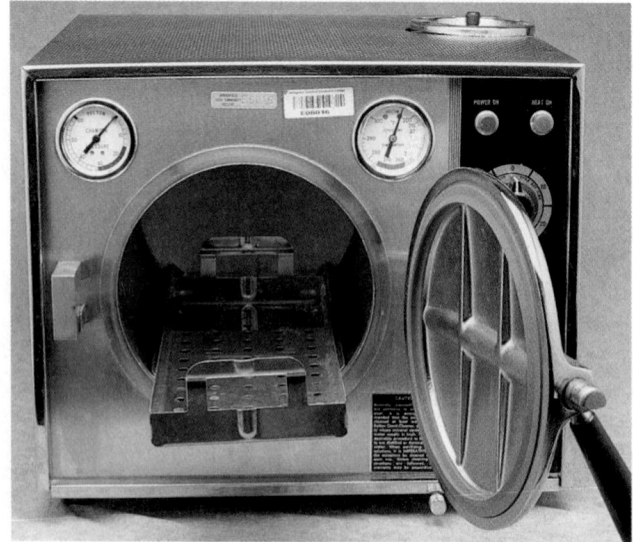

Figure 10-23   Commonly found in physician's offices, autoclaves are used for sterilization by steam pressure, usually at 250–254°F (121°C) for a specified length of time.

The recommended temperature for effective sterilization in an autoclave is 250–254°F. Unwrapped items should be sterilized for 20 minutes, loosely wrapped items for 30 minutes, and tightly packed items for at least 40 minutes. When uncertain about the proper amount of time necessary, the medical assistant should refer to the manufacturer's recommendations. The overall effectiveness of the autoclave in sterilizing contents is totally dependent on the medical assistant following proper operating procedure.

How to Load Packages. It is of extreme importance that instruments and materials be positioned properly in the autoclave in order for the steam to circulate through and between packs and penetrate them. Do not overload the autoclave. Place items as loosely as possible inside the chamber. Leave a one- to three-inch space between packs and the walls of the autoclave. Correct positioning and spacing allows sterilization to take place provided the medical assistant adheres to proper temperature, pressure, and time requirements.

Autoclave Maintenance and Cleaning. The autoclave, like any piece of equipment in the medical office, needs regular cleaning and maintenance. Frequency of cleaning the autoclave will depend somewhat on its usage. If the autoclave is used every day, the inner chamber should be washed with a mild detergent and cloth, rinsed, and dried on a daily basis. The outer jacket should be wiped clean of dust and soil. Follow the manufacturer's instructions and recommendations for cleansers. Omni cleanser is a well-known brand of autoclave cleanser.

At least once a week the autoclave should be drained of water and cleaned thoroughly. Cleaning the autoclave requires that it be drained, filled with cleaning solution, run through a 20-minute heated cycle, drained of solution, filled with distilled rinse water, run through another 20-minute heated cycle, drained of rinse solution, and filled with distilled water again. Then the inner shelves are removed and scrubbed and the inner chamber is wiped clean. Since this process is fairly time-consuming and will certainly put the autoclave out of use for a while, consideration should be given to scheduling the weekly cleaning at a time when personnel can devote the time and when the autoclave is not in demand for sterilization processes.

Distilled water is inexpensive, readily available, and always recommended to prevent mineral build-up. During the cleaning process, attention should be given to inspecting the rubber seal for cracks or wear. An extra replacement

General rules to ensure proper sterilization using an autoclave:

- Articles placed into the autoclave must have been sanitized and dried.
- The articles are wrapped and placed to allow adequate exposure of all surfaces (Figure 10-24). Instrument hinges should be opened and serrations exposed inside packages.
- To avoid trapped air pockets, containers should be placed on their sides with lids loosely in place.
- Any wrapping material used must be approved for autoclave use.
- Timing should not start until the gauges reach 15 pounds of pressure and 254°F.
- When the cycle is complete, the door must be opened slightly to allow steam to escape. The sterile wrapped articles will be hot and damp and should be left in the autoclave to cool and dry. Microorganisms can contaminate the sterile articles through the damp wrapping if the door is opened too wide or if articles are handled while damp.

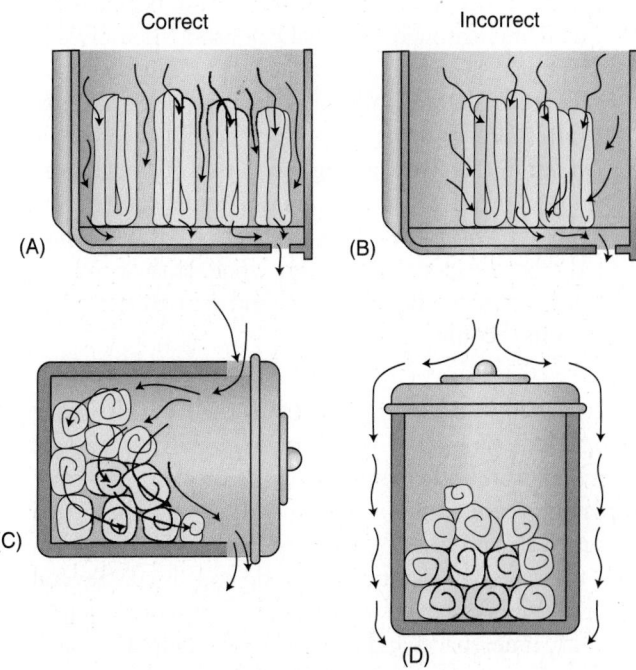

Correct   Incorrect

(A)   (B)

(C)

(D)

Figure 10-24 (A) Proper placement of instruments in the autoclave allows steam to circulate and penetrate from all sides. (B) Packages incorrectly loaded in autoclave. (C) When placed correctly, the jar should lay on its side with the cover loosely in place to allow steam to freely circulate through the jar and properly sterilize the dressings. (D) Incorrect method. (Courtesy of Steris Corporation, Mentor, OH) rubber seal should always be kept on hand. The seals are available through medical supply sources. Refer to the manufacturer's instructions for regularly scheduled replacement of the rubber seal and other recommended maintenance procedures.

Quality Control and Assurance for Autoclave.

Quality control when using an autoclave consists of proper maintenance, proper operation, and observation of the temperature and pressure gauges. Equally important is the regular use of sterilization indicators and culture tests. Several types of sterilization indicators and culture methods are available:

- *Sterilization strips.* Contain a **thermolabile** dye that darkens when exposed to steam at the proper temperature and pressure for the proper amount of time. These indicators are placed in the center of the wrapped article (Figure 10-25).

- *Culture tests.* Available as a culture strip containing heat-resistant spores. The strip is placed in the center of a wrapped article and placed in a fully loaded autoclave. After processing is complete, the article is unwrapped and the strip is placed into a culture medium. If the autoclave is functioning properly and the medical assistant has followed proper operating procedure, no growth should occur. Also available through Becton-Dickinson Microbiology Systems is an ampule called the Kilit Ampule. These biological indicators are ampules that contain spores of the thermophile "Bacillus stearothermophilus." After being processed through the autoclave, the Kilit Ampule is sent to a cooperating laboratory for week-long observation for survival of the bacilli spores. A written report of the results is generated by the laboratory and sent to the office for its records.

Autoclave Wrapping Material and Packaging Supplies.

Wrapping or otherwise packaging surgical instruments and other surgical and medical articles prior to placing them in the autoclave will extend their shelf life up to six months. Before these articles are wrapped, they must first be sanitized, rinsed, and dried. Several materials are available for wrapping. Cost, convenience, visibility, time, space, and ease of use will help determine which to use. Many offices will utilize a combination of materials.

- Muslin is a cloth wrap available in several sizes and colors. Even with the cost of the initial purchasing, occasional replacements, autoclave tape, and laundering, muslin is still a very economical option. Besides these cost-effective advantages, many surgi-

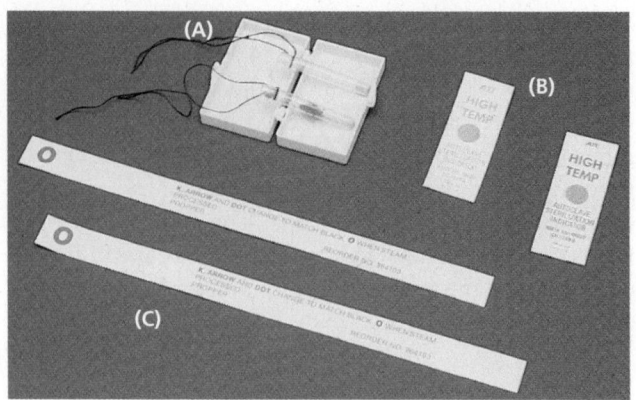

Figure 10-25 Types of sterilization indicators. (A) Commercially available pellets sealed in a glass container with string attached. Pellets melt when placed inside a package in the autoclave when proper temperature time and pressure have been attained. (B) Indicators are inserted into a holder and then placed into the center of a package to be sterilized. Indicator changes color when proper time, temperature, and pressure have been obtained. (C) Sterilization strips are placed in the center of packages to be sterilized. Strips change color when proper temperature, time, and pressure have been attained.

cal instruments may be wrapped together in muslin, making up a convenient surgery/procedure set. One of the main disadvantages of muslin is the inability to view the contents. Another disadvantage is the need for constant examination for holes, tears, and wearing out of the cloth. Patching is not a reasonable option since iron-on patches impede penetration of steam and sewn-on patches create their own set of perforations. A defective muslin cloth should be discarded. Wrapping space and training of personnel are necessary when using cloth.

- Paper sterilization wrapping squares are available in many different sizes and types. This disposable type of material requires that a new paper be used each time autoclave tape is needed, but eliminates the need for laundering. Similar to cloth wrapping, paper wraps also lend themselves to larger sets of articles being wrapped together for surgery or procedural packs. As with muslin cloth, wrapping space and some personnel training are necessary. Paper wraps are opaque, making viewing of the contents impossible.

- Sterilization pouches or bags may be either plastic or paper or a combination (Figure 10-26). They are fairly inexpensive and very easy to use. Since no wrapping is involved, additional work space is not required. Another advantage of bags is the visibility of the items inside. Some pouches are packaged on a continuous roll and are available in a variety of

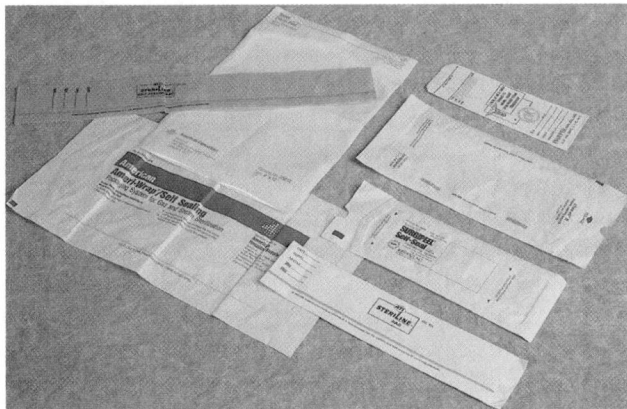

Figure 10-26   Various types and sizes of self-sealing bags for sterilization.

widths. This allows the medical assistant to cut the bag to fit the article. Since both ends need to be taped closed, it is very difficult to remove the article while maintaining its sterility. Probably the best bag-type option is individual bags with the top end open for instrument placement and the bottom end factory closed with a peel-apart seal. The article is inserted into the top opening, the bag is taped closed, and the package is sterilized (Figure 10-27). When needed, the sterile article is removed through the factory-sealed bottom end in a peel-apart sterile fashion. These bags need to be purchased in several individual sizes and are expensive

but have the advantages of ease of use and item visibility and are probably the preferred method for most medical offices today.

Autoclave Tape. Autoclave tape is chemically treated to become "striped" when exposed to heat. The striped pattern indicates exposure to high temperature but does not measure pounds of pressure or duration of exposure. Because of these limitations, autoclave tape does not assure that the wrapped package is sterile, only that it has been heated. Since it is placed on the outside of the package, it does not assure that steam has penetrated to the inner article but does help to determine if a package has been processed (Figure 10-28).

Labeling Packages for Autoclave. Surgical packages should be clearly labeled. Clear bags usually have a designated place for labeling, and muslin- or paper-wrapped packages may be labeled across the autoclave tape. Proper labeling should include the names of the articles in the pack, the date of sterilization, and the initials of the medical assistant responsible for the wrapping. The name of the instrument or article should be as specific as possible, especially when using the opaque cloth or paper wraps. If many instruments have been wrapped together for a specific surgery or for a specific physician, the label should clearly state which surgery or surgeon. For example, a "laceration repair set" could contain all the necessary instruments for repairing a laceration. "Dr. Peterson's vasectomy set" would contain all the instruments Dr.

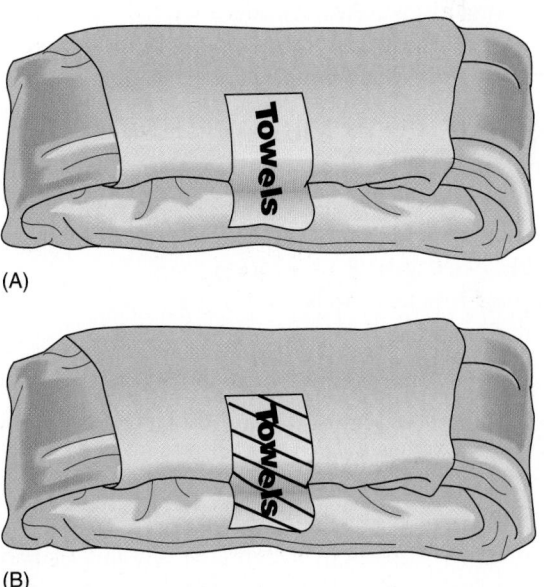

(A)

(B)

Figure 10-28   Package of towels (A) before and (B) after autoclaving. Note that the autoclave tape has a striped pattern indicating that the package was exposed to a high temperature. This does not assure sterility, however.

Figure 10-27   The medical assistant is placing a sanitized instrument into a sterilization bag for autoclaving by inserting the tips of the hemostat in first.

Peterson needs to perform a vasectomy, including, perhaps, personal preference instruments. The date of sterilization will help determine the expiration of sterility and determine a "pull date" for resterilizing. Initialing the package allows for accountability if necessary. Labels should always be written with a permanent marker. Ballpoint pen should never be used because the ink will smear when wet. Caution should be taken to avoid puncturing through the package during labeling.

Wrapping Techniques. Articles must be wrapped in a specific way in order to ensure they remain sterile when opened. Wrapped surgical instruments need to be double wrapped. Some methods advocate placing both layers of wrapping material together and double wrapping the pack in one process. A much more useful method is the "wrap-ping twice" technique (see Procedure 10-5). The wrapping twice technique allows for additional options at the time of opening. Wrapping twice allows for a completely wrapped inner sterile package to be applied to the surgical tray. This wrapping twice technique eliminates struggling to control multiple instruments during the unwrapping process; and, if the inner package becomes contaminated during the unwrapping, the medical assistant has the additional option of unwrapping the inner package using the same technique without having to start over. All packs should be neatly and securely wrapped; firm enough to prevent the instruments from movement, but loose enough to permit adequate steam penetration.

See Procedure 10-5, Wrapping Instruments for Sterilization in Autoclave, and Procedure 10-6, Instrument Steam Sterilization (Autoclave).

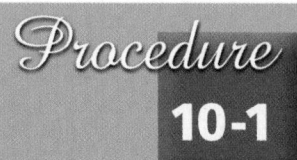

Procedure 10-1   Medical Asepsis Handwash

STANDARD PRECAUTIONS:

PURPOSE:
To reduce pathogens on the hands and wrists, thereby decreasing direct and indirect transmission of infectious microorganisms. Average duration is two minutes before beginning to work with patients, 30 seconds following each patient contact.

EQUIPMENT/SUPPLIES:
Sink (preferably with foot-operated controls)
Soap (preferably liquid soap in foot-operated container; bar soap discouraged)
Water-based antibacterial lotion
Disposable paper towels
Nail stick or brush

PROCEDURE STEPS:
1. Remove all jewelry (plain wedding band is only acceptable jewelry). RATIONALE: Jewelry harbors microorganisms on the hands.
2. Prepare disposable paper towel (if using pull-down dispenser, prepare the amount of paper towel necessary for drying hands following wash; if using folded towels, have accessible). RATIONALE: Following the handwashing, you may not touch any contaminated surface, such as the

handle on a paper-towel dispenser or the water faucets.
3. Never allow your clothing to touch the sink; never touch the inside of the sink with your hands. RATIONALE: The sink is considered contaminated at all times (Note: sinks must be sanitized and disinfected at the end of each day).
4. Turn on the faucet with a dry paper towel (Figure 10-29A). Discard paper towel. Adjust water temperature to lukewarm. RATIONALE: Lukewarm water is best for handwashing because excessively hot water may overdry the skin.
5. Wet hands and apply soap using a circular motion and friction; rub into a lather (Figure 10-29B). RATIONALE: This initial handwash is to remove visible soil and some microorganisms. Interlace fingers to clean between them (Figure 10-29C).
6. Use an orange stick or brush at the first hand-washing of each day (Figures 10-29D and E). RATIONALE: Nails harbor excessive numbers of microorganisms. Even with trimmed nails, this step must be performed on a daily basis.
7. Rinse hands with hands pointed down and lower than elbows (Figure 10-29F). RATIONALE: When hands are held lower than elbows, pathogens and contaminated water run off the hands and not up on the forearms.

(continues)

Procedure 10-1 (continued)

8. Repeat soap application and lather; interlace fingers well, wash with vigorous, circular motions all parts of hands including wrists; wash for at least one minute or longer depending on degree of contamination. RATIONALE: Appropriate length of handwashing is required to provide enough friction to remove soil and pathogens.

9. Rinse well, keeping hands pointed downward. RATIONALE: Rinsing removes microorganisms, contaminated water, and soap from the hands.

10. Repeat handwashing for the first handwashing of the day or if necessary for contaminated or visibly soiled hands. Lather wrists using a circular motion and friction. Rinse arms and hands. RATIONALE: When the hands are excessively contaminated or soiled, two handwashings may be necessary to remove microorganisms from the hands.

11. Dry hands and wrists with disposable paper towel; do not touch towel dispenser following handwashing; blot instead of rubbing with towel; if sink is not foot operated, use a clean disposable towel to turn off water faucet. RATIONALE: Touching the towel dispenser contaminates the hands. Blotting the hands dry reduces drying of the skin. Turning faucet off with paper towel prevents recontamination from dirty faucet.

12. Discard paper towel in waste container. Do not leave contaminated towels for repeated use. NOTE: Repeat handwashing procedure prior to and following each patient contact, procedure, or meal. RATIONALE: Handwashing must be performed on a regular and frequent basis to ensure the reduction of microorganisms transmitted by hands.

    Water-based antibacterial lotion can be applied to prevent chapped, excoriated skin. If skin is excoriated, the medical assistant may not be able to work due to breaks in the skin.

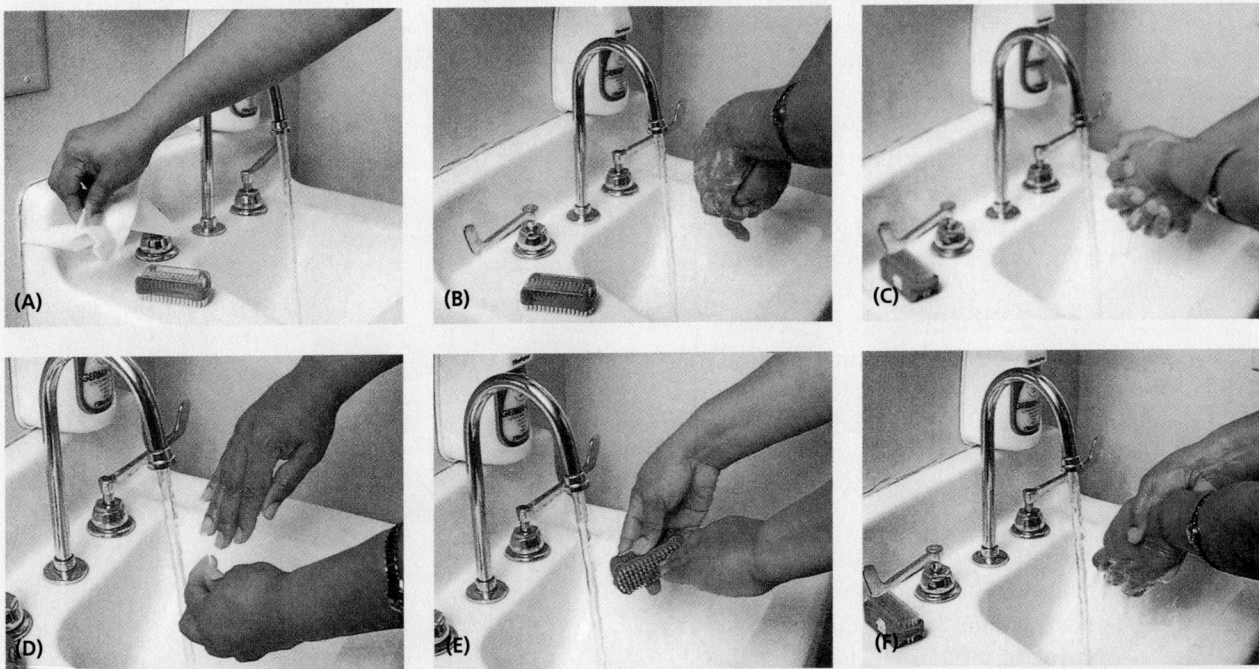

Figure 10-29 (A) Prepare towels for use. Turn on the faucet and adjust water to a lukewarm temperature. (B) Wet hands. Let water flow downward off hands and fingertips. (C) Use a circular motion to create friction and wash the palms and backs of hands. Interlace the fingers to clean between them. (D) Use an orange stick to clean under fingernails. (E) A hand brush may also be used to clean under fingernails. (F) Rinse hands thoroughly letting the water flow downward off your hands and fingertips.

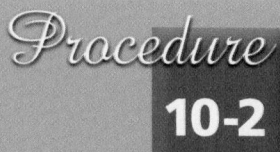

10-2 **Sanitization of Instruments**

STANDARD PRECAUTIONS:

PURPOSE:
To properly clean contaminated instruments to remove tissue or debris.

EQUIPMENT/SUPPLIES:
Sink (or ultrasonic cleaner: follow manufacturer's instructions)
Sanitizing agent (low-sudsing detergent, approved chemical disinfectant, or blood solvent)
Brush
Disposable paper towels
Plastic apron
Disposable gloves, heavy-duty if cleaning sharps
Goggles
Biohazard waste container

PROCEDURE STEPS:
1. Wear disposable gloves, goggles, and apron. RATIONALE: Contaminated instruments pose a blood and body fluid precaution as indicated by OSHA standards. Disposable gloves must always be worn to sanitize instruments. Wear heavy-duty gloves if cleaning sharp instruments. Goggles are worn to protect eyes from splashing of contaminated debris during scrubbing procedure. A plastic apron provides protection from splashing of clothing.

2. As soon as possible following a procedure in which an instrument is contaminated, rinse the instrument in water and disinfectant solution; rinse again under running water. RATIONALE: Rinsing contaminated instruments as soon as possible following use removes debris and tissue that could quickly dry onto the instrument, making sanitization more difficult.

3. If contaminated instrument must be carried from one place to another for sanitization, place the instrument in a basin labeled "Biohazard." RATIONALE: Do not carry contaminated instruments in your hands. Biohazard basins must be sanitized and disinfected daily according to procedures for Standard Precautions.

4. Scrub each instrument well with detergent and water; scrub under running water, and be sure to scrub inside any edges and all surfaces (Figure 10-30). RATIONALE: Thorough scrubbing removes tissue and debris from all aspects of the contaminated instrument. If all tissue is not removed with scrubbing, the instrument may not be sterilized during sterilization procedures.

5. Rinse well with hot water. RATIONALE: Tissue and debris, as well as detergent, must be completely removed. Hot water will help remove all residue and aid in the drying process while rust and water spots will be eliminated.

6. After they are rinsed, place instruments on muslin or disposable paper towel until all instruments have been scrubbed and rinsed. RATIONALE: Often more than one instrument is sanitized; do not place sanitized instrument in the bottom of the sink or on a countertop without a disposable paper towel.

7. Dry instruments with muslin or disposable paper towels. RATIONALE: Wet instruments may rust or corrode. When preparing instruments for the sterilization procedures, they should be dry. Check instruments for working condition.

8. Remove gloves, wash hands.

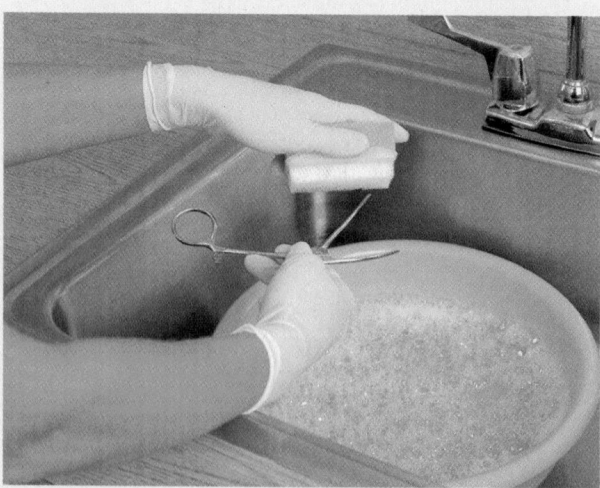

Figure 10-30 Medical assistant is using a scrub brush, plastic basin, and protein solvent detergent to sanitize surgical instruments. Note the medical assistant also is wearing gloves.

Procedure 10-3 Removing Contaminated Gloves

STANDARD PRECAUTIONS:

PURPOSE:
To carefully remove and dispose of contaminated gloves in order to contain exposure.

EQUIPMENT/SUPPLIES:
Biohazard waste container

PROCEDURE STEPS:
1. Grasp the palm of the used left glove with the right hand to begin removing the first glove.

Notice hands are held away from the body and pointed downward (Figure 10-31A and B). RATIONALE: Holding the hands away from the body will further prevent exposure to biological contaminants.
2. Turn the used left glove inside out and hold it in the right gloved hand (Figure 10-31C, D, and E). RATIONALE: Turning the glove inside out helps isolate the biological contaminants.
3. Holding the glove that has been removed with the hand that still has the glove on, the medical assistant inserts two fingers of the ungloved hand between her arm and the inside of the dirty glove (Figure 10-31F).

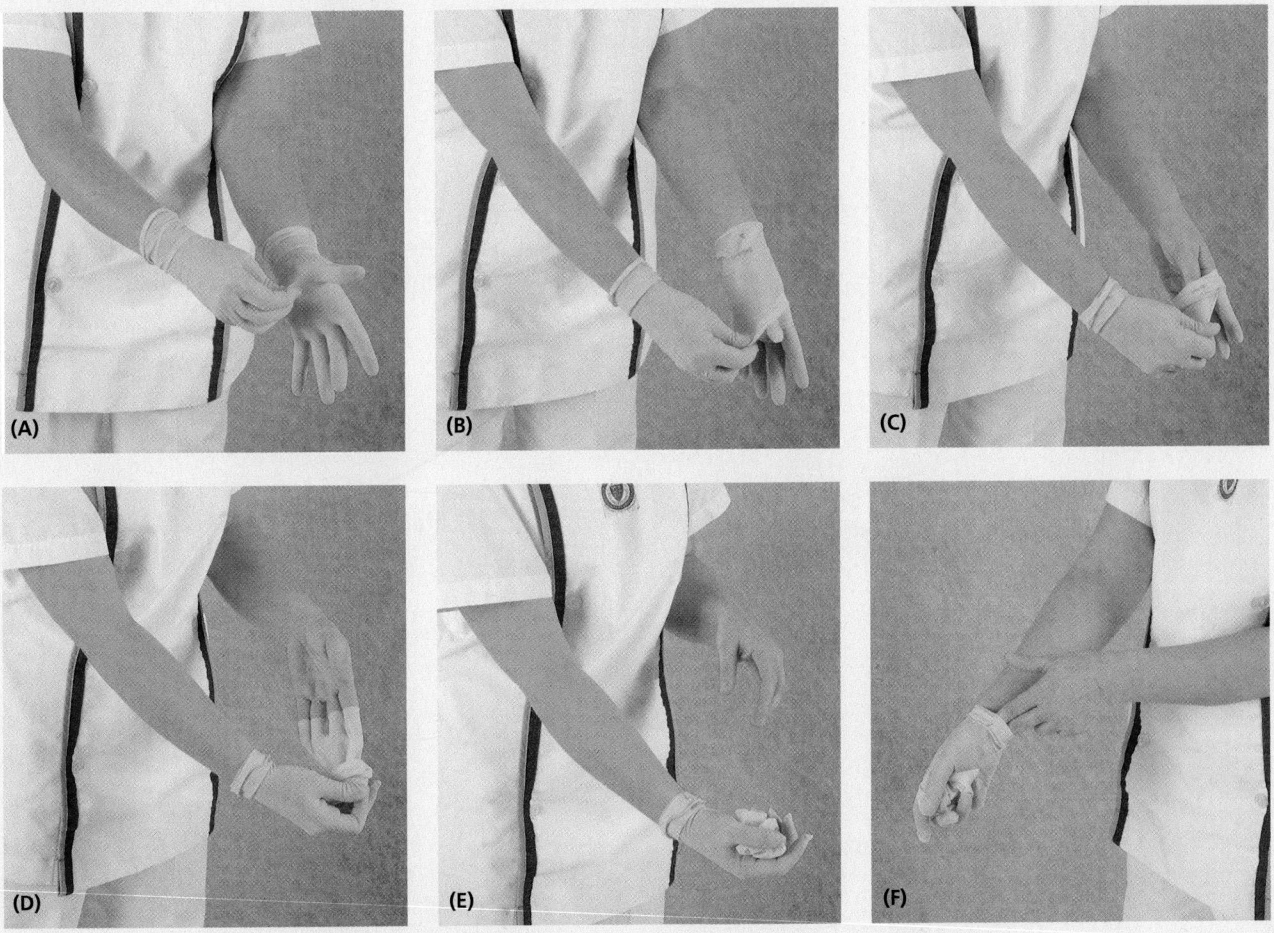

Figure 10-31 (A) Grasp the palm of the used left glove with the right hand. (B) Begin removing the first glove. (C and D) Turn the used left glove inside out. (E) Hold it in the right hand. (F) Hold the removed glove with the hand that is still gloved.

(continues)

Procedure 10-3 *(continued)*

4. Turn the right dirty glove inside out over the other. One glove is inside the other and the medical assistant can handle the gloves because the dirty, contaminated area is inside the gloves (Figure 10-31G and H). RATIONALE: Both gloves are inverted with the biological contaminates isolated.

5. Dispose of the inverted gloves into a biological waste receptacle (Figure 10-31I). RATIONALE: All biological waste should be placed into a red biohazard bag.

6. Wash hands thoroughly. RATIONALE: Immediate washing of hands is an additional precaution.

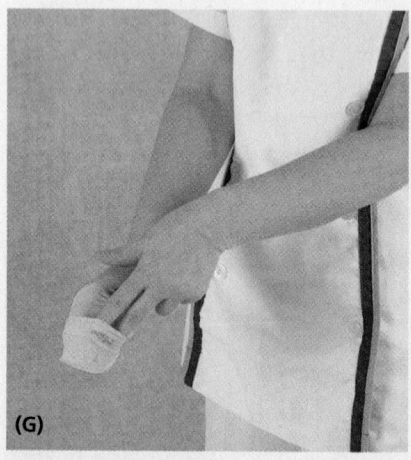 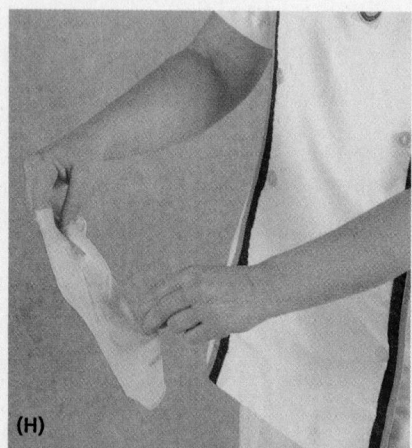 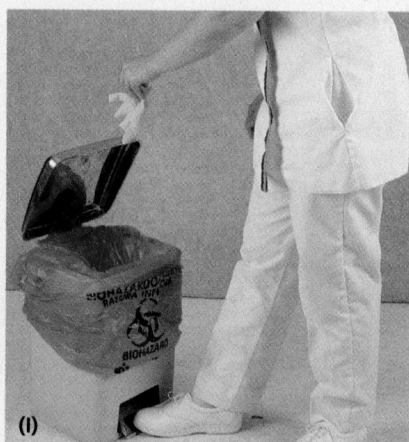

Figure 10-31 *(continued)* (G) Insert two fingers of the ungloved hand inside the dirty glove and turn it inside out over the other. (H) One glove is now inside the other. (I) Dispose of gloves in biohazard container.

Procedure 10-4   **Chemical Disinfection of Instruments**

STANDARD PRECAUTIONS:

PURPOSE:

Chemical disinfection is used to achieve medical asepsis for instruments that will be used during *external* physical examinations or procedures (i.e., thermometers, percussion hammers, nasal and aural specula).

EQUIPMENT/SUPPLIES:

Container with airtight lid (Figure 10-32A)

Disinfectant chemical solution (various brands and instructions for specific use)

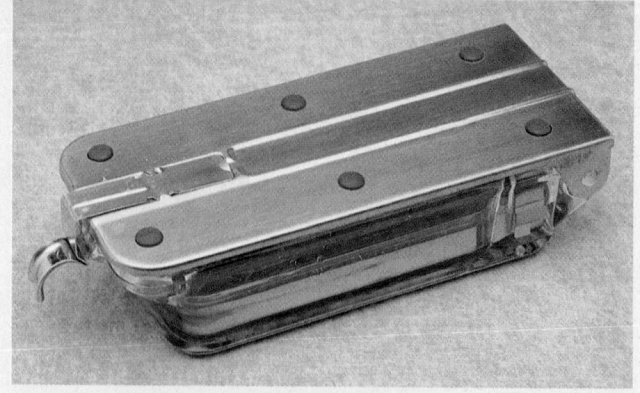

Figure 10-32 (A) Closed Bard-Parker® tray.

(continues)

Procedure 10-4 *(continued)*

Timer or clock
Water for rinsing following disinfection
Heavy-duty gloves
Biohazard waste container

PROCEDURE STEPS:

Chemical Disinfection:

1. Sanitize instruments that require medical aseptic chemical disinfection. RATIONALE: Recall that medical asepsis is not sterile and should not be used for instruments that will be used in invasive procedures requiring sterile technique.

2. Read the manufacturer's instructions on the original container of chemical disinfection solution. RATIONALE: Each brand of chemical disinfection solution has specific preparation instructions and germicidal properties; choose the solution that best fits the needs of the ambulatory care setting. Keep the solution in the original container to reduce chances of accidental poisoning.

3. Put on gloves. RATIONALE: Chemical disinfectant solutions are harsh on skin.

4. Prepare the solution as indicated by the manufacturer; place the date of opening or preparation on the container with your initials. RATIONALE: Following the manufacturer's instructions ensures proper germicidal properties. Note the expiration date of the prepared solution.

5. Pour the prepared solution into a container with an airtight lid; avoid splashing the solution (Figure 10-32B). RATIONALE: Disinfectant chemical solutions should not be left exposed to open air in order to prevent accidental inhalation or poisoning. Splashing solution may cause inhalation, skin, or mucous membrane contact and could cause injury.

6. Place sanitized instruments into solution; instruments must be completely covered; avoid splashing solution when putting instruments in tray. RATIONALE: If instruments are not covered with solution, disinfection cannot occur.

7. Close lid of container; label container with name of solution, exposure time, and initials. RATIONALE: Exposure time is the required time indicated by the manufacturer to achieve

disinfection. Initialing work ensures accountability and responsibility.

8. Do not open or add additional instruments during disinfection period. RATIONALE: Adding instruments during a disinfection procedure limits the overall effectiveness of the disinfectant solution.

9. Following required exposure time, lift items from the container tray and rinse well under distilled water or tap water (according to the manufacturer's instructions). Do not use instruments without rinsing off chemical disinfectant solution; often solution is caustic and may corrode instruments over time.

10. Remove instruments and place on muslin or disposable paper towel.

11. Dry instruments with muslin or paper towel.

CAUTION: Use disinfection solution for only as many days as recommended by the manufacturer. Disinfectant properties will only last as long as reported by the manufacturer's instructions. (NOTE: Dispose of used solution as recommended by the manufacturer's instructions.)

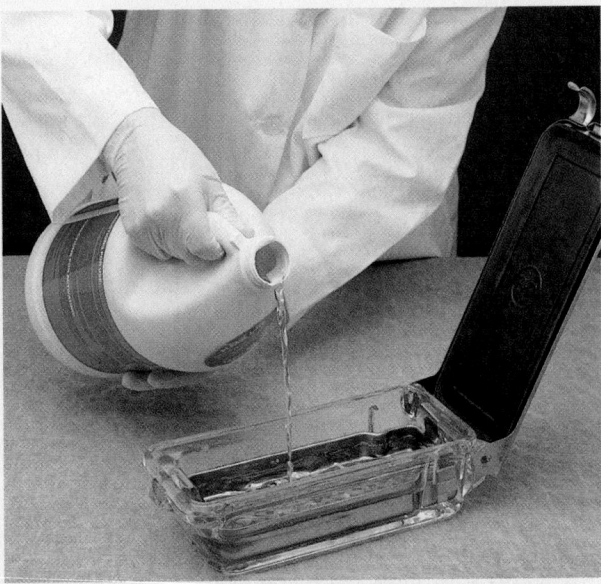

Figure 10-32 *(continued)* (B) With gloves on, carefully pour disinfectant solution into Bard-Parker® tray in preparation for soaking a sanitized instrument for disinfection.

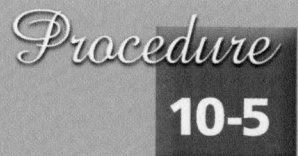

Wrapping Instruments for Sterilization in Autoclave

10-5

PURPOSE:
To properly wrap sanitized instruments for sterilization in an autoclave.

EQUIPMENT/SUPPLIES:
Sanitized instruments
Wrapping material (muslin or disposable wrapping paper)
Sterilization indicator
2 × 2 gauze or cotton balls (if instrument has hinges)
Autoclave wrapping tape
Permanent marker or felt-tip pen (Figure 10-33A)

PROCEDURE STEPS:
1. Prepare a clean, dry, flat surface of adequate size to lay the wrapping material. RATIONALE: A clean area reduces risk of contamination. Adequate space is required for proper wrapping.
2. Select two wraps of adequate size in which to wrap instruments.
3. Place one square of wrapping material at an angle in front of you on the dry surface with one corner pointed directly toward you.
4. Place the sanitized instrument or articles to be placed in the autoclave just below the center of the wrap. Open instruments with hinges as wide as possible and place a 2 × 2 gauze or cotton ball in the opening (Figure 10-33B). RATIONALE: Instruments with hinged parts that are not spread open prior to autoclaving may not be properly sterilized.
5. Place one sterilization indicator with the instrument. RATIONALE: Sterilization indicators inside packages ascertain sterilization of each individual package. Indicators change colors when the required temperature has been reached, documenting the effectiveness of the sterilization. NOTE: quality control for autoclave operation can be evaluated with sterilization indicators.
6. Bring the corner of the wrap closest to you up and over the article toward the center. Bring the tip of the same corner back toward you until it reaches the folded edge, creating a fan-

fold effect. Smooth the edges of the fold. The article should remain completely covered (Figure 10-33C).
7. Fold one side edge toward the center line; fan-fold back to side, and crease (Figure 10-33D).
8. Repeat step 7 for the other side edge (Figure 10-33E).
9. Fold the package up from the bottom (Figure 10-33F).
10. Fold the top edge down and over the entire package (Figure 10-33G). RATIONALE: Final edge should wrap entire package for assurance of adequate coverage and protection once contents are sterilized. If wrap does not cover adequately, unwrap and start over with larger wrapping material.
11. To "wrap twice," place this package into the center of a second wrap (Figure 10-33H). Repeat steps 7 through 10. RATIONALE: Double wrapping allows more control of multiple instruments when setting up a surgical tray.
12. Tape with autoclave tape across the point left exposed. RATIONALE: Autoclave tape indicates whether or not the package has been through the autoclave; it is not a form of sterilization indicator or quality control.
13. Label the tape with the name of the instrument or type of pack (i.e., laceration repair pack), date of sterilization, and your initials (Figure 10-33I). RATIONALE: Proper instrument labeling is required to identify wrapped sterilized instruments. Instruments wrapped and sterilized in paper or cloth wrappers are considered sterile for four weeks from the date of sterilization. Initialing packages ensures accountability and responsibility.
14. Place wrapped instruments in autoclave. RATIONALE: If wrapped instruments are not to be immediately autoclaved, do NOT date the package. Leave the package on a clean, dry surface and date the package just prior to autoclaving.
15. Document the procedure.

(continues)

Procedure

10-5 *(continued)*

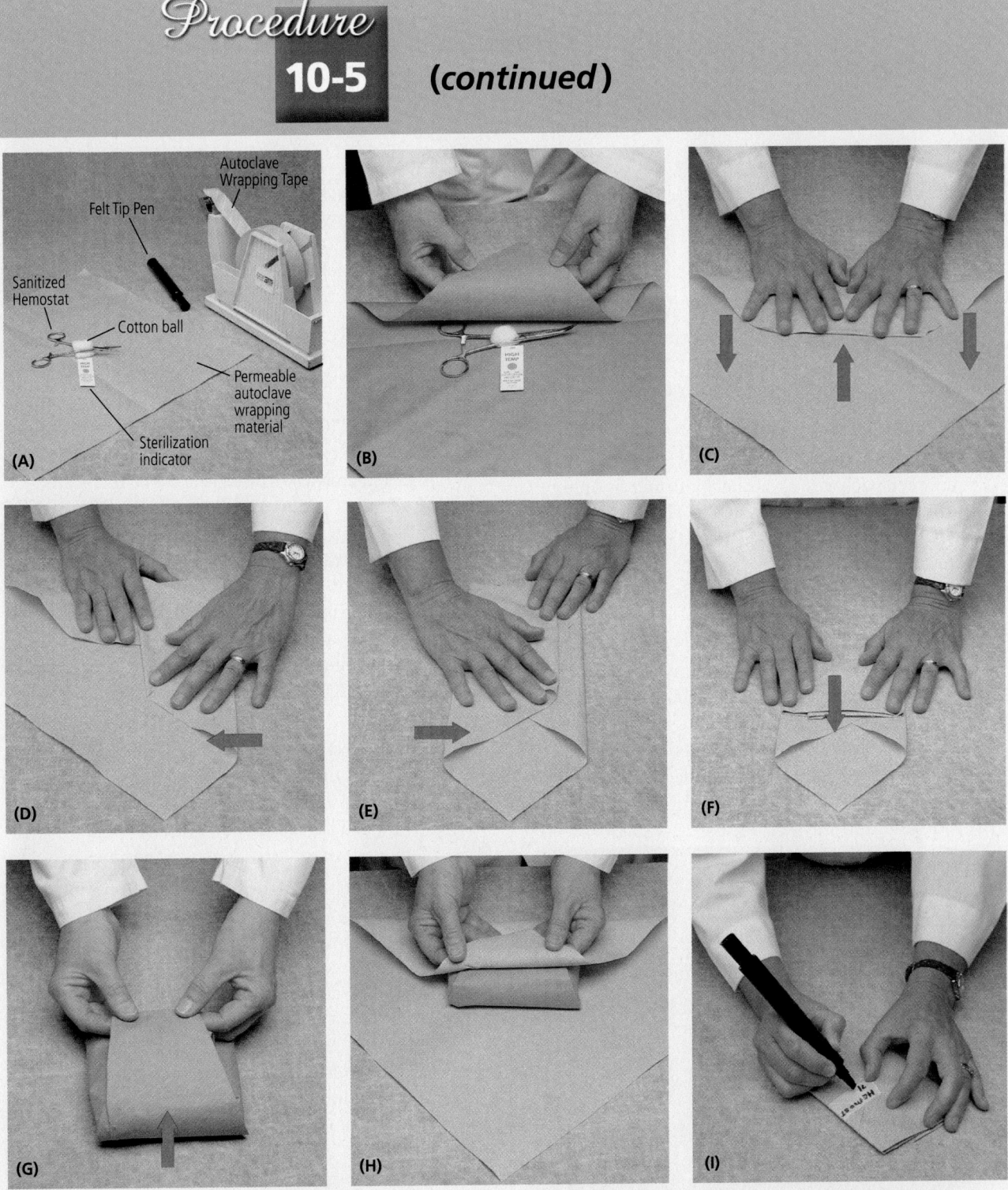

Figure 10-33 (A) Equipment needed to wrap surgical instruments or equipment for sterilization in an autoclave. (B) Place a cotton ball between the hinge joints of sharp instruments and a sterilization indicator in with the instruments to be wrapped. (C) The wrapping paper is folded toward center. A small corner is turned back on itself. (D) Fold one side toward center leaving a small corner turned back on itself. (E) Fold other side toward center leaving small corner turned back on itself. (F) The package is folded up from the bottom and secured. (G) Fold top down over package. (H) Wrap first package in another wrap. Double wrapping allows more control of multiple instruments when setting up a surgical tray. (I) Wrapped package is secured with heat-sensitive autoclave tape and labeled with the date, contents, and medical assistant's initials.

Procedure 10-6

Steam Sterilization of Instruments (Autoclave)

PURPOSE:
To rid instruments of all forms of microbial (microorganism) life for use in invasive procedures.

EQUIPMENT/SUPPLIES:
Steam sterilizer (autoclave)
Autoclave manufacturer procedure manual
Wrapped sanitized instrument package(s) with sterilization indicators placed inside package (or unwrapped item if removed with sterile transfer forceps)

PROCEDURE STEPS:
1. Load packages into autoclave tray; allow 3 inches between packages; avoid stacking directly on top of other packages (Figure 10-34). RATIONALE: Steam circulates in predictable patterns in an autoclave. When packages are loaded too closely or improperly, proper sterilization will not occur in individual packages.
   A. Load jars of dressings or cups on their sides, with tops ajar or loosely in place. RATIONALE: Steam is trapped within a jar when it is right side up; containers and goods will not be sterilized if loaded sitting up vertically.
   B. Load cloth or dressing packages vertically 3 inches apart.

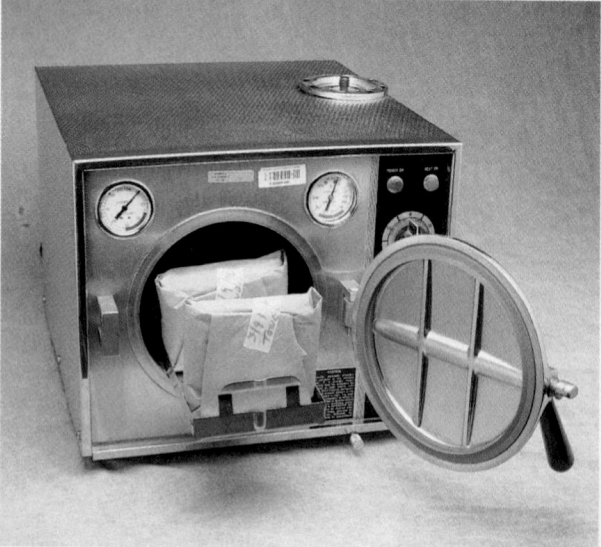

Figure 10-34 Carefully load packages into the autoclave so that the steam is able to penetrate all sides of the package allowing proper sterilization.

C. Load unwrapped items in similar fashion, not allowing item to touch any other item.
   D. Load unwrapped instruments flat with handles opened.
2. Close autoclave door and seal. RATIONALE: Pressure cannot be achieved without a proper seal.
3. Turn on autoclave and set temperature to achieve 250–254°F (121°C) and 15 pounds of pressure according to the manufacturer's guidelines. RATIONALE: Proper heat and pressure levels must be achieved in order to kill all microorganisms within the autoclave.
4. When the temperature dial indicates 250–254°F (121°C) and 15 pounds of pressure has been achieved inside the autoclave, begin necessary exposure time by setting timer. RATIONALE: Exposure time is required to kill all microorganisms. Careful note should be given to setting exposure time only after the proper temperature and pressure settings have been achieved.

Item	Required exposure time
wrapped instrument packages or trays	30 minutes
unwrapped items	15 minutes
unwrapped items covered with cloth	20 minutes

5. Do not attempt to open the door during the autoclave cycle. RATIONALE: Opening the door prematurely will allow the steam under pressure to cause injury.
6. Following completion of the autoclave cycle, exhaust steam pressure from the autoclave by following the manufacturer's instructions. RATIONALE: Read the manufacturer's instructions carefully.
7. Open the door approximately one inch after the pressure gauge indicates zero (0) pressure and the temperature gauge indicates a decrease to at least 212°F. RATIONALE: Do not open the door until these standards have been reached; injury may occur upon premature opening of the door.

(continues)

Procedure 10-6 *(continued)*

8. Allow the contents to completely dry, approximately 10–15 minutes; do NOT touch contents until completely dry. RATIONALE: If packages are still wet or damp, microorganisms can enter a wrapped package, rendering it contaminated. Liquids travel along paper or cloth by capillary action and will be contaminated by microorganisms on countertops or from hands.

9. Remove wrapped contents with dry, clean hands and store in clean, dry area for sterilized packages only. RATIONALE: Sterilized wrapped packages can be held with clean hands, since only the interior contents require maintenance of sterility. If the outer wrapper is required to remain sterile, remove with sterile transfer forceps and place on a sterile field or in sterile storage areas.

10. Remove unwrapped contents with sterile transfer forceps; resanitize and resterilize the transfer forceps following use. RATIONALE: Sterile transfer forceps must have been sterilized immediately prior to or along with the unwrapped item.

11. Perform quality control on a regular basis, based on usage. RATIONALE: Quality control and maintenance of an autoclave is critical to assurance of proper operation. Accountability and responsibility to monitor quality control should be the responsibility of the medical assistant(s) most often responsible for sterilization.
    A. Monitor sterilization indicators with each use of sterilized instruments.
    B. Weekly perform quality control by documenting sterilization indicator outcome on a log; date and initialize quality control log entries.

12. Service the autoclave regularly according to the manufacturer's guidelines. When sterilization is not being achieved, take equipment out of service and contact a service agency for repair. RATIONALE: It is the responsibility of the medical assistant to take out of service any equipment that is not operating properly as a component of risk management.

13. Document the procedure.

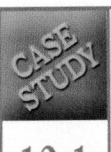 **10-1** Your physician employer asks you to help develop an exposure control plan. Include the measures the employer must take to eliminate or lessen an employee's risk of exposure to blood or OPIM. How often will the plan be reviewed?

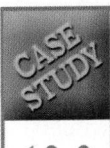 **10-2** Considering the growth requirements for pathogens, describe how to discourage bacterial growth in the clinical area of the ambulatory care setting.

SUMMARY

Effective infection control measures are the first defense against the transmission of infectious diseases in the ambulatory care setting. Reliance on standard and transmission-based precautions, protective barriers, and basic principles of disinfection and sterilization promotes professional and responsible clinical care for patients. When the processes of infection control are applied to all clinical procedures, the chain of infection may be broken by many varied means. Remember that an infectious disease will not spread to another person if the chain is broken at any stage.

Infectious diseases and accidents occur through lack of education and carelessness. Medical assistants must understand the importance of the regulations and guidelines set forth by the federal government and follow through by helping employers implement them. In doing so, the health and safety of patients and health care workers can be protected, the spread of infectious diseases can be kept under control, and the risk of contracting an infectious disease such as AIDS or hepatitis B will be greatly minimized.

Every medical office and ambulatory care setting must, by law, have clearly written and readily available manuals containing information about Standard Precautions and OSHA for the safe handling, storage, and disposal of blood, body fluids, and chemicals.

Through consistent use of Standard Precautions and adherence to OSHA laws, health care providers can acquire the behaviors and techniques needed to safeguard themselves and their patients.

Because of frequent changes in the laws, it is necessary for medical assistants and all other health care providers to keep abreast of the government mandates.

REVIEW QUESTIONS

Multiple Choice

1. The bloodborne virus considered to pose the greatest threat to health care workers is:
   a. hepatitis B (HBV)
   b. human immunodeficiency virus (HIV)
   c. hepatitis A
   d. hepatitis C
2. Standard Precautions are issued by:
   a. HHS
   b. CDC
   c. HCFA
   d. OSHA
3. The Bloodborne Pathogen Standard is primarily concerned with:
   a. reducing the transmission of HIV and hepatitis B infections
   b. protecting the employer
   c. regulating the use of personal protective equipment
   d. taking blood samples from patients
4. In the chain of infection, the location of the infectious agent is known as the:
   a. reservoir
   b. portal of exit
   c. portal of entry
   d. means of transmission
5. The stage in infectious disease in which symptoms are vague and undifferentiated is called the:
   a. incubation stage
   b. prodromal stage
   c. acute stage
   d. onset of disease stage
6. An autoclave is an instrument used during:
   a. chemical sterilization
   b. steam sterilization
   c. dry heat sterilization
   d. gas sterilization

Critical Thinking

1. Analyze the importance of infection control and give five examples of how a medical assistant would practice responsible infection control in the ambulatory care setting.
2. Identify and describe the steps in the chain of infection.
3. Describe four types of infectious agents.
4. Explain sanitization and its function in the ambulatory care setting.
5. Describe three autoclave wrapping materials and packaging supplies.
6. Give eight examples of body fluids considered to be biohazardous substances. Explain how medical assistants could become exposed to blood and/or body fluids.
7. Describe needlestick and its relevance to HIV and HBV infection.
8. Discuss infectious waste and its disposal.
9. What is the purpose of OSHA's standard for bloodborne pathogens and who does it cover?
10. What is PPE? Name several types of PPE. Who is responsible for providing it?

WEB ACTIVITIES

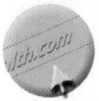

Go online to the Centers for Disease Control and Prevention and find the most current information about Standard Precautions. What is the procedure that must be followed in the event of a needlestick?

REFERENCES/BIBLIOGRAPHY

Bonewit, K. (2000). *Clinical procedures for medical assistants* (8th ed.). Philadelphia: W. B. Saunders Company.

Hegner, B., & Caldwell, E. (1999). *Nursing assistant: A nursing process approach* (8th ed.). Albany, NY: Delmar.

Ignatavicius, D. D., Workman, M., & Mishler, M. (1999). *Medical-surgical nursing: A nursing process approach* (3rd ed.). Philadelphia: W. B. Saunders Company.

Kinn, M. E., & Woods, M. A. (1999). *The medical assistant: Administrative and clinical* (8th ed.). Philadelphia: W. B. Saunders Company.

Lewis, M. A., & Tamparo, C. D. (1998). *Medical law, ethics, and bioethics in the medical office* (3rd ed.). Philadelphia: F A. Davis Company.

Marshall, J. (1995). *Fundamental skills for the clinical laboratory professional*. Albany, NY: Delmar.

Marshall, J. (1997) *Medical laboratory assistant*. New Jersey: Brady, Prentice Hall Division.

Occupational Safety and Health Administration Bloodborne Pathogen Regulation Section 1910.1030.

PDR generics (1st ed.). (1995). Montvale, NJ: Medical Economics Data Production Co.

Phipps, W. J., Sands, J., & Marek, J. F. (1999). *Medical-surgical nursing: Concepts and clinical practice* (6th ed.). St. Louis, MO: Mosby-Year Book, Inc.

Rice, J. (1999). *Principles of pharmacology for medical assisting*. (3rd ed.). Albany, NY: Delmar.

Smeltzer, S. C., & Bare, B. G. (2000). *Brunner and Suddarth's textbook of medical-surgical nursing* (9th ed). Philadelphia: J.B. Lippincott Company.

Taber's cyclopedic medical dictionary (18th ed.). (1999). Philadelphia: F.A. Davis Company.

Thompson, J. M., McFarland, G. K., Hirsch, J. E., & Tucker, S. M. (1998). *Mosby's clinical nursing* (4th ed.). St. Louis: C. V. Mosby.

U.S. Department of Health and Human Services, Centers for Disease Control and Prevention. (1997, November 7). *Draft guideline for isolation precautions in hospitals*. (Federal Register). Washington, DC: U.S. Government Printing Office.

Zakus, S. (1995). *Clinical procedures for medical assistants* (3rd ed.). St. Louis: Mosby-Year Book Inc.

TAKING A MEDICAL HISTORY, THE PATIENT'S CHART, AND METHODS OF DOCUMENTATION

KEY TERMS

Allergy

Chart

Chief Complaint

Clinical Diagnosis

Debridement

Objective

Problem-Oriented Medical Record (POMR)

SOAP

Source-Oriented Medical Record (SOMR)

Subjective

OUTLINE

The Function of the Medical History

The Cross-Cultural Model

Patient Information Forms

    Administrative or Demographic Data Forms

    Medical Forms

Computerized Health History

The First Office Contact

    Telephone Contact

    Personal Visit

    Emergency Visit

Completing the Medical History Forms

    Interacting with the Patient

    Displaying Cultural Awareness

    Handling a Difficult Patient

    Dealing with Sensitive Topics

Parts of the Medical History

    Chief Complaint

    Present Illness

    Past Medical History

    Family History

    Social History

    Review of Systems

The Patient's Record and Its Importance

    Contents of Medical Records

Methods of Charting/ Documentation

    Source-Oriented Medical Records

    Problem-Oriented Medical Records

    Computer Modified Records

    SOAP Method of Charting

    Abbreviations Used in Charting

    Correcting an Error

    Chart Organization

OBJECTIVES

The student should strive to meet the following performance objectives and demonstrate an understanding of the facts and principles presented in this chapter through written and oral communication.

1. Define the key terms as presented in the glossary.

2. Understand the necessity and function of the medical history in patient treatment.

3. Define the parts of the medical history.

4. Identify and use effective methods of interacting with a patient.

5. Obtain a medical history from the patient.

6. Explain the different methods of charting/documentation.

(continues)

7. Define the meaning and function of SOAP.
8. Understand some issues of cultural sensitivity in taking a medical history.
9. Describe the contents of a medical record.
10. State five reasons why the medical record is important.
11. Document accurately.

ROLE DELINEATION COMPONENTS

CLINICAL
Patient Care
- Adhere to established triage procedures
- Recognize and respond to emergencies

GENERAL (TRANSDISCIPLINARY)
Professionalism
- Project a professional manner and image
- Adhere to ethical principles

Communication Skills
- Treat all patients with compassion and empathy
- Recognize and respect cultural diversity
- Adapt communications to individual's ability to understand
- Use professional telephone technique
- Use effective and correct verbal and written communications
- Recognize and respond to verbal and nonverbal communications
- Use medical terminology correctly
- Receive, organize, prioritize, and transmit information
- Serve as liaison   (*continues*)

SCENARIO

When clinical medical assistant Audrey Jones, CMA, of Doctors Lewis & King takes a patient history, she typically uses a form custom-designed for the office. Audrey uses the form as a guideline to be sure she gathers all pertinent information. However, she has learned that she must tailor her questions to the patient and sometimes will rearrange the order of the questions if necessary. While Audrey is adept at gathering specific and necessary patient information, she also is aware of patient concerns and sensitivities and adapts her approach to accomplish the task while making the patient feel at ease.

INTRODUCTION

In order to treat a patient effectively, the physician must know the patient's past medical history. If the patient is already established in the ambulatory care setting, the physician can work from the existing chart (record) with additional information obtained at the time of the office or clinic visit.

For a new patient, however, or for an established patient who has not been in for some time, an updated medical history form is of vital importance. Information contained in this history includes past medical problems, current medications and medication allergies, as well as other factors contributing to the patient's health.

Often the family practice clinic will have a broad questionnaire for patients to complete or the physician may tailor the medical history form to a particular specialty. The specialist physician will often mail the form to the patient prior to the appointment so that the patient can answer the questions in a quiet environment and have access to some of the information requested such as names and addresses of other physicians that they have seen.

The role of the medical assistant in taking the patient history is to be as thorough as possible while being as sensitive as possible. Respect for the patient's privacy must be balanced with the need for the kind of complete information that results in informed medical treatment and care.

The patient chart or medical record is a legal document that is a collection of confidential patient information. Should a patient's medical record be introduced in court, it becomes a legal record of care given. It is important that charting in the record be accurate, clear, concise, and complete.

THE FUNCTION OF THE MEDICAL HISTORY

The medical history is the basis for all treatment rendered by the physician, any on-call physician, and any specialist consulted to treat the patient. During the history-taking process, the physician often will discover information that helps guide treatment for the patient. The medical history in the **chart**, or record, makes it easier for the physician to recall previous treatment. Notes and laboratory results in the chart quickly show the progress of the treatment. In addition, the charts give a base for statistical analysis: for the physician's own research, for insurance records, and for the health department, especially for infectious diseases. The health history and chart notes also become a legal record of the treatment rendered to the patient. This is especially important if the patient is making an injury claim against another party or if the patient makes a malpractice claim against the physician. If the records in the chart are precise and correct, the chart becomes a good defense; however, if the charting or documentation is sloppy or incomplete, the entire record could be set aside as an insufficient or incorrect record of treatment. The best procedure is to document everything concerning a patient including all treatment rendered, telephone calls, missed appointments, and discussions with other specialists regarding the patient's treatment.

THE CROSS-CULTURAL MODEL

It is important for the medical assistant to understand that every physician-patient interview is a cross-cultural one. Physicians and patients view the gathering of the patient history and the personal visit quite differently. Health and illness are inseparable from social and cultural beliefs. Who patients are—their background, their belief system, their family orientation, and their cultural heritage—influences their choices in health care. Physician and patient have different concerns and anticipations and the medical assistant conducting the interview needs to be aware of these varying perspectives. Consider the following perspectives.

- *Patient's chief concern:* The illness. The personal and social significance and the problems created by a perceived illness are important to the patient.

- *Physician's chief concern:* Disease. The physician is concerned with the malfunctioning and maladaptation of biological and psychological processes.

- *Patient's idea of treatment success:* Being able to successfully manage an illness and its problems is often more important to the patient than the curing of the disease.

- *Doctor's idea of treatment success:* Treatments, medications, and procedures that control disease problems and evaluating outcomes in these terms.

The medical assistant may find it helpful to ask certain questions of patients to help them move across cultures:

1. What do you think caused your problem?
2. When do you think it started?
3. What does it do to your body?
4. What do you expect from the course of this problem?
5. What do you fear from this problem?
6. What kind of treatment do you expect?

All these questions involve and respect the patient's perception. When conducting an interview with a patient, it is also wise to remember that the dominant form of care in the world is not the physician or medical staff but the family.

PATIENT INFORMATION FORMS

There are two sets of information forms in the medical office.

Administrative or Demographic Data Forms

The first set of forms includes the patient demographic data form and the financial information form. The demographic data form (Figure 11-1) registers the patient's full name, address, mailing address if different, home and work telephone numbers, date of birth, social security number and all insurance information, person to be contacted in case of emergency, and a release of information signature. Some medical offices include a second form, the financial information form (Figure 11-2), to be signed regarding the financial policy of the practice including billing, insurance billing, copayment billing, and any finance charges added to monthly billings.

PATIENT INFORMATION

TODAY'S DATE _____
   Patient's name (Last) _____ (First) _____ (M.I.) _____
   Address _____
   Phone (home) _____ (work) _____ (message) _____
   Please circle: Single/Married/Divorced/
                     Widowed   Male/Female
   Date of Birth ____ / ____ / ____
   Social Security # _____ / _____ / _____
   Occupation _____ Employer _____
   Spouse or Guardian Name _____

PRIMARY INSURANCE:
   Insurance Company Name _____
   Insurance Company Address _____
   Subscriber's Name _____
   Subscriber's Social Security # _____ / _____ / _____
   Group # _____

SECONDARY INSURANCE:
   Insurance Company Name _____
   Insurance Company Address _____
   Subscriber's Name _____
   Subscriber's Social Security # _____ / _____ / _____
   Group # _____

_____
Person to notify in case of emergency
   Name _____ Phone (_____) _____

ASSIGNMENT AND RELEASE: I authorize my insurance benefits be paid directly to the physician. I understand that I am financially responsible for any balance due. I authorize the physician or insurance company to release any information required for this claim.

   Signed _____ **Date** _____

Figure 11-1   Patient information forms typically include demographic data, insurance information, emergency contact, and patient's signature for acceptance of financial responsibility.

Medical Forms

The second set of forms is the medical history form, which can be as short as one page (8½″ × 11″) or as long and detailed as six to eight pages. This form includes information on:

1. The current problem (chief complaint or CC) for which the patient is being seen
2. The patient's past medical history
3. The patient's family medical history
4. Social history including marital status or sexual orientation and occupation

FINANCIAL POLICY

In order to reduce confusion and misunderstanding between our patients and the clinic, we have adopted the following financial policy. If you have any questions about this policy, please discuss them with our Billing Manager. We are dedicated to providing the best possible care and service to you and we regard your complete understanding of your financial responsibilities as an essential element of your care and treatment.

Unless other arrangements have been made in advance by yourself or your health coverage carrier, <u>full payment is due at time of service</u>. For your convenience, we accept Visa, MasterCard, or we can arrange a payment schedule.

YOUR INSURANCE:

We accept assignment of benefit from Medicare. We also have direct billing agreements with many insurance companies. We will bill those plans for whom we have an agreement and will only require that you pay the copayment at the time of service.

If your medical plan determines a service is "not covered," you will be responsible for the entire charge. Payment is due upon receipt of statement from this office.

MINOR PATIENTS:

The adult accompanying the patient and the parent or guardian with custody will be billed for all services rendered to minor patients.

MISSED APPOINTMENTS:

In order to provide the best service and availability to our patients, we ask you to notify us 24 hours in advance if you know that you will be unable to keep the appointment. We reserve the right to charge for missed appointments.

I have read the financial policy and I understand it and agree to be bound by its terms.

_____   Date _____

Figure 11-2   A sample financial information form. Ambulatory care settings will have different financial policies depending on their practice and the insurance companies they work with.

The best form is neither too long nor too complicated. Patients may feel overwhelmed with a long form and will not finish it or will give up, stating they cannot remember all the information. The form that is simple and brief can provide the most information. Some patients find a history form too intimidating. It is easier for these patients to talk directly with the medical assistant or the physician about social history, feeling a one-to-one exchange is more personal and private.

A sample of a short history form is included in Figure 11-3. This form asks the reason for the visit (chief

Please take a moment to fill out this form. It will give us more detailed information about your medical history than would be obtainable in a normal office visit, and will also free up time to discuss the more current problems, and answer any questions about your health that you may have. This information is entirely confidential.

NAME _____

Why you are here today (chief complaint) _____

Please circle any of the following symptoms that you have experienced recently:

Chest pain		Cough	
Chest pressure		Phlegm	
Chest heaviness		Coughing up blood	
Circulation problems		Shortness of breath	
Palpitations		Wheeze	
Rapid heartbeat		Change in exercise tolerance	
Irregular heartbeat			
Ankle swelling		Burning or pain on urination	
		Difficulty starting or stopping urination	
Change in appetite		Dribbling after urination	
Unexpected weight loss		Incontinence of urine	
Nausea		Blood in urine	
Vomiting		Cloudiness of urine	
Difficulty swallowing			
Belly pains		Skin rash	
Gas pains		New or changing moles	
Change in bowel habit:		Excess bruising or bleeding	
change in frequency		Mouth sores	
change in shape		Denture problems	
change in color		Sinus drainage or stuffiness	
change in consistency		Facial pain	
size of stool			
Blood, mucus or slime		Panic attacks	
Rectal pain or discomfort		Anxiety	
Hemorrhoids		Depression	
		Sadness	
Disturbance of sleep		Seizures	
Insomnia		Problems with concentration or memory	
Early wakefulness			
		Dizziness	
Fatigue		Fainting	
Fever/chills/sweat		Lightheadedness on standing	
Change in energy level		Vision problems	
Swollen glands		Hearing problems	
Sinusitis or chronic allergies		Numbness or tingling in arms or legs	
		Weakness in arms or legs	

PLEASE TURN PAGE OVER

Figure 11-3 Sample medical history form. *(continues)*

Have you ever had an allergic reaction to any medication?   YES   NO

If yes, what was/were the name/s of the medication/s? _____

What was/were the reaction/s? _____

_____

Past Medical History

Health Problem List	When first identified	Is the problem active?

List of surgeries	When performed?

Current Medications	Dose	Frequency	Date Started

Family History: Does any family member have the following conditions?			
Condition	Who?	Age at onset?	Age now?
Heart disease before age 60			
High cholesterol			
High blood pressure			
Diabetes			
Tuberculosis			
Cancer			
Other illness			
Depression			
Suicide			
Other psychiatric illness			

Social History:

Occupation: _____ Employer: _____

Marital status: **single**   **married**   **widowed**   **divorced**

Children: **male** ages now _____   **female** ages now _____

Do you smoke? _____ How many cigarettes per day? _____

Do you drink alcohol? _____ How many drinks per day? _____

Do you use recreation drugs or chemical substances? _____ Which ones? _____

          How often? _____

Do you have a sexual preference? _____   Male _____   Female _____

Do you have any sexual problems? _____   What kind(s)? _____

Figure 11-3   *(continued)*

complaint); symptoms the patient may be experiencing; past medical history including allergies to medications, past medical problems and surgeries, current medications; family history; and social history. Depending upon the ambulatory care setting, this form can be tailored to include vaccines and immunizations, usage of recreational drugs, exercise and diet regimens, accident information (especially if patient was hurt on the job), and any other information suited to the practice's specialty.

COMPUTERIZED HEALTH HISTORY

Some health care facilities use computerized health histories. These can be of two types: patient-generated and health care provider-generated. In patient-generated health histories, the patient responds on the computer to various questions, and then reviews information with the medical assistant for completeness. When using a health care provider-generated health history, the medical assistant completes the information on the screen after the patient interview. Frequently these programs are user-friendly and save time for both the patient and medical assistant. Some patients may not want to use a computer, however, and should be given the option of answering questions face to face.

THE FIRST OFFICE CONTACT

Telephone Contact

The first contact with a medical assistant in the ambulatory care setting is usually a telephone call. The patient or a relative of the patient calls to get information about the physician and the practice. When this occurs, primary administrative information is obtained including the patient's full name, telephone number, medical problem, insurance company, and sometimes the address as well. The administrative and medical history forms are given to the patient to complete upon coming into the office. If there is a long period of time between the telephone contact and the actual office visit, these forms may be mailed to the patient for completion.

Personal Visit

At times a physician will refer a patient to a specialist. When this happens, the patient may come to the specialist's office in person to bring records, X rays, or a referral and to make an appointment. If the patient is a member of a health maintenance organization, a referral from the primary care physician is usually mandatory. When the patient has a referral, the information forms are given to the patient to fill out in the office or to take home to complete in a quiet, undisturbed environment where the patient has access to records of past medical care.

Emergency Visit

When an acutely ill patient is referred by another physician to be seen immediately, or if an office or urgent care center accepts new patient emergency visits, the medical assistant usually knows about the visit in advance. In order to facilitate the history-taking process, the medical assistant may take the patient directly to an examination room where the atmosphere is quieter and private. This puts the patient at ease, which helps in preparing the forms. Depending upon the nature of the emergency, the medical assistant can help by asking the questions on the forms and writing down the patient's responses.

COMPLETING THE MEDICAL HISTORY FORMS

Interacting with the Patient

When the medical assistant is taking the medical history, the first responsibility is to put the patient at ease. A comfort level must be developed between medical assistant and patient. The medical assistant must guide the conversation, keeping it on track in order to obtain the most information for the physician. Allowing conversation to wander, talking about other people, or letting the patient tell anecdotes does not help to complete the history. Explaining a term or concept that the patient does not understand is helpful to the patient. The medical assistant must remain professional and not be embarrassed or made uncomfortable by the patient's answers, whether regarding illness, actions, or lifestyle. Refer to Table 11-1.

If the patient is already an established patient but has not seen the physician for several months or longer,

TABLE 11-1	GENERAL APPROACH TO THE HISTORY

1. Ensure an appropriate environment that is well-lighted, at a comfortable temperature, quiet, private, and free of distractions.
2. Sit facing the patient at eye level; the patient should be seated. Ensure that the patient is as comfortable as possible, since obtaining the health history can be a lengthy process. Figure 11-4 illustrates an appropriate setting.
3. Ask the patient if there are any questions about the interview before you begin.
4. Avoid the use of medical jargon. Use terms the patient can understand.
5. Reserve asking intimate and personal questions (social history) until rapport is established.
6. Remain flexible in obtaining the health history. It does not need to be obtained in the exact order it is presented in this chapter or on the form.
7. Remind the patient that all information will be treated confidentially.

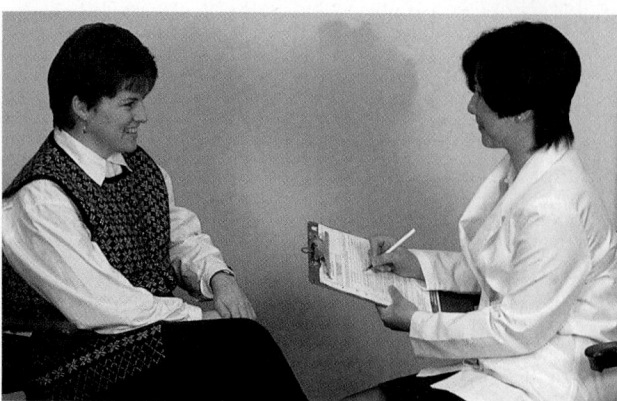

Figure 11-4   Showing concern for the patient's well-being can put the patient at ease while the medical assistant takes the medical history.

update the medical history by asking if any illnesses have occurred in the months elapsed, if any new allergies to any medications or other substances have occurred and the reaction to each. The chief complaint for the current visit should always be documented. The chief complaint is the problem that brings the patient to the physician this particular visit. Sometimes when patients know they are going to be seen, they save several problems to discuss. Depending on the appointment schedule for the day, the medical assistant may need to remind patients that an appointment for a specific problem was made and that the physician can see them for only that particular problem this visit. Another appointment can be made to discuss the remaining concerns on the list if necessary. The medical assistant should always note the chief complaint before the physician sees the patient to assure the main problem is addressed.

Displaying Cultural Awareness

As the medical assistant begins the encounter with the patient, awareness of cultural differences and other problems that may inhibit communication is important. Any number of situations may arise which the medical assistant must be prepared to address. The medical assistant has already overcome major obstacles if it is known that the patient does not speak English as a first language or needs an interpreter, if the patient is deaf and needs an interpreter, if the patient is from a culture in which the female patient does not disrobe for the physician, or if the patient has a mental disorder making communication difficult.

If there is a language difficulty, the medical assistant may be required to arrange for an interpreter. There are language interpreters in most areas; especially in large urban areas, an interpreter might be found for nearly any language. If the patient is receiving medical care through

Medicaid, special arrangements can be made for an interpreter through the state agency administering the program. Often the patient will bring a family member to interpret; however, if the matter is intensely personal, the patient may not want to reveal personal matters with the family member present and may prefer an outside, objective interpreter.

The medical assistant should be accessible and should listen to the patient. Sometimes the patient will be uneasy talking to the physician but may be more comfortable telling the medical assistant about the problem. Medical assistants can play a very important part in the medical practice by listening and communicating both with the patient and with the physician.

Handling a Difficult Patient

Some patients are frightened, hostile, or depressed. It is important to be open to nonverbal as well as verbal communication in answer to questions. Some patients react positively to a hand placed gently on the forearm; it calms and reassures them. Other patients have a negative response, pulling away from any such contact.

The medical assistant needs to know when to touch the patient appropriately, always with permission either expressed or implied. (If the medical assistant tells the patient a blood pressure reading is next and reaches for the patient's arm and the patient extends an arm, permission to take the reading is implied. If, however, the patient pulls away and states no blood pressure is to be taken, permission is not given and the reading must not be done at that time.)

Trying to get information from a reluctant patient can be difficult and requires patience and understanding. If the patient is hesitant to discuss a problem with the medical assistant, it is better not to press for information. Pressing for information may make the patient become defensive or angry and can impair communication altogether.

A patient may come to the office upset and crying. This patient must be made to feel more in control, that no one is going to rush care being given. Sometimes just taking a few moments to sit with such patients until they feel more settled is enough to calm them and enable the history-taking interview to proceed.

Uncommunicative patients may require some special questioning techniques. The medical assistant may have to supply a sample of problems to get these patients to acknowledge the health concerns they have. Or they may shrug their shoulders at every question and be unresponsive. Some patients may simply say, "I don't know. I

just don't feel well." If a relative has accompanied the patient to the appointment, it may be appropriate initially to have the relative present with the patient. In this way the patient has a familiar face in the unfamiliar, often frightening, physician's office. It is always the patient's decision if anyone else is to be in the room.

Some patients may have particular needs which they often will state to the medical assistant. These may be as simple as not wanting to sit or wanting the door ajar. Meeting these needs is usually a minor matter and makes patients feel more comfortable.

Dealing with Sensitive Topics

Alcohol, drug use, and sexual practices are some of the most sensitive areas that are addressed in the health history. Some consideration in dealing with these sensitive topics include:

- Ask these questions in the later stages of the interview after rapport has been established.

- Use direct eye contact; this demonstrates the importance of the topic to the patient and your lack of embarrassment.

- Pose questions in a matter-of-fact tone.

- Adopt a nonjudgmental demeanor.

- Utilize the communication technique of "normalizing" when appropriate (e.g., "Some high school students drink alcohol/use drugs/engage in sexual relationships on a regular basis. Does this happen at your school? With you?").

- Observe an experienced medical assistant elicit sensitive information from patients; note the medical assistant's verbal and nonverbal behavior.

If the medical assistant can enhance communication with the patient, communication between physician and patient will be more effective.

PARTS OF THE MEDICAL HISTORY

The components of the patient's medical history include:

- Personal data contained on the administrative form
- Chief complaint, which is noted at each visit by the medical assistant
- Present illness
- Past medical history
- Family history
- Social and occupational history
- Review of systems

Chief Complaint

The **chief complaint** (usually abbreviated CC) is the specific reason that brought the patient to see the physician. It should be noted in as few words as possible but be very specific. It can be a direct quote from the patient.

A good example of a chief complaint notation might be "nausea and vomiting × 3 days." This is a **subjective** complaint in that it is known by the patient but cannot be seen or measured by the physician. It is specific, however, in relating the patient's condition. The "×" is an abbreviation for the length of time since the symptom first occurred. Another example is "hurt ankle when tripped over curb yesterday." Again this is subjective but specific about cause, time of onset, and complaint. The ankle is visibly swollen and very painful to touch. The swelling is an **objective** sign, a manifestation that can be seen, heard, or measured by any observer.

On the other hand, a poor example of a chief complaint is "has not been feeling well." This notation tells the physician nothing about what symptoms or problems the patient has been experiencing. It gives no specific clue as to what the problem is from the patient's perspective. The medical assistant should try to pinpoint a complaint to a body system, to a time frame, to pain in a specific area. The patient usually will respond to questions that offer several options.

Nine characteristics of each chief complaint should be ascertained for a complete history. These characteristics are:

1. Location
2. Radiation
3. Quality
4. Quantity
5. Associated manifestations
6. Aggravating factors
7. Alleviating factors
8. Setting
9. Timing

Note that all chief complaints may not have all nine qualifiers; hoarseness, for example, may not be characterized by quantity.

Present Illness

The present illness is usually reflected in the chief complaint. Then the chief complaint is expanded upon to determine the onset of the illness, what the patient has done to treat the illness, and any current medications. In the preceding example of nausea and vomiting, the patient may indicate inability to eat or take fluids. This would alert the physician to possible dehydration. Often the present illness is based upon a prior health problem. For instance, a history of congestive heart failure gives a patient's symptoms of fluid retention, wheezing, and shortness of breath more importance since these are very common complications. Without this knowledge of the patient's past history, these symptoms could be confused with bronchitis, asthma, or pneumonia.

Past Medical History

The past medical history includes all health problems, major illnesses, and surgeries that the patient has had, all current medications including dosages and reasons for taking them, all allergies to any medications and the specific allergic reaction to each. These are very important to the present illness, for many health problems can overlap and affect the patient in several areas. A patient with a long history of diabetes mellitus may present with an ulcer on his foot. While the same ulcer in an otherwise healthy patient will heal with little intervention, the diabetic patient will require major treatment and attention including **debridement** (removal of dead or damaged tissue or foreign debris), antibiotics, and close monitoring.

Medications have side effects and contraindications that can affect patients. **Allergies** to medications can be serious and need to be noted in a readily visible part of the chart. Usually a red sticker is placed in a conspicuous area on the outside of the chart noting medication allergies. A notation is added inside the chart as well. The information needs to be updated at least annually. Also document herbal, vitamin, and mineral supplements the patient is taking.

Patients may be asked to complete a Release of Information form (Figure 11-5). This form is sent to their former physicians to obtain past medical records.

**AUTHORIZATION TO RELEASE
HEALTH CARE INFORMATION**

Patient _____ Date of Birth _____
SSN _____ Previous Name _____
I request and authorize _____ to
release the health care information of the patient named
above to:
  Name _____
  Address _____
This request and authorization applies to:
(Please initial the appropriate box)
___ Health care information relating to the following treat-
  ment, condition, or dates of treatment:
  _____
___ All health care information **EXCLUDING** specific infor-
  mation relating to sexually transmitted diseases (including HIV/AIDS), alcohol or drug use, or visits related
  to psychiatric disorders or mental health.
___ All health care information **INCLUDING** specific information relating to sexually transmitted diseases (including HIV/AIDS), alcohol or drug use, or visits related
  to psychiatric disorders or mental health.
___ Other: _____
I understand that my express consent is required to
release any health care information relating to testing,
diagnosis, and/or treatment of HIV (AIDS virus), sexually
transmitted disease, psychiatric disorders/mental health,
or drug and/or alcohol use. If I have been tested, diagnosed, or treated for HIV (AIDS virus), sexually transmitted disease, psychiatric disorders/mental health, or drug
and/or alcohol use, you are specifically authorized to
release all health care information relating to such diagnosis, testing, or treatment.

_____ / _____
Signature of patient or patient's   Relationship
authorized representative   to patient

_____
Date

Figure 11-5   Sample release of information form.

If the patient has several physicians, the examining physician will encourage the patient to
choose one physician to manage primary med-
ical care so that all medical care and records are concentrated in one office. Under most managed care insurance
policies, patients have one primary care physician
(women may also have an obstetrician/gynecologist) who
coordinates the patient's health care.

Family History

The family history can provide clues to the patient's present condition. By asking open-ended questions about

Patient Teaching Tip

Patients who are adopted may have limited information about their biological parents. Encourage adopted patients to be frank with
their family health history. If the family health
history of the biological parents is unknown,
this is documented. It is not uncommon for
patients to seek out their birth parents in an
attempt to learn more about their family
health history.

The family health history of adoptive parents can be equally important. Certain environmental factors (smoking, drug and alcohol
use, sanitation) can influence the health of the
adopted child.

medical problems of siblings, parents, and grandparents,
the physician will be alerted to hereditary and familial diseases and disorders such as coronary artery disease, hypertension, breast cancer, and so forth. Present ages of
siblings, parents, and grandparents, or cause of their death
and age at time of death are noted. For instance, a family
history of diabetes together with the patient's symptoms of
frequent urination and thirst may make a diagnosis of diabetes mellitus a possibility.

Social History

The social history of patients includes their marital status,
sexual orientation, occupation, hobbies, and use of alcohol, tobacco, and recreational drugs or other chemical
substances. This part of the history includes those
lifestyles and behaviors that may put the patient at greater
risk for injury or disease than would normally be found
from factors in the family history and past medical history.
If the patient's usage of alcohol exceeds an average
amount and a hobby the patient pursues is auto racing,
the physician will counsel the patient about the danger of
the combination of these two behaviors.

Be aware that patients may refuse to answer questions pertaining to sexual history; attempt to return to
these questions later. Ask the patient if a medical assistant
of a different gender would make the patient more comfortable in discussing sexual practice.

For instance, the adolescent patient may refuse to
answer questions of a sexual matter or provide false
answers if the parent or caregiver is present. It may be best
to ask the caregiver to leave the room at the completion
of the health history so you can ask the patient if there is
anything else to note in the sexual history.

Be alert for cues that demonstrate the patient's desire for knowledge of sexual education, such as questions or requests for written information. Answer the patient's questions, provide educational materials, and refer the patient to a specialist when indicated.

It may be necessary to inquire about the patient's home environment. You need to be attentive for clues that signal the necessity of performing an in-depth home environment assessment. Some clues include, but are not limited to, poor hygiene, frequent infections, smoke inhalation, burns, malnutrition, and falls (especially in the elderly).

Review of Systems

After the history is taken by the medical assistant, the review of systems (ROS) is performed by the physician during the physical examination. This is an orderly and systematic check of each part of the body and is recorded. The physician asks questions concerning each organ and system of the body during the examination of the patient. The ROS, in conjunction with the physical examination,

helps elicit information that is essential to the diagnosis of disease. The physician usually begins with an overall assessment and proceeds to check each body system in an organized manner. The order in which this is done may vary from one physician to another, but all will check the cardiovascular, respiratory, gastrointestinal, genitourinary, and neurological systems as well as the extremities, the musculoskeletal system, and the skin.

Both positive and pertinent negative findings are documented in the ROS. When a response is positive, the physician asks the patient to describe it as completely as possible. Table 11-2 lists the symptoms and diseases that can be ascertained during the ROS. Many ambulatory care settings have preprinted ROS sheets. These are convenient, as positive findings can be circled and noted. Negative responses are not circled.

By the completion of this portion of the history, the physician usually has an idea about the patient's condition.

To complete the exam, the physician usually orders laboratory tests depending on the findings and the probable diagnosis. These results, together with the history,

---

TABLE 11-2 REVIEW OF SYSTEMS

General
Patient's perception of general state of health at the present time; difference from usual state; vitality and energy levels

Neurological
Headache, change in balance, incoordination, loss of movement, change in sensory perception/feeling in an extremity, change in speech, change in smell, fainting, loss of memory, tremors, involuntary movement, loss of consciousness, seizures, weakness, head injury

Psychological
Irritability, nervousness, tension, increased stress, difficulty concentrating, mood changes, suicidal thoughts, depression

Skin
Rashes, itching, changes in skin pigmentation, black and blue marks, change in color or size of mole, sores, lumps, change in skin texture, odors, excessive sweating, acne, loss of hair, excessive growth of hair or growth of hair in unusual locations, change in nails, amount of time spent in the sun

Eyes
Blurry vision, visual acuity, glasses, contacts, sensitivity to light, excessive tear-

ing, night blindness, double vision, drainage, bloodshot, pain, blind spots, flashing lights, halos around objects, glaucoma, cataracts

Ears
Hearing deficits, hearing aid, pain, discharge, lightheadedness, ringing in the ears, earaches, infection

Nose and Sinuses
Frequent colds, discharge, itching, hay fever, postnasal drip, stuffiness, sinus pain, polyps, obstruction, nosebleed, change in sense of smell

Mouth
Toothache, tooth abscess, dentures, bleeding/swollen gums, difficulty chewing, sore tongue, change in taste, lesions, change in salivation, bad breath

Throat/Neck
Hoarseness, change in voice, frequent sore throats, difficulty swallowing, pain/stiffness, enlarged thyroid

Respiratory
Shortness of breath, shortness of breath on exertion, phlegm, cough, sneezing, wheezing, coughing up blood, frequent upper respiratory tract infections, pneumonia, emphysema, asthma, tuberculosis

Cardiovascular
Shortness of breath that wakes you up in the night, chest pain, heart murmur, palpitations, fainting, sleep on pillows to breathe better, swelling, cold hands/feet, leg cramps, myocardial infarction, hypertension, valvular disease, pain in calf with walking, varicose veins, inflammation of a vein, blood clot in leg, anemia

Breasts
Pain, tenderness, discharge, lumps, change in size, dimpling

Gastrointestinal
Change in appetite, nausea, vomiting, diarrhea, constipation, usual bowel habits, black, tarry stools, vomiting blood, change in stool color, excessive gas, belching, regurgitation or heartburn, difficulty swallowing, abdominal pain, jaundice, hemorrhoids, hepatitis, peptic ulcers, gallstones

Urinary
Change in urine color, voiding habits, painful urination, hesitancy, urgency, frequency, excessive urination at night, increased urine volume, dribbling, loss in force of stream, bedwetting, change in urine volume, incontinence, pain in lower abdomen, kidney stones, urinary tract infections

(continues)

TABLE 11-2 *(continued)*		
Musculoskeletal Joint stiffness, muscle pain, back pain, limitation of movement, redness, swelling, weakness, bony deformity, broken bones, dislocations, sprains, gout, arthritis, osteoporosis, herniated disc *Female Reproductive* Vaginal discharge, change in libido, infertility, sterility, pain during intercourse, menses (last menstrual period, age period started, regularity, duration, amount of bleeding, premenstrual symptoms, intermenstrual bleeding, painful periods), menopause (age of onset, duration, symptoms, bleeding),	obstetrical (number of pregnancies, number of miscarriages/abortions, number of children, type of delivery, complications), type of birth control, estrogen therapy *Male Reproductive* Change in libido, infertility, sterility, impotence, pain during intercourse, age at onset of puberty, testicular pain, penile discharge, erections, emissions, hernias, enlarged prostate, type of birth control *Nutrition* Present weight, usual weight, food intolerances, food likes, food dislikes, where meals are eaten	*Endocrine* Bulging eyes, fatigue, change in size of head, hands, or feet, weight change, heat/cold intolerances, excessive sweating, increased thirst, increased hunger, change in body hair distribution, swelling in the anterior neck, diabetes mellitus *Lymph Nodes* Enlarged, tenderness *Hematological* Easy bruising/bleeding, anemia, sickle cell anemia, blood type

examination, and patient symptoms, help to lead to a **clinical diagnosis.**

All of the components of the patient's medical history document integral parts of the patient's health. If any part is lacking, the current understanding of the patient's health is not complete. By using all the components, the physician can evaluate the patient's health completely and more easily.

See Procedure 11-1 for steps in taking a medical history.

THE PATIENT'S RECORD AND ITS IMPORTANCE

The patient's chart or record is a collection of confidential information that concerns the patient, care given to the patient, patient progress, and laboratory and other diagnostic test results that have been completed. This information is arranged in a file folder or a binder, or is held together by other suitable means. It is used for a variety of purposes, but primarily it is used to provide a foundation for planning patient care and making decisions about patient care. Other purposes for a medical record include using it as a basis for communication among care givers, for statistical analysis in research, and for reporting infectious diseases to the health department. It is also a legal document and belongs to the physician or the agency in which the physician is employed. See Chapter 7 regarding legal guidelines and medical records. Since it is a legal document, the medical record can be used to determine if patient care has been given according to the standards of care that the law recognizes; therefore, it must be complete, concise, accurate, and legible. Many important items of information must be written in the patient record and the medical assistant will be one of the professionals making chart entries.

Contents of Medical Records

Each patient has his or her own medical record. All patients' records hold standard information. In addition to the patient information forms previously mentioned, other important components of the record include:

- Informed consent forms
- Physical examination outcomes
- Laboratory and diagnostic test results
- The physician's diagnosis and plan of treatment
- Surgical reports
- Progress reports
- Follow-up care
- Telephone calls
- Discharge summary
- Other communications (from other physicians, laboratories, or agencies)
- Patient records from other physicians
- Medication history

METHODS OF CHARTING/ DOCUMENTATION

There are three primary ways to maintain chart notes. They are:

- Source-oriented medical records
- Problem-oriented medical records
- Computer-generated/modified records.

Source-Oriented Medical Records

The traditional or conventional method of charting, **source-oriented medical record (SOMR),** consists of a chronological set of notes for each visit beginning with the patient's first visit (Figure 11-6). This form of charting makes it difficult to follow or track a specific patient problem. The caregiver must search through the record to locate information about a particular patient problem. Source-oriented notes may be typed by the medical transcriptionist from dictation after the physician has seen the patient.

The example of handwritten chart notes shows the complete history taken at the time of examination including the present illness (if any), the past medical history, allergies, family history, habits (social history), and review of systems. The physical examination follows with each area noted. Impressions and changes in medications and plan finish the examination notes.

Problem-Oriented Medical Records

A more efficient way of keeping chart notes is the **problem-oriented medical record (POMR)**. This method is used extensively today, especially by clinics or any medical practice where more than one physician may see the patient. This method calls for a list of problems to be made, dated, and numbers assigned to them. When a patient is seen, the problems are identified by number throughout the record. This system makes it easier for the physician to follow the patient's progress.

The problem-oriented medical record has four major components:

- *The database:* The patient's medical history, results from laboratory and other diagnostic tests, and results of physical examination are the core of the record.

- *The problem list:* Each problem is listed individually and assigned a number and dated.

- *The diagnostic and treatment plan:* This component addresses the laboratory and other diagnostic tests completed and the physician's plan for treating the patient.

- *Progress notes:* These notes are entered on every problem initially recorded. Documentation is done chronologically and includes patient's complaints, problems, condition, treatment, and responses to treatment and care given.

Physicians may dictate their notes to be typed by a medical transcriptionist and then filed in the chart (Figure 11-7). These notes may follow the form seen in the handwritten chart note or as in Figure 11-7.

Computer-Modified Records

The final example (Figure 11-8), shows a computer chart note that ties both methods together: the problems are

---

04/01/_ abdominal pain × 3 weeks
WT 192   BP 152/88   T 97.6   P78   R18
Pt complaining severe abdominal pain for 2 wks getting progressively worse. Describes as burning, pressure.
Past Med. Hist.   chronic Peptic Ulcer Disease
                  quit smoking 3 yr ago – now back
                  to 2 ppd
Allergies–penicillin–hives 1950s
Family Hist   noncontributory
Habits   smokes 2 ppd
            beer–several daily
ROS
HEENT noncontributory–PERRLA OU correct to 20/20
        CR–clear, no rales, ronchi; murmurs
        GI–some guarding. No masses, tenderness lower
        abdomen. No nausea, vomiting, diarrhea
        GU–clear
PE alert; oriented to time & place
      HEENT–pupils   nat teeth
      fundi   thyroid   } ∅
      carotids
      chest–clear
      heart–no murmurs or enlargement
      abdomen–∅ masses
      rectal–soft brown stool in vault
      extremities–neg.
      neuro–reg.
      skin–clear
Impression–Chronic Peptic Ulcer Disease
            Hypertension, mild
Plan–Lab–CBC, Chem 7, UA, barium swallow
Rx–Omeprazole 20 mg qd
Return 3 days
M. Woo, MD

Figure 11-6   Sample of a handwritten chart note.

Leo McKay
Date of Birth 01/22/49
Office visit 04/01/__

This 52-year-old patient is seen after a several year absence because of abdominal pain which began approximately 2 weeks ago with progressively worsening abdominal pain. He has stopped eating to see if pain would improve, which it did not. Finally yesterday he stopped taking fluids as well. Until this episode, he was drinking several beers daily and smoking approximately 2 ppd.

Weight is 192. BP 152/88 P 78 R 18 T 97.6. He is a well-developed, moderately obese male in moderate distress. Abdomen is tense with some guarding at RUQ.

Abdominal pain - pt needs barium swallow, CBC, Chem 7 and UA. To restrict diet to clear liquids until seen in 2 days, omeprazole 20 mg qd.
      JW/tlm

Figure 11-7   Example of dictated and transcribed chart note.

Patient: Leo McKay
Date of Birth: 01/22/49
Visit Date: 04/01/__

Chief Complaint: Abdominal pain
History: Has been ill over the last 2 weeks with progressively worsening abdominal pain.
Review of Symptoms: Patient denies the following:
- Chest pain, Chest pressure, Chest heaviness, Circulation problems, Palpitations, Rapid heartbeat, Irregular heartbeat, Ankle swelling
- Cough, Phlegm, Coughing up blood, Shortness of breath, Wheeze, Change in exercise tolerance
- Burning or pain on urination, Difficulty starting or stopping urination, Dribbling after urination, Incontinence of urine, Blood in urine, Cloudiness of urine
- Change in appetite, Unexpected weight loss, Nausea, Vomiting, Difficulty Swallowing, Belly pains, Gas pains, Change in bowel habit: change in frequency, shape, color, consistency, size of stool; Blood, Mucus, or Slime, Rectal pain or discomfort, Hemorrhoids
- Skin rash, New or changing moles, Excess bruising or bleeding
- Mouth sores, Denture problems, Sinus drainage or stuffiness, Facial pain
- Panic attacks, Anxiety, Depression, Sadness, Seizures, Problems with concentration or memory, Disturbance of sleep, Insomnia, Early wakefulness
- Dizziness, Fainting, Lightheadedness on standing, Headaches, Vision problems, Hearing problems, Numbness or tingling in arms or legs, Weakness in arms or legs

Medications, including Herbal, Vitamin, and Mineral Supplements

Drug	Dose	Freq.	Started
none			

Medical Problem List

Problem	When Dx'd	Active?
Peptic Ulcer	1985	no

List of Surgeries

Surgical Procedure	When
none	

Family History: Parents deceased, father died of heart attack, mother of breast cancer.
Social History: Divorced, no children
Habits: Smokes 2 ppd, Several beers daily
Allergies: Penicillin _____

Physical Examination

GENERAL: Well developed and well nourished gentleman in no distress. No jaundice, cyanosis, clubbing, or edema.
VITALS: Weight = 192, Temp = 97.6, Pulse = 78, R = 18, BP = 152/88
HEENT: Normocephalic and without evidence of trauma, tympanic membranes and external auditory canals are normal. Pharynx and mouth are normal.
NECK: supple, no masses or thyromegaly.
NODES: No cervical nodes palpable. No axillary or inguinal adenopathy.
CARDIOVASCULAR SYSTEM: Heart sounds: no murmurs, rubs or gallops, carotids with good upstrokes, no bruits heard. Peripheral pulses including radials, brachials, and femorals intact. Posterior tibial, and dorsalis pedis pulses intact.
RESPIRATORY SYSTEM: resps 18/min, trachea central, expansion, fremitus, resonance, and breath sounds normal.
ABDOMEN: soft, no masses, organomegaly, or tenderness. No loin or costo-vertebral angle tenderness. Inguinal canals are intact without herniae. Bowel sounds active.
GENITOURINARY: Penis without lesions or discharge, scrotum, testicles, epididymis and cords all normal
RECTAL: no masses, tenderness, or hemorrhoids. Soft brown stool in vault. Prostate normal in size, and shape without nodules or tenderness.
MUSCULOSKELETAL SYSTEM: Joints with full ROM, no joint tenderness or swelling. Muscle bulk symmetric and normal.
SKIN: without masses, skin tags, rash, blisters or ulcerations. Nails are normal without splinter hemorrhages.
NEUROLOGICAL SYSTEM: Alert and oriented to place, person, and time. Communicates with good word recognition and appropriate word usage. Cranial nerves and spinal nerves grossly intact.

Assessment and Plan

Problem	Plan/Status
Abdominal pain	Reports about two weeks of epigastric and retrosternal chest pain radiating up and to the left. Episodes of pain occur usually during the day and last for 3-4 hours. No associated dyspnea, palpitations, sweats, dizziness. No nausea, vomiting or diarrhea. No blood in the stool. To get barium swallow, CBC, Chem 7 and UA. Begin omeprazole 20 m qd.

Follow-up appointment: 3 days
Mark Woo MD

Figure 11-8   Sample of computer-generated medical history and physical examination.

Leo McKay
Date of Birth 01/22/49
Visit Date: 04/04/___

S: Patient returns after undergoing barium swallow. He is not in as much discomfort as last visit. States he has been taking clear liquids only and is hungry.
O: Lab results are back. Chem 7 shows slightly elevated glucose at 133. CBC and UA normal. Barium swallow shows two small areas of ulceration.
A: Gastric ulcer.
P: Reduce omeprazole to 10 mg qd. Recheck glucose at return visit in 4 weeks.

MW/tlm

Figure 11-9 Sample of a dictated and transcribed SOAP follow-up visit note.

Leo McKay
Visit Date: 04/04/___

| Symptoms: | Feeling somewhat better. Abdominal pain is less on the Omeprazole. |
| Exam: | Weight = 185   BP = 150/84 Patient had barium swallow showing two areas of ulceration. Lab tests show normal findings for CBC and UA. Chem 7 shows slightly elevated glucose at 133. |

Assessment	Plan
Gastric ulcer	Omeprazole 10 mg qd. Recheck glucose at return visit.

Follow-up appointment: 4 weeks.

Mark Woo, MD

Figure 11-10 Sample of computer-generated follow-up visit note.

stated, but the record grows in chronological order. Note that the past health problems are shown at the top of each entry and all current medications are shown on each entry. Computer-modified records are advantageous if an agency has computer terminals in a network connected to a main computer. Records can be brought up on a terminal by a physician and reviewed, updated, and saved whenever the physician wants to do so. Records are available 24 hours a day and therefore can be accessed by the physician on a home computer. Protecting patient's confidentiality must always be a priority when medical records are computerized.

SOAP Method of Charting

Charting under SOMR and POMR techniques for follow-up visits is accomplished most efficiently using a method with the acronym **SOAP**. In this method, the *subjective* complaint (patient's symptoms) is listed. This is the patient's description of the current problems. These problems are not discernible to an observer. The *objective* findings are those made by the physician during the physical examination, vital signs, and laboratory and other test results. These findings can be seen, felt, or measured, and the findings are observable. *Assessment* of the problem is next. The physician weighs the objective findings with the subjective information the patient has given and forms a diagnosis. The physician then formulates a *plan*. The plan includes further laboratory tests, X rays, medications, and instructions to the patient. Usually there is a follow-up appointment made for a few days or two to three weeks for a new problem, followed by a several month follow-up for the problem once it has been brought under control.

Examples of the transcribed (Figure 11-9) and the computer-generated (Figure 11-10) follow-up visit notes are shown here.

Abbreviations Used in Charting

Abbreviations are used extensively in charting to document information. Some are used as a short-hand to save time and space, while other abbreviations are used to give an exact meaning to a finding. For instance, the abbreviation N&V indicates "nausea and vomiting" without having to write out the entire expression. See Table 11-3 for commonly used abbreviations.

Correcting an Error

When an error has been made in the chart and it needs to be corrected, the proper procedure is to draw a line through the error, note "error" just above the line, and sign your initials and the date (Figure 11-11). Then enter the correct information. Do not erase, obliterate, or otherwise try to change the error because that will invalidate the legal and medical value of the patient's chart. As a medical assistant, you will be responsible for entering information in a patient's record and keeping it confidential. Remember that a patient's medical record is a legal document and it may be necessary to use it as evidence in a court of law.

TABLE 11-3	ABBREVIATIONS COMMONLY USED IN CHARTING
BP or B/P	blood pressure
c̄	with
CBC	complete blood count
CC	chief complaint
CPE	complete physical exam
D&C	dilation and curettage
dx	diagnosis
ECG, EKG	electrocardiogram
EEG	electroencephalogram
ER	emergency room
GI	gastrointestinal
GU	genitourinary
GYN	gynecology
HEENT	head, eyes, ears, nose, and throat
I&D	incision and drainage
L	left
MI	myocardial infarction
N&V	nausea and vomiting
NVD	nausea, vomiting, and diarrhea
OPD	outpatient department
OR	operating room
P	pulse
PERRLA	pupils equal, round, reactive to light and accommodation
PT	physical therapy
R	right
R	respiration
ROM	range of motion
ROS	review of systems
s̄	without
SOAP	subjective, objective. assessment, plan
SOB	short of breath
T	temperature
T&A	tonsillectomy and adenoidectomy
UCHD	usual childhood diseases
URI	upper respiratory infection
UTI	urinary tract infection
WNL	within normal limits
XR	X ray
>	greater than
<	less than
↑	increase
↓	decrease
Δ	change

Chart Organization

The chart notes are kept in chronological order for the primary physician. The laboratory tests, hospital notes, consultations by other physicians, and any correspondence should be kept in an orderly fashion. Figure 11-12 shows a chart with information easily found.

The chart order presents current medications on the left side of the chart with the laboratory reports and pathology reports underneath, each in chronological order. In the POMR system, often the list of medical problems is found above the current medications.

On the right side of the chart, the physician's notes are in chronological order with the most recent on top. The X rays and EKGs follow, including MRIs, mammograms, CT scans, exercise tolerance tests (ETTs), echocardiograms, and other similar tests. Following these are the hospital notes, including the history and physical, hospital consultations, and discharge summary. Consultations by other physicians are grouped next, again in chronological order.

The miscellaneous section may include anything from referrals for insurance companies to orders and updates from nursing homes or home health services. Finally, the correspondence section includes letters, insurance claim forms, and requests for prior medical records.

If a chart is kept in a specific order, information needed is easily gleaned by the medical assistant, the physician, or the front office administrative assistant.

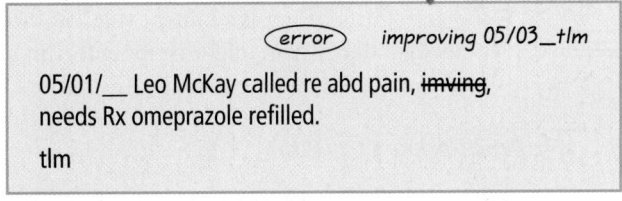

Figure 11-11   Correcting a charting error.

Current Medications	Primary Physician's Notes
Laboratory Results	EKGs - X RAYS
Pathology Reports	Hospital Notes
	Consultations
	Miscellaneous
	Correspondence

Figure 11-12   Sample chart organization.

Procedure

11-1   Taking a Medical History

PURPOSE:
To obtain a medical history from a patient new to the ambulatory care setting.

EQUIPMENT/SUPPLIES:
Patient history forms
Clipboard
Pens

PROCEDURE STEPS:
1. Introduce yourself to the new patient. Confirm identity of the patient and escort to the examination room or private area.
2. Make eye contact and use positive body language to put patient at ease.
3. Explain the purpose and importance of obtaining the patient information. Ask the questions on the form, trying to get as much information as possible without letting the patient wander from the subject.
4. Ask each question clearly. Be sure patient understands all questions. Ask about allergies.
5. Repeat patient answers when needed to confirm. Be specific when documenting answers. Do not just write "yes" for tobacco use. List "2 packs per day." Be specific.
6. Write legibly using dark ink (blue or black).
7. Recheck the medical history form to be sure all parts are complete. Note any additional information provided by patient. Make sure numbers, dates, spelling, and other information are accurate and legible.
8. Prepare the patient for the review of systems and physical examination if this is indicated.
9. Document the procedure.

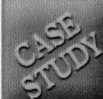

CASE STUDY 11-1

Maria Jover, a patient of Dr. Elizabeth King at Doctors Lewis & King, has finally convinced her teenage son to make an appointment for a physical. Adam Jover is 17, outgoing, fun loving, and apparently healthy. But Maria is concerned that he may be engaging in harmful social activities and hopes that by seeing Dr. Winston Lewis, Adam may discover ways to protect himself and his health. Adam agreed to the appointment but is adamant that his mother not accompany him. At the ambulatory care setting, it is decided that Adam might be more forthcoming with a male medical assistant, so Joe Guerrero is scheduled to take Adam's medical history before Dr. Winston does a review of systems.

CASE STUDY REVIEW

1. When Joe Guerrero first sits down with Adam to take the history, he notices that Adam is very ill at ease and nervous. What can Joe do to reassure Adam that his privacy will be protected?

2. When Joe attempts to take the social history, Adam seems evasive about answering Joe's questions and finally admits that he doesn't want his mother, Maria, to know about his social activities. What is Joe's response?

3. By the end of the interview, it becomes apparent that Adam may be engaging in some behaviors that put him at high risk for contracting the HIV virus. How can Joe provide Adam with guidance without alienating him?

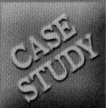

Harvey DiAntonio is a 46-year-old patient who lives at 45 W. Smith Avenue, Baltimore, Maryland, 21208. His date of birth is July 8, 1954. His phone number is 667-1870. He is a Baltimore City fire fighter and has been for 21 years. He has union medical insurance and Blue Cross/Blue Shield (BC/BS) is his carrier. His number is 211-67-87-56. He also carries major medical and his policy is Diagnostic #4. He has been referred by the fire department physician, Dr. Alan Byers. Mr. DiAntonio's complaint is severe "gripping" pain in the anterior mid-chest sometime radiating to the abdomen, neck, and both arms. Pain seems to occur with strenuous exercise, when walking uphill. Pain usually lasts 20 minutes with each episode. Pain does "ease up" when he ceases activity. Mr. DiAntonio states his episodes have occurred while he was shaving, climbing stairs at work, after a heavy meal, and during sexual intercourse. One episode last week was accompanied with dizziness, nausea, and fatigue. The episodes have been going on now once or twice a month for five months. Mr. DiAntonio's past history is essentially noncontributory. It is questionable whether this is due to good health or the fact that the patient has not had a physical examination for eight years. Surgeries include tonsillectomy and adenoidectomy, T & A, 1958, and appendectomy in 1964. Fractured rib, left side, in 1984 due to fire fighting incident. Usual childhood diseases. Hospitalized for observation, 1962, Sinai Hospital, for an unusually long episode of bronchitis. Social history shows that the patient is a pump operator on the job with much heavy exertion. Smokes 1½ to 2 packs of cigarettes per day and is a moderate drinker. He has a weight problem off and on and tends to eat too much while on duty. Lives in a one story home. Hobbies include carpentry and music. Some family problems and tension exist as both of his children are in adolescence. Patient describes himself as "fun-loving" with a "quick temper" and worries about meeting financial needs of the family. Is in a position to retire from active duty, but states he could not tolerate the boredom.

Family history shows both parents deceased—mother of heart attack, age 59, and father of unknown cause at age 49. Has two siblings, one brother with history of hypertension and one sister living and in good health. Has two children both living and well. Family history otherwise negative.

Physical examination revealed a well-nourished, well-developed male in no acute distress at this time. Patient does seem a bit anxious about this examination. T. 98.6 - P. 94 - R. 24 - BP 175/104. Ht. 69″, Wt. 198 pounds. HEAD, EYES, EARS, NOSE, THROAT—normal. NECK—supple. Trachea in midline. CHEST—normal in contour. Calcium deposit on left sixth rib probably due to history fracture. HEART—after careful examination with the patient recumbent and the scope placed lightly on the chest wall near the apex, a left atrial sound was heard (presystolic gallop). ABDOMEN—negative. EXTREMITIES—negative. GENITALIA—negative. SKIN—negative. NEUROLOGICAL—negative. Laboratory tests performed show a hemoglobin of 11.0 Gms. Awaiting results of serum cholesterol, calcium, phosphorus, and blood urea nitrogen. Chest X ray essentially negative. EKG report showed atrial sounds occurring presystolically with long P-R intervals. DIAGNOSIS: 1)Angina Pectoris. 2)Anemia 3)Hypertension. TREATMENT: Nitroglycerin tabs, sublingually as needed. To return to office in two weeks to follow medication effects. In consultation with patient, the patient was advised to control physical activity and quantity of food intake. Avoid extreme cold, 8 hours of sleep/night. Avoid emotional upsets. Attempt 4 meals/day. Low fat 1600 calorie diet. No smoking, moderate alcohol intake.

CASE STUDY REVIEW

1. Identify the following parts of the case study above and extract from the case study the portion that matches the appropriate medical history component.

   - Personal data
   - Chief complaint
   - Present illness
   - Past medical history
   - Family history
   - Social history
   - Review of systems

2. Using appropriate terminology and abbreviations, make a charting entry for Mr. DiAntonio by using the SOAP method of charting.

SUMMARY

The patient's medical chart or record is the mainstay of the medical practice. The history contained within it is the rationale for all decisions made by the physician for a patient. The more complete that information is, the better the physician can serve the patient. The more easily accessible the information in the chart is, the more efficiently the physician can treat the patient. The medical assistant must recognize the importance of documenting in the medical record information that concerns the patient, such as patient progress, care given, laboratory tests performed, prescription refills, and missed appointments. This collection of information must be accurate, concise, and complete and it must remain confidential.

REVIEW QUESTIONS

Multiple Choice

1. If the patient has difficulty with English, the medical assistant should:
   a. set up the appointment for the patient and obtain the services of an interpreter to be present as well
   b. not set the appointment until contact is made with the interpreter
   c. speak more loudly so the patient will understand
   d. suggest that the patient find a physician who speaks this language

2. If the patient's social history reflects exposure to sexually transmitted diseases including HIV, the medical assistant should:
   a. use standard precautions for this particular patient
   b. let the laboratory assistants know that there is a problem with this patient
   c. treat the patient the same as all other patients
   d. mark the chart somehow to alert to possible HIV patient

3. A helpful question to ask the returning patient is:
   a. Are you feeling bad today?
   b. Didn't you get better with the treatment prescribed last visit?
   c. Have you noticed any changes in your condition since your last visit?
   d. Do you realize you have gained six pounds since your visit last week?

4. When the patient complains of not feeling well, the medical assistant should:
   a. mark the chief complaint as "patient not feeling well"
   b. ask helpful questions to help the patient express specific problems or symptoms
   c. pin down the symptoms by guessing what the problem could be
   d. let the physician work with the patient

5. Source-oriented medical records:
   a. are chronological, and usually over a long period of time
   b. use lists such as lists of problems or lists of medications
   c. are the best for finding information quickly
   d. are best when many physicians see the patient

Critical Thinking

1. Name the sections of a medical history.
2. Define each section and state its importance.
3. What are the three main ways that new patients set up a first appointment?
4. How can a medical assistant help a patient provide a medical history?
5. What avenues of help are available to a medical assistant and physician for a patient with special needs?
6. What kinds of barriers should a medical assistant be prepared to encounter?
7. Name the methods of charting and compare them.
8. Where in a chart would you find a discharge summary? A follow-up visit for a consultation? A copy of the worker's compensation claim form?
9. What should be noted on the outside of the chart as well as in the chart notes?
10. What is the proper way to make a correction in a chart?

WEB ACTIVITIES

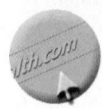

Using Case Study 11-2, go into the World Wide Web to research the treatment of Mr. Harvey DiAntonio's three diagnoses: coronary artery disease, hypertension, and anemia, using the National Institutes of Health as a resource.

REFERENCES/BIBLIOGRAPHY

Bonewit-West, K. (1995). *Clinical procedures for medical assistants* (4th ed.). Philadelphia: W. B. Saunders.

Frew, M. A., Lane, K., & Frew, D. (1995). *Comprehensive medical assisting: Competencies for administrative and clinical practice* (3rd ed.). Philadelphia: F. A. Davis.

Keir, L., Wise, B. A., & Krebs, C. (1998). *Medical assisting: Administrative and clinical competencies* (4th ed.). Albany, NY: Delmar.

Kinn, M. E., & Woods, M. A. (1999). *The medical assistant: Administrative and clinical* (8th ed.). Philadelphia: W. B. Saunders.

Prinkett-Ramutrowski, B., Barrie, A., Keller, C., Dazarow, L., & Abel, C. (1999). *Medical assisting: A patient-centered approach to administrative and clinical competencies*. New York: McGraw Hill.

Zakus, S. (1995). *Clinical procedures for medical assistants* (3rd ed.). St. Louis: Mosby LifeLine, Mosby-Year Book, Inc.

KEY TERMS

Afebrile
Apical
Apnea
Arrhythmia
Baseline
Bradycardia
Bradypnea
Cheyne-Stokes
Diastole
Dyspnea
Emphysema
Eupnea
Febrile
Frenulum
Hyperpnea
Hypertension
Hyperventilation
Hypotension
Hypoventilation
Orthopnea
Pyrexia
Rales
Rhonchi
Stertorous
Stridor
Systole
Tachycardia
Tachypnea
Wheezes

OUTLINE

The Importance of Accuracy
Temperature
    Terms Used to Describe Body
      Temperature
    Types of Thermometers
    Recording Temperature
    Measuring Temperature
    Cleaning and Storage of
      Thermometers
Pulse
    Pulse Sites
    Measuring a Pulse
    Normal Pulse Rates
    Pulse Abnormalities
    Recording Pulse Rates

Respiration
    Respiration Rate
    Abnormalities
Blood Pressure
    Equipment for Measuring Blood
      Pressure
    Measuring Blood Pressure
    Recording Blood Pressure
      Measurement
    Normal Blood Pressure Readings
    Blood Pressure Abnormalities
Height and Weight
    Height
    Weight
    Significance of Weight
Measuring Chest Circumference

OBJECTIVES

The student should strive to meet the following performance objectives and demonstrate an understanding of the facts and principles presented in this chapter through written and oral communication.

1. Define the key terms as presented in the glossary.

2. Discuss normal and abnormal temperatures, including factors affecting temperature.

3. Identify and explain the procedures for using, caring for, and storing of the various types of thermometers.

4. Describe the locations and procedure for obtaining pulse rate.

5. Explain the procedure for obtaining respiration rates.

6. Identify and describe normal and abnormal pulse and respiratory rates and the factors affecting each.

7. Describe the appropriate equipment and procedure for obtaining a blood pressure measurement. *(continues)*

8. Identify normal and abnormal blood pressure, including factors affecting blood pressure.

9. Describe the procedures for obtaining height, weight, and chest measurements of adults.

10. Accurately record measurements on the patient chart.

ROLE DELINEATION COMPONENTS

CLINICAL

Fundamental Principles

- Apply principles of aseptic technique and infection control
- Comply with quality assurance practices

Patient Care

- Obtain patient history and vital signs
- Prepare and maintain examination and treatment areas
- Prepare patient for examinations, procedures, and treatments
- Assist with examinations, procedures, and treatments

GENERAL (TRANSDISCIPLINARY)

Legal Concepts

- Document accurately

SCENARIO

At Doctors Lewis & King, clinical medical assistant Joe Guerrero, CMA, assists both physicians in taking patients' vital signs. One of his favorite patients is Abigail Johnson, a friendly woman in her seventies who always has a kind disposition despite her financial and medical difficulties. Abigail is overweight and suffers from hypertension, so her blood pressure is monitored on a regular basis to be certain that it is under control. In reviewing Abigail's chart, Joe notices that her blood pressure has been quite stable for the last few visits. He also checks her weight and notices that Abigail is slowly losing weight. Abigail's chart, with its history of blood pressure and other measurements, informs Joe's perspective and is a helpful record when evaluating the progress Abigail has made since she became a patient three years ago.

INTRODUCTION

One of the most important and commonly performed tasks of a medical assistant is obtaining and recording patient vital signs. Vital signs, also sometimes referred to as cardinal signs, include temperature, pulse, respiration, and blood pressure, abbreviated TPR B/P. They are indicative of the general health and well-being of a patient, and with regular monitoring, may measure patient response to treatment. Vital signs, in total or in part, are an important component of each patient visit. Height and weight measurements, while not considered vital signs are often a routine part of a patient visit.

Patients will exhibit vital sign readings that are uniquely their own. As a result, baseline assessments of vital signs are usually obtained during the patient's initial visit. These baseline results are used as a reference point for future readings, differentiating between what is normal and abnormal for the patient.

 Two extremely important habits must be developed by the medical assistant before taking a patient's vital signs: aseptic technique in the form of hand washing and recognition and correction of factors that may influence results of vital signs. Proper hand washing before taking vital signs will assist in preventing cross contamination of patients. Refer to the discussion on standard precautions and medical asepsis in Chapter 10. Also, emotional factors of patients must be recognized and addressed. Explaining procedures and allowing the patient the opportunity to relax will ease apprehension that may affect readings.

THE IMPORTANCE OF ACCURACY

Vital signs may be altered by many factors. Medical assistants must recognize and correct factors that may produce inaccurate results. For example, patients may exhibit anxiety over potential test results or findings of the physician. They may be angry or may have rushed into the office. A patient may have had something to eat or drink prior to the visit or may have had a long wait in the reception area. Patient apprehension and mood must always be considered by the medical assistant, for these factors can affect vital signs. The medical assistant may be required to take vital signs more than once during an office visit to ascertain a baseline and obtain an impression of overall well-being of the patient.

Accuracy in taking vital signs is necessary because treatment plans are developed according to the measurement of the vital signs. Variations can indicate a new disease process or the patient's response to treatment. They may also indicate the patient's compliance with a treatment plan. Although taking vital signs is a task commonly performed by the medical assistant, it is never to be taken casually or lightly, and should never be rushed or incompletely performed. Concentration and attention to proper procedure will help assure accurate measurements and quality care of the patient. The following text will discuss procedures used to measure the vital signs of children and adults. Procedures used for infant examinations will be discussed in Chapter 15.

TEMPERATURE

Body temperature is maintained and regulated by two processes functioning in conjunction with one another: heat production and heat loss.

Body heat is produced by the actions of voluntary and involuntary muscles. As the muscles move, they use energy which, in response, produces heat. Cellular metabolic activities such as the process of breaking food-sugars down to simpler components (catabolism), are another source of heat.

The body loses heat by a combination of five processes:

1. *Convection.* The process by which heat is lost through the skin by being transferred from the skin by air currents flowing across it; such as a fan used on a hot day for cooling purposes.
2. *Conduction.* The transfer of heat from within the body to the surface of the skin and then to surrounding cooler objects touching the skin, such as clothing.
3. *Radiation.* Body heat lost from the surface of the skin to a cooler environment, much like a cool room becoming warm when occupied by many people.
4. *Evaporation.* A heat loss mechanism that uses heat absorption through vaporization of perspiration.

5. *Elimination.* Heat that is lost through the normal functioning of the intestinal, urinary, and respiratory tracts.

The delicate balance between heat production and heat loss is maintained by the hypothalamus in the brain. The hypothalamus monitors blood temperature and will trigger either the heat loss or heat production mechanism with as little as 0.04°F change in blood temperature.

Body temperature is measured in degrees and is influenced by several factors.

● An increase of temperature may result from a bacterial infection, increased physical activity or food intake, exposure to heat, pregnancy, drugs that increase metabolism, stress and severe emotional reactions, and age. Age becomes a factor in that infants have an average body temperature that is one to two degrees higher than adults.

● Decrease in temperature may result from viral infections, decreased muscular activity, fasting, a depressed emotional state, exposure to cold, drugs that decrease metabolic activities, and age. Age in this instance refers to the elderly, in that the elderly have decreased metabolic activity resulting in a decrease in body temperature.

● Another factor that can increase or decrease body temperature is time of day. During sleep and early morning the temperature is at its lowest, while later in the day with muscular and metabolic activity the temperature increases.

Due to the many factors influencing body temperature and the uniqueness of individuals there is no "normal" temperature. The medical assistant must think of temperatures in terms of the "average," which for an adult is 98.6°F, or 37.0°C.

Terms Used to Describe Body Temperature

The following terms are used to describe body temperature:

- afebrile: absence of fever

- febrile: fever is present

- *fever:* body temperature elevated beyond normal range. Pyrexia is another term for fever.

- *onset:* time when fever begins

- *lysis:* body temperature gradually returns to normal following a period of fever

- *crisis:* body temperature drops suddenly to normal levels, the patient may perspire profusely (diaphoresis)

- *intermittent:* a fluctuating fever that returns to or below baseline, then rises again

- *remittent:* a fluctuating fever that does not return to the baseline temperature. It fluctuates, but remains elevated.

- *continuous:* a fever that remains above the baseline. It does not fluctuate, but remains fairly constant.

Figure 12-1 depicts types of fever.

Types of Thermometers

There are four types of thermometers available for use in the ambulatory care setting:

- mercury (or clinical)

- disposable

- digital

- tympanic

Mercury or Clinical Thermometers. These thermometers are made of glass with a bulb end containing mercury. As temperature increases, the mercury expands and rises in a column located within the thermometer. These have been used for many years. There are two types of mercury thermometers. One, commonly used in the United States, measures temperature in Fahrenheit (F) while the other measures in Celsius (C). There are charts

available that convert one scale to the other; however, the medical assistant can quickly and accurately calculate the conversion by using the following formulas:

To convert °F to °C = F temperature, subtract 32, then multiply by ⅝

To convert °C to °F = C temperature, multiply by ⅝, then add 32

Mercury thermometers are available in three styles: oral with a slender and elongated tip and blue color-coded end; rectal with a rounded tip and red color-coded end; and security for axillary measurement with a rounded tip with no color coding on the end. See Figure 12-2. Mercury thermometers are cleaned and disinfected with soap and cool water, rinsed, dried, and soaked in a disinfectant solution for at least thirty minutes. Oral and rectal thermometers are never placed in the same solution nor cleansed together as cross contamination with microorganisms from rectal to oral can occur.

 To prevent patient-to-patient cross contamination, a disposable plastic sheath is placed on all clinical thermometers when in use.

Disposable Thermometers. These are individually wrapped strips with heat-sensitive dots that change color to indicate temperature. They are used once and then discarded. There are strips for use on the forehead and others for oral use. Although strips are easy to use and prevent patient cross contamination, accuracy is questionable.

Digital Thermometers. These are widely used handheld battery-operated units that have easy-to-read digital display screens to indicate results (Figure 12-3). Digital thermometers are available in Fahrenheit or Celsius scales. Probes are attached and are color coded blue for oral, and red for rectal. The probes have disposable plastic covers. The plastic cover acts as a barrier to prevent contamination of the probe and is replaced for each patient to prevent cross contamination of the patient. An accurate result can be obtained in approximately ten seconds.

Tympanic Thermometers. The use of tympanic thermometers is becoming more popular as they are fast, provide no discomfort to the patient, can be used on infants as well as adults, and are usually accurate. They consist of a handheld unit with a probe tip that is inserted into the ear securely to make a seal. Disposable tips are used to prevent cross contamination. Accurate results are obtained in less than two seconds. With the tympanic method of measuring body temperature, the procedure is complete in a few seconds. It is comfortable for the

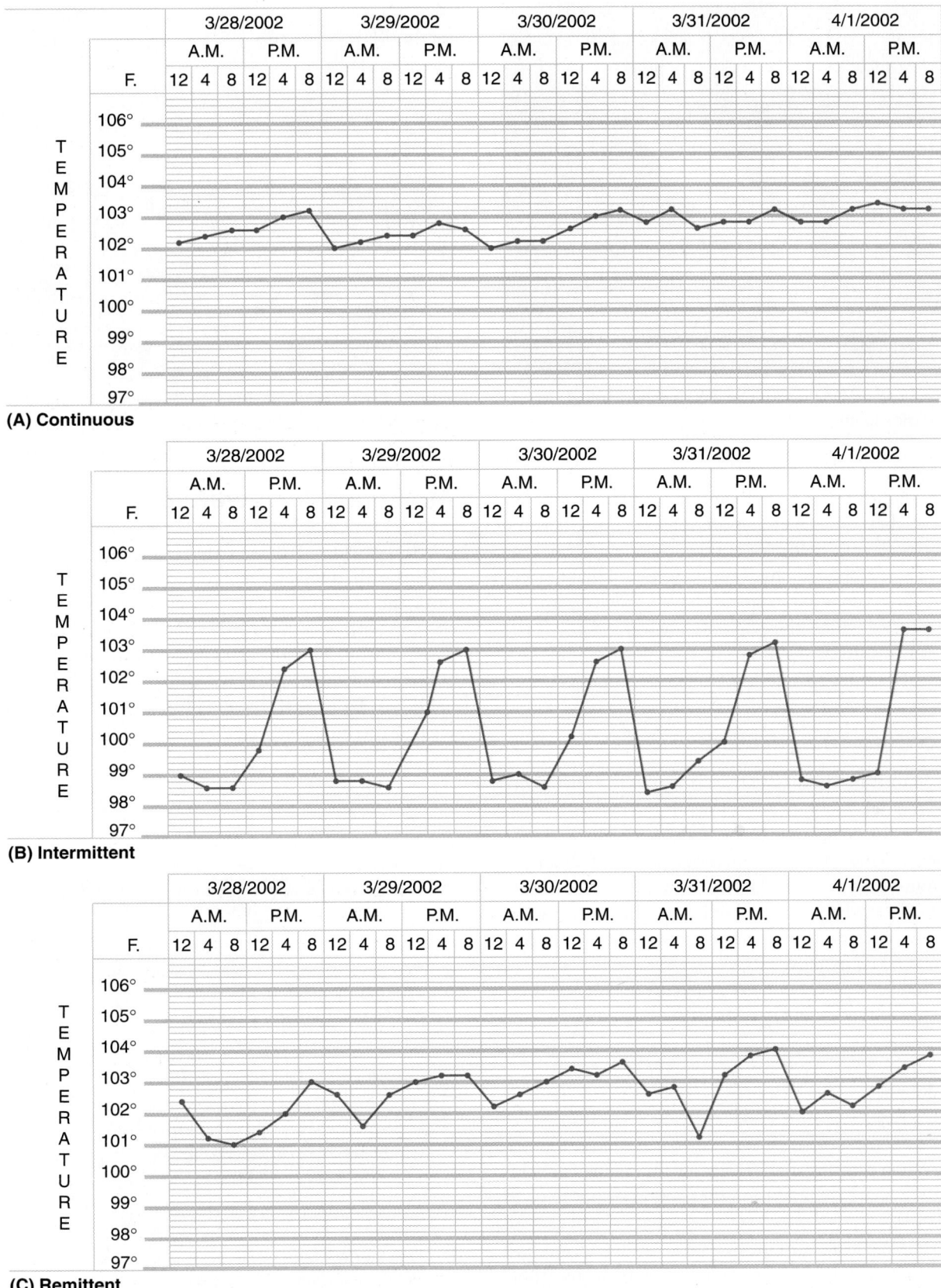

Figure 12-1 Types of Fevers. (A) Continuous—remains above baseline. Does not fluctuate. (B) Intermittent—a fluctuating fever. Returns to or below baseline, then rises again. (C) Remittent—a fluctuating fever, but does not return to baseline temperature. Remains elevated, but fluctuates.

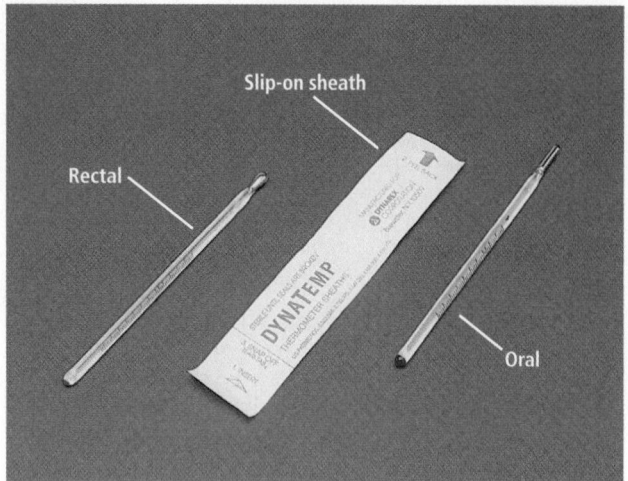

Figure 12-2 Mercury reusable thermometers with disposable plastic slip-on sheath.

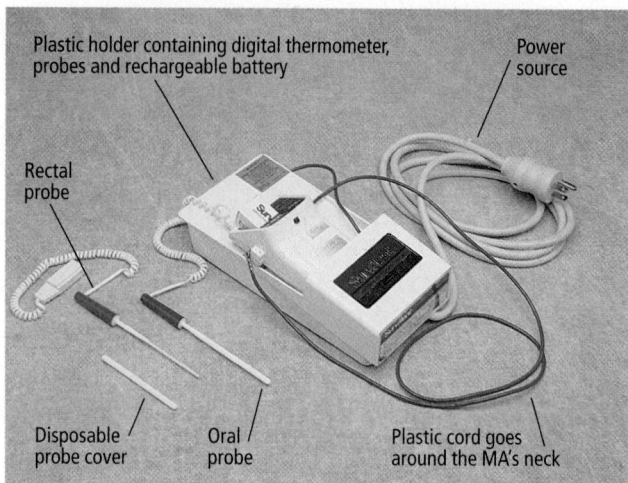

Figure 12-3 Digital thermometers have interchangeable oral and rectal probes attached to a battery-operated portable unit.

patient, nonthreatening to infants and children, and may be used when other methods are inappropriate. It is the thermometer of choice for pediatric patients over two years of age. However, physicians have found that inaccurate readings can result if patients have impacted cerumen in the ear of which they may be unaware. Also, if the patient has otitis media, a middle ear infection, the reading tends to be inaccurate.

Recording Temperature

Temperature may be taken on each visit to the physician's office in order to obtain a baseline for the patient. When recording the temperature, the scale used for the results must be designated (F) for Fahrenheit and (C) for Celsius. The route used must be labeled as well; methods other than oral must be labeled according to the route used as there is a difference in the measurement. Use (R) for rectal, and (A) for axillary.

Temperatures obtained by mercury and digital thermometers will be recorded as shown:

Oral   T 98.6°F
Rectal   T 99.6°(R) F
Axillary   T 97.6°(A) F

When a facility uses a tympanic thermometer exclusively, the route is known and therefore does not have to be labeled.

The medical assistant must read all manufacturer's instructions before using any digital or tympanic thermometer. Each may have a slight difference in operating procedure.

Procedures 12-1 through 12-7 detail steps involved in taking temperature by various routes.

Measuring Temperature

Oral Temperatures. To read a mercury thermometer, hold the thermometer at eye level and move it slightly until the mercury column can be seen. Note where the mercury is in relation to the numbers and lines on the thermometer. The longer lines on a Fahrenheit scale are calibrated by one full degree while the smaller lines are calibrated by two-tenths of a degree (Figure 12-4). On a Celsius thermometer, each long line represents a degree.

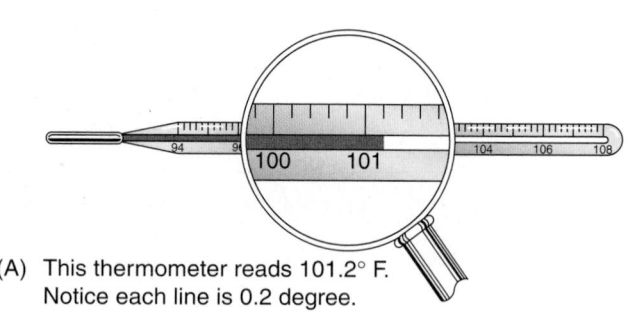

(A) This thermometer reads 101.2° F.
     Notice each line is 0.2 degree.

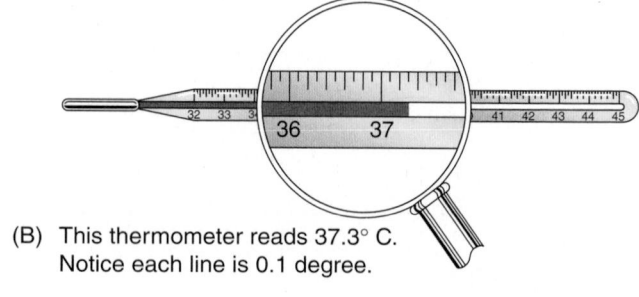

(B) This thermometer reads 37.3° C.
     Notice each line is 0.1 degree.

Figure 12-4 (A) Fahrenheit thermometer. (B) Celsius thermometer.

They are numbered consecutively, with nine lines between numbers, each line representing one-tenth of a degree. See Procedure 12-1 to take an oral temperature using a mercury thermometer.

To use an oral strip for taking a temperature, follow the same steps as with a mercury thermometer. Make certain that the package is not damaged then peel it back to reveal the strip. The strip is then inserted into the patient's mouth. After the appropriate time interval has elapsed, the thermometer is removed and the dots that have changed color are read using the scale located on the strip. While convenient to use, accuracy is not always assured with the strips and therefore they may not be appropriate for clinical use. See Procedure 12-2 to take an oral temperature using a disposable oral strip.

The procedure for obtaining an oral temperature with a digital thermometer (see Procedure 12-3) follows the same steps as when using a mercury thermometer. The digital thermometer is stored on a recharging base. When it is removed from the base, it is turned on and ready for use. A disposable cover is placed over the blue probe for oral temperatures. The probe is placed in the patient's mouth following the same procedures as used with a mercury thermometer. When the temperature has been obtained, the thermometer will beep at which time the temperature will be displayed on the screen. The probe cover is ejected into a biohazard container and the unit is returned to the base. The temperature is then recorded in the patient chart. Always read and follow the manufacturer's directions for use and care of a digital unit.

Aural Temperature.

Taking a temperature with a tympanic thermometer is a fast, safe method for obtaining a patient's temperature. This is becoming quite common in ambulatory care settings. Tympanic temperature can be obtained without discomfort for the patient whether elder, infant, or reluctant.

The tympanic thermometer measures the patient's temperature by measuring the infrared waves produced by the tympanic membrane and recording the temperature in less than two to three seconds on a digital screen. The tympanic membrane and the hypothalamus of the brain share the same blood supply, thus an accurate measurement of the body temperature can be obtained.

The greatest benefits of the tympanic thermometer are that it

- gives nearly instant results

- does not come into contact with mucous membranes, thereby minimizing cross contamination

- uses a site that is readily accessible

- is not affected by the patient smoking or drinking hot or cold liquids

- does not require that the patient be conscious

- is an easy instrument to use. The unit is battery operated and uses a disposable probe cover or ear speculum

Drawbacks to the tympanic thermometer have been demonstrated in pediatric patients with ear conditions such as otitis media. An inaccurate recording can result because the fluid buildup in the inner ear limits infrared wave transmission.

The tympanic thermometer is a handheld unit that is inserted into the outer third of the ear canal. See Procedure 12-4 to obtain an aural temperature using a tympanic thermometer.

Rectal Temperature.

The rectal method of obtaining a temperature is used on infants and young children and patients who are unable or incapable of cooperating with the oral method of temperature taking. Pediatric procedures are covered in Chapter 15. Patients experiencing breathing difficulties, such as an upper respiratory infection, asthma, or emphysema, or unable to follow instructions, as seen with senility, mental retardation, or Alzheimer's disease, will require a rectal temperature method. Rectal temperatures will have a reading that is approximately one degree higher than oral temperatures because the rectum is a closed body cavity. See Procedure 12-5 to measure a rectal temperature using a mercury thermometer.

See Procedure 12-6 for using a digital thermometer to measure the rectal temperature. The red probe is covered with a plastic cover and lubricated. Insert gently ½ inch for infants, 1 inch for a child, and 1½ inches for an adult. When the temperature registers, the thermometer will beep and provide a readout on the screen. The plastic cover is ejected into a biohazard container.

Axillary Temperature.

An axillary temperature may be used when the patient is an infant or for other reasons is unable to have an oral or rectal temperature taken. This method may be used for patients who display breathing difficulties or who are unable to follow directions as a result of mental incapacity. This is the least accurate method of obtaining a patient's temperature and should be used when other routes are unavailable or inappropriate. An axillary temperature is approximately one degree lower than an oral temperature because the axilla is an open body cavity.

Cleaning and Storage of Thermometers

Oral and rectal mercury thermometers must always be kept separated. Axillary security thermometers may be cleaned with the oral thermometers. The thermometer is rinsed immediately after use, then cleansed in a mild soap and cool water solution. Then the thermometer is dried and placed in a disinfectant solution, such as 70 percent isopropyl alcohol or solution of Zephiran Chloride for thirty minutes. Before storage or use, the thermometer must be rinsed and carefully dried. Storage will depend upon the policy of the facility. Containers used to store clean and uncleaned thermometers must be labeled to prevent possible improper use and cross contamination. Containers must be emptied and cleaned daily. New solution will be added according to the manufacturer's direction and at each cleaning.

Digital and tympanic thermometers are cleaned according to the manufacturer's directions. The covers protect the probes from contamination. Each type of thermometer will have a storage case or a wall-mounted base made specially for storing the unit. Disinfect these types of thermometers by wiping with a solution of 70 percent alcohol.

PULSE

The pulse rate consists of two phases of the heart action and can be felt when compressing an artery. As the heart contracts it increases pressure on the arterial walls. The increased pressure passes through the arteries in a wave-like movement resulting in a slight expansion in the arterial wall. When the heart relaxes, the pressure is decreased in the arteries, resulting in the wall returning to its previous position. One contraction and relaxation of the heart is equal to one heart cycle or heart beat. The pulse and heartbeat rate should be the same.

Pulse Sites

The pulse can be felt in those areas of the body where an artery is close to the surface and an underlying solid structure such as a bone. The common pulse sites include the radial, carotid, temporal, brachial, femoral, popliteal, and dorsalis pedis arteries (Figure 12-5). An apical pulse, located at the apex of the heart, may also be taken. Although the radial, brachial, and carotid arteries are the most frequently used sites for pulse rates, it is important to recognize pulse beats because circulation may be monitored by palpating the other sites. Pulse sites are also used when necessary as pressure points for controlling severe bleeding.

- The *radial* pulse is located at the thumb side of the wrist approximately one inch above the base of the thumb. This is the most commonly used site for obtaining a pulse rate.

- The *carotid* pulse, used during emergency situations and when performing CPR, is found between the larynx and sternocleidomastoid muscle in the front side of the neck on either side of the trachea.

- The *brachial* pulse is found in the inner aspect of the elbow called the antecubital space. This pulse site is the most commonly used site to obtain blood pressure measurements.

- The *temporal* pulse is located at the temple area of the head. It is rarely used to obtain a pulse rate but may be used to monitor circulation or control bleeding from the head and scalp.

- The *femoral* pulse is located in the groin area. It is a deep artery and must be compressed firmly to be felt.

- The *popliteal* pulse is located at the back of the knee. The patient must be in a supine position with the knee flexed for it to be felt as the artery is deep within the knee. This artery is the one used for leg blood pressure measurements and to monitor circulation.

- The *dorsalis pedis* pulse is felt on the top of the foot slightly to the side of midline next to the extensor ligament of the great toe, between the first and second metatarsal bones. It is commonly used to monitor lower limb circulation.

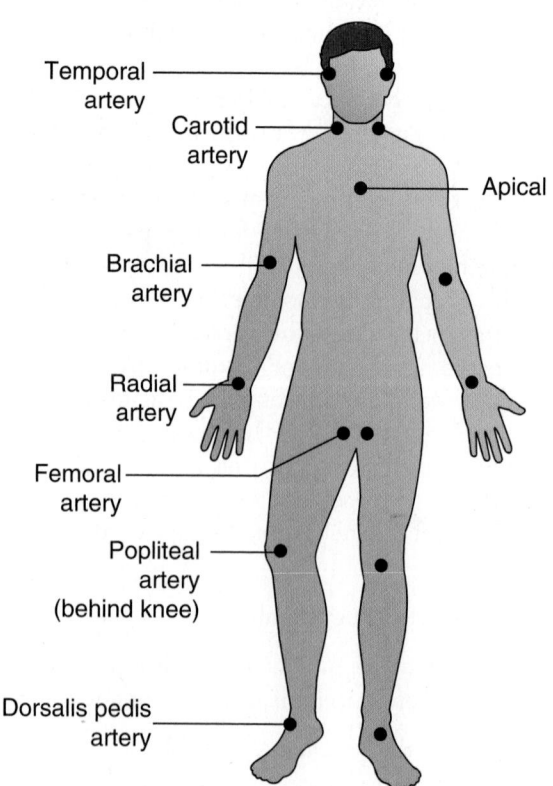

Temporal artery
Carotid artery
Apical
Brachial artery
Radial artery
Femoral artery
Popliteal artery (behind knee)
Dorsalis pedis artery

Figure 12-5   Pulse sites in the body.

● *Apical pulse* is found at the apex of the heart, located at the fifth intercostal space left side, mid-clavicular line. That is, between the fifth and sixth ribs in the middle of the clavicle (usually below the nipple), left of the sternum. A stethoscope is required to obtain an apical pulse. Apical pulse is used on cardiac patients and to obtain infant pulse rates as they are difficult to obtain by the usual methods.

Measuring a Pulse

When measuring a pulse rate, other characteristics besides the rate must also be noted. These characteristics include rhythm, volume of pulse, and condition of the arterial wall.

The rate is the number of pulsations or beats felt for one minute. Pulse rates may vary according to age, activities, general health, gender, emotions, pain, and medications. The rate is lower when sleeping and higher when active or exercising. Rates for infants and children are higher than for adults. Well-conditioned athletes will have a lower than average resting rate as their cardiovascular system has been developed to function more efficiently.

Rhythm of the pulse refers to the time between pulsations and regularity of the beat. Normal rhythm occurs when the beats are felt at regular intervals. Abnormal rhythms, arrhythmias, are those rhythms in which the interval between pulsations is altered by either an increased or decreased time span. Arrhythmias must be noted and reported as they may indicate heart disease.

The volume of the pulse refers to the strength of the beat that is felt. The pulsations may feel full, strong, hard, soft, thready, or weak. A pulse may have a regular rate and yet have a variation in intensity or volume. Volume should be noted and reported.

Condition of the arterial wall can be felt as the pulse is taken. The normal artery feels soft and elastic. The abnormal artery may feel hard, knotty, wiry, or a combination of these. These should be noted and reported as they may indicate cardiac disease.

Normal Pulse Rates

Average pulse rates vary from birth to adulthood. At birth the pulse rate is much higher; as we age it generally decreases. Average rate by age group:

Birth	130–160 beats per minute
Infants	110–130 beats per minute
Children (between 1 and 7 years)	80–120 beats per minute
Children over 7 years	80–90 beats per minute
Adults	60–80 beats per minute

Pulse Abnormalities

Abnormalities may be in the rate, rhythm, and feel of the arterial wall.

Common pulse rate abnormalities include bradycardia, a pulse rate less than 60 beats per minute, and tachycardia, a pulse rate greater than 100 beats per minute. Common arrhythmias would include a pulsation felt before expected, which is called a premature ventricular contraction or PVC, and sinus arrhythmia. An occasional premature contraction can occur in response to stress, caffeine, nicotine, alcohol, or lack of sleep. Sinus arrhythmia is a variation of rhythm during respiration and may be found in children and young adults. The rate increases with inspiration and decreases with expiration. This usually does not require treatment.

When any pulse rate abnormalities or arrhythmias are felt, they must be noted, recorded, and the physician alerted. See Chapter 25 for information on electrocardiography.

Recording Pulse Rates

Pulse rates are normally recorded after the temperature, for example: T 98.6° P 72 regular. Any unusual findings should be recorded and reported to the physician.

Procedure 12-8 describes measuring a radial pulse; Procedure 12-9 describes measuring an apical pulse.

RESPIRATION

The function of respiration (breathing) is the exchange of gases: oxygen and carbon dioxide. External respiration occurs when oxygen is drawn into the lungs and carbon dioxide is expelled from the lungs. Internal respiration occurs when oxygen is used by the cells for cellular function. Carbon dioxide is a byproduct of cellular function and is expelled as a waste product. Respiration is an involuntary act controlled by the medulla oblongata of the brain. The medulla oblongata measures blood levels of carbon dioxide and triggers a respiration when the level of carbon dioxide increases. Although it is an involuntary act, respiration may be altered by holding the breath or when hyperventilation occurs. One inspiration (inhalation) drawing in of air, and one expiration (exhalation) expelling air, equals one respiration.

Characteristics of respiration such as rate, rhythm, and depth are noted when measuring respiration.

Respiratory rate is the number of respirations per minute. The normal respiratory rate, eupnea, varies with age, activities, illness, emotions, and drugs. The normal respiration rate to pulse rate is 1:4, one respiration to four pulse beats.

Respiratory rhythm refers to the pattern of breathing. This can vary with age, with adults having a regular pattern while infants have an irregular pattern. Rhythm may be altered by laughing and sighing.

> ## Normal respiratory rates:
>
> | | |
> |---|---|
> | Infants | 30–60 respirations per minute |
> | Children (1–7 years) | 18–30 respirations per minute |
> | Adults | 12–20 respirations per minute |

Depth of respiration is the amount of air that is inspired and expired with each respiration. In the resting state, the amount should be consistent. Depth is noted by watching the degree of rise and fall of the chest wall when measuring respiration rate.

Respiration Rate

Procedure 12-10 describes steps involved in measuring respiration rate.

Abnormalities

Abnormalities of the respiration rate may be found in the rate, depth, rhythm, and sounds of respiration.

Rate abnormalities include apnea, tachypnea, bradypnea, and Cheyne-Stokes.

Apnea is the temporary complete absence of breathing. This may be a result of a reduction in stimuli to the respiratory center of the brain. Apnea will occur when the breath is voluntarily held and in Cheyne-Stokes respiration. It can be a serious symptom of other conditions of the cardiovascular and renal systems. It also can result from a head injury such as a concussion.

Tachypnea is a respiratory rate greater than 40 respirations per minute. It may be caused by hysteria or be transient in the newborn. Excessive loss of carbon dioxide may occur if tachypnea is prolonged; there is a potential for this to lead to more serious problems.

Bradypnea is a decrease in the number of respirations and is commonly seen during sleep or due to certain diseases.

Cheyne-Stokes is a regular pattern of irregular breathing rate. The cycle starts with a period of apnea lasting 10 to 60 seconds followed by increasing depth and rate of respiration, which is then followed by a decrease in rate with apnea starting the cycle once again. This cycle may be normal for children, but may indicate brain dysfunction.

Orthopnea is a respiratory condition of severe dyspnea (labored breathing). Breathing is difficult in any position *other* than sitting erect or standing. This may be seen in patients with heart failure, angina pectoris, asthma, pulmonary edema, emphysema, pneumonia, and spasmodic coughing. Patients who experience orthopnea must be examined in a sitting position. Other positions will cause discomfort and not be possible.

Abnormalities in the depth of respiration may be divided into shallow abnormalities, such as hypoventilation, and deep abnormalities, such as hyperpnea and hyperventilation.

Hypoventilation occurs when respiration is decreased in rate and shallow in depth, and may result from a depression of nervous stimuli of the respiratory center in the brain.

Hyperpnea is respiration that is increased both in depth and rate. This is commonly seen with activities such as physical exercise. It can also be associated with pain, respiratory diseases, cardiac diseases, hysteria, and some drugs.

Hyperventilation is a type of breathing in which the amounts of oxygen drawn in during inspiration are greatly increased; this results in a decrease in the amount of blood carbon dioxide. Hyperventilation may be associated with asthma, pulmonary embolism or edema, and acute anxiety. The patient may be treated by reducing the amount of oxygen inhaled during an inspiration. The patient may be instructed to hold one nostril closed while breathing or may be instructed to breathe into a paper bag. Either procedure will reduce the amount of inspired oxygen and bring the oxygen and carbon dioxide blood levels back to within normal range.

Breath Sounds. The presence or absence of breath sounds can be indicative of respiratory problems. Sounds should be listened for and noted when taking the patient's respiratory rate.

Rales and rhonchi are rattling sounds heard during inspiration and expiration when the lung passageways contain secretions. The physician uses a stethoscope to listen for rales, which are associated with some lung diseases. Rhonchi are sounds similar to snoring, usually produced by a rattle in the throat.

Wheezes are high-pitched musical sounds heard on expiration. They can be the result of an obstruction in the bronchi and bronchioles of the lungs. Wheezes are commonly associated with asthma and emphysema, a chronic pulmonary disease characterized by dilated and damaged alveoli.

Stridor is a crowing sound heard on inspiration as a result of an obstruction of the upper airway. It is associated with laryngitis, a foreign body obstruction, and croup in children.

Stertorous respiration is described as a snoring sound with labored breathing. The sound is created by obstruction of air passages in the head.

BLOOD PRESSURE

Blood pressure measures cardiovascular function by measuring the force of blood exerted on peripheral arteries during the cardiac cycle or heartbeat. The measurement consists of two components. The first is the force exerted on the arterial walls during cardiac contraction and is called systole. The second is the force exerted during cardiac relaxation and is called diastole. They represent the highest (systole) and lowest (diastole) amount of pressure exerted during the cardiac cycle. Blood pressure is recorded as a fraction with the systolic measurement written, followed by a slash, and then the diastolic measurement.

Example: systole/diastole or 120/80

Blood pressure may be affected by many factors including blood volume, peripheral resistance, vessel elasticity, condition of the muscle of the heart, genetics, diet and weight, activity, and emotional state.

- Blood volume is the amount of blood in the arteries. Increased volume increases blood pressure, while a decrease in volume will decrease blood pressure as in the case of a hemorrhage.

- Peripheral resistance is the resistance to blood flow in the arteries. The resistance is in direct relationship to the lumen of the arteries. The smaller the lumen, the more pressure needed to push blood through, while the reverse is true: the larger the lumen, the less resistance and less pressure needed to push the blood through. The size of the lumen can become smaller from deposits of fatty cholesterol, resulting in an increase in blood pressure.

- Vessel elasticity refers to the ability of arteries to expand and contract to provide a steady flow of blood. As a person ages, elasticity of the vessels is reduced. It can cause an increase in arterial wall resistance resulting in an increase in blood pressure.

- The condition of the heart muscle is extremely important to blood flow and blood pressure. A strong heart muscle provides a forceful pump resulting in efficient blood flow and normal blood pressure. A weak heart muscle results in an inefficient pumping action of the heart leading to a decrease in blood pressure and blood flow. See Chapter 25, Electrocardiography.

Equipment for Measuring Blood Pressure

Blood pressure is measured by the auscultatory (listening) method using a sphygmomanometer and a stethoscope (Figure 12-6). There are two types of sphygmomanometers commonly used in the ambulatory care setting: mercury manometer and aneroid manometer (Figures 12-7 and 12-8).

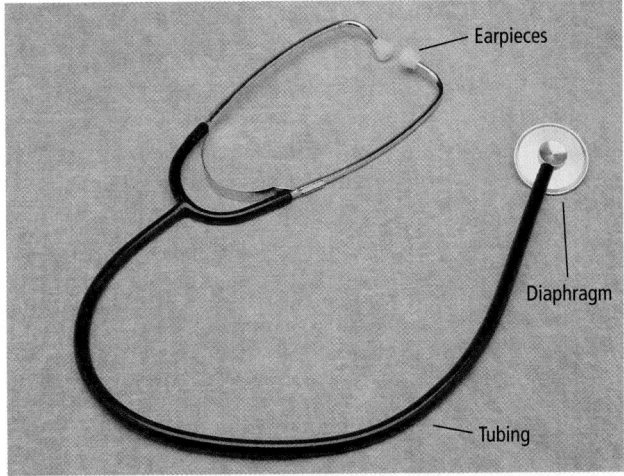

Figure 12-6 A single-head stethoscope. Used with a sphygmomanometer to measure blood pressure.

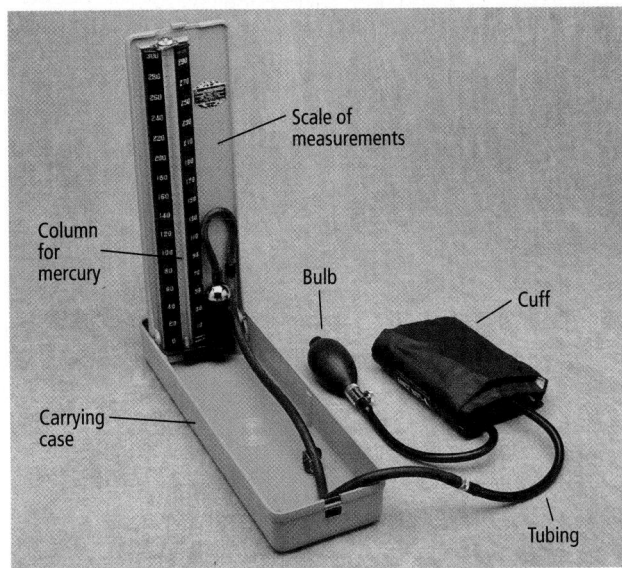

Figure 12-7 Mercury sphygmomanometer with cuff.

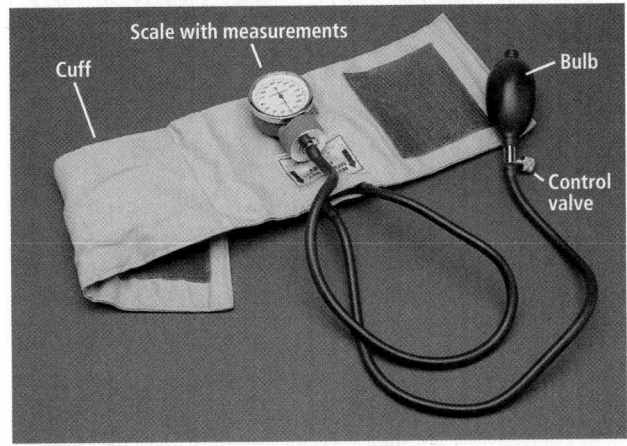

Figure 12-8 Aneroid sphygmomanometer.

The mercury manometer consists of a cuff containing a rubber bladder attached by rubber tubing to a glass column of mercury. The blood pressure is read at the meniscus of the mercury as it descends the column. Mercury manometers are the most accurate method of blood pressure measurement and are considered the standard as blood pressure is measured in millimeters of mercury. Although the most accurate, mercury manometers do have disadvantages: they are not as portable as aneroid manometers, and there is always the danger of a mercury spill should the glass column break. Mercury manometers need to be cleaned and checked regularly for accuracy by a professional technician. Care in handling and storage is important to prevent air bubbles and dirt from forming in the column or breaking the glass containing the mercury.

The aneroid manometer is a cuff containing a rubber bladder attached to a dial. The blood pressure is read at the level of the needle descending the dial. Aneroid manometers need to be calibrated regularly as they do not maintain calibration easily. Care in handling and storage will decrease the loss of calibration. While not as accurate as a mercury manometer, aneroid manometers are easily portable and there is no danger of a mercury spill.

Cuff sizes in both mercury and aneroid manometers range from the smallest cuff to the largest obese and thigh cuff (Figure 12-9). The appropriate cuff size is necessary in order to obtain an accurate blood pressure measurement. A cuff that is too small will give an artificially high blood pressure reading, while a cuff that is too large will give an artificially low reading. The selection of the cuff size depends upon the size of the arm, not the age of the patient. Due to the size of the arm, it may be necessary to use an adult-size cuff on a child or a pediatric-size cuff on an adult. Adult cuffs should have a width that covers one-third to one-half the circumference of the arm. The

length of the bladder should cover approximately 80 percent of the arm (about twice the size of the width). The cuff for a child should cover two-thirds of the upper arm.

Measuring Blood Pressure

The sounds heard during blood pressure measurement are named the Korotkoff sounds. The cause of the sounds is not known. They may be a result of distention of the vessels or the sound of the blood passing through the vessels. In either case, Korotkoff sounds have five distinct phases.

- *Phase I.* Begins with the first sound heard when deflating the cuff. It is a sharp tapping sound. Note this first sound as this will be the *systolic reading* of the blood pressure.

- *Phase II.* This sound is the result of more blood passing through the vessels as the cuff is deflated. The sound is that of a soft swishing sound.

- *Phase III.* More blood continues to pass through the vessels as the cuff is deflated. The sound is a rhythmic tapping sound. If blood pressure measurements are not carefully followed and Phases I and II are missed, Phase III may erroneously be reported as the systolic pressure.

- *Phase IV.* Blood is now passing through the vessels fairly easily as the cuff is deflated. The sounds heard will be a muffling and fading of the tapping sounds. This phase may be used to record the diastolic pressure in children and in those patients where a tapping sound is heard to zero.

- *Phase V.* Blood is flowing freely at this time, consequently all sounds disappear. The disappearance of sounds is noted and recorded as the *diastolic pressure*.

The procedure for taking blood pressure is a two-step method called the palpatory method. Step one of the method establishes the peak inflation level and is performed by placing the cuff on the patient's arm, palpating the radial pulse, and with a smooth pumping action inflating the cuff until the radial pulse can no longer be felt. The number where the radial pulse disappears is noted. The cuff is then deflated and the arm allowed to rest for a minute or two. The peak inflation level is then calculated by taking that number and adding 30 millimeters to it. This gives an indication as to the level to which to inflate the cuff when ausculating or listening to the sounds for the systolic and diastolic measurements. The purpose of this method is twofold: (1) patient comfort is assured as the cuff is not unnecessarily overinflated; (2) this procedure eliminates the possibility of missing an auscultatory gap. Auscultatory gap is heard in some patients. It is a time, usually between Phase I and II or III,

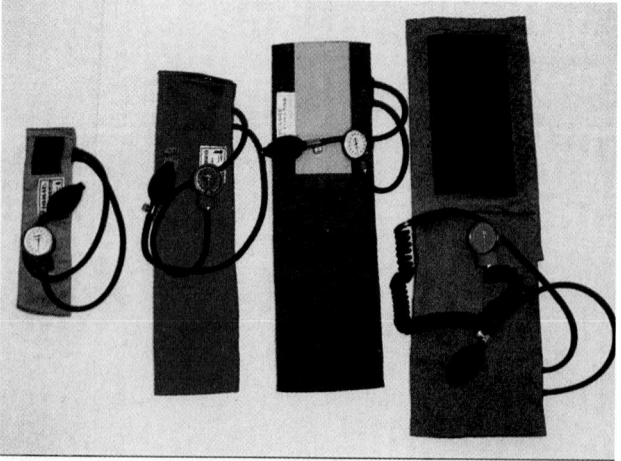

Figure 12-9 Blood pressure cuffs in sizes to fit the arm of a small child to an adult thigh. It is important to have the correct size to obtain an accurate reading.

when all sounds disappear. Within 20 to 30 millimeters, the sounds reappear. If the procedures are not followed carefully, the auscultatory gap is missed and the blood pressure measurement is incorrect in that systolic and diastolic readings may be in error according to the length of the gap. See Table 12-1.

Pulse pressure is the difference between the systolic and diastolic measurements. The normal range for pulse pressure is 30 to 50 mm. The difference should be no more than one-third of the systolic reading.

Recording Blood Pressure Measurement

The blood pressure is recorded on the patient chart in a fraction format. The position of the patient (sitting or lying down) may be noted. The arm used is also noted, particularly if the blood pressure has been taken in both arms.

Example: 120/80, rt. arm, supine

For children and those patients whose blood pressure can still be heard to zero, the beginning of Korotkoff Phase IV and zero are both recorded.

Example: 120/70/0

Procedure 12-11 outlines the procedure for measuring blood pressure.

Normal Blood Pressure Readings

Normal blood pressure is low at birth and gradually increases with age until adulthood, at which point it should remain fairly constant.

Newborn	50–52/25–30
Child 6 years	95/62
Child 10 years	100/65
Adolescent 16 years	118/75
Adult	Systolic below 140
	Diastolic below 89

Blood Pressure Abnormalities

There are only two possible blood pressure abnormalities: hypertension, blood pressure that is consistently above normal; and hypotension, blood pressure that is consistently below normal in which the patient is unable to function.

Hypertension. There are four types of hypertension: primary or essential, secondary, benign, and malignant.

TABLE 12-1	**ERRORS IN BLOOD PRESSURE MEASUREMENT PROCEDURES**

Errors in measuring blood pressure must be avoided. Common errors include:

1. Improper cuff size.
2. The arm is not at heart level. Do not hold the arm up or let the patient hold up the arm. Pressure is altered when this is done.
3. Cuff is not completely deflated before use or after palpatory method, resulting in a higher pressure measurement.
4. Deflation of the cuff is faster than 2 to 4 millimeters per second. Sounds are missed if this happens.
5. Reinflating the cuff during the procedure without allowing the arm to rest for 1 to 2 minutes.
6. Patient is not relaxed and comfortable. An anxious, apprehensive patient will have a reading that is higher than the actual blood pressure.
7. Improper cuff placement. Cuff is too loose, too tight, or not positioned correctly over the brachial artery.
8. Defective equipment in which there are air leaks in the bladder or valve, the mercury column is dirty, or air bubbles are present. Mercury and aneroid sphygmomanometers are not calibrated at zero.

All of these errors are easily corrected by following careful procedure and by having the manometers calibrated and/or cleaned according to a regular maintenance schedule.

● The most commonly seen form of hypertension is primary or essential. It is hypertension with no apparent cause or cure, but is treatable. Treatment is designed to control hypertension and is a lifelong process. It will not be cured, just controlled.

● Secondary hypertension is the result of some underlying problem such as renal disease, pregnancy, endocrine imbalances, obesity, arteriosclerosis, or atherosclerosis. Once the underlying problem has been removed, the blood pressure returns to normal. Secondary hypertension can be successfully treated.

● Hypertension that has a slow progression but may progress to the same endpoint as in malignant hypertension, is referred to as benign hypertension.

● Malignant hypertension progresses rapidly with severe damage to the cardiovascular system, possibly to the point of death.

Hypotension. Hypotension is blood pressure persistently below normal, usually below 90/60, although this may be normal for some healthy adults. Hypotension is defined as a blood pressure so low that the patient is unable to function normally. It is usually a result of various shock-like conditions such as hemorrhage, traumatic or emotional shock, central nervous system disorders, or chronic wasting diseases. With treatment for the underlying problems, the blood pressure usually will be in the range of normal readings.

Orthostatic hypotension occurs when a person rapidly changes position from supine to standing, when standing in one position for too long, or as a side effect of certain medications. In this instance, the blood pressure has momentarily dropped and the person will experience vertigo and may have blurred vision. These symptoms usually last only a few seconds, just long enough for the blood pressure to return to normal. Care should be taken when helping patients to an upright position from a supine position as orthostatic hypotension can lead to syncope and injury from falling.

HEIGHT AND WEIGHT

Although not considered a vital sign, height and weight are routinely measured if warranted by the age and the physical condition of the patient. Many physicians prefer that height and weight be measured as part of a yearly physical examination and otherwise may vary the frequency of patient height and weight measurements. Height and weight are normally measured simultaneously.

For children, height and weight are typically measured during each physician visit. The height of adults may be obtained on the initial visit only and weight taken on all visits. An adolescent or young adult may have height measured more frequently in order to plot body changes. Because elderly patients tend to lose the cushioning between vertebrae as part of aging, they may need to have their height measured more frequently to check the stage of any degeneration.

 Elderly patients require special attention by the medical assistant when measuring height and weight. It is especially important to assist elderly patients both on and off the scale, for the scale platform is movable and elderly patients may lose their balance and fall if unassisted.

Height

To measure a patient's height, a scale with a measuring bar is necessary (Figure 12-10). A paper towel is placed on the scale as the patient's shoes should be removed for accurate measuring. The patient is asked to step on the scale and face away from the measuring bar. Assist patient onto the scale; the scale platform is movable and the patient could fall.

There are two reasons for having the patient's back to the scale. When the measuring bar is lifted, it could cause face or eye injuries if the patient were facing the

bar. Lifting the measuring bar prior to the patient stepping on the scale can also lead to eye and face injuries in that the patient could inadvertently walk into the bar. Another reason to have the patient's back to the scale is if the patient does not look straight ahead, the head is not level, which could result in a less than accurate measurement.

After the patient is on the platform, the measuring bar is placed firmly on the patient's head and the line between where the solid bar and sliding bar meet is read. The bars are measured in quarter inches (Figure 12-11). Children's heights may be recorded in inches, while adults will be recorded in feet and inches. Conversion from inches to feet is accomplished by taking the number of inches and dividing by twelve.

See Procedure 12-12 to measure height.

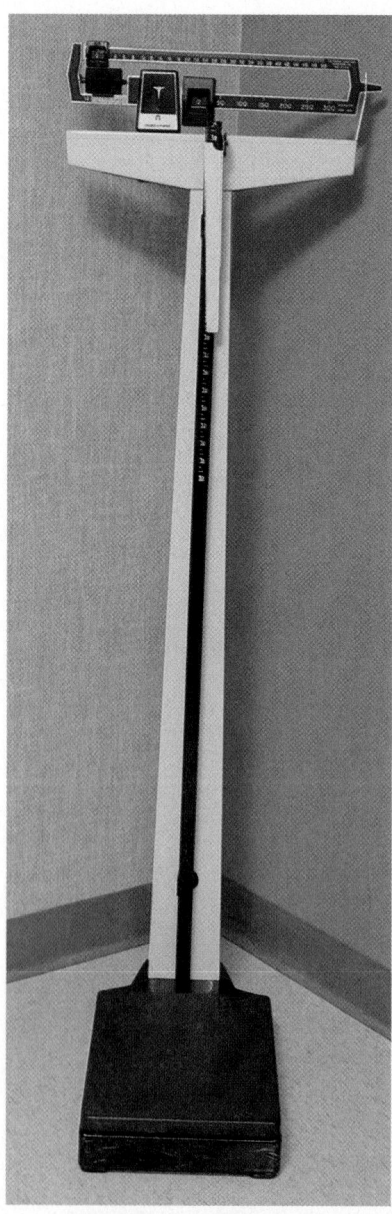

Figure 12-10
Traditional beam balance scale with measuring bar.

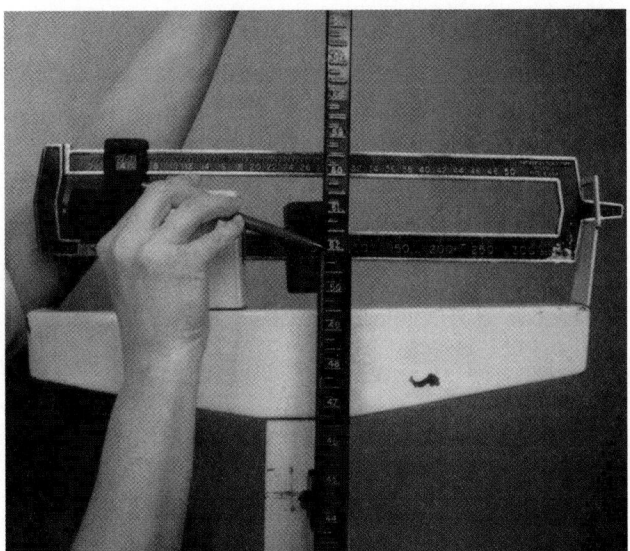

Figure 12-11 Read the height at the movable point of the ruler. The bars are measured in quarter inches.

Weight

Physician preference and patient health will dictate the frequency of measuring an adult's weight. Some physicians require the patient's weight measured on each visit while others do not if there are no health problems that require weight monitoring. Some health conditions that do require weight monitoring include obesity, eating disorders, hormone disorders such as diabetes and thyroid malfunction, hypertension, pregnancy, cancer, and some digestive disorders.

When measuring the weight of a patient, the medical assistant must maintain the patient's privacy. Most people are very conscious of their weight and may become embarrassed if the measurement is taken where others may see and hear. Privacy is important and often overlooked. The medical assistant must also be careful of comments regarding a patient's weight particularly with the obese patient and with those being treated for eating disorders. Encouragement for weight loss for the dieting patient is beneficial but must be done in privacy. Other comments are inappropriate.

Occasionally a patient will be instructed by the physician to monitor weight at home. It is important for the patient to understand the necessity of weighing at the same time each day as weight may vary significantly throughout the day. A normal routine is to measure weight before breakfast.

Before an accurate weight can be obtained, the scale must be calibrated. The point of the balance beam must be floating in the center when no weight is applied to the scale. Some scales are equipped with a screw at the end that can be turned slightly until the beam is in the correct floating position. Once it is centered, it is calibrated and ready for use.

The patient will wear normal indoor clothing, rather than disrobing, for weight measurement. Heavy coats or other outerwear should be removed. Heavy objects and purses should not be held during the procedure. A chair or counter should be provided to place these objects on while the procedure is being performed. Shoes should be removed.

See Procedure 12-13 for measuring adult weight.

Occasionally, as in the case of medication dosage, the medical assistant may be required to convert pound weight into kilogram weight.

1 kilogram = 2.2 pounds
To convert pounds to kilograms:
Take the number of pounds and divide by 2.2
Example: 130 pounds divided by 2.2 = 59.09 kg
To convert from kilograms to pounds:
Take the number of kilograms and multiply by 2.2
Example: 40 kilograms multiplied by 2.2 = 88 lb.

Significance of Weight

The careful monitoring of a patient's weight may provide an insight into metabolic, nutritional, and emotional problems.

MEASURING CHEST CIRCUMFERENCE

Occasionally, the medical assistant may be instructed to measure the chest of an adult. This procedure is done on patients with emphysema and as a requirement for insurance and truck driver licenses. Two measurements will be taken, one on the deepest inspiration and one on the deepest expiration. A comparison is then made to ascertain chest capacity. To perform the procedure, ask the patient to disrobe from the waist up. Place a tape measure around the chest at nipple level. Instruct the patient to inhale deeply while you measure, then ask the patient to exhale completely while you take the second measurement. Record the results as inspiration number and expiration number. The physician performs any necessary comparison.

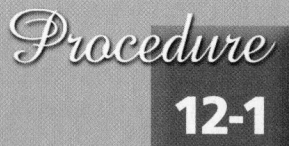

Measuring an Oral Temperature Using a Mercury Thermometer

Procedure 12-1

STANDARD PRECAUTIONS:

PURPOSE:
To obtain an oral temperature.

EQUIPMENT/SUPPLIES:
Thermometer
Disposable thermometer sheaths
Gloves
Paper towels
Biohazard waste container

PROCEDURE STEPS:

1. Wash hands and follow standard precautions.
2. Assemble equipment.
3. Identify patient.
4. Position the patient in a comfortable position.
5. Determine if the patient has ingested hot or cold drinks or food or has been smoking within the previous half hour. RATIONALE: Ingesting hot or cold substances or smoking can result in an arbitrary increase or decrease in temperature results.
6. Explain the procedure. RATIONALE: To obtain patient cooperation and consent.
7. Shake the thermometer with a quick flip of the wrist until it reads below 96.0°F. RATIONALE:

To obtain an accurate result, the mercury must be below 96.0°F.

8. Cover thermometer with the sheath (Figure 12-12). RATIONALE: To prevent microorganism cross contamination.
9. Apply gloves.
10. Insert thermometer under the tongue to the side of the mouth. RATIONALE: Under the center of the tongue is the frenulum which impedes placement in this area.
11. Instruct patient to close mouth without placing teeth on thermometer (Figure 12-13). RATIONALE: To prevent air leakage and to avoid patient biting on thermometer.
12. Leave in place for 3 to 5 minutes.
13. Remove thermometer after appropriate time has elapsed.
14. Remove and discard sheath in biohazard waste container (Figure 12-14).
15. Holding the thermometer at eye level, read the thermometer (Figure 12-15).
16. Wash thermometer in cool water using friction, rinse, and dry. Place on clean paper towel.
17. Remove gloves and discard in biohazard waste container.
18. Wash hands.
19. Document on patient record.

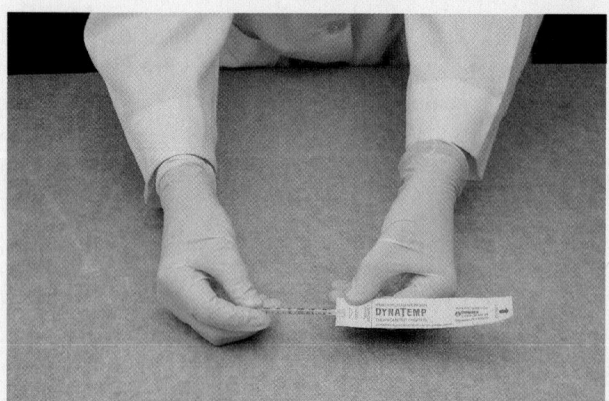

Figure 12-12 Cover the mercury thermometer with the disposable sheath.

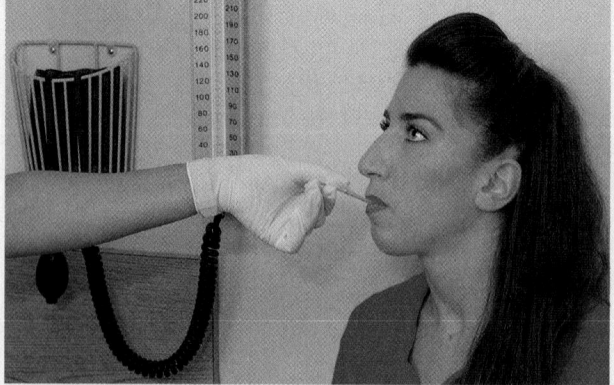

Figure 12-13 Place mercury oral thermometer sublingually (to the side of the mouth) in a heat pocket and ask patient to close mouth without placing teeth on thermometer.

(continues)

Procedure 12-1 (continued)

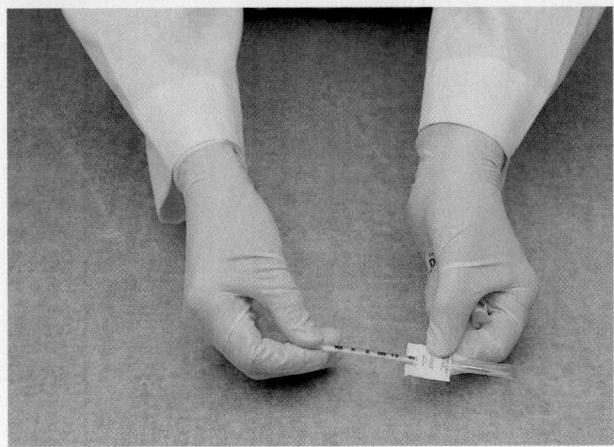

Figure 12-14 Remove the plastic sheath and discard in biohazard container before reading the thermometer.

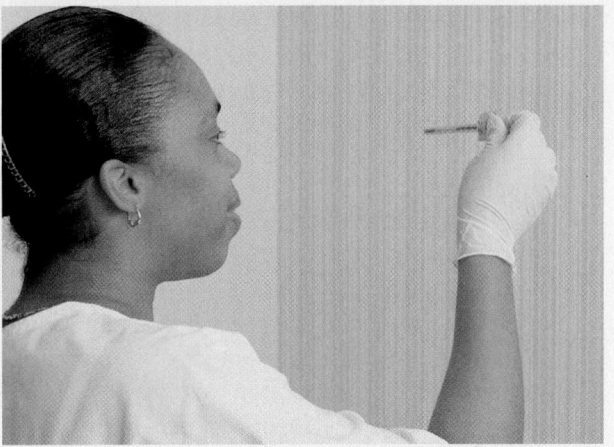

Figure 12-15 Rotate the stem slightly back and forth until you can see the silver mercury column in the middle. The point where the mercury stops is the reading to record.

Procedure 12-2 Measuring an Oral Temperature Using a Disposable Oral Strip Thermometer

STANDARD PRECAUTIONS:

PURPOSE:
To obtain an oral temperature.

EQUIPMENT/SUPPLIES:
Oral strip thermometer (Figure 12-16)
Gloves
Biohazard waste container

PROCEDURE STEPS:
1. Wash hands and follow standard precautions.
2. Assemble equipment.
3. Identify patient.
4. Position the patient in a comfortable position.
5. Determine if the patient has ingested hot or cold drinks or food or has been smoking within the

(*continues*)

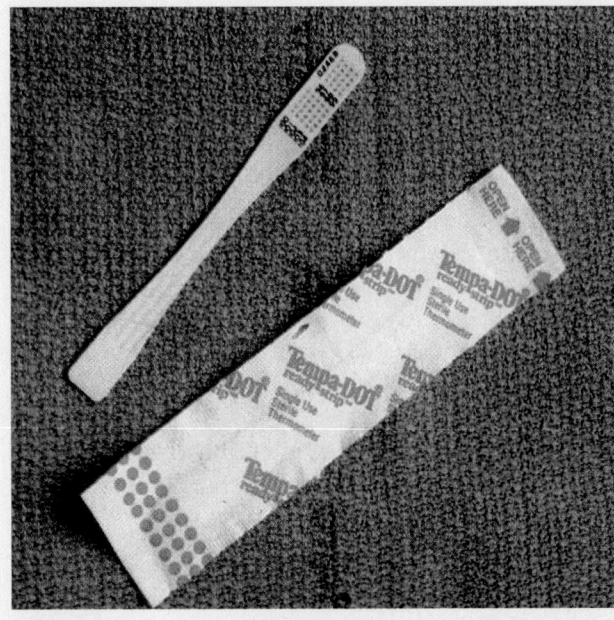

Figure 12-16 Disposable oral strip thermometer.

Procedure 12-2 *(continued)*

previous half hour. RATIONALE: Ingesting hot or cold substance or smoking can result in an arbitrary increase or decrease in temperature results.

6. Explain the procedure. RATIONALE: To obtain patient cooperation and consent.
7. Apply gloves.
8. Insert disposable oral strip thermometer under the tongue to the side of the mouth. RATIONALE: Under the center of the tongue is the frenulum, the fold of mucus membrane that attaches the tongue to the floor of the mouth, which impedes placement in this area.
9. Instruct patient to close mouth tightly. RATIONALE: To prevent air leakage.
10. Leave in place for 60 seconds.
11. Remove thermometer after appropriate time has elapsed.
12. Wait 10 seconds to read the dots.
13. Read temperature by locating the last dot that has changed color (Figure 12-17).
14. Discard strip in biohazard waste container.
15. Remove gloves and discard in biohazard waste container.
16. Wash hands.
17. Record temperature.
18. Document the procedure.

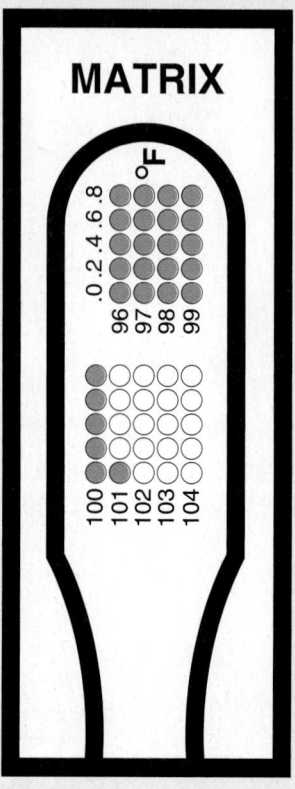

Figure 12-17 The reading on this disposable oral thermometer is 101°F.

Procedure 12-3 **Measuring an Oral Temperature Using a Digital Thermometer**

STANDARD PRECAUTIONS:

PURPOSE:
To obtain an oral temperature.

EQUIPMENT/SUPPLIES:
Digital thermometer
Probe covers
Biohazard waste container

PROCEDURE STEPS:
1. Wash hands and follow standard precautions.
2. Assemble equipment.
3. Identify patient.
4. Position the patient in a comfortable position.
5. Determine if the patient has ingested hot or cold drinks or food or has been smoking within the previous half hour. RATIONALE: Ingesting hot or cold substance or smoking can result in an arbitrary increase or decrease in temperature results.

(continues)

Procedure

12-3   (*continued*)

6. Explain the procedure. RATIONALE: To obtain patient cooperation and consent.
7. Select blue (oral) probe.
8. Cover with probe cover (Figure 12-18). RATIONALE: To prevent microorganism cross contamination.

9. Insert under the tongue to either side of the mouth (Figure 12-19). RATIONALE: Under the center of the tongue is the frenulum which impedes placement in this area.
10. Instruct patient to close mouth without placing teeth on thermometer. RATIONALE: To prevent air leakage.
11. Leave in place until the beep is heard.
12. Remove thermometer after appropriate time has elapsed.
13. Read the results on the digital display window.
14. Discard probe cover in biohazard waste container (Figure 12-20).
15. Replace digital thermometer in the base holder.
16. Wash hands.
17. Record temperature.
18. Document the procedure.

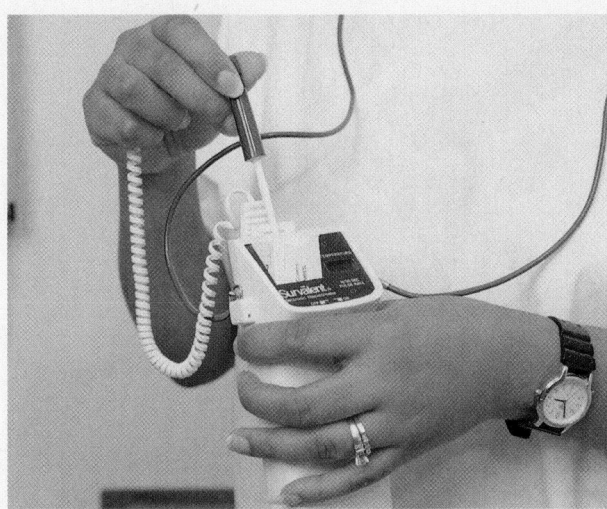

Figure 12-18   Slide the probe into the disposable cover, adjusting if necessary.

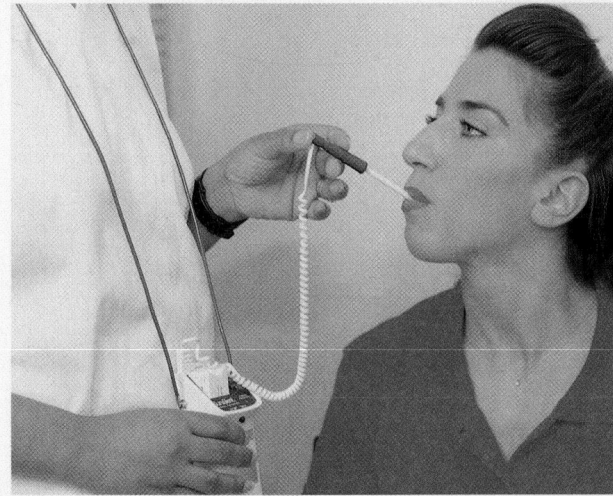

Figure 12-19   Insert the thermometer under tongue to either side of mouth.

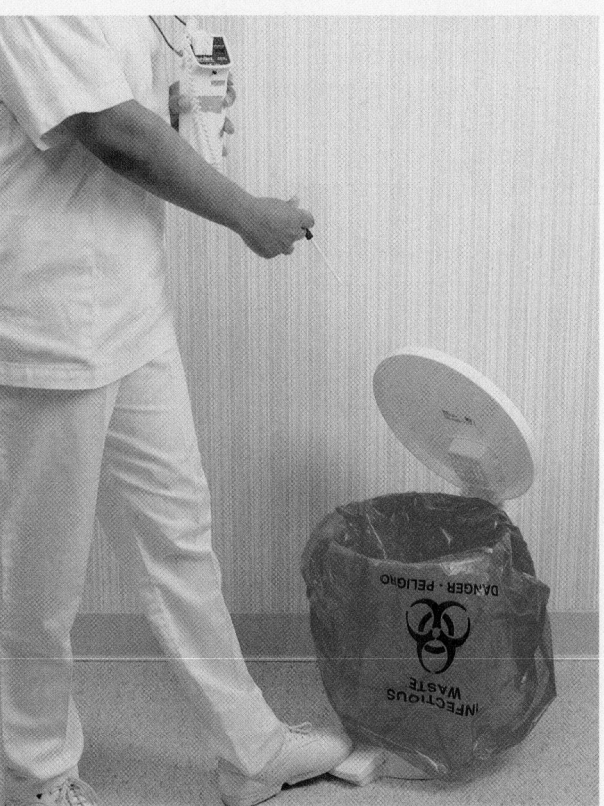

Figure 12-20   Discard probe cover in biohazard waste container.

Procedure 12-4

Measuring an Aural Temperature Using a Tympanic Thermometer

STANDARD PRECAUTIONS:

PURPOSE:

To obtain an aural temperature using a tympanic thermometer.

EQUIPMENT/SUPPLIES:

Tympanic thermometer (Figure 12-21)
Covers or ear speculum
Waste container

PROCEDURE STEPS:

1. Wash hands following standard precautions.
2. Assemble equipment.
3. Identify the patient.
4. Explain procedure. RATIONALE: This will help gain patient's cooperation and consent.
5. Place cover on thermometer (Figure 12-22).
6. Set thermometer to start.
7. Gently place probe into ear canal to seal the area and activate the system (Figure 12-23). RATIONALE: Air leaks will occur if the ear canal is not sealed.
8. Wait until the temperature is displayed on the screen.
9. Remove from the ear.
10. Discard cover into waste container by pressing the release button.
11. Wash hands.
12. Replace thermometer.
13. Record temperature in patient chart.

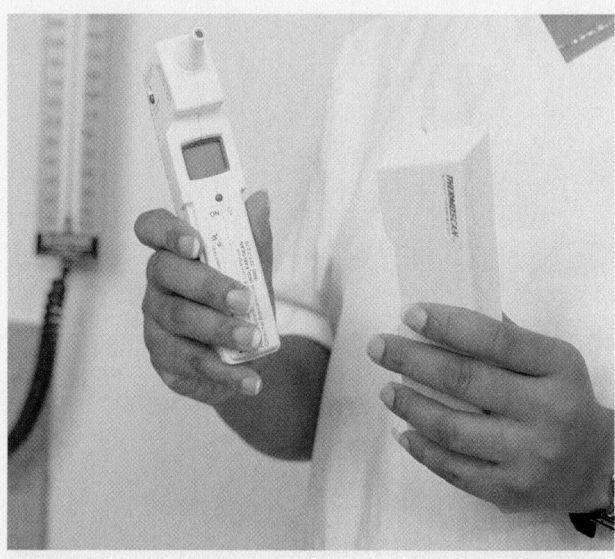

Figure 12-22   Attach the disposable speculum or cover to the tympanic thermometer to prevent spread of microorganisms between patients.

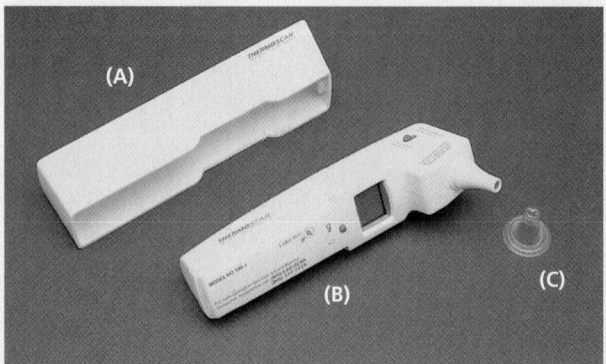

Figure 12-21   Tympanic thermometer: (A) holder, (B) tympanic thermometer, and (C) disposable speculum or cover.

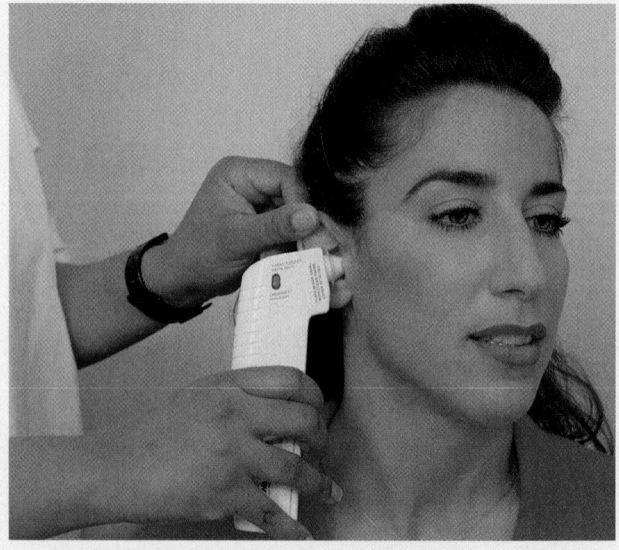

Figure 12-23   Pull up on the ear to straighten the auditory canal for an accurate reading.

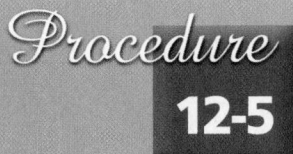

Procedure 12-5

Measuring a Rectal Temperature Using a Mercury Thermometer

STANDARD PRECAUTIONS:

PURPOSE:
To obtain a rectal temperature using a mercury thermometer.

EQUIPMENT/SUPPLIES:
Rectal thermometer (red tip)
Sheath
Lubricating jelly
Gloves
Clean paper towels
Biohazard waste container

PROCEDURE STEPS:
1. Wash hands, following standard precautions.
2. Assemble equipment.
3. Identify patient.
4. Explain procedure to patient. RATIONALE: Ensures understanding and gains patient cooperation and consent.
5. Remove clothing from the waist down, drape as necessary. RATIONALE: Maintains patient modesty, privacy, and warmth.
6. Position patient in Sims' position.
7. Place sheath on thermometer. RATIONALE: To prevent microorganism cross contamination.

8. Lubricate with lubricating jelly (Figure 12-24). RATIONALE: Easier insertion of thermometer and safety for patient.
9. Apply gloves.
10. Spread buttocks, gently insert thermometer into the rectum past the sphincter (1½ inches) for adult (Figure 12-25).
11. Hold buttocks together and keep the thermometer in place for 5 minutes. Do not let go of it. RATIONALE: Patient movement can cause thermometer to move in patient's rectum and cause injury.
12. Remove from rectum.
13. Place thermometer on gauze or tissue that was used to help lubricate thermometer.
14. Wipe lubricant from patient's anal area or offer tissue to patient. Place tissue in biohazard container.
15. Ensure patient's comfort and safety.
16. Remove sheath and place in biohazard container.
17. Read thermometer.
18. Wash, rinse, and dry thermometer.
19. Place thermometer on clean paper towel on shelf.
20. Remove gloves. Place in biohazard container.
21. Wash hands.
22. Immerse thermometer in container with alcohol marked "rectal" for thirty minutes.
23. Document on patient record, indicating a rectal temperature.

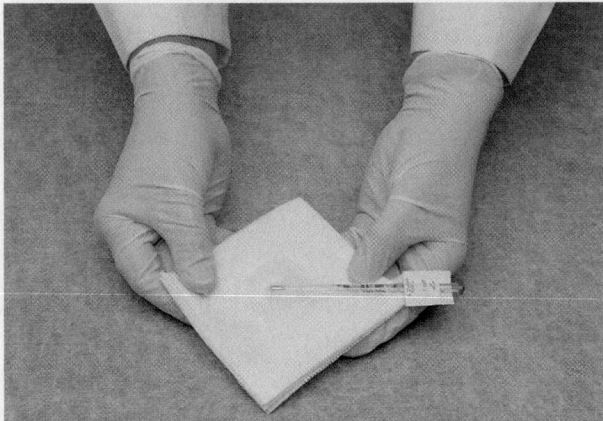

Figure 12-24 Lubricate thermometer by putting lubricant on tissue or gauze, then place first inch or two of the thermometer into the lubricant.

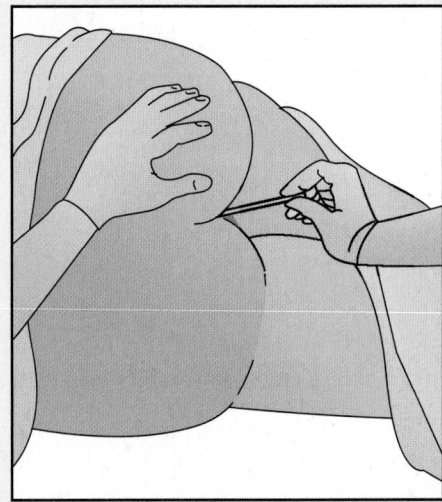

Figure 12-25 Gently insert thermometer into the rectum.

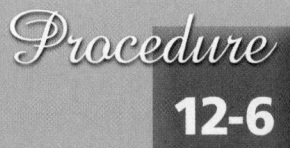

Measuring a Rectal Temperature Using a Digital Thermometer

12-6

STANDARD PRECAUTIONS:

PURPOSE:
To obtain a rectal temperature using a digital thermometer.

EQUIPMENT/SUPPLIES:
Digital thermometer with red probe
Probe cover
Lubricating jelly
Gloves
Biohazard waste container

PROCEDURE STEPS:
1. Wash hands and glove, following standard precautions.
2. Assemble equipment.
3. Identify patient.
4. Explain procedure to patient. RATIONALE: Ensures understanding and gains patient cooperation and consent.
5. Remove clothing from the waist down, drape as necessary. RATIONALE: Maintains patient modesty, privacy, and warmth.

6. Position patient in Sims' position.
7. Place probe cover on red probe (rectal). RATIONALE: To prevent microorganism cross contamination. Red probe indicates rectal thermometer.
8. Lubricate with lubricating jelly. RATIONALE: Easier insertion of thermometer and safety for patient.
9. Spread buttocks, gently insert thermometer into the rectum past the sphincter (1½ inches) for adult.
10. Hold buttocks together while holding the thermometer. Do not let go of thermometer. RATIONALE: Holding buttocks together prevents air leaks and inaccurate recording. Holding onto thermometer ensures patient safety.
11. Hold in place until the beep is heard.
12. Read results on digital display window.
13. Remove from rectum.
14. Discard probe cover into biohazard waste container by pushing the release button.
15. Replace thermometer on holder base.
16. Remove gloves, discard in biohazard waste container, and wash hands.
17. Offer tissue to patient to wipe anus. Assist patient in dressing and position as necessary.
18. Record on the patient chart labeled with (R) indicating a rectal temperature.

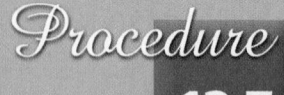

Measuring an Axillary Temperature

12-7

STANDARD PRECAUTIONS:

PURPOSE:
To obtain an axillary temperature using a mercury thermometer.

EQUIPMENT/SUPPLIES:
Mercury thermometer
Sheath

Towelettes
Paper towels

PROCEDURE STEPS:
1. Wash hands, following standard precautions.
2. Assemble equipment, place sheath on thermometer.
3. Identify patient.
4. Explain procedure. RATIONALE: This elicits patient cooperation and consent.

(continues)

Procedure

12-7 *(continued)*

5. Ask patient to remove clothing to provide access to axilla.
6. Gown as necessary to maintain patient modesty and warmth.
7. Wipe axillary area with dry towel or towelette to remove moisture. RATIONALE: Moisture in the axilla will cause inaccurate reading.
8. Place thermometer in axilla.
9. Ask patient to fold arm against chest or abdomen (Figure 12-26).
10. Leave in place for 10 minutes.
11. Carefully remove.
12. Remove sheath and discard.
13. Read thermometer.
14. Wash, rinse, and dry thermometer.
15. Place clean thermometer on clean paper towel or shelf.
16. Wash hands.
17. Immerse thermometer in container marked "oral" with alcohol for thirty minutes.
18. Document temperature in patient's record, indicating axillary temperature.

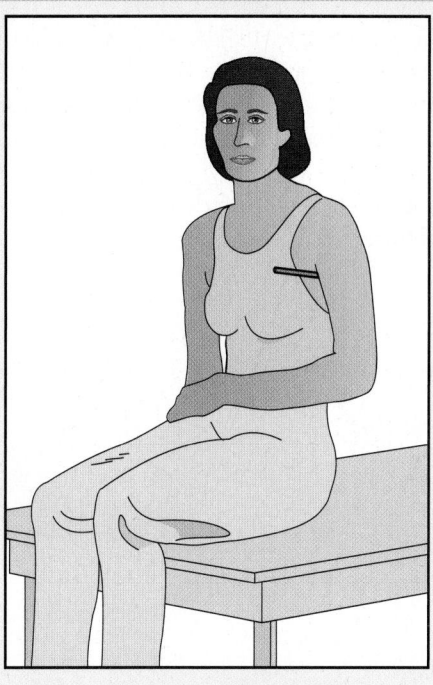

Figure 12-26 After placing thermometer in axilla, ask patient to fold arm against chest or abdomen.

Procedure

12-8 **Measuring a Radial Pulse**

STANDARD PRECAUTIONS:

PURPOSE:
To obtain a pulse rate.

EQUIPMENT/SUPPLIES:
Watch with a second hand

PROCEDURE STEPS:
1. Wash hands.
2. Identify patient.
3. Explain procedure. RATIONALE: Ensures patient cooperation and consent.

(continues)

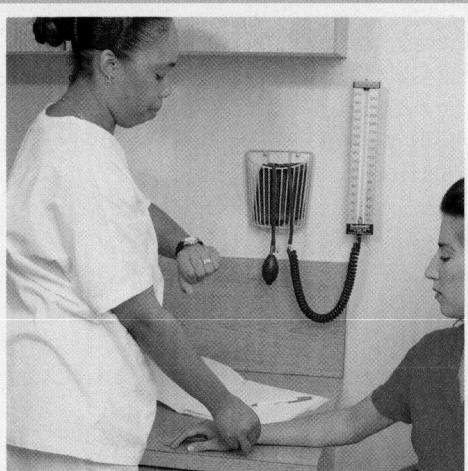

Figure 12-27 Position patient with wrist resting on table or lap.

Procedure

12-8   (*continued*)

4. Position patient with the wrist resting either on a table or on lap (Figure 12-27).
5. Locate the radial pulse with the pads of your first three fingers. Do not use thumb; it has its own pulse.
6. Gently compress the radial artery enough to feel the pulse.

7. Count the pulsations for one full minute.
8. Note any irregularities in rhythm, volume, and condition of artery.
9. Wash hands.
10. Record the pulse in the patient chart following the temperature, noting any irregularities.

Procedure

12-9   Taking an Apical Pulse

STANDARD PRECAUTIONS:

PURPOSE:
To obtain an apical pulse rate.

EQUIPMENT/SUPPLIES:
Stethoscope
Watch with second hand

PROCEDURE STEPS:
1. Wash hands.
2. Assemble equipment.
3. Identify patient.
4. Explain procedure. RATIONALE: Ensures patient cooperation and consent.
5. Assist patient in disrobing, removing clothing from the waist up.
6. Provide a gown or drape for patient modesty and warmth.
7. Position the patient in a supine position. RATIONALE: Easier access to apex of heart.
8. Locate the fifth intercostal space, midclavicular, left of sternum (Figure 12-28). RATIONALE: Location of apex of heart.
9. Place stethoscope on the site and listen for the lub-dup sound of the heart.
10. Count the pulse for one minute; each lub-dup equals one pulse.
11. Assist the patient to sit up and dress.

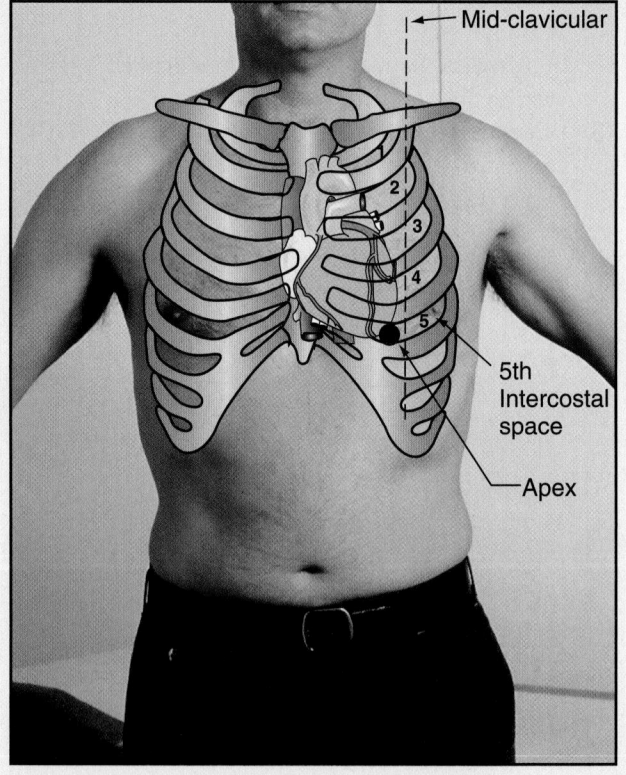

Figure 12-28   Locate the apical pulse by counting intercostal spaces. Locate the fifth intercostal space.

(*continues*)

Procedure 12-9 (*continued*)

12. Wash hands.
13. Record the pulse in the patient chart with the designation of (AP) to denote method of obtaining the pulse and note any arrythmias.

NOTE: Apical pulse and radial pulse are frequently taken simultaneously, with the radial pulse taken by another individual (Figure 12-29). Both pulse rates should be identical. A discrepancy may indicate a cardiac problem.

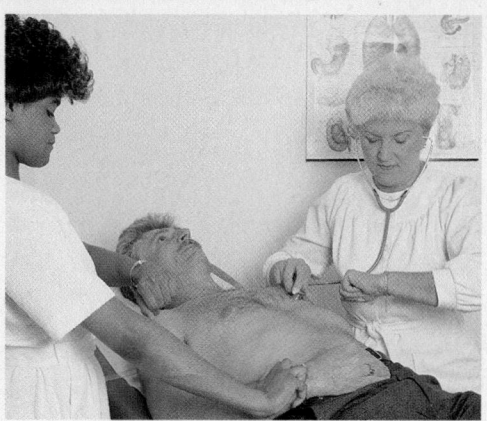

Figure 12-29 Sometimes apical and radial pulses are taken simultaneously.

Procedure 12-10 Measuring the Respiration Rate

STANDARD PRECAUTIONS:

NOTE: The respiration rate is normally taken immediately before or after the pulse rate. It should be taken without patient knowledge, as respiration can voluntarily be altered. While counting respiration, it is best to continue grasping the wrist as if still taking the pulse. This procedure will assist in preventing alteration of breathing by the patient.

PURPOSE:
To obtain an accurate respiratory rate.

EQUIPMENT/SUPPLIES:
Watch with second hand

PROCEDURE STEPS:
1. Wash hands.
2. Identify the patient.
3. Position patient in a comfortable position.
4. Watch the rise and fall of the chest wall for one minute, or, while holding the patient's arm, place it across the chest and feel for the rise and fall of chest wall. Alternatively, place a hand on the patient's shoulder and feel and watch for the rise and fall of the chest wall (Figure 12-30).
5. Note depth, rhythm, and breath sounds while counting.
6. Wash hands.
7. Record respiration rate in patient chart, noting any irregularities and sounds.

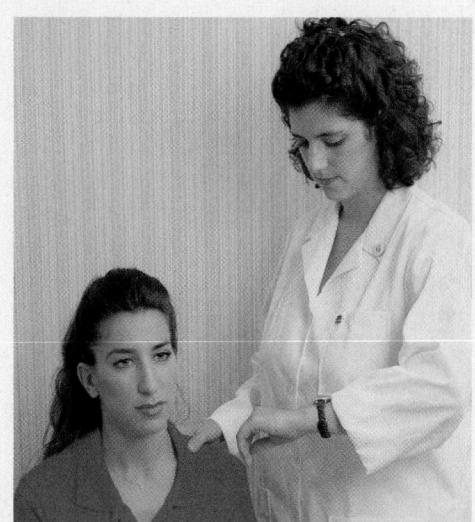

Figure 12-30 Place hand on patient's shoulder. Feel and watch for rise and fall of the chest wall.

Procedure

12-11   Measuring a Blood Pressure

STANDARD PRECAUTIONS:

PURPOSE:
To measure blood pressure.

EQUIPMENT/SUPPLIES:
Stethoscope
Sphygmomanometer
Alcohol wipes

PROCEDURE STEPS:
1. Wash hands.
2. Assemble equipment, making sure that cuff size is correct. RATIONALE: Inappropriate cuff size will result in inaccurate measurement.
3. Clean earpieces of stethoscope with alcohol wipe.
4. Identify patient.
5. Explain procedure. RATIONALE: May be the first instance where blood pressure is measured; to allay anxiety and ensure cooperation and consent.
6. Position patient comfortably; if sitting, feet flat on the floor, arm resting at heart level on the lap or a table. RATIONALE: Legs crossed may arbitrarily increase blood pressure; arm above heart level may result in inaccurate reading.
7. Bare the upper arm. If clothing is restricting, have patient remove it. RATIONALE: Tight clothing on the arm can produce inaccurate results.
8. Palpate brachial artery.
9. Securely center the bladder of the cuff over the brachial artery above the bend of the elbow. RATIONALE: Cuff should be high enough so stethoscope does not touch it. Extraneous sounds may be heard.
10. Palpate the radial pulse and smoothly inflate cuff until the pulse is no longer felt; note the number.
11. Quickly deflate the cuff and allow arm to rest for about 1 minute. Calculate peak inflation level. RATIONALE: This ensures that an auscultatory gap is not missed.
12. Make sure cuff is completely deflated.
13. Position stethoscope over the brachial artery and hold in position with the fingers only.

14. Inflate cuff smoothly and quickly to the peak inflation level (Figure 12-31).
15. Deflate the cuff at a rate of 2 to 4 millimeters of mercury per second.
16. Listen for Korotkoff Phase I; note when it appears.
17. Continue deflation, noting the Korotkoff Phases.
18. Note when all sounds disappear, Korotkoff Phase V.
19. Continue deflating the cuff at the same rate for at least another 10 millimeters after sounds have disappeared. RATIONALE: To hear an auscultatory gap should one be present.
20. The cuff may then be deflated quickly.
21. Remove the cuff.
22. Clean earpieces and diaphragm of stethoscope with alcohol wipes.
23. Wash hands.
24. Record the measurement in patient's chart.

NOTE: On a patient's initial visit and in hypertensive patients, the physician may want the blood pressure taken in both arms. There is normally a slight variation in pressure between the arms. If it is necessary to repeat the procedure, wait approximately five minutes before doing so.

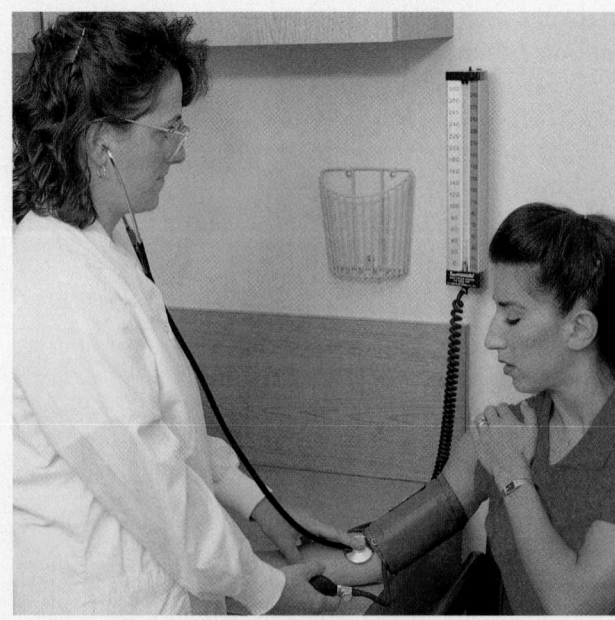

Figure 12-31   Inflate cuff smoothly and quickly.

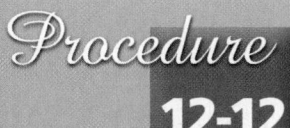

12-12   Measuring Height

STANDARD PRECAUTIONS:

PURPOSE:
To obtain the height of a patient.

EQUIPMENT/SUPPLIES:
Scale with measuring bar
Paper towel

PROCEDURE STEPS:
1. Wash hands.
2. Identify patient.
3. Explain the procedure to patient to ensure understanding, cooperation, and consent.
4. Instruct patient to remove shoes and stand on paper towel on scale with back against scale, looking straight ahead. RATIONALE: Back against scale aids patient safety.
5. Assist patient onto scale. RATIONALE: Scale platform is movable and patient may become unsteady and lose balance and fall.
6. Lower measuring bar until firmly resting on top of head (Figure 12-32).
7. Assist patient to step off of the scale. Allow patient to sit and help with shoes if necessary.

8. Read line where measurement falls.
9. Lower measuring bar to its original position.
10. Wash hands.
11. Record height in patient chart.

   Example: Ht. 5'6"

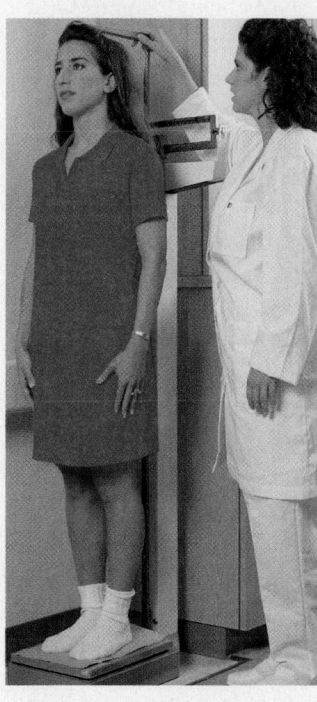

Figure 12-32
To measure height, have the patient stand with back against scale and keep head level.

12-13   Measuring Adult Weight

STANDARD PRECAUTIONS:

PURPOSE:
To obtain the weight of the patient.

EQUIPMENT/SUPPLIES:
Balance beam scale
Paper towels

PROCEDURE STEPS:
1. Wash hands.
2. Identify patient.
3. Explain the procedure to patient to ensure understanding and cooperation.
4. Place a paper towel on scale. RATIONALE: Paper towel protects patient's feet.
5. Instruct the patient to place heavy objects on the area provided, including heavy objects that may be in their pockets.

(continues)

Procedure
12-13   *(continued)*

6. Instruct the patient to remove shoes, jackets, and heavy sweaters and step on the scale. Assist patient to the center of the scale. RATIONALE: The scale platform is movable and the patient may become unsteady, lose balance, and fall.

7. Move the lower weight bar (measured in 50-pound increments) to the estimated number (the patient may be asked for approximate weight).

8. Slowly slide the upper bar until the balance beam point is centered (Figure 12-33).

9. Read the weight by adding the upper bar measurement to the lower bar measurement.

10. Assist the patient to step off of the scale.

11. Provide a chair for the patient to sit to put on shoes. Return objects to the patient.

12. Return the weights to zero.

13. Wash hands.

14. Record measurement in the patient chart.

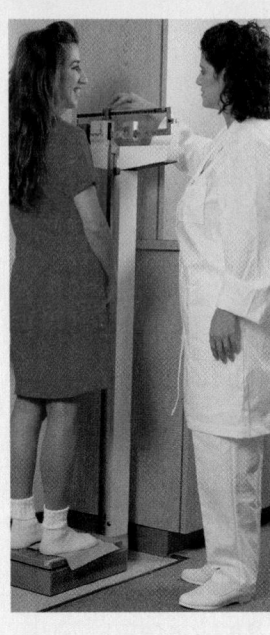

Figure 12-33 When weighing the patient, slide the upper bar until the balance beam point is centered.

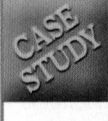

Herb Fowler, a regular patient of Dr. Lewis at Doctors Lewis & King, is an African-American man in his fifties. He has smoked for many years and only recently has thought about quitting smoking because of a chronic cough. Herb is also significantly overweight but has a hard time making the decision to give up smoking *and* change his diet. While his blood pressure has been stable for the last few years, clinical medical assistant Audrey Jones, CMA, is concerned when she takes Herb's vital signs during his most recent checkup. His weight is slightly up and his blood pressure has jumped from 140/90 to 156/100.

CASE STUDY REVIEW

1. Why is a blood pressure reading of 156/100 a cause for concern? Should Audrey take a second reading?

2. In addition to alerting the physician to the change in Herb's blood pressure and weight, Audrey feels she may be able to provide advice to the patient (with physician's permission). How can Audrey use her communication and medical assisting knowledge to counsel Herb Fowler on lifestyle changes?

3. To follow up, Audrey reviews her knowledge of hypertension and discusses the four types with the physician. What are the four kinds of hypertension and what are their characteristics?

SUMMARY

Throughout life, a patient will undergo various measurements to ascertain growth, development, and general health and well-being. The normal range for each of these measurements will vary according to the stage of life of the patient at the time of examination. The medical assistant must be aware of what to expect when measuring a patient in each life stage. Awareness of normal expectations for each stage of life will assist the medical assistant to perform the procedures in a more effective and efficient manner and aid in observing any abnormal signs and measurements.

Along with differences seen with age, the medical assistant will see differences in patients because each patient has unique medical problems.

The medical assistant has a great responsibility when performing patient measurements and must ensure patient safety and comfort while obtaining accurate results.

REVIEW QUESTIONS

Multiple Choice

1. The average adult oral temperature is:
   a. 96.2°F   c. 98.6°F
   b. 97.8°F   d. 99.5°F
2. The artery commonly used for taking a patient's pulse is:
   a. carotid   c. radial
   b. brachial   d. popliteal
3. A blood pressure cuff that is too small will:
   a. have no effect on the results
   b. give an arbitrarily low result
   c. give an arbitrarily high result
   d. have an effect on certain patients only
4. Rectal thermometers should be cleansed with:
   a. hot soapy water
   b. cool soapy water
   c. alcohol
   d. 10 percent bleach solution
5. The term used to indicate a pulse rate significantly above the average is:
   a. bradycardia   c. arrhythmia
   b. tachycardia   d. sinus rhythm

Critical Thinking

1. Discuss methods the medical assistant may use to obtain patient cooperation when taking vital signs.
2. Describe and demonstrate the appropriate charting procedure for normal vital sign results.
3. Discuss the responsibilities of the medical assistant in measuring vital signs.
4. Describe the care and use for each of the various types of thermometers.
5. Describe the procedure for converting temperatures from one scale to the other and calculate the following conversions:
   a. 98.6°F = _____ °C
   b. 39.1°C = _____ °F
6. Discuss the rationale for not using the thumb for taking the pulse rate of a patient.
7. Discuss the reasons for taking the respiratory rate of a patient without the patient's knowledge.

8. Discuss the importance of using the appropriate blood pressure cuff size when measuring a patient's blood pressure.
9. Discuss the normal vital signs differences expected between an infant and an adult.
10. Describe the following:
    a. hypertension   c. apnea
    b. tachycardia   d. remittent fever

WEB ACTIVITIES

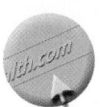

1. Access information on the Internet from the American Heart Association regarding essential hypertension and answer the following:
   a. What population of Americans is at greatest risk for essential hypertension?
   b. List four patient education tips for lowering blood pressure without the aid of medication.
   c. Check the list of normal blood pressure readings in this chapter and compare it to what the American Heart Association says are normal blood pressure measurements at various ages.
2. Access information on the Internet from the National Research Council and list its recommendations for weight of the following females:

Height	Age	Weight in Pounds
5' 2"	19–34 years	?
5' 4"	19–34 years	?
5' 6"	19–34 years	?

REFERENCES/BIBLIOGRAPHY

Keir, L., Wise, B. A., & Krebs, C. (1998). *Medical assisting: Administrative and clinical competencies* (4th ed.). Albany, NY: Delmar.

Kinn, M. E., & Woods, M. A. (1999). *The medical assistant: Administrative and clinical* (8th ed.). Philadelphia: W. B. Saunders.

Taber's cyclopedic medical dictionary. (18th ed.) (1999). Philadelphia: F. A. Davis.

Zakus, S. (1995). *Clinical procedures for medical assistants* (3rd ed.). St. Louis: Mosby-Year Book.

Chapter

13

THE PHYSICAL EXAMINATION

KEY TERMS

Ataxia
Bruits
Catheterization
Cyanosis
Fenestrated Drape
Jaundice
Labyrinthitis
Pallor
Pyorrhea
Scleroderma
Symmetry
Tinnitus
Vertigo
Vitiligo

OUTLINE

Methods of Examination
  Observation or Inspection
  Palpation
  Percussion
  Auscultation
  Mensuration
  Manipulation
Positioning and Draping
  Examination Positions
Equipment and Supplies for the
  Physical Examination

Basic Components of a Routine
  Physical Examination
  Patient Appearance
  Gait
  Stature
  Posture
  Body Movements
  Speech
  Breath Odors
  Nutrition
  Skin and Appendages
  The Physical Examination
    Sequence

OBJECTIVES

The student should strive to meet the following performance objectives and demonstrate an understanding of the facts and principles presented in this chapter through written and oral communication.

1. Define the key terms as presented in the glossary.
2. Describe the six methods used in physical examinations.
3. Name and describe eight positions used for physical examinations.
4. Discuss the purpose of draping and demonstrate the appropriate draping procedure for each type of position.
5. Identify at least ten instruments and supplies used for examination of various parts of the body.
6. Identify eight basic components of a physical examination.
7. Describe the sequence followed during a routine physical examination.
8. Recall method of examination, instrument used, and position for examination of at least eight body parts.

CLINICAL

Fundamental Principles

- Apply principles of aseptic technique and infection control
- Comply with quality assurance practices

Patient Care

- Obtain patient history and vital signs
- Prepare and maintain examination and treatment areas
- Prepare patient for examinations, procedures, and treatments
- Assist with examinations, procedures, and treatments
- Maintain medication and immunization records

GENERAL (TRANSDISCIPLINARY)

Legal Concepts

- Document accurately

At the multiphysician Inner City Health Care facility, five physicians are employed on a rotating basis, with two or three working at any one time. Clinical medical assistants Wanda Slawson, CMA, and Bruce Goldman, CMA, have developed a clear understanding of what each physician prefers in both room and patient preparation. Wanda and Bruce also coordinate with each other and with office managers Jane O'Hara and Walter Seals, both CMAs, to ensure patient comfort. Depending on the patient and the type of examination, Wanda will often assist with patient preparation when the patient is female and Walter will assist when the patient is a male.

INTRODUCTION

Physical examinations are performed to obtain a picture of the health and well-being of the patient. An initial examination will provide a baseline reference for future examinations. The examination follows a standard routine, usually starting at the head and following through the entire body, including all major organs and body systems. Although the sequence of events for the physical examination is relatively standard, variations will occur according to physician preference, type of practice, and patient's chief complaint. Diagnostic procedures such as laboratory and X rays may be ordered or performed in the facility or sent to an outside laboratory. At the conclusion of the physical examination, the physician will have an impression of the patient's general health, diagnosis if possible, and treatment plans. The physician uses information from three major sources to aid in making a diagnosis: the health history, the physical examination, and laboratory tests and diagnostic procedures.

The role of the medical assistant throughout the physical examination will greatly depend upon the physician. Some physicians will delegate many duties to the medical assistant, while others will require little assistance. Commonly performed medical assisting duties can be divided into two cate-

gories: patient preparation and room preparation. Patient preparation includes patient explanation and preparation, positioning, draping, vital signs, specimen collection such as urine and blood, and electrocardiogram (ECG). Room preparation includes assembling the appropriate instruments and equipment for the physician and assuring patient privacy and comfort.

Additional medical assisting duties include handing the physician instruments and equipment as required and taking notes dictated by the physician. Throughout and following the examination, the medical assistant will adhere to the principles of medical asepsis and standard precautions as required by OSHA. The effective medical assistant will establish an efficient but flexible routine providing for the needs of both the patient and physician.

METHODS OF EXAMINATION

There are six methods used by the physician to examine the body. They include observation or inspection, palpation, percussion, auscultation, mensuration, and manipulation. The physician will use all in total or in part depending upon the type of examination being performed.

Observation or Inspection

This is the process of observing the patient. The general health, posture, body movements, skin, mannerisms, and care in grooming are all noted. Closer observation will be focused on body **symmetry** (correspondence in shape and size of body parts located on opposite sides of the body) and contour. Deformities and skin rashes will be observed. Skin color is also noted (Figure 13-1).

Palpation

This is an examination of the body using touch and may be used to help verify observations. A body part or organ may be felt for size and condition. Abdominal masses may be felt through the abdominal wall. Skin texture, moisture, and temperature can be felt. The contour of limbs and rigidity and position of bones and joints may be felt. Palpation may be performed with the use of fingertips, one or both hands, or the palm of the hand (Figure 13-2).

Percussion

This is the process of eliciting sounds from the body by tapping with either a percussion hammer or fingers. The vibrations and sounds from underlying organs and cavities can be felt and heard. Using this method can determine the presence of air or solid material in the organ or cavity being checked. Healthy structures that are dense, such as the liver, produce a dull sound. Hollow structures such as the lungs should produce a more hollow sound. There are two methods used to perform percussion. The direct method is by tapping directly on the surface of the skin. The indirect method is performed by placing a finger or hand on the surface of the skin and tapping the hand (Figure 13-3).

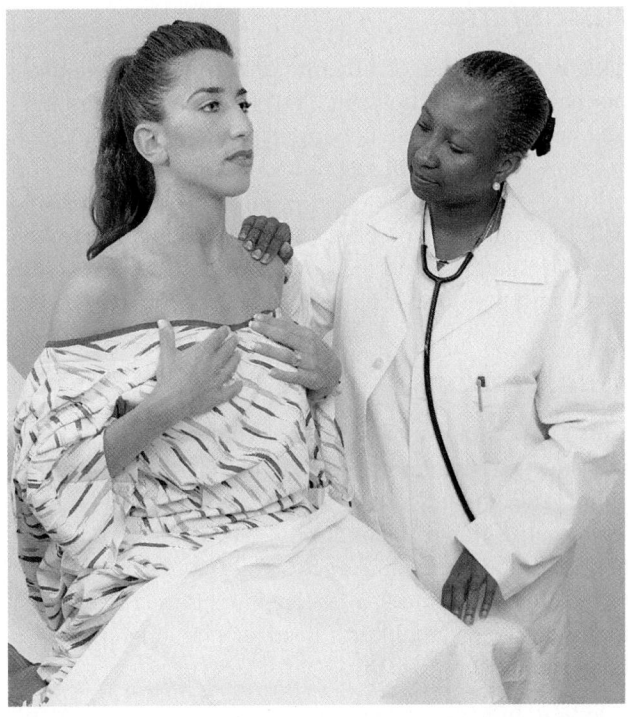

Figure 13-1 The physician observes the patient for signs of disease. This method of examination is known as observation or inspection.

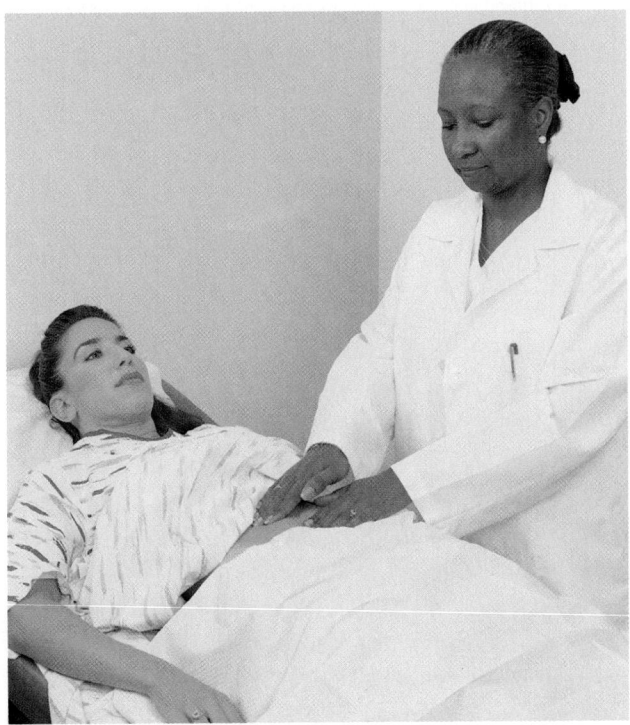

Figure 13-2 The physician palpates the abdomen during the physical examination to feel for abnormalities.

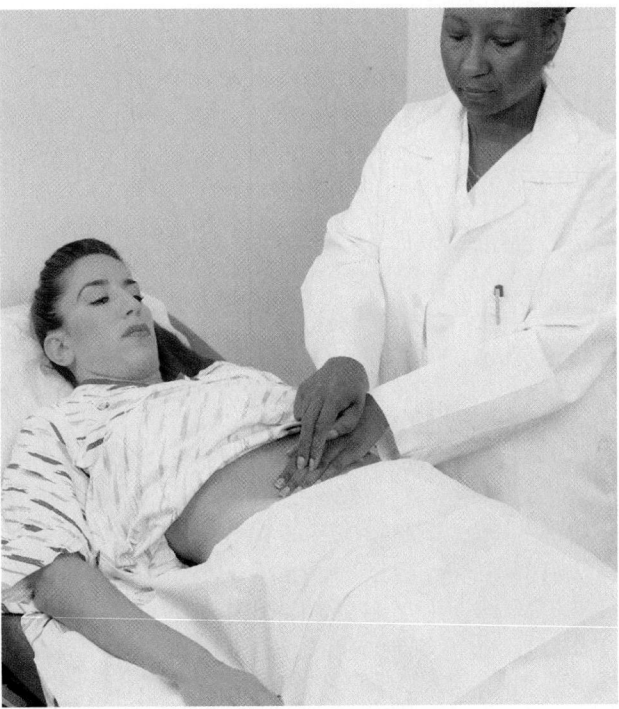

Figure 13-3 The physician uses percussion during the physical examination to tap the body to produce sounds that may indicate disease.

Auscultation

This is the process of listening directly to body sounds, normally with a stethoscope. The physician listens for lung and heart sounds such as murmurs, rales, or **bruits**, which generally are abnormal sounds heard on auscultation of an organ or vessel such as a vein or an artery. The abdomen will be examined for bowel sounds which include the clicks and gurgles of normal bowel activity, the sounds that occur with peristalsis (Figures 13-4 and 13-5).

Mensuration

This method of examination uses the process of measuring. The measurement of height and weight, the length of a limb, the amount of flexion and extension of an extremity are all forms of mensuration. Measurement of chest and infant head circumference are also forms of mensuration. In most instances, a tape measure is used to perform mensuration of an infant's head or circumference of a body part (Figure 13-6).

Manipulation

This method checks the amount of flexion and extension of a joint by applying forceful passive movement on the joint. Range of motion of some joints may be checked using this method. See Chapter 21 for information on range of motion.

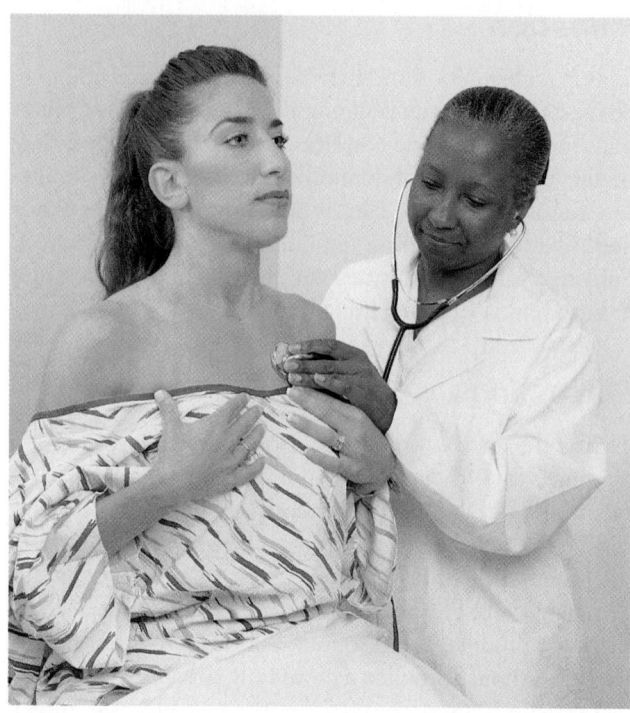

Figure 13-4   The physician uses a stethoscope to listen to sounds from the patient's body. This method of physical examination is known as auscultation.

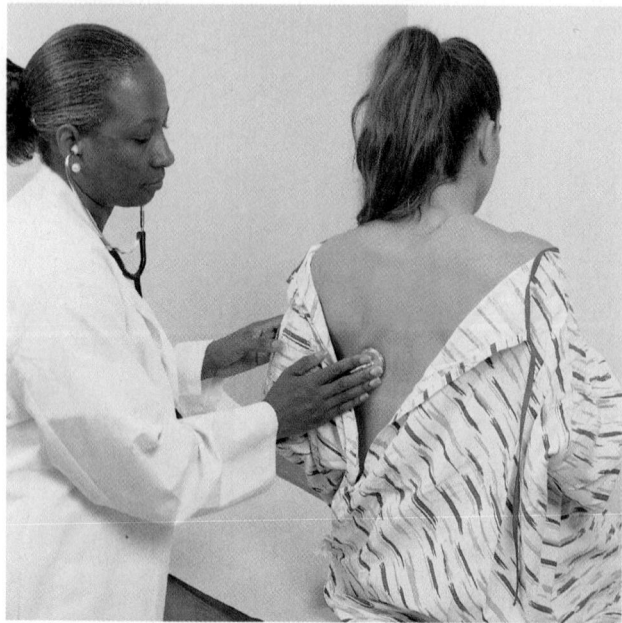

Figure 13-5   Auscultation is performed on the anterior and posterior portion of the body.

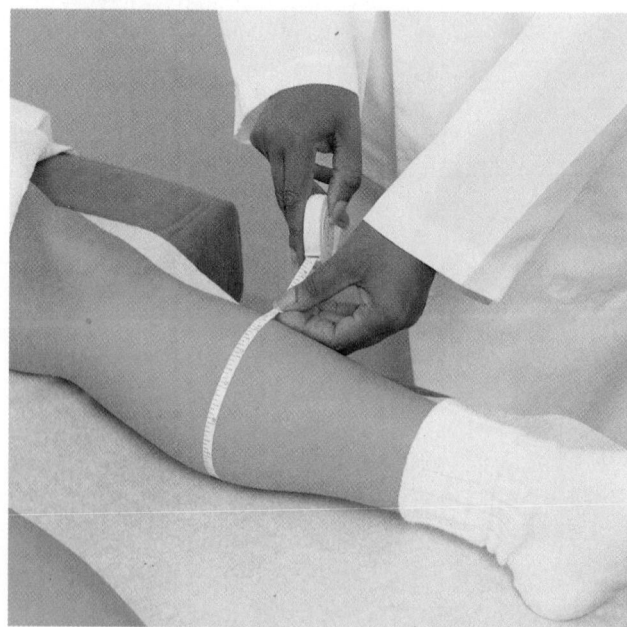

Figure 13-6   A tape measure may be used to measure the circumference of the calf of the patient's leg or other body part. This method of physical examination is known as mensuration.

POSITIONING AND DRAPING

Physical examinations may require the patient to be placed in various positions. Each position is designed to make examination of a particular area of the body easier and more efficient. The medical assistant may assist the patient in disrobing and will provide the appropriate drape and/or gown. The medical assistant also instructs the patient about the appropriate position required for the examination and may assist the patient into position by providing support and guidance. The patient experiencing pain should be allowed to assume the position with minimal help, as too much assistance by another may increase the pain. Always provide for patient safety.

Proper draping to protect modesty and prevent embarrassment is essential. If patients are capable of helping themselves, the medical assistant should leave the room while the patient disrobes and puts on a drape or a gown. If the patient is disoriented or extremely ill, the medical assistant must stay in the room; patient privacy can be provided by discreetly removing clothing and covering the patient as quickly as possible. When the patient is a child, the medical assistant should note the comfort level of the child while the child is getting disrobed. Children develop modesty at an early age and may be embarrassed by sitting on the examination table wearing only underwear. Respect a child's right to privacy by offering a gown or drape. The elderly will need assistance with disrobing and draping. Care must be taken to provide as much modesty and privacy as possible as you assist patients of all ages.

 Never turn your back on seriously ill or disoriented patients or young children. Ensure patient safety at all times.

Examination Positions

There are a number of positions that may be required of the patient during the physical examination. The position used will depend on the type of examination. Eight common positions are outlined in Procedures 13-1 through 13-8. These include:

1. Supine (horizontal recumbent) (Procedure 13-1)
2. Dorsal recumbent (Procedure 13-2)
3. Lithotomy (Procedure 13-3)
4. Fowler's (Procedure 13-4)
5. Knee-Chest (Procedure 13-5)
6. Prone (Procedure 13-6)
7. Sims' (Procedure 13-7)
8. Trendelenburg (Procedure 13-8)

Supine (Horizontal Recumbent). This position is assumed when lying flat facing up (Figure 13-7). It is used for examination of the anterior surface of the body from head to toe. When the physician is performing a physical examination on a female, she should be provided with a gown and instructed to wear it with the opening in the front. A drape is then placed over the lap or from the waist down.

Dorsal Recumbent. The patient lies on her back (dorsal) face up, legs separated, knees flexed with feet flat on the table (Figure 13-8). This is the most comfortable position for patients with back and abdominal problems. Examinations performed in this position include rectal, vaginal, head, neck, and chest, as well as abdominal palpation. It can also be used for urinary **catheterization**. Preteen and early teen girls requiring a pelvic examination may be placed in this position and will require careful instructions and procedure explanations. The patient is covered with a drape that is diamond shaped. One edge of the diamond can be lifted to examine the genitalia without exposing the rest of the body.

Lithotomy. The patient is assisted to lie on her back similar to the dorsal recumbent position except the buttocks should be as close to the bottom edge of the table as

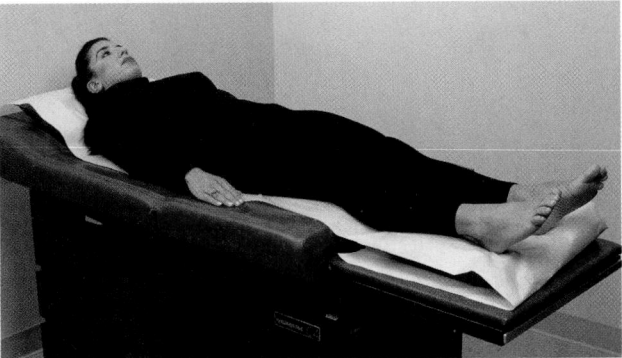

Figure 13-7 Supine or horizontal recumbent position.

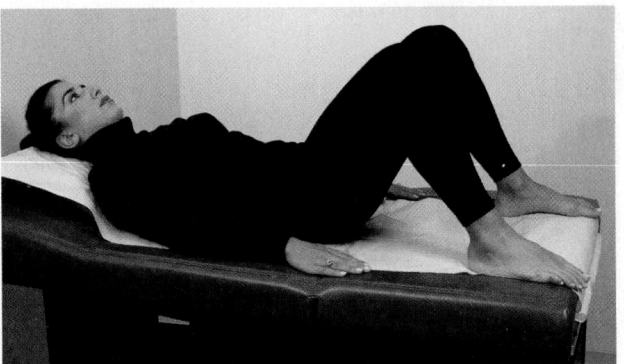

Figure 13-8 Dorsal recumbent position.

possible and feet placed in stirrups attached to the foot of the table (Figure 13-9). The lithotomy position is used for genital and pelvic examinations. It can also be used for urinary catheterization. At the conclusion of the examination, the patient should slide toward the head of the table before getting up from this position. Patients with special needs, such as the elderly and those physically challenged as with severe arthritis, may not be able to assume this position. If this is the case, assist patient into Sims' position (see Procedure 13-7) and the sigmoidoscopy, proctoscopy, or pelvic exam can be done in this position for these patients.

Fowler's. The patient sits in a position with the back of the examination table raised to either 45 degrees (Semi-Fowler's) (Figure 13-10) or 90 degrees (High-Fowler's) (Figure 13-11). Legs rest flat on the table. A pillow may be placed under the knees. This position is used for patients having cardiovascular or respiratory problems to facilitate their breathing, and for examination of the upper body and head.

Knee-Chest. This position puts the weight of the body on the knees and chest (Figure 13-12). The patient is instructed to kneel on the table and spread the knees shoulder width apart. The buttocks should be elevated, back straight with the chest resting on the table. The head is positioned to one side, with arms flexed on the side of the head and hands under the head. This is not a comfortable position and the patient may need assistance. If the position is too uncomfortable or difficult, have the patient rest on the elbows. This position is used primarily for proctologic examinations, sigmoidoscopy procedures, and in some instances vaginal examinations. Draping will require a large drape to cover the entire body. It may be necessary to use two smaller drapes, holding them together with towel clamps. A diamond- or triangle-shaped drape allows for one edge to be lifted to expose only the rectal area. Do not place the patient in knee-chest position until the physician is ready to begin the procedure.

Proctologic. This position requires the use of a specialized table known as a proctologic examination table (Figure 13-13). The patient is instructed to disrobe and to kneel on the knee board of the table. The patient then bends at the hips and rests the chest on the table. The head is supported by a head board. The table is then turned to elevate the buttocks. A triangular, diamond-shaped, or **fenestrated drape**

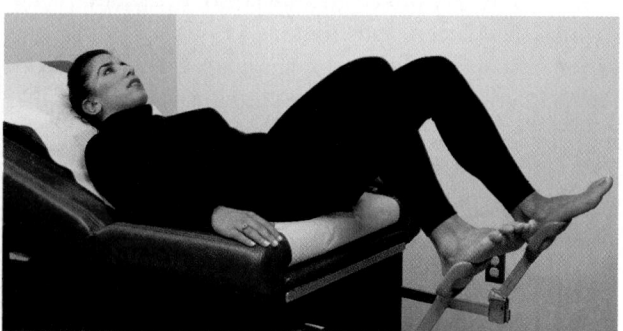

Figure 13-9   Lithotomy position.

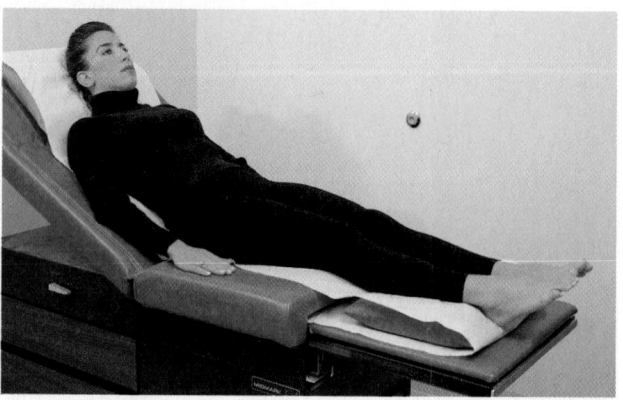

Figure 13-10   Semi-Fowler's position (45-degree angle).

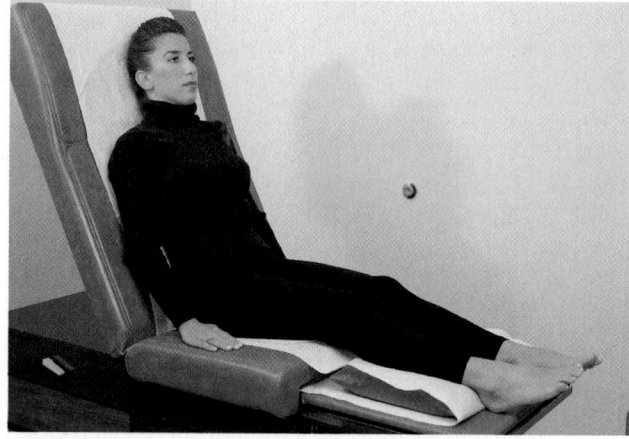

Figure 13-11   High Fowler's position (90-degree angle).

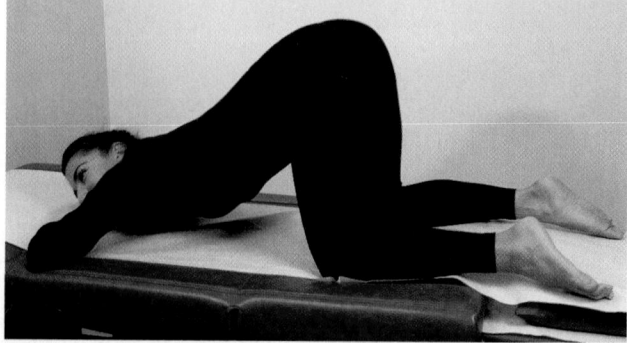

Figure 13-12   Knee-chest position.

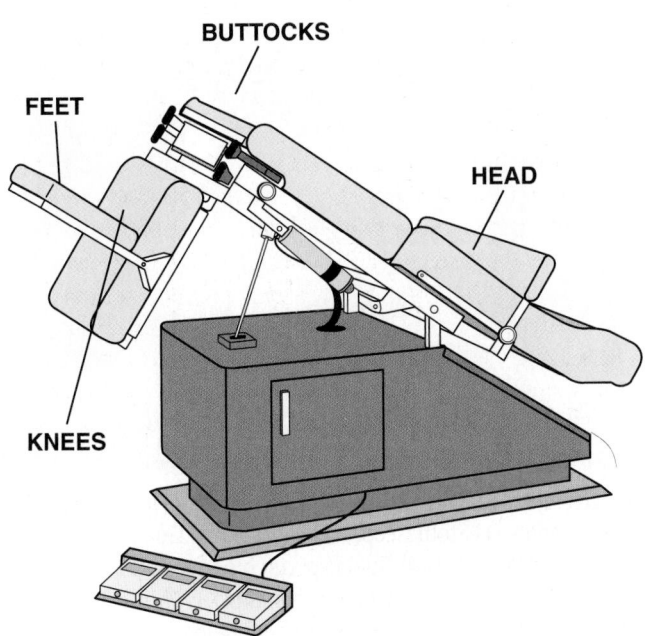

FEET

BUTTOCKS

HEAD

KNEES

Figure 13-13 Proctologic table.

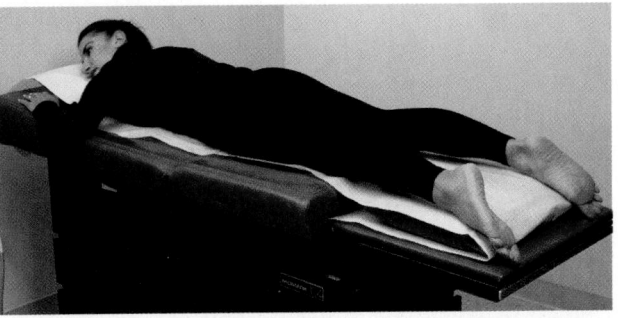

Figure 13-14 Prone position.

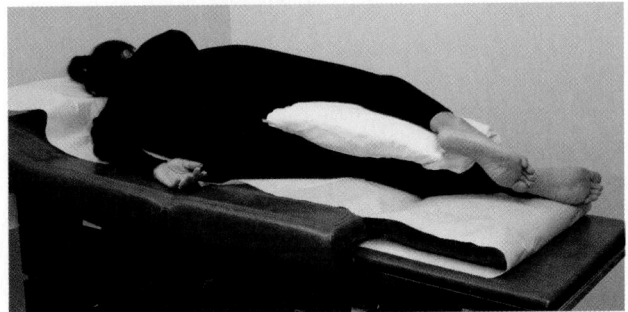

Figure 13-15 Sims' or lateral position.

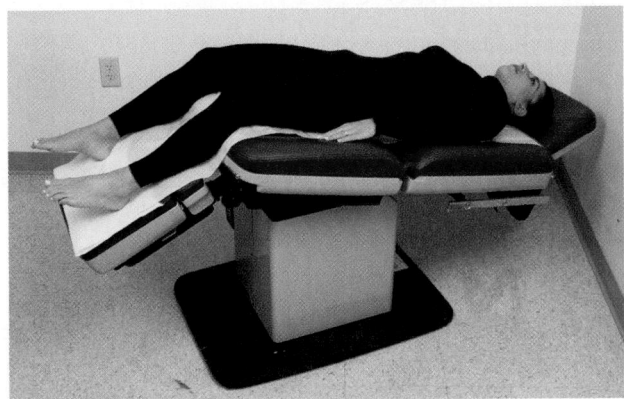

Figure 13-16 Trendelenburg position.

will cover the patient from the shoulders to the knees. This position is used for proctologic examinations.

Prone. The patient is instructed to lie face down on the table with head turned to side, arms may be placed above head or along side of body (Figure 13-14). The drape must cover from the mid-chest area to the legs. This position may be used for examining the posterior aspect of the body, including the back or spine.

Sims' (lateral). The patient is instructed to lie on the left side; the left arm and shoulder may be drawn back behind the body (Figure 13-15). The left knee is slightly flexed to support the body and the right knee is flexed sharply. A small pillow is provided for under the patient's head and a pillow may also be placed between the patient's legs if it does not interfere with the examination being performed. The drape should be large enough to cover the patient from the shoulders to the knees (triangle or diamond shape to expose rectum). This position may be used for vaginal or rectal examination, for rectal temperatures, sigmoidoscopy, or for enemas.

Trendelenburg. The patient lies flat on the back, face up, with the knees flexed and the legs hanging off the end of the table. Legs and feet are supported by a footboard (Figure 13-16). The table is positioned with the head 45 degrees lower than the body. The drape covers from the shoulders to the knees. This position is primarily used for surgical procedures of pelvis or abdomen. Variation of this position may be used for a patient in shock. (See Chapter 9 for information about emergency procedures.)

EQUIPMENT AND SUPPLIES FOR THE PHYSICAL EXAMINATION

Equipment and supplies used for physical examinations should be properly cleaned and ready for the physician's use. Refer to Chapters 10 and 19 for proper cleaning and care of instruments. The list of instruments and supplies in Table 13-1 includes those that may be used in the physical examination. However, this is a limited list. Actual equipment and supplies needed will vary with the physician and with the type of examination. Figure 13-17 shows some common instruments that may be used in the physical examination. For instruments used in specialty examinations, see Chapter 18.

TABLE 13-1	INSTRUMENTS AND SUPPLIES NEEDED FOR A PHYSICAL EXAMINATION	
Balance beam scales	Laryngeal mirror	
Tape measure	Pharyngeal mirror	
Thermometer	Examination lights	
Stethoscope	Penlight	
Sphygmomanometer	Gloves	
Alcohol swabs	Emesis basin	
Cotton balls	Percussion hammer	
Gauze sponges	Patient gown	
Otoscope	Drape	
Tuning fork	Tissues	
Ophthalmoscope	Specimen bottles/slides— request forms	
Tonometer		
Nasal speculum	Biohazard and regular waste containers	
Tongue depressors		

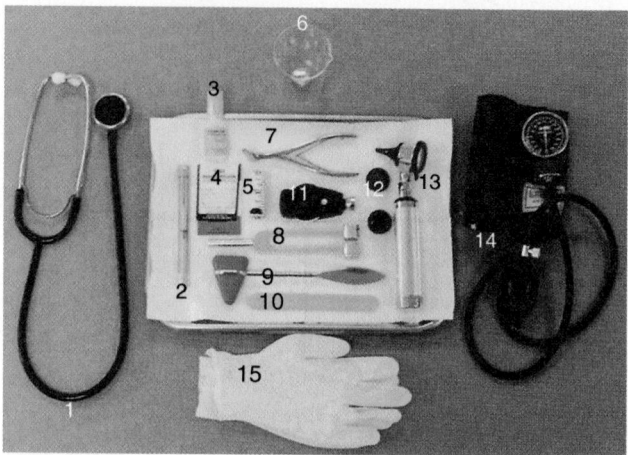

Figure 13-17 Instruments and supplies used in the physical examination: (1) Stethoscope. (2) Penlight. (3) Guaiac/occult blood test developer. (4) Guaiac/occult blood test. (5) Flexible tape measure. (6) Urine specimen container. (7) Metal nasal speculum. (8) Tuning fork. (9) Percussion hammer. (10) Tongue depresser. (11) Ophthalmoscope (head). (12) Okastic ear/ nose speculum. (13) Otoscope head attached to base handle. (14) Sphygmomanometer. (15) Latex gloves.

BASIC COMPONENTS OF A ROUTINE PHYSICAL EXAMINATION

The physical examination of the patient begins as soon as the patient enters the office. While the physical examination is performed by the physician, it is important for the medical assistant to be aware of the various examination components and the significance of each as an indicator of patient well-being.

Patient Appearance

General appearance and actions are noted as the patient is received by the medical assistant and during the patient history (see Chapter 11). Skin color is checked, general grooming, ease of conversation, and answers to questions are noted. The medical assistant should be alert to a patient with abnormal skin color, confusion or disorientation, or difficulty in movement. Such a patient may have a serious problem and should be placed in an examination room and the physician contacted immediately.

The following aspects of the patient's health are evaluated by the physician through the method of physical examination known as observation.

Gait

Gait pertains to the manner or style of walking. The patient may have a limp, walk with feet wide apart, appear to be dragging one leg, or have difficulty maintaining balance. The physician will observe the patient's gait by instructing the patient to walk on a designated straight line. Abnormal gait can include **ataxia**, uncoordinated

wide-based walk; steppage, in which the leg stepping forward is raised high enough to raise the toes off the ground; drag-to, in which the feet are dragged forward rather than lifted and moved; and spastic, in which the legs are held stiffly together and the feet are slightly dragged forward. Each of these gaits can indicate a disease process or health problem associated with neurological functioning.

Stature

The height of the patient is measured. The physician will look for height, trunk, and limb proportion.

Posture

Since normal posture is erect with the head held up, a patient in pain may exhibit postural differences. The spine might be in a fixed position, or there may be limited motion in an extremity. The physician will observe spine movement and alignment as the patient performs prescribed movements. Abnormalities can include kyphosis (humpback), which may be seen in the elderly, particularly women with osteoporosis; lordosis, abnormal curvature of the lumbar area, and scoliosis, curvature of the upper spine.

Body Movements

These may be either voluntary or involuntary. Voluntary body movements describe those movements intended to be made by the patient. Involuntary body movements are movements not controlled by the patient. Tremors are a form of involuntary movement that may be seen in the mouth, fingers, hands, arms, and legs of a patient. Tremors can indicate a neurological health problem. Involuntary body movements are usually easily observed.

Speech

The patient's speech may reveal abnormal conditions. Abnormalities include aphonia, loss of voice usually due to laryngitis, but which may have other causes; aphasia, the inability to express oneself through speech or writing, which may indicate brain injury or disease; and dysphasia, an inability to use appropriate speech patterns, such as using words in the wrong order. This may indicate a brain lesion.

Breath Odors

These may be detected when speaking with the patient or when obtaining vital signs. A sweet fruity odor may indicate acidosis. This may result from diabetes mellitus, starvation, or renal disease. A musty odor may indicate liver disease and an ammonia odor may indicate uremia.

Nutrition

There are various published charts containing guidelines for normal weight established by height and age. Overweight and underweight are defined as being above or below the published charts. Obesity and underweight have previously been mentioned in Chapter 12. Edema is a condition that causes weight gain and is an excessive accumulation of fluids in the body tissues. To test for edema, the physician will press a finger against the skin of the patient in an area over a bony prominence such as the ankle. If edema is present, pitting will be evident when the finger is removed. Fat tissue will not leave an indentation when pressed.

Skin and Appendages

Skin problems include abnormal skin color such as redness, **pallor**, **cyanosis**, **jaundice**, and **vitiligo**. Pallor is defined as lack of color or paleness; cyanosis is a slightly blue or gray discoloration of the skin, often seen in patients with severe anemia; jaundice is a yellowing of the skin, often due to obstructed bile ducts or liver disease; and vitiligo is characterized by white patches on the skin, observed against normal pigmentation. Other skin conditions are lesions, ulcers, and bruises. Texture may be smooth, rough, and scaly and have loss of elasticity. These findings may indicate health problems and/or excessive exposure to the sun. The nails can also indicate some forms of health problems. Infections, either local or sys-

SPOTLIGHT ON AAMA ESSENTIALS THROUGH CAAHEP

- Listening to how a patient says he or she feels is just as important as observing an irregularity during a physical examination.
- Always strive to maintain the patient's dignity and privacy by knocking before entering the examination room.
- Maintaining the patient's confidentiality will enable him or her to open up more readily and provide you with a better account of his or her chief complaint.

temic, may be observed in nails that are brittle, grooved, or lined. The appearance of the fingertips can be indicators of disorders as seen in a clubbing, which may indicate congenital heart disease; and spooning, which may be seen in severe iron deficiency anemias. Abnormal hair distribution as in facial hair on a female may indicate hormonal changes.

The Physical Examination Sequence

There is a sequence followed for a physical examination, although physician preference and the patient's chief complaint can produce a variation to this sequence.

The physical examination begins with the medical assistant taking and recording the patient's vital signs, height, weight, and visual acuity and auditory ability when appropriate. Additional laboratory procedures, such as urinalysis and blood analysis or electrocardiography, may be performed as directed by the physician prior to the physical examination. Prior to the examination, a patient will be instructed to empty the bladder saving a urine specimen for analysis. The patient is then told about the examination and what to expect during the examination. Any questions the patient might have should be answered by the medical assistant or referred to the physician. The patient should be instructed about disrobing (a private area should be provided for disrobing). The medical assistant should be explicit as to what clothing is to be removed and what can be left on. If a complete physical examination is required, all clothing should be removed. A gown and drape are provided for the patient. The medical assistant may leave the room while the patient disrobes unless the patient asks for help or is unable to manage alone. It is appropriate to knock before reentering the room.

It is customary for the medical assistant to remain in the room when the physician is examining a patient for patient comfort and as a deterrent to potential lawsuits.

The medical assistant will place the instruments for the examination on the counter or Mayo stand, according to physician preference, but usually in order of use. When lamps are used for the examination, the medical assistant may turn them on and have them ready for the physician. Make sure that the light is not directed into the patient's eyes. Inform the physician that the patient is ready when the patient is comfortably positioned on the examination table. Normally the physical examination will start at the head and proceed downward. See Table 13-2 for a detailed review of the components of the physical examination.

TABLE 13-2 COMPONENTS OF THE PHYSICAL EXAMINATION

Body Part	Position	Instrument Used	Method of Exam	Physician's Findings Normal	Abnormal
General appearance	Standing	—	Inspection	Patient is cooperative, good hygiene, good skin color, ease of gait.	Uncooperative, behavior inappropriate, unkempt appearance.
Skin	Supine	Flashlight	Inspection Palpation	Good color, warm to touch. No lesion such as warts, moles, abscesses, rashes.	Jaundice, cyanosis, pallor, redness, flakiness of skin, lesions, rashes.
Head and neck	Supine or Semi-Fowler's or sitting on edge of table	Light source	Inspection Palpation	Symmetry of head. Hair not dry or oily and distributed evenly. Scalp free of lesions and not dry.	Asymmetry of head. Alopecia, dry, flaky scalp. Swelling, lumps or pain in head or neck.
Eyes	Supine or Semi-Fowler's or sitting on edge of table	Flashlight Ophthalmoscope	Inspection Mensuration	Snellen test shows accurate visual acuity. Able to identify color plates. No tearing. Pupillary reaction to light equal. Retina pink and blood vessels healthy. Tonometer measurement of intraocular pressure within normal limits. No bulging of eyeballs.	Poor visual and color ability. Dull appearing eyes. Drainage. Unequal pupils. Clouded lens. Unequal papillary reaction. Intraocular pressure increased. Torturous, unhealthy retinal blood vessels. Bulging eyeballs.
Ears	Supine or Semi-Fowler's or sitting on edge of table	Otoscope Flashlight Tuning fork and/or audiometer	Inspection Percussion	Cerumen not impacted on tympanic membrane. Tympanic membrane gray and intact. No discharge or pain. Able to hear tuning fork or audiometer.	Impacted cerumen. Red, bulging tympanic membrane. Discharge (pus or blood). Inability to hear sound from tuning fork. Poor auditory ability when checked with audiometer.
Nose	Supine or Semi-Fowler's or sitting on edge of table	Nasal speculum Flashlight	Inspection	Mucous membranes moist and pink. Able to detect specific odors. Septum straight. Nostrils equal in size. No abnormal discharge. No lesions.	Dry, red swollen mucous membranes. Unable to detect odors. Deviated septum. Nostrils nonflaring. Discharge, polyps noted.
Mouth and throat	Supine or Semi-Fowler's or sitting on edge of table	Flashlight Tongue depressors Laryngeal and pharyngeal mirrors	Inspection	Gag reflex present. Mucous membranes moist and pink. Teeth intact, pink tongue. Tonsils nonswollen, pink.	No gag reflex. Tongue rough. Pallor of mucous membranes. Dental caries. Swollen tonsils.
Arms and hands	Supine or Semi-Fowler's or sitting on edge of table	Percussion hammer	Inspection Palpation	Good muscle tone. Normal range of motion. Nails pink, smooth. Ability to squeeze doctor's hands with equal strength.	Poor muscle tone. Poor range of motion. Nails cyanotic. Brittle, ridged nails.
Chest and lungs	Supine or Semi-Fowler's or sitting on edge of table	Stethoscope Tape measure	Inspection Palpation Auscultation Mensuration Percussion	Axillary lymph nodes not palpable. Lungs clear. No cough. Ribs nontender. Symmetrical chest wall. Respirations and heart rate normal. Normal chest sounds.	Enlarged axillary lymph nodes. Asymmetry of chest wall. Respiration and heart rate abnormal. Abnormal chest sounds.

(continues)

Head. The patient will be in a sitting position for this examination. The face will be checked for puffiness especially around the eyes. Facial skin will be checked for **scleroderma**, a tight and atrophied skin. The elderly patient may have fatty patches that appear raised and yellowish on the eyelids. The hair and scalp are checked. The head and neck are palpated for lumps and swelling.

Eyes. The appearance of the eyes is examined. The pupils of the eyes will then be checked for light accommodation. When a penlight or flashlight is placed in front of the pupil, the pupil will constrict. The other pupil should constrict equally. If they do not constrict and return to normal equally, it may indicate a problem in the brain. A tonometer may be used to measure the intraocular eye pressure of patients over the age of 35 years. Normal eye

TABLE 13-2 *(continued)*

Body Part	Position	Instrument Used	Method of Exam	Physician's Findings Normal	Abnormal
Heart	Supine or Semi-Fowler's or sitting on edge of table	Stethoscope ECG	Auscultation Palpation Mensuration	Normal heart function per ECG. Regular rhythm, rate of heart sounds. No murmurs. Blood pressure normal range. Pulse points good quality.	Abnormal heart function per ECG. Irregularity of rhythm, rate. Murmurs. Blood pressure outside normal ranges. Poor pulse quality.
Breasts	Supine	—	Inspection Palpation	No lumps, tenderness, swelling, or thickening. No sores or lesions. No bleeding or discharge from nipples. No lymph node swelling in axilla. No dimpling or "orange peel" appearance.	Lumps, tenderness, swelling, thickening. Sores or lesions. Bleeding or discharge from nipple. Lymph node enlargement in axilla. "Orange peel" appearance to breast tissue. Dimpling of skin.
Abdomen	Supine	Stethoscope Measuring tape	Inspection Palpation Auscultation Mensuration Percussion	Liver, spleen not palpable. Symmetry to abdomen. No abnormal bowel sounds. No abnormal sounds from organs in abdomen. Abdomen soft. No abdominal or inguinal hernias.	Liver, spleen enlarged. Asymmetrical abdomen. Increased or decreased bowel sounds. Unusual sounds elicited from percussion of abdominal organs. Abdominal distention. Ascites. Presence of abdominal, umbilical, or inguinal hernia.
Female genitalia and rectum	Lithotomy or dorsal recumbent or Sims'	Vaginal speculum Light source	Inspection Palpation	External genitalia without lesions, sores, ulcerations. Vaginal mucosa pink and without discharge. Nontender ovaries. Cervix smooth, noneroded, noninflamed. Good muscle tone in perineal floor and rectum. Negative stool for occult blood. Non-palpable lymph nodes in groin.	Lesions, sores, ulcerations. Discharge from vagina, cervix. Painful ovaries. Cervix ulcerated, inflamed. Poor muscle tone in perineal and rectum floor. Prolapse of uterus or bladder into vagina. Hemorrhoids. Positive hemocult. Enlarged inguinal lymph nodes.
Male genitalia	Supine Standing	—	Inspection Palpation	Penis pink, no discharge. No lesions, sores, ulcers. Testicles firm, nontender, and movable. Rectal musculature intact. Nonpalpable prostate. Nonpalpable lymph nodes in groin.	Discharge from penis. Ulcers, sores, other types of lesions. Testicles tender, swollen. Relaxed anal sphincter. Hemorrhoids. Positive hemocult slide. Enlarged prostate. Enlarged lymph nodes in groin.
Legs and feet	Supine Prone	Tape measure	Inspection Mensuration Palpation	Normal muscle tone and range of motion. No edema. Pulses normal. No varicosities. Toenails smooth, no signs of fungus or other infection. Calves equal in size.	Muscle weakness. Poor range of motion. Edema. Diminished pulse. Varicose veins. Toenails ridged, infected. Unequal calf measurements.
Neurological exam	Supine	Percussion hammer Safety pin Cotton ball	Percussion Inspection	Normal reflexes oriented to time and place. Appropriate responses. Normal responses to sensation. Alert. Steady gait. No vertigo or syncope.	All reflexes disoriented. Inappropriate responses. Dulled response to pain and sensation. Lethargic. Unsteady gait. Poor coordination. Vertigo. Syncope.

pressure is 20 to 25 mm Hg. An increase above normal will be found in glaucoma. The physician will use an ophthalmoscope to view the retina of the eye. This is done by turning out the lights in the room allowing pupils to dilate. The patient is instructed to look straight ahead while the physician looks into the eye. Retinal changes indicate disease.

Ears. An otoscope is used by the physician to examine the ears. The external ear is checked for redness in the ear canal and buildup of cerumen. A healthy tympanic membrane has a pearly gray appearance. A red appearance to the tympanic membrane may indicate infection in the middle ear, known as otitis media. **Vertigo** may indicate that the patient has an inner ear infection or **labyrinthitis**. **Tinnitus** or ringing in the ears may indicate inner ear problems. Other symptoms of ear problems include pain, discharge, and deafness. The tuning fork is used in testing the sensations of hearing, including bone conduction and air conduction.

Nose. The nasal cavity will be visualized by the physician with the use of a nasal speculum. Discharge from the nose may indicate a postnasal drip in which the sinuses may be draining into the nose and throat. Other abnormalities may include obstruction due to a deviated septum. Polyps and ulcerations may be found in the nasal cavity. Epistaxis or nosebleed may be seen when the capillaries rupture on the surface of the nasal mucosa.

Mouth and Throat. The physician will use a tongue blade or depressor and a light source. The teeth and gums will be checked for dental hygiene such as caries and the gums will be checked for signs of **pyorrhea** (discharge of pus from the gums around the teeth). If the tonsils are present, they will be checked for signs of infection such as redness or white pockets of pus. The larynx and pharynx are examined in the same manner, using laryngeal and pharyngeal mirrors to look for abnormal redness and patches indicating a disease. The floor of the mouth is examined both visually and by palpation for indications of swollen glands and ulcerations.

Neck. The physician palpates the neck looking for swollen lymph nodes. The thyroid gland is palpated anteriorly and posteriorly for size, symmetry, and texture. The patient will be asked to swallow several times while the physician feels the thyroid gland. A small glass of water may be given to the patient to aid in swallowing. Range of motion will be checked by having the patient turn the head in each direction. Care must be taken with the elderly. The patient should be instructed to move the head slowly.

Chest. The symmetry of the chest is observed, both anteriorly and posteriorly. Chest measurement may have been performed prior to the examination. The chest of a patient with emphysema will appear barrellike in shape. While the patient is sitting, the physician will listen to the lungs with a stethoscope. The patient may be instructed to take several deep breaths during this process.

 Carefully monitor the patient, particularly the elderly, as deep breathing may cause dizziness. The physician will be listening for abnormal lung sounds previously discussed. The physician may examine the lungs by percussion. Heart sounds will be auscultated both anteriorly and posteriorly. In cases of heart disease, the medical assistant may have been instructed to obtain an electrocardiogram.

Breast. The patient will be placed in a supine position and instructed to place the hand behind the head on the side on which the examination is taking place. The physician will examine the breast for masses by using a circular motion starting at the outer edge of the breast and working toward the center. The nipple will then be gently squeezed to see if there is any discharge. The patient is then instructed to change arm positions so that the other breast may be examined. With the patient in a sitting position, the physician will observe the breasts for symmetry. Female patients should be instructed on the procedure to follow for performing monthly breast self-examination. This may be an embarrassing procedure for the female. Maintain as much modesty as possible by carefully draping and giving emotional support. See Chapter 14 for more detailed information on breast examination.

Abdomen. The patient is placed in a dorsal recumbent or supine position with the arms at the sides for examination of the abdomen. The drape is lowered to just above the pubic hair. The female patient will wear a gown open in the front which can be pulled to the sides while still covering the breast. The physician will normally stand on the right side of the patient while performing this part of the examination. The abdomen will be examined by palpation, percussion, and auscultation. Following the quadrants of the abdomen, the physician will gently palpate the organs in each quadrant working from side to side. The physician will feel for organ size and location as well as the presence of masses, percuss the abdomen listening for sounds from abdominal organs, use the stethoscope to listen for presence of abdominal sounds, and will visually inspect the abdominal area for changes in skin color, scars, or other abnormalities. The contour of the abdomen may be flat or slightly convex. The presence of hernias will be checked both in the supine and standing positions. Patients with abdominal disorders may give a history of dyspepsia, dysphagia and/or excessive flatulence, nausea, and vomiting.

Genitalia. Also refer to Chapters 14 and 16 for more detailed information.

Female Genitalia. The patient is placed in the lithotomy position. The physician will examine both the external genitalia and reproductive organs. The rectum may be examined and a hemoccult test done at the conclusion of the pelvic examination. See Chapter 18 for information regarding the hemoccult slide test. After the examination, the patient is instructed to slide toward the head of the table and may be allowed to sit up slowly. Haste may cause orthostatic hypotension and dizziness.

Male Genitalia. Care must be taken to protect patient modesty and privacy. The physician will begin the examination by inspecting and retracting the foreskin of the penis if the patient is uncircumcised. The glans penis will be inspected for discharge and redness. The penis and scrotum will then be palpated for possible tenderness and masses. Due to the seriousness of testicular cancer, the patient will be instructed, usually by the physician, in the procedure to perform monthly testicular examinations. Refer to Chapter 16.

Rectal Examinations. The physician may examine the rectum as a part of the male genitalia exam. The patient is placed in either the Sims' or knee-chest position. The physician will perform a manual examination. The prostate gland is then examined by palpation. The physician inserts the gloved index finger into the rectum and palpates the prostate gland for any masses or swelling.

(See Chapter 16 for more information.) A lubricated rectal speculum may then be inserted for visual examination. Since this is uncomfortable for the patient, emotional support is important. The physician can visualize the rectum for any bleeding, fissures, polyps, or lesions.

Reflexes. The patient's reflexes are observed by the physician in both the supine and sitting positions. A percussion hammer is used. While sitting with the arm flexed, the elbow will be lightly tapped to elicit movement from the biceps. The patellar or knee-jerk reflex is tested by tapping the area just below the patella at the knee. The Achilles reflex or ankle-jerk is tested by tapping the Achilles tendon. The Babinski reflex is tested on the sole of a relaxed foot (the great toe will flex) with the patient in a supine position. Reflexes determine the integrity of the neurological system.

Procedure 13-9 outlines the steps in assisting with the physical examination.

Once the examination has been completed, the patient will be instructed to dress. The patient should be given privacy while dressing. Assist the patient as needed. Do not remain in the room to clean it while the patient is dressing. Remain in the room if the patient requires assistance. Further instructions regarding other testing procedures and treatment plans will be provided by the physician. Be specific with instructions to patients regarding what they should do after they are completely dressed.

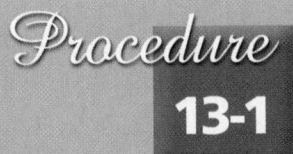

Positioning Patient in the Supine Position

STANDARD PRECAUTIONS:

PURPOSE:
To safely and properly assist patient into supine position for examination of anterior surface of the body from head to toe.

EQUIPMENT/SUPPLIES:
Drape
Gown

PROCEDURE STEPS:
1. Wash hands and follow standard precautions.
2. Assemble supplies.

3. Assist patient to sit on end of table.
4. Assist patient to lie back on table as you pull out the table extension. Support patient's feet and back while extending foot of table.
5. Cover patient with drape from shoulders to ankles.
6. Place small pillow under patient's head.
7. Upon completion of a procedure, assist patient to sitting position. RATIONALE: Allowing patient to remain seated helps to prevent dizziness caused by orthostatic hypotension.
8. Push table extension back into place while supporting patient's feet.
9. Once patient is stable (check color of skin, pulse), give further instructions as required.

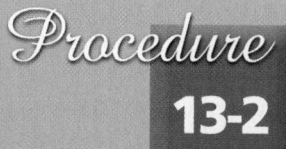

Positioning Patient in the Dorsal Recumbent Position
13-2

STANDARD PRECAUTIONS:

PURPOSE:
To safely and properly assist patient to dorsal recumbent position for catheterization or pelvic exam, head, neck, chest, abdominal, or lower limb examination.

EQUIPMENT/SUPPLIES:
Drape
Gown

PROCEDURE STEPS:
1. Wash hands and follow standard precautions.
2. Assist patient to sit on end of table.

3. Assist patient to lie back on table; extend the foot of the table while you support patient's feet and back.
4. Assist patient to bend knees and place feet flat on the surface of the table. Push in foot extension.
5. Cover patient with drape (diamond shape) from shoulders to ankles.
6. Place small pillow under patient's head.
7. Upon completion of procedure, assist patient to sitting position while you push table extension back into place and support patient's feet.
8. Have patient sit at end of table for a few minutes. RATIONALE: This helps prevent dizziness and possible fall from low blood pressure due to orthostatic hypotension.
9. Once patient is stable (check color of skin, pulse), give further instructions as required.

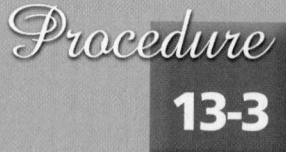

Positioning Patient in the Lithotomy Position
13-3

STANDARD PRECAUTIONS:

PURPOSE:
To safely and properly assist patient in lithotomy position for genital or pelvic examination or for urinary catheterization.

EQUIPMENT/SUPPLIES:
Drape
Gown

PROCEDURE STEPS:
1. Wash hands and follow standard precautions.
2. Have patient disrobe from waist down and put on gown.

3. Assist patient to sit on end of table. Cover patient's lap and legs with drape.
4. Assist patient to lie back on table as you support patient's feet and back while extending foot of table.
5. Position stirrups level with the table and approximately one foot from edge of table. Lock stirrups into position. RATIONALE: Facilitates patient examination and ensures patient safety.
6. Have patient slide down on table. Have patient move as close to edge of examination table as possible.
7. Assist patient to bend knees and assist her in placing feet in stirrups. Move drape to diamond shape to ensure privacy.
8. Place small pillow under patient's head.

(continues)

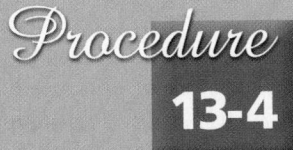

Procedure **13-3** (continued)

9. Upon completion of procedure, extend foot extension of table.
10. Place feet on foot extension and assist patient to slide toward head of table.
11. Assist patient to sitting position while replacing foot extension.

12. Have patient sit at end of table for a few minutes. RATIONALE: This helps prevent dizziness and possible fall from low blood pressure due to orthostatic hypotension.
13. Once patient is stable (check color of skin, pulse), give further instructions as required.

Procedure **13-4** Positioning Patient in the Fowler's Position

STANDARD PRECAUTIONS:

PURPOSE:
To safely and properly assist patient into the Fowler's position for examination of upper body and head; often used for patients with cardiovascular or respiratory problems.

EQUIPMENT/SUPPLIES:
Drape
Gown

PROCEDURE STEPS:
1. Wash hands and follow standard precautions.
2. Provide gown and assist to disrobe if necessary.
3. Assist patient to sit on end of table. Cover lap and legs with drape.

4. Assist patient to slide back on table leaning against the back rest which has been raised slightly.
5. Support patient's feet while extending foot of table.
6. Position head of table at a 90° angle (45° for Semi-Fowler's).
7. Place pillow under patient's knees for comfort.
8. Cover patient with drape from shoulders to ankles.
9. Upon completion of procedure, replace foot extension.
10. Have patient sit at end of table for a few minutes. RATIONALE: This helps prevent dizziness and possible fall from low blood pressure due to orthostatic hypotension.
11. Once patient is stable (check color of skin, pulse), give further instructions as required.

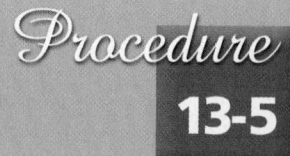

Procedure 13-5

Positioning Patient in the Knee-Chest Position

STANDARD PRECAUTIONS:

PURPOSE:

To safely and properly assist patient in knee-chest position for examination of the rectum, sigmoid colon, and in some instances the vagina.

EQUIPMENT/SUPPLIES:

Drape
Gown

PROCEDURE STEPS:

1. Wash hands and follow standard precautions.
2. Have patient completely undress. Provide gown.
3. Instruct patient to sit on end of table with drape over lap and legs.
4. Instruct patient to lie back on table while you support patient's feet and back and extend foot of table.
5. Assist patient to turn onto abdomen by turning toward you and being careful to stay in center of table to avoid a fall. Support patient by placing your left hand on patient's back and guide the patient toward you. Adjust drape.
6. Assist patient to rise to knees while bending at hips to place chest on table, keeping covered with drape.
7. Arms are bent to side of head with hands under head.
8. If this position is uncomfortable, have patient rest on elbows. Adjust drape from shoulders to ankles.
9. Upon completion of procedure, assist patient to lie flat on abdomen and then turn onto the back toward you and then return to sitting position.
10. Have patient sit at end of table for a few minutes. RATIONALE: This helps prevent dizziness and possible fall from low blood pressure due to orthostatic hypotension.
11. Once patient is stable (check color of skin, pulse), give further instructions as required.

NOTE: Since this is an embarrassing and uncomfortable position, it is best that the patient not be placed into this position until the physician is ready for the examination.

Procedure 13-6

Positioning Patient in the Prone Position

STANDARD PRECAUTIONS:

PURPOSE:

To safely and properly assist patient into the prone position for examination of posterior aspect of the body including the back, spine, or legs.

EQUIPMENT/SUPPLIES:

Drape
Gown

PROCEDURE STEPS:

1. Wash hands and follow standard precautions.
2. Have patient undress. Provide gown.
3. Assist patient to sit on end of table. Place drape over lap and legs.
4. Assist patient to lie back on table while you support patient's feet and back and extend foot of table.
5. Assist patient to turn toward you, then onto abdomen being careful to stay in center of table to avoid a fall. Place pillow under feet and head.
6. Adjust patient drape from shoulders to ankles.

(continues)

Procedure 13-6 (continued)

7. Upon completion of procedure, assist patient to turn toward you, then assist to sitting position.
8. Have patient sit at end of table for a few minutes. RATIONALE: This helps prevent dizziness and possible fall from low blood pressure due to orthostatic hypotension.
9. Once patient is stable (check color of skin, pulse), give further instructions as required.

Procedure 13-7 Positioning Patient in the Sims' Position

STANDARD PRECAUTIONS:

PURPOSE:
To safely and properly assist patient into Sims' position for rectal examination, rectal temperature, proctoscopy, sigmoidoscopy, for an enema, and in some instances for vaginal examination.

EQUIPMENT/SUPPLIES:
Drape
Gown

PROCEDURE STEPS:
1. Wash hands and follow standard precautions.
2. Have patient undress. Provide gown.
3. Assist patient to sit on end of table. Place drape over lap and legs.
4. Assist patient to lie back on table while you support patient's feet and back and extend foot of table.
5. Assist patient to turn toward you onto the left side with left arm behind body, placing body weight on chest. Adjust drape.
6. Assist patient to slightly flex left knee and flex right knee to a 90° angle for support.
7. Right arm is bent in front of body with hand toward head at an angle to provide support.
8. Adjust drape from shoulders to ankles creating triangle or diamond shape.
9. Upon completion of procedure, instruct patient to turn toward you, then onto back, and then to sitting position.
10. Have patient sit at end of table for a few minutes. RATIONALE: This helps prevent dizziness and possible fall from low blood pressure due to orthostatic hypotension.
11. Once patient is stable (check color of skin, pulse), give further instructions as required.

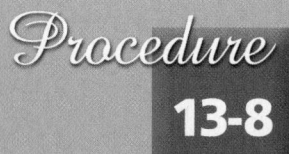

Positioning Patient in the Trendelenburg Position

13-8

STANDARD PRECAUTIONS:

PURPOSE:
To safely and properly assist patient into Trendelenburg position for certain abdominal and pelvic surgical procedures.

EQUIPMENT/SUPPLIES:
Drape
Gown

PROCEDURE STEPS:
1. Wash hands and follow standard precautions.
2. Assist patient to undress. Provide gown.
3. Assist patient to sit on end of table. Place drape over lap and legs.
4. Assist patient to lie back on table, with head at head board. Adjust drape.
5. Patient's feet are flexed over the end of the table.
6. Head of table may be lowered to a 45° angle.
7. Adjust drape from shoulders to ankles to ensure privacy.
8. Upon completion of procedure, assist patient to return to sitting position.
9. Allow patient to sit at end of table for a few minutes. RATIONALE: This helps prevent dizziness and possible fall from low blood pressure due to orthostatic hypotension.
10. Once patient is stable (check color of skin, pulse), give further instructions as required.

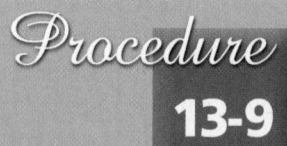

Assisting with a Complete Physical Examination

13-9

STANDARD PRECAUTIONS:

PURPOSE:
To assist physician in a complete physical examination.

EQUIPMENT/SUPPLIES:

Balance beam scales	Tape measure
Pharyngeal mirror	Thermometer
Lubricant	Stethoscope
Examination lights	Sphygmomanometer
Penlight	Alcohol wipes
Gloves	Cotton balls
Emesis basin	Gauze sponges
Percussion hammer	Safety pins
Patient gown	Otoscope
Drape	Tuning fork
Tissues	Ophthalmoscope
Specimen bottles/ slides—request forms	Tonometer Nasal speculum
Biohazard and regular waste container	Tongue depressors Laryngeal mirror

PROCEDURE STEPS:
1. Wash hands. Adhere to Standard Precautions.
2. Assemble equipment.
3. Place instruments in easily accessible sequence for physician use. RATIONALE: Efficient use of time and space.
4. Greet and identify patient.
5. Explain procedure to patient. RATIONALE: To obtain patient cooperation and allay apprehension.
6. Review medical history with patient. Refer to Chapter 11 for obtaining patient history. RATIONALE: To assure complete history has been obtained and is current.

(continues)

Procedure
13-9 *(continued)*

7. Take and record patient vital signs, visual acuity, and hearing test results.
8. Obtain a urine specimen. Refer to Chapter 30 for urine collection procedures.
9. Obtain all required blood samples. Refer to Chapters 28 and 29 for blood specimen collection procedures.
10. Perform electrocardiogram if directed by physician. Refer to Chapter 25 for ECG procedure.
11. Provide patient with appropriate gown and drape.
12. Assist patient to disrobe completely; explain where the opening for the gown is to be placed. RATIONALE: To assist patient in maintaining modesty, privacy, and warmth.
13. Assist patient in sitting at the end of the table; drape patient across lap and legs. RATIONALE: Always drape patient to maintain modesty.
14. Inform physician when patient is ready.
15. When the physician arrives, remain by the patient ready to assist patient and physician.
16. Position patient in a sitting or supine position for the head, throat, eye, ear, and neck examination.
17. Lights may be turned off to allow pupils to dilate for retinal examination.
18. Hand the physician instruments as required (some physicians will not require the medical assistant to hand the instruments).
19. The sitting position will be maintained for auscultation of the chest and heart.
20. Assist the patient into a supine position and drape for examination of the chest. Breast examination is discussed in Chapter 14.
21. Maintain a quiet atmosphere to enhance the ability of the physician in hearing heart and lung sounds. RATIONALE: Quiet is necessary to hear heart and chest sounds accurately.
22. Position patient in supine position and drape for abdominal examinations and examination of extremities.
23. Gynecological examination may then be performed. Refer to Chapter 14. Assist patient into lithotomy position for gynecological examination. Male genitalia examined.
24. If rectal examination is necessary, assist patient into Sims' position.
25. Place patient in prone position for examination of posterior aspect of body.
26. Upon completion of the examination, assist patient to sitting position and allow to sit at end of table for a few minutes. RATIONALE: Allows patients to recover from potential dizziness.
27. Assure patient stability (check color of skin, pulse) before allowing patient to stand up. RATIONALE: Prevents the possibility of a patient fainting from orthostatic hypotension.
28. Assist patient in dressing; provide privacy.
29. Chart any notes or patient instructions per physician orders.
30. Escort patient to physician's office for discussion of examination results.
31. Put on disposable gloves.
32. Dispose of gown and drape in biohazard waste container. RATIONALE: Prevent microorganism cross contamination; gown and drape may have body secretions on them.
33. Dispose of contaminated materials in biohazard container. RATIONALE: Prevent microorganism cross contamination of bloodborne pathogens and other potentially infectious materials (OPIM).
34. Remove table paper and dispose in biohazard waste container. RATIONALE: Prevent microorganism cross contamination.
35. Disinfect counters and examination table with a solution of 10 percent bleach. RATIONALE: Prevent microorganism cross contamination by blood and OPIM.
36. Clean, disinfect, or sterilize reusable instruments as appropriate (refer to Chapters 10 and 19). RATIONALE: Prevent microorganism cross contamination.
37. Remove gloves, discard in biohazard waste container. RATIONALE: Prevent microorganism cross contamination by blood and OPIM.
38. Wash hands.
39. Replace table paper and equipment in preparation for the next patient.
40. Document the procedure.

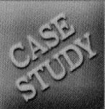

At Inner City Health Care, clinical medical assistant Wanda Slawson is helping Liz Corbin, a part-time administrative/clinical medical assistant, learn to prepare the examination room and patients for the physical examination. In addition to alerting Liz to physician preferences, Wanda wants to be sure that Liz has a solid understanding of the methods of examination, positions and draping, and the components of the physical exam.

13-1

CASE STUDY REVIEW

1. In reviewing with Liz the methods of examination used by physicians, what six primary methods would Wanda have Liz describe?

2. What patient positions would Liz need to know?

3. Wanda asks Liz to recall the various examination components and their significance. How should Liz respond?

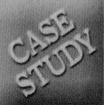

Mrs. Mason, a 72-year-old somewhat frail female with arthritis and hypertensive heart disease has an appointment today for a complete physical exam. It will include a basic physical exam and an exam of the pelvis because she has had bright red vaginal spotting.

13-2 ### CASE STUDY REVIEW

1. Discuss positions and draping for the physical exam including pelvic for this patient.

2. Discuss any special safety needs for Mrs. Mason.

3. What additional supplies and/or equipment should be available for the physician?

SUMMARY

A complete physical examination should be performed on the initial visit of the patient. Findings at this examination, both normal and abnormal, provide a baseline for future examinations.

The role of the medical assistant throughout the examination is twofold. The assistant assembles the necessary instruments and may hand them to the physician when requested. The medical assistant will also prepare specimens as required by the examination and physician. Responsibilities to the patient include explanations and careful positioning, protecting modesty by careful draping and, most important, providing comfort, emotional support, and safety ensurance. By performing these duties, the medical assistant can assure patient compliance and physician efficiency.

REVIEW QUESTIONS

Multiple Choice

1. The method of examination that is the process of listening directly to body sounds is called:
   a. percussion
   b. auditory
   c. auscultation
   d. the direct method

2. The supine position is also known as:
   a. horizontal recumbent
   b. dorsal recumbent
   c. knee-chest
   d. Sims'

3. During the physical examination, ataxia might be observed, which relates to:
   a. stature
   b. posture

c. body movement

d. speech

4. When the patient asks a question of the medical assistant, the medical assistant should:

   a. refer all questions to the physician

   b. try to answer all questions, even if uncertain

   c. answer questions to the extent of knowledge; refer others to the physician

   d. ask the patient to please hold all questions until the examination is complete

5. When the abdomen is being examined, the patient is typically in a:

   a. supine position

   b. prone position

   c. Fowler's position

   d. Sims' position

Critical Thinking

1. Discuss the responsibilities of the medical assistant during a physical examination.

2. Review the six methods used in the physical examination.

3. Give two reasons why positioning and draping are done.

4. Describe a type of examination that may be performed while the patient is placed in each of the following positions:

   a. lithotomy:

   b. Sims':

   c. knee-chest:

   d. supine:

5. List and describe the various components of a physical examination.

6. Explain the sequence for a physical examination.

7. List the instruments and/or supplies needed for examining the following body areas:

   a. head:

   b. reflexes:

   c. chest:

   d. abdomen:

8. Describe the cleaning process that the following instruments will need after their use in an examination:

a. nasal speculum

b. tuning fork

c. percussion hammer

d. reusable otoscope speculum

9. List and describe the three sources of information the physician uses to aid in making a diagnosis.

10. List two procedures or tests the medical assistant might perform as part of the patient's physical examination.

WEB ACTIVITIES

1. Using one of the "gateways" for general health and medical information and its links to other sites, gather information about the U.S. government's guidelines for average adult height and weight measurements. According to the government tables, what is considered an appropriate weight for your height?

2. Explore the Web for information about the following conditions and their possible causes:

   - changes in retinal blood vessels
   - enlarged liver
   - ascites
   - varicose veins
   - vertigo

REFERENCES/BIBLIOGRAPHY

Fremgen, B. F. (1998). *Essentials of medical assisting: Administrative and clinical competencies* (1st ed.). Upper Saddle River, NJ: Prentice Hall/Simon & Schuster.

Keir, L., Wise, B. A., & Krebs, C. (1998). *Medical assisting: Administrative and clinical competencies* (4th ed.). Albany, NY: Delmar.

Kinn, M. E., & Woods, M. A. (1999). *The medical assistant: Administrative and clinical* (8th ed.). Philadelphia: W. B. Saunders.

Taber's cyclopedic medical dictionary (18th ed.). (1999). Philadelphia: F. A. Davis.

Thibodeau, G., & Patton, K. (1996). *The human body in health & disease* (2nd ed.). St. Louis: Mosby Year Book.

Zakus, S. (1995). *Clinical procedures for medical assistants* (2nd ed.). St. Louis: Mosby Year Book.

ASSISTING WITH SPECIALTY EXAMINATIONS AND PROCEDURES

OBSTETRICS AND GYNECOLOGY

KEY TERMS

Abortion
Amniocentesis
Bartholin Gland
Braxton-Hicks
Candidiasis
Carcinoma in situ
Cervical Punch Biopsy
Cesarean Section
Chlamydia
Colposcopy
Condylomata
Congenital Anomalies
Coupling Agent
Cryosurgery
Dilation
Dysmenorrhea
Dyspareunia
Dysplasia
Eclampsia
Ectopic
Effacement
Endometriosis
Fulgarated
Genitalia
Gestation
Gestational Diabetes
Gravidy
Human Chorionic Gonadotrophin
Hyperemesis Gravidarum
Hysterosalpingogram
Involution
Lamaze
Lochia   (*continues*)

OUTLINE

Obstetrics
Initial Prenatal Visit
Subsequent or Return Prenatal
    Visits
Complications of Pregnancy
Parturition
Postpartum Period

Gynecology
The Gynecological Examination
Gynecological Diseases and
    Conditions
Other Diagnostic Tests Used to
    Detect Female Reproductive
    System Diseases

OBJECTIVES

The student should strive to meet the following performance objectives and demonstrate an understanding of the facts and principles presented in this chapter through written and oral communication.

1. Explain the importance of prenatal care, and discuss what examinations will be performed as part of the initial visit.

2. Explain why the initial prenatal visit is important.

3. Describe what laboratory tests and procedures are performed during the initial prenatal visit.

4. List 12 conditions and/or diseases that can cause a pregnant woman and her fetus to be at greater risk for problems during the pregnancy.

5. List signs and symptoms and their possible corresponding conditions that the physician searches for during the prenatal history and physical examination.

6. Calculate an EDC (or EDB) using Nagele's Rule.

7. Explain the purpose of ultrasonography and amniocentesis.

8. List and describe six types of abortion.

9. Explain what occurs in each of the three stages of labor.

10. Describe what takes place during the postpartum examination.

11. List and describe the diseases and disorders that can affect the female.

12. Describe the laboratory tests and procedures that can help diagnose the diseases and disorders that can affect the female.   (*continues*)

KEY TERMS (*continued*)

Multigravida
Nagele's rule
Neonatal
Nullipara
Oxytoxin
Parity
Parturition
Patent
Pelvic Inflammatory Disease
Placenta Abruptio
Placenta Previa
Polycystic
Pre-eclampsia
Prenatal
Primigravida
Prostaglandin
Puerperium
Sickle Cell Anemia
Tay-Sachs
Thalassemia
Titer
Trichomoniasis
Trimester
Ultrasonography
Viable

OBJECTIVES (*continued*)

13. Describe seven sexually transmitted diseases.
14. Explain the medical assistant's responsibilities with a gynecological exam.
15. Describe breast self-examination and method of teaching patient breast self-examination.
16. Discuss menopause.
17. Explain hormone replacement therapy.
18. Describe several methods of contraception.
19. Explain reasons for impaired fertility.
20. Describe three therapies to assist in reproduction.

ROLE DELINEATION COMPONENTS

CLINICAL

Fundamental Principles

- Apply principles of aseptic technique and infection control
- Screen and follow up patient test results

Patient Care

- Obtain patient history and vital signs
- Prepare patient for examinations, procedures and treatments

Diagnostic Orders

- Collect and process specimens
- Perform diagnostic tests

(*continues*)

SCENARIO

At Inner City Health Care in the obstetrical department, Wanda Slawson and Bruce Goldman, both certified medical assistants, are preparing for the day's appointments. Both take responsibility for being certain all rooms have appropriate equipment and supplies needed for today's patients. There are three ultrasonograms in addition to the pelvic exams, Pap smear, and breast exams scheduled for the afternoon. Wanda is responsible for assisting the physician with each of them. She is careful to follow all safety precautions before, during, and after assisting with exams and procedures. She is careful to explain procedures to the patients and to direct any questions to the physician.

INTRODUCTION

Obstetrics is the medical specialty in which the physician treats the female from the prenatal period through labor, delivery, and during the six-week postpartum period. Gynecology is the specialty that treats the medical and surgical disorders and diseases of the female reproductive tract. Both specialties are usually combined, and the physician who practices them is known as an obstetrician/gynecologist, or simply, an OB/GYN physician. Knowledge of

ROLE DELINEATION COMPONENTS (continued)

GENERAL (TRANSDISCIPLINARY)

Legal Concepts

● Document accurately

Instruction

● Instruct individuals according to their needs

● Teach methods of health promotion and disease prevention

the female anatomy, the laboratory tests and procedures for both specialties, the diseases and disorders that affect the female during her nonpregnant and pregnant states, and patient education are essential for the medical assistant who will care for these patients. The goal of the OB/GYN specialty is to promote the health and well-being of the woman and her baby.

OBSTETRICS

Obstetrics is the branch of medicine that provides care to the mother and fetus during pregnancy, labor, delivery, and the postpartum period known as the **puerperium**. Pregnancy is a period of approximately forty weeks from the day that conception takes place (Figure 14-1). The puerperium is the period of six weeks following delivery when the mother's body is returning to its prepregnant state. Visits to the physician for pre- and postnatal care are the initial **prenatal** visit, return visits, and the six-week postpartum checkup.

Initial Prenatal Visit

The initial prenatal visit is of utmost importance and usually occurs after a woman has missed a second menstrual period or after an at-home pregnancy test is positive. It is a time of health promotion for the expectant mother and her baby. It is also the time for diagnosis and treatment of maternal disorders that may have been present before the pregnancy or that may have developed during the course of the pregnancy. Growth and development of the fetus are followed and identification of problems that may impede a normal labor are sought. There is ongoing assessment of the expectant mother and the fetus. Any abnormalities can indicate a problem or complication necessitating further testing and assessment. Early detection and management of conditions such as **gestational diabetes**, urinary tract infections, anemia, and **preeclampsia** can prevent serious complications.

The initial visit requires more time than subsequent visits because a thorough history and physical examination are done, including breast, abdominal, pelvic, and vaginal exams. Pelvic measurements are taken to help

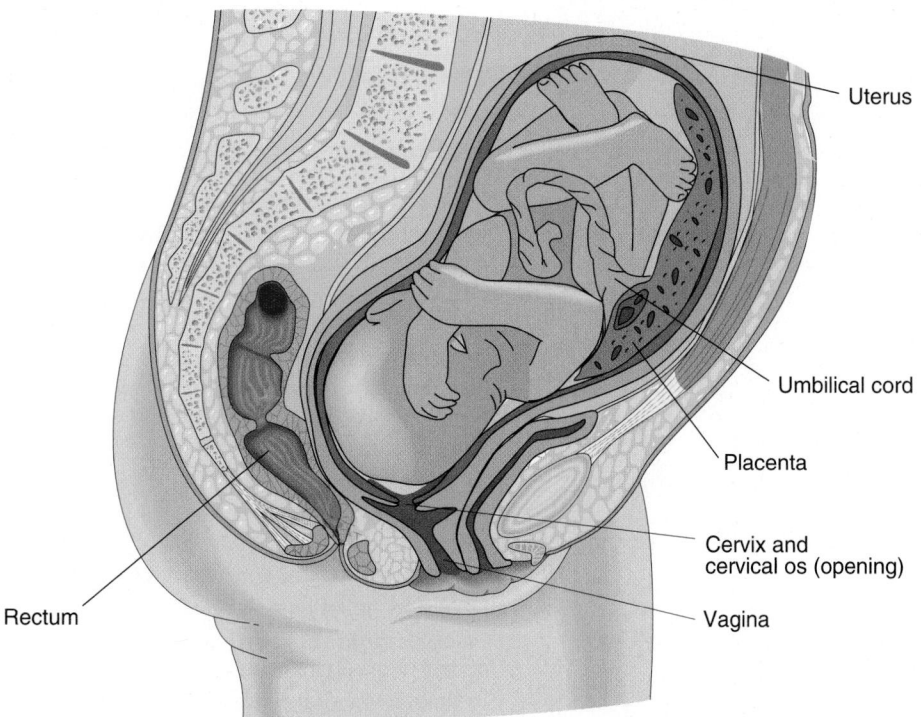

Figure 14-1 Normal uterine pregnancy.

ascertain if the pelvis is adequate for a fetus to be delivered vaginally.

The initial visit is followed by monthly visits and then weekly visits beginning about the twenty-eighth week. The routine visits consist of checking weight, blood pressure, testing blood and urine, education about nutrition, activity and rest, and preparing for childbirth.

Many groups of women do not receive prenatal care. Lack of financial resources, lack of transportation, and poor communication by health care providers are some of the reasons that some women do not participate in prenatal care. Modesty may deter some women from seeking prenatal care. Exposing the body to a male is viewed as a major violation of modesty in some cultures. This is why protecting the privacy of all patients is critical.

Certain cultures expect their women to observe practices believed to ensure a favorable pregnancy. Mexican women are advised not to watch an eclipse of the moon; the belief is that the baby will be born with congenital anomalies. Some Spanish women in the United States wear a braided cord around the midsection to ward off nausea and to ensure safe birth. Medals and beads, often worn by women, are believed to ward off evil spirits. Other cultures believe that inactivity during pregnancy will safeguard the mother and baby. There are also many dietary influences within different cultures. (See Chapter 22 for more information about culture and diet and food choices.) Respect for all cultures is of great importance and judgments should not be made that some women are ignorant or lazy.

All women should be fully involved in their care. Women with physical or emotional disabilities must have their particular needs addressed. When necessary, make adaptations whenever possible for women who are mentally challenged, blind, deaf, or physically incapacitated.

Laboratory Tests. The laboratory tests that are part of the initial prenatal visit are described in Table 14-1.

Patient Education. Patient education includes such topics as nutrition, dental care, rest, and exercise as well as discussion about over-the-counter (OTC) and prescription medications. Alcohol and tobacco and their dangers and potential harm to fetus and mother should also be discussed. Medications, alcohol, cigarettes, and mind-altering substances taken by the mother have deleterious effects on the fetus and should not be used.

Before the birth, the expectant couple is encouraged to choose a method of feeding the infant. During the initial prenatal visit, benefits of breast-feeding the newborn are discussed. Breast-feeding is encouraged because it offers many nutritional, psychological, and immunologic benefits. Because the immune system of newborns is not fully developed, the high level of immunoglobulins in breast milk gives them protection against some pathogenic diseases of the respiratory and gastrointestinal tracts. Close contact between mother and newborn is certain with breast-feeding, and bonding can readily take place. Breast-fed infants seem to have fewer allergic reactions. For the mother, one benefit of breast-feeding is that

---

TABLE 14-1   LABORATORY TESTS AT THE INITIAL PRENATAL VISIT

Laboratory Test	Disease or Condition
Complete blood count (CBC)	To detect anemia or infection
Urinalysis with microscopic examination (pH, specific gravity, color, glucose, albumin, proteins, WBC, RBC, casts, ocetone, human chorionic gonadotrophin [HCG])	To detect diabetes mellitus, renal disease, infection, hypertensive disease, pregnancy
Blood type, Rh factor	To detect Rh incompatibility
Rubella titer	To determine immunity to rubella
Renal function	Renal impairment evaluation in women with history of diabetes mellitus, hypertension, or kidney disease
Tuberculin skin test	Screens for tuberculosis
Venereal disease research lab (VDRL) and rapid plasma reagin (RPR)	To detect syphilis
Human Immunodeficiency Virus (HIV) with patient permission	Screens for HIV antibodies
Hepatitis B+C virus	Screens for hepatitis B and hepatitis C viruses
Glucose Tolerance Test (GTT)	Screens for gestational diabetes
Cardiac evaluation electrocardiogram (ECG), chest x ray, and/or echocardiogram	Evaluates cardiac function in women with history of heart disease or hypertension
Pap smear	To check for cervical dysplasia, herpes simplex virus 2
Vaginal and/or rectal smear or culture	To check for gonorrhea, chlamydia, human papilloma virus (HPV)

the uterus **involutes**, or returns more quickly to the non-pregnant state.

Formal childbirth education classes given in various languages teach the fundamentals of labor, delivery, and newborn care and feeding.

Prenatal History. The prenatal history will be comprehensive and include much of the same information that is obtained during the taking of a regular medical history. However, emphasis will be on identification of the high-risk patient. Particular attention is given to women who have a history of one or more of the following situations or conditions because they may place women at greater risk during pregnancy:

- Use of legal drugs (OTC, prescription, tobacco, caffeine, alcohol), illegal drugs (marijuana, cocaine), and herbal products

- Age under 16 and over 35 years

- Rh negative blood (particularly if father has Rh positive blood)

- A history of repeated premature labors and deliveries, abortions, or stillbirths

- Genetic diseases in the family

- Previous **Cesarean section**

- Diabetes

- Hypothyroidism or hyperthyroidism

- Sexually transmitted disease

- Hypertension

- Nutritional deficiencies

- Cardiac problems

- Kidney conditions

- Epilepsy

- Headaches

Any of these conditions or diseases place the woman and fetus at risk for serious complications.

During the initial prenatal visit, an obstetrical history is taken, which includes the **gravidy**, or total number of pregnancies, including the present pregnancy, regardless of duration. The history also includes the **parity**, the number of pregnancies carried to the point of viability regardless of whether the baby was born alive or dead. Multiple births, twins, and triplets count as one pregnancy (gravida) and one delivery (para). For example, a woman pregnant for the first time is referred to as Gravida 1, Para 0. After this woman delivers, regardless if the baby is born alive or dead, if it reached the age of **viability**, the history of the woman is Gravida 1, Para 1. Viability is the ability to grow and develop after birth. The term **multigravida** refers to a woman who has been pregnant more than once. **Nullipara** describes a woman who has not carried a pregnancy to viability.

The present prenatal history includes information about the present pregnancy. The physician searches for problems indicative of high-risk factors. Identifying high-risk patients helps to limit maternal and newborn deaths and diseases. Some factors that indicate that a patient is at high risk are inadequate nutrition; use of drugs such as alcohol, tobacco, or cocaine; existing medical conditions such as high blood pressure or diabetes; sexually transmitted disease; and poverty. The physician watches for signs and symptoms that indicate a potentially serious condition. Examples are listed in Table 14-2.

TABLE 14-2	SIGNS AND SYMPTOMS OF POTENTIALLY SERIOUS CONDITIONS
Signs and Symptoms	**Possible Condition**
Rapid weight gain	Pre-eclampsia
Headaches	Pre-eclampsia
Hypertension	Pre-eclampsia
Vision changes	Pre-eclampsia
Severe nausea and vomiting	Hyperemesis gravidarum/ dehydration
Bleeding, discharge, abdominal pain/cramping	Threatened abortion
Edema	Pre-eclampsia
One sided pelvic or abdominal pain	Ectopic pregnancy (Figure 14-2)
Chills, fever	Vaginal infection, sexually transmitted disease

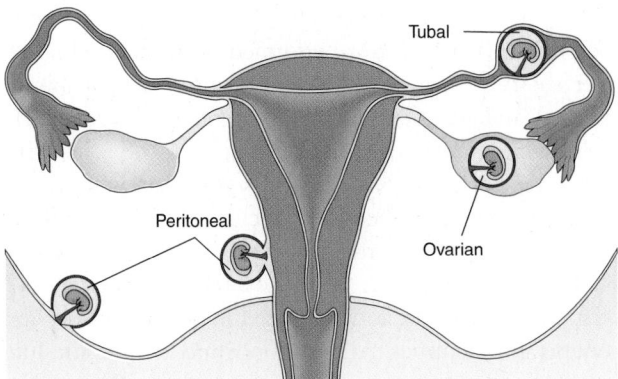

Figure 14-2 Sites of ectopic pregnancy.

Subsequent or Return Prenatal Visits

Each subsequent visit includes weight, blood pressure, urinalysis, complete blood count with hemoglobin and hematocrit, measurement of the height of the uterine fundus (a tape measure is used by placing it on the anterior symphysis pubis and the crest of the uterus), and fetal heart measurements. Generally, it is not possible to determine with accuracy the exact date of conception. Many formulas have been used for calculating the EDB (expected date of birth) or EDC (expected date of confinement). While none is foolproof, **Nagele's rule** is the usual method used because it is reasonably accurate. Nagele's rule is to add seven days to the first day of the last menstrual period (LMP), subtract three months, and add one year. An example is:

> the first day of LMP = July 10, 2000
> add 7 days = July 17
> subtract 3 months = April 17
> add one year = April 17, 2001

Another method to calculate EDB or EDC is to add seven days to LMP and count forward nine months. Most women give birth seven days before or after the EDB or EDC.

Vaginal exams are only done periodically up to two to three weeks prior to the EDB or EDC. Patients are encouraged to attend classes in the **Lamaze** method of childbirth as well as classes in the care of the newborn.

Tests and Procedures

Alpha Fetal Protein (AFP). Another test that may be done during a subsequent visit is a blood test known as alpha fetal protein blood test (AFP). It is done about the sixteenth week of pregnancy. It is a screening test only, done to rule out neural tube defects, abdominal wall defects, and chromosomal problems such as Down syndrome. If the test is positive, additional testing such as an **aminocentesis** or an ultrasound will be used to help make a diagnosis.

Chorionic Villi Sampling (CVS). Chorionic villi sampling (CVS) is a test performed on women who are over age thirty-five, have a history of chromosomal abnormalities, and are known carriers of a genetic disorder such as **thalassemia**, **sickle cell anemia**, or **Tay-Sachs**. The test is done at about 8 to 10 weeks **gestation** and has an advantage over amniocentesis because the latter cannot be done before the fourteenth week. For the CVS test, a sample of tissue that surrounds the fetus is taken by means of suction. The sample is analyzed in the laboratory for genetic abnormalities. An ultrasonogram is done simultaneously with an amniocentesis in order to avoid possible injury to the fetus or placenta.

Ultrasonography/Amniocentesis. Two tests can be done that can supply vital information: **ultrasonography**, or ultrasound, and amniocentesis. Ultrasound can be performed in the first, second, or third **trimester**. It uses high-frequency sound waves to produce an image of the fetus. A **coupling agent** is spread onto the mother's abdomen to enhance penetration of sound waves through the tissue, and the scanning mechanism is moved over the abdomen. An image of the fetus can be viewed on a screen similar to a television screen. Photos are taken during the exam. The technique usually takes about one half hour. There are no known side effects to the fetus or mother, and ultrasound uses no X rays. There is no pain involved, but slight discomfort can occur due to a full bladder. (A quart of fluid should be consumed one hour prior to the test and finished within 15 or 20 minutes.) A full bladder is essential to a good-quality ultrasound because it supports the uterus in position for good imaging. This procedure may be used to identify the number of fetuses, check the age of the fetus (number of weeks gestation), and detect some fetal abnormalities.

An amniocentesis is the surgical puncturing, with a long, thin needle, of the amniotic sac through the woman's abdomen. The purpose of this test is to obtain, by aspiration, a sample of amniotic fluid that contains fetal cells. The procedure can be done as early as fourteen weeks and helps to diagnose genetic mishaps, **congenital anomalies** (present at birth), and chromosomal defects. It also can be used to determine the lung capacity of the fetus.

Ultrasonography is performed while the physician is doing the amniocentesis to identify the position of the fetus and placenta, thereby avoiding injury to either. The procedure is not without risk and is not universally accepted. There can be bleeding, leaking of amniotic fluid, and infection.

Fetal heart rate is another test. Monitoring can be done in one of two ways: a nonstress test monitors the fetus's heart rate while it is moving spontaneously or a stress test monitors the fetal heart rate while the mother is stimulated with medication to have mild uterine contractions. Normally, the fetal heart rate will accelerate to a certain safe limit while it is being stressed.

Complications of Pregnancy

Abortion/Interruption of Pregnancy. The interruption of pregnancy before the fetus is viable is known as **abortion**. There are six types of abortion.

1. *Spontaneous:* Unknown etiology.
2. *Complete:* Expulsion of all products of conception, fetus, and placenta with no surgical intervention.
3. *Missed:* Fetus dies in the uterus and must be removed. Usually a dilation and curettage (D and C) is the surgical procedure performed.

4. *Incomplete:* Only parts of the fetus and placenta are expelled. Tissue remains in the uterus and a D and C usually must be performed.
5. *Threatened:* Bleeding from the uterus, but there are no contractions or dilation of cervix. Pregnancy continues.
6. *Induced:* Evacuation of the fetus and placenta from the uterus at the mother's request or because mother's health is in jeopardy.

Eclampsia. Eclampsia syndrome, also known as toxemia of pregnancy, can occur in pregnancy and result in convulsions unrelated to epilepsy or other brain conditions. It is a potentially life-threatening disorder characterized by hypertension, generalized edema, and proteinuria. It can put the woman and her fetus in grave danger. Pre-eclampsia is less severe. The symptoms are the same, except there are no convulsions. This is why weight is measured, blood pressure checked, and a urinalysis (including a check for protein) are routinely performed. Sudden significant weight gain, rise in blood pressure, and the presence of protein in the urine can indicate possible pre-eclampsia. The cause is unknown. The problem is seen more often in women who have received inadequate prenatal care, especially poor nutrition, in **primigravida** (pregnant for the first time) under age eighteen, in women with pre-existing cardiovascular and renal conditions, as well as in women who are diabetic.

Gestational Diabetes. Gestational diabetes first appears during the second or third trimester of the pregnancy and usually disappears after the woman has delivered her baby or when the pregnancy terminates for any other reason. This type of diabetes is usually a milder form of the disease. Prompt detection (through blood and urine glucose testing) and therapy are essential to avoid fetal and **neonatal** (newborn) illness and death.

Hyperemesis Gravidarum. Hyperemesis gravidarum, or excessive vomiting during pregnancy, can be very harmful and is more than morning sickness, which is a common complaint during the first trimester. The cause of the condition is not known, but it is thought to be related to the cells that become the placenta and to the production of pregnancy hormones. The symptoms include uncontrollable nausea and vomiting, inability to eat and exhaustion from inability to sleep. Severe dehydration can result and starvation may ensue. This complication is usually not fatal, but it is a severe problem that warrants immediate treatment. Treatment includes intravenous fluids to replace those lost through vomiting and mild sedation to aid rest and sleep.

Placenta Previa. Placenta previa occurs when the placenta implants low in the uterus and partially or com-

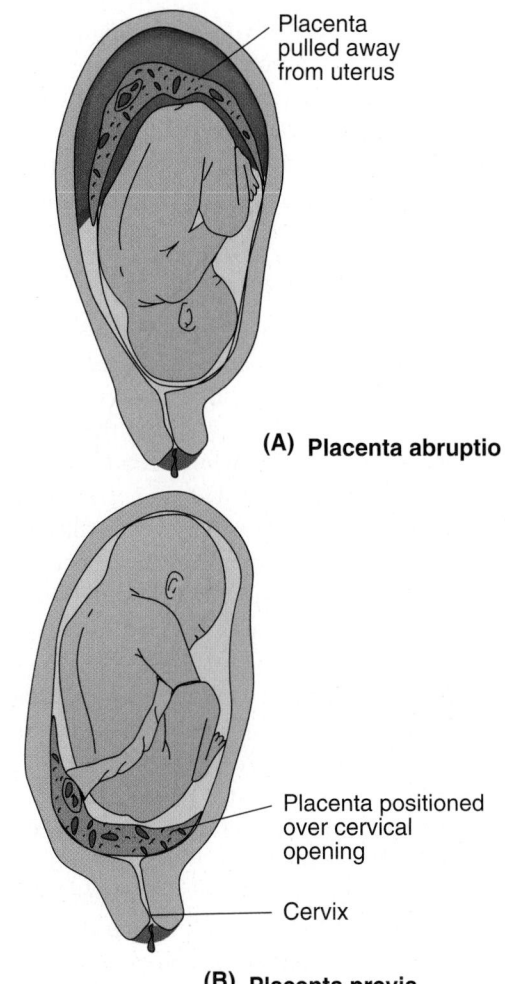

Figure 14-3   (A) Placenta abruptio. (B) Placenta previa.

pletely covers the cervical os. It is an emergency. The cause is unknown. When labor ensues and the cervix begins to dilate, the placenta is pulled away from the wall of the uterus and causes bleeding. On occasion, the bleeding, which comes on suddenly and is painless, will stop spontaneously. If it continues, significant maternal blood is lost, and the fetus may suffer anoxia and die when the placenta separates from the blood supply (Figure 14-3).

Ultrasonography will determine where the placenta is attached at which time the diagnosis can be made and treatment begun. Treatment depends on the gestational age of the fetus and the percent of placenta that covers the cervical os. Cesarean section may be necessary to remove the placenta, control bleeding, and deliver the fetus safely.

Placenta Abruptio. Placenta abruptio occurs when the placenta prematurely and abruptly separates from the uterine lining (see Figure 14-3A). It can result in fetal distress and death, and maternal shock. It usually occurs late in pregnancy but can occur during labor.

Factors that contribute to this complication are multiple pregnancies, chronic hypertension, trauma to the uterus, and sudden release of amniotic fluid. Delivery as soon as possible either vaginally or by Cesarean section is indicated. The prognosis of the newborn depends on the extent of hypoxia suffered during labor and delivery.

Impaired Fertility. The inability to conceive and bear a child after a period of unprotected sex is known as impaired fertility. Some reasons for this problem can be that many couples delay pregnancy until later in life when fertility is naturally lower. The increase in the incidence of **pelvic inflammatory disease** (PID), the increase in substance abuse, and environmental conditions such as pesticides and lead all can contribute to impaired fertility.

Diagnosis and treatment of impaired fertility requires a physical, emotional, and financial investment over a long period of time. To diagnose impaired fertility in the female, a complete history and physical exam are performed. Endocrine system and anatomic and physiologic abnormalities are sought. Laboratory tests on urine and blood are performed. Proof of ovulation can be determined by retrieving an ovum from the uterine tube, performing an endometrial biopsy, assessing mucus characteristics, and taking the basal body temperature. Levels of estrogen, progesterone, follicle-stimulating hormone, and lutenizing hormone are also measured. A **hysterosalpingogram**, an X ray of the uterus and tubes after the injection of dye, reveals defects in either the uterus or tubes.

Laparoscopy can be performed to visualize the internal pelvic structures. Tubal patency, **endometriosis**, pelvic adhesions, or **polycystic** ovaries can be seen. Endometrial biopsy is done to examine the tissue to determine whether the endometrium is capable of accepting a fertilized ovum for implantation. Ultrasonography, either abdominal or transvaginal, can assess pelvic organs for abnormalities.

Tests that can be performed on a male to diagnose impaired fertility are semen analysis, hormone analysis, and biopsy of a testicle. Once a diagnosis of impaired fertility has been made, a number of therapies are available to assist in reproduction. Some of them are:

- In vitro fertilization (IVF), indicated for fallopian tube blockage and endometriosis: Eggs are retrieved from ovaries, fertilized with sperm in the laboratory, then transferred to her uterus.

- Gamete intrafallopian transfer (GIFT): Eggs are retrieved from ovaries. An egg and sperm are aspirated into a special catheter then placed into the fallopian tube where fertilization can occur naturally.

- In vitro fertilization and gamete intrafallopian transfer (IVF + GIFT) with donor sperm: Eggs are retrieved from ovaries, fertilized with donor sperm in the laboratory, aspirated into a special catheter, then placed into the fallopian tube where fertilization can take place naturally.

 In some cultures, a woman is deemed the responsible party for impaired fertility, and the impairment is thought to be caused by her sins, evil spirits, or her own deficiencies. The virility of a male is questioned unless he is able to manifest his sexual potency by having a child.

Parturition

Parturition or labor is the process during which the uterus, through contractions, expels the fetus and placenta. There are three stages of labor:

Stage I Dilation: From onset of labor until complete **dilation** (expansion) and **effacement** (thinning and shortening) of cervix

Stage II Expulsion: From complete dilation and effacement through the birth of fetus (expulsion)

Stage III Placental: From birth of fetus through expulsion of the placenta

Labor is believed to be triggered by the release of **oxytoxin** and **prostaglandins** after the level of other hormones drop. When the oxytoxin is released, it causes the muscles of the uterus to contract. **Braxton-Hicks** contractions, often referred to as false labor, can usually be differentiated from real labor because of their irregularity and tendency to disappear when the woman moves about and changes positions.

Signs and symptoms to watch for during labor that indicate complications are heavy vaginal bleeding, sudden rise or drop in blood pressure, increased activity by the fetus, headache, extreme restlessness, and visual changes. Meconium in the vaginal discharge can indicate fetal distress.

Postpartum Period

The postpartum period is the time known as the puerperium during which the body returns to nonpregnant state. It is usually 4 to 6 weeks after delivery. The body undergoes changes during this time. The uterus involutes (returns to normal size) and healing of any injuries takes place.

A vaginal discharge, known as lochia, appears during the puerperium. It consists of tissue, blood, white blood cells, mucus, and bacteria. It can be described by its appearance. Lochia rubra is bright red and appears the first three days following delivery. Lochia serosa is pink or brown in color and is indicative of less blood. By about 10 days, the flow decreases, becomes whitish-yellow, and is known as lochia alba. Lochia usually disappears by the third week postpartum but may last for up to 6 weeks. Menstruation usually begins in a nursing mother 3 to 6 months after delivery, 2 months for non-nursing mothers. The mother is told to avoid heavy lifting, not to become fatigued, to eat a well-balanced diet, and to continue to take her prenatal tablets. An appointment in six weeks will evaluate the mother's general health, and the physician will discuss infant care, breast feeding, the importance of exercise and good nutrition, and birth control. The medical assistant can stress the importance of yearly Pap smears and of monthly breast self-examinations as these are important aspects of patient education.

Contraception. Voluntary prevention of pregnancy is known as contraception. The opportune time to discuss contraception with the mother is soon after delivery and before discharge from the hospital. She should know what method of contraception she and her partner will use before resuming sexual activity. To discuss contraception at the six-week postpartum checkup can be too late. Sexually transmitted disease (STD) protection should also be reviewed before discharge.

Written instructions about methods of contraception are important and help the patient understand options that are available.

Some nonprescription kinds of contraception are the various barrier methods: latex condoms, contraceptive foam, spermicide (nonoxynol-9) used with a condom to help prevent STDs, vaginal sponges that contain a spermicide, and abstinence.

Prescription methods of contraception include hormonal contraception in the form of oral birth control pills or Norplant®, a surgical implant of progestin in the upper arm, which provides up to five years of contraception. Other prescription methods include a diaphragm used with a spermicide, a cervical cap to fit over the cervix, and an intrauterine device (a small device made of copper or progesterone-medicated plastic).

Sterilization is a surgical procedure that renders the individual infertile. The woman's uterine tubes are **fulgarated** (destroyed by means of an electric current) or bands and clips are placed around the tubes to block them (ligation). Both fulgaration and ligation are considered to be permanent methods. Female sterilization can be performed immediately after birth or any time afterward during any phase of the menstrual cycle. Laparoscopic surgery is the usual approach.

The surgical procedure performed on a male to render him sterile is a vasectomy. It can be performed on an outpatient basis under local anesthesia. Small incisions are made into the scrotum above and to the side of each testicle. Each vas deferens is identified, ligated twice, and then severed. It is important for the patient to realize that sterility is not immediate because some sperm remain in the sperm ducts following vasectomy. One week to several months may elapse before the ducts are sperm free. Some form of contraception is necessary until two consecutive sperm counts are zero. (See Chapter 16.)

Another method of contraception recently approved by the Food and Drug Administration is a medication known as RU 486, which is used to cause or induce an abortion. It prevents a fertilized egg from implanting in the uterus.

GYNECOLOGY

Gynecology is the specialty that studies diseases of the female reproductive tract and the breasts. The gynecological examination is routinely performed in an office or clinic and usually includes abdominal, pelvic and breast examination, and a Pap smear. It can be done as part of the female's complete physical exam, or it can be a separate exam performed in the gynecologist's office or gynecology clinic. Early diagnosis and treatment of problems associated with the female reproductive organs helps the female to achieve optimum health of these organs and is the goal of the OB/GYN physician.

The Gynecological Examination

It is recommended that a gynecological exam and Pap smear be done annually on all women beginning when they become sexually active or by age 20. It is done to assess the female's health and to screen for cancer of the reproductive organs. It includes a breast examination by the physician and instructions for the patient about how to perform her own breast self-examination (BSE). It also includes a pelvic examination and Pap smear. Pap tests are done to detect cervical cancer. Women should be especially conscientious in scheduling annual Pap tests if they have a family history of uterine or cervical cancer. Early detection of cervical cancer and appropriate treatment can cure the disease. Others feel that in healthy women a Pap test done every 1 to 3 years is sufficient. The American Cancer Society recommends that females have a Pap test at least every 3 years, beginning when they become sexually active, or at age 20, if there have been two initial negative Pap test results 1 year apart. Encourage patients to have regular Pap tests. Women at high risk should have a Pap test every 6 months. If the patient is experiencing a vaginal discharge and there is a suspicion of a vaginal infection, smear(s) and cultures of discharge will be done to aid in diagnosis. See Chapter 31, Basic Microbiology, for more information.

Other gynecologic problems that may arise between annual gynecological examinations may require that an appointment, in addition to the annual gynecological checkup that is routinely done, be made and may include such symptoms and problems as severe **dysmenorrhea** (painful menses), lower abdominal pain, bleeding between menstrual periods, **dyspareunia** (painful intercourse), sexual dysfunction, infertility, and discomfort from menstrual symptoms. Women experiencing these problems will have a gynecological examination, and the physician will determine a diagnosis based upon the examination, patient's history, symptoms, signs, and laboratory data.

Breast Examination. The physician performs a breast examination on the patient as part of a gynecological examination. The physician looks for redness, dimpling, and puckering, and palpates each breast and axilla feeling for lumps or thickening. Part of the medical assistant's responsibility is to teach patients how to perform the BSE. Figure 14-4 provides illustrations for performing the BSE. The physician may also provide several pamphlets and/or a breast model with lumps and thickening for enhancing patient education and awareness about the importance of the examination (Figure 14-5A and B). (See Procedure 14-2.)

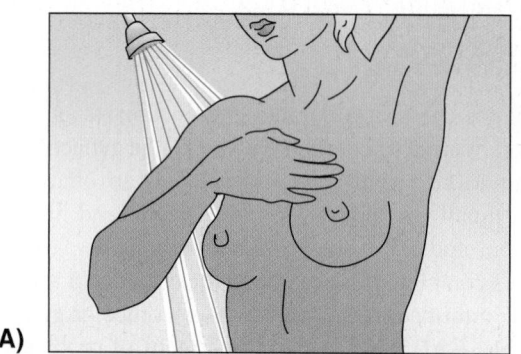

(A)

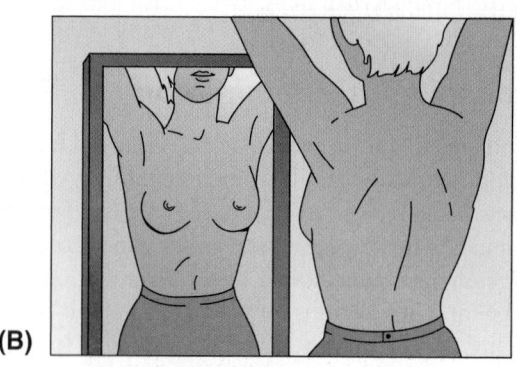

(B)

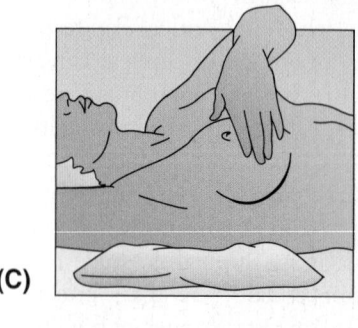

(C)

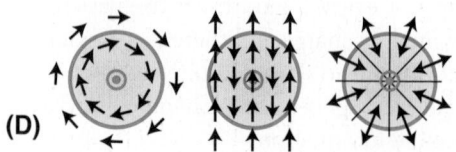

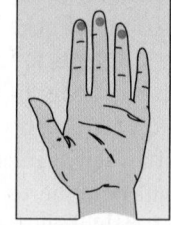

(D)

Finger pads

Figure 14-4   (A–D) Breast self-examination. (Courtesy of American Cancer Society)

Patient Teaching Tip

Breast Self-Examination
1. Breast self-examination (BSE) should be done in three different positions.
   a. In a warm shower (soaping each breast) checking for lumps, thickening, or changes that differ from previous self-exam. Refer to Figure 14-4A.
   b. In front of a mirror, checking for changes in appearance. Refer to Figure 14-4B.
   c. Lying flat in a supine position helps breast tissue spread allowing better palpation of outer tissue. Refer to Figure 14-4C. Use pads of fingers.
   d. Examine the breasts in a circular motion starting at 12 o'clock and moving around the breast clockwise. Use an up and down motion or an inward and outward motion from nipple outward or chest wall inward (Figure 14-4D).
2. Do the breast self-examination at the same time each month, 7 to 10 days after menses. Repeating the exam the same time each month provides familiarity with the contours of the body and allows for hormonal levels to return to premenstrual status. The breasts may be swollen, tender, and have thickening due to hormonal influence around the time of the menstrual cycle and for 7 to 10 days following menses.

Physician Breast Examination. The American Cancer Society recommends that:
a. Women ages 20 to 39 have a breast physical examination by a physician every 3 years and women age 40 and over have one yearly.
b. Women without symptoms of breast cancer ages 40 to 49 should have a mammogram every 1 to 2 years, and women age 50 and over, once a year (Figure 14-6 and 14-7). A tumor or mass can often be seen with a mammography up to 2 years before either the physician or patient notices or feels a tumor.

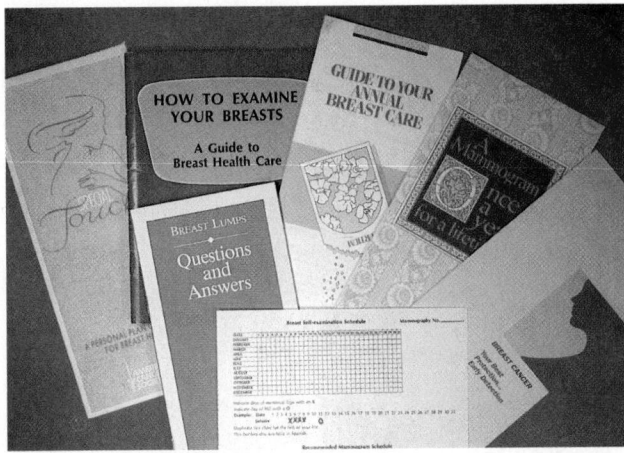

Figure 14-5A Informational pamphlets detailing the breast self-examination and its importance can be very helpful to patients.

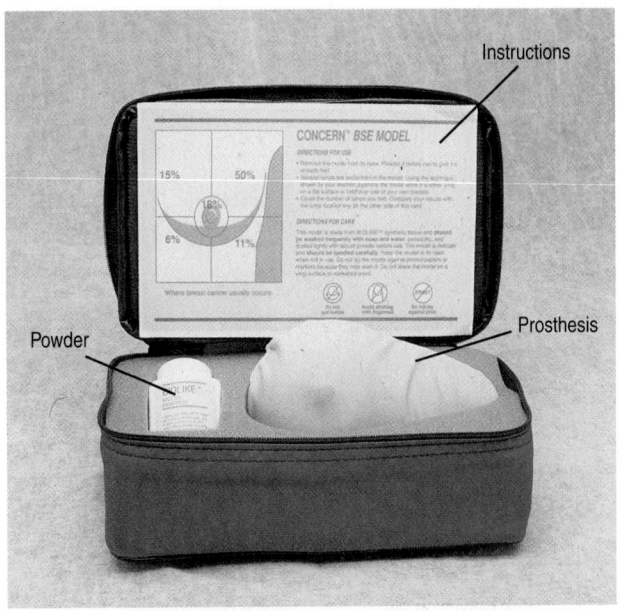

Figure 14-5B Breast self-examination model kit contains instructions for breast self-examination and powder to aid fingers in gliding over the breast prosthesis. The prosthesis contains lumps and thickened areas for identification and location.

Assisting with a Gynecologic Examination.

The gynecologic (GYN) exam consists of either four or five parts depending on whether the Pap test is done with the GYN exam. These parts include:

1. Inspection of external **genitalia** (labia minora, labia majora, urinary meatus, clitoris, **Bartholin glands,** and vagina) for swelling, lesions, or ulcerations.
2. Pelvic examination of cervix, uterus, tubes, and ovaries including a bimanual examination.
3. Rectal examination.
4. Breast examination.

5. The gynecologic pelvic examination can be performed with or without a Pap test. A Pap smear is taken during the gynecologic examination (Figure 14-8). The patient must refrain from sexual intercourse, using vaginal medication, and douching for 24 hours prior to the Pap test. These activities can interfere with obtaining a good sample of cervical

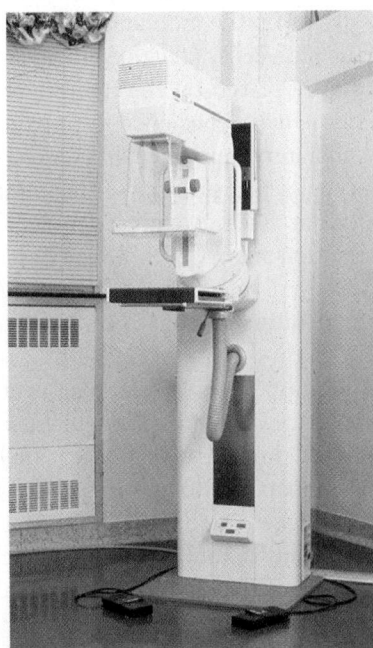

Figure 14-6 Breasts are compressed by the plates of mammographic x-ray unit.

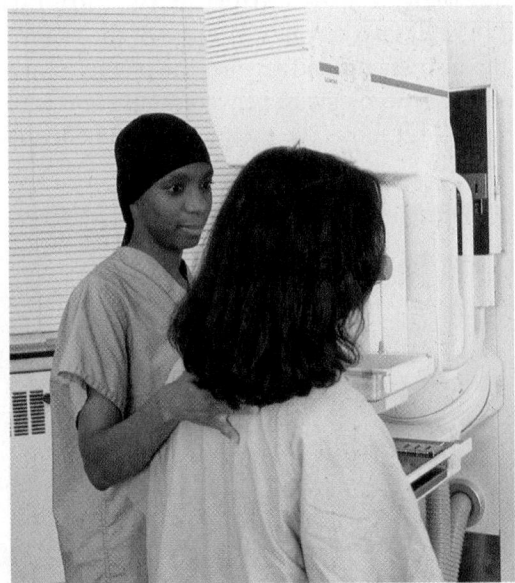

Figure 14-7 The technologist positions the patient for a mammography. The procedure requires the patient to move into various positions so different angles of the breast tissue may be x-rayed.

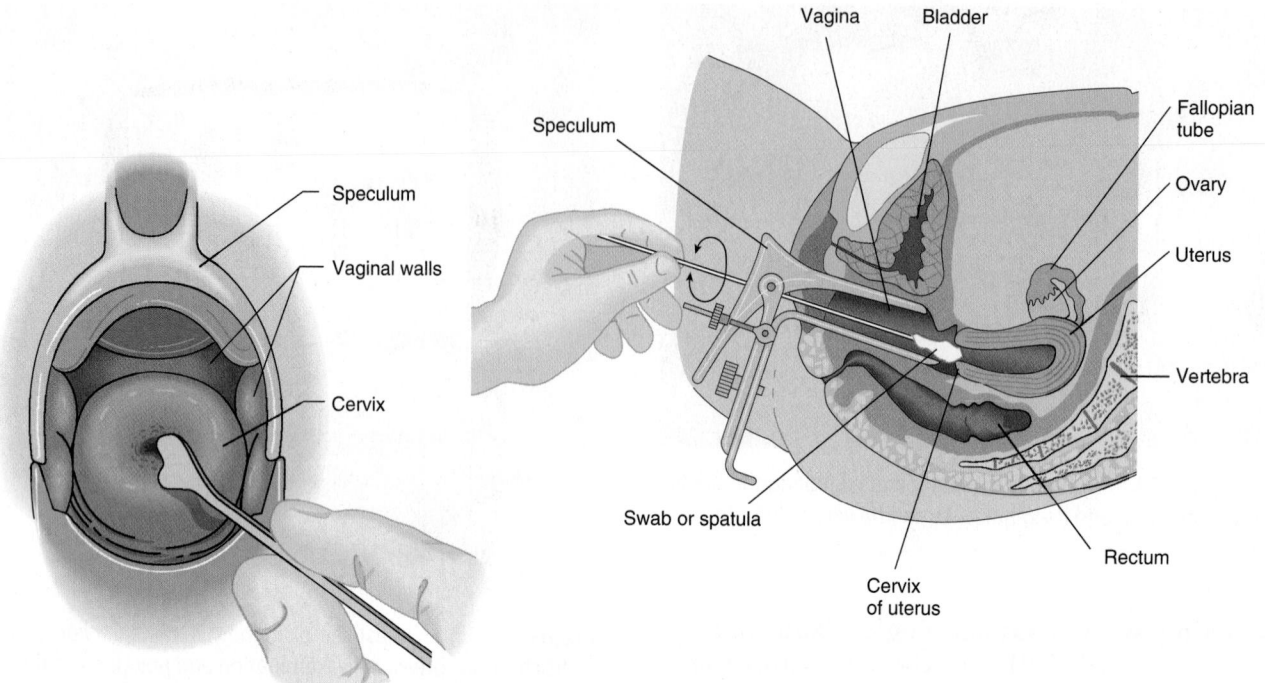

Figure 14-8   Use of speculum and obtaining a Pap smear.

cells. Also, a Pap smear cannot be done during menstruation because the red blood cells obscure the cervical cells.

The medical assistant should prepare the patient, equipment, and room prior to the examination.

Gynecologic Examination with Pap Equipment. On a Mayo tray near the end of the exam table, place the instruments and supplies the physician needs to perform the gynecologic or pelvic examination with Pap test. Figure 14-9 shows the equipment commonly needed

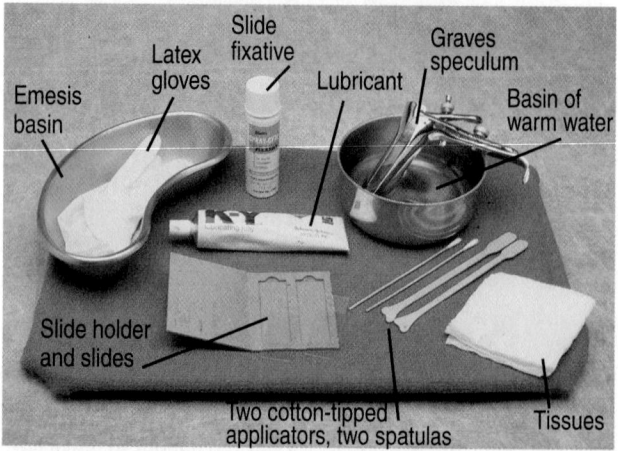

Figure 14-9   Setup for gynecologic examination including Pap smear.

for the examination. To aid in the inspection portion of the examination, a gooseneck lamp should be placed at the foot of the table behind the stool on which the physician will sit. (See Procedure 14-3.)

Pap Smear. The federal government regulates laboratories that perform testing on Pap smears. There are requirements placed on the individuals who test the specimens for malignant cells, and they include specialized training. Limits are placed on the number of slides that can be read in one day. Proficiency testing, mandated by the Clinical Laboratory Improvement Act of 1988 (CLIA '88) ensures accuracy and precision of test results and is a requirement for Pap smear examination. See Chapter 26 for more information about CLIA '88.

A computerized method, known as PAPNET, is used to retest Pap smears that have been analyzed by technologists. The method duplicates the process that the technologists perform. It is hoped that eventually the PAPNET will replace Pap smears done manually.

Another test, known as Virapap, can be used to screen for the human papiloma virus (HPV) in a Pap smear. There is higher incidence of cervical cancer in women who have HPV, and the test can help identify these women who are at greater risk for cervical cancer.

A system for cytologic reporting of a Pap smear is a descriptive report that tells the physician exactly what cellular changes have taken place. The classification includes the grades of cervical intraepithelial neoplasia (CIN).

- Problems ovulating
- Chronic stress
- Scar tissue from surgery, infection, or ectopic pregnancy
- Tumors

A woman who is having difficulty conceiving and has a history of any of the above will have a physical examination by a physician who specializes in infertility. The specialist will decide what tests and/or procedures are necessary. Hormone levels may be measured to look for hypothyroidism and ovarian function determined through a surgical procedure, such as laparoscopy. A test for **patency** (openness) of the fallopian tubes can be performed by a hysterosalpingogram, a radiographic procedure done following injection of dye into the vagina, through the cervix, into the uterus, and out the fallopian tubes. The dye will pass through all of these organs if there is no blockage in any of them. (See Impaired Fertility, page 264.)

Menopause. The period of time that marks permanent cessation of menstrual activity is known as menopause. It usually occurs between the ages of 35 and 58. There may be a gradual decline in monthly menstrual flow, or a woman may suddenly cease to menstruate. Natural menopause occurs when the ovaries produce less and less estrogen. This causes the ovaries to cease ovulation and, therefore, menstruation stops. Surgical menopause is caused by the surgical removal of both ovaries (bilateral oophorectomy). Symptoms occur soon after ovulation ceases with both natural and surgical menopause. Symptoms may last for a few months to several years and include mild to severe symptoms. Hot flashes, chills, nervousness, fatigue, apathy, mental depression, crying episodes, insomnia, palpitations, and headache are some common symptoms experienced by some women. The long-term effects on lower estrogen levels are osteoporosis and atherosclerosis. Hormone replacement therapy (HRT) helps to prevent these diseases and reduce patient symptoms. There is some controversy regarding HRT benefits. Some studies show an increase in cancers of the female reproductive system in patients using HRT. Many authorities recommend HRT for most women unless they have a family history of breast cancer. Physicians believe that the benefits outweigh the risks for most women. When HRT is combined with a healthy lifestyle, well-being and health improve.

Endometriosis. This painful, common condition is characterized by endometrial tissue adhering to tissue and organs outside of the uterus. It is primarily found in the pelvis, adhering to an ovary, fallopian tube, or pelvic peritoneum. It also can be found outside of the pelvis, even in

---

SPOTLIGHT ON AAMA ESSENTIALS THROUGH CAAHEP

- Being sensitive to a female patient's physiological as well as emotional needs during a gynecologic and breast examination is extremely important and can make the difference between a patient returning for a follow-up checkup and not coming back.

- Part of the role of the medical assistant during a pelvic examination is to provide the patient with reassurance that the procedure is painless, especially if it is the first gynecological examination she has had.

- The best way a medical assistant can assist the physician in identifying obstetrical and gynecological problems in her female patients is to listen to her complaints, fears, and concerns, and then follow up in the appropriate manner.

CIN 1 = mild **dysplasia** (abnormal tissue development)

CIN 2 = moderate dysplasia

CIN 3 = severe dysplasia or **carcinoma in situ**

Pap Smear Results. The Pap smear will usually be sent to a reference laboratory where a pathologist will examine it and record the results on the cytology report form. The form will be returned to the physician.

Gynecological Diseases and Conditions

The female reproductive system is affected by many diseases and conditions caused by hormonal imbalance, cysts, infection, and tumors. Some of the more common disorders and diseases are covered here.

Infertility. Most women, with unprotected intercourse, will be able to conceive within a year. The inability to conceive can be caused by a problem with either the male or the female. Some common causes of infertility in a female are:

- Endometriosis
- Certain medications
- Blocked fallopian tubes

the abdomen adhering to tissue and organs, such as the bowel. The cause is unknown. The abnormal and engorged endometrial tissue responds to hormonal stimulation (estrogen) and builds up along with the normal endometrium of the menstrual cycle. It sloughs off at time of menstruation and is very painful. The blood has not had a way to leave the body and is discharged into the pelvic or abdominal cavities.

Endometriosis symptoms may respond to contraceptive medication because these pills suppress menstruation and no further treatment is necessary (see Figure 14-10). However, long-term hormonal treatment may help alleviate symptoms. Hysterectomy may be necessary if the woman does not respond to hormonal therapy.

Ovarian Cysts.

Cysts that appear on the ovary are common. As part of the menstrual cycle, the ovarian follicles enlarge and become graafian follicles. Only one of these graafian follicles ruptures at the time of ovulation. The follicles that do not rupture, but remain, are filled with fluid. They may enlarge and become cysts (Figure 14-11).

Ultrasonography will aid in viewing the ovaries. Most ovarian cysts resolve without treatment. Laparoscopy can be done to either drain or remove the cyst. Contraceptive therapy many times is helpful in resolving the cyst without surgery.

Direct viewing of the ovaries and surgery may be necessary because cancer of the ovary must be ruled out.

Ovarian Cancer.

Because the symptoms of ovarian cancer do not appear until the disease has had an opportunity to become established, it is difficult to make a diagnosis early in the disease process. Therefore, if a woman has any symptoms, the cancer has been present for some time. Symptoms may be pressure in the pelvis, lower abdominal discomfort, weight loss, and fluid in the abdomen. Diagnosis can be made by laparoscopic surgery and a biopsy. Hysterectomy and bilateral salpingo-oophorectomy are done followed by radiation therapy and/or chemotherapy. The cause is not known.

Pelvic Inflammatory Disease (PID).

This disease involves some or all of the female reproductive tract and can be a mild to serious infection. The causative microorganism is usually a sexually transmitted pathogen. The microorganism enters through the vagina and ascends through the cervix into the body of the uterus. It can spread out through the fallopian tubes into the pelvic cavity. Culture and sensitivity of the vaginal discharge are performed, and appropriate antibiotics are prescribed. Early treatment helps to lessen damage caused by scar tissue that forms in the pelvis and organs. Delayed treatment can cause septic shock, which can be life-threatening. Infertility and ectopic pregnancy are long-range problems that can occur (see Tables 14-3, 14-4, and 14-5).

Other Diagnostic Tests and Treatments for Reproductive System Diseases

Colposcopy.

Colposcopy is the examination of the vagina and cervix by means of a lighted instrument that has a three-dimensional magnifying lens called a col-

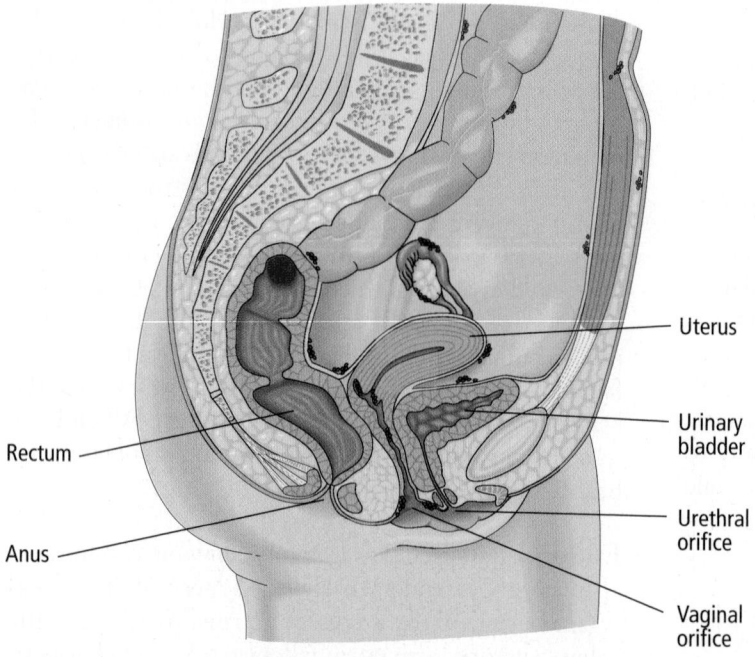

Figure 14-10 Endometriosis—common sites of endometrial implants.

Uterus

Urinary bladder

Urethral orifice

Vaginal orifice

Rectum

Anus

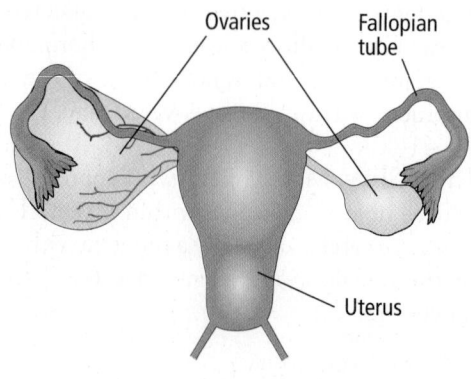

Ovaries

Fallopian tube

Uterus

Figure 14-11 Ovarian cyst.

TABLE 14-3 FEMALE REPRODUCTIVE SYSTEM

Disease/ Disorder	Laboratory Diagnostic Tests			Radiography	Surgery	Medical Tests or Procedures
	Blood	Urine	Other			
Bartholin Gland Infection			Exudate culture and sensitivity		Incision and drainage	Pelvic exam
Breast Cancer	Breast cancer gene detection BRCAI			Mammography Ultrasonography	Biopsy of breast lesion	Monthly breast self-exam
Cervical Cancer			Pap smear		Cone biopsy Dilation & curettage (D&C)	Pelvic exam Colposcopy
Endometriosis		Urinalysis		Abdominal ultrasonography Chest x-ray	Laparoscopy Hysterectomy	Pelvic exam
Fibrocystic Breasts				Mammography Ultrasonography	Biopsy	Monthly breast self-exam
Pelvic Inflammatory Disease	Complete blood count and differential (CBC)	Urinalysis	Culture and sensitivity of vaginal discharge	Pelvic ultrasonography	Laparoscopy	Pelvic exam
Sexually Transmitted Diseases						
• Chlamydia	Serology	Urinalysis	Direct urethral and/or cervical smear using monoclonal antibodies			Pelvic exam
• Condylomata (genital warts)		Urinalysis		Excisional biopsy		Pelvic exam Pap smear
• Neisseria Gonorrhea	Complete blood count and differential (CBC)	Urinalysis	Direct smear of vaginal discharge, anal canal, and oropharynx Thayer-Martin culture	Pelvic ultrasonography		Pelvic exam
• HBV and HIV						
Vaginitis						
• Candidiasis	Blood glucose	Urinalysis	Wet mount: direct vaginal smear with potassium hydroxide (1 drop)			Pelvic exam
• Trichomoniasis		Urinalysis	Wet mount: direct vaginal smear with isotomic saline (1 drop)			Pelvic exam

TABLE 14-4 DESCRIPTION OF FEMALE REPRODUCTIVE SYSTEM DISORDERS AND CONDITIONS

- Bartholin Gland Infection. Infection of the gland(s) that open near the vaginal opening.
- Breast Cancer. Most common site of cancer in females. A genetic cause has been identified for some breast cancers. Some symptoms are lump, thickening, swelling, dimpling, pain, and nipple discharge.
- Cervical Cancer. A carcinoma of the cervix of the uterus caused by a progressive cervical dysplasia. Most common in women aged 30 to 40. A significant risk factor is seen in women who become sexually active early in their lives and who have multiple sex partners.
- Endometriosis. Presence of endometrium in sites other than inside the uterus. May be found on the ovaries, fallopian tubes, large bowel, lungs, and pleura. Causes pelvic pain, dysmenorrhea, and infertility.

(continues)

TABLE 14-4 *(continued)*

- Fibrocystic Breasts. Benign cysts in breast tissue that increase or decrease in size during menses. Thought to be a normal variation in breast tissue due to monthly hormonal influence prior to onset of menses.
- Pelvic Inflammatory Disease (PID). Pelvic reproductive organs become inflamed and infected by bacteria, viruses, or parasites. An ascending infection can ensue involving the vagina, cervix of uterus, body of uterus, fallopian tubes, and ovaries. Causes vaginal discharge, pain, fever. May cause infertility.
- Premenstrual Syndrome (PMS). Cluster of symptoms that occur monthly prior to the onset of menses thought to be caused by progesterone-estrogen imbalance. Symptoms include fluid retention, weight gain, irritability, and mood swings.
- Sexually Transmitted Diseases (STDs). Several diseases caused by bacteria, viruses, protozoa that are transmitted through sexual intercourse (vaginal, anal, oral).
  - Chlamydia. An invasion by an intracellular parasite causing urethritis, cervicitis, pelvic inflammatory disease, proctitis, infant pneumonia, and conjunctivitis.
  - Condylomata (Human Papilloma Virus). Genital warts caused by a virus. Grow around the external genitalia, rectum, cervix. Associated with abnormal Pap smears.
  - Neisseria Gonorrhea. An infection by a bacterium that can involve the cervix, urethra, fallopian tubes and ovaries, rectum, mouth.
- Vaginitis. Inflammation of the vagina may be caused by bacteria, fungus, protozoa, chemical irritants, irritation from foreign bodies, vitamin deficiency, uncleanliness, and intestinal worms.
  - Candidiasis. A yeast (fungal) infection of the vagina caused by prolonged antibiotic therapy, pregnancy, or diabetes which can change the normal vaginal flora leading to overgrowth of the fungus.
  - Trichomoniasis. An infection by a protozoan most commonly spread through sexual intercourse or may come from fecal contamination of the vagina.

TABLE 14-5   COMMON SEXUALLY TRANSMITTED DISEASES

Pathology	Symptoms	Test	Treatment
AIDS	Flu-like, lymphadenopathy, infections, malignancies, pneumonia	HIV	Medication—AZT, DDI—but disease is fatal
Chlamydia	Usually asymptomatic	Culture	Doxycyline
Condylomata	Warts on external and internal genitalia	Visual exam	Cryocautery or chemocautery preferred but electrocautery can be used Keratolytic agents used such as Podofilox
Gonorrhea	Usually asymptomatic; yellowish-green discharge with dysuria in advanced stages	Gram stain or Thayer-Martin culture	Penicillin
Herpes Simplex II	Itching and soreness followed by genital vesicles, which heal in 10 to 14 days	Visual exam with blood test for confirmation	Acyclovir®
Syphilis	Stage I: papule develops into ulcer, which develops into chancre of vulva Stage II: fever, general malaise, dermal and mucosal lesions Stage III: degeneration of CNS, lesions of internal structures	VDRL, RPR, FTA, or TPI	Penicillin
Trichomonas	Milky white, frothy, malodorous discharge with genital burning and itching	Potassium wet hydroxide mount for microscopic exam	Oral Flagel®, partner(s) must also be treated

poscope. The examination is done to determine if areas in the vagina or the cervix contain precancerous cells or tissue. The procedure is performed following an abnormal Pap test. It can also be performed to evaluate a lesion noted during a pelvic examination and to follow up after treatment of cervical cancer. Because the instrument has the ability to magnify tissue, the cervix can be more readily examined and a biopsy taken.

The patient is placed in lithotomy position and is prepared as she would be for a gynecologic examination. A nonlubricated speculum is inserted into the vagina. The vagina is swabbed with a long cotton-tipped applicator that has been moistened with saline. (This provides better visualization of the cervical tissue.) The cervix is then swabbed with acetic acid to dissolve mucus and provide a good contrast between normal and abnormal tissue. A staining medium can be used as another means of identifying abnormal cells. If the physician finds an area of abnormal tissue, a biopsy can be performed using cervical punch biopsy forceps. The specimen is examined by a pathologist to determine whether or not malignant cells are present.

Cervical Punch Biopsy.

The **cervical punch biopsy** is usually done in conjunction with a colposcopy to obtain a sample of cervical tissue for pathological examination. The specimen is examined for malignant cells and the biopsy usually follows an abnormal Pap smear report.

The procedure is performed with the patient in lithotomy position and with a vaginal speculum in place. The physician may stain the cervix to aid in identifying abnormal tissue. If the colposcope is being used, it illuminates and magnifies the cervical tissue and the physician will take several tissue samples using the cervical punch biopsy forceps. If bleeding ensues, it can be controlled with a vaginal packing, or the area can be cauterized to stop the bleeding. The specimen is placed in a container with formalin, a completed requisition form is attached to the container, and it is sent to the pathology laboratory for examination. The patient may expect a small amount of bleeding and should notify the physician if bleeding ensues that is greater than a menstrual period. A discharge that has a strong, foul odor is to be expected and can last for up to one month following the procedure.

Cryosurgery.

Cryosurgery is used to treat tissue by freezing temperatures. Chronic cervicitis and cervical erosion are two common problems treated in this manner. (Also refer to Chapter 19 for information on cryosurgery.) The freezing temperature causes cells to die and they are

Patient Teaching Tip

Post Cryosurgery of Cervix
1. Expect a clear, watery, heavy discharge for up to one week, tapering off for up to four weeks.
2. Use only sanitary pads, not tampons. Change often, cleansing perineal area with each pad change.
3. Report signs of infection: fever, foul discharge, pain, nausea, or vomiting.
4. Do not engage in sexual intercourse, douche, or use tampons for four weeks.
5. Expect a heavier than usual menstrual period the following month.

then cast off from the cervix and eventually replaced with healthy cells about a month following the procedure.

The procedure is performed with the patient in lithotomy position and the cervix is swabbed to remove mucous. The probe is placed against the affected area of the cervix and the machine is turned on. The liquid nitrogen flows over the area for about three minutes and freezes the tissue. The patient may have some pain similar to dysmenorrhea that may last for about one-half hour. There should be no strong, foul odor but there can be a discharge for up to one month. Patients should report any foul smelling discharges as this may indicate an infection. Healing usually takes 4–6 weeks.

Patient Teaching Tip

Post Cervical Biopsy
1. Rest for 24 hours following the procedure.
2. Do not lift heavy objects for two weeks.
3. Leave packing in place for 24 hours or as directed. Do not insert another tampon unless told to do so by the physician.
4. Report any bleeding greater than a normal menstrual period.

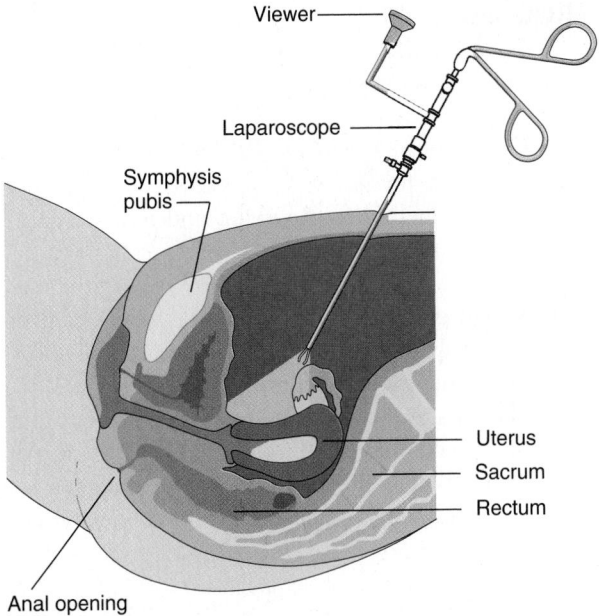

Figure 14-12   Laparoscopy.

Laparoscopy. Laparoscopy is a procedure in which a lighted instrument is used to view the inside of the pelvic cavity. It can be helpful in diagnosing endometriosis and ovarian cysts. A tubal ligation, severing of the fallopian tubes, can be done laparoscopically (Figure 14-12).

Dilation and Curettage (D and C). Dilation and curettage (D and C) is a surgical procedure that involves the dilating and scraping of the endometrial tissue. It is commonly performed to remove any remaining tissue following an incomplete abortion or to examine the tissue if the female has had abnormal uterine bleeding.

Diseases and conditions of the female reproductive tract and their appropriate tests and procedures are listed in tables 14-1 and 14-2.

Procedure 14-1 — Assisting with Routine Prenatal Visits

STANDARD PRECAUTIONS:

PURPOSE:
To monitor the progress of the pregnancy.

EQUIPMENT/SUPPLIES:
Scale
Disposable gloves
Tape measure
Sphygmomanometer
Stethoscope
Doppler fetoscope and coupling agent
Urine specimen container
Biohazard waste container

PROCEDURE STEPS:
1. Wash hands.
2. Set up equipment.
3. Identify patient.
4. Obtain urine specimen. RATIONALE: A urine specimen for analysis is necessary. An empty bladder facilitates the exam and is more comfortable for the patient.
5. Measure blood pressure.
6. Weigh patient. RATIONALE: Assesses gain or loss of weight to help determine fetal development and maternal nutrition.
7. Have patient disrobe from waist down and put on a gown open in the front. RATIONALE: An open gown facilitates access to the abdomen for exam and measurement of the fundal height.

8. Test the urine specimen while waiting for the physician. RATIONALE: Urinalysis is done for detection of glucose and/or protein, which can indicate disease.
9. Assist patient onto exam table and drape her. RATIONALE: The patient may be off balance and unsteady on her feet due to the enlargement of the abdomen. Provide for her safety.
10. Assist the physician as the exam is performed.
    • Hand the physician the tape measure to measure height of fundus
    • Hand the physician the Doppler fetal pulse detector for measurement of fetal heart rate. The medical assistant may spread the coupling agent onto the patient's abdomen.
11. After the exam, assist patient to sit for a few moments. Assess her color, pulse. RATIONALE: Orthostatic hypotension can occur when a patient rises from a recumbent position. Give the patient time for the blood pressure to go back to normal so she will not experience dizziness from lowered blood pressure.
12. Provide any instruction or clarification of physician's orders.
13. Apply gloves. Discard disposable supplies per OSHA guidelines. Disinfect equipment used.
14. Remove gloves.
15. Wash hands.
16. Set up for the next patient.
17. Record all information in patient's record.

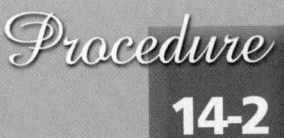

Instructing Patient in Breast Self-Examination

Procedure 14-2

PURPOSE:
To properly instruct a woman in the procedure for performing a breast self-examination.

EQUIPMENT/SUPPLIES:
Breast model
Breast self-exam pamphlets
Pamphlet on breast self-examination

PROCEDURE STEPS:
Shower:
1. Examine breasts in a warm bath or shower. RATIONALE: Warm water softens the skin and hands glide easily over wet skin.
2. Using the flat pads of the three middle fingers moving in a circular motion, use the right hand to examine the left breast and left hand to examine the right breast. Beginning at the top outside edge using a circular, clockwise motion, examine part of each breast, ending at the nipple.
3. Check for lumps, thickening, and anything that is different from previous exams.

Mirror:
1. Inspect the breasts with arms at sides.
2. Raise arms high overhead.
3. Look for any change in contour of each breast.
4. Observe for swelling, hard lump, dimpling of skin (orange skin), or changes in nipple (retracting, swelling, or discharge).
5. Rest both hands on hips and pressing down flex chest muscles.

Lying Down:
1. Place a pillow or towel under right shoulder with the right hand behind the head to examine the right breast.
2. With left hand and fingers flat, press gently in small circular motions, starting at the top of the breast and moving toward the nipple.
3. Examine every part of the right breast tissue.
4. Repeat the procedure on the left breast using a pillow or a towel under the left shoulder and examine using the right hand.
5. Squeeze the nipple of each breast gently between thumb and index finger.
6. Report any abnormalities to the physician.

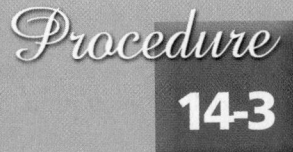

Assisting with Gynecologic or Pelvic Examination and a Papanicolaou (Pap) Test

Procedure 14-3

STANDARD PRECAUTIONS:

PURPOSE:
To assist the physician in collecting cervical cells for laboratory analysis for early detection of malignant cells of the cervix and to assess the health of the reproductive organs to detect diseases leading to early diagnosis and treatment.

EQUIPMENT/SUPPLIES:
2 pair nonsterile gloves
2–3 frosted end glass slides
Vaginal speculum
  (plastic or metal)
Basin of warm water
Long cotton-tipped
  applicator or cytology
  brush
Cervical scrapers
Fixative

Light source
Drape sheet
Marking pencil
Lubricant
Slide holder
Lab requisition
Urine specimen container
Tissues
Biohazard waste container

(continues)

Procedure

14-3   *(continued)*

PROCEDURE STEPS:

1. Wash hands and assemble necessary supplies near patient.
2. Request that patient empty her bladder. (Instruct patient to save urine specimen and provide specimen container if ordered by physician.) RATIONALE: An empty bladder facilitates examination of the uterus and a urine specimen is frequently used for a urinalysis.
3. Provide patient with gown and request her to completely undress.
4. Explain procedure to patient.
5. Instruct patient to sit at end of table when ready. Drape patient for privacy. Label the frosted end of the slide with a marking pencil. Include patient's name on slide. Indicate site from where specimen is collected c = cervix, v = vagina, e = endocervical.
6. Assist patient into lithotomy position. Patient's knees should be relaxed and thighs rotated out as far as comfortable. Drape for privacy and warmth.
7. Encourage patient to breathe slowly and deeply through the mouth during exam. RATIONALE: Allows for relaxation of pelvic muscles and easier insertion of vaginal speculum.
8. Warm stainless steel vaginal speculum with warm water or place on a heating pad. Note: Do not lubricate speculum. Lubricant obscures exfoliated cervical cells when Pap test is being performed.
9. Hand speculum and spatula or cytology brush to physician.
10. Apply gloves.
11. Hold slides for physician to apply smear of exfoliated cells, one for vaginal (v), one for cervical (c), and one for endocervical (e) in that order.
12. Spray fixative over slide within 10 seconds at a distance of about 6 inches. Allow to dry for at least 10 minutes. RATIONALE: This maintains

cell appearance and avoids contamination of cells. Avoid getting too close to slide with spray since this may destroy or damage cells. Slides must be fixed before they dry to protect the appearance of the cells.

13. Place lubricant on physician's gloved fingers without touching gloves, for bimanual and rectal exams. The physician will insert the index and middle fingers into the vagina. The other hand is placed on the lower abdomen. The size, shape, and position of the uterus and ovaries are palpated.
14. The physician will insert one gloved finger into the rectum to check the tone of the rectal and pelvic muscles. Hemorrhoids, rectal fissures, or other lesions may be palpated.
15. Assist patient to wipe genitalia and rectum.
16. Help patient to a sitting position, allowing her to rest awhile. Check her pulse and skin color. RATIONALE: Some patients, especially elderly, can experience orthostatic hypotension.
17. Discard disposable supplies per OSHA guidelines. If stainless steel speculum was used, soak in cool water. Sanitize and sterilize as soon as convenient.
18. Remove gloves and wash hands.
19. Assist patient down and off the table if necessary.
20. Instruct patient to dress. Inform patient of how and when test results will be reported to her.
21. Prepare laboratory requisition (cytology request) form. Include physician name and address, date, source of specimen, patient's name, address, date of last menstrual period (LMP), and hormone therapy. Place slides in slide container, attach requisition to container, and send to laboratory.
22. Wash hands.
23. Document procedure in the patient's chart.

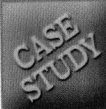

Maria Rodriguez has an appointment to see Dr. King today. It is her initial prenatal visit. She tells Liz Corbin, the medical assistant, as she is escorted from the reception area that she has been feeling, "pretty good."

14·1 CASE STUDY REVIEW

1. Explain the importance of the initial prenatal visit. Discuss.
2. Name five specific diseases and conditions for which Dr. King will be on the alert during Maria's pregnancy.
3. What laboratory and other procedural tests may be performed at the initial visit?
4. Discuss areas of patient education and health promotion that Liz will discuss with Maria at the initial visit.

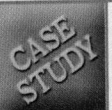

Emily Harris is scheduled to have a cervical punch biopsy.

CASE STUDY REVIEW

14·2

1. Explain the postbiopsy instructions she will need.

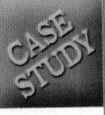

Annette Sanderson has made an appointment with Dr. King because she has had symptoms of vaginitis. When she arrives at the clinic, you take her chief complaint and history. She tells you that she has a milky-white, frothy, vaginal discharge and that she itches in the genital area.

14·3 CASE STUDY REVIEW

1. What tests/procedures will you prepare for Dr. King in consideration of Annette's symptoms?
2. What is the most likely causative microorganism for these symptoms?
3. Describe the treatment that Dr. King may prescribe.

SUMMARY

Obstetrics and gynecology are two specialties that are usually practiced by the same physician. The OB/GYN physician will care for the health and well-being of the female in her pregnant and nonpregnant states. Knowledge of the numerous tests and procedures that are performed to diagnose and treat problems in the female patient are essential. Health promotion and patient education are of extreme importance whether the patient is an obstetrical patient and scheduled for her initial prenatal visit or a gynecological patient scheduled for yearly pelvic, Pap, and breast examinations.

REVIEW QUESTIONS

Multiple Choice

1. Which of the following conditions or diseases that a obstetrical patient experiences is considered to place her in the high-risk category?
   a. urinary tract infection
   b. 19 years of age
   c. both partners Rh negative
   d. poor nutritional habits
   e. poor hygiene

2. Using Nagele's Rule, calculate the expected date of confinement (EDC) of a patient whose last menstrual period (LMP) was August 20, 2000.
   a. November 27, 2001
   b. December 13, 2001
   c. May 27, 2001
   d. April 20, 2001

3. The primary test performed at about the sixteenth week to check the fetus for neural tube defects is known as:
   a. alphafetal protein analysis (AFP)
   b. amniocentesis
   c. chorionic villi sampling (CVS)
   d. rubella titer
   e. Rh factor

4. The release of which of the following hormones is thought to cause labor to begin?
   a. progesterone
   b. estrogen
   c. oxytoxin
   d. thyroxine

5. Ultrasonography is done to check for which of the following?
   a. gestational diabetes
   b. pre-eclampsia
   c. degree of effacement
   d. number of weeks of gestation

6. Following a cervical punch biopsy, it is normal for the patient to experience which of the following?
   a. bleeding greater than a normal menstrual period
   b. no odor to vaginal discharge
   c. a strong, foul odor to vaginal discharge
   d. severe abdominal cramps

7. To make the diagnosis of trichomoniasis, the medical assistant will need to prepare for which of the following?
   a. Pap smear
   b. ultrasonography
   c. wet mount
   d. culture and sensitivity
   e. blood glucose

8. To diagnose pelvic inflammatory disease (PID), the physician may order which of the following?
   a. wet mount
   b. Pap smear
   c. urinalysis
   d. rubella titer
   e. ultrasonography

9. Which of the following is/are primarily associated with abnormal Pap smears?
   a. endometriosis
   b. Bartholin cyst
   c. condylomata
   d. ovarian cysts
   e. pelvic inflammatory disease

10. The primary purpose of colposcopy is to:
   a. treat advanced cancer of the vagina and cervix
   b. detect dysplastic cells of cervix following a positive Pap smear
   c. detect an ectopic pregnancy in the fallopian tube
   d. treat endometriosis of the pelvic cavity

Critical Thinking Questions

1. A pregnant woman who has had no prenatal care has not had a period for six months. She has called the OB/GYN clinic to schedule an appointment because she has had vaginal bleeding. She continues to feel fetal movement. a) What laboratory tests or procedures will the doctor order? b) What diagnosis is the physician most likely to make?

2. A 17-year-old female has missed her period and has called the clinic complaining of sharp right quadrant pain. What tests/procedures will help the physician make a diagnosis?

3. A 38-year-old woman has been diagnosed with human papilloma virus (HPV) infection. What is the significance of this infection?

4. A 27-year-old woman wants to schedule an appointment because she has had some bright red bleeding following intercourse.

5. Lower abdominal and back pain that increases just prior to and during menses may be caused by what condition?

WEB ACTIVITIES

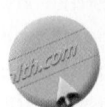

Obstetrics

Access a web site for expectant parents to locate information about the following:

1. Obtain fact sheets about each trimester.
2. Compile a list of tests, complications, and postpartum recovery.

Gynecology

Locate a web site specific to cancer of the female reproductive tract to complete the following:

1. What treatment options are available for cancer of the endometrium?
2. What tests are available to help diagnose the cancer?
3. Print a list of local support groups for women with endometrial cancer.

REFERENCES/BIBLIOGRAPHY

Bobak, I., Lowdermilk, D., Jensen, M., & Perry, S. (1999). *Maternity Nursing* (5th ed.). St. Louis, MO: Mosby-Year Book, Inc.

Damjanov, I. (1996). *Pathology for the health related profession* (1st ed.). Philadelphia: W. B. Saunders Company.

Ehrlich, A., & Schroeder, C. L. (1997). *Medical terminology for health professions* (4th ed.). Albany, NY: Delmar.

Frazier, M. S., Drzymkowski, J. A., & Doty, S. J. (1996). *Essentials of human diseases and conditions* (1st ed.). Philadelphia: W. B. Saunders Company.

Health Ink and Vitality. (August 2000). Your tour guide to health web sites, *Vitality, 14*(8), 12.

Health Ink and Vitality. (September 2000). Your tour guide to health web sites. *Vitality, 14*(9), 12.

Miller, B. F., & Keane-Brackman, C. (1992). *Encyclopedia and dictionary of medicine, nursing and allied health* (5th ed.). Philadelphia: W. B. Saunders Company.

Taber's cyclopedic medical dictionary. (18th ed.). (1999) Philadelphia: F. A. Davis Company.

Tamparo, C., & Lewis, M. (2000). *Diseases of the human body* (3rd ed.). Philadelphia: F. A. Davis Company.

Zakus, S. (1995). *Clinical procedures for medical assistants* (3rd. ed.). St. Louis: Mosby-Year Book, Inc.

PEDIATRICS

KEY TERMS

Exudate
Myringotomy
Suppurative
Tympanostomy

OUTLINE

What Is Pediatrics?
    Preparation of Vaccines for
      Administration
    Recommended Vaccination
      Schedule
Growth Patterns
    Developmental Patterns
Measuring the Infant or Child
    Height and Weight Measurements
    Height and Weight Measuring
      Devices
    Measuring Head Circumference
    Measuring Chest Circumference
Pediatric Vital Signs
    Temperature
    Pulse

    Respirations
    Blood Pressure
**Collecting a Urine Specimen from
  an Infant**
**Screening Infants for Hearing
  Impairment**
**Screening Infant and Child Visual
  Acuity**
Common Disorders and Diseases
    Otitis Media
    The Common Cold
    Tonsillitis
    Pediculosis
    Asthma
    Child Abuse

OBJECTIVES

*The student should strive to meet the following performance objectives and demonstrate
an understanding of the facts and principles presented in this chapter through written and
oral communication.*

1. Define the key terms as presented in the glossary.

2. Describe pediatric care including measuring height, weight, head, chest
   circumference, and vital signs.

3. Explain the process of collecting a urine specimen.

4. Describe common pediatric diseases and disorders.

5. Explain the importance of immunizations and scheduling of them.

CLINICAL

Fundamental Principles

- Apply principles of aseptic technique and infection control
- Comply with quality assurance practices
- Screen and follow up patient test results

Diagnostic Orders

- Collect and process specimens
- Perform diagnostic tests

Patient Care

- Obtain patient history and vital signs
- Prepare and maintain examination and treatment areas
- Prepare patient for examinations, procedures and treatments
- Assist with examinations, procedures and treatments
- Prepare and administer medications and immunizations
- Maintain medication and immunization records
- Coordinate patient care information with other health care providers

GENERAL
(TRANSDISCIPLINARY)

Legal Concepts

- Document accurately

Instruction

- Instruct individuals according to their needs
- Teach methods of health promotion and disease prevention

At Inner City Health Care, clinical assistant Bruce Goldman is responsible for encouraging parents to keep track of their children's immunization records. Bruce teaches parents the importance of immunizations for long-term health protection and the importance of following recommended vaccination schedules for maximum benefit.

INTRODUCTION

New techniques and developments occur frequently in medicine and medical assistants must refine existing skills and learn new ones to be knowledgeable and proficient and to provide the most current, up-to-date quality care to patients. The medical assistant who works in a pediatrician's office or a pediatric ambulatory care setting that treats infants and children will need additional skills when providing pediatric care to patients.

Knowledge of the developmental stages and diseases of infants and children, the ability to gain the child's confidence and trust, and the caregivers' cooperation are all skills required to provide for the physiological, emotional, and psychological needs of the pediatric patient. This chapter covers the specialty examination and the appropriate clinical procedures in pediatrics.

WHAT IS PEDIATRICS?

Pediatrics is the branch of medicine that cares for newborns, infants, children, and adolescents. Pediatricians are physicians who diagnose and treat health problems and diseases specific to these age groups. This patient population has special needs, and medical assistants must be knowledgeable about the growth and development phases of life and diseases unique to pediatric patients. Children form judgments and have fears about health care providers. They need an atmosphere that is comfortable and one in which their physiological, emotional, and psychological needs are recognized and addressed.

Medical assistants must gain the confidence and trust of the child, allay fear, and help to promote positive relationships between the child and the physician and must themselves develop a positive relationship with the child. Children are likely to be cooperative when being examined or during a procedure if good rapport has been established. It is important to be honest with young patients and approach them at their level of understanding. Allow children to touch and hold a "safe" instrument, such as a stethoscope, and explain its purpose to them. By doing so anxiety and fear can be reduced (Figure 15-1).

The first physical examination of a newborn is performed immediately after delivery. The pediatrician

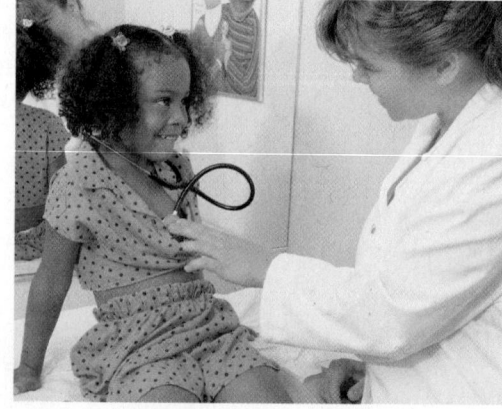

Figure 15-1 The medical assistant is making a game of a procedure to gain the child's cooperation.

will assess the infant's ability to exist outside of the mother's uterus. A scoring system is used to determine the infant's physical condition at one minute and five minutes after birth. It is known as the APGAR score. Muscle tone, skin color, respiration, heart rate, and response to stimuli are given a score 0, 1, 2, and so on, with the highest score 10. Infants with low APGAR scores need immediate attention, such as stimulation, oxygen, medication, and so on. Their condition is closely monitored.

Many patients seen in the pediatric setting are babies or children who are not ill. They are considered "well-baby" or "well-child" patients and are having routine checkups. Ill babies or children seen in the pediatrician's office or pediatric clinic are often called "sick-child" or "sick-baby" patients. Well-baby appointments are regularly scheduled appointments during which time the physician examines the child and evaluates the growth and development of the child. Most offices schedule well-baby appointments after birth according to the following time frame: 1, 2, 4, 6, 9, 12, 15, 18, 24 months, and yearly thereafter.

The goal of well-baby visits or checkups is prevention of health problems and diseases. Typically, immunizations are given during these appointments. The chart shown in Figure 15-2 includes immunization schedules

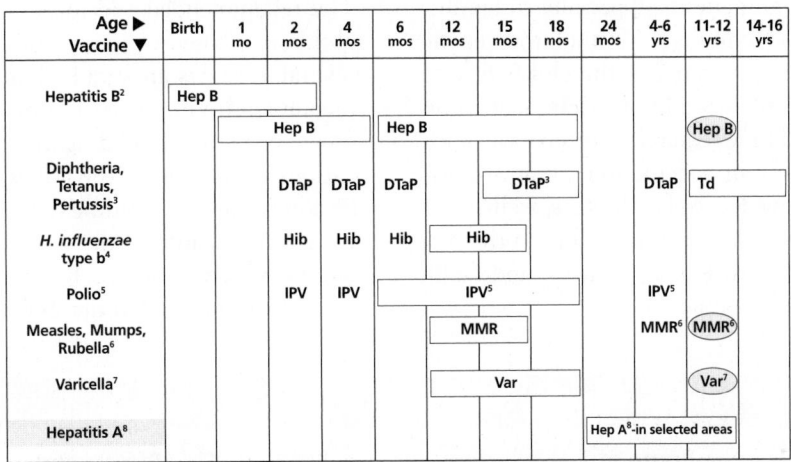

Recommended Childhood Immunization Schedule
United States, January – December 2000

Vaccines[1] are listed under routinely recommended ages. Bars indicate range of recommended ages for immunization. Any dose not given at the recommended age should be given as a "catch-up" immunization at any subsequent visit when indicated and feasible. Ovals indicate vaccines to be given if previously recommended doses were missed or given earlier than the recommended minimum age.

Age ▶ Vaccine ▼	Birth	1 mo	2 mos	4 mos	6 mos	12 mos	15 mos	18 mos	24 mos	4-6 yrs	11-12 yrs	14-16 yrs
Hepatitis B[2]	Hep B	Hep B			Hep B						Hep B	
Diphtheria, Tetanus, Pertussis[3]			DTaP	DTaP	DTaP		DTaP[3]			DTaP	Td	
H. influenzae type b[4]			Hib	Hib	Hib	Hib						
Polio[5]			IPV	IPV		IPV[5]				IPV[5]		
Measles, Mumps, Rubella[6]						MMR				MMR[6]	MMR[6]	
Varicella[7]						Var					Var[7]	
Hepatitis A[8]									Hep A[8]-in selected areas			

Approved by the Advisory Committee on Immunization Practices (ACIP), the American Academy of Pediatrics (AAP), and the American Academy of Family Physicians (AAFP).

IS 5081

(For **necessary footnotes** and important information, see reverse side.)

On October 22, 1999, the Advisory Committee on Immunization Practices (ACIP) recommended that Rotashield (RRV-TV), the only US-licensed rotavirus vaccine, no longer be used in the United States (MMWR Morb Mortal Wkly Rep. Nov 5, 1999;48(43):1007). Parents should be reassured that their children who received rotavirus vaccine before July are not at increased risk for intussusception now.

1 This schedule indicates the recommended ages for routine administration of currently licensed childhood vaccines as of 11/1/99. Additional vaccines may be licensed and recommended during the year. Licensed combination vaccines may be used whenever any components of the combination are indicated and its other components are not contraindicated. Providers should consult the manufacturers' package inserts for detailed recommendations.

2 <u>Infants born to HBsAg-negative mothers</u> should receive the 1st dose of hepatitis B (Hep B) vaccine by age 2 months. The 2nd dose should be at least 1 month after the 1st dose. The 3rd dose should be administered at least 4 months after the 1st dose and at least 2 months after the 2nd dose, but not before 6 months of age for infants.
   <u>Infants born to HBsAg-positive mothers</u> should receive hepatitis B vaccine and 0.5 mL hepatitis B immune globulin (HBIG) within 12 hours of birth at separate sites. The 2nd dose is recommended at 1 to 2 months of age and the 3rd dose at 6 months of age.
   <u>Infants born to mothers whose HBsAg status is unknown</u> should receive hepatitis B vaccine within 12 hours of birth. Maternal blood should be drawn at the time of delivery to determine the mother's HBsAg status; if the HBsAg test is positive, the infant should receive HBIG as soon as possible (no later than 1 week of age).
   <u>All children and adolescents (through 18 years of age)</u> who have not been immunized against hepatitis B may begin the series during any visit. Special efforts should be made to immunize children who were born in or whose parents were born in areas of the world with moderate or high endemicity of hepatitis B virus infection.

3 The 4th dose of DTaP (diphtheria and tetanus toxoids and acellular pertussis vaccine) may be administered as early as 12 months of age, provided 6 months have elapsed since the 3rd dose and the child is unlikely to return at age 15 to 18 months. Td (tetanus and diphtheria toxoids) is recommended at 11 to 12 years of age if at least 5 years have elapsed since the last dose of DTP, DTaP, or DT. Subsequent routine Td boosters are recommended every 10 years.

4 Three *Haemophilus influenzae* type b (Hib) conjugate vaccines are licensed for infant use. If PRP-OMP (PedvaxHIB or ComVax [Merck]) is administered at 2 and 4 months of age, a dose at

6 months is not required. Because clinical studies in infants have demonstrated that using some combination products may induce a lower immune response to the Hib vaccine component, DTaP/Hib combination products should not be used for primary immunization in infants at 2, 4, or 6 months of age unless FDA-approved for these ages.

5 To eliminate the risk of vaccine-associated paralytic polio (VAPP), an all-IPV schedule is now recommended for routine childhood polio vaccination in the United States. All children should receive four doses of IPV at 2 months, 4 months, 6 to 18 months, and 4 to 6 years. OPV (if available) may be used only for the following special circumstances:
   1. Mass vaccination campaigns to control outbreaks of paralytic polio.
   2. Unvaccinated children who will be traveling in <4 weeks to areas where polio is endemic or epidemic.
   3. Children of parents who do not accept the recommended number of vaccine injections. These children may receive OPV only for the third or fourth dose or both; in this situation, health care professionals should administer OPV only after discussing the risk for VAPP with parents or caregivers.
   4. During the transition to an all-IPV schedule, recommendations for the use of remaining OPV supplies in physicians' offices and clinics have been issued by the American Academy of Pediatrics (see *Pediatrics*, December 1999).

6 The 2nd dose of measles, mumps, and rubella (MMR) vaccine is recommended routinely at 4 to 6 years of age but may be administered during any visit, provided at least 4 weeks have elapsed since receipt of the 1st dose and that both doses are administered beginning at or after 12 months of age. Those who have not previously received the second dose should complete the schedule by the 11- to 12-year-old visit.

7 Varicella (Var) vaccine is recommended at any visit on or after the first birthday for susceptible children, ie, those who lack a reliable history of chickenpox (as judged by a health care professional) and who have not been immunized. Susceptible persons 13 years of age or older should receive 2 doses, given at least 4 weeks apart.

8 Hepatitis A (Hep A) is shaded to indicate its recommended use in selected states and/or regions; consult your local public health authority. (Also see *MMWR Morb Mortal Wkly Rep.* Oct 01, 1999;48(RR-12); 1-37).

Immunization Protects Children
Regular checkups at your pediatrician's office or local health clinic are an important way to keep children healthy.
   By making sure that your child gets immunized on time, you can provide the best available defense against many dangerous childhood diseases. Immunizations protect children against: hepatitis B, polio, measles, mumps, rubella (German measles), pertussis (whooping cough), diphtheria, tetanus (lockjaw), *Haemophilus influenzae* type b, and chickenpox. All of these immunizations need to be given before children are 2 years old in order for them to be protected during their most vulnerable period. Are your child's immunizations up-to-date?

The chart on the other side of this fact sheet includes immunization recommendations from the American Academy of Pediatrics. Remember to keep track of your child's immunizations—it's the only way you can be sure your child is up-to-date. Also, check with your pediatrician or health clinic at each visit to find out if your child needs any booster shots or if any new vaccines have been recommended since this schedule was prepared.
   If you don't have a pediatrician, call your local health department. Public health clinics usually have supplies of vaccine and may give shots free.

American Academy of Pediatrics

Figure 15-2 Recommended vaccination schedule for infants and children. (Courtesy of American Academy of Pediatrics)

from the American Academy of Pediatrics. The Academy urges that all children be immunized because the vaccines provide the best defense against many dangerous childhood diseases. Immunizations protect children against hepatitis B, polio, measles, mumps, rubella, pertussis, diphtheria, tetanus, haemophilus influenza type b, and chicken pox. All of these need to be given before age two to protect children during the period of their lives when they are more susceptible to infectious diseases.

Preparation of Vaccines for Administration

Careful attention to both proper storage of vaccines and thorough patient preparation for immunization will promote effective vaccination results. Access to vaccination should be available to all patients, especially to families with young infants and children. Most of the recommended vaccines are administered in the child's first 15 months of life. Access involves cost of vaccines, appointment requirements, and time required to receive vaccines. Some offices permit walk-in vaccination administration with free or low co-pay fee only. Routine well-infant examinations should be scheduled according to the recommended vaccination schedule to promote and facilitate maintenance of the schedule.

Vaccine storage should follow specific manufacturer's guidelines. Some vaccine preparations require refrigeration or protection from light.

Vaccines stimulate the immune system to produce antibodies against pathogens. Some patients may have conditions or pre-existing conditions that would contraindicate vaccine administration. Safe vaccine administration requires assessment and recognition of conditions that would contraindicate vaccine administration at any specific time. Contraindications for each vaccine are presented in Table 15-1. When any vaccine is not given because of an existing contraindication, careful documentation and notification of the physician are required.

Recommended Vaccination Schedule

The recommended vaccination schedule for infants and children is based on the premise that repeated doses for several vaccines are required and vaccine manufacturers recommend administering only compatible vaccines at any one visit to avoid drug interactions. If no contraindications are present at the following ages, vaccines should be administered according to the schedule to ensure complete vaccination by the age of 15 to 18 months, with booster vaccines upon school entry and again every ten years throughout adult life. Should any vaccine be missed

TABLE 15-1 VACCINE ADMINISTRATION GUIDELINES

Vaccine	Disease	Route of Administration	Contraindications	Side Effects and Adverse Reactions	Comments
DTP	Diptheria, tetanus, pertussis	IM	Fever, inconsolable or high-pitched crying, neurological disorders or family history of neurological disorders, acute polio outbreak	Mild fever, drowsiness, anorexia, fretfulness. **Risk of severe neurological damage is 4.2% within 3 days of administration.**	Boosters required
MMR	Measles, mumps, rubella	SC (needle free of alcohol) (use only supplied diluent)	Immunosuppression, allergy to eggs, active untreated TB, febrile illness, pregnancy	Fever, few side effects	Vaccine promotes immunity in 95 to 99% of patients
Inactive Polio Virus (IPV)	Poliomyelitis	IM	Immunosuppression, acute illness, debilitated condition	Rare	Vaccine does not protect from pre-existing or incubating polio
Hib	Meningitis caused by H. influenza b	IM (use only supplied diluent)	Acute illness	Minimal side effects	Immunity not attained for several days to a week
HBV	Hepatitis B Vaccine	IM	Allergy to yeast, serious active infection, severe cardiovascular disease	Malaise, headache, nausea, vomiting, pain at site, upper respiratory infections, fever	Antibody response greater in children and young adults than in older adults (99% for children under 1 year)
Varicella	Chicken pox	IM	Avoid if allergic to eggs or neomycin		Need for booster unknown at this time

Patient Teaching Tip

Encourage patients to be aware of different vaccines and keep track of vaccination schedules by posting recommended schedules in visible locations in the ambulatory care setting.

Figure 15-2 illustrates the recommended vaccination schedule for infants and children, which is supported by the American Academy of Pediatrics, the Advisory Committee on Immunization Practices (ACIP), the Committee on Infectious Diseases (COID), the Commission of Public Health and Scientific Affairs (COPHSA), and the American Academy of Family Physicians (AAFP).

for any reason, vaccine schedules are available to ensure adequate vaccine administration.

Sick-baby or sick-child visits are those appointments that have been arranged for ill babies or children who will be examined by the pediatrician in order to determine a diagnosis and appropriate treatment for a particular problem.

Clinical responsibilities for medical assistants during either type of visit include the same or similar procedures as the adult examination. The instruments used for the pediatric physical exam are similar to those used for an adult physical exam. Vital signs are taken, visual acuity is measured, a urine specimen may be obtained, blood drawn and processed, height and weight measurements are taken, and head circumference is measured. To gain the child's confidence, begin the exam at the feet and work up to the head. These are some of the skills and procedures medical assistants will perform or with which they will assist during the pediatric office or clinic visit.

GROWTH PATTERNS

Growth patterns provide valuable information to the pediatrician regarding the infant's physical progress. They are also used to calculate pediatric doses of medication. Height and weight and head circumference are measured at each regularly scheduled appointment at the pediatric facility. The measurements are then plotted on a physical growth percentile chart that is part of the patient's permanent record (Figure 15-3).

Developmental Patterns

Infants develop very quickly in their first year of life. Motor skills progress rapidly and children also learn to speak. Children's vocabulary increases quickly, and they learn not only how to talk, but also how to walk. They are becoming toilet trained by about age three.

As preschoolers, children have been able to master many motor skills and are exhibiting signs of developing social skills.

School-age children have perfected their motor skills and their intelligence is growing quickly. Self-worth and a sense of achievement are developing. Social skills continue to improve.

By the time children become adolescents, they attempt to establish an identity as adults. Peer pressure is powerful and is important to adolescents. They may be torn between parental values versus peer values. This stage of development is the time when most adolescents mature emotionally and are becoming more capable of making beneficial choices and decisions. See Figure 15-4 for an illustration of growth and development of infants and toddlers.

Infant/Child Failure to Thrive. The failure of an infant or a child to grow and thrive may have many organic and inorganic causes. There may be social and emotional causes. Many of the causes for an infant or a child failing to grow and thrive may be treated if found in time. The emotionally deprived infant needing affection will not grow, as there will be a lack of growth hormone production. Once this child is given physical and emotional warmth, the growth hormone is produced and the child will grow. Other reasons for an infant failing to thrive may be because the infant has a chronic disease, a diet that is inadequate in calories and proteins, a disorder of the heart, brain, or kidneys, or has been improperly fed.

MEASURING THE INFANT OR CHILD

Careful measuring of the infant or child and monitoring of growth pattern are essential and should be done in a consistent and accurate manner.

Height and Weight Measurements

To record or plot height and weight measurements, first locate one growth value either length (highlighted yellow) or weight (highlighted red) in the vertical columns of the Physical Growth Percentile Chart in Figure 15-5. Find the child's age in months in the horizontal rows (highlighted green). Locate the area where the growth value lines intersect on the graph and plot the height and weight by marking with a dot. Connect dots from previous examination with a ruler to provide a neat and accurate graphic recording. The date, age, measurements, and

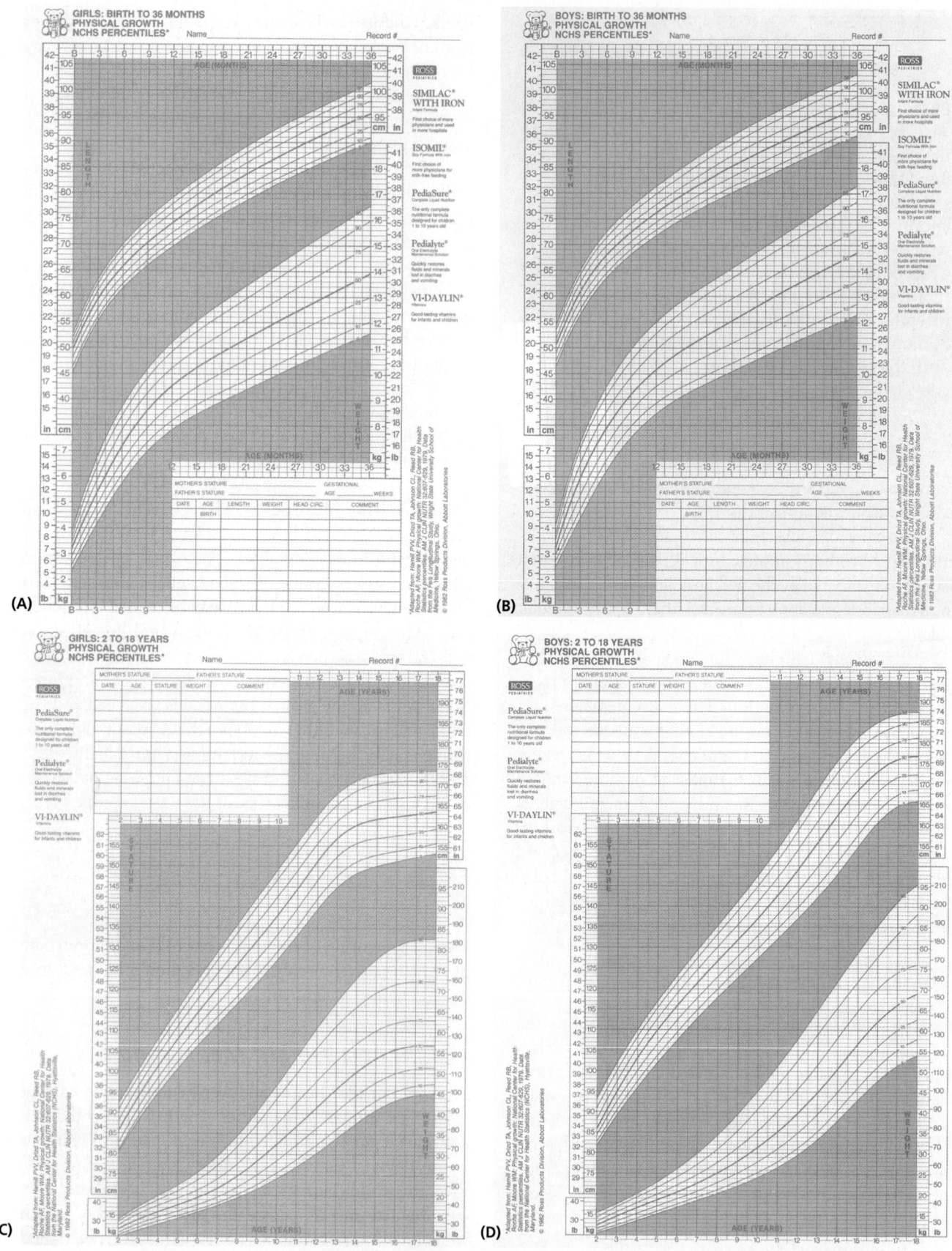

Figure 15-3   (A) Growth chart for girls' height and weight, age birth to 36 months. (B) Growth chart for boys' height and weight, age birth to 36 months. (C) Growth chart for girls' height and weight, age 2 to 18 years. (D) Growth chart for boys' height and weight, age 2 to 18 years. (Reprinted with permission of Ross Laboratories, Columbus, OH 43216, from NCHS Growth Charts)

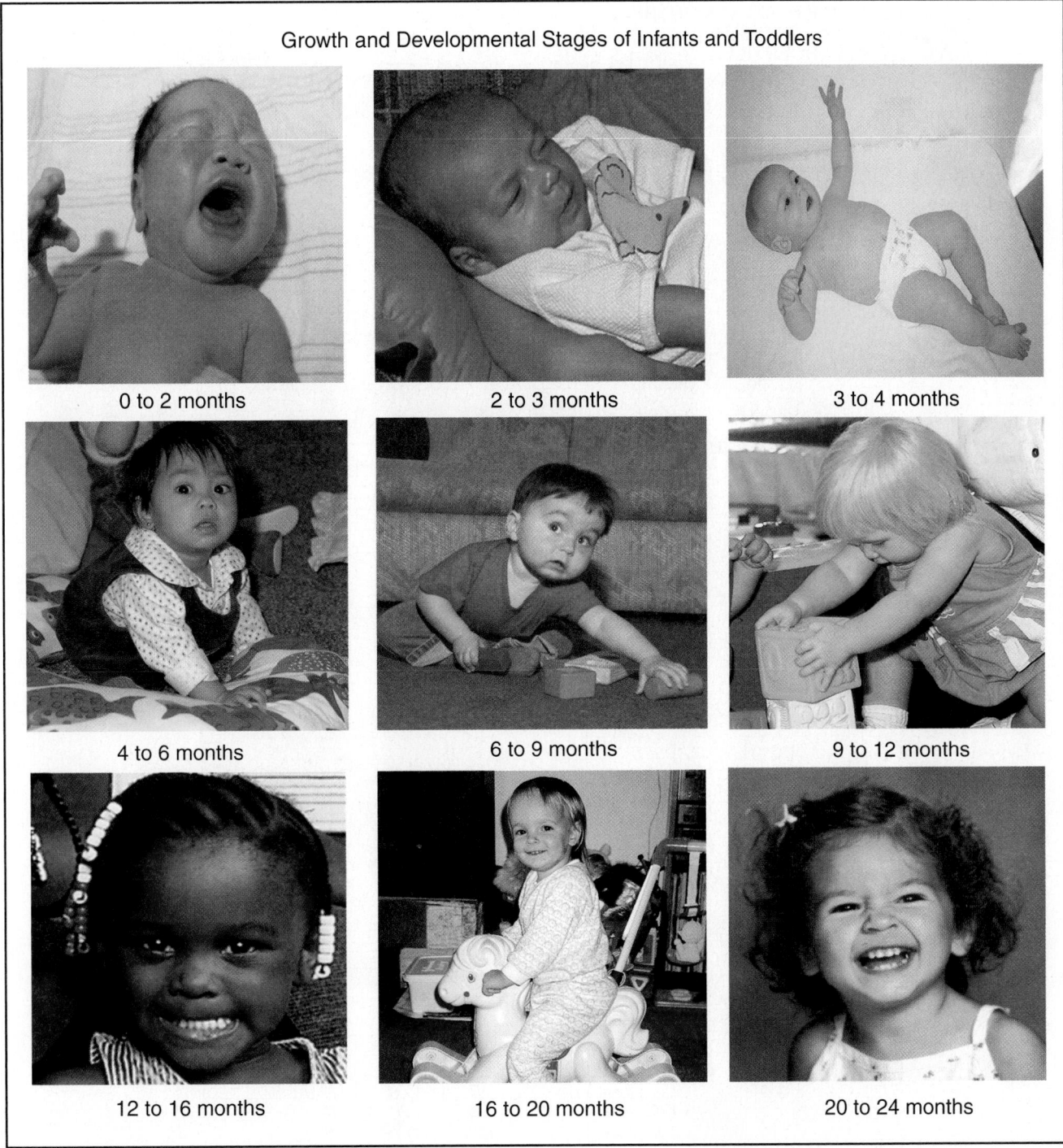

Growth and Developmental Stages of Infants and Toddlers

0 to 2 months

2 to 3 months

3 to 4 months

4 to 6 months

6 to 9 months

9 to 12 months

12 to 16 months

16 to 20 months

20 to 24 months

Figure 15-4   Growth and developmental stages of infants and toddlers.

comments should also be indicated at the bottom of the chart.

The curved lines printed across the growth charts show the normal range of growth of infants and children in the United States. The numbers on the right side of the chart, in the vertical boxes between age 34 and 35 months, show the percentiles of other children the same age. To determine into which percentile the infant falls in relation to other infants of the same age, follow the line (percentile) upward to the percentage values along the edge of the graph. The National Center for Health Statistics (NCHS) growth charts become a permanent record of the child's development. These give the physician a quick way to check the child's growth in relation to that of other children the same age. Growth charts aid in the diagnosis of growth abnormalities and nutritional disorders

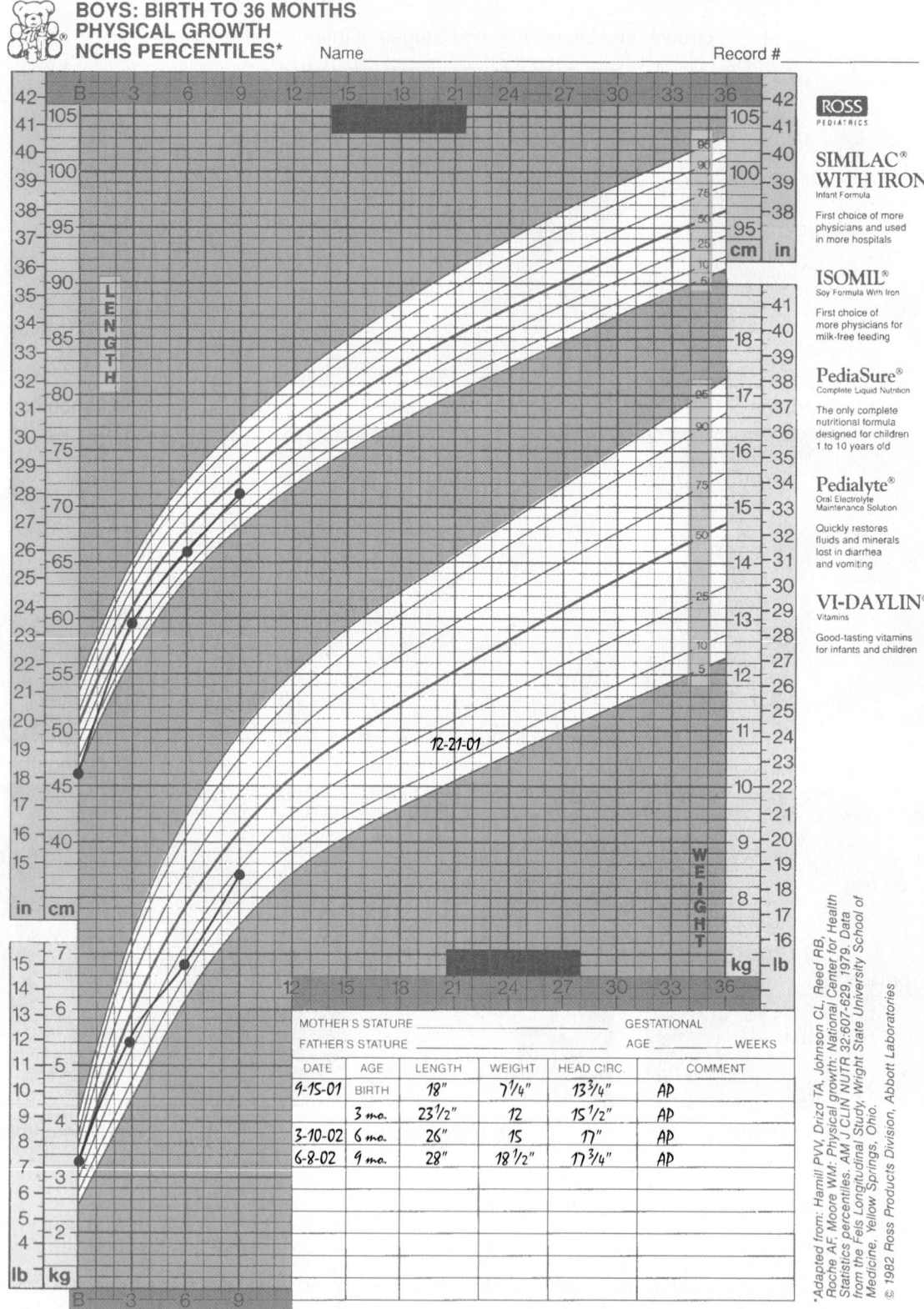

Figure 15-5   Sample growth chart with information plotted at birth, 3, 6, and 9 months. Sections in this figure have been highlighted to help you locate the values: length (yellow), weight (red), age (green), and percentiles (white). (Reprinted with permission of Ross Laboratories, Columbus, OH 43216, from NCHS Growth Charts)

and disease. Hereditary factors also influence growth patterns; therefore, having the family's history is important.

Height and Weight Measuring Devices

Various devices are available for measuring height and weight in children. Infants and small children are weighed on an infant platform scale, which provides a measurement in pounds and ounces and kilograms and grams (Figure 15-6). The scale has a platform with curved sides in which the child may sit or lie. Weigh the infant or child in as few clothes as possible, removing the diaper and shoes or slippers. A small sheet, cloth diaper, or paper towel should be placed on the scale before weighing the infant or child, to avoid the transfer of microorganisms from bare skin.

Infant length can be measured using an infant measuring board, which consists of a rigid headboard and movable footboard. Place the measuring board on a table and position the infant on his back on the board, with the head touching the headboard. Move the footboard up until it touches the bottom of the infant's feet.

An infant can also be measured on a pad by placing a pin into the pad or making a pencil mark at the top of the head and a second pin or mark at the heel of the extended leg. The length is the distance between the two pins. A tape measure can also be used. Note: 1 inch = 2.54 cm

A stature-measuring device may be used to measure height once the child is able to stand erect without support. The device consists of a movable headpiece attached to a rigid measuring bar and platform (Figure 15-7). A paper towel should be placed on the platform before use to avoid the potential transmission of microorganisms from bare feet.

Measuring Head Circumference

Head circumference measurement is routinely recorded on an infant's chart to alert the physician to any abnormal development. This procedure should be performed during routine visits until the child is 36 months old. Thereafter it should be measured on a yearly basis until the age of 6 years. Head circumference measurement requires a flexible paper or metal measuring tape. A cloth tape may stretch and give a false measurement. Head circumference is plotted similarly to height and weight but on separate Growth Percentile Charts for head measurements (Figure 15-8). Generally, head and chest circumference are equal at about 1 to 2 years of age. Rapid growth above the normal percentile may indicate hydrocephalus, a disorder in which excessive fluid accumulates around the brain causing an increase in intracranial pressure and possible brain damage. This could lead to mental and physical problems. Conversely, the growth of the head which falls below the normal percentile may indicate microencephaly caused by a premature closure of the fontanels. In this instance, there is not enough room for the development of the brain, and mental retardation can result. Head circumference for a newborn should be between 12.5 to 14.5 inches or 31.75 to 36.83 cm.

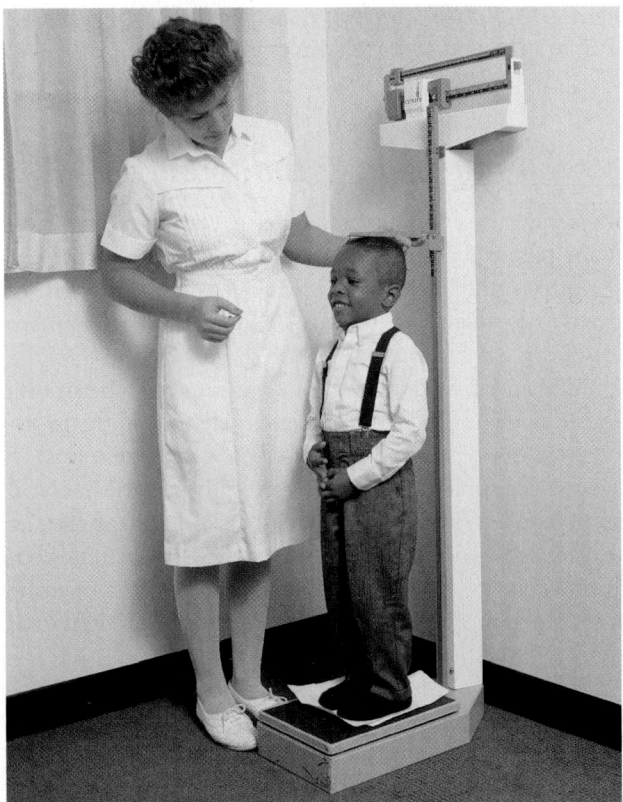

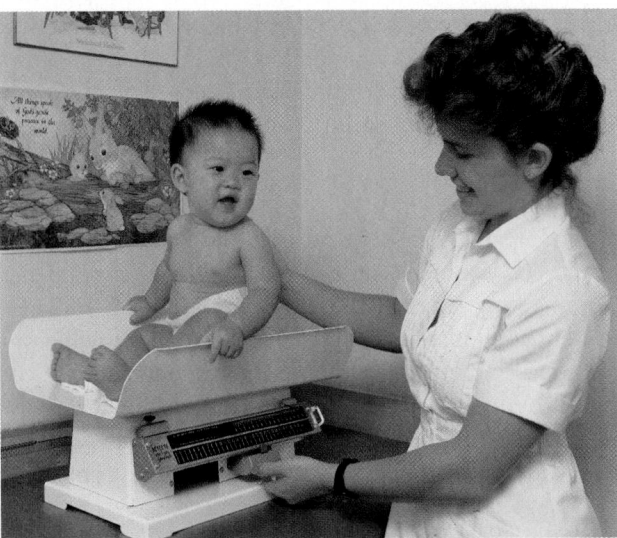

Figure 15-6 Infants who are able to sit and small children can be weighed on a platform scale.

Figure 15-7 Young children who are able to stand erect without support can be measured on a scale that has a stature-measuring device attached.

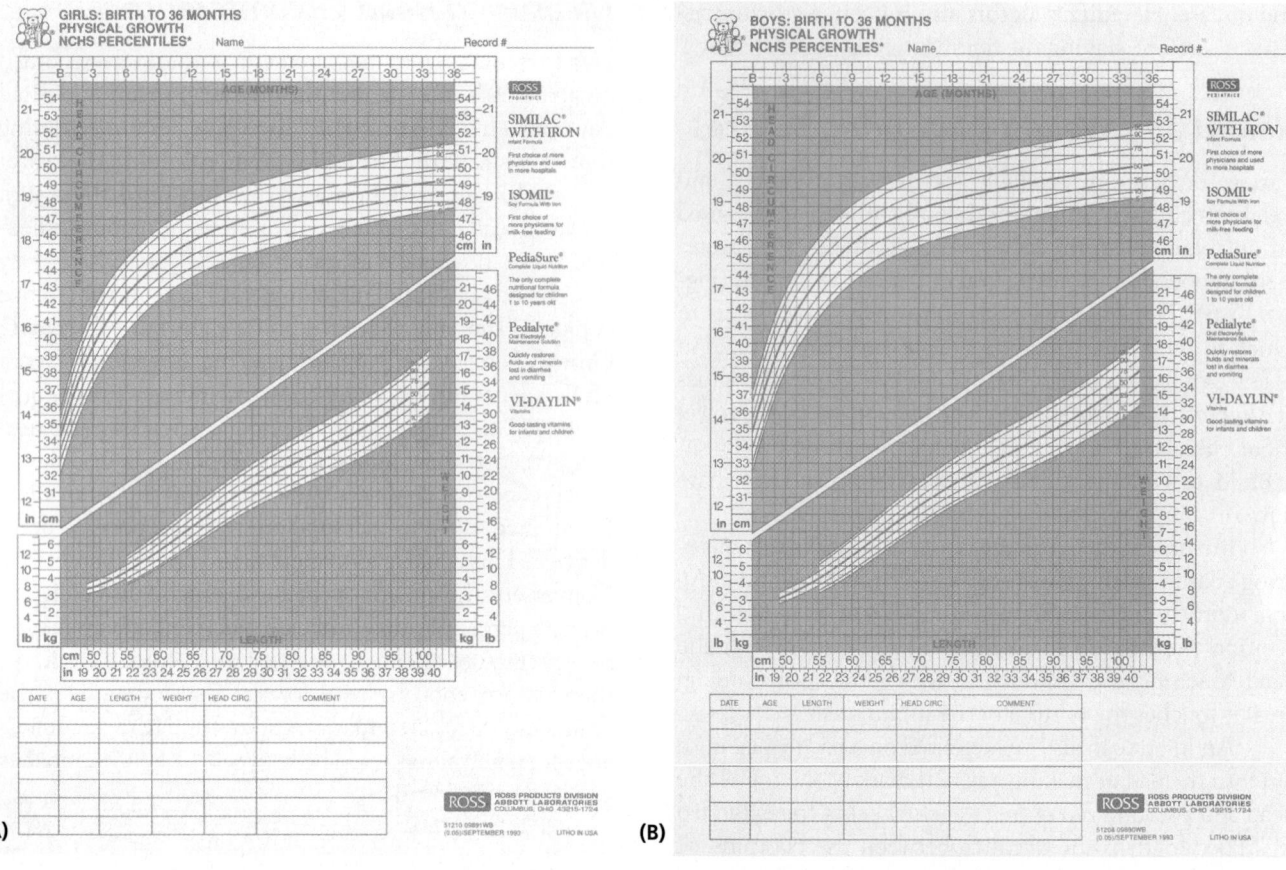

Figure 15-8 (A) Growth chart for girls' head circumference, birth to 36 months. (B) Growth chart for boys' head circumference, birth to 36 months. (Reprinted with permission of Ross Laboratories, Columbus, OH 43216, from NCHS Growth Charts)

Measuring Chest Circumference

Measuring the chest circumference of an infant is not normally performed during routine examinations. It may be performed and monitored when there is a suspicion of overdevelopment or underdevelopment of the heart and/or lungs, or calcification of rib cartilage. To measure the chest of an infant, snugly wrap the measuring tape around the chest at nipple level. It is preferable to read the measurement during the resting phase between respirations.

Occasionally it may be necessary for the medical assistant to convert measurement results into inches or centimeters. To accomplish the task accurately, note that 1 inch equals 2.54 cm. (See Procedure 15-1 for measuring infant chest and head circumference and weight and height.)

To convert inches to centimeters, multiply the number of inches by 2.54:

Inches × 2.54 = Centimeters

To convert centimeters to inches, divide the number of centimeters by 2.54:

Centimeters ÷ 2.54 = Inches

PEDIATRIC VITAL SIGNS

As with older children and adults, pediatric vital signs are commonly taken by the medical assistant. The vital signs are more fully covered in Chapter 12 for adult patients; however, specific procedures for taking an infant's temperature, pulse, respiration, and blood pressure are explained here. These procedures are done very differently for infants than for older children and adults.

Temperature

Body temperature may be measured in Fahrenheit (F) or Celsius (C) through oral, rectal, axillary, or tympanic routes. Many types of thermometers are used. Mercury (glass) thermometers have been replaced in ambulatory care areas and most offices by digital thermometers, electronic thermometers, and tympanic membrane sensors or aural, which provide accurate temperature readings in less time. Broken mercury thermometers release vapors into the air, which are toxic when inhaled and lead to mercury poisoning. Proper disposal of the mercury is regulated by the health department and varies from state to state. Electronic and digital thermometers can display temperature within 15 to 60 seconds, depending on the model used. A reading can be obtained by infrared tympanic membrane sensor in as little as 2 seconds.

Oral Temperature. The oral route is used for children over 5 years of age. Caution the child against biting down on the thermometer. If a mercury thermometer is used, wait about 3 minutes before removing the thermometer. Do not take an oral temperature if the child has a history of seizures.

Aural Temperature. The aural route uses the tympanic membrane thermometer. It is used on children over the age of two because it is considered less accurate for children under two years. Otitis media and impacted cerumen are two other reasons why this route may not be selected. A reading can be obtained in a matter of seconds.

Rectal Temperature. Rectal temperatures may be taken with caution in infants and toddlers when other methods or routes are not advised. Place the child prone or on the side, with the knees flexed. An infant can also lie prone on a parent's lap. Do not force the thermometer. When using a mercury thermometer, allow approximately 3 to 5 minutes to obtain an accurate reading. Rectal temperatures are not indicated for children who have had rectal surgery or for those who have diarrhea. (See Procedure 15-2.)

Axillary Temperature. Axillary temperatures are often preferable to rectal or oral temperatures for toddlers and preschoolers because they are safe and nonintrusive to take. Place the mercury thermometer or probe of the digital thermometer in the axillary space and have the child hold the arm close to the trunk. If a mercury thermometer is used, keep in place for 5 minutes before reading (Figure 15-9).

Pulse

The apical pulse is heard at the apex of the heart, located at the fifth intercostal space left side, midclavicular line.

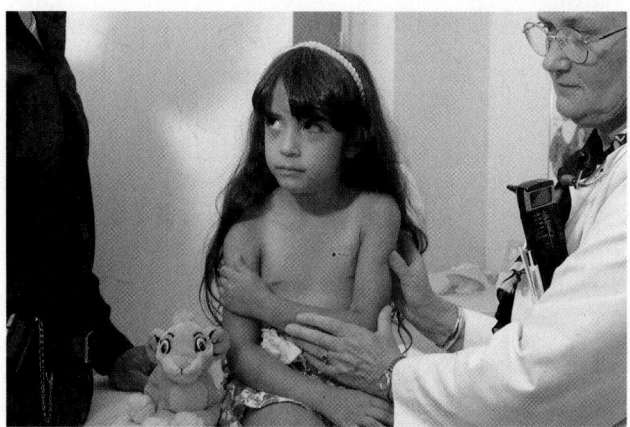

Figure 15-9 Taking an axillary temperature of a young child.

TABLE 15-2	NORMAL HEART RATE RANGES FOR CHILDREN	
Age	Heart Rate Range	Average Heart Rate
Infants to 2 years	100–160	110
2 to 6 years	70–120	100
6 to 10	70–110	90
10 to 16 years	60–100	85

That is, between the fifth and sixth ribs in the middle of the clavicle (usually below the nipple), left of the sternum. A stethoscope is required to obtain an apical pulse. The apical pulse is generally preferred over other pulse locations for infants and small children (under 5 years of age). Each "lub-dub" sound is counted as 1 heart beat. The pulse is counted for 1 full minute. (See Procedure 15-3.)

The normal pulse rate varies with age, decreasing as the child grows older (Table 15-2). The heart rate may also vary considerably among children of the same age and size. The heart rate increases in response to exercise, excitement, anxiety, and fever and decreases to a resting rate when the child is still.

Listen to the heart rate, noting whether the heart rhythm is regular or irregular. Children often have a normal cycle of irregular rhythm associated with respiration called sinus arrhythmia. In sinus arrhythmia, the child's heart rate is faster on inspiration and slower on expiration. Record whether the pulse is normal, bounding, or thready.

Respirations

In older children and adolescents, respiratory rate is counted in the same way as in an adult. In infants and young children (under 6 years of age), however, the respiratory rate is assessed by observing the rise and fall of the abdomen. Inspiration, when the chest or abdomen rises, and expiration, when the chest or abdomen falls, are counted as 1 respiration. Because these movements are often irregular, they should be counted for 1 full minute for accuracy. Normal respiratory rate varies with the child's age (Table 15-3). (See Procedure 15-4.)

TABLE 15-3	NORMAL RESPIRATORY RATE RANGES FOR CHILDREN
Age	Respiratory Rate per Minute
1 year	20–40
3 years	20–30
6 years	16–22
10 years	16–20
17 years	12–20

Blood Pressure

The blood pressure of an infant is not normally taken unless requested by the physician. In children 3 years of age and older, blood pressure should be measured annually as part of a routine vital sign assessment.

Blood pressure may be measured using mercury gravity, electronic, or aneroid equipment and a pediatric cuff. The size of the blood pressure cuff is determined by the size of the child's arm or leg. A general rule of thumb is that the width of the inflatable bladder should be 40 percent of the circumference of the extremity used. If the cuff is too small, pressure will be falsely high; if too large, falsely low. Sometimes it is difficult to hear the blood pressure in an infant or small child. Use a pediatric stethoscope over pulse sites if possible.

If the pulse still cannot be auscultated, the blood pressure can be measured by touch. Palpate for the pulse. Keeping your fingers on the pulse, pump up the cuff until the pulse is no longer felt. Slowly open the air valve, watching the column of mercury, and note the number where the pulse is again palpated. This is called the palpated systolic blood pressure.

COLLECTING A URINE SPECIMEN FROM AN INFANT

Occasionally the medical assistant may be required to obtain a urine specimen from an infant for laboratory testing. Special procedures and equipment are required for this procedure. The collection bag is clear plastic with adhesive tabs for application to the perineum of the infant (Figure 15-10). (See Procedure 15-5.)

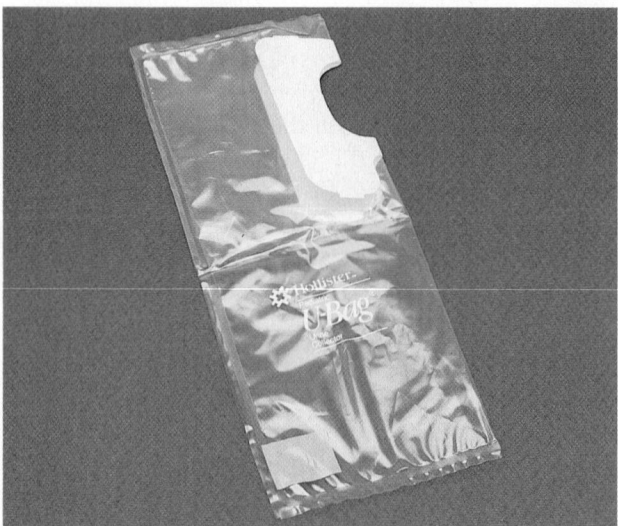

Figure 15-10   Pediatric urine collector. The collector is opened, and the paper backing is removed exposing the adhesive surface. The collector is firmly attached over the child's cleansed genitalia to prevent leakage.

SCREENING INFANTS FOR HEARING IMPAIRMENT

In some hospitals, infants are screened for hearing impairment immediately following delivery. An automated system for checking hearing ability is used by some clinics. It is a more complex screening requiring the use of sensors. As the infant moves in response to sounds produced by the system and recorded by sensors attached to the infant. This procedure is a more definitive screening process. The medical assistant must maintain a quiet environment while these screening procedures are being performed as extraneous sounds may invalidate the results.

SCREENING INFANT AND CHILD VISUAL ACUITY

Measuring the visual acuity of an infant is difficult and is not usually performed unless visual impairment is suspected. Newborns will respond to light by tightly shutting their eyes, keeping them closed until the light is removed. Older infants will follow an object up and down when it is placed directly in front of the eyes. It is estimated that a newborn has the vision equivalent to 20/150 which will reach the adult level of 20/20 by the age of 6 months. The medical assistant will be required to maintain a nonstimulating environment while the physician is screening the infant, as any interference may invalidate results.

The kindergarten chart is used to test visual acuity in young children. It contains pictures in descending size and the lines are labeled in the same manner as the Snellen Chart. The child is asked to identify the picture as the medical assistant points to it (Figure 15-11).

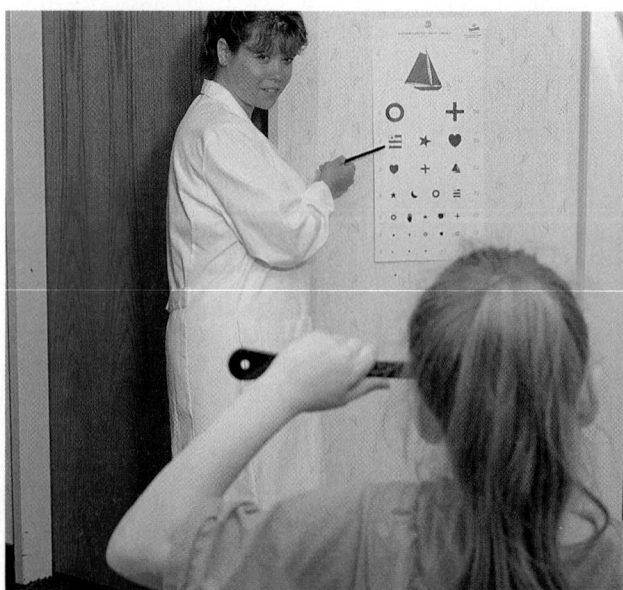

Figure 15-11   Measuring distance visual acuity of a child using a kindergarten vision screening chart.

The E chart is a series of "E"s pointing in different directions in descending size. The size and labeling are the same as the Snellen chart. This chart is used for older children. The child will be asked to point in the direction of the E as the medical assistant points to it (Figure 15-12).

Make a game out of measuring young children's visual acuity as their attention span is very limited.

COMMON DISORDERS AND DISEASES

Young children grow and physically change very quickly. Their immune systems develop normally when they are healthy infants and children. Immunizations, together with their own developing immune system give them protection from dangerous childhood diseases. Many life-threatening illnesses have been controlled because of scheduled immunization, the child's own developing immune system, and the use of antibiotics for infections.

Otitis Media

Otitis media is a commonly occurring disorder of infants and young children. It is characterized by inflammation of the middle ear. Fluid accumulates behind the tympanic membrane with a degree of temporary hearing loss. It is commonly known as a middle ear infection. Because of the infant and young child's eustachian tubes' connection to the nose and throat, bacteria that causes throat and res-

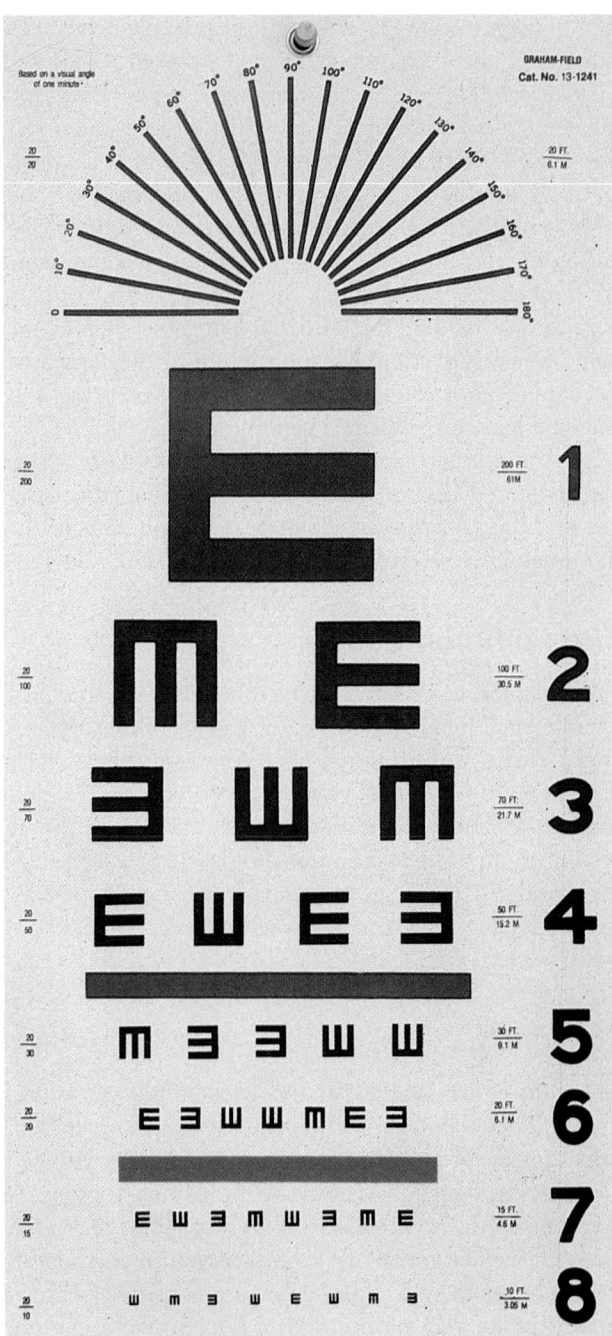

Figure 15-12 Snellen "E" or "Big E" chart for testing distance visual acuity of children.

piratory infections can easily access the inner ear via the eustachian tube. The fluid in the middle ear can become infected by the bacteria present in the nose and throat. The fluid turns to pus and is known as **suppurative** otitis media. Pain and loss of hearing are common symptoms. Many young children have eustachian tubes that are horizontal and narrow, which predisposes them to otitis media. As children develop physically, they can "outgrow" otitis media.

SPOTLIGHT ON AAMA ESSENTIALS THROUGH CAAHEP

- Gaining a child's confidence and trust during a pediatric examination will help to promote a positive relationship among the child, the physician, and the members of the medical staff.

- Protecting a child's space and modesty during an examination will help to encourage a more positive experience during the examination.

- Making a game out of a procedure and encouraging the child to take part in the examination will help to provide a more positive relationship between the child and the medical assistant.

The physician can diagnose otitis media by visually examining the tympanic membrane with an otoscope. The membrane will be bulging and appear red and inflamed. If **exudate** or an oozing of pus is present, a culture and sensitivity can be done. The treatment for otitis media is antibiotics. To avoid antibiotic overuse and pathogen resistance, physicians will attempt to prescribe antibiotic therapy only when necessary. Decongestants are helpful in some children. For chronic otitis media, a **myringotomy**, incision into the tympanic membrane, may be necessary to avoid the rupture of the tympanic membrane and the scarring that results. Scarring can cause permanently impaired hearing ability.

Tympanostomy is a surgical procedure in which pediatric ear tubes are placed through the tympanic membrane to promote ongoing drainage. Chronic otitis media that is left untreated can result in permanent hearing loss.

The Common Cold

The common cold is aptly named because it is the most common and frequent disease that young children experience. Viruses are the usual microorganism that cause a cold, and they are spread by direct contact and droplets through the air when children cough and sneeze. Some symptoms are inflammation of the nasopharynx, coughing, nasal discharge, sneezing, and fever. Treatment consists of getting sufficient rest, forcing fluids, and eating a well-balanced diet.

Tonsillitis

The tonsils are located in the back of the nose and throat. They aid in protecting the respiratory tract from infection but frequently become inflamed and infected while doing their job. The cause most often is group A beta-hemolytic streptococcus. Fever, cough, sore throat, and red, swollen tonsils are common symptoms. Diagnosis can be made by doing a culture and sensitivity of tonsillar exudate. Antibiotics will rid the child of infection. Tonsillectomy is considered for older children who have chronic tonsillitis.

Pediculosis

Infestation with the head louse is known as pediculosis capitis and is common among school-age children. The parasites suck blood from humans and are highly contagious. Diagnosis can be made by visual examination of the hair and scalp and observing the eggs (known as nits) on the hair. Special medications applied to the hair is an effective treatment. Care should be taken to launder bed linens and clothing every day.

Asthma

Asthma has increased dramatically in the general population but especially in children. The cause of asthma is not known, but it can be brought on by environmental substances, such as pollen, chemicals, cigarette smoke, mold, and dog and cat hair. Its symptoms include wheezing, coughing, and shortness of breath. It is a serious chronic respiratory disease. Spasms of the bronchi trap air and mucus in the lungs. The child will complain of a tight chest and will have shallow respirations and a nonproductive cough. The asthma attack may become an emergency situation. The pediatrician may refer the child to an allergy specialist who will test the child for various allergies. Respiratory therapy is helpful for some children.

Child Abuse

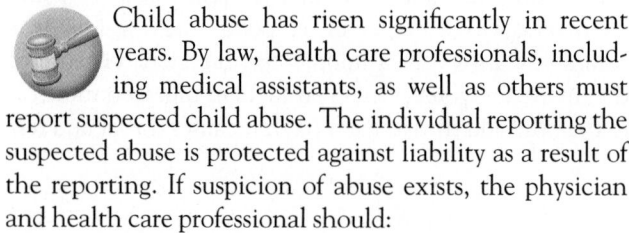 Child abuse has risen significantly in recent years. By law, health care professionals, including medical assistants, as well as others must report suspected child abuse. The individual reporting the suspected abuse is protected against liability as a result of the reporting. If suspicion of abuse exists, the physician and health care professional should:

- Treat child's injuries
- Send child to hospital if necessary
- Inform parents of the diagnosis
- Inform parents that the incident will be reported to the public and social service agency
- Notify child protective agency
- Document all information
- Provide court testimony if requested

Some injuries commonly seen in child abuse include poor hygiene, bruises, welts, malnutrition, burns, fractures, head injuries, dislocated joints and neglected well-baby appointments.

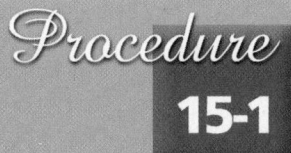

Procedure 15-1 Measuring the Infant: Weight, Height, Head, and Chest Circumference

STANDARD PRECAUTIONS:

PURPOSE:

To obtain an accurate measurement of an infant's weight, height, head, and chest circumference for medical records and to screen for growth abnormalities.

EQUIPMENT/SUPPLIES:

Infant scale	Patient's chart
Paper protector	Pen
Flexible measuring	Ruler
tape	Biohazard waste
Growth chart	container

PROCEDURE STEPS:

Measuring Infant Weight

1. Wash hands. Explain procedure to parent(s).
2. Undress infant (including the diaper).
3. Place all weights to left of scale to check balance.
4. Place a clean utility towel on scale, check balance scale for accuracy being sure to compensate for the weight of the towel. RATIONALE: The protection that the paper utility towel affords helps to reduce transmission of microorganisms and will provide warmth because the scale will be cool.

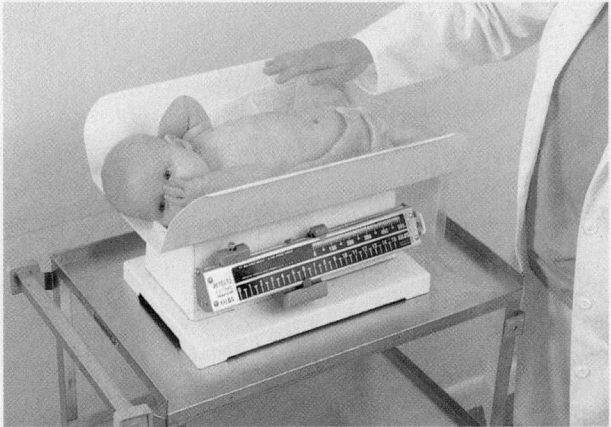

Figure 15-13 Infants who are unable to sit erect should be weighed on their back on a platform scale.

5. Gently place infant on her back on the scale. Place your hand slightly above the infant's body to ensure safety (Figure 15-13). RATIONALE: This will safeguard the infant from falling.
6. Place the bottom weight to its highest measurement that will not cause the balance to drop to the bottom edge.
7. Slowly move upper weight until the balance bar rests in the center of the indicator. A balanced scale will provide an accurate weight. Read the infant's weight while she is lying still.
8. Return both weights to their resting position to the extreme left.
9. Gently remove infant and apply diaper. (Parent can help with diapering and holding infant.)
10. Discard used protective paper towel per OSHA guidelines.
11. Sanitize scale.
12. Wash hands.
13. Document results according to office policy (pounds and ounces or kilograms) on growth chart, patient's chart, and parent's booklet if available. Connect dot from previous examination with a ruler to complete graph.

Measuring Infant Length/Height

1. Wash hands. Explain procedure to parent(s).
2. Remove infant's shoes.
3. Gently place infant on her back on the examination table. If the pediatric table has a headboard, ask parent to hold infant's head against (end) headboard of table at zero mark of ruler while you place infant's heels against footboard. Gently straighten infant's back and legs to line up along ruler. If there is no footboard (to place infant's feet against), use your right hand as a guide (Figure 15-14). If necessary, gently place your left hand over the child's legs at the knees to secure the child in place and straighten the legs so you can read the recumbent length from the head to the heel. RATIONALE: Sometimes it is difficult to straighten the legs.
4. Read length on the measuring device in inches or centimeters.
5. Wash hands.

(continues)

Procedure

15-1   (continued)

6. Document measurement on growth chart, patient's chart, and parent's booklet if available. Connect dot from previous examination with a ruler to complete graph.

Measure Head Circumference

1. Wash hands and explain procedure to parent(s).
2. Talk to infant to gain cooperation. Infant may be held by parent or lie on examination table for procedure. Older children of 2 or 3 years may stand or sit if they will remain still.
3. Place the measuring tape snugly around the head from the occipital protuberance to the supraorbital prominence. This is the largest part of the head (Figure 15-15).

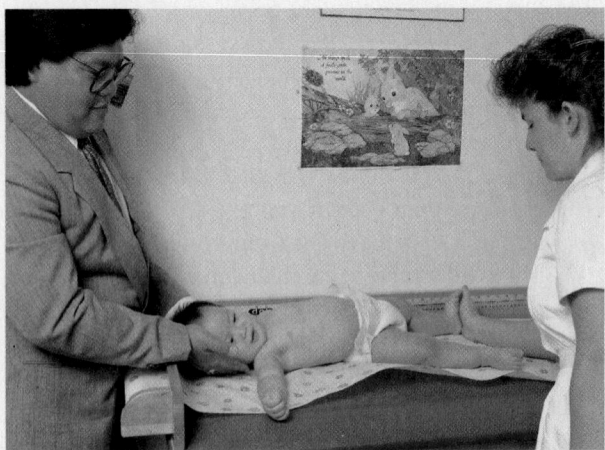

Figure 15-14   Measuring the recumbent length of an infant.

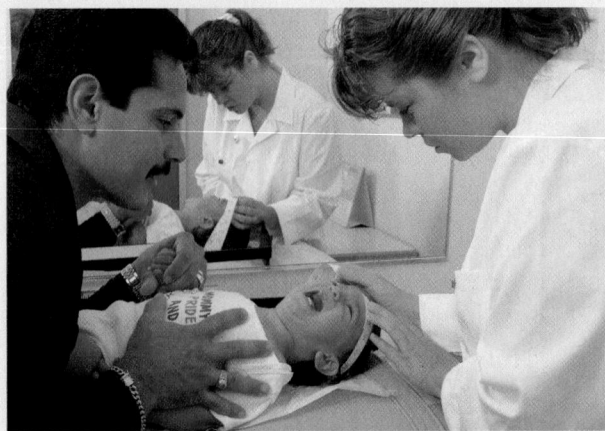

Figure 15-15   Measuring infant's head circumference.

4. Read the measurement which will be in either inches (to nearest ½ inch) or centimeters (to nearest 0.01 cm).
5. Wash hands.
6. Document results according to office policy on growth chart, patient's chart, and parent's booklet if available. Connect dot from previous examination with a ruler to complete graph.

Measure Infant's Chest Circumference

1. Wash hands and explain procedure to parent(s).
2. Use one thumb to hold tape measure with zero mark against the infant's chest at the midsternal area. With the other hand, bring the tape around/under the back to meet the zero mark of the tape in front. Take the measurement of the chest just above the nipples with the tape fitting around the child's chest under the axillary region. If you need assistance in holding the child still, ask the parent or another assistant. The measurement should be taken when the child is breathing normally and during the resting phase between respirations (Figure 15-16).
3. Read measurement to the nearest 0.01 cm or $\frac{1}{16}$ inch.
4. Wash hands.
5. Document results in patient's chart.

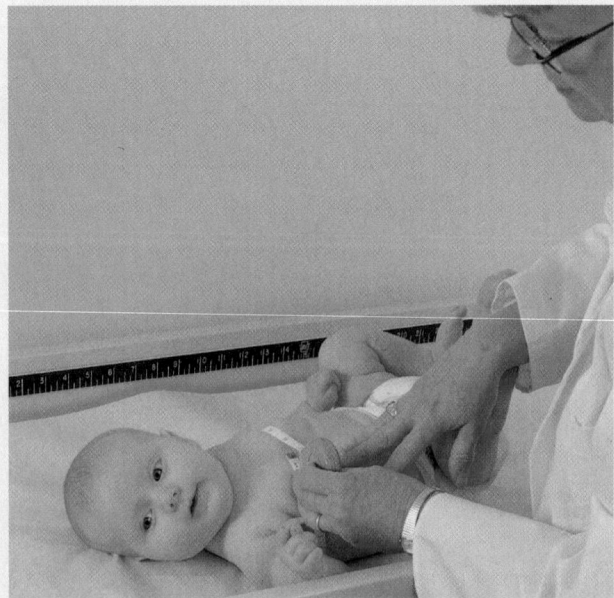

Figure 15-16   Measuring infant's chest circumference.

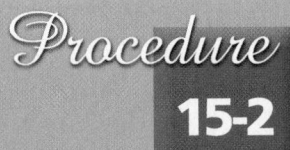

Procedure 15-2 — Taking an Infant's Rectal Temperature with a Mercury or Digital Thermometer

STANDARD PRECAUTIONS:

PURPOSE:

To obtain a rectal temperature using a mercury or digital thermometer.

EQUIPMENT/SUPPLIES:

Mercury rectal thermometer (red tip) and sheath
 or
Digital thermometer (red probe) and probe cover
Lubricating jelly
4 × 4 gauze sponges
Gloves
Biohazard waste container

PROCEDURE STEPS:

1. Wash hands.
2. Assemble equipment.
3. Identify patient.
4. Explain procedure to parent(s). RATIONALE: Gain cooperation and assistance in disrobing infant and positioning properly.
5. Remove infant's diaper.
6. Position infant in a prone position having parent or another medical assistant safeguard infant.
7. Place sheath on thermometer. RATIONALE: Prevents microorganism cross contamination.
8. Lubricate with lubricating jelly. (Place lubricant on a 4 × 4 gauze sponge and place tip of thermometer in lubricant.) RATIONALE: Easier insertion of thermometer.
9. Apply gloves.
10. Spread buttocks, insert thermometer gently into the rectum past the sphincter; for an infant this is ½ inch (Figure 15-17).
11. Hold buttocks together while holding the thermometer. If necessary, restrain infant movement by placing your arm across infant's back. Parent can immobilize infant's legs. RATIONALE: Ensure infant's safety and comfort.
12. Hold in place for five minutes. Do not let go of the thermometer. RATIONALE: Movement by infant can cause thermometer to move and injure the infant.
13. Remove from rectum. Have parent attend to infant.
14. Remove sheath and place in biohazard container.
15. Read thermometer.
16. Wash, rinse, and dry thermometer. Place on clean paper towel.
17. Remove gloves, discard in biohazard waste container.
18. Wash hands.
19. Place thermometer in a disinfectant solution for rectal thermometers.
20. Assist parent in dressing infant if necessary.
21. Record on the patient chart labeled with (R) indicating a rectal temperature.

Using Digital Thermometer

1. Follow steps 1 through 11 for taking temperature with mercury thermometer.
2. Hold digital thermometer in place until the beep is heard.
3. Read results on digital display window.
4. Remove thermometer from rectum.
5. Discard probe cover into biohazard waste container by pressing the eject button on probe end.
6. Replace thermometer on holder base.
7. Remove gloves, discard in biohazard waste container, and wash hands.
8. Assist patient in dressing and position as necessary.
9. Record on the patient chart labeled with (R) indicating a rectal temperature.
10. Wash hands.

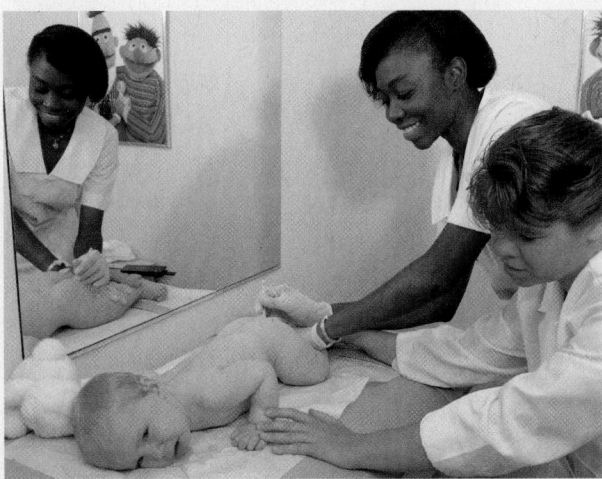

Figure 15-17 Taking the rectal temperature of an infant in the prone position.

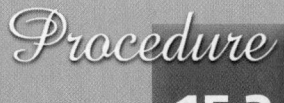

Procedure 15-3   Taking an Apical Pulse on an Infant

STANDARD PRECAUTIONS:

PURPOSE:
To obtain an apical pulse rate.

EQUIPMENT/SUPPLIES:
Stethoscope
Watch with second hand
Alcohol wipes

PROCEDURE STEPS:
1. Wash hands.
2. Assemble equipment.
3. Identify patient.
4. Explain procedure to parent.
5. Assist in disrobing infant if necessary.
6. Provide a drape for infant's warmth if necessary.
7. Position the infant in a supine position or sitting in the parent's lap. RATIONALE: The supine position may offer easier access to apex of heart if the child is calm.
8. Locate the fifth intercostal space, midclavicular line, left of sternum. RATIONALE: Location of apex of heart.
9. Place warmed stethoscope on the site and listen for the lub-dup sound of the heart.
10. Count the pulse for one minute; each lub-dup equals one heartbeat or pulse.
11. Wash hands.
12. Record the pulse in the infant's chart with the designation of (AP) to denote method of obtaining the pulse.
13. Note any arrhythmias.
14. Assist patient as needed.
15. Clean earpieces and diaphragm of stethoscope with alcohol wipes. RATIONALE: Prevents cross contamination of microbes between patients.
16. Wash hands again.

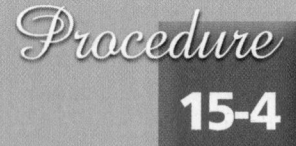

Procedure 15-4   Measuring Infant's Respiration Rate

STANDARD PRECAUTIONS:

PURPOSE:
The respiration rate is normally taken immediately before or after the pulse rate to obtain an accurate respiratory rate.

EQUIPMENT/SUPPLIES:
Watch with second hand

PROCEDURE STEPS:
1. Wash hands.
2. Identify the patient.
3. Position infant in a supine position.
4. Place hand on the chest to feel the rise and fall of the chest wall for one minute.
5. Note depth, rhythm, and breath sounds while counting.
6. Wash hands.
7. Record respiration rate in patient chart, noting any irregularities and sounds.

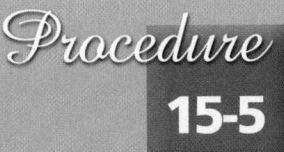

Obtaining a Urine Specimen from an Infant or Young Child

15-5

STANDARD PRECAUTIONS:

PURPOSE:
To obtain a specimen of urine from an infant or young child.

EQUIPMENT/SUPPLIES:
Urine collection bag
Laboratory request form
Gloves
Washcloth
Soap
Water
Towel
Biohazard waste container

PROCEDURE STEPS:
1. Wash and glove hands following standard precautions.
2. Assemble equipment.
3. Identify patient and explain procedure to parent(s).
4. Instruct parent to remove diaper.
5. Wash and dry perineal area. RATIONALE: Cleaning area reduces microorganism level and provides better quality urine specimen.
6. Apply collection bag, secure with adhesive tabs.
   a. Females: spread perineum, place bag over labia (Figure 15-18).
   b. Males: place bag over penis and scrotum.
7. Replace diaper carefully.
8. Frequently check bag for urine.
9. Once specimen has been collected, remove bag carefully.
10. Prepare specimen as required. Send to laboratory in a specimen container with a requisition or process the specimen in the office laboratory.
11. Remove gloves and discard in biohazard waste container.
12. Wash hands.
13. Record collection in patient's chart.

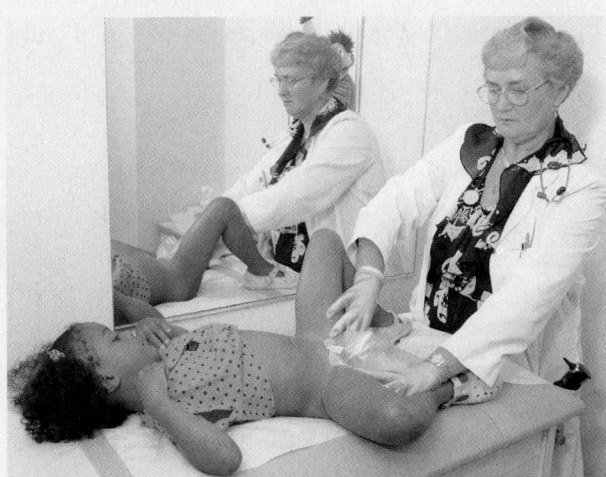

Figure 15-18 Applying the pediatric urine collector on a female. The opening of the bag should be directly over the urinary meatus. On a male, the scrotum and penis should project through the round opening of the bag.

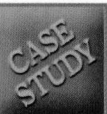

After examining Joey Little, Dr. King confirms the diagnosis of otitis media.

CASE STUDY REVIEW

15-1

1. Explain otitis media, the most common reason for its occurrence, and its treatment.
2. How can parents and caregivers be educated to help prevent otitis media?

SUMMARY

Caring for the health and well-being of infants and children through their various developmental stages and into adolescence is the responsibility of the pediatric practice.

Careful observation of the parent or caregiver and the child is helpful to the treatment and care given to the child. The medical assistant is responsible for reporting to the physician any suspicion of child abuse.

Opportunities abound for educating parents about topics that will keep their children healthy throughout life and include nutrition, sleep, immunization, and exercise. Pamphlets are available to share with parents and caregivers.

Children need respect and should be treated with empathy and love, and in doing so, a positive relationship can be developed with the child.

REVIEW QUESTIONS

Multiple Choice

1. At what age should the first polio vaccine be given?
   a. birth
   b. 1 month
   c. 2 months
   d. 3 months
   e. 6 months
2. One procedure done to treat otitis media is:
   a. suppuration
   b. tympanostomy
   c. ear irrigation
   d. otoscopy
   e. myringectomy
3. The pathogen usually responsible for causing tonsillitis is:
   a. staphylococcus aureus
   b. meningiococcus
   c. beta-hemolytic streptococcus group A
   d. beta-hemolytic streptococcus group B
4. Head circumference is measured on the child until what age?
   a. 1 year
   b. 2 years
   c. 4 years
   d. 6 years

5. An apical pulse is taken over which of the following sites?
   a. 3rd intercostal space on the left side
   b. 4th intercostal space on the left side
   c. 5th intercostal space on the left side
   d. 6th intercostal space on the left side

Critical Thinking Questions

1. You notice when you undress a two-year-old child to prepare for a physical examination that there are bruises on the buttocks and what appear to be burns on the feet. What course of action do you take?
2. Explain the importance of head circumference measurement.
3. Explain the importance of growth charts.
4. Describe the appropriate position in which to place an infant for a rectal temperature.
5. Describe the appearance of the pediatric urine collector bag. What is the best way to make certain it will adhere to the child's body?
6. Explain the type of chart used to test visual acuity in young children.
7. When is it appropriate to use the tympanic thermometer while taking a child's temperature?
8. When taking an infant's rectal temperature, what precautions should be taken?

9. Chest circumference measurements on an infant are performed for what purpose?
10. What do the curved lines printed across growth charts indicate?

WEB ACTIVITIES

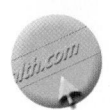

Search for the American Pediatric Academy on the World Wide Web to answer the following:

1. What information is available about immunization for Hepatitis B?
2. What is the most recent recommendation that the American Academy of Pediatrics has made regarding varicella immunization?

REFERENCES/BIBLIOGRAPHY

Damjanov, I. (1996). *Pathology for the health related profession* (1st ed.). Philadelphia: W. B. Saunders Company.

Frazier, M. S., Drzymkowski, J. A., & Doty, S. J. (1996). *Essentials of human diseases and conditions* (1st ed.). Philadelphia: W. B. Saunders Company.

Fremgen, B. (1998). *Essentials of medical assisting: Administrative and clinical competencies*. Upper Saddle River, NJ: Brady-Prentice Hall.

Keir, L., Wise, B., & Krebs, C. (1998). *Medical assisting: Administrative and clinical competencies* (4th ed.). Philadelphia: W. B. Saunders Company.

Kinn, M. E., & Woods, M. A. (1999). *The medical assistant: Administrative and clinical* (8th ed.). Philadelphia: W. B. Saunders Company.

Tamparo, C., & Lewis, M. (2000). *Diseases of the human body* (3rd ed.). Philadelphia: F. A. Davis Company.

MALE REPRODUCTIVE SYSTEM

KEY TERMS

Cryptorchidism
Intravenous Pyelogram
Orchiectomy
Residual
Retention
Transilluminator
Transurethral Resection

OUTLINE

Testicular Examination
Disorders of the Male
   Reproductive System
   Benign Prostatic Hypertrophy
   Prostatitis
   Prostate Cancer
   Testicular Cancer
   Sexually Transmitted Diseases

Assisting with the Male
   Reproductive Examination
Diagnostic Tests and Procedures
   Vasectomy
   Semen Analysis

OBJECTIVES

The student should strive to meet the following performance objectives and demonstrate an understanding of the facts and principles presented in this chapter through written and oral communication.

1. Define key terms.
2. Describe common disorders and diseases of the male reproductive system.
3. Explain benign hyperplasia of the prostate.
4. Identify signs and symptoms of the various disorders and diseases of the male reproductive system.
5. Describe the common diagnostic tests and procedures used in the male reproductive system.
6. Explain testicular self-examination.

CLINICAL

Fundamental Principles

- Apply principles of aseptic technique and infection control
- Comply with quality assurance practices
- Screen and follow up patient test results

Diagnostic Orders

- Collect and process specimens
- Perform diagnostic tests

Patient Care

- Obtain patient history and vital signs
- Prepare and maintain examination and treatment areas
- Prepare patients for examinations, procedures, and treatments
- Assist with examinations, procedures, and treatments
- Coordinate patient care information with other health care providers

GENERAL (TRANSDISCIPLINARY)

Legal Concepts

- Document accurately

Instruction

- Instruct individuals according to their needs
- Teach methods of health promotion and disease prevention

SCENARIO

Joe Geurro, CMA, finds many situations daily to educate patients because he knows how important it is. He keeps abreast of the latest techniques and procedures about diseases and problems of the male reproductive system. He attends lectures, workshops and seminars when possible, and uses the World Wide Web for the latest information from the American Cancer Society about prostate cancer as a resource for people with prostate cancer. With Dr. Woo's permission, Joe shares that information with patients.

INTRODUCTION

The male reproductive system consists of a pair of testes in which sperm and hormones are produced, a system of tubes that transport the sperm to the outside of the body, and a penis that transports the sperm into the female reproductive tract. There are glands such as the prostate that secrete fluid and become part of the semen. The testes are suspended in the scrotum. Sperm are developed in tubules in the testes. Upon maturity, the sperm enter the epididymis, a convoluted tube resting on the surface of the testes. The epididymis leads to the vas deferens that passes into the abdominal cavity. The ejaculatory duct opens into the urethra. Semen is expressed through the urethral opening. Diagnostic tests, procedures, disorders, and conditions common to the male reproductive system are shown in Tables 16-1 and 16-2.

TESTICULAR EXAMINATION

Early detection of testicular cancer relies heavily on the patient's willingness to perform self-examination of these body parts on a regular basis. Patient teaching is valuable when used to educate the patient about self-examination for detection of abnormalities such as lumps or thickenings. Figure 16-1 illustrates a testicular self-examination and Procedure 16-1 outlines steps for instructions usually given by the medical assistant.

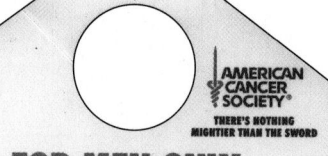

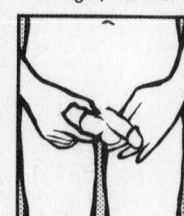

FOR MEN ONLY

How to do TSE (a self-exam)

Cancer of the testicle can be cured if you find it early.

Use the shower check.

1. Check your testicles once a month.

2. Roll each testicle between your thumb and finger, like this:

Feel for hard lumps or bumps.

3. If you notice a change or have aches or lumps, tell your doctor right away so something can be done about it.

Testicular cancer can be cured.

You should also know that prostate cancer is the most common cancer in men. Men over age 50 should have an annual health check-up that includes a prostate examination.

FOR MORE INFORMATION CALL THE AMERICAN CANCER SOCIETY TOLL FREE: 1-800-ACS-2345

Figure 16-1
Testicular self-examination.
(Courtesy of American Cancer Society)

Patient Teaching Tip

1. Testicular cancer is one of the leading causes of death in men under the age of 40.
2. Risk factors include an undescended testicle, cryptorchidism, and childhood mumps.
3. Prognosis is good when found in the early stages.

TABLE 16-1   MALE REPRODUCTIVE SYSTEM

| Disease/Disorder | Laboratory Diagnostic Tests | | | Radiography | Surgery | Medical Tests or Procedures |
	Blood	Urine	Other			
Benign Hyperplasia of Prostate	• PSA (rules out or detects prostate cancer)	• Urinalysis		• Intravenous pyelogram • Pelvic ultrasound	• Biopsy of prostate gland	• Rectal exam • Cystoscopy
Cancer of Prostate	• PSA (detects prostate cancer) • Acid phosphotase	• Urinalysis		• Intravenous pyelogram • Pelvic ultrasound	• Biopsy of prostate gland	• Rectal exam • Cystoscopy
Epididymitis	• Complete blood count	• Urinalysis • Culture and sensitivity of urine	• Culture and sensitivity of urethral discharge	• Intravenous pyelogram • Pelvic ultrasound		
Prostatitis	• Complete blood count	• Urinalysis • Culture and sensitivity of urine				• Rectal exam
Sexually Transmitted Diseases						
• Chlamydia		• Urinalysis	• Direct urethral smear using monoclonal antibodies			
• Genital Herpes (male or female)		• Urinalysis	• Culture of living tissue • Tzanck smear test			
• Gonorrhea	• Complete blood count	• Urinalysis • Culture and sensitivity of urine	• Direct smear of urethral discharge, anal canal, and oropharynx • Thayer-Martin culture	• Pelvic Ultrasound • Laparoscopy		• Cystoscopy
• Syphilis	• VDRL (Venereal disease research laboratory) • Treponema Pallidum Hemagglutination Test • Rapid plasma reagin	• Urinalysis • Culture and sensitivity of urine	• Culture of chancre			
• HVB and HIV See Chapter 4.						
Testicular Cancer					• Biopsy of testicle	

TABLE 16-2 DESCRIPTIONS OF MALE REPRODUCTIVE DISORDERS AND CONDITIONS

- Benign Hyperplasia of Prostate (BHP). Common in men over sixty years of age probably due to disturbance in sex hormones as the reproductive period of life declines. Because the gland surrounds the urethra, urinary flow is obstructed and can lead to urinary retention and urinary tract infection.
- Cancer of Prostate. Common malignancy. Most frequent cause of cancer in men after lung and colon cancers. Symptoms similar to BHP because the cancer causes the prostate to harden and obstruct the flow of urine.
- Epididymitis. Inflammation of the epididymis usually caused by gonorrhea. Epididymis becomes enlarged, hard, and painful.
- Prostatitis. Inflammation of the prostate gland that can result from an infection in an adjacent structure such as gonococcus of the urethra or *E-Coli* from the bladder. Seen in patients with frequent urinary tract infections (UTI) and sexually transmitted disease.

- Sexually Transmitted Disease (STD).
  - Chlamydial Infection. Common in males and females. A prevalent STD that often coexists with gonorrhea.
  - Genital Herpes. Painful, viral disease which is dormant and recurs periodically. There is no cure. Characterized by blisters similar to chicken pox. Common in men and women.
  - Gonorrhea. Caused by a bacterium and the infection can spread producing a stricture of the urethra or the vas deferens. Sterility can result if both vas deferens become involved.
  - Syphilis. Caused by a spirochete. Chancres develop. Can heal. If untreated, the disease progresses to stages two and three. Severe damage to the cardiovascular system, brain, vision, and hearing loss occur. General paralysis and death can result.
  - HVB & HIV see Chapter 4.
- Testicular Cancer. Primarily seen in males aged 15 to 35 and can be highly malignant.

DISORDERS OF THE MALE REPRODUCTIVE SYSTEM

Benign Prostatic Hypertrophy

Benign hypertrophy of the prostate gland or benign hypertrophic prostate gland also known as benign prostatic hyperplasia (BPH) is common in men age 50 or older. Symptoms include **retention** (the inability to completely empty the bladder), a diminished flow of urine, and difficulty starting to urinate. It is thought that the cause is aging and may be related to hormonal changes. The prostate enlarges and, because it surrounds the urethra, it causes constriction of the urethra and the associated symptoms. The physician can palpate the enlarged prostate gland when performing a rectal examination. This helps in making a diagnosis. Other tests may include a blood test known as prostate specific antigen (PSA), a urinalysis, and an **intravenous pyelogram** (an x-ray of the kidneys, ureters, and bladder using a contrast medium). If **residual** urine stays in the bladder, infections can develop, and kidneys may cease functioning because they can't drain urine properly into the bladder when it is full (Figure 16-2).

The PSA blood test is used to detect abnormally high levels of a protein substance that may indicate prostate cancer. The American Cancer Society recommends that men age 50 and over have an annual PSA blood test.

Ultrasound can be used to view the prostate, bladder, or kidneys. A biopsy of the prostate, done in conjunction with an ultrasound, can help diagnose either benign prostatic hypertrophy or cancer.

Treatment of BPH, in some cases, consists of medi-cation that can relax prostate muscles, hormones that block prostate growth, or bladder relaxants. **Transurethral resection** of the prostate (removal of prostate tissue using a device inserted through the urethra) is the most common surgical treatment. Instruments are inserted through the penis and a laser can be used to remove the excess tissue (Figure 16-3).

Prostatitis

Prostatitis, or inflammation of the prostate, occurs primarily in men over age 50. The prostate may enlarge and cause pain and discomfort, such as burning while urinating. There can be pain in the back, muscle aches, and urinary frequency. The cause may be bacterial, such as from gonorrhea, or may be caused by another pathogen that produced a urinary tract infection. Urinalysis, urine culture, and rectal exam (to palpate the prostate) help in making a diagnosis. Treatment is usually medication, such as penicillin and pain medication, and the patient will be told to force fluids by increasing fluid intake significantly.

Prostate Cancer

Prostate cancer is the third leading cause of cancer death in men, after lung and colon cancer. Metastasis to the spine or pelvis is not unusual. The symptoms, if present, are similar to urinary obstruction, difficulty urinating, frequency of urination, and inability to urinate. It is of value to check the blood level of PSA, but a biopsy is necessary to be certain. An ultrasonogram and CAT scan can help to determine if there has been any metastasis. Treatment consists of prostatectomy, hormonal therapy, radiation, and chemotherapy.

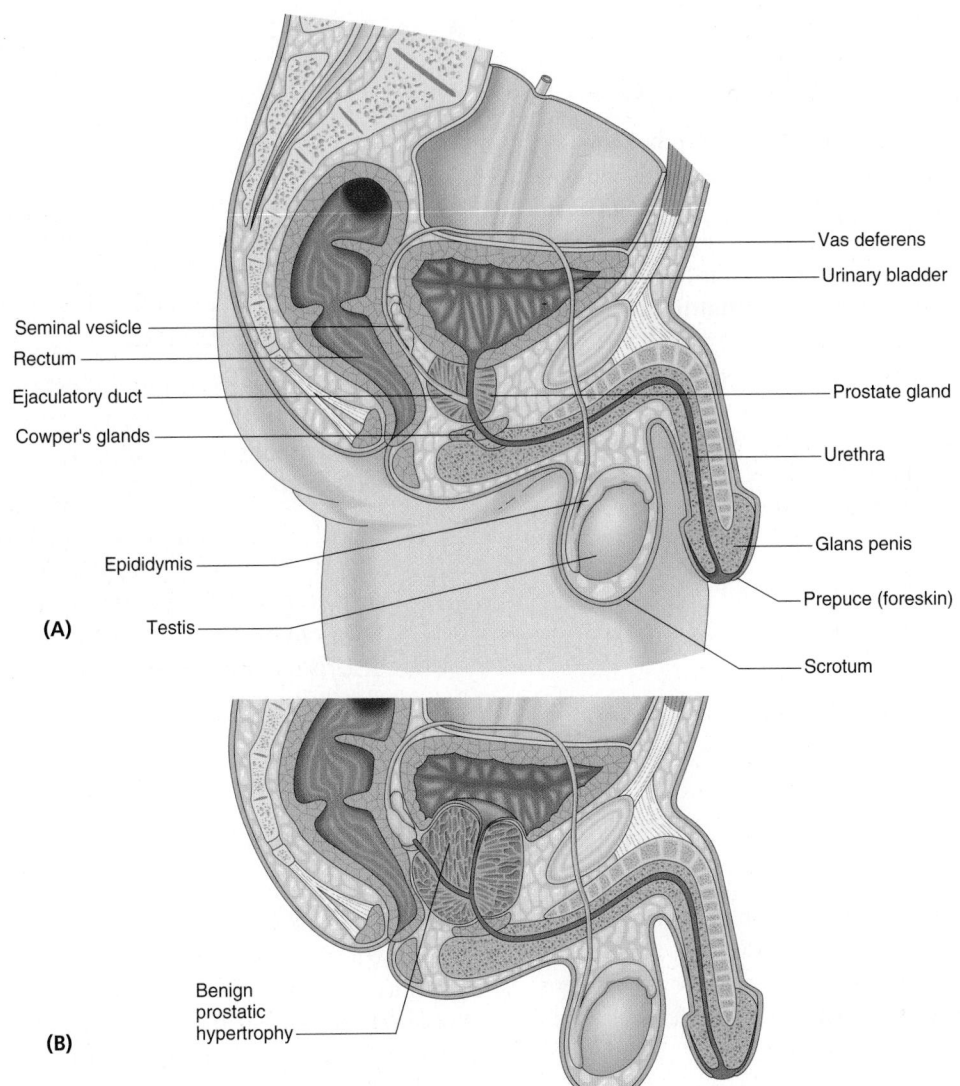

Seminal vesicle

Rectum

Ejaculatory duct

Cowper's glands

Vas deferens

Urinary bladder

Prostate gland

Urethra

Glans penis

Prepuce (foreskin)

Epididymis

Scrotum

(A) Testis

Benign prostatic hypertrophy

(B)

Figure 16-2   Normal and enlarged prostate: (A) Normal; (B) Benign prostatic hypertrophy or hyperplasia.

Testicular Cancer

Testicular cancer is the most common kind of cancer in males between the age of 20 and 35 years, otherwise it is rarely seen. Usually a painless lump is found in a testicle. An undescended testicle, cryptorchidism, and a history of mumps are predisposing factors. Diagnosis can be made by performing a biopsy after palpation of the testicle finds a mass. Surgery to excise the testicle, **orchiectomy**, followed by radiation and chemotherapy is the usual course of action. Monthly testicular examinations are recommended by the American Cancer Society for all men and are considered the best preventive measure for testicular cancer. See Figure 16-1 and Procedure 16-1.

Sexually Transmitted Diseases

Sexually transmitted diseases (STDs) affect men and women, can damage health, and become life-threatening. Refer to Tables 16-1 and 16-2. Also see information in Chapter 14 regarding STDs.

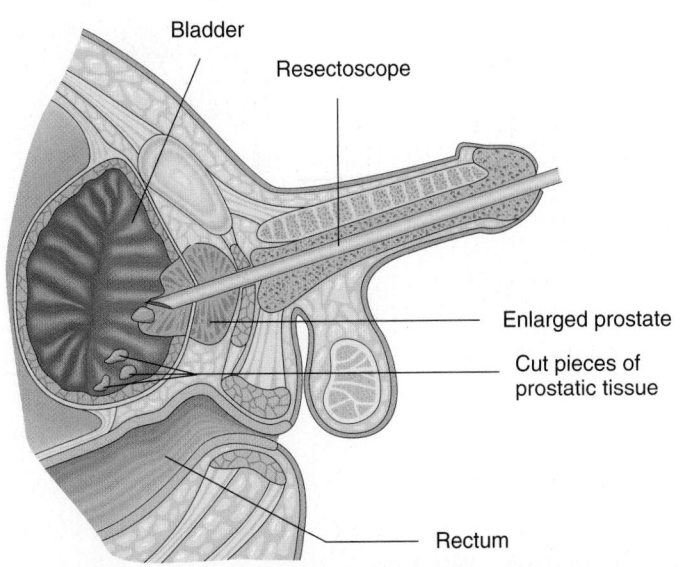

Bladder

Resectoscope

Enlarged prostate

Cut pieces of prostatic tissue

Rectum

Figure 16-3   Transurethral resection of prostate (TURP).

ASSISTING WITH THE MALE REPRODUCTIVE EXAMINATION

A female medical assistant may or may not be requested to assist the physician with the examination of the male reproductive system. The physician will examine the penis and the foreskin of the penis in an uncircumcised patient. The penis and testes are examined for swelling, masses, or discomfort. A **transilluminator** may be used by the physician to check the prostate gland. A lighted instrument used to inspect a cavity or organ, the transilluminator would be passed through the rectum to illuminate the prostate gland through the walls of the rectum. The physician will do a digital rectal examination to check the size of the prostate and will also check for an inguinal hernia.

DIAGNOSTIC TESTS AND PROCEDURES

Tests and procedures, in addition to those previously addressed, include vasectomy and a semen analysis.

Vasectomy

A vasectomy is performed to surgically sterilize the male. The vas deferens extends up into the abdomen where it connects to create the ejaculatory duct that opens into the urethra. By removing a portion of each vas deferens, sperm cannot travel to mix with semen, thereby causing the male to be sterile (Figure 16-4).

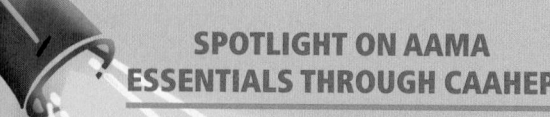

SPOTLIGHT ON AAMA ESSENTIALS THROUGH CAAHEP

● Being sensitive to the male patient's needs and emotions during an examination will help to provide a more positive relationship between the patient and the medical assistant.

● Helping the male patient establish a good rapport with the physician will promote a more positive experience during the examination process.

● Being aware of a patient's cultural diversity is extremely important and necessary to assist the patient in dealing with "old wives' tales" and rumors regarding disorders and illnesses affecting the male reproductive system.

Semen Analysis

Semen testing is frequently performed in the physician's office or clinic to determine sperm cell counts before referring patients to a specialist, such as a physician who treats infertility. It is also done as part of a complete fertility workup and to evaluate the effectiveness of a vasectomy. See Chapter 32 for extensive information about semen analysis.

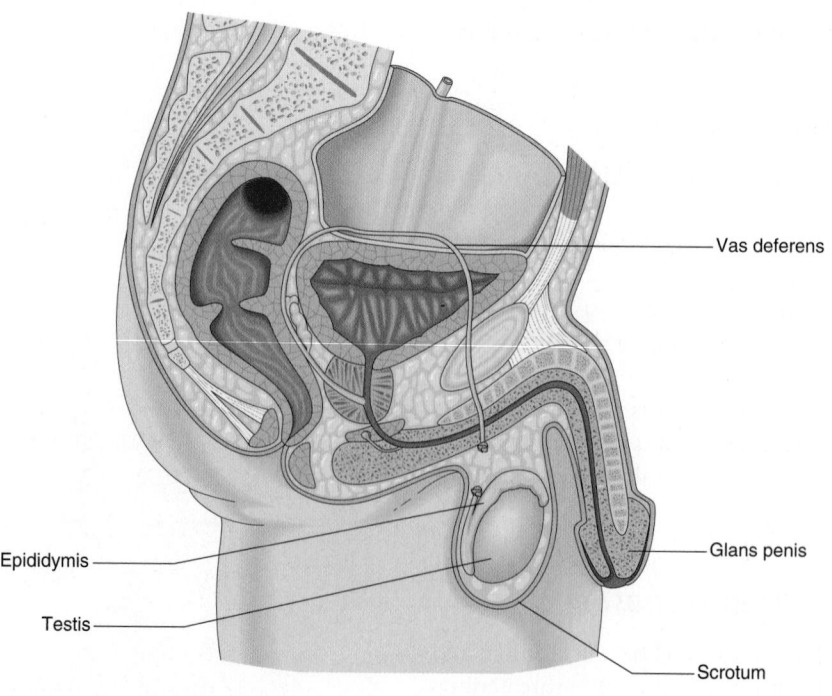

Figure 16-4 Vasectomy.

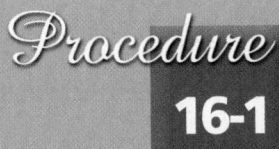

Instructing Patient in Testicular Self-Examination

PURPOSE:
To provide a patient with information concerning testicular screening for the presence of a painless mass in the scrotum.

EQUIPMENT/SUPPLIES:
Testicular self-examination card

PROCEDURE STEPS:

1. Instruct patient to examine his testicles in a warm shower. RATIONALE: The warmth causes the scrotal skin to relax.
2. Examine each testicle separately with both hands.
3. Place the index and middle fingers underneath the testicle and the thumbs on top. Roll the testicle gently between the fingers.
4. Locate the epididymis. Provide a chart to the patient that illustrates the testes and epididymis. RATIONALE: A lump can be similar in size to the epididymis and needs to be distinguished from the epididymis.
5. Look for swelling or changes in the scrotal area.
6. Encourage the patient to report anything unusual to the physician.

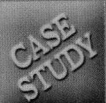

16-1

Adam Desmond has an appointment today in the clinic for a physical examination, and his chief complaint is that he has been having trouble sitting through ball games or movies without having to go to the bathroom to urinate several times.

CASE STUDY REVIEW

1. How can Dr. Woo make a diagnosis of benign prostatic hypertrophy?
2. What preliminary tests might Dr. Woo order for Mr. Desmond today?

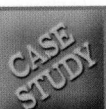

16-2

John Toomey called to say that he discovered "something hard in his right testicle, like a marble."

CASE STUDY REVIEW

1. What will Dr. King's examination consist of?

SUMMARY

A thorough knowledge of the diseases and disorders of the male reproductive system and the diagnostic tests and procedures that are performed for this specialty will enhance the quality of care given by the medical assistant.

REVIEW QUESTIONS

Multiple Choice

1. Cancer of the prostate may be detected early by which of the following?
   a. prostate-specific antigen
   b. transurethral resection
   c. semen analysis
   d. urine culture
2. The best preventive measure for testicular cancer is which of the following?
   a. yearly physical examination
   b. yearly intravenous pyelogram
   c. monthly self-examination
   d. monthly urinalysis with cultures
3. Benign prostate hypertrophy (BPH) is thought to be caused by:
   a. excessive consumption of alcohol
   b. aging and hormonal changes
   c. recurrent epididymitis
   d. chronic chlamydia infections
4. Which of the following is a symptom of prostatitis?
   a. painful urination
   b. low sperm count
   c. eruptions on the scrotum
   d. high testosterone level
5. The most definitive way to diagnose cancer of the prostate is by which of the following?
   a. ultrasonography
   b. intravenous pyelogram
   c. biopsy of the prostate
   d. semen analysis

Critical Thinking

1. Describe how a male should perform a self-testicular examination.
2. What is the purpose of severing the vas deferens?
3. List several symptoms of benign prostatic hypertrophy, and explain why the symptoms occur.

4. Describe the blood test that is helpful to diagnose prostate cancer.
5. Explain why benign prostatic hypertrophy is more common in men age 50 and over.
6. What age group is afflicted by testicular cancer, and how can the patient take action to detect it?
7. Describe two reasons why the physician orders a semen analysis.
8. List several sexually transmitted diseases that a male can contract.
9. How is a rectal examination on a patient useful to the physician in determining a diagnosis for a patient who has nocturia?
10. How is benign hypertrophy of prostate treated?

WEB ACTIVITIES

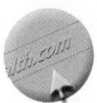

Search for information on the Internet regarding benign prostatic hypertrophy. Describe two surgical procedures that can be done for this condition.

REFERENCES/BIBLIOGRAPHY

Damjanov, I. (1996). *Pathology for the health related profession* (1st ed.). Philadelphia: W. B. Saunders Company.

Ehrlich, A. (1997). *Medical terminology for health professionals* (3rd ed.). Albany, NY: Delmar.

Frazier, M. S., Drzymkowski, J. A., & Doty, S. J. (1996). *Essentials of human diseases and conditions* (1st ed.). Philadelphia: W. B. Saunders Company.

Kinn, M. E., & Woods, M. A. (1999). *The medical assistant: Administrative and clinical* (8th ed.). Philadelphia: W. B. Saunders Company.

Neighbors, M., & Tannehill-Jones, R. (2000). *Human diseases.* Albany, NY: Delmar.

Taber's cyclopedic medical dictionary (18th ed.). (1999). Philadelphia: F. A. Davis Company.

Tamparo, C., & Lewis, M. (2000). *Diseases of the human body* (3rd ed.). Philadelphia: F. A. Davis Company.

Chapter

17

GERONTOLOGY

KEY TERMS

Arteriosclerosis
Cognitive Functioning
Cystitis
Dementia
Empathy
Geriatrics
Gerontology
Hyperthermia
Hypothermia
Incontinence
Macular Degeneration
Pernicious Anemia
Presbycusis
Residual Urine
Senile
Transient Ischemic Attack

OUTLINE

Societal Bias
Facts about Aging
Physiologic Changes
    Senses
    Integumentary System
    Nervous System
    Musculoskeletal System
    Respiratory System
    Cardiovascular System
    Gastrointestinal System
    Urinary System
    Reproductive System
Prevention of Complications
Psychological Changes
The Medical Assistant and the
    Geriatric Patient
    Memory-Impaired Older Adults
    Visually Impaired Older Adults
    Elder Abuse

OBJECTIVES

The student should strive to meet the following performance objectives and demonstrate an understanding of the facts and principles presented in this chapter through written and oral communication.

1. Define the key terms.
2. Identify expected physiological changes that occur as part of the aging process.
3. List five common functional changes that can occur.
4. Describe prevention techniques for complications arising from age-related disorders.
5. Explain two myths about aging.
6. Explain the importance of communication with the elderly.

CLINICAL

Fundamental Principles

- Apply principles of aseptic technique and infection control
- Screen and follow up patient test results

Patient Care

- Obtain patient history and vital signs
- Prepare and maintain examination and treatment areas
- Assist with examinations, procedures, and treatments
- Coordinate patient care information with other health care providers

Diagnostic Orders

- Collect and process specimens
- Perform diagnostic tests

GENERAL (TRANSDISCIPLINARY)

Legal Concepts

- Maintain confidentiality
- Practice within the scope of education, training, and personal capabilities
- Document accurately
- Follow federal, state, and local legal guidelines
- Comply with established risk management and safety procedures

SCENARIO

Mrs. Johnson is an 82-year-old patient of Dr. King, and she is scheduled for an appointment in the cardiac clinic. She is being evaluated for congestive heart disease and has had hypertension for many years. It was difficult to control, but now it responds to medication. She has become a volunteer at the gift shop at St. Louis Hospital. She is an example of an elderly person with chronic illnesses who has changed some long-time behaviors that were harmful to her health.

INTRODUCTION

Gerontology is the scientific study of the problems associated with aging. **Geriatrics** is the branch of medicine that specializes in all aspects of aging: physiological, pathological, psychological, economic, and sociological. The importance of studying gerontology is becoming more recognized because the expected lifespan is increasing. Thousands of people are living to be 100 years old or older. The aging population is growing rapidly and according to the U.S. Census Bureau, by the year 2030, there will be 60 million people older than age 65. The 80 and above age group is currently the fastest growing group. As a medical assistant, you will be experiencing the impact on the health care system of this growing population of people.

Through knowledge of the physical and psychological changes that occur as an individual ages, as a medical assistant you will be better able to recognize the special needs of this group of people. You will draw upon and use effective communication skills and provide quality health care to the geriatric patients.

SOCIETAL BIAS

In our culture, there is a deeply ingrained bias about aging. Elderly people are systematically stereotyped, and there is much discrimination because of age. Myths and stereotypes are common and the medical assistant can be an advocate for the elderly and can be sensitive to these myths and stereotypes. Accurate information and useful concepts about aging must be communicated to the general public. Elderly oftentimes are viewed as sick, frail, powerless, sexless, and burdensome. As a society, we are obsessed with the negative aspects of aging rather than the positive. The most popular myth is, "to be old is to be sick." Recent studies indicate that older Americans are generally healthier than their counterparts of nearly a decade ago. Even in advanced old age, a majority of the older population has little functional disability. Years of research have debunked this myth. Because of better education about the practice of healthier lifestyles, to be old in America does not mean to be sick and frail. Thousands of people are living to be over 100 years old because of the recognition that healthy lifestyles are the most important factor in helping people to live long, healthy, productive lives. Such factors as good nutrition, regular exercise, stress reduction, yearly physical examinations, not smoking, and today's technology help suppress the aging process.

FACTS ABOUT AGING

- Aging is progressive and universal.

- There are no diseases specific to aging.

- As people age, not all functional changes are related to disease. Interest, personal, and financial resources, family structure, genetics, and attitude all play a part. The individual's lifestyle is also a factor. For example, smoking, misuse of chemicals such as alcohol or drugs, type of diet, and exercise all play a part in how people age.

- There is a wider range of what is considered "normal" function among older people than among younger people. There is a greater variability among older people in their physical abilities, sizes, and characteristics than among younger groups (Figure 17-1).

- All old age is not alike. People in their 60s, 70s, 80s, and 90s are all different.

PHYSIOLOGICAL CHANGES

Although aging is a normal process, not all individuals age in the same way or at the same rate, because no two people have exactly the same genetic inheritance, personal lifestyle, or experiences in life. All of these factors strongly influence the ways in which we grow older. Some believe that the body endures wear and tear and stress during life and that because of this, eventually the body loses its ability to function as well as it had. Others believe that as people grow older, the body produces smaller and smaller amounts of various hormones and other chemicals that keep the body functioning. The fewer of these kinds of substances that are produced, the more susceptible an individual becomes to disease.

Every body system undergoes changes as we age. The changes are physiological and psychological. As individuals move into their 60s and beyond, they will show physiological changes that are part of the aging process. As people age, their body systems function less effectively, causing them to have difficulty performing their ordinary, everyday tasks of living. Also, as people grow older, they become more susceptible to disorders and diseases. When taking the medical history of an older patient, it is evident that many have one or several chronic illnesses. Heart disease, diabetes, arthritis, hypertension, and vision and auditory impairments are common.

Although it is important to be knowledgeable about the physiological changes that occur as part of aging, it is important to realize that the majority of the elderly are free of serious, chronic health problems.

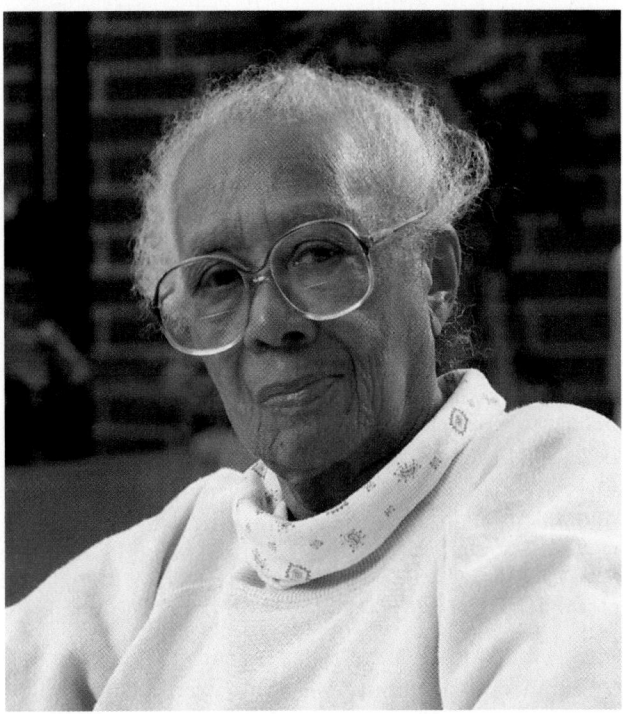

Figure 17-1 Note the many signs of aging.

Senses

Vision. Many changes occur in the eye's ability to function. Pupil size diminishes limiting the amount of light that can go through it to reach the retina. There is a diminished production of tears so the eye is dry, red, and irritated. The lens may become cloudy and the cornea thickens. There is increased sensitivity to glare. Several problems can occur as a result of these changes. There is less ability to see clearly at any distance and to discern various shades of colors. Older people will need eyeglasses to help correct their vision loss, but reading small print can remain very difficult. Glare can be minimized by incorporating a process known as polarization into corrective lenses.

Cataracts, **macular degeneration**, and glaucoma are common findings in the elderly. Cataracts can be surgically excised if they are large. Glaucoma can be treated medically or surgically, but if left untreated can lead to blindness. Macular degeneration can lead to vision impairment. The macular of the retina is an important area in the visualization of fine details. Degeneration of it is the leading cause of visual impairment over age 50, making it difficult to do fine work or such activities as threading a needle. Laser surgery may halt the progression of the degeneration.

Hearing. Loss of hearing in the aging process is not uncommon. It usually occurs over a period of years, and the older person may not be aware of the loss. Loss of hearing ability begins at about the third decade of life. Many times, individuals with hearing loss seem inattentive or confused and are thought to be mentally weak or **senile**. Presbyacusia or **presbycusis** is the progressive loss of hearing ability caused by the normal aging process.

Taste and Smell. Taste and smell diminish, making food less appealing because it no longer tastes as good as it once did (Figure 17-2). Taste buds decrease in size. Detecting odors becomes difficult and impaired and further lessens the desire for food. It is not unusual for older people to lose weight and even to become malnourished because of the loss of the ability to taste and smell. Lacking the sense of smell can be dangerous because of the inability to smell smoke or gas and other dangerous fumes.

Integumentary System

Aging individuals' skin becomes more fragile with less subcutaneous and connective tissue. Exposure to sunlight is the major cause of wrinkled skin, "liver spots," and leathery-looking skin.

Sweat glands become smaller and the body becomes nonsensitive to heat and cold. **Hyperthermia**, an unusually high fever, and **hypothermia**, an unusually low body temperature, are serious problems, and exposure to excessive hot or cold temperatures should be avoided. See Chapter 21, Rehabilitation and Therapeutic Modalities.

Hair loses color and becomes thinner. The skin dries and is less elastic. Fingernails and toenails thicken.

Nervous System

The brain shrinks in size as an individual ages because brain cells do not continue to divide throughout life as other cells do. Some loss of memory or delay in memory can be expected in many, but not all, aging people. Mental competence is the rule rather than the exception for older people. Sudden loss of memory accompanied by confusion and inability to do tasks once able to be performed could be an indication of an organic problem, such as **transient ischemic attack**, a temporary interference of the blood supply to the brain, or a brain lesion.

Problems with balance, temperature regulation, diminished pain sensation, and insomnia can occur as part of the physical changes of aging that affect the nervous system.

Chronic illnesses from which many elderly people suffer many times require several different medications to keep under control. Side effects of medication (over-the-counter and prescription) can cause decreased mental capacity as can malnutrition and substance abuse.

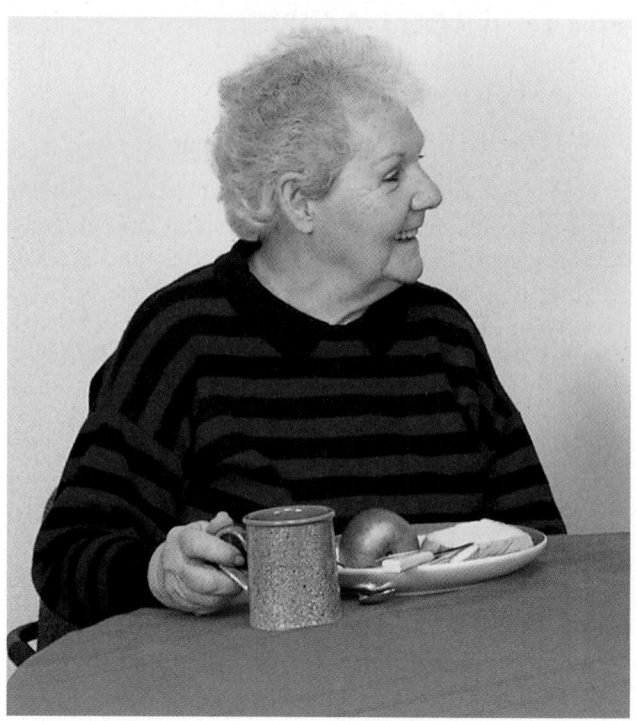

Figure 17-2   The elderly may tend to add more salt and sugar to their food to compensate for their diminished sense of taste.

Musculoskeletal System

The musculoskeletal system changes are evident because elderly people have less muscle strength. This results in loss of mobility and the activities of daily living (ADL) become more difficult. There is less flexibility and joints can stiffen. Loss of height and a stooped appearance can result. Arthritis and osteoporosis are not unusual, and the aging can suffer fractured bones more easily. Poor nutrition, malnourishment, and lack of exercise all contribute to these conditions and prolong healing time as well. See Chapter 21.

Respiratory System

Breathing capacity diminishes, and oxygen and carbon dioxide exchange is lessened. The rib and chest muscles become smaller and less efficient. Lungs lose their elasticity, and the older person may be dyspneic, short of breath (SOB), and more prone to pneumonia.

Cardiovascular System

Heart disease and blood vessel disorders are the major cause of death in the United States. Lifestyle has been implicated as the most significant cause of cardiovascular disease. Blood vessels lose their elasticity, become narrower, build up with plaque, and the arteries harden. This is known as **arteriosclerosis**. The myocardium loses some of its ability to pump effectively. This, together with narrowed and plaque-filled arteries, causes the heart to pump harder. Hypertension, or sustained high blood pressure, is a direct result of these factors. Hypertension can contribute to the accumulation of plaque in artery walls. Congestive heart failure is the inability of the heart to pump effectively to meet the body's demand for blood. Myocardial infarction, or heart attack, is another result of arteriosclerotic heart disease.

Gastrointestinal System

Stomach secretions and mobility slow as part of aging. Peristalsis slows and food moves through the gastrointestinal tract more slowly. **Pernicious anemia** is a disorder that can occur when cells of the stomach lining fail to secrete the intrinsic factor. Associated with the absence of hydrochloric acid, pernicious anemia affects the nervous system and red blood cell formation. Fewer calories are needed in the aging process because metabolism slows. Many overeat if they are lonely, gain weight, and may become obese. Eating is a social as well as physiological event, and if there is no one to eat with, many elderly will not prepare a meal or eat properly to have good nutrition. Loss of vigor and vitality occur. Malnourishment is not uncommon.

Poor eating habits, poor nutrition, overeating, or undereating can also lead to dental problems. Poor dental hygiene leads to gum disease and loss of teeth, many times making the chewing of food difficult and discouraging.

Urinary System

The kidneys decrease in size making urine production and output less. With cardiovascular arteriosclerosis, blood flow to the kidney is less. Filtering waste products from the blood is impaired. Medications are not excreted as quickly as they are in a young, healthy person. Levels of medication may rise to a dangerous level with poor filtration. The bladder walls become more inelastic, and the ability to empty the bladder completely becomes difficult. **Residual urine** remains in the bladder, and microorganisms can cause an infection. **Cystitis** is an inflammation of the bladder. Urinary **incontinence**, the uncontrollable loss of urine, can be the result of many factors, such as relaxed muscles in the female pelvic floor, cystitis, hypertrophy of prostate gland, and diabetes.

Reproductive System

Women experience menopause at about age 55. Estrogen produced by the ovaries ceases, and changes in the female genitalia are noticed. Hot flashes are not uncommon because of blood vessel dilation and contraction. Vaginal secretions diminish, the vagina becomes smaller, and infections are more likely. Estrogen replacement therapy helps to lessen symptoms and helps to protect women from heart disease and osteoporosis.

Men continue to produce sperm well after 50 years of age; however, testosterone levels diminish and may be the reason that many men over 50 suffer from benign hypertrophy of the prostate. Medication may help in some cases; otherwise surgery, a prostatectomy, may be performed.

Aging men and women maintain their sexual desires and many enjoy sexual intercourse more when there are no longer children in the home. There is more privacy and time to relax.

PREVENTION OF COMPLICATIONS

The elderly are at risk for complications as a result of changes in the structure and function of their body systems.

Accidents can happen because of impaired vision and the inability to see well or to hear a warning sound, such as a fire alarm.

Malnutrition and anemia can develop because of poor nutrition or poor absorption of food. This can be caused by lack of interest in food because of lack of sense of taste or smell.

Elderly people may have diminished sensitivity and lack the ability to feel pain as well as a younger person does. Heat and cold applications can injure an aging person if not watched carefully. Also, simple fractured bones may go unnoticed for some time. Loss of balance, disorientation, and confusion may be signs of impaired nervous system function.

Because many elderly suffer from osteoporosis, bones are more easily fractured. Falls are more common because of a loss of vision ability and balance.

Respiratory tract infections are not unusual. Pneumonia is a serious complication in this group of people. Encourage fluid intake and activity to keep the lungs healthy.

Urinary infections are more common. Adequate fluid intake (eight 8-ounce glasses of liquid per day) help keep infections at bay. Incontinence occurs when pelvic floor muscles are relaxed following childbirth.

Circulatory problems because of cardiovascular disease can cause poor circulation to the extremities, especially the legs. Fluid retention with noticeable edema are a common complication along with hypertension and congestive heart failure.

Vaginitis is more common because of vaginal dryness and irritation caused by lack of estrogen. The prostate gland enlarges making urination difficult for males.

PSYCHOLOGICAL CHANGES

There is a great deal of variation in the psychological functioning of the elderly. Among the factors that contribute are the person's health, psychosocial history, race, gender, and environmental aspects, such as education, support system, and social class.

The level of decline in an elderly person's intelligence is affected by social factors. People who maintain their intelligence tend to be in better health, have had more education, are in a high socioeconomic group, and are involved with others and in their community.

Dementia affects memory, personality, and cognitive functioning (awareness, reasoning, judgment, intuition). Alzheimer's is a common form of dementia. Some research has shown that there may be a genetic, as well as environmental, link to the cause of Alzheimer's disease. People who have had a stroke may suffer from dementia, impairing brain functioning.

Depression in the elderly can occur from loss of a spouse, chronic illness, or financial problems.

Personality seems to help determine how individuals adapt to changes that they experience as they grow older.

THE MEDICAL ASSISTANT AND THE GERIATRIC PATIENT

Many elderly suffer from dementia, mental illness, depression, stress, boredom, fear of the unknown, loss of independence, feelings of rejection and worthlessness, low self-esteem, loneliness, dependence, failed expectations, and disappointments. All of these factors coupled with the physiological changes that can occur offer a special challenge to the medical assistant caring for the health and needs of this group of patients. Allow patients time to ventilate and express their concerns, allow for private and confidential discussion, and empathize with their situation by being aware of their feelings, emotions, and behavior. Good communication is essential for quality care of the elderly. Do not talk to the elderly as if they are children. Speak slowly and clearly. Face the individual while talking. Write instructions in addition to verbalizing them.

Memory-Impaired Older Adults

Geriatric care poses challenges when attempting to communicate with impaired older adults. The inability to communicate on a meaningful level can be frustrating and challenging, especially for the older person who is struggling to communicate but can't find the right words. Following are some techniques that can be effective in improving verbal communication with older people experiencing memory impairment.

SPOTLIGHT ON AAMA ESSENTIALS THROUGH CAAHEP

- Being sensitive to a person's aging process also means being sensitive to their individual needs, such as loss of visual acuity, loss of hearing, and in some cases, loss of independence.

- By practicing good communication skills, the medical assistant can help to enhance the older person's self-esteem and self-worth.

- Holding a person's hand or just giving him or her a soft touch often helps to lessen the older patient's fears and thus helps facilitate the overall care and treatment by the physician.

1. Talk to the person in a nondistracting place. It can be very difficult for an older person to concentrate or to sort things out when there are environmental distractions, such as other conversations, equipment noises, or people walking by.
2. Begin conversations with orientating information. Identify yourself, and call the older person by his/her preferred name. Explain the purpose of your visit.
3. Use short words and short, simple sentences with no pronouns.
4. Speak slowly and say individual words clearly.
5. Never "talk down" or be condescending. This is demeaning. Speak in an adult manner as you would a co-worker or friend. Provide the dignity and respect you wish to receive yourself.
6. Lower the tone (pitch) of your voice. A raised pitch is a signal that one is upset. A lower pitch is also easier for people with hearing impairments.
7. Talk to the person in a warm and pleasant manner. Use nonverbal cues, such as facial expression, tone of voice, or touch, to show your feelings of affection and concern. Smiling, taking the older person's hand, or touching the person on the arm can vividly communicate that you are interested and really care.
8. When giving instructions, allow plenty of time for the information to be absorbed.
9. Give clear and simple instructions.
10. Ask the person to do one task at a time.
11. Listen actively. If you do not understand, apologize to the person by saying that you did not understand

exactly what was said. It is extremely important to phrase responses in a way that does not damage the self-esteem of the older person.

12. Avoid asking direct questions that require the person to remember a fact.

13. Focus on well behavior or things that we know the patient can still do.

14. Use humor when appropriate. If expressed naturally, humor brings much needed laughter, a dimension which is often lost in the health care setting.

15. Let the person know when you leave and if you are returning.

16. When discussing a case with another staff member, do so in private to protect patient confidentiality.

Visually Impaired Older Adults

Visually impaired people need to know you are present, but don't approach the individual until you make your presence known. Help by explaining his location, and identify others who may also be present (Figure 17-3).

Making Contact
Introduce yourself. Ask the visually impaired patient if he would like assistance. If he does, offer your arm by saying so and by touching your hand or forearm against his.

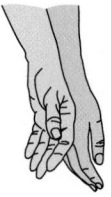

Pace
The pace should be comfortable for both of you. If the patient tightens his grip or pulls on your arm, slow down; your pace may be too fast or he may be anxious. You should alert the patient to obstacles such as curbs, stairs, doors, and thresholds. Be specific, but do not confuse him with too much information.

Grip
The patient grips your arm just above the elbow. The grip must be firm but not so tight that it becomes uncomfortable.

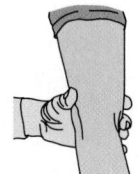

Stance
The patient stands next to you, slightly behind. His arm is bent and held close to his side. Relax your arm and let it hang naturally at your side.

Stairs
When approaching stairs, tell the patient. Let him know whether you are going to go up or down. Be sure you approach the stairs directly, not at an angle. Have the patient stand next to the handrail if there is one.

Pause at the top (or bottom) of the stairs and describe anything unusual about them. The patient will find the handrail and reach forward with his foot to locate the edge of the first step. Start down (or up) the stairs, keeping yourself one step ahead. Keep a steady pace.

When you reach a landing, stop immediately. (Do not take an extra step.) Doing so lets the patient know that there are no more steps, and he can then match his stride with yours.

The same procedure should be used when approaching curbs. Point out any changes in the terrain, even small ones.

Sitting
When guiding someone to a chair, walk up to it and place your hand on the back of the chair. Let the patient trail your arm down to its back. Tell him which way the chair is facing, and he can then seat himself.

If the chair lacks a back or is very large, bring the patient up to the chair so that his legs are against the front of it. He can then reach down to locate the arms and seat of it before he sits.

If the chair is at a table, describe the relationship of the chair, the table, and the patient. Place one of his hands on the chair and the other hand on the table.

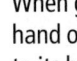

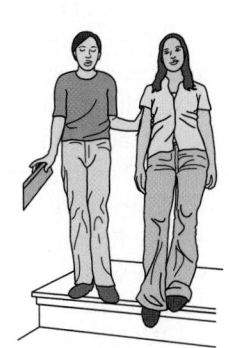
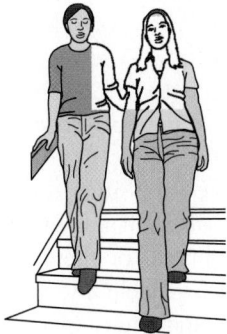
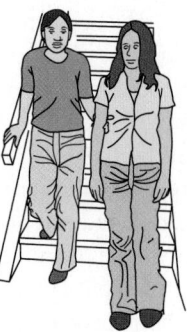

Figure 17-3 Sighted guide techniques.

(continues)

Doors

When approaching a closed door, tell the patient its position when open. For example, "The door opens away and to the left." Or say, "Take the door with your left hand." After you open the door and begin to walk through, the patient will have his hand ready to help hold it open as you walk through together. The patient will move his arm across the front of his body to find the door with the palm of his hand. He should close it behind you if it is not a self-closing door. Use the narrow passage technique in addition to this technique if the doorway is narrow.

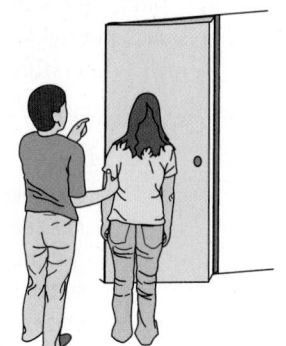

Narrow Passage Technique

When coming to a narrow passage, tell the patient. Move your guiding arm to the center of your back. Slow your pace. He will move behind you and extend his arm, placing you in a single-file position. Once you pass through the narrow passage, bring your arm forward and return to the normal stance.

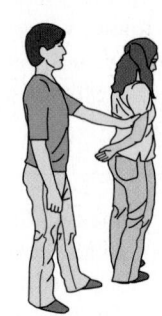

Figure 17-3   (*continued*)

Elder Abuse

What is elder abuse? Massachusetts law defines elder abuse as the committing or omitting of an act that results in serious physical or serious emotional injury to an elderly person. All states have elder abuse laws. Abuse includes physical abuse, emotional abuse, and neglect. The law protects elders abused or neglected by caretakers.

All persons age 60 and over living in the community are protected under the law. Who must report elder abuse? Physicians, medical interns, dentists, nurses, family counselors, police officers, psychologists, homemakers, licensed home health care aids, and many more are required to report abuse. Agencies are also liable. Any person required to report abuse who fails to do so is subject to a fine. Anyone who has reasonable cause to believe an elder has been abused may report and has a moral obligation to protect elders. In most states, the department responsible for elder affairs has established an elder abuse hotline to receive reports of abuse. Reports may also be made to the designated protective service agency in your community. Once reports are received by the elder protective services program, if appropriate, a caseworker will assess the situation to determine the nature and extent of the abuse. If abuse is confirmed, services will be provided to eliminate or alleviate abuse. Many social services are usually available. Mental health, legal, homemaker services, and alternative living arrangements may be provided. See Chapter 7.

Some signs and symptoms of mistreatment or abuse include:

Psychological Signs and Symptoms

- Increasing depression
- Anxiety
- Withdrawn/timid
- Hostile
- Unresponsive
- Confused
- New poverty
- Longing for death
- Vague health complaints
- Anxious to please

Physical Signs and Symptoms

- Lack of personal care
- Lack of supervision
- Bruises
- Welts
- Lack of food
- Beatings
- Neglect
- Unsatisfactory living conditions

There are many other signs and symptoms and not all of those listed by themselves indicate mistreatment, neglect, or abuse. If any seem to increase in number or severity, it may indicate a problem. By observing closely, you may be able to initiate corrective action or reduce or prevent the situation from deteriorating.

Usually the victim is frail (weak), physically and/or emotionally, and dependent upon the abuser for basic survival needs. The victim may be afraid to speak out for fear of retaliation.

Where should one call for information? Contact elder protective services programs in the Yellow Pages of your phone book, or call the Eldercare Locator toll free at (800) 677-1116.

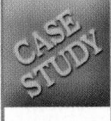

Adelaide Robinson, 83 years old, has an appointment Thursday morning for a re-check of her most recent complaint. She tells you that she is moving slower than she did just six months ago, and she has noticed less flexibility as well.

CASE STUDY REVIEW

1. What are the possible causes of Mrs. Robinson's complaints?
2. What effect will these problems have on Mrs. Robinson's daily routine?
3. What might Dr. King suggest Mrs. Robinson do to help alleviate symptoms?

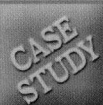

Sally Donovan, age 92, is in the gerontology clinic today. Her main concern, problem, and reason for appointment is that she "cannot taste or smell much anymore and food doesn't taste good." She wants suggestions from the physician about how to improve her taste and smell so she can enjoy food more freely.

CASE STUDY REVIEW

1. What are some reasons for the elderly to lose their sense of taste and smell?
2. Describe any dangers that can be associated with loss of taste and smell.

SUMMARY

Many aging people live well into their 80s, 90s, and even to 100 years of age. They remain physically and mentally stimulated. They learn a foreign language, learn to play a musical instrument, love to read, garden, and volunteer. Elderly are more aware today, than ever before, of the importance of a healthy lifestyle and of its significant contribution to their long and healthy lifespan.

Other elderly, due to genetic inheritance, wear and tear, stress, and loss of chemicals and hormones, seem to age quickly but have little control over these factors.

Many others practice poor health habits, some by choice and others by circumstance. These habits contribute to chronic diseases, disability, and a shorter and unhealthy lifespan.

Above all, dispel myths about the elderly. Be patient, kind, consistent, and thoughtful.

REVIEW QUESTIONS

Multiple Choice

1. The most chronic condition associated with the elderly is:
   a. arteriosclerotic heart disease
   b. cystitis
   c. presbycusis
   d. pernicious anemia
2. An eye disease common to the elderly that is characterized by fluid pressure buildup is:
   a. macular degeneration
   b. presbyopia
   c. cataract
   d. glaucoma
3. Why do joints in the elderly become worn?
   a. cartilage erodes in the joints
   b. osteoporosis makes bones brittle
   c. muscle fibers decrease
   d. vertebrae become thinner
4. Inability to cough deeply and raise mucous makes elders more susceptible to which of the following?
   a. emphysema
   b. asthma
   c. pneumonia
   d. bronchitis
5. Residual urine refers to:
   a. catheterized urine for urinalysis
   b. first-voided specimen
   c. amount of urine left in bladder after voiding
   d. total amount of urine in the bladder when full

Critical Thinking

1. How can an elder's food be made more appealing?
2. What are some strategies that seniors can do to keep mentally and physically stimulated?
3. What are some ways that the elderly can keep bones from becoming brittle?
4. Describe a vision problem that leaves the elderly having difficulty seeing color intensity.
5. What are four causes of urinary incontinence?
6. What is the most common myth about seniors?
7. What are your thoughts about this myth?
8. Give three ways to enhance communication with the elderly.
9. What is the best way to approach a visually impaired person?
10. Older Americans are generally healthier today than older Americans of 10 years ago. What are some of the reasons for this?

WEB ACTIVITIES

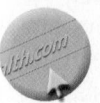 Search for a website that provides information publications about health issues surrounding the elderly.

1. Find the Patient's Bill of Rights. Summarize these rights.
2. Search for information about advanced directives. Find and describe two major types.

REFERENCES/BIBLIOGRAPHY

Cox, H. (2001). *Later life: The realities of aging* (5th ed.). Upper Saddle River, NJ: Prentice Hall.

Hegner, B., Caldwell, E., & Niedham, B. (1998). *Assisting in long-term care* (4th ed.). Albany, NY: Delmar.

Kinn, M. E., & Woods, M. A. (1999). *The medical assistant: Administrative and clinical* (8th ed.). Philadelphia: W. B. Saunders Company.

Markson, E., & Hollis-Sawyer, G. (2000). *Readings in social gerontology.* Los Angeles, CA: Roxbury Publishing Co.

Quadagno, J. (1999). *Aging and the life course.* New York: McGraw-Hill College.

Taber's cyclopedic medical dictionary (18th ed.). (1999). Philadelphia: F. A. Davis Company.

EXAMINATIONS AND PROCEDURES OF BODY SYSTEMS

18

KEY TERMS

Alimentary Canal
Allergen
Alveoli
Aphasia
Appendicular Skeleton
Aseptic
Auricle
Axial Skeleton
Biopsy
Bronchi
Calculi
Carbuncle
Catheterization
Closed Fracture
Colonoscopy
Comedone
Cystoscopy
Demyelination
Dislocation
Dysuria
Emaciation
Endoscopy
Equilibrium
Erosion
Erythema
External Respiration
Frequency
Furuncle
Gait
Guaiac
Hematemesis
Hematochezia
Hematuria
Hydronephrosis

(continues)

OUTLINE

Urinary System
  Signs and Symptoms of Urinary
    Conditions and Disorders
  Diagnostic Tests
  Urinary Catheterization
Digestive System
  Signs and Symptoms of Digestive
    Conditions and Disorders
  Diagnostic Tests
Sensory System
  The Eye
  The Ear

Respiratory System
  Spirometry
Musculoskeletal System
  Fractures, Casting, and Cast
    Removal
  Cast Care Guidelines
Neurological System
  Components of a Neurological
    Screening
Circulatory System
Blood and Lymph System
Integumentary System
  Allergy Skin Testing

OBJECTIVES

The student should strive to meet the following performance objectives and demonstrate an understanding of the facts and principles presented in this chapter through written and oral communication.

1. Define the key terms as presented in the glossary.
2. Describe how to perform a urinary catheterization.
3. State the proper protocol when collecting urine for a drug screening.
4. Describe patient preparation for occult blood testing.
5. Discuss patient instructions for three diagnostic digestive system tests: The upper GI series, a barium enema, and a cholecystogram.
6. Differentiate between an instillation and an irrigation.
7. Discuss the different types of visual acuity charts and how to use them appropriately.
8. Explain the medical assistant's role when assisting with audiometry.
9. Describe how to perform a nasal irrigation.
10. Describe the proper use of a metered dose nebulizer.

(continues)

KEY TERMS
(*continued*)

Ingestion
Internal Respiration
Lesion
Malabsorption
Malaise
Melena
Nebulizer
Nitrogenous
Nocturia
Obturator
Occluder
Oliguria
Ophthalmoscope
Otoscope
Perforation
Peripheral Nerve
Peritonitis
Polycystic
Polyp
Proteinuria
Pyuria
Spirometry
Stratum Corneum
Uremia
Urgency
Wheal

OBJECTIVES (*continued*)

11. Briefly discuss the role of the medical assistant during spirometry.
12. Explain the medical assistant's role in cast application and cast removal and the guidelines for cast care.
13. List items required by a physician for a neurological exam and explain the medical assistant's role in the exam.
14. Identify patient education information for sputum collections.
15. Explain oxygen administration using a nasal cannula.

ROLE DELINEATION COMPONENTS

CLINICAL
Fundamental Principles

● **Apply principles of aseptic technique and infection control**

● **Comply with quality assurance practices**

● **Screen and follow up patient test results**

Diagnostic Orders

● **Collect and process specimens**

● **Perform diagnostic tests**

Patient Care

● **Obtain patient history and vital signs**

(*continues*)

SCENARIO

At Inner City Health Care, a number of specialty examinations are scheduled for Tuesday the 8th. Administrative medical assistant Jane O'Hara, who is office manager, is careful to schedule patients requiring specialty procedures so that times do not overlap; before she schedules, Jane makes certain examination rooms are available with an extra margin of time between patients. Clinical medical assistants Wanda Slawson and Bruce Goldman take responsibility to ensure that all supplies and equipment are assembled, that both physician and patient are comfortable with the physical environment, and that all safety precautions are followed before, during, and after the examination or procedure.

INTRODUCTION

New techniques and developments occur frequently in medicine and medical assistants must refine existing skills and learn new ones in order to be knowledgeable and proficient and to provide the most current, up-to-date quality care to patients. The medical assistant who works in a specialist's office or an ambulatory care setting that treats a variety of patient problems will need additional skills when providing specialty care to patients. Patients with complaints specific to a particular body system or body part need specialized care.

- **Prepare and maintain examination and treatment areas**
- **Prepare patient for examinations, procedures, and treatments**
- **Assist with examinations, procedures, and treatments**
- **Coordinate patient care information with other health care providers**

GENERAL (TRANSDISCIPLINARY)

Legal Concepts

- **Document accurately**

Instruction

- **Instruct individuals according to their needs**
- **Teach methods of health promotion and disease prevention**

The medical assistant will assist the physician with a multitude of clinical procedures that are an integral part of each specialty examination.

This chapter covers specialty and body system examinations and the appropriate clinical procedures in urology; endoscopy; and the sensory, respiratory, musculoskeletal, neurological, circulatory, blood and lymph, and integumentary systems.

Each specialty description includes tables that contain information on diseases, disorders, and diagnostic tests and procedures used to confirm diagnoses. Other diseases and disorders and procedures related to each specialty are addressed in the body of the text.

URINARY SYSTEM

The urinary system includes the kidneys, ureters, and bladder. The main function of the kidneys is to form and excrete urine, which contains waste products harmful to body tissues. The kidneys also regulate water balance in the body and help maintain the acid base balance of body fluids.

Collecting and processing urine for laboratory analysis is covered in Chapter 30, Urinalysis. Several other clinical and diagnostic procedures of the urinary system will be covered in this section including urinary catheterization and performing a urine drug screen and a diagnostic X ray known as an intravenous pyelogram (IVP) used to diagnose disorders of the urinary tract.

Diagnostic tests, procedures, disorders, and conditions common to the urinary system are shown in Tables 18-1 and 18-2.

Signs and Symptoms of Urinary Conditions and Disorders

Signs and symptoms of urinary tract diseases include any abnormality in urine or in the ability to urinate. Some common signs and symptoms are: **dysuria**, **proteinuria**, **hematuria**, **pyuria**, **frequency**, **urgency**, **oliguria**, and **nocturia**. Patients may complain of flank or low back pain or experience fever, nausea, vomiting, general **malaise**, and fatigue.

Urinary tract infection (UTI) is the most common disorder of the system as it manifests itself with many of the above signs and symptoms. Urinary tract infection is a broad diagnosis covering any infection of the urinary tract including the urethra, bladder, and kidneys. UTIs may be caused by virus and fungus, but by far the most common infection is due to bacteria.

Bacteria may reach the urinary tract through the blood (hematogenous infection) or by entering the tract through the urethra (ascending infection). Hematogenous infection is less common and is usually the result of septicemia. In this case, the urinary tract is a site of secondary infection. Primary infection may begin in the respiratory or gastrointestinal tract and be carried to the urinary tract throughout the blood.

Diagnostic Tests

The most commonly performed test to diagnose urinary system disorders is a urinalysis. Many different disorders of the urinary system can be identified, making this test extremely valuable. A specimen of urine can be analyzed for many components such as pH, specific gravity, protein, glucose, leukocytes, and blood. The specimen can be further analyzed by examination under the microscope to look for bacteria, white and red blood cells, crystals, and cysts.

Urine culture and sensitivity can be performed and will indicate if a urinary tract infection is present so the appropriate antibiotic can be prescribed by the physician. To obtain a urine specimen for culture, there are two ways to collect the specimen, clean catch or by **catheterization**. See Procedures 18-1 and 18-3 and Chapter 30, Urinalysis.

Blood tests can be done to determine whether waste products are being adequately filtered out of the circulatory system. A test for kidney function confirms the status of glomeruli function.

Two **nitrogenous** waste products normally filtered from the blood are urea and creatinine. A blood urea nitrogen (BUN) test will check for levels of these two

TABLE 18-1 URINARY SYSTEM DISORDERS

| Disease/ Disorder | Laboratory Diagnostic Tests | | | Radiography | Surgery | Medical Tests or Procedures |
	Blood	Urine	Other			
Cancer of Urinary Bladder	• Complete blood count	• Urinalysis • Culture and sensitivity of urine		• Intravenous pyelogram • Pelvic ultrasound	• Biopsy of bladder	• Cystoscopy
Cystitis	• Complete blood count	• Nitrate • Urinalysis • Culture and sensitivity of urine		• Intravenous pyelogram		• Cystoscopy
Glomerulo-nephritis	• Blood urea nitrogen • Creatinine • Blood culture • Sedimentation rate • Electrolytes	• Urinalysis • Culture and sensitivity of urine		• Intravenous pyelogram • Ultrasound of kidneys		• Biopsy of kidney(s)
Polycystic Kidneys	• Blood urea nitrogen • Creatinine • Electrolytes	• Urinalysis		• Intravenous pyelogram • Ultrasound of kidneys • Computerized tomography (CT Scan)		
Pyelonephritis	• Blood urea nitrogen • Creatinine • Blood culture • Electrolytes	• Urinalysis		• Intravenous pyelogram • Ultrasound of kidneys		
Renal Calculi	• Complete blood count • Uric acid	• Urinalysis		• X ray of kidney, ureters, and bladder • Ultrasound of kidneys, ureters, and bladder • Intravenous pyelogram	• Lithotripsy	• Cystoscopy
Urinary Tract Infection (UTI)	• Complete blood count	• Urinalysis • Culture and sensitivity of urine				• Cystoscopy

TABLE 18-2 DESCRIPTION OF URINARY DISORDERS AND CONDITIONS

• Cancer of Urinary Bladder. Linked to cigarette smoking, industrial chemicals. Microscopic hematuria one of the first symptoms.

• Cystitis. Inflammation of the urinary bladder. More common in females due to the short length of the urethra. *E. coli* may travel from the rectum to the bladder. Infectious organisms can invade the bladder during sexual intercourse. Frequency, burning, urgency are common symptoms.

• Glomerulonephritis. Seen in children and young adults post streptococcal infection; strep throat, scarlet fever. Causes degenerative inflammation of glomeruli. Chills, fever, weakness are common symptoms. Edema and albumin in urine are common.

• Polycystic Kidneys. A congenital anomaly. Kidneys contain multiple cysts and greatly dilated tubules do not open into renal pelvis. Hypertension, kidney failure, and death can result.

• Pyelonephritis. Caused by pyogenic bacteria such as *E. coli*, streptococci, or staphylococci. May originate in the bladder and ascend to the kidneys. Pyuria, chills, fever, sudden back pain are symptoms. Dysuria is common.

• Renal Calculi. May be present with or without symptoms. Cause intense pain when they lodge in the ureter(s). Formed by certain salts (perhaps calcium).

wastes. High levels of waste products can result in **uremia**, a toxic condition of the blood that, if not reversed, leads to death. (See Chapter 30, Urinalysis.)

An intravenous pyelogram (IVP), a kidneys-ureters-bladder (KUB), and cystogram are radiologic examinations of the urinary tract.

Intravenous Pyelogram (IVP). An intravenous pyelogram (IVP) is used to examine the urinary tract (kidneys, ureters, and bladder) for blockage, narrowing, growths, and calculi. This urinary tract diagnostic X ray is also used to diagnose disorders such as lesions, **hydronephrosis**, and **polycystic** kidneys.

Patient Preparation for IVP. In studies of the urinary system, the IVP requires that the patient prepare with laxatives, enemas, and fasting (Table 18-3). The IVP consists of an intravenous injection of an iodine-based contrast medium that is used to define the structures of the urinary system. A retrograde pyelogram is a study of the urinary tract done by inserting a sterile catheter into the urinary meatus. Radiopaque contrast medium then flows upward into the kidneys. This diagnostic test is usually done in conjunction with cystoscopy. Patients should have iodine-sensitivity tests prior to the examination to determine the possibility of an allergic reaction. A voiding cystogram may be ordered in conjunction with an IVP. In this case, the contrast medium is injected into the bladder by catheter and no special patient preparation is needed. See Chapter 20, Diagnostic Imaging.

Cystoscopy. Cystoscopy is a procedure that uses a lighted scope (cytoscope) to view the urethra and bladder. Inflammation, **calculi**, and **polyps** can be seen using a cystoscope. A biopsy of the bladder can be done while performing a cystoscopy. See Figure 18-1.

Biopsy of the Kidney. Biopsies of the kidney will help confirm a diagnosis. Using radiology, a fine-gauge

> ## Patient Teaching Tip
>
> 1. Inform the patient not to flush the toilet after voiding into the specimen container.
> 2. The urine sample should remain in full view of the donor until it is secured for transport to the laboratory.

needle is inserted through the flank to remove a piece of kidney tissue for analysis and possible malignancy.

Urinary Drug Screening (Urine Toxicology Screening). There may be circumstances when it is necessary to check a patient's urine specimen for traces of drugs. At times, employees and athletes are required to have their urine tested to qualify for employment or sports activities.

It is legally necessary to have a signed consent form from patients for all drug screening tests performed. It may also be necessary to identify the patient or donor before a test is performed by requesting a photo ID which can be copied and filed with the consent form.

Depending on the drug collection kit used, the urine sample volume can vary from 1 mL to 40 mL. Some kits may also supply a bluing agent that the medical assistant will need to place in the toilet and toilet tank prior to the urine collection. The collector should wait immediately outside the collection area to receive the sample directly from the donor. (See Procedure 18-1.)

TABLE 18-3	INTRAVENOUS PYELOGRAM	
Purpose	**Patient Education**	**Precautions**
To examine the urinary tract: kidneys, ureters, bladder, for blockage, narrowing, growths, calculi.	1. Light evening meal night before 2. Cathartic (laxative) 3. NPO after 9:00 P.M. 4. Cleansing enema(s) in A.M.	Contrast medium of iodine used for visualization (check with patient regarding seafood or iodine allergies) *Warn patients of possible warm flushed sensation when dye is injected and that they may experience a metallic taste.

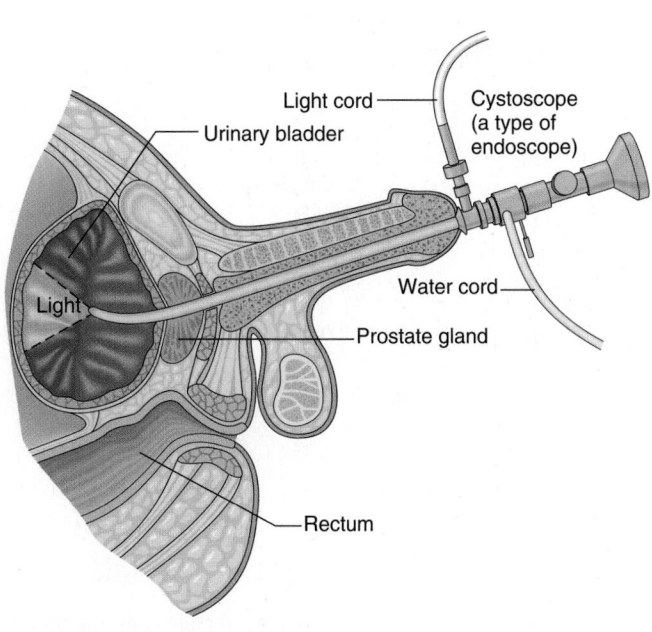

Figure 18-1 Cystoscopy.

Urinary Catheterization

The medical assistant may either perform or assist with the urinary bladder catheterization, which is the introduction of a sterile catheter (tube) through the urethra into the bladder for withdrawal of urine. See Figure 18-2 for male and female anatomy for catheterization. There are basically three reasons for catheterizing patients:

1. To obtain a sterile urine specimen for analysis
2. For relief of urinary retention
3. To instill medication into the bladder, after the bladder is emptied

In some cases, this procedure is done by a urologist; however, some physicians in obstetrics-gynecology and general and family practice may perform or have the medical assistant perform the catheterization. Catheterizing male patients is generally performed by physicians themselves. The physician may order a culture and sensitivity of the urine obtained from catheterization if the patient is experiencing dysuria, frequency, and urgency. This is done to determine if microorganisms are present and if so, what the causative microorganism is, in order to prescribe the appropriate antibiotics.

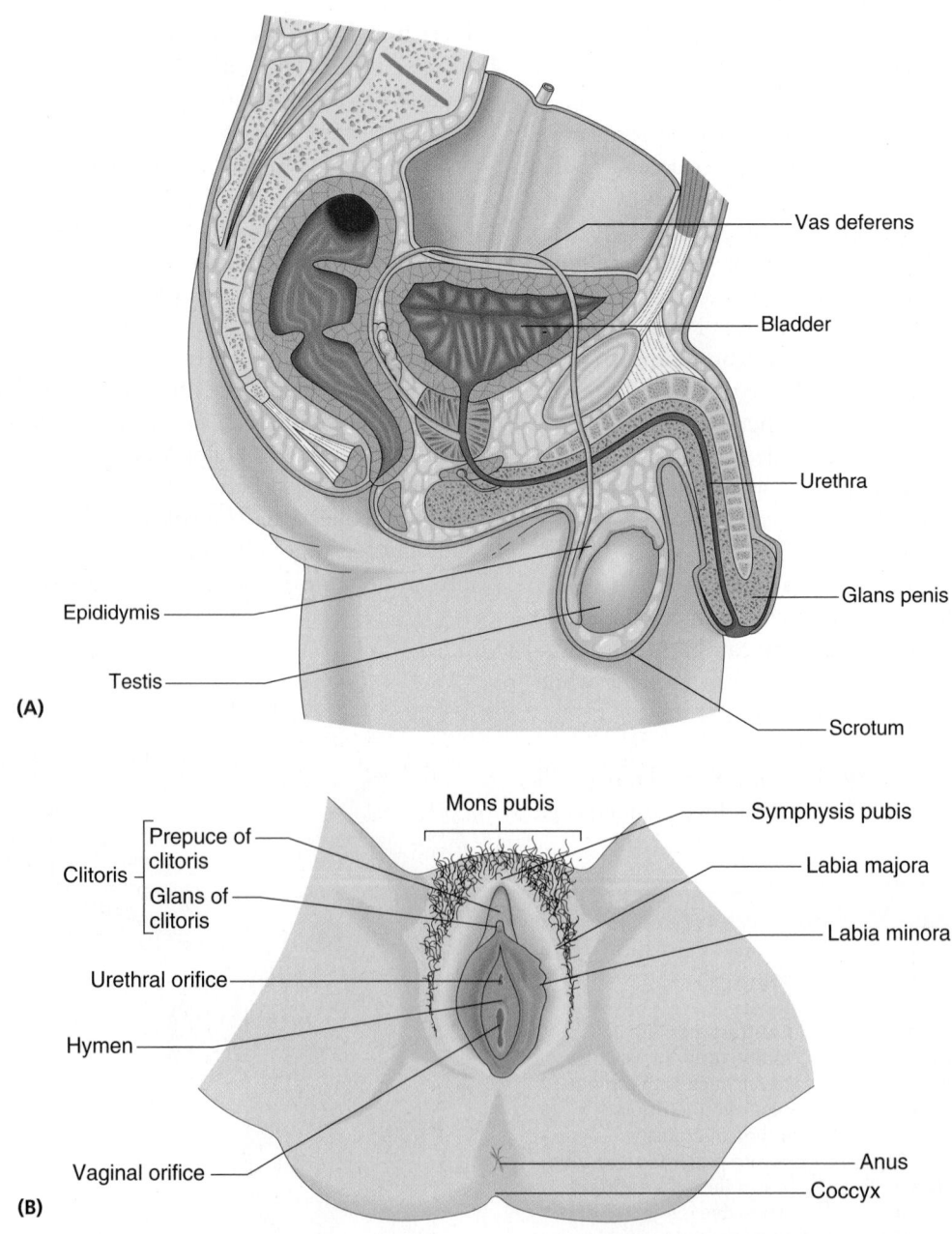

(A)

(B)

Figure 18-2   (A) Cross-sectional view of male anatomy showing urethra and bladder for catheterization. (B) External genitalia of the female.

SPOTLIGHT ON AAMA ESSENTIALS THROUGH CAAHEP

- Maintaining a smile and offering a kind word can allay a patient's fears and do a lot to win a permanent customer and patient.

- Whenever the medical assistant is required to perform an examination or procedure, she or he should be friendly, outgoing, and explain the procedure to the patient.

- Concern for patients generally results in happier patients who return in the future for care.

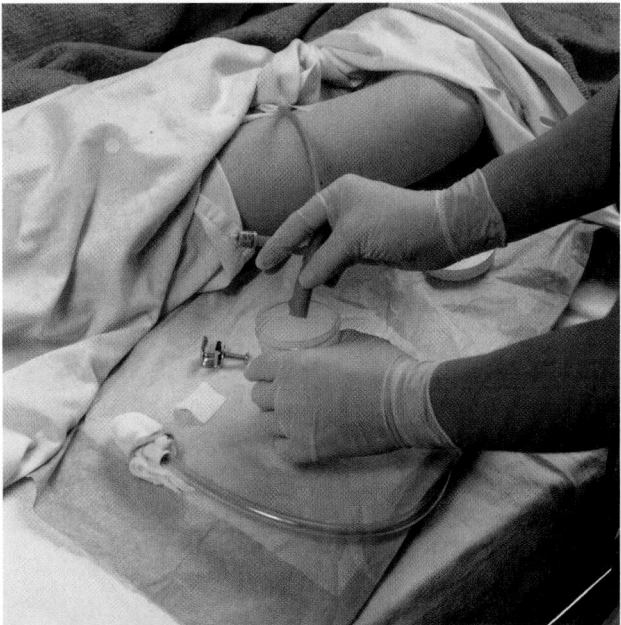

Figure 18-3 Urinary catheterization can be performed using a straight catheter, which is removed immediately after a urine specimen has been obtained, or it can be performed using a Foley catheter (an indwelling catheter). The indwelling catheter remains in the patient's bladder by means of a small inflated balloon at the bladder end of the catheter. A urine specimen can be obtained by disconnecting the tubing, being careful to make certain that asepsis is maintained.

SAFETY Sterile technique must be maintained throughout the catheterization. Contamination of any items during the procedure requires discarding the item and obtaining new sterile equipment before continuing the procedure (Figure 18-3).

See Procedure 18-2 to perform a urinary catheterization on a female patient and Procedure 18-3 for male catheterization.

Catheterization Equipment. French catheters are used in performing catheterizations in which the catheter is removed following the procedure. The Foley catheter is used when the catheter will remain in the urinary bladder

(indwelling catheter). Sterile, disposable catheterization kits are available that contain all necessary items to perform the procedure. See Figure 18-4 for types of urinary catheterizations.

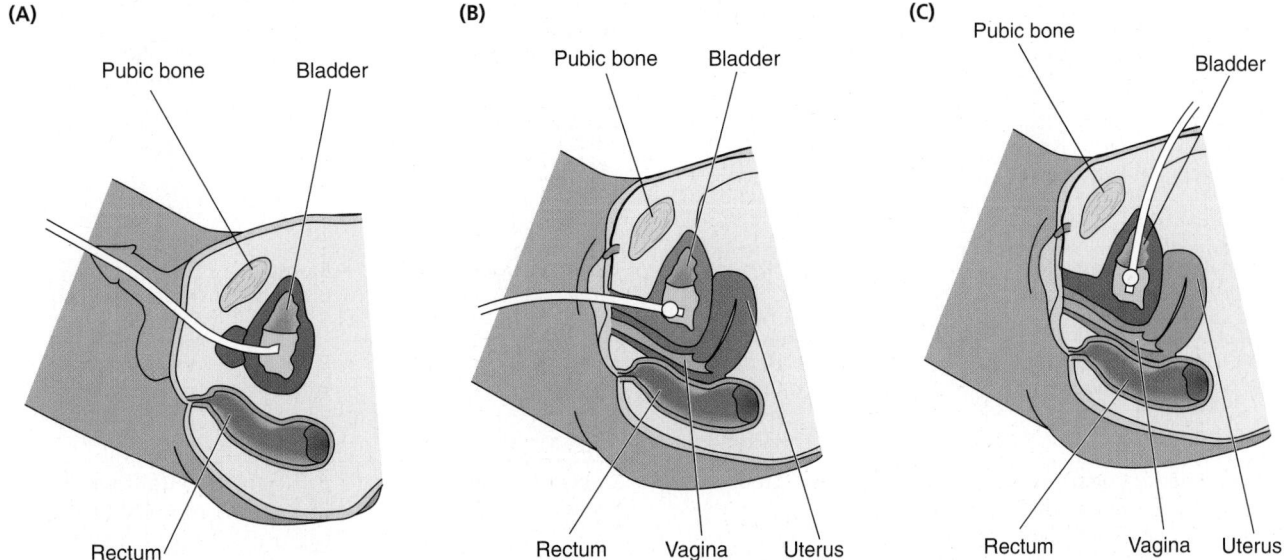

Figure 18-4 Types of urinary catheterizations: (A) In and out catheter. (B) Indwelling catheter. (C) Suprapubic catheter.

DIGESTIVE SYSTEM

The gastrointestinal system performs five functions which include:

1. **Ingestion** of food and breaking it into smaller particles
2. Passage of food through the digestive system (peristalsis)
3. Digestion through secretions of digestive enzymes
4. Absorption of nutrients into the bloodstream
5. Defecation of the solid waste products of digestion

When any of these functions is hindered, the digestive system malfunctions.

The digestive process begins in the mouth and concludes at the anus. As food passes through the **alimentary canal**, or digestive tract, it is mixed with gastric juices and enzymes allowing it to break down into smaller nutrients which allows absorption through the walls of the small intestine. Contents that have not been absorbed travel through the large intestine and are excreted through the anus. See Tables 18-4 and 18-5 for the common tests, procedures, disorders, and conditions of the digestive system. Figure 18-5 shows the major organs of the digestive system.

TABLE 18-4   DIGESTIVE SYSTEM DISORDERS

| Disease/ Disorder | Laboratory Diagnostic Tests | | | Radiography | Surgery | Medical Tests or Procedures |
	Blood	Urine	Other			
Anorexia Nervosa	• Complete blood count • Electrolytes • Blood glucose	• Urinalysis				• Electrocardiography
Appendicitis	• Complete blood count	• Urinalysis • Pregnancy test		• Abdominal ultrasound		• Rectal exam
Bulimia	• Complete blood count • Electrolytes	• Urinalysis				• Electrocardiography
Cholecystitis	• Complete blood count • Serum bilirubin	• Urinalysis		• Cholecystogram • Ultrasound of gall bladder		
Cholelithiasis	• Complete blood count • Serum bilirubin			• Cholecystogram • Ultrasound of gall bladder • I.V. cholangiogram		
Colon Cancer	• Complete blood count • Electrolytes			• Barium enema • Abdominal ultrasound	• Biopsy of colon	• Sigmoidoscopy • Colonoscopy
Crohn's Disease	• Complete blood count • Electrolytes			• Abdominal ultrasound • Barium enema	• Biopsy of colon	• Sigmoidoscopy • Colonoscopy • Stool culture
Diverticulitis	• Complete blood count • Erythrocyte sedimentation rate			• Barium enema		• Sigmoidoscopy • Colonoscopy
Duodenal Ulcer	• Complete blood count		• H. pylori	• Upper gastrointestinal series	• Biopsy duodenum	• Gastroscopy • Stool for occult blood
Gastric Ulcer	• Complete blood count		• H. pylori • Culture stomach secretions	• Upper gastrointestinal series	• Biopsy stomach lining	• Gastroscopy
Gastroenteritis	• Complete blood count • Electrolytes		• Stool culture	• Upper gastrointestinal series		• Gastroscopy • Colonoscopy

(continues)

TABLE 18-4 *(continued)*

| Disease/ Disorder | Laboratory Diagnostic Tests | | | Radiography | Surgery | Medical Tests or Procedures |
	Blood	Urine	Other			
Gastritis	• Complete blood count			• Upper gastrointestinal series		• Gastroscopy
Hemorrhoids	• Complete blood count				• Hemorrhoidectomy	• Physical exam • Proctoscopy
Hepatitis	• Protein • Bilirubin • Liver functions • Alkaline phosphotase • Gamma globulin	• Urinalysis			• Liver biopsy	• Liver scan
Hiatal Hernia				• Upper gastrointestinal series • Chest X ray	• Biopsy	• Esophagoscopy
Pinworms	• Complete blood count		• Stool sample for ova and parasites			• Perianal exam

TABLE 18-5   DESCRIPTION OF DIGESTIVE DISORDERS AND CONDITIONS

- Anorexia Nervosa. A disease of psychological origin. The individual does not eat and becomes emaciated and malnourished because of the need to avoid weight gain.
- Appendicitis. Acute inflammation of the appendix usually caused by infection or obstruction. Characterized by pain, nausea, vomiting, and fever.
- Bulimia. A syndrome in which an individual binges on food and then purges by inducing vomiting. The reason individuals engage in this behavior is to avoid weight gain, and it is of psychological origin.
- Cholecystitis. Inflammation of the gallbladder. Usual cause is gall stones, but other causes may be bacteria or chemical irritants.
- Colon Cancer. Common malignancy characterized by change in bowel habits, diarrhea or constipation and abdominal discomfort as tumor grows.
- Crohn's Disease. Chronic disease which exhibits inflammation of the ileum resulting in diarrhea, right lower quadrant pain and attacks of diarrhea and frequent blood in the stools.
- Diverticulitis. Inflammation of diverticula usually caused by impacted feces or bacteria in the sacs. Pain, cramp-like, usually in left side of abdomen. Obstruction can develop.
- Diverticulosis. Diverticula in colon without symptoms.
- Duodenal Ulcer. Lesion in the mucous membrane of the small intestine usually caused by hyperacidity.
- Gastric Ulcer. Caused by bacteria H. pylori.
- Gastroenteritis. Inflammation of the stomach and intestinal tract. Causes nausea, vomiting, diarrhea. May be caused by ingestion of pathogen.
- Gastritis. Inflammation of the stomach lining usually caused by an undefined irritant including alcohol, bacteria, or viruses. It can result in stomach discomfort, nausea and/or vomiting.
- Hepatitis. Inflammation of the liver caused by infection from a virus resulting in hepatomegaly, anorexia, and jaundice.
    Hepatitis A. Spread by fecal contamination of food or water.
    Hepatitis B. Spread by blood and body fluids contamination or sexual contact, contaminated needles, perinatal fluids, semen.
    Hepatitis C. Spread by blood (i.e., transfusion), contaminated needles, sexual contact.
    Hepatitis D. Intimate and sexual contact with intravenous drug users.
    Refer to Chapter 10 for more information about hepatitis.
- Hiatal Hernia. Congenital or traumatic protrusion of stomach through the diaphragm into the chest cavity (Figure 18-6).
- Pinworms. Intestinal parasites causing intestinal and rectal infection.

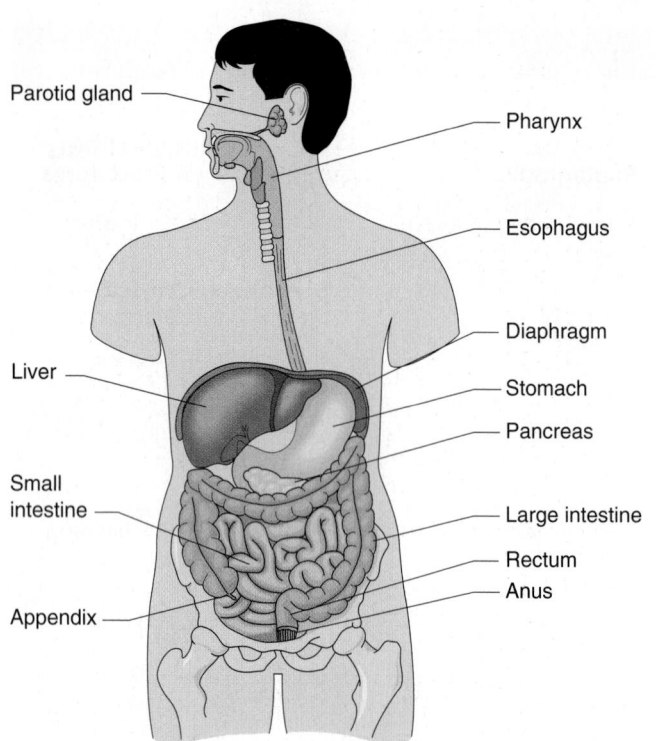

Figure 18-5   The digestive system.

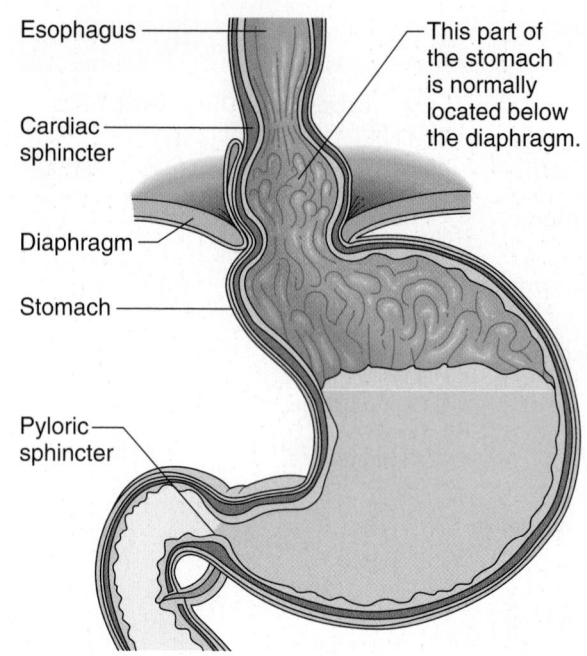

Figure 18-6   Hiatal hernia.

Signs and Symptoms of Digestive Conditions and Disorders

Common signs and symptoms of disorders and diseases of the digestive tract include nausea, vomiting, stomach cramping, diarrhea, heartburn, loss of appetite, weight loss, indigestion, fatigue, **hematemesis**, **melena**, and **hematochezia**.

There are many disorders and diseases of the digestive tract that can cause these signs and symptoms. Gastritis, a common ailment of the stomach, can be caused by caffeine, aspirin and other medication, spicy foods, and alcohol, and is characterized by epigastric pain, nausea, and vomiting of blood (hematemesis). Gastroenteritis, inflammation of the stomach and small intestine, another common ailment, is also known as food poisoning, intestinal flu, or traveler's diarrhea. It can be caused by infections from contaminated food or water, drug reactions, and allergic reactions to particular foods. Peptic ulcers found in the stomach are called gastric ulcers and can be caused by the action of pepsis, an enzyme. It is an **erosion** of the mucous lining of the stomach. Salicylates (such as aspirin), alcohol, smoking, oversecretion of hydrochloric acid, and stress seem to be implicated in this disease. Some gastric ulcers may be caused by the bacteria *H. pylori* and require antibiotic treatment. Ulcers found in the duodenum are called duodenal ulcers and are similar to gastric ulcers. A duodenal ulcer is an erosion of the mucous lining of the duodenum, a part of the small intestine. If determined that the ulcer is caused by the bacteria, antibiotics will be prescribed. Both types of ulcers seem to run a chronic course and if they are not controlled, the ulcerated area can **perforate** and hemorrhage ensues. Contents of the stomach or intestine can spill out into the abdominal cavity and cause a serious complication called **peritonitis** (infectious organisms enter the membrane covering the internal organs). See Figures 18-7 and 18-8.

Diarrhea is characterized by frequent liquid bowel movements. Diarrhea and vomiting may have many causes such as allergic reactions, infections from food or water,

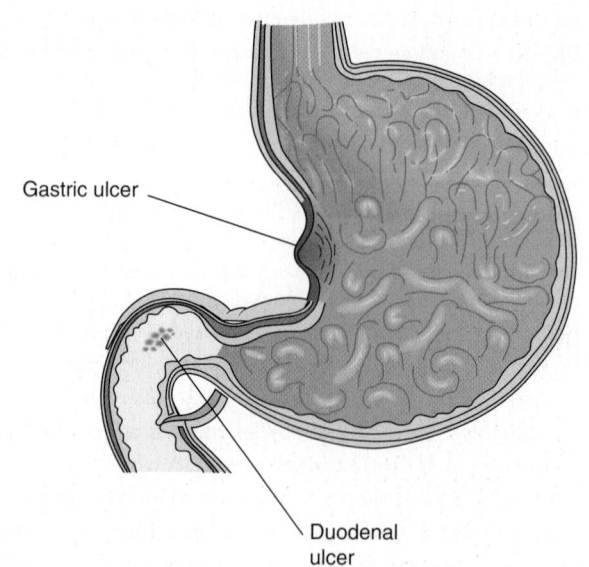

Figure 18-7   Peptic ulcers.

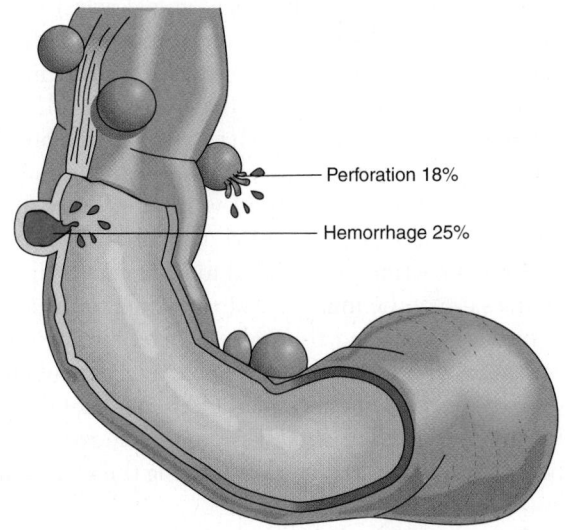

Figure 18-8   Diverticulosis.

or from stress. Dehydration can become a problem if diarrhea continues for several days. Infants, children, and the elderly are especially vulnerable to dehydration from vomiting and diarrhea.

Diagnostic Tests

Diagnostic tests for the digestive system commonly include radiography and **endoscopy**. An upper GI series

(barium swallow) is done to visualize the esophagus, stomach, and upper portion of the small intestine. A lower GI series (barium enema) will visualize the large intestine. See Figures 18-9, 18-10, and Chapter 20, Diagnostic Imaging.

Endoscopy allows the physician to look directly into the digestive organs with a lighted scope. Some examples of endoscopies used in the digestive tract are named by the organ being scoped:

> stomach: gastroscopy
>
> colon: colonoscopy
>
> sigmoid colon: sigmoidoscopy
>
> entire upper GI area: esophagogastro-duodenoscopy (EGD). (See Figure 18-11.)

Biopsies can be taken during an endoscopic procedure.

Sigmoidoscopy. Sigmoidoscopy is a diagnostic examination of the interior of the sigmoid colon. It is a useful aid in the diagnosis of cancer of the colon, ulcerations, polyps, tumors, bleeding, and other lower intestinal disorders. The sigmoidoscope is a metal or plastic (disposable) instrument with a light source and a magnifying lens, which permits the mucous membrane of the sigmoid colon to be seen.

The metal and plastic types of scopes may still be used in some offices (Figure 18-12), but the instrument

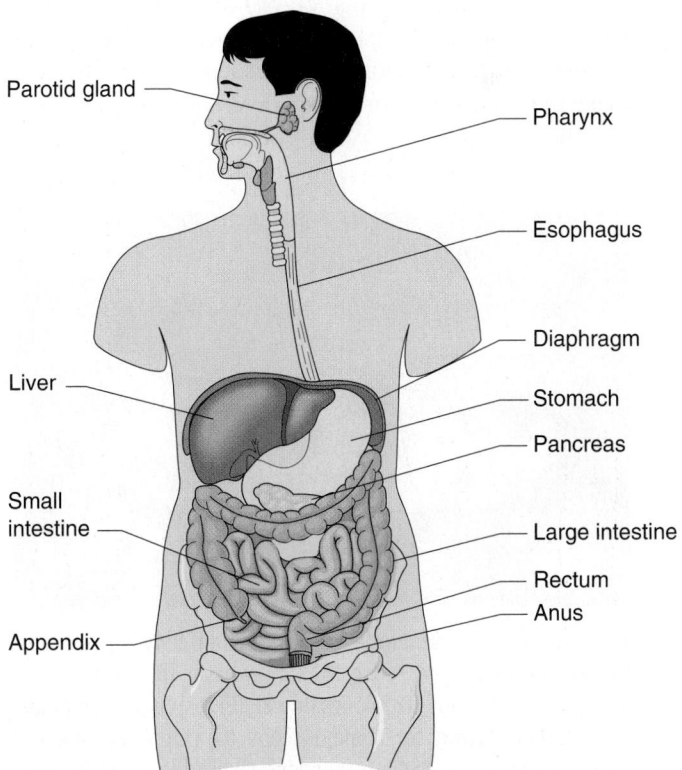

Figure 18-9   Lower GI; highlighted area is visualized.

Figure 18-10   Upper GI; highlighted area is visualized.

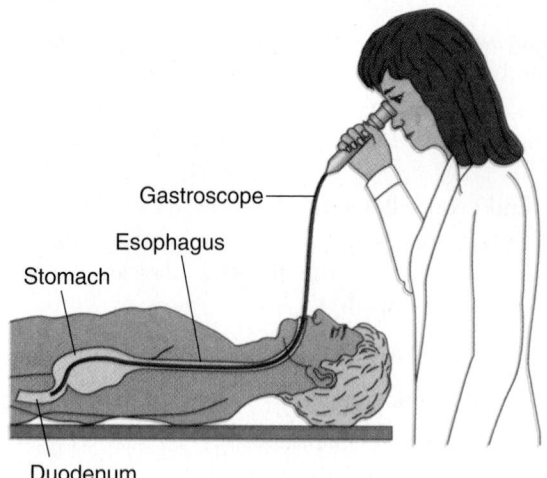

Figure 18-11 Esophagogastro-duodenoscopy procedure (EGD).

most commonly used by physicians is the flexible sigmoidoscope, which is shown assembled with items necessary for the procedure. Since it is flexible, it can be inserted much farther into the colon. This instrument makes it possible to view more of the mucous membranes of the intestines (Figure 18-13).

An **obturator** is inserted into the sigmoidoscope. The tip of the obturator and scope are lubricated and carefully inserted into the rectum. Then the obturator is removed so that the sigmoid colon can be seen. Patients find this an unpleasant procedure.

As with any examination of the abdominal cavity, you should advise the patient to empty the bladder and evacuate the bowel before the procedure begins. This will make the exam easier for both patient and examiner. During the procedure the patient should be instructed to

breathe through the mouth deeply and slowly to relax abdominal muscles. Patients may feel the urge to defecate during a colon examination because of the stretching of the intestinal wall from the instrument passing through and air being introduced with it. If patients use the breathing technique mentioned, this discomfort can be relieved. The procedure should last only a few minutes, especially if patients have followed preparation instructions.

Air is sometimes introduced into the colon (by the examiner's use of the inflation bulb attached to the scope with tubing) to distend the wall of the colon for easier placement of the lumen of the endoscope. Patients find this to be uncomfortable and sometimes painful. The physician may need to use suction to remove mucus, blood, or fecal material that is obstructing the view of the colon.

Assistance in handing necessary items to the physician and giving support to the patient are the medical assistant's roles during these exams.

It will also most often be the medical assistant who tells the patient how to prepare for the sigmoidoscopy and explains how the test is performed. For successful examination, proper preparation is essential. In addition to having patients restrict dairy products, raw fruits and

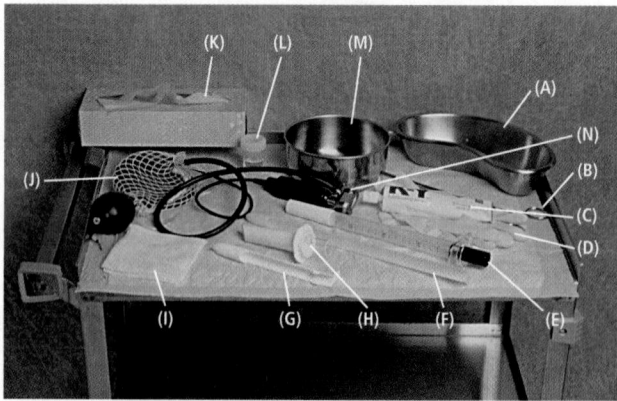

Figure 18-12 Setup for a proctosigmoidoscopy with a rigid sigmoidoscope and anoscope. (A) Kidney basin. (B) Sponge forceps. (C) Lubricant. (D) Gloves (latex). (E) Disposable sigmoidoscope. (F) Obturator for sigmoidoscope. (G) Obturator for anoscope. (H) Anoscope. (I) Gauze sponges. (J) Insufflator. (K) Tissues. (L) Biopsy container. (M) Basin of water. (N) Magnifying lens.

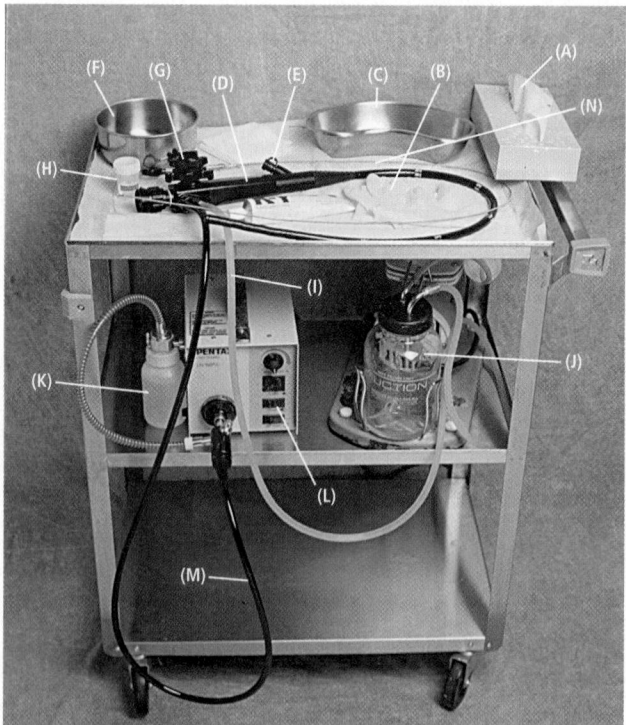

Figure 18-13 Setup for a proctosigmoidoscopy with a flexible sigmoidoscope. (A) Tissues. (B) Latex gloves. (C) Kidney basin. (D) Flexible sigmoidoscope insertion tube. (E) Eye lens. (F) Basin for water. (G) Control head. (H) Biology container with formalin. (I) Suction tubing. (J) Suction apparatus. (K) Water bottle. (L) Sigmoidoscope control panel. (M) Power cord.

vegetables, and grains and cereals from their diet, they should be encouraged to drink plenty of clear liquids and eat lightly the day before the scheduled appointment for the sigmoid colon exam. A plain commercial enema should be self-administered at home approximately 2 hours before the exam. Physicians may vary the instructions according to the patient's condition. If patients are not completely informed about preparations and the exam is attempted with unsatisfactory results, it will have to be repeated, which is both costly and inconvenient. Satisfactory results are obtained by giving patients both oral and written instructions.

There are occasions, during an appointment for which the patient was "worked in" to the schedules, when the physician feels that the patient's condition warrants the examination of the sigmoid colon. In this case, the physician will order an enema to be given to the patient in the office.

It is not a common procedure to administer an enema to a patient in the medical office or clinic, but is sometimes a necessity in the successful completion of a sigmoidoscopy or other rectal examination. Even though a patient may have received proper instructions and carried them out before the scheduled appointment, there is no guarantee that the patient achieved success. In the event that the patient comes in for the appointment and the colon is not sufficiently evacuated of feces for a sigmoidoscopy, the physician may order a cleansing enema so that the exam can be completed. It is generally best to proceed with the planned procedure, even with the delay of the enema. Usually this works out well for patient and staff, because rescheduling presents difficulties for everyone.

Often the patient did follow the list of instructions, but was not able to retain the enema solution long enough to get satisfactory results. You will more likely be able to encourage the patient to retain the contents of the enema longer. You may want to explain that the longer the contents are retained, the more successful the results will be. Otherwise, it may have to be repeated, or the exam rescheduled. Be certain that you use an examination room that is close to the rest room for the patient's convenience when you administer an enema. Your patience and understanding are needed, because many patients are embarrassed to have an enema administered to them. The procedure that follows will provide the information you need to carry out this procedure.

Some exams, such as diagnostic sigmoidoscopy and X rays, require the use of laxatives by the patient the day before or the morning of the exam. This may present a problem in the patient's personal or employment schedule if instructions are not made clear before the appointment is scheduled. Most patients are fearful of what the diagnostic examination will disclose. Helping them

Patient Teaching Tip

When patients come in for rectal or sigmoidoscopy examinations, here are a few informative topics that you may discuss with them with the physician's direction.

1. Remind them that laxatives and enemas should only be used by direction of the physician.
2. Constipation may be avoided/relieved by including fresh fruits and vegetables, cereals, and grains in the diet, drinking plenty of liquids (water), and getting regular exercise.
3. Instruct them that if they have any of the following symptoms persistently it could mean that a disease or an abnormal condition is present and consulting the physician is strongly advised: heartburn or indigestion, nausea and/or vomiting, constipation or diarrhea, excessive gas or bloating, stool that is tarry (black) or other than a normal brown color.
4. Inform patients who are age 40 and over that they should routinely test their stool for occult blood every 2 years for detection of cancer of the colon, or more often if advised by the physician (if family history indicates). All patients over age 50 should test annually.
5. Advise patients to include high-fiber foods in their diets, avoid fat (especially saturated fats) and cholesterol, and eat red meats very sparingly.
6. Urge patients to eat from a variety of foods (from the food pyramid) and to eat 4 to 6 small meals rather than 1 or 2 large meals daily to promote better utilization of nutrients and more energy.
7. Suggest to patients that it is better to select snacks and beverages wisely such as fruits, vegetables, and juices over coffee/tea/pop and high-calorie sweets or chips.

choose a convenient appointment time and explaining the reasons for the preparations they must undergo is usually appreciated.

Proper positioning of the patient during the sigmoidoscopy is important for both the physician's viewing of the rectum and sigmoid colon and the patient's comfort. Proctology tables are designed especially for this procedure (Figure 18-14). They provide support of the patient's chest and head with the arm resting against the head-

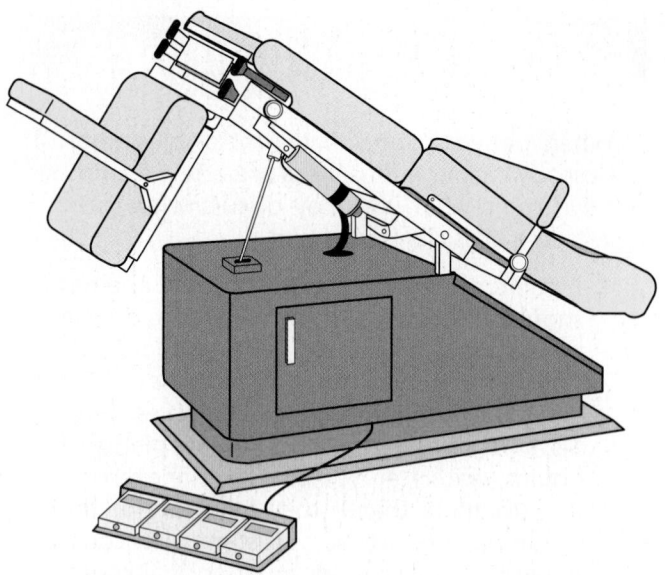

Figure 18-14   Proctologic table.

board as the table is tilted to the knee-chest position. Those who cannot tolerate this position are assisted into Sims' position for the exam. Many physicians find this acceptable and it is more comfortable for the patient. You should ask about the physician's preference in patient position since there are many variations.

The physician may wish to view the intestinal mucosa following a normal bowel movement. More often, the patient is instructed to eat a light diet containing plenty of clear liquids and avoiding dairy products for 24 hours before the exam, and to have a plain cleansing enema the morning of, or 2 hours before, the exam. Still other physicians may wish patients to use laxatives the day before and an enema the night before and also the morning of the exam. Patients have usually eaten little within the past few days because of their abdominal distress.

In the diagnosis of hemorrhoids, fissures, and ulcerations, the physician usually begins investigative procedures by examining the anus and the interior of the rectum with a proctoscope. During the sigmoidoscopy, the physician may want to take a biopsy of questionable tissue from the sigmoid colon to aid in confirming the diagnosis. It is a good rule to have all possible necessary items available. When the patient has been prepared and the physician is ready to begin the exam, the medical assistant hands the necessary instruments and supplies to the physician as needed. Remember to advise patients to report any problems, such as bleeding, discharge, swelling, or any other unusual discomfort following any procedure. A biopsy lab request form must be completed and accompany the tissue to the lab. Containers for biopsy specimens have a formaldehyde solution to preserve the tissue until the analysis is done.

Patient Teaching Tip

Following sigmoidoscopy, patients should drink plenty of clear fluids to help relieve the usual abdominal discomfort and flatulence. Patients may also find relief in lying in a prone position with a pillow across their midabdominal area to aid in the passage of gas.

See Procedure 18-4 to assist with a proctosigmoidoscopy.

While the proctosigmoidoscope examines the rectum and sigmoid colon with either a flexible or rigid (metal) scope, a procedure known as a **colonoscopy** can be scheduled in the outpatient department of the hospital or performed in the office or clinic. A flexible fiberoptic instrument is used and the entire length of the large intestine (colon) can be examined for lesions such as tumors, polyps, fissures, and so on. Biopsies which consist of small tissue pieces can be removed with a snare-type instrument inserted through the colonoscope. The tissue is microscopically examined by a pathologist to determine whether or not a malignancy is present in the colon. The patient receives a muscle relaxant/tranquilizer to facilitate the examination.

Fecal Occult Blood Test

Patients may be instructed to obtain three stool specimens at home to allow examination of a fecal sample for occult (hidden) blood. **Guaiac** slides, applicators, and envelopes will be given to the patient to take home (Figure 18-15). The patient will need to obtain a small stool sample from three separate bowel movements. Three separate samples are used to allow detection of blood from gastrointestinal lesions that exhibit intermittent bleeding. The medical assistant's role is to instruct the patient on how to properly collect the stool specimens on the test slides and care and store the slides until they are returned to the office. (See Procedure 18-5).

For patients who have daily bowel movements, this will not be a problem. For patients who have difficulty with daily elimination, it may take several days to collect the samples. Patients should not use laxatives unless directed by the physician.

Positive tests for occult blood require further testing such as sigmoidoscopy and colonoscopy to identify the source of bleeding. If a lesion is found either in the rectum or colon, a biopsy can be performed and sent to the laboratory for examination of cells for malignancy. (See Procedure 18-5.)

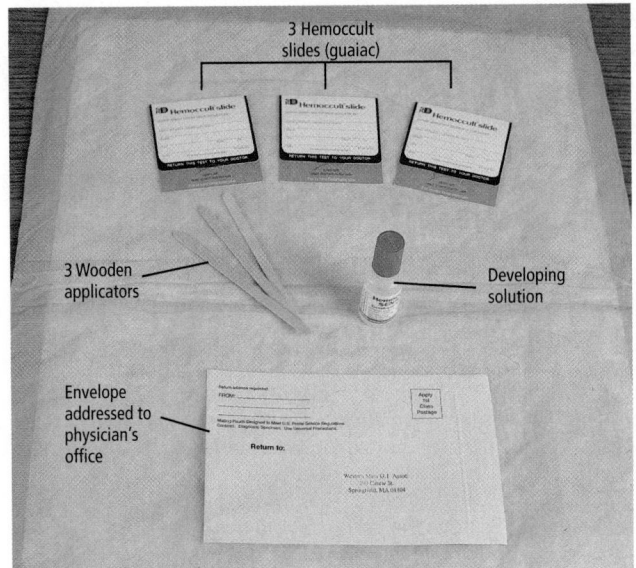

Figure 18-15 Supplies needed for the guaiac hemoccult test for fecal occult blood. The patient will take all supplies home except the developing solution.

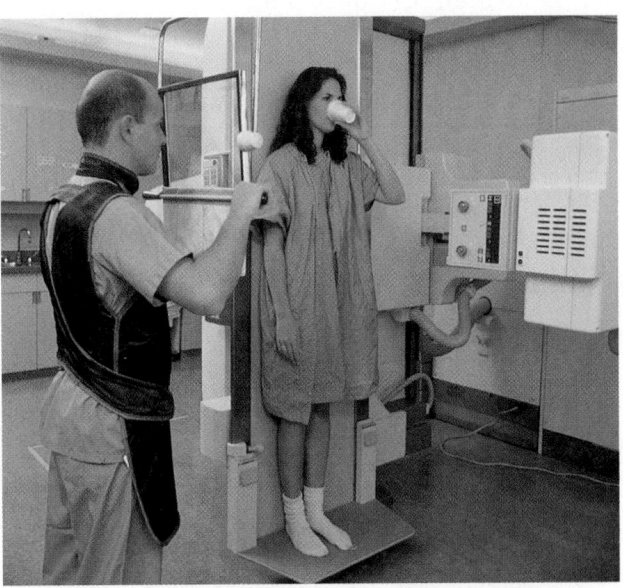

Figure 18-16 In a barium swallow test, barium sulfate is swallowed and X rays are taken of the esophagus, stomach, and small intestine. This is also known as an upper GI series.

Patient Teaching Tip

The following steps should be followed two days before the fecal occult blood test and continued until three slides have been prepared:

1. Avoid red meats, processed meats, and liver. These release hemoglobin which can produce a false positive result.
2. Avoid turnips, broccoli, cauliflower, and melons. These foods may contain a substance, peroxibase, that will cause a false positive result.
3. Avoid aspirin, iron supplements, and large doses of vitamin C for seven days prior to test. These substances may cause gastric bleeding that can mask bleeding from a lesion.
4. Consume a high-fiber diet. Fiber provides roughage to promote bowel movement and encourage bleeding from any lesion that may be present.
5. Do not begin test during menses, for three days after menses, or if bleeding from hemorrhoids.
6. Drink plenty of fluids to help avoid constipation.
7. Store slides at room temperature and protect from heat, sun, and fluorescent lights.

X-Ray Studies of the Digestive System. There are several diagnostic X-ray studies that can be performed to study digestive structures and functions for disease. They include the upper GI series (barium swallow) (Figure 18-16), lower GI series (barium enema), and the cholecystogram. Table 18-6 presents the purpose, patient preparation, and procedures for each of these studies.

SENSORY SYSTEM

The special senses of vision, hearing, **equilibrium**, smell, and taste permit the body to detect information about the environment. The eyes, ears, nose, and taste buds are all sense organs which contain specialized receptor organs. See Table 18-7 for diseases and disorders and diagnostic tests and procedures for eyes, ears, and nose.

The Eye

The eye is the primary organ for sight and is one of the few organs of the body externally exposed. Its accessory structures—the eyelids, eyelashes, lacrimal ducts, and extrinsic muscles—provide protection for the eye. The anterior portion of the eyeball protrudes outward and the remainder is protected by the orbit.

The intraocular structures consist of some parts of the eye visible externally and parts visible only through an ophthalmoscope. The intraocular structures include the following:

● Sclera: white area covering the outside of the eye except over the pupil and iris

TABLE 18-6	PATIENT PREPARATION AND PROCEDURE FOR X-RAY STUDIES OF THE DIGESTIVE SYSTEM			
Test	**Purpose**	**Patient Prep**	**Procedure**	**Time**
Barium swallow (upper GI series)	To study the esophagus, stomach, duodenum, and small intestine for disease (ulcers, tumors, hiatal hernia, esophageal varices)	Day prior to X ray: 1. Light evening meal 2. NPO after midnight Day of test: 1. NPO Postprocedural: 1. Increase fluid intake 2. Take laxative as prescribed	1. The patient is asked to drink a flavored barium mixture while standing in front of the fluoroscope. 2. The radiologist observes the passage down the digestive tract 3. The patient is turned to various positions to allow good visualization of the intestine 4. X rays are taken	1 hr
Barium enema (lower GI series)	To study the colon for disease (polyps, tumors, lesions)	Clear liquid one day prior (allowed: carbonated beverages, clear gelatin, clear broth, coffee & tea with sugar). No milk or milk products 8 oz of water every hour until bedtime Prep kit: (usually supplied by physician's office) to include bottle of magnesium citrate, Dulcolax tab(s) Day prior to X ray: 1. Late afternoon drink bottle of magnesium citrate 2. Early evening take Dulcolax tab(s) as prescribed 3. Light eve. meal. NPO except water, after dinner Morning of procedure: 1. NPO 2. Cleaning enema Postprocedural instructions: 1. Increase fluid intake and dietary fiber 2. Report to physician if no bowel movement within 24 hours of test	1. The colon is filled with a barium sulfate mixture 2. The patient is turned in various positions to allow the barium to fill the colon. Air is injected to move the barium along the colon 3. When the colon is full, X rays are taken	1–2 hrs
Cholecystogram	To study the gallbladder for disease (stones, duct obstruction), inflammation	1. Evening before test fat-free dinner 2. Patient takes dye tablets with 8 oz water 3. Cathartic or cleansing enemas may be prescribed 4. NPO after dinner and tablets	1. A series of radiographs is taken 2. A fatty meal may be given to stimulate the gallbladder to empty 3. Other radiographs can then be taken to check gallbladder function	1 hr

- Cornea: clear tissue covering the pupil and iris

- Iris: round disk of smooth and radial muscles giving the eye its color.

- Pupil: round opening in the iris that changes size as the iris reacts to light and dark

- Anterior chamber: space between cornea and iris/pupil filled with clear fluid called aqueous humor

- Posterior chamber: space between the iris and lens that is filled with aqueous humor

- Lens: clear fibers enclosed in a membrane that refract and focus light to the retina

- Posterior cavity: the space in the posterior part of the eyeball filled with thick, gelatinous material called vitreous humor

- Posterior sclera: white opaque layer covering the posterior part of the eyeball

- Choroid layer: the layer between the sclera and retina containing blood vessels

- Retina: the inside layer of the posterior part of the eye that receives the light rays (visual stimuli)

The mechanism of vision occurs after impulses leave the retina and travel through the optic nerves to the

TABLE 18-7 SENSORY SYSTEM DISORDERS

| Disease/ Disorder | Laboratory Diagnostic Tests | | | Radiography | Surgery | Medical Tests or Procedures |
	Blood	Urine	Other			
Cataract						• Ophthalmologic exam
Chalazion					• Excision	
Color-Blindness						• Ishihara color plates
Conjunctivitis			• Culture and sensitivity of eye discharge			
Corneal Abrasion						• Fluorescein sodium
Diabetic Retinopathy					• Laser	• Fluorescein • Angiogram
Epistaxis	• Complete blood count					• Blood pressure
External Otitis	• Complete blood count		• Culture and sensitivity of exudate			
Glaucoma						• Ophthalmologic exam including intraocular pressure
Ménière's Disease						• Audiometry
Myopia						• Ophthalmologic exam
Hyperopia						• Astigmatoscopy
Presbyopia						• Snellen chart
Astigmatism						• Jaeger chart
Nasal Polyps					• Biopsy of polyp (lesion)	• Nasal exam
Otitis Media	• Complete blood count		• Culture and sensitivity of exudate		• Myringotomy • Tympanostomy	• Tympanography
Otosclerosis						• Audiometry • Rinne test
Retinal Detachment					• Laser or surgery to reattach	
Sinusitis	• Complete blood count		• Culture and sensitivity of exudate	• Sinus X rays		
Stye (Hordeolum)			• Culture and sensitivity if exudate present		• Incision and drainage	

brain. At the optic chiasm the nerve fibers cross and continue to the thalamus. These fibers synapse with other neurons that send the impulses to the right and left visual area of the occipital lobe of the brain. Since the tracts cross at the optic chasm, the stimuli coming from the right visual fields are translated in the visual area of the left occipital area, and the stimuli coming from the left visual fields are translated in the visual area of the right occipital lobe. See Table 18-8 for Common Eye Disorders. See Figure 18-17 and 18-18 for anatomy of the eye.

Signs and symptoms that are common to eye diseases and disorders are pain or burning in or around the eye, decreased visual acuity, any visual changes such as seeing sudden flashes of light, and eye redness.

Measuring Visual Acuity. A procedure commonly performed by the medical assistant is the measuring of a patient's visual acuity. This is only a screening process used when errors in refraction are suspected. The procedure must be performed in a well-lighted quiet area.

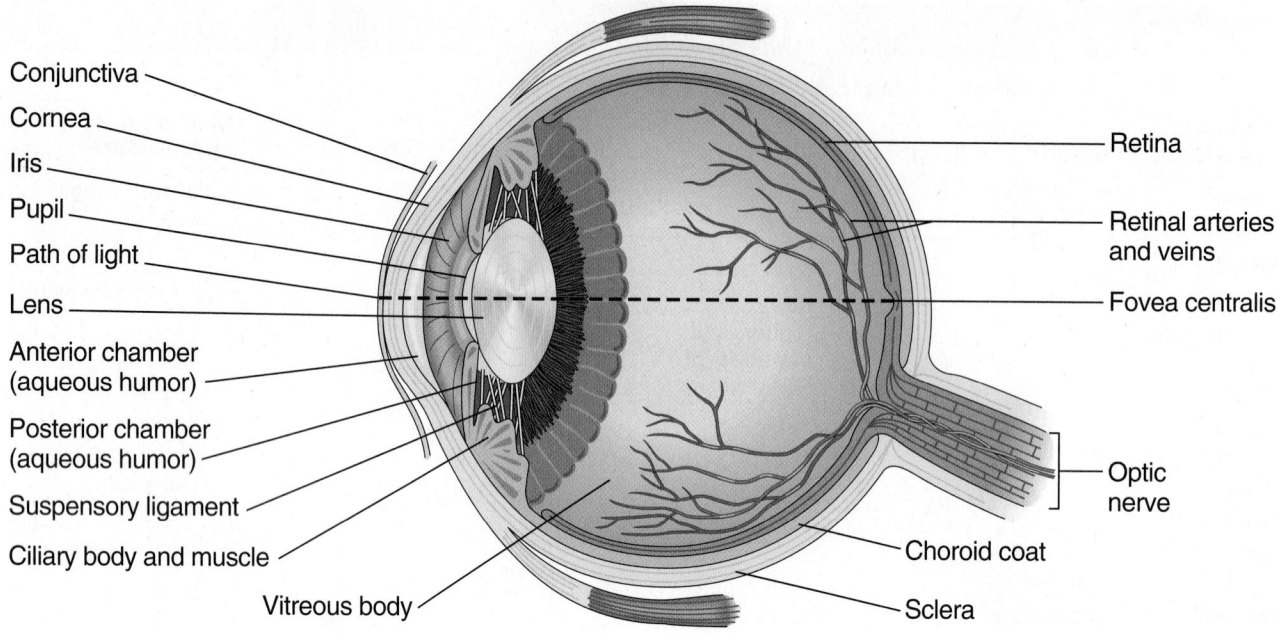

Conjunctiva
Cornea
Iris
Pupil
Path of light
Lens
Anterior chamber (aqueous humor)
Posterior chamber (aqueous humor)
Suspensory ligament
Ciliary body and muscle
Vitreous body

Retina
Retinal arteries and veins
Fovea centralis
Optic nerve
Choroid coat
Sclera

Figure 18-17   The eyeball—cross section view.

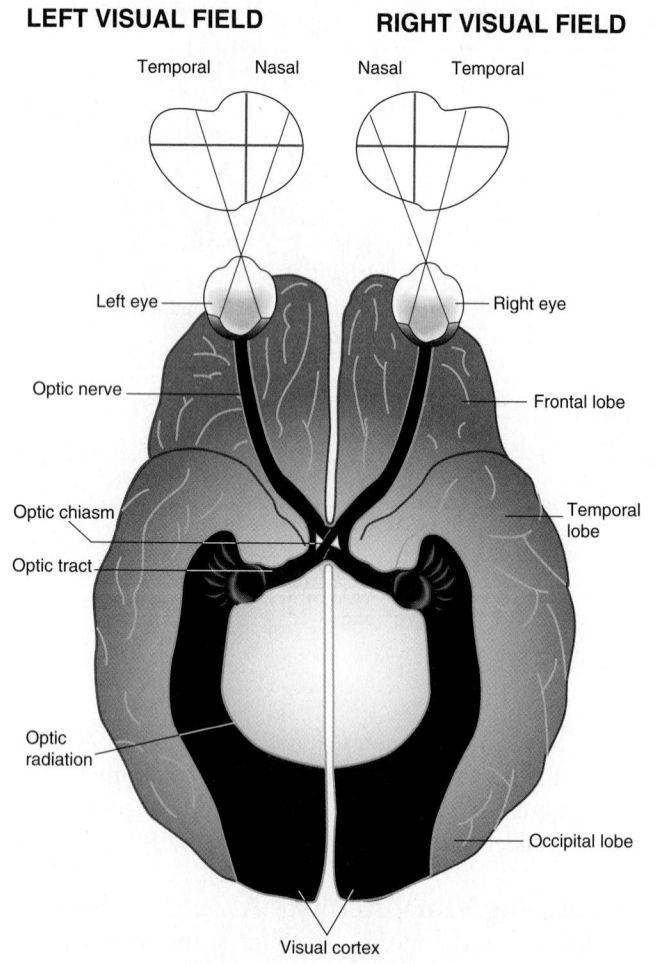

LEFT VISUAL FIELD   **RIGHT VISUAL FIELD**

Temporal   Nasal   Nasal   Temporal

Left eye   Right eye
Optic nerve   Frontal lobe
Optic chiasm   Temporal lobe
Optic tract
Optic radiation
                                  Occipital lobe
Visual cortex

Figure 18-18   The visual pathways of the eye.

TABLE 18-8   DESCRIPTION OF EYE DISORDERS

Refraction and Other Disorders:

- Astigmatism. Irregular lens curvature or cornea shape causing improper focusing of objects.
- Cataract. Lens loses its transparent nature due to changes in its proteins. Usually brought on by aging.
- Color blindness. Inability to distinguish among colors. Caused by an absence of a cone photopigment, a genetic disorder.
- Conjunctivitis. Caused by a bacterial infection or irritant resulting in irritated and reddened conjunctiva. If caused by bacteria, conjunctivitis is highly contagious. See Figure 18-19.
- Corneal Abrasion. Caused by an injury to the cornea by a foreign body resulting in pain, tearing, redness, and possible infection.
- Glaucoma. Condition caused by increased intraocular pressure due to a buildup of aqueous humor. This results in mild visual disturbances with little or no pain but can lead to blindness if untreated.
- Nearsightedness (Myopia). Caused by an elongated eyeball and the image is focused in the front of the retina resulting in the inability to focus on objects at a distance.
- Farsightedness (Hyperopia). Caused when the eyeball is shortened and the image is focused behind the retina causing distance vision to be fuzzy.
- Presbyopia. Attributed to the aging process when the lens loses its elasticity, and the ability to accommodate. Vision is hampered when items are close.
- Stye (Hordeolum). Inflamed sebaceous gland of the eyelid caused by bacterial infection. Erythema, tenderness at site are common symptoms. See Figure 18-20.

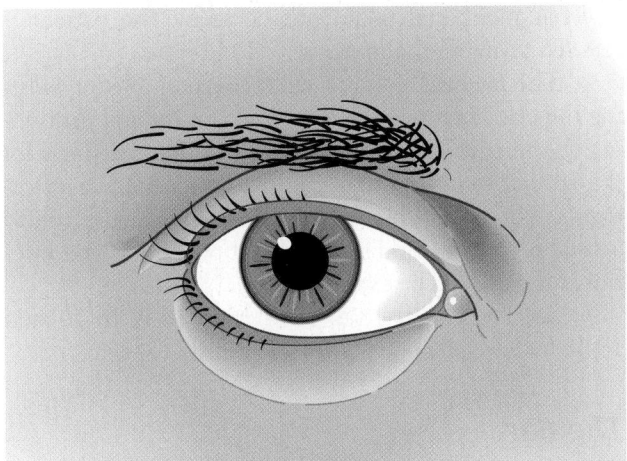

Figure 18-19   Conjunctivitis.

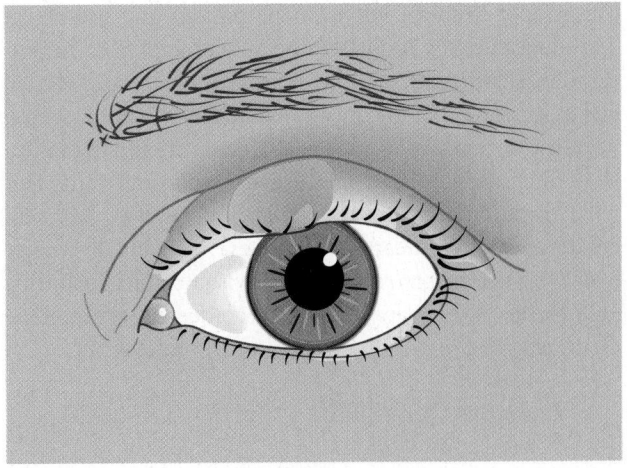

Figure 18-20   Stye (hordeolum).

While performing the procedure, the medical assistant must observe the patient for any action that may indicate difficulty with vision. These actions would include squinting, wiping of the eyes, or leaning toward the chart. In near-vision acuity, these actions would include holding the card nearer or farther than the stated position. The commonly used chart for distance visual acuity is the Snellen chart for the adult. Near-vision is commonly checked by using the Jaeger card.

The Jaeger chart used for checking clear vision is a small card that is held by the patient between 14 and 16 inches from the eye. The medical assistant measures the distance for accuracy. This is the distance from which a person with normal vision is able to read printed material such as a newspaper. The Jaeger test consists of a series of reading material, the letters of which gradually become smaller. Record the last line number that the patient can easily read. The patient is checked with and without corrective lenses and each eye is checked separately.

Errors in refraction is the term used to designate visual acuity abnormalities. The common visual abnormalities include: myopia (nearsightedness), the ability to see only near objects clearly; hyperopia (farsightedness), the ability to see only distant objects clearly; and astigmatism, uneven curvature of the cornea resulting in a scattering of light rays producing blurry vision. Presbyopia (associated with the aging process) is an increase in farsightedness and a loss of lens elasticity that is necessary to accommodate for near vision and is seen primarily in the older patient. (See Figure 18-21.)

The Snellen chart consists of the alphabet letters in various combinations starting at the top with a large E, and descending sized Es by line toward the bottom. Each line is labeled with the visual acuity measurement.

Recording Visual Acuity. Visual acuity, both near and far, is recorded in a fraction format. The numerator indicates

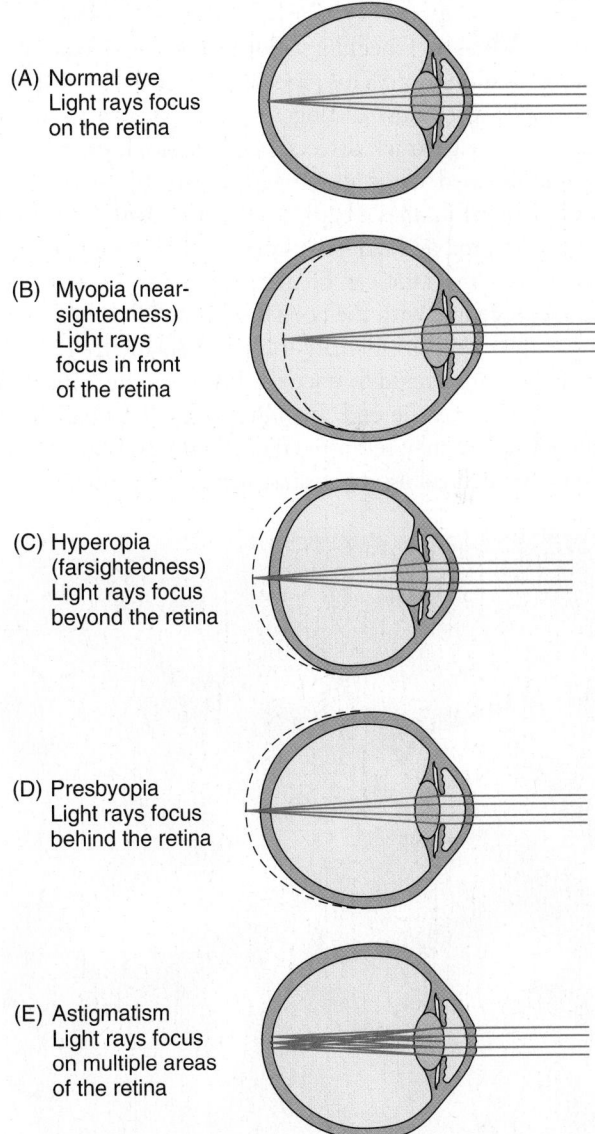

Figure 18-21   (A) Normal eye vision. (B) Myopia. (C) Hyperopia. (D) Presbyopia. (E) Astigmatism.

the 20-foot distance between the patient and the chart. The denominator indicates the visual acuity of the patient in relationship to the normal seeing eye. Normal vision is 20/20. This means that at 20 feet the eye is seeing what the normal eye would see at 20 feet. Should the vision be 20/20, this indicates that the eye is seeing at twenty feet what the normal eye would see at 30 feet away. A visual acuity of 20/15 indicates that the eye is seeing at twenty feet what the person with normal visual acuity would be able to see at 15 feet. Vision is recorded on the patient chart as right eye OD and left eye OS, both eyes OU.

Example: OD 20/20   OS 20/20   OU 20/20

Patients should be screened with and without their corrective lenses and results recorded as such in patients' records.

Color Vision. Checking color vision is not part of a routine examination. This procedure is usually performed on people who must distinguish color as part of their occupation, e.g., truck drivers, pilots, and salespeople. A commonly used color vision test is the Ishihara color graph. The Ishihara is a book containing pages comprised of varying sized and colored circles. Inside the circles are numbers or lines that can be traced. The patient is seated for the procedure with the book held 14 to 16 inches away and is instructed to identify the numbers as the page is turned or is instructed to trace the line from the indicated starting point to the end. Inability to see the number or follow the line may indicate color blindness. Should this occur the medical assistant must inform the physician as

to what number(s) could not be seen. The patient is referred to an ophthalmologist.

The medical assistant will be responsible for assisting the physician in ophthalmologic exams and performing the tests for visual acuity. Diagnostic procedures for the special senses involve the use of specialized instruments. The use of the **ophthalmoscope** (Figure 18-22) assists in identifying disease-related problems. The interior of the eye can be examined.

See Procedures 18-6, 18-7, 18-8, 18-9, 18-10, and 18-11 for specialty procedures for the eye.

The Ear

The structures of hearing and equilibrium are divided into the external ear, the middle ear, and the inner ear. The external ear includes the pinna (**auricle**) and the external auditory canal. The pinna is mostly cartilaginous tissue with a small amount of adipose tissue in the earlobe. The external auditory canal is about one inch in length and contains hair and wax (cerumen)-producing glands. The external ear and middle ear are separated by the tympanic membrane (eardrum).

The middle ear, also called the tympanic cavity, is a small space containing three bones, the malleus (hammer), incus (anvil), and stapes (stirrup). Next to the stapes is the oval window that leads to the inner ear. The eustachian tube connects the middle ear to the throat.

The inner ear is the most sophisticated part of the ear. It is responsible for both hearing and equilibrium (balance). The inner ear consists of a fluid-filled space housing the vestibule, the semicircular canals, the round

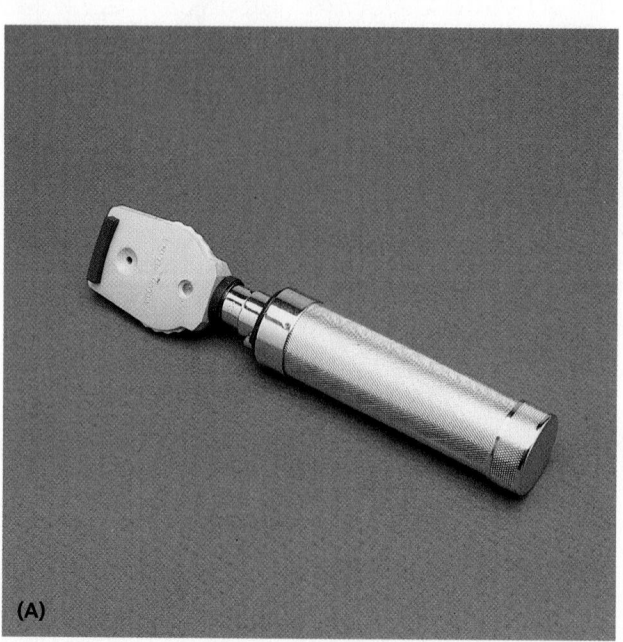

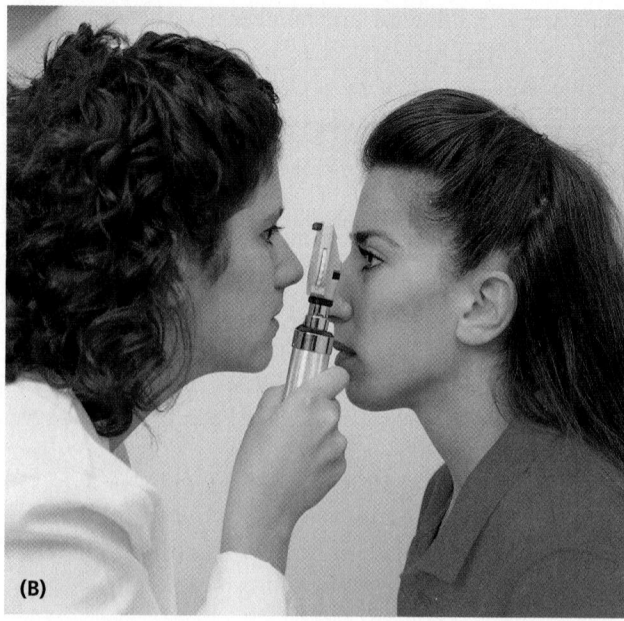

Figure 18-22   (A) The ophthalmoscope is used to identify eye disorders. (B) Here, the physician uses the ophthalmoscope to view the interior of the patient's eye.

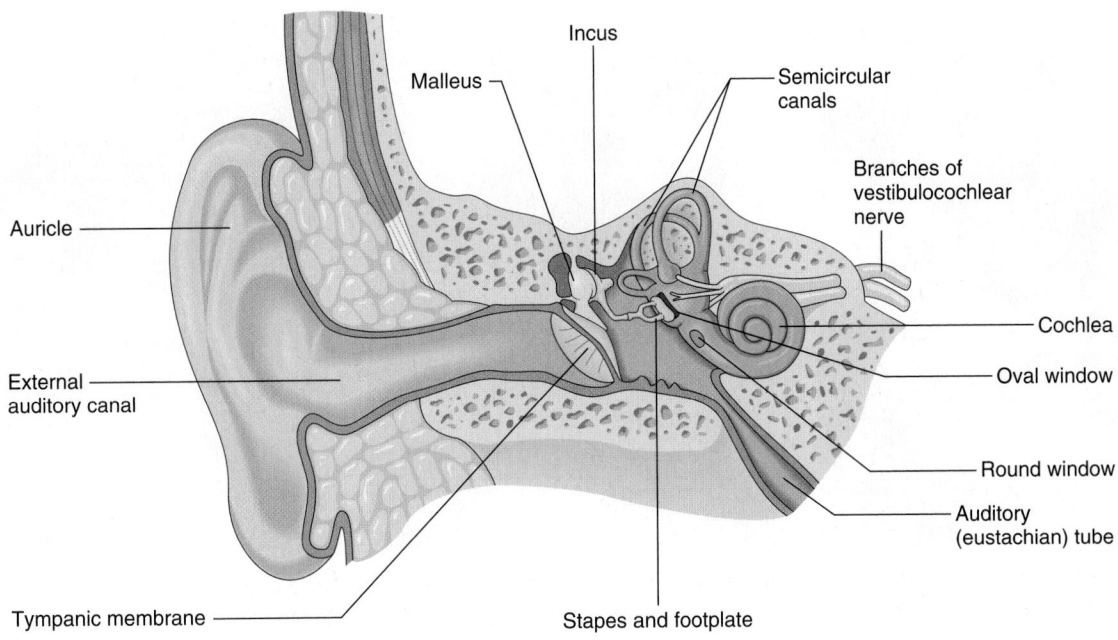

Figure 18-23   The ear.

window, and the cochlea. The structures in the vestibule are responsible for maintaining equilibrium during movement of the head. The semicircular canals assist the body to adjust to changes in direction. The movement of fluid in this area can cause symptoms of dizziness. The cochlea is the organ of hearing.

The outer ear (pinna) picks up sound waves that are sent through the external auditory canal to the tympanic membrane. The membrane vibrates in reaction to the sound striking it. These vibrations pass through the three tiny middle ear bones through the oval window and into the fluid in the cochlea. Receptor cells respond and transfer the sounds into electrical impulses that travel to the brain via the acoustic nerve. The receiving area of the brain for auditory impulses is in the temporal lobe. (See Figure 18-23.)

Diseases or conditions of the ear, if left untreated, can cause damage to nerves and tissues and can result in some degree of hearing impairment, from mild to deafness. Table 18-9 describes common diseases of the ear.

Measuring Auditory Ability. The simple methods of measuring hearing (gross hearing) are usually performed by the physician. The patient may be instructed to place a finger in one ear while the physician whispers one or two words in the other. The patient is then asked to repeat the words. A ticking watch may be placed by the patient's ear to ascertain hearing. A vibrating tuning fork may be placed on the mastoid process behind the ear and then on top of the head. The patient is asked if the sound vibrations could be heard or felt. This procedure will identify nerve or conduction deafness (Figure 18-24).

TABLE 18-9   EAR DISORDERS
• *External Otitis (swimmer's ear).* A buildup of fluid with inflammation of the surface of the eardrum. Symptoms are pain, fever, and decreased hearing acuity.
• *Otitis Media.* Acute infection of the middle ear usually caused by bacteria. Symptoms are pain, fever, discharge, and decreased hearing acuity.
• *Otosclerosis.* Conduction deafness caused by hardening of the stapes.
• *Ménière's Disease.* Characterized by deafness, vertigo, and tinnitus. Probable cause is edema of the labyrinth.
• *Impacted Cerumen.* Caused by accumulation of hardened cerumen that has built up against the tympanic membrane. Impaired hearing and tinnitus can result.

Conduction deafness occurs when the sound wave is not transmitted to the middle ear. This type of deafness may be a result of the presence of ear wax (cerumen) in the ear canal or a scarred tympanic membrane. Nerve deafness is a result of injury along the course of the nerves leading from the inner ear to the auditory centers of the brain.

A more complex procedure may be performed by the medical assistant using an audiometer. A quiet room with no distractions is required for the procedure to be accurate. The patient is seated facing away from the medical assistant and the audiometer, then ear phones are placed over the ears. The patient is instructed to raise a hand when a sound is heard. The audiometer has two dials, one for the various wave lengths and the other for wave intensity. Starting at the lowest pitch, the intensity is increased until the patient responds to the sound. The

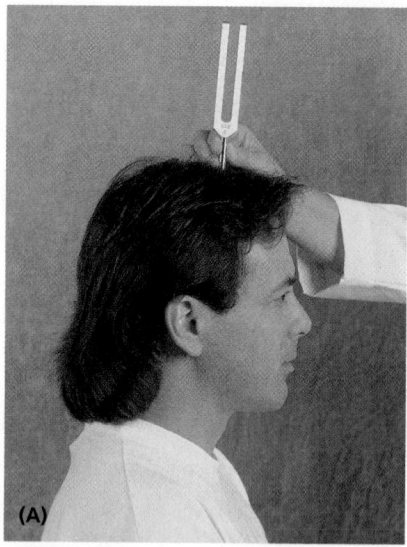
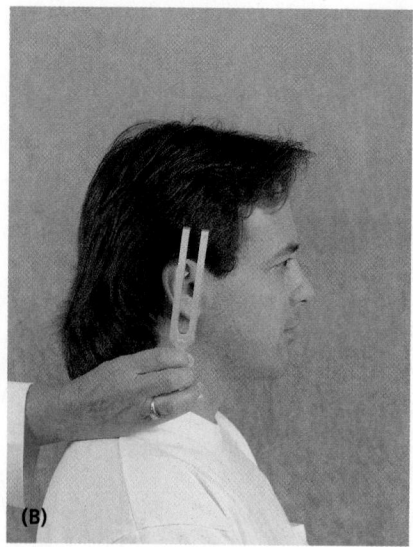
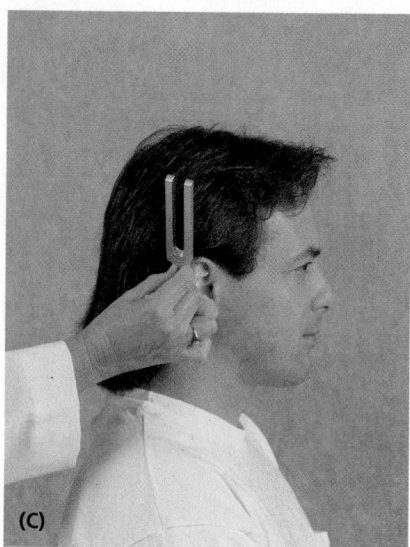

Figure 18-24 (A) The physician holds the tuning fork against the crown of the patient's head to determine which ear can hear the sound. (B) To check air conduction of sound, the physician holds the tuning fork one inch from the patient's auditory meatus. (C) The physician places the tuning fork on the bony prominence (mastoid bone) behind the patient's ear to check bone conduction of sound.

next pitch is then tested in the same manner. This process continues until the highest pitched sound is tested. The results are obtained by noting the number of intensity at which the sound was heard. When performing the procedure, the medical assistant must not develop a pattern that can be detected by the patient. The ears should be tested in an alternating fashion to ensure accuracy. (See Procedure 18-12.)

The medical assistant employed in an industrial medical facility may be required to monitor hearing of some employees. If this is the case, care must be taken to have the hearing test performed before the employee goes to work for the day. Hearing loss may result from the day's activities in some noisy facilities even when ear plugs are worn.

Tympanometry is a procedure used to ascertain the ability of the middle ear to transmit sound waves and is commonly performed on children to diagnose middle ear infections. A probe is inserted into the ear canal to measure the air pressure of the ear canal in relationship to the air pressure found in the middle ear. Tympanogram is the recording produced by this procedure. The waves and peaks are measured providing an indication of possible middle ear abnormalities.

During auditory testing, the medical assistant provides equipment to the physician and may perform irrigation or instillation to the external canal of the ear. Diagnostic procedures for the special senses involve the use of specialized instruments, including the otoscope, which assists in identifying disease-related ear problems (Figure 18-25).

Procedures 18-12, 18-13, and 18-14 describe steps in audiometry and ear irrigation and instillation.

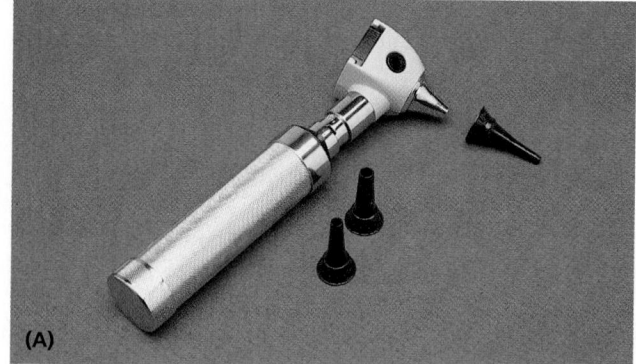

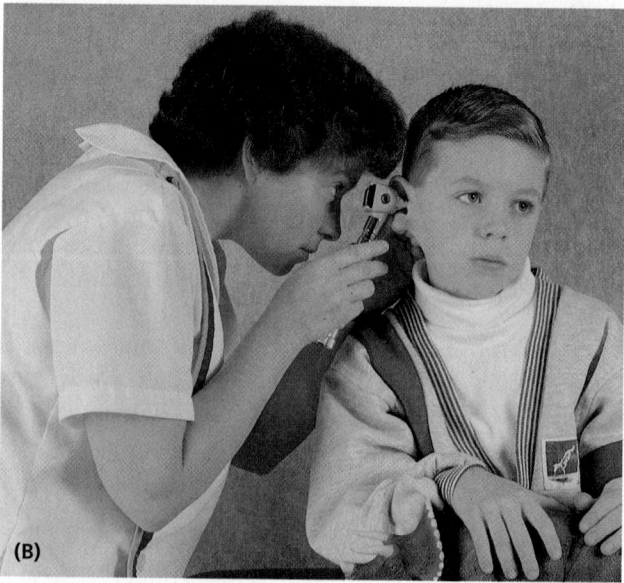

Figure 18-25 (A) An otoscope with three different sizes of reusable specula. (B) The otoscope is used to examine the patient's tympanic membrane.

RESPIRATORY SYSTEM

The respiratory process is all important to the life process. **External respiration** allows for the exchange of carbon dioxide and oxygen across the cell walls into the airspaces of the lungs. **Internal respiration** is the exchange of these gases at the cellular levels of the organs.

The respiratory process begins with air entering the nose or mouth, where it passes through the pharynx, down into the trachea, into the **bronchi**, and then enters the lungs. Gas exchange takes place when the blood filters through the **alveoli**. See Table 18-10 for respiratory diseases and disorders diagnostic procedures and Table 18-11 for a description of respiratory disorders.

Respiratory disorders are diagnosed with various X rays, bronchoscopy, blood studies, and pulmonary function studies. Cultures of sputum and the pharynx are widely used diagnostic tests. Irrigations of the nose, collection of sputum specimens, and assisting with pulmonary tests are the roles of the medical assistant. See Procedures 18-15, 18-16, 18-17, 18-18, 18-19, 18-20 and 18-21 for specialized respiratory examinations and procedures.

Spirometry

A commonly used tool in the medical office or clinic, **spirometry** assists the physician in the evaluation of signs and symptoms of pulmonary disease by measuring the air capacity of the lungs. Three components of lung functions are measured:

1. Forced virtual capacity (FVC), which represents the volume of air that can be exhaled from the lung after the lung is filled with air to meet its total capacity.
2. Forced expiration volume at 1 second (FEV), which is the volume of gas forcibly exhaled from the lungs the first second of expiration.
3. Mean expiration flow (FEF) rate, which is a measure on a volume-time curve.

Most spirometers are computerized and thus automatically calculate the lung functions.

See Procedure 18-21 to assist with spirometry.

TABLE 18-10   RESPIRATORY SYSTEM DISORDERS

| Disease/ Disorder | Laboratory Diagnostic Tests | | | Radiography | Surgery | Medical Tests or Procedures |
	Blood	Urine	Other			
Asthma	• Complete blood count • Arterial blood gases		• Sputum analysis	• Chest X ray		• Pulmonary function tests • Skin testing for allergies
Bronchitis	• Complete blood count		• Sputum culture and analysis	• Chest X ray		• Bronchoscopy
Emphysema	• Complete blood count • Arterial blood gases			• Chest X ray		• Pulmonary function tests
Influenza	• Complete blood count			• Chest X ray		
Laryngitis			• Throat culture			• Laryngoscopy
Lung Cancer	• Complete blood count		• Sputum cytology	• Chest X ray	• Biopsy of lung tissue	• Bronchoscopy
Pharyngitis	• Complete blood count		• Throat culture			
Pneumonia	• Complete blood count		• Blood culture • Sputum smear	• Chest X ray		
Pleurisy	• Complete blood count			• Chest X ray		
Tonsillitis	• Complete blood count • Streptococcal antibody test		• Throat culture			
Tuberculosis	• Complete blood count		• Sputum culture • Acid fast smear of sputum	• Chest X ray	• Biopsy of lung tissue	• Tuberculin skin test: Mantoux tine

TABLE 18-11   DESCRIPTION OF RESPIRATORY DISORDERS

- **Asthma.** Spasm of the smooth muscle of the bronchi brought on by an allergen and/or emotional upsets. Characterized by dyspnea and wheezing.
- **Bronchitis.** Inflammation of the bronchi, caused by viral or bacterial infection with a dry, painful cough, progressing to a productive cough of greenish-yellow sputum. Symptoms: cough, slight fever, chills, malaise, soreness under the sternum.
- **Emphysema.** Enlargement of the alveoli due to lost elasticity, usually brought on by a long-time irritant, such as cigarette smoking. Results in dyspnea, chronic cough, weight loss, and the appearance of a "barrel chest."
- **Influenza.** A viral infection of various strains of the upper respiratory tract (URI). Sudden onset of chills, fever, cough, sore throat, gastrointestinal disorders are common. Can range from mild to life-threatening.
- **Laryngitis.** Hoarseness, cough, aphonia caused by infections from nose or throat.
- **Lung Cancer.** Cancer that may appear in trachea, air sacs, and other lung tubes.
- **Pharyngitis.** Inflammation of the pharynx caused by a bacteria, virus, or an irritant. Difficulty in swallowing, pain, redness, and inflammation of the pharynx are some of the symptoms. Streptococcus is the most common bacterial infection, influenza virus and the common cold virus are the most common viruses involved. May be accompanied by fever, malaise, headache.
- **Pneumonia.** Inflammation of the lungs caused by bacteria, fungi, viruses, and chemical irritants. Usually has sudden onset and is characterized by chills, fever, chest pain, cough, purulent sputum. Symptoms include sore throat, fever, lymphadenopathy.
- **Pleurisy.** Inflammation of the pleura caused by bacteria or viruses. Symptoms include pain, fever, cough, chills and dyspnea.
- **Tonsillitis.** Inflammation of the tonsils usually caused by streptococcus. Tonsils become red and enlarged causing severe pharyngitis, fever.
- **Tuberculosis.** Inflammatory infiltrations, formation of tubercles, abscesses, fibrosis, and calcification. Can lead to infection of other body systems.

MUSCULOSKELETAL SYSTEM

The muscular system and the skeletal system interact to coordinate the supporting framework and movements of the body. The musculoskeletal system includes bones, joints, muscles, and surrounding tissue. The skeletal system provides support, protection for vital organs, and allows for the attachment of ligaments, tendons, and muscles. The muscular system gives the body form and shape and is responsible for the coordination of movement.

Bones of the skeletal system store minerals for later use by the body. They are classified according to their shape. Characteristics of bones are their marking, which provides for the attachment of muscles, joining of another bone, and which allows for the passage of nerves and blood vessels. The skeletal system is divided into two parts, the **appendicular skeleton** (126 bones) and the **axial skeleton** (80 bones).

One of the top four reasons a patient visits a physician is for back pain. During the visit, the physician will evaluate the patient for contributory factors for the pain by assessing the patient for any deformities, asymmetry, and/or signs of restricted motion. The physician will do a functional assessment by observing the patient's **gait** for indications of decreased mobility and postural changes associated with aging or injury. Flexion tests are done with a goniometer to detect the degree of resistance applied to a given force, thus defining restricted motion and the amount of discomfort associated with movement. Supine straight leg raising (SLR) tests are done to detect the amount of hamstring flexibility and can assess sciatic nerve damage.

There are over 600 muscles in the body. Muscles are comprised of bundles of muscle fibers, each with the ability to contract and relax. Any disease process that disrupts the balance between these two systems severely hampers a person's ability to move effectively and painlessly. See Tables 18-12, 18-13, and 18-14.

TABLE 18-12   MUSCULOSKELETAL SYSTEM DISORDERS

| Disease/ Disorder | Laboratory Diagnostic Tests | | | Radiography | Surgery | Medical Tests or Procedures |
	Blood	Urine	Other			
Carpal Tunnel Syndrome	• Erythrocyte sedimentation rate • Uric acid • Complete blood count				• Surgical repair	• Electro-myography

(continues)

TABLE 18-12 (*continued*)

Disease/ Disorder	Laboratory Diagnostic Tests			Radiography	Surgery	Medical Tests or Procedures
	Blood	**Urine**	**Other**			
Dislocation				• X ray		
Gout	• Uric acid • Complete blood count • Erythrocyte sedimentation rate	• Urinalysis	• Synovial fluid analysis	• Skeletal X rays		
Herniated disk				• Computerized tomography • Magnetic resonance imaging		
Osteoarthritis	• Complete blood count • Sedimentation rate			• Skeletal X rays including vertebrae		
Osteoporosis	• Serum calcium • Alkaline phosphatase • Estrogen level • Total protein • Creatinine	• Calcium • Creatinine		• Bone scan		
Rheumatoid Arthritis	• Rheumatoid factor • Antinuclear antibody test • Lupus erythematosis test • Erythrocyte sedimentation rate • Complete blood count		• Synovial fluid analysis			
Rickets	• Serum phosphorus • Vitamin D • Creatinine	• Calcium • Phosphorus • Creatinine				
Spinal Curvatures Scoliosis Lordosis Kyphosis				• X rays of spine		

TABLE 18-13 MUSCULAR/CONNECTIVE TISSUE DISORDERS

Disease/ Disorder	Laboratory Diagnostic Tests			Radiography	Surgery	Medical Tests or Procedures
	Blood	**Urine**	**Other**			
Back Pain		• Urinalysis		• X ray		• Computerized tomography (CT) • Magnetic resonance imaging (MRI)
Bursitis				• X ray affected joint for calcium deposits		
Fibromyalgia	• Rheumatoid arthritis antibody			• Skeletal X rays		• Electromyography
Strain, Sprain				• X ray affected body part to rule out fracture		
Tendonitis				• Arthrogram		

TABLE 18-14 DESCRIPTION OF SKELETAL AND MUSCULAR DISORDERS

Bone

- Carpal Tunnel Syndrome. Causes pain and weakness of hand and fingers. May cause paresthesia of hand and fingers. Caused by compression of the median nerve against the carpal bones. Usually results from repetitive tasks (such as typing or rolling hair).
- Cleft palate. Congenital disorder caused by nonunion of the maxillary bones. Surgical repair needed to close palate.
- Fractures. Break in a bone classified according to angle, usually caused by trauma or pathology.
- Herniated Disk. A rupture of the cushioning mass between two intervertebrae disks of the spine most often caused by injury. Causes back pain that may radiate into buttock(s) and down leg.
- Osteoporosis. Diminished bone mass caused by lack of calcium deposits in the bone, predisposing patients to fracture.
- Paget's Disease. Chronic disease marked by a high rate of bone destruction and irregular bone repair. The new bone fractures easily. Cause unknown, but may be hereditary.
- Rickets. Abnormal bone softening caused by inadequate utilization of vitamin D, inadequate intake or loss of calcium. One symptom is night fever.
- Spinal Curvatures. Spinal defects with exaggerated curves caused by diseases of the spine, faulty posture and/or congenital malformations.
  - Scoliosis—right or left sideways curvature of the spine.
  - Lordosis—inward curvature of the spine (swayback).
  - Kyphosis—outward curvature of the spine (hunchback).

Joints

- Dislocation. A bone forcibly displaced from its joint usually caused by trauma.
- Gout. Form of arthritis caused by metabolic disturbances in purine metabolism resulting in uric acid crystal deposits in the joints. Causes periodic attacks of arthritis pain and joint inflammation.
- Osteoarthritis. Common, chronic inflammatory process of the joints, with overgrowth of bone and spur formation. Accompanies aging. Causes swollen joints and pain.
- Rheumatoid Arthritis. More serious and crippling form caused by inflammation of the synovial tissues of several joints, may be caused by antigen-antibody reaction. Systemic symptoms include fatigue, temperature elevation, sensory disturbances, pain, and joint deformities.

Muscle Disorders

- Back Pain. Localized discomfort in the lumbar area caused by stretching or straining of a muscle.
- Bursitis. Inflammation of the cavity found in connective tissue of a joint that is lined with synovial fluid usually caused by trauma.
- Fibromalgia. Discomfort of muscles, tendons, ligaments, and soft tissues brought on by trauma, strain, and emotional stress.
- Strain. Trauma to a muscle from violent contraction.
- Spasm. Sudden involuntary muscle contraction.
- Sprains. Caused by trauma to a joint with torn ligament if severe.
- Tendonitis. Inflammation of tendons and attachments caused by trauma such as strain.

Diagnostic procedures involving the skeletal system involve the extensive use of various forms of X rays and visual examination techniques. A bone biopsy may be ordered when additional diagnostic data are required. The muscular system employs the use of electrical stimulation to measure the neuromuscular activity and strength of muscles.

Therapeutic treatment of muscular system injuries caused by trauma is clinically handled by the use of hot and cold therapy and ultrasound therapy. These procedures are discussed in Chapter 21.

Fractures, Casting, and Cast Removal

A **closed fracture** or **dislocation** of the wrist, forearm, or upper arm is often treated in the ambulatory care setting. (See Table 18-15 for other types of fractures. Also refer to Chapter 9.)

Types of casting materials used are the plaster-of-Paris, synthetic or plastic cast, and the air cast. Plaster-of-Paris casts are formed by wetting bandage rolls impregnated with calcium sulfate and molding it to the injured body part. Synthetic casts (Figure 18-26) are formed by using tapes with either a polyester, cotton combination, fiberglass, or plastic resin imbedded in the tape. Air casts are a type of inflatable immobilizer and are used for sprains and postcast support. The type of casting material used is dependent upon physician preference and the body part to which a cast is being applied. Synthetic casts are lighter, stronger, and more water resistant.

- *Short arm cast.* Extends from the fingers to just below the elbow. (Fracture or dislocation of wrist and forearm.)

TABLE 18-15 TYPES OF FRACTURES
Fractures can be simple, or closed, so called because the bone is broken with no penetration of the skin; or they can be compound, or open, so called because the broken bone has protruded through the skin and there is an open wound in addition to the fracture. Two of the most common fractures are both simple fractures: Colles fracture and Potts fracture. Colles fracture is a fracture of the lower end of the radius. Potts fracture is a fracture of the lower part of the fibula and the malleolus of the tibia. Fractures are described by their characteristics: Greenstick. The bone is bent on one side and fractured on the other. Oblique. The bone is fractured and runs obliquely to the axis of the bone. Transverse. The bone is fractured at a right angle to the axis of the bone. Comminuted. The bone is splintered into fragments. Impacted. The bone is fractured into fragments and the fragments have been driven into the interior of another bone.

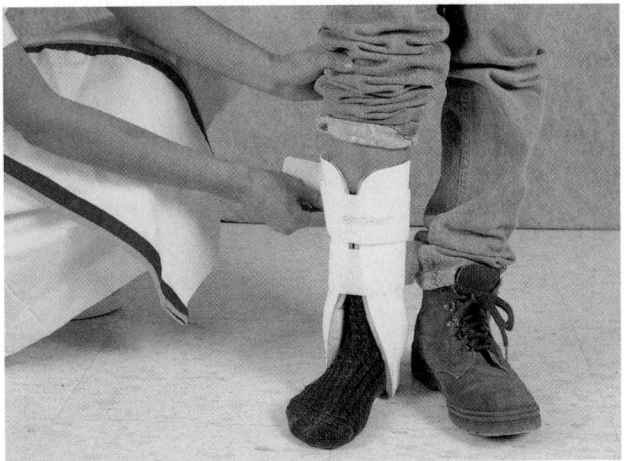

Figure 18-26 A synthetic cast being adjusted.

Long arm cast. Extends from the fingers to the axilla, with a bend at the elbow. (Fracture of the upper arm.)

The medical assistant's role in cast application and removal is to offer assistance to the physician and to provide the required equipment and supplies. Patient teaching of cast care is also a primary function of the medical assistant. Procedures 18-22 and 18-23 outline steps in applying a plaster-of-Paris cast and assisting in cast removal.

Cast Care Guidelines

The medical assistant should instruct the patient on managing and caring for a cast.

- Allow the casting material to dry by exposing it to the air and keeping it uncovered, even during the night. Applying pressure to the cast prior to drying can result in tissue damage under the pressure area.

- Elevate the casted extremity to aid in reducing swelling and pain. This allows for a better fitting cast, and thus less discomfort.

- Observe the fingers or toes for changes in color, temperature changes, and decreased sensation and tingling. This could indicate the cast is too tight.

- Do not place objects into the cast to scratch irritated skin. A break in the skin will provide a breeding ground for bacteria. Do not use powder or creams.

- Do not get the cast wet. This could lead to a malformation of the cast, thus misalignment of the extremity. Cover with waterproof covering when bathing. If the cast gets wet, dry it with a hair dryer.

- Cleaning a cast can be accomplished by using a damp cloth.

- When decorating a cast, use only water-soluble paints or marking pens. This allows the cast to breathe, thus avoiding tissue damage.

- Do not cut or trim the cast. Use a type of masking tape if there is a sharp edge.

- Notify the physician if any of the following occurs:

  1. A bad odor coming from the cast. This may indicate an infection.
  2. Numbness, tingling, severe pain, difficulty moving, severe swelling, or cold fingers or toes. The cast may be too tight.
  3. A burning sensation over a bony area. The cast may be too tight.
  4. Bleeding or pink to red discoloration on the cast. There may be bleeding from a wound under the cast.

NEUROLOGICAL SYSTEM

The nervous system functions to coordinate the activities of body systems and allows for the body to adapt to its internal and external environment. Diagnosis and treatment of the brain, spinal cord, and **peripheral nerve** disorders are often difficult because of the interdependence of one part of the system on another.

The physician will screen the patient during a physical examination for neurological signs and symptoms. The medical assistant's role in a neurological screening is to observe and evaluate the patient's mental status and to assist or perform other tests as directed by the physician. Most of the exam is performed in conjunction with the

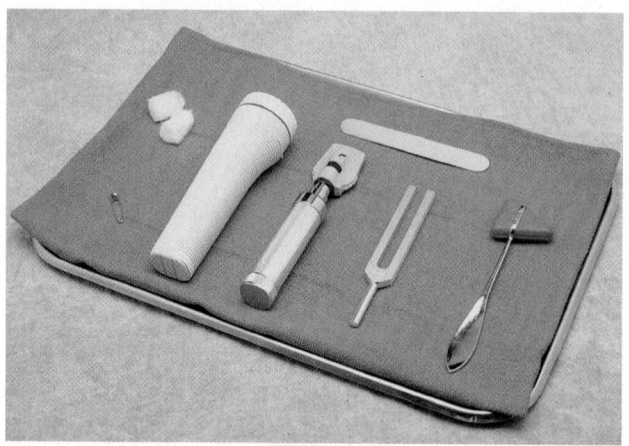

Figure 18-27 Equipment and supplies are used in the neurological screening to test reflexes, touch, smell, and coordination.

complete physical examination, but it can also be done when a patient is exhibiting specific signs and symptoms of a neurological problem such as lack of sensation, seizures, confusion, paralysis, or **aphasia**.

The equipment and supplies used in a neurological screening are those that test the patient's reflexes, touch, sense of smell, and degree of coordination to name a few (Figure 18-27). The physician pays particular attention to symmetrical strength and notes unequal weakness on either side of the body. A patient's gender and body build will be considered when examining muscle mass and tone. Table 18-16 describes neurological diagnostic procedures; Table 18-17 outlines neurological disorders.

Procedures performed to confirm a diagnosis of a neurological problem or disease are limited to the use of various X-ray and electrical impulse studies. The medical assistant will assist the physician during the procedures. Patient teaching by the medical assistant prior to a proce-

TABLE 18-16 NEUROLOGICAL SYSTEM DISORDERS

Disease/ Disorder	Laboratory Diagnostic Tests			Radiography	Surgery	Medical Tests or Procedures
	Blood	**Urine**	**Other**			
Bell's Palsy	• Complete blood count					
Cerebral Vascular Accident				• Cerebral angiography • Computerized tomography • Magnetic resonance imaging		• Electroencephalography • Lumbar puncture
Epilepsy				• Computerized tomography • Magnetic resonance imaging		• Electroencephalography
Herpes Zoster	• Varicella-Zoster antibody					• Culture of cell scrapings from lesion
Multiple Sclerosis				• Computerized tomography • Magnetic resonance imaging		• Lumbar puncture
Rabies	• Complete blood count					
Reye's Syndrome	• Complete blood count • Serum ammonia		• Liver function studies		• Liver biopsy	• Lumbar puncture • Exam of cerebral spinal fluid
Sciatica				• Computerized tomography • Magnetic resonance imaging		
Tic Douloureux					• Biopsy of trigeminal nerve	

TABLE 18-17 DESCRIPTION OF NEUROLOGICAL DISORDERS

- Bell's Palsy. Paralysis of seventh cranial nerve caused by an acute inflammation. Usually characterized by unilateral facial paralysis and pain, but can be bilateral.
- Cerebral Vascular Accident (CVA). Loss of blood supply to the brain (anoxia). May be caused by a ruptured or clogged blood vessel in the brain and hypertension. Symptoms include sudden loss of consciousness and paralysis. Also referred to as a stroke.
- Epilepsy. Episodes of seizures caused by changes in electrical brain potentials which result in disturbed brain impulses or function.
- Headache. Diffuse pain in different parts of the head. May be acute or chronic with varying degree of pain and may be caused by a variety of reasons.
- Herpes Zoster. An acute infectious disease caused by varicella zoster virus. Painful vesicular eruptions.
- Meningitis. Inflammation of the membranes of the spinal cord or brain. Symptoms include a stiff neck, headache, anorexia, and irregular fever.
- Multiple Sclerosis. Chronic progressive disease characterized by demyelination of nerve fibers. The cause is unknown. First symptoms are visual disturbances and muscle weakness.
- Parkinson's. A slowly progressive disease, usually occurring in later life, caused by a degeneration of brain cells due to lack of dopamine in the brain. Muscle rigidity and akinesia are common symptoms.
- Rabies. Caused by a virus and transmitted to humans by scratches or bites from animals infected with the virus. The disease infects the brain and spinal cord and causes acute encephalitis.
- Reye's Syndrome. A neurologic illness usually seen in young children following a viral infection such as influenza, varicella, Epstein-Barr. There may be a connection between the viral infection and aspirin. Cause is unknown, but characteristic symptoms include vomiting, rash, lethargy and neurologic involvement, seizures and coma.
- Sciatica. Severe pain in the leg along the course of the sciatic nerve felt at the back of the thigh and running down the inside of the leg. Caused by compression of the nerve by a ruptured intervertebral disk or osteoarthritis. Characterized by sharp, shooting pain running down back of thigh. Leg movement aggravates the pain.
- Tic Douloureux. Degeneration of or pressure on the trigeminal nerve (fifth cranial) causing severe stabs of pain that radiate from the angle of the jaw along one of the branches. Pain may be felt in the eye, lip, nose, tongue. Pain may come and go for hours.

dure and active reinforcement during a procedure will promote patient cooperation. Procedure 18-24 outlines steps involved in removing cerebrospinal fluid from the lumbar area.

Components of a Neurological Screening

During the neurological screening examination, various functions are observed. Procedure 18-25 outlines the steps involved in a neurological screening examination.

- Mental status:
  Level of consciousness (alert)
  Memory (recall of past and present)
  Cognition (ability to calculate and remember current events)
  Mood (is it appropriate for the conversation)
  Ideational content (hallucinations)
- Cranial nerve function:
  Cranial nerve I   Cranial nerve II
  Aroma identification   Visual acuity
                           Visual fields
                           Optic disc
  Cranial nerves III, IV, and VI extraocular eye muscles

Cranial nerve V sensations of the face, scalp, teeth
Cranial nerve VII facial expressions, taste
Cranial nerve VIII ear—hearing and equilibrium
Cranial nerve IX and X gag reflex, saliva secretion, voice, slowing of heartbeat
Cranial nerve XI neck and shoulder muscle
Cranial nerve XII tongue

The physician continues with the neurological examination by checking the patient for the following:

- Cerebral function:
  Memory
  Muscle coordination
  Sensory interpretation
  Posture and gait
- Motor function:
  Muscle tone
  Strength
  Muscle mass
  Twitching
- Sensory function:
  Touch (pain, light touch, vibration, position sense)

● Deep tendon reflexes:

Extremities:

Upper—biceps, triceps

Lower—quadriceps, achilles

Additional Tests:

Angiography provides visualization of the circulation of the blood throughout the brain.

Computerized tomography (CT) helps to diagnose hemorrhage and tumors.

Electroencephalography (EEG) records the electrical activity of the brain and helps to diagnose seizures and tumors.

Magnetic resonance imaging (MRI) helps to diagnose tumors and hemorrhage. (See Chapter 20.)

CIRCULATORY SYSTEM

The circulatory system is comprised of the heart and a complex network of blood vessels. Their function is to pump and transport the blood to all parts of the body, thus supplying oxygen and removing waste products from body tissues. Table 18-18 reviews circulatory system disorders and diagnostic procedures; Table 18-19 provides a description of disorders of the circulatory system.

The variety of diagnostic procedures used to determine the patient's diagnosis are necessary because of the complexity of the cardiovascular system. The medical assistant assists with and performs some of the procedures used for clinical diagnosis. Electrocardiogram (ECG) procedure is found in Chapter 25.

TABLE 18-18 CIRCULATORY SYSTEM DISORDERS

| Disease/ Disorder | Laboratory Diagnostic Tests | | | Radiography | Surgery | Medical Tests or Procedures |
	Blood	Urine	Other			
Angina Pectoris				• Ultrasonography		• Electrocardiography • Stress test
Congestive Heart Failure				• Chest X ray		• Electrocardiography • Venous pressure
Coronary Artery Disease	• Electrolytes • Chemistry LDL, HDL, Cholesterol			• Angiography • Thallium stress test • Cardiac catheterization		
Essential Hypertension	• Electrolytes	• Urinalysis	• Kidney Function	• Chest X ray		• Electrocardiography
Mitral Valve Stenosis				• Echocardiography • Cardiac catheterization		• Electrocardiography
Myocardial Infarction	• Cardiac enzymes • Complete blood count			• Thallium stress test • Cardiac catheterization • Ultrasonography		• Electrocardiography
Pericarditis	• Complete blood count • Erythrocyte sedimentation rate • Cardiac enzymes • Bacterial antibodies	• Urinalysis	• Blood culture	• Chest X ray		• Electrocardiography
Rheumatic Fever	• Complete blood count • Streptococcal antibodies • Sedimentation rate • Cardiac enzymes • Kidney function • Liver function		• Throat culture	• Echocardiography		• Electrocardiography
Thrombo-phlebitis	• Bleeding and clotting time • Complete blood count	• Urinalysis		• Doppler ultrasonography • Angiography • Radioactive fibrinogen		
Varicose Veins				• Venography		

TABLE 18-19   DESCRIPTION OF CIRCULATORY SYSTEM DISORDERS

- Angina Pectoris. Chest pain caused by lack of oxygen to the myocardium. Usual cause is coronary arteriosclerosis.
- Congestive Heart Failure. A syndrome characterized by the heart's inability to pump blood adequately to the body tissues. Characterized by congestion in the lungs, or edema of lower extremities, dyspnea on exertion, cough and related edema.
- Coronary Artery Disease. Arteriosclerosis of the coronary arteries leading to impaired blood flow to the myocardium. Complete occlusion leads to myocardial infarction. May also be caused by thrombus in a coronary artery. Angina pectoris is the name of the chest pain that occurs due to lack of oxygen to the myocardium.
- Essential Hypertension. Consistently elevated blood pressure with no apparent cause.
- Mitral Valve Stenosis. Narrowing of mitral valve obstructing flow from atrium to ventricle. Usual cause is a rheumatic heart disease as a result of a streptococcal infection (throat or scarlet fever). Thrombi can form.
- Myocardial infarction. Death of myocardial tissue caused by anoxia to the myocardium. Symptoms include: dyspnea, chest pain, nausea, vomiting, diaphoresis.
- Pericarditis. Inflammation of the pericardium. Caused by tuberculosis, pyogenic organisms, uremia, myocardial infarction. Characterized by fever, dry cough, dyspnea, palpitations.
- Rheumatic Fever. A systemic disease affecting the heart, joints, and central nervous system following a Group A beta-hemolytic streptococcal infection. May occur without symptoms. Symptoms include fever, migratory joint pain, pericarditis, heart murmur.
- Thrombophlebitis. An inflammation of a vein with thrombus formation, may be caused by trauma. Symptoms: pain and swelling in affected vein.
- Varicose Veins. Enlarged, twisted and engorged veins, commonly occurring in the saphenous veins but may occur in any vein in the body. Caused by conditions that hamper venous return, such as pregnancy, standing for long periods of time and obesity. Symptoms: pain in feet and ankles, swelling, leg ulcers.

BLOOD AND LYMPH SYSTEM

The blood and lymph are excellent indicators of many underlying diseases. As blood circulates through body tissues and organs, it deposits nutrients and removes wastes. Failure to accomplish this leaves the body in a disease state. Blood cells include erythrocytes, leukocytes, and platelets and each has its own function. Studying the results of laboratory findings assists the physician in making a diagnosis.

Lymph is important because of its filtering properties. The body's immune system relies heavily on the fact that the lymph passes through the lymph glands and bacteria and other substances are filtered out. Table 18-20 describes diseases and disorders diagnostic procedures for

TABLE 18-20   BLOOD AND LYMPH SYSTEM DISORDERS

Disease/ Disorder	Laboratory Diagnostic Tests			Radiography	Surgery	Medical Tests or Procedures
	Blood	Urine	Other			
Anemias	• Serum iron • Complete blood count • Red blood cell count • Serum B_{12}		• Gastric analysis	• Ferrokinetic studies • Radioactive B_{12}		• Bone marrow
Hodgkin's Disease	• Complete blood count • Liver function			• Chest X ray • Lymphangiography	• Lymph node biopsy	• Bone marrow
Infectious Mononucleosis	• Complete blood count • Monoscreen • Heterophile antibody • Epstein-Barr virus • Liver Function					
Leukemia	• Complete blood count • Liver function • Platelet count • Bleeding time					• Bone marrow
Lymphedema			• Lymphangiography			

TABLE 18-21   DESCRIPTION OF BLOOD/LYMPH SYSTEM DISORDERS

- *Anemias.* All anemias are manifested by a reduction in circulating red blood cells and the amount of hemoglobin, which is the volume of packed red blood cells per 100 ml of blood. Symptoms include pallor of the skin, nailbeds, and mucous membranes; weakness; vertigo; headache; drowsiness; and general malaise.

    Iron Deficiency. Lack of reserve iron in the body and in red blood cells that lack hemoglobin resulting from inadequate dietary intake of iron, iron malabsorption, blood loss, or pregnancy.

    Pernicious anemia. Lack of intrinsic factor in the stomach secretions (hydrochloric acid). Vitamin B_{12} cannot be absorbed. Red cells cannot develop properly.

    Sickle cell anemia. A hereditary chronic anemia characterized by abnormal red blood cells causing lysis of the cells and the formation of clumps in the blood vessels, impairing circulation.

- *Hodgkin's Disease.* An idiopathic malignancy of the lymphatic system causing enlargement of lymphatic tissue, spleen, and liver. Symptoms include fever and night sweats.

- *Leukemia.* Overproduction of abnormal and immature white blood cells. Cause is unknown. Symptoms include anemia, fatigue, fever, and joint pain.

- *Lymphedema.* Abnormal accumulation of lymph in the extremities caused by obstruction of the lymphatics. Symptoms include edema in arms or legs.

blood and lymphatic system; Table 18-21 describes blood and lymph system disorders.

Common laboratory and diagnostic procedures requested by the physician include some of the following:

- *Complete Blood Count* (CBC). A routine test that includes a hemoglobin, hematocrit, and red and white blood cell count.

- *Differential.* Distinguishes among the various types of white blood cells.

- *Erythrocyte Sedimentation Rate* (SED Rate or ESR). Done to time the speed of red blood cells settling to the bottom of a test tube.

- *Platelet Count.* The number of platelets in a blood specimen.

- *Liver Function Studies.* Measure coagulation factors, prothrombin, and fibrinogen necessary for blood coagulation.

- *Schilling Test.* Radioactive vitamins B_{12} and intrinsic factor measured in 24-hour urine specimen.

Procedures to collect blood specimens and laboratory procedures are covered in Chapter 28, Venipuncture, and Chapter 29, Hematology.

INTEGUMENTARY SYSTEM

The integumentary system consists of the skin and its associated structures, such as hair, nails, nerve endings, and the sebaceous and sudoriferous glands. This system provides protection for the body against invasion of microorganisms and trauma and helps regulate body temperature. Nerve endings sense pressure, touch, and pain. Structurally, the skin consists of two layers (Figure 18-28),

which function differently from one another to perform specific activities.

- Epidermis is the outer layer of the skin that is comprised of squamous epithelium and produces keratin and the pigment melanin.

- Dermis is the inner layer of the skin made up of connective tissue and contains blood vessels, nerve endings, and glands. Provides strength and elasticity.

- Subcutaneous connective tissue (hypodermis) is the layer on which the skin and muscles lie and consists of elastic and fibrous connective tissue and adipose tissue. Guards against heat loss and provides insulation.

Skin disorders frequently produce a **lesion** unique to a specific skin disease, thus allowing for the diagnosis to be based on the appearance of the lesion, the patient's history, allergies, emotional well-being and inherited diseases. If the lesion appears suspicious, the physician may perform a **biopsy** for tissue analysis. This procedure aids in the diagnosis and treatment of specific skin disorders. Table 18-22 describes integumentary system diseases and diagnostic procedures; Table 18-23 describes skin disorders of the integumentary system.

Diagnostic procedures involving the skin range from the simple to the complex. Simple observations such as skin color, texture, size and shape of a lesion, and patient history can lead to a quick diagnosis. Confirmatory procedures such as clinical studies of urine and blood, culture of a purulent lesion, X rays, and biopsies of the affected tissues can further delineate the disease.

The clinical procedures most commonly performed by the medical assistant concerning the skin are obtaining wound cultures, the application of a sterile dressing to the wound site, and allergy skin testing.

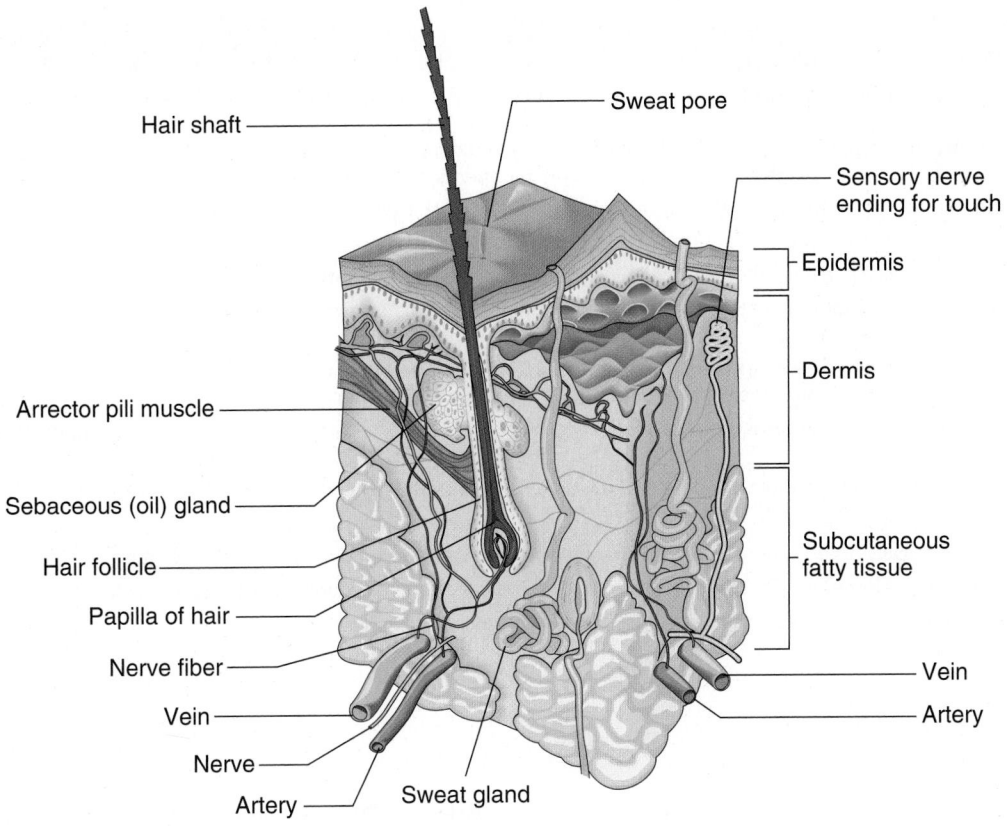

Figure 18-28   Cross section of skin.

TABLE 18-22	INTEGUMENTARY SYSTEM DISORDERS					
	Laboratory Diagnostic Tests					
Disease/ Disorder	**Blood**	**Urine**	**Other**	**Radiography**	**Surgery**	**Medical Tests or Procedures**
Abscess (Furuncle Carbuncle)	• Complete blood count • Blood glucose		• Culture and sensitivity of wound exudate		• Incision and drainage	
Acne			• Culture of skin lesions			
Corn, Callus, Wart (Verucca) Mole (nevus)					• Excisional Biopsy • Electrocautery	
Dermatitis	• Serum IgE				• Biopsy of lesion	
Dermato-phytosis			• Culture			• Wood's rays
Impetigo	• Complete blood count		• Gram stain of discharge from lesion			
Melanoma				• Chest X ray	• Biopsy of lesion	
Psoriasis					• Skin biopsy	
Scleroderma	• Sedimentation rate • Rheumatoid arthritis factor • Antinuclear antibodies	• Urinalysis • Kidney function		• Gastrointestinal • Chest		
Skin Cancer					• Biopsy of lesion	

TABLE 18-23   DESCRIPTION OF SKIN DISORDERS

- Abscess. Furuncle "Boil". Acute circumscribed infection of the subcutaneous tissues and surrounding tissues caused by staphylococci.
  Carbuncle. A circumscribed inflammation and infection of the skin and deeper tissues accompanied by fever, leukocytosis, and sometimes prostration. Caused by staphylococcus and common in patients with diabetes.
- Acne. Chronic inflammatory disease caused by blocked sebaceous glands, characterized by comedones, papules, and pustules.
- Corn and Callus. Thickening and hyperplasia of the stratum corneum caused by pressure or friction to the affected area.
- Dermatitis. Caused by a specific irritant characterized by erythema or redness as in inflammation.
- Dermatophytosis. A highly contagious infectious fungus infection of the skin. Common on hands and feet. When feet are infected, it is known as athlete's foot or tinea pedis.
- Herpes Zoster. An acute infectious disease caused by varicella-zoster virus. Characterized by inflammation of the ganglia of the spinal or cranial nerves. Painful, vesicular eruptions occur along the course of the nerves.
- Impetigo. Contagious small pustules caused by a staphylococci or streptococci or a combination of both and spread by direct contact.
- Melanoma. A malignant pigmented mole. Virulent and invasive. Can be caused by ultraviolet light exposure.
- Nevus. A mole. Usually congenital.
- Psoriasis. Chronic, genetically determined dermatitis, characterized by flat reddened areas with silvery scales.
- Scleroderma. Progressive thickening of the skin involving collagen tissue. Systemic involvement occurs. Cause is unknown.
- Skin Cancer. Malignant lesions on the skin surface caused by exposure to ultraviolet rays.
- Verruca. A wart. Caused by a virus.

Allergy Skin Testing

When performing allergy skin tests, the likelihood of severe allergic reaction is a distinct possibility. Emergency treatment must be available immediately and consists of the following: 1) notify physician immediately; 2) have patient lie down; 3) apply constriction band above the site of allergen application to suppress absorption of allergen; 4) have epinephrine injection ready to be administered; 5) check patient's vital signs. See Chapter 9, Emergency Procedures and First Aid.

Scratch Test. The back and arms are used for this type of allergy testing. The skin surface is numbered in rows approximately 2 inches apart so that they can be identified. A small scratch is made on the surface of the skin and the allergen is placed on the scratch. As many as 50 allergens can be used at one time. A reaction to the allergen usually occurs within a half-hour. If the patient is allergic to a substance, a wheal or hive will develop at the scratch site. The site is compared to a scratch test with no allergens introduced into it, but rather an allergy-free fluid. The physician will read the results, which are graded on a scale from 2 to 4. A number 2 reaction indicates a wheal larger than the control scratch reaction (which is minimal). A number 3 is given to a larger reaction and a 4 is given to a reaction in which there are extensions of the wheal beyond the usual circumscribed area of the wheal. The allergen extract should be wiped away from the scratch area that is exhibiting a number 4 reaction.

Patch Test. The suspected allergen is placed on the skin and is covered with a square of cellophane and held in place by tape. As many as 25 tests can be done at one time and results are read in 24 to 96 hours.

Intradermal Test. A small dose (0.1cc) of an allergen is injected intradermally. Ten to fifteen tests can be done simultaneously on each arm, and the patient can suffer a severe reaction more quickly. This test is always done on the patient's forearm.

Radioallergosorbent Test (RAST). This laboratory test is obtained by venipuncture and uses radioisotopes to measure minute, specific antibodies present in the circulating blood. Scratch, patch, and intradermal testing provide immediate information about allergies and is less expensive.

Following any type of allergy skin test, the patient is told to remain in the office for 20 to 30 minutes in order to watch for an allergic reaction. If a reaction occurs, emergency medications and supplies must be readily available.

Common procedures with which the medical assistant can assist the physician are the cutaneous punch biopsy and wart and mole removal. The prime responsibilities of the medical assistant are to follow the principles of surgical aseptic technique, infection control, and standard precautions; provide the physician with the required supplies as needed; safely handle and transport the biopsy specimen; and document in patient record that biopsy was sent to the laboratory.

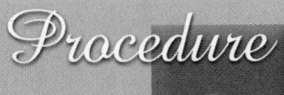

18-1 Performing a Urine Drug Screening

STANDARD PRECAUTIONS:

PURPOSE:
To accurately obtain a urine specimen from a patient for traces of drugs.

EQUIPMENT/SUPPLIES:
Urine Drug Kit (provide at least 2 choices)
Gloves
Biohazard waste container

PROCEDURE STEPS:
1. Ask patient to show a photo ID and have patient sign a consent form, keeping copies for the patient file. RATIONALE: Only the person scheduled to take the test will be able to do so.
2. Wash hands and explain procedure to the patient.
3. Supply at least two (2) collection kits from which the patient can choose one.
4. Have patient remove unnecessary outer garments, empty pockets, and wash and dry hands. RATIONALE: Patient cannot substitute another specimen.
5. Instruct patient to collect at least 40 mL of urine in the collection container.
6. Put on gloves. Record temperature of specimen, volume, and any contamination. RATIONALE: If fresh, specimen should be at least 98.6°F.
7. Label specimen and have patient initial specimen lid.
8. Seal specimen kit bag and have patient initial. RATIONALE: Kit bags are tamper-proof.
9. Secure sample in a locked container until pickup.
10. Collector and donor will need to sign off on the test collection procedure to document all procedure steps were followed.
11. Remove gloves and dispose of in biohazard waste container.
12. Wash hands.
13. Document procedure in patient's chart.

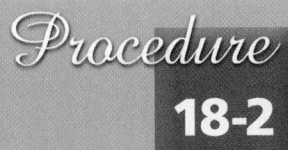

18-2 Performing a Urinary Catheterization on a Female Patient

STANDARD PRECAUTIONS:

PURPOSE:
To obtain a sterile urine specimen for analysis or to relieve urine retention.

EQUIPMENT/SUPPLIES:
Catheter kit (commercially available)
Sterile gloves
Antiseptic solution (Betadine®)
Waxed paper bag
Lubricant
Sterile cotton balls
Sterile urine container with label
Sterile 2 × 2 gauze sponges
Forceps
Sterile absorbent plastic pad
Sterile catheter (size and type as ordered by physician)
Biohazard waste container
Laboratory requisition form

PROCEDURE STEPS:
1. Identify the patient and explain the procedure.
2. Instruct patient to breathe slowly and deeply during procedure. RATIONALE: This helps the

(continues)

Procedure 18-2 *(continued)*

patient relax the abdominal and pelvic muscles and facilitates easier insertion of the catheter.

3. Wash hands and assemble supplies.
4. Place catheter kit on Mayo stand near the patient.
5. Provide adequate lighting.
6. Have patient disrobe below the waist; provide a drape.
7. Position patient into a dorsal recumbent position on an exam table. RATIONALE: This allows for access to the urinary meatus.
8. Drape patient with sheet exposing only external genitalia.
9. Open outer wrapping of sterile kit.
10. Place sterile absorbent plastic pad under patient's buttocks. Place catheter tray between patient's legs.
11. Ask patient to keep knees apart. RATIONALE: This position provides good visualization of the urinary meatus.
12. Wash hands and put on sterile gloves.
13. Pour Betadine® over three cotton balls in appropriate compartment of the kit.
14. Open urine specimen container.
15. Apply sterile lubricant to a gauze sponge and place tip of catheter in lubricant and other end of catheter into the sterile basin.
16. Remind patient to breathe slowly. Spread labia with nondominant hand. Dominant hand remains sterile. With dominant hand and sterile forceps, wipe genitalia with each of the three antiseptic soaked cotton balls, with a front to back motion. First, wipe the right labia using front to back motion. Discard cotton ball into waxed paper bag that is placed away from sterile area. Second, wipe the left labia repeating procedure and last, wipe down the center discarding cotton ball after each wipe. Discard forceps. Continue to hold labia apart until catheter is inserted. RATIONALE: Holding labia open will keep urinary meatus from becoming contaminated from labia while inserting catheter.

17. Using sterile gloved hand, pick up catheter and hold it about 3 to 4 inches from lubricated end.
18. Gently insert lubricated tip of catheter into urinary meatus approximately 6 inches or until urine begins to flow. Move nondominant hand to hold catheter in place.
19. Interrupt urine flow by clamping off. RATIONALE: Stop flow of urine while specimen container is positioned.
20. Position end of catheter into urine specimen container.
21. Collect specimen by releasing clamp and collecting approximately 60 ml of urine.
22. Allow remaining urine to flow into basin until flow ceases. Pinch catheter closed.
23. Remove catheter gently and slowly.
24. Dry area with remaining cotton balls.
25. Tighten lid on the urine specimen container.
26. Remove procedure items.
27. Position patient for comfort.
28. Assist patient in sitting up or relaxing in a horizontal recumbent position.
29. Allow patient to remain lying down. Help patient to sit on edge of table. Check patient's color and pulse.
30. Discard disposable items per OSHA guidelines.
31. If collecting specimen for analysis, label specimen container and attach to completed laboratory requisition form.
32. Assist patient from exam table.
33. Clean room and table. Remove gloves and discard in biohazard waste container.
34. Wash hands.
35. Document procedure in patient's chart including the amount of urine collected. Document that specimen was sent to outside laboratory (if appropriate).

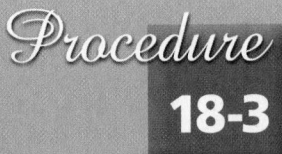

Performing a Urinary Catheterization on a Male Patient

18-3

STANDARD PRECAUTIONS:

PURPOSE:

To obtain a sterile urine specimen for analysis or to relieve urine retention.

EQUIPMENT/SUPPLIES:

Catheter kit (commercially available)
Sterile gloves
Antiseptic solution (Betadine®)
Waxed paper bag
Lubricant
Sterile cotton balls
Sterile urine container with label
Sterile 2 × 2 gauze sponges
Forceps
Sterile absorbent plastic pad
Sterile catheter (size and type as ordered by physician)
Biohazard waste container
Laboratory requisition form

PROCEDURE STEPS:

1. Identify the patient and explain the procedure.
2. Instruct patient to breathe slowly and deeply during procedure. RATIONALE: This helps the patient relax the abdominal and pelvic muscles and facilitates easier insertion of the catheter.
3. Wash hands and assemble supplies.
4. Place catheter kit on Mayo stand near the patient.
5. Provide adequate lighting.
6. Have patient disrobe below the waist; provide a drape.
7. Position patient into a dorsal recumbent position on an exam table. RATIONALE: This allows for access to the urinary meatus.
8. Drape patient with sheet exposing only external genitalia.
9. Open outer wrapping of sterile kit.
10. Place sterile underpad under patient's penis. Figure 18-29A. RATIONALE: Provides sterile field.
11. Wash hands. Put on sterile gloves.
12. Open fenestrated drape and, being careful not to contaminate drape or gloves, position drape opening over penis. Figure 18-29B.
13. Place sterile pad on table top or onto Mayo stand and empty contents of kit onto it.
14. Apply sterile lubricant to a sterile gauze sponge and place tip of catheter in lubricant and the end of catheter into sterile kit.
15. With nondominant hand, hold the penis below the glans. In uncircumcised males, the glans must be pulled pack to expose the meatus. This is done entirely with the nondominant hand. RATIONALE: The dominant hand remains sterile so as not to contaminate remaining sterile equipment.

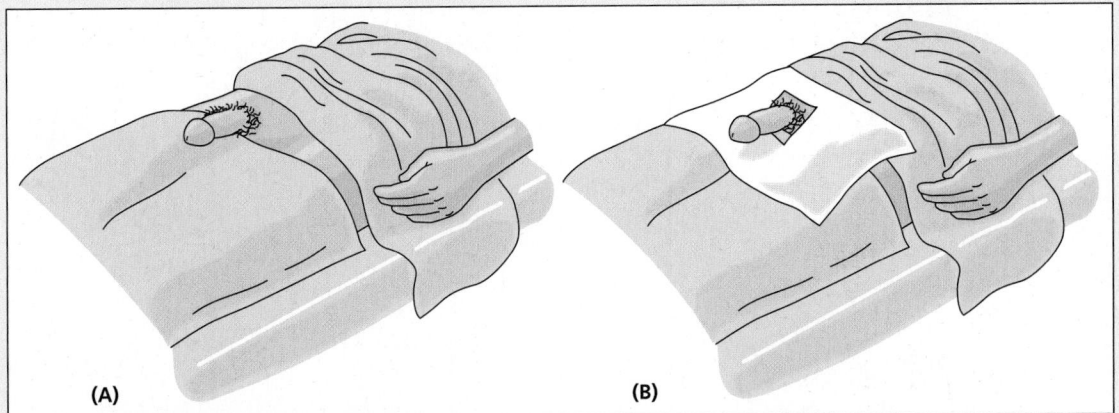

Figure 18-29   (A) Place sterile underpad under patient's penis. (B) Open fenestrated drape. Being careful not to contaminate drape or gloves, position drape opening over penis.

(continues)

Procedure 18-3 *(continued)*

16. With the dominant hand, take the sterile forceps and a cotton ball that has been dipped in Betadine®, clean around the meatus in a circular motion from center toward outside. Use all three cotton balls and Betadine®. Figure 18-30.
RATIONALE: Assures that as many microorganisms as possible will be removed from the meatus and surrounding areas before insertion of sterile catheter.

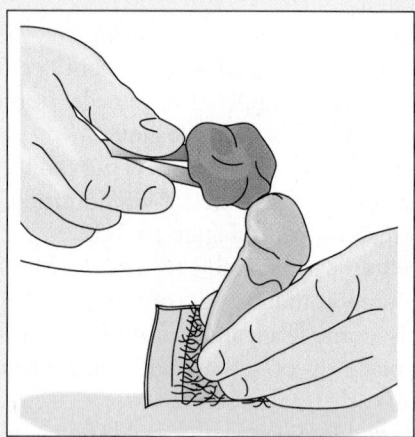

Figure 18-30   With the dominant hand, take the sterile forceps and a cotton ball dipped in Betadine® and clean around the meatus in a circular motion from center toward outside. Use all three cotton balls and Betadine®.

17. With the dominant hand, take catheter out of lubricant and while holding the penis upright and straight with the nondominant hand, insert the catheter approximately 6″ until the urine flows into the sterile kit. Figure 18-31A.
RATIONALE: Holding the penis upright and straight facilitates insertion of the catheter.
CAUTION: Do not force catheter. If problems arise attempting insertion, do not continue with procedure.
18. Obtain a specimen if ordered. Figure 18-31B.
19. After urine flow ceases, remove catheter gently and slowly.
20. Dry penis with remaining cotton ball(s).
21. Position patient for comfort.
22. Discard disposable items per OSHA guidelines.
23. If collecting specimen for analysis, label specimen container and attach to completed laboratory requisition form.
24. Assist patient from exam table.
25. Clean room and table. Remove gloves and discard in biohazard waste container.
26. Wash hands.
27. Document procedure in patient's chart including the amount of urine collected. Document that specimen was sent to outside laboratory (if appropriate).

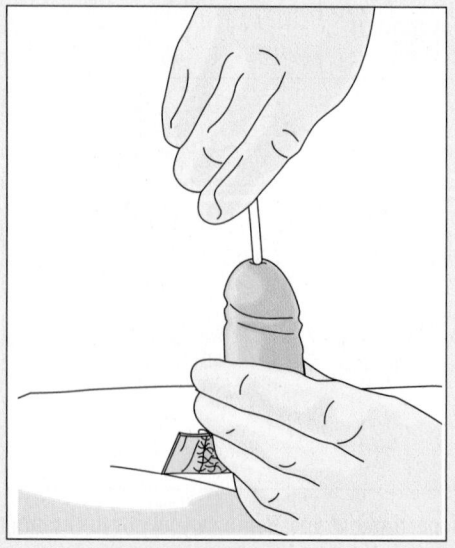

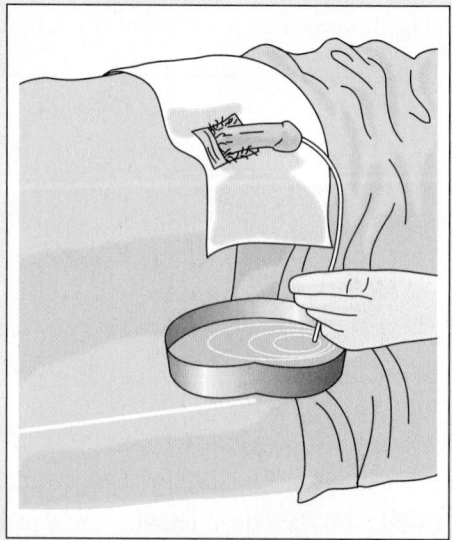

(A)   (B)

Figure 18-31   (A) With the dominant hand, take catheter out of lubricant and while holding the penis upright and straight with the nondominant hand, insert the catheter approximately 6″ until the urine flows into the sterile kit. (B) Obtain a specimen if ordered.

Procedure

18-4 Assisting with Proctosigmoidoscopy

STANDARD PRECAUTIONS:

PURPOSE:

To assist the physician in assessing the status of the sigmoid colon and rectum for signs of disease such as tumors, polyps, ulcerations, hemorrhoids, or rectal bleeding.

EQUIPMENT/SUPPLIES:

Sigmoidoscope with obturator, either a flexible fiber-optic sigmoidoscope or a rigid sigmoidoscope
Sterile biopsy forceps
Patient gown
Sterile specimen container w/preservative
Laboratory requisition form
Tissues
Biohazard waste container
Patient drape
Small pillow
Anoscope
Rectal speculum
Insufflator
Suction machine and tip
Probe with bulb tip
Gloves
Finger cots
Long cotton applicators
Lubricating jelly
Basin of water
4 × 4 gauze sponges

PROCEDURE STEPS:

1. Wash hands and prepare equipment and supplies.
2. Check the lights on the illuminated instruments for loose bulbs by turning the bulb clockwise. Turn the switch to the on position to verify the light is working. Turn off light.
3. Label specimen container with patient's name, address, date, and source.
4. Check to see that obturators are correctly positioned.
5. Have a basin ready to receive used instruments.
6. Prepare a basin of water to rinse out suction tubing.

7. Test suction machine.
8. Prepare patient. Be sure patient has been properly prepared; i.e., necessary laxative taken, enema administered, and adequate results obtained from enema.
9. Identify patient.
10. Verify consent form has been signed.
11. Explain procedure to the patient. RATIONALE: Reassuring the patient promotes relaxation and reduces apprehension.
12. Ask patient to empty bladder and save specimen (if required). RATIONALE: Facilitates examination and is more comfortable for patient.
13. Ask patient to disrobe and put on gown.
14. Assist patient into the knee-chest position or Sims' lateral position which assures accessibility to the rectum and sigmoid colon. Some physicians have special proctologic tables that tilt the patient into knee-chest position. RATIONALE: Abdominal contents tip forward and away from pelvic area, making it easier to insert the sigmoidoscope.
15. Drape the patient and place small towel directly over the anus and under the perineal area or use a fenestrated drape over the anus.
16. Apply gloves and assist the doctor during examination.
17. Place lubricant on physician's gloves for digital examination.
18. Warm metal scope by placing in warm water for a few minutes.
19. Lubricate scope tip.
20. Plug in scope when physician is ready to use. RATIONALE: Plugging in too soon allows the light source to get too hot and may harm the patient.
21. Remind the patient to take slow deep breaths to promote relaxation of muscles to facilitate insertion of the sigmoidoscope.
22. Attach inflation bulb.
23. Attach light source.
24. Observe patient throughout procedure. Provide support and reassurance.
25. Take instruments from physician as needed.

(continues)

Procedure 18-4 (continued)

26. Pass long cotton-tipped applicators to the physician and assist with suction equipment.
27. Place suction tubing in basin of water.
28. Place instruments in basin.
29. Assist with collection of biopsy by handing biopsy forceps to the physician. Do not touch inside of specimen container. RATIONALE: Container is sterile and will become contaminated if inside is touched. Inaccurate results may occur.
    a. Receive and care for specimen. Label properly.
30. Clean patient's anus with tissue.
31. Remove gloves. Wash hands.
32. Assist patient to supine position after examination. Do not let patient rise too rapidly because of the possibility of dizziness. Check patient's blood pressure. RATIONALE: Vagal nerve stimulation may cause shocklike symptoms, or orthostatic hypotension can occur from lying flat for extended period.
33. Assist patient to dress if needed.
34. Apply gloves.
35. Transport specimen with completed lab requisition form.
36. Clean room and equipment following OSHA guidelines. Flexible sigmoidoscope should be sanitized and subjected to cold sterilization according to manufacturer's directions. Metal (rigid) sigmoidoscope must be sanitized and sterilized in the autoclave.
37. Remove gloves and wash hands.
38. Document procedure in patient's chart.

Procedure 18-5 Fecal Occult Blood Test

STANDARD PRECAUTIONS:

PURPOSE:
To test feces for occult blood.

EQUIPMENT/SUPPLIES:
3 guaiac slide test kits containing three slides, applicators, and envelope

PROCEDURE STEPS:
1. Check expiration dates on occult slides. RATIONALE: Outdated slides can give an inaccurate reading.
2. Identify the patient.
3. Fill out all information on the front flap of all three slides (Figure 18-32).
4. Explain the stool collection process; the patient will need to:

a. Keep slides at room temperature away from sunlight. RATIONALE: Sunlight destroys effectiveness of guaiac paper and could result in an inaccurate result.
b. Open the front flap of the first slide.

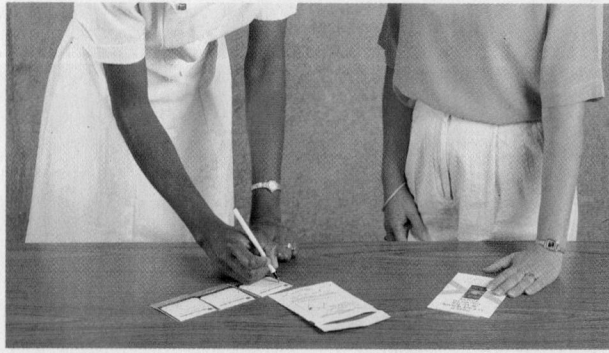

Figure 18-32 Medical assistant writes patient name, date, and specimen numbers on each hemoccult slide.

(continues)

Procedure
18-5 *(continued)*

c. Use one end of the wooden applicator to apply a thin smear of the stool sample from the toilet to Box "A." Note: *Do not collect during menstrual cycle or if hemorrhoids are present.*

d. Repeat the procedure using the other end of the applicator, taking a specimen from a different section of the same stool and applying a thin smear to Box "B." RATIONALE: Occult blood may be distributed differently throughout the bowel movement.

e. Dispose of the applicator in a waste container.

f. Close the cover after air drying overnight.

g. Date the front flap.

h. Repeat the process with the next two bowel movements, on subsequent days.

5. Provide the patient with an envelope to return the slides to the physician's office (Figure 18-33).

6. Record that the test kit and instructions were given to patient.

Developing the fecal occult slide

When the patient returns the fecal occult samples to the office, the medical assistant will be responsible for developing the slides. Although most slides may be stored for up to 14 days before developing, the medical assistant should develop them as soon as possible because the patient may have already stored them for several days. Test results are important to ensure prompt treatment should a problem be discovered.

EQUIPMENT/SUPPLIES:
Prepared fecal slides from patient
Occult blood developer
Reference card that accompanies kit
Gloves
Biohazard waste container

PROCEDURE STEPS:
1. Check the expiration date on the developer.
2. Apply gloves.
3. Open the window flap on the back of the slide.
4. Apply two drops of the developer to each Box "A" and "B," directly over each smear (Figure 18-34). RATIONALE: Paper contains the chemical guaiac, which will help identify occult blood.
5. Interpret the results within 30 to 60 seconds. Record the results.
6. A positive reaction will have a blue halo appear around the perimeter of the specimen.

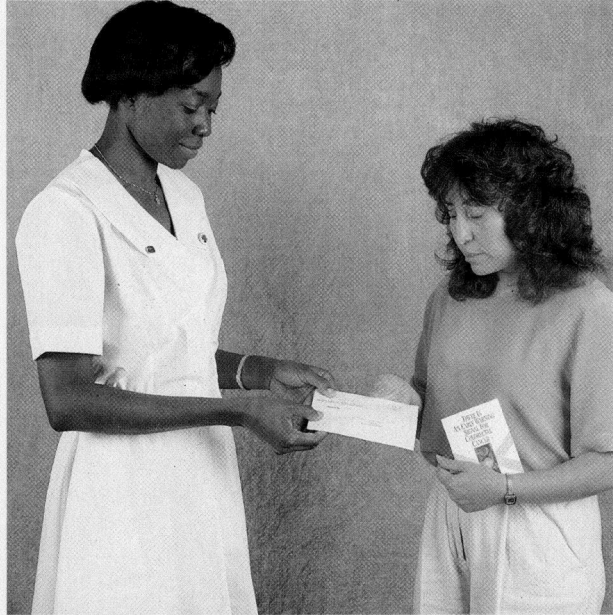

Figure 18-33 Medical assistant has put the three hemoccult slides and wooden applicators into a preaddressed envelope which the patient will use to return slides to the office. Patient also has been given instructions for collecting the three samples, which can be obtained at home.

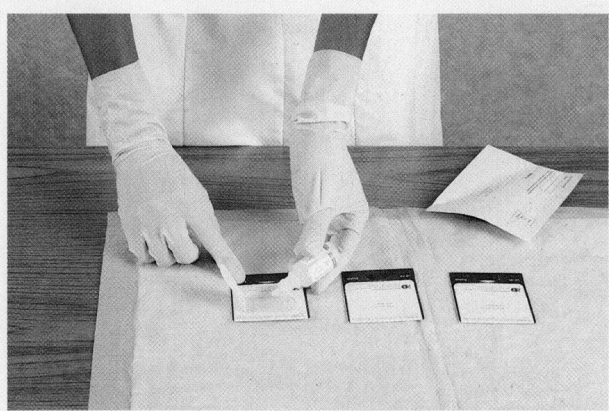

Figure 18-34 The medical assistant has removed three hemoccult slides from envelope received from a patient and places developing solution on the slide.

(continues)

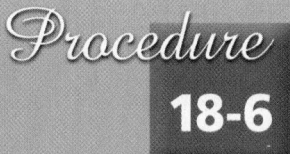

Procedure 18-5 *(continued)*

7. Perform the quality control procedure by processing the positive and negative monitor strip on each slide to confirm the test system is functional. RATIONALE: Failure of the positive strip to turn blue or negative strip to remain neutral indicates faulty supplies. Recheck expiration dates on slide and developer. Repeat test if necessary.

8. Dispose of all supplies according to OSHA guidelines.
9. Remove gloves and dispose in biohazard waste container.
10. Wash hands.
11. Document results in patient's chart.

Procedure 18-6 **Performing Visual Acuity Testing Using a Snellen Chart**

STANDARD PRECAUTIONS:

PURPOSE:
To perform a visual screening test to determine a patient's distance visual acuity.

EQUIPMENT/SUPPLIES:
Snellen eye chart placed at eye level (appropriate for age and reading ability of patient)
Pointer
Occluder
Alcohol wipes

PROCEDURE STEPS:
1. Wash hands and assemble equipment.
2. Prepare a well-lighted room, free from distractions and with a distance mark 20 feet from the eye chart.
3. Explain the procedure to the patient. Patients should be tested with their glasses or contact lenses, unless otherwise indicated by the physician.
4. Instruct the patient to stand behind the mark and cover the left eye with the occluder (Figure 18-35). Instruct the patient to keep the left eye open under the occluder and not to apply pres-

sure to the eyeball. RATIONALE: Closing of the eye not being tested may cause the person to squint when reading the chart.
5. Stand next to the chart and point to row 3 instructing the patient to read each letter with the right eye, verbally identifying each letter read (Figure 18-36). If unable to read line 3, go

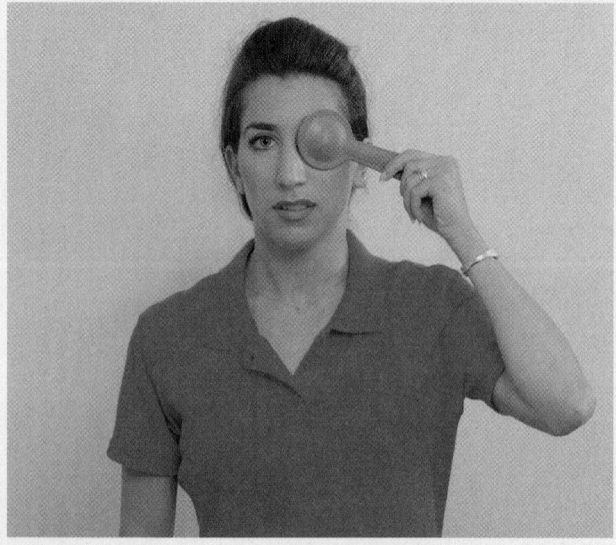

Figure 18-35   The patient covers the left eye with the occluder, keeping the eye open under the occluder.

(continues)

Procedure 18-6 *(continued)*

to line 2 or 1. RATIONALE: Pointing to each row helps the patient to focus on one row of letters at a time. Beginning at row 3 saves time.

6. Record the results at the smallest line the patient can read with two or fewer errors. Vision is recorded as right eye, left eye, both eyes.

   Examples: OD 20/25; OS 20/20; OU 20/20

   RATIONALE: Visual acuity is recorded as a fraction. The number above the line on the chart is the distance the patient is standing from the chart. The number below the line on the chart is the distance from which a person with normal vision can read that row of letters.

7. Record the patient's reaction during the test. RATIONALE: Leaning forward, squinting or straining, or eye tears may indicate eye problems.

8. When finished with the examination of the right eye, use the same procedure to test the left eye.

9. Wipe occluder with alcohol. Wash hands. Record the results.

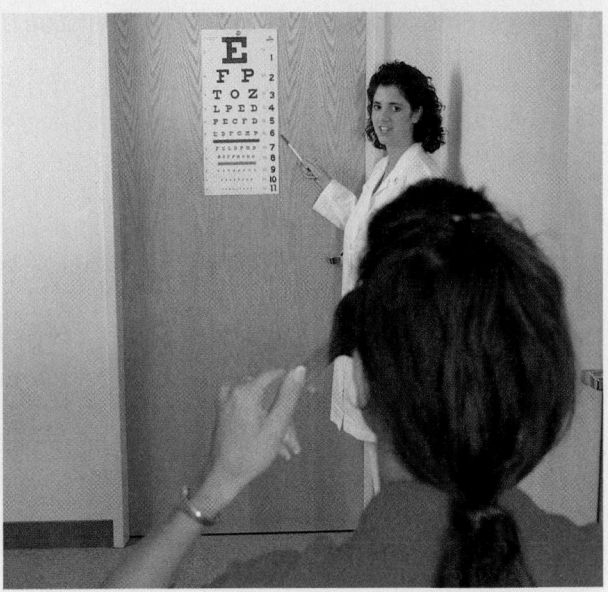

Figure 18-36 The patient uses the right eye to read the letters on the chart. The patient is instructed to start with row 3. Here she is reading row 6.

Procedure 18-7 **Measuring Near Visual Acuity**

STANDARD PRECAUTIONS:

PURPOSE:
To measure the near vision of the patient.

EQUIPMENT/SUPPLIES:
Appropriate near visual acuity chart
3 × 5 cards or occluder

PROCEDURE STEPS:

1. Wash hands.
2. Identify patient.
3. Explain procedure to patient; provide occluder. RATIONALE: To obtain patient cooperation.

4. Position patient in a comfortable position.
5. Position the near visual acuity card 14 inches from the patient by measuring with a tape measure. RATIONALE: To obtain accurate results.
6. Have patient lightly (no pressure) cover the left eye with the occluder. RATIONALE: Pressure will cause blurring of the other eye.
7. Have patient read the paragraphs printed on the card.
8. Once patient has reached a line where more than two mistakes are made, note the visual acuity for that eye (allow the patient to repeat the line to verify acuity).

(continues)

Procedure
18-7 (*continued*)

9. Repeat the process to measure the left eye.
10. Repeat the process to measure both eyes.
11. Record the result in the patient chart. Results are charted 14/14 for normal near visual acuity.

12. Discard the 3 × 5 card or disinfect the occluder. RATIONALE: To prevent microorganism cross-contamination.
13. Wash hands.
14. Record results.

Procedure
18-8 Performing Color Vision Test Using the Ishihara Plates

STANDARD PRECAUTIONS:

PURPOSE:
To assess a patient's ability to distinguish between the colors red and green.
Patient Education:

1. Explain that the purpose of the test is to determine if the patient has a color vision deficiency.
2. Show patient plate number twelve as an example of the test process.

EQUIPMENT/SUPPLIES:
Ishihara plates (1–12) (Figure 18-37)

PROCEDURE STEPS:

1. Wash hands and assemble the equipment in a room lighted by daylight. RATIONALE: Direct sunlight or electric light may produce errors in the results because of an alteration in the appearance of shades of color.

2. Hold each plate 75 cm or 30 inches from the patient and tilted so that the plane of the plate is at a right angle to the line of the patient's vision (Figure 18-38).
3. Record the number given by the patient on each plate.

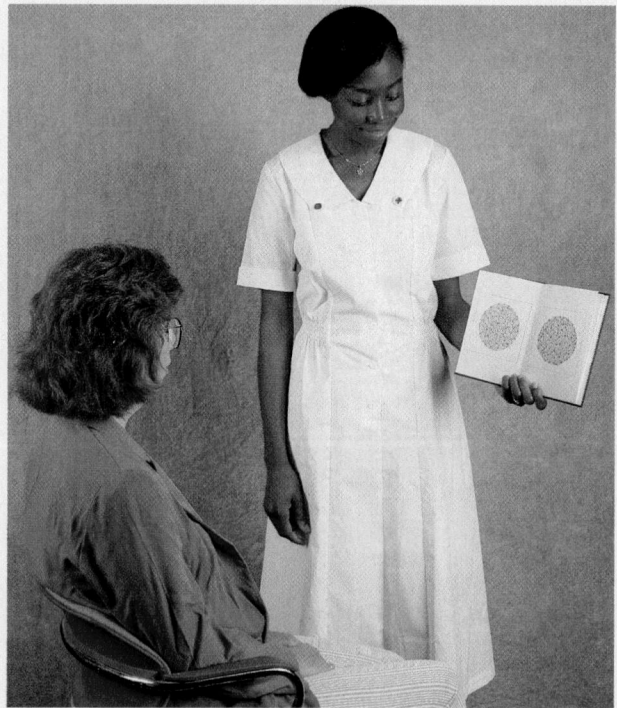

Figure 18-38 The medical assistant holds the plate 30 inches, or 75 cm, from the patient and tilts the card so that the plane of the plate is at a right angle with the line of the patient's vision.

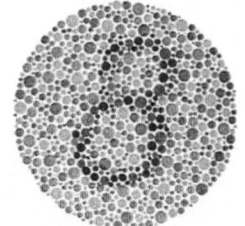 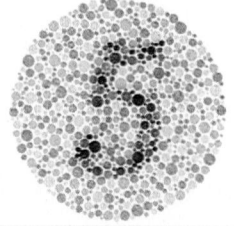

Figure 18-37 Ishihara plates are used to assess the patient's ability to distinguish between the colors red and green.

(*continues*)

Procedure 18-8 (*continued*)

4. Assess the patient's readings and record. RATIONALE: If ten or more plates are read correctly, the color vision is regarded as normal.
   Source for Error: Test plates should be kept covered when not in use. Undue exposure to sunlight causes a fading of the color plates, thus leading to inaccurate test interpretation.

Procedure 18-9 Performing Eye Instillation

STANDARD PRECAUTIONS:

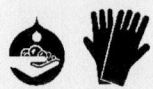

PURPOSE:
To treat eye infections, soothe irritation, anesthetize, and dilate pupils. Ophthalmic medication is supplied in liquid or ointment form. Use separate medication for each eye, if both are affected.

EQUIPMENT/SUPPLIES:
Sterile eye dropper
Sterile ophthalmic medication as ordered by the physician, either drops or ointment
Sterile cotton balls
Sterile gloves

PROCEDURE STEPS:
1. Wash hands.
2. Assemble supplies using sterile technique.
3. Check medication carefully as ordered by the physician, including expiration date. Read label three times.
4. Identify patient.
5. Explain procedure to the patient and inform the patient that instillation may temporarily blur vision.
6. Position the patient in a sitting or lying position.
7. Instruct the patient to stare at a fixed spot during instillation of the drops.
8. Prepare medication using either drops or ointment.
9. Have the patient look up to the ceiling and expose the lower conjunctival sac of the affected eye by using fingers over a tissue to pull down (Figure 18-39).
10. Place the number of drops ordered in the center of the lower conjunctival sac or a thin line of ointment in the lower surface of the eyelid being careful not to touch the eyelid, eyeball, or eyelashes with the tip of the medication applicator. Carefully replace dropper in bottle to avoid contamination.
11. Have the patient close the eye and roll the eyeball. RATIONALE: Movement distributes the medication evenly.
12. Blot excess medication from eyelids with cotton ball from inner to outer canthus.
13. Dispose of supplies.
14. Wash hands.
15. Record procedure in patient's chart.

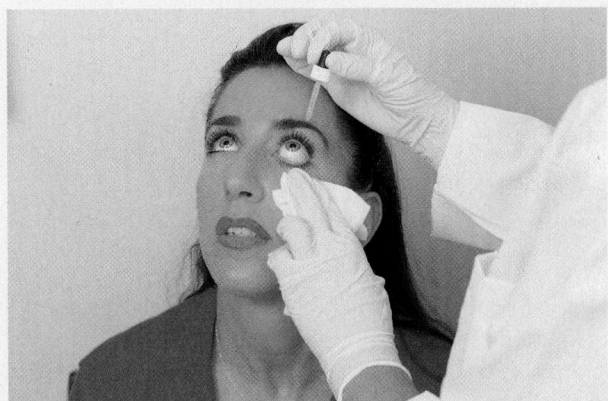

Figure 18-39 When instilling medication into the patient's eye, the patient should look up to the ceiling and the medical assistant should pull down on the lower lid. Contact with the eyeball should be avoided.

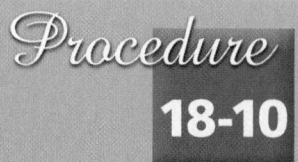

Performing Eye Patch Dressing Application

Procedure 18-10

STANDARD PRECAUTIONS:

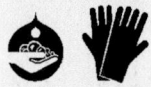

PURPOSE:
To apply a sterile eye patch.

EQUIPMENT/SUPPLIES:
Tape
Sterile eye patch
Sterile gloves

PROCEDURE STEPS:
1. Wash hands and assemble supplies.
2. Identify patient.
3. Explain the procedure.
4. Position the patient in a sitting or supine position.
5. Instruct the patient to close both eyes during the application of the patch. Prepare sterile area by opening the sterile package and using the inside of the package as a sterile field. Apply sterile gloves.
6. Place the patch over the affected eye using sterile gloves.
7. Secure the patch with 3 to 4 strips of transparent tape diagonally from mid-forehead to below the ear.
8. Remove gloves.
9. Wash hands.
10. Document the procedure and provide verbal and written care instructions to the patient.

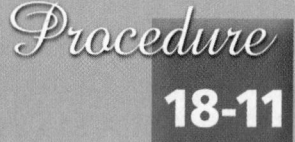

Performing Eye Irrigation

Procedure 18-11

STANDARD PRECAUTIONS:

PURPOSE:
To irrigate the patient's affected eye.
 a. To cleanse of a foreign object
 b. To cleanse discharge
 c. To remove chemicals
 d. To apply antiseptic
 e. To apply heat

EQUIPMENT/SUPPLIES:
Sterile irrigation solution as ordered by the physician
Sterile bulb syringe (rubber)
Kidney-shaped basin to catch irrigation solution
Sterile cotton balls
Sterile gloves
Biohazard waste container
Towel
Pillow

PROCEDURE STEPS:
1. Wash hands and assemble supplies. Note: If both eyes need to be irrigated, use separate equipment for each eye. RATIONALE: Avoid cross-contamination.
2. Identify patient.
3. Explain the procedure to the patient.
4. Position the patient in a supine position.
5. Check expiration date on solution bottle.
6. Check label three times. Warm solution to body temperature (98.6°F).
7. Tilt head toward affected eye. Place towel on patient shoulder. RATIONALE: Avoid cross-contamination of unaffected eye by allowing the solution to flow from the affected eye into the kidney basin.
8. Place the basin beside the affected eye. RATIONALE: Allows for the solution to drain into a catch receptacle.
9. Put on sterile gloves.

(continues)

Procedure 18-11 *(continued)*

10. Moisten 2 to 3 cotton balls with irrigation solution and clean the eyelids and eyelashes of the affected eye from inner to outer canthus. Discard after each wipe.
11. Expose the lower conjunctiva by separating the eyelid with your index finger and thumb.
12. Have the patient stare at a fixed spot.
13. Irrigate the affected eye with sterile solution by resting the sterile bulb syringe on the bridge of the patient's nose being careful not to touch the eye or conjunctival sac with the syringe tip. Allow the stream to flow from the inside canthus to the outer corner of the eye (Figure 18-40). RATIONALE: This avoids a flow of solution into the unaffected eye causing cross contamination.
14. After irrigation, dry the eyelid and eyelashes with sterile cotton balls.
15. Discard supplies in biohazard container if discharge or exudate is present.
16. Remove gloves.
17. Wash hands and document procedure.

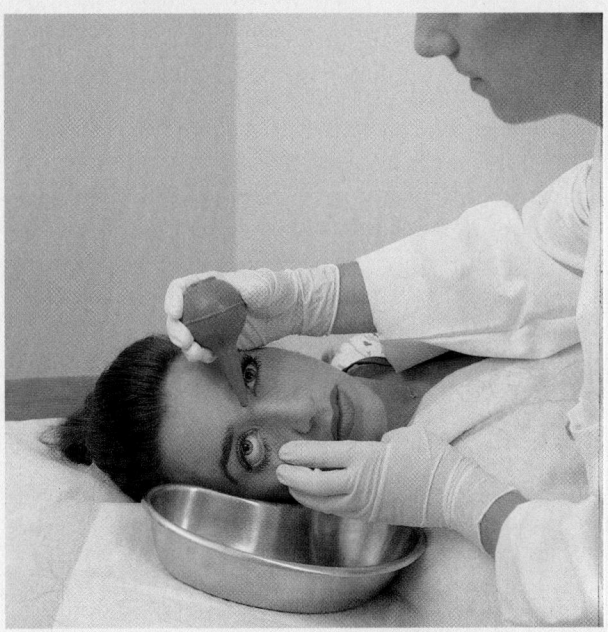

Figure 18-40 The medical assistant irrigates the patient's eye. Note that the solution will go from inner to outer canthus. The patient is turned toward the affected eye.

Procedure 18-12 **Assisting with Audiometry**

STANDARD PRECAUTIONS:

PURPOSE:
To assist in testing patient for hearing loss.
Patient Education:
1. Explain the use and purpose of the audiometer and that the test measures frequency of sound waves and ability of patient to hear various frequencies of sound waves (one frequency at a time).
2. When the patient hears a new frequency, he is to signal the tester.

EQUIPMENT/SUPPLIES:
Audiometer with head phones
Quiet room

PROCEDURE STEPS:
1. Wash hands and assemble equipment and supplies.
2. Prepare room. Test must be held in a room without outside noises. RATIONALE: Outside interference may cause inaccurate test results, especially in the lower frequencies which are more difficult to hear.
3. Explain procedure to patient.

(continues)

Procedure

18-12 (continued)

4. Position patient in a comfortable sitting position.
5. Have patient put on head phones. The procedure is done on each ear separately.
6. If the medical assistant has been thoroughly trained to do the procedure, the physician will allow the medical assistant to perform the audiometry. The audiometer is started at low frequency. The patient indicates when the sound is heard and the medical assistant plots it on the graph (the audiogram) (Figure 18-41).
7. The frequencies gradually increase until completed.
8. The other ear is checked in the same manner.
9. The results are given to the physician for interpretation.
10. Equipment is cleaned following manufacturer's instructions.
11. Wash hands.
12. Document procedure on patient's chart.

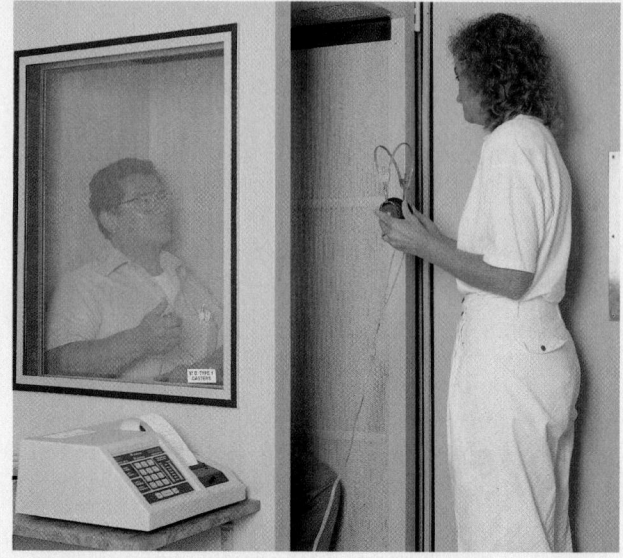

Figure 18-41   The patient presses the handheld control button each time he hears a sound. The medical assistant plots sounds heard on the audiogram.

Procedure

18-13 Performing Ear Irrigation

STANDARD PRECAUTIONS:

PURPOSE:

To remove impacted cerumen, discharge, or foreign materials from the ear canal as directed by the physician.

EQUIPMENT/SUPPLIES:

Irrigation solution as ordered by the physician warmed to body temperature (98.6°F).
Ear syringe or bulb
Ear basin or emesis basin
Basin for warmed solution
Towel
Cotton balls
Otoscope

PROCEDURE STEPS:
1. Wash hands and assemble equipment.
2. Identify patient.
3. Explain the procedure and inform the patient that during the procedure a minimal amount of discomfort and dizziness may be experienced caused by solution coming into contact with the tympanic membrane.
4. Place the patient in a sitting position with head tilted toward affected ear and use an otoscope to visualize the affected ear.
5. Cleanse the outer ear with a wet cotton ball moistened with irrigation solution.
6. Gently pull the auricle upward and back in order to straighten the ear canal.

(continues)

Procedure

18-13 (continued)

7. Tilt the patient's head slightly forward and to the affected side (Figure 18-42). RATIONALE: This position allows the solution to flow into the basin by gravity.

8. Place towel on the patient's shoulder of the affected side.

9. Place the ear basin under the affected ear and have the patient hold the basin in place.

10. Check label of solution three times for correctness and also check the expiration date of the solution.

11. Pour the solution into a basin and fill the syringe with the warmed irrigation solution as prescribed by the physician. Use about 30 to 50 cc of solution at a time. (Repeat Step 5.)

12. Straighten the external auditory canal by pulling back and upward on the auricle for adults.

13. Expel air from syringe and gently insert the syringe tip into the affected ear, being careful not to insert too deeply. Do not occlude external auditory canal. Direct the flow of the solution upward toward roof of canal. RATIONALE: This will avoid injury to the tympanic membrane and prevent occlusion of external auditory canal, allowing solution to drain out.

14. Repeat the irrigation allowing the solution to drain from the ear, noting the return. Allow for free flow of return each time.

15. Dry the outer ear and visualize the inner ear with the otoscope to verify the procedure has removed or dislodged the foreign body.

16. Notify the physician the procedure has been completed.

17. When the procedure is completed, remove the ear basin and towel.

18. Have patient lie on affected side on exam table for ear to continue draining.

19. Provide dry cotton balls to the patient to catch any further drainage if directed by the physician.

20. Dispose of supplies.

21. Wash hands.

22. Document the procedure noting return and amount. Provide postcare instructions:

    a. Report any pain or dizziness to the physician.

    b. Do not insert any foreign object (i.e., cotton applicator) into the ear canal.

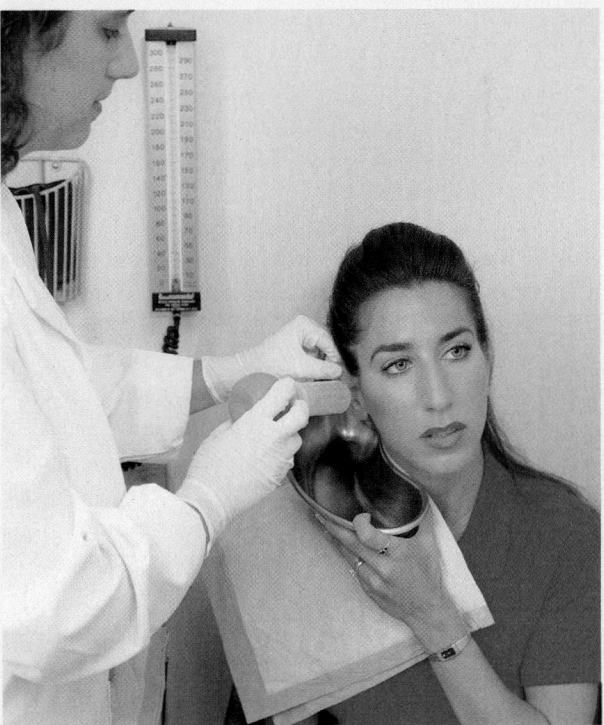

Figure 18-42 When irrigating the patient's ear, the affected ear is tipped to facilitate the flow of solution. The tip of the syringe does not occlude the opening to the external auditory canal.

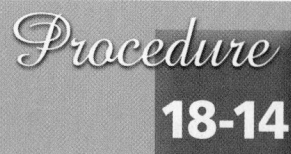

18-14   Performing Ear Instillation

STANDARD PRECAUTIONS:

PURPOSE:
To soften impacted cerumen, fight infection with antibiotics, or relieve pain.

EQUIPMENT/SUPPLIES:
Otic medication as prescribed by the physician
Sterile ear dropper
Cotton balls
Gloves

PROCEDURE STEPS:
1. Wash hands and assemble supplies.
2. Identify patient.
3. Explain procedure to the patient.
4. Position patient to either lie on unaffected side or sitting position with head tilted toward unaffected ear. RATIONALE: Facilitates flow of medication.
5. Check otic medication three times against the physician's order and check expiration date of the medication. RATIONALE: Only otic medication can be used in the ear. Checking the medication three times minimizes medication error.
6. Draw up the prescribed amount of medication.
7. Gently pull the top of the ear upward and back (adult) or pull earlobe downward and backward (child) (Figure 18-43).

8. Instill prescribed dose of medication (number of drops) by squeezing rubber bulb on dropper into the affected ear.
9. Have the patient maintain the position for about 5 minutes to retain medication.
10. When instructed by the physician, insert moistened cotton ball into external ear canal for 15 minutes. RATIONALE: Moistened cotton ball will not absorb medication and will help retain medication in ear.
11. Dispose of supplies.
12. Wash hands.
13. Document procedure.

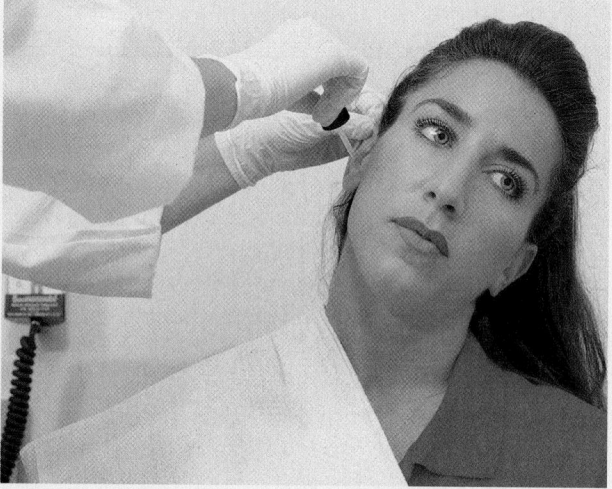

Figure 18-43   When instilling drops into patient's ear, have the patient tilt head so the affected ear is uppermost.

18-15   Assisting with Nasal Examination

STANDARD PRECAUTIONS:

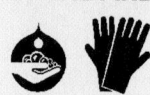

PURPOSE:
To assist the physician with the nasal exam when looking for polyps, engorged superficial blood vessels, and to assist in the possible removal of a foreign body.

(continues)

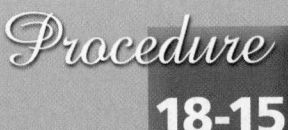

18-15 *(continued)*

Patient Education:
When a foreign object is involved, instruct the patient not to blow the nose or to attempt to remove the object because this could cause tissue damage or push the object deeper into the nasal passage.

EQUIPMENT/SUPPLIES:
Nasal speculum
Light source
Gloves
Bayonet forceps
Kidney basin

PROCEDURE STEPS:
1. Wash hands and assemble supplies.
2. Identify patient.
3. Explain the procedure to the patient.
4. Place the patient in a sitting position.
5. Reassure the patient.
6. Hand the physician equipment and supplies as needed.
7. Clean equipment and dispose of supplies per OSHA guidelines.
8. Wash hands.
9. Document procedure noting foreign object if applicable.

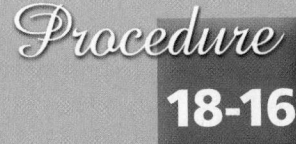

18-16 Performing Nasal Irrigation

STANDARD PRECAUTIONS:

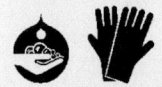

PURPOSE:
To remove a foreign body, relieve inflammation, or increase drainage.
Patient Education:
Instruct the patient not to blow the nose for 5 minutes after the procedure. RATIONALE: Blowing the nose could force the solution into the sinuses or ears.

EQUIPMENT/SUPPLIES:
Bulb-tip syringe
Emesis basin
Basins for irrigation solution
Towels
Nonsterile gloves

PROCEDURE STEPS:
1. Wash hands and assemble supplies.
2. Identify patient.
3. Explain the procedure to the patient.
4. Warm irrigation solution to 98.6°F.
5. Position the patient with head slightly tilted in a sitting position. RATIONALE: Promotes nasal drainage.
6. Place towel across patient's chest and shoulders to absorb solution that may splash.
7. Have the patient hold the emesis basin under the nose.
8. Pour warmed irrigation solution into a basin and withdraw the irrigating solution into the bulb syringe.
9. Insert the tip of the syringe into the affected nostril and gently squeeze the bulb. Do not occlude nostril.
10. Repeat until the required amount of solution has been used.
11. When complete, assist the patient. Give the patient a towel to wipe the face.
12. Dispose of supplies per OSHA guidelines.
13. Wash hands.
14. Document the procedure.

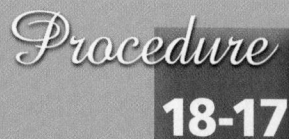

Procedure 18-17 — Performing Nasal Instillation

STANDARD PRECAUTIONS:

PURPOSE:

To provide medication to the nose as ordered by the physician.

Patient Education:

1. Instruct the patient to keep the head tilted back during the procedure to allow the medication to cover the nasal tissues.
2. Do not blow nose immediately following treatment. Medication will be forced out of nose.

EQUIPMENT/SUPPLIES:

Medication as ordered by physician
Medicine dropper
Cotton balls or 2 × 2 gauze sponges

PROCEDURE STEPS:

1. Wash hands and assemble equipment.
2. Identify patient.
3. Explain procedure to the patient.
4. Position the patient with the head lower than the shoulders.
5. Draw medication into dropper after checking medication three times and checking expiration date.
6. Place the dropper over the center of the outside of the affected nostril. Care should be taken not to touch the inside of the nostril. RATIONALE: Touching the inside of the nostril will lead to contamination of the dropper.
7. Repeat the procedure for the other nostril if required.
8. Instruct the patient to remain in position for 5 minutes.
9. Provide cotton balls or gauze sponges to the patient when the patient returns to a sitting position. RATIONALE: Medication may still drain from the nostrils.
10. Dispose of the supplies per OSHA guidelines.
11. Wash hands.
12. Document the procedure.

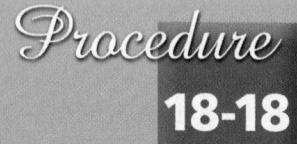

Procedure 18-18 — Obtaining a Sputum Specimen

STANDARD PRECAUTIONS:

PURPOSE:

To collect a quality sputum specimen for laboratory analysis to assist in diagnosing disease.

Patient Education:

1. If specimen must be collected at home, the container must be closed, labeled with date, time, and patient's name.
2. Encourage the patient to drink plenty of fluids. RATIONALE: Increased fluid intake keeps mucus moist.

EQUIPMENT/SUPPLIES:

Tissues
Small plastic bag to deliver specimen to laboratory
Sterile sputum container & label
Laboratory requisition
Nonsterile gloves
Goggles
Gown
Biohazard waste container

PROCEDURE STEPS:

1. Wash hands, assemble supplies, and label container.

(continues)

Procedure 18-18 *(continued)*

2. Explain procedure to the patient. If specimen is to be collected for AFB (acid-fast bacillus), three specimens are needed on three different days.
3. Identify patient.
4. Put on gloves, goggles, and gown.
5. Instruct patient to cough deeply and to expectorate directly into the sterile container (Figure 18-44). RATIONALE: The cough must be deep since this will bring up secretions from the lungs and bronchial tubes. Tell the patient to take several deep breaths in order to cough up sputum (not saliva).
6. Secure the top of the container.
7. Fill out laboratory requisition and secure it to the specimen container. Place in plastic bag and deliver to laboratory within 30 minutes after collection.
8. Dispose of supplies per OSHA guidelines.
9. Wash hands.
10. Document the procedure.

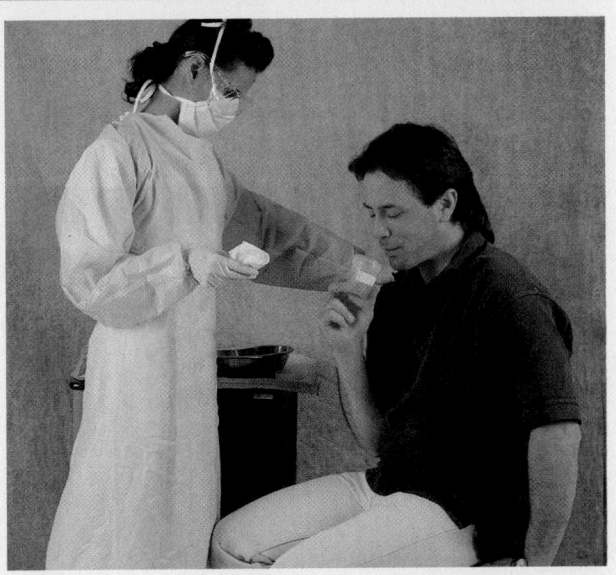

Figure 18-44 The patient should cough deeply and expectorate directly into the sterile container. Note medical assistant is wearing personal protective equipment.

Procedure 18-19 Administer Oxygen by Nasal Cannula for Minor Respiratory Distress

STANDARD PRECAUTIONS:

PURPOSE:
To provide a low dose of concentrated oxygen to a patient during periods of respiratory distress (e.g., chronic obstructive pulmonary disease).
Patient Education:
1. Demonstrate the position of the nasal prongs of the cannula into the nose. They face upward and the tab rests above the upper lip.
2. Describe how to clear the oxygen cylinder valve by turning it counterclockwise.
3. Oxygen supports combustion and a fire can start with oxygen in use. Friction, static electricity, or a lighted cigarette or cigar can cause ignition.

EQUIPMENT/SUPPLIES:
Portable oxygen tank with stand
Disposable nasal cannula with connecting tube
Flowmeter
Pressure regulator

PROCEDURE STEPS:
1. Wash hands and explain procedure to the patient.
2. Identify patient.
3. Open the cylinder one full turn, counterclockwise.
4. Check the pressure gauge. RATIONALE: This will determine the amount of pressure in the cylinder.
5. Attach the nasal cannula to the tubing and then to the flowmeter.

(continues)

Procedure 18-19 (continued)

6. Adjust the flow rate according to the physician's order.
7. Check for oxygen flow through the cannula.
8. Place the tips of cannula into the nares no more than 1 inch.
9. Adjust the tubing around the patient's ears (Figure 18-45) and secure it under the chin.
10. Answer patient's questions.
11. Wash hands.
12. Document the procedure.
    Note: Oxygen is usually humidified to prevent drying of respiratory mucosa.

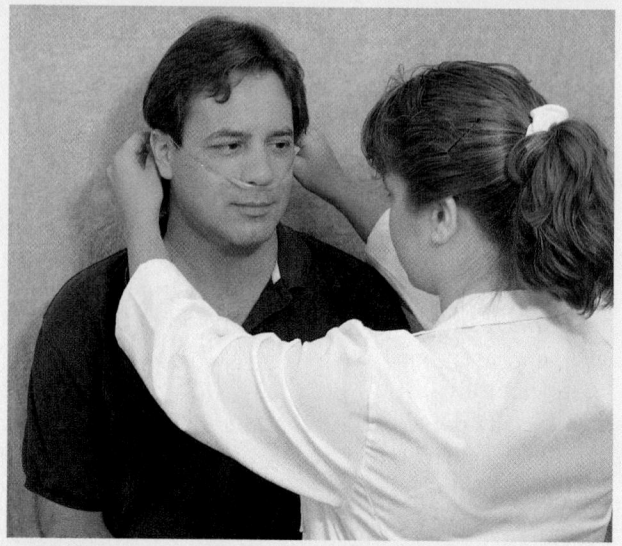

Figure 18-45   Position the nasal cannula, adjusting the tubing around the patient's ears and securing the cannula under the chin.

Procedure 18-20 Instructing Patient in Use of Metered Dose Nebulizer

STANDARD PRECAUTIONS:

PURPOSE:
To instruct a patient in the correct use of a handheld nebulizer, a device that delivers a fine mist of medication with or without the use of oxygen to the respiratory tract including the lungs.
Patient Education:
1. Remind the patient to inhale slowly.
2. Close the mouth and lips around the mouthpiece.
3. Clean the inhaler by rinsing the mouthpiece in warm water.
4. Adhere to prescribed dose.

EQUIPMENT/SUPPLIES:
Handheld nebulizer containing medication ordered by the physician

PROCEDURE STEPS:
1. Wash hands and assemble equipment.
2. Identify patient.
3. Demonstrate the use of the equipment to the patient and then have the patient return the demonstration.
4. Instruct the patient to exhale fully.
5. Holding the nebulizer upside down, close the mouth, lips, and teeth around the mouthpiece.
6. Tilting the head back, instruct the patient to take a deep breath and at the same time push the bottle against the mouthpiece.

(continues)

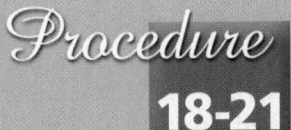

Procedure 18-20 *(continued)*

7. Instruct the patient to continue to inhale until the lungs are full.
8. Remove the mouthpiece and slowly exhale.
9. Repeat steps 4 through 7 if the physician has ordered more than one dose.

10. Wash hands.
11. Document patient was given instructions and has demonstrated to you the use of the nebulizer.

Procedure 18-21 Spirometry Testing

STANDARD PRECAUTIONS:

PURPOSE:

To prepare a patient for a spirometry to obtain optimum test results.

Patient Education:

1. Reinforce the importance of good posture during the process.
2. When blowing into the mouthpiece, the lips must seal tightly around it.
3. Explain the parameters needed for successful completion of the test.

   Parameters:

   - Patient must inhale deeply and quickly and exhale quickly and forcibly until no air can be expelled.
   - Patient must refrain from the use of bronchodilators for 24 hours prior to test.
   - Explain to the patient that maximum effort is required for accurate test results.

EQUIPMENT/SUPPLIES:

Spirometer
Disposable mouthpiece

PROCEDURE STEPS:

1. Wash hands and assemble equipment.
2. Identify the patient.
3. Explain the procedure and equipment to the patient. Allow the patient to breathe into the machine to become acquainted with the equipment.
4. Place the patient in a comfortable position (sitting/standing). Loosen tie or collar.
5. Instruct the patient not to bend at the waist when blowing into the mouthpiece.
6. Reinforce the inhalation process (deep breaths to fill the lungs to maximum capacity).
7. Instruct the patient to continue to blow into the mouthpiece until instructed to stop.
8. Be supportive and encouraging throughout the test.
9. Wash hands.
10. Attend to patient's needs.
11. Place the test results on the patient's chart after being reviewed by the physician.

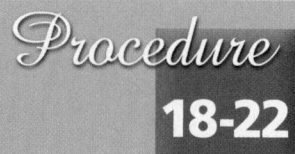

Assisting with Plaster-of-Paris Cast Application

Procedure 18-22

STANDARD PRECAUTIONS:

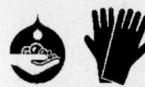

PURPOSE:
To assist physician in cast application.
Patient Education:
1. Instruct patient how to cover cast when bathing. Showersafe® is a type of waterproof material that can be used to cover a cast while showering.
2. Provide patient with dietary information for bone healing. Protein and high-calcium foods help the bone to heal.

EQUIPMENT/SUPPLIES:
Cast material:
Plaster bandage roll or synthetic tape
Container of 75°F water, which is lined with plastic or cloth to catch loose plaster
Water
Stockinette (3-inch width for arms, 4 inch for leg casts)
Webril (Sheet wadding)
Bandage
Scissors
Rubber gloves
Sponge rubber for padding

PROCEDURE STEPS:
1. Provide the patient with an explanation of the procedure.
2. Answer any questions about the injury or cast application within the scope of the medical assistant's training.
3. Wash hands and assemble the equipment and supplies.
4. Position the patient in a sitting position or as required by the physician.
5. Put on gloves.

6. Clean and dry the area to be casted, as directed by the physician. Chart any areas of bruising, redness, or open areas. RATIONALE: Appropriate documentation of skin condition is needed to assist in evaluation of the extremity at a later time.
7. Pad bony prominence with sponge rubber. RATIONALE: To protect from pressure.
8. Provide the correct width of stockinette for the area on which cast is being applied. RATIONALE: A stockinette that is too large will form creases, thus allowing for injury to tissues.
9. Provide physician with correct width of webril. RATIONALE: Webril provides protection to the patient's skin preventing pressure sores. Folds in the padding could lead to irritation of the skin.
10. Place the bandage in the container of warm water for 5 seconds. Remove from water and gently squeeze to remove excess water. Do not wring.
11. Assist with the application of the cast material as requested by the physician.
12. Reassure patient as needed.
13. After cast application, review cast care instructions and provide written instructions for cast care and isometric exercises (if prescribed by the physician). Reinforce any precautions given by the physician. RATIONALE: Reviewing possible complications with the patient enhances the immediate reporting of circulatory impairment and infection.
14. Discard water down the sink drain being cautious to keep plaster from going down the drain. Discard plaster in trash receptacle.
15. Clean work area.
16. Remove gloves and wash hands.
17. Schedule patient for next appointment to have cast checked.
18. Document the procedure.

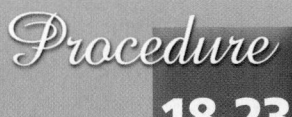

18-23 Assisting with Cast Removal

STANDARD PRECAUTIONS:

PURPOSE:
To assist the physician with the removal of a cast.

EQUIPMENT/SUPPLIES:
Cast cutter
Cast spreader
Bandage scissors
Bag for disposing of cast materials

PROCEDURE STEPS:
1. Wash hands.
2. Explain the cast removal process to the patient. The cutter vibrates and does not spin. Some pressure and warmth may be experienced.

RATIONALE: Explaining the procedure reduces apprehension and fears about being cut with the blade.
3. Reassure the patient that skin color and muscle tone will improve with therapy.
4. Hand the physician the equipment as requested.
5. After the procedure provide written instructions for postcare.
6. Clean equipment.
7. Wash hands.
8. Document cast removal and appearance of body part from which cast was removed.

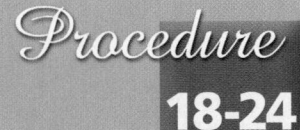

18-24 Assisting the Physician During a Lumbar Puncture

STANDARD PRECAUTIONS:

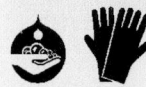

PURPOSE:
To assemble supplies and position the patient for removal of cerebrospinal fluid from the lumbar area which will be sent to the laboratory for analysis.
Patient Education:
1. Review post-spinal tap instructions.
   a. The patient should remain in a prone position for 2 to 3 hours to allow tissues to close over the puncture site and minimize cerebrospinal fluid leakage.
   b. Reinforce the need to increase fluid intake since this helps to replace fluid loss.
   c. Report any severe headaches or alterations in neurological status (paralysis, numbness, tingling, and so on).

EQUIPMENT/SUPPLIES:
Drape
Xylocaine 1%–2%
Syringe and needle for anesthetic
Sterile gloves
Disposable sterile lumbar puncture tray (to include):
  Skin antiseptic with applicator
  Band-Aid
  Spinal puncture needle
  3 test tubes with corks or tops
  Drape
  Manometer
  Laboratory requisition
  Examination light

PROCEDURE STEPS:
1. Reinforce physician's explanation of the procedure and answer questions.
2. Verify the patient has signed a consent form.

(continues)

Procedure **18-24** *(continued)*

3. Patient should be instructed to empty the bladder and bowel.
4. Wash hands and set up sterile field for the physician.
5. Cleanse the puncture site with antiseptic soap and water. Rinse.
6. Position the patient in a lateral recumbent position with the back at the edge of the exam table and a small pillow under the head. RATIONALE: Patient's alignment of the spine is best achieved in a horizontal position.
7. Drape patient for warmth and privacy.
8. Have the patient draw the knees up to the abdomen and grasp onto knees (Figure 18-46A) and flex chin on chest. RATIONALE: Position allows for easier needle insertion into the subarachnoid space of the spinal cord because this position widens the spaces between the lumbar vertebrae. Procedure is performed at the fourth intervertebral space of the lumbar region (Figure 18-46B).
9. The physician will swab the puncture site with antiseptic such as Betadine®.
10. The physician drapes area with fenestrated drape.
11. Assist physician to aspirate anesthetic.
12. Help the patient maintain this position until the needle has reached the subarachnoid space. RATIONALE: Movement by the patient could produce trauma to the spinal cord area.
13. Remind patient to breathe evenly, not to hold his breath or talk, since this may interfere with the pressure reading.
14. At the physician's direction, have the patient straighten his legs. RATIONALE: Muscle tension can give false pressure reading.

15. After the procedure has been completed, the physician will apply a Band-Aid to the puncture site. The patient is placed in a prone position for 2 to 3 hours, or as directed by the physician. RATIONALE: This helps prevent cerebrospinal fluid from leaking through the puncture site.
16. Apply gloves. Cap specimens tightly.
17. Label samples with date, patient's name, and number CSF #1, #2, #3.
18. Send the labeled specimen to the laboratory with the appropriate laboratory requisition. Store in incubator.
19. Clean area using standard precautions.
20. Remove gloves.
21. Wash hands.
22. Document procedure in patient's chart.

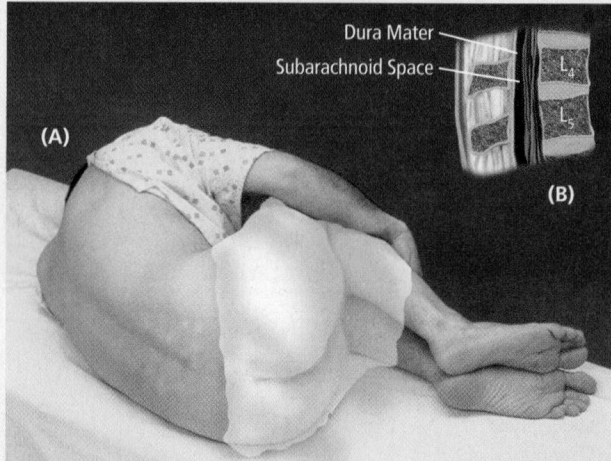

Figure 18-46   (A) Have the patient draw up the knees to the abdomen and grasp onto knees. Chin should flex on chest. (B) The site for the lumbar puncture.

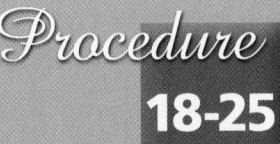

Assisting the Physician with a Neurological Screening Examination

STANDARD PRECAUTIONS:

PURPOSE:
To determine a patient's neurological status.
Patient Education:
Inform the patient the purpose of the exam is to assess her response to pain and touch reflexes and other neurological functions.
a. The physician will use several supplies to test the functioning of each cranial nerve and to test the reflexes and the coordination of the patient.

EQUIPMENT/SUPPLIES:
Percussion hammer
Safety pin
Material for odor identification
Cotton ball
Tuning fork

Flashlight
Tongue blade
Ophthalmoscope

PROCEDURE STEPS:
1. Wash hands.
2. The mental status examination can be done by the medical assistant when taking the patient's medical history by observing the following:
   a. When taking patient's history, pay special attention to level of awareness, memory, cognition, and mood. When the patient answers questions during the history taking, note if behavior is appropriate for the circumstances.
3. The physician will evaluate the cranial nerve functions by using the results of the visual acuity tests as well as other tests.
4. Assist the patient as needed during and after the exam.
5. Document procedure in patient's chart.

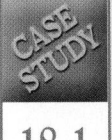

Corey Bayer is a fifteen-year-old patient at City Health Care. He sustained an injury to his right wrist today during soccer practice. Dr. Rice has examined him and ordered an X ray of the right forearm. The results show that Corey has sustained a Colles' fracture of the right wrist. Dr. Rice asks you to prepare the equipment to apply a cast.

18-1 CASE STUDY REVIEW

1. Describe assisting in cast application. What are the medical assistant's responsibilities?
2. Following Corey's cast application, describe the cast care instructions that will be given to Corey and his mother.

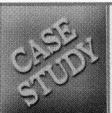

Dr. Rice has scheduled Anita Blanchette for a spirometry test and wants you to telephone her the day before the test to prepare her for it so that optimal results are obtained.

18-2 CASE STUDY REVIEW

1. What information can you give to Anita prior to her spirometry to obtain the best test results?

SUMMARY

Medical assistants are a vital link in the team of health care providers. A thorough knowledge and understanding of the various body system examinations and clinical procedures routinely performed as part of patient care will enhance the quality of care given.

Some of the specialty procedures will be performed on a routine basis in the ambulatory care setting; others will only be performed occasionally and perhaps only in the larger settings that offer special-

ized as well as primary care. Sometimes, in order to feel comfortable assisting with the less common procedures, medical assistants may need to broaden their base of knowledge by conducting independent research. Medical assistants who are willing to constantly expand their clinical understanding will not only fine-tune their professional skills but will derive greater satisfaction from their job performance.

REVIEW QUESTIONS

Multiple Choice

1. What are the elevated skin lesions affecting the epidermis caused by the papilloma viruses called?
   a. scleroderma
   b. moles
   c. calluses
   d. warts
2. What is the disorder that is characterized by discomfort of the muscles, tendons, ligaments, and soft tissues brought on by trauma, strain, and emotional stress?
   a. carpal tunnel syndrome
   b. bursitis
   c. gout
   d. fibromyalgia
3. What type of fracture has its bone fragments driven into each other?
   a. greenstick
   b. impacted
   c. oblique
   d. comminuted
4. What disease is caused by a degeneration of brain cells caused by lack of dopamine, bringing about muscle rigidity and akinesia?
   a. multiple sclerosis
   b. Bell's palsy
   c. Parkinson's
   d. tic douloureux
5. An acute circumscribed infection of the subcutaneous tissues caused by staphylococcus is a:
   a. comedone
   b. carbuncle
   c. furuncle
   d. psoriasis

Critical Thinking

1. Describe how to perform a urinary catheterization.
2. Why are the rules of evidence always followed during a drug screen?
3. Phyllis Lomeli, a new patient of Dr. Reynolds, has been experiencing gastrointestinal problems. Dr. Reynolds has ordered fecal occult blood tests for the patient. What diet instructions does the medical assistant give to the patient? What directions and supplies does the medical assistant give to the patient? When the guaiac slides are returned, how does the medical assistant develop and interpret them?
4. List the patient preparation instructions for the following tests:
   a. barium enema
   b. upper GI
   c. cholecystogram
   d. intravenous pyelogram
5. List the steps the medical assistant must follow when performing the visual acuity test on an adult, a 9-year-old child, and a 4-year-old toddler.
6. What is the use and purpose of the audiometer? How is the test administered?
7. Explain the rationale when doing an eye irrigation that the flow of the irrigating solution is from the inside canthus to the outer canthus of the eye.
8. Differentiate among bronchitis, emphysema, and asthma.
9. Discuss how to obtain a sputum specimen.
10. What is the medical assistant's role when assisting in spirometry?
11. List the various types of casting material used in a physician's office. What are the cast care guidelines that the medical assistant gives to the patient?

12. List the components of a neurological screening.
13. When a mental status exam is given, what five areas are being reviewed?
14. Explain the medical assistant's role when assisting with a lumbar puncture.

WEB ACTIVITIES

Use the Internet to search for information from a medical site to find answers to the following:

1. What is the most current treatment for kidney stones?
2. What are the long-term harmful effects of cigarette smoking?
3. What recommendations does the surgeon general of the United States have for quitting smoking cigarettes?

REFERENCES/BIBLIOGRAPHY

Bonewit-West, K. (2000). *Clinical procedures for medical assistants* (5th ed.). Philadelphia: W. B. Saunders Co.

Campeau, F. & Fleitz, J. (1999). *Limited radiography* (2nd ed.). Albany, NY: Delmar.

Damjanov, I. (1996). *Pathology for the health-related professions.* Philadelphia: W. B. Saunders Co.

Ehrlich, A. (1997). *Medical terminology for health professionals* (3rd ed.). Albany, NY: Delmar.

Frazier, M. S., Drzymkowski, J. A., & Doty, S. J. (1996). *Essentials of human diseases and conditions.* Philadelphia: W. B. Saunders Co.

Keir, L., Wise, B. A., & Krebs, C. (1998). *Medical assisting: Administrative and clinical competencies* (8th ed.). Albany, NY: Delmar.

Kinn, M. & Woods, M. (1999). *The medical assistant: Administrative and clinical* (8th ed.). Philadelphia: W. B. Saunders Co.

Neighbors, M., & Tannehill-Jones, R. (2000). *Human diseases.* Albany, NY: Delmar.

Taber's cyclopedic medical dictionary (1999) (18th ed.). Philadelphia: F. A. Davis Company.

Tamparo, C., & Lewis, M. (2000). *Diseases of the human body* (3rd ed.). Philadelphia: F. A. Davis Company.

Tortora, G., & Grabowski, S. (1996). *Principles of anatomy and physiology.* New York: Harper Collins.

Travaline, J., & Criner, G. J. (1994, August). Pulmonary function testing using a spirometer. *Hospital Medicine, 57.*

White, G. (1998). *Basic clinical lab competencies for respiratory care* (3rd ed.). Albany, NY: Delmar.

Wojciechowski, W. (2000). *Respiratory care sciences: An integrated approach* (3rd ed.). Albany, NY: Delmar.

Zakus, S. (1995). *Clinical procedures for medical assistants* (3rd ed.). St. Louis: Mosby-Year Book, Inc.

ADVANCED TECHNIQUES AND PROCEDURES

ASSISTING WITH MINOR SURGERY

KEY TERMS

Allergy
Anesthesia
Antibacterial
Approximate
Bandage
Betadine®
Cautery
Contamination
Dressing
Epinephrine
Exudate
Fenestrated
Friable
Hibeclens®
Hydrogen Peroxide
Infection
Inflammation
Informed Consent
Isopropyl Alcohol
Ligature
Liquid Nitrogen
Mayo Stand/Instrument Tray
Ratchets
Silver Nitrate
Sitz Bath
Sodium Hydroxide
Strictures
Surgery Cards
Surgical Asepsis
Suture
Swaged
Volatile

OUTLINE

Surgical Asepsis
   Handwashing for Surgical Asepsis
Sterile Principles
**Common Surgical Procedures
   Performed in Physicians'
   Offices and Clinics**
Alternative Surgical Methods
   Electrosurgery
   Cautery
   Cryosurgery
   Laser Surgery
Suture Materials and Supplies
   Suture/Ligature
   Suture Needles
Instruments
   Structural Features
   Categories and Uses
   Care of Instruments
   Chemical "Cold" Sterilization

Supplies and Equipment
   Sponges and Wicks
   Solutions/Creams/Ointments
   Dressings and Bandages
   Anesthetics
Patient Care and Preparation
   Patient Preparation and Education
   Informed Consent
   Medical Assisting Considerations
   Postoperative Instructions
   Wounds, Wound Care, and the
     Healing Process
Basic Surgery Set-Up
   Basic Rules and Concepts for
     Setup of Surgical Trays
Minor Surgery Process
Preparation for Minor Surgery
   Using Dry Sterile Transfer Forceps

OBJECTIVES

The student should strive to meet the following performance objectives and demonstrate an understanding of the facts and principles presented in this chapter through written and oral communication.

1. Define the key terms as presented in the glossary.
2. Define surgical asepsis and differentiate between surgical asepsis and medical asepsis.
3. List eight basic rules to follow to protect sterile areas.
4. Explain the sizing standards of suture material and the criteria used to select the most appropriate type and size.
5. Given a variety of surgical instruments, be able to identify each and describe its intended use. *(continues)*

6. Demonstrate the ability to select the most appropriate type of dressings for a given situation.

7. State advantages and disadvantages of Betadine®, Hibeclens®, isopropyl alcohol, and hydrogen peroxide when each is used as a skin antiseptic.

8. Define anesthesia, and explain the advantages and disadvantages of epinephrine as an additive to injectable anesthetics.

9. List five preoperative issues to be addressed in patient preparation and education.

10. List five postoperative concerns to be addressed with the patient and the caregiver.

11. Demonstrate applying sterile gloves.

12. Demonstrate setting up a surgical tray, including laying the field, applying supplies and instruments, pouring a sterile solution, using transfer forceps, and covering the sterile tray.

13. Explain what is meant by alternative surgical methods.

ROLE DELINEATION COMPONENTS

CLINICAL

Fundamental Principles

- **Apply principles of aseptic technique and infection control**
- **Comply with quality assurance practices**

Patient Care

- **Obtain patient history and vital signs**
- **Prepare and maintain examination and treatment areas**
- **Prepare patient for examinations, procedures and treatments**
- **Assist with examinations, procedures and treatments**
- **Maintain medication and immunization records**

(*continues*)

SCENARIO

It might be instructive to compare two different ambulatory care settings. At the multiphysician Inner City Health Care, minor surgery is performed on a routine basis. Certain days are dedicated to certain procedures. Because of the high volume of patients and different physician preferences, Inner City maintains two special rooms for minor surgery and has a large selection of instruments. At the smaller two-physician Lewis and King, however, minor surgical procedures are less frequent and are conducted in the patient examination rooms.

INTRODUCTION

Minor office surgery differs greatly from major surgery, not only in complexity but in the supplies, equipment, instruments, and personnel needed. Some minor office surgery is performed by the physician alone; some require the assistance of the medical assistant. Most ambulatory care settings do not need a large variety of surgical instruments, but will often need more than one of the more frequently used instruments. As a personal preference, special instruments may be purchased and maintained for a specific physician to use during a particular surgical procedure. These particular instruments are generally not used by any other physician.

The equipment and supplies used in minor office surgery are usually portable and easily maintained. It is the larger practices that perform many minor office surgeries that can afford the space and expense of maintaining a special room just for that purpose. Often patient examination rooms serve as small surgical suites with portable **Mayo stands/instrument trays**, supplies, and equipment brought into the room for the procedure.

Whether assisting with minor surgery is a routine or an infrequent event for the medical assistant, it is nonetheless important to be knowledgeable about the use and care of instruments and room as well as patient preparation for minor surgery. Medical assistants should also understand the preference of each physician on staff in order to make the minor surgical procedure comfortable and effective for both patient and physician.

SURGICAL ASEPSIS

Regardless of the number and complexity of minor surgical procedures performed in the office or ambulatory care center, surgical asepsis must be strictly maintained. Surgical asepsis uses practices known as sterile techniques. The primary purpose of surgical asepsis is to prevent microorganisms from entering the patient's body during an invasive procedure. Some examples of invasive procedures include creating an opening in the skin such as a surgical incision, closing a wound such as a laceration, giving an injection, or inserting a sterile catheter into a sterile body cavity such as the urinary bladder.

Because microorganisms are on virtually every surface such as skin, instruments, surgical instrument trays, clothing, and even in the air, it is necessary to destroy as many as possible before any surgical procedure. Surgical asepsis or sterile technique prevents microorganism entry into the body during an invasive procedure and, therefore, protects the patient from infection. Once the items and areas are sterilized, every precaution must be taken to prevent contamination of the sterile items or areas either from a nonsterile surface or from airborne contamination.

Living tissue surfaces such as skin cannot be sterilized but can be made as free of pathogens as possible before the use of a sterile covering. One example of this concept is the use of the surgical handwashing technique prior to applying sterile gloves (see Procedure 19-1). Another example of asepsis is preparing the patient's skin with a surgical scrub solution prior to applying sterile drapes around the intended surgical site.

Refer to Chapter 10 for more complete information on the concepts of asepsis and aseptic techniques including handwashing for medical asepsis and methods of sterilization for surgical asepsis.

The differences between handwashing for medical asepsis as discussed in Chapter 10 (see Procedure 10-1) and handwashing for surgical asepsis are addressed in the following section.

Handwashing for Surgical Asepsis

Handwashing for medical asepsis is defined as removing pathogenic microorganisms from the hands after contamination. Medical handwashing is used many times throughout the day to cleanse the skin after removing contaminated gloves, assisting with patient care, and touching unclean surfaces. Handwashing for surgical asepsis is defined as removal of as many microorganisms as possible prior to performing surgery or a sterile procedure. Handwashing for surgical asepsis consists of meticulously washing hands prior to applying sterile gloves. Both medical and surgical aseptic handwashing techniques are designed to prevent exposing patients, health care workers, and the public to potentially harmful microorganisms.

Proper protocol when assisting with minor surgery requires the use of surgical handwashing at the beginning of each workday as well as prior to sterile techniques, with the complementary use of medical handwashing before leaving the office and when returning and between patients and procedures. Any opening in the medical assistant's skin should be covered with a sterile adhesive dressing and gloves are worn during any direct patient contact. See Chapter 10 for information on standard precautions.

For a summary of how surgical handwashing differs from medical handwashing see Table 19-1.

STERILE PRINCIPLES

Sterile principles are a set of guidelines designed to designate what items and areas are considered sterile and what actions cause contamination. Some areas are logical and clear, some are subtle and less clear. It has already been noted that some surfaces, such as skin, cannot be sterilized. In addition, large items such as instrument stands and their trays cannot fit into an autoclave for sterilization. To create sterile areas and surfaces where sterility is not possible, sterile gloves can be worn over the hands and sterile drapes can be applied to trays once both have been washed with soap and water, rinsed, and dried.

TABLE 19-1 DIFFERENCE BETWEEN MEDICAL AND SURGICAL HANDWASHING	
Medical Handwashing	**Surgical Handwashing**
• 2 minute duration	• 5–6 minute duration
• Wash hands and wrists	• Wash hands, wrists, and forearms to the elbows
• Hands should be held down during rinsing	• Hands should be held up during rinsing
• Scrub nails with brush; clean under nails with cuticle stick	• Scrub nails with brush and clean under each nail with cuticle stick
• Apply lotion*	• Do not apply lotion*
• Glove for protection	• Glove for sterility and personal protection

*The use of lotions is encourage to help prevent chafing of the skin, especially with frequent hand washings. Nevertheless, recent studies have determined that lotions containing petroleum or mineral oil can break down latex and should be avoided if latex gloves are going to be worn within one hour after applying the lotion. If lotions are applied immediately prior to gloving, the use of water-based lotions is recommended. Of special interest to persons with latex sensitivities (see Chapter 10) is the fact that using lotions and creams actually increases the amount of latex protein that is transferred from the gloves into the skin, thereby increasing the symptoms of latex sensitivity.

Guidelines to protect sterile items and areas include:

● A sterile object may not touch a nonsterile object.

● Sterile objects must not be wet. Moisture will draw microorganisms into the sterile object.

● An acceptable border between a sterile area and a nonsterile area is one inch. The portion of a drape that hangs over the edge is considered nonsterile, no matter what its size. Sterile articles should be placed in the center of the sterile field and away from the edge as much as possible.

● Do not turn your back on a sterile field. If you cannot see the field, you cannot be aware of what touched it.

● Anything below the waist is considered contaminated. In support of this principle, all surgery trays should be positioned above the waist. All articles are to be held above the waist.

● All sterile objects (such as gloved hands) must be held in front and away from the body and above waist level.

● Do not cough, sneeze, or talk over a sterile field. Airborne particles may fall onto the sterile area and contaminate it.

● Do not reach over the sterile area. Clothing may touch and thereby contaminate the area. Spend as little time as possible reaching into the sterile area.

● Do not pass contaminated dressings or instruments over the sterile field.

● Arrange for the physician to place contaminated instruments into a separate container or area.

● Always be aware of actions in order to determine whether the sterile field has been contaminated. When in doubt, err on the side of safety.

● When opening sterile packages, the outer wrapper is contaminated. It should be opened without touching the inner contents, and the contents are then dropped onto the sterile field. Double wrapping can be used. (Refer to Chapter 10, Procedure 10-4.)

● Sterile solutions in bottles should be poured into sterile basins or cups on the sterile field without touching the rim of the bottle and without splashing solution onto the sterile field. If the sterile field is not polylined and becomes wet, it is considered contaminated, because when a field is wet it acts as a wick and draws microorganisms into the article. Using polylined drapes as sterile fields protects against contamination.

COMMON SURGICAL PROCEDURES PERFORMED IN PHYSICIANS' OFFICES AND CLINICS

All minor surgery has commonalities as well as specifics. The following specific minor surgery includes lists of needed instruments, supplies, and equipment as well as basic patient preparation and postoperative instructions for some of the more frequently performed minor surgery. The following procedures are suggested protocol only, as each physician will have preferences and techniques unique to them and their practices.

This section includes a general procedure for assisting with minor surgery and is followed by specific minor surgical procedures, including:

● Assisting with Minor Surgery (Procedure 19-2)

● Suturing of Laceration or Incision (Procedure 19-3)

- Dressing Change (Procedure 19-4)

- Suture Removal (Procedure 19-5)

- Application of Sterile Adhesive Skin Closure Strips (Procedure 19-6)

- Sebaceous Cyst Excision (Procedure 19-7)

- Incision and Drainage of Localized Infections (Procedure 19-8)

- Aspiration of Joint Fluid (Procedure 19-9)

- Hemorrhoid Thrombectomy (Procedure 19-10)

ALTERNATIVE SURGICAL METHODS

Alternative surgical methods refer to those methods not requiring the use of a surgical knife or scalpel, but which use other methods of cutting or destroying, such as electric current, heat, freezing, chemicals, or laser beam. Which method is used is determined by the physician's preference.

Electrosurgery

Electrosurgery uses an electric current in a concentrated area to either cut or destroy tissue whenever pathological examination is not required. The equipment for electrosurgery consists of a power source, usually a small boxed unit, and a detachable handheld applicator with removable tips. The tips are available in various sizes and are removable for cleaning and sterilizing.

Electrosurgery is very useful in removing benign skin tags and warts. The main advantage of electrosurgery is that the bleeding is controlled through the cauterization of the blood vessels as the electric current is applied. The terms *electrocoagulation, electrofulguration, electrodessication, electroscission,* and *electrosection* all refer to various uses of electric current to either coagulate blood vessels, destroy tissue either with a spark or by drying, or cut tissue.

Cautery

The word **cautery** comes from the term *caustic* and means the application of a caustic chemical or destructive heat. The burning of tissue, either chemically or electrically, is known as cauterization. Sometimes during surgical procedures unnecessary bleeding can be controlled by use of an electrocautery machine (Figure 19-1). Tissues that do not need to be pathologically examined, such as benign skin tags, can be destroyed using cauterization. Some common chemicals used to destroy tissue and stop bleeding are **silver nitrate, liquid nitrogen,** and **sodium hydroxide.**

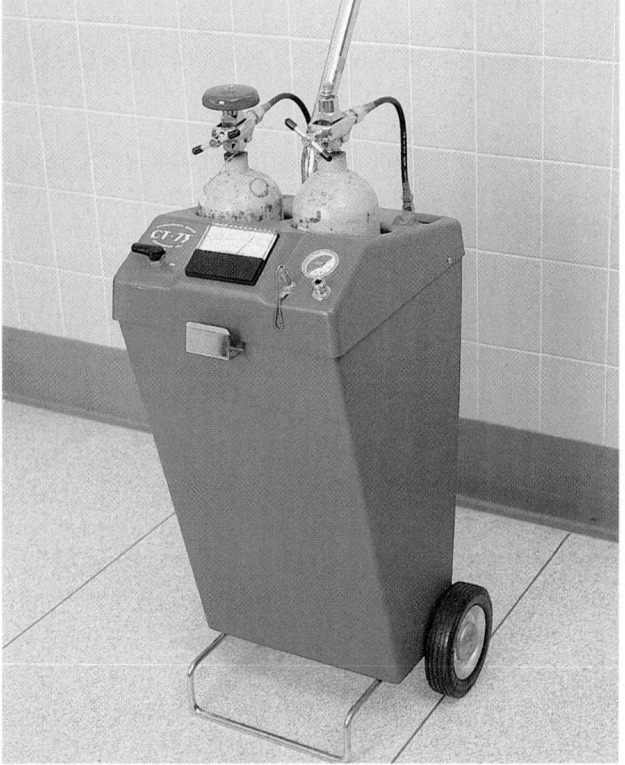

Figure 19-1 Electrocautery machines are used to burn tissue with electric current. This is done to destroy tissue, such as warts or polyps, or to cauterize small blood vessels to decrease blood loss during surgery.

Chemical Tissue Destruction. Silver nitrate is available in a solid form, impregnated on the end of a wooden applicator stick. Silver nitrate is especially useful inside the nose to cauterize **friable,** easily broken, blood vessels in the treatment of epistaxis (nosebleed).

Liquid nitrogen, often incorrectly referred to as dry ice is extremely **volatile,** easily evaporated, and must be kept in a covered insulated canister. Liquid nitrogen is obtained when nitrogen gas is compressed under very cold temperatures into a liquid. It is most often used to destructively "freeze" warts.

Liquid chemical caustic agents such as sodium hydroxide are used to permanently destroy the growth plates of toenails whenever total and permanent removal of the toenail is necessary.

Electrical Tissue Destruction. Electrical burning of tissue is performed with the use of an electrical instrument called an electrocautery. A wand on the end of a handheld apparatus is electrically heated and applied to tissues. The adjustable current is controlled by a foot pedal. Disposable battery-operated cautery units designed for one-time use are also available.

Cryosurgery

Cryosurgery refers to the destruction of tissue by freezing. Some types of tissues react differently to heat than cold in the rate of healing and level of scarring. The cryogenic substance most often used to destructively freeze tissue is liquid nitrogen. Liquid nitrogen may be applied to cervical erosions to facilitate the healing growth of normal tissue.

The cryogenic properties of solid carbon dioxide make it useful for freezing warts and nevi as well. Histo-freezer is the trade name of an aerosol spray canister containing imethyl ether as the freezing agent. Hollow disposable cotton-tipped applicators attach to the Histo-freezer canister. The applicator tip is placed on the lesion and the imethyl ether passes through the hollow core of the applicator and freezes the target tissue. More extensive tank units are available for more complex procedures. The tank units have a pistol-type adaptor with stainless steel tips of various sizes.

Laser Surgery

Laser is an acronym for Light Amplification by Stimulated Emission of Radiation. The laser instrument converts light into a very intense beam. By focusing the laser beam onto the target, the application can be extremely precise without damaging surrounding tissue. Over the past two decades, laser surgery has become less expensive, more readily available, and consequently much more widespread as a treatment of choice for surgery in dermatology, ophthalmology, and plastic surgery. Most specialty surgery is now using laser in various ways. With the advent of many physicians utilizing laser technology in the ambulatory care setting, the medical assistant must be familiar with the dangers involved with laser surgery and safety precautions must be implemented. Attending a laser education and safety workshop is recommended for all personnel intending to work with lasers.

The following precautions are designed to heighten awareness and serve as a safety guide:

- When the laser beam is focused on the target tissue, the cells explode and vaporize. Care should be taken not to inhale the vapors.

- Whenever high levels of electricity are used, care should be taken to avoid burns and to assure that the equipment is always in good working order.

- Safety glasses should be worn by the physician, medical assistant, and, if possible, the patient.

- The patient should not have the skin prepared with flammable products such as alcohol-based antiseptics.

- Sterile water should be readily available to extinguish any fire if the beam accidently ignites cloth or paper in the area.

SUTURE MATERIALS AND SUPPLIES

Suture/Ligature

The word **suture** can be used as a verb to describe the motion of sewing or as a noun to describe the material—the thread—used to sew. Suturing, or sewing, a wound is a common procedure in physicians' offices. The purpose is to **approximate**, or bring together the edges of a wound. Suturing hastens healing and lessens scarring. Whether the wound is an accidental laceration or a surgical incision, the suturing process is basically the same. When thread is used for tying (e.g., ends of blood vessels during surgery) rather than sewing, it is termed **ligature**. The terms *suture* and *ligature* both refer to thread, but they are named according to their uses.

Most suture material, or thread, used in minor surgical procedures comes already fused, or **swaged**, to a needle and packaged in various lengths (see Figure 19-2). Eighteen inches is a preferred length because it is short enough to be manageable yet long enough to complete most suturing procedures. Combinations of sizes and types of suture materials and sizes and shapes of needles are endless, but most physicians will use a select few. Selection of the many different suture materials and needles is based on size, strength, and purpose. Suture ranges in size on a scale from the smallest gauge below 0 (aught) to the

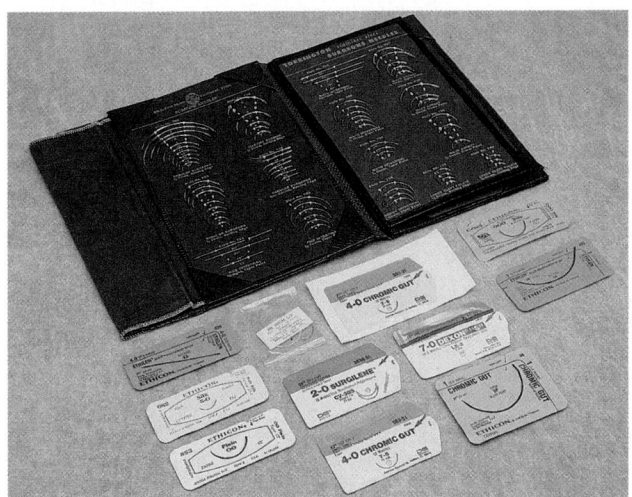

Figure 19-2　Top case displays a variety of curved and straight surgical needles. Bottom packages display a variety of prepackaged suture materials with needles of various sizes and shapes.

largest gauge above 0. The scale from 6-0 to 4 includes all sizes from the smallest to the largest:

6-0, 5-0, 4-0, 3-0, 2-0, 0, 1, 2, 3, 4

Sometimes 2-0 is labeled 00, 3-0 labeled 000, 4-0 labeled 0000, and so on.

If the tissue being sutured is delicate, as on the face or neck, the smaller suture material is used; the finer the stitch, the less scarring. Some sutures are made from materials that dissolve when they come in contact with the tissue enzymes. These are referred to as absorbable sutures. Surgical gut (also called cat gut) is made from sheep intestinal tissue. Left "natural" or uncoated, it is called plain gut suture and will dissolve or be absorbed in about one to two weeks. If more time is needed to heal, surgical gut may be coated with chromion salts. It is then called chromion gut and allows for a longer period of healing to take place before dissolving. Absorbable gut suture is used for underlying tissues where removal is not reasonable and areas where suture removal is inconvenient. Individual body chemistries will influence the exact absorption rate of both plain and treated gut suture. (Gut is rarely used now and has been replaced by an artificial absorbable suture called vicryl.) Suture is also made of nonabsorbable materials such as stainless steel, silk, cotton, nylon, and Dacron. Each type of suture material comes in a variety of options such as different colors for ease of visualization, braiding for additional elasticity and strength, and coatings for lubrications and to lessen irritability to tissues.

Suture Needles

The needles swaged to the suture material are also varied (Figure 19-2). In minor office surgery the needles are usu-

ally curved. They are categorized according to size, shape, radius of curve, and type of point. Needles may be termed cutting needles, round taper point needles, or blunt point needles.

INSTRUMENTS

Structural Features

Rarely does the phrase "form determines function" have as much meaning as when discussing surgical instruments. One can almost always correctly imagine function simply by close examination of the instrument's design. Handles designed to be squeezed between the thumb and finger are called "thumb" handles. "Ring" handles are designed for the insertion of the thumb and finger into rings. **Ratchets** are locking mechanisms located between the rings of the handles and are used for locking the instrument closed. Ratchets are designed to close in varying degrees of tightness. Serrations are the crevices etched into the surfaces of the jaws of hemostats, some forceps, and needle holders. The serrations provide a more secure grip during use with slippery tissues without actually puncturing the tissue. For the purposes of puncturing tissue, forceps with teeth are an option. Teeth may be numerous or few but are always sharp and should approximate tightly when the instrument is closed. To help delicate tips match up properly, some thumb instruments may have a guide pin built into the handle. Box-lock is the name given to a special type of hinge found on most ring-handled instruments, especially grasping instruments such as hemostats, forceps, and needle holders. Since the box-lock provides strength and aids in the prevention of warping, most instruments with ratchets also need the box-lock hinge. Other features include prongs, hooks, and loops (Figure 19-3).

Categories and Uses

Several companies publish and distribute large pictoral catalogs of well over 30,000 medical-surgical instruments. A glance through these references shows the many choices available. For ease of discussion, learning, and cataloging, most surgical instruments are placed according to their uses into three basic categories.

Cutting	Scissors and scalpels
Grasping/Clamping	Hemostats, forceps, clamps, and needle holders
Dilating/Probing	Specula, scopes, probes, retractors, and dilators

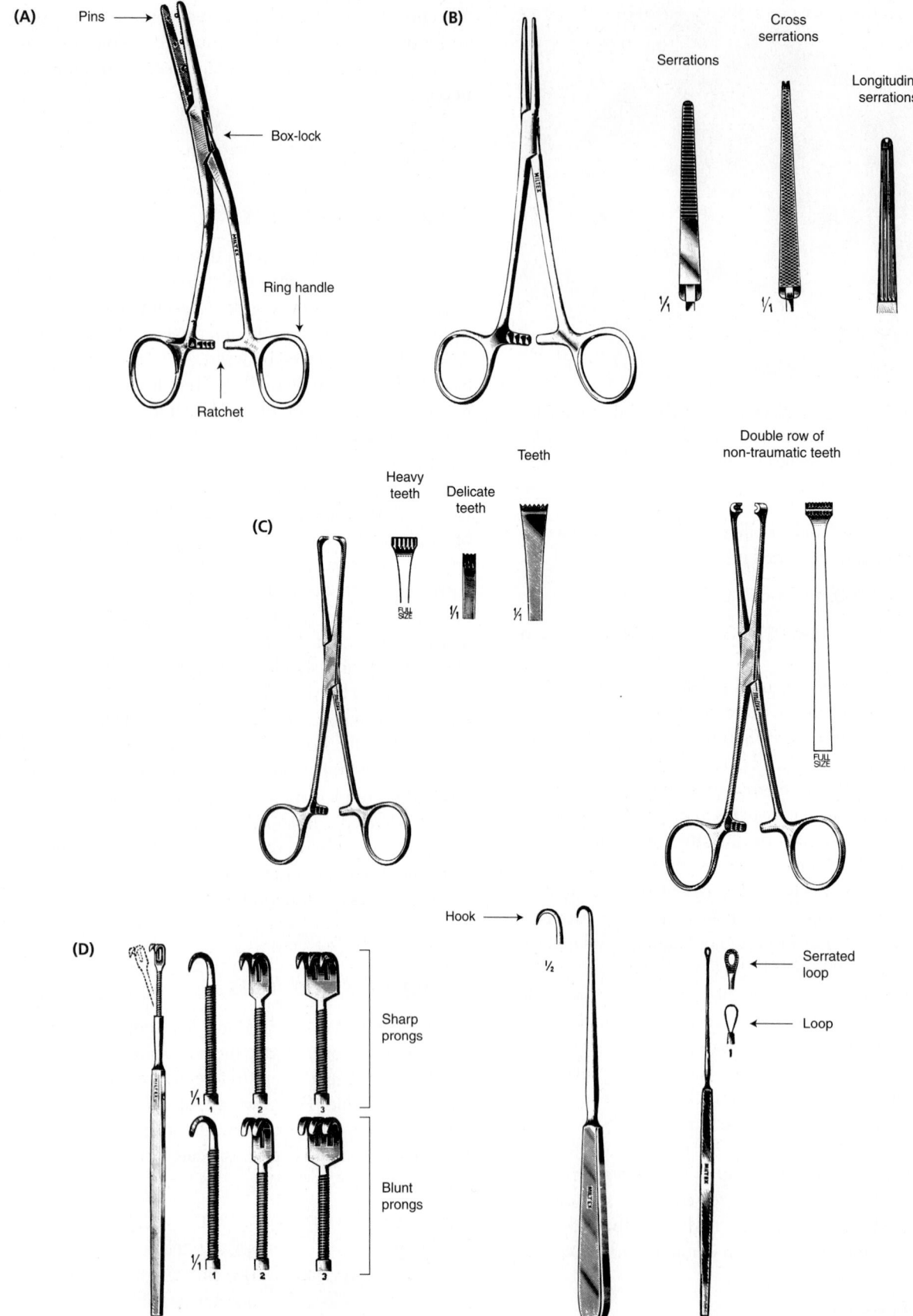

(A) Pins → Box-lock Ring handle Ratchet

(B) Serrations Cross serrations Longitudinal serrations

(C) Heavy teeth Delicate teeth Teeth Double row of non-traumatic teeth

(D) Sharp prongs Blunt prongs Hook → Serrated loop Loop

Figure 19-3 Structural features of instruments include (A) ratchets, box-locks, pins, and ring handle; (B) serrations; (C) teeth; (D) prongs, hooks, and loops. (Courtesy of Miltex Instrument Company, Inc.)

Instruments designed for specific purposes within medical specialties often do not readily fit into any one group and are called specialty instruments. This group includes long-handled gynecological instruments as well as other instruments designed to meet specific needs within specialty practices.

Scissors and Scalpels. Most of the cutting instruments are scissors. Scissors have ring handles, two blades, and vary in size, shape, and function. Because scissors have two blades, the word *scissors* is always plural. Bandage scissors have one rounded tip to allow insertion under a bandage without causing injury to the patient. The two most common styles are the Lister bandage scissors and the finer finger bandage scissors (Figure 19-4).

Operating scissors are used to cut tissues and generally have very sharp blades. The blades may be curved or straight, and the tips may be sharp, blunt, or a combination of each. They are described as sharp/sharp (s/s), blunt/blunt (b/b), or sharp/blunt (s/b) (Figure 19-5A). A special type of scissors, the Mayo dissecting scissors, may be straight or curved, but are never described as sharp or blunt since the tips are specifically designed to be neither but have a beveled edge with slightly rounded points (Figure 19-5B). Very useful, delicately bladed scissors are iris scissors, originally named for usefulness in eye surgery but now widely used in many procedures. Iris scissors may be either curved or straight (Figure 19-6A). Suture scissors, also called stitch or stitch removal scissors, have a distinctively

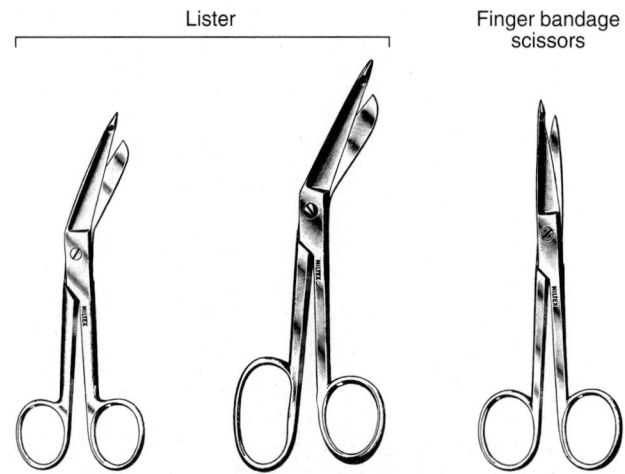

Figure 19-4 Bandage scissors: (A) Lister bandage scissors, small. (B) Lister bandage scissors, large, with one large finger ring. (C) Knowles finger bandage scissors, straight. (Courtesy of Miltex Instrument Company, Inc.)

notched blade to facilitate the insertion of one tip under a suture (Figure 19-6B).

Another common instrument in the cutting category is the scalpel. The scalpel is actually a blade secured to a handle which, when combined, becomes a surgical knife or scalpel. Disposable one-piece units are also available. The most common blade sizes are #10, #11, and #15, with #11 often referred to as a "stab blade" due to its sharp point (Figure 19-7A). Handles vary in size but the most popular are the sturdy #3 and #3L (long) and the more delicate #7 (Figure 19-7B).

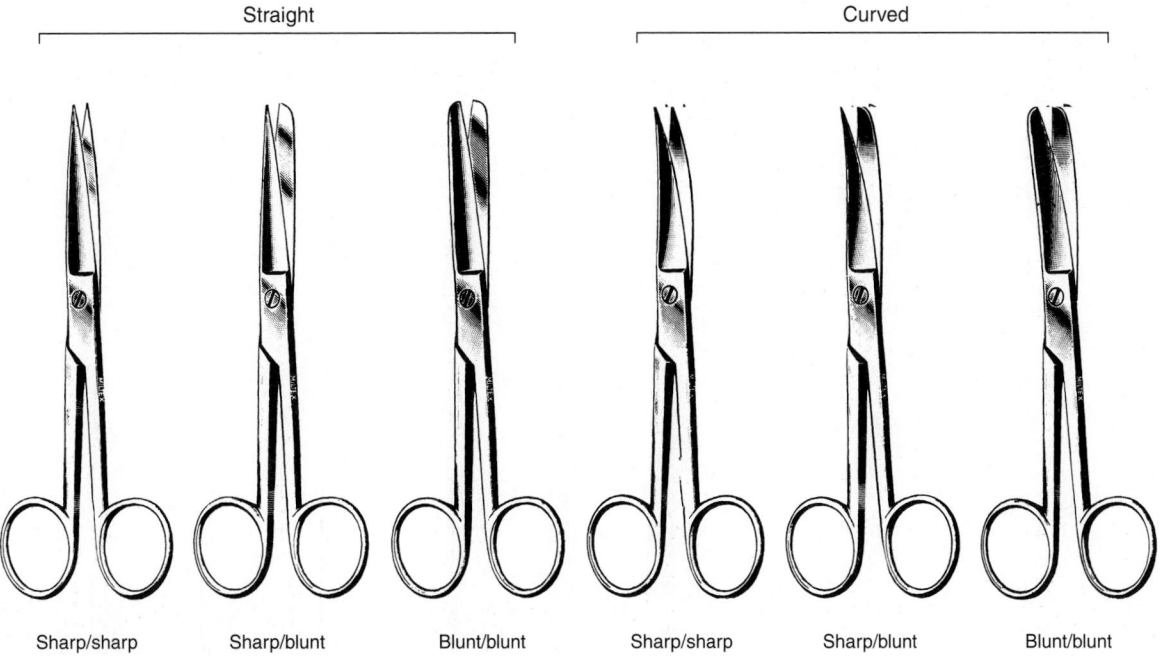

Figure 19-5A   Standard operating scissors. (Courtesy of Miltex Instrument Company, Inc.)

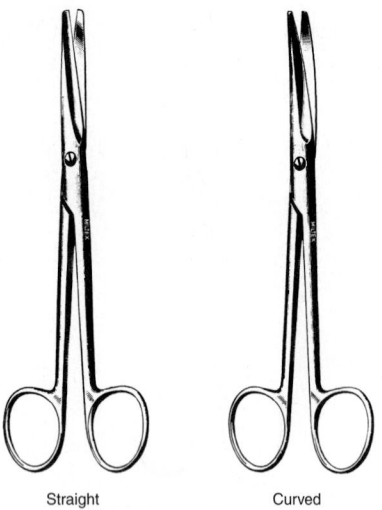

Figure 19-5B   Mayo dissecting scissors. (Courtesy of Miltex Instrument Company, Inc.)

Hemostats, Forceps, Clamps, and Needle Holders. Grasping and clamping instruments are the largest of the instrument categories. These instruments are used for many different tasks. Included in this category are the towel clamps or clips, needle holders, and forceps. Forceps designed to hold tissue often have teeth and serrations in order to grasp firmly. Many forceps also have locking mechanisms called ratchets. Forceps may have ring handles or use a squeeze concept like a tweezer. Forceps number in the hundreds, but most offices need only a select few. Like the word *scissors*, the word *forceps* is always plural. Hemostatic forceps, or hemostats, are used to grasp and clamp blood vessels. Their name means literally to "stop blood." Since blood vessels are slippery, hemostatic forceps have serrations for grasping and ratchets for locking tightly. Mosquito hemostatic forceps have fine tips, with serrations along the entire length of the tips. The Kelly hemostats

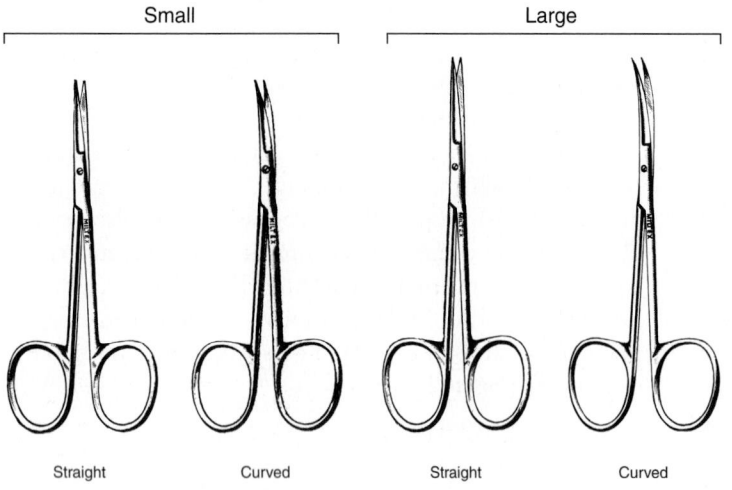

Figure 19-6A   Iris scissors. (Courtesy of Miltex Instrument Company, Inc.)

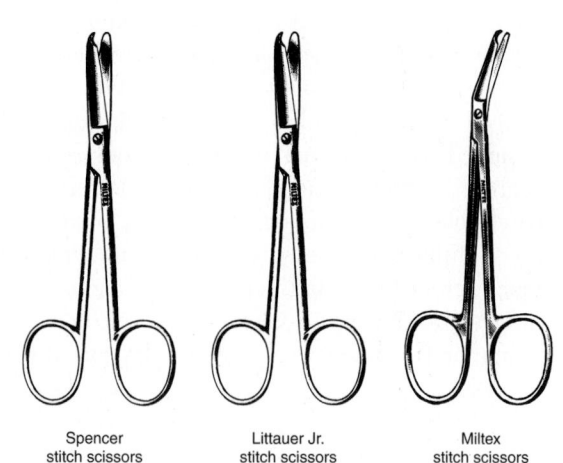

Figure 19-6B   Suture or stitch scissors. (Courtesy of Miltex Instrument Company, Inc.)

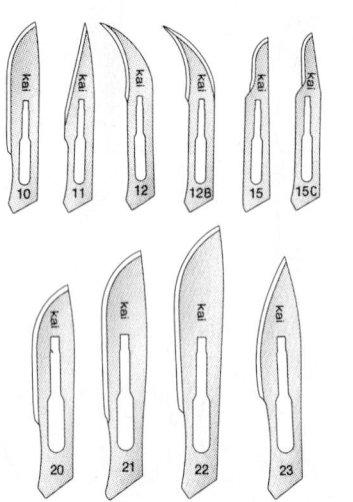

Figure 19-7A   Surgical blades: #10, #11, #12, #12B, #15, #15C, #20, #21, #22, and #23. (Courtesy of Miltex Instrument Company, Inc.)

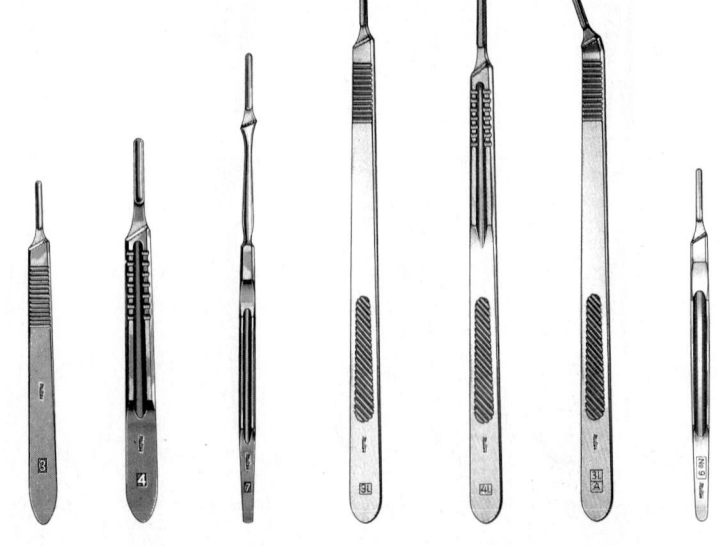

Figure 19-7B   Scalpel handles: #3, #4, #7, #3L, #3LA (angled), and #9. (Courtesy of Miltex Instrument Company, Inc.)

have serrations only along partial length of the tips. Both the Kelly and Crile hemostatic forceps are sturdier, and the Rochester Ochsner hemostatic forceps have teeth. All types may be straight or curved (Figure 19-8).

Allis tissue forceps are of a similar design to hemostatic forceps but have unique angular jaws with teeth. Another type of grasping instrument are thumb forceps, sometimes referred to as "pick-ups." Thumb forceps do not have ring handles or ratchets but are more like the common tweezers. Thumb forceps with teeth are called tissue forceps because of their ability to grasp tissue. Dressing forceps do not have teeth and are very useful for dressing wounds and applying sterile skin closure strips. Dressing forceps are also used to insert sterile gauze packing strips into wounds to facilitate drainage. The Adson, a special type of thumb forceps, is easily differentiated by the shape. Adsons may have teeth or be plain.

The Lucae bayonet-type forceps, used in nose and ear procedures, have a thumb handle and are curved to allow the simultaneous use of other instruments and scopes and to facilitate viewing. In contrast, the Hartman ear forceps, Duckbill ear alligator-type forceps, and the Hartman nasal dressing forceps have ring handles but also are bent for ease in ear and nose procedures. See Figure 19-9 for examples of each.

Splinter forceps do not have teeth and are used for pulling splinters. Many splinter forceps such as the plain splinter forceps and the Walter are of the thumb-handled style, but the Physician's splinter forceps have ring handles and the Virtus have a spring-type handle (Figure 19-10).

Sponge forceps such as the Foerster may have rings on the tips and, as the name implies, are used to hold surgical gauze sponges. The sponge forceps may have long handles making them very useful for gynecological procedures and are then called uterine sponge forceps. Many medical offices will use the uterine sponge forceps as transfer forceps (Figure 19-11). See Basic Surgery Setup also in this chapter.

Towel clamps are used to attach surgical field drapes to each other and in some situations, such as when bisecting the vas deferens in a vasectomy, to clamp onto dissected tissue. In the case of a vasectomy, the Backhaus towel clamp is used to hold the dissected section of the vas deferens (Figure 19-12).

Needle holders are ratcheted instruments similar to hemostats but with a wider and more stout jaw. Often called needle drivers, they are designed to hold the needle firmly without crushing it. Most needle holders have a vertical ditch in the center of the jaw to disperse tension and help prevent slipping of the needle. Needle holders such as the Crile-Wood may have a special groove in which to place the needle during suturing. Some needle holders come equipped with a cutting edge which eliminates the need for a separate scissors to cut the suture material (Figure 19-13).

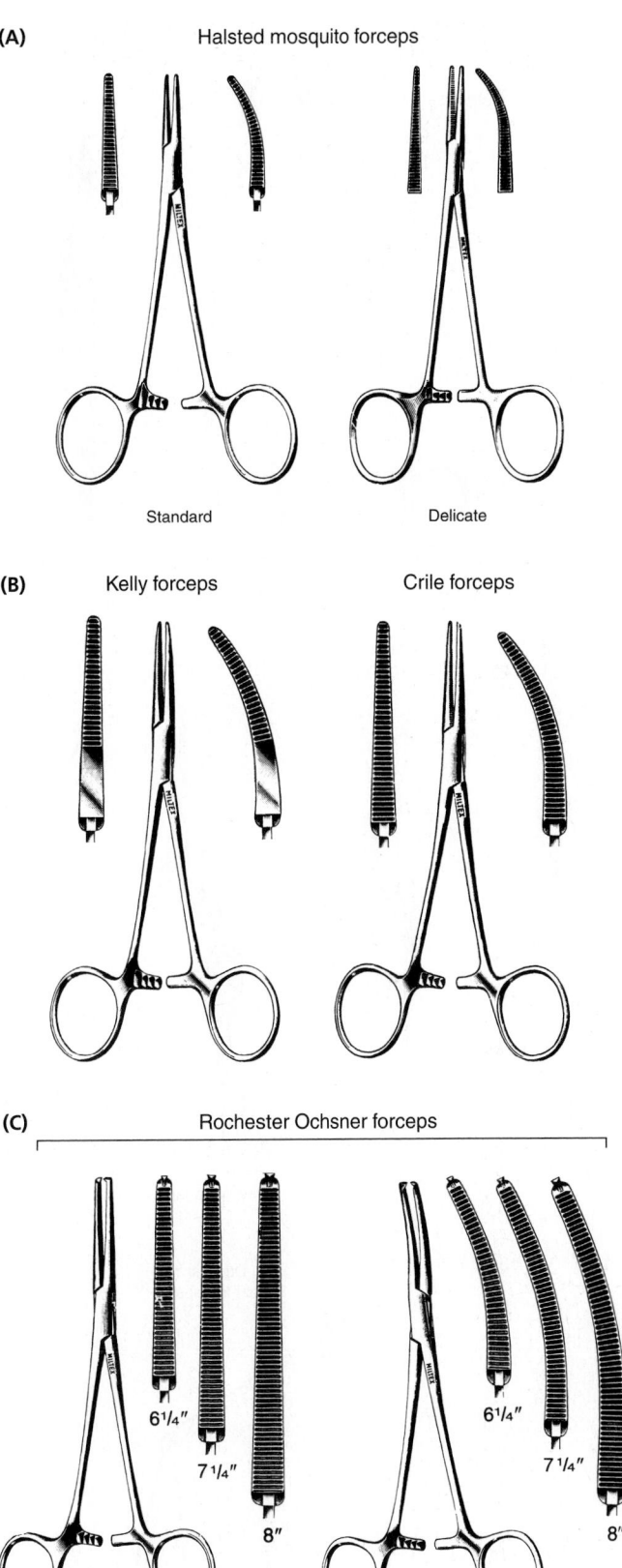

Figure 19-8 Hemostatic forceps include (A) Halsted mosquito forceps; (B) Kelly and Crile forceps; (C) Rochester Ochsner forceps. (Courtesy of Miltex Instrument Company, Inc.)

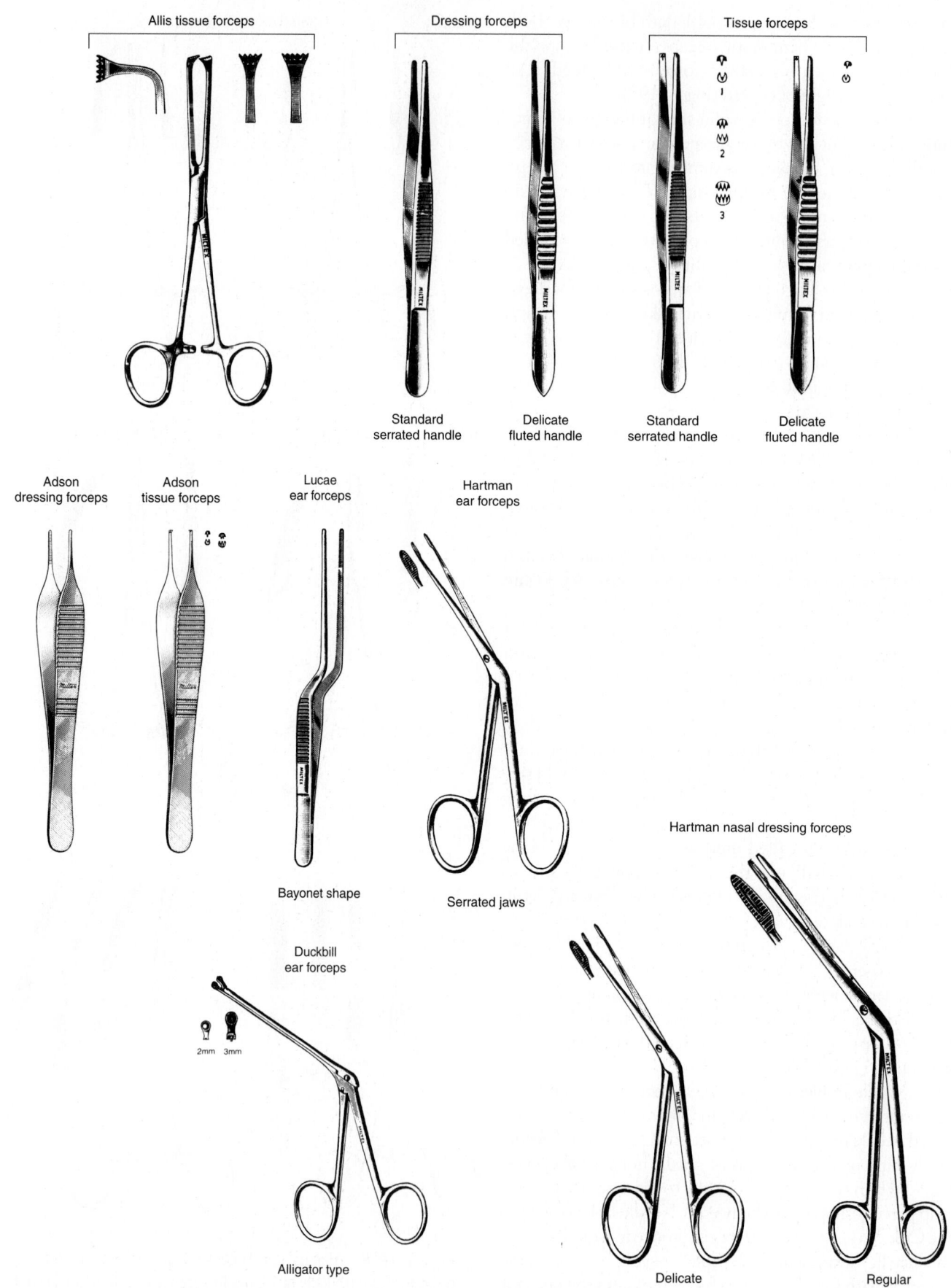

Figure 19-9 Tissue and dressing forceps. (Courtesy of Miltex Instrument Company, Inc.)

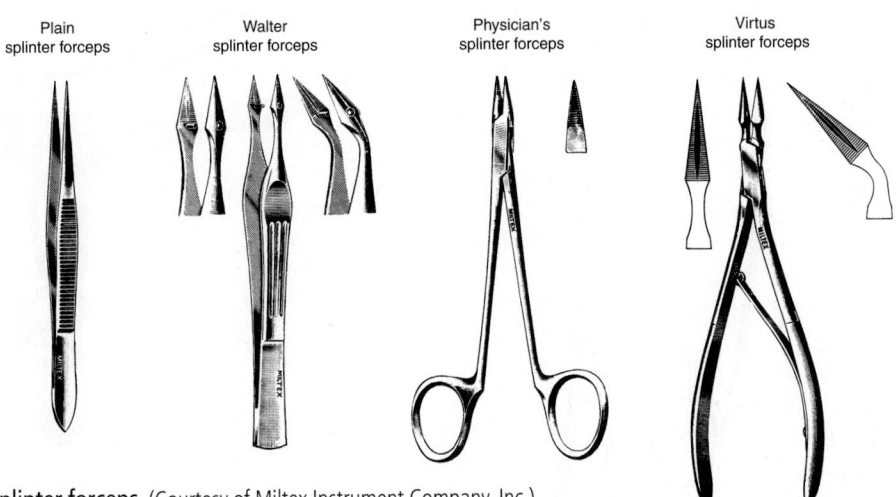

Figure 19-10 Splinter forceps. (Courtesy of Miltex Instrument Company, Inc.)

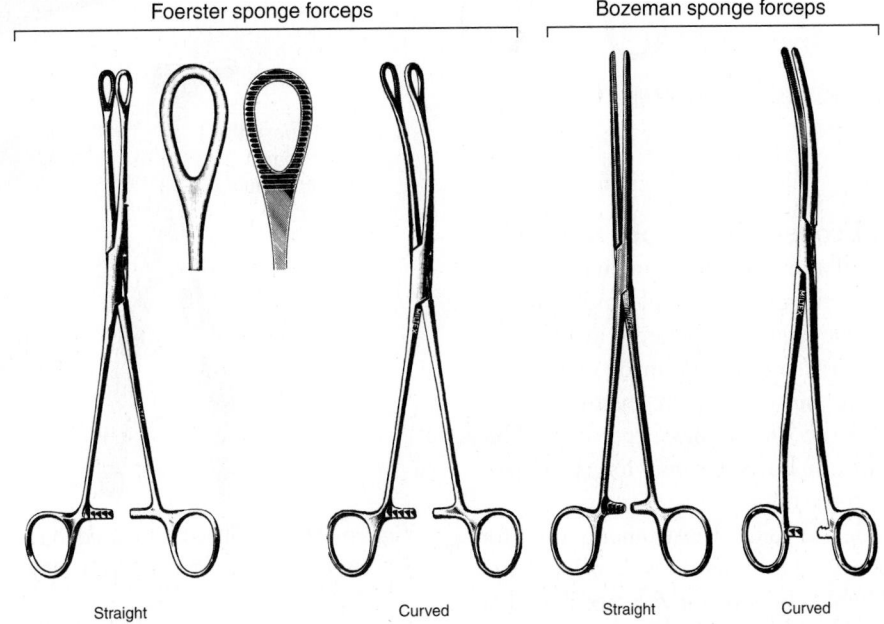

Figure 19-11 Sponge forceps. (Courtesy of Miltex Instrument Company, Inc.)

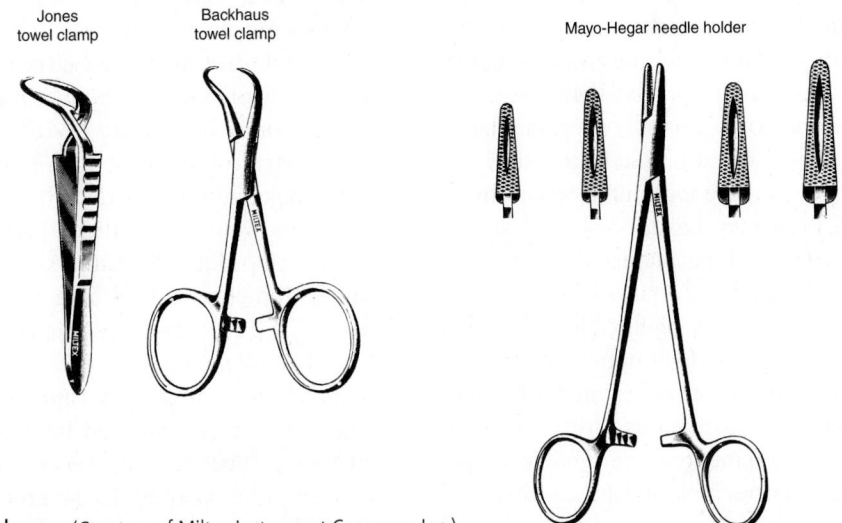

Figure 19-12 Towel clamps. (Courtesy of Miltex Instrument Company, Inc.)

Crile-Wood needle holder   Olsen-Hegar needle holder

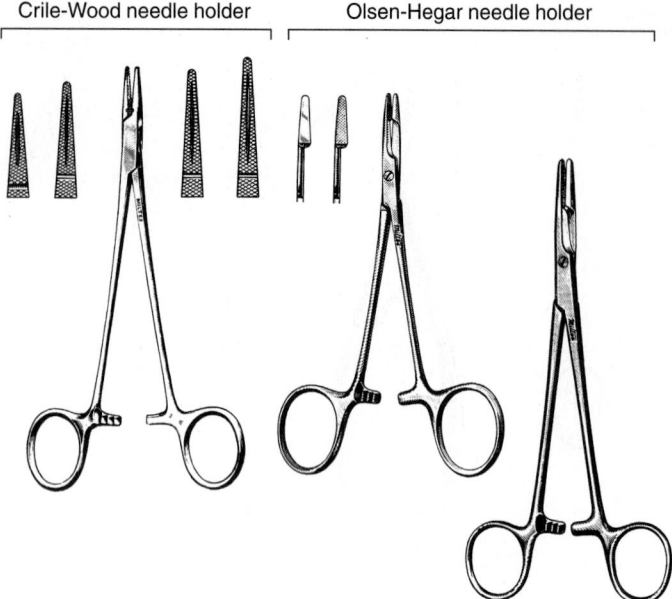

Figure 19-13 Needle holders. (Courtesy of Miltex Instrument Company, Inc.)

Specula, Scopes, Probes, Retractors, and Dilators.

The category of dilators and probes includes specula which are designed for enlarging and exploring body orifices (Figure 19-14). The vaginal speculum is available in various lengths and widths and may be made of metal or disposable plastic. The most common instrument for enlarging the nostril is the Vienna nasal speculum. This instrument is used with the Lucae bayonet forceps to perform procedures within the nose.

Scopes are defined as lighted instruments used for viewing. The otoscope, used to visualize the ear canal and eardrum, has a small light aimed into an ear speculum. Ear specula may be disposable or reuseable. If reused, they are sanitized, chemically disinfected, rinsed, and dried before reuse. Proctoscopes, anoscopes (Figure 19-15), and rigid sigmoidoscopes are used for viewing the rectum, anus, and the sigmoid portion on the large intestine and have guides called obturators to ease insertion. The light source for the proctoscopes and anoscopes is usually a separate lamp. Although the light sources cannot be sterilized, they can be meticulously disinfected. The speculum portion that is inserted into the rectum may be disposable plastic or made of metal. Both the metal speculum and its obturator may be sanitized and sterilized in the autoclave.

There is another group of long flexible scopes that are much more complex and use fiber-optic light sources. Fiber-optic scopes are considered to be medical equipment rather than surgical instruments. Although considered to be medical equipment, these flexible scopes are inserted into body cavities and must be sanitized and sterilized.

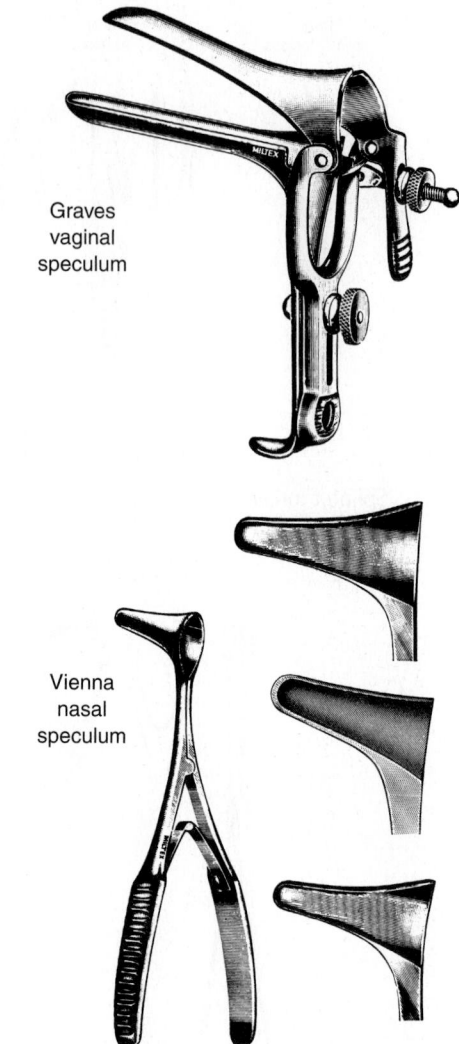

Graves vaginal speculum

Vienna nasal speculum

Figure 19-14 Specula are used to explore body canals. (Courtesy of Miltex Instrument Company, Inc.)

Probes are slender instruments used to probe into a hidden area, body cavity, or wound. Sounds are long, slender probing instruments used to determine the size and shape of the area being probed or to detect the presence of an unseen foreign body. Sounds may be calibrated in centimeters or inches (Figure 19-16).

Retractors used in minor surgery are often called skin hooks and are used to hook onto and retract the edges of a wound to facilitate better viewing. Skin hooks are fine-tipped and delicate. As with all of the finer surgical instruments, special care should be taken to avoid damaging the delicate tips (Figure 19-17).

Dilators are double-ended metal rods with smooth rounded tips, ranging in calibrated sizes from small to large. Dilators are inserted into narrowed or constricted ducts and tubes for the purpose of gradually dilating or enlarging the opening. Hegar uterine dilators are used to dilate the cervix to gain access to the inside of the uterus.

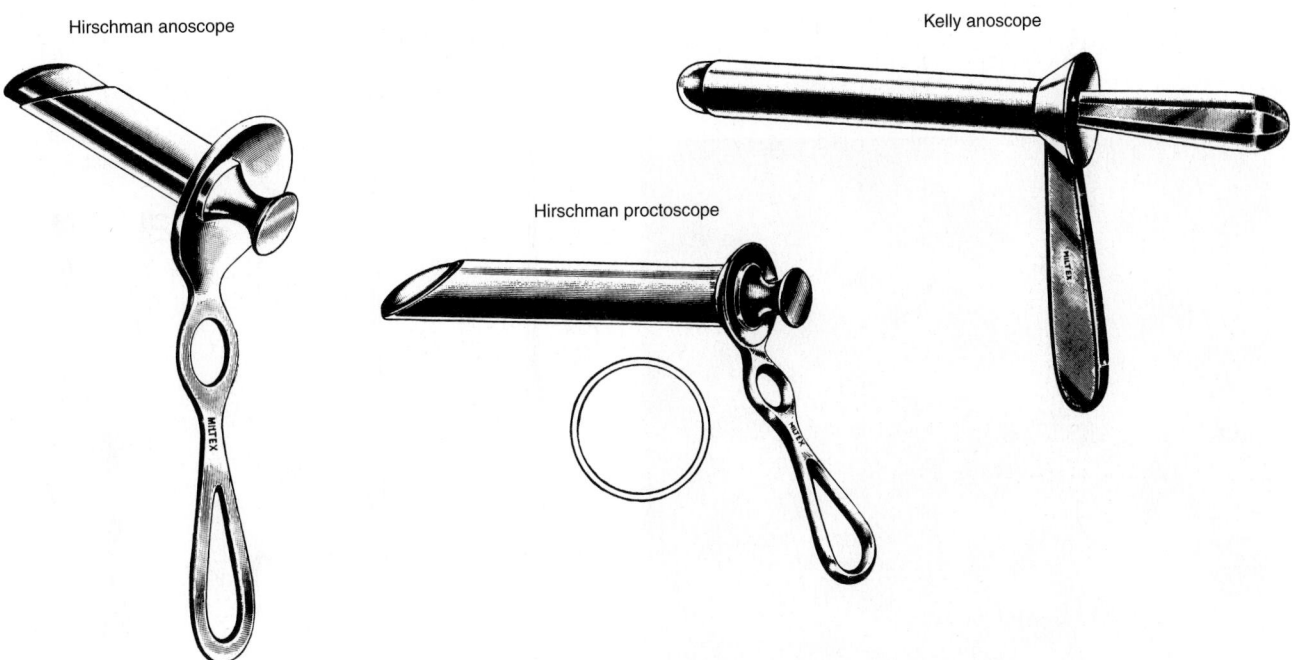

Hirschman anoscope

Kelly anoscope

Hirschman proctoscope

Figure 19-15 Scopes are used for viewing body orifices. (Courtesy of Miltex Instrument Company, Inc.)

Larry probe, groved director

Pratt rectal probe

Walther urethral sound

Sims uterine sound (maleable)

Volkman retractors

Miltex skin hooks

½

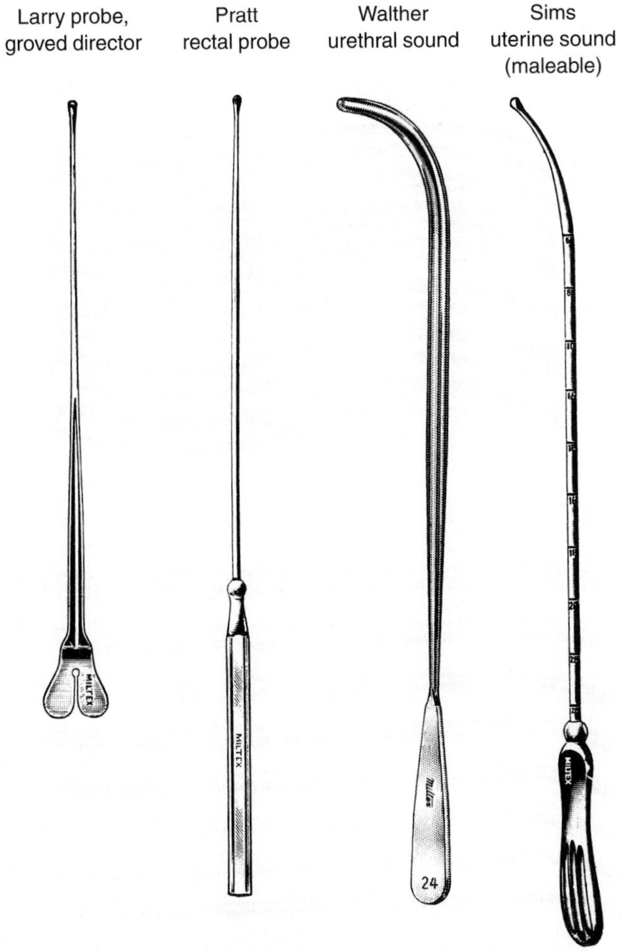

Figure 19-16 Various types of probes and sounds. (Courtesy of Miltex Instrument Company, Inc.)

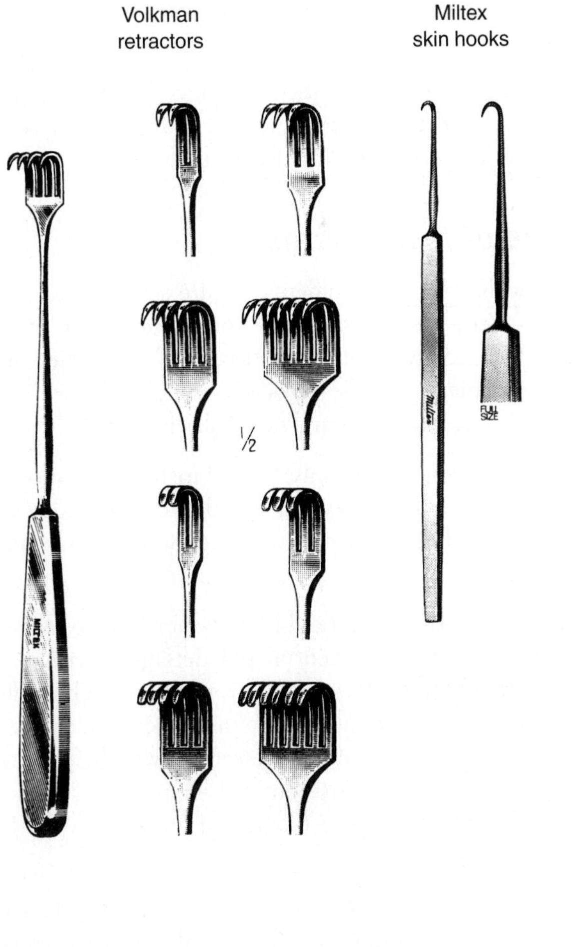

Figure 19-17 Various types of retractors. (Courtesy of Miltex Instrument Company, Inc.) (*continues*)

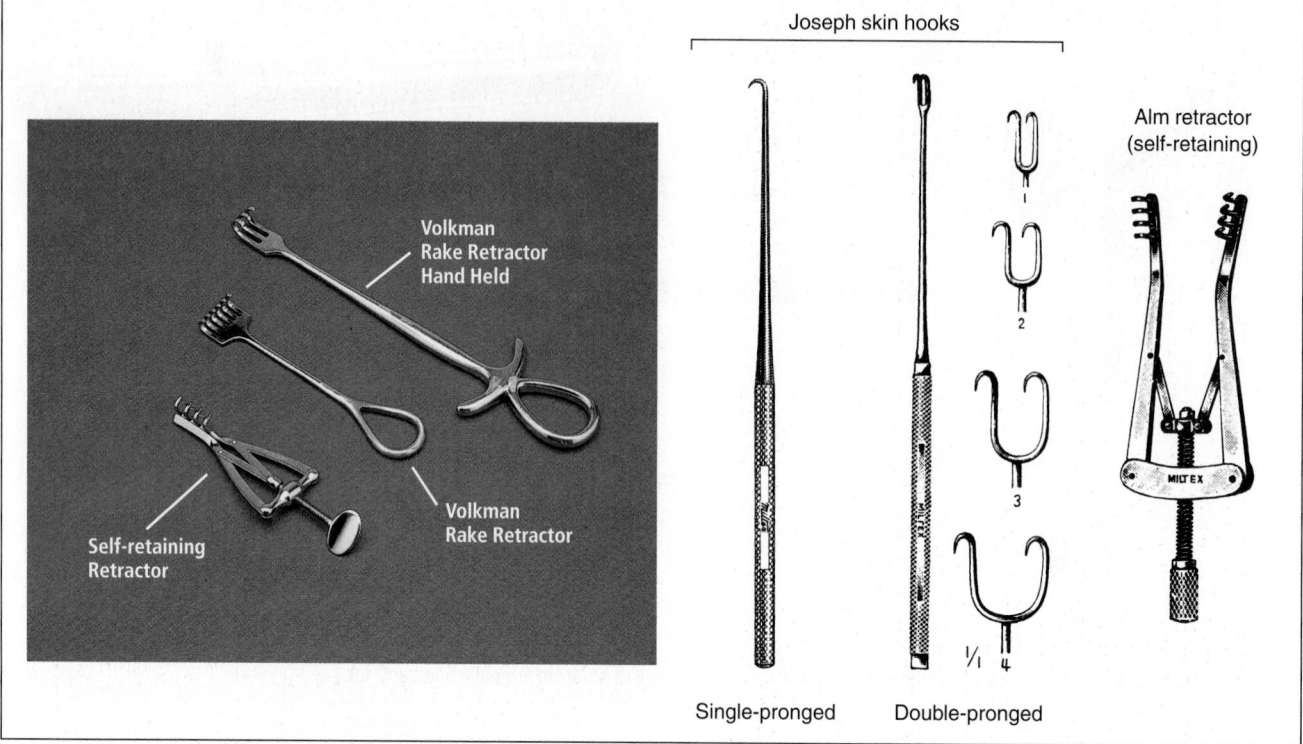

Figure 19-17   Various types of retractors. (*continued*)

Esophageal dilators are used to relieve **strictures**, or narrowing, of the esophagus. Urethral dilators are used to relieve strictures of the urethra (Figure 19-18).

Care of Instruments

Medical/surgical instruments require special care to prevent excessive wear and tear and unnecessary damage. Careful and frequent inspections will determine when instruments need to be replaced or repaired.

Some basic rules and rationales include:

- Immediately after use, soiled instruments should be soaked. This prevents blood and other body fluids from drying onto the working surfaces of the instruments.

- Soak solutions should be about room temperature and contain a neutral pH detergent with a protein/blood solvent. The proteins in the body fluids will not coagulate on the instruments in cool water and the neutral pH detergent will help prevent spotting and corrosion of the metals. Solvents will help break up the blood and proteins in the body fluids.

- Soak basins should be plastic to prevent damaging of points and edges. If a metal soak basin is used, placing a towel on the bottom as padding will help prevent damage to the instruments.

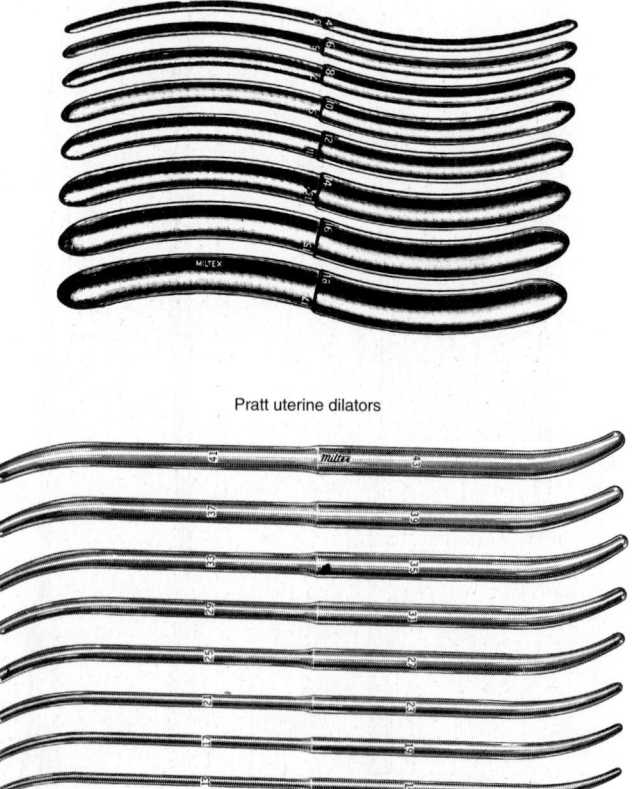

Figure 19-18   **Two types of dilators.** (Courtesy of Miltex Instrument Company, Inc.)

- Heavy-duty rubber gloves should be worn when cleaning instruments to lessen the likelihood of being stuck or cut with the sharp points and edges.

- Delicate instruments should be separated from heavier instruments to prevent the delicate instruments from being bent or otherwise damaged.

- Sharp instruments should be carefully separated from the other instruments and washed with extreme caution. The danger of being cut or punctured is greater when cleaning sharp instruments than at most other times and the sharp instruments are usually the most contaminated.

- A soft bristle brush should be used to scrub hinges, ratchets, and serrations. The brush should be firm enough to clean crevices thoroughly yet soft enough to prevent scratching instruments.

- Immediately after sanitization, instruments should be thoroughly rinsed and dried to prevent spotting and water damage.

- Carefully inspect all surfaces, edges, and points. Check for nicks, dulling, and warping. Test blades for sharpness. Be sure the instrument is not bent or pitted. Handles should also be checked for nicks that may snag and tear surgical gloves, thus disrupting the protective barrier and causing contamination.

- Damaged or malfunctioning instruments should be repaired or replaced.

Ultrasonic Cleaning. Surgical instruments can be cleaned (sanitized) by using an ultrasonic cleaner. Instruments are placed into a tank of water and detergent. Sound waves vibrate to loosen debris and contaminants. Place instruments with ratchets or hinges into the cleaner in an open position. The articles, when finished, are rinsed well, dried, and wrapped for sterilization. The process of sanitizing contaminated instruments by ultrasound is safe for all instruments including delicate instruments. Follow manufacturer's directions for use and care of the ultrasonic cleaner.

Sanitization by use of an ultrasonic cleaner eliminates cleaning instruments by hand, thereby reducing the risk of contamination to the medical assistant.

- Instruments should be processed in the cleaner for the full recommended cycle time—usually 5 to 10 minutes.

- Place instruments in open position into the ultrasonic cleaner. Make sure that "sharps" (scissors, knives, osteotomes) blades do not touch other instruments.

- All instruments have to be fully submerged.

- Do not place dissimilar metals (stainless, copper, chrome plated) in the same cleaning cycle.

- Change solution frequently—at least as often as the manufacturer recommends.

- Rinse instruments with water after ultrasonic cleaning to remove ultrasonic cleaning solution.

Chemical "Cold" Sterilization

This type of sterilization is sometimes referred to as "cold" sterilization which indicates that heat-sensitive items such as fiber-optic endoscopes and delicate cutting instruments can be immersed in a chemical solution. The chemicals used are reliable and capable of destroying bacteria and their spores and, used in strict accordance with the manufacturer's instructions regarding length of immersion time, sterility can be assured.

See Procedure 19-11. Also, see Chapter 10 for disinfection and sanitization procedures.

SUPPLIES AND EQUIPMENT

The supplies necessary for minor office surgery are often disposable and should be replenished as needed. Most medical/surgical supply companies have catalogs available for ordering and many companies have sales representatives who make regular stops or are available by telephone to assist in the ordering process. Sales representatives are familiar with the products their company markets and are extremely useful as a resource. Samples of new products are often available for trial, and optional choices are always offered. Medical/surgical supply companies frequently offer special prices for larger quantity purchases. If a medical/surgical supply item is being used frequently and storage space is available, buying in larger quantities might be more cost-effective. If a product currently being used is not meeting expectations, requesting optional trial products is usually the first step toward finding a better product. Following are some of the more commonly used supplies associated with minor surgery.

Sponges and Wicks

Surgical sponges are prepackaged squares of folded gauze used in surgery. Within the physician's office, sponges are more often referred to by their size. A gauze square measuring four inches by four inches is called a 4×4 (Figure 19-19). The other most useful sizes are 3×3 and 2×2. The 4×4s are either packaged in individual peel-apart packages of two or may be purchased in nonsterile bulk packages of one hundred. The individual packages are

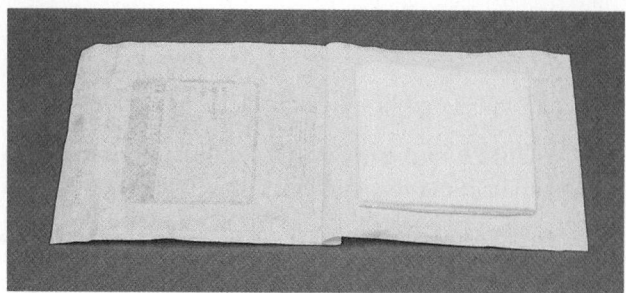

Figure 19-19 Peel-apart sterile open package of 4 × 4 gauze. These are also referred to as 4 × 4s or, in surgery, as surgical sponges.

convenient, sterile, and very useful for most purposes, but cost more per sponge than the non-sterile bulk packages. For larger surgical needs, the medical assistant may package bulk sponges in a canister and sterilize several sponges for later use (see Chapter 10). Most sponges are simply folded gauze, but some have cotton or rayon pads embedded in them to increase absorption ability and to create a softer texture. The medical assistant using the sponge will probably have a preference among the different types and uses. Gauze sponges are used in wound cleansing, in skin preparation, as absorbable sponges during surgery, as dressings and coverings, and for padding. The ambulatory care setting may prefer to have different sizes and types in stock to meet different needs.

Sterile surgical wicks or wound packing strips are used when an infected wound needs to remain open for drainage. The wicking material is made of narrow strips of gauze packaged in long lengths in opaque glass bottles. The most recognizable trade name is Iodoform®. The bottles are sterile and packaged for multiple-use purposes. Extreme care should be taken to prevent contamination during removal of individual lengths. The bottle is opened using sterile technique, sterile dressing forceps are inserted into the bottle, the strip is cut to the desired length using sterile scissors, and the lid is applied without compromising the sterility of the remaining wicking material in the bottle.

Solutions/Creams/Ointments

Many different soaps and solutions are available and effective as skin cleansers, preoperative scrubs, paints, soaks, and antiseptics. **Betadine®** (povidone-iodine) is a well-known antiseptic and is available as a surgical soap called a "scrub" and as a nonsoap solution for preoperative skin preparation/paint. **Hibeclens®** is another very effective antiseptic that does not have the staining tendencies of iodine. Medical/surgical supply companies will have names and samples of other products. Consideration should be made to cost, effectiveness, ease of use, shelf life, and personal preferences. **Isopropyl alcohol**, a 70 percent alcohol solution, is of limited medical/surgical use although due to its rapid volatility rate and its ability to dissolve oils, it is still preferred for skin preparation prior to injections and venipuncture. Isopropyl alcohol is available in bottles for use with cotton/rayon balls or in convenient individually packaged pledgets. Isopropyl alcohol can be irritating and is not effective as a preoperative skin preparation. **Hydrogen peroxide** is a noncaustic mildly effective skin antiseptic. It bubbles on contact with mucous membranes and other moist skin surfaces, dissolving blood and proteins, and seems to have a mechanical cleansing action. Hydrogen peroxide is ineffective as a skin prep prior to surgery but is useful for cleaning after surgery.

Antibacterial creams and ointments are sometimes applied topically on wounds to aid healing. Antibacterial creams are usually white, water-based, and nongreasy. Antibacterial ointments are usually clear and oil based. If a wound requires thorough cleaning between dressing changes, an antibacterial cream is preferred due to the ease of removal.

Some examples of sterile solutions are sterile saline, sterile distilled water, and Betadine® solution.

Dressings and Bandages

Dressings are defined as the sterile material applied directly onto the surface of a wound or surgical site. **Bandages** are defined as the supportive material applied over the top of dressings and are nonsterile. A dressing, being sterile, should be handled with care to avoid contamination of the wound. Often a nonstick pad or topical medication will be applied to the wound to prevent the dressing from adhering to the wound.

Dressings are usually made of gauze and need to completely cover the wound. Dressings must be adequately absorbent.

Bandages are used to keep dressings in place, to provide padding and protection, and to immobilize. Bandaging may consist of rolled gauze wrapped around the wound area with an additional sturdier wrap applied overall. An elastic bandage may provide additional support, and a triangular bandage or sling even more. A unique type of bandage is the tubular gauze bandage. Tubular gauze bandages are used to cover appendages such as fingers, arms, toes, and legs and come in various sizes according to the size of the body part being covered. Refer to Chapter 9 for further information about bandages. See Figure 19-20 for examples and illustrations of various bandage-wrapping techniques.

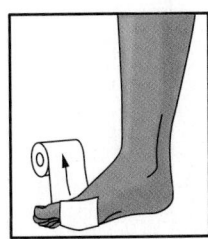

Foot and ankle Use 3-inch width. Hold foot at right angle to leg. Start bandage on ridge of foot just back of the toes.

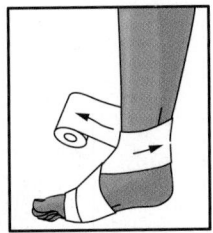

Pass bandage around foot from inside to outside. After two or three complete turns around foot, ascending toward the ankle on each turn, make a figure eight turn by bringing bandage up

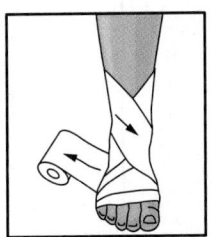

over the arch–to the inside of the ankle–around the ankle–down over the arch–and under the foot.

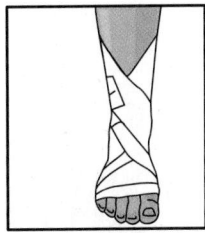

Repeat the figure eight wrapping two to three times. Fasten end by pressing the last 4 to 6 inches of unstretched bandage to the preceding layer.

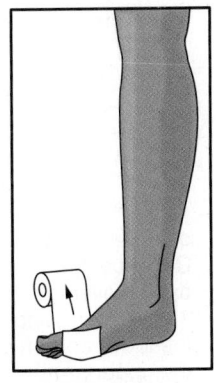

Lower leg: Use 3-4 inch width depending on the size of the leg. A leg wrap requires two rolls of bandage. Hold foot at right angle to leg. Start bandage on ridge of foot just back of the toes.

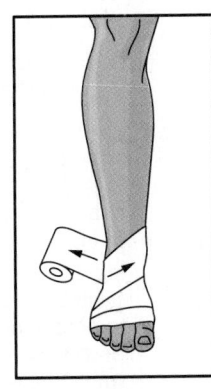

Pass bandage around foot from inside to outside. After two complete turns around foot, make a figure eight turn by bringing bandage up over the arch–to the inside of the ankle– around the ankle–

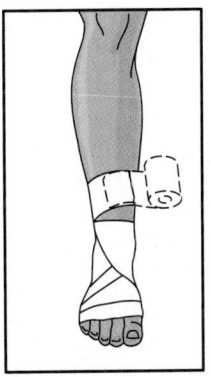

down over the arch–and under the foot. Start circular bandaging, making the first turn around the ankle. To begin the second roll of bandage, simply overlap the unstretched ends by 4 to 6 inches, press firmly, and continue wrapping.

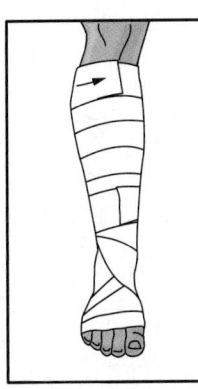

Wrap bandage in spiral turns to just below the kneecap. Fasten end by pressing the last 4 to 6 inches of unstretched bandage to the preceding layer.

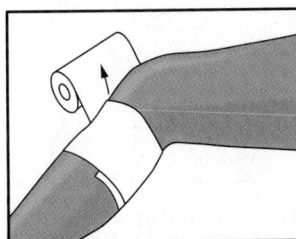

Knee: Use 4 inch width. Bend knee slightly. Start with one complete circular turn around the leg just below the knee.

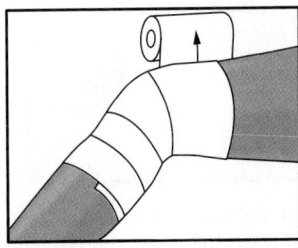

Start circular bandaging, applying only comfortable tension. Cover kneecap completely.

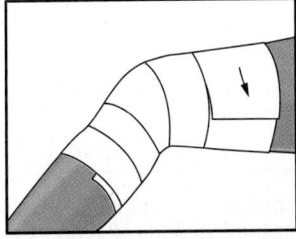

Continue wrapping to thigh just above the knee. Fasten end by pressing the last 4 to 6 inches of unstretched bandage to the preceding layer.

Figure 19-20 Bandage-wrapping techniques illustrating the circular, spiral, and figure-eight turns. The Peg Self-Adhering elastic bandage is used in these illustrations. (Courtesy Becton-Dickinson Division, Becton, Dickinson, and Co., Rutherford, NJ)   *(continues)*

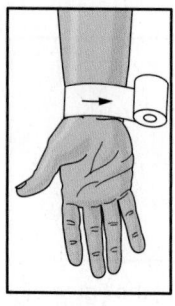 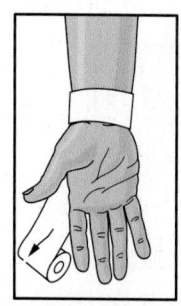 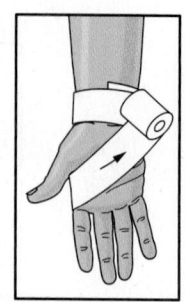 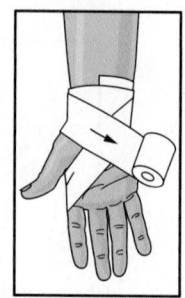 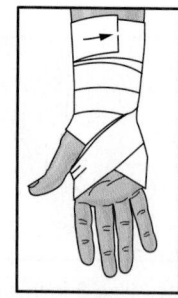

Wrist Use 2- or 3-inch width. Anchor bandage loosely at the wrist with one complete circular turn.

Carry the bandage across the back of the hand, through the web space between the thumb and index finger

and across palm to the wrist, Make a circular turn around

the wrist and once more carry the bandage through the web space and back to the wrist.

Start circular bandaging, ascending to the wrist. Fasten the end by pressing the last 4 to 6 inches of unstretched bandage to the preceding layer.

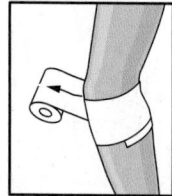 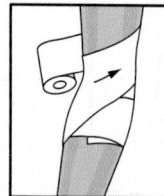 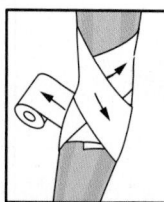 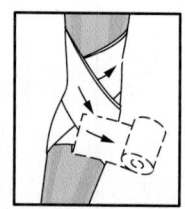 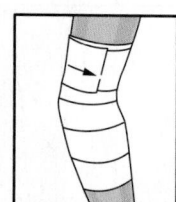

Elbow Use 3- or 4-inch width, depending on the size of the arm. Two rolls of bandage are required to complete the wrap. Start with a complete circular turn just below the elbow.

Wrap bandage in loose figure eights

to form a protective bridge across the front of the elbow joint.

Fasten end by pressing 4 to 6 inches of unstretched bandage to preceding layer. Start second bandage with a circular turn below the elbow

over the first wrap. Continue spiral bandaging over the elbow, ascending to the lower portion of the upper arm. Fasten end with circular turn.

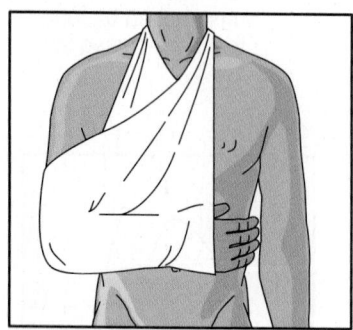 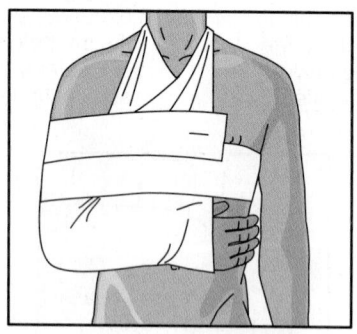 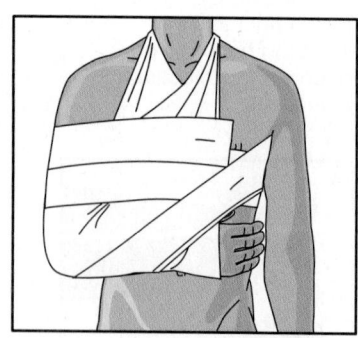

Shoulder A shoulder wrap is used to provide additional support for an arm in a sling. Use 4- or 6-inch width. One or two rolls of bandage may be used. Start under the free arm.

Carry the bandage across the back, over the arm in the sling, across the chest and back under the free arm in complete circular, overlapping turns. Fasten the end by pressing 4 to 6 inches of unstretched bandage to underlying bandage.

Additional support can be obtained with a second bandage. Start at the back just behind the flexed elbow in the sling. Carry the bandage under the elbow, up over the forearm, around the chest and back, and repeat. Fasten end.

Figure 19-20 *(continued)*

Anesthetics

The word **anesthesia** means the loss of feeling or sensation. An anesthetic is any mechanism that causes this loss of feeling. The application of extreme cold can be an anesthetic because it causes numbness to nerve endings and thus the loss of feeling. Anesthetics may be inhaled, topically applied or sprayed, or injected either directly into a vein (intravenously), the spinal column (intrathecally), or locally (subcutaneously) into the tissues at the site of the surgical procedure.

Injectable Anesthetics. Most anesthetics used in minor surgery are administered locally through injection into the subcutaneous tissues. The nerves exposed to the anesthetic become temporarily unable to conduct sensations and feelings to the brain, thereby causing a lack of pain sensation in the area during minor surgery. All synthetic local anesthetics have names that end in "caine." Some of the most common are Xylocaine (lidocaine), Novacaine (procaine), Marcaine, and Carbocaine. Local anesthetics are available in single-dose vials or ampules of 10 mL, but most medical offices prefer the cost-effectiveness of multiple-dose vials containing 30 to 50 mL. Local anesthetics are also available in varying strengths such as 0.5 percent, 1 percent, and 2 percent.

Injectable anesthetics may contain an additive called **epinephrine**. Epinephrine causes vasoconstriction and is used when reduced blood flow to the area is desired. The medical assistant is often delegated the responsibility of filling the syringe with the prescribed amount and strength of the ordered anesthesia or may assist the physician in drawing up the medication.

Drawing Techniques. If the physician plans to inject the anesthesia prior to applying sterile gloves, either the medical assistant or the physician may draw up the medication. The filled syringe is then placed on the side, rather than directly on the sterile field. This allows the physician to anesthetize the patient prior to beginning the sterile procedure. After the anesthesia has taken effect, the physician will perform a surgical handwash, apply sterile gloves, and begin the surgery.

When the physician applies sterile gloves prior to injecting the anesthesia, the sterile syringe may be placed directly on the sterile field either empty or filled. One person wearing sterile gloves may handle the syringe and draw up the medication while another person not wearing sterile gloves holds the vial. This method requires either that the syringe and needle be applied directly to the sterile tray or handed directly to a "sterile" person. Refer to Chapter 24 for the specific techniques for drawing up medications.

Topical Spray Anesthetics. Not all anesthesia is injectable. Topical (applied to the surface) anesthetics are available in liquid and spray. The most common topical anesthetic used in the medical office is ethyl chloride spray. Ethyl chloride freezes the skin to allow for simple piercing or lancing. The anesthetic action usually only lasts for a few seconds; therefore, the procedure must be performed quickly. One example for the use of ethyl chloride spray is to briefly numb an area prior to an injection. A lesion that is infected is extremely painful to inject with a local anesthetic; however, by using ethyl chloride spray before the injection, the patient is able to remain still. Ethyl chloride spray may also be used prior to installing intravenous lines.

See Table 19-2 for a summary of supplies and equipment.

TABLE 19-2	SUPPLIES AND EQUIPMENT COMMONLY USED IN MINOR SURGERY
Item	**Use/Description**
Sponges	Used in wound cleansing, skin preparation, as absorbable sponges during surgery, as dressings and coverings, and for padding. Also called 4 × 4s. Typically made of folded gauze, though some have cotton or rayon pads embedded in them to increase absorption.
Wicks	Used when an infected wound needs to remain open for drainage. Wicking material is made of narrow strips of gauze packaged in long lengths in opaque glass bottles, which should be opened using sterile technique.
Solutions	Used as skin cleansers, preoperative scrubs, paints, soaks, and antiseptics. Most common are Betadine, an antiseptic often used in soap form as a scrub; Hibeclens, an effective antiseptic without iodine's staining properties; isopropyl alcohol, a 70 percent alcohol solution favored for skin preparation prior to injections and venipuncture but not effective as a preoperative skin preparation; hydrogen peroxide, a mildly effective noncaustic skin antiseptic.
Creams and ointments	Antibacterial. May be used topically on wounds to promote healing.
Dressings	Sterile material applied directly onto surface of a wound or surgical site. Usually made of gauze. Must be adequately absorbent and completely cover the wound.
Bandages	Nonsterile supportive materials applied over dressings to keep the dressing in place. May be rolled gauze, elastic bandage, or tubular gauze bandage.
Anesthetics	A mechanism used to cause the loss of feeling. May be inhaled, topically applied, sprayed, or injected directly into a vein, the spinal column, or locally into the tissues at the site of the surgical procedure.

PATIENT CARE AND PREPARATION

Patient Preparation and Education

If the patient is having a planned surgical procedure performed, an opportunity for patient preparation and education is available. Patients may need to modify their diet, adjust medication, acquire special supplies, adjust their personal home and work situations, obtain prior approval from their insurance, and prepare for the postoperative period. If the patient is having an urgent procedure performed, such as a laceration repaired, there is less time for preparation. In either case, the medical assistant will need to follow an established protocol covering wound care, patient education, patient health consideration, and consent. In the case of an accidental wound, the medical assistant needs to determine the cause of the wound and the date of the last tetanus injection. See Chapter 10 for specific information about immunization schedules. The medical assistant must also check to determine whether or not the patient has allergies or sensitivities of any kind, in particular to medication.

Diet modifications include abstaining from eating and/or drinking for several hours prior to the surgical procedure as well as restricting the types and amounts of certain foods or liquids consumed prior to and directly after the procedure. When patients are aware of special dietary needs after surgery, they can shop early and be prepared. An example of a medication treatment includes prescribing an antibiotic to be taken as a precaution against acquiring an infection following surgery or adjusting anticoagulant medications to prevent excessive bleeding during surgery. Each clinic, physician, procedure, and patient will have individual requirements and preferences. The patient might be required to obtain special supplies for the convalescent period. For instance, immediately after a vasectomy a scrotal support is usually recommended. Crutches or special foot coverings might be necessary following foot or leg surgery. Specific wound dressing and bandages might need to be purchased prior to the surgery in anticipation of the postoperative need. Having another person accompany the patient to the clinic for the surgery is required for the safe return home. Knowing the planned period of time for recovery allows the patient to make the necessary arrangements for work, child care, and other personal situations.

Informed Consent

Prior to a surgical procedure, the patient's written consent must be obtained. In many medical and all surgical procedures, a written, informed consent form must be signed. An informed consent is a document that may be created specifically for a particular procedure or that may be an established document available for duplication. An informed consent document informs the patient of the medical or surgical procedure to be performed; describes to the patient, in lay terms, the actual procedure; cites alternative treatments; and lists the possible undesirable outcome and risks involved in the procedure. See Chapter 7 for additional information on informed consent.

The cost of the procedure is also important information. Any questions the patient has about the surgery should be answered completely by the physician and an assessment should be made that the patient understands the answers. Even in the best of circumstances, results cannot be guaranteed. Most of the difficult situations between physicians' practices and patients come from misunderstandings about unexpected outcomes. If patients are informed completely, even unplanned results are better tolerated.

Medical Assisting Considerations

The general health and condition of the patient prior to surgery is very important when planning the recovery. A frail, weak man living alone may need home health care following even a simple surgical procedure. Some people may not be able to follow standard preoperative or postoperative instructions. The recovery may depend on the availability of supplies beyond what the patient can financially afford. If difficult circumstances can be identified prior to the surgery, arrangements can be made with home health care services, community assistance services, or friends and family. This can help avoid complications. Prior medical history should also be established and questions should be asked regarding **allergies** and sensitivities to medications and medical substances.

Postoperative Instructions

Postoperative instructions should be written and clearly understood by the patient. If the patient has a caregiver at home, the postoperative instructions should be clearly understood by the caregiver as well. The telephone number of the clinic and an after-hours number should be written on the postoperative instructions and brought to the attention of the patient and caregiver. It is good practice to plan to call patients within the first postoperative day to check on their condition.

Wounds, Wound Care, and the Healing Process

There are many different types of wounds based on the type of injury incurred. Wounds may be classified as open or closed, accidental or intentional (surgical).

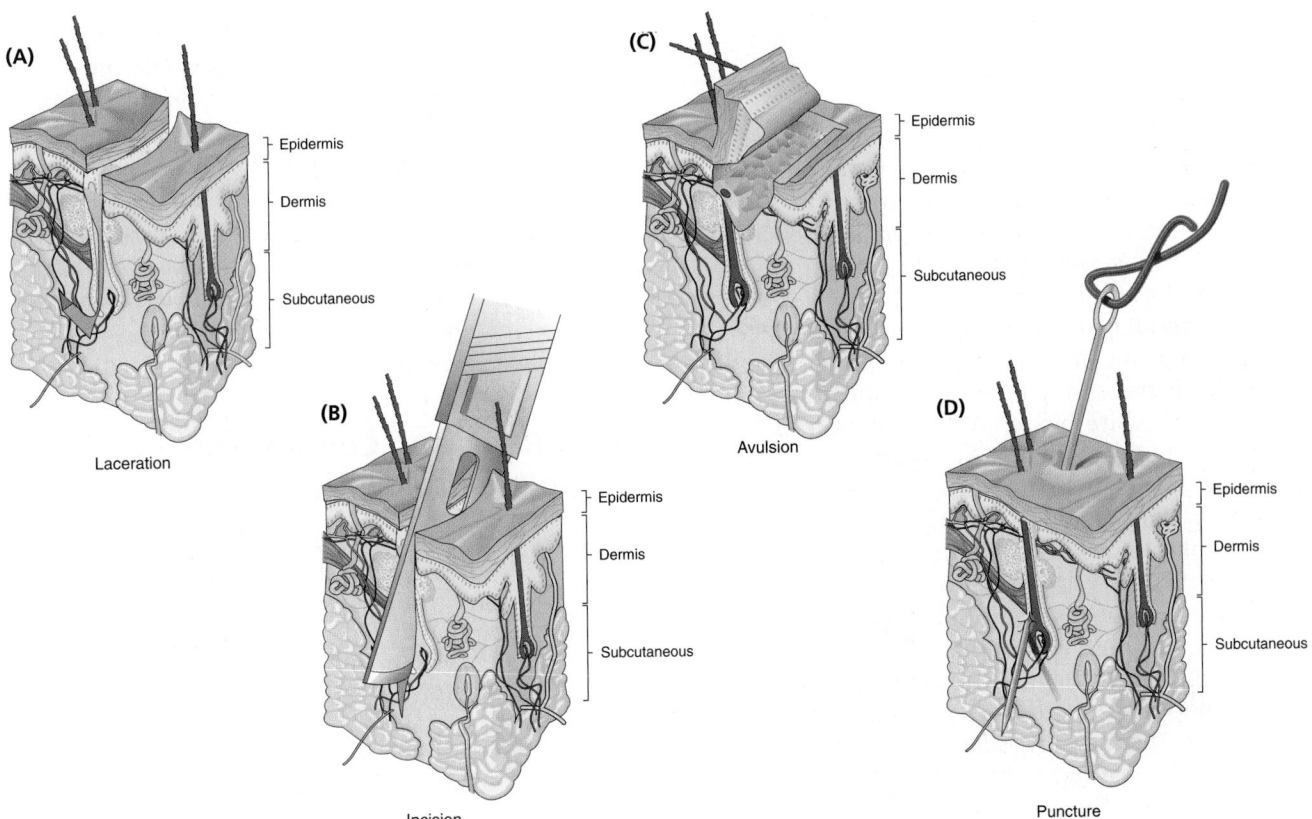

Figure 19-21 Open wounds. (A) Lacerations are accidental tearing of the body tissue usually made by sharp objects. The torn flesh may be smooth or jagged and is usually difficult to clean and suture properly. There is typically extensive bleeding. Paper cuts are examples of lacerations. (B) Incisions are intentional cuts typically made with a scalpel for surgical procedures. (C) Avulsions are accidental tearing away of a part or structures of the skin. (D) Punctures are holes or wounds made by a pointed object and can be either accidental or intentional. Puncture wounds have little bleeding because the point of entry is small. These wounds are typically not much larger than the instrument entering the skin. A puncture wound may also be the result of a bite or a gunshot wound.

Lacerations, incisions, avulsions, and punctures are all examples of open wounds (Figure 19-21). They are a result of tearing or cutting of the skin.

Ecchymosis (bruise), contusion, and hematoma are all examples of closed wounds. They are due to a blunt trauma that damages underlying tissues but leaves the skin intact (Figure 19-22).

Wounds are classified as superficial if the injury does not extend deeper than the subcutaneous tissues. Deep wounds extend beyond the subcutaneous layer. The size and location as well as the depth of the wound are all important descriptors both for the medical record and for proper insurance reimbursement. A typical description of a patient wound that is an intermediate laceration might be, "patient sustained a deep 3.5 cm laceration to the anterior surface of the right knee caused by a fall onto a rock." A puncture wound might be described as, "patient presents with a 2 cm deep puncture wound on the plantar surface of the left foot obtained from stepping on a rusty nail." Both statements describe not only the size, depth, location, and type of wound, but also the causative factor.

Inflammation is the body's natural reaction to trauma. Inflammation is also a normal process of wound healing. Occasionally inflamed tissue will become infected if the trauma is caused by a pathogen. While a certain degree of inflammation is expected, prevention of infection is a primary goal (see Chapter 10).

See Chapter 9 for further description of wounds and emergency care of wounds.

The best treatment for infection is prevention. Instructing the patient about proper wound care is

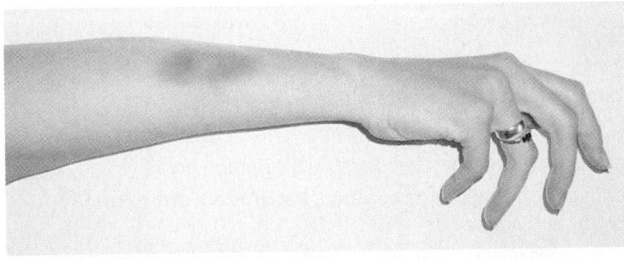

Figure 19-22 Closed wounds include contusions, ecchymoses, and hematomas. This photograph shows an ecchymosis.

Patient Teaching Tip

The basic signs of inflammation are redness, heat, swelling, pain, and loss of function. Any one or more of these may be present in varying intensities during an inflammatory process. Most wounds will have a mild inflammation described as slightly red or pink, mild warmth, slightly tender to the touch, and mildly swollen. The symptoms are caused by increased blood supply to the traumatized area and the infiltration of white blood cells in reaction to the trauma. Patients should be taught to watch for an increase in the intensity of redness, pain, swelling, and heat or any drainage, fever, or lymph gland swelling which indicates an infection from invading pathogens. The patient should be given instructions as to what actions to take if these symptoms of infection are noticed. The instructions should include a name and telephone numbers to call during the day or night. The medical assistant should reassure the patient not to hesitate to contact the center or physician if infection is suspected.

extremely important. Encourage the patient to keep the wound clean and dry. In certain circumstances, the physician may prescribe a warm soak solution or the application of a topical antibacterial medication. Protecting the wound from further trauma and contamination will also aid in the healing process. Opinions will differ on whether a wound is best left open to air or covered with a dressing. Most health care providers will agree that covering a wound is preferred whenever contamination is likely. (See Procedure 19-4.)

BASIC SURGERY SETUP

Preparing for surgery includes assembling supplies and equipment, setting up the surgery tray, getting the patient and room ready, and preparing to assist during surgery. The specific instruments, supplies, and equipment needed for each surgery should be listed on individual **surgery cards**. These cards may be 3×5 or 5×7 cards stored in a card file or full sheets of procedures compiled in a manual or notebook. Each physician will have individual sets for each surgical procedure performed. Information on the surgery card should include physician glove size, standing preoperative and postoperative instructions, and any additional information specific to the physician's needs or to the surgical procedure.

Basic Rules and Concepts for Setup of Surgical Trays

In addition to basic sterile principles, the guidelines in Table 19-3 will help ensure the sterile field remains sterile.

MINOR SURGERY PROCESS

For ease in understanding the individual tasks involved in minor office surgery, Table 19-4 provides generic steps for setting up the surgical tray, preparing the room, preparing the patient, assisting with the surgery, and the cleanup process. Table 19-4 is intended as a quick checklist only and does not include all the specific details necessary for each surgery. Refer to the individual surgical procedures that follow for more details.

PREPARATION FOR MINOR SURGERY

The following section includes the following procedures used in preparation for minor surgery:

- Applying Sterile Gloves (Procedure 19-1)

- Preparation of Patient Skin for Minor Surgery (Procedure 19-12)

- Setting Up and Covering a Sterile Field (Procedure 19-13)

TABLE 19-3 GUIDELINES FOR STERILE TRAY SETUPS
• Set up the sterile surgery tray just prior to the surgery to allow less chance of accidental contamination.
• Immediately after the tray is set up, cover it with a sterile drape.
• Once the tray is prepared and covered, move it directly into the surgery area rather than leaving it in a common area.
• Inform the patient and others in the surgery room that the tray is sterile and should not be touched. Patients are often curious about instruments and may attempt to look under the covers if not cautioned against it.
• If the medical assistant is interrupted while preparing the tray and it becomes necessary to leave the tray unattended, cover the tray and move it out of traffic paths to prevent it from being bumped.

TABLE 19-4 PREPARATIONS FOR MINOR SURGERY

Tray Setup

1. Wash hands.
2. Reference surgery card.
3. Gather equipment and supplies.
4. Sanitize and disinfect Mayo instrument tray.
5. Set up sterile field.
6. Place sterile instruments and supplies on the sterile field.
7. Apply sterile gloves.
8. Arrange instruments and supplies in an organized and logical manner.
9. Medication may be drawn up with assistance (optional).
10. Recheck tray for accuracy and completeness.
11. Remove gloves.
12. Cover and transport tray.
13. Add sterile solution (skin antiseptic) to tray if required.

Room Preparation

In preparing a room for a surgical procedure, all equipment should be clean and in good working order. Be certain to have spare parts such as light bulbs and filters readily available. Turn on equipment prior to the procedure to make sure all is working properly.

1. Check room equipment (light, stool, machinery, examination table, waste receptacle).
2. Check room supplies (tissue, extra gloves, and so on).
3. Arrange accessory supplies on the side counter in a logical order (pathology specimen bottle containing preservative, lab requisition, sterile glove package, dressings/bandages, postoperative medications).

Patient Preparation

1. Wash hands.
2. Greet patient and ensure identity.
3. Escort the patient to the procedure room and offer restroom facilities.
4. Discuss the patient's compliance to preoperative instructions.
5. Explain the procedure again and address any questions.
6. Review postoperative instructions.
7. Check for signed informed consent form.
8. Have the patient remove appropriate clothing and position the patient on the examination table. Offer a drape, gown, pillow, and blanket for comfort.
9. Prepare the skin for the surgical procedure (Procedure 19-12).

Assisting with Minor Surgery

1. Remove the sterile cover from the surgical tray while the physician applies sterile gloves.
2. Assist the physician with stool and lamp adjustment as needed.
3. If the medical assistant did not perform the skin preparation, assist the physician as needed during skin preparation and draping. The equipment and supplies for skin preparation are separate from the surgery tray and equipment (see Procedure 19-12).
4. Adjust the instrument tray and equipment around the physician.
5. Assist with drawing up local anesthetic or other medication as needed.
6. Apply clean gloves for protection or sterile gloves to assist.
7. Surgery begins.
8. The medical assistant either assists with sterile procedure or supports the patient as needed.
9. After surgery, assist with or perform dressing of wound.
10. Clean patient if necessary.
11. Dispose of biohazardous waste materials.
12. Remove contaminated gloves, wash hands.
13. Assist the patient postoperatively.

Assisting the Patient Postoperatively

1. Check patient vital signs.
2. Remain with patient to ensure patient safety. Allow to rest if necessary.
3. Assist patient off examination table and assist with clothing as necessary.
4. Review written postoperative instructions with patient and caregiver. Dressing should be kept clean and dry. Patient should report any signs of infection.
5. Clarify any medication orders with patient and caregiver.
6. If not previously arranged, schedule follow-up appointment.
7. Document postoperative instructions in patient record.

Room and Equipment Cleanup

1. Apply barrier gloves.
2. Dispose of drapes, table cover, pillowcase, and so on. Use biohazardous waste receptacle whenever appropriate.
3. Transfer contaminated surgical tray to cleanup area.
4. Using forceps, isolate sharps from surgical tray and dispose of them into designated sharps container.
5. Place instruments into a soak solution.
6. Sanitize Mayo instrument tray and all surfaces (examination table, stool, counter, lamp, machinery, and equipment).
7. Dispose of contaminated barrier gloves and apply protective gloves.
8. Disinfect all surfaces (examination table, stool, counter, lamp, machinery, and equipment).
9. Allow to dry.
10. Sanitize, dry, rewrap, and sterilize instruments.

Note: During most surgical procedures, if tissue is excised, it is placed in a biopsy specimen jar containing formalin (a preservative) and sent to the pathology laboratory with an appropriately completed requisition (Figure 19-23).

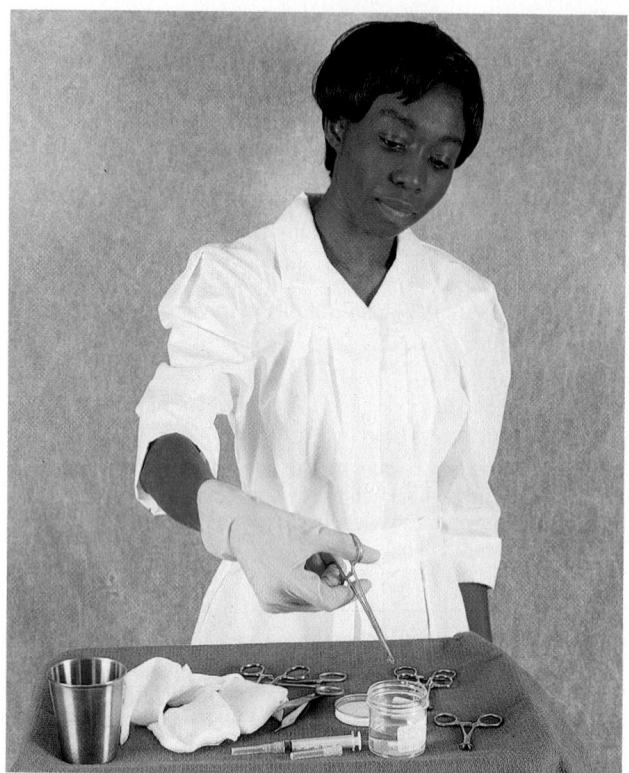

Figure 19-23   Medical assistant placing tissue for biopsy into specimen jar with formalin. The specimen will be sent to the pathology lab for examination.

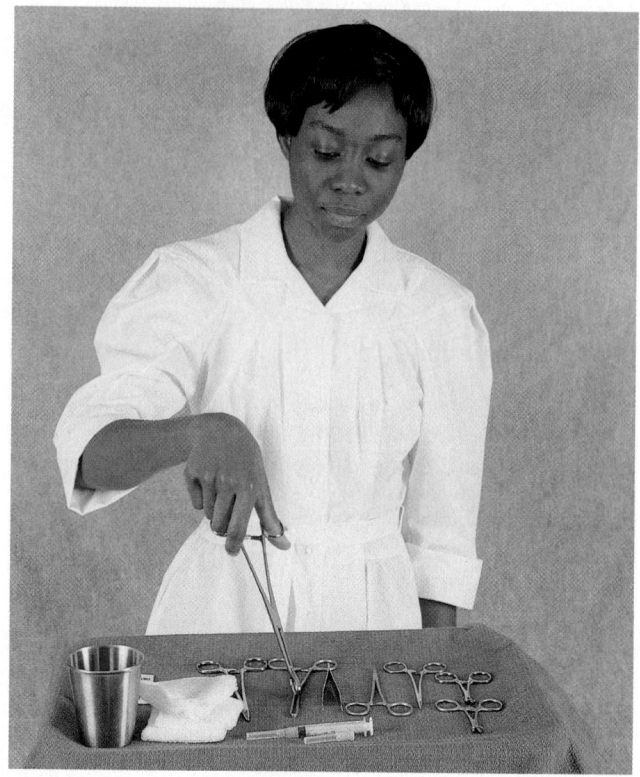

Figure 19-24   If sterile gloves have been removed, use dry sterile transfer forceps to apply or rearrange sterile items on the tray.

● Opening Sterile Packages of Instruments and Supplies and Applying Them to a Sterile Field (Procedure 19-14)

● Pouring a Sterile Solution into a Cup on a Sterile Field (Procedure 19-15)

Setting up surgical trays for specific surgeries will be addressed in a later section of this chapter.

A sterile tray is set up in the surgical area for immediate use. Therefore, a solution will be poured just prior to the tray being used because it will not have to be moved.

Using Dry Sterile Transfer Forceps

Occasionally after a sterile tray has been set up and sterile gloves removed, an additional item needs to be applied to the tray. The use of dry sterile transfer forceps allows sterile items to be applied or sterile items on the tray to be rearranged without the application of another pair of sterile gloves (Figure 19-24). The practice of using wet sterile transfer forceps is no longer recommended. Instead, when the use of sterile transfer forceps is needed, dry sterile transfer forceps are unwrapped, used only once, and then reprocessed for sterilization and subsequent use.

Procedure

19-1 Applying Sterile Gloves

STANDARD PRECAUTIONS:

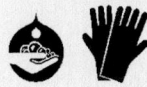

PURPOSE:

Since hands cannot be sterilized, everyone performing sterile procedures must wear sterile gloves. This procedure provides direction on how to apply sterile gloves without compromising sterility.

EQUIPMENT/SUPPLIES:

Packaged pair of sterile gloves

PROCEDURE STEPS:

1. Remove rings and watch. Wash hands using surgical asepsis. RATIONALE: Rings and watches can snag and tear gloves and therefore interfere with barrier protection.
2. Inspect glove package for tears or stains. RATIONALE: Tears and stains indicate that the gloves are no longer considered sterile and must be disposed of or used for a nonsterile purpose.
3. Place the glove package on a clean, dry, flat surface above waist level. RATIONALE: Using a contaminated surface could compromise the sterility of the sterile package.

4. Peel open the package taking care not to touch the sterile inner surface of the package. Do not allow the gloves to slide beyond the sterile inner border. RATIONALE: Care must be taken to maintain the sterility of the gloves.
5. The gloves should be opened with the cuffs toward you, the palms up, and the thumbs pointing outward. If the gloves are not positioned properly, turn the package around, being careful not to reach over the sterile area or touch the inner surface or the gloves. RATIONALE: Sterile gloves are packaged in this position for ease in application.
6. With the index finger and thumb of the nondominant hand, grasp the *inner* cuffed edge of the opposite glove. The glove should be picked straight up off the package surface without dragging or dangling the fingers over any nonsterile area (Figure 19-25A). RATIONALE: Picking up the glove by grasping the inner cuff prevents the outer glove from becoming contaminated. Strict adherence must be made to the sterile principles listed in the beginning of this chapter.
7. With the palm up on the dominant hand, carefully slide the hand into the glove. Do not allow the outside of the glove to come in contact with anything. Always hold the hands above the waist

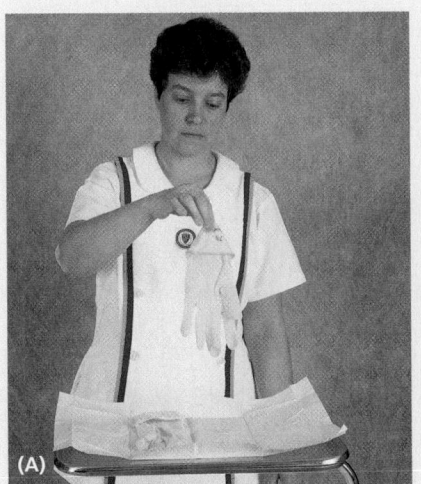
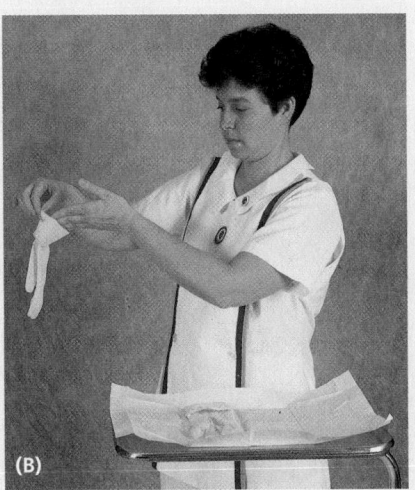
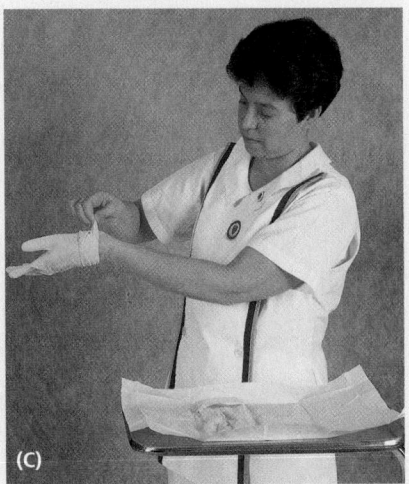

Figure 19-25 To apply sterile gloves: (A) With the nondominant hand, grasp the *inner* cuffed edge of the opposite glove. (B) With palm up on the dominant hand, slide the hand into the glove. (C, D) Hold the hand above the waist and away from the body.

(continues)

Procedure

19-1   (continued)

and away from the body (Figure 19-25B, C, D). RATIONALE: Keeping the palm up allows the glove to remain sterile in the palm area if it rolls slightly on the back of the hand.

8. With the gloved hand, pick up the glove for the remaining hand by slipping four fingers under the *outside* of the cuff. Lift the second glove up, keeping it held above the waist and away from the body. Do not allow the glove to drag across the package or touch nonsterile surfaces (Figure 19-25E). RATIONALE: The outside of the second glove is sterile

and may only be touched by another sterile surface.

9. With the palm up, slip the second hand into the glove. Do not allow the outside of the gloves to touch nonsterile skin (Figure 19-25F).

10. Adjust the gloves on the hands as needed, but avoid touching the wrist area. Keep gloved hands above the waist and away from the body. Do not touch nonsterile surfaces with the gloved hands (Figure 19-25G, H, I).

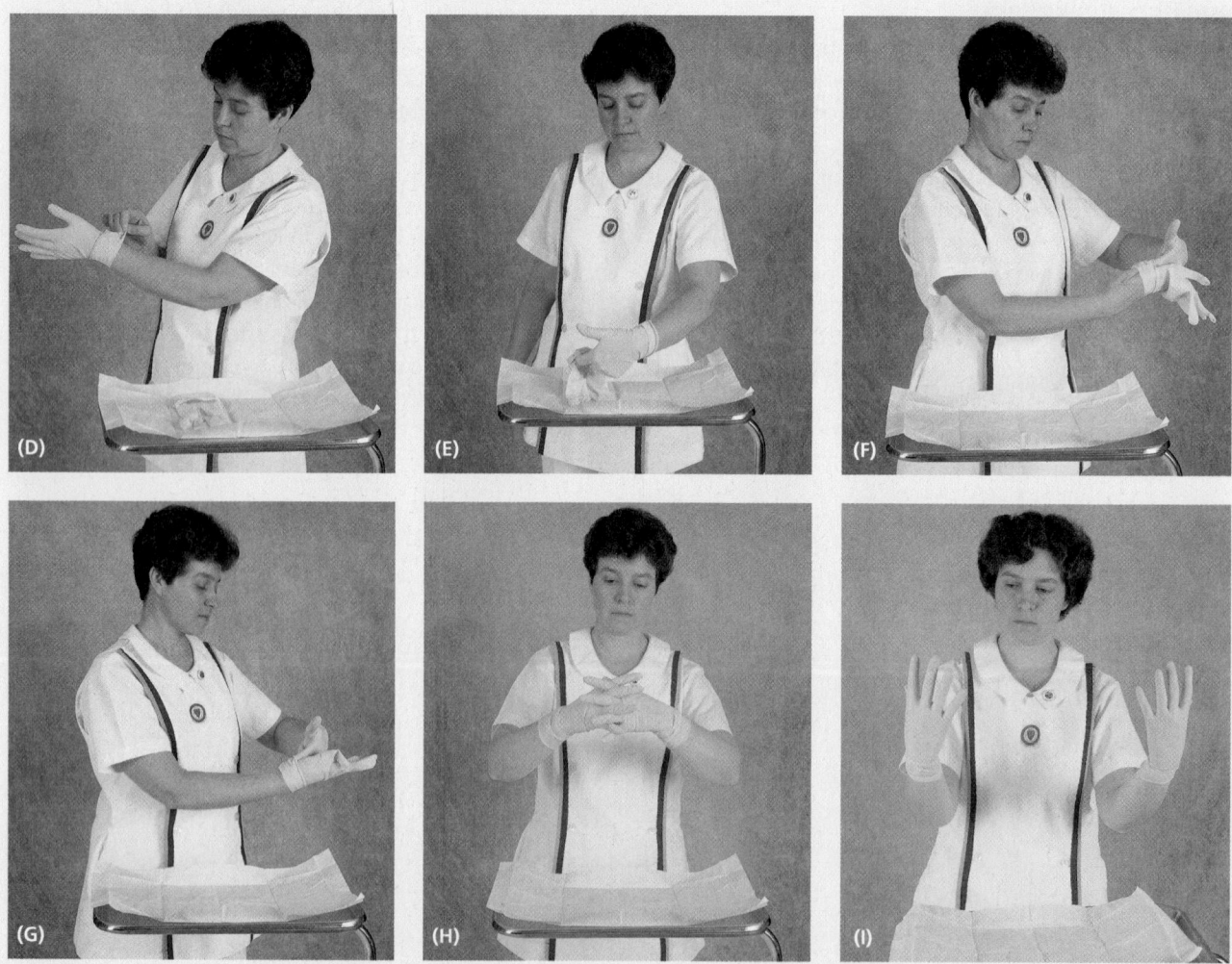

Figure 19-25 *(continued)* (E) With the gloved hand, pick up the glove for the remaining hand by slipping four fingers under the *outside* of the cuff. (F) With palm up, slip the second hand into the glove. (G, H, I) Adjust gloves. Avoid touching wrist area. Keep gloved hands above the waist and away from the body.

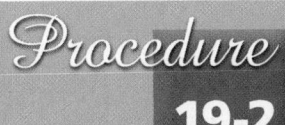

19-2 Assisting with Minor Surgery

STANDARD PRECAUTIONS:

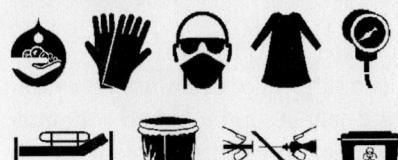

PURPOSE:
To maintain sterility during minor surgical procedures that require surgical excision of a neoplasm.

EQUIPMENT/SUPPLIES:
Mayo stand on which to create a sterile field that includes:

Needles and syringe	Tissue forceps
Bowl	Needle holder
Betadine solution	Skin retractor
Gauze sponges	Transfer forceps
Scalpel and blades	Side table:
Dissecting scissors	Sterile gloves
Operating scissors	Labeled biopsy containers
Forceps that hold	with formalin
the drapes or 4	Appropriate laboratory
sterile towels and	requisition
4 clamps	Anesthesia
Hemostats (2 curved	Alcohol wipes
and 2 straight)	Dressing tape, bandages
Thumb forceps	Biohazard container
Suture material	

PROCEDURE STEPS:

1. Check room for readiness and equipment for cleanliness.
2. Wash hands.
3. Set up side table of nonsterile items. RATIONALE: Nonsterile items cannot be placed onto a sterile field because they will contaminate it.
4. Perform surgical asepsis handwash.
5. Set up sterile field on a Mayo stand or on a clean dry flat surface.
   A. Use a commercially prepared sterile setup that is appropriate for the surgical procedure. Open the setup creating a sterile field from the inside of the sterile wrap. Add other articles such as instruments and supplies by using sterile transfer forceps or peel-apart packages that can be opened in a sterile fashion. (Refer to Procedure 19-14 on opening sterile packages.)

or

   B. Remove a sterile fanfolded towel from a canister of sterile towels using sterile transfer forceps. Hold one edge of the sterile towel and allow it to become unfolded by gently shaking it. Grasp the other edge and gently place the towel on the Mayo stand from the farther side to the side nearest you. Add sterile articles as described in A. RATIONALE: This maneuver prevents leaning over the sterile towel and contaminating it as you lay it down.
6. Apply sterile gloves. Arrange instruments according to use.
7. Cover the sterile field with a sterile towel if not being used immediately. Gently place towel from the side nearest you to side farthest from you.
8. Identify patient, explain the procedure, and prepare the patient. Refer to patient preparation in Table 19-3.
9. Prepare patient's skin. Refer to Procedure 19-12.
10. Remove the sterile cover from the sterile setup as the physician applies sterile gloves. Lift the towel by grasping the tips of the corners farthest away from you and lifting toward you. Do not allow arms to pass over sterile field. RATIONALE: Avoids crossing over sterile field.
11. Assist the physician as necessary, being certain to follow the principles of surgical asepsis.
    - The physician will inject the local anesthetic, apply Betadine or other antiseptic to the surgical site, apply sterile drapes, and begin the surgery.
    - The medical assistant will hold the vial of anesthesia while the physician withdraws the appropriate dose.
    - Adjust the instrument tray and equipment around the physician.
    - Assure a good light source.
    - Comfort and support patient emotionally.
    - Assist with the surgery as directed by the physician (sterile gloves must be worn).
    - Hand instruments to the physician and receive used intruments from the physician and place in a basin or container out of patient's sight.

(continues)

Procedure 19-2 *(continued)*

- If necessary, hold biopsy container to receive specimen being excised.
- Do not contaminate the inside of the container.
- Hold the cover facing down. Tightly place cover on the container.
- Assist with or apply sterile dressing to the operative site.
12. Assist patient as necessary. Refer to Assisting the Patient Postoperatively in Table 19-4.
13. The specimen container must be handled with disposable gloves as recommended by standard precautions. The container must be tightly covered, labeled with the patient's name, date, type, and source of specimen and sent to the laboratory accompanied by the appropriate laboratory requisition.
14. Wearing appropriate personal protective equipment (PPE), clean surgical or examination room.
    - Dispose of used sponges in biohazard container and knife blades and other disposable sharps in puncture-proof sharps container.
    - Rinse used surgical intruments; soak, sanitize, and sterilize for reuse.
    - Remove gloves and other PPE and dispose of per OSHA guidelines.
15. Wash hands.
16. Document in the patient's record that the specimen was sent to the laboratory.

Procedure 19-3 **Suturing of Laceration or Incision Repair**

STANDARD PRECAUTIONS:

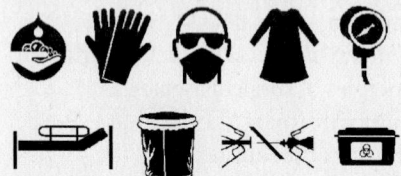

PURPOSE:

Suturing is recommended if a laceration or incision is gaping, bleeding uncontrolledly, or is located on the face, neck, or a bend of a body part or extends deep into underlying tissue. Suturing facilitates healing by approximating the edges. Suturing decreases scarring, helps decrease the likelihood of infection, and promotes healing. The wound and the surrounding area must be meticulously cleaned of any dirt and debris. Many physicians have standard orders for wound cleaning prior to suture repair of either a laceration or incision-type wound.

EQUIPMENT/SUPPLIES:

Surgical tray:
  Syringe and needle for anesthetic
  Hemostats (curved)
  Adson or tissue forceps
  Iris scissors (curved)
  Suture material and needle
  Needle holder
  Gauze sponges
Side table:
  Anesthetic as ordered by the physician
  Dressings, bandages, and tape
  Splint/brace/sling (optional)
  Sterile gloves

PROCEDURE STEPS:

1. Wash hands.
2. Identify the patient and explain the procedure. Check for signed consent forms.
3. Reassure and comfort the patient as needed.
4. Assess cause of wound and its severity.
   - Determine any known allergies and last tetanus booster.
   - Identify any health concerns to avoid possible complications.

(continues)

Procedure 19-3 (continued)

- Soak wound in an antiseptic solution as ordered by physician.
- Clean and dry wound.
- Position patient comfortably, lying down.
5. Assist the physician as needed.
6. Support the patient as needed.

Give postoperative care:
7. Apply sterile gloves.
8. Clean area around the wound.
9. Dress/bandage/splint wound following physician's preference.
10. Remove gloves.

11. Wash hands.
12. Check patient's vital signs.
13. Explain wound care to the patient (and caregiver) and provide written instructions including symptoms of infection.
14. Assist the patient with any concerns or questions.
15. Arrange for follow-up appointment and medication as ordered.
16. Dispose of supplies per OSHA guidelines. Clean room, sanitize instruments, sterilize for reuse.
17. Wash hands.
18. Document the procedure.

Procedure 19-4 Dressing Change

STANDARD PRECAUTIONS:

NOTE: After most minor surgical procedures have been completed, the wound is usually covered with a dry sterile dressing that may need to be removed periodically so that the wound can be checked for healing or for suture removal. Another dry sterile dressing may then be applied.

PURPOSE:
To remove a wound dressing and apply a dry sterile dressing.

EQUIPMENT/SUPPLIES:
Sterile field:
  Several sterile gauze sponges and other dressing material as needed
  Sterile bowl with Betadine solution
  Sterile dressing forceps
  Sponge forceps
Side area:
  Nonsterile gloves
  Sterile gloves
  Container of hydrogen peroxide or sterile water

Cotton-tipped applicators
Sterile adhesive strips
Antibacterial ointment/cream as ordered
Tape
Sponge forceps
Bandage scissors (2)
Waterproof waste bag
Biohazard waste container

PROCEDURE STEPS:
1. Wash hands.
2. Prepare sterile field. Add gauze sponges, bowl with solution, and forceps.
3. Position a waterproof bag away from sterile area.
4. Pour Betadine solution into sterile bowl.
5. Identify the patient and explain the procedure.
6. Reassure and comfort the patient as needed.
7. Loosen tape on dressing by pulling tape toward wound, or cut off bandage if necessary.
8. Put on nonsterile gloves or use forceps.
9. Carefully remove bandage, place in biohazard waste container. Do not pass over sterile field.
10. Remove dressing, taking care not to cause stress on the wound (Figure 19-26A).

(continues)

Procedure

19-4   *(continued)*

A. If stuck to the wound, pour small amounts of sterile water or hydrogen peroxide over dressing; allow to soak for a short time. Remove dressing when loose enough to remove without resistance. Note type and amount of drainage if present.

11. Place used dressing in waterproof bag without touching inside or outside of bag.

12. Assess wound and note any drainage or signs of infection. Remove and discard gloves in waterproof bag.

13. Wash hands.

14. Apply sterile gloves.

15. Clean the wound with Betadine solution (Figure 19-26B).

16. Dispose of used gauze in waterproof bag.

17. Using forceps, apply sterile gauze sponge(s) to wound (Figure 19-26C and D).

18. Remove gloves, dispose of in waterproof bag.

19. Secure dressing with adhesive tape (Figure 19-26E), roller bandage, or elastic bandage.

20. Dispose of waterproof bag in biohazard container.

21. Wash hands.

22. Document procedure and describe wound appearance (i.e., discharge, signs of infection, healing, etc.)

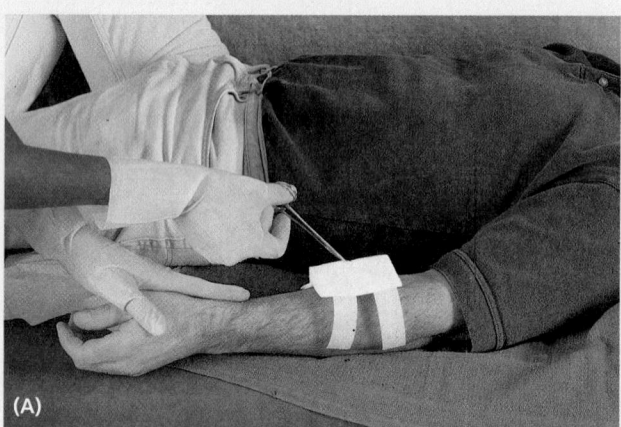
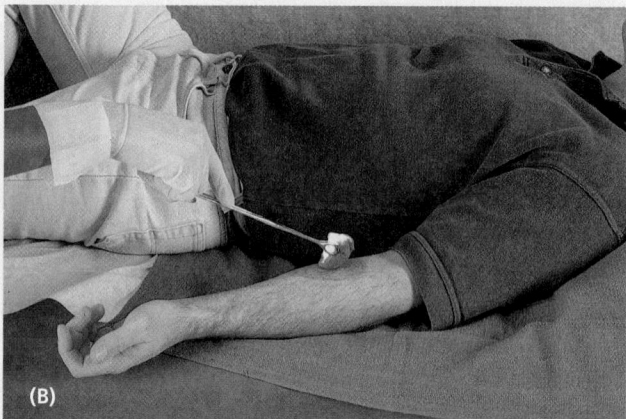
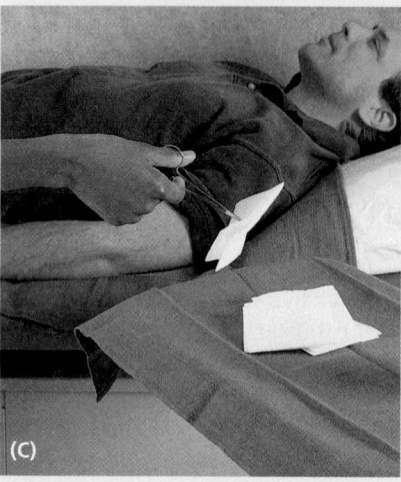
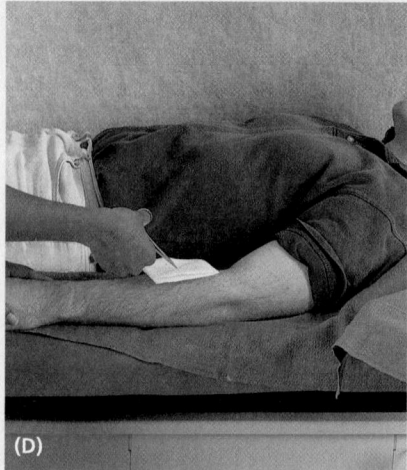
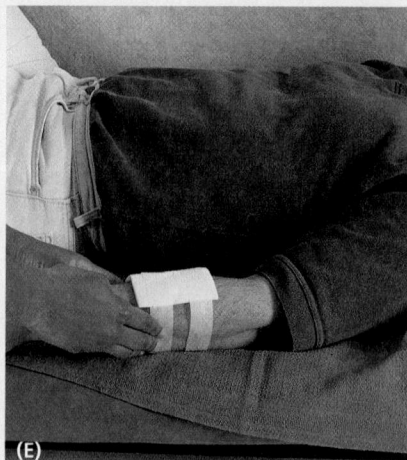

Figure 19-26   To change a dressing: (A) Gently remove dressing. Do not cause stress on wound. (B) Clean wound with Betadine solution. (C, D) Using dressing forceps, apply sterile gauze sponge(s) to wound. (E) Secure dressing with adhesive tape, roller bandage, or elastic bandage.

Procedure

19-5 | Suture Removal

STANDARD PRECAUTIONS:

NOTE: Many minor surgical procedures require that suturing be done to approximate the skin edges to promote healing. Since these sutures are nonabsorbable, they must be removed when the wound has healed. The patient will return to the office or clinic to have the sutures removed. The medical assistant will remove the dressing and check the wound. The physician will also check the wound for degree of healing and determine that the sutures can be removed.

PURPOSE:
To remove sutures from a healed minor surgical wound (as per physician).

EQUIPMENT/SUPPLIES:
(See Figure 19-27.)
Gauze sponges
Bandage scissors
Biohazard waste container
Tape
Sponge forceps
Suture removal kit (suture scissors or staple remover, thumb forceps, and 4 × 4s)
Sterile latex gloves
Betadine solution or wash

PROCEDURE STEPS:
1. Identify patient.
2. Wash hands.
3. Open suture removal kit.
4. Apply sterile gloves.
5. Using thumb forceps, gently pick up one knot of a suture. Gently pull upward toward suture line. RATIONALE: Less pressure is exerted on suture line.
6. Using suture removal scissors, cut one side of the suture as close to skin as possible (Figure 19-28A and B). RATIONALE: Holding knot with forceps and cutting suture as close to skin as possible, the suture will be pulled out from under the skin, avoiding contamination of the wound.
7. Remove all sutures in the same manner, noting number of sutures removed. Dispose of the sutures on a sterile gauze sponge.
8. Examine the wound to be certain all sutures have been removed.
9. Apply Betadine solution to area.
10. Apply dry sterile dressing if ordered by the physician (see Procedure 19-4).
11. Remove gloves.
12. Dispose of used items per OSHA guidelines.
13. Wash hands.
14. Check patient's vital signs if indicated.
15. Explain wound care, provide written instructions to patient.
16. Arrange follow-up appointment if necessary.
17. Document the procedure.

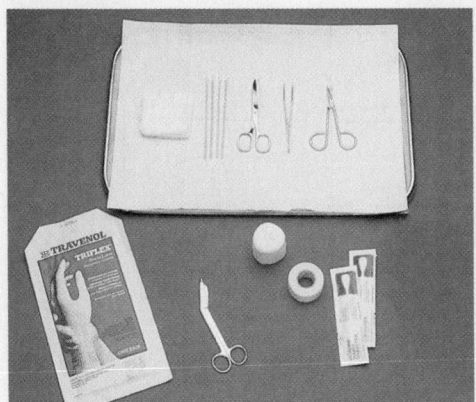

Figure 19-27 Equipment and supplies for suture removal.

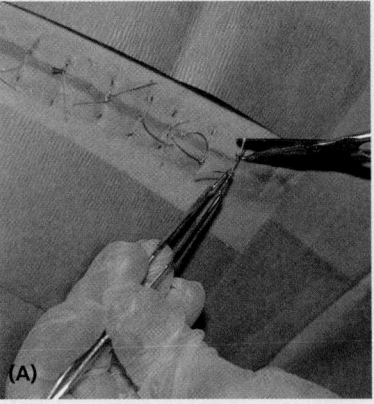
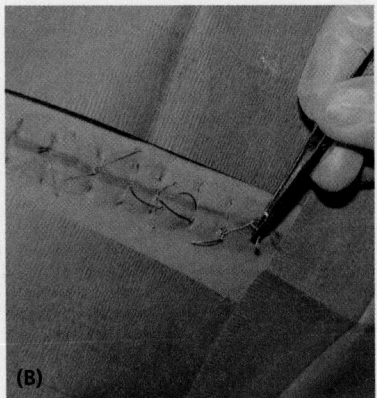

Figure 19-28 To remove sutures: (A) Grasp suture knot with thumb forceps. Place curved tip of suture removal scissors just next to skin under the suture. Clip. (B) Gently pull the suture knot up and toward the incision with thumb forceps to remove.

Procedure 19-6 — Application of Sterile Adhesive Skin Closure Strips

STANDARD PRECAUTIONS:

NOTE: On occasion, a superficial wound does not require sutures. However, the edges of the wound can be drawn together and sterile strips of adhesive are used to hold the edges of the wound together to facilitate healing.

PURPOSE:

To approximate the edges of a wound after the removal of sutures. Sometimes used in lieu of sutures or to give additional support along with sutures.

EQUIPMENT/SUPPLIES:

Sterile field:
  Suture removal instruments (as indicated)
  Sterile adhesive skin closure strips
  Iris scissors (straight)
  Tincture of benzoin (optional)
  Sterile cotton-tipped applicators (for tincture of benzoin)
Side area:
  Sterile gloves
  Dressings, bandages, and tape

PROCEDURE STEPS:

1. Identify the patient and explain the procedure.
2. Position patient comfortably.
3. Wash hands and apply gloves.
4. Remove bandages and dressings. See Procedure 19-4.
5. Clean and dry wound. See Procedure 19-4.
6. Assess the need for skin closure strips and alert the physician as indicated.
7. Remove gloves, wash hands, open container of tincture of benzoin, apply sterile gloves.

8. Apply tincture of benzoin to edges of wound if directed. Use sterile cotton-tipped applicator, taking care not to let it come into contact with the actual wound.
9. Remove strips from packaging one at a time. Apply one end of a skin closure strip to one side of the wound. Place the first strip over the center of the wound (Figure 19-29A).
10. Secure the end to the skin by carefully pressing.
11. Stretch the strip across the edge of the wound and secure on the other side in the same manner. This motion should bring the edges together without puckering the skin.
12. Apply the next two closure strips at halfway points between the first strip and each end of the wound (Figure 19-29B and C).
13. Continue in this manner until the edges are approximated. Keep wound edges in alignment.

Give postoperative care:

14. Dress and bandage if necessary.
15. Dispose of used items per OSHA guidelines.
16. Remove gloves and wash hands.
17. Check the patient's vital signs.
18. Explain wound care to the patient (and caregiver) and provide written instructions including symptoms of infection.
19. Assist the patient with any concerns or questions.
20. Arrange for follow-up appointment and medication as ordered.
21. Document the procedure.

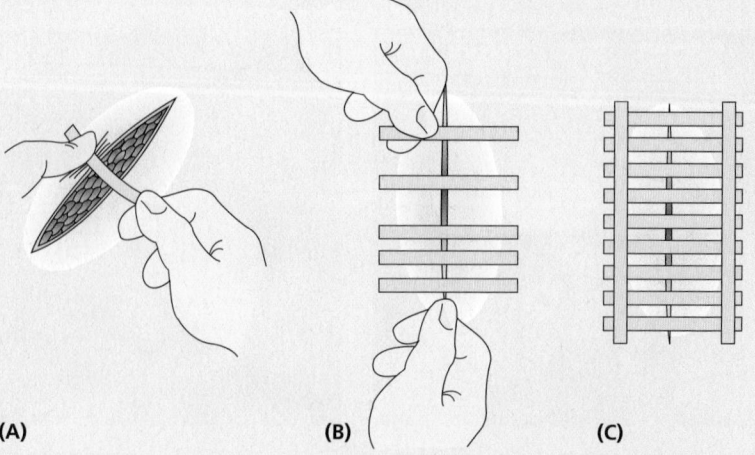

(A) (B) (C)

Figure 19-29 To apply skin closure strips: (A) Apply first strip in center of incision. (B) Apply closures to each side of center. (C) Apply closures parallel to incision.

Procedure 19-7 Sebaceous Cyst Excision

STANDARD PRECAUTIONS:

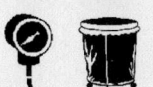

NOTE: A sebaceous cyst is a benign retention cyst, sometimes called a "wen." Sebaceous cysts are caused by an oil duct becoming "plugged" which causes the sebum (oil) to accumulate in the gland. Eventually the oil gland becomes distended. Sebaceous cysts that become inflamed or infected need to be removed. The patient may also elect to have a noninflamed sebaceous cyst removed if it is unsightly or located in a bothersome area. Incision and drainage of a sebaceous cyst is usually not the treatment of choice because they tend to recur if the entire cyst is not completely excised. Ideally, the entire cyst sac is removed intact, but occasionally the sac ruptures during removal and large amounts of foul-smelling biohazardous sebum can be expelled. In preparation for this occurrence, extra gauze sponges and gloves should be available.

PURPOSE:

To remove an inflamed or infected sebaceous cyst. To remove a sebaceous cyst that is not inflamed or infected but is located on an area of the body where the cyst is unsightly or where it may become irritated from rubbing.

EQUIPMENT/SUPPLIES:

Surgical tray:
 Syringe/needle for anesthesia
 Iris scissors (curved)
 Mosquito hemostat (curved)
 Scalpel blades and handle
 Suture material with needle
 Mayo scissors (curved)
Side area:
 Skin prep supplies
 Tissue forceps (2)
 Gauze sponges (many)
 Needle holder
 Fenestrated drape (a drape with openings)
 Antiseptic solution (Betadine)
 Gloves (sterile and nonsterile)
 Personal protective equipment
 Anesthesia as directed

Dressing, bandages, tape
Specimen container/requisition (optional)
Biohazard waste container
Extra gauze sponges
Safety razor (optional)
Alcohol pledgets
Culturette (optional)

PROCEDURE STEPS:

1. Wash hands.
2. Identify the patient and explain the procedure.
3. Reassure and comfort the patient as needed.
4. Determine any known allergies and last tetanus booster.
5. Check for signed consent form.
6. Identify any health concerns to avoid possible complications.
7. Position the patient comfortably, lying down.
8. Perform the skin preparation as directed. (See Procedure 19-12.)
9. Wear appropriate PPE if cyst is infected. RATIONALE: Purulent material may drain out of the wound.
10. Assist physician to inject the anesthesia by holding the vial while the physician withdraws the appropriate amount of anesthesia. Continue to assist while the physician incises the cyst, removes it, and sutures the surgical incision. The physician will place the specimen in a container with a preservative to be sent to the pathology lab for analysis.
11. Support patient during surgery.

Give postoperative care:

12. Apply sterile gloves.
13. Clean area around the wound.
14. Dress and bandage as directed.
15. Dispose of items per OSHA guidelines. Remove gloves.
16. Wash hands.
17. Check the patient's vital signs.
18. Explain wound care to the patient (and caregiver) and provide written instructions including symptoms of infection.
19. Assist the patient with any concerns or questions.
20. Arrange for follow-up appointment and medication as ordered.
21. Document the procedure and that specimen sent to laboratory if appropriate.

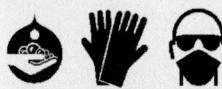 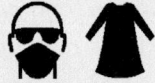

Incision and Drainage of Localized Infections

19-8

STANDARD PRECAUTIONS:

NOTE: An abscess is a localized accumulation of pus surrounded by inflamed tissue. The body attempts to isolate pus into a pocket or abscess as a means of protecting itself by walling off the pathogens and preventing them from spreading throughout the body. Incision and drainage is the procedure of cutting into an area (often an abscess) for the purposes of draining the fluid/material. A culture of the exudate can be done to identify microorganisms. Rather than suturing or otherwise closing the wound, the physician may place a gauze wick or a penrose drain into the wound to facilitate continued drainage. The most commonly used type of wick is Iodoform. Iodoform is available in 5-yard lengths and widths of ¼ inch, ½ inch, and 1 inch. Iodoform is packaged sterile in glass bottles under the Johnson & Johnson brand name of Nu Gauze. Care must be taken when removing the desired length from the bottle to avoid contaminating the remaining gauze. To accomplish this, the medical assistant might hold the bottle and remove the lid to allow the physician to reach into the bottle with a sterile thumb forceps and pull out the desired length. Sterile scissors are then used to cut the strip without contaminating the remaining wick. The Iodoform is packed into the wound with a short length exposed. After several hours or days of continued draining, the wick may be removed, and the wound allowed to heal. The patient may be put on an appropriate antibiotic.

The medical assistant should exercise caution by wearing appropriate PPE when assisting with this procedure since the exudate can be heavy and contains pathogenic microorganisms.

PURPOSE:

To incise and drain an abscess or other localized infection.

EQUIPMENT/SUPPLIES:

Surgical tray:
  Syringe/needle for anesthesia
  Scalpel blades and handle
  Thumb forceps
  Mosquito hemostat (optional)
  Gauze sponges (many)
  Fenestrated drape
  Tissue forceps (2)
  Mayo scissors
  Iris scissors
  Antiseptic solution such as Betadine in sterile cup
Side area:
  Skin prep supplies
  Gloves (sterile and nonsterile)
  Personal protective equipment
  Anesthesia as directed
  Dressing, bandages, and tape
  Specimen container with preservative/requisition
    (optional)
  Biohazard waste container
  Extra gauze sponges
  Iodoform gauze wick or penrose drain
  Alcohol pledget
  Antiseptic solution
  Culturette (optional)

PROCEDURE STEPS:

1. Wash hands.
2. Identify the patient and explain the procedure.
3. Reassure and comfort the patient as needed.
4. Determine any known allergies and last tetanus booster.
5. Check for signed consent form.
6. Identify any health concerns to avoid possible complications.
7. Position the patient comfortably, lying down.
8. Put on PPE.
9. Perform the skin preparation as directed. (See Procedure 19-12.)
10. Assist the physician as needed to inject the anesthesia by holding the vial while the appropriate amount is aspirated for injection. The physician will incise the abscess and either Iodoform gauze or a penrose drain will be inserted into the wound to encourage drainage.
11. Support the patient as needed.

Give postoperative care:

12. Apply sterile gloves.
13. Clean area around the wound.

(continues)

Procedure

19-8 (continued)

14. Dress and bandage as directed. Several thicknesses of dressing material may be needed to absorb **exudate**, or the accumulated fluid in a cavity.
15. Dispose of items per OSHA guidelines. Remove gloves.
16. Wash hands.
17. Check the patient's vital signs.
18. Explain wound care to the patient (and caregiver) and provide written instructions such as to apply warm moist compresses to wound. Explain to watch for symptoms of infection.
19. Assist the patient with any concerns or questions.
20. Arrange for follow-up appointment and medication as ordered.
21. Document the procedure.

Procedure

19-9 Aspiration of Joint Fluid

STANDARD PRECAUTIONS:

NOTE: The most common reason for aspirating fluid is to remove excess fluid from a joint, often the knee. A long sturdy needle is inserted into the joint capsule and fluid is removed. Often a long-acting anesthetic and cortisone are injected at the same time. The fluid can be diagnostically examined for blood, pus, and fatty substances and also cultured for infective pathogens. Postoperatively, the patient may be placed on anti-inflammatory medications to treat the inflammation and antibiotics if the culture is positive for pathogens.

PURPOSE:
To remove excess synovial fluid from a joint following injury.

EQUIPMENT/SUPPLIES:
Surgical tray:
  Syringe/needle for anesthesia
  Gauze sponges
  Sterile basin for aspirated fluid
  Fenestrated drape (optional)
  Syringe/needle for drainage

Side area:
  Skin prep supplies
  Gloves (sterile and nonsterile)
  Personal protective equipment
  Anesthesia as directed
  Cortisone medication as directed
  Culturette (optional)
  Pathology requisition
  Specimen container
  Biohazard waste container
  Extra gauze sponges (sterile, unopened)
  Alcohol pledgets
  Dressing and bandages

PROCEDURE STEPS:
1. Wash hands.
2. Identify the patient and explain the procedure.
3. Reassure and comfort the patient as needed.
4. Determine any known allergies and last tetanus booster.
5. Check for signed consent form.
6. Identify any health concerns to avoid possible complications.
7. Position the patient comfortably, lying down.
8. Put on PPE if needed.
9. Perform the skin preparation as directed. (See Procedure 19-12.)

(continues)

Procedure 19-9 *(continued)*

10. Assist the physician by holding the vial as anesthesia is aspirated. The physician will inject anesthesia and then insert a needle into the synovial sac and aspirate fluid with the syringe. The aspirated fluid will be put into a sterile bowl as the syringe fills with fluid. The process continues until excess fluid is removed.
11. Support the patient as needed.

Give postoperative care:

12. Apply sterile gloves.
13. Clean area around the wound.
14. Dress and bandage as directed.
15. Dispose of items per OSHA guidelines. Remove gloves.

16. Wash hands.
17. Check the patient's vital signs.
18. Explain wound care to the patient (and caregiver) and provide written instructions including symptoms of infection.
19. Assist the patient with any concerns or questions.
20. Arrange for follow-up appointment and medication as ordered.
21. Apply gloves and eye/mouth protection. Place aspirated fluid into a sterile container and cover tightly.
22. Send labeled specimen to the pathology lab if directed.
23. Document the procedure.

Procedure 19-10 Hemorrhoid Thrombectomy

STANDARD PRECAUTIONS:

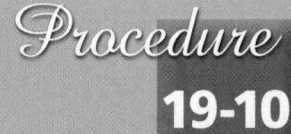

NOTE: Hemorrhoids are dilated or varicose veins in the rectum, either internal or external. Sometimes a blood clot can form in a protruding portion of the hemorrhoid and the vessel can become inflamed. The hemorrhoid is incised with a scalpel blade and the clot removed with a hemostat forceps. Suturing is not usually necessary. Soaking the area in a **sitz bath** can aid in healing.

PURPOSE:

To excise inflamed hemorrhoids.

EQUIPMENT/SUPPLIES:

Surgical tray:
  Syringe/needle for anesthesia
  Mosquito hemostat (curved)
  Sterile basin
  Gauze sponges

Fenestrated drape
Side area:
  Skin prep supplies
  Gloves (sterile and nonsterile)
  Personal protective equipment
  Anesthesia as directed
  Biohazard waste container
  Extra gauze sponges
  Soft absorbent pad, similar to sanitary napkin
  T-bandage (to hold pad in place)

PROCEDURE STEPS:

1. Wash hands.
2. Identify the patient and explain the procedure.
3. Reassure and comfort the patient as needed.
4. Determine any known allergies and last tetanus booster.
5. Check for signed consent form.
6. Identify any health concerns to avoid possible complications.
7. Position the patient comfortably, according to physician preference; usually lithotomy position is used.
8. Assist with adequate draping for patient comfort.

(continues)

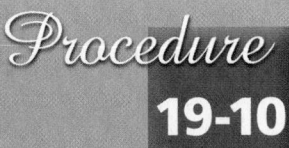

19-10 *(continued)*

9. Apply PPE if necessary.
10. Perform the skin preparation as directed. (See Procedure 19-12.)
11. Assist the physician to aspirate the appropriate amount of local anesthesia. After administering the anesthesia, the physician will excise the hemorrhoids with a scalpel. Suturing is usually not necessary.
12. Support the patient as needed.

Give postoperative care:
13. Apply sterile gloves.
14. Assist the physician in placing the soft absorbent pad against the wound. It may be held in place with a T-shaped bandage.

15. Dispose of used items per OSHA guidelines. Remove gloves and wash hands.
16. Assist the patient as needed.
17. Check the patient's vital signs.
18. Explain wound care to the patient (and caregiver) per physician. Sitting in a tub of warm water is soothing and aids healing. Provide written instructions including signs of complications such as excessive bleeding or pain.
19. Assist the patient with any concerns or questions.
20. Arrange for follow-up appointment and medication as ordered.
21. Document the procedure.

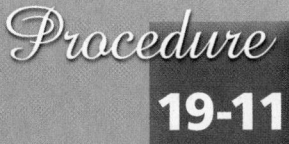

19-11 Chemical "Cold" Sterilization

STANDARD PRECAUTIONS:

PURPOSE:
To sterilize heat-sensitive items such as fiber-optic endoscopes and delicate cutting instruments using appropriate chemical solution.

EQUIPMENT/SUPPLIES:

Chemical solution	Timer
such as Cidex	Sterile water
Steris System®	Gloves—heavy duty
(Percacetic acid)	Sterile towel
Airtight container	Plastic-lined sterile drapes

PROCEDURE STEPS:

1. Sanitize items (see Chapter 10) that require chemical sterilization. Rinse and dry. RATIONALE: Recall that debris and body proteins must be scrubbed from items prior to sterilization.

2. Read manufactuer's instructions on original container of chemical sterilization solution. RATIONALE: Each brand of chemical sterilization solution has specific preparation instructions and germicidal properties; choose the solution that best fits the needs of the ambulatory care setting. Keep the solution in its original container to reduce chances of accidental poisoning.

3. Put on gloves. RATIONALE: Heavy-duty gloves help protect from sharp items puncturing the skin. Chemicals are harsh on the skin.

4. Prepare solution as indicated by manufacturer, place the date of opening or preparation on the container and initial it. RATIONALE: Following manufacturer's instructions ensures sterility. Note the expiration date of solution.

5. Pour solution into a container with an airtight lid, avoid splashing. RATIONALE: Chemicals should not be left exposed to open air in order to prevent evaporation and loss of potency, exposure to environmetal contaminants, accidental inhalation, or

(continues)

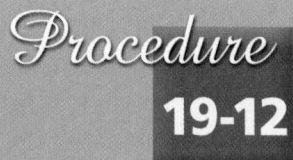

Procedure 19-11 *(continued)*

poisoning. Splashing may cause skin or mucous membrane contact and result in injury.

6. Place sanitized and dried items into the solution, completely submersing item(s). Avoid splashing when placing items into airtight container. RATIONALE: Total immersion is necessary for sterility to be achieved.

7. Close lid of container, label with name of solution, exposure time required per manufacturer, and initial. RATIONALE: Exposure time is the required time indicated by the manufacturer to achieve sterility. Initialing work ensures accountability and responsibility.

8. Do not open lid nor add additional items during the processing time. RATIONALE: Adding to the container interrupts the sterilization process and limits the effectiveness of the chemical.

9. Following the recommended processing time, lift item(s) from the container using sterile gloved hands or sterile transfer forceps. Carefully hold item above sterile basin and pour copious amounts of sterile water over it and through it (endoscopes) until adequately rinsed of chemical solution.

RATIONALE: Item(s) once processed are sterile and must be handled appropriately. Using sterile gloved hands or sterile transfer forceps ensures sterile-to-sterile contact and no contamination of the item(s). Sterile water is poured through the inner channels of endoscopes to rinse chemicals from the inside as well as the outside.

10. Hold item(s) upright for a few seconds to allow excess sterile water to drip off.

11. Place the sterile item on a sterile towel (which has been placed on a sterile field) and dry it with another sterile towel. The towel used for drying is removed from sterile field. The use of sterile drapes that have a plastic polylined barrier layer between two layers of paper is recommended for the sterile field. RATIONALE: Plastic-lined sterile drapes create a barrier to prevent moisture from drawing contaminants from the metal surgical instrument tray or countertop up into the sterile area.

Procedure 19-12 **Preparation of Patient Skin for Minor Surgery**

STANDARD PRECAUTIONS:

NOTE: The skin contains many microorganisms and the patient's skin must be prepared prior to minor surgery to remove as many of the microorganisms as possible. Wound infection results when microorganisms enter the body. Since it is impossible to sterilize the skin, the operative site and an area surrounding it are scrubbed, shaved (hair harbors microorganisms), washed, and painted with an antiseptic such as Betadine solution.

PURPOSE:
To remove as many microorganisms as possible from patient's skin prior to surgery.

EQUIPMENT/SUPPLIES:
Absorbent pad
Drape
Disposable prep kit (includes: antiseptic soap, several sponges, razor, and a container for water)
Sterile water
Antiseptic solution
Sterile bowl

(continues)

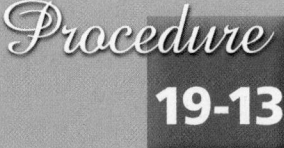

Procedure 19-12 *(continued)*

Sterile gloves for medical assistant and physician (2 pairs)
If kit is unavailable, equipment needed is:
Sterile bowls (2)
Antiseptic soap
Sterile gauze sponges
Sterile razor
Basin for soiled sponges

PROCEDURE STEPS:

1. Wash hands.
2. Assemble equipment.
3. Identify patient.
4. Explain procedure, provide privacy, and drape patient if appropriate.
5. Provide good light source.
6. Position patient for comfort and exposure of site.
7. Wash hands.
8. Protect area under preparation site with an absorbent pad.
9. Put on sterile gloves or use sterile transfer forceps.
10. Apply antiseptic soap (Betadine) with 4 × 4 sponges, beginning at operative site and moving outward in a circular motion from the center to away from center of prepared area. RATIONALE: Work from cleaner to least clean areas to prevent contamination.
11. Discard used sponges as necessary.

12. Using razor and holding skin taut, shave hair away from operative site, following hair growth pattern. RATIONALE: This prevents accidental nicks. Nicked skin can cause infection.
13. When hair has been removed, scrub again in a circular fashion as in step 10 for about 2 to 5 minutes.
14. Rinse shaved area with sterile water and dry with a sterile 4 × 4 gauze sponge.
15. Remove and appropriately discard absorbent pad, 4 × 4 sponges, disposable prep kit, and gloves. RATIONALE: This removes used supplies and equipment from prepped skin area and avoids contamination.
16. Wash hands.
17. Using sterile transfer forceps, remove a sterile towel to place under operative site. RATIONALE: Placing a sterile towel under the operative area keeps site free from contamination.
18. Cover with a sterile towel. Instruct patient not to touch the area.
19. Pour antiseptic solution (Betadine) into the sterile bowl. Physician will put on sterile gloves or will use sterile transfer forceps and using a sterile 4 × 4 gauze sponge will paint the operative site with the antiseptic solution. Let dry, drape patient with sterile drapes, and commence with the surgical procedure.

Procedure 19-13 Setting Up and Covering a Sterile Field

STANDARD PRECAUTIONS:

PURPOSE:

Disposable sterile field drapes or sterile towels are used to isolate a sterile area or field as well as to cover the sterile field for use in minor surgery and sterile procedures. They are available in convenient peel-apart packages, fanfolded for ease of use, and often are two-tone in color to aid in differentiating one side from the other. Sterile towels are fanfolded and stored in canisters.

NOTE: A variety of materials, both disposable and nondisposable, can be used to set up and cover a sterile

(continues)

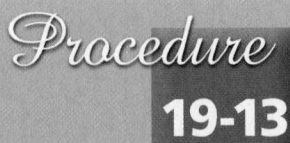

Procedure

19-13   *(continued)*

field. All material must contain certain criteria to be safe for use and all have advantages and disadvantages. For example, woven textile fabrics are moisture retardant and are effective barriers to microbial penetration. A combination of paper and plastic disposable drapes is an excellent barrier against microorganisms and moisture. Many times medical office preference is determined by financial consideration.

EQUIPMENT/SUPPLIES:

Disposable sterile field drapes (2) or sterile towels (2) (muslin or linen with water-repellent finish)
Mayo instrument tray/stand
Sterile transfer forceps (if needed)

PROCEDURE STEPS:

1. Wash hands.
2. Sanitize and disinfect a Mayo instrument tray.
3. Select an appropriate disposable sterile field drape and place the drape package on a clean, dry, flat surface, or remove a fanfolded sterile cloth towel from a canister using sterile transfer forceps.
4. If using disposable drape, peel open the package exposing the fanfolded drape. Assure that the cut corners of the drape are toward you; turn the package if necessary. Or: remove sterile towel from canister using sterile transfer forceps. RATIONALE: Sterile field drapes are fanfolded and positioned within the package to facilitate ease of use. Sterile towels are fanfolded and positioned within the canister for ease of use.
5. With thumb and forefinger of one hand, carefully grasp the top cut corner without touching the rest of the drape or towel and pick the drape or towel up high enough to assure that as it unfolds it does

not drag across a nonsterile area. RATIONALE: The drape or towel will naturally unfold as it is lifted, so care must be taken to assure that it is lifted quickly and allowed to unfold without touching a nonsterile surface.

6. Holding the drape or towel above waist level and away from the body, grasp the opposing corner so that both corners along the long edge of the drape are being held.
7. Keeping the drape or towel above waist level and away from the body, reach over the Mayo tray with the drape or towel. Take care that the lower edge of the drape or towel does not drag across the tray. RATIONALE: Sterile principles state that sterile items should be kept above the waist.
8. Gently pull the drape or towel toward you as it is laid onto the tray. If adjustment is needed to center the drape or towel, do not touch the center of the drape or towel, or reach over the sterile field. Walk around or reach underneath the tray to move it or make adjustments. RATIONALE: The edges that hang over the tray are no longer considered sterile.
9. To cover the sterile field with a second sterile drape or towel, follow steps 4 through 7; then instead of pulling the drape or towel toward you (as described in step 8), which would necessitate reaching over the sterile field, apply the covering drape or towel by holding it up in front of the field. Adjust the lower edge so it is even with the lower edge of the field drape or towel. With a forward motion, carefully lay the cover over the sterile field. RATIONALE: Reaching over the sterile field would contaminate the tray.

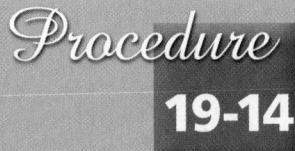

Opening Sterile Packages of Instruments and Supplies and Applying Them to a Sterile Field

Procedure 19-14

STANDARD PRECAUTIONS:

NOTE: Sterile instruments and supplies are packaged in a manner that allows them to be opened and accessed without compromising sterility. Refer to other sections of this chapter for the specific steps of wrapping techniques, sterile gloving, and setting up sterile fields. The "wrapping twice" method of double wrapping was used in preparing the surgical packs for the following procedure.

PURPOSE:

To open sterile packages of surgical instruments and supplies and place them onto a sterile field using sterile technique.

EQUIPMENT/SUPPLIES:

Mayo instrument tray
Sterile field drapes (2) or sterile towels (2)
Sterile gloves
Wrapped-twice sterile surgical instruments
Prepackaged sterile surgical supplies

PROCEDURE STEPS:

1. Assemble supplies.
2. Wash hands and set up sterile field.

3. Position package of surgical instruments on palm of nondominant hand with outer envelope flap on top. RATIONALE: This will facilitate opening the pack while protecting its sterile contents.
4. Grasping the taped end of the top flap, open the first flap away from you. Do not touch the inside of the flap (Figure 19-30A).
5. Grasping just the folded back tips of the side flaps, pull the right-sided flap to the right. Then pull the left-sided flap to the left, taking care not to reach over the package (Figure 19-30B and C). RATIONALE: Pulling the tips of the flaps toward each side allows the inner portion of the package to be exposed without contamination.
6. Pull the last flap toward you by grasping the folded-back tip taking care not to touch the inner contents of the package. RATIONALE: Pulling the last tip toward you allows you to avoid reaching over the inner contents of the package.
7. Gather all of the loose edges together to obtain a snug covering over your nondominant hand. Close your covered hand over the inner package and carefully apply the inner package to the sterile field (Figure 19-30D and E). RATIONALE: Gathering the loose edges prevents them from being dragged across the sterile field.

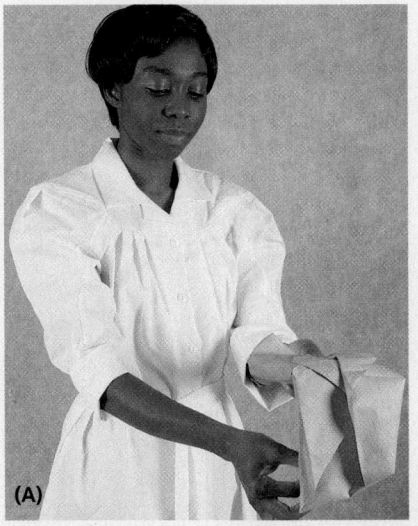
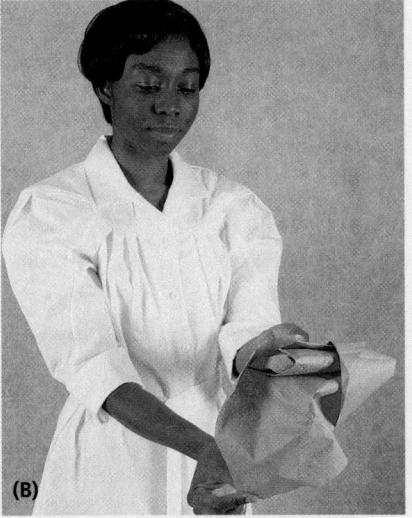
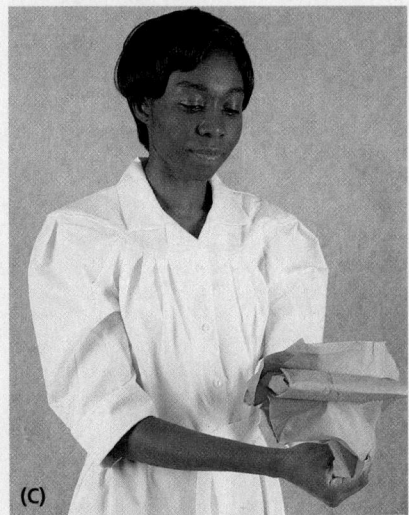

Figure 19-30 To open sterile packages: (A) Grasp the taped end of the top flap, and open the first flap away from you. Do not touch the inside of the flap. (B) Grasp just the folded back tips of the side flaps, and pull the right-sided flap to the right. (C) Now pull the left-sided flap to the left. Do not reach over the package. *(continues)*

Procedure 19-14 *(continued)*

8. Open peel-apart packages using sterile technique by grasping both edges of the flaps and pulling them apart in a rolling down motion, keeping both hands together. The sterile item should be exposed gradually between the two peel-apart edges. The sterile inner contents may then be offered to the sterile-gloved physician or applied to the sterile field using a flipping motion (Figure 19-30F), taking care not to contaminate either the package contents or the field.

9. Apply sterile gloves. Arrange instruments and supplies in an organized and logical manner according to the physician's preference (Figure 19-30G and H). RATIONALE: Instruments should be arranged in the order of use. All handles should be pointed toward the user. Instruments should be

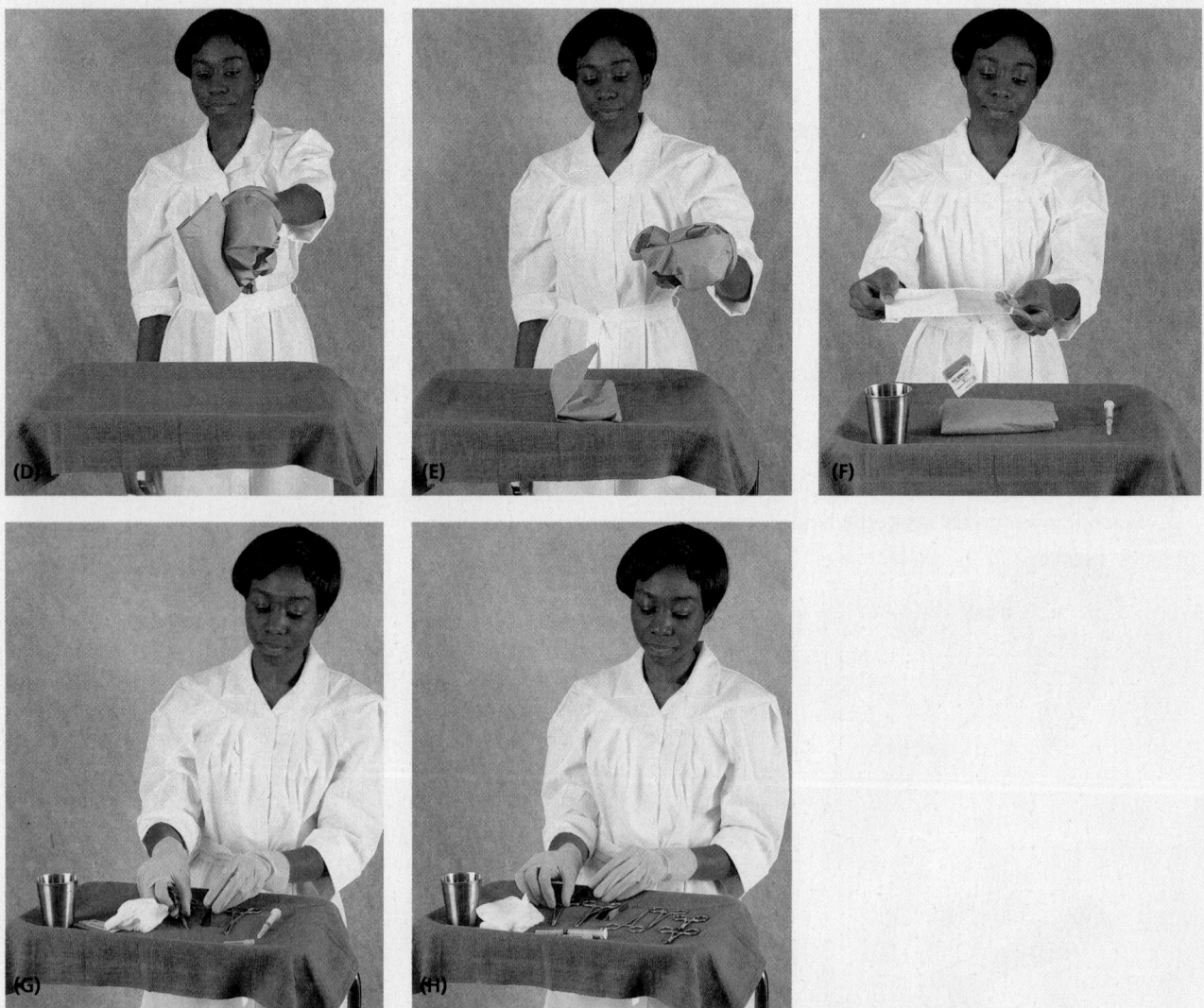

Figure 19-30   To open sterile packages: *(continued)* (D) Gather the loose edges together to obtain a snug covering over your nondominant hand. (E) Close the covered hand over the inner package, and apply the inner package to the sterile field. (F) Open peel-apart packages using sterile technique, exposing sterile item gradually. (G and H) Arrange instruments and supplies according to physician preference.   *(continues)*

Procedure 19-14 *(continued)*

separated as much as possible within the space of the field so entanglement of instruments is not a problem.

10. Apply the sterile field cover (Figure 19-30I and J). RATIONALE: A sterile cover will need to be

applied if the surgical tray will not be used immediately, needs to be moved, or if the medical assistant leaves the tray unattended.

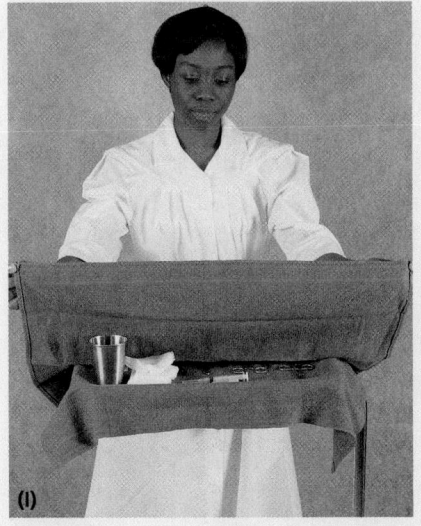
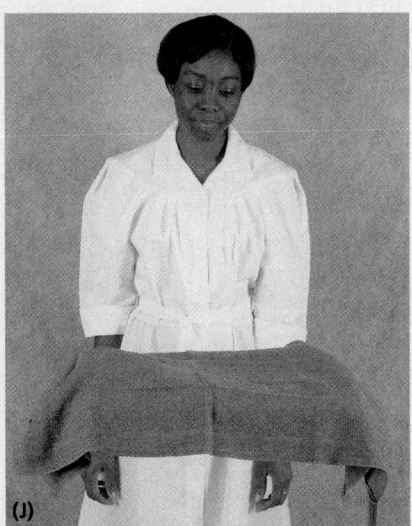

Figure 19-30 To open sterile packages: *(continued)* (I and J) Apply the sterile field cover.

Procedure 19-15 Pouring a Sterile Solution into a Cup on a Sterile Field

NOTE: Occasionally, sterile solutions will need to be poured into a sterile cup which has been placed onto the sterile tray. The solution is sterile, but the outside of the container is not; therefore special precautions need to be taken in order to pour the solution into the cup without contaminating the sterile field. The solution is always poured after the tray has been moved into the surgical area to avoid spilling during the movement.

STANDARD PRECAUTIONS:

PURPOSE:
To pour a sterile solution into a cup on a sterile tray in a sterile manner.

EQUIPMENT/SUPPLIES:
Covered sterile surgical tray with a sterile cup in upper right corner
Container of sterile solution

PROCEDURE STEPS:
1. Wash hands.
2. Transport the surgical tray into the surgical area before pouring the solution. Or: the surgical tray can be set up for immediate use in the surgical area. RATIONALE: The solution may tip and spill during transport.
3. Read the label of the solution container three times and check the expiration date. RATIONALE: To eliminate the possibility of pouring the wrong solution or an outdated solution.

(continues)

Procedure
19-15 (continued)

4. Remove the cap from the solution container taking care not to touch the inner surface of the cap. Place the cap upside down on a nonsterile surface to avoid touching the inner surface of the cap with a nonsterile surface. When the cap is held in the hand, hold it right side up. RATIONALE: Touching the inside of the cap with either your hand or a nonsterile surface will contaminate the inside of an otherwise sterile container.

5. Read the label again to assure accuracy. Place palm over the label to protect the label from stains. Pour a small amount of the solution into a bowl or cup that is outside the sterile field. RATIONALE: This action will cleanse the lip of the container. NOTE: If the surgical tray is set up in a surgical area, the solution can be poured prior to covering the surgical tray with a sterile drape or towel.

6. Carefully pull back the upper right corner of the tray cover to expose the cup. Take care to only touch the corner tip of the cover and not reach over the exposed field. RATIONALE: Touching the underside of the cover or reaching over the exposed sterile field will contaminate the sterile surgical tray.

7. Approaching from the corner of the tray, and using the cleansed side of the lip of the container, pour the needed amount of solution into the sterile cup (Figure 19-31). Precaution should be taken

to avoid splashing, spilling, reaching over the field, or touching any of the sterile surfaces. RATIONALE: Splashing or spilling of the solution would cause the sterile field drape to become wet, which could cause contaminants to "wick" from the metal tray into the sterile field. Use of a polylined sterile field drape will create a barrier.

8. Replace the cap of the solution container using sterile technique.

9. Replace the corner of the drape cover using sterile technique or cover with a sterile drape or towel.

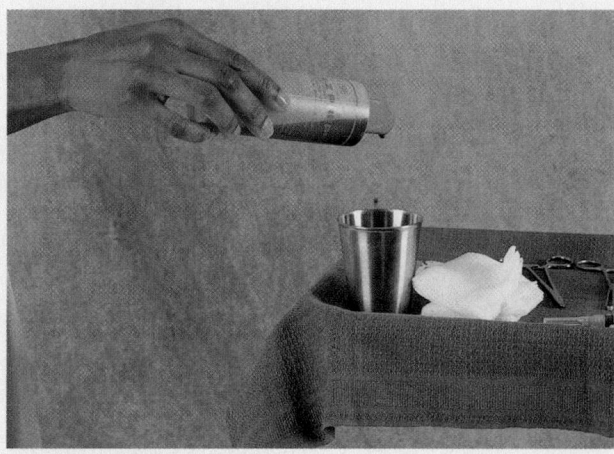

Figure 19-31 Approaching from the corner of the tray, pour the needed amount of solution into the sterile cup. Use the cleansed side of the container lip for pouring.

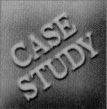

19-1

Cele Little, an eighty-something patient at Inner City Health Care, is having minor surgery performed on Thursday morning. Her sister, Dottie Tate, also a patient and also in her eighties, will come with Cele; a friend from the local senior citizen center has offered to drive them to the center and home again. Dottie is more nervous about the procedure, the removal of a bothersome cyst, than Cele. After talking with the sisters about the procedure, medical assistant Wanda Slawson, CMA, MLT, realizes this and wants to reassure Dottie but also wants her to be prepared to be caregiver to Cele.

CASE STUDY REVIEW

1. Where should Wanda begin in her communication with the two sisters?
2. What specific advice should Wanda give Cele and Dottie before the procedure?
3. What instructions should Wanda give the sisters to follow after the procedure?

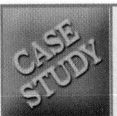

CASE STUDY

19-2

Letisha Brown has been scheduled to have a nevus excised from her upper back.

CASE STUDY REVIEW

1. Explain how you would prepare her for the surgery.
2. Explain how you would care for her postoperatively.
3. What will become of the excised nevus? Explain your actions.

SUMMARY

In assisting with minor surgery in the ambulatory care setting, the medical assistant needs to know sterile principles and understand the difference between medical and surgical asepsis. Knowledge of suture materials, instruments, and other supplies such as dressings and bandages is also critical. In preparing for minor surgical procedures, the medical assistant's communication skills will be needed, for patients can be apprehensive and will require both reassurance and education. In addition to understanding the basic process and preparations for assisting with minor surgery, the medical assistant should also be aware of the steps involved in some of the more common minor surgical procedures.

REVIEW QUESTIONS

Multiple Choice

1. Which of the following describes the primary purpose of surgical asepsis?
   a. to prevent microorganisms from collecting on the Mayo stand
   b. to prevent microorganisms from causing inflammation
   c. to prevent microorganisms from entering the body during an invasive procedure
   d. to prevent microorganisms from multiplying
2. A basic rule to follow to protect sterile items is:
   a. a sterile object may touch a nonsterile object under certain circumstances
   b. it is safe to turn your back on the sterile field if you leave plenty of room between you and the field
   c. provide the physician a separate container for contaminated instruments
   d. gloved hands are held at the same height as the hip bone
3. Which of the following is the smallest size suture material?
   a. 0
   b. 2-0
   c. 4-0
   d. 1

4. Which of the following is an example of absorbable suture material?
   a. gut
   b. chromium salts
   c. silk
   d. Dacron
5. What is the purpose of adding epinephrine to the local anesthetic?
   a. to prevent an allergic reaction
   b. to reduce blood flow in the operative site through vasoconstriction
   c. to reduce patient discomfort during the procedure
   d. to maintain patient vital signs
6. Which of the following actions might the physician take if a sebaceous cyst were infected?
   a. remove the cyst
   b. do a biopsy of the cyst
   c. perform cryosurgery on the cyst
   d. incise and drain the cyst

Critical Thinking

1. You have just removed a double-wrapped instrument pack from the autoclave and notice a small tear in the outermost wrap. The inner wrap appears to be intact. What would your action be? Why?

2. You are setting up a sterile surgical tray and have already applied your sterile gloves before you realize you forgot to place the suture package on the tray. You have several options. What are they and what are the advantages and disadvantages of each?

3. What would be the rationale behind leaving a wound open rather than suturing it? On what basis would this decision be made?

4. While you are preparing a patient for surgery, he confides in you that he doesn't have anyone to drive him home, but he only lives three miles away and plans to drive himself. How do you respond?

5. You have thoroughly explained the postoperative instructions to the patient and caregiver. Are written instructions also necessary? Why or why not?

6. While pouring a sterile solution into a bowl on the sterile field, you accidentally splash a very tiny amount of the solution onto the field. What is your next step? Explain your actions.

7. Dr. Woo asks you to assist him in repairing the laceration on Jaime Carrera's hand. Though you are un-

sure, you think you may have noticed a tiny hole in the palm of your left glove. What is your next step?

8. While assisting during an incision and drainage of a localized infection on Abigail Johnson's left leg, you notice there is a large amount of exudate that discharges from the incisional site. What, if any, precautions should you take?

WEB ACTIVITIES

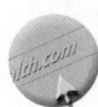 Search the Internet to explore the most current outpatient surgical procedures for hemorrhoids, cataracts, and cholelithiasis.

REFERENCES/BIBLIOGRAPHY

Bonewit-West, K. (2000). *Clinical procedures for medical assistants* (5th ed.). Philadelphia: W. B. Saunders Company.

Taber's cyclopedic medical dictionary (18th ed.). (1999). Philadelphia: F. A. Davis Company.

20

DIAGNOSTIC IMAGING

KEY TERMS

Claustrophobia
Dosimeter
Echocardiogram
Esophageal Varices
Fluoroscope
Ionizing Radiation
Noninvasive
Oscilloscope
Palliative
Radioactive
Radiograph
Radiolucent
Radionuclides
Radiopaque
Radiopharmaceuticals
Stomatitis
Transducer

OUTLINE

X-Ray Machine
Radiation Safety
Contrast Media
Patient Preparation
Positioning of the Patient
Fluoroscopy
Diagnostic Imaging
   Ultrasonography
   Positron Emission Tomography
    (PET)

Computerized Tomography
   (CT)
Magnetic Resonance Imaging
   (MRI)
Flat Plates
Filing Films and Reports
Radiation Therapy
Nuclear Medicine

OBJECTIVES

The student should strive to meet the following performance objectives and demonstrate an understanding of the facts and principles presented in this chapter through written and oral communication.

1. Define key terms as presented in the glossary.
2. Describe safety precautions for personnel and patients as they relate to ionizing radiation treatments.
3. Explain how fluoroscopy is used and explain its benefits.
4. Describe the various positions used during X-ray procedures.
5. Describe four X-ray procedures that require patient preparation.
6. Discuss the uses of ultrasonography, positron emission, tomography, computerized tomography, magnetic resonance, and flat plates.
7. Discuss how radiographs are stored.
8. Explain the differences among radiology, radiation therapy, and nuclear medicine.
9. Recall four side effects of radiation.

ROLE DELINEATION COMPONENTS

ADMINISTRATIVE

Administrative Procedures

- Schedule, coordinate, and monitor appointments
- Schedule inpatient and outpatient admissions and procedures

CLINICAL

Fundamental Principles

- Screen and follow up patient test results

Patient Care

- Prepare patients for examination, procedures, and treatments
- Coordinate patient care information with other health care providers

GENERAL (TRANSDISCIPLINARY)

Professionalism

- Project a professional manner and image
- Adhere to ethical principles

Communication Skills

- Adapt communication to individual's ability to understand

Legal Concepts

- Maintain confidentiality
- Practice within the scope of education, training, and personal capabilities
- Comply with established risk management and safety procedures

Instruction

- Instruct individuals according to their needs

SCENARIO

In the radiology department of Inner City Hospital, there are several patients waiting to have their procedures performed. Wanda Shawson brings Don Waite to the department for an intravenous pyelogram. She is careful to make certain that Mr. Waite has been properly prepared for the procedure. She does not want the procedure to have to be repeated due to the inconvenience and anxiety it may cause Mr. Waite, nor does she want there to be additional expense and time spent repeating the procedure.

INTRODUCTION

X rays were named when a German physicist, Wilhelm Roentgen, discovered them in 1895. He noticed that the X rays were able to pass through human skin, paper, wood, and other solid materials. Because he did not know what they were, he called them X rays.

X rays or **radiographs** are a valuable diagnostic tool used to visualize internal organs and structures when searching for diseases and disorders. They are also a valuable therapeutic tool because they can be used to treat cancerous neoplasms.

Radiology uses X rays, radioactive substances, and ultraviolet rays. There are three specialties into which radiology can be classified: diagnostic radiology, radiation therapy, and nuclear medicine.

X rays are often not taken in an office setting; rather, they are taken in the radiology department of a hospital or a free-standing X-ray service outside of the hospital. Some X rays, such as those looking for a fractured bone, require no preparation, while others, such as an intravenous pyelogram, require special preparation.

In some states, medical assistants and other health care professionals who are not licensed to take radiographs are not allowed by law to assist with radiologic procedures. The medical assistants must have a basic understanding of radiology and radiology safety in order to instruct patients in proper preparation for radiologic procedures and to protect themselves from X-ray exposure.

X-RAY MACHINE

There are three main parts to an X-ray machine: the table, the X-ray tube, and the control panel. The tube is where the X rays are produced and then come out as a beam of X ray. Lead surrounds the tube except for the area where the beams of X ray are sent out. The table on which the patient lies is movable in several directions, even upright or angled. The control panel is positioned behind a lead wall especially designed for shielding the radiographer from X rays when an X ray is being taken (Figure 20-1).

RADIATION SAFETY

X rays, though invisible to the human eye, are extremely powerful and can be dangerous and harmful. Exposure to radiation can destroy tissue and permanently damage the eyes, bone marrow, and the skin. They are also harmful to the developing embryo and fetus, causing severe anomalies and death.

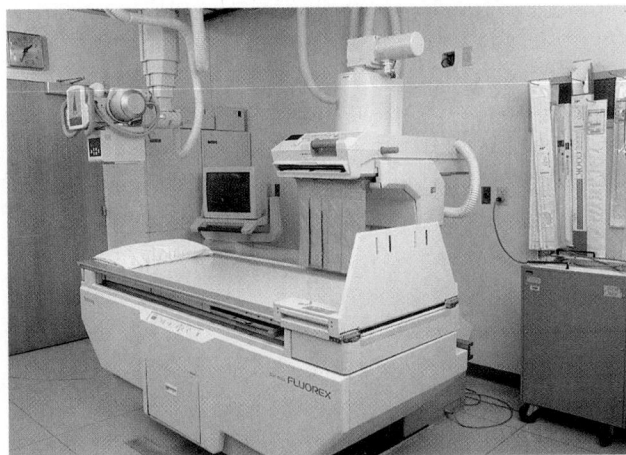

Figure 20-1 Radiographic room prepared for procedure.

Personnel in the X-ray department and others who are exposed to X rays must wear a **dosimeter**, a small badge-like device worn above the waist. The dosimeter contains a strip of film that measures the amount of X ray a person is exposed to. The dosimeter film is read on a regular basis and radiation exposure is reported to a supervisor. Exposure can come from the X-ray beam itself or from scattered rays that are produced when going through the patient's body.

Patients must wear lead aprons over the reproductive organs, and technicians must shield themselves with lead aprons and gloves if they are assisting, but shields are not necessary when standing behind the lead wall working the control panel. Additionally, walls in rooms where X rays are taken are lead-lined to absorb scattering rays.

CONTRAST MEDIA

Various body structures are of different densities. Bone is denser than skin and, therefore, can absorb more X rays leaving fewer to be picked up by the X-ray film. Thus, an X ray of bone will appear white. A lung is less dense, and the X rays can penetrate lung tissue. The lung appears black on the radiograph. If X rays do not penetrate a structure easily, it is termed **radiopaque**, if they penetrate readily, it is termed **radiolucent**. Contrast media are radiopaque and help to obtain a radiographic image of an internal organ or structure that ordinarily would be difficult to see because the contrast media cause the organs or structures of the body to absorb more radiation.

Some commonly used contrast media are barium sulfate, iodine compounds, air, and carbon dioxide. Barium is a chalky compound, and when mixed with water, can be swallowed by the patient or administered as an enema by a radiologic technician. It is used for upper and lower gastrointestinal series of X rays. The patient is told

to drink extra fluids to flush out barium. Iodine salts are radiopaque and are used for kidney, gallbladder, and thyroid exams. Some individuals are allergic to the iodine salts used as contrast media. Patients are asked whether they have any allergies, but in particular, allergies to foods that contain iodine, such as fish.

Air and carbon dioxide are used to visualize the spinal cord and joints, but have been replaced by use of the magnetic resonance imaging (MRI) machine.

PATIENT PREPARATION

By law, without special education and training about X rays, the medical assistant's role in X-ray procedures in most states will be limited to patient preparation information and explanations about what the patient can anticipate. A thorough knowledge of the procedure that the physician has ordered is essential, and the medical assistant must be certain that patients understand the preparation they are about to undertake. Verbal explanations should be followed up with written instructions. Many patients, fearful of what the ordered X ray will show, are anxious and frightened and can easily forget verbal instructions. Proper preparation is essential for the best results on the radiographs. Repeating a procedure because of inadequate preparation results in increased patient anxiety, time, expense, and inconvenience (Table 20-1).

TABLE 20-1   PATIENT PREPARATION AND PURPOSE OF X-RAY PROCEDURES

Test	Purpose	Patient Preparation	Procedure
Angiography	To visualize the inside of blood vessel walls. Helps to diagnose heart attacks, stroke, and aneurysm (Figure 20-2).	NPO 6–8 hours prior to exam.	1. Contrast medium (iodine) injected into an artery or vein. 2. Catheter threaded to the appropriate site. 3. Digital angiography can be done and stored on computer disk.
Barium swallow (upper GI series)	To study the esophagus, stomach, duodenum, and small intestine for disease (ulcers, tumors, hiatal hernia, esophageal varices) (Figure 20-3A).	Day prior: Light evening meal. NPO after midnight. Day of test: NPO. Postprocedural: Increase fluid intake. Take laxative as prescribed.	1. The patient is asked to drink a flavored barium mixture while standing in front of the fluoroscope. 2. The radiologist observes the passage down the digestive tract. 3. The patient is turned to various positions to allow good visualization of the intestines. 4. X rays are taken.
Barium enema (lower GI series)	To study the colon for disease (polyps, tumors, lesions).	Prep kit (usually supplied by physician's office) to include bottle of magnesium citrate and Dulcolax tablet(s). Day prior: 1. Clear liquid allowed: carbonated beverages, clear gelatin, clear broth, coffee and tea with sugar. No milk or milk products. 2. 8 oz. of water every hour until bedtime. 3. Late afternoon, drink bottle of magnesium citrate. 4. Early evening, take Dulcolax tablet(s) as prescribed. 5. Light evening meal. NPO except water after dinner. Morning procedure: NPO, cleaning enema Postprocedural: 1. Increase fluid intake and dietary fiber. 2. Report to physician if no bowel movement within 24 hours of test.	1. The colon is filled with a barium sulfate mixture. 2. The patient is turned in various positions to allow the barium to fill the colon. Air is injected to move the barium along the colon. 3. When the colon is full, X rays are taken.
Cholangiography	To view the bile ducts for possible calculi or lesions.	May have cleaning enema one hour before exam. Meal preceding exam is withheld.	Contrast medium injected and radiograph of bile ducts is taken.
Cholecystography	To study the gallbladder for disease (stones, duct obstruction), inflammation.	1. Evening before test, fat-free dinner. 2. Patient takes dye tablets with 8 oz. of water. 3. Cathartic or cleansing enemas may be prescribed. 4. NPO after dinner and tablets.	1. A series of radiographs is taken. 2. A fatty meal may be given to stimulate the gallbladder to empty. 3. Other radiographs can then be taken to check gallbladder function.
Cystography	To view the urinary bladder for lesions, calculi.	Day prior: Light evening meal. NPO after midnight.	Contrast medium injected and radiograph of the urinary bladder is taken.
Hysterosalpingography	To view the uterus and fallopian tubes for blockage and lesions. To check for pelvic masses.	Laxative evening before. Cleansing enema day of exam. Meal prior to exam is withheld.	Contrast medium injected and radiographs taken of uterus and fallopian tubes. Carbon dioxide may also be used.
Intravenous Pyelography (IVP)	Visualization of kidneys, ureters, and bladder to detect kidney stones, lesions, strictures of urinary tract.	Eat a light evening meal and nothing after midnight. A laxative and enema are used to clean out the intestines to prevent a blocked view of the ureters behind the intestines.	A contrast medium of iodine salts is given intravenously after it has been determined that the patient is not allergic to iodine. (See Chapter 18.)
Mammography	To detect abnormalities in the breast, especially breast cancer.	Do not wear lotion, deodorant, or powders. Remove clothing from waist up. No contrast medium required.	Breast is positioned on the mammograph and compressed to flatten it. Two radiographs are taken of each breast, from the side and from above.
Retrograde Pyelography	To view the kidneys and urinary tract for abnormalities.	Drink 4–5 glasses of water prior to examination unless sedated, then NPO.	Contrast medium injected and radiographs taken of the kidneys and urinary bladder.

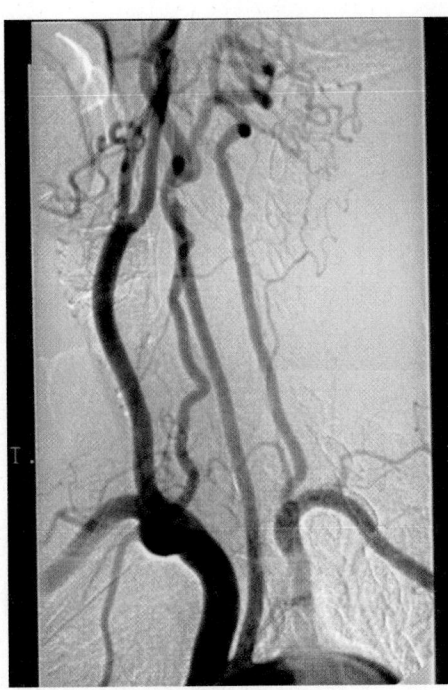

Figure 20-2   Carotid angiography.

POSITIONING THE PATIENT

The correct patient position is important for obtaining the best quality X ray and the type of examination that is necessary will determine patient position. Some basis views are:

- Anterioposterior view (AP)–the anterior surface of the body faces the X-ray tube and X rays are directed from the front toward the back of the body.

- Posteroanterior view (PA)–the posterior surface of the body faces the X-ray tube and X rays are directed from back to front (Figure 20-4A and 20-4B).

- Lateral view–X rays pass through the body from one side to the opposite side.

- Right lateral view (RL)–X rays are directed through the body from the left to the right side. The right side of the body is next to the film.

- Left lateral view (LL)–X rays are directed through the body from the right to the left side. The left side of the body is next to the film.

- Oblique view–the body is positioned at an angle.

- Supine view–the body is lying face up, on the back.

- Prone view–the body is lying face down, on the abdomen.

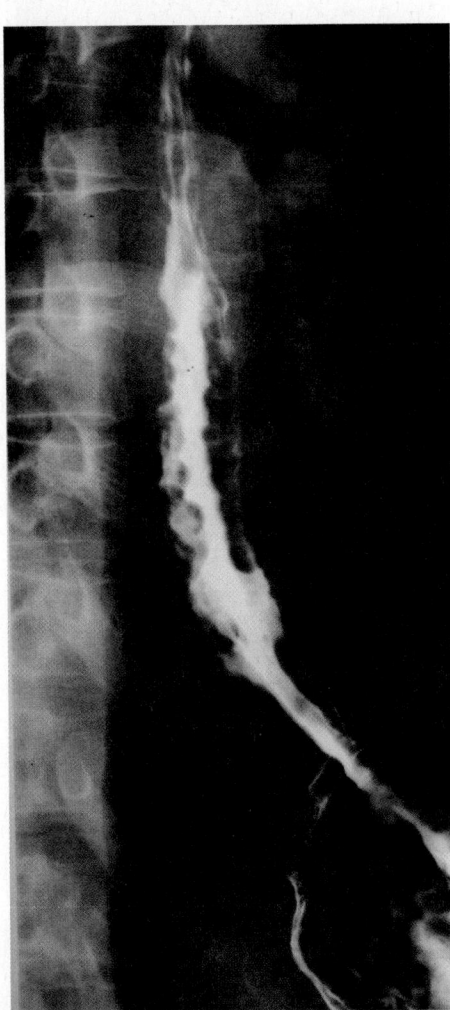

Figure 20-3A   Esophageal varices.

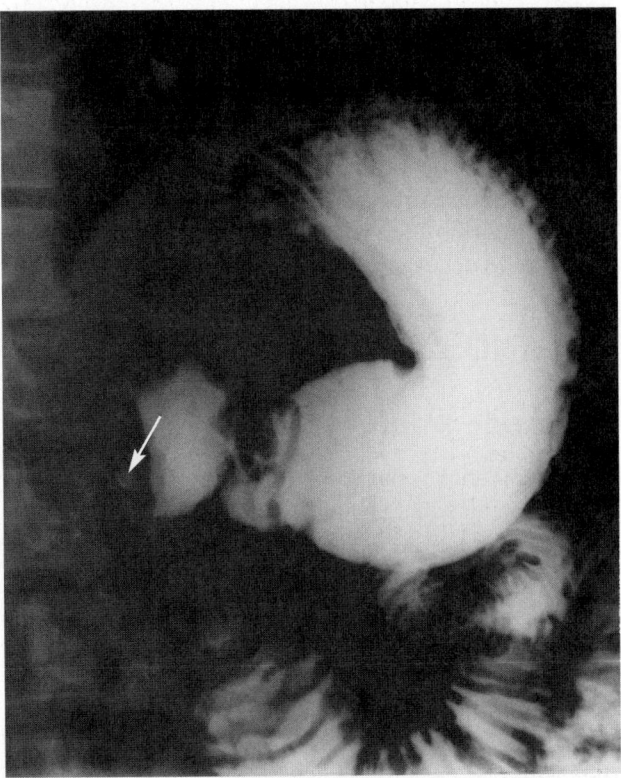

Figure 20-3B   Duodenal ulcer.

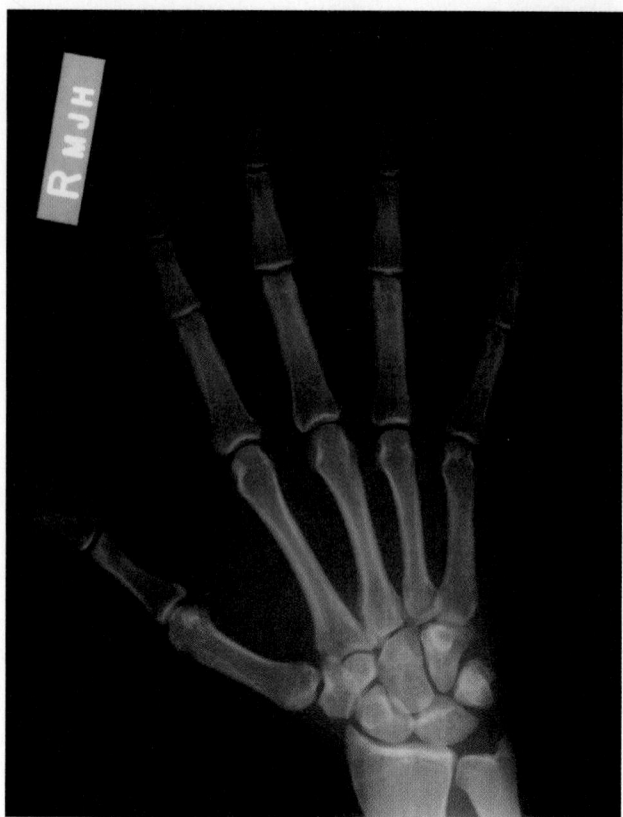

Figure 20-4A   PA hand.

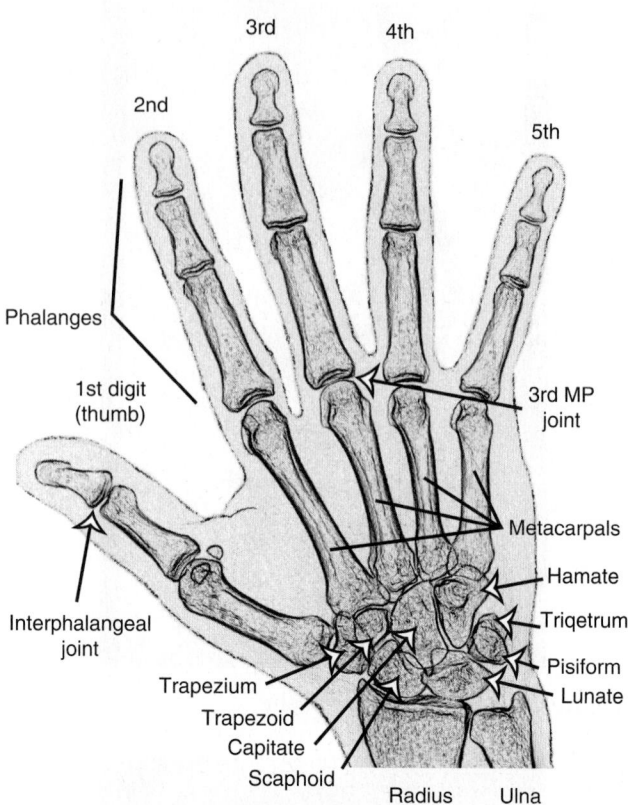

Figure 20-4B   PA hand.

FLUOROSCOPY

Fluoroscopy is the process of using a **fluoroscope** to view internal organs and structures of the body so that they may be seen in motion immediately by the radiologist. The patient is usually given a contrast medium and placed between the X-ray tube and the fluoroscope. Fluoroscopy is used for procedures such as cardiac catheterization and for viewing the function of the stomach and intestinal structures to detect any abnormalities (Figure 20-5).

DIAGNOSTIC IMAGING

Ultrasonography

Ultrasonography, computerized tomography, and magnetic resonance imaging allow for greater imaging detail than conventional radiographs. Ultrasonography, or ultrasound, has been available longer than the others. High-frequency sound waves (inaudible to the human ear) are used to image internal soft tissues. It can be used to help diagnose problems in the abdominal organs, the liver, and gallbladder. It cannot be used for skeletal structures or the lungs. An **echocardiogram**, an ultrasound of the heart, can view it and determine the size, shape, and position of the heart and the motion made by the valves

opening and closing. Ultrasound has advantages over other methods of viewing internal organs and structures in that it uses no X rays and allows for continuous viewing while organs and structures are in motion.

During ultrasound, a **transducer** is used with a coupling agent and sound waves are emitted from the head of the transducer. The transducer is placed firmly on the patient's body over the organ to be examined. The sound waves pass through the skin and bounce off the body's tissues and are reflected back to the transducer. These

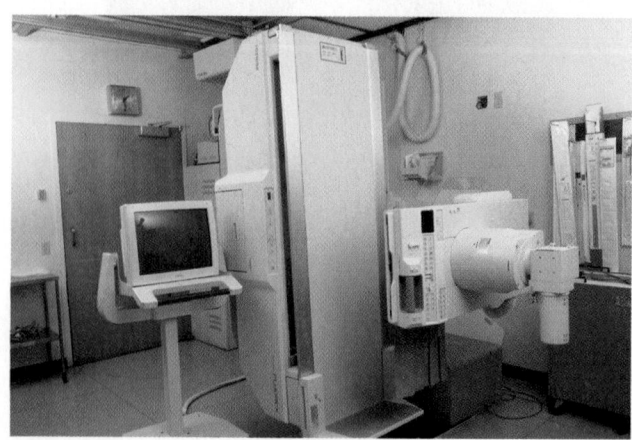

Figure 20-5   Fluoroscopic room ready for upper GI study.

echoes are displayed on an oscilloscope, showing a visual pattern or picture. The image or record produced is known as a sonogram or echogram. A permanent film for the patient's record and videotape can also be made.

Ultrasonography, because it is noninvasive, is widely accepted for obstetrical use. Gestational age can be determined, congenital anomalies detected, multiple fetuses noted, ectopic pregnancy diagnosed, and fetal size and position determined.

Ultrasound takes 15 to 45 minutes and the preparation depends on the body part being examined. An obstetrical ultrasound may require the patient to have a full bladder in order to push aside the intestines. An ultrasound of the gallbladder and liver require the patient to have had nothing to eat or drink for eight to 12 hours prior to the exam. The patient must remain still unless requested to change positions. Therapeutic ultrasonography is discussed in Chapter 21 (Figure 20-6).

Positron Emission Tomography (PET)

Positron emission tomography, or PET, is a radiographic procedure using a computer and a radioactive substance. The radioactive substance is injected into the patient's body and gives off charged particles. They combine with particles in the patient's body to produce color images that tell the amount of metabolic activity there is in an organ or structure.

PET imaging is primarily a diagnostic medical imaging modality. It makes use of specialized, intravenously injected radiopharmaceuticals that emit positrons, which can be detected out of the body due to high energy releases. Specialized detectors arranged around the patient sense the energy and map the location from which it originated inside the body. These radiopharmaceuticals can be chemically designed to localize in the heart, brain, or certain types of tumors throughout the body. A clinical image is formed by the accumulation of positron emissions in a target organ. The patient's emission pattern forms a clinical image. This image is compared to the normal distribution by the nuclear medicine physician.

Generally, low to moderate doses are used to diagnose disease in patients. Certain nuclear medicine treatment studies use specialized radiopharmaceuticals that will isolate in the area to be treated. These agents emit their energy locally, irradiate tissue, and usually do not leave the body, unlike diagnostic radiopharmaceuticals. The properties and intent of diagnostic radiopharmaceuticals are different from therapeutic radiopharmaceuticals (Figure 20-7).

Computerized Tomography (CT)

A computerized tomograph uses a small amount of radiation. The beams penetrate body tissues to produce a series of cross-sectional images of the body part being examined. It allows images of structures that cannot be seen with regular X rays. It is a noninvasive test that usually requires no preparation and uses the computer with a minimal amount of radiation. It rotates 360 degrees around the patient to obtain cross-sectional images that can be viewed on a monitor and on film. It is ideal for early detection of tissue tumors such as childhood cancers and abdominal tumors, and it helps in directing radiation therapy for tumor masses. On occasion, a contrast medium is injected for a better view of internal structures. If contrast medium is used, the patient must be NPO (have nothing by mouth) for four hours before the patient is placed onto a motorized table that moves the body part to be examined into a scanner that surrounds that part of the patient. In 15 to 20 minutes, an entire body can be scanned (Figures 20-8A, 20-8B and 20-8C).

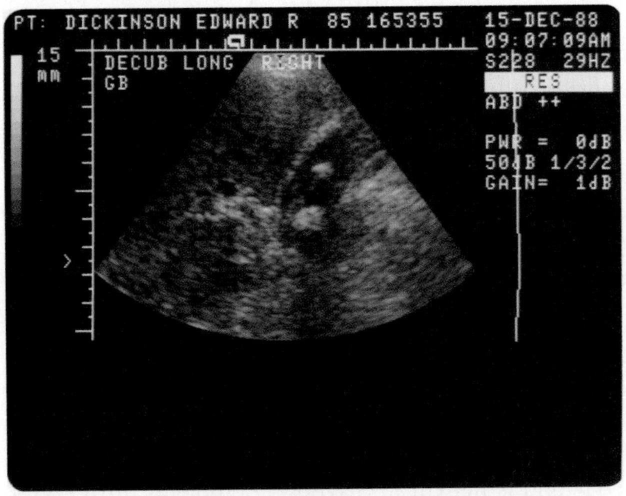

Figure 20-6 Sonogram of gallbladder with gallstones.

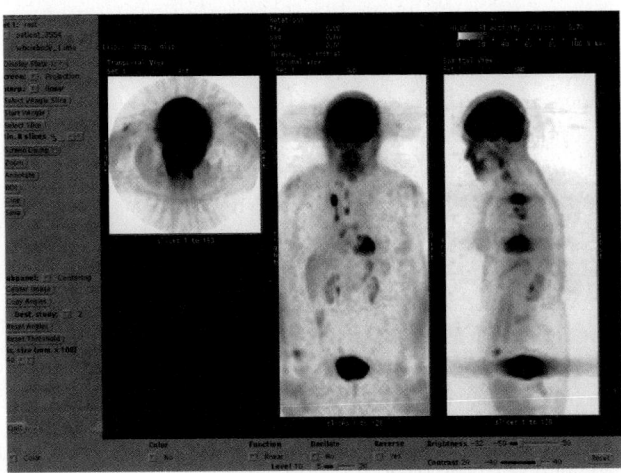

Figure 20-7 PET body scan demonstrates a tumor in the right lung.

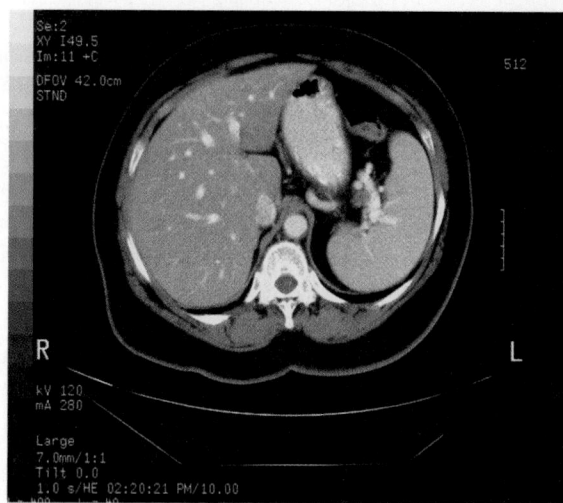

Figure 20-8A   The positive contrast seen in the text and the highlighted hepatic vessels, inferior vena cava, aorta, and splenic artery denotes the administration of IV contrast media in this CT scan.

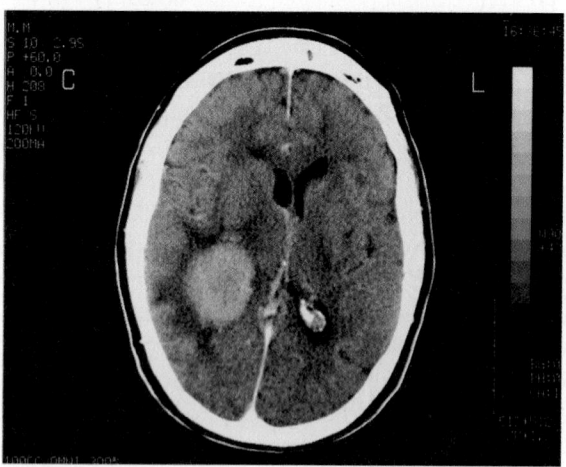

Figure 20-8B   Axial CT scan demonstrates a meningioma surrounded by edema.

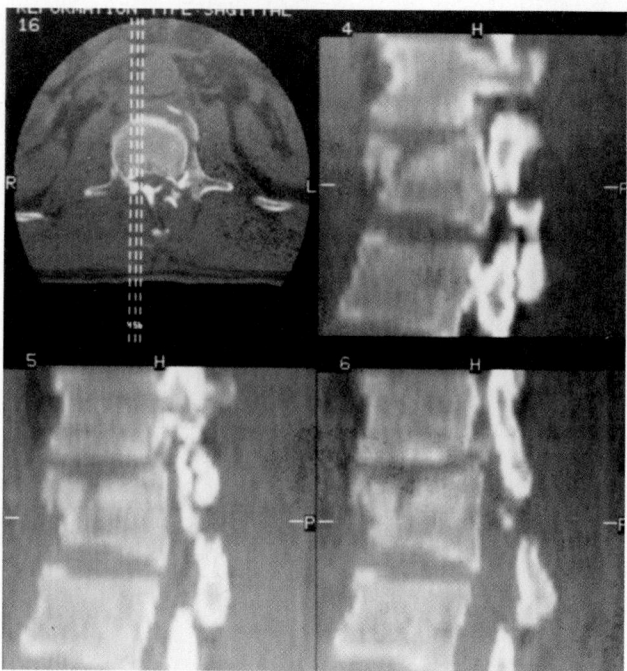

Figure 20-8C   Axial scan showing a fractured thoracic vertebra. The three sagittally reconstructed images depict the area denoted by the dotted lines.

Magnetic Resonance Imaging (MRI)

Images produced by magnetic resonance imaging are of exceptionally high quality. No **ionizing radiation** is used, and it is noninvasive, safe, and painless procedure. All body areas can be viewed by the MRI, but it is especially helpful for soft tissues. It is very good for the spine, pelvis, and joints and is superior for visualizing the brain. The examiner can see through fluid-filled tissue with exceptional detail using an MRI machine. The computer forms the visual image.

The patient lies on a table inside a cylinder-shaped machine in which there is an electromagnet. The machine is sealed with the patient inside. Some patients who suffer from **claustrophobia** may need medication to help relieve symptoms of anxiety. Open MRI machines are now available and are particularly useful for those patients who are too apprehensive to be sealed in the traditional MRI machine.

Some drawbacks to the MRI are that it cannot be used for patients who have pacemakers or other metal clips left in place on internal structures or organs as part of a surgical procedure. An MRI is not as useful as conventional X rays or a CT scan for diagnosing fractured bones.

Patients are told to remove all objects that have metal: watches, belts, hairpins, rings, other metal jewelry, and credit cards because of the strong magnet in the MRI machine. Loose, comfortable clothing without zippers or snaps should be worn. The procedure takes about 45 minutes to an hour, during which time the patient must remain still. The technician, while not in the room with the patient, has a camera and microphone with which to communicate with the patient. An intermittent tapping sound can be heard throughout the procedure and earphones are available if the patient wants them (Figures 20-9 and 20-10).

Flat Plates

Flat plates are also known as "plain" films because they require no special technique or the use of contrast medium. This type of X ray is used on various parts of the body and is helpful in diagnosing problems in the skull, abdomen, chest, sinuses, and bone.

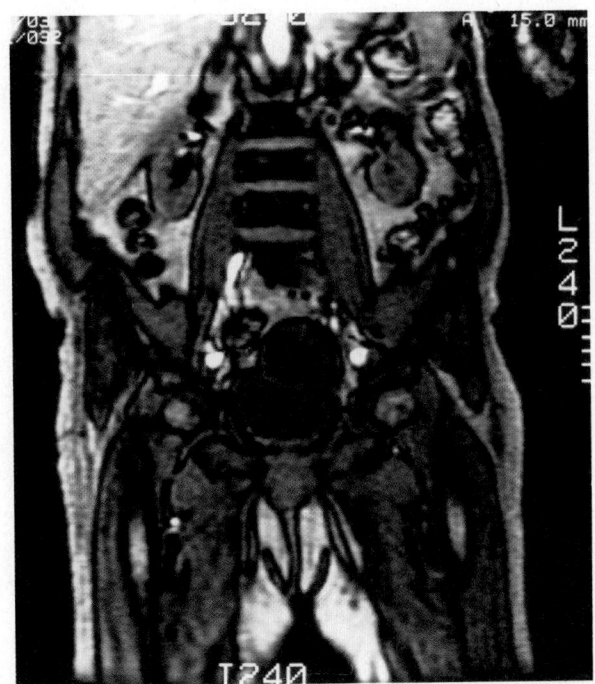

Figure 20-9 Coronal image of abdomen acquired during a breath hold in this MRI.

Filing Films and Reports

Because radiographs are part of the patient's permanent record, they must be safeguarded from the environment. Such conditions as heat, moisture, and light can damage them. Processed films are stored in special envelopes with the patient's name, date, and identification number marked on the outside. They are stored in a cool, dry place. The films are the property of the hospital or other facility where the films were taken and usually remain where they were taken. Storage on-site makes them accessible for future use for comparison purposes and eliminates the possibility of their being lost if they were allowed to be taken away from the facility where they were taken. Written reports of the findings are prepared by the radiologist and sent to the patient's physician(s) (Figure 20-11).

RADIATION THERAPY

Radiation therapy is generally used to treat tumors that cannot be surgically removed or are inaccessible for surgical removal, and for treatment of a malignant tumor that was surgically excised, but a portion of the tumor remains.

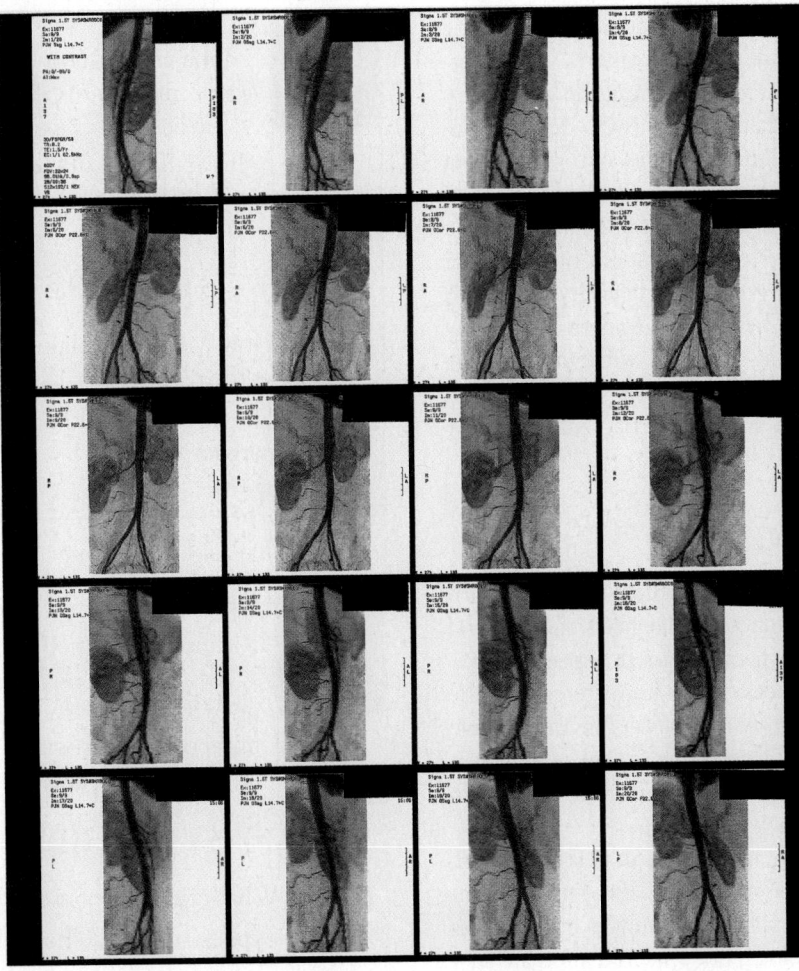

Figure 20-10 Magnetic resonance angiography.

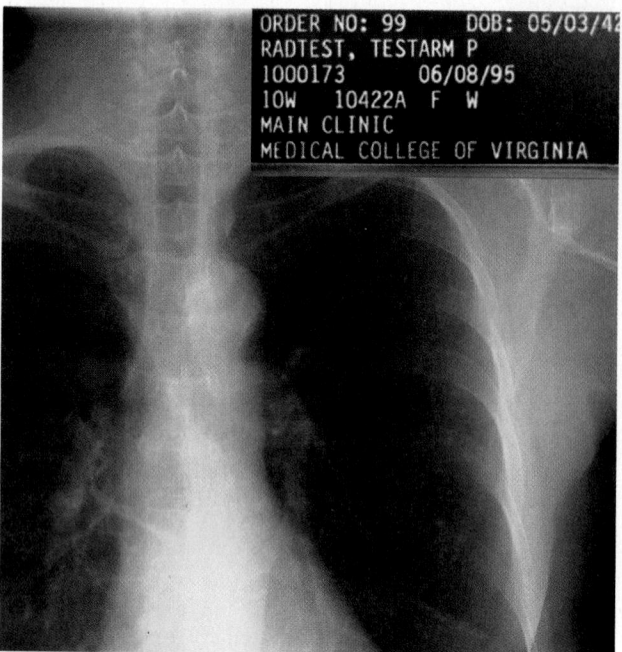

Figure 20-11A Radiograph showing patient identification information.

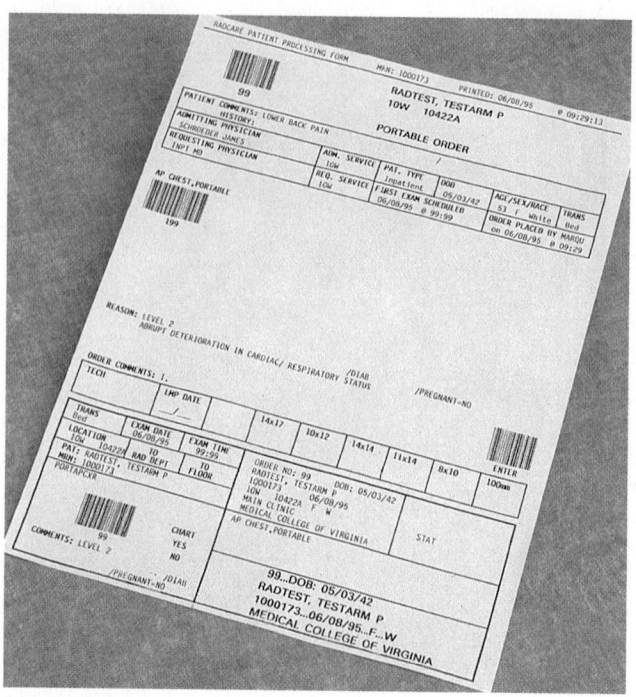

Figure 20-11B Sample requisition form.

When used to treat inaccessible or inoperable tumors, the treatment is considered **palliative** treatment. The treatments shrink the tumor, thereby lessening the symptoms. The treatments can be either external, with direct radiation aimed through the surface of the skin to an area within the body, or internal, using various applications of radioactivity such as seeds or beads that are planted inside the body and left there for a certain amount of time. The aim with radiation therapy is to interfere with cell growth and to disrupt the DNA. The object is to destroy as many of the malignant cells as possible without harming healthy cells surrounding the tumor. The side effects can be nausea, vomiting, hair loss, anorexia, bone marrow suppression, and **stomatitis**.

NUCLEAR MEDICINE

Nuclear medicine is the branch of medicine involved with the use of **radioactive** substances for diagnosis, therapy, and research. Specific training is necessary for this speciality.

Radioactive substances are administered to the patient either by mouth or by injection. The radioactive compounds, known as **radionuclides**, travel to an organ or area in the body that attracts them and creates an image of that area.

If the radionuclide is in an area that is abnormal, such as a tumor, it is referred to as "hot." If it does not concentrate in the abnormality, but surrounds it instead, this is known as a "cold" area. Both hot and cold areas are suggestive of abnormalities.

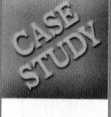

CASE STUDY

20-1

Gloria McDermott is scheduled to have a gastrointestinal (GI) series of X rays next week because of persistent complaints of stomach pain that is unrelieved by the prescription medication Dr. King has prescribed for her.

CASE STUDY REVIEW

1. How will you explain to her the purpose of the test?

2. How will you tell her about how to prepare for the exam?

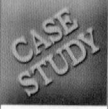

CASE STUDY

20-2

Raymond Brunnelle has had a series of X rays, a GI series, a cholecystogram, and an MRI of his abdomen. He has scheduled an appointment with a gastroenterologist and asks you to get all of the films for him.

CASE STUDY REVIEW

1. What is your response to his request?

2. Explain why they should be kept on-site.

SUMMARY

Radiology and diagnostic imaging are helpful in the diagnosis and treatment of diseases and conditions because procedures can be done to visualize internal structures and their functions. Radiation is not without its risks to personnel and patients, but by follow-ing specific safety precautions, the health and safety of all involved can be safeguarded.

The three specialty areas are radiology, radiation therapy, and nuclear medicine.

REVIEW QUESTIONS

Multiple Choice

1. Which of the following radiologic procedures does *not* require a contrast medium?
   a. hysterosalpingogram
   b. mammogram
   c. cholecystogram
   d. angiogram
2. A cholecystogram requires which type of contrast medium?
   a. air
   b. tablets
   c. carbon dioxide
   d. radionuclides
3. A cholangiogram will examine:
   a. upper GI tract
   b. lower GI tract
   c. bile ducts
   d. kidneys and ureters
4. In which of the following positions does the posterior aspect of the body face the X-ray tube and the anterior face the film?
   a. oblique
   b. anterioposterior
   c. posteroanterior
   d. prone
   e. supine
5. The radiologic procedure of choice for brain imaging is:
   a. computerized tomography
   b. positron emission tomography
   c. magnetic resonance imaging
   d. ultrasonogram
   e. thermography

Critical Thinking Questions

1. Describe the purpose of a lead apron and lead-lined walls in the radiology department.
2. For what is thermography used?
3. How are X rays used to diagnose?
4. How are X rays used to treat patient diseases or conditions?
5. Describe four types of contrast media.

6. What are the effects of radiation on an embryo or fetus?
7. To whom do X-ray films belong once they are taken and processed?
8. Describe how radiation therapy helps to destroy malignant neoplasms.
9. What special precautions should be taken when a patient is having an intravenous pyelogram, especially the initial time?
10. What do some state laws require of personnel who take X rays?

WEB ACTIVITIES

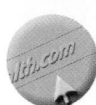

Access a web site regarding the radiologic technology profession to determine which states allow medical assistants to take and process X rays.

REFERENCES/BIBLIOGRAPHY

Bonewit-West, K. (2000). *Clinical procedures for medical assistants* (5th ed.). Philadelphia: W. B. Saunders Company.

Cornuelle, A., & Gronefeld, D. (1998). *Radiographic anatomy positioning: An integrated approach.* Stanford, CT: Appleton and Lange.

Cowling, C. (1998). *Radiographic positioning procedures, Volume II: Advanced imaging procedures.* Albany, NY: Delmar.

Early, P. J., & Sodee, D. B. (1995). *Principles and practice of nuclear medicine* (2nd ed.). St. Louis: Mosby-Year Book.

Fregmen, B. (1998). *Essentials of medical assisting administrative and clinical competencies.* Upper Saddle River, NJ: Brady-Prentice Hall.

Greathouse, J. (1998). *Radiographic positioning procedures, Volume I: Basic positioning and procedures.* Albany, NY: Delmar.

Kinn, M. E., & Woods, M. A. (1999). *The medical assistant: Administrative and clinical* (8th ed.). Philadelphia: W. B. Saunders Company.

Metler, F. A., Jr., & Guiberteau, M. J. (1997). *Essentials of nuclear medicine imaging* (4th ed.). Philadelphia: W. B. Saunders Company.

Taber's cylopedic medical dictionary. (18th ed.). (1999). Philadelphia: F. A. Davis Company.

KEY TERMS

Abduction

Activities of Daily Living (ADL)

Adduction

Ambulation

Assistive Device

Atrophy

Body Mechanics

Circumduction

Contracture

Cryotherapy

Dorsiflexion

Eversion

Extension

Flexion

Gait

Gait Belt

Goniometer

Goniometry

Hemiplegia

Hyperextension

Inversion

Modalities

Muscle Testing

Plantar Flexion

Pronation

Range of Motion (ROM)

Rehabilitation Medicine

Rotation

Supination

Thermotherapy

Ultrasound

Vasoconstriction

Vasodilation

OUTLINE

The Role of the Medical Assistant in Rehabilitation

Principles of Body Mechanics

Posture

Using the Body Safely and Effectively

Lifting Techniques

Transferring Patients

Assisting Patients to Ambulate

Assistive Devices

Walkers

Crutches

Canes

Wheelchairs

Therapeutic Exercises

Range of Motion

Muscle Testing

Types of Therapeutic Exercise

Electromyography

Electrostimulation of Muscle

Range of Motion Exercises

Therapeutic Modalities

Heat and Cold

Moist and Dry Heat Modalities

Moist and Dry Cold Modalities

Deep Tissue Modalities

OBJECTIVES

The student should strive to meet the following performance objectives and demonstrate an understanding of the facts and principles presented in this chapter through written and oral communication.

1. Define the key terms as presented in the glossary.

2. Define rehabilitation medicine and explain its importance in patient care.

3. Discuss the importance of correct posture and body mechanics, and demonstrate how to safely transfer patients and lift or move heavy objects using proper body mechanics.

4. Describe safety precautions and techniques used when helping a patient to ambulate and demonstrate how to assist the patient to safely stand and walk.

5. Demonstrate how to safely care for the falling patient.

6. Describe assistive devices and the importance of each in helping patients to ambulate.

(continues)

OBJECTIVES (*continued*)

7. Demonstrate how to measure patients for a walker, crutches, and a cane and help them ambulate safely with each device.

8. Describe the ambulation gaits used with crutches.

9. Discuss the safety precautions and techniques used when pushing a wheelchair.

10. Explain the importance of joint range of motion and the method used to measure joint movement.

11. Explain the importance of therapeutic exercise and the types of therapeutic exercises used in patient rehabilitation.

12. Describe electromyography and its purpose.

13. Explain the purpose of the electrostimulation of muscle.

14. Identify by name the body movements used in range of motion (ROM) exercises.

15. Explain the body's physiological reactions to heat and cold therapeutic modalities.

16. Be able to identify and describe the various types of hot and cold modalities, and describe how ultrasound works.

ROLE DELINEATION COMPONENTS

CLINICAL

Patient Care

- Prepare patient for examinations, procedures and treatments
- Assist with examinations, procedures and treatments

GENERAL (TRANSDISCIPLINARY)

Legal Concepts

- Document accurately

Instruction

- Instruct individuals according to their needs
- Teach methods of health promotion and disease prevention

SCENARIO

In a large urgent care center like Inner City Health Care, a team of therapists is responsible for providing patients with a high level of rehabilitative care. However, the clinical medical assistants at Inner City also are involved on a daily basis in the care of patients who have suffered injuries such as fractures or severe back pain. Clinical medical assistant Wanda Slawson, CMA, MLT and clinical medical assistant Bruce Goldman, CMA are often responsible for transferring patients and getting them safely from the reception area to the examination room and from wheelchair to examination table. While being acutely aware of the needs and safety of the patient, Wanda and Bruce also make sure they protect themselves by using proper body mechanics, by observing good posture, by using their arm and leg muscles and not their back muscles, and by always bending from the hips and knees, not the waist. Wanda's and Bruce's observation of these important principles protects their health and ensures the safety of their patients.

INTRODUCTION

Physical disability affects millions of people in the United States, regardless of age, race, or socioeconomic status. Every year thousands of people survive strokes, head or spinal cord injury, or other debilitating illness or injury that leaves them unable to perform complete independent function. Some of these individuals recover completely. Others recover to their fullest ability, living the rest of their lives with some type of disability. Still other patients suffer from chronic conditions such as arthritis or severe back pain that incapacitates them to the extent they cannot work or completely care for themselves.

Rehabilitation medicine is a field of medical disciplines that uses physical and mechanical agents to aid in the diagnosis, treatment, and prevention of diseases or bodily injuries. Its goal is to aid in the restoration of those functions that have been affected by the patient's condition. For those who have suffered permanent loss of ability, it seeks to find practical substitutions for that loss while assisting patients to make the most of their remaining abilities.

Most rehabilitation services are prescribed by the physician in charge of a patient's care and, depending upon the patient's condition, can include a recommendation to one or several rehabilitation specialists. Most likely, that specialist will be a physical therapist, occupational therapist, speech therapist, or sports medicine specialist, although the field of rehabilitation medicine is certainly not limited to these four areas of specialty.

Professional rehabilitation therapists, in whichever field they practice, are specifically trained and licensed in their field of expertise to assess, plan, and execute the patient's treatment in an overall effort to restore that patient to the highest level of physical and social independence possible. The medical assistant, as a member of an interdisciplinary health team, can use medical assisting skills to enable patients to regain normal or near normal function after an illness or injury.

THE ROLE OF THE MEDICAL ASSISTANT IN REHABILITATION

As a medical assistant, you may find yourself working in one of the rehabilitation fields. Such opportunities might include an ambulatory care setting with a specialty in physical therapy or sports medicine, an orthopedic surgeon's practice, the occupational or speech therapy department of a large suburban hospital, or other outpatient clinic or medical office. For the more chronically ill, nursing homes and rehabilitation hospitals also focus on restoring patients to as much independence as possible.

Whatever the rehabilitation setting, you will most likely find that you are a member of an interdisciplinary team of health care professionals who bring a broad knowledge base to patient care (Table 21-1). However, the physician is responsible for prescribing any type of rehabilitative medicine.

It is important to remember that patients seeking rehabilitation treatment may have suffered a tremendous loss of physical ability, leaving them vulnerable to feelings of helplessness. They may be able to perform only limited **activities of daily living (ADL)** or normal daily self-care

TABLE 21-1	SOME OF THE SPECIALIZED FIELDS OF REHABILITATION MEDICINE
Physical Therapy/ Physiotherapy	The treatment of disorders with physical and mechanical agents and methods to restore normal function after injury or illness.
Occupational Therapy	The use of activities to help restore independent functioning after an injury or illness.
Speech Therapy	The diagnosis and treatment of speech disorders.
Sports Medicine	A branch of medicine that specializes in the treatment and prevention of injuries caused by athletic participation.

such as brushing their teeth, getting dressed, and eating. Perhaps they cannot even do the simple tasks we take for granted every day, leaving them completely dependent on another person for help.

Understanding and encouragement are vital to the recovery process of these patients. While working with disabled persons, remember that certain tasks may be very challenging to them. More than likely they are acutely aware of their impairment and feel frustrated at their loss of function and discouraged about the future. Some patients may also suffer some speech impairment, making communication difficult or impossible. Respect for their dignity will build their self-esteem and have a positive effect on their treatment.

PRINCIPLES OF BODY MECHANICS

Much of the medical assistant's work with disabled persons will require great physical effort, particularly if patients are incapable of lifting or moving themselves. Moving patients or heavy, awkward objects can be hazardous for the patient as well as the caregiver if not performed correctly.

Body mechanics is the practice of using certain key muscle groups together with good body alignment and proper body positioning to reduce the risk of injury to both patient and caregiver. Always be conscious of using proper body mechanics, not just on the job, but in everything that requires moving, lifting, pushing, or pulling heavy or awkward objects.

Posture

Practicing good body mechanics starts with good posture. Good posture protects the entire body, particularly the back, whether standing, sitting, or lying down.

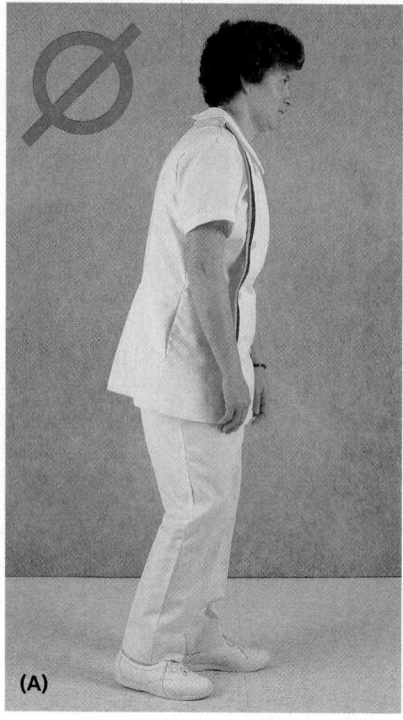
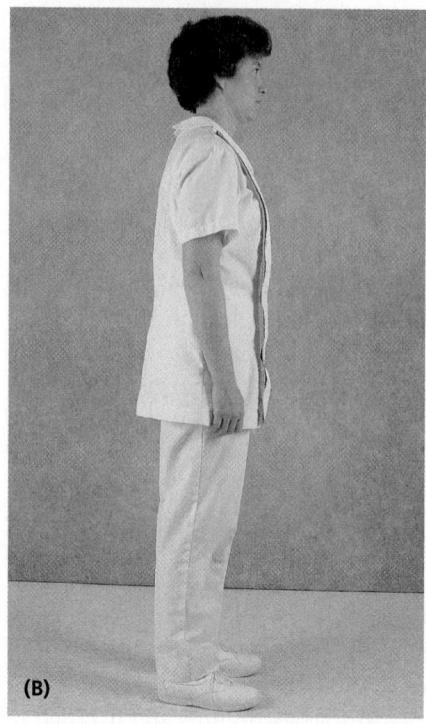

Figure 21-1 (A) A medical assistant demonstrating poor posture. (B) Good posture not only looks more professional but can prevent back injuries.

Glance at yourself sideways in a full-length mirror. When standing, does your posture most resemble that in Figure 21-1A or Figure 21-1B? When the body's muscle groups and body parts are in proper alignment, as shown in Figure 21-1B, the body is said to be in balance. Good balance is important for your body to function at its best. It enables you to lift, push, and pull easily and safely.

Frequently check your posture by reminding yourself to keep your chin and chest up, shoulders back, pelvis tilted slightly inward, feet straight and shoulder-width apart, and weight evenly distributed to both legs with a slight bend in your knees.

Using the Body Safely and Effectively

The spine is a flexible rod, designed to bend in many directions and hold the back steady. However, the muscles of the back are small and not meant for lifting heavy loads. They can be easily damaged if called upon to work beyond their natural ability. The muscles in the arms and legs, however, are large and were designed for heavy work. Rely on these muscles when lifting and carrying heavy objects, bending over or bending down, or moving patients.

It is important to keep several basic rules in mind whenever performing any task:

● Keep the back as straight as possible and feet shoulder-width apart to provide a good base of support (Figure 21-2).

● Always bend from the hips and knees, which enables the largest muscles of the legs to do the hard work, but *never* bend from the waist (Figure 21-3).

● Pivot the entire body instead of twisting it.

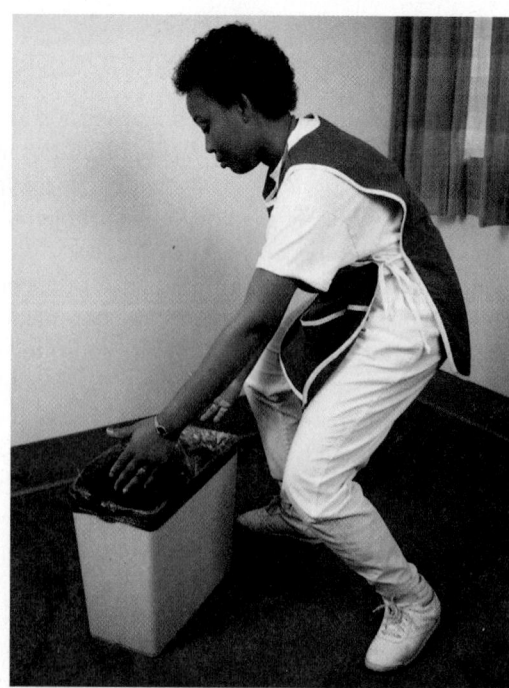

Figure 21-2 Provide a good base of support by keeping the back straight and feet apart.

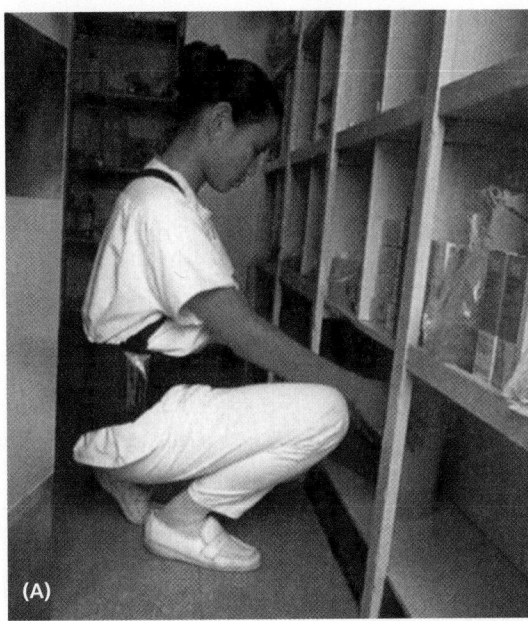
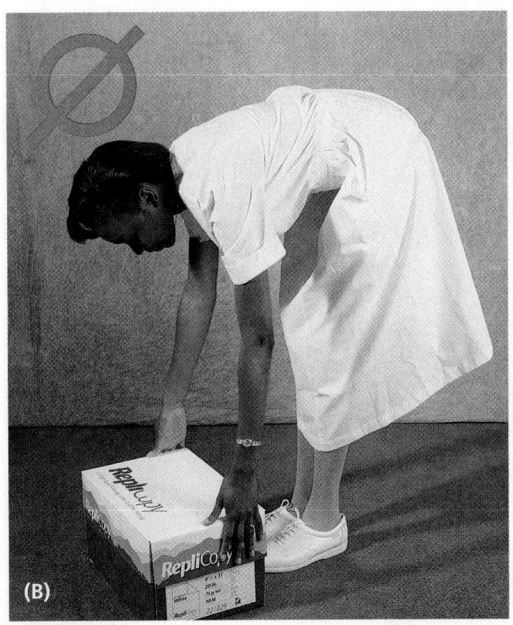

Figure 21-3   (A) Always bend from the hips and knees. (B) Never bend from the waist.

- Use the body's weight to push or pull any heavy object.
- Obtain help if unable to move a patient or object that is too heavy.

- Hold heavy objects close to the body (Figure 21-4).
- Make sure the path is clear and the area to receive the object is ready before lifting or moving it.
- Get into the habit of wearing a body support if a job includes much lifting (Figure 21-5).

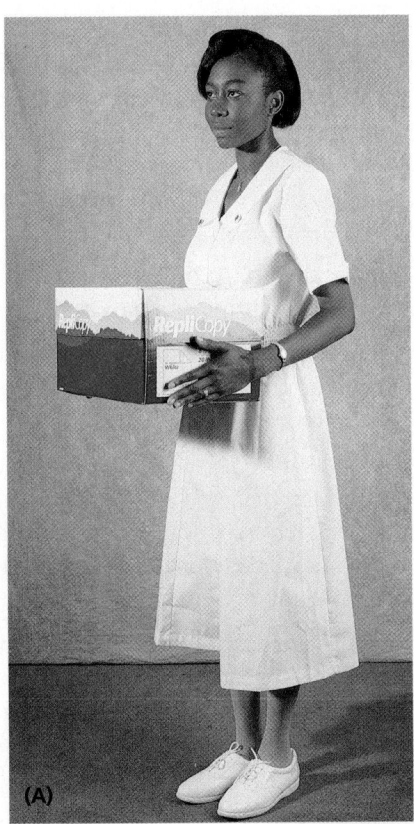
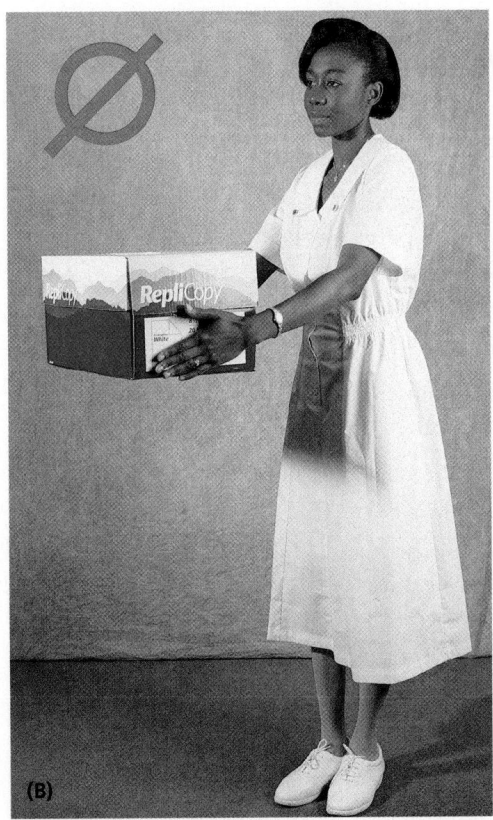

Figure 21-4   (A) When carrying heavy objects, hold them close to the body. (B) Never carry heavy objects out in front.

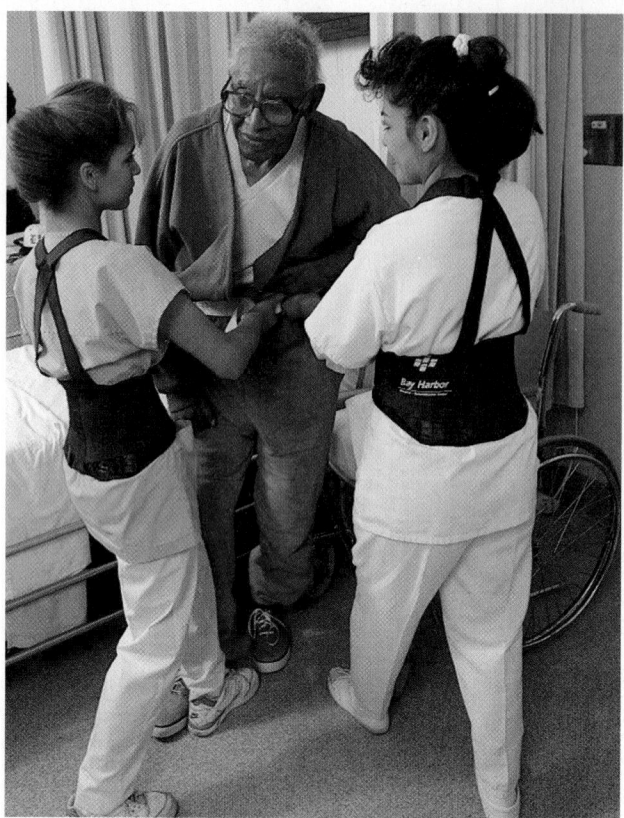

Figure 21-5 When a patient or object is too heavy, get help if necessary. Consider wearing a body support to protect the back if a job requires frequent lifting.

Lifting Techniques

When lifting patients or moving or lifting heavy objects, certain techniques should be used to prevent back injury:

- Get as close as possible to the object or person being lifted, since this allows the center of gravity to be maintained over the base of support.

- Keep the feet apart, one slightly in front of the other, and knees slightly bent.

- Use the large muscles of the legs and arms to lift, not back muscles.

- Keep the back straight to transfer the workload to larger arm and leg muscles.

- Bend from the hips and knees, squat down, and push up with leg muscles.

TRANSFERRING PATIENTS

It may be necessary to transfer patients if they cannot walk or lift themselves. Such patients may have a wide variety of disabilities, from severe back pain to **hemiplegia**, or paralysis of one side of the body resulting from a stroke, accident, or other condition. The

frail elderly also require particular care when being transferred, as they are more prone to bruising and broken bones.

As a safety precaution, it is important to remember good body mechanics when transferring patients. The act of lifting and moving someone can throw off one's center of gravity and therefore the base of support. Provide a wider base of support by moving the feet further apart and bending slightly, using strong arm and leg muscles to lift.

Before beginning any transfer, observe certain precautions:

- Make sure the equipment is stable and firm. Lock the brakes of the wheelchair and make sure the exam table or other surface will not move during the transfer.

- Check that there are no obstructions to trip over when making the transfer.

- Take small shuffling steps, and avoid crossing the feet.

- It is best if the transfer surfaces being used are close to the same height. If possible, lower the examination table or bed to the height of the wheelchair.

- Position the equipment according to the patient's physical limitations or disability. If the patient is stronger on one side, make sure that is the side on which the transfer will take place. It not only makes the transfer easier, it gives the patient more confidence.

- Always use a **gait belt**, a safety belt worn around the patient's waist, when transferring a patient. Lift the patient by grasping the belt from underneath and lifting up. Never lift a patient by the arms, or under the armpits, as this could cause injury to you and the patient.

- Take advantage of any assistance the patient can provide in lifting and moving.

- Never have patients put their arms around your neck or on your shoulders as it could cause you to be injured.

- Make sure both you and the patient are wearing footwear that will not slip or hinder the transfer process in any way. If a prosthesis or brace is involved, make sure it is secure and will not present a problem.

- Thoroughly explain to the patient what you intend to do, and make sure the patient understands what to expect during the transfer. Instructions need to be simple and repeated when necessary.

- Practice good body mechanics. Get close enough to the patient so you can lift with your legs. Always bend at the hips instead of the waist.

- Ascertain beforehand whether or not assistance will be needed with the transfer.

- Finally, take sufficient time when completing each step. Many patients will want to help themselves. Respect their courage, but remember that safety is of the utmost importance.

See Procedure 21-1 for proper steps in transferring patients from a wheelchair to an examination table. Procedure 21-2 outlines steps for transfer from examination table to wheelchair.

ASSISTING PATIENTS TO AMBULATE

In spite of the great strides that have been made in recent years to provide access for disabled persons, **ambulation**, or walking, is a functional activity that still provides the ultimate level of independence and freedom. For many patients, being able to ambulate again gives them tremendous satisfaction because the act of walking more than anything else signifies their return to wellness. Some patients take months to walk again by undergoing exercises and treatment designed to strengthen specific muscles.

Before assisting with any type of ambulation, there are several safety issues to remember:

- Make sure the patient is ready to walk. If a patient has trouble sitting well, or cannot balance once standing up, walking should not be attempted.

- The patient should be wearing good shoes that are flat, supportive, and have a rubber sole.

- Check to be certain there are plenty of handholds or railings within easy reach should the patient become unstable during walking.

- A gait belt provides a firm hold on the patient should the patient require assistance with stability at any time. For the patient just starting to walk, this device should be used and held by the caregiver throughout the session.

- Monitor the patient when standing and throughout the ambulation session for signs of fatigue and vertigo.

- Ambulate only as long as the patient has strength. Never push the patient beyond endurance.

- Never hurry a patient.

- Be ready should a patient start to fall. Generally, patients will fall toward their weaker side, but sometimes their legs lose stability and they go straight down.

Procedures 21-3 and 21-4 detail the steps involved in assisting patients to stand and walk and caring for a falling patient.

ASSISTIVE DEVICES

For some patients, the extent of their physical disability may determine that ambulation is only possible with the help of an **assistive device**, or walking aid such as a walker, crutches, or cane. For others, their physical disability is such that mobility is not possible at all without the use of a wheelchair.

Some assistive devices provide stability and support, while others require more coordination. Depending upon the patient's condition, one assistive device may be used until the patient has gained enough strength and coordination to move on to another type of assistive device, with the ultimate goal of walking unaided. The device a patient needs depends both on the disability and the patient's recuperation curve and is prescribed after careful evaluation by the attending physician or other health professional (Table 21-2).

Whatever device a patient will be using, medical assistants may be called upon to measure the patient for the correct size and provide instruction in its proper use and care. Once the patient has become proficient on level surfaces, provide instruction on sitting, standing, turning around, and negotiating stairs, curbs, ramps, doors, and other obstacles. Additionally, patients should be taught how to protect themselves should they fall and how to get back up.

Walkers

Walkers are best used for patients who require maximum assistance with balance and coordination, as they provide stability and support when the patient is standing or walking. They provide patients with the ability to ambulate independently with confidence. In order to use one, patients must be strong enough to be able to hold themselves upright while leaning on the walker.

Various styles of walkers are available. The two most widely used walkers are those that have rubber tips on the legs (stationary walkers), and those with wheels on the bottom of the legs (rolling walkers). Walkers that have wheels can be easily pushed ahead by the patient while walking and are best for patients who primarily need a walker for balance.

Most walkers are made of aluminum and are lightweight; most can be easily folded for storage or transport. The major disadvantage is that they must be used on level ground and cannot be used on stairs. Walkers are also difficult to use when attempting to go through doorways and in small areas around the house.

TABLE 21-2 TYPES OF ASSISTIVE DEVICES

Assistive Device	Features	Patient Requirements
Walkers		
Standard	• Adjustable • Rubber tips	• Requires upper body strength • Provides maximum stability and support • Excellent for older persons
Rolling	• Legs have wheels • Otherwise same as regular walker	• Good for patients who need walker only for balance and not support
Crutches		
Axillary	• Wooden or steel • Worn under axillae	• Requires good upper body strength and balance • Not recommended for older persons • Best for younger persons with lower extremity or hip fractures that will heal in a short time • Provides greatest range of ambulation
Forearm (Lofstrand or Canadian)	• Shorter than axillary crutches • Has metal cuff worn around forearm	• Less stable than axillary crutches • Best for long-term crutch use • Reduces stress on axillary vessels and nerves • Requires upper body strength and more stability and coordination • Provides most maneuverability of all crutches
Platform	• Platform affixed to a crutch • Patient bears weight on forearm	• Best for patients with severe arthritis or poor use of hands • Does not require as much upper body strength • Requires good balance
Canes		
Standard	• Single leg • Curved handle • Rubber tip	• Good for patients with only one good arm, lateral instability, or balance conditions
Quad (four-point)	• Single cane resting on a platform with four legs • Rubber tips on legs	• Better for patients with more severe conditions • Does not require as much coordination, but still requires balance and upper body strength in one arm
Walkcane or Hemiwalker	• Has four legs that come all the way up to a handlebar • Rubber tips on all legs	• Provides most stability of all canes • Best for hemiplegic patients who require extra support on one side

Fitting a Walker. Most walkers can be adjusted for a proper fit. The height of the handgrip should be adjusted to the individual patient just below the patient's waist, or at the top of the femur so the elbow can be bent at a 30° angle when the patient is standing with hands on the handgrip (Figure 21-6).

Procedure 21-5 provides steps for assisting a patient to ambulate with a walker.

Crutches

Crutches provide the ambulating patient with a great deal more mobility and flexibility. They provide good stability and support, while allowing for a broad range of gait patterns and ambulating speeds.

Three basic types of crutches are prescribed, depending upon the patient's physical limitations and abilities: axillary crutches, forearm crutches (also called Lofstrand or Canadian crutches), and platform crutches (Figure 21-7).

Axillary crutches are made of wood or aluminum and are used primarily for persons who need crutches tem-

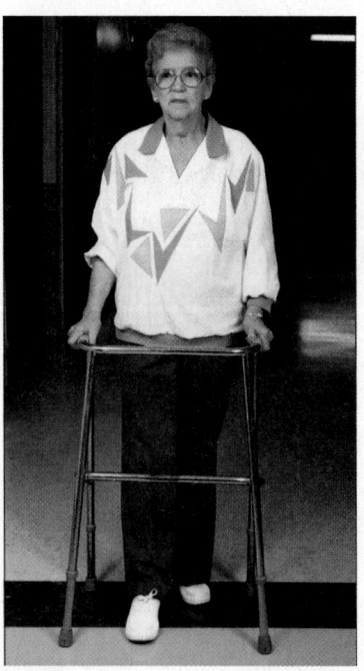

Figure 21-6 Proper fit for a walker. Note the patient's elbows are flexed at a 30° angle.

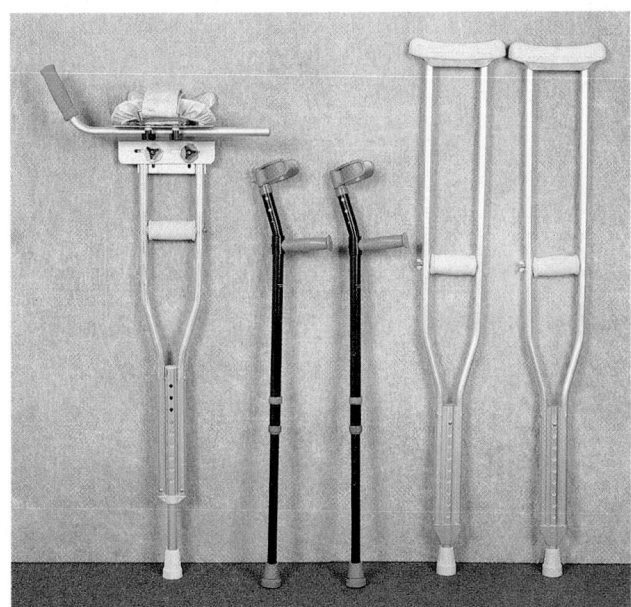

Figure 21-7 Types of crutches, from left to right: platform, forearm or Lofstrand, and axillary.

porarily while a lower extremity heals. Axillary crutches are ideal for stronger patients and pediatric patients who have minor injuries, but are not recommended for the frail elderly since upper body strength and balance are both required in order to use them (Figure 21-8). These crutches are easily transported and can be used to maneuver on stairs or in tight places.

Forearm crutches, or Lofstrand or Canadian crutches as they are also known, are shorter and provide less stability than axillary crutches. Forearm crutches are fixed with a metal or hard plastic cuff that fits around the patient's forearm. The weight is borne almost exclusively on the hand grip, requiring a great deal of upper body strength and coordination to use. This type of crutch is generally recommended for patients who will need crutches permanently or for a long period of time since they do not put any pressure on the axillary vessels and nerves (Figure 21-9).

The *platform crutch* is a third type of crutch that is recommended for patients who cannot grip the handles of other types of crutches or bear weight through their wrists or hands. The crutch has a platform attached to the top that includes a hand grip. It is high enough for the patient to use with the elbow bent at a right angle. The patient bears his weight completely on the forearm, which requires stability, strength, and coordination. The platform crutch is an ideal substitute for a cane when a patient only requires minimal weight transfer, but cannot bear weight on or grip with the hands (Figure 21-10).

Measuring a Patient for Axillary Crutches. To determine the right height of the crutches, have the patient stand tall. Be sure the patient is wearing good walking shoes. Adjust the height of the crutch so it is about two to three fingers, or two inches below the patient's axillae, or armpits (Figure 21-11). Adjust the

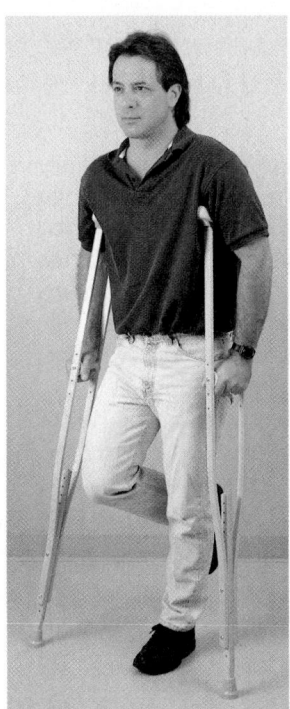

Figure 21-8 Patient using axillary crutches.

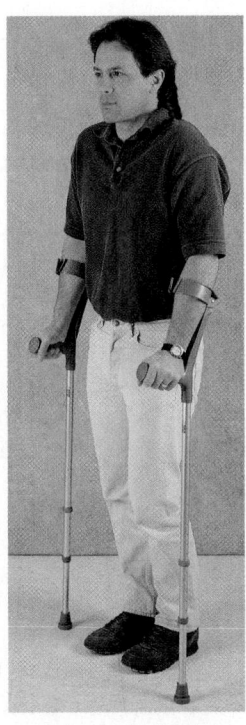

Figure 21-9 Patient using Lofstrand or forearm crutches.

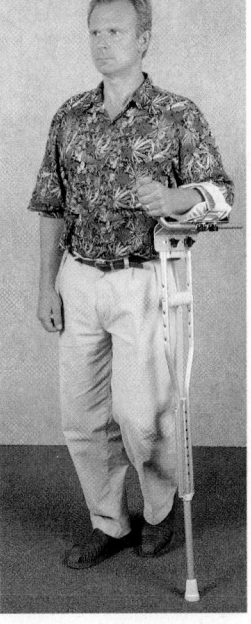

Figure 21-10 Patient using a platform crutch. This crutch is an ideal substitute for a cane if the patient cannot bear weight in his upper arm or on his hand.

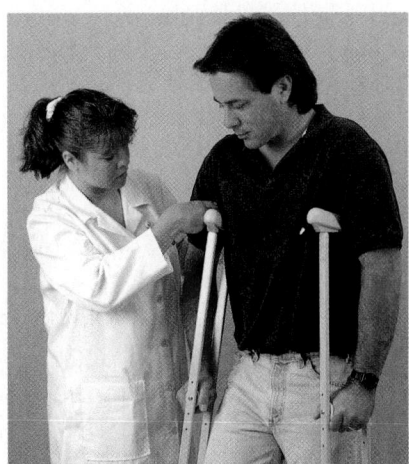

Figure 21-11 Measuring for axillary crutches. Note the height is about two to three fingers below the patient's armpit.

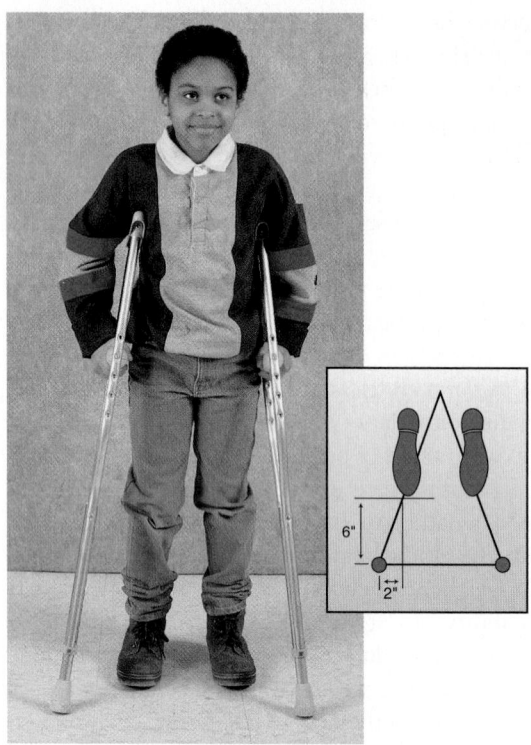

Figure 21-12   The distal end of the crutch should be 2 inches lateral and 6 inches anterior to the foot to form a triangle.

hand grips so the patient's elbows are bent at about a 20° to 30° angle. Position the crutch tips about 2 inches lateral and 6 inches anterior to the foot. When the patient is standing correctly, the crutch tips and patient's feet should form a triangle (Figure 21-12).

Procedure 21-6 indicates steps for teaching patients to ambulate with axillary crutches.

Crutch-Walking Gaits. The type of **gait**, or walk, a patient uses depends on the patient's injury and condition and is determined by the physician or licensed therapist. In crutch-walking gaits, each time the patient's foot or crutch touches the ground it is called a *point*. There are five gaits that are commonly used in crutch ambulation. The number of points in the gait relates to the number of feet and crutch tips that are on the ground at the same time.

Common crutch-walking gaits include two-point, three-point, four-point, swing-to, and swing-through gaits.

Two-Point Gait. There are two types of two-point gaits:

1. The first type is a nonweight-bearing gait. The patient places the crutch tips about 18 inches in front of him. He pushes off, taking the weight off his body and transferring it to his hands, then brings his strong leg forward past the crutches.
2. The second gait, called the two-point alternating gait, is used when the patient can bear weight on

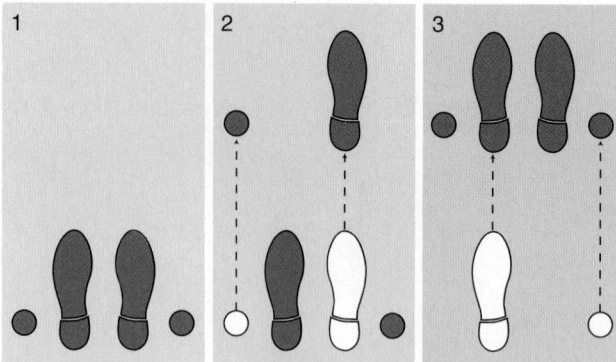

Figure 21-13   Two-point gait. The patient is bearing weight on both legs.

both legs. The opposite foot and crutch are advanced forward at the same time (Figure 21-13). This gait is a more advanced gait, and is used after the four-point gait has been mastered.

Three-Point Gait. This gait is used when the patient can only bear partial weight on one leg, or just touch that foot to the floor. Both the crutches and the weak leg are advanced at the same time. The body weight is then transferred forward to the crutches, and the stronger leg is advanced and placed slightly in front of the crutches (Figure 21-14).

Four-Point Alternating Gait. This is a slower gait that is used for patients who can bear weight on both legs and

---

Patient Teaching Tip

When instructing patients in the use of axillary crutches, impress upon them the importance of putting all their weight on their hands, not on the armpits. Many patients using crutches for the first time mistakenly put the pressure on their armpits, which can damage the axillary nerve. Also reinforce the need for wearing flat, nonskid shoes when using crutches.

Throw rugs and other obstacles in the home or work area are a danger to patients on crutches. Remind them to have such hazards removed. Teach patients to check crutches daily for the following:

- Check that the wing nuts that adjust the crutches are tight.
- Check the crutch tips for wear and tear.
- Check the foam pads of the hand grips and armpit rests for tears.

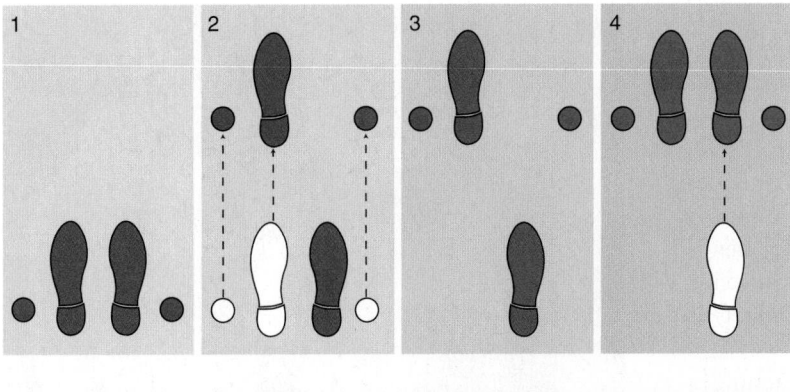

Figure 21-14   Three-point gait. The left leg is the weaker leg and bears no weight.

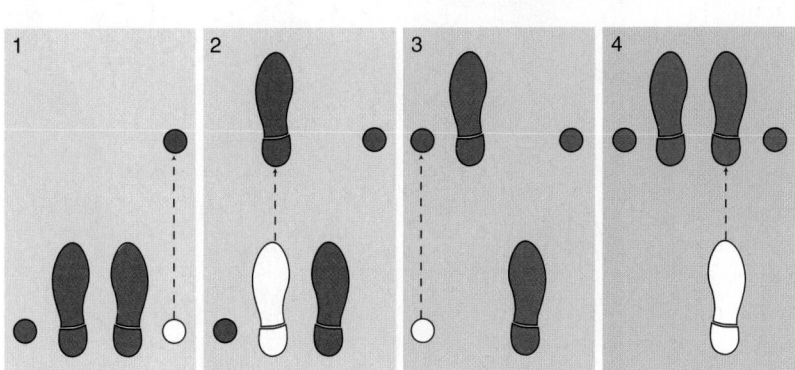

Figure 21-15   Four-point gait. The patient is bearing weight on both legs.

move each leg separately. The patient moves one crutch forward, then the opposite foot. The patient then moves the other crutch forward, then the opposite foot (Figure 21-15).

Swing-To Gait. The patient starts with the crutches at his side. He moves both crutches forward, transfers his weight forward, and swings both feet together up to the crutches.

Swing-Through Gait. Start with the crutches at the side. Move both crutches forward. Transfer the weight and swing both feet through the crutches, stopping slightly in front of the crutches.

Sitting. The patient backs into a straight chair with armrests until the seat of the chair touches the back of the legs. Crutches are held in the hand on the strong side and opposite the weak leg. With the other hand the patient can grasp the armrest of the chair and lower slowly into the chair.

Standing. The patient holds both crutches in the hand on the strong side, moves forward in the chair, grasps the armrest with the hand on the weaker side, then pushes up to a standing position.

Canes

A cane is used when the patient has one weak side and will need this assistive device for a longer period of time than crutches. It is also useful for patients who have a general but minor weakness on one side or those who have poor balance.

Canes come in three basic types, are made of either aluminum or wood, and have rubber tips. Some are adjustable and some are not (Figure 21-16). The first type of cane is called a *standard*, or single-tipped cane. It has a curved handle for gripping, and the newer canes have a hand grip attached. The standard cane is used for patients with less severe walking conditions and needs a small amount of support.

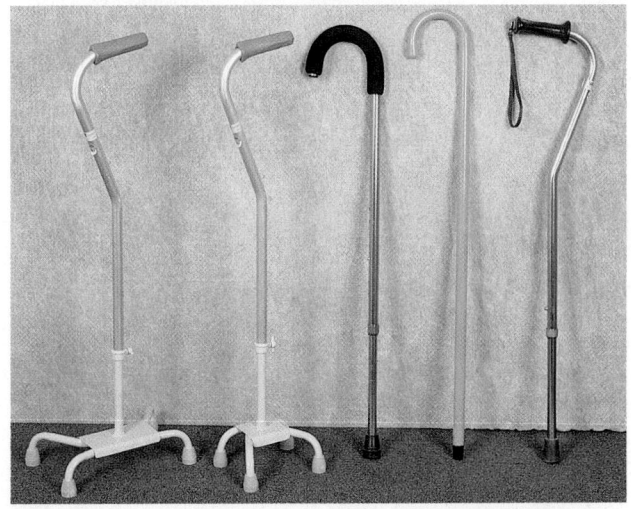

Figure 21-16   Types of standard canes: (A) Quad canes. (B) Single-tip canes.

The second type of cane is a four-legged, or *quad* cane. It is a single cane that rests on a four-legged platform, provides stability and a wide base of support, and is for patients with more severe walking difficulties.

The third type of cane is a *walkcane* (Figure 21-17). It has four legs and a handlebar for gripping, and provides the best support of all canes. This type of cane is also referred to as a Hemiwalker because it is ideal for hemiplegic patients who need the extra stability of this wide base. When the cane is the correct height, the elbow is flexed at a 20 to 30° angle.

Procedure 21-7 outlines the steps for teaching a patient how to walk safely with a cane.

Wheelchairs

Wheelchairs are mobile chairs that enable patients with severe ambulation conditions, or no ability to ambulate at all, to otherwise get around. Some must be moved manually, either by the patient or by someone else. Others are motorized and can be controlled completely by the patient (Figure 21-18).

Many advancements in wheelchair design over the years have enabled patients with chronic conditions to longer be restricted to a home or hospital environment. Today, all public buildings and many private ones have handicapped access ramps as an alternative to stairs, remote-controlled doors, elevators that can accommodate a wheelchair, and other amenities that enable wheel-

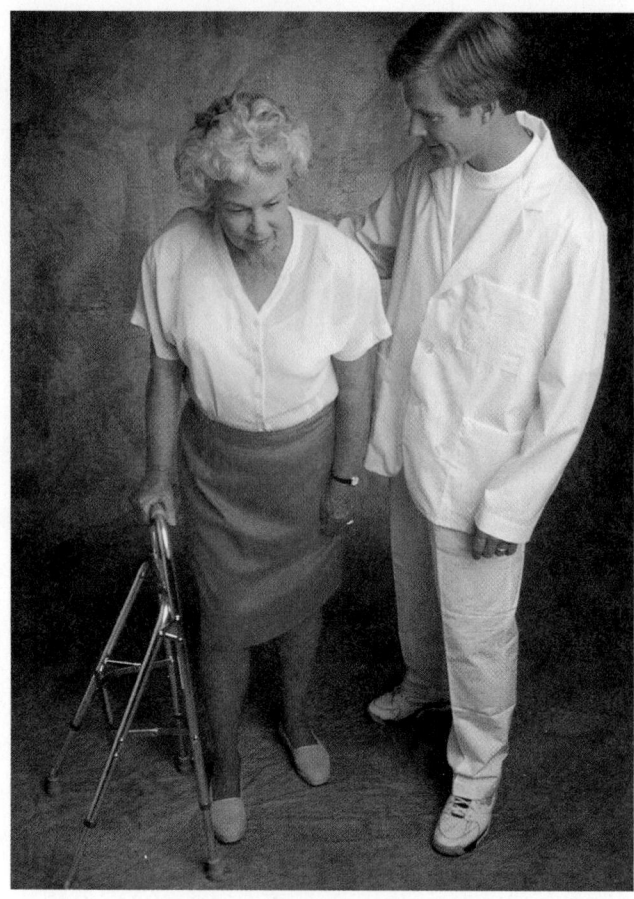

Figure 21-17 A walkcane being used by a hemiplegic patient. (Courtesy of Guardian Products)

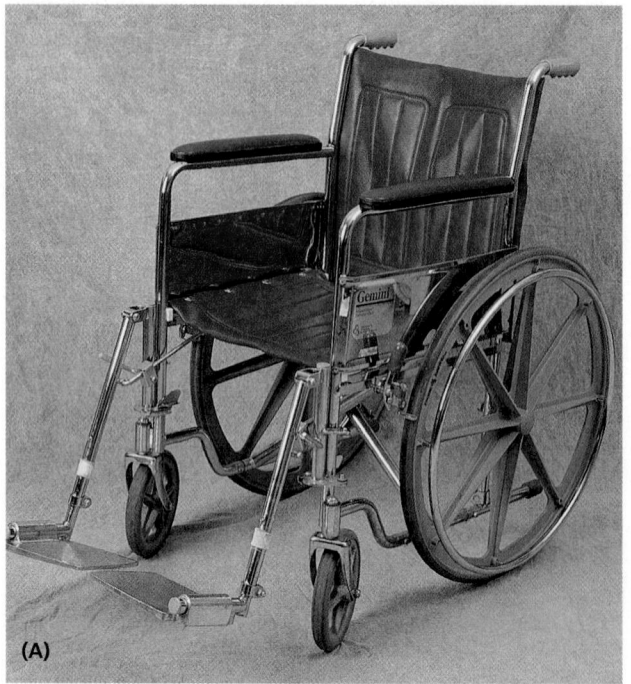

(A)

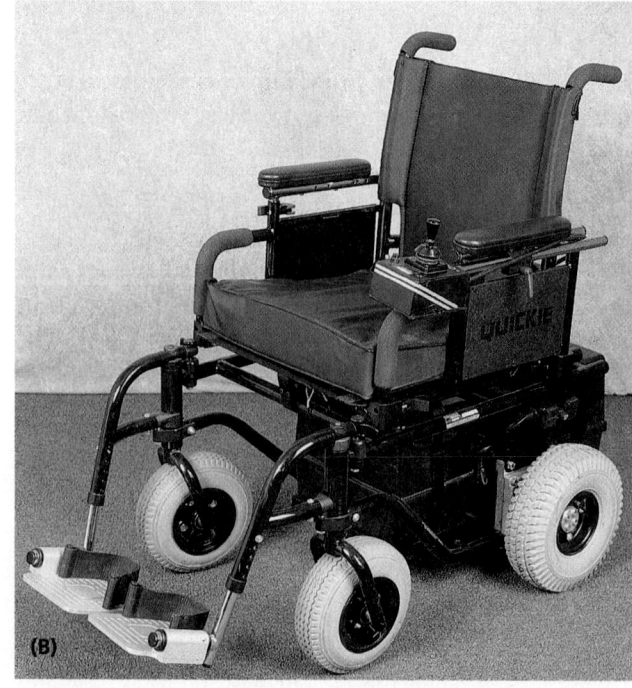

(B)

Figure 21-18 (A) A manual wheelchair. (B) A motorized wheelchair.

chair patients to get around almost as well as if they were ambulating.

There are many types of wheelchairs and modifications that can be tailored to suit a patient's particular disability and lifestyle. There are even wheelchairs that enable patients to take part in sports activities. Many car manufacturers can modify a van to accommodate a wheelchair, and some are equipped to allow wheelchair patients to drive.

Patients who will be using a wheelchair for a long time are taught how to maintain it. Depending upon their abilities, they check it regularly to make sure all the parts are working correctly, and, if they are able, to make any necessary repairs. Patients are taught to use the wheelchair safely and maneuver into and out of difficult spaces.

If a patient is being pushed by someone else, that individual must learn basic safety rules for transporting a patient:

- Make sure that the brakes are locked when transferring a patient into and out of a wheelchair and if a patient must be left alone in the wheelchair for any length of time, lock the brakes.
- Make sure the patient's feet are placed on the footrests when the wheelchair is in use.
- Guide the wheelchair from behind and use your weight to help push it (Figure 21-19).
- Always back into and out of elevators.
- Stay to the right in corridors.
- Back down slanted ramps.

THERAPEUTIC EXERCISES

Range of Motion

The musculoskeletal system is a complex joining of bones, joints, ligaments, and tendons. Not only does it give structure to the body and protect the body's vital organs, it allows for movement so we can carry out a multitude of activities.

The bones of almost all the joints of the body are designed to move as well, each joint having its own **range of motion (ROM)**. Range of motion refers to the amount of movement that is present in a joint.

Normal ROM varies between people and depends upon several factors, such as age, gender, and whether the motion being performed is passive (assisted motion) or active (voluntary motion). There is a standard range of motion for all movable joints, and it is this standard that is used when evaluating the joint movement of a particular patient.

The measurement of joint motion is called **goniometry**. Joint movement is measured with an instrument called a **goniometer** and is always expressed in degrees. For example, the average person lying flat with arms to the sides can move the elbows from a 20° hyperextension (extending the arm beyond its normal limits) to 0° extension, through to 150° of flexion, or bending (Figure 21-20).

Range of motion evaluation is one of several tools used when developing a therapeutic program for a patient.

Muscle Testing

The other tool used for evaluating the movement abilities of a patient is muscle testing. While goniometry focuses on joint movement, **muscle testing** evaluates the motion,

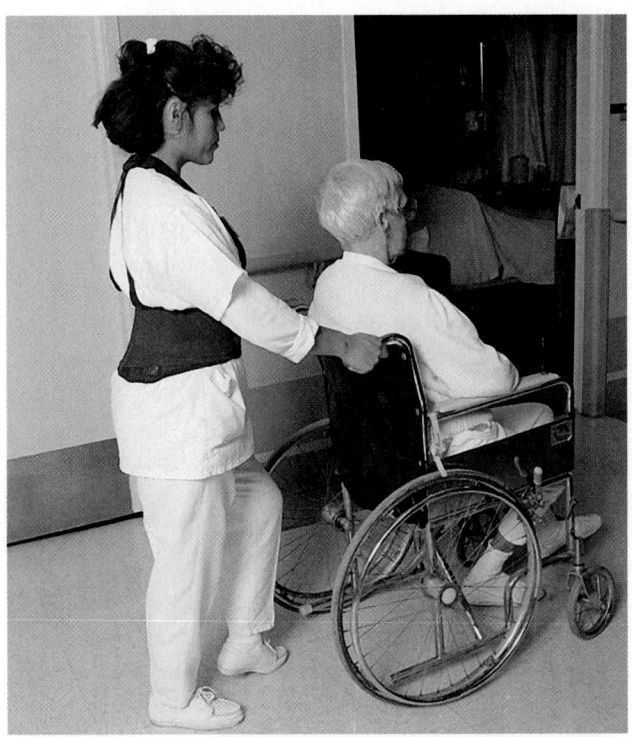

Figure 21-19 Guide the wheelchair from behind.

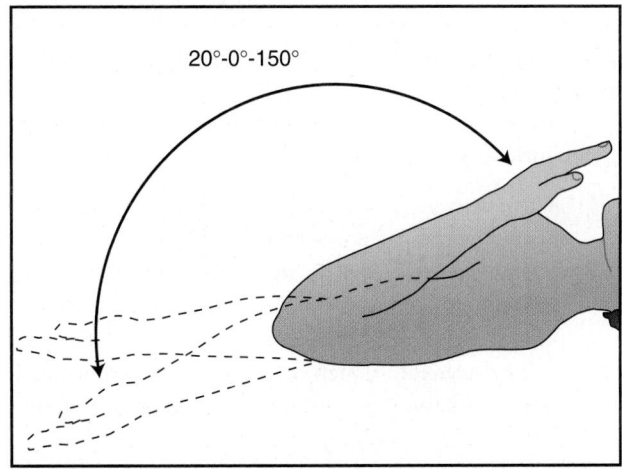

Figure 21-20 Joint mobility is measured against standard ranges of motion (ROM) and is always expressed in degrees.

strength, and task potential of a given muscle. *Range of motion* testing for muscles determines how flexible and resilient a muscle may be. *Strength testing* shows how hard a muscle can work. *Task potential* of a muscle means how well a muscle can aid in accomplishing a given activity. As a medical assistant, you may assist with testing the patient for joint mobility, posture, and strength of muscles.

Types of Therapeutic Exercise

Without constant exercise, the musculoskeletal system would deteriorate. Joints would become stiff and **contractures**, or deformities, could develop. Muscles would **atrophy**, or shrink and lose strength. Bones would lose vital minerals such as calcium and phosphorus. And the body's overall circulation would decrease, which would in turn create a separate set of unhealthy conditions.

Like drugs, exercise has a powerful and systemic effect on the body. It involves the function of joints, bones, muscles, nerves, tendons, ligaments, as well as the circulatory and respiratory systems. Therapeutic exercises are prescribed after careful evaluation by a trained specialist and are tailored to each patient depending upon that patient's individual condition and rehabilitation goals. It is the role of the medical assistant to understand the goals and objectives of the therapeutic exercise program in order to better support and encourage patients to complete their program.

While an athlete uses exercise to build strength and endurance in order to attain a certain level of performance, therapeutic exercises are prescribed for a variety of therapeutic and preventive effects. They are used most commonly for therapeutic reasons to correct or prevent deformities, regain body movement after an accident or disease, restore joint motion after immobility, improve neuromuscular coordination, and improve or develop activities of daily living.

Exercise is also used for another important reason. It can prevent many common problems brought on by inactivity, such as those problems associated with respiration and circulation.

A variety of exercise programs are employed for therapeutic or preventive purposes.

1. *Active exercises*, which are self-directed and performed by the patient without assistance.
2. *Passive exercises*, which are performed by another person with no voluntary participation from the patient.
3. *Assisted exercises*, which help the patient voluntarily move weakened muscles with the use of an assistive device, such as a therapy pool.
4. *Active resistance exercises*, which provide voluntary movement against various types of manual or mechanical pressure to increase muscle strength.

Electromyography

Electrical activity of a muscle can be recorded on a graph or film to help to determine how well muscles contract. An electromyograph is the instrument used to test the electrical activity of a muscle. An electrode (using a small gauge needle) is inserted through skin into the muscle, and measurements can be made as to muscle strength.

Electrostimulation of Muscle

An electric current of low voltage can help to stimulate muscles to exercise by innervating the sensory and motor nerves for that muscle. It is helpful for a patient who has nerve damage to the muscle and cannot voluntarily move the muscle. The purpose is to prevent atrophy of the muscle and help to restore muscle function.

The low current of electricity passing through the patient's muscle acts similarly to the patient's own nerves causing the muscle to contract and relax. The stimulation is helpful to retrain a patient after suffering an injury to a muscle or muscle group.

Range of Motion Exercises

As a medical assistant, you may be called upon to perform range of motion exercises. Range of motion exercises are designed to maintain joint mobility and are either performed passively (someone else does the movement) or actively (the patient does the movement).

Joint movement has a special vocabulary. It will be helpful when learning range of motion exercises to consult the terms and their definitions, as shown in Table 21-3.

TABLE 21-3	TERMINOLOGY OF JOINT MOVEMENT
Abduction	Motion away from the midline of the body
Adduction	Motion toward the midline of the body
Circumduction	Circular motion of a body part
Dorsiflexion	Moving the foot upward at the ankle joint
Eversion	Moving a body part outward
Extension	Straightening of a body part
Flexion	Bending of a body part
Hyperextension	A position of maximum extension, or extending a body part beyond its normal limits
Inversion	Moving a body part inward
Plantar Flexion	Moving the foot downward at the ankle
Pronation	Moving the arm so the palm is down
Rotation	Turning a body part around its axis
Supination	Moving the arm so the palm is up

Before performing range of motion exercises on a patient, you will need to observe some general precautions:

- Always move the patient's limbs gently, within pain tolerance and the flexibility of the limb.

- Use slow, careful movements that allow the muscles time to adjust to the movement.

- Always support the limb above and below the joint.

- It is best to perform passive ROM with the patient in the supine position.

- ROM should never cause pain. If the patient reports pain at any time, the ROM exercises should be discontinued until a physician or other health care professional can determine the source of pain.

- Repeat each movement several times or as prescribed by the physician.

Procedure 21-8 provides ROM exercises for various parts of the upper body. Procedure 21-9 provides ROM exercises for lower extremities.

THERAPEUTIC MODALITIES

Sometimes, therapeutic exercise is not the best or only way to restore injured or painful joints and tissues. A patient's condition may respond equally well to certain physical agents, called **modalities**, which take advantage of the properties of heat, cold, electricity, light, and water to improve circulation, minimize pain, and correct or alleviate muscular and joint malfunction.

Many modalities have been around for centuries, and some can easily be performed by the patient or caregiver at home. Modalities can be used locally to treat a small area at a time or systemically to alter a patient's temperature or soothe many groups of painful muscles or joints. The patient's condition and rehabilitation program both influence the modality or combination of modalities used.

Heat and Cold

Heat, or **thermotherapy**, acts on the body by causing **vasodilation** (dilation of the blood vessels). The effect of heat increases circulation to an area and acts to speed up the repair process. Heat can be used to:

- Relax muscle spasms

- Relieve pain in a strained muscle or sprained joint

- Relieve localized congestion and swelling

- Increase drainage from an infected area

- Increase tissue metabolism and repair

However, because heat dilates the blood vessels and increases circulation, it also acts to speed up the inflam-

matory process, which can lead to more serious problems, such as increased bleeding and swelling. Heat should never be used on pregnant or menstruating women, as it can induce uterine contractions. Also, heat should not be used longer than its prescribed length of time.

Cold applications, or **cryotherapy**, are used to constrict blood vessels and slow or stop the flow of blood to an area. This process, also called **vasoconstriction**, slows down the inflammatory process, which can reduce or prevent swelling of inflamed tissues, reduce bleeding, numb the pain sensation by acting as a topical anesthetic, and reduce drainage to an area.

By understanding how heat and cold affects the body, it is easier to observe whether or not they are having the desired therapeutic effect. Heat and cold modalities can be extremely effective, which is why they are so widely used for treating certain physical conditions. However, the effects of heat and cold modalities depend on several conditions: the type of modality used, the length of time it is applied, the patient's condition, and the area or areas being treated.

 Precautions for Heat and Cold Applications. When applying either heat or cold modalities, you need to take certain precautions to avoid injury. If misused, any therapeutic modality can actually cause more damage to the site that is trying to heal. Prior to starting any treatment, keep the following precautions in mind:

- Infants and patients who cannot report a burning sensation should be watched carefully. Infants and the elderly are particularly susceptible to burns.

- Heat and cold sensitivity varies with the patient; check patients frequently and never leave them alone.

- Never have a patient lie on a heating pad, as severe burning can result. Place a rubber cover over the heating pad if using with moist dressings.

- Always wrap appliances with cloth before applying them to the skin.

- Only soak or immerse patients in water between 104°F to 113°F (40°C to 45°C). Temperatures of 116°F (47°C) or above can cause burning.

- Heat can cause uterine contractions in menstruating or pregnant women.

- Never use heat within the first 48 hours of an acute inflammatory process and never apply heat to newly burned skin.

- Watch carefully persons with impaired circulation, or cardiovascular, renal, sensorineural, or respiratory conditions, or osteoporosis.

- Lack of sensation to a therapy may mean impaired circulation to an area and the patient may be unable to report a burning sensation.

- As heat concentrates in metal materials, have patients remove all jewelry and other metal objects, and administer the treatment on nonmetal tables and chairs.

Moist and Dry Heat Modalities

Moist Heat Therapies. Moist heat refers to heat modalities that feel moist against the skin. Moist heat penetrates better than dry heat and aids in improving circulation, relaxation, and mobility.

Hot Soaks. Hot soaks are generally used for soaking the extremities and can easily be administered at home by the patient or caregiver. The patient's body part is gradually immersed in plain or medicated water no hotter than 110°F (44°C) for a short time, usually no more than about 15 minutes. The patient should be positioned to be comfortable. Observe the patient's skin for excessive redness and, if noticed, remove the limb at once. Always dry the skin carefully by patting, not rubbing it.

Total body immersion in hot water can be administered in a whirlpool bath or special Hubbard tank. This treatment is often prescribed to promote relaxation, circulation, and movement of limbs in preparation for exercise. The mechanical action of agitating water moving over the body in a whirlpool is called hydromassage and can

both relax muscles and stimulate circulation. The Hubbard tank is a bit larger and provides room for limited body exercise without the effects of gravity.

Hot Compresses and Packs. A hot compress is usually applied to a small area, and is prepared by soaking and wringing out either a square of gauze or other absorbent material (like a clean washcloth) and applying it for a limited time to the affected area (Figure 21-21). Hot compresses can easily be administered at home. A hot pack is used for a larger area and generally involves the use of a professional hot pack administered in the clinical setting. This type of hot pack is soaked in hot water, removed with tongs and drained, and placed over larger areas such as the back or shoulders.

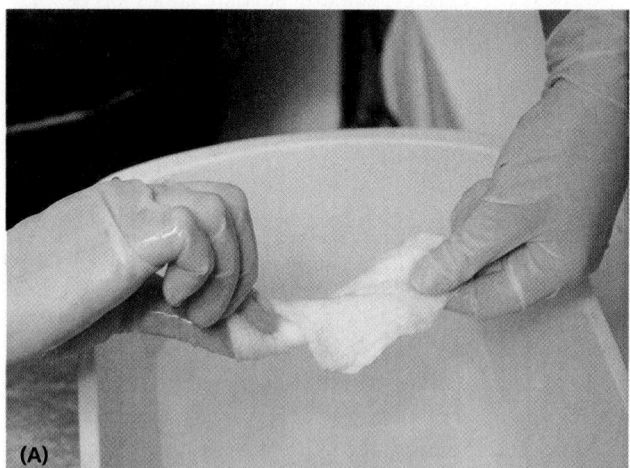

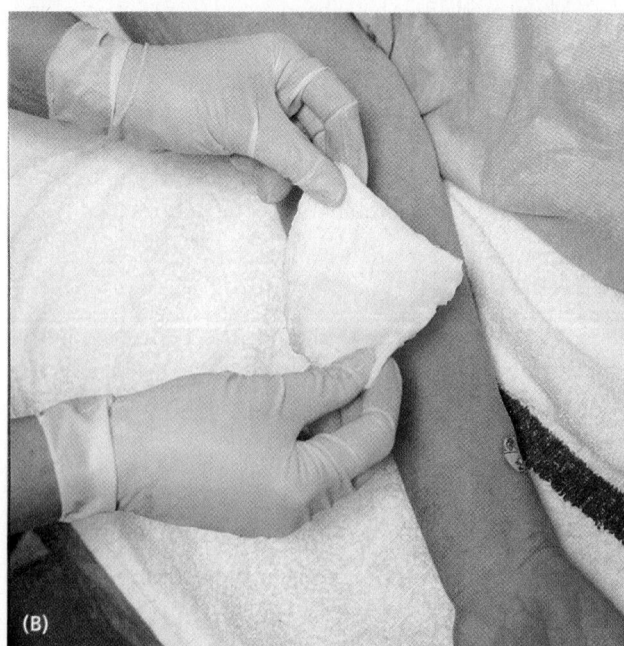

Figure 21-21 (A) Dip hot compresses frequently into a basin of hot water to keep them warm. (B) Apply compresses directly to the skin.

Paraffin Wax Bath. This type of treatment is most often used for chronic joint disease, such as rheumatoid arthritis. The bath mixture of seven parts paraffin to one part mineral oil is heated to melting (about 127°F) and the body part dipped in the mixture several times until a thick coat of wax builds up. The body part is then wrapped in foil, cloth, or plastic wrap to help insulate the heat, then left on for 30 minutes or less. Once peeled off, the circulatory effects of this treatment can last up to several hours. It is an excellent modality for warming up joints prior to range of motion or other exercises. This modality, ordered by a physician, will be carried out in the physical therapy department by a professional therapist.

Dry Heat Therapies. Dry heat applications feel dry against the skin and do not penetrate like moist heat. They are used more to improve circulation for the purposes of relieving swelling and healing wounds, as well as to relax muscles and reduce muscle spasms. Most dry heat modalities can also be performed easily by the patient or caregiver at home.

Heating Pads and Packs. Heating pads and commercially prepared packs are used for smaller areas and should always be covered with a cloth prior to applying against the skin. Never let a patient lie directly on a heating pad, as burns can result. Set the switch on the heating pad to a low or medium setting and observe the proper time of exposure.

If you are using a hot water bottle, fill the bottle with water that does not exceed 125°F (52°C) (Figure 21-22) and expel the excess air so the bottle can be more pliable and fit to the contour of the body part being treated. Reduce the water temperature to between 115°F and 125°F (46° to 52°C) for children over two and 105°F and 115°F (41° to 46°C) for children under two and elderly patients. Make sure the outside of the bottle is dry, and cover it with a cloth before applying it (Figure 21-23). Check the temperature often and refill it periodically to maintain the proper heat level.

An Aquamatic K-Pad® is a commercial pad that is safer to use than a heating pad or hot water bottle because you can maintain a constant temperature and regulate that temperature more carefully. It is a pad with tubes that are filled with distilled water and heated by a control unit (Figure 21-24). The pad must be covered and left on the patient for no more than about 30 minutes.

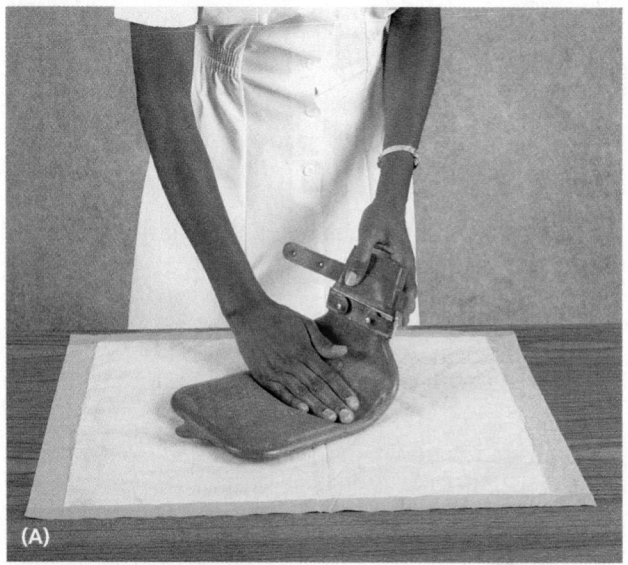

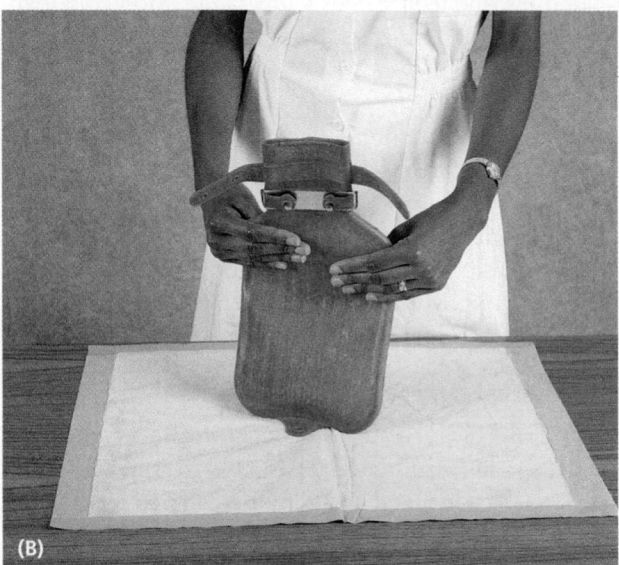

Figure 21-23 (A) Before filling it, expel the air from the hot water bottle by flattening it on the table. (B) After filling, hold the water bottle upright until the water reaches the neck to expel air. Dry the bag, and place in a protective cover.

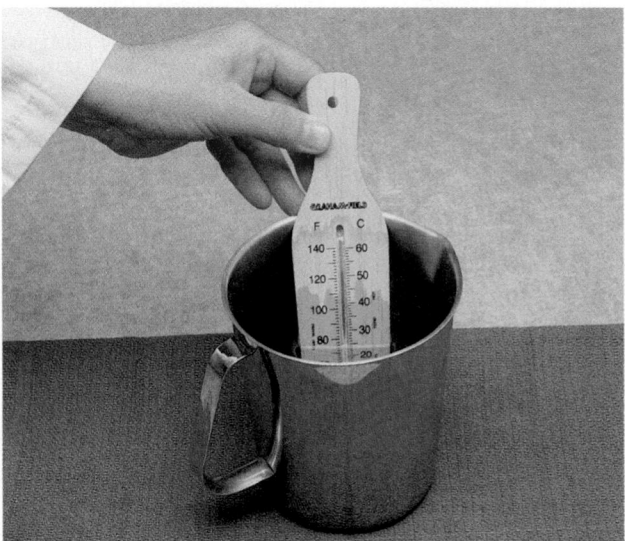

Figure 21-22 When using a water bottle, the water temperature should not exceed 125°F (52°C) or 115°F (46°C) for children under two and elderly patients.

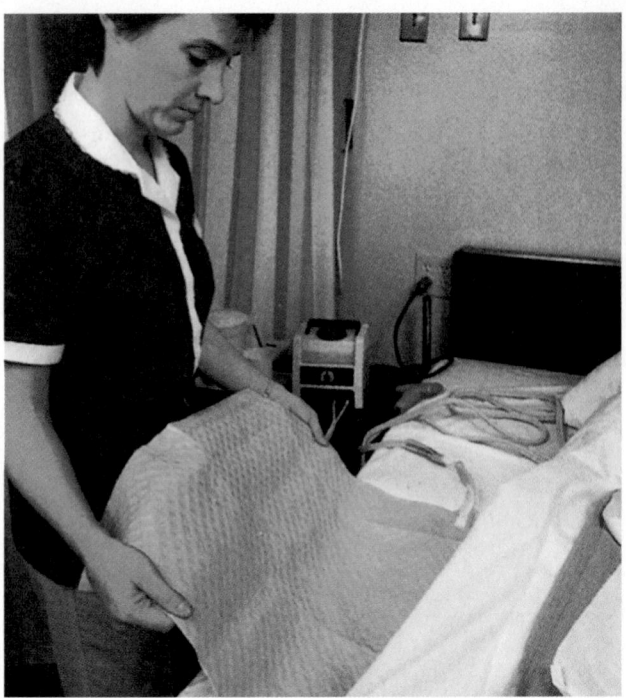

Figure 21-24 Use the Aquamatic K-Pad to maintain a constant temperature of heat.

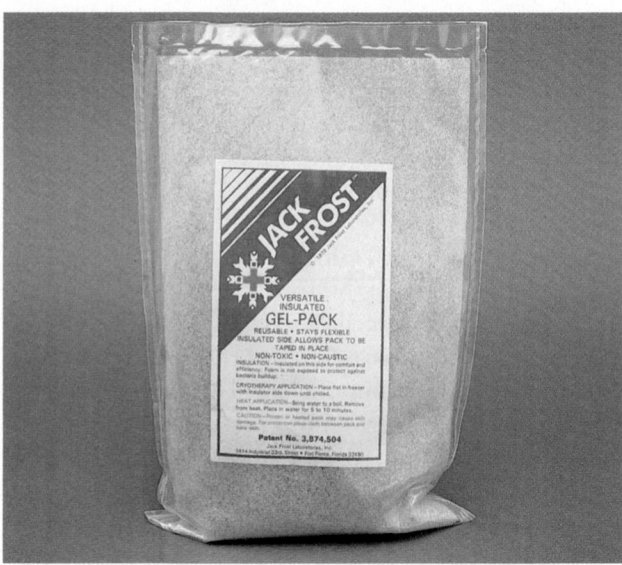

Figure 21-25 A chemical ice pack. These should be covered with a cloth before applying it to the skin.

Moist and Dry Cold Modalities

Moist Cold Therapies. Moist cold therapies refer to cold modalities that feel moist against the skin. Moist cold, as with moist heat, penetrates better than dry cold and is used to prevent swelling or edema, relieve pain or tenderness, and reduce body temperature. Most cold therapies can be performed easily at home by the patient or caregiver.

Cold Compresses and Packs. Cold compresses are used for smaller areas, and cold packs for larger areas. For a cold compress, immerse the cold cloth, gauze, or other clean material in a basin filled with ice and cold water. Wring out the cloth and apply it to the affected area. Keep the cloth cold by immersing it several times throughout the treatment. Cold or ice packs are administered in the same manner.

Dry Cold Therapies. Dry cold treatments are used for all the same reasons as a moist cold treatment, but are better for bleeding and acute injuries. Dry cold is also an excellent therapy for sprains, strains, burns, or bruises.

The temperature used depends on the area being treated and the method used, as well as the patient's tolerance for cold temperatures. In general, the colder the temperature, the shorter the duration of exposure.

Ice Packs. Dry cold treatments include ice packs and commercially prepared chemical ice packs. Always cover the pack with cloth before applying it to the skin (Figure 21-25). Generally, ice packs can be kept on the body longer than heat packs, about 30 minutes. See also Chapter 9. A commercial ice pack can be used for smaller areas and can usually be chilled in the freezer. Since they do not freeze and become solid, these ice packs are pliable, making them ideal for contouring to the body part being treated.

Deep Tissue Modalities

Ultrasound. Ultrasound is a high-frequency acoustic vibration that is part of the electromagnetic spectrum, and its frequencies are beyond the perception of the human ear. This type of treatment uses high-frequency

Patient Teaching Tip

Neither heat nor cold applications should be left on the skin for prolonged periods for both can have counterproductive effects if not monitored carefully. When applying heat or cold, periodically check the skin for signs of paleness or redness. If the patient experiences any tingling reaction, discontinue the application. Report the observations, and document.

sound waves that are converted to heat in the deeper tissues.

Ultrasound is an effective form of treatment for chronic pain or acute injuries such as sprains or strains. It relaxes muscle spasms, increases the elasticity of tissue such as tendons and ligaments, and stimulates circulation, which in turn speeds up the healing process.

 Ultrasound waves travel best in tissue that has a high concentration of water, such as muscles, but they cannot penetrate and move through tissue such as bone that has a low water content. In fact, ultrasound treatment must be used carefully near bones, particularly those near the surface, as their waves are capable of concentrating in one area and causing damage.

Since ultrasound waves cannot be conducted through air, a special gel is applied to the skin surface that acts as a conduit. The sound waves are generated through an applicator that is rubbed over the gel. This applicator must be kept moving to prevent any internal damage caused by too high a concentration of sound waves. The duration of treatment lasts anywhere from 5 to 15 minutes, depending upon the condition being treated and the recommendation of the physician or other health care provider. It is important to note that, because of its potential dangers, ultrasound treatment should only be administered if the medical assistant or other caregiver is specially trained in its safe and effective use.

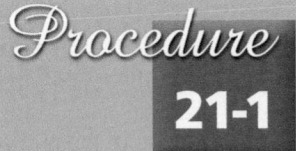

Transferring Patient from Wheelchair to Examination Table

STANDARD PRECAUTIONS:

PURPOSE:
To move a patient safely from a wheelchair to the examination table.

EQUIPMENT/SUPPLIES:
Stool with rubber tips and a handle for gripping
Gait belt

PROCEDURE STEPS:
1. Wash hands.
2. Identify the patient and introduce yourself. Explain to the patient what you are going to do.
3. Place the wheelchair next to the examination table and lock the brakes. **CAUTION:** The side nearest the examination table should be the patient's stronger side to allow the patient to balance on that leg during the transfer.
4. Place the gait belt snugly around the patient's waist and tuck the excess end under the belt (Figure 21-26A).
5. Move the footrests up and out of the way. Have the patient place feet on the floor. Newer wheelchairs have removable footrests. Taking them off enables you to put the wheelchair closer to the examination table. There is also less chance of being bumped or bruised by the wheelchair.

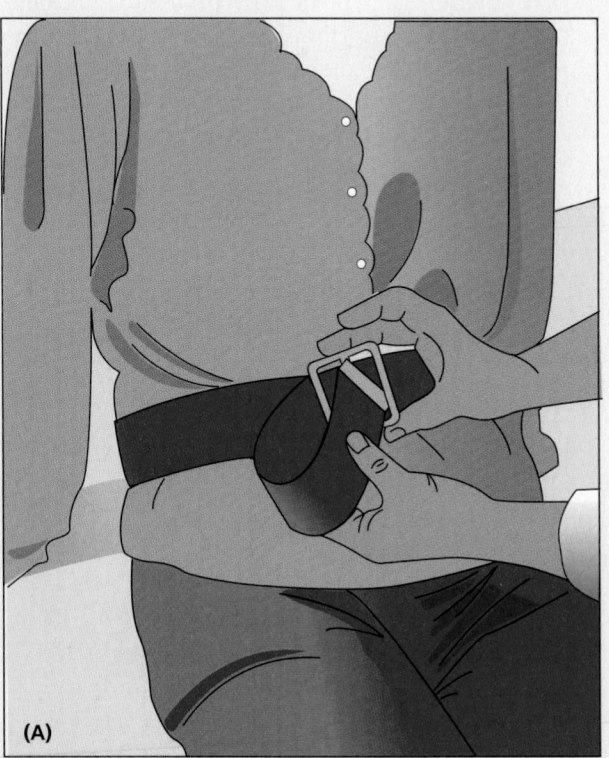

(A)

Figure 21-26 (A) A gait belt is always applied snugly around the patient's waist before attempting to move or ambulate with patients. *(continues)*

Procedure 21-1 (continued)

6. Position the stool in front of the examination table as close to the wheelchair as possible (Figure 21-26B).
7. Have the patient move to the edge of the wheelchair.
8. Stand directly in front of the patient with your feet slightly apart. Bending at the hips and knees, grasp the gait belt and have the patient place his hands on the armrests of the wheelchair so he can push up when you give the signal (Figure 21-26C). If the patient doesn't have the upper body strength to push off, simply let his arms rest in front of him.
9. Give a signal and lift the gait belt upward, pushing with your knees. If the patient has the strength in his good leg, he should push up with that leg in addition to pushing up with his arms.
10. Still grasping the gait belt, have the patient step onto the stool with the foot closest to the examination table, and pivot so his back is to the examination table (Figure 21-26D). Make sure the buttocks are lifted slightly higher than the bed. Support the patient's weaker, outer leg with your leg furthest from the examination table.

11. Have the patient grasp the stool handle and place his other hand on the examination table.
12. Gently ease the patient to a sitting position on the examination table.
13. Position the patient on the examination table as necessary.
14. Move the wheelchair and stool out of the way.

Modification: Two-Person Transfer
1. Place the gait belt snugly around the patient's waist and tuck the excess end under the belt.
2. Have one person stand in front of the patient and the other to the side, next to the examination table.
3. Both persons should grasp the gait belt from underneath. Have the patient place his hands on the armrests of the wheelchair.
4. On one person's signal, both persons pull the patient straight up. The patient should also push up with his hands, but if he doesn't have the upper body strength to push off, simply let his arms rest in front of him (Figure 21-27).

(continues)

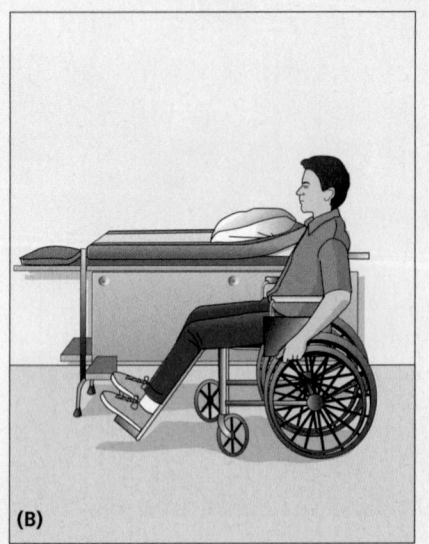

(B)

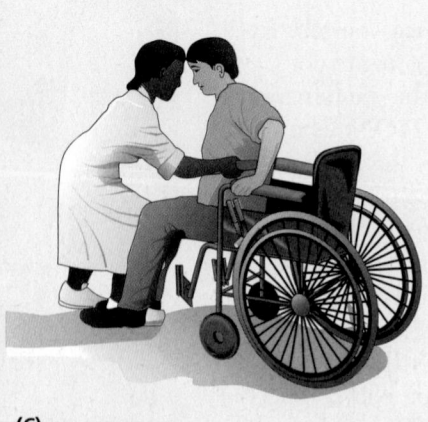

(C)

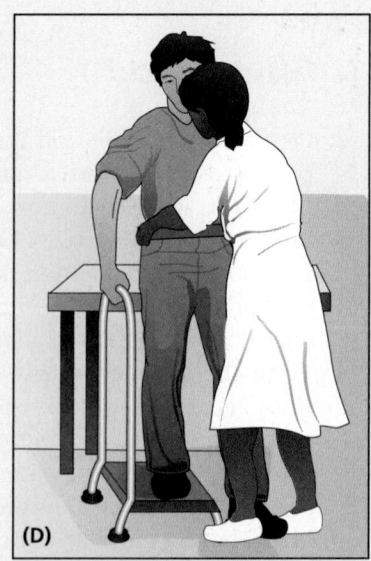

(D)

Figure 21-26 *(continued)* (B) Position the stool in front of the examination table and as close to the wheelchair as possible. (C) Before lifting, observe proper body mechanics to avoid injuring yourself or the patient. (D) Check that the patient's foot is firmly placed on the stool before completing the transfer.

Procedure 21-1 (continued)

5. The person nearest the examination table moves the wheelchair out of the way, while the other pivots the patient and has the patient place his stronger leg on the stool. If the patient has the upper body strength, he should also grasp the handle of the stool.
6. On one person's signal, both persons lift the patient onto the examination table.
7. Position the patient on the examination table as necessary.

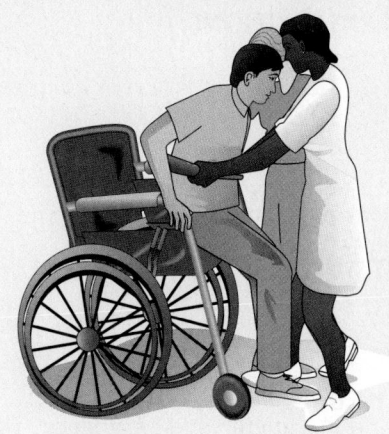

Figure 21-27 A two-person transfer when the patient does not have the upper-body strength to help move himself.

Procedure 21-2 Transferring Patient from Examination Table to Wheelchair

STANDARD PRECAUTIONS:

PURPOSE:
To move a patient safely from the examination table to a wheelchair.

EQUIPMENT/SUPPLIES:
Stool with rubber tips and a handle for gripping
Gait belt

PROCEDURE STEPS:
1. Wash hands.
2. Identify the patient and introduce yourself. Explain to the patient what you are going to do.
3. Position the wheelchair next to the examination table and lock the brakes. NOTE: Place the wheelchair so it is closest to the patient's stronger side so he can transfer his weight onto the stronger foot as he gets down.
4. Position the stool next to the wheelchair.
5. Assist the patient to rise to a sitting position. Place the gait belt snugly around the patient's waist and tuck the excess end under the belt.

6. Place your arm under the patient's arm and around his shoulders, and your other arm under his knees. Pivot the patient so his legs are dangling over the side of the examination table.
7. Keeping a hand on the patient, move so you are directly in front of him.
8. Grasp the patient by placing your hands under the gait belt. Plant your feet shoulder's width apart and bend your knees so you will have a strong base of support.
9. On your signal, pull the patient slightly toward you so his feet come down onto the stool. The patient should push off the examination table and grasp the stool handle for support.
10. Still grasping the gait belt, have the patient step onto the floor with his strong leg, and pivot at the same time so his back is to the wheelchair.
11. Have the patient grasp the armrests of the wheelchair.
12. Bending from your knees and hips, gently lower the patient into the wheelchair and make sure he is comfortably seated.
13. Lower the footrests and place his feet on them.

Procedure 21-3 Assisting the Patient to Stand and Walk

STANDARD PRECAUTIONS:

PURPOSE:
To help a patient ambulate safely.

EQUIPMENT/SUPPLIES:
Gait belt

PROCEDURE STEPS:
1. Wash hands.
2. Identify the patient and introduce yourself. Explain to the patient what you are going to do.
3. Lock the brakes on the wheelchair, if the patient is using one. Place the patient's feet on the floor and move the foot plates out of the way.
4. Instruct the patient to slide forward in the chair.
5. Place the gait belt around the patient's waist and tuck the excess end under the belt.
6. Standing directly in front of the patient, grasp the gait belt from underneath and assist her to stand on your signal. At the same time, have the patient push up on the armrests of the wheelchair.
7. Steady the patient momentarily and watch for balance, strength, and skin color. If necessary, take her pulse.
8. If the patient appears steady and has balance, strength, and good skin color, proceed by standing slightly behind and to the side of the patient's weaker side.
9. Grasp the gait belt with one hand and place the other hand on the patient's bent arm for support. Note the gait belt is grasped with your fingers under the belt, palm up and elbow bent (Figure 21-28).
10. Start with the same foot as the patient and keep in step with her.
11. Document the procedure including date, time, duration of ambulation, response of patient, and instructions given.

Modification: Two-Person Assist with Ambulation
1. Perform the preceding steps 1 through 5.
2. Have a person stand on either side of the patient. Grasp the gait belt from underneath with one hand, and place the other hand on the patient's back for support.
3. During ambulation, there should be a person on either side of the patient and slightly behind (Figure 21-29). Both persons should be grasping the gait belt throughout the ambulation session.
4. Document the procedure including date, time, duration of ambulation, response of patient, and instructions given.

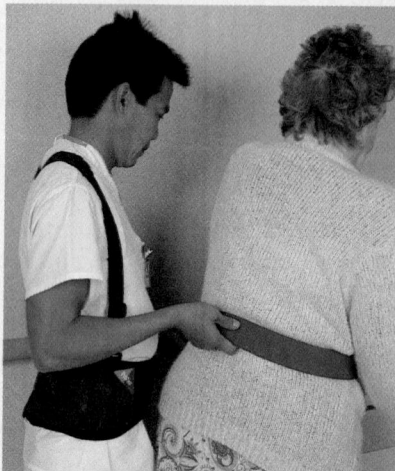

Figure 21-28 Firmly grasp the gait belt from underneath, with the palm up and elbow bent.

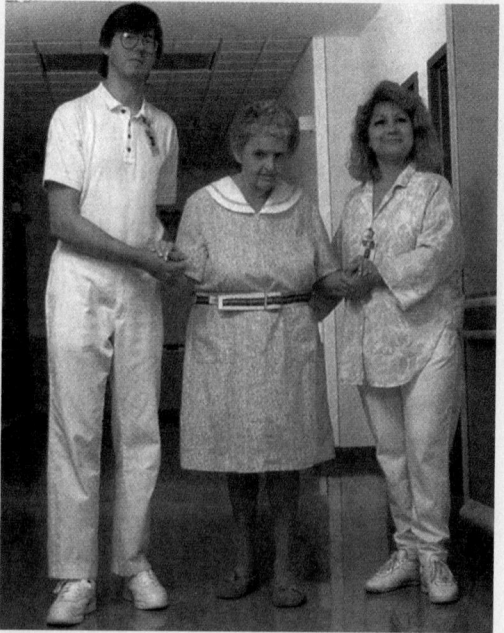

Figure 21-29 When two persons are assisting with ambulation, have them stand on either side of the patient.

Procedure

21-4   **Care of the Falling Patient**

PURPOSE:
To help the patient fall safely to avoid injury.

EQUIPMENT/SUPPLIES:
Gait belt (should already be on patient)

PROCEDURE STEPS:
1. Keep a firm hand on the gait belt. **CAUTION:** Never grab clothing, as it can shift and become unstable.
2. If the patient falls backwards, widen your stance to become a more stable base of support for her to fall against (Figure 21-30). Gently guide the patient to the floor, call for assistance, and take her pulse.
3. If the patient falls to either side, steady her back onto her feet. To do this, you will need to move your foot in the direction she is falling. Inquire whether the patient would like to terminate the ambulation session and check for signs of fatigue. If necessary, call for assistance. Check blood pressure and pulse.
4. Should the patient fall forward, support her around the waist. Step forward with your outer leg and gently lower her to the floor, making sure to protect her from injury (Figure 21-31). Call for assistance and take blood pressure and pulse.
5. Have the patient examined by a nurse or doctor prior to moving her again.
6. Document the fall in an incident report.

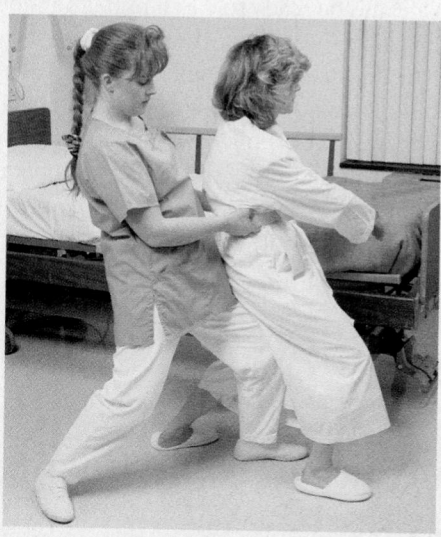

Figure 21-30   Support a falling patient with a wide base of support.

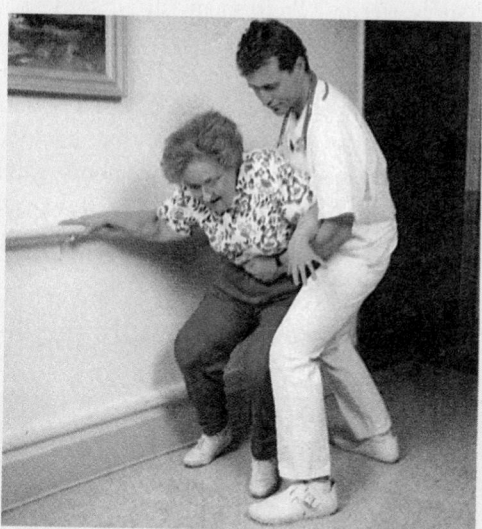

Figure 21-31   Ease the falling patient to the floor, and try to protect the head.

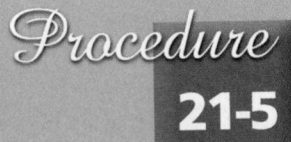

Assisting a Patient to Ambulate with a Walker

21-5

STANDARD PRECAUTIONS:

PURPOSE:
To allow a patient to ambulate independently and safely with a walker.

EQUIPMENT/SUPPLIES:
Walker
Gait belt

PROCEDURE STEPS:
1. Wash hands.
2. Identify the patient and introduce yourself. Explain to the patient what you are going to do.
3. Apply the gait belt snugly around the patient's waist and tuck the excess end under the belt.
4. Check the walker to be sure the rubber suction tips are secure on all the legs. Check the handrests for rough or damaged edges that could cut or pinch the patient. The adjustments should be tightened so they will not slip.
5. Be sure the patient is wearing good walking shoes with a rubber sole.

6. Check the height of the walker. The handrests should be level with the tip of the patient's femur, and the elbows should be flexed at a 30° angle.
7. Position the patient inside the walker, and instruct the patient to hold onto the handles while keeping the walker in front of him.
8. Position yourself behind and slightly to the side of the patient.
9. Have the patient lift the walker and place all four legs of the walker in front of him so the back legs are even with the patient's toes.
10. Instruct the patient to lean forward and transfer his weight so that he steps into the walker, first with his stronger leg, then the weaker leg. Make sure he brings his stronger leg past the weaker leg.
11. Monitor the patient carefully. Be alert for signs of fatigue and be ready to catch him if he should fall.
12. If the walker has rollers, the patient simply rolls the walker ahead a comfortable distance, then walks into it. The patient can also walk normally with a rolling walker by simply rolling it in front and leaning into the gait, using the walker for support.
13. Document the date, time, duration of ambulation, response of patient, and instructions given. Initial the report.

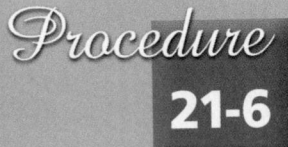

Teaching the Patient to Ambulate with Axillary Crutches

21-6

STANDARD PRECAUTIONS:

PURPOSE:
To teach the patient how to ambulate safely using axillary crutches.

EQUIPMENT/SUPPLIES:
Axillary crutches
Gait belt

PROCEDURE STEPS:
1. Wash hands.
2. Identify the patient and introduce yourself. Explain to the patient what you are going to do.
3. Assemble the axillary crutches and be sure they are in good working order. Make sure there are rubber suction tips on the bottom ends and that they are not worn or torn. Check the axillary bar and handrest to be sure they are covered with padding, and that the padding is not cracked or worn. Be sure the wing nuts are tight.

(continues)

Procedure **21-6** *(continued)*

4. Check the measurement of the crutches. Pediatric crutches must be used for pediatric patients.
5. Apply the gait belt and assist the patient to stand and place the crutches under the armpits.
6. Instruct the patient to carry his weight completely on his hands and not on his armpits.
7. Have the patient put all his weight on his good leg, and bend the weak leg slightly so it will not drag on the floor as he walks.
8. Assist the patient with the required gait.
9. Wash hands.
10. Document the date, time, duration of ambulation, and instructions given.

Procedure **21-7** Assisting a Patient to Ambulate with a Cane

STANDARD PRECAUTIONS:

PURPOSE:
To teach patients how to walk safely with a cane.

EQUIPMENT/SUPPLIES:
Appropriate cane for patient
Gait belt

PROCEDURE STEPS:
1. Wash hands.
2. Ascertain what type of cane the physician or therapist indicates your patient is to be using and assemble the equipment.
3. Identify the patient and introduce yourself. Explain to the patient what you are going to do.
4. Check the cane to be sure the bottom has a rubber suction tip. If a quad or walkcane is to be used, make sure all the legs have rubber suction tips.
5. Apply the gait belt snugly around the patient's waist if needed and tuck the excess end under the belt. Assist the patient to a standing position.
6. Place the cane relatively close to the body to the side of the foot of the strong leg. Adjust the cane so the handle is at the level of the patient's hip joint (Figure 21-32).
7. During weightbearing, the patient's elbow should be flexed 20° to 30°.

8. The cane and the involved leg are advanced simultaneously.
9. Have the patient move the weak leg forward while transferring the weight to the cane.
10. Have the patient move the strong leg forward past the cane.
11. Follow along behind and to the side of the patient's weak side.
12. Wash your hands.
13. Document the date, time, duration of ambulation, response of patient, and instructions given.

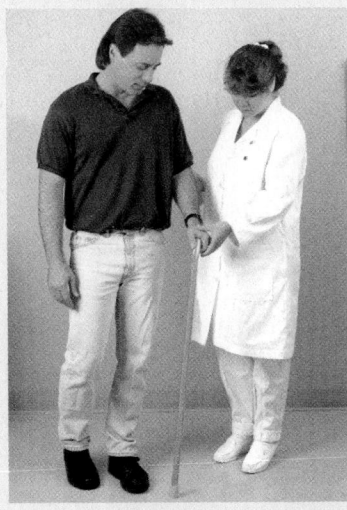

Figure 21-32 In placing the cane, be sure the handle comes to the top of the patient's hip and elbow is flexed 20 to 30°.

Procedure 21-8   Range of Motion Exercises, Upper Body

STANDARD PRECAUTIONS:

PURPOSE:
To maintain or increase joint mobility in the upper extremities and prevent contractures.

EQUIPMENT/SUPPLIES:
None
NOTE: This procedure is best done with the patient in the supine position (see Chapter 13). Repeat each movement several times.

PRE-PROCEDURE STEPS:
1. Wash hands.
2. Identify the patient and introduce yourself. Explain to the patient what you are going to do.

PROCEDURE STEPS:

Shoulder Flexion
1. Keep the patient's arm straight and hold the arm at the wrist and elbow.
2. Lift the patient's arm straight over his head until it rests flat on the bed or table above the patient's head (Figure 21-33).
3. Bend the patient's elbow if there is not enough room on the bed.
4. Bring the arm back to the patient's side.

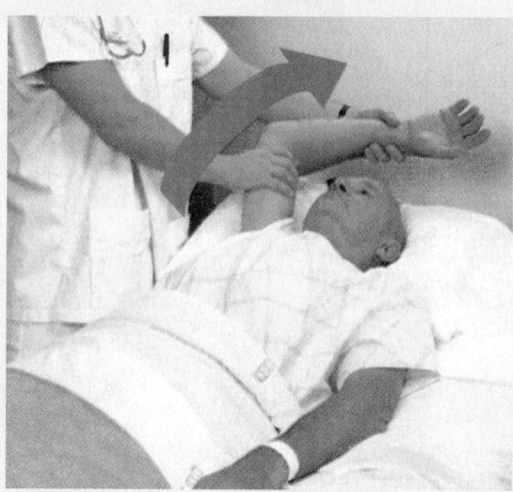

Figure 21-33   Shoulder flexion.

Shoulder Abduction and Adduction
1. Keep the patient's arm straight by his side, with the palm of his hand facing up. Support the arm at the wrist and elbow.
2. Keeping the patient's arm straight, bring it out at a right angle to his body (Figure 21-34A).
3. Bring the arm back to the patient's side. Keeping the arm straight, bring it across the body (Figure 21-34B).
4. Return the patient's arm to a position parallel to the body.   (*continues*)

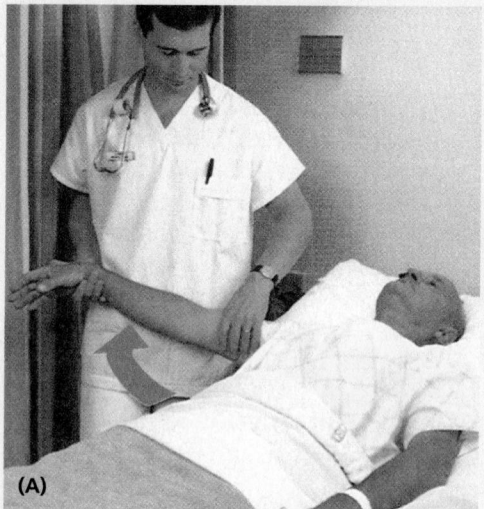

(A)

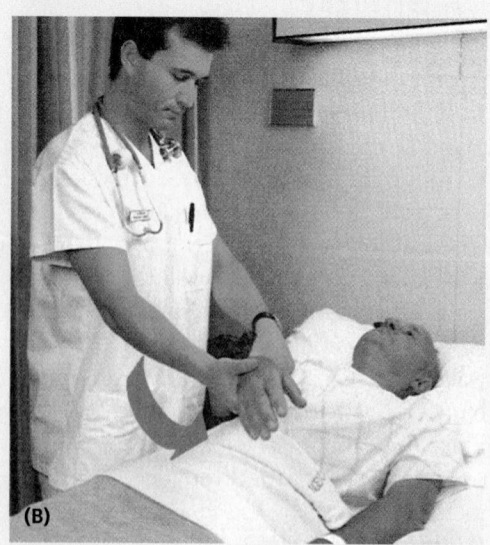

(B)

Figure 21-34   (A) Shoulder abduction. (B) Shoulder adduction.

Procedure

21-8 *(continued)*

Internal and External Shoulder Rotation
1. Bring the arm out at a right angle from the body.
2. Bend the elbow at a right angle, keeping the upper arm on the bed.
3. Keeping the patient's arm at a right angle, gently press down on the shoulder with one hand while holding the patient's wrist with the other.
4. Move the hand gently back until it touches the bed next to the patient's head.
5. Bring the hand back down until the palm of the patient's hand touches the bed.

Elbow Flexion and Extension
1. With the patient's arm by his side and his palm up, flex and extend the elbow (Figure 21-35).

Wrist Extension and Flexion
1. Support the patient's arm above the wrist.

2. Holding the palm of the patient's hand, extend the wrist, then straighten it (Figure 21-36A).
3. Place your hand over the patient's hand while still supporting the wrist. Bend or flex the hand (Figure 21-36B).

Wrist Inversion and Eversion
1. Grasp the patient's wrist with one hand and grasp his hand with the other.
2. Slowly bend the patient's hand toward his body, then away from his body (Figure 21-37).

Wrist Supination and Pronation
1. Grasp the patient's wrist with one hand and his hand with the other.
2. Slowly turn the patient's hand toward his feet, then toward his face.   *(continues)*

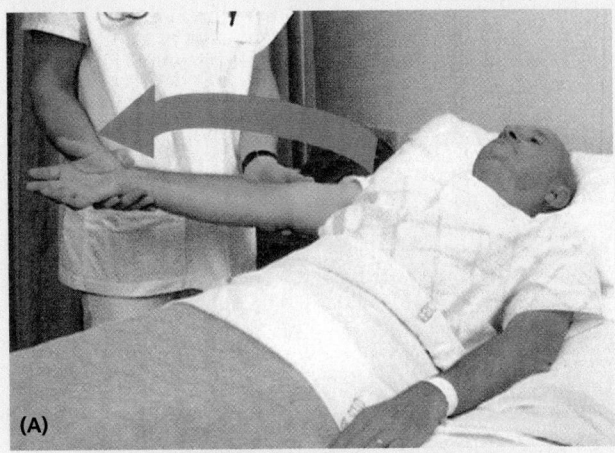

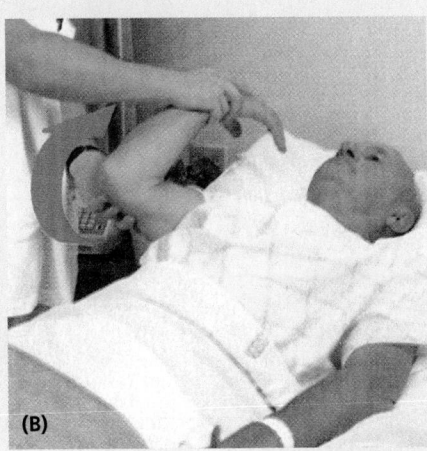

Figure 21-35   (A) Elbow extension. (B) Elbow flexion.

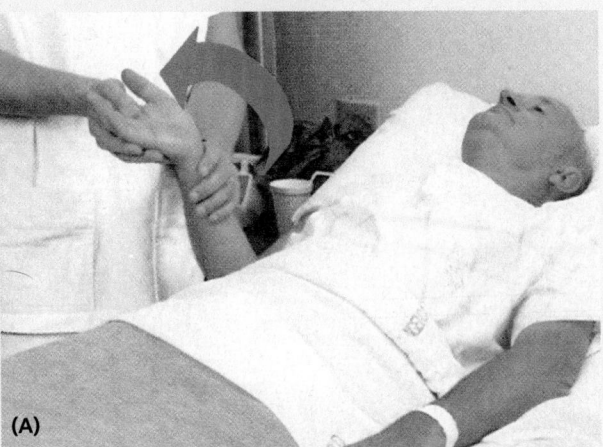

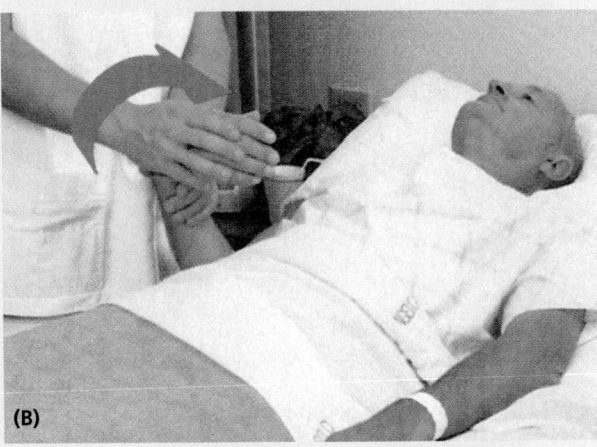

Figure 21-36   (A) Wrist extension. (B) Wrist flexion.

Procedure
21-8   *(continued)*

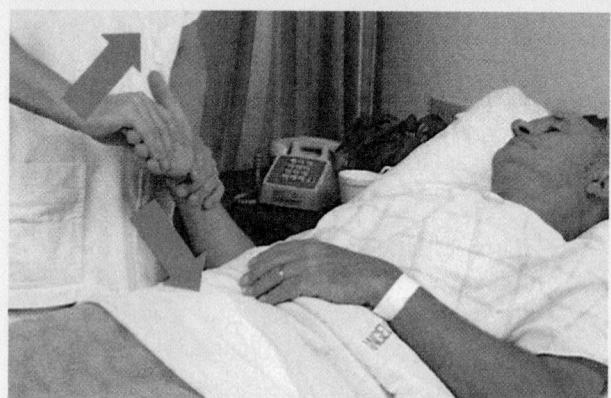

Figure 21-37   Wrist inversion and eversion.

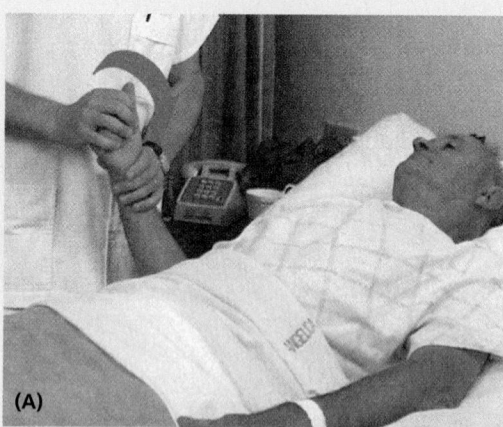

(A)

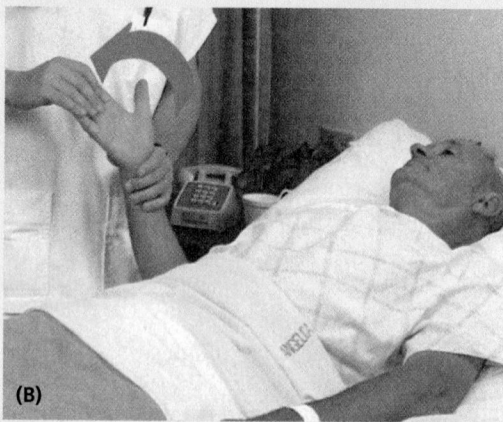

(B)

Figure 21-38   (A) Finger flexion. (B) Finger extension.

Finger Flexion and Extension
1. Support the patient's wrist with one hand. Cover his finger with the other hand and curl them over to make a fist (Figure 21-38A).
2. Uncurl the patient's fingers and straighten them (Figure 21-38B).

Finger and Thumb Abduction and Adduction
1. Hold the patient's hand flat. Slowly pull each finger away from the thumb (Figure 21-39A), then pull it back straight (Figure 21-39B).
2. Pull the thumb away from the rest of the fingers, then pull it back straight (Figure 21-40).

Thumb Opposition
1. Support the patient's hand.
2. Touch each finger with the thumb (Figure 21-41).

POST-PROCEDURE STEPS:
1. Wash hands.
2. Document the date, time, limbs given ROM, and response of patient. Initial the report.

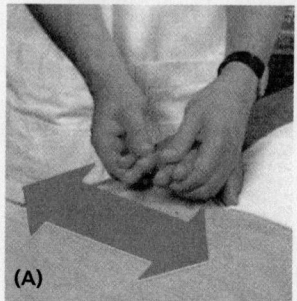

(A)

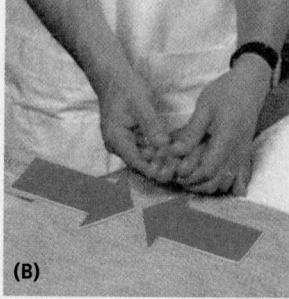

(B)

Figure 21-39   (A) Finger abduction. (B) Finger adduction.

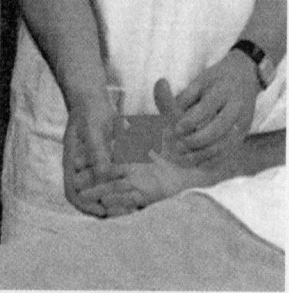

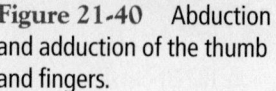

Figure 21-40   Abduction and adduction of the thumb and fingers.

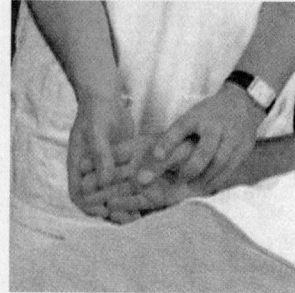

Figure 21-41   Thumb opposition.

Range of Motion Exercises, Lower Body

STANDARD PRECAUTIONS:

PURPOSE:

To maintain or increase joint mobility in the lower extremities and prevent contractures.

EQUIPMENT/SUPPLIES:

None

NOTE: This procedure is best done with the patient in the supine position. Repeat each movement several times.

PRE-PROCEDURE STEPS:

1. Wash hands.
2. Identify the patient and introduce yourself. Explain to the patient what you are going to do.

PROCEDURE STEPS:

Hip Abduction and Adduction

1. Support the patient's knee and ankle.
2. Keeping the patient's leg straight, move the entire leg away from the body (Figure 21-42A).

3. Move the patient's leg back, toward the midline of the body (Figure 21-42B).

Hip and Knee Flexion and Extension

1. Support the patient's knee and ankle.
2. Bend the patient's knee and raise it as far toward the patient's chest as his tolerance and comfort will allow (Figure 21-43A).
3. Lower and straighten the patient's leg (Figure 21-43B).

Hip Rotation

1. Support the patient's leg at the knee and ankle.
2. Roll the patient's leg in a circular motion, away from the body.
3. Roll the patient's leg in a circular motion, toward the body.

Ankle Dorsiflexion and Plantar Flexion

1. Keep the patient's leg flat on the bed. NOTE: It may be more comfortable if the patient's knee is slightly bent. Grasp his ankle with one hand and the heel of his foot with the other.

(continues)

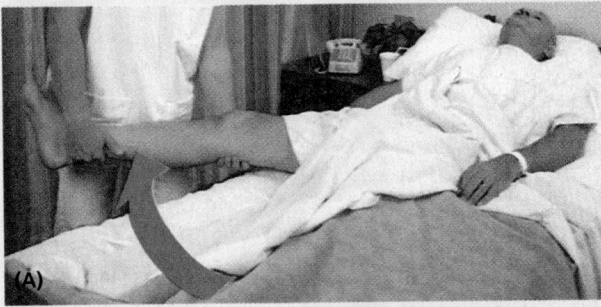

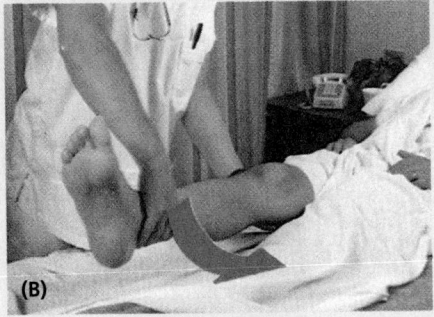

Figure 21-42 (A) Hip abduction. (B) Hip adduction.

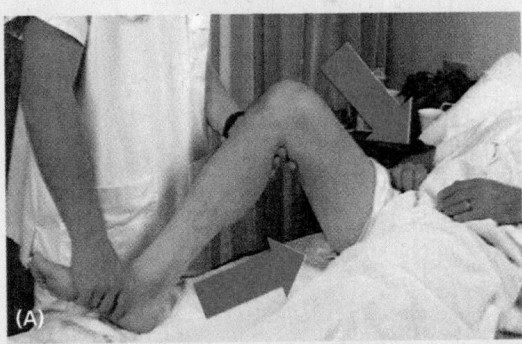

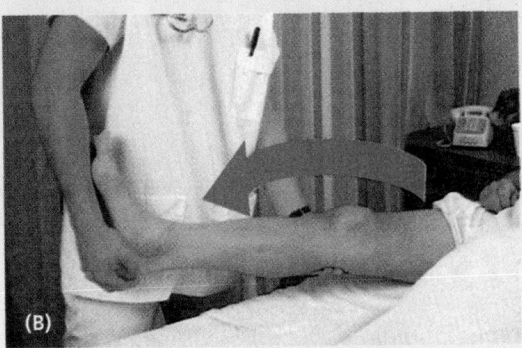

Figure 21-43 (A) Hip and knee flexion. (B) Knee extension.

Procedure

21-9 (*continued*)

2. With the hand holding the patient's heel, flex the patient's foot and rest the bottom of his foot against your forearm. Keep your elbow straight (Figure 21-44A).
3. Dorsiflex the ankle by pushing the foot toward the patient's knee with your arm.
4. Return the foot to its flexed position against your forearm.
5. Keeping your one hand on the patient's ankle, plantar flex the ankle by drawing the foot down toward the foot of the bed (Figure 21-44B).

Foot Inversion and Eversion
1. Grasp the patient's ankle with one hand and the arch of his foot with the other.
2. Gently turn the patient's foot inward (Figure 21-45A).
3. Return the patient's foot to the midline, then gently turn it outward (Figure 21-45B).

TOE FLEXION AND EXTENSION
1. Hold the patient's ankle in one hand and place your fingers over the patient's toes with the other hand.
2. Bend the toes, then straighten them.

TOE ABDUCTION AND ADDUCTION
1. Move each toe one at a time away from the second toe (Figure 21-46A).
2. Move each toe one at a time toward the second toe (Figure 21-46B).

POST-PROCEDURE STEP:
1. Wash hands.
2. Document the date, time, limbs given ROM, and response of patient. Initial the report.

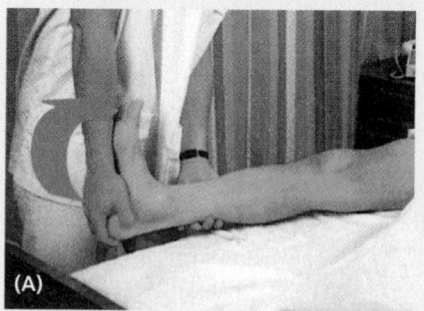
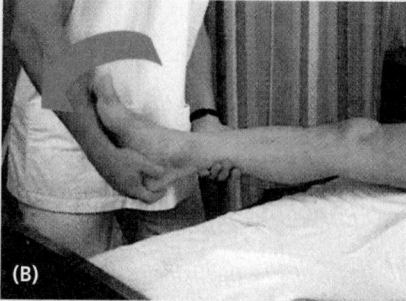
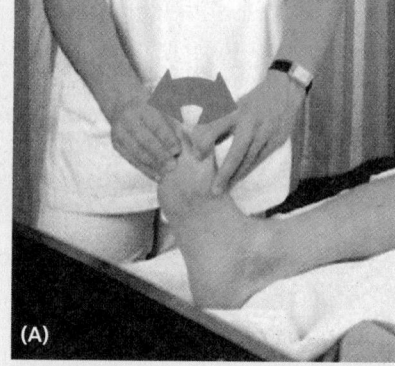

Figure 21-44   (A) Ankle dorsiflexion. (B) Plantar flexion.

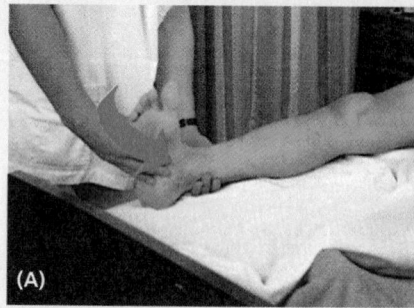
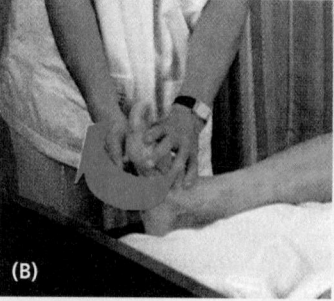
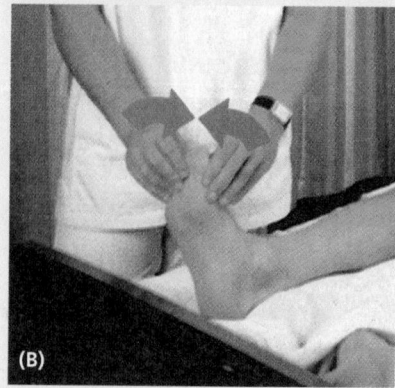

Figure 21-45   (A) Foot inversion. (B) Foot eversion.

Figure 21-46   (A) Toe abduction. (B) Toe adduction.

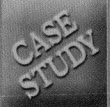

It is a mild summer afternoon in the city of Carlton, the home of Inner City Health Care. The softball season is in full swing, and Inner City has treated its share of players and spectators who have suffered minor injuries. On this particular Tuesday, Bill Schwarz, a regular patient, comes in late in the day in obvious pain. Bruce Goldman, the clinical medical assistant on duty, quickly gets the patient into a wheelchair. From the patient's description of the situation and the pain, Bruce suspects a sprained ankle. Dr. Woo is on call and available to examine the patient immediately and asks Bruce to transfer Bill from the wheelchair to the examination table.

CASE STUDY REVIEW

1. What are some of the general principles the medical assistant should observe during any transfer?
2. Summarize the steps involved in transferring the patient from the wheelchair to the examination table.
3. Summarize the steps involved in transferring the patient from the examination table to the wheelchair.

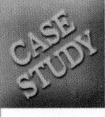

After diagnosing Mr. Schwarz with a sprained left ankle, Dr. Woo has prescribed an ace bandage to the ankle, crutches, and an ice pack to be applied to the ankle. He has also given Mr. Schwarz a prescription for pain relievers and has recommended that Mr. Schwarz stay off his feet as much as possible. He is to keep the leg elevated with an ice pack on it.

CASE STUDY REVIEW

1. Explain what you would tell Mr. Schwarz about applying the ice pack to his ankle at home.

SUMMARY

Rehabilitation medicine is a field of medical disciplines that specializes in both preventing disease or injury and restoring physical function. It uses a combination of physical and mechanical agents to aid in the diagnosis, treatment, and prevention of diseases or bodily injury, including exercise and a variety of treatment modalities.

Much of what a medical assistant might do on the job in this field involves some form of lifting or moving of heavy objects. It is important to remember to use good body mechanics in order to prevent back or other injury. When transferring patients, good body mechanics ensures the safety of both caregiver and patient. If necessary, get someone to help with the transfer.

Helping the patient to ambulate safely following a period of sedentary recuperation is an important part of a rehabilitation program. If they are not able to ambulate on their own, patients can be fitted for a variety of assistive walking devices, including walkers, crutches, and canes. Crutch walking, by far the most common use of an assistive device, can be done using one of several walking patterns, or gaits, depending

upon the patient's condition, strength, and stability. Whatever assistive device is used, it is important that the patient be measured correctly for that device and taught how to periodically check it for safety.

In addition to ambulation, there are a number of other types of therapeutic exercises. Depending upon the patient's condition, an exercise program can be prescribed after evaluating the patient's joint range of motion and muscle strength. Joints and muscles must be exercised regularly in order to avoid muscle atrophy or joint contractures, as well as improve circulation and maintain or improve overall health. Range of motion and other exercises can be performed either by the caregiver, the patient, or a combination of the two.

In addition to exercise, a variety of therapeutic modalities might also be used as part of the patient's rehabilitation program. The various properties of heat, cold, light, electricity, and water act on the body to improve circulation, minimize pain, or correct or alleviate joint and muscle malfunction. Heat dilates the blood vessels, thereby increasing circulation to an area and speeding up the repair process. Cold constricts the blood vessels, slowing circulation and therefore the inflammatory process. Ultrasound and other electrical diathermies use an electrical current to create heat in the deeper tissues of the body. It is important to understand how each modality affects the physiological functioning of the body and observe certain safety precautions to avoid injuring the patient.

REVIEW QUESTIONS

Multiple Choice

1. Brushing teeth, getting dressed, and eating are referred to as:
   a. rehabilitation medicine
   b. activities of daily living (ADL)
   c. body mechanics
   d. occupational therapy
2. Hemiplegia is defined as:
   a. inability of the patient to ambulate properly
   b. severe back pain
   c. paralysis of one side of the body
   d. confinement to a wheelchair
3. Ambulatory assistive devices include:
   a. gait belts
   b. walkers, canes, and crutches
   c. wheelchairs
   d. stools with handholds
4. Motion away from the midline of the body is called:
   a. adduction
   b. pronation
   c. extension
   d. abduction
5. Supination involves:
   a. placing the patient in the supine position
   b. moving the arm so the palm is up
   c. bending a body part
   d. straightening a body part

Critical Thinking

1. Define rehabilitation, and explain its importance in patient care.
2. If a patient should fall to the side, what action would you take to ensure safety?
3. Describe the procedure for measuring for axillary crutches.
4. What kind of patient would need a forearm crutch?
5. In crutch-walking gaits, what is a *point*?
6. Describe the five different types of crutch gaits.
7. List the six safety rules for transporting a patient in a wheelchair.
8. What is joint range of motion, how is it measured, and how is the measurement expressed?
9. How do heat and cold affect the body's physiology and for what conditions should each be used?
10. Describe how ultrasound works and identify the patient conditions for which it is an effective treatment.

WEB ACTIVITIES

Access information online about the Americans with Disabilities Act of 1990.

1. To what group of people does the act apply?
2. What does the act provide for these individuals?
3. Does the act have any influence over access to physicians' offices and clinics? Explain.

REFERENCES/BIBLIOGRAPHY

Bonewit-West, K. (2000). *Clinical procedures for medical assistants* (5th ed.). Philadelphia: W. B. Saunders Company.

Frey, R., & Shearer Cooper, L. (1996). *Introduction to nursing assisting: Building language skills.* Albany, NY: Delmar.

Hegner, B., & Caldwell, E. (1999). *Nursing assistant: A nursing process approach* (8th ed.). Albany, NY: Delmar.

Keir, L., Wise, B. A., & Krebs, C. (1998). *Medical assisting: Administrative and clinical competencies* (4th ed.). Albany, NY: Delmar.

Medical assisting video series: Administrative and clinical procedures. (1997). Albany, NY: Delmar.

Norkin, C. C., & White, D. J. (1995). *Measurement of joint motion: A guide to goniometry* (2nd ed.). Philadelphia: F. A. Davis Company.

O'Sullivan, S. B., & Schmitz, T. (2000). *Physical rehabilitation: Assessment and treatment* (4th ed.). Philadelphia: F. A. Davis Co.

Simmers, L. (1998). *Diversified health occupations* (3rd ed.). Albany, NY: Delmar.

Taber's cyclopedic medical dictionary. (18th ed.). (1999). Philadelphia: F. A. Davis Company.

Weiss, R. C. (1999). *The physical therapy aide: A work text.* Albany, NY: Delmar.

Zakus, S. (1995). *Clinical procedures for medical assistants* (3rd ed.). St. Louis, MO: Mosby-Year Book, Inc.

NUTRITION IN HEALTH AND DISEASE

KEY TERMS

Amino Acid
Antioxidant
Ascorbic Acid
Basal Metabolic Rate
Calorie
Carotene
Catalyst
Cellulose
Cholecalciferol
Cobalamin
Coenzyme
Digestion
Diuretic
Electrolytes
Extracellular
Fat-Soluble
Folic Acid
Glycogen
Homeostasis
Kwashiorkor
Major Mineral
Marasmus
Metabolism
Niacin
Nutrient
Nutrition
Oxidation
Preservative
Processed Food
Pyridoxine
Riboflavin
Saturated Fat
Thiamin
Tocopherol
Trace Mineral
Water-Soluble

OUTLINE

Nutrition and Digestion
Types of Nutrients
    Energy Nutrients
    Other Nutrients
Reading Food Labels
    Items on the Nutrition Label
    Comparing Labels
Nutrition at Various Stages of Life
    Pregnancy and Lactation
    Infancy
    Adolescence
    Elderly

Therapeutic Diets
    Weight Control
    Diabetes Mellitus
    Cardiovascular Disease
    Cancer
Diet and Culture

OBJECTIVES

The student should strive to meet the following performance objectives and demonstrate an understanding of the facts and principles presented in this chapter through written and oral communication.

1. Define the key terms as presented in the glossary.
2. Describe the relationship of nutrition to the functioning of the digestive system.
3. Identify the seven basic nutrient types.
4. Explain the relationship and balance between the three energy nutrients.
5. Distinguish between water-soluble and fat-soluble vitamins.
6. Explain the reason for nutrition labels on food packaging.
7. Read and interpret nutrition facts and ingredients on three food packages.
8. Discuss various therapeutic diets, and explain how each can help to control a particular disease state or accommodate a change in the life cycle.

**GENERAL
(TRANSDISCIPLINARY)**

Instruction

- **Instruct individuals according to their needs**
- **Teach methods of health promotion and disease prevention**
- **Locate community resources and disseminate information**

This morning at Inner City Health Care, clinical medical assistant Wanda Slawson, CMA, was conferring with Dr. Rice on three of the center's patients whose diets needed modification. With the help of Dr. Rice, Wanda was putting together dietary changes for patient Edith Leonard, who is in her early seventies and losing weight because she is not eating well enough or often enough; Corey Boyer, in the prime of adolescence and capable of eating large quantities of food with little nutritional value; and Annette Samuels, who recently discovered she was pregnant. All these patients have different nutritional requirements, and Wanda wants to encourage all to review and modify their diets.

INTRODUCTION

The human body is in a constant state of fluctuation. The outside environment is constantly changing, and the body requires **homeostasis**, or a continual internal environment, which, in turn, gives us a requirement for nutrients. The nutrients we take into our bodies replenish the materials we have used. In this way, homeostasis is maintained and our bodies have a relatively balanced internal environment. **Nutrition** is the study of the taking of nutrients into the body and how the body uses them.

The normal healthy individual will consume and use close to what the body needs in order to stay healthy. However, some individuals either do not consume enough nutrients or consume too much of a particular type of nutrient. These are poor diets that can cause particular

disease states and the diet must be modified to return the patient to good health. In addition, specific disease states, such as diabetes mellitus, warrant a change from a normal diet in order to control the progress of the disease. The human body also goes through many changes in a lifetime and with these changes come new nutritional needs.

This chapter explores the balance of nutrients required for good health and examines therapeutic modifications to the diet that should take place at various life stages or in the presence of disease. The astute medical assistant will recognize the role of nutrition in maintaining health and use a knowledge of nutritional principles to encourage patients to adopt a healthy lifestyle.

NUTRITION AND DIGESTION

Nutrition includes ingestion, digestion, absorption, and metabolism of food. It is known that good nutrition has resulted in longer life spans and healthier individuals through the control of preventable diseases. The food eaten by an individual is used to build and repair cells and tissues of the body. Therefore, it is important to have knowledge and information about nutrition and to make appropriate food choices for optimum health. The well-nourished individual is less susceptible to infection and disease.

Patient education is important especially when the normal diet must be modified to treat the patient's illness. The medical assistant can answer questions only through a knowledge of good nutrition and what constitutes the therapeutic diets prescribed by the physician.

Digestion involves the physical and chemical changes that the body makes to food to make it absorbable. Absorption is the transfer of the nutrients from the gastrointestinal tract into the blood stream. Without absorption, the body would not receive the nutrients. Figure 22-1 shows the digestive system and its basic functions.

TYPES OF NUTRIENTS

Nutrients serve many purposes in the body. Some nutrients can provide energy in order for the body to perform activities such as the pumping of the heart, the division of cells, or the contraction of muscles. Nutrients also provide building blocks so that proteins or phospholipids can be made within the body or they can act as catalysts to help processes such as the clotting mechanism proceed at a

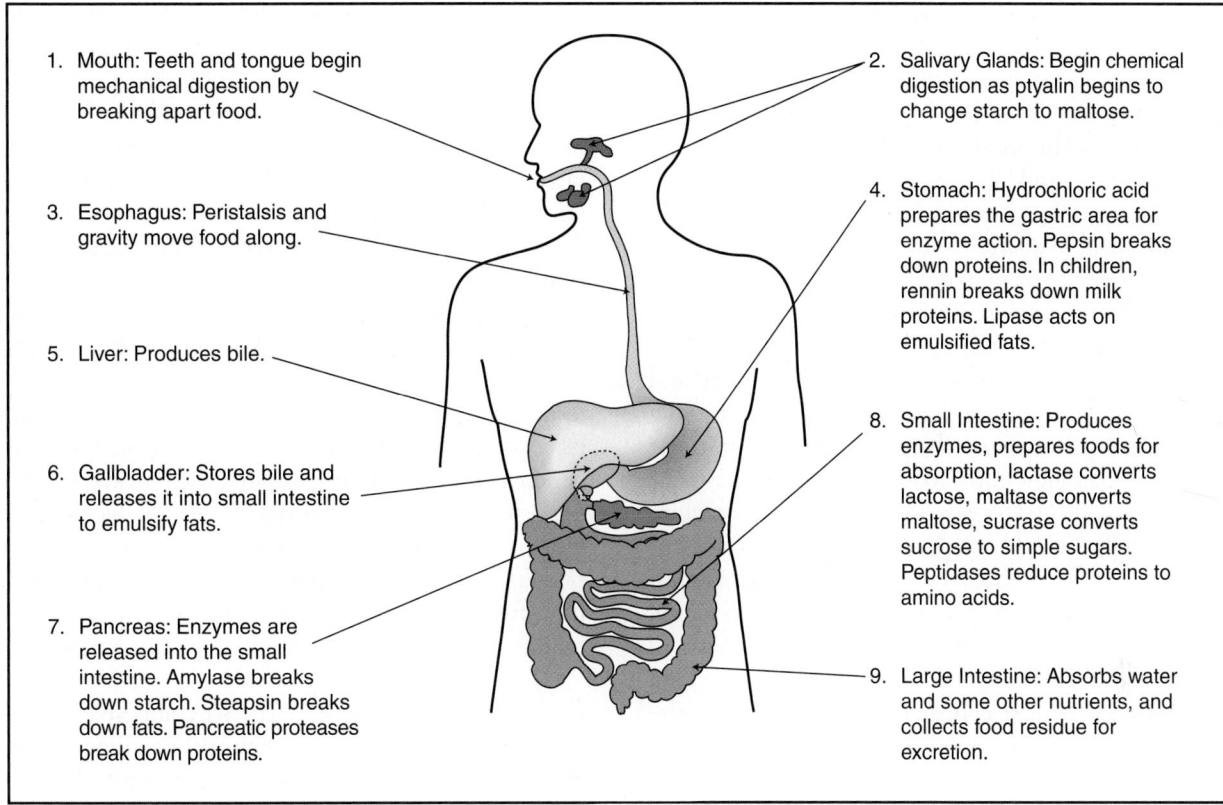

1. Mouth: Teeth and tongue begin mechanical digestion by breaking apart food.

2. Salivary Glands: Begin chemical digestion as ptyalin begins to change starch to maltose.

3. Esophagus: Peristalsis and gravity move food along.

4. Stomach: Hydrochloric acid prepares the gastric area for enzyme action. Pepsin breaks down proteins. In children, rennin breaks down milk proteins. Lipase acts on emulsified fats.

5. Liver: Produces bile.

6. Gallbladder: Stores bile and releases it into small intestine to emulsify fats.

7. Pancreas: Enzymes are released into the small intestine. Amylase breaks down starch. Steapsin breaks down fats. Pancreatic proteases break down proteins.

8. Small Intestine: Produces enzymes, prepares foods for absorption, lactase converts lactose, maltase converts maltose, sucrase converts sucrose to simple sugars. Peptidases reduce proteins to amino acids.

9. Large Intestine: Absorbs water and some other nutrients, and collects food residue for excretion.

Figure 22-1   The digestive system.

faster rate. Essentially, ingested substances that help the body stay in its homeostatic state can be called **nutrients**.

Nutrients can be divided into two groups: those that provide energy and those that do not. Table 22-1 shows examples of each of these two groups. Those that provide energy are comprised of three types: carbohydrates, fats (lipids), and proteins. Each of these three substances is used in ways other than making energy, but it is important to remember that these are the only substances from which the body can derive energy. Nutrients that do not provide energy are also important and perform other vital functions as described previously. These nutrients include vitamins, minerals, water, and fiber.

TABLE 22-1 TYPES OF NUTRIENTS	
Nutrients are divided into two groups: those that provide energy and those that do not. Both groups are essential to good health	
Energy Nutrients	**Other Nutrients**
Carbohydrates	Vitamins
Lipids (Fats)	Minerals
Proteins	Water
	Fiber

Energy Nutrients

The three energy nutrients, carbohydrates, fats, and proteins, have one thing in common: all can be converted into energy.

Carbohydrates. Carbohydrates are made up of carbon, hydrogen, and oxygen. Although many compounds are made up of these three elements, it is the ratio of these elements that is important. Carbohydrates are made up of units called sugars. The scientific term for sugar is saccharide, and carbohydrates can exist as monosaccharides, disaccharides, or polysaccharides.

A monosaccharide is composed of a single unit of sugar while disaccharides have two units of sugar. Together, monosaccharides and disaccharides are known as simple sugars. Examples of monosaccharides are glucose, fructose, and galactose. Glucose is the sugar that the body uses most efficiently, so most ingested sugar is broken down in the intestines and converted to glucose in the liver. Fructose is found largely in fruits, while galactose is a product of lactose digestion. Examples of disaccharides are lactose, maltose, and sucrose. Lactose is found primarily in milk or milk products. Maltose is a product of starch breakdown. Sucrose is one of the sweetest sugars and is what we commonly refer to as table sugar. It occurs naturally in many fruits and vegetables as well as sugar cane and the sugar beet, which are commercial sources of refined sugar.

Polysaccharides are also known as complex carbohydrates. They are made up of many units of sugar connected together. The most common polysaccharides are starches, glycogen, and fiber. Starches are the most important dietary complex carbohydrate. **Glycogen** is only ingested in small quantities, but is an important carbohydrate form for storage of glucose in the body. Fiber is a special polysaccharide because it cannot be digested.

Because the simple sugars are composed of only one or two units of sugar, their digestion takes little time and absorption occurs soon after ingestion. The body initially experiences a large increase in sugar concentration in the blood which is brought down to within a normal range by the release of insulin. The complex carbohydrates require more time to digest, and as a result there is a slow absorption of the single carbohydrate units as the larger starch molecule is broken down. This is demonstrated in Figure 22-2. In this case, there would be a moderate increase in the sugar levels in the blood and this would continue for a longer period of time. A continuous level of sugar in the bloodstream is necessary for a constant energy supply.

Fats. Fats, also called lipids, are also composed of carbon, hydrogen, and oxygen, but in a ratio different from carbohydrates. They exist as triglycerides in the body. A triglyceride has three fatty acids attached to a glycerol molecule (Figure 22-3). The fatty acid component of a triglyceride has several important characteristics. The first is whether or not it is essential to the diet. The only true essential fatty acid in the human diet is linoleic acid, and all other fatty acids the body requires can be derived from this. Another important characteristic of fatty acids is saturation. When a fatty acid is saturated, every carbon molecule on the fatty acid holds as many hydrogens as possible. If it does not hold all the hydrogens possible, it is called unsaturated. The more unsaturated the fatty acid, the more liquid the fat. For example, lard has very saturated fatty acids and a thick consistency compared to corn oil, which has relatively unsaturated fatty acids and a thin consistency. If an **unsaturated fat** is hydrogenated, combined with hydrogen, it becomes more saturated. Saturated fats are more common in foods from animal sources than from plant sources. Generally, saturated fatty acids tend to raise the level of fats and cholesterol in the blood.

Proteins. While protein is also composed of carbon, hydrogen, and oxygen, it contains one more important element: nitrogen. The basic structural unit of protein is the **amino acid**. There are twenty-two amino acids in proteins. Eight of these are needed in the diet in order for the body to function normally. One more, histidine, is essential only during childhood. The rest of the amino acids can be synthesized from the eight, provided that they are present in adequate quantities. A complete protein is so named because it has all eight of the essential amino acids. An incomplete protein does not contain all of these. The best sources for complete proteins are meats and animal products such as milk and eggs. Most plants

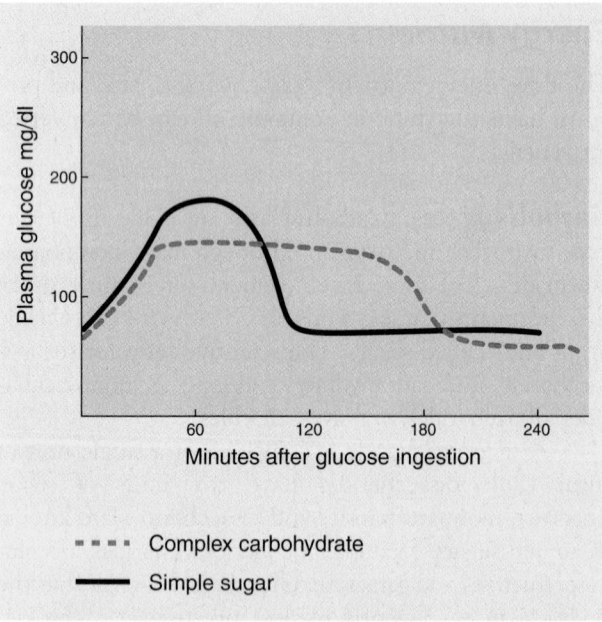

Figure 22-2 This graph shows how complex carbohydrates (red broken line) and simple sugar (black line) are used by the body (in minutes) after glucose ingestion. Simple sugar peaks to approximately 120–160 mg/dl in 60 minutes and returns to a normal level with 120 minutes. Complex carbohydrates (red broken line) never rise above approximately 130–140 mg/dl during a 60-minute period; that level is maintained for the next 120 minutes and then returns to normal.

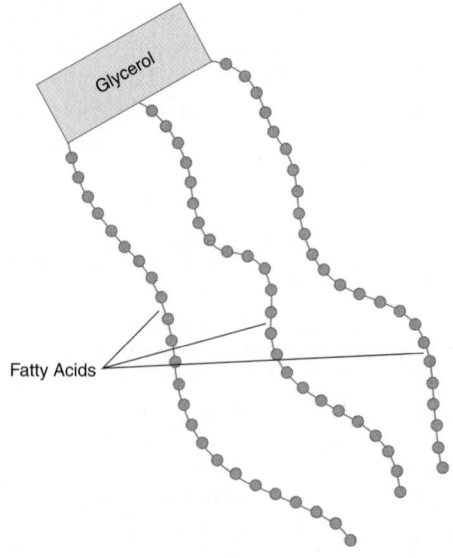

Figure 22-3 A triglyceride has three fatty acids attached to a glycerol molecule.

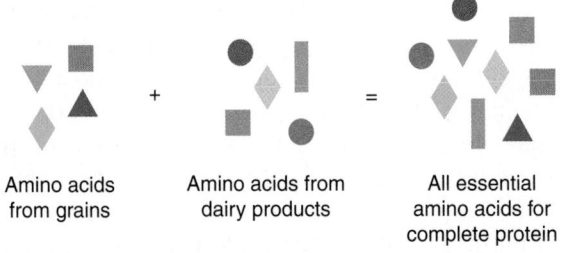

| Amino acids from grains | Amino acids from dairy products | All essential amino acids for complete protein |

Figure 22-4 Some foods, such as grains and dairy products, may not have all the essential amino acids when considered separately. Combined, however, these form a complete protein and therefore are considered complementary.

provide only incomplete proteins and must be combined with complementary incomplete proteins to obtain all eight amino acids (Figure 22-4).

Although protein is described as an energy nutrient, its main function is not to provide energy but to provide amino acids to be used as building components of body proteins, which can be used as enzymes, hormones, and as the basic structural unit in all body tissues and cells. The body uses carbohydrates and fats as its primary energy sources; however, when these are in short supply, the body diverts its use of protein for structural purposes to use it as an energy source. This has detrimental effects on the body.

Deficiencies in protein usually occur along with deficiencies in total Calories. The disease associated with these deficiencies is called protein-energy malnutrition (PEM). Another disease, marasmus, also includes deficiencies in minerals and vitamins but is often used interchangeably with PEM. The symptoms of marasmus include severe wasting, wrinkling of the skin, and growth failure. Another disease, kwashiorkor, was originally thought to be the result solely of protein deficiency, but now its cause is debated. The symptoms of kwashiorkor include edema, irritability, and growth failure. Both occur in infants and young children.

Energy Balance. While all of the energy nutrients are capable of supplying energy to the body, they do so in different ways and in varying amounts. The amount of energy that a substance is able to supply can be measured in large Calories. Nutrition is discussed in terms of the large Calorie, which is always capitalized to distinguish it from the small calorie. The large Calorie (abbreviation: C or Cal) is also expressed as a kilocalorie (abbreviation: kcal). One thousand small calories equal one large Calorie or one kilocalorie.

Carbohydrates and proteins both give four Calories for each respective gram. So, if ten grams of pure carbohydrate were ingested, it would yield forty Calories.

$$10 \text{ grams of carbohydrate} \times \frac{4 \text{ Calories}}{\text{gram of carbohydrate}} = 40 \text{ Calories}$$

Similarly, if ten grams of protein were used for energy, it would yield forty Calories.

$$10 \text{ grams of protein} \times \frac{4 \text{ Calories}}{\text{gram of protein}} = 40 \text{ Calories}$$

Fats, in comparison, yield nine Calories for every gram of fat. Fats, therefore, are a more energy-rich food source than carbohydrates or proteins because they give more Calories for every gram used. If ten grams of fat were used, it would yield ninety Calories.

$$10 \text{ grams of fat} \times \frac{9 \text{ Calories}}{\text{gram of fat}} = 90 \text{ Calories}$$

The total of all changes, chemical and physical, that take place in the body is called metabolism. The metabolic rate concerns itself with the changes in the body with respect to energy. It is the balance between the energy that is brought into the body and the energy used by the body. Energy is used during every action of the body, including voluntary activities such as walking or riding a bicycle and involuntary activities such as breathing and cellular repair.

The level of energy required for activities that occur when the body is at rest is called basal metabolism. The basal metabolic rate (BMR) will vary according to several factors. For example, the BMR will be higher in individuals with leaner body mass because it takes more energy to fuel the muscles than it does to store fat. BMR will also be higher for individuals in a period of high growth rate such as children and pregnant women.

Ideally, an individual will take in as many Calories as the body will use each day. When a person takes in more Calories than will be used, the body will store the excess energy in the form of fat. When a person uses more energy than is brought into the body, the body breaks down these stores. When the stores of fat are depleted, the body will start to break down its protein structures.

For an optimal energy balance in the body, the largest percentage of Calories in the diet should come from carbohydrates. Ideally, the percentage should be 50 to 60 percent of total calories consumed. The percentage of Calories attributable to fat should not be higher than 30 percent, with a percentage closer to 20 percent being preferred. Proteins should make up 10 to 20 percent of Calories in the diet.

Take note that these values are the percentage of the total Calories derived from each energy nutrient—not the percentage of grams. This distinction is important because of the difference in Calories derived from each energy nutrient. Figure 22-5 gives an example of these calculations.

The emphasis on carbohydrates was recently demonstrated with the U.S. Department of Agriculture's new

Label for Mystery Food:	Amount Per Serving
Calories	149
Total Fat	9g
Total Carbohydrate	14g
Total Protein	3g

The first calculation to make is one that converts grams to Calories.

$$9 \text{ grams of fat} \times \frac{9 \text{ Calories}}{\text{gram}} = 81 \text{ Calories due to fat}$$

$$14 \text{ grams of carbohydrate} \times \frac{4 \text{ Calories}}{\text{gram}} = 56 \text{ Calories due to carbohydrate}$$

$$3 \text{ grams of protein} \times \frac{4 \text{ Calories}}{\text{gram}} = 12 \text{ Calories due to protein}$$

The next calculation is to find the percentage of total Calories due to each of the energy nutrients.

$$\frac{81 \text{ Calories due to fat}}{149 \text{ total Calories}} = 54\%$$

$$\frac{56 \text{ Calories due to carbohydrate}}{149 \text{ total Calories}} = 38\%$$

$$\frac{12 \text{ Calories due to protein}}{149 \text{ total Calories}} = 8\%$$

Figure 22-5 Calculations of percentages of total calories due to fat, carbohydrate, or protein.

pyramid shape for the ideal diet, which has a base of foods from the breads, rice, and pasta groups (Figure 22-6).

In many cultures outside of the United States, rice, bread, and noodles are the basis of the diet.

In the United States, we have available great amounts of food from the dairy and meat groups. Unfortunately, dairy products and meats, while containing many good nutrients, also contain a great deal of fat. Studies have shown that many Americans are obese (as defined as weight being at least 20% greater than what their ideal weight should be). The American diet is too high in fat, has too many calories, salt, and cholesterol and insufficient amounts of complex carbohydrates and fiber. As a result, many illnesses and diseases occur, such as heart disease, high blood pressure, diabetes, and cancer. It is hoped that learning about nutrition by using this pyramid will help Americans make healthier food choices.

Other Nutrients

There are many other nutrients essential to maintaining good health. Although they do not provide the body with energy, they perform a variety of necessary functions. They include vitamins, minerals, water, and fiber.

Vitamins. Vitamins are a class of nutrient in which each specific vitamin has a function entirely its own. They are complex molecules and are required by the body in minute quantities. Vitamins were first named as letters of the alphabet. These names have been supplemented

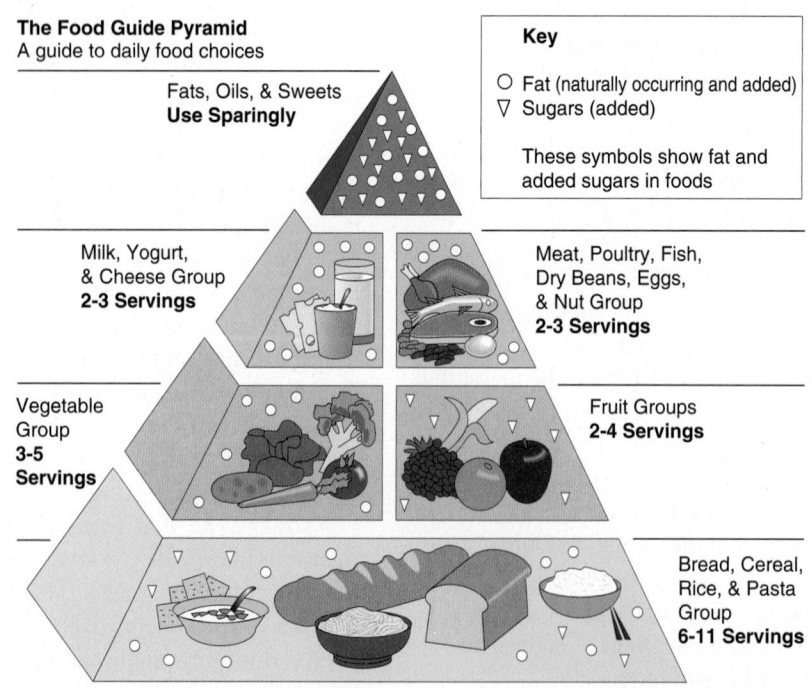

Figure 22-6 The U.S. Department of Agriculture's guide to a balanced diet takes the shape of a pyramid. The foundation of a good diet is made up of carbohydrate-rich foods; the fats, oils, and sugars represent the tip of the pyramid and should be used sparingly. (Courtesy of U.S. Department of Agriculture)

with chemical names and both should be learned. Vitamins generally have one of two functions: to facilitate cellular metabolism by acting as a coenzyme with a catalyst, and to act as a component of tissue structure. A **catalyst** allows a chemical reaction to proceed at a much quicker rate and without as much energy input, and the **coenzyme** is the nonprotein part that acts with it. Neither a catalyst nor its coenzyme is used in the reaction and so each can be used again and again. Vitamins that work with catalysts are only needed in minute quantities.

Vitamins are divided into two classes based on water solubility. The vitamins that are not soluble in water are said to be fat soluble. This is important because the **fat-soluble** vitamins are not carried into the bloodstream easily and are stored in fatty tissue, especially the liver. The **water-soluble** vitamins are not so easily stored and blood levels must be maintained by constant dietary intake. Toxicity can occur with high doses of either type of vitamin but is more likely to occur with the fat-soluble vitamins because they are stored in the body. The vitamins are listed in Table 22-2.

There are four fat-soluble vitamins, which include vitamin A, vitamin D, vitamin E and vitamin K. The first one, vitamin A, has two forms. The form that is used by

TABLE 22-2   VITAMIN SOURCES AND FUNCTIONS

Vitamins are divided into two classes based on water solubility: fat-soluble vitamins and water-soluble vitamins.

Name	Food Sources	Functions	Deficiency/Toxicity
Fat-Soluble Vitamins			

Vitamin A (carotene or retinol)	Animal
	  Liver
	  Whole milk
	  Butter
	  Cream
	  Cod liver oil
	Plants
	  Dark green leafy vegetables
	  Deep yellow or orange fruit
	  Fortified margarine
		Dim light vision
		Maintenance of mucous membranes
		Growth and development of bones
			Deficiency
			  Night blindness
			  Xerophthalmia
			  Respiratory infections
			  Bone growth ceases
			Toxicity
			  Cessation of menstruation
			  Joint pain
			  Stunted growth
			  Enlargement of liver

Vitamin D (cholecalciferol)	Animal
	  Eggs
	  Liver
	  Fortified milk
	Plants
	  None
		Bone growth	Deficiency
			  Rickets
			  Osteomalacia
			  Poorly developed teeth
			  Muscle spasms
			Toxicity
			  Kidney stones
			  Calcification of soft tissues

Vitamin E (alphatocopherol)	Animal
	  None
	Plant
	  Margarines
	  Salad dressing
		Antioxidant	Deficiency
			  Destruction of RBCs
			Toxicity
			  Hypertension

Vitamin K (phytonadione)	Animal
	  Egg yolk
	  Liver
	  Milk
	Plant
	  Green leafy vegetables
	  Cabbage
		Blood clotting	Deficiency
			  Prolonged blood clotting
			Toxicity
			  Hemolytic anemia
			  Jaundice

Water-Soluble Vitamins			

Thiamin (Vitamin B$_1$)	Animal
	  Liver
	  Eggs
	  Fish
	  Pork
	  Beef
	Plants
	  Whole and enriched grains
	  Legumes
		Coenzyme in oxidation of glucose	Deficiency
			  Gastrointestinal tract, nervous and cardiovascular system problems
			Toxicity
			  None

(continues)

TABLE 22-2 *(continued)*

Name	Food Sources	Functions	Deficiency/Toxicity

Riboflavin (Vitamin B_2)	Animal
	  Milk
	Plants
	  Green vegetables
	  Cereals
	  Enriched bread
		Aids release of energy from food	Deficiency
			  Cheilosis
			  Glossitis
			  Photophobia
			Toxicity
			  None

Pyridoxine (Vitamin B_6)	Animal
	  Pork
	  Milk
	  Eggs
	Plants
	  Whole grain cereals
	  Legumes
		Synthesis of nonessential amino acids
		Conversion of tryptophan to niacin
		Antibody production
			Deficiency
			  Cheilosis
			  Glossitis
			Toxicity
			  Liver disease

Vitamin B_{12} (cobalamin)	Animal
	  Seafood
	  Meat
	  Eggs
	  Milk
	Plants
	  None
		Synthesis of RBCs
		Maintenance of myelin sheaths
			Deficiency
			  Degeneration of myelin sheaths
			  Pernicious anemia
			Toxicity
			  None

Niacin (Vitamin B_3, nicotinic acid)	Animal
	  Milk
	  Eggs
	  Fish
	  Poultry
		Transfers hydrogen atoms for synthesis of ATP	Deficiency
			  Pellagra
			Toxicity
			  Vasodilation of blood vessels

Folacin	Animal
	  None
	Plants
	  Spinach
	  Asparagus
	  Broccoli
	  Kidney beans
		Synthesis of RBCs	Deficiency
			  Glossitis
			  Macrocytic anemia
			Toxicity
			  None

Biotin	Animal
	  Milk
	  Liver
	Plants
	  Legumes
	  Mushrooms
		Coenzyme in carbohydrate and amino acid metabolism
		Niacin synthesis from tryptophan
			Deficiency
			  None
			Toxicity
			  None

Pantothenic acid (Vitamin B_5)	Animal
	  Eggs
	  Liver
	  Salmon
	Plants
	  Mushrooms
	  Cauliflower
	  Peanuts
	  Yeast
		Metabolism of carbohydrates, lipids, and proteins
		Synthesis of acetylcholine
			Deficiency
			  None
			Toxicity
			  None

Vitamin C (ascorbic acid)	Fruits
	  All citrus
	Plants
	  Broccoli
	  Tomatoes
	  Brussel sprouts
	  Potatoes
		Prevention of scurvy
		Formation of collagen
		Healing of wounds
		Release of stress hormones
		Absorption of iron
			Deficiency
			  Scurvy
			  Muscle cramps
			  Ulcerated gums
			Toxicity
			  Raise uric acid level
			  Hemolytic anemia
			  Kidney stones
			  Rebound scurvy

the body is retinol, which is found in animal foods. The form found in plants is carotene. **Carotene** is converted into retinol in the body. Vitamin A is part of the pigment rhodopsin found in the eye and is responsible in part for vision, especially night vision. Vitamin A also gives strength to epithelial tissue and is required for healthy skin and mucous membranes. Sources of vitamin A include animal fats, butter, and cheese.

Vitamin D, also called **cholecalciferol**, is the fat-soluble vitamin involved in the metabolism of calcium in the body. It not only helps with absorption of this important mineral, but also with formation and maintenance of bone tissue. Vitamin D can be made in the body with exposure to sunlight. Rickets and osteomalacia are diseases caused by a deficiency in vitamin D. When deficiencies occur, especially during childhood, malformation of the skeleton is seen. Sources of vitamin D include milk, cod liver oil, and egg yolk.

Another fat-soluble vitamin is vitamin E, or **tocopherol**. It belongs to a group of compounds called **antioxidants**, which reduce the likelihood of **oxidation** of substances. This ability to reduce oxidation has recently led to suggestions that vitamin E may slow the aging process, but its true effectiveness is yet to be demonstrated. Vitamin E is found in lettuce and other green leafy vegetables, wheat germ, and rice.

Vitamin K is a fat-soluble vitamin required for the production of prothrombin. Prothrombin is one agent responsible for the clotting of blood. Deficiencies can result in prolonged blood clotting time and hemorrhage. Vitamin K is synthesized by intestinal bacteria, and bile is required for its absorption. About half of the body's requirement for vitamin K is fulfilled in this way. Sources of vitamin K include fats, fishmeal, oats, alfalfa, wheat, and rye.

Vitamin C, or **ascorbic acid**, is a water-soluble vitamin. Vitamin C is a constituent of connective tissue and acts to hold cells together. A deficiency of vitamin C causes scurvy, in which the walls of the capillaries become so weakened that they burst. Vitamin C also helps with wound healing and with the absorption of iron. Sources include most fresh fruits (especially citrus fruits) and vegetables (especially tomatoes).

The last group of water-soluble vitamins is the B-complex vitamin. It is important to remember that each vitamin in the B-complex is a separate vitamin with distinct functions. Vitamin B_1, or **thiamin**, helps in the conversion of glucose to energy. The disease beriberi is caused by thiamin deficiency and is characterized by neuritis edema, and cardiovascular changes. Sources include whole grain cereals, peas, beans, vegetables, and brewer's yeast. Vitamin B_2, or **riboflavin**, is also involved in energy production and is important in the production of proteins and necessary for normal growth. Sources include eggs, liver, milk, brewer's yeast, and green vegetables. A third

B-complex vitamin, **niacin**, works with both thiamin and riboflavin in the production of energy. Lack of niacin results in gastrointestinal and central nervous system disturbances. All three of these vitamins are important throughout the body.

Vitamin B_6, or **pyridoxine**, has an important role in protein metabolism, especially the synthesis of proteins. It is also important in the metabolism of fats and carbohydrates. Vitamin B_6 is found in rice, beans, and yeast. Another B-complex vitamin, **folic acid**, is involved in the formation of DNA and the formation of red blood cells. Folic acid is found in liver, yeast, and green leafy vegetables. Vitamin B_{12}, or **cobalamin**, is another vitamin important to the functioning of red blood cells. This vitamin is responsible for the synthesis of the heme portion of hemoglobin, and deficiencies in vitamin B_{12} result in the disease pernicious anemia. Because vitamin B_{12} is only found in animal foods such as liver, kidney, and dairy products, pernicious anemia may be a problem for some vegetarians. Pernicious anemia may also occur when there is decreased production of a factor required for vitamin B_{12} absorption. Other B-complex vitamins, pantothenic acid, vitamin B_5, and biotin, are generally responsible for energy metabolism.

Minerals. Minerals differ from vitamins in two distinct ways. While vitamins are complex molecules, minerals are singular elements. Another way that minerals differ from vitamins is that while vitamins are only required in minute quantities, some minerals are required in larger amounts. The foundation of the classification of minerals falls into two groups: major and trace minerals. No matter how small the quantity required of either a mineral or vitamin, all are vital to a healthy body. Some minerals are considered **electrolytes**, in that they become ionized and carry a positive or negative charge. The levels of these minerals in the bloodstream must be carefully balanced for the body to function in a healthy state.

There are seven **major minerals** (Table 22-3). They are calcium, phosphorus, sodium, potassium, magnesium, chlorine, and sulfur.

Calcium (Ca) is the mineral present in the largest quantity in the body because of its involvement in the structure of bone and teeth. It is also important in blood clotting, muscle contraction, and nerve conduction. Its levels in the blood must be kept at very narrow limits to ensure that the nervous and muscular tissues can function. This is especially important for the beating heart tissue. When there is a deficiency of calcium in the diet, calcium is taken from the bones to keep the blood calcium levels constant. The resulting deficient peak bone mass may put a person at risk for osteoporosis. This condition develops when there is not enough calcium in the bones and the bones become porous and easily broken.

TABLE 22-3   THE SEVEN MAJOR MINERALS AND THEIR FOOD SOURCES

Name	Food Sources	Functions	Deficiency/Toxicity
Calcium (Ca)	Milk exchanges Milk, cheese Meat exchanges Sardines Salmon Vegetable exchanges Green vegetables	Development of bones and teeth Permeability of cell membranes Transmission of nerve impulses Blood clotting	Deficiency Osteoporosis Osteomalacia Rickets
Phosphorus (P)	Milk exchanges Milk, cheese Meat exchanges Lean meat	Development of bones and teeth Transfer of energy Component of phospholipids Buffer system	(Same as calcium)
Potassium (K)	Fruit exchanges Oranges, bananas Dried fruits	Contraction of muscles Maintaining water balance Transmission of nerve impulses Carbohydrate and protein metabolism	Deficiency Hypokalemia Toxicity Hyperkalemia
Sodium (Na)	Table salt Meat exchanges Beef, eggs Milk exchanges Milk, cheese	Maintaining fluid balance in blood Transmission of nerve impulses	Toxicity Increase in blood pressure
Chloride (Cl)	Table salt Meat exchanges	Gastric acidity Regulation of osmotic pressure Activation of salivary amylase	Deficiency Imbalance in gastric acidity Imbalance in blood pH
Magnesium (Mg)	Vegetable exchanges Green vegetables Bread exchanges Whole grains	Synthesis of ATP Transmission of nerve impulses Activator of metabolic enzymes Relaxation of skeletal muscles	
Sulfur (S)	Meat exchanges Eggs, poultry, fish	Maintaining protein structure Formation of high-energy compounds	

Phosphorus (P) is another mineral important in bone formation. Phosphorus also is involved in numerous activities associated with energy metabolism, as well as maintaining a proper pH balance in the blood.

Sodium (Na) and potassium (K) are two minerals that act as electrolytes. Together they work to maintain proper water balance. They also help in maintenance of proper pH balance and are involved in nerve and muscular conduction and excitability. In addition, potassium is involved in protein synthesis and release of insulin from the pancreas.

Magnesium (Mg) is another mineral that is involved with energy metabolism. It also functions in nerve and muscle excitability and is stored in bone.

Chloride (Cl) is very important in pH balance and is the major **extracellular** (outside the cell) anion. It is also a major component of gastric secretions in the form of hydrochloric acid.

The last major mineral is sulfur (S). It is a component of one of the amino acids and therefore is found in protein. It is also involved in energy metabolism.

The **trace minerals** are required in smaller quantities but are as important as the major minerals. Some of the more important trace minerals include iron, copper,

chromium, molybdenum, selenium, manganese, iodine, zinc, cobalt, and fluorine.

Iron is vital to life because of its role in the heme molecule, which carries oxygen to every cell in the body. Iron-deficiency anemia results when the diet is low in iron and is characterized by small, pale red blood cells. Iron is also part of the molecule myoglobin, found in muscle cells, and is involved in a number of metabolic reactions.

Copper, chromium, molybdenum, selenium, and manganese are trace minerals important as factors in a number of metabolic reactions. Selenium acts as an antioxidant and has been receiving much of the recent publicity that vitamin E has. Iodine is also involved in metabolism but is unique in that the only place that iodine is found is in the thyroid hormones. Without it, the thyroid gland would be unable to regulate the overall metabolism of the body.

Zinc is an important constituent of many parts of the body but most notable is its involvement with the immune system and growth of tissues. Deficiencies lead to decreased ability to heal and lower immune resistance. Cobalt is part of vitamin B_{12} and is therefore important for the functioning of red blood cells. Fluorine is involved in calcified tissues. Its involvement in strengthening teeth has led to the fluoridation of most public water supplies. Its role in the prevention of osteoporosis has been suggested but is still under investigation.

Water. Water is the most important nutrient. The human body can go far longer without food than it can without water. Water has a multitude of functions in the body. It is the major solvent of the body and is the medium in which most biochemical reactions of the body take place. As a solvent, water also is essential for the removal of toxic waste from the body. In addition, it is an important component of many structures, the body being composed of 50 to 60 percent water. Being the major component of blood, water serves as a transporter. Another function of water is its lubricating role, especially in joints and in the digestive system. In addition, water helps control temperature within the body by eliminating excess heat through the evaporation of water secreted in the form of perspiration.

Because the body cannot store water, water that is lost daily must continually be replenished. Water is lost through perspiration, fecal material, urine, and respiration. Water can be replenished in part from foods that are ingested, but additional water should also be consumed. It is suggested that eight glasses of water be taken in per day. While other beverages are important sources of water, it should be considered that caffeine and alcohol are **diuretics** and will cause the body to lose water through increased urinary output. Beverages containing these substances should not be counted in the eight glasses of water.

Fiber. Although most fiber is carbohydrate in composition, it is included in its own section because of its special characteristics. Fiber comes only from plant sources. An adequate supply of fruits, vegetables, and grains is necessary to ensure enough fiber in the diet. Fiber cannot be digested and therefore is not absorbed into the body. Although fiber is not digested, it is important for the proper functioning of the gastrointestinal tract because it adds bulk to the fecal material as it is passed through the intestines; therefore, it gives the muscles of the tract something against which to work. Lack of fiber in the diet has been implicated in such gastrointestinal disorders as diverticulitis and colorectal cancer.

There are several types of fiber. Most are carbohydrates and include **cellulose**, gums, mucilages, algal polysaccharides, pectins, and hemicellulose. Another important fiber, lignin, is not a carbohydrate. It is suggested that the diet contain 15 to 20 grams of fiber per day. The American diet tends to be far below this suggestion, in part due to the consumption of processed foods. During processing, fiber is often removed. This is true with polished, or white, rice where the husk has been removed. Fiber levels should be increased gradually to prevent gastrointestinal distress, which can include diarrhea or flatulence.

READING FOOD LABELS

When assisting patients to change or modify their diets, the medical assistant must be knowledgeable not only about types of nutrients, but about how these nutrients are expressed in the foods we eat. The nutritional analysis presented on a package's food label is a helpful guide to understanding levels of fat, cholesterol, sodium, carbohydrate, protein, and vitamins contained in a particular food.

Many of the foods we eat are **processed foods**, which are cooked or packaged with parts removed or ingredients added. We rely on the labels on the cans, bottles, and boxes to tell us what nutrients are inside. The government wants to make it easier for people to understand the labels.

The government also wants to prevent food companies from fooling people into thinking something has good nutrition when it really does not. Food companies often put words on their labels to make people believe a product is healthy. Words like "healthy" and "light" or "lite" are not adequately descriptive. To discover what is in the package and if it is healthy, it is important to read the nutrition label (Figure 22-7).

Nutrition Facts

Serving Size: 1/2 Cup
Servings Per Container: 4

Amount Per Serving

Calories 100 Calories from Fat 30

	% Daily Value*
Total Fat 3g	**5%**
Saturated Fat 0g	0%
Cholesterol 0mg	**0%**
Sodium 340mg	**14%**
Total Carbohydrate 15g	**5%**
Dietary Fiber 1g	4%
Sugars 0g	
Protein 2g	

Vitamin A 0% • Vitamin C 0%
Calcium 0% • Iron 2%

*Percent Daily Values are based on a 2,000 calorie diet. Your daily values may be higher or lower depending on your calorie needs:

	Calories	2,000	2,500
Total Fat	Less than	65g	80g
Sat Fat	Less than	20g	25g
Cholesterol	Less than	300mg	300mg
Sodium	Less than	2,400mg	2,400mg
Total Carbohydrate		300g	375g
Dietary Fiber		25g	30g

Calories per gram:
Fat 9 • Carbohydrate 4 • Protein 4

Ingredients: Flour, Water, Yeast, Vegetable Oil, Salt, Artificial Flavor and Color.

Figure 22-7 Labels on food packages give facts about the ingredients and nutrition of the food in the package.

Items on the Nutrition Label

Serving Size. The nutrition information given is for one serving of the food. In this case, one serving is one-half cup of the food. This package contains four servings.

Calories. The label lists the number of calories per serving as well as the number of calories from fat per serving. This number should be less than 30 percent of the total calories. For example, if the total calories is 100, the calories from fat should be 30 or less.

The % Daily Value. The % daily value is the amount of a nutrient obtained by eating one serving of the product. The amount is given in a percentage based on a diet of 2,000 calories a day. For example, if the packaged food has 3 grams of fat, the total fat from eating one serving is 5% of the total fat that should be ingested in an entire day.

Fat and Cholesterol. Because it is important to eat a low-fat diet, the nutrition labels list both the total amount of fat and the amount of saturated fat per serving. Saturated fat comes from an animal source and contains more cholesterol than unsaturated fats, which come from vegetable sources. The cholesterol content is also listed.

Sodium. The amount of sodium per serving is listed. This category is especially important for patients on a sodium-restricted diet.

Carbohydrates. The total amount of carbohydrates per serving is listed along with the amount of carbohydrates that come from simple sugar. These two types of carbohydrates are separated for individuals who are trying to eat more complex carbohydrates and less simple sugar.

Other Information. The amount of fiber, protein, and only some vitamins and minerals are listed.

Ingredients. The ingredients contained in a packaged food are listed on the label. The item that is in the largest quantity is listed first. For example, if a product lists flour first and water second, there is more flour than water in the product. Preservatives, or chemicals added to food to keep it fresh longer, and artificial flavors and colors are often added to processed floods.

Comparing Labels

Look at some labels from snack foods that people eat when they want something crunchy and salty. Figure 22-8 (A), (B), and (C) show labels from potato chips, pretzels, and snack crackers. When comparing products, compare equal amounts. These products list the serving as 30 or 28 grams. That is close enough to compare the labels.

Patient Teaching Tip

Encourage patients to read and evaluate food labels. Typically, they should look for:

- No fat or the lowest amount of fat and saturated fat. Calories from fat should not be more than 30 percent of total calories.
- No cholesterol or low cholesterol. Total cholesterol should be less than 300 milligrams (mg) per day.
- Low sodium content. Total sodium should be less than 2,400 mg per day.
- High fiber. Fiber intake should be as high as possible.
- Vitamins and minerals. Some vitamins and minerals occur naturally and sometimes they are added to food during processing.

In reviewing these labels, note the amount of fat and saturated fat in each item. It might be assumed that potato chips, which are fried, would be high in fat. It may be surprising that the snack crackers have high fat content. Pretzels are the clear winner for a low-fat snack.

In terms of sodium, calories, and sugar, pretzels have the most sodium, but all three are high in sodium.

All three are low in sugar. Their calories are nearly the same as are the amounts of fiber and protein. The pretzels have the most carbohydrates and the crackers have the most artificial flavors, colors, and preservatives.

NUTRITION AT VARIOUS STAGES OF LIFE

As nutrients were discussed in the preceding sections, ranges of suggested normal requirements were offered. These ranges should be used as a guide, remembering that each individual is unique and there will be variations for requirements.

Pregnancy and Lactation

Pregnancy and lactation both cause marked changes in a woman's body and both require an increase in various nutrients. During pregnancy, not only does the growth of the fetus require additional nutrients, but the growth of the placenta, the increase in adipose tissue in the mother, the increased volume of blood, and the growth of breast tissue also require additional nutrients.

The increased demand for nutrients is not just a demand for Calories, but also for other specific nutrients to be increased, most notably protein. Protein require-

Potato Chips
Nutrition Facts

Serving Size: 1oz.
(28g/About 19 Chips)
Servings Per Container: 6

Amount Per Serving

Calories 150

Calories from Fat 90

% Daily Value*

Total Fat 10g	**15%**
Saturated Fat 2.5g	**13%**
Cholesterol 0mg	**0%**
Sodium 340mg	**14%**
Total Carbohydrate 15g	**5%**
Dietary Fiber 1g	**4%**
Sugars 1g	
Protein 2g	

Vitamin A 0% • Vitamin C 10%

Calcium 0% • Iron 2%

*Percent Daily Values are based on a 2,000 calorie diet. Your daily values may be higher or lower depending on your calorie needs:

	Calories	2,000	2,500
Total Fat	Less than	65g	80g
Sat Fat	Less than	20g	25g
Cholesterol	Less than	300mg	300mg
Sodium	Less than	2,400mg	2,400mg
Total Carbohydrate		300g	375g
Dietary Fiber		25g	30g

Calories per gram:

Fat 9 • Carbohydrate 4 • Protein 4

Ingredients: Potatoes, Vegetable Oil (Contains one or more of the following: Canola, Corn, Cottonseed, or Partially Hydrogenated Canola, Soybean or Sunflower Oil), Salt.

(A)

Pretzels
Nutrition Facts

Serving Size: 7 Pretzels
(30g)
Servings Per Container: 9.4

Amount Per Serving

Calories 120

Calories from Fat 10

% Daily Value*

Total Fat 1g	**2%**
Saturated Fat 0g	**0%**
Cholesterol 0g	**0%**
Sodium 360mg	**15%**
Total Carbohydrate 24g	**8%**
Dietary Fiber 1g	**4%**
Sugars 1g	
Protein 3g	

Vitamin A 0% • Vitamin C 0%

Calcium 0% • Iron 2%

*Percent Daily Values are based on a 2,000 calorie diet. Your daily values may be higher or lower depending on your calorie needs:

	Calories	2,000	2,500
Total Fat	Less than	65g	80g
Sat Fat	Less than	20g	25g
Cholesterol	Less than	300mg	300mg
Sodium	Less than	2,400mg	2,400mg
Total Carbohydrate		300g	375g
Dietary Fiber		25g	30g

Calories per gram:

Fat 9 • Carbohydrate 4 • Protein 4

Ingredients: Unbleached Wheat Flour, Water, Corn Syrup, Partially Hydrogenated Vegetable Oil (Soybean), Yeast, Salt, Bicarbonates and Carbonates of Sodium.

(B)

Wheat Snack Crackers
Nutrition Facts

Serving Size: 25 Cracker
(30g)
Servings Per Container: 7

Amount Per Serving

Calories 150

Calories from Fat 70

% Daily Value*

Total Fat 7g	**11%**
Saturated Fat 2g	**10%**
Cholesterol 0mg	**0%**
Sodium 310mg	**13%**
Total Carbohydrate 16g	**5%**
Dietary Fiber 1g	**4%**
Sugars 2g	
Protein 3g	

Vitamin A 0% • Vitamin C 0%

Calcium 0% • Iron 4%

*Percent Daily Values are based on a 2,000 calorie diet. Your daily values may be higher or lower depending on your calorie needs:

	Calories	2,000	2,500
Total Fat	Less than	65g	80g
Sat Fat	Less than	20g	25g
Cholesterol	Less than	300mg	300mg
Sodium	Less than	2,400mg	2,400mg
Total Carbohydrate		300g	375g
Dietary Fiber		25g	30g

Calories per gram:

Fat 9 • Carbohydrate 4 • Protein 4

Ingredients: Enriched Flour, Partially Hydrogenated Soybean and/or Cottonseed Oil, Dehydrated Potatoes, Steamed Crushed Wheat, Sugar, Salt, Natural and Artificial Flavors, Corn Syrup, Monosodium Glutamate, Dehydrated Cheddar Cheese, Dextrose, Nonfat Dry Milk, Artificial Color (Yellow 5, Yellow 6).

(C)

Figure 22-8   (A) An example of food label from potato chips. (B) An example of food label from pretzels. (C) An example of food label from snack crackers.

ments are nearly double during pregnancy. Because of the role vitamins play in metabolism and structure, they are needed in higher quantities than usual. In addition, calcium, phosphorus, and iron are needed in such high amounts that usually a vitamin supplement is prescribed. It is important that diet modifications are not simply an increase in Calories but include quality foods high in minerals, vitamins, and protein.

Pregnancy is an important time for both fetus and mother. It is normal and healthy for the mother to gain weight, and Calories should not be skimped at this time. During lactation there is still a requirement for higher levels of nutrients; however, overall, it is not as high as during pregnancy. A baby is more likely to be healthy and develop normally if the mother has good nutritional habits during pregnancy and breast-feeding.

Infancy

Infancy is a time of continuous growth, and many of the mother's nutritional requirements during pregnancy are still required by the baby after birth. In the first year of life, the baby will triple birth weight. The infant will need two to three times more Calories per kilogram (kg) of body weight than the normal adult. This is true for protein as well, and most of the vitamins and minerals are required at higher levels per kg. Most of these can be furnished with breast milk or formula; however, once iron stores have been used up, the infant will require an iron supplement, which is why pediatricians prescribe infant liquid iron supplement. Because of the high rate of growth, especially of the nervous system, infancy is a very important time to be sure nutritional requirements are met.

Adolescence

During adolescence, individuals experience the greatest levels of growth. The period of growth varies from person to person, but generally begins sooner with females. Except for times of pregnancy and lactation, the need for total nutrients is greatest at this stage of growth. At the end of the growth spurt, nutrient requirements decrease, and young adults must then also decrease the amount of food they consume.

Two particular nutrients that especially need to be altered during adolescence are iron and calcium. Iron requirements increase for the female as she begins menstruation. Calcium requirements increase for both males and females as bone development is occurring at a rapid rate.

Elderly

Aging is a natural process of the body. While aging occurs in different stages and at different rates for each individual, some generalities can be made. As we age, our cellular metabolism tends to slow. Coupled with a general decline in physical activity, this results in a decreased requirement for Calories. At the same time, there may be an increase in nutrient requirement in special circumstances. There is always an increased requirement for nutrients, vitamins, and protein in particular during illness, especially the prolonged illness that may occur in the elderly. With aging, there may be increased breakdown of cells, and as a result there is an increased requirement for nutrients that repair and builds cells and tissues. There is also a need to ingest more nutrients because of decreased absorption within the digestive tract. So while there is less need for Calories, there is more need for nutrient-rich foods.

This may become difficult for elderly individuals for several reasons. One may be an individual's psychological state. Loneliness and depression affect many elderly, especially after the loss of a spouse. Elderly may not like the idea of eating alone. The economic status of the individual also may present problems, as after retirement income will generally fall. Physiologically, taste tends to diminish with age and interest in food may decrease. In addition, problems with teeth and a decrease in salivary gland secretions may make eating painful. Many medications will cause a decrease in saliva production. Also, decreased motility in the gastrointestinal tract may lead to constipation, making eating uncomfortable. All these, as well as a general unwillingness to break old habits may make it difficult to change the diet to keep up with the body's aging process.

THERAPEUTIC DIETS

Thus far this chapter has examined the nutrient requirements of the body under normal conditions. There are times, however, when the body becomes diseased and nutrient requirements change. These changes may be due to disease states such as diabetes mellitus or conditions resulting from a poor diet such as obesity. Therapeutic diets are designed to overcome or control these conditions.

The diet can be modified in a number of ways. The number of overall Calories can be adjusted or one type of nutrient may be restricted or encouraged. The consistency, texture, and spiciness of food may be varied. The frequency of eating may be increased or decreased. When counseling patients, remember that habits are hard to change. The medical assistant should be supportive and encouraging.

Weight Control

Overweight and underweight are both weight disorders. The problem in defining overweight or underweight stems from the fact that there is no ideal weight for an entire population. There is only an ideal weight for the individual. Ideal weight can depend on many factors including age, gender, lean muscle mass, bone structure, and physical activity. Obesity is generally considered more than 20 percent overweight. Height-weight tables now generally give ranges that vary more than twenty pounds. The ratio of fat tissue to lean muscle mass is a better indicator of whether individuals are at their ideal weight than a specific weight.

Individuals will gain weight if they consume more Calories than they need. Conversely, individuals will lose weight if they use more Calories than they ingest. In either case, the individual must bring the amount of Calories ingested into balance with the amount used. For the overweight individual, this means either decreasing Calorie consumption, or increasing Calorie usage, or both. For the underweight individual, it usually entirely involves increasing Calorie consumption.

Weight loss has become a big business. However, individuals do not need to spend tremendous amounts of money to lose weight; patient education about low-Calorie, low-salt foods and a moderate exercise program are basic starting points for weight loss. Because losing more than 1 to 2 pounds a week can put an individual into nutritional deficiency, goals should not be set higher than this. Modifications made to the diet should then be maintained even after the weight is lost and should be continued throughout life. Losing weight takes much effort, and the patient needs constant encouragement and support from medical personnel and family.

Diabetes Mellitus

Diabetes mellitus is a disease in which there is either reduced or no production of insulin, or in which there is reduced or no response to insulin. Approximately 5 percent of the population has diabetes mellitus in some form. Most patients with this disease are not dependent on insulin and can control their condition by monitoring diet and weight.

Normally, after a meal, the body secretes the hormone insulin which makes its way to all cells of the body. Insulin signals the cells that the glucose is available and should be brought in so that it can be converted to energy. If the cells do not receive this signal, or do not respond to it, their ability to use glucose is markedly reduced. Because the body uses glucose as its main energy source, the ramifications of this affect almost every tissue of the body. In addition, the high levels of glucose that remain in the bloodstream put a tremendous strain on the kidney and other major body organs causing problems such as myocardial infarction, vascular diseases, neuropathy, and infections.

The effects of diabetes mellitus can be controlled with a general goal of maintaining a regular level of glucose in the bloodstream, avoiding large fluctuations between high and low levels. There are several ways suggested to accomplish this. Total Calories need not be altered, unless the diabetic patient is overweight. However, the ratio of carbohydrate, fat, and protein must be closely monitored. Total carbohydrates should be increased, but simple sugars should be avoided. Because of the longer rate of digestion and absorption of complex carbohydrates, these will be released over a longer period of time and prevent a sudden high level of glucose in the bloodstream, and are the type of carbohydrates diabetics need. Increasing fiber content also increases the time of absorption and decreases the likelihood of sudden increases in glucose levels in the bloodstream. Regular snacks may be added between meals to maintain levels of glucose. The trend is for patients to take charge of their own care. The role of educator for the medical assistant will be

an important one to facilitate patient self-management. See Chapter 24 for more information about diabetes and insulin.

Cardiovascular Disease

Cardiovascular disease is currently the leading cause of death in the United States. The unfortunate aspect is that much of it is preventable. Cardiovascular disease encompasses a variety of problems. Two of these problems, hypertension and atherosclerosis, often work hand in hand to perpetuate one another until a myocardial infarction occurs. It is important to remember that the conditions leading up to a myocardial infarction do not occur overnight. They have been developing slowly over many years, often asymptomatically. These conditions can be reduced or prevented with lifestyle modifications such as a healthy diet, moderate exercise, cessation of smoking, and weight management. The focus of this section will be on a healthy diet to prevent cardiovascular disease.

Hypertension, or elevated blood pressure, is often of unknown etiology. Sometimes it has a familial connection. When the blood pressure is only moderately increased, certain diet modifications can be used to lower it. If it is severe, drug therapy may be used in conjunction with diet therapy. The largest diet factor in controlling elevated blood pressure is restricting sodium because it plays such an important role in maintenance of water levels in the body. An increased volume of blood and water will increase the pressure on the blood vessel walls. Eliminating sodium includes more than simply eliminating use of table salt. Foods that are particularly high in sodium include smoked meats, luncheon meats, olives, pickles, chips, crackers, catsup, and cheese. In some cases, eliminating foods with only moderate salt levels may be indicated. These may include certain meats, breads containing baking powder or baking soda, shellfish, and some vegetables.

Atherosclerosis is another condition that can lead to a myocardial infarction. Atherosclerosis is hardening of the arteries due to deposits of fatty substance. It should not be confused with arteriosclerosis, which is a hardening of the arteries due to loss of the elasticity of the arterial wall. Atherosclerosis leads to arteriosclerosis which generally occurs because of a lack of exercise and elevated blood cholesterol levels. The elasticity can be regained by increasing activity, although it should be started slowly and under a physician's guidance. Atherosclerosis and arteriosclerosis often occur together. Smoking and hypertension will increase the likelihood of developing both of these conditions.

The conditions of atherosclerosis and arteriosclerosis facilitate each other. The fatty deposits associated with atherosclerosis tend to occur at points of damage to the inner walls of the artery. One of the causes of this damage is high pressure at points where there may be narrowing due to deposits that are already there, or due to the constriction of blood vessels due to nicotine. Carbon monoxide brought into the bloodstream during smoking also causes damage to the arterial walls. The deposits and hardening increase the blood pressure which in turn causes more damage and more deposits. It is a cycle that is difficult to stop. The best solution is prevention.

Fats and cholesterol in the diet have been strongly implicated in atherosclerosis. It is not only total fat that is important, but also types of fat ingested. The effect of high levels of fats and cholesterol in the diet will vary among individuals, and the factor in atherosclerosis is the levels of these substances in the bloodstream. Some individuals are able to ingest high amounts of fat and cholesterol without the body maintaining high levels of it in the blood. Unfortunately, this is not the case for everyone, and fat and cholesterol levels in the bloodstream must be closely monitored. Fat levels are measured by looking at triglycerides and lipoproteins. Lipoproteins are a complex made of fatty acids and proteins and are used to carry fat and cholesterol in the bloodstream. Low-density lipoproteins (LDL) are used by the body to transport fats and cholesterol to the body tissues. These are the lipoproteins more likely to deposit cholesterol and fat into the arterial wall. High-density lipoproteins (HDL) carry fats and cholesterol to the liver to be broken down and used. These lipoproteins are more likely to remove fats and cholesterol from the deposits in the arterial walls. HDL levels can be increased by exercise.

If total serum cholesterol and LDL levels are found to be elevated, the individual must modify the diet, and if severe enough, drug therapy may be indicated. The percentage of Calories from fat should be kept below 30 percent of total daily dietary intake, with less than a third of these coming from saturated fats. Cholesterol consumption should be less than 300 mg per day.

If a person suffers a myocardial infarction, it is important that the heart muscle be allowed to rest to facilitate proper healing. This includes bed rest, initially with a gradual progression to limited activity over about a two-week period. Then the patient is allowed to resume full activity. Rehabilitation consists of cessation of smoking, control of hypertension, weight reduction through a low-fat, low-calorie diet, and a program of exercise. All help to improve myocardial function.

Cancer

Cancer is a disease that comes in a variety of forms. It generally means that normal regulatory mechanisms within a cell have broken down. The result is that cells continue to grow in an unrestrained manner, diverting energy and nutrients from the patient's body to the cells' uncontrolled growth. There are many stages through which these cells may go, and they will go through them at varying rates. The ramifications of this new growth will vary depending on what types of cells are affected.

For these reasons, each cancer patient will have varying nutritional requirements. However, there are some generalities that can be made. First, there is definitely a need for increased Calories. Because the new growth has the ability to divert nutrients to itself, the result is the body receives fewer nutrients. It will then break down its own tissue. In addition, there is an increased need for nutrients to supply the immune system with energy and nutrients in its attempt to destroy the cancerous cells.

If the patient receives chemotherapy or radiation treatment, there is an even greater need for increased nutrients. These therapies are directed at killing cells that are rapidly dividing. This includes not only the cancerous cells, but also healthy cells such as those of the lining of the gastrointestinal tract and hair follicles. Increased nutrients are needed for repair and replacement of the lost cells, and protein levels in particular should be increased. Because of the disturbance of the gastrointestinal lining, digestion and absorption may also be decreased. It is important that the patient maintain as healthy a nutritional status as is possible rather than having to make up for nutritional deficiencies.

The patient will likely experience loss of appetite as well as nausea and vomiting. There are several ways to

SPOTLIGHT ON AAMA ESSENTIALS THROUGH CAAHEP

- In cases in which a patient does not want to eat, recommending that he or she share a meal with someone else may improve the appetite.

- Being aware of a patient's dietary needs, likes, and dislikes can help the medical assistant develop a nutritional plan that is both pleasant to the person's taste buds and appropriate for dietary needs.

- A medical assistant who has some knowledge of ethnic food choices can be reassuring to patients who may need to make some dietary changes but would like to make them within the parameters of their own cultures.

cope with this. First, food should be made as appealing as possible. Also, if the patient has difficulty swallowing, food can be liquefied in a food processor. Generally, food will be better tolerated if it is slightly chilled; extremes of temperature should be avoided. Several smaller meals may be easier to eat than three large meals.

DIET AND CULTURE

 Medical assistants are likely to come into contact with patients from many different ethnic groups. Many of these patients will have diets based upon traditional cultures, and some of the foods they eat, or the way they combine foods, may be unfamiliar to the medical assistant. Often, diets in other cultures are sensible ones, with foods chosen or combined to make up a complete protein. The medical assistant who has some knowledge of ethnic food choices can help reassure patients that the dietary changes they need to make are within the parameters of their own cultures. Table 22-4 presents some highlights of the food choices of different ethnic groups.

Vegetarian diets are also fairly common around the globe including the United States. With a good variety of

TABLE 22-4 SAMPLE FOOD CHOICES OF VARIOUS CULTURAL, RELIGIOUS, AND ETHNIC GROUPS	
Culture/Region/Group	**Diet and Food Choices**
Native American	It is thought that approximately half of the edible plants commonly eaten in the United States today originated with the Native Americans. Examples are corn, potatoes, squash, cranberries, pumpkins, peppers, beans, wild rice, and cocoa beans. In addition, they used wild fruits, game, and fish. Foods were commonly prepared as soups and stews, and dried. The original Native American diets were probably more nutritionally adequate than their current diets, which frequently consist of too high a proportion of sweet and salty, snack-type, empty calorie foods. Native American diets today may be deficient in calcium, vitamins A, C, and riboflavin.
U.S. Southern	Hot breads such as corn bread and baking powder biscuits are common in the U.S. South because the wheat grown in the area does not make good quality yeast breads. Grits and rice are also popular carbohydrate foods. Favorite vegetables include sweet potatoes, squash, green beans, and lima beans. Green beans cooked with pork are commonly served. Watermelon, oranges, and peaches are popular fruits. Fried fish is served often, as are barbecued and stewed meats and poultry. There is a great deal of carbohydrate and fat in these diets and limited amounts of protein in some cases. Iron, calcium, and vitamins A and C may sometimes be deficient.
Mexican	Mexican food is a combination of Spanish and Native American foods. Beans, rice, chili peppers, tomatoes, and corn meal are favorites. Meat is often cooked with the vegetable as in chili con carne. Corn meal is used in a variety of ways to make tortillas and tamales, which serve as bread. The combination of beans and corn makes a complete protein. While tortillas filled with cheese (called enchiladas) provide some calcium, the use of milk should be encouraged. Additional green and yellow vegetables and vitamin C-rich foods would also improve these diets.
Puerto Rican	Rice is the basic carbohydrate food in Puerto Rican diets. Vegetables commonly used include beans, plantains, tomatoes, and peppers. Bananas, pineapple, mangoes, and papayas are popular fruits. Favorite meats are chicken, beef, and pork. Milk is not used as much as would be desirable from the nutritional point of view.
Italian	Pastas with various tomato or fish sauces, and cheese are popular Italian foods. Fish and highly seasoned foods are common to Southern Italian cuisine while meat and root vegetables are common to northern Italy. The eggs, cheese, tomatoes, green vegetables, and fruits common to Italian diets provide excellent sources of many nutrients, but additional milk and meat would improve the diet.
Northern and Western European	Northern and Western European diets are similar to those of the U.S. Midwest, but with a greater use of dark breads, potatoes and fish, and fewer green vegetable salads. Beef and pork are popular as are various cooked vegetables, breads, cakes, and dairy products.
Central European	Citizens of Central Europe obtain the greatest portion of their calories from potatoes and grain, especially rye and buckwheat. Pork is a popular meat. Cabbage cooked in many ways is a popular vegetable as are carrots, onions, and turnips. Eggs and dairy products are used abundantly.
Middle Eastern	Grains, wheat, and rice provide energy in these diets. Chickpeas in the form of hummus are popular. Lamb and yogurt are commonly used as are cabbage, grape leaves, eggplant, tomatoes, dates, olives, and figs. Black, very sweet (Turkish) coffee is a popular beverage.
Chinese	The Chinese diet is varied. Rice is the primary energy food and is used in place of bread. Foods are generally cut into small pieces. Vegetables are lightly cooked and the cooking water is saved for future use. Soybeans are used in many ways, and eggs and pork are commonly served. Soy sauce is extensively used, but it is very salty and could present a problem with patients on low-salt diets. Tea is a common beverage, but milk is not. This diet may be low in fat.

(continues)

TABLE 22-4   (*continued*)

Culture/Region/Group	Diet and Food Choices
Japanese	Japanese diets include rice, soybean paste and curd, vegetables, fruits, and fish. Food is frequently served tempura style, which means fried. Soy sauce (shoyu) and tea are commonly used. Current Japanese diets have been greatly influenced by Western culture.
Southeast Asian	Many Indians are vegetarians who use eggs and dairy products. Rice, peas, and beans are frequently served. Spices, especially curry, are popular. Indian meals are not typically served in courses as Western meals are. They generally consist of one course with many dishes.
Thailand, Vietnam, Laos, and Cambodia	Rice, curries, vegetables, and fruit are popular in Thailand, Vietnam, Laos, and Cambodia. Meat, chicken, and fish are used in small amounts. The wok (a deep, round fry pan) is used for sautéing many foods. A salty sauce made from fermented fish is commonly used.
Jewish	Interpretations of the Jewish dietary laws vary. Those who adhere to the Orthodox view consider tradition important and always observe the dietary laws. Foods prepared according to these laws are called kosher. Conservative Jews are inclined to observe the rules only at home. Reform Jews consider their dietary laws to be essentially ceremonial and so minimize their significance. Essentially the laws require the following: • Slaughtering must be done by a qualified person, in a prescribed manner. The meat or poultry must be drained of blood, first by severing the jugular vein and carotid artery, then by soaking in brine before cooking. • Meat or meat products may not be prepared with milk or milk products. • The dishes used in the preparation and serving of meat dishes must be kept separate from those used for dairy foods. • A specified time, six hours, must elapse between consumption of meat and milk. • The mouth must be rinsed after eating fish and before eating meat. • There are prescribed fast days—Passover Week, Yom Kippur, and Feast of Purim. • No cooking is done on the Sabbath—from sundown Friday to sundown Saturday. These laws forbid the eating of: • the flesh of animals without cloven (split) hooves or that do not chew their cud • hind quarters of any animal • shellfish or fish without scales or fins • fowl that are birds of prey • creeping things and insects • leavened (contains ingredients that cause it to rise) bread during the Passover Generally, the food served is rich. Fresh smoked and salted fish, and chicken are popular, as are noodles, egg, and flour dishes. These diets can be deficient in fresh vegetables and milk.
Roman Catholic	Although the dietary restrictions of the Roman Catholic religion have been liberalized, meat is not allowed its adherents on Ash Wednesday and Fridays during Lent.
Eastern Orthodox	Followers of this religion include Christians from the Middle East, Russia, and Greece. Although interpretations of the dietary laws vary, meat, poultry, fish, and dairy products are restricted on Wednesdays and Fridays and during Lent and Advent.
Seventh Day Adventist	Generally, Seventh Day Adventists are ovolacto-vegetarians, which means they use milk products and eggs, but no meat, fish, or poultry. They may also use nuts, legumes, and meat analogues (substitutes) made from soybeans. They consider coffee, tea, and alcohol to be harmful.
Mormon (Latter Day Saints)	The only dietary restriction observed by Mormons is the prohibition of coffee, tea, and alcoholic beverages.
Islamic	Adherents of Islam are called Muslims. Their dietary laws prohibit the use of pork and alcohol, and other meats must be slaughtered according to specific laws. During the month of Ramadan, Muslims do not eat or drink during daylight hours.
Hindu	To the Hindus, all life is sacred and small animals contain the souls of ancestors. Consequently, Hindus are usually vegetarians. They do not use eggs as they represent life.
Vegetarians	There are several vegetarian diets. The common factor among them is that they do not include red meat. Some include eggs, some fish, some milk, and some even poultry. When carefully planned, these diets can be nutritious. They can contribute to a reduction of obesity, high blood pressure, heart disease, some cancers, and possibly diabetes. They must be carefully planned so they include all needed nutrients. Lacto-ovo vegetarians use dairy products and eggs but no meat, poultry, or fish. Lacto-vegetarians use dairy products but no meat, poultry, or eggs.

(*continues*)

TABLE 22-4 *(continued)*

Culture/Region/Group	Diet and Food Choices
Vegans	Vegans avoid all animal foods. They use soybeans, chickpeas, and meat analogues made from soybeans. It is important that their meals be carefully planned to include appropriate combinations of the nonessential amino acids to provide the needed amino acids. For example, beans served with corn or rice, or peanuts eaten with wheat, are better in such combinations than any of them would be if eaten alone. Vegans can show deficiencies of calcium, zinc, vitamins A, D, and B_{12} and, of course, proteins.
Zen Macrobiotic Diets	The macrobiotic diet is a system of ten diet plans developed from Zen Buddhism. Adherents progress from the lower number diet to the higher, gradually giving up foods in the following order: desserts, salads, fruits, animal foods, soups, and ultimately vegetables, until only cereals—usually brown rice—are consumed. Beverages are kept to a minimum and only organic foods are used. Foods are grouped as Yang (male) or Yin (female). A ratio of 5 : 1 Yang to Yin is considered important. Most macrobiotic diets are nutritionally inadequate. As the adherents give up foods according to plans, their diets become increasingly inadequate. These diets can be especially dangerous because avid adherents promise medical cures from the diets that cannot be attained, and so medical treatment may be delayed when needed.

grains, vegetables, fruits, and dairy products, a vegetarian diet can supply an individual with all the required nutrients. Pernicious anemia, a disease caused by lack of cobalamin (vitamin B_{12}), is sometimes associated with vegetarian diets that do not contain enough animal product (see the section on vitamins in this chapter). One type of vegetarian, vegan, does not eat any product associated with animals, including milk or eggs. This type of diet is particularly susceptible to nutritional deficiencies.

In speaking with patients about diet and dietary changes, it is important to remember that patients choose their diets for a variety of reasons, including cultural, religious, or ethical beliefs. The medical assistant should respect the patient's reasons for following a certain diet while encouraging any modifications.

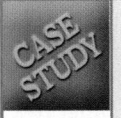

Anita Ferguson is a new patient at Inner City Health Care. She is a sixteen-year-old who is four months pregnant and came to the urgent care center only a couple of weeks ago. After Wanda Slawson, CMA, took Anita's medical history, and after Anita was examined by the physician, Wanda set aside time to answer any questions Anita might have about her pregnancy. Anita is obviously scared, wants the baby, but does not want her life to change. According to the history, Anita has lost a few pounds in the last two weeks.

22-1

CASE STUDY REVIEW

1. What patient education can Wanda provide to alert Anita to the importance of diet and weight gain during pregnancy?
2. What foods should Wanda encourage Anita to eat?
3. If Anita resists Wanda's suggestions and has not gained any weight by the next visit, how should Wanda proceed?

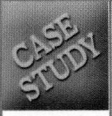

Dr. Lewis prescribed a diabetic diet for Mrs. Johnson.

CASE STUDY REVIEW

22-2

1. Describe what is included in a diabetic diet.
2. Describe the patient education you would employ to help Mrs. Lewis understand the diet and to help her reach her goal of improved health.

SUMMARY

Seven types of nutrients are required by the body for maintenance of good health. Carbohydrates, fats, and proteins provide energy for the body. Vitamins, minerals, fiber, and water cannot provide energy but are responsible for many vital processes within the body.

Nutritional needs change at various points in the life cycle. During pregnancy, lack of nutrients can be detrimental to the development of the fetus and the health of the expectant mother. The need for nutrients is great during infancy and childhood, with the greatest need for total nutrients occurring during adolescence. During adulthood, the requirement for Calories decreases. With the decrease in basal metab-olism that occurs with aging, the requirement for Calories decreases even more.

At times of disease, the diet of the individual must be modified to help relieve stress put on the body by the disease, to give energy to fight the disease, and, in cases where the disease is diet-related, to lessen the severity of the disease.

It is important to have adequate nutritional intake during every stage of life. The healthier one is, the better one feels. Nutritional status should be examined and adjustments made if necessary with the goal of helping patients maintain a healthy body.

REVIEW QUESTIONS

Multiple Choice

1. The transfer of nutrients from the gastrointestinal tract into the bloodstream is:
   a. ingestion
   b. digestion
   c. absorption
   d. elimination
2. Fats are considered a(n):
   a. mineral
   b. vitamin
   c. energy nutrient
   d. fiber
3. The total of all chemical and physical changes that take place in the body is called:
   a. homeostatis
   b. metabolism
   c. a catalyst
   d. an antioxidant
4. According to the USDA food pyramid, you should:
   a. have 3 to 5 servings of vegetables a day
   b. severely limit the number of servings of pasta
   c. never use fats, oils, and sugars
   d. consider meat the foundation of the pyramid
5. Another name for vitamin E is:
   a. tocopherol
   b. caratene
   c. biotin
   d. pyridoxine

Critical Thinking

1. Evaluate your own diet. Write down every item you ingest for a day and find the values of the nutrients contained in the foods. A medical dictionary is a good source for listing the nutrient value of selected foods. If you are eating prepared foods, read the package food label. Remember, you are trying to get an idea of your average daily diet, so don't change your diet for your analysis unless you plan to maintain it. What is the balance of your energy nutrients? Are you getting enough vitamins and minerals? Are you getting adequate fiber? What modifications could be made?
2. For each of the following vitamins and minerals, suggest some symptoms that might appear if there were a deficiency.
   vitamin A
   vitamin K
   vitamin C
   thiamin
   riboflavin
   cobalamin (vitamin B_{12})
   calcium
3. Consider the functions of the various regions of the digestive system, and look up in a medical dictionary each of the following procedures. Describe the problems that might exist with the following procedures if diet modifications do not take place.
   colostomy
   gastroileostomy
   gastrectomy

4. Explain why a breakfast high in complex carbohydrates is an important goal.
5. Discuss why the new pyramid shape is an accurate portrayal of the ideal diet.
6. Write a response to a teenage woman who refuses to gain weight during her pregnancy.
7. What are some things to consider when assessing the diet of an elderly person?
8. Find five things a person can do to decrease the risk of heart disease. Compile a list from the class. How many of the items are associated with diet? How many of the items involve you?
9. Describe how the diet can be used to control diabetes mellitus. When a person becomes dependent on insulin, should the diet continue to be used?
10. Following is information from a label for peanut butter. Calculate the percentage of calories due to fat, protein, and carbohydrate.

Serving size	2 tbs.
Calories	204
Protein	9 grams
Carbohydrates	6 grams
Fat	16 grams

WEB ACTIVITIES

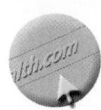

Search the Web for information about the U.S. Department of Agriculture's Food Guide Pyramid.

1. Is the pyramid appropriate for all ages?
2. Are the daily food choices the same for a child as for an adult?

Search community agencies on the Web for information about the following diseases and the role nutrition plays in prevention of the disease:

1. diabetes mellitus
2. arteriosclerotic heart disease
3. hypertension

REFERENCES/BIBLIOGRAPHY

Frey, R., & Shearer-Cooper, L. A. (1996). *Introduction to nursing assisting: Building language skills*. Albany, NY: Delmar.

Lankford, T. R. (1994). *Foundations of normal and therapeutic nutrition* (2nd ed.). Albany, NY: Delmar.

Mahan, L. K., & Arlin, M. (1999). *Krause's food, nutrition & diet therapy* (10th ed.). Philadelphia: W. B. Saunders.

Townsend, C. E. (2000). *Nutrition and diet therapy* (7th ed.). Albany, NY: Delmar.

Williams, S. R. (2001). *Basic nutrition and diet therapy* (11th ed.). St. Louis: Mosby-Year Book, Inc.

Chapter

23

BASIC PHARMACOLOGY

KEY TERMS

Abuse
Administer
Anaphylaxis
Contraindication
Dispense
Pharmacology
Prescribe
Pruritus
Urticaria

OUTLINE

Medical Uses of Drugs
Drug Names
History and Sources of Drugs
   Plant Sources
   Animal Sources
   Mineral Sources
   Synthetic Drugs
   Genetically Engineered Pharma-
     ceuticals
Drug Regulations and Legal
  Classifications of Drugs
   Controlled Substance Act of 1970
   Prescription Drugs
   Nonprescription Drugs
   Proper Disposal of Drugs
   Administer, Prescribe, Dispense

Drug References and Standards
   How to Use the PDR
   Other Reference Sources
Classification of Drugs
Principal Actions of Drugs
   Factors That Affect Drug Action
   Undesirable Actions of Drugs
Drug Routes
Forms of Drugs
   Liquid Preparations
   Solid and Semisolid Preparations
   Other Drug Delivery Systems
Storage and Handling of
  Medications
Emergency Drugs and Supplies
Drug Abuse
   Effects of Drug Abuse

OBJECTIVES

The student should strive to meet the following performance objectives and demonstrate an understanding of the facts and principles presented in this chapter through written and oral communication.

1. Define the key terms as presented in the glossary.
2. Recall five medical uses for drugs.
3. Describe three types of drug names and give an example, for one drug, of all three names.
4. List five sources of drugs.
5. Describe the Federal Foods, Drug, and Cosmetic Act and the Controlled Substance Act of 1970.
6. Name the five controlled substances schedules and describe appropriate storage of the substances. *(continues)*

497

7. Define the law in terms of administering, prescribing, and dispensing drugs.
8. Describe the four most commonly used sections of the *Physician's Desk Reference* (PDR).
9. Describe the principal actions of drugs and three undesirable reactions.
10. Describe routes of drug administration and drug forms.
11. Describe handling and storing of drugs.
12. List emergency drugs and supplies.
13. Recall commonly abused drugs and describe their physical and emotional effects.
14. Critique the legal role and responsibilities of the medical assistant.

ROLE DELINEATION COMPONENTS

CLINICAL

Fundamental Principles

- **Comply with quality assurance practices**

Patient Care

- **Maintain medication and immunization records**

GENERAL (TRANSDISCIPLINARY)

Legal Concepts

- **Document accurately**
- **Follow federal, state and local legal guidelines**
- **Maintain awareness of federal and state health care legislation and regulations**
- **Maintain and dispose of regulated substances in compliance with government guidelines**
- **Comply with established risk management and safety procedures**

SCENARIO

Policy at Doctors Lewis & King dictates that a patient medication history is taken on the first appointment, routinely updated, and reviewed whenever medication is prescribed, dispensed, or administered. Both administrative and clinical medical assistants work together to ensure that this policy is carried out. When making a patient appointment, administrative medical assistants ask patients to bring with them any medications (keeping them in the labeled container) that they are currently using. When taking or updating a patient history, clinical medical assistants Audrey Jones and Joe Guerrero ask a number of questions of patients regarding medications and gently probe to assure that the patient includes all medications in the history and describes any allergy or hypersensitivity they may have to certain drugs.

INTRODUCTION

Pharmacology is the study of drugs, the science that is concerned with the history, origin, sources, physical and chemical properties, uses, and effects of drugs upon living organisms. Medical assistants in the ambulatory care setting need to understand basic pharmacology including the uses, sources, forms, and delivery routes of drugs; must know and be able to implement the intent of the law regarding controlled substances and other medications; and must have a knowledge of drug classifications and actions in order to be able to caution patients when taking prescription or nonprescription drugs. In addition, the medical assistant must be able to educate patients about a drug's intended purpose and the correct way to take the drug for maximum effectiveness. In this chapter, you will learn how to translate the doctor's prescription (℞) for the patient and calculate and administer drugs if this is legally allowed by the state in which you will practice as a medical assistant.

In this chapter, an overview of pharmacology is given; it is considered a review for medical assistants who have had a formal course in the subject. Information on dosage calculation and medication administration can be found in Chapter 24.

MEDICAL USES OF DRUGS

A drug is defined as a medicinal substance that may alter or modify the functions of a living organism. There are five medical uses for drugs.

- *Therapeutic*. Used in the treatment of a condition to relieve symptoms. An example is an antihistamine that may be used in the treatment of an allergy.

- *Diagnostic*. Used in conjunction with radiology and other diagnostic imaging procedures to allow the physician to pinpoint the location of a disease process. An example is dye tablets used in the X-ray study of the gallbladder.

- *Curative*. Used to kill or remove the causative agent of a disease. An example is an antibiotic.

- *Replacement*. Used to replace substances normally found in the body. Hormones and vitamins are examples of replacement drugs.

- *Preventive or Prophylactic*. Used to ward off or lessen the severity of a disease. Examples are immunizing agents such as vaccines.

DRUG NAMES

Most drugs have three types of names: chemical, generic, and trade or brand name.

- The chemical name describes the drug's molecular structure and identifies its chemical structure.

- The generic name is the drug's official name and is assigned to the drug by the United States Adopted Names Council. A generic drug can be manufactured by more than one pharmaceutical company. When this is the case, each company markets the drug under its own unique trade or brand name.

- A trade or brand name is registered by the U.S. Patent and Trademark Office and is approved by the U.S. Food and Drug Administration (FDA). The ® symbol following a drug's trade or brand name indicates that the name is registered and protected for 17 years. No other manufacturer can make or sell the drug during that time. Once the patent expires, any manufacturer can sell the drug under its generic name or a new trade name. The original trade name can not be reused.

Example:
Chemical name: 1, 4, 3, 6-dian hydrosorbitol-2, 5 dinitrate
Generic name: isosorbide dinitrate
Trade/Brand name: Sorbitrate®

When physicians prescribe a drug, they may use either the generic or trade name. It is not uncommon for physicians to prescribe the generic form of a drug because it is usually less costly for the patient. Sometimes physicians specify drugs by their trade names. Some states allow patients to request that their pharmacist dispense the generic drug equivalent unless the physician has specified that the drug be dispensed by its trade name. Also, in some states, a pharmacist may select a generic form of a drug if not specifically directed otherwise by the physician. Generic and trade name drugs have the same chemical composition and must adhere to identical FDA standards; therefore, according to most state laws, they can be used interchangeably. The drug label reflects the drug products dispensed.

HISTORY AND SOURCES OF DRUGS

Drugs prepared from roots, herbs, bark, and other forms of plant life are among the earliest known pharmaceuticals. Their origin can be traced back to primitive cultures where they were first used to evoke magical powers and to drive out evil spirits. Having discovered that certain plants were pharmacologically useful, a search was begun for sources of drugs.

Today this search continues. In addition to plants, drugs are derived from animals, minerals, and produced in laboratories utilizing chemical, biochemical, and biotechnological processes.

Plant Sources

The leaves, roots, stems, or fruit of certain plants may contain medicinal properties. For example, the dried leaf of the foxglove plant (*Digitalis purpurea*) is a source of digitalis, a cardiac glycoside used in the treatment of certain heart conditions.

Animal Sources

A number of essential extracts are obtained from tissues such as the pancreas and adrenal glands of animals. An example of a drug obtained from animals is insulin, a hormone that can be extracted from the pancreas of cows and hogs, though it is also made synthetically and by genetic engineering. Insulin is used in the treatment of diabetes mellitus. Two common compounds extracted from the adrenal glands of animals are adrenalin and cortisone.

Mineral Sources

Some naturally occurring mineral substances are used in medicine in a highly purified form. One such mineral is sulfur which has been used as a key ingredient in certain bacteriostatic drugs. It is now prepared synthetically and used in the treatment of urinary and intestinal tract infections.

Synthetic Drugs

These drugs are artificially prepared in pharmaceutical laboratories. By combining various chemicals, scientists can produce compounds that are identical to a natural drug or create entirely new substances. Thousands of drugs are now produced synthetically. Examples are Motrin® (ibuprofen) and Feldene® (piroxician).

Genetically Engineered Pharmaceuticals

Scientists are now capable of creating new strains of bacteria using a technique known as gene splicing. Through this process, hybrid forms of life have been created that benefit human beings by providing an alternative source of drugs, such as Humulin® (insulin) for the diabetic patient and interferon for use in treatment of cancer. These drugs can be manufactured in large quantities; thus, they are less expensive than natural substances.

DRUG REGULATIONS AND LEGAL CLASSIFICATIONS OF DRUGS

  Qualified medical practitioners who prescribe, dispense, or administer drugs must comply with federal and state laws. The laws govern the manufacture, sale, possession, administration, dispensing, and prescribing of drugs. All drugs available for legal use are controlled by the Federal Food, Drug, and Cosmetic Act. The law protects the public by ensuring the purity, strength, and composition of foods, drugs, and cosmetics. It also prohibits the movement in interstate commerce of altered and misbranded food, drugs, devices, and cosmetics. Enforcement of the act is the responsibility of the Food and Drug Administration (FDA), which is part of the Department of Health and Human Services (HHS).

Controlled Substance Act of 1970

One category of drugs—those with potential for abuse or addiction—is regulated by the Controlled Substance Act of 1970. It controls the manufacture, importation, compounding, selling, dealing in, and giving away of drugs that have the potential for abuse and addiction. The drugs are known as controlled substances and include heroin and cocaine and their derivatives and narcotics, stimulants, and depressants. The Drug Enforcement Agency (DEA) of the U.S. Justice Department monitors and enforces the act, which is also known as the Comprehen-

sive Drug Abuse Prevention and Control Act. Under federal law, physicians who prescribe, administer, or dispense controlled substances must register with the DEA and renew their registration as required by state law.

Applications for registration are made directly to the DEA Registration Section, P.O. Box 28083, Central Station, Washington, DC 20038-8083. A licensed physician is issued a registration that must be renewed at regular intervals (Figure 23-1). The renewal form is sent approximately two months prior to the expiration date.

Controlled Substances Schedules. Controlled substances are classified according to five schedules:

- Schedule I specifies drugs that have a high potential for abuse and are not accepted for medical use within the United States. Examples are heroin and lysergic acid diethylamide (LSD).

- Schedule II drugs include those that also have a high abuse potential but that do have an accepted medical use within the United States. Examples are amphetamines and cocaine. Because of their high potential for abuse, a special DEA Form #222 must be used to order these drugs. The form is not necessary for Schedule III and IV drugs. A written prescription is required for Schedule II drugs and it can not be renewed.

- Schedule III drugs have a low-to-moderate potential for physical dependence, yet have a high potential for psychological dependency. Some examples are barbiturates and various drug combinations containing codeine and paregoric. Prescriptions for Schedule III drugs can be either written or oral. They can be refilled, but only five times within six months.

- Misuse or abuse of Schedule IV drugs can lead to limited physical or psychological dependency. Examples of these drugs include chloral hydrate and diazepam. Prescriptions for Schedule IV drugs may include refills, but refills are limited to five times within six months.

- Schedule V drugs have the lowest abuse potential of controlled substances. Some examples from this schedule are Lomotil® and Donnagel®. Some drugs from Schedule V may include refills, but refills are limited to five times within six months.

On occasion, the DEA will reclassify drugs and move them from one schedule to another.

So they can be readily identified, controlled substances are labeled with a large C with a Roman numeral inside it to indicate from which schedule the drug has come, for example, Ⓒ.

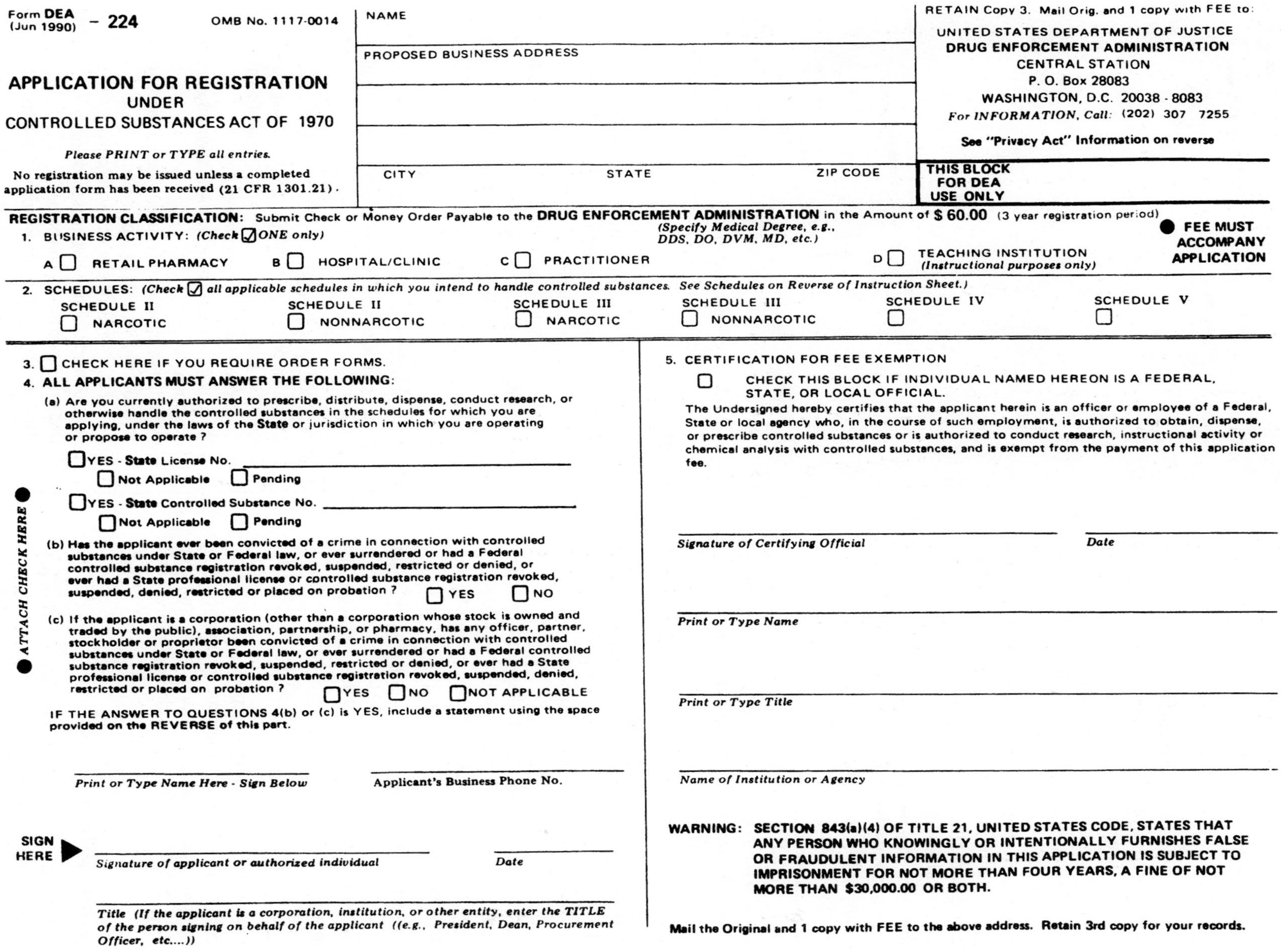

Form **DEA** (Jun 1990) – **224** OMB No. 1117-0014

APPLICATION FOR REGISTRATION
UNDER
CONTROLLED SUBSTANCES ACT OF 1970

Please PRINT or TYPE all entries.

No registration may be issued unless a completed application form has been received (21 CFR 1301.21).

NAME

PROPOSED BUSINESS ADDRESS

CITY STATE ZIP CODE

RETAIN Copy 3. Mail Orig. and 1 copy with FEE to:

UNITED STATES DEPARTMENT OF JUSTICE
DRUG ENFORCEMENT ADMINISTRATION
CENTRAL STATION
P. O. Box 28083
WASHINGTON, D.C. 20038 - 8083
For INFORMATION, Call: (202) 307 7255

See "Privacy Act" Information on reverse

THIS BLOCK FOR DEA USE ONLY

REGISTRATION CLASSIFICATION: Submit Check or Money Order Payable to the **DRUG ENFORCEMENT ADMINISTRATION** in the Amount of **$ 60.00** (3 year registration period)

● FEE MUST ACCOMPANY APPLICATION

1. BUSINESS ACTIVITY: *(Check ☑ ONE only)*

A ☐ RETAIL PHARMACY B ☐ HOSPITAL/CLINIC C ☐ PRACTITIONER *(Specify Medical Degree, e.g., DDS, DO, DVM, MD, etc.)* D ☐ TEACHING INSTITUTION *(Instructional purposes only)*

2. SCHEDULES: *(Check ☑ all applicable schedules in which you intend to handle controlled substances. See Schedules on Reverse of Instruction Sheet.)*

SCHEDULE II ☐ NARCOTIC SCHEDULE II ☐ NONNARCOTIC SCHEDULE III ☐ NARCOTIC SCHEDULE III ☐ NONNARCOTIC SCHEDULE IV ☐ SCHEDULE V ☐

3. ☐ CHECK HERE IF YOU REQUIRE ORDER FORMS.
4. **ALL APPLICANTS MUST ANSWER THE FOLLOWING:**

(a) Are you currently authorized to prescribe, distribute, dispense, conduct research, or otherwise handle the controlled substances in the schedules for which you are applying, under the laws of the **State** or jurisdiction in which you are operating or propose to operate?

☐ YES - **State** License No.
☐ Not Applicable ☐ Pending

☐ YES - **State** Controlled Substance No.
☐ Not Applicable ☐ Pending

● ATTACH CHECK HERE ●

(b) Has the applicant ever been convicted of a crime in connection with controlled substances under State or Federal law, or ever surrendered or had a Federal controlled substance registration revoked, suspended, restricted or denied, or ever had a State professional license or controlled substance registration revoked, suspended, denied, restricted or placed on probation? ☐ YES ☐ NO

(c) If the applicant is a corporation (other than a corporation whose stock is owned and traded by the public), association, partnership, or pharmacy, has any officer, partner, stockholder or proprietor been convicted of a crime in connection with controlled substances under State or Federal law, or ever surrendered or had a Federal controlled substance registration revoked, suspended, restricted or denied, or ever had a State professional license or controlled substance registration revoked, suspended, denied, restricted or placed on probation? ☐ YES ☐ NO ☐ NOT APPLICABLE

IF THE ANSWER TO QUESTIONS 4(b) or (c) is YES, include a statement using the space provided on the **REVERSE** of this part.

Print or Type Name Here - Sign Below Applicant's Business Phone No.

SIGN HERE ▶ *Signature of applicant or authorized individual* *Date*

Title (If the applicant is a corporation, institution, or other entity, enter the TITLE of the person signing on behalf of the applicant ((e.g., President, Dean, Procurement Officer, etc....))

5. CERTIFICATION FOR FEE EXEMPTION

☐ CHECK THIS BLOCK IF INDIVIDUAL NAMED HEREON IS A FEDERAL, STATE, OR LOCAL OFFICIAL.

The Undersigned hereby certifies that the applicant herein is an officer or employee of a Federal, State or local agency who, in the course of such employment, is authorized to obtain, dispense, or prescribe controlled substances or is authorized to conduct research, instructional activity or chemical analysis with controlled substances, and is exempt from the payment of this application fee.

Signature of Certifying Official *Date*

Print or Type Name

Print or Type Title

Name of Institution or Agency

WARNING: SECTION 843(a)(4) OF TITLE 21, UNITED STATES CODE, STATES THAT ANY PERSON WHO KNOWINGLY OR INTENTIONALLY FURNISHES FALSE OR FRAUDULENT INFORMATION IN THIS APPLICATION IS SUBJECT TO IMPRISONMENT FOR NOT MORE THAN FOUR YEARS, A FINE OF NOT MORE THAN $30,000.00 OR BOTH.

Mail the Original and 1 copy with FEE to the above address. Retain 3rd copy for your records.

Figure 23-1 Licensed physicians who prescribe, administer, or dispense controlled substances must register with the Drug Enforcement Agency (DEA) of the U.S. Justice Department. The registration must be renewed at regular intervals.

The physician's DEA number must appear on each prescription for controlled substances.

A copy of the federal law and a complete list of controlled substances and their schedules are available from any DEA office.

Storage of Controlled Substances. Federal law requires that all controlled substances be kept separate from other drugs. They must be stored in a well-constructed metal box or compartment that has a double lock. Controlled substances must be protected from possible misuse and abuse, and persons who administer controlled substances must record them in a separate record book. The book must be maintained on a daily basis and kept for a minimum of two to three years, depending on state laws. Patient name, address, date of administration of the controlled substance, drug name, dose, and route and method of administration must be included in the record. Record keeping applies only to persons who administer or dispense controlled substances.

Controlled substances stored and used on the premises must be counted at the end of each workday, verified by two individuals for accuracy of count, and recorded on an audit sheet. An inventory record of Schedule II drugs must be submitted to the DEA every two years.

Due to the increase in office and clinic drug theft and substance abuse, as well as the stringent federal laws that apply to storing, dispensing, and administration of controlled substances, many offices and clinics do not keep controlled substances on the premises.

Medical Assistant Role and Responsibilities. Medical assistants are required to know the legalities that surround controlled substances. Medical assistant responsibilities may include:

1. Monitor the physician's DEA registration renewal date
2. Maintain legally designated records and inventories of drugs (Figure 23-2)
3. Provide security for all drugs, in particular controlled substances
4. Provide security for prescription pads
5. Properly destroy expired drugs and document
6. Know and understand federal and state laws that regulate drugs, including controlled substances

Prescription Drugs

State laws require that licensed practitioners who prescribe drugs must write and sign an order for the dispensing of drugs. This process is known as writing a prescription. Some examples of drugs that require a prescription are all of the controlled substances (except for

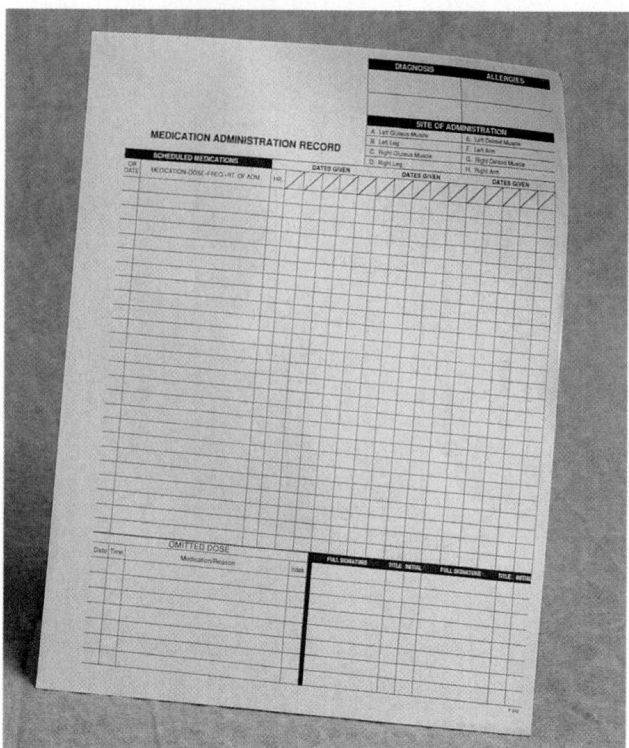

Figure 23-2 It is important to maintain patient medication records both for the safety of the patient and to protect the practice.

Schedule I) such as meperidine and pentobarbital, and other categories such as digoxin, a cardiac drug, and epinephrine, a vasoconstrictor.

Medical assistants need to advise patients after the physician prescribes a drug. See Figure 23-3 for a list of patient education considerations. Patients should also read warning labels on medication containers (Figure 23-4).

Guidelines for patients who take prescription medications include:

1. Take exactly as directed.
2. Inform the physician of unusual or adverse reactions.
3. Continue to take the medication for the duration of the prescribed number of days, weeks, etc.
4. If you want to discontinue the medication, inform your physician.
5. Do not take other medications or herbs concurrently without checking with your physician.
6. Do not take someone else's prescribed medication.
7. Store all medications away from children.
8. Discard unused medication properly.
9. Heed warning labels on medication containers.

Figure 23-3 Guidelines for patients when taking prescription medications.

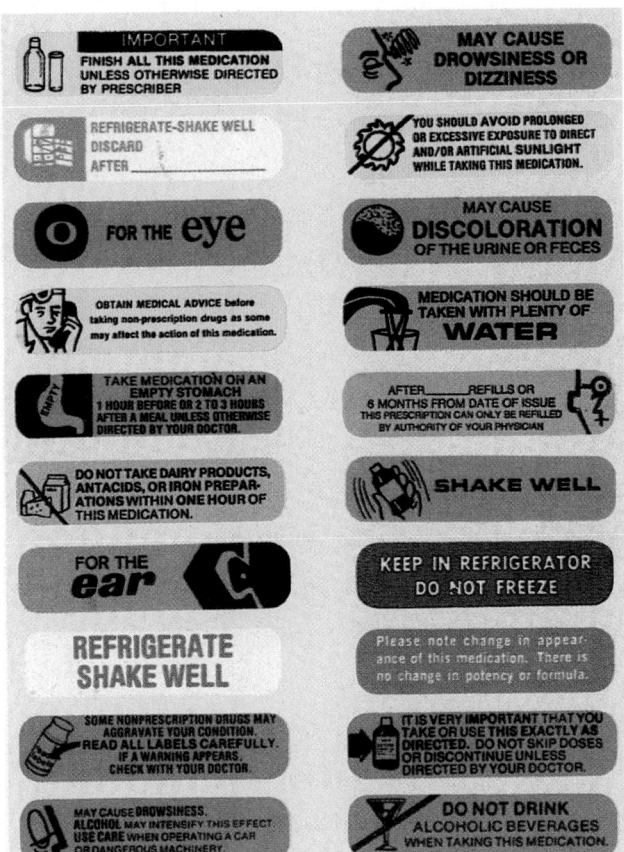

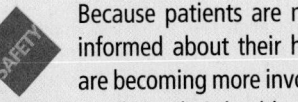

Figure 23-4 Warning labels are placed on prescription medication containers, and patients should be advised to read and adhere to the precautions or instructions.

Nonprescription Drugs

Drugs that are frequently referred to as over-the-counter (OTC) drugs fall into the category of nonprescription drugs. These drugs are readily accessible to the public. They do not require a prescription because the FDA considers them safe to use without a physician's advice. Examples of OTC drugs are aspirin, ibuprofen, and vitamins such as vitamin C. While over-the-counter drugs are considered safe, it is useful for the medical assistant to offer patients some guidelines (Figure 23-5).

Proper Disposal of Drugs

All drug labels contain an expiration date. When that date has been reached, the drug must be removed from the shelf and destroyed (Figure 23-6).

An expired drug cannot be dispensed nor administered because it could be harmful.

To destroy expired drugs, liquids and ointments can be rinsed down the drain and will be destroyed by the sewage system. Powdered drugs can be mixed with water and disposed of in the same manner. Pills and capsules can

Because patients are more aware and better informed about their health care needs, they are becoming more involved in making choices and decisions about their health care. When they choose to take over-the-counter (OTC) drugs, they need information and guidance. Over the past few years, some previous prescription drugs have been changed to OTC drugs. The safety of these drugs can only be assured if patients take them as directed.

Patients need to realize that OTC medications:

1. Can interact with other drugs (either prescribed or other OTCs) and cause undesirable or adverse reactions or complications
2. May be used in lieu of seeking professional help and thereby interfere with the need for medical care
3. Can mask symptoms and exacerbate an existing condition
4. May have several active ingredients, which may be found to be undesirable
5. Have a safe minimum dose, which may not have the desired therapeutic effect

Figure 23-5 Guidelines for patients when taking non-prescription (over-the-counter) medications.

be flushed down the toilet. Vials and ampules of liquid drugs are opened and their contents poured down the drain.

If a medication is removed from its original container, it should not be used (for example, the patient refused the medication); do not replace it in the container. Dispose of it as outlined earlier.

Outdated and expired controlled substances are handled differently. They must be returned to the pharmacy (as required by law). If a controlled substance has been either dropped onto the floor (and is thus unfit to be

Patient Teaching Tip

Many patients keep unused medications past their expiration date. This presents a potential health hazard, as some medications lose their potency after a period of time, while others become toxic. It is best to inform patients to discard any unused portion of medication by the stated date. Encourage patients to check their medicine cabinets at the same time every year so it becomes a routine practice.

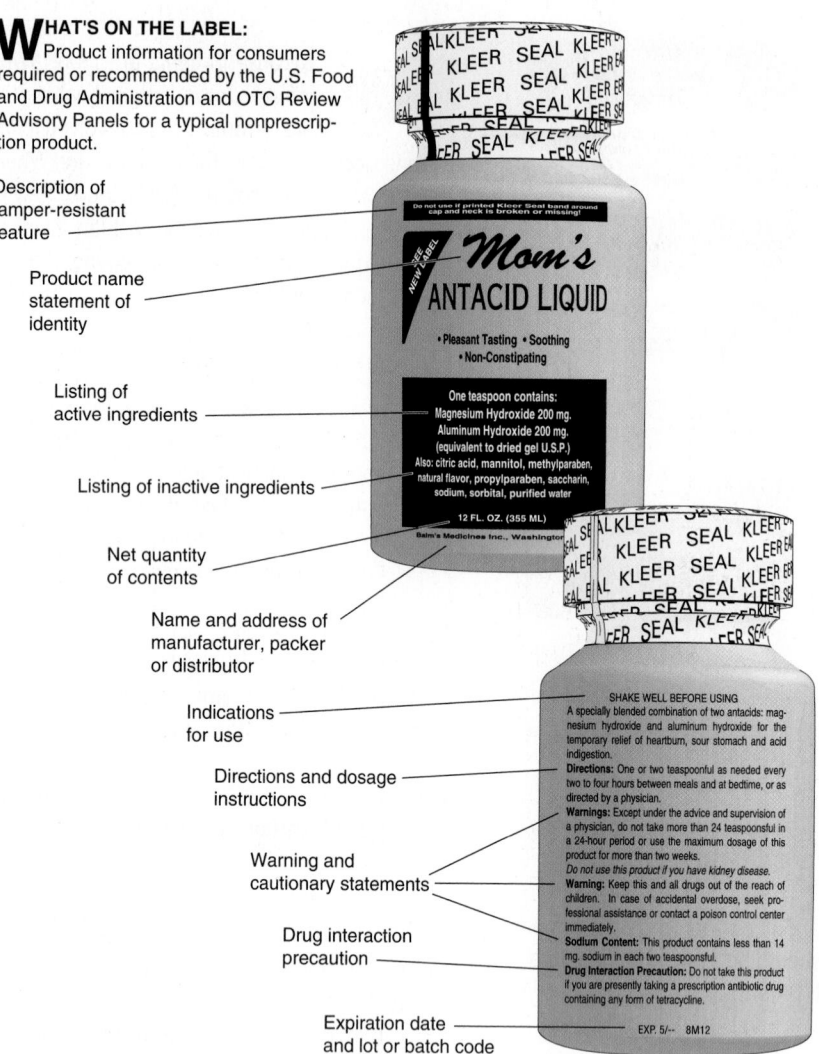

WHAT'S ON THE LABEL:
Product information for consumers required or recommended by the U.S. Food and Drug Administration and OTC Review Advisory Panels for a typical nonprescription product.

Description of tamper-resistant feature

Product name statement of identity

Listing of active ingredients

Listing of inactive ingredients

Net quantity of contents

Name and address of manufacturer, packer or distributor

Indications for use

Directions and dosage instructions

Warning and cautionary statements

Drug interaction precaution

Expiration date and lot or batch code

Figure 23-6   Medication labels contain valuable information essential to the safe and effective use of the drug.

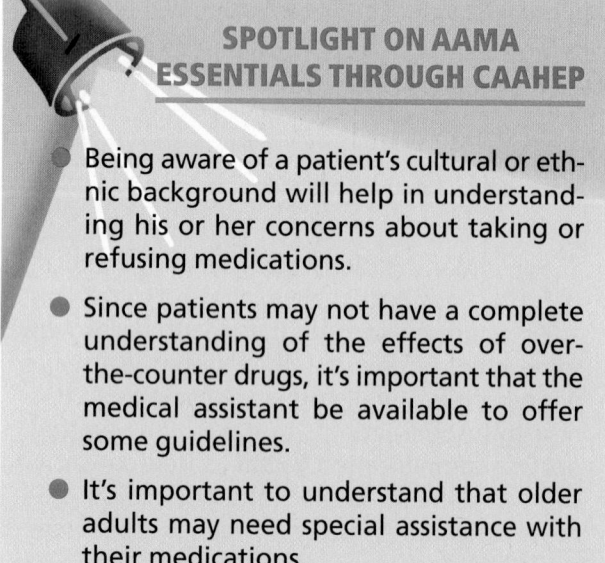

SPOTLIGHT ON AAMA ESSENTIALS THROUGH CAAHEP

● Being aware of a patient's cultural or ethnic background will help in understanding his or her concerns about taking or refusing medications.

● Since patients may not have a complete understanding of the effects of over-the-counter drugs, it's important that the medical assistant be available to offer some guidelines.

● It's important to understand that older adults may need special assistance with their medications.

given to a patient) or has spilled (if in liquid form), a witness should verify the action and proper documentation must take place.

The local DEA office and local police must be notified and the appropriate paperwork completed if there has been a loss or theft of a controlled substance.

Administer, Prescribe, Dispense

There are three ways to handle drugs in the physician's office or clinic: by prescribing, dispensing, or administering them. To **prescribe** a drug means that the licensed practitioner (physician, physician assistant, or nurse practitioner) gives a written order to be taken to the pharmacist to be filled. To **dispense** a drug means to give the medication (either prescription or OTC) to the patient to be taken at another time. To **administer** a drug means to give it to the patient by mouth or injection or any other method of administration.

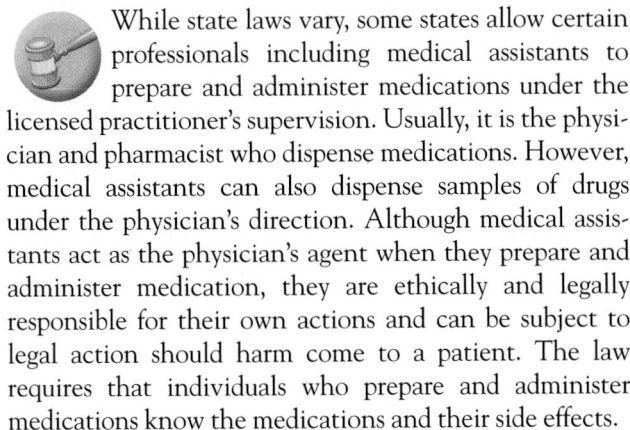 While state laws vary, some states allow certain professionals including medical assistants to prepare and administer medications under the licensed practitioner's supervision. Usually, it is the physician and pharmacist who dispense medications. However, medical assistants can also dispense samples of drugs under the physician's direction. Although medical assistants act as the physician's agent when they prepare and administer medication, they are ethically and legally responsible for their own actions and can be subject to legal action should harm come to a patient. The law requires that individuals who prepare and administer medications know the medications and their side effects.

DRUG REFERENCES AND STANDARDS

The strength, purity, and quality of drugs differ depending on how they are manufactured. To control the differences, standards have been set. By law, the various drug products must meet standards that are set forth by the U.S. Food and Drug Administration (FDA). A special reference book, *United States Pharmacopeia/National Formulary*, lists the drugs for which standards have been established. The book is recognized by the U.S. government as the official list of drug standards, which are enforced by the FDA. Every five years the book is updated in an attempt to include all drug products in the United States.

Other useful books used as references include the *Compendium of Drug Therapy* and *Desk Reference for Nonprescription Drugs*, and the *Physician's Desk Reference* (PDR), which is published annually by Medical Economics Company in cooperation with pharmaceutical companies. It is one of the most widely used reference books and is found in most offices and clinics. It is divided into seven sections of drug information, which are followed by other useful drug information such as a list of products, poison control 800 telephone numbers, conversion tables, and a guide to management of drug overdose (Figure 23-7).

How To Use the PDR

The four most commonly used sections of the PDR list drugs according to:

- Brand name and generic name (pink section), section 2
- Classification or category (blue section), section 3
- Product information (white section), section 5
- Alphabetical arrangement by manufacturers (white section), section 1

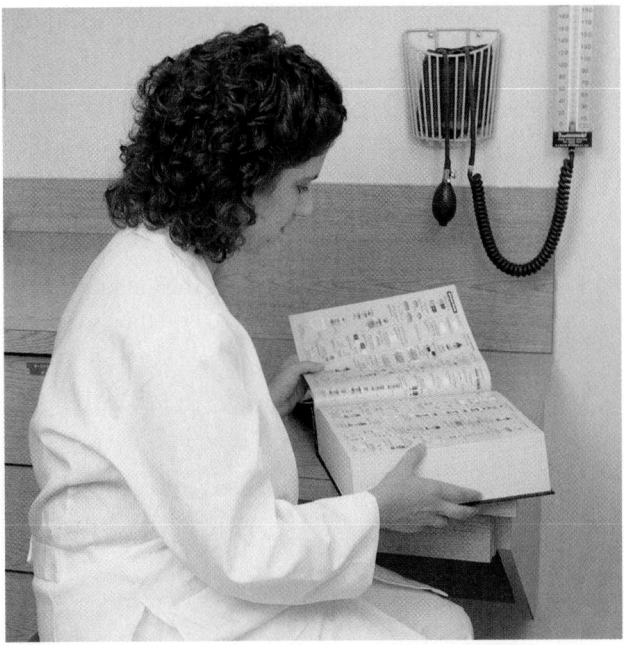

Figure 23-7 The *Physicians' Desk Reference* (PDR) is a valuable resource for the medical assistant who wishes to obtain information about a specific medication.

The following guidelines will assist you as you learn to use the PDR.

1. If you know the brand name of the drug, turn to the pink section and locate the drug in the alphabetical listing. The manufacturer's name will be in parentheses, followed by a page number or two page numbers. The first number is the product identification page number. The second number is the product information section (white).

Example: Look up Achromycin V capsules in a current PDR. This example is based on the 2000 edition.

Achromycin V®

[a-kro-mi-cin]

tetracycline HCl

for ORAL USE

Turn to page 1528 of the PDR (2000 edition) and note all the information provided about the drug.

- *Description*. Gives the origin and chemical composition of the drug.
- *Clinical Pharmacology*. Indicates the effect of the drug upon the body and the process by which the drug exerts this effect.
- *Indications*. States the various conditions, diseases, types of microorganisms, etc., for which the drug is used.

- *Contraindications*. States when the drug should not be given to a specified person.

- *Warnings*. Gives the potential dangers of the drug.

- *Precautions*. States the possible unfavorable effects that the drug may have upon a patient.

- *Adverse Reactions*. Lists the side effects of the drug.

- *Dosage and Administration*. States the amount (usual daily dose for adults and children) and time sequence of administration.

- *How Supplied*. Lists the various forms of the drug and their dosages.

2. If you know the classification of the drug, turn to the blue section and locate the category of the drug.

   Example: Antibiotics, systemic

   Tetracyclines

   Achromycin V® capsules (Lederle)
   p. 1528

NOTE: All controlled substances listed in the PDR are indicated with the symbol C with the Roman numeral II, III, IV, or V printed inside the C to designate the schedule in which the substance is classified.

Example: Duramorph® Ⓒ, morphine sulfate USP.

Other Reference Sources

On occasion you may not find the drug that you are looking for listed in the PDR. When this happens:

- Refer to another drug reference book

- Ask a pharmacist about the drug

- Refer to the packet insert that comes in the drug package

The package insert that most manufacturers provide with their products is an important source of information about a particular drug. This is a brief description of the drug, its clinical pharmacology, indications and usage, contraindications (any symptom or circumstance that indicates that the use of a particular drug is inappropriate when it would otherwise be advisable), warnings, precautions, drug interactions, adverse reactions, overdose, dosage, and administration. The package insert can be a valuable source of information about drugs that might not be listed elsewhere.

Information about some older medications, such as digoxin, can be found in the package insert since they may have been deleted from the current PDR. The package insert also is a useful tool in the absence of a PDR.

CLASSIFICATION OF DRUGS

Drugs can be classified (arranged in groups) in a number of ways. Some examples are:

- Drugs used to treat or prevent disease (examples are hormones and vaccines)

- Drugs that have a principal action on the body (examples are analgesics and anti-inflammatory drugs)

- Drugs that act on specific body systems or organs (examples are respiratory and cardiovascular drugs)

- Drug preparation (examples are suppository, liquid)

Table 23-1 shows a list of common drug classifications. See the Appendix for the most widely prescribed generic and brand name medications.

PRINCIPLE ACTIONS OF DRUGS

In general, drugs may be grouped as follows: those that act directly upon one or more tissues of the body; those that act upon microorganisms; and those that replace body chemicals.

Certain drugs have selective action, such as stimulants, which increase cell activity, and depressants, which decrease cell activity.

Other drugs may have what is known as:

1. *Local action*. The drug acts on the area to which it is administered.
2. *Remote action*. A drug affects a part of the body that is distant from the site of administration.
3. *Systemic action*. The drug is carried via the bloodstream throughout the body.
4. *Synergistic action*. One drug increases the action of another.

Factors that Affect Drug Action

The four principal factors that affect drug action are: absorption, distribution, biotransformation, and elimination. These factors depend upon the individual patient, the form and chemical composition of the drug, and the method of administration.

1. *Absorption* is the process whereby the drug passes into the body fluids and tissues.
2. *Distribution* is the process whereby the drug is transported from the blood to the intended site of action, site of biotransformation, site of storage, and site of elimination.
3. *Biotransformation* is the chemical alteration that a drug undergoes in the body.
4. *Elimination* is the process whereby the drug is excreted from the body. Elimination occurs via the

TABLE 23-1 COMMON CLASSIFICATIONS OF DRUGS AND THEIR ACTIONS

Classification (with Phonetic Spelling)	Action	Examples of Drugs Commonly Used in Ambulatory Care Setting
Analgesic (an"al-je'sik)	An agent that relieves pain without causing loss of consciousness.	acetaminophen (Tylenol) acetylsalicylic acid (aspirin) ibuprofen (Advil, Motrin)
Anesthetic (an"es-thet'ik)	An agent that produces a lack of feeling. May be local or general depending upon the type and how administered.	lidocaine HCl (Xylocaine) procaine HCl (Novacaine)
Antacid (ant-as'id)	An agent that neutralizes acid.	Amphojel, Gelusil, Mylanta, Milk of Magnesia
Antianemic	An agent that replaces iron.	iron (imferon), ferrous sulfate
Antianxiety (an"ti-ang-zi'e-te)	An agent that relieves anxiety and muscle tension.	benzodiazepines: diazepam (Valium) chlordiazepoxide HCl (Librium) alprazolam (Xanax)
Antiarrhythmic (an"te-a-rith'mik)	An agent that controls cardiac arrhythmias.	lidocaine HCl (Xylocaine) propranolol HCl (Inderal)
Antibiotic (an"ti-bi-ot'ik)	An agent that is destructive to or inhibits growth of microorganisms.	penicillins (Pentids, Duracillin, Polycillin, Pipracil, Augmentin)
Anticholinergic (an"ti-ko"lin-er'jik)	An agent that blocks parasympathetic nerve impulses.	atropine, scopolamine, trihexyphenidyl HCl (Artane)
Anticoagulant (an"ti-ko-ag'u-lant)	An agent that prevents or delays blood clotting.	heparin sodium, Dicumarol, warfarin sodium (Coumadin)
Anticonvulsant (an"ti-kon-vul'sant)	An agent that prevents or relieves convulsions.	carbamazepine (Tegretol) phenytoin (Dilantin) ethosuximide (Zarontin)
Antidepressant (an"ti-dep-res'ant)	An agent that prevents or relieves the symptoms of depression.	monamine oxidase (MAO) inhibitors: isocarboxazid (Marplan), phenelzine sulfate (Nardil), amitriptyline HCl (Elavil), imipramine HCl (Tofranil), trazodone (Desyrel), fluoxentine (Prozac)
Antidiarrheal (an"ti-di-a-re'al)	An agent that prevents or relieves diarrhea.	Pepto-Bismol, Kaopectate, Diphenoxylate HCl (Lomotil)
Antidote (an-ti'dot)	An agent that counteracts poisons and their effects.	naloxone (Narcan)
Antiemetic (an"ti-e-met'ik)	An agent that prevents or relieves nausea and vomiting.	Tigan, Dramamine, Phenergan, Reglan, Marinol
Antihistamine (an"ti-his'ta-min)	An agent that acts to counteract histamine.	Dimetane, Benadryl, Seldane
Antihypertensive (an"ti-hi"per-ten'siv)	An agent that prevents or controls high blood pressure.	methyldopa (Aldomet) clonidine HCl (Catapres) metoprolol tartrate (Lopressor)
Anti-inflammatory (an"ti-in-flam'a-to-re)	An agent that counteracts inflammation.	naproxen (Naprosyn) aspirin, ibuprofen (Advil, Motrin)
Antimanic (an"ti-man'ik)	An agent used for the treatment of the manic episode of manic-depressive disorder.	lithium
Antineoplastic (an"ti-ne"o-plas'tik)	An agent that kills or destroys malignant cells.	busuflan (Myleran) cyclophosphamide (Cytoxan)
Antipsychotic	An agent that helps in schizophrenia and chronic brain syndrome.	haloperdol (Haldol) chlorpromazine (Thorazine)
Antipyretic (an"ti-pi-ret'ik)	An agent that reduces fever.	aspirin, acetaminophen (Tylenol)
Antitussive (an"ti-tus'iv)	An agent that prevents or relieves cough.	codeine, dextromethorphan (Pertussin, Romilar)
Antiulcer (an"ti-ul'ser)	An agent that relieves and heals ulcers.	cimetidine (Tagamet) ranitidine (Zantac)
Bronchodilator (brong"ko-dil-a'tor)	An agent that dilates the bronchi.	isoproterenol HCl (Isuprel) albuterol (Proventil)

(continues)

TABLE 23-1 *(continued)*

Classification (with Phonetic Spelling)	Action	Examples of Drugs Commonly Used in Ambulatory Care Setting
Contraceptive (kon"tra-sep'tiv)	Any device, method, or agent that prevents conception.	Envid-E 21, Ortho-Novum 10/11-21; 10/11-28 Triphasil-21
Decongestant (de"con-gest'ant)	An agent that reduces nasal congestion and/or swelling.	oxymetazoline (Afrin) phenylephrine HCl (Neo-Synephrine) pseudoephedrine HCl (Sudafed)
Diuretic (di"u-ret'ik)	An agent that increases the excretion of urine.	chlorothiazide (Diuril) furosemide (Lasix) mannitol (Osmitrol)
Expectorant (ek-spek'to-rant)	An agent that facilitates removal of secretion from broncho-pulmonary mucous membrane.	guaifenesin (Robitussin)
Hemostatic (he"mo-stat'ik)	An agent that controls or stops bleeding.	Humafac, Amicar, vitamin K
Hypnotic (hip-not'ik)	An agent that produces sleep or hypnosis.	secobarbital (Seconal); chloral hydrate; ethchlorvynol (Placidyl)
Hypoglycemic (hi"po-gli-se'mik)	An agent that lowers blood glucose level.	insulin; chlorpropamide (Diabinese)
Laxative (lak'sa-tiv)	An agent that loosens and promotes normal bowel elimination.	Metamucil powder, Dulcolax
Muscle relaxant (mus'el re-lak'sant)	An agent that produces relaxation of skeletal muscle.	Robaxin, Norflex, Paraflex, Skelaxin, Valium
Sedative (sed'a-tiv)	An agent that produces a calming effect without causing sleep.	amobarbital (amytal) butabarbital sodium (Buticaps) phenobarbital
Tranquilizer (tran"kwi-liz'er)	An agent that reduces mental tension and anxiety.	Thorazine, Mellaril, Haldol
Vasodilator (vas"o-di-la'tor)	An agent that produces relaxation of blood vessels; lowers blood pressure.	isorbide dinitrate (Isordil) nitroglycerin
vasopressor (vas"o-pres'or)	An agent that produces contraction of muscles of capillaries and arteries; elevates blood pressure.	metaraminol (Aramine) norepinephrine (Levophed)

gastrointestinal tract, respiratory tract, skin, mucous membranes, and mammary glands.

Undesirable Actions of Drugs

Most drugs have the potential for causing an action other than their intended action. For example:

1. *Side Effect.* An undesirable action of the drug that may limit the usefulness of the drug.
2. *Drug Interaction.* Occurs when one drug potentiates—increases—or diminishes the action of another drug. These actions may be desirable or undesirable. Drugs may also interact with various foods, alcohol, tobacco, and other substances.
3. *Adverse Reaction.* An unfavorable or harmful unintended action of a drug, such as an allergic reaction.

A patient may experience an allergic reaction to a drug after administration. It is often mild and may exhibit itself in the form of a rash, **urticaria**, or **pruritus**. On occasion, a severe reaction or **anaphylaxis** can occur, which is hypersensitivity to a drug or other foreign protein. It is the least common allergic reaction, but can become severe very quickly and result in dyspnea and shock. Loss of consciousness and death can result. To help prevent an allergic reaction or minimize its risk, the medical assistant should attempt to ascertain prior to administration of every drug whether the patient has any known allergies. The medical assistant should be aware of signs and symptoms of allergic reaction and notify the physician immediately so that appropriate emergency treatment can be given. One or two injections of epinephrine usually reverses the life-threatening symptoms of anaphylaxis and is followed by administration of an antihistamine such as Benadryl®.

DRUG ROUTES

Drugs are manufactured in a variety of forms and for various purposes. The route of a drug refers to how it is administered to the patient and thereby transported into the patient's body. Certain medications can be administered by more than one route, while others must be administered via a specific route.

The route of administration is determined by a number of factors. One factor is the action of the medication on the body, either local or systemic. Intravenous medication reaches the systemic circulation rapidly via the bloodstream and quickly becomes effective. Injections of medication and medications absorbed through mucous membranes are absorbed quickly. Oral medications take longer to act since they must be digested by the stomach and then be absorbed into the bloodstream.

Another factor in route selection is the physical and emotional state of the patient. The patient's consciousness level, emotional status, and physical restrictions are considered when selecting a route to administer medication.

A third factor to consider is the characteristics of the drug. An example is insulin. Insulin is destroyed by digestive enzymes; therefore, the route of administration must be by injection.

The most frequently utilized routes of administering medication to the patient are oral and parenteral routes: oral medications are taken by mouth; parenteral generally by injection. Other routes of administration include:

- Direct application to the skin (lotions, creams, liniments, ointments, and transdermal systems)
- Sublingual (tablets, liquid, drops)
- Buccal (tablets)
- Rectal (suppositories, ointments)
- Vaginal (suppositories, creams, tablets, applications)
- Inhalation (sprays, aerosols)
- Instillation (liquid, drops)

FORMS OF DRUGS

Drugs are compounded in three basic types of preparations: liquids, solids, and semisolids. The ease with which a drug's ingredients can be dissolved largely determines the variety of forms manufactured. Some drug agents are soluble in water, others in alcohol, and others in a mixture of several solvents.

The method for administering a drug depends upon its form, its properties, and the effects desired. When given orally, a drug may be in the form of a liquid, powder, tablet, capsule, or caplet. If it is to be injected, it must be in the form of a liquid. For topical use, the drug may be in the form of a liquid, powder, or semisolid. Oral and injectable medications are examples of preparations designed for internal use.

Liquid Preparations

Liquid preparations are those containing a drug that has been dissolved or suspended. Depending upon the solvent used, the drug may be further classified as an aqueous (water) or alcohol preparation. When prescribed for internal use, liquid preparations other than emulsions are rapidly absorbed through the stomach or intestinal walls.

Solid and Semisolid Preparations

Tablets, capsules, caplets, troches or lozenges, suppositories, and ointments are examples of solid and semisolid preparations. These products offer great flexibility as a means of dispensing different dosages of drugs (Figure 23-8).

Other Drug Delivery Systems

Technological advances have introduced new ways by which drugs can be introduced into the patient. In addition to the conventional preparations, the following miniature therapeutic systems offer special delivery of medication to targeted areas.

Transdermal System. The transdermal system of medication delivery consists of a small adhesive patch that may be applied to intact skin near the treatment site. For example, Transderm Scop® used for preventing motion sickness, may be applied behind the ear; Nitro-Dur® (Figure 23-9), used for preventing angina pectoris, may be applied to the chest; Estraderm®, used to treat menopausal symptoms, may be applied to the trunk, and Nicoderm®, used to relieve the body's craving for nicotine, may be applied to any area above the waist. A transdermal system generally consists of four layers (Figure 23-10):

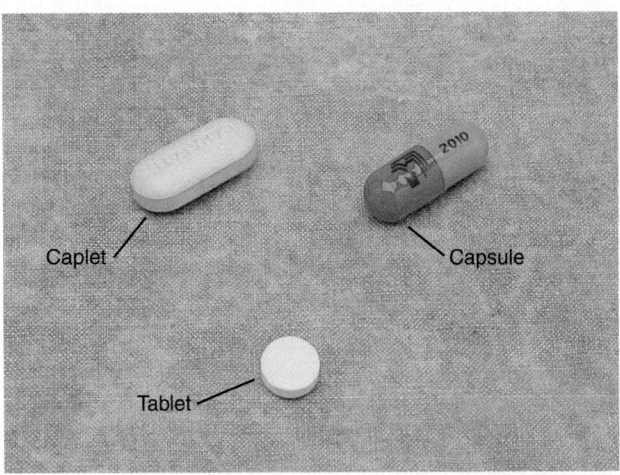

Figure 23-8 Drugs are manufactured in various forms, including solid preparations like this caplet, capsule, and tablet.

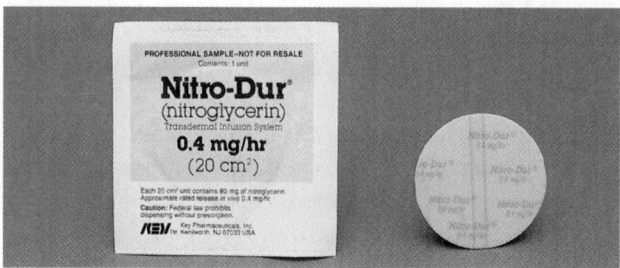

Figure 23-9 Nitro-Dur® is a transdermal system of delivering medication used for preventing and for long-term management of angina pectoris. It may be applied to the chest.

1. An impermeable backing that keeps the drug from leaking out of the system
2. A reservoir containing the drug
3. A membrane with tiny holes that controls the rate of drug release
4. An adhesive layer or gel that keeps the device in place

Eye-Curing Lens. Another innovative drug delivery system is one in which a drug, contained between two ultrathin plastic membranes, is placed inside the lower eyelid. It appears to cause little or no discomfort and provides a controlled release of the medication for an extended period of time. Pilocarpine, a miotic that causes contraction of the pupils, is being used in this method for the treatment of glaucoma.

Implantable Devices. These devices are available in several shapes and sizes and are positioned just beneath the skin near blood vessels that lead directly to the area to be medicated. For example, an infusion pump that is about the size of a hockey puck can be implanted below the skin near the waist to provide continuous delivery of chemotherapy to patients with liver cancer. This device, which has a refillable drug reservoir, is connected by an outlet catheter to the patient's blood vessel. In addition to providing a continuous supply of medication, these devices have the advantage of delivering higher doses with fewer side effects than can be realized through the systemic route.

STORAGE AND HANDLING OF MEDICATIONS

Certain precautions should be followed if the ambulatory care setting keeps medications on the premises. The goal should be to store all medications in their original containers in a separate room in a locked cabinet. Many medications require storage in a certain manner, such as a dark area or in a dark container (to keep light away from them) or in the refrigerator. Some must be kept in glass containers only because

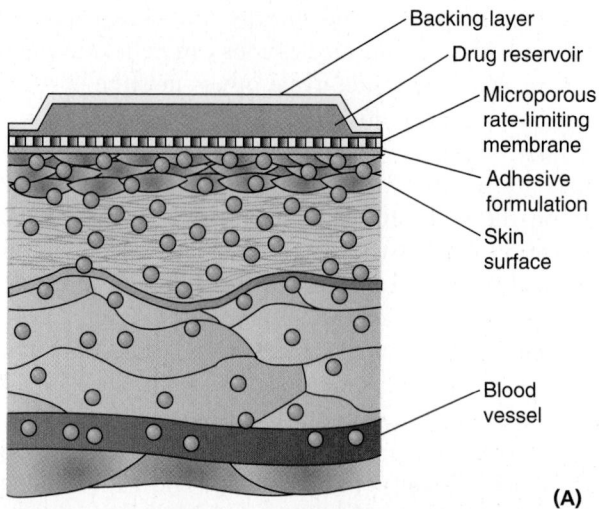

Backing layer
Drug reservoir
Microporous rate-limiting membrane
Adhesive formulation
Skin surface

Blood vessel

(A)

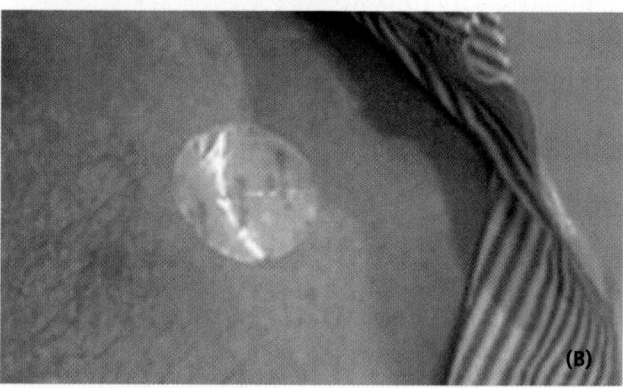

(B)

Figure 23-10 (A) The multilayer unit comprising Transderm-Nitro® delivers nitroglycerin into the bloodstream in a consistent, controlled manner for 24 hours. The very thin unit contains a backing layer, a reservoir of nitroglycerin, a unique rate-limiting membrane, and an adhesive layer that has a priming dose of nitroglycerin. (B) The patch is applied to the skin. (Courtesy of CIBA Pharmaceutical Company)

plastic may react with the medication's chemical composition. The drug label indicates proper storage and handling for each medication.

Keep medications that are for internal use separated from those intended for external use.

Access to medications is simplified if they are organized in the storage area either according to their classification (diuretic, hormones) or according to the alphabet.

EMERGENCY DRUGS AND SUPPLIES

The ambulatory care setting should maintain a tray, box, cabinet, or crash cart (see Chapter 9) especially and solely for drugs and supplies needed in an emergency such as anaphylaxis or other form of shock. The drugs listed in Table 23-2 are a sample of some general drugs to keep readily available for emergencies.

TABLE 23-2	EXAMPLES OF COMMON EMERGENCY DRUGS

Adrenalin (a-dren'a-lin) or **epinephrine** (ep-i-nef-rin)
A vasoconstrictor. Relieves anaphylactic shock.

Aminophylline (am-in-off'ilin)
A bronchodilator. Relaxes smooth muscle of the respiratory tract.

Benadryl (ben'a-dril)
An antihistamine that relieves allergic symptoms.

Compazine (com-pa'zeen)
An antiemetic. Relieves symptoms of nausea and vomiting.

Dextrose (deks'trose) 50%
Used for hypoglycemia to counteract hyperinsulinism.

Digoxin (di-jox'in)
Cardiac drug. Used for congestive heart failure, arryhthmias. Slows and strengthens heartbeat.

Diuril (di'ur-il)
Promotes excretion of urine.

Hydrocortisone (hi"dro-cort'i-zon)
An anti-inflammatory. Used to suppress swelling and shock.

Ipecac Syrup (i'pe-kak)
Emetic. Used to induce vomiting in certain types of poisonings.

Narcan (nar'can)
Antidote. Used in narcotic overdose.

Nitroglycerin (ni"tro-glis'er-in)
Vasodilator. Dilates coronary arteries. Used in treatment of angina pectoris.

Valium (val'e-um)
Antianxiety, muscle relaxant. Used to calm very anxious patients and to relax muscles. Valium is a Schedule IV drug and therefore must be kept in a locked cabinet.

Other supplies and equipment to keep along with the drugs on the emergency cart are:

- Intravenous materials such as IV fluids, needles, syringes, alcohol, swabs, constriction band, and tape
- Sphygmomanometer
- Stethoscope
- Oxygen and mask
- Airways
- Defibrillator
- Suction equipment (nasopharyngeal)

Check the tray on a regular basis (weekly, monthly, depending on use) according to need. Check the oxygen tank and gauge. Replace items that have been used as soon as possible and discard drugs and supplies that have reached their expiration dates. Document that the tray has been checked and updated. (See Chapter 9 for more information about emergencies in the office and other ambulatory areas.)

DRUG ABUSE

  There has been an enormous increase in the **abuse**, or misuse, of legal and illegal drugs. Any drug can be abused, whether it is penicillin, alcohol, or a controlled substance such as cocaine. Medical assistants, while caring for patients, may unexpectedly come in contact with patients who abuse or misuse drugs.

Medical assistants must be able to recognize the symptoms of drug abuse in a patient or coworker and report it to the physician. Health professionals including physicians are among the individuals who may have a problem with drug or alcohol abuse and this must be reported to the proper professional association. Refer to Chapter 7 for more information on drug abuse.

There are many programs available for treatment of drug abuse. Detoxification and rehabilitation are examples of treatment programs.

Following are examples of drug types most commonly abused:

- Marijuana, LSD ("acid"), Mescaline
- Narcotics: Cocaine, Heroin
- Amphetamines: Dexedrine®, Ritalin®
- Depressants: Valium®, alcohol
- Barbiturates ("barbs," "downers," "red devils") Nembutal®, Seconal®

Effects of Drug Abuse

When an individual is directly under the influence of a particular substance, acute effects of drug abuse are evident. For example, the acute effects of amphetamines may include symptoms that affect the central nervous system, such as euphoria, excitement, anorexia, or insomnia. Dilated pupils, nervousness, talkativeness, agitation, tachycardia, fever, and chills are other symptoms of amphetamine abuse.

As an abused substance, cocaine is usually sniffed or snorted into the nose or smoked in a form called crack or freebase. It is absorbed through the mucous membrane. Effects begin within a few minutes and then subside within an hour. Dilated pupils, elevated blood pressure, tachycardia, and increased body temperature are symptoms of the acute effects of cocaine. Euphoria and excitement are probable reasons for its high abuse potential. Death comes from respiratory and circulatory failure.

Barbiturates are used medically as sedatives to relieve anxiety. Abuse effects include slurred speech, confusion, poor motor coordination, and impaired judgment. Coma and death result from very high doses. Abrupt withdrawal can be fatal and symptoms include apprehension, weakness, tremors, delirium, and convulsions.

LSD (lyseric acid diethylamide) is a hallucinogenic agent with no medicinal benefit. It is an extremely potent drug causing altered perception and mood changes that range from euphoria to deep depression. Long-term use can cause chromosomal changes and prolonged adverse psychological effects such as suicide attempts.

Marijuana is usually used by smoking it in the form of a hand-rolled cigarette. Feelings of euphoria, relaxation, and drowsiness are the primary effects of the drug. Individuals lose inhibitions and may exhibit inappropriate behavior, poor coordination, and poor judgment. Hallucinations are possible. Tachycardia, increased appetite, and decreased pulmonary function are other symptoms that can occur and aggravate existing medical conditions such as heart disease or hypertension. Although marijuana has been shown to have some limited medicinal uses, in most states it remains classified as a Schedule I drug under the Federal Controlled Substance Act.

The same social pressures that influence young people to try alcohol are responsible for introducing people of all ages to the previously mentioned drugs and other chemical substances. Because it is easier to prevent drug abuse than it is to break an established habit, most efforts to combat drug abuse are directed at the young. However, people of all ages, including older people, may be or become abusers.

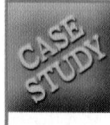

CASE STUDY 23-1

Maria Jover complains of vaginal discharge and discomfort. Dr. King confirms the diagnosis of a yeast infection by performing a smear and identifying the microorganism. Dr. King prescribes over-the-counter vaginal suppositories. After asking Maria if she has any questions, medical assistant Audrey Jones proceeds to help Maria understand the self-administration of this particular medication.

CASE STUDY REVIEW

1. The patient, Maria, asks Audrey Jones whether she can use some vaginal suppositories she bought last year. How should Audrey respond?

2. Maria tells Audrey that the last time she had a vaginal yeast infection she only used part of the recommended number of suppositories because the infection cleared up. How should Audrey respond?

3. Maria does not really like using suppositories. Should Audrey ask Dr. King to prescribe another form of medication for the yeast infection? What other forms might be available?

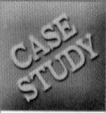

CASE STUDY 23-2

Dr. Lewis keeps a small quantity of various controlled substances on the premises for use in an emergency situation.

CASE STUDY REVIEW

1. What are the legalities that surround controlled substances in so far as Joe Guerrero, the medical assistant, is concerned?

2. What are his responsibilities?

SUMMARY

Medical assistants must know state and federal laws that govern the distribution and administration of medications and understand their role and responsibilities in light of these laws. Knowledge of drug regulations, the legal classifications of drugs including controlled substances, and prescribing, administering, and dispensing of drugs is essential to ensure compliance with the law.

Available resources and reference books will provide valuable information about pharmaceutical products, their classifications, routes, forms, storage and handling, and side effects.

Emergency drugs and supplies should be available on a crash cart or a tray or cabinet for the sole use in an office emergency.

With the increase of drug abuse and misuse, it is important for medical assistants to recognize the signs of drug abuse in patients and coworkers and to report abuse to the physician or supervisor.

REVIEW QUESTIONS

Multiple Choice

1. Which of the following drugs is commonly used in an emergency such as anaphylactic shock?
   a. lomotil
   b. interferon
   c. cytoxan
   d. epinephrine
2. Which of the following types of drugs do physicians prescribe most frequently?
   a. generic
   b. official
   c. chemical
   d. brand
3. An example of a drug that can be obtained from an animal is:
   a. digitalis
   b. insulin
   c. imferon
   d. sulfur
4. Which of the following is an example of a controlled substance?
   a. Nembutal
   b. Keflin
   c. Inderal
   d. Aldomet
5. After you have poured a medication and taken it to the patient, he refuses to take it. You should:
   a. give it to another patient who has the same medication prescribed
   b. return the refused medication to its original container
   c. save it for the next time the patient is due for another dose
   d. dispose of it down the sink and document

Critical Thinking

1. Drugs are derived from various sources. List five sources of drugs.
2. How does the Federal Food, Drug, and Cosmetic Act protect the public?
3. The _____ is recognized by the United States government as the official list of standardized drugs.
4. Describe the principal factors that affect drug action.
5. While preparing an injection of Demerol® (meperidine), you accidentally drop and break the ampule spilling its contents. Describe what actions you would take.

6. Name five emergency drugs that may be found on a crash cart or emergency tray. Describe the use and actions of each.
7. Under what circumstances can a medical assistant dispense stock medication?
8. Audrey Jones is considering taking a new position with a physician who is opening an office in another state. Audrey will be responsible for the clinical aspect of the practice. Where can Audrey find information about laws that apply to her in regard to administering medications? Where can she get information about the storage and handling on the premises of narcotics?
9. List several drug references and briefly describe the contents of the PDR.
10. After lunch, a newly hired medical assistant is helping you get Lenore McDonell back into her wheelchair following her physical examination. You strongly suspect that the medical assistant has been drinking alcohol because she is uncoordinated in her movements and there is a strong odor of what seems to be alcohol on her breath. Describe your next action.

WEB ACTIVITIES

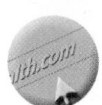

Explore on the Internet for information regarding the Drug Enforcement Agency.

1. Print a copy of Schedules I-V of the controlled substances.

REFERENCES/BIBLIOGRAPHY

Bonewit-West, K. (2000). *Clinical procedures for medical assistants* (5th ed.). Philadelphia: W. B. Saunders Company.

Physicians' desk reference. (2000). Montvale, NJ: Medical Economics.

Prickett-Ramutkowski, B., Barrie, A. T., Keller, C., Dazarow, L., & Abel, C. (1999). *Glencoe medical assisting: A patient-centered approach to administrative and clinical competencies.* New York: Glencoe/McGraw-Hill.

Rice, J. (1999). *Principles of pharmacology for medical assisting* (3rd ed.). Albany, NY: Delmar.

Taber's cyclopedic medical dictionary (18th ed.). (1999). Philadelphia: F. A. Davis Company.

Zakus, S. (2001). *Mosby's clinical skills for medical assistants* (4th ed.). St. Louis: Mosby-Year Book.

KEY TERMS

Administering

Apnea

BSA

Compounding

Dispensing

Hypoxemia

Meniscus

Nomogram

Parenteral

Precipitate

Retrolental Fibroplasia

Status Asthmaticus

Taut

Unit Dose

OUTLINE

Legal and Ethical Implications of Medication Administration
Ethical Considerations
The Medication Order
The Prescription
Drug Dosage
Age
Weight
Gender
Other Factors
The Medication Label
Calculation of Drug Dosages
Understanding Ratio
Understanding Proportion
Weights and Measures
Medications Measured in Units
How to Calculate Unit Dosages
Insulin
Diabetes
Calculating Adult Dosages
The Proportional Method
The Formula Method
Calculating Children's Dosages
Body Surface Area
Kilogram of Body Weight
Administration of Medications
The "Six Rights" of Proper Drug Administration

Medication Error
Patient Assessment
Administration of Oral Medications
Equipment and Supplies for Oral Medications
Administration of Parenteral Medications
Hazards Associated with Parenteral Medications
Reasons for Parenteral Route Selection
Parenteral Equipment and Supplies
Site Selection and Injection Angle
Marking the Correct Site for Intramuscular Injection
Basic Guidelines for Administration of Injections
Z-Track Method of Intramuscular Injection
Administration of Allergenic Extracts
Inhalation Methods of Medication Administration
Implications for Patient Care
Administration of Oxygen

OBJECTIVES

The student should strive to meet the following performance objectives and demonstrate an understanding of the facts and principles presented in this chapter through written and oral communication.

1. Define the key terms as presented in the glossary.
2. Discuss the legal and ethical implications of medication administration.
3. Describe the medication order.
4. Describe the parts of a prescription.
5. Define drug dosage.
6. State what information is found on a medication label.
7. Understand ratio and proportion.
8. Use the metric, household, and apothecary systems of measurement and convert between metric and apothecary systems.
9. Understand units of medication dosage.
10. Correctly calculate adult and children's dosages.
11. List the guidelines to follow when preparing and administering medications.
12. Describe safe disposal of syringes, needles, and biohazard materials.
13. Describe site selection for administration of injections.
14. Understand allergenic extracts.
15. Describe inhalation medication and its administration.

ROLE DELINEATION COMPONENTS

CLINICAL

Fundamental Principles

- Apply principles of aseptic technique and infection control
- Comply with quality assurance practices

Patient Care

- Prepare patient for examinations, procedures, and treatments
- Assist with examinations, procedures, and treatments
- Prepare and administer medications and immunizations
- Maintain medication and immunization records

(continues)

SCENARIO

At Doctors Lewis & King, office policy dictates that a medicine card must be written out prior to the administration of any medication to a patient. Clinical medical assistant Joe Guerrero, CMA, is very careful to check the physician's order, then prepare the medicine card before preparing and administering medication. He notes that the card contains the patient's name, the physician's order, and the date, time, and route the medication is to be administered. After giving the medication to the patient, Joe documents the fact in the patient file and then, according to procedure, tears up the medicine card.

INTRODUCTION

Despite the fact that many ambulatory care centers use what is known as the unit dose type of medication preparation, there remains a responsibility for medical assistants to know and understand how to calculate dosages of medication and to safely administer them to patients.

This chapter addresses calculation of adult and pediatric dosages of medication using the metric and apothecaries' systems. It also emphasizes the legal aspects of medication administration and discusses oral and parenteral medication administration.

ROLE DELINEATION
COMPONENTS (*continued*)

GENERAL
(TRANDISCIPLINARY)

Legal Concepts

- Document accurately
- Follow federal, state, and local legal guidelines
- Maintain awareness of federal and state health care legislation and regulations
- Maintain and dispose of regulated substances in compliance with government guidelines
- Comply with established risk management and safety procedures

LEGAL AND ETHICAL IMPLICATIONS OF MEDICATION ADMINISTRATION

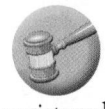 Members of the health care profession who prepare and administer medications are ethically and legally responsible for their own actions. Under law, these individuals are required to be licensed, registered, or otherwise authorized by a physician.

Each state has enacted laws governing the practice of medicine, nursing, and pharmacy. These laws vary from state to state; therefore, it is essential that medical assistants become familiar with the laws of the state in which they are employed before administering any medication. In some states, the only health professional authorized to give injections, other than a physician, is the registered nurse. In other states, legislation gives physicians broad authority to delegate responsibility for administering medication to other health care workers such as medical assistants. Laws have been passed in some states specifying which qualified and properly educated and trained persons may perform certain medical acts.

Regardless of the differences in state authorization laws, the courts will not permit the careless action of health care workers to go unpunished, especially when such actions result in harm or death to the patient. Under the law, those administering medications are expected to be knowledgeable about the drugs that they administer and the effects the drug(s) may and/or will have on the patient. Never administer a medication without thorough knowledge of the drug. It is the medical assistant's responsibility to know the information about a medication listed in Figure 24-1 before administering it to a patient.

Ethical Considerations

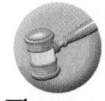 Anyone who has access to medications may be tempted to use them for personal benefit. To do so is not only unethical, it is considered to be illegal. The conversion to personal use of medications intended for another is unethical and may cause harm to the patient. It is also unethical and illegal to take any medication that belongs to your employer, even aspirin or drug samples, without proper authorization.

The Medication Order

The medication order is given by the physician. It is for a specific patient and denotes the drug to be given, the dosage, the form of the drug, the time for or frequency of administration, and the route by which the drug is to be given.

The Prescription

The prescription is a written legal document that gives directions for compounding, dispensing, and administering a medication to a patient. There are nine parts to a prescription (Figure 24-2).

The purpose of a prescription is to control the sale and use of drugs that can be safely and effectively used only under the supervision of a licensed physician. Federal law divides medicines into two main classes: prescription medicines and over-the-counter (OTC) medicines. The prescription is written by the physician and signed with an ink pen. The pharmacist fills the prescription according to the physician's order. Once the prescription has been filled, the assigned prescription number and all other information may be entered into a computer. The hard copy of the prescription is filed and kept for a minimum of seven years. Schedule II controlled substances prescriptions (see Chapter 23) are kept separate from other prescriptions and are

---

1. Drug name (generic and brand)
2. Action
3. Uses
4. Contraindications
5. Warnings when indicated
6. Adverse reactions
7. Dosage and route
8. Implications for patient care
9. Patient teaching
10. Special considerations

Figure 24-1 Medical assistants should have a thorough knowledge of any medication they administer to a patient and should consult references such as the *Physician's Desk Reference (PDR)*.

Parts of a Prescription

1. The physician's name, address, telephone number, and registration number.
2. The patient's name, address, and the date on which the prescription is written.
3. The *superscription* that includes the symbol Rx ("take thou").
4. The *inscription* that states the names and quantities of ingredients to be included in the medication.
5. The *subscription* that gives directions to the pharmacist for filling the prescription.
6. The *signature* (Sig) that gives the directions for the patient.
7. The physician's signature blanks. Where signed, indicates if a generic substitute is allowed or if the medication is to be dispensed as written.
8. REPETATUR 0 1 2 3 p.r.n. This is where the physician indicates whether or not the prescription can be refilled.
9. □ LABEL Direction to the pharmacist to label the medication appropriately.

[1]
[2]
[3]
[4]
[5]
[6]
[7]
[8]
[9]

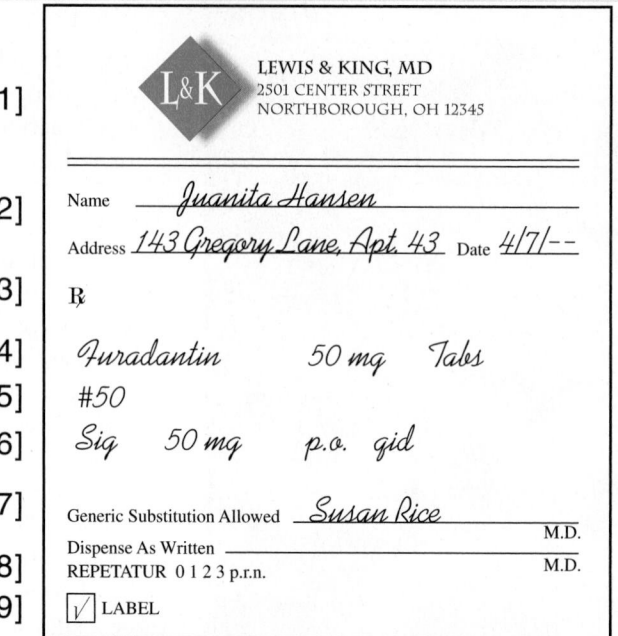

Figure 24-2   Prescriptions are written legal documents that give directions for compounding, dispensing, and administering a medication. Prescriptions have nine distinct elements.

stamped with a red C. Schedule III through V prescriptions are stamped with a red C and filed.

Prescriptions for Controlled Substances.
Federal laws require that specific procedures be followed by the physician when prescribing controlled substances. See Table 24-1.

All prescriptions for controlled substances must be dated and signed on the date issued, bearing the full name and address of the patient and the name, address, and DEA number (see Chapter 23) of the physician. The prescription must be written in ink or typewritten and signed by the physician's own hand.

Prescription Abbreviations and Symbols.
It is important to be knowledgeable of the most common abbreviations used by the physician when an order for a prescription drug is given. The abbreviations are a clear and concise means of writing orders. This medical shorthand is an international language used by professional and nonprofessional people involved with patient care. All abbreviations in Table 24-2 should be memorized to enable medical assistants to prepare medications safely and accurately for administration.

DRUG DOSAGE

The dosage or dose is the amount of medicine that is prescribed for administration. It is determined by the physician or qualified practitioner who considers the following important factors: age, weight, gender, and other factors as well.

Age

The usual adult dose is generally suitable for the 20 to 60 age group. Infants, young children, adolescents, and the elderly require an individualized dosage regimen.

Weight

The average adult dosage is based upon 150 pounds (about 68 kilograms). Individuals who weigh less or more

TABLE 24-1	REQUIREMENTS FOR PRESCRIPTIONS FOR CONTROLLED SUBSTANCES		
	Verbal Order or Prescription	**Written Prescription**	**Refills**
Schedule I	NOT FOR MEDICINAL USE		
Schedule II	no	yes	no
Schedule III	yes	yes	5× or 6 months
Schedule IV	yes	yes	5× or 6 months
Schedule V	yes	yes	yes

TABLE 24-2	COMMON PRESCRIPTION ABBREVIATIONS AND SYMBOLS
Abbreviation or Symbol	**Meaning**
aa	of each
ac	before meals
AD	right ear
ad lib	as desired
AS	left ear
aq	water
AU	both ears
bid	twice a day
c	with
cc	cubic centimeter
caps	capsules
dil	dilute
ʒ	dram
elix	elixir
Gm	gram
gr	grain
gt or gtt	drop (drops)
h	hour
hs	at bedtime
IM	intramuscular
IU	international units
IV	intravenous
kg	kilogram
L	liter
liq	liquid
m or min	minim
mg	milligram
ml or ML	milliliter
mm	millimeter
NPO	nothing by mouth
non rep	do not repeat
OD	right eye
OS	left eye
OU	both eyes
℥	ounce
pc	after meals
per	by or with
po	by mouth
prn	as needed
pt	patient
q	every
qd	every day
qh	every hour
q (2, 3, 4) h	every (2, 3, 4) hours
qid	four times a day
qod	every other day
qs	of sufficient quantity
Rx	take
s	without
sc	subcutaneous
sol	solution
ss	one-half
stat	at once
tab	tablet
Tbs	tablespoon
tsp	teaspoon
tid	three times a day
tr	tincture
ung	ointment

than this should have the dosage based upon **BSA** (body surface area) or kilogram of body weight.

Gender

Many medications are contraindicated during pregnancy and breastfeeding. It is important that these two factors be known before any dose of medication is prescribed.

Other Factors

There are other factors that determine the dosage of a medication including:

1. Physical and emotional condition of patient
2. Disease process, especially kidney disease because of impaired excretion
3. Presence of more than one disease process
4. Causative microorganism(s) and the severity of the infection
5. Patient's past medical history, allergies, and idiosyncrasies
6. The safest method, route, time, and amount to effect the desired maximum result

THE MEDICATION LABEL

The medication label can be a source of valuable information to medical assistant and patient. Regardless of whether administering a prescription drug or taking a nonprescription product, an understanding of the information provided on the label is essential to the safe and effective use of any medicine. In addition to the name and address of the manufacturer, other important items of information on a medication label include:

- The trade or brand name for the medication
- The generic name (or listing of active and inactive ingredients)
- The National Drug Code (NDC) numbers that can be used to identify the manufacturer, the product, and the size of the container
- The dosage strength in a given amount of the medication
- The usual dosage and frequency of administration
- The route of administration
- Precautions and warnings
- The expiration date for the medication

Other information that may be on a medication label includes directions for storage and directions for mixing or reconstituting a powdered form of the drug. (See Figure 24-3.)

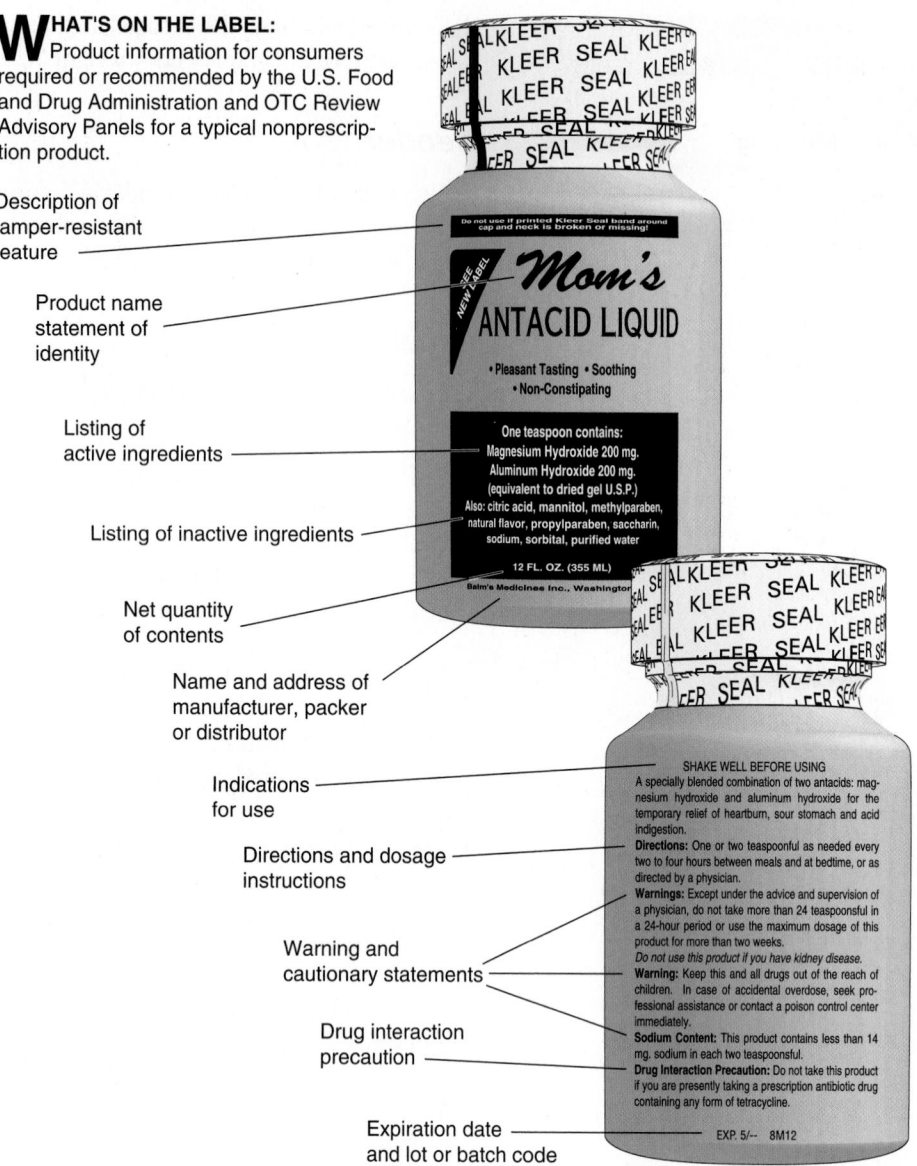

WHAT'S ON THE LABEL:
Product information for consumers required or recommended by the U.S. Food and Drug Administration and OTC Review Advisory Panels for a typical nonprescription product.

Description of tamper-resistant feature

Product name statement of identity

Listing of active ingredients

Listing of inactive ingredients

Net quantity of contents

Name and address of manufacturer, packer or distributor

Indications for use

Directions and dosage instructions

Warning and cautionary statements

Drug interaction precaution

Expiration date and lot or batch code

Figure 24-3 Medication labels contain valuable information essential to the safe and effective use of the drug.

CALCULATION OF DRUG DOSAGES

The preparation and administration of medications is one of the most important and critical tasks that medical assistants perform. Today, drugs are more potent and more likely to cause physiological changes in the body; therefore, anyone who administers medications must do so with extreme care.

Incorrectly calculated or measured dosages are the leading cause of error in the administration of medications. A drug error is a violation of a patient's rights. It is important that medical assistants develop a working knowledge of mathematics in order to calculate or measure accurately a medication that is to be administered to a patient.

Understanding Ratio

Ratio is a method of expressing the relationship of a number, quantity, substance, or degree between two similar components. For example, the relationship of one to five is written 1:5. Note that numbers are side by side and separated by a colon.

In mathematics, a ratio may be expressed as a quotient, a fraction, or a decimal.

Ratio Expressed as a Quotient. A quotient is the number found when one number is divided by another number. The ratio one to five written as a quotient is $1 \div 5$.

Ratio Expressed as a Fraction. A fraction is the process of dividing or breaking a whole number into parts. The ratio one to five written as a fraction is $\frac{1}{5}$.

Ratio Expressed as a Decimal. A decimal is a linear array of numbers based upon ten or any multiple of ten. To express the ratio one to five as a decimal, divide the denominator (5) into the numerator (1).

$$\text{(denominator)} \quad 5\overline{)1.0}^{\,0.2} \quad \text{(numerator)}$$

The ratio may be expressed as:

A *quotient*	A *fraction*	A *decimal*
$1 \div 5$	⅕	0.2

Understanding Proportion

Proportion is a process of expressing the comparative relationship between a part, share, or portion with regard to size, amount, or number. In mathematics, a proportion expresses the relationship between two ratios. In setting up a proportion, the ratios are separated by : or an = sign. In this text, the equal sign (=) is used to separate ratios.

Example: $3 : 4 = 1 : 2$
Read: Three is to four equals one is to two.

The four terms of a proportion are given special names. The *means* are the inner numbers or the second and third terms of the proportion.

Example: $3 : 4 = 1 : 2$ (4)   (1)
                        means

The *extremes* are the outer numbers or the first and fourth terms of the proportion.

Example: $3 : 4 = 1 : 2$ (3)   (2)
                        extremes

In a true proportion, the product of the means equals the product of the extremes.

Example: *means*   (16)   (1)
                  $8 : 16 = 1 : 2$
        extremes   (8)   (2)
                $16 \times 1 = 16$ (*means*)
                $8 \times 2 = 16$ (*extremes*)

Solving for X. The proportion is a very useful mathematical tool. When a part, share, or portion of the problem is unknown, then *x* represents the unknown factor. You can determine the unknown by solving for *x*. The unknown factor *x* may appear any place in the proportion.
     Now solve for *x* in the problem: $3 : 4 = x : 12$.

1. Multiply the terms that contain the x and place the product to the left of the equal sign (4x).

2. Multiply the other terms and place the product to the right of the equal sign (36).
3. To find *x*, divide the product of *x* into the product of the other terms.

$$4x = 36$$
$$x = \frac{36}{4} \text{ or } 36 \div 4$$
$$x = 9$$

After finding the unknown factor, check your mathematical skills by determining if you have a true proportion. This technique is called proof or proving your answer. To prove your answer:

1. Place the answer you found for *x* back into the formula where *x* was.

$$3 : 4 = 9 : 12$$

2. Now multiply the means by the means, and the extremes by the extremes.
3. The results will equal each other.

Formula: $3 : 4 = x : 12$

Proof: $3 : 4 = 9 : 12$

                $4 \times 9 = 36$
                $3 \times 12 = 36$

Weights and Measures

There are three systems of measurement used in pharmacology to calculate dosage. These systems are metric, household, and apothecary. The metric system is used throughout the world as the official language of communication in scientific and technical fields. It is based upon the decimal system: the number 10 or multiples of 10.

Metric System Guidelines. The following guidelines are helpful when learning basic facts about the metric system:

1. Arabic numbers are used to designate whole numbers; e.g., 1, 250, 500, 1000.
2. Decimal fractions are used for quantities less than one; e.g., 0.1, 0.01, 0.001, 0.0001.
3. To ensure accuracy, place a zero before the decimal point; e.g., 0.1, 0.001, 0.0001.
4. The Arabic number precedes the metric unit of measurement; e.g., 10 grams, 2 millimeters, 5 liters.
5. The abbreviation for gram should be capitalized (Gm) or written as (g) to distinguish it from grain (gr).
6. The abbreviation for liter is capitalized (L).

7. Prefixes are written in lowercase letters; e.g., milli, centi, deci, deka.
8. Capitalize the measurement and symbol when it is named after a person; e.g., Celsius (C).
9. Periods are no longer used with most abbreviations or symbols.
10. Abbreviations for units are the same for singular and plural. An "s" is not added to an abbreviation to indicate a plural.

The Seven Common Metric Prefixes. It is important to know common metric prefixes to have a solid foundation for determining metric equivalents. When a metric prefix is combined with a root of physical quantity, you arrive at multiples or submultiples of the metric system.

Example:

- **milli** (prefix): one-thousandth of a unit
  meter (root): a measure of length
  millimeter: one-thousandth of a meter

- **kilo** (prefix): one thousand units
  liter (root): a measure of volume
  kiloliter: one thousand liters

- **micro** (prefix): one-millionth of a unit
  gram (root): a measure of mass and/or weight
  microgram: one-millionth of a gram

Prefixes:

micro (mi'kro)	=	one millionth of a unit written as 0.000001
milli (mil'i)	=	one-thousandth of a unit written as 0.001
centi (sen'ti)	=	one-hundredth of a unit written as 0.01
deci (des'i)	=	one-tenth of a unit written as 0.1
deka (dek'a)	=	ten units written as 10
hecto (hek'to)	=	one hundred units written as 100
kilo (kil'o)	=	one thousand units written as 1000

Fundamental Units:

Following are the fundamental units of the metric system:

meter (m)	length
liter (L)	volume
gram (Gm, g)	mass and/or weight

The meter is the fundamental unit of length in the metric system and originally formed the foundation for the entire system. A meter is equal to 39.37 inches, which is slightly more than a yard, or 3.28 feet.

A millimeter is about the width of the head of a pin. It takes approximately 2½ centimeters to make an inch; a decimeter is approximately 4 inches.

Meter (m)	=	Length
1 millimeter (mm)	=	0.001 meter
1 centimeter (cm)	=	0.01 meter
1 decimeter (dm)	=	0.1 meter
1 meter (m)	=	1 meter
1 dekameter (dam)	=	10 meters
1 hectometer (hm)	=	100 meters
1 kilometer (km)	=	1000 meters

The liter is the metric unit of volume. A liter is equal to 1.056 quarts, which is 0.26 gallon or 2.1 pints.

A milliliter is equivalent to one cubic centimeter (cc), because the amount of space occupied by a milliliter is equal to one cubic centimeter. The weight of one milliliter of water equals approximately one gram. It takes approximately 15 milliliters to make 1 tablespoon. It takes 15 or 16 minims to make one milliliter.

Liter (L)		Volume
1 milliliter (mL)	=	0.001 liter
1 centiliter (cL)	=	0.01 liter
1 deciliter (dL)	=	0.1 liter
1 liter (L)	=	1 liter
1 dekaliter (daL)	=	10 liters
1 hectoliter (hL)	=	100 liters
1 kiloliter (kL)	=	1000 liters

The gram is the metric unit of mass and/or weight. It equals approximately the weight of 1 cubic centimeter or 1 milliliter of water. A gram is equal to approximately 15 grains or 0.035 ounce.

Gram (Gm, g)		Mass and/or Weight
1 microgram (μg)	=	0.000001 gram
1 milligram (mg)	=	0.001 gram
1 centigram (cg)	=	0.01 gram
1 decigram (dg)	=	0.1 gram
1 gram (Gm, g)	=	1 gram
1 dekagram (dag)	=	10 grams
1 hectogram (hg)	=	100 grams
1 kilogram (kg)	=	1000 grams

The metric equivalents most frequently used in the medical field are:

Length	Volume
2½ centimeters (cm) = 1 inch	1000 milliliters (mL) or 1000 cubic centimeters (cc) = 1 liter (L)

Weight

1000 micrograms (μcg)	=	1 milligram (mg)
1000 milligrams (mg)	=	1 gram (Gm, g)
1000 grams (Gm, g)	=	1 kilogram (kg)
1 kilogram	=	2.2 pounds (lb)

TABLE 24-3 COMMON HOUSEHOLD MEASURES

Drop (gt) = approximate liquid measure depending on kind of liquid measured and the size of the opening from which it is dropped.

60 drops (gtt)	is equal to:	1 teaspoon (t or tsp)
1 dash	is equal to:	Less than ⅛ teaspoon
3 teaspoons (tsp)	is equal to:	1 tablespoon (T or tbsp)
2 tablespoons (tbsp)	is equal to:	1 ounce (oz)
4 ounces (oz)	is equal to:	1 juice glass
6 ounces (oz)	is equal to:	1 teacup
8 ounces (oz)	is equal to:	1 glass or cup
16 tablespoons or 8 ounces	is equal to:	1 measuring cup (c)
2 cups (c)	is equal to:	1 pint (pt)
2 pints (pt)	is equal to:	1 quart (qt)
4 quarts (qt)	is equal to:	1 gallon (gal)

Household Measurements. Household measurements are approximate measurements. They are more frequently used in the home than in the medical field, but the medical assistant should be familiar with the common household measurements listed in Table 24-3.

Apothecary Measurements. Apothecary measurements are rarely used today, but there are still some medications ordered in grains, drams, and minims; therefore, it is important that medical assistants learn some basic apothecary equivalents as listed in Table 24-4. Note that some of the apothecary measurements are also household measures. However, in the apothecary system, 12 ounces is equal to 1 pound; in the household system, 16 ounces is equal to 1 pound.

Because medications can be prescribed in either metric, apothecary, or household measurements, it is important

TABLE 24-4 BASIC APOTHECARY MEASUREMENTS

Apothecary Units of Weight

60 grains (gr)	is equal to	1 dram (dr)
8 drams (dr)	is equal to	1 ounce (oz)
12 ounces (oz)	is equal to	1 pound (lb)

Apothecary Units of Liquid Volume

60 minims (m)	is equal to	1 fluidram (fldr)
8 fluidrams (fldr)	is equal to	1 fluid ounce (fl oz)
16 fluid ounces (fl oz)	is equal to	1 pint
2 pints (pt)	is equal to	1 quart
4 quarts (qt)	is equal to	1 gallon (gal)

TABLE 24-5 APPROXIMATE EQUIVALENTS AMONG METRIC, APOTHECARY, AND HOUSEHOLD SYSTEMS

Metric	Apothecary	Household
DRY		
60 mg	1 gr	
1 Gm	15 gr	¼ tsp
15 Gm	4 dr	1 tbsp (3 tsp)
30 Gm	1 oz	1 oz (2 tbsp)
	12 oz	1 lb (16 oz)
1 kg		2.2 lb
LIQUID		
	1 m	1 gt
1 mL (1 cubic centimeter)	15 m	15 gtt
5 mL	1 fldr	1 tsp
15 mL	4 fldr	1 tbsp (3 tsp)
30 mL	1 oz (8 fldr)	1 fl oz (2 tbs)
500 mL	(1 pt)	(1 pt or 2 cups)
1000 mL	(1 qt or 2 pts)	4 cups (1 qt)
LENGTH		
2.5 cm		1 in
1 m		39.37 in

to know equivalents among all three in order to calculate the dose of prescribed medication. See Table 24-5.

Metric System Conversion. The process of changing into another form, state, substance, or product is known as conversion. In the metric system, changing from one unit to another involves multiplying or dividing by 10, 100, 1000, and so forth. This can be done by the proportional method or by moving the decimal in the correct direction.

Proportional Method for Converting Metric Equivalents. There are six basic steps in the proportional method, plus an additional step to prove the answer. The following example will serve as a model for future applications of the proportional method of converting metric equivalents.

Example:
Convert 1500 milligrams to grams.

$$1500 \text{ mg} = _____ \text{ Gm, g}$$

Step 1. Since the unknown factor in the given formula is the number of grams contained in 1500 milligrams, substitute the symbol *x* for grams in the equation.

Step 2. Setting up the proportion requires that you know metric equivalents. For example, in this problem you have to know that 1000 milligrams (mg) = 1 gram (Gm, g).

Step 3. Since you know that 1000 mg is equal to 1 Gm, you can create one-half of the equation. Write the equivalent and place it on the left of the equal sign.

$$1000 \text{ mg} : 1 \text{ Gm} =$$

Step 4. Now that you have the left side of the equation, set up the right side by using the designated metric value 1500 mg : *x* Gm. Always write the smallest equivalent as to the largest equivalent, e.g., mg : Gm. By being consistent, it is less likely errors will occur.

$$1000 \text{ mg} : 1 \text{ Gm} = 1500 \text{ mg} : x \text{ Gm}$$

Step 5. Note that you have an equal equation:

$$\text{mg} : \text{Gm} = \text{mg} : \text{Gm}$$

The first values on either side of the equal sign are milligrams, and the second values on either side are grams.

Step 6. Now solve for the unknown (*x*) by multiplication and division. Multiply the means by the means and the extremes by the extremes. **NOTE:** Once the proportion is correctly set up, simply use the numbers as you multiply and divide.

$$1000 : 1 = 1500 : x$$

$$
\begin{aligned}
1000x &= 1500 \\
x &= 1500 \div 1000 \\
x &= 1.5
\end{aligned}
\qquad
\begin{aligned}
& 1.5 \\
1000 & \overline{)1500.0} \\
& \underline{1000} \\
& 500.0 \\
& \underline{500}
\end{aligned}
$$

Step 7. To make sure the answer is correct, prove the work: Place the answer 1.5 Gm into the formula where *x* once was. Now multiply the means by the means and the extremes by the extremes.

$$1000 \text{ mg} : 1 \text{ Gm} = 1500 \text{ mg} : 1.5 \text{ Gm}$$
$$1500 = 1500$$

MEDICATIONS MEASURED IN UNITS

Medications such as insulin, heparin, some antibiotics, hormones, vitamins, and vaccines are measured in units (U). These medications are standardized in units based on their strengths. The strength varies from one medicine to another, depending upon the source, condition, and method by which it is obtained.

How to Calculate Unit Dosages

When calculating medications that are ordered in units, use either the proportional method or the formula method.

The Proportional Method

Example:
The physician orders 4000 USP units of heparin given deep subcutaneously. On hand is heparin 500 USP units per milliliter.

Step 1. Use the following proportion to calculate the dose:

Known unit on hand		Known dosage form		Dose ordered		Unknown amount to be given
5000 U	:	1 mL	=	4000 U	:	*x* mL

$$
\begin{aligned}
5000x &= 4000 \\
x &= \tfrac{4}{5} = \tfrac{4}{5} \text{ mL or } 0.8 \text{ mL}
\end{aligned}
$$

Use a tuberculin syringe to draw up 0.8 mL, or convert ⅘ mL to minims.

Step 2. Convert ⅘ mL to minims. **NOTE:** There are 15 or 16 minims per milliliter.
Multiply:

$$\frac{4}{\overset{}{\underset{1}{\cancel{5}}}} \times \frac{\overset{3}{\cancel{15}}}{1} = \frac{4}{1} \times \frac{3}{1} = 12 \text{ minims}$$

Administer 12 minims (of 5000 U/ML for correct dose of 4000 units) to the patient.

The Formula Method

Example:
The physician orders 450,000 units of Bicillin 1M. On hand is Bicillin 600,000 units per milliliter.

Step 1. Use the following formula to calculate the dose:

$$\frac{\text{Dose ordered (desired)}}{\text{Dose on hand}} \times \text{Quantity} = \text{Amount to give}$$

$$\frac{450,000 \text{ U}}{600,000 \text{ U}} \times 1 \text{ mL} = \frac{\overset{3}{\cancel{450,000}}\text{U}}{\underset{4}{\cancel{600,000}}\text{U}} \times 1 \text{ mL} = \tfrac{3}{4} \text{ mL}$$

Step 2. You may convert to minims. If you do, multiply ¾ by 16.

$$\frac{3}{\underset{1}{\cancel{4}}} \times \frac{\overset{4}{\cancel{16}}}{1} = 12 \text{ minims}$$

The patient will receive 12 minims of Bicillin 600,000 U for the ordered dose of 450,000 U.

Insulin

Insulin is a chemical substance (hormone) secreted by the beta cells of the islets of Langerhans in the pancreas. Insulin is necessary for the proper metabolism of blood glucose and maintenance of the correct blood sugar level. Inadequate secretion of insulin, as in the disease diabetes mellitus, results in hyperglycemia and subsequent excessive production of ketone bodies. Eventual coma can ensue.

Patients' needs are individualized according to the severity of their disease; treatment includes taking insulin, controlling diet, and exercise. The diet is well-balanced and consists of the correct number of calories distributed among carbohydrates, fats, and proteins. Patients are taught to monitor blood and urine glucose levels at home throughout the day, for the dosage of insulin taken depends on the amounts of glucose detected. Uncontrolled diabetes mellitus can result in serious complications such as circulatory problems, especially in the feet and legs, bedsores, infection, and gangrene. Special care of the feet is essential. The mouth and teeth require excellent oral hygiene.

Diabetes

The National Diabetes Data Group of the National Institutes of Health organized the various forms of diabetes into the following categories:

Type I   Insulin-dependent diabetes mellitus (IDDM)
Type II   Noninsulin-dependent diabetes mellitus (NIDDM)
Type III Women who developed glucose intolerance in association with pregnancy

Patient Teaching Tip

Encourage patients with diabetes to enroll in diabetic education classes, which are offered at most local hospitals. Patients also need to realize that treatment of diabetes is a lifelong commitment and that they must abide by everything that the hospital teaches.

Type IV   Other types of diabetes associated with pancreatic disease, hormonal changes, adverse effects of drugs, or genetic or other anomalies.

Individuals with Type I diabetes must take insulin injections on a regular basis to maintain life. The dosage of insulin is expressed in units and is individualized by the physician for each patient. The amount of insulin that a person must take is based on blood and urine glucose levels, diet, exercise, and the individual's needs (Tables 24-6 and 24-7).

It is *extremely important* that the *exact dosage of insulin be taken by the patient.* Too little or too much insulin can cause serious problems ranging from a blood sugar level too low or too high, to coma, and even death. It may be the medical assistant's responsibility to administer insulin and/or to teach patients or their families how to administer insulin.

When administering insulin, the U-100 syringe (1 cc or LO-DOSE® ½ cc) is preferred. U-100 means there are 100 units of insulin per milliliter or cubic centimeter. Insulin dosage should always be expressed in units rather than in milliliters or cubic centimeters. For example, if the physician orders 30 units of U-100 NPH insulin, use a U-100 syringe and draw up 30 units of U-100 NPH insulin.

TABLE 24-6 RAPID-ACTING INSULIN: INSULIN PREPARATIONS U-100				
Rapid-Acting	**Onset of Action**	**Peak**	**Duration**	**Appearance**
Regular	½ hour	2½ to 5 hours	8 hours	Clear, colorless
Crystalline zinc	½ to 1 hour	2 to 4 hours	8 hours	Clear, colorless
Semilente	1½ hour	5 to 10 hours	16 hours	Cloudy
Humulin R	15 minutes	1 hour	6 to 8 hours	Clear, colorless
Mixtard	½ hour	4 to 8 hours	24 hours	Cloudy
Velosulin	½ hour	1 to 3 hours	8 hours	Clear
Novolin	½ hour	2½ to 5 hours	8 hours	Clear

TABLE 24-7   INTERMEDIATE-ACTING AND LONG-LASTING INSULIN: INSULIN PREPARATIONS U-100

	Onset of Action	Peak	Duration	Appearance
Intermediate-Acting				
NPH	½ hour	4 to 12 hours	24 hours	Cloudy
Lente	2½ hours	7 to 15 hours	24 hours	Cloudy
Insulatard NPH	½ hour	4 to 12 hours	24 hours	Cloudy
Novolin L	2½ hours	7 to 15 hours	22 hours	Cloudy
Novolin N	1½ hours	4 to 12 hours	24 hours	Cloudy
Humulin N	1 hour	4 hours	24 hours	Cloudy
Long-Acting				
Ultralente	4 hours	10 to 30 hours	36 hours	Cloudy
PZI (protamine zinc insulin)	4 to 8 hours	14 to 20 hours	36 hours	Cloudy

Precautions to Observe When Administering Insulin

- Be sure to use the proper insulin, the one ordered by the physician. Refer to Tables 24-6 and 24-7 for various insulin preparations.

- Do not substitute one insulin for another.

- Use the correct syringe, U-100.

- Dosage of insulin is always measured in units and is individualized for each patient.

- Check the label for the name and type of insulin, strength, and expiration date.

- Make sure the insulin has the proper appearance. Refer to Tables 24-6 and 24-7 for proper appearance of various insulins.

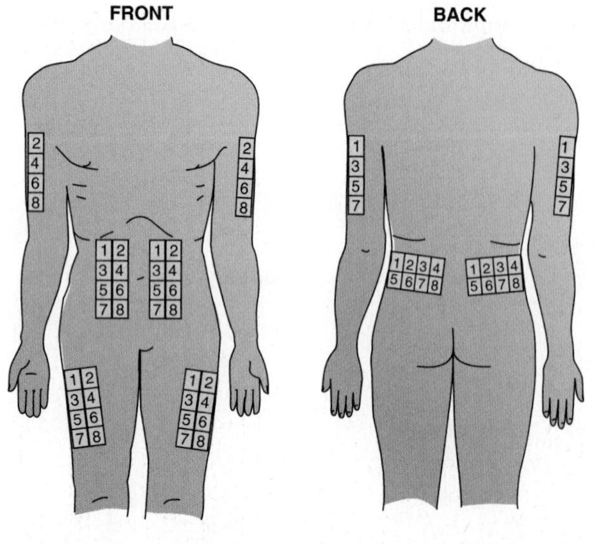

- When insulin is not in use, store it in a cool place and avoid freezing.

- When mixing insulins in one syringe, be certain they are compatible.

- Avoid shaking the insulin bottle. Roll gently in palms of hand to mix. This method prevents bubbles in the medication.

- Use a subcutaneous needle, but inject at a 90° angle.

- Use a site rotation system and select an appropriate site. Insulin injection sites must be rotated to prevent tissue damage. Record site used (Figure 24-4).

- Do not massage after injection.

- Always follow the physician's order and office policy when mixing insulins.

CALCULATING ADULT DOSAGES

Two measures, weight and volume, are used to determine the amount of medication that is to be administered. The weight of a medication may be expressed as any of the following:

- milliequivalent (mEq)

- microgram (mcg)

- milligram (mg)

- gram (Gm, g)

- grain (gr)

- unit (U)

The volume of a medication may be expressed as a:

- milliliter (ml)

- cubic centimeter (cc)

Figure 24-4   Sites and rotation for insulin administration.

- minim (m)

- dram (dr)

- ounce (oz)

- by a variety of household measures, such as the teaspoon (tsp)

Many different methods can be used when calculating the dosage to be administered. Two of the most useful methods, the proportional method and the formula method, are described.

The Proportional Method

Example:
The physician orders 0.2 Gm of Equanil tabs. The dose on hand is 400 mg tabs.

Step 1. Determine whether the medication ordered and the medication on hand are available in the same unit of measure.

Step 2. If the medication ordered and the medication on hand are not in the same unit of measure, convert so that both measures are expressed using the same unit of measure.
Conversion: To change 0.2 Gm to mg

$$1000 \text{ mg} : 1 \text{ Gm} = x \text{ mg} : 0.2 \text{ Gm}$$
$$x = 200 \text{ mg}$$
$$\text{or}$$
$$\text{multiply } 0.2 \times 1000 = 200$$

Step 3. Now use the following proportion to calculate the dosage. Remember that 0.2 Gm was converted to 200 mg.

Known *unit* *on hand*	:	*Known* *dosage* *form*	=	*Dose* *ordered*	:	*Unknown* *amount to* *be given*
400 mg	:	1 tab	=	200 mg	:	*x* tab

$$400 : 1 = 200 : x$$

$$400x = 200$$

$$x = \frac{\overset{1}{\cancel{200}}}{\underset{2}{\cancel{400}}} \text{ (Reduce fraction to lowest terms)}$$

$$x = \tfrac{1}{2} \text{ tab of 400 mg.}$$

Step 4. Prove your answer. Place your answer in the original formula in the *x* position.

$$400 \text{ mg} : 1 \text{ tab} = 200 \text{ mg} : \tfrac{1}{2} \text{ tab}$$
$$200 = \tfrac{1}{2} \text{ of } 400$$
$$200 = 200$$

The Formula Method

Example:
The physician orders 0.2 Gm of Equanil tabs. The dose on hand is 400 mg tabs.

Step 1. Determine whether the medication ordered and the medication on hand are available in the same unit of measure.

Step 2. If the medication ordered and the medication on hand are not in the same unit of measure, convert so that both measures are expressed using the same unit of measure.
Conversion: To change 0.2 Gm to mg

$$1000 \text{ mg} : 1 \text{ Gm} = x \text{ mg} : 0.2 \text{ Gm}$$
$$x = 200 \text{ mg}$$
$$\text{or}$$
$$\text{multiply } 0.2 \times 1000 = 200$$

Step 3. Now use the following formula to calculate the dosage.

$$\frac{\text{Dose ordered (desired)}}{\text{Dose on hand}} \times \frac{\text{Quantity}}{1} = \frac{\text{Amount to give}}{\text{(form of drug)}}$$

$$\frac{D}{H} \times Q = \text{Amount to give}$$

The physician ordered 0.2 Gm of Equanil tabs (0.2 Gm converts to 200 mg). The dose on hand is 400 mg tabs.

$$\frac{200 \text{ mg}}{400 \text{ mg}} \times 1 \text{ tab} = \frac{200}{400} \text{ or } \tfrac{1}{2} \text{ tab}$$

Give ½ tab of 400 mg.

CALCULATING CHILDREN'S DOSAGES

Each child is an individual with differences in age, size, and weight. In the past, formulas such as Young's, Clark's, and Fried's rules were used to calculate pediatric dosages. These formulas determined what fraction of an adult dose was appropriate for a child. Since each child does not develop in the same way during a given time span, these formulas have been replaced by more exact methods of determining the correct dosage of medication for a child.

Today, there are two basic methods used to calculate children's dosages:

- According to kilogram of body weight

- According to body surface area (BSA)

The body weight method is generally the method of choice, since most medications are ordered in this way and it is easier to calculate. The body surface area (BSA) is an exact method, but one must use a formula and a **nomogram** (a device-graph that shows relationship among numerical values) to determine a correct dosage.

Body Surface Area

The body surface area (BSA) is considered to be one of the most accurate methods of calculating medication dosages for infants and children up to 12 years of age. This method requires the use of a nomogram that estimates the body surface area of the patient according to height and weight (Figure 24-5).

The body surface area is determined by drawing a straight line from the patient's height to the patient's weight. Intersection of the line with the surface area column is the estimated BSA. This figure is then placed in the following formula:

$$\frac{\text{BSA of child (m}^2)}{1.7 \text{ (m}^2)} \times \text{adult dose} = \text{child dose}$$

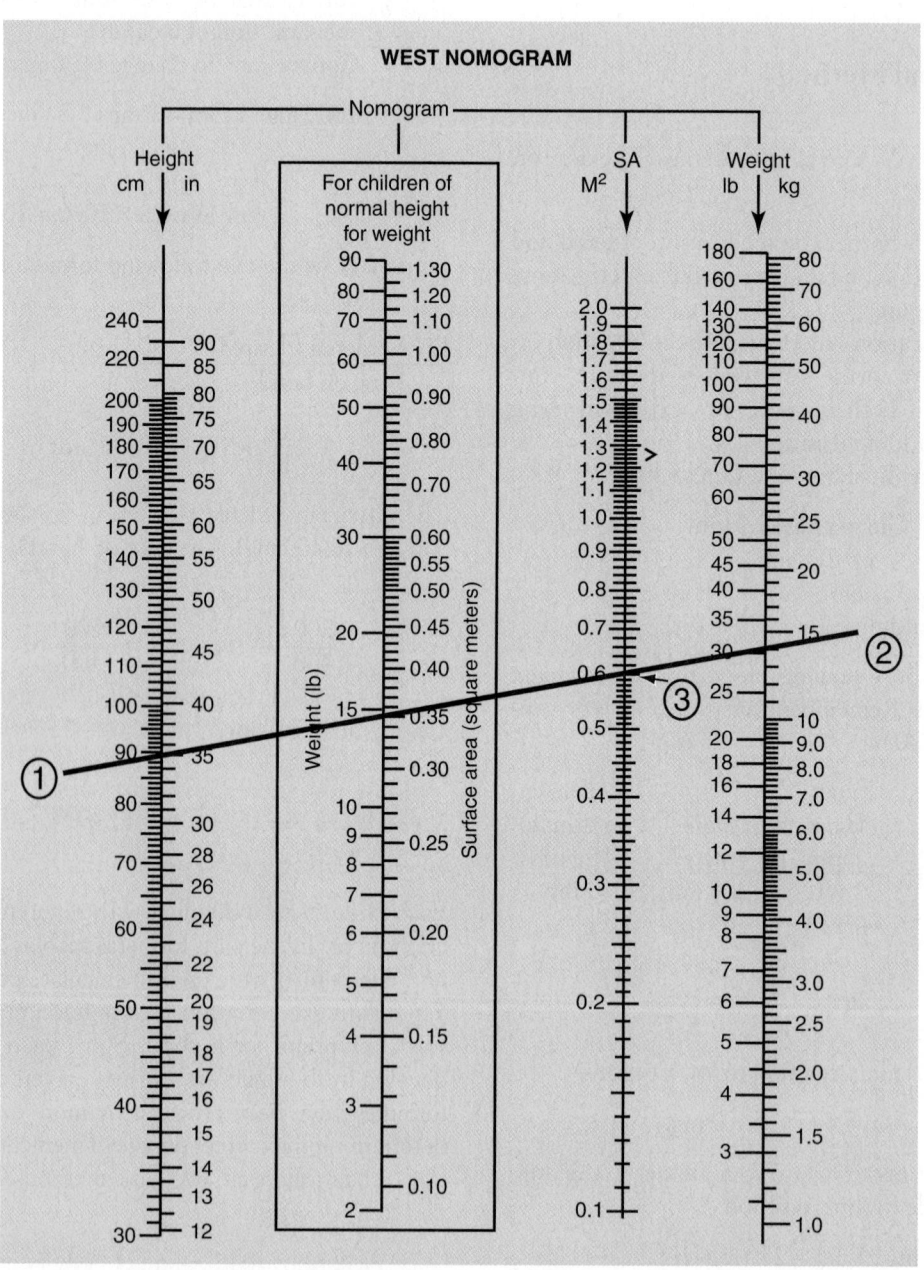

Figure 24-5   Body surface area (BSA) is determined by drawing a straight line from the patient's height (1) in the far left column to his or her weight (2) in the far right column. Intersection of the line with body surface area (BSA) column (3) is the estimated BSA (m²). For infants and children of normal height and weight BSA may be estimated from weight alone by referring to the enclosed area. (From *Nelson Textbook of Pediatrics* (15th ed.) by R. E. Behrman, R. M. Kleigman, & A. M. Arvin, 1996, Philadelphia: Saunders. Reprinted with permission.)

This formula is based on the average adult who weighs 140 pounds and has a body surface area of 1.7 square meters (1.7 m^2).

Example:
Marion Carrera is a 4-year-old child who is 40 inches tall and weighs 38 lbs. (BSA 0.7). The physician has ordered Demerol for pain. The average adult dose of Demerol is 50 mg per ml. What dosage will be given to Marion according to the BSA method?

$$\frac{0.7 \ (\text{m}^2)}{1.7 \ (\text{m}^2)} \times \frac{50 \ \text{mg}}{1} = \text{child's dose}$$

$$\frac{0.7 \ (\text{m}^2)}{1.7 \ (\text{m}^2)} \times \frac{50}{1} = \frac{35}{1.7} = 20.5 \ \text{mg} = 20.5 \ \text{or} \ 21 \ \text{mg}$$

Now use the formula $\frac{\text{Desired}}{\text{Have}} \times$ Quantity to convert mg to ml.

$$\frac{21 \ \text{mg}}{50 \ \text{mg}} \times 1 = x \ \text{mL}$$

$$\frac{21}{50} = 0.42 \ \text{mL administered in a tuberculin syringe}$$

Kilogram of Body Weight

It may be the responsibility of the medical assistant to calculate the amount of dosage ordered by the physician according to the patient's body weight. Today, many medications are ordered in this manner; therefore, it is essential that you learn how to calculate dosage according to this method. The following example will guide you step by step through the mathematical process of calculating dosage according to kilogram of body weight.

There are 2.2 pounds in one kilogram.

Example:
The physician ordered an antiepileptic agent, Depakene (valproic acid) 15 mg/kg/day capsules for Clark Kipperley, who weighs 110 pounds. The medication is to be given in three divided doses.

Step 1. To express pounds in kilograms, divide the weight in pounds by 2.2. Convert the patient's weight to kilograms:

$$110 \div 2.2 = 50 \ \text{kilograms}$$

Step 2. Now, calculate the prescribed dosage by placing 50 in the appropriate place:

$$15 \ \text{mg/50/day}$$
$$15 \times 50 = 750 \ \text{mg/day}$$

Step 3. To determine the amount of each dose, divide 750 by 3 (divided doses).

$$750 \ \text{mg} \div 3 = 250 \ \text{mg}$$

Depakene is available in 250 mg capsules and 250 mg/5 cc syrup. The physician ordered the medication in capsules, so Clark will receive a 250 mg capsule every 8 hours for a total of three doses a day.

In the same example, use the proportional method to calculate kilogram of body weight.

Step 1. To convert 110 pounds to kilograms, set up the proportion as follows:

$$2.2 \ \text{1b} : 1 \ \text{kg} = 110 \ \text{1b} : x \ \text{kg}$$

Step 2. Now, solve for x.

$$2.2 : 1 = 110 : x$$
$$2.2x = 110$$
$$x = 50$$

Step 3. Now, calculate the prescribed dosage by placing 50 in the appropriate place: mg/50 kg/day

$$15 \times 50 = 750 \ \text{mg/day}$$

Step 4. To determine the amount of each dose, divide 750 by 3 (divided doses).

$$750 \div 3 = 250 \ \text{mg per dose}$$

ADMINISTRATION OF MEDICATIONS

Regardless of a medication's form or the route by which it is administered, certain basic guidelines must be followed. These guidelines are:

1. Practice medical asepsis. (See Chapter 10.) Wash your hands before and after administering a medication. Remember OSHA guidelines and standard precautions (Chapter 10).
2. Work in a well-lighted area that is free from distractions.
3. Follow the "Six Rights" of proper drug administration (see following section).
4. Always check for allergies before administering any medication.
5. Give only drugs ordered by a licensed physician or practitioner who is authorized to prescribe medications.
6. Never give a medication if there is any question about the order.
7. Be completely familiar with the drug that you are administering before giving it to the patient. Look it up in the *PDR*.
8. Always check the expiration date on the medication label.
9. Never give a drug if its normal appearance has been altered in any way (color, structure, consistency, or odor).

10. Make out a medicine card (Figure 24-6) for medications, dose, route, and time exactly as ordered by the physician using the physician's order from the patient's record as a guide.

11. Give only those medications that you have actually prepared for administration.

12. Do not allow someone else to give a medication that you have prepared.

13. Once you have prepared a medication for administration, do not leave it unattended.

14. Be careful in transporting the medication to the patient.

15. When administering oral medications, stay with the patient until you are certain that the medication has been taken.

16. Shake (to mix) all liquid medications that contain a **precipitate** before pouring. A precipitate is a substance that separates from a solution if allowed to stand.

A medicine card is written out prior to administration of any medication to the patient in the ambulatory care setting. The information is taken directly from the physician's order sheet of the patient's record. An example follows.

Information needed:

Patient name: Abigail Johnson

Physician's order: Cardizem (diltiazem hydrochloride) 180 mg po stat. Winston Lewis, MD.

The medicine card is then used to document the information on Mrs. Johnson's record. Following documentation, tear up the medicine card and discard.

> Room 3
>
> Johnson, Abigail
>
> Cardizem
>
> 180 mg
>
> po
>
> stat
>
> 10/24/_ - 10 A.M.

Figure 24-6 A medicine card is used to prepare, administer, and record medications, dose, route, and time as ordered by the physician.

17. When pouring a liquid medication, hold the measuring device at eye level or place it on a flat surface and squat down so you can observe it at eye level. Read the correct amount at the lowest level of the **meniscus**, which is the top surface of the column of liquid.

18. Do not contaminate the cap of a bottle while pouring a medication. Place the cap with the rim pointed upward to prevent contamination of that portion that comes into contact with the medication.

19. Keep all drugs not being administered in a safe storage place.

20. Carefully follow the procedural steps for the type of medication that you are giving or the type of procedure you are performing.

21. Always keep safety precautions in mind. The United States Department of Health and Human Services, Public Health Service, and Centers for Disease and Prevention Control recommend following standard precautions for prevention of HBV, HIV, and other bloodborne diseases (refer to Chapter 10).

The "Six Rights" of Proper Drug Administration

The "Six Rights" have been developed as a checklist of activities to be followed by those who give medications. This easy-to-remember list should always be followed to ensure the proper administration of any drug:

1. *Right Drug.* To be sure that the correct drug has been selected, compare the medication order with the label on the medication. A frequent check of the medication label is a good way to avoid a medication error. One should make a practice of reading the label on each of the following three occasions:

   First: When the medication is taken from the storage area.

   Second: Just before removing it from its container.

   Third: Upon returning the medication container to storage or prior to discarding the empty container.

2. *Right Dose.* It is essential that the patient receive the right dose. If the dose ordered and the dose on hand are *not the same*, carefully determine the correct dose through mathematical calculation. When calculating dosage, it is advisable to have another qualified person verify the accuracy of your calculations before the medication is administered.

3. *Right Route.* Check the medication order to be sure that you have the right route of administration (Figure 24-7A).

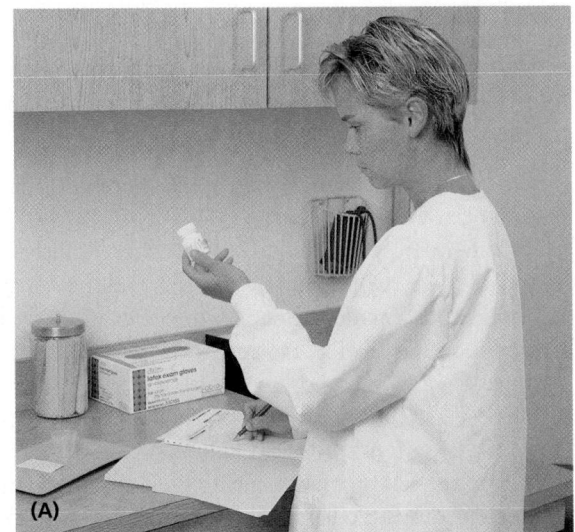

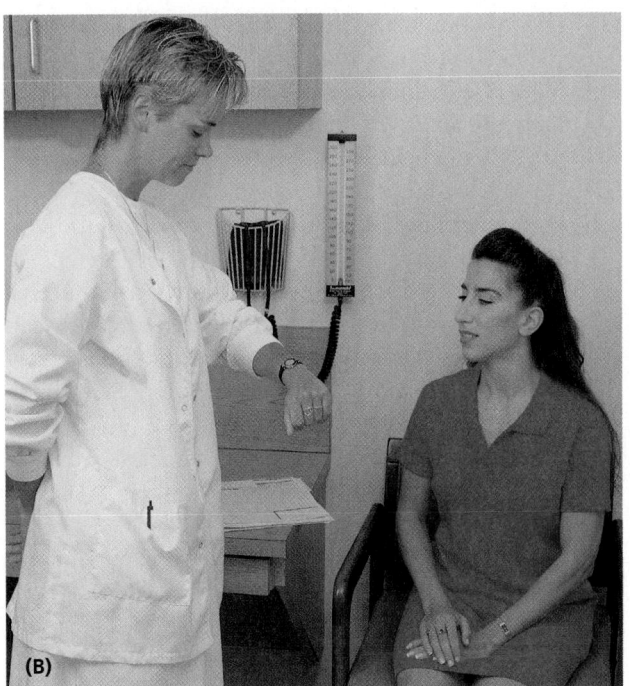

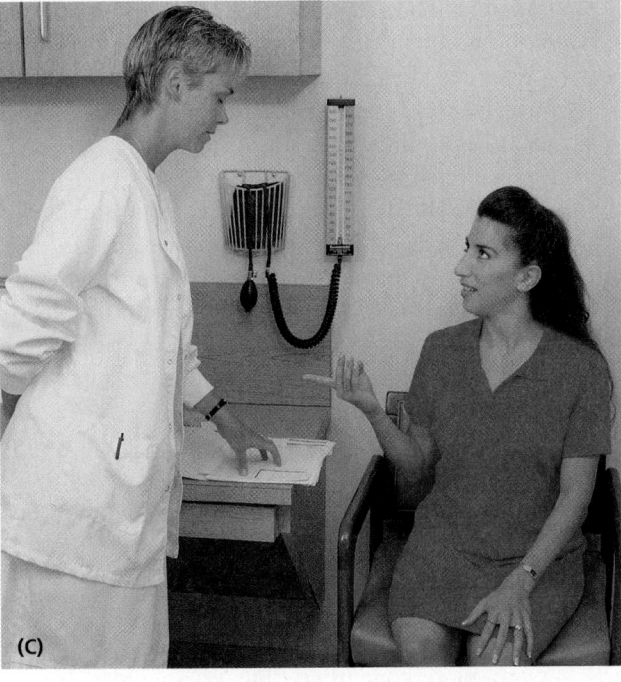

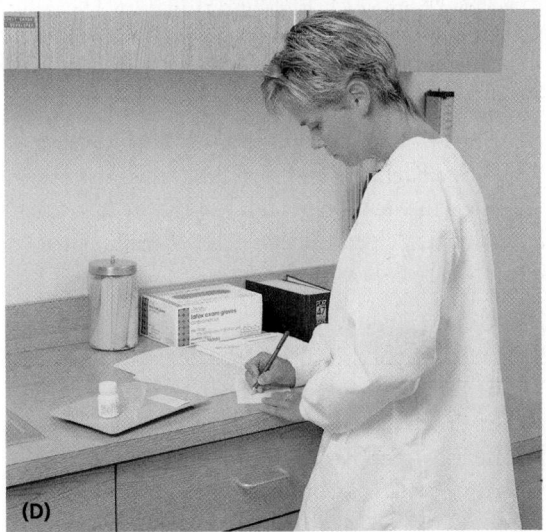

Figure 24-7 (A) Medical assistant checks the right drug, the right route, and the right dose of medication to administer. (B) Medical assistant checks for the right time to administer medication to the patient. (C) Medical assistant assesses patient before administering the medication. The medical assistant ascertains she has the right patient and asks the patient if she has any allergies. (D) Medical assistant documents administration of medication in patient's record.

4. *Right Time.* You are responsible for medicating the patient at the proper time. Check the medication order to ensure that a drug is administered according to the time interval prescribed. For a drug to be maintained at the proper blood level, care must be taken to administer it at the right time (Figure 24-7B).

5. *Right Patient.* Before administering any medication, always be sure that you have the right patient. A good safety practice is to correctly identify the patient on each occasion when you administer a medication. In a hospital, always check the patient's identification bracelet. In the ambulatory care facility, call the patient by name or ask the patient to state her name (Figure 24-7C).

6. *Right Documentation:* The recording process is the vital link between physician, patient, and medical assistant. It is an account of the essential data that are collected and preserved. The patient's chart is a legal document; therefore, all data should be

recorded in ink or typed. The data should be accurate and clearly stated. It is important that certain data about drug administration be entered in the patient's chart (Figure 24-7D):

- Patient's name
- Date and time of administration
- Name of the medication and the amount (dosage) administered
- Route by which the medication was administered
- Any unusual reactions experienced by the patient
- Any complications in administering the drug (patient refusing to take the medication, difficulty in swallowing)
- If the medication was *not* given, state why and dispose of the medication according to agency policy
- Patient data, such as blood pressure, pulse, respirations, when appropriate
- Effectiveness of the drug (for example, a patient with Parkinson's disease shows improvement after three weeks of treatment with Levodopa)
- Your name or initials and title

Medication Error

Medication errors should not happen when personnel follow the "Six Rights" of proper drug administration and the essential medication guidelines; however, honest mistakes will be made periodically. A medication error occurs when any of the following happen:

1. A drug is given to the wrong patient.
2. The incorrect drug is given.
3. The drug is given via an incorrect route.
4. The drug is given at the incorrect time.
5. The incorrect dose is administered.
6. Incorrect data are entered on the patient's chart.

When a medication error occurs, follow standard procedure:

a. Recognize that an error has been made.
b. Stay calm. Assess the patient's condition and/or reactions to the medication.
c. Report the error immediately to the physician. Give the details of the mistake and the patient's reactions.
d. Follow the physician's order for correcting the error.
e. Document the error in the patient's record or the facility's record form.
   - Describe the type of error.
   - Describe the patient's reactions.
   - Describe the steps taken to correct the error.
   - State date, time, and your name.

Patient Assessment

Before administering any medication, carefully assess the patient's condition. An assessment should include, but is not limited to, the following conditions:

1. *Age.* Is the medication and route suitable for the patient at a particular stage in life? The stages of life include infancy, childhood, adolescence, adulthood, and old age. During infancy, early childhood, and old age, a smaller dose of medication may be required than would be appropriate for the other stages in life.

2. *Physical Conditions.* Potential problems associated with the patient's physical condition must be considered. Female patients during pregnancy or while breastfeeding should not be given certain contraindicated medications.

3. *Body Size.* The amount of medication given and size of the needle used are directly related to the size of the patient. Pediatric and geriatric patients usually have less subcutaneous and/or muscular tissue per body surface area than the average adult (see Body Surface Area, pages 528–529). Small, thin patients usually require less medication, and a shorter needle may be used to reach the appropriate tissue level. On the other hand, the large or obese patient may require more medication than the average adult and a longer needle to reach the appropriate tissue level.

4. *Gender.* Consider differences that are related to the gender of the patient.
   - *Muscular Build.* Male patients are generally more muscular than female patients. Always inspect and palpate muscle tissue with this in mind when determining the appropriate needle length to reach muscle tissue.
   - *Skin Texture.* Male patients usually have tougher skin than females. A young person's skin usually has more tone than that of an older person. Slightly more force is required to penetrate skin that is tough or lacking in tone.

5. *Injection Site.* Always inspect and palpate the skin before administering an injection. The following body areas should be avoided when choosing the site for an injection:
   - Any type of skin lesion
   - Burned areas
   - Inflamed areas
   - Previous injection sites
   - Any traumatized area
   - Scar tissue (vaccination, keloid)
   - Moles, warts, birthmarks, tumors, lumps, hard nodules
   - Nerves, large blood vessels, bones
   - Cyanotic areas

- Edematous areas
- Paralyzed areas
- Arm on same side as mastectomy

Correct injection sites are illustrated later in this chapter.

ADMINISTRATION OF ORAL MEDICATIONS

Oral medications are easily and economically administered with a high degree of safety. There are, however, several disadvantages associated with the oral route. For instance, the drug may:

- Have an objectionable odor
- Have an objectionable taste
- Cause discoloration of the teeth, mouth, and tongue
- Irritate the gastric mucosa
- Be altered by digestive enzymes
- Be poorly absorbed from the digestive system due to illness or nature of the medication
- Not be taken by the patient
- Have less predictable effects upon the body when given orally than when given by the parenteral route (by injection)
- Not be able to be swallowed if in tablet, capsule, or caplet form

Equipment and Supplies for Oral Medications

Three measuring devices commonly used in the administration of oral medications are the medicine cup, the water cup, and the medicine dropper. The medicine cup (Figure 24-8) comes in various sizes and shapes, depend-

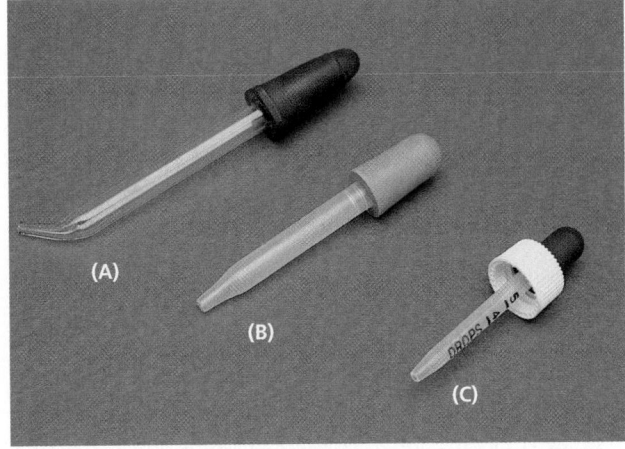

Figure 24-9 Various types of medicine droppers: (A) Glass. (B) Plastic. (C) Plastic calibrated.

ing upon its manufacturer and its intended use. Cups may be calibrated in fluid ounces, fluidrams, cubic centimeters (cc), milliliters (mL), and tablespoons.

The water cup is a small plastic or paper cup that is disposable. The average water cup holds 3 ounces of liquid.

The medicine dropper (Figure 24-9) may be calibrated in milliliters, minims, or drops. Medicine droppers are often included with the bottle of medication. Uncalibrated droppers may be provided when the medicine is administered only in drops. The size of the drop varies with the size of the dropper opening, the angle at which it is held, the force exerted on the rubber bulb, and the viscosity of the medication.

It is important that the appropriate measuring device be selected for a medication and the prescribed dosage accurately measured. The selection of the measuring device depends upon the physical structure of the medication (solid or liquid), the amount of medication prescribed, the size of the measuring device, and the calibrations on the container.

See Procedure 24-1 for administration of oral medications.

ADMINISTRATION OF PARENTERAL MEDICATIONS

The term **parenteral** is used to describe the injection of a liquid substance into the body via a route other than the alimentary canal. The most frequently used parenteral routes are:

- *Subcutaneous.* Just below the surface of the skin. A subcutaneous injection is usually given at a 45-degree angle.

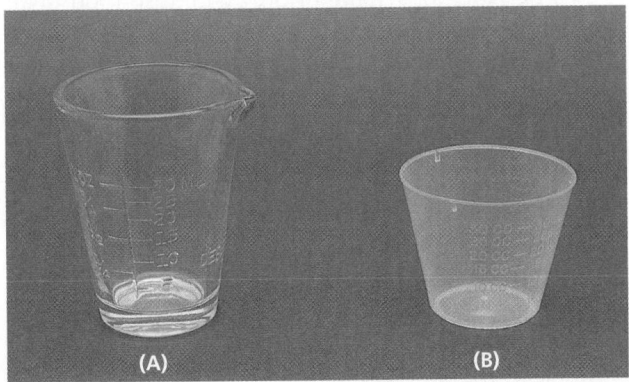

Figure 24-8 Medicine cups: (A) Glass. (B) Plastic.

● *Intramuscular.* Within the muscle. An intramuscular injection is given at a 90-degree angle, passing through the skin and subcutaneous tissue, and penetrating deep into muscle tissue.

● *Intradermal.* Within the dermal layer of the skin. An intradermal injection is given at an angle between 10 degrees and 15 degrees.

Medications that have been prepared for use by injection are available in multiple dose form (vials) and in unit dose form (ampules and cartridge-needle units). (See Figure 24-10.) **Unit dose** forms are premeasured amounts, packaged on a per-dose basis.

● *Ampule.* A small, sterile, prefilled container that usually holds a single dose of a hypodermic solution.

● *Cartridge-Needle Unit.* A disposable sterile cartridge containing a premeasured amount of medication. This unit is designed for use in a nondisposable cartridge-holder syringe such as the Tubex® or Carpuject®.

● *Vial.* A small, sterile, prefilled glass bottle containing a hypodermic solution.

Hazards Associated with Parenteral Medications

Injections of medications must be done with extreme care. Sterile technique must be used because the needle and medication are being introduced into the patient's body and microorganisms must not be transmitted. Appropriate site selection and proper technique assure effectiveness of the medication.

Additional dangers to be aware of when administering medications parenterally (by injection) include:

1. Allergic reaction (if present) will be swift
2. Injury to bone, nerve, or blood vessel
3. Breaking of needle in tissue (rare)
4. Injecting into a blood vessel instead of tissue. (This is avoided by checking for blood return, or aspiration.)

Reasons for Parenteral Route Selection

The parenteral route is selected because of:

1. Rapid response time to medication
2. Accuracy of dosage
3. Need to concentrate medication in a specific body part or area (joint or local anesthetic)
4. Inability to administer orally because the medication is destroyed by gastric juices or the patient is incapable of taking medication orally

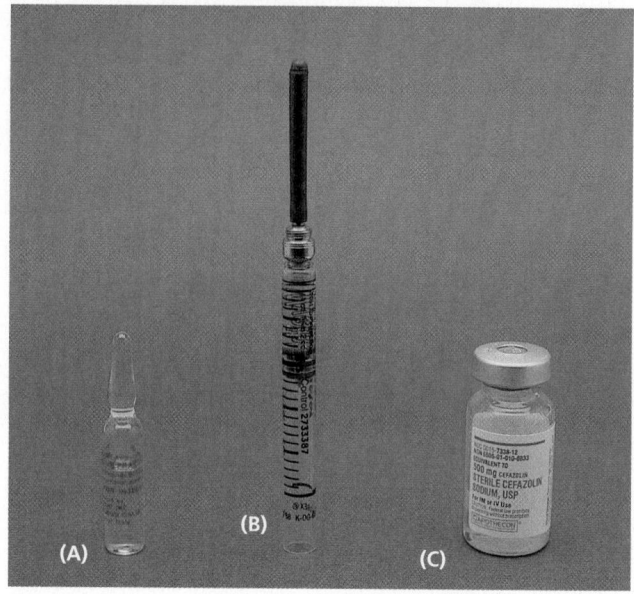

Figure 24-10   Medications given parenterally: (A) Ampule. (B) Sterile cartridge with premeasured medication. (C) Vial of powder for reconstitution.

Because parenteral medications are intended for use by injection, they must be supplied as liquids. Some medications are supplied in powder form and must be reconstituted to a liquid form for injection. See Procedure 24-8.

Because they must be in liquid form, the amount of parenteral medications is expressed in terms of volume (cubic centimeters, milliliters, minims, or ounces). The strength of the drug contained in the liquid is usually expressed in terms of its weight (milliequivalents, micrograms, milligrams, grams, grains, or units). Therefore, medications ordered for parenteral use are often ordered by both weight and volume.

Example:
Atropine sulfate injection (gr = weight; mL = volume)

$$0.4 \text{ mg (gr } \frac{1}{150} \text{) per mL}$$

The parenteral route of drug administration offers an effective mode of delivering medication to a patient when a rapid and direct result is desired. Since the effect of a parenteral medication is faster than by the oral route, the accuracy of dosage calculation is very important.

Parenteral Equipment and Supplies

Syringes. Syringes are classified as disposable, nondisposable, and as combinations of these two types. They also may be classified according to their intended use. In addition to the standard hypodermic syringes that are in general use, there are special-purpose syringes for irrigations and/or oral feedings, tuberculin syringes, and insulin syringes.

Disposable Syringes. Disposable syringes are those that are sterilized, prepackaged, nontoxic, nonpyrogenic, and ready for use. They are available as a syringe-needle unit and are generally enclosed in individual peel-apart packages of durable paper or clear plastic. They are available in sizes from ½ cubic centimeter to 50 cubic centimeters. The 1-cc, 3-cc, and 5-cc syringes are the ones most often used when parenteral medications are administered.

A disposable syringe-needle unit consists of a syringe with an attached needle. The needle is covered by a hard plastic sheath to prevent it from accidentally penetrating the package or sticking the user. The unit may be sealed within a peel-apart package or encased in a rigid plastic container that has been heat-sealed to ensure sterility. Labeling usually includes the manufacturer's name, type and size of the syringe, gauge and length of the needle, and a reorder number. Packages are usually color-coded for ease of identification. Disposable syringes are generally preferred for the administration of parenteral medications because they ensure sterility and sharp needles. Also, disposable syringes eliminate the need for resterilizaton, which is costly, time-consuming, and possibly unsafe if not done properly.

Nondisposable Syringes. Nondisposable syringes are usually made of specially strengthened glass resistant to thermal shock. These units, consisting of round glass barrels with individually fitted plungers, are manufactured to exacting specifications.

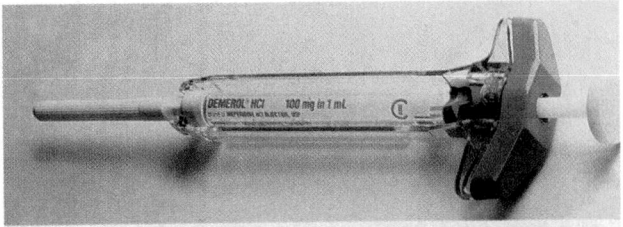

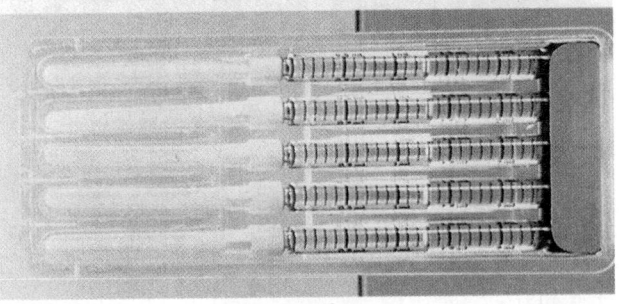

Figure 24-11 The Carpuject® is another kind of cartridge-injection system. This unit is shown with a package of prefilled cartridges. (Courtesy Sanofi Withrop Pharmaceuticals.)

Nondisposable glass syringes are available in sizes from 1 cubic centimeter to 50 cubic centimeters. These syringes are not often used for the administration of injections. They may be used by physicians to perform special procedures such as paracentesis, thoracentesis, thoracotomy, and tracheotomy.

Combination Disposable/Nondisposable Cartridge-Injection Syringes. A cartridge-injection system, such as the Carpuject® (Figure 24-11) or Tubex® (Figure 24-12A–E) consists of a disposable cartridge-needle unit and

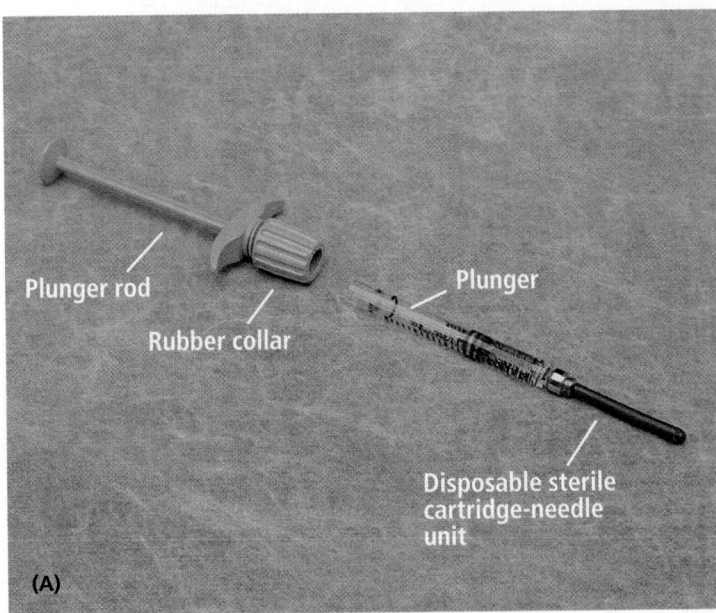

(A)

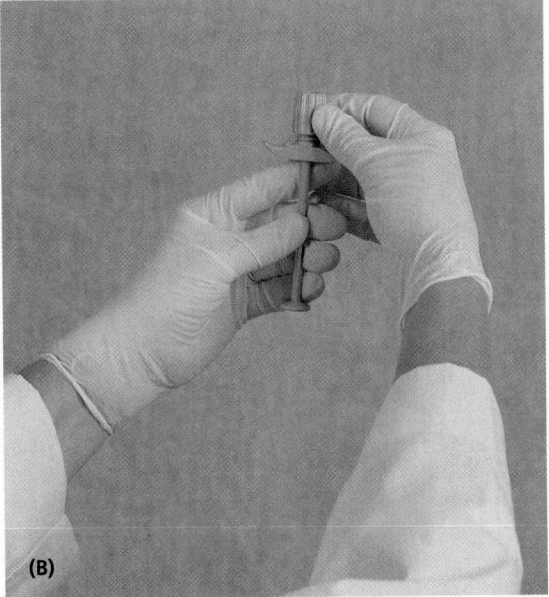

(B)

Figure 24-12 (A) Tubex® injector. Reusable cartridge holder with disposable sterile cartridge needle unit. (B) Turn ribbed collar to open position. *(continues)*

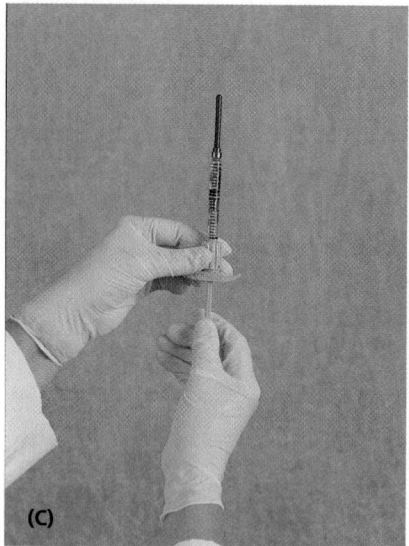
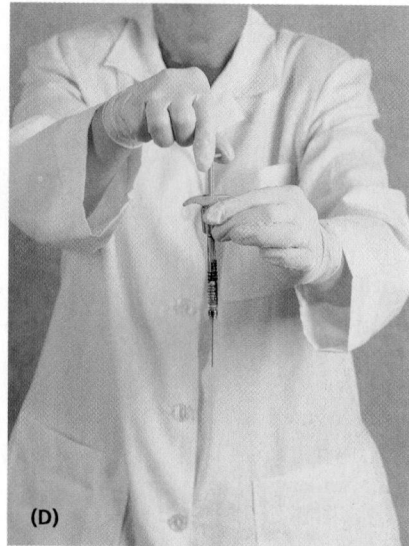
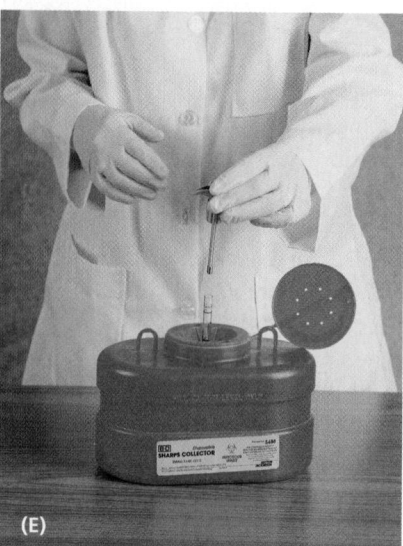

Figure 24-12 (*continued*) (C) Insert the sterile cartridge-needle unit into the open end of the injector. The ribbed collar is firmly tightened. The plunger of the injector and the plunger of the cartridge-needle unit are tightened and ready for use. (D) The medical assistant prepares to dispose of the cartridge-needle unit. The needle is not recapped. The plunger rod is disengaged by unscrewing. The ribbed collar is loosened. (E) The medical assistant holds the cartridge-needle unit over a sharps container and the unit drops into the container.

a nondisposable cartridge-holder syringe. The cartridge-needle unit is factory-sealed and sterile and contains a precisely measured unit dose of medicine. The cartridge-holder syringe may be made of durable chrome-plated brass or of plastic. These reusable syringes are designed for quick and safe loading and unloading of cartridge-needle units, which are manufactured in various sizes and dosage capacities, and contain a wide range of medications.

The combination of disposable/nondisposable syringe system is easy to use and convenient. When using this system, be careful to read the label and compare the medication order with the label. For example, the physician may order Demerol® 25 mg and the cartridge is 50 mg/cc. Give ½ cc and properly discard the other ½ cc according to office policy. Another person must witness the disposal of the Demerol®, which is a controlled substance.

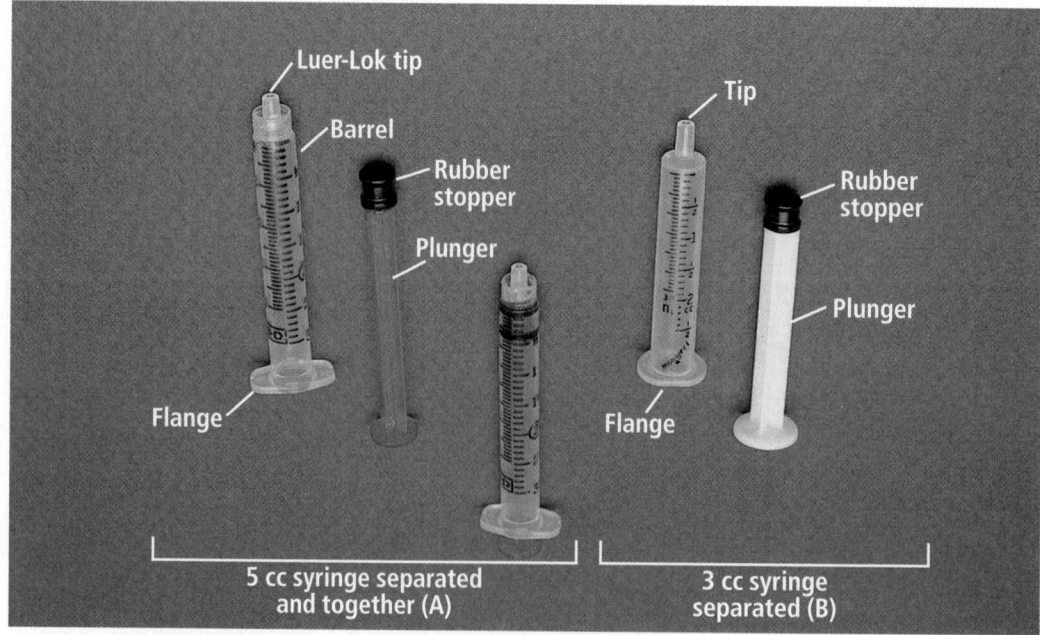

Figure 24-13 Parts of a syringe: (A) A 5-cc syringe separated and unseparated with Luer-Lok® tip. (B) A 3-cc syringe separated with plain tip.

TABLE 24-8	THE MOST FREQUENTLY USED SYRINGES FOR PARENTERAL MEDICATIONS	
Type of Syringes	**Size and Calibration**	**Typical Uses**
Hypodermic	3 cc Calibrated 0.1 15/16 minims/cc	Intramuscular and subcutaneous injections
Hypodermic	5 cc Calibrated 0.2	Venipuncture and intramuscular injections
Hypodermic	Larger sizes (10 cc, 30 cc, and 60 cc)	Medical/surgical treatments, aspirations, irrigations, venipunctures, gavage (tube-to-stomach) feedings
Tuberculin	1 cc Calibrated 0.1 and 0.01 16 minims/cc	To inject minute amounts for intradermal injections, allergy testing, allergy injections
Insulin	U-100 (0.5 cc) U-100 (1 cc)	Lo-Dose® administration of insulin Insulin administration

Parts of a Syringe. The component parts of a syringe consist of a barrel, plunger, flange, and tip (Figure 24-13).

- The *barrel* is the part that holds the medication and has graduated markings (calibrations) on its surface for use in measuring medications.

- The *plunger* is a movable cylinder designed for insertion within the barrel, and provides the mechanism by which a medication (or other substance) is drawn into or pushed out of the barrel.

- The *flange* is at the end of the barrel where the plunger is inserted. It forms a rim around the end of the barrel where the plunger is inserted and has appendages against which one places the index and middle fingers when drawing up solution for injection. The flange also prevents the syringe from rolling when laid on a flat surface.

- The *tip* is at the end of the barrel where the needle is attached.

The parts of a syringe that must remain sterile during the preparation and administration of a parenteral medication are the inside of the barrel, the section of the plunger that fits inside the barrel, and the syringe tip to which the needle is to be attached.

Types of Syringes and Uses. Syringes are named according to their sizes and uses. Table 24-8 lists the types, sizes, calibrations, and uses of syringes used in the administration of parenteral medications. Figure 24-14 shows various sizes of disposable syringes.

One should always choose a needle with sufficient length to reach the desired tissue level (see Table 24-9). A large person may require a longer needle to reach the correct body tissue than would be required for a smaller person. The delivery of medication to the proper tissue level is very important. A concentrated or irritating medication that is intended for deep intramuscular injection could be delivered instead into the subcutaneous tissue of an obese

patient if one selects a needle that is too short. Such an inappropriate injection may cause a sterile abscess. This unnecessary complication can be avoided by considering the size of the patient when choosing the length of the needle.

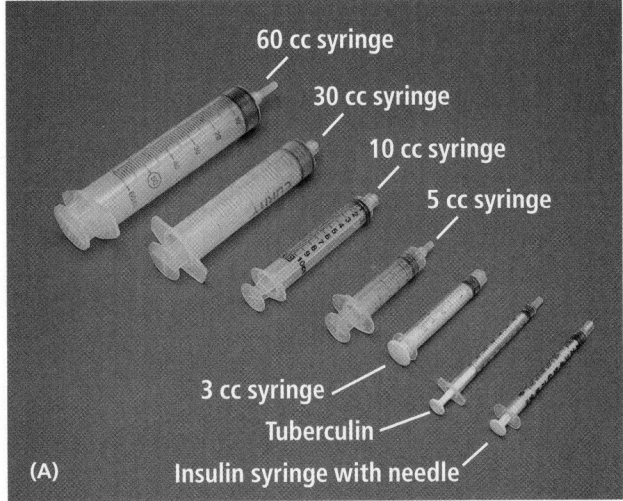

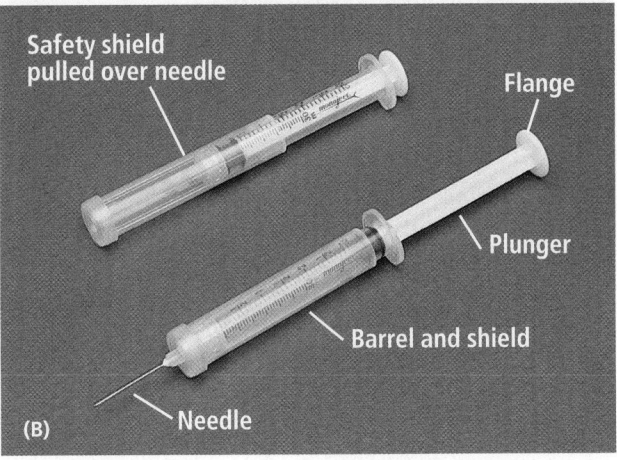

Figure 24-14 (A) Various sizes of disposable syringes. Note tuberculin and insulin syringes. (B) A type of safety syringe.

TABLE 24-9	SYRINGE-NEEDLE COMBINATIONS FOR VARIOUS PARENTERAL ROUTES	
Subcutaneous Injection	**Intramuscular Injection**	**Intradermal Injection**
3-cc syringe/25G, ⅝ inch needle	3-cc syringe/23G, 1 inch needle	1-cc syringe/25G, ⅝ inch needle
3-cc syringe/26G, ⅜ inch needle	3-cc syringe/22G, 1½ inch needle	1-cc syringe/26G, ⅜ inch needle
3-cc syringe/27G, ½ inch needle	3-cc syringe/21G, 1½ inch to 2 inch needle	1-cc syringe/27G, ½ inch needle
U-100 (1 cc)/26G, ½ inch needle		

Needles. Both disposable and nondisposable needles are available for use with syringes. Of these, the most frequently used are disposable needles, which are individually packaged in sterile paper or plastic containers. Disposable needles and syringe-needle units are available with a color-coded sheath. The sheath protects the needle and identifies its gauge and length. Needle gauges (G) range from 16 to 30, and their lengths vary from ⅜ inch to 2 inches. The needle's gauge is determined by the diameter of the lumen or opening at its beveled tip. The larger the gauge, the smaller the diameter of its lumen. For example, a 30-gauge needle is much smaller than a 16-gauge needle.

Nondisposable needles are made of high-quality stainless steel. They are equipped with a mounting hub that has a cylindrical opening designed to slip over the lock onto the tip of a syringe, such as a Luer-Lok®. See Figure 24-15 for various sizes and types of needles.

Parts of a Needle. Figure 24-16 shows the parts of a needle used to administer parenteral medications.

- The *point* is the sharpened end of the needle. The point is formed when the end of the shaft is ground away to form a flat, slanted surface called the *bevel*.

- The hollow core of the needle, when exposed at the beveled point, forms an oval-shaped opening called the *lumen*.

- The hollow steel tube through which the medication passes is the *shaft*.

- The other end of the shaft attaches to the *hub*, which is part of the needle unit that is designed to mount onto the syringe.

- The point at which the shaft attaches to the hub is called the *hilt*.

The Safe Disposal of Needles and Syringes. The careless disposal of used needles and syringes may present a health risk to any person coming into contact with the used equipment. An accidental stick by a contaminated needle could transmit diseases such as hepatitis B, syphilis, Rocky Mountain spotted fever, tuberculosis, malaria, varicella zoster, and acquired immunodeficiency syndrome (AIDS). Used needles and syringes should be discarded in a rigid, puncture-proof container (Figure 24-17). Do not recap the needle after giving the injection. Most needlesticks occur at this time. Refer to Chapter 10 for OSHA regulations.

Sharps Collectors. The B-D point-of-use Sharps Collector System eliminates the need to reshield the needle, thereby reducing the risk of an accidental needlestick.

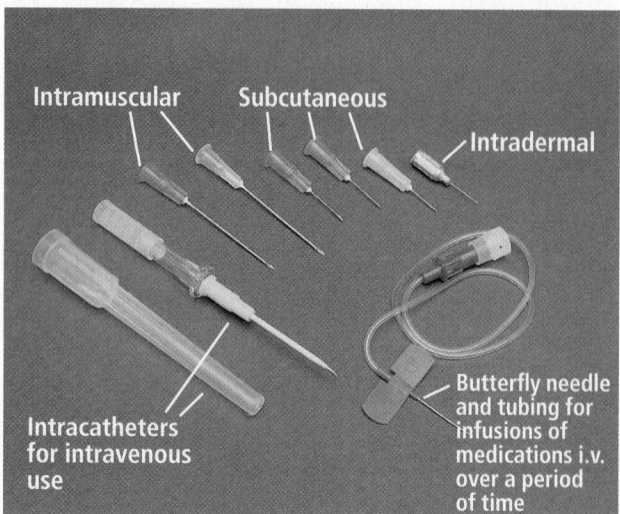

Figure 24-15 Various sizes and types of needles. Different colored hubs denote needle gauges.

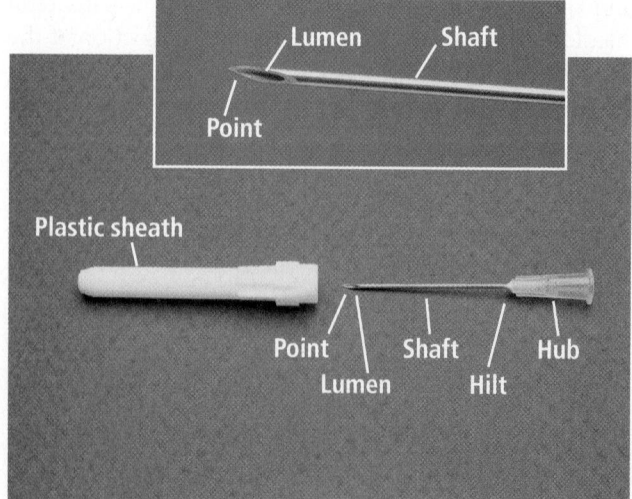

Figure 24-16 Parts of a needle and needle sheath. Inset shows point, lumen, and shaft.

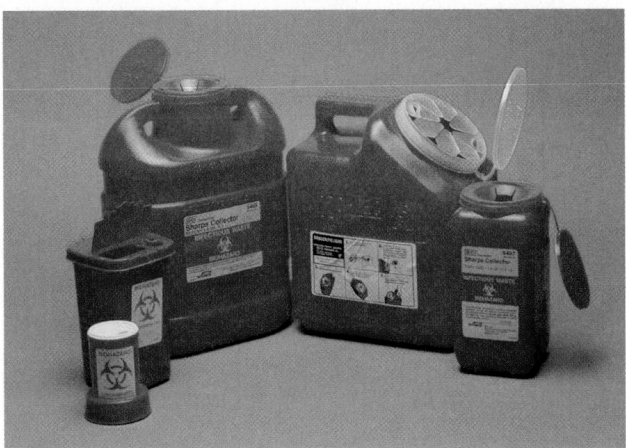

Figure 24-17 Place used needles, point down, in puncture-proof sharps containers.

Needles are placed point downward, away from the fingers. The disposable inner container is clearly marked and may be incinerated or autoclaved according to facility policy.

SITE SELECTION AND INJECTION ANGLE

The selection of a proper site for a subcutaneous, intramuscular, or intradermal injection and the correct angle of insertion for each will assure that the medication is delivered to the correct tissue type (see Figure 24-18).

A subcutaneous injection is given at an angle of 45 degrees just below the surface of the skin wherever there is subcutaneous tissue. The shaded areas in Figure 24-19A are usually used for subcutaneous injections because they are located away from bones, joints, nerves, and large blood vessels.

An intramuscular injection is given at a 90-degree angle, passing through the skin and subcutaneous tissue and penetrating deep into muscle tissue. Body areas normally used for intramuscular injections are the dorsogluteal area, ventrogluteal area, deltoid muscle, and vastus lateralis.

Intradermal injections are given at an angle between 10 degrees and 15 degrees into the dermal layer of the skin. The body areas used for intradermal injections are the inner forearm and the middle of the back (Figure 24-19B). The reasons for the use of these two sites are that the skin is thin and there is very little hair.

Marking the Correct Site for Intramuscular Injection

To give a safe injection, it is necessary to become familiar with the anatomical structures associated with the injection site. With knowledge of where such structures are located, it is easier to mark injection sites that avoid bones, nerves, and large blood vessels.

Dorsogluteal Site. The dorsogluteal site is the traditional location for giving most (adult) deep intramuscular injections (Figure 24-20). Commonly referred to as the "upper outer quadrant of the buttocks," this description can be easily misinterpreted and result in an injection into the inappropriate area. To locate the correct site for a

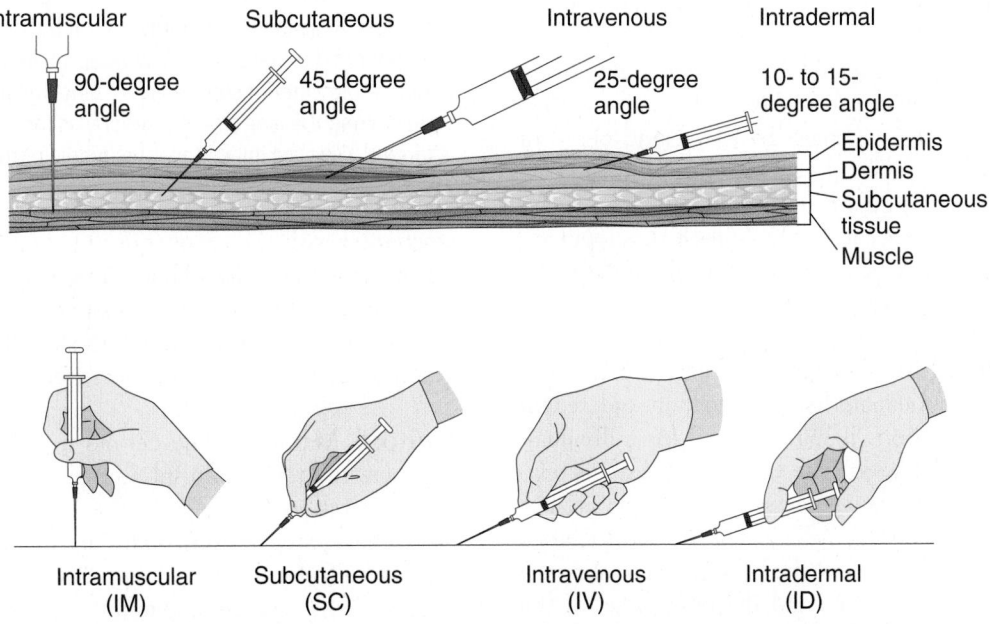

Figure 24-18 Angles of injection for intramuscular, subcutaneous, intravenous, and intradermal injections.

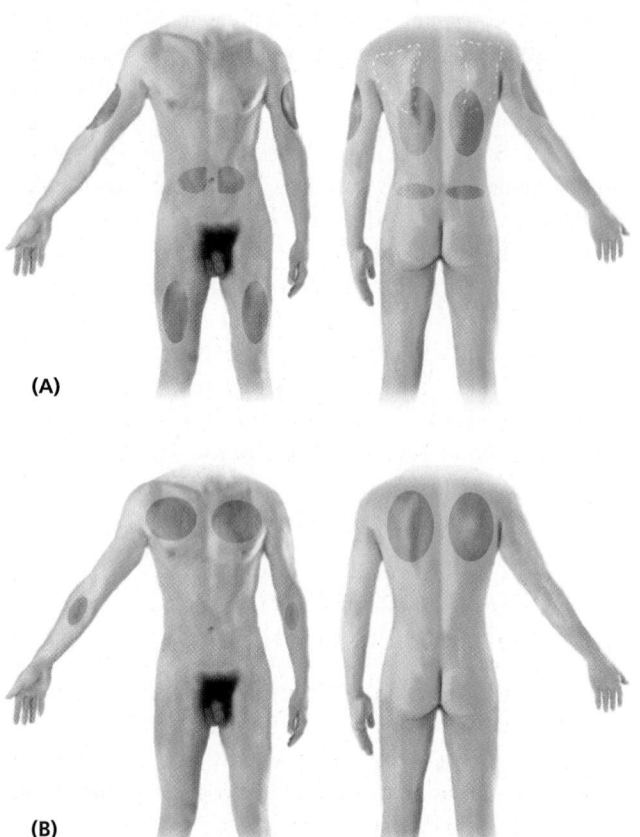

(A)

(B)

Figure 24-19 Injection sites: (A) Subcutaneous. (B) Intradermal.

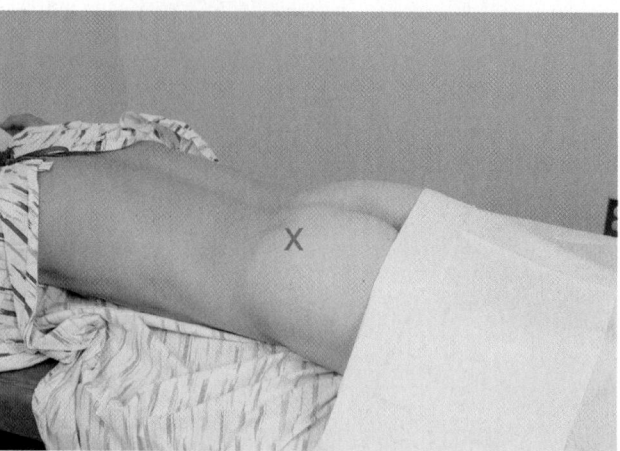

Figure 24-20 The dorsogluteal intramuscular injection site. Locate the posterior iliac spine and the greater trochanter. Draw an imaginary line between the two locations. The area above and outside this line is the injection site.

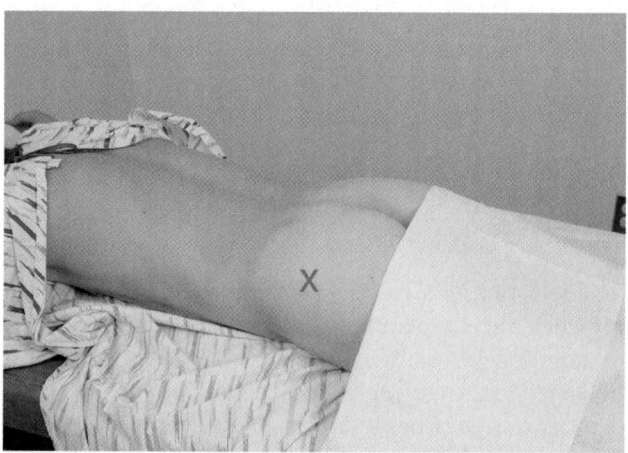

Figure 24-21 The ventrogluteal intramuscular injection site. Palpate the greater trochanter, iliac crest, and anterior superior iliac spine. If given into the patient's left buttock, the palm of the right hand is placed on the greater trochanter and the index finger on the anterior superior iliac spine. The middle finger is spread along the iliac crest posteriorly as far as possible. A "V" is formed. Give the injection in the middle of the V.

dorsogluteal injection, locate the posterior iliac spine and place a small x on this spot. Then locate the greater trochanter of the femur and mark this spot. Draw (or imagine) a diagonal line between the two locations. The area above and outside this line and about 3 inches below the iliac crest is the correct location of the dorsogluteal site.

Extreme caution should be used when giving intramuscular injections in the dorsogluteal area. Improper site selection can result in damage to the sciatic nerve or injection into the superior gluteal artery or vein. This site is contraindicated for infants and is used only as a site of last resort in children because of less muscle development. The muscle mass may be degenerated in the elderly, the nonwalking, or the emaciated patient.

Ventrogluteal Site. The ventrogluteal site can generally accommodate the majority of medications ordered for intramuscular injection. It may be used for individuals from infancy to adulthood. The ventrogluteal site is relatively free of major nerves and vessels, thereby making it a choice site for IM injections. To locate the ventrogluteal injection site, palpate to find the greater trochanter, the anterior superior iliac spine, and the bony ridge of the iliac crest (Figure 24-21). With these three locations identified, place the palm of your hand against the greater

trochanter with the tip of your index finger on the anterior superior iliac spine. Then spread your middle finger as far from the index finger as possible. Place an X in the center of the triangle formed by the middle and index fingers to mark the correct injection site.

Deltoid Muscle. The deltoid muscle is a small but adequate site for certain intramuscular injections. These IM preparations include vaccines, narcotics, sedatives, and vitamin preparations. The site should not be used for an infant. To locate the deltoid injection site, place your fingers on the shoulder and find the acromion (lateral triangular projection of the spine of the scapula forming the point of the shoulder) and the deltoid tuberosity that lies

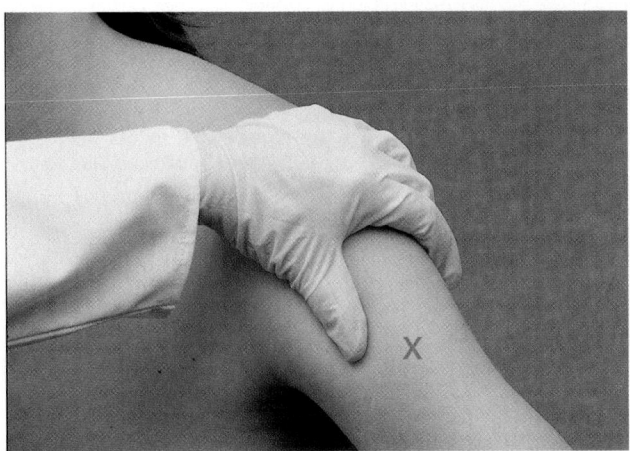

Figure 24-22 The deltoid intramuscular injection site is located on the upper outer aspect of the arm, below the lower edge of the acromion.

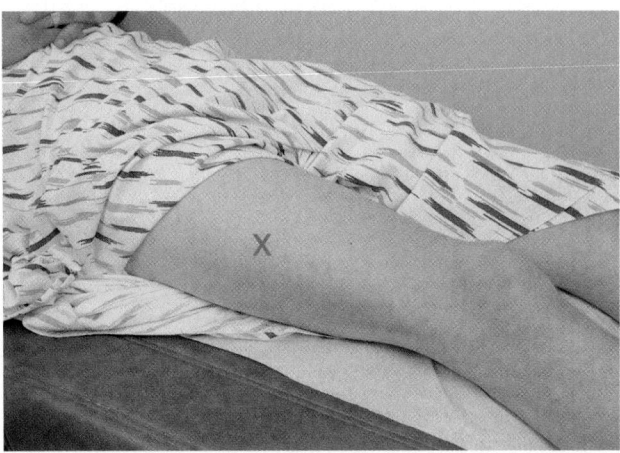

Figure 24-23 The vastus lateralis intramuscular injection site is located by dividing the leg into thirds by palpating the greater trochanter and the patella. The injection is given into the middle third of the area.

lateral to the side of the arm, opposite the axilla (Figure 24-22). The correct injection site is 1 to 2 inches (about the width of three fingers) below the acromion.

CAUTION: Do not inject medicine into the upper and lower aspects of the deltoid muscle. Care should be taken to avoid brachial and axillary nerves and blood vessels, the radial nerve, acromion, and the humerus.

Vastus Lateralis Site. The vastus lateralis is the preferred site for intramuscular injections in infants and children. It is also used for IM injections in adults. This site generally accommodates the majority of IM injections

ordered and is a relatively safe site as the nerves and vessels supplying the area are not generally endangered. The vastus lateralis is a part of the quadriceps femoris. The muscle is located on the anterolateral aspect of the patient. For infants and children, the site lies below the greater trochanter of the femur and within the upper lateral quadrant of the thigh (Figure 24-23).

For the adult patient, the correct injection site is within the middle third of the muscle.

Figures 24-24A through 24-24E review the four injection sites.

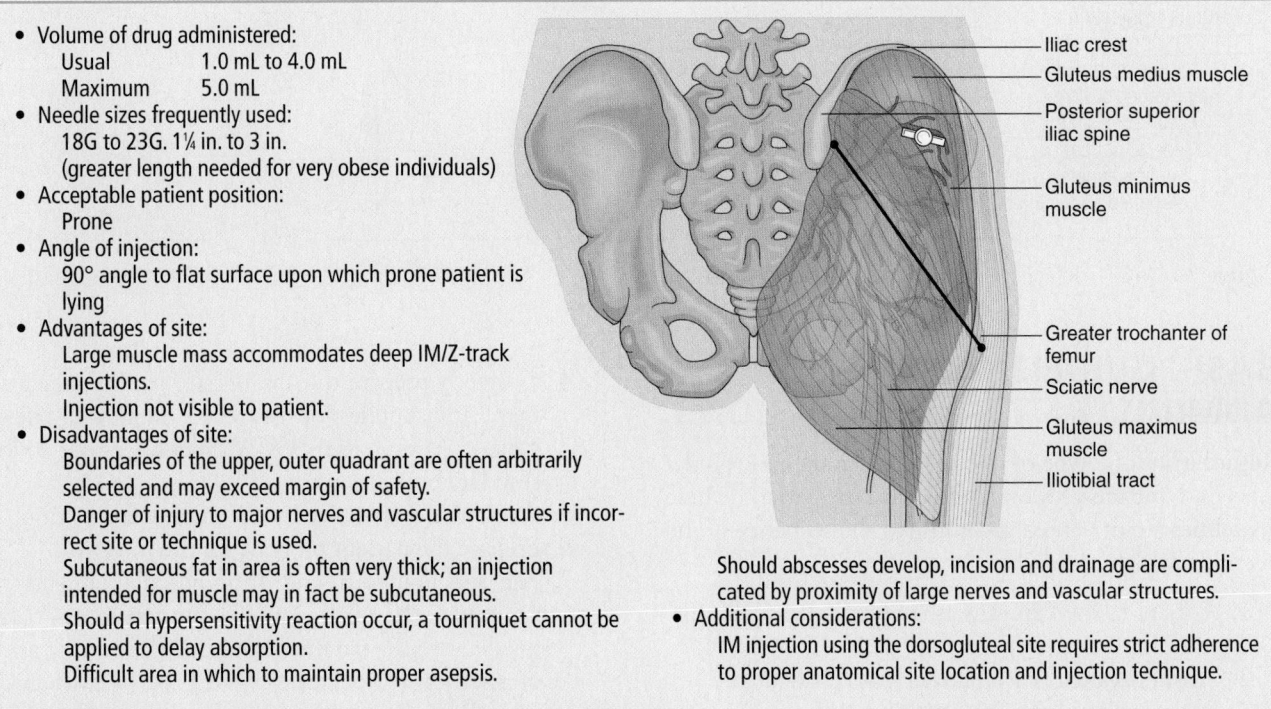

- Volume of drug administered:
  Usual   1.0 mL to 4.0 mL
  Maximum   5.0 mL
- Needle sizes frequently used:
  18G to 23G. 1¼ in. to 3 in.
  (greater length needed for very obese individuals)
- Acceptable patient position:
  Prone
- Angle of injection:
  90° angle to flat surface upon which prone patient is lying
- Advantages of site:
  Large muscle mass accommodates deep IM/Z-track injections.
  Injection not visible to patient.
- Disadvantages of site:
  Boundaries of the upper, outer quadrant are often arbitrarily selected and may exceed margin of safety.
  Danger of injury to major nerves and vascular structures if incorrect site or technique is used.
  Subcutaneous fat in area is often very thick; an injection intended for muscle may in fact be subcutaneous.
  Should a hypersensitivity reaction occur, a tourniquet cannot be applied to delay absorption.
  Difficult area in which to maintain proper asepsis.

Labels on figure: Iliac crest; Gluteus medius muscle; Posterior superior iliac spine; Gluteus minimus muscle; Greater trochanter of femur; Sciatic nerve; Gluteus maximus muscle; Iliotibial tract

Should abscesses develop, incision and drainage are complicated by proximity of large nerves and vascular structures.
- Additional considerations:
  IM injection using the dorsogluteal site requires strict adherence to proper anatomical site location and injection technique.

Figure 24-24A Injection technique for dorsogluteal site, adult.

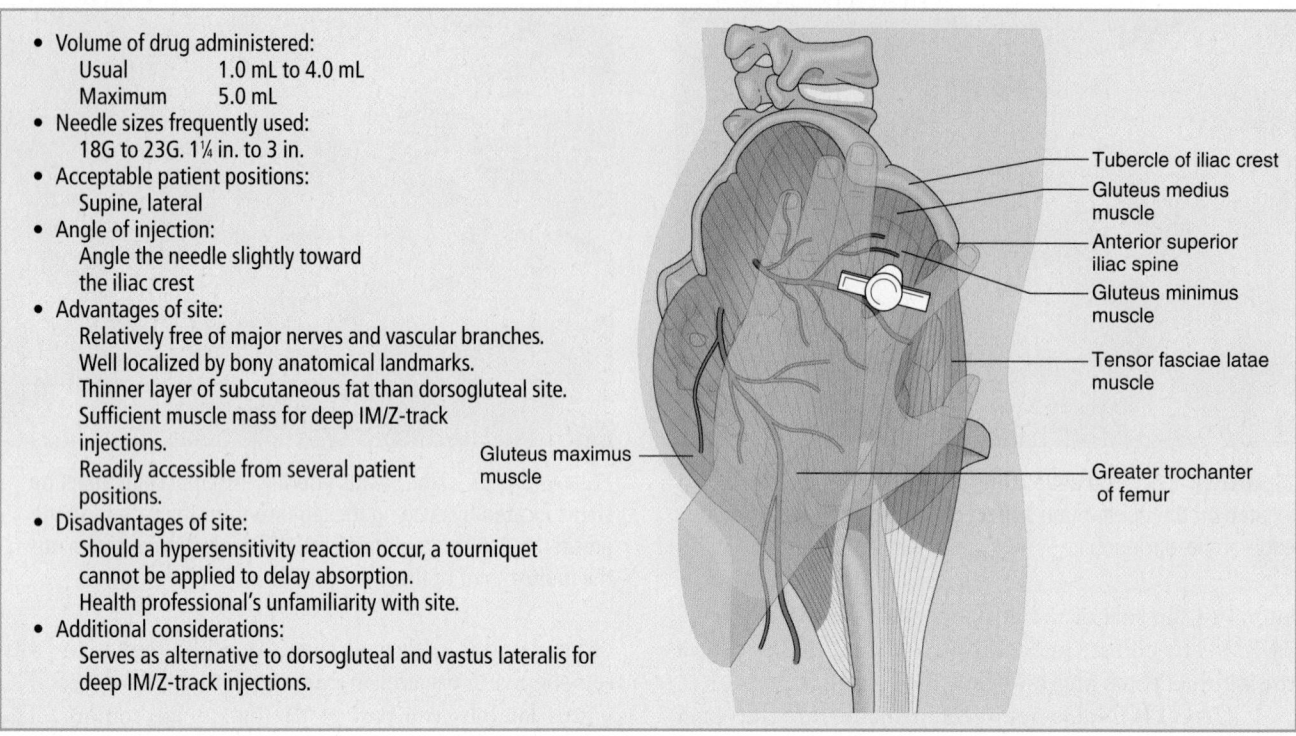

- Volume of drug administered:
    Usual   1.0 mL to 4.0 mL
    Maximum   5.0 mL
- Needle sizes frequently used:
    18G to 23G. 1¼ in. to 3 in.
- Acceptable patient positions:
    Supine, lateral
- Angle of injection:
    Angle the needle slightly toward
    the iliac crest
- Advantages of site:
    Relatively free of major nerves and vascular branches.
    Well localized by bony anatomical landmarks.
    Thinner layer of subcutaneous fat than dorsogluteal site.
    Sufficient muscle mass for deep IM/Z-track
    injections.
    Readily accessible from several patient
    positions.
- Disadvantages of site:
    Should a hypersensitivity reaction occur, a tourniquet
    cannot be applied to delay absorption.
    Health professional's unfamiliarity with site.
- Additional considerations:
    Serves as alternative to dorsogluteal and vastus lateralis for
    deep IM/Z-track injections.

Tubercle of iliac crest
Gluteus medius muscle
Anterior superior iliac spine
Gluteus minimus muscle
Tensor fasciae latae muscle
Gluteus maximus muscle
Greater trochanter of femur

Figure 24-24B   Injection technique for ventrogluteal site, adult.

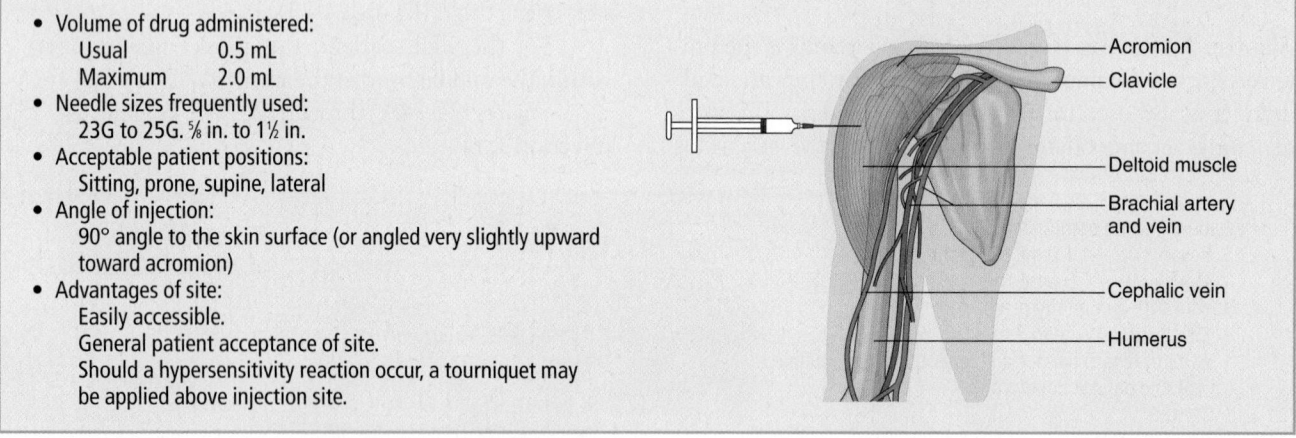

- Volume of drug administered:
    Usual   0.5 mL
    Maximum   2.0 mL
- Needle sizes frequently used:
    23G to 25G. ⅝ in. to 1½ in.
- Acceptable patient positions:
    Sitting, prone, supine, lateral
- Angle of injection:
    90° angle to the skin surface (or angled very slightly upward
    toward acromion)
- Advantages of site:
    Easily accessible.
    General patient acceptance of site.
    Should a hypersensitivity reaction occur, a tourniquet may
    be applied above injection site.

Acromion
Clavicle
Deltoid muscle
Brachial artery and vein
Cephalic vein
Humerus

Figure 24-24C   Injection technique for deltoid site, adult.

BASIC GUIDELINES FOR ADMINISTRATION OF INJECTIONS

Regardless of the type of injection, there are basic guidelines that one must follow to safeguard the patient. These guidelines are presented according to the sequence of the events to which they relate:

1. Adhere to the "Six Rights" of proper drug administration.
2. Always evaluate each patient as an individual.
3. Select a needle-syringe unit that is the appropriate size for the proper administration of a parenteral medication.

4. Correctly prepare the appropriate parenteral equipment and supplies for use. Wash hands and put on gloves. Always use OSHA guidelines and follow standard precautions.
5. Select the correct site for the intended injection.
6. Prepare the patient properly for the injection.
7. For subcutaneous and intramuscular injections, use a smooth, quick, dart-like motion to insert the needle into the patient's skin. Use the correct angle of insertion (45 degrees or 90 degrees) for the injection. Once the needle is inserted, gently pull back on the plunger (aspirate) to ensure that the needle is not in a blood vessel.

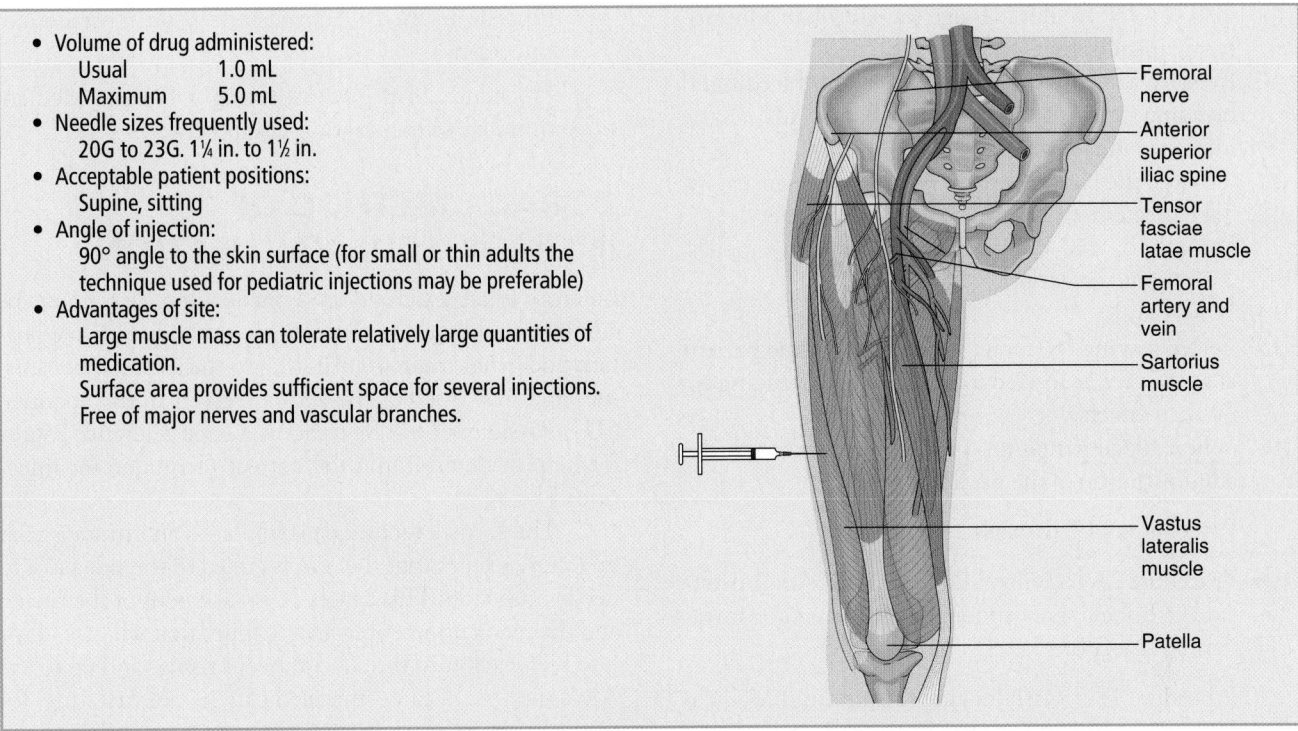

- Volume of drug administered:
    Usual   1.0 mL
    Maximum   5.0 mL
- Needle sizes frequently used:
    20G to 23G. 1¼ in. to 1½ in.
- Acceptable patient positions:
    Supine, sitting
- Angle of injection:
    90° angle to the skin surface (for small or thin adults the technique used for pediatric injections may be preferable)
- Advantages of site:
    Large muscle mass can tolerate relatively large quantities of medication.
    Surface area provides sufficient space for several injections.
    Free of major nerves and vascular branches.

Labels: Femoral nerve; Anterior superior iliac spine; Tensor fasciae latae muscle; Femoral artery and vein; Sartorius muscle; Vastus lateralis muscle; Patella

Figure 24-24D   Injection technique for vastus lateralis site, adult.

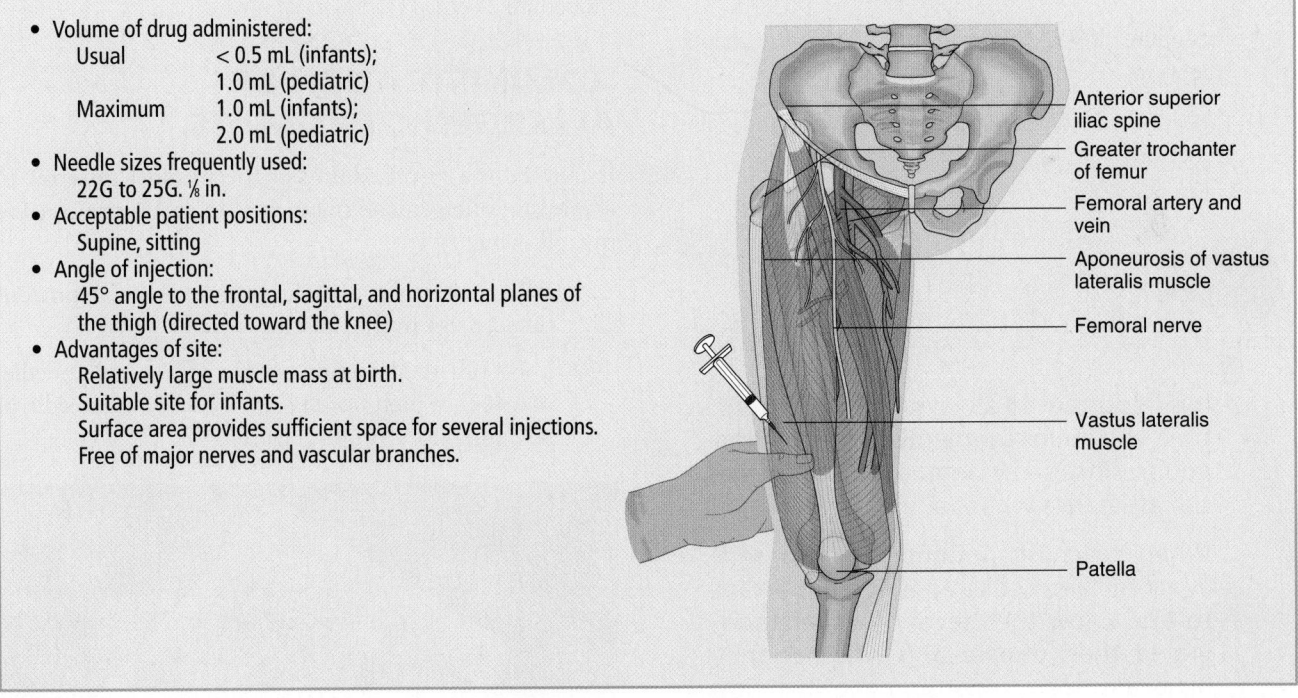

- Volume of drug administered:
    Usual   < 0.5 mL (infants);
                        1.0 mL (pediatric)
    Maximum   1.0 mL (infants);
                        2.0 mL (pediatric)
- Needle sizes frequently used:
    22G to 25G. ⅝ in.
- Acceptable patient positions:
    Supine, sitting
- Angle of injection:
    45° angle to the frontal, sagittal, and horizontal planes of the thigh (directed toward the knee)
- Advantages of site:
    Relatively large muscle mass at birth.
    Suitable site for infants.
    Surface area provides sufficient space for several injections.
    Free of major nerves and vascular branches.

Labels: Anterior superior iliac spine; Greater trochanter of femur; Femoral artery and vein; Aponeurosis of vastus lateralis muscle; Femoral nerve; Vastus lateralis muscle; Patella

Figure 24-24E   Injection technique for vastus lateralis site, pediatric.

CAUTION: If blood appears in the syringe upon aspiration, smoothly withdraw the needle, properly discard the used unit, and prepare another injection for administration. Repeat the preceding steps.

8. Slowly inject the medication into the patient.

9. With a quick, smooth motion, remove the needle from the injection site. Discard the syringe needle unit in a puncture-proof container. Cover the injection site with a dry, sterile cotton swab and gently massage the site.

CAUTION: Do not massage the site when administering insulin, Imferon, or heparin.

10. Remove the cotton swab and check for bleeding. If bleeding occurs, apply a sterile Band-Aid® to the injection site. Remove gloves.

11. Observe the patient for any signs of hypersensitivity.

12. Take precautions to ensure the patient's safety.

13. Properly discard the used equipment and supplies. This should be done as soon as possible.

14. Wash hands.

15. Before leaving the room, make sure that the patient is given proper instructions and is experiencing no unusual effects.

16. Follow documentation procedures to record the administration of the medication.

Procedures 24-2 through 24-8 include:

- Procedure 24-2 General Procedure for Administration of Subcutaneous, Intramuscular, and/or Intradermal Injections

- Procedure 24-3 Withdrawing (Aspirating) Medication from a Vial

- Procedure 24-4 Withdrawing (Aspirating) Medication from an Ampule

- Procedure 24-5 Administering a Subcutaneous Injection

- Procedure 24-6 Administering an Intramuscular Injection

- Procedure 24-7 Administering an Intradermal Injection

- Procedure 24-8 Reconstituting a Powder Medication for Administration Equipment

Z-TRACK METHOD OF INTRAMUSCULAR INJECTION

Imferon is an example of a medication that must be administered by using the Z-track method. This medication and others that are irritating to the subcutaneous tissues and may discolor the skin are given in this manner. (The *Physician's Desk Reference* is a good reference source for help in determining the correct technique for injections.)

The Z-track technique is similar to an intramuscular injection, except that the skin is pulled to the side prior to needle insertion. This causes a displacement of the tissues and the medication enters in a manner that will not allow it to seep back into the subcutaneous tissues and up to the skin's surface. Because the medications are irritating, for the comfort of the patient, change the needle on the syringe after aspirating the medication from the ampule or vial before injecting the patient with the medication. See Procedure 24-9.

ADMINISTRATION OF ALLERGENIC EXTRACTS

It may be the responsibility of the medical assistant to administer allergenic extracts. It is important to observe the following:

- Allergic extracts are *always* given in subcutaneous tissue, *never* in the muscle.

- Use a tuberculin syringe with a 25G, ⅝ inch needle, or a 26G, ⅜ inch needle, or a 27G, ½ inch needle or ICC allergist syringes (Figure 24-25).

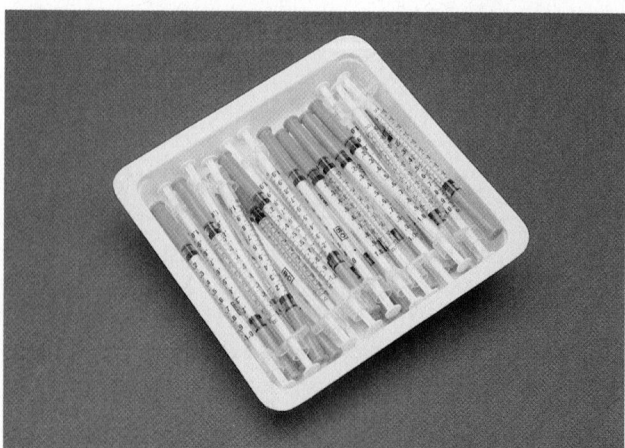

Figure 24-25 Allergist syringes.

- Use a site rotation system for each injected extract.

- Correctly document the procedure.

- Allergenic extracts should be refrigerated; they should retain potency for 10 to 12 weeks.

- Adverse reactions such as itching, swelling, and redness should be reported immediately to the physician.

- Severe reactions such as anaphylactic shock have occurred; therefore, emergency equipment and supplies must be available for use (see Chapter 23 for emergency supplies).

- Allergy testing can only be done when physician is present.

Example:
Patient's Name:

Date	Dose	Site
6/24/__	1st 0.05 cc s.c.	Lt. arm
6/27/__	2nd 0.10 cc s.c.	Rt. arm
6/30/__	3rd 0.15 cc s.c.	Lt. arm

 The patient should be observed for 15 to 30 minutes following the injection of an allergenic extract.

Susceptible individuals can develop allergic reactions to many foreign substances. It is prudent that the allergic person be totally aware of those substances and/or things that are known allergens.

INHALATION METHODS OF MEDICATION ADMINISTRATION

The act of drawing breath, vapor, or gas into the lungs is known as inhalation. Inhalation therapy may involve the administration of medicines, water vapor, and such gases as oxygen, carbon dioxide, and helium.

An inhaler may be used to deliver medications to the lungs. Medications that utilize an inhaler include bronchodilators, mucolytic agents, and steroids. Inhalers are useful in the delivery of treatment for chronic obstructive pulmonary disease (COPD) and/or reversible obstructive airway disease. An inhaler is a small, handheld apparatus, usually an aerosol unit, that contains a microcrystalline suspension of medication. When activated, it produces a fine mist or spray containing the medication. This suspension is then drawn into the respiratory tract, settling deep into the lungs and alveoli.

Implications for Patient Care

- Patients should be instructed to follow the prescribed medication regimen. The prescribed medicine and the type of inhaler to be used will

determine the method of administration. A handheld inhaler may be utilized for oral or nasal inhalation, depending on the type ordered by the physician.

Inhalation therapy may be contraindicated in patients with delicate fluid balance, cardiac arrhythmias, **status asthmaticus**, and hypersensitivity to the medication. As with any medication, the physician will determine the treatment regimen for each patient.

Administration of Oxygen

Oxygen is a colorless, odorless, tasteless gas that is essential for life. When the body does not have an adequate supply of oxygen, a state of **hypoxemia** (lack of oxygen in the blood) develops, and the irreversible damage to vital organs is possible. When a lack of oxygen threatens a person's survival, supplemental oxygen must be prescribed and administered immediately, and arterial blood gas analysis will have to be made after oxygen administration has been started. If it is not an emergency or life-threatening situation, an arterial blood gas analysis will be made before the physician prescribes the dosage and method of administration. The normal range for oxygen in the arterial blood is 80 to 100 mm Hg (millimeters mercury). Oxygen is supplied in tanks (Figure 24-26) for use in the ambulatory care setting, but in a hospital setting oxygen is piped in through a wall pipe system.

Dosage. When oxygen is to be administered, dosage is based on individual needs. Since oxygen is a drug, the

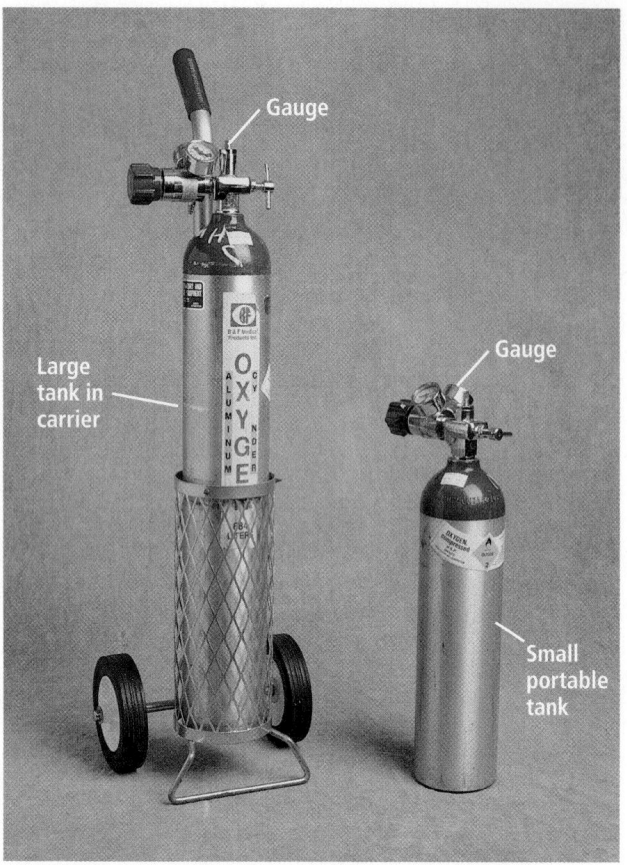

Figure 24-26   Oxygen tanks. Note gauge at top of tanks.

physician will prescribe the flow rate, concentration, method of delivery, and length of time for administration. Oxygen is ordered as liters per minute (LPM) or L/min and as percentage of oxygen concentration (%).

It is the medical assistant's responsibility to follow physician orders and adhere to the guidelines for proper drug administration. Always assess the patient as an individual, explain the procedure, and carefully observe the patient for signs of improvement or symptoms of oxygen toxicity.

CAUTION: Oxygen toxicity may develop when 100 percent oxygen is breathed for a prolonged period. As with any other drug, toxicity depends upon dose, time, and the patient's response. The higher the dose, the shorter the time required to develop toxicity. Symptoms of oxygen toxicity are substernal pain, nausea, vomiting, malaise, fatigue, numbness, and a tingling of the extremities.

High concentrations of inhaled oxygen cause alveolar collapse, intra-alveolar hemorrhage, hyaline membrane formation, disturbance of the central nervous system, and **retrolental fibroplasia** in newborns.

NOTE: **Apnea** (absence of breathing) can result when giving oxygen at a flow-rate greater than 2 liters per minute to COPD patients, especially those with emphysema.

Methods of Oxygen Delivery. Many methods are available today for the delivery of oxygen. The more commonly prescribed methods include the use of nasal cannulas, nasal catheters, and masks. Other methods of delivery involve the use of isolettes, hoods, and tents.

Nasal Cannula. When a low concentration of oxygen is desired, the nasal cannula (Figure 24-27) is the simplest and most convenient method for the administration of oxygen. Made of plastic, the nasal cannula consists of two hollow prongs through which oxygen passes, and a strap or other device to secure it to the patient's head (Figure 24-28). Do not place the direct flow of O_2 against the patient's nasal mucosa, as this causes tissue dehydration.

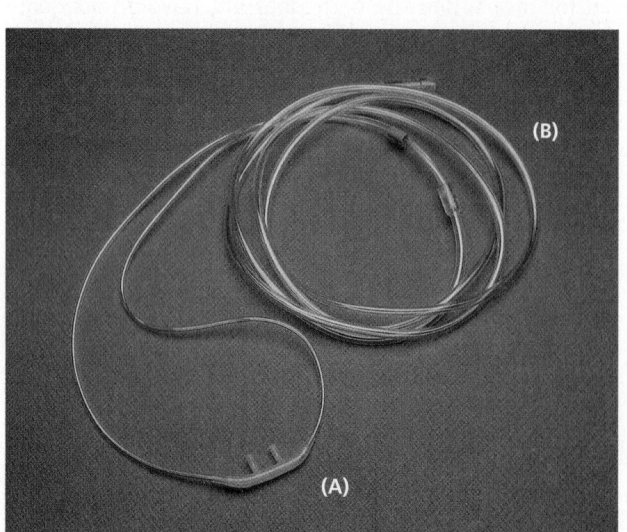

Figure 24-27   (A) Oxygen cannula. (B) Tubing.

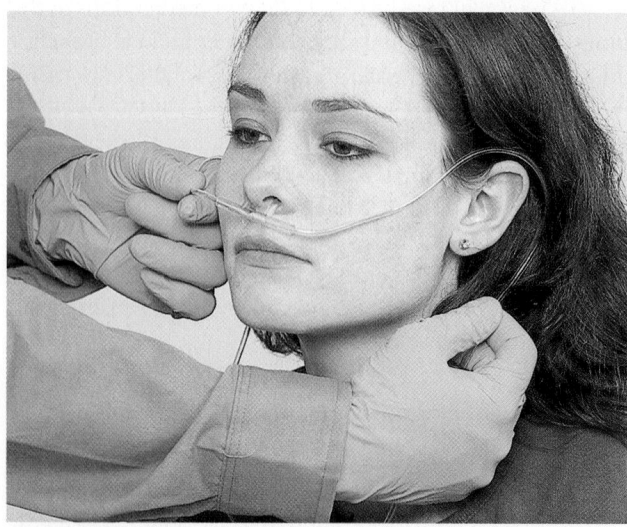

Figure 24-28   Medical assistant adjusts nasal cannula around patient's head for oxygen administration.

Flow rates greater than 2 to 4 liters per minute require humidification.

Nasal Catheter. The nasal catheter is a disposable plastic tube that has small holes at the inserted end. These holes diffuse the flow of oxygen for better distribution to lung tissue with minimum dehydration. The nasal catheter is seldom used today, because it causes mucus membrane irritation and has to be changed every 8 hours. Due to the discomfort caused to the patient by the catheter, the nasal cannula is the preferred method for the delivery of oxygen.

Mask. The common types of masks used for inhalation therapy include plastic disposable, partial rebreather, non-rebreather, and Venturi (Figure 24-29). These devices are employed when the patient requires high humidity and a precise amount of oxygen. To be effective, the mask must be fitted snugly to the patient (Figure 24-30).

   CAUTION: Oxygen must be humidified before delivery to the patient in order to prevent drying of the respiratory mucosa.

Oxygen Safety Precautions. Oxygen supports combustion; thus, there is the danger of a fire being started when oxygen is in use. Extreme caution should be exercised because ignition can be caused by friction, static electricity, or a lighted cigar or cigarette when O_2 is being administered. In the physician's office, oxygen is generally stored in tanks. These tanks must be checked on a regular basis and replaced as necessary.

Patient Teaching Tip

Explain safety measures to the patient who uses oxygen at home. Cigarettes, lighters, candles, and other smoking materials should not be used in the room where oxygen is used. Instruct the patient to wear nonstatic-producing clothing, such as cotton.

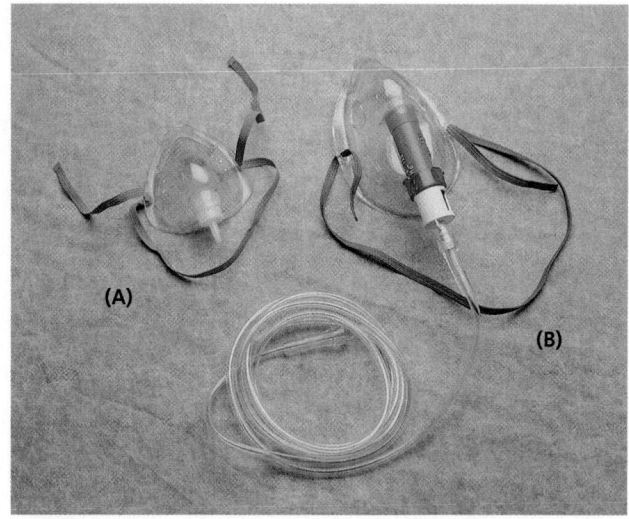

Figure 24-29   Oxygen masks: (A) Without tubing. (B) With tubing.

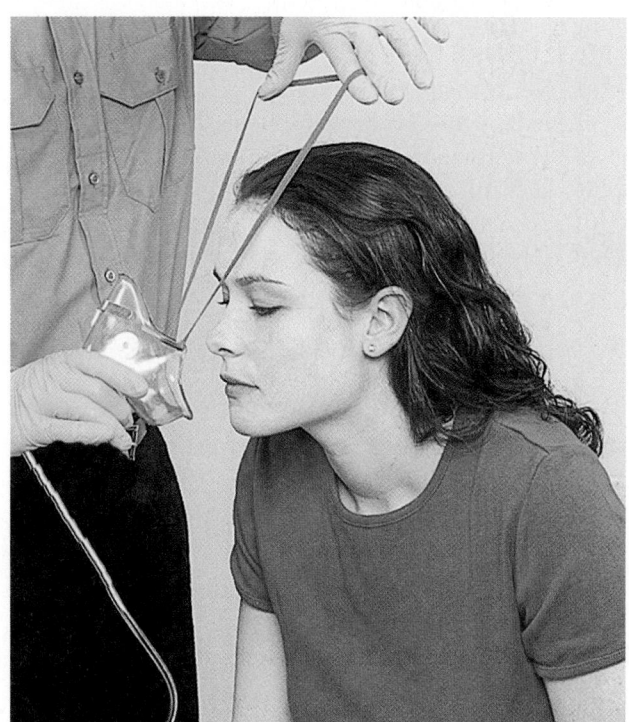

Figure 24-30   Medical assistant adjusts oxygen mask around patient's head.

Procedure

24-1   Administration of Oral Medications

STANDARD PRECAUTIONS:

PURPOSE:
Correctly administer an oral medication after receiving a physician's order and assembling the necessary equipment and supplies.

EQUIPMENT/SUPPLIES:
Proper medication
Medicine card
Water, milk, or juice for patient

PROCEDURE STEPS:
1. Verify the physician's order.
2. Follow the "Six Rights" (Figure 24-31A).
3. Perform medical asepsis handwash.
4. Work in a well-lighted, quiet, clean area.
5. Assemble equipment and supplies.
6. Obtain the correct medication using the medicine card.
7. Compare the medication label with the medicine card (first time).
8. Check the expiration date.
9. Calculate dosage if necessary.
10. Correctly prepare (a, b, or c) (Figure 24-31B).
    a. Multiple dose solid medication
    b. Unit dose medication
    c. Liquid medication
11. Compare medicine label with medicine card (second time).
12. Return medication to shelf and check label (third time).
13. Properly transport the medicine.
14. Identify the patient. Explain the procedure.
15. Assess patient. Take vital signs if indicated.
16. Assist patient to a comfortable position.
17. Provide water, milk, or juice (unless contraindicated).
18. Administer the medication. Be certain that the patient takes the medicine (Figure 24-31C).
19. Provide for the patient's safety: Observe the patient for any adverse reactions.
20. Care for equipment and supplies according to OSHA guidelines.
21. Wash hands.
22. Document the procedure in the patient chart using the medicine card (Figure 24-31D).

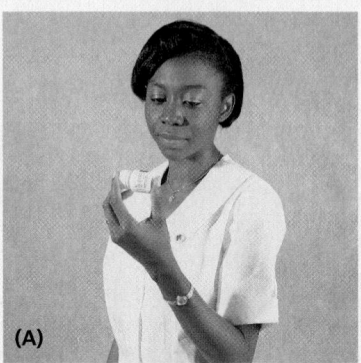

(A)

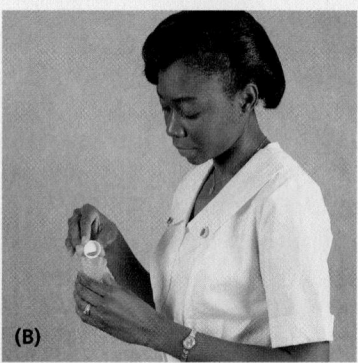

(B)

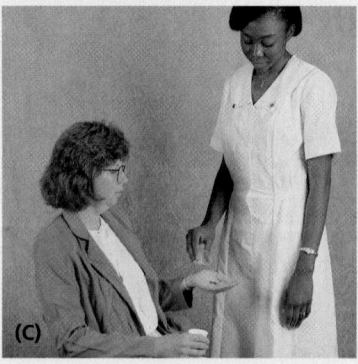

(C)

Figure 24-31   (A) Medical assistant checks for right drug, right dose, right route, and expiration date before pouring medication. (B) Medical assistant pours capsules from the cover of the medicine container into a medicine cup prior to administering medicine to the patient. The medication is poured into cover to avoid contamination of medicine. (C) Medical assistant administers the medication, being certain that patient takes the medicine.   *(continues)*

Procedure

24-1   *(continued)*

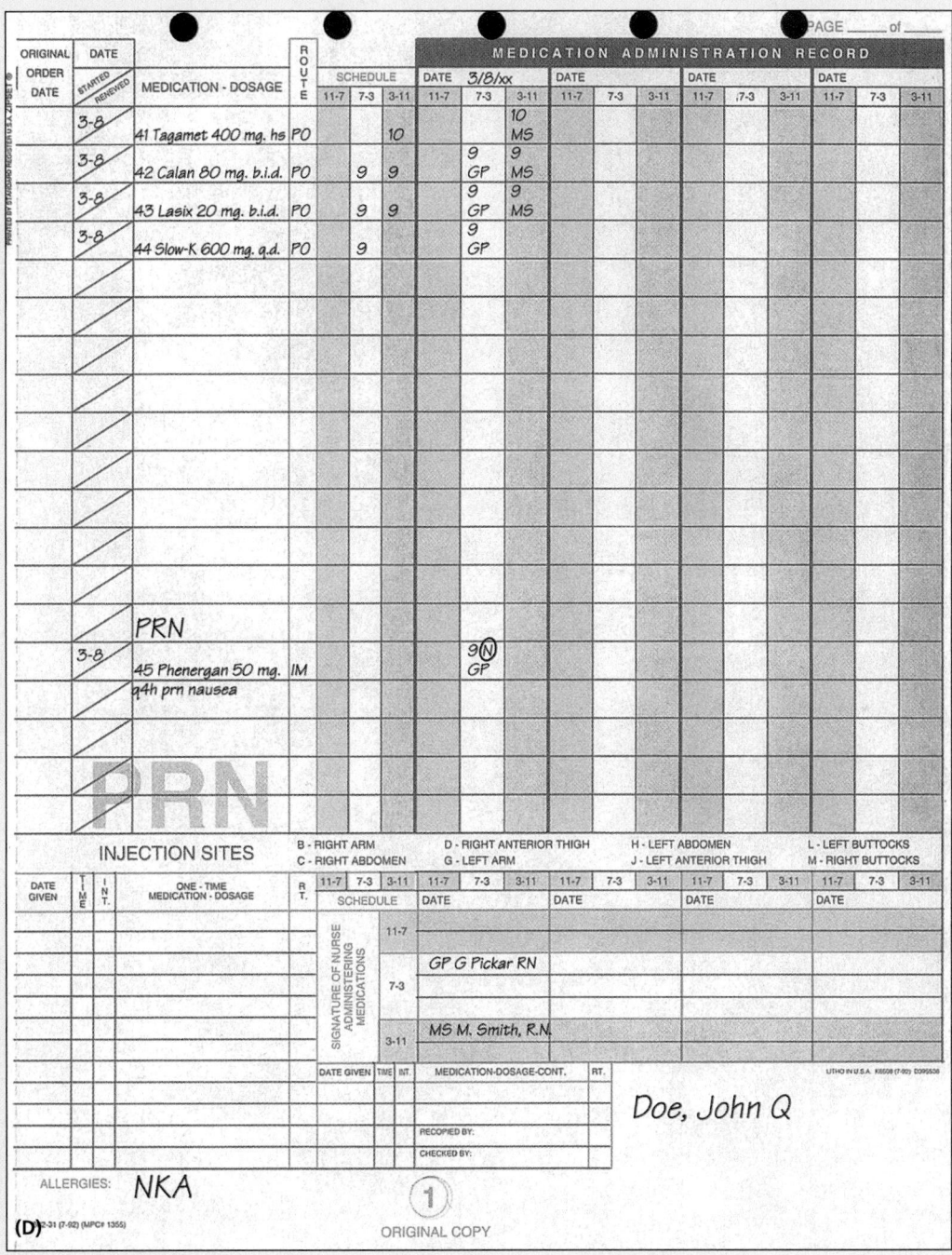

Figure 24-31 *(continued)* (D) Example of a medication administration record for patient's chart.

Procedure 24-2

Administration of Subcutaneous, Intramuscular, and Intradermal Injections

STANDARD PRECAUTIONS:

PURPOSE:

To properly administer subcutaneous, intramuscular, and intradermal injections.

EQUIPMENT/SUPPLIES:

Medication as ordered by the physician and medicine card
Appropriately sized needle-syringe unit
Alcohol wipes
Disposable gloves
Sharps container

PROCEDURE STEPS:

1. Verify the physician's order. Make out medicine card taking information from physician's order sheet from patient record.
2. Follow the "Six Rights."
3. Perform medical asepsis handwash. Adhere to OSHA guidelines.
4. Work in a well-lighted, quiet, clean area.
5. Obtain the appropriate syringe-needle unit and alcohol wipe.
6. Obtain the correct medication.
7. Compare the medication label with the medicine card (first time).
8. Check expiration date on medicine.
9. Calculate dosage, if necessary.
10. Prepare syringe-needle unit for use (Figure 24-32A–E).
11. Withdraw medication from container.
12. Compare medicine label with the medicine card (second time).
13. Place filled syringe-needle unit on the medicine tray with medicine card. Check the medication label with the medicine card (third time).
14. Correctly transport the medicine to the patient.
15. Identify the patient. Explain the procedure.
16. Assess the patient. Put on gloves.
17. Prepare the patient for the injection (drape, position, allay apprehension).

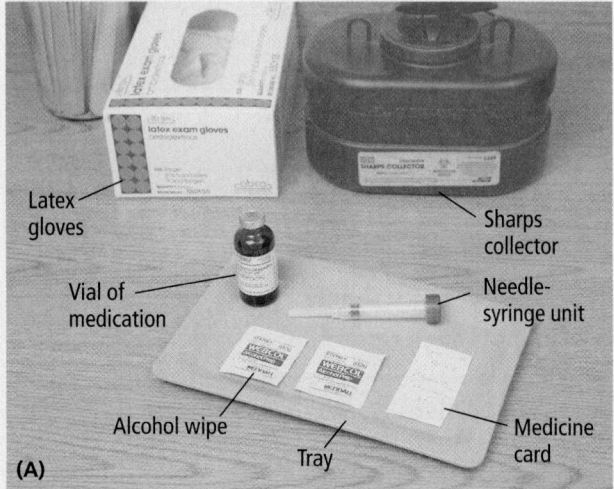

(A)

Latex gloves — Vial of medication — Alcohol wipe — Tray — Sharps collector — Needle-syringe unit — Medicine card

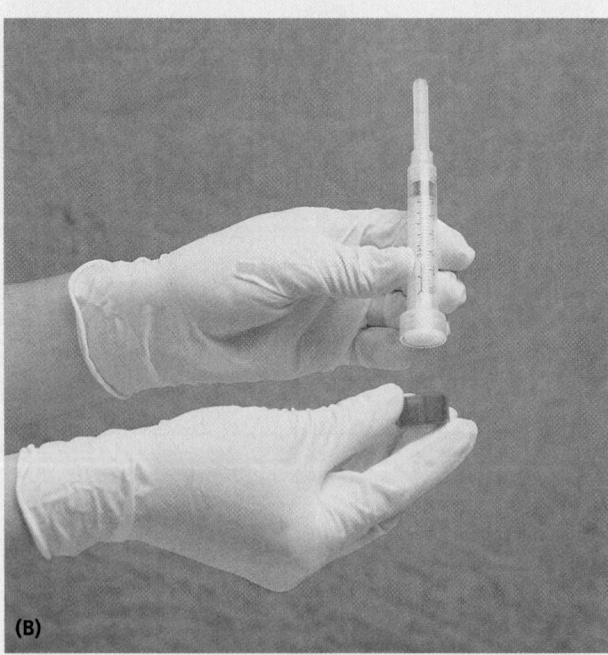

(B)

Figure 24-32   Preparing the syringe-needle unit for use: (A) Assemble the equipment and supplies needed to draw up medication from a vial. (B) Remove the cap from the cover of the sterile syringe-needle unit. *(continues)*

Procedure

24-2   *(continued)*

18. Select an appropriate injection site. Follow a rotating schedule if appropriate.
19. Cleanse the injection site with a sterile alcohol wipe. Use a circular motion, working from the center out to about 2 inches beyond the planned injection site.
20. Allow the skin to dry.
21. Administer the injection. Aspirate to be certain needle is not in a blood vessel (except for intradermal injection). Immediately dispose of syringe-needle unit in a puncture-proof container.
22. Massage injection site unless contraindicated (insulin, Imferon, heparin).
23. Observe the patient for signs of difficulty.
24. Inspect the injection site for bleeding, apply Band-Aid if necessary.

25. Properly dispose of used equipment and supplies. Remove gloves.
26. Perform medical asepsis handwash.
27. Correctly document the procedure.

Procedure to follow should the medical assistant sustain an accidental needlestick after the injection:

- Thoroughly wash the site where the stick occurred.
- Cleanse the skin with an antiseptic.
- Report the incident.
- Document the incident and retain a copy for yourself.
- Obtain medical attention. Be tested for HBV and HIV.
- Fill out appropriate OSHA paperwork (200 form).

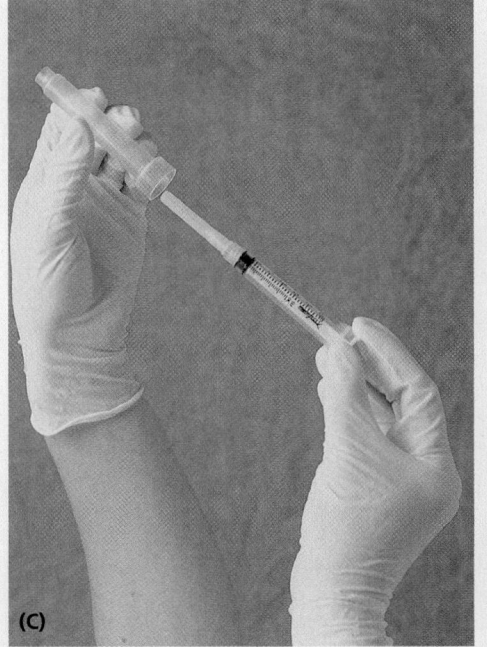
(C)

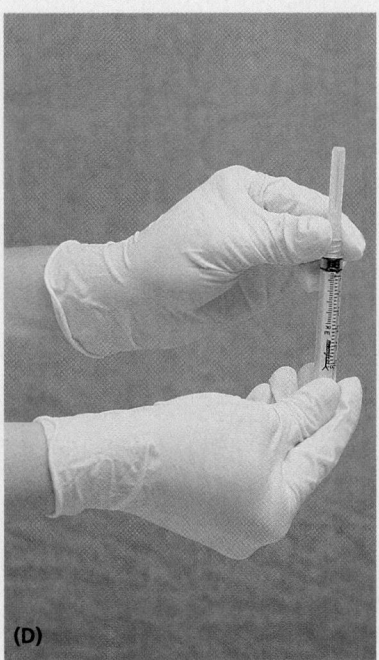
(D)

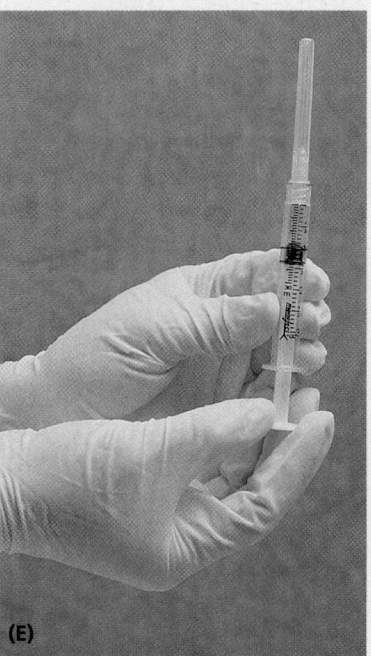
(E)

Figure 24-32   *(continued)* (C) Pull the sleeve of the cover off and remove the syringe-needle unit. (D) Secure the needle by twisting it clockwise. (E) Pull the plunger to check for ease of gliding operation.

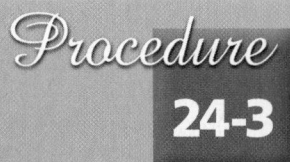

Withdrawing (Aspirating) Medication from a Vial

Procedure 24-3

STANDARD PRECAUTIONS:

PURPOSE:

Medication is supplied in a variety of packaging. Medication from a vial must be aspirated into a syringe for parenteral injection.

EQUIPMENT/SUPPLIES:

Medication order	Vial of medication
Medicine card	Alcohol wipes
Appropriate syringe and needle with cover	Disposable gloves
	Sharps container

PROCEDURE STEPS:

1. Read the medication order and assemble equipment. Check for the "Six Rights." Read the vial label by holding it next to the medicine card (first time).
2. Wash hands. Apply gloves.
3. Select the proper size needle and syringe for the medication and the route (e.g., for subcutaneous injection of insulin, 100-U insulin syringe and 25G, ⅝ inch needle). If necessary, attach the needle to the syringe.
4. Check the vial label against the medicine card (second time).
5. Remove the metal or plastic cap from the vial. If the vial has been opened previously, clean the rubber stopper by applying an alcohol wipe in a circular motion (Figure 24-33A).
6. Remove the needle cover—pull it straight off.
7. Inject air into the vial as follows:
   a. Hold the syringe pointed upward at eye level. Pull back the plunger to take in a quantity of air that is equal to the ordered dose of medication.
   b. Hold the vial upright (inverted) according to personal preference. Take care not to touch the rubber stopper.
   c. Insert the needle through the rubber stopper of the vial. Inject the air by pushing in the plunger (Figure 24-33B).
8. Withdraw the medication: Hold the vial and the syringe steady. Pull back on the plunger to with-

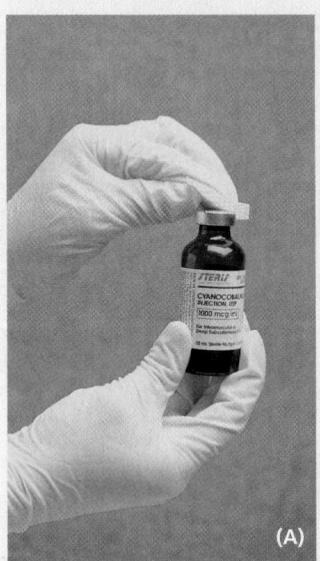

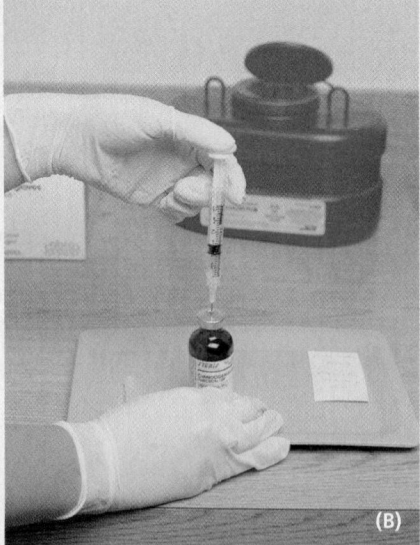

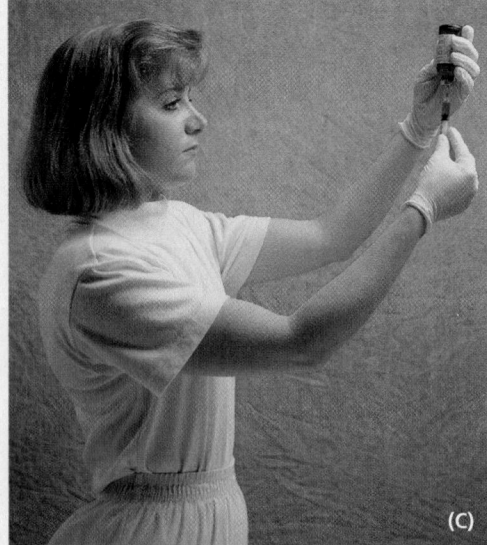

Figure 24-33 (A) Disinfect the rubber stopper on the medication vial with an alcohol wipe. (B) Keeping the bevel of the needle above the fluid level, inject an amount of air equal to medication quantity to be withdrawn. (C) Hold syringe pointed upward at eye level and with the bevel of the needle in the medication. Pull back plunger and aspirate the quantity of medication ordered.

(continues)

draw the measured dose of medication. Measure accurately. Keep the tip of the needle below the surface of the liquid; otherwise, air will enter the syringe. Keep syringe at eye level (Figure 24-33C).

9. Check the syringe for air bubbles. Remove them by tapping sharply on the syringe (Figure 24-33D). Check measurement for accuracy.

10. Remove the needle from the vial. Replace the sterile needle cover (Figure 24-33E).

11. Check the vial label against the medicine card (third time).

12. Place the filled needle and syringe on a medicine tray or cart with an alcohol wipe and the medicine card. The dose is now ready for injection.

13. Return multiple-dose vials to the proper storage area (cabinet or refrigerator). Dispose of unused medication in a single-dose vial according to facility procedure. (Remember, disposal of a controlled substance must be witnessed and the proper forms signed.)

14. If medication is a tissue irritant, change to another sterile needle. RATIONALE: Tissue irritants can cause tissue necrosis.

15. Discard used syringe-needle unit immediately after use in a sharps container.

16. Remove gloves and dispose in biohazard waste container.

17. Wash hands.

18. Document the procedure.

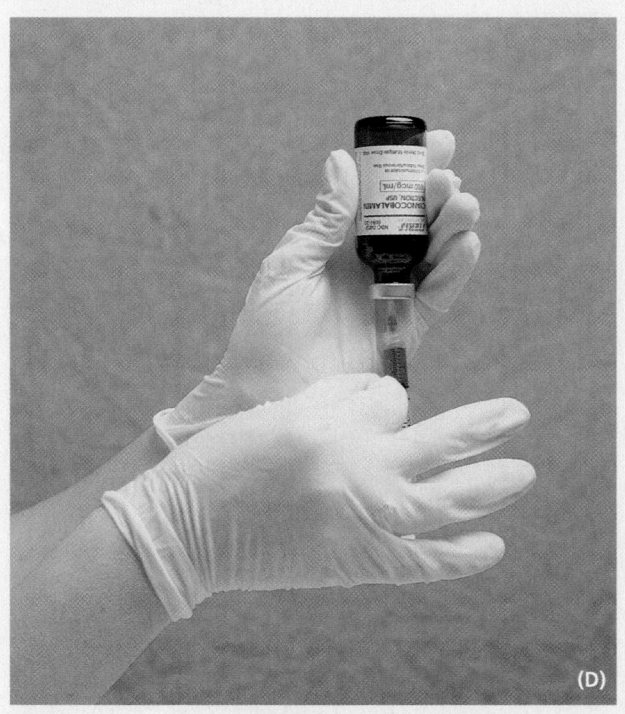

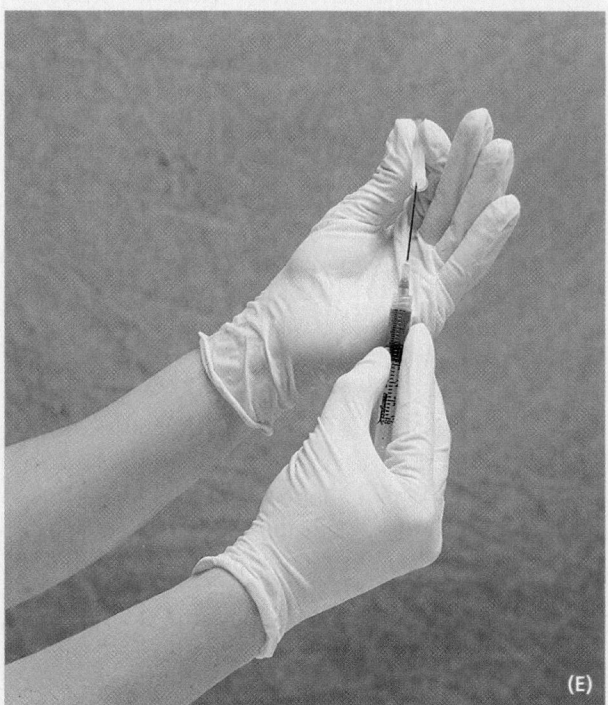

Figure 24-33 *(continued)* (D) Tap syringe to eliminate air bubbles. Hand should hold syringe while tapping it. (E) After the correct dose has been withdrawn, recover the sterile needle. Place medication on a tray along with medication card and an alcohol wipe and safely transport to the patient.

Procedure 24-4

Withdrawing (Aspirating) Medication from an Ampule

STANDARD PRECAUTIONS:

PURPOSE:

Medication is supplied in a variety of packaging. An ampule is a sterile, glass, single-dose container of liquid medication. It is aspirated into a syringe for parenteral injection.

EQUIPMENT/SUPPLIES:

Medicine tray and medicine card
Ampule of medication
Alcohol wipes
Sterile gauze sponges
Sharps container
Sterile needle-syringe unit
Gloves

PROCEDURE STEPS:

1. Check the physician's order. Write out medicine card.
2. Wash hands and gather equipment. Put on gloves.
3. Obtain ampule of medication. Read label and check medicine card for correct medication, dose, route, and time (first time). Check medication expiration date.
4. Flick ampule of medication (medication will often get "trapped" above the neck of the ampule). A sharp flick of the wrist will help force all of the medication down below the neck of the ampule into the body of the ampule (Figure 24-34A). RATIONALE: This is important to ensure all medication is available in the body of the ampule in order to calculate the correct dose. If some of the medication remains trapped above the neck in the top of the ampule, some medication will not be available for use and it is possible to give an incorrect dose, especially if the patient is to receive the entire contents of the ampule.
5. Thoroughly disinfect the neck with an alcohol swab. Check label (second time). RATIONALE: The needle will enter the opening of the ampule

and wiping the neck of the ampule prior to removal of the top ensures disinfection of the neck or opening of the ampule.

6. With a sterile gauze, wipe dry the neck of the ampule. Completely surround the ampule with the gauze and forcefully snap off the top of the ampule by pushing the top away from you (Figure 24-34B). RATIONALE: Ensure medical assistant safety from possible injury from broken glass. Discard top in sharps container.
7. Place opened ampule down on medicine tray. Check label (third time).
8. With a prepared sterile syringe-needle unit that has a filter on the needle, aspirate the required dose into the syringe (Figure 24-34C). Cover needle with sheath and transport to patient on the medicine tray. RATIONALE: Filtered needles prevent glass particles from being aspirated with medication.
9. Identify the patient.

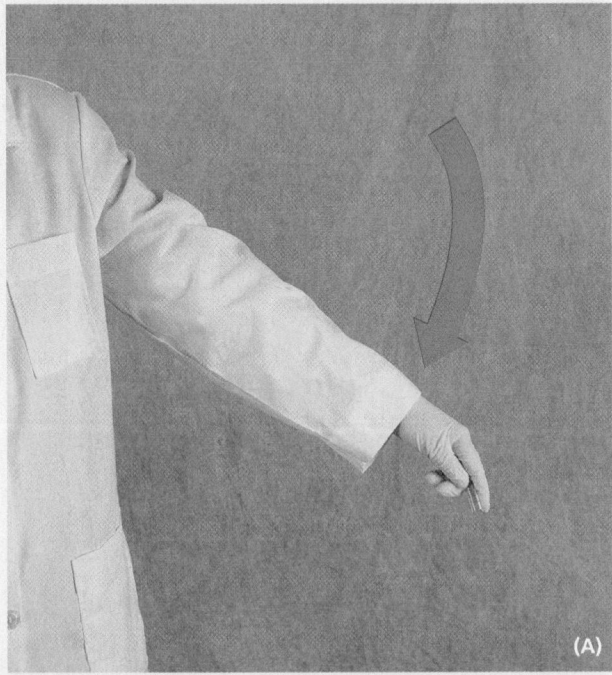

(A)

Figure 24-34 (A) Hold ampule by the top and force all the medication into the bottom of the ampule by a snap of the arm and wrist. *(continues)*

Procedure

24-4 **(continued)**

10. Administer medication.
11. Discard syringe-needle unit into sharps container. Alcohol wipes and gauze are discarded in biohazard waste container.

12. Remove gloves and dispose in biohazard waste container.
13. Wash hands.
14. Document the procedure.

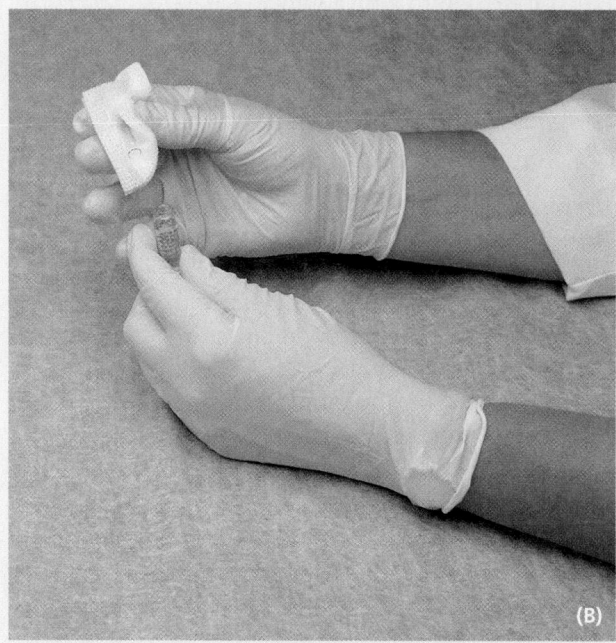

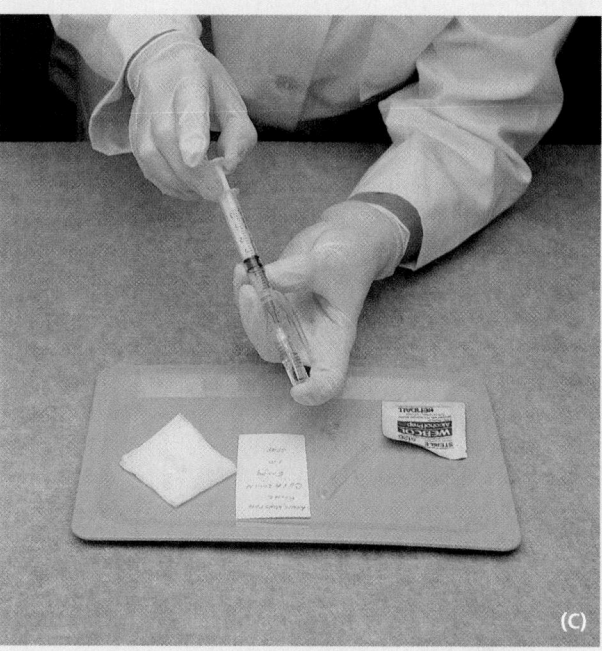

Figure 24-34 *(continued)* (B) Remove top from ampule. Turn hand up and out simultaneously. (C) Aspirate required dose into syringe.

Administering a Subcutaneous Injection
24-5

STANDARD PRECAUTIONS:

PURPOSE:
Correctly administer a subcutaneous injection after receiving a physician's order and assembling the necessary equipment and supplies.

EQUIPMENT/SUPPLIES:
Medication ordered   Alcohol wipes
   by physician   Disposable gloves
Medicine card   Sharps container
Appropriately sized
   needle-syringe unit

PROCEDURE STEPS:
1. Verify the physician's order. Make out a medicine card.
2. Follow the "Six Rights."
3. Perform medical asepsis handwash. Adhere to OSHA guidelines.
4. Work in a well-lighted, quiet, clean area.
5. Obtain the appropriate equipment and supplies.
6. Obtain the correct medication.
7. Compare the medication label with the medicine card (first time).
8. Check expiration date on medicine.
9. Calculate dosage, if necessary.
10. Correctly prepare the parenteral medication.
11. Compare medication label with the medicine card (second time).
12. Replace medication in appropriate area (shelf, refrigerator). Compare the medication label (third time).
13. Correctly transport the medicine to the patient.
14. Identify the patient. Explain the procedure.
15. Assess the patient. Put on gloves.
16. Prepare the patient for the injection (drape, position, allay apprehension).
17. Select an appropriate injection site.
18. Correctly cleanse the site using a circular motion starting with the injection site and moving outward to a 2-inch diameter. Allow skin to dry.
29. Remove needle guard.
20. Grasp skin to form a 1-inch fold.
21. Insert needle quickly at a 45-degree angle (Figure 24-35).
22. Aspirate to be certain needle is not in a blood vessel.
23. Slowly inject the medicine.
24. Correctly remove the needle and syringe.
25. Immediately dispose of needle and syringe in a sharps container.
26. Cover site. Massage (unless contraindicated as with insulin, Imferon, and heparin).
27. Provide for patient's safety.
28. Remove gloves and wash hands.
29. Document the procedure. Example: 12/16/2001 10 AM NPH insulin 8 units S.C. (L) deltoid area. S. Jones, CMA.

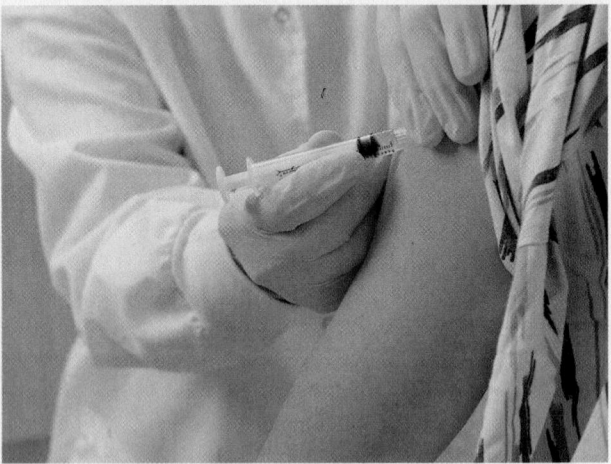

Figure 24-35   Insert needle at 45-degree angle into upper arm.

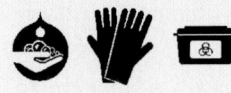

Administering an Intramuscular Injection

24-6

STANDARD PRECAUTIONS:

PURPOSE:

Correctly administer an intramuscular injection after receiving a physician's order and assembling the necessary equipment and supplies.

EQUIPMENT/SUPPLIES:

Medication ordered by physician with medication
   card
Appropriately sized needle-syringe unit
Alcohol wipes
Disposable gloves
Sharps container

PROCEDURE STEPS:

1. Verify the physician's order. Make out a medicine card.
2. Follow the "Six Rights."
3. Perform medical asepsis handwash. Adhere to OSHA guidelines.
4. Work in a well-lighted, quiet, clean area.
5. Obtain the appropriate equipment and supplies.
6. Obtain the correct medication.
7. Compare the medication label with the medicine card (first time).
8. Check expiration date.
9. Calculate dosage, if necessary.
10. Correctly prepare the parenteral medication.
11. Compare medicine label with the medicine card (second time).
12. Replace medication on appropriate shelf and compare medication label with medicine card (third time).
13. Correctly transport the medicine to the patient.
14. Identify the patient. Explain the procedure.
15. Assess the patient. Put on gloves.
16. Prepare the patient for the injection (drape, position, allay apprehension).
17. Select an appropriate injection site.

18. Correctly cleanse the site using a circular motion and covering a 2-inch diameter. Allow the skin to dry.
19. Remove needle guard.
20. Stretch the skin **taut**, pulling it tight.
21. Using a dart-like motion, insert needle to the hub at a 90-degree angle (Figure 24-36).
22. Release the skin.
23. Aspirate to check for blood.
24. Slowly inject the medicine.
25. Correctly remove the needle and syringe.
26. Immediately dispose of needle and syringe in a sharps container.
27. Cover site. Massage (unless contraindicated as with insulin, Imferon, and heparin).
28. Dispose of equipment. Remove gloves.
29. Wash hands.
30. Observe the patient for signs of difficulty.
31. Provide for patient's safety.
32. Document the procedure. Example: 12/16/2001 10 AM Demerol 75 mg I.M. (L) deltoid area. S. Jones, CMA.

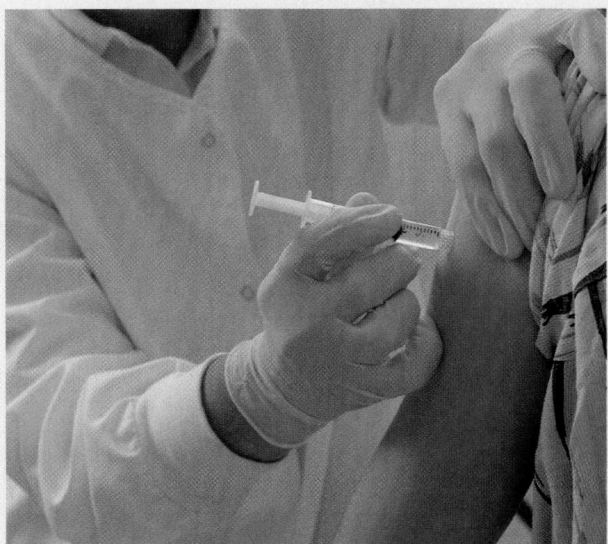

Figure 24-36   Using deltoid area of upper arm, insert needle to the hub at a 90-degree angle.

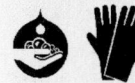

Procedure
24-7

Administering an Intradermal Injection

STANDARD PRECAUTIONS:

PURPOSE:
Correctly administer an intradermal injection after receiving a physician's order and assembling the necessary equipment and supplies.

EQUIPMENT/SUPPLIES:
Medication as ordered by physician with medication card
Appropriately sized needle-syringe unit
Alcohol wipes
Disposable gloves
Sharps container

PROCEDURE STEPS:
1. Verify the physician's order. Make out a medicine card.
2. Follow the "Six Rights."
3. Perform medical asepsis handwash. Adhere to OSHA guidelines.
4. Work in a well-lighted, quiet, clean area.
5. Obtain the appropriate equipment and supplies.
6. Obtain the correct medication.
7. Compare the medication label with the medicine card (first time).
8. Check expiration date.
9. Calculate dosage, if necessary.
10. Correctly prepare the parenteral medication.
11. Compare medication label with the medicine card (second time).
12. Replace medication on appropriate shelf and compare medication label with medicine card (third time).
13. Correctly transport the medicine to the patient.
14. Identify the patient. Explain the procedure.
15. Assess the patient. Put on gloves.
16. Prepare the patient for the injection (drape, position, allay apprehension).
17. Select an appropriate injection site (Figure 24-37A). For other sites, refer back to Figure 24-19B.

18. Correctly cleanse the site using a circular motion and covering a 2-inch diameter. Allow the skin to dry.
19. Remove needle guard.
20. Pull the skin tissue taut.
21. Carefully insert the needle at a 10- to 15-degree angle, bevel upward to about ⅛ inch. Do not aspirate.
22. Steadily inject purified protein derivative (PPD) (Figure 24-37B). Within 24 to 72 hours, a bleb, or slight elevation of the skin, will be produced at the injection site.
23. Correctly remove the needle after a brief delay. RATIONALE: Minimizes leakage.
24. Immediately dispose of needle and syringe in a sharps container.

(continues)

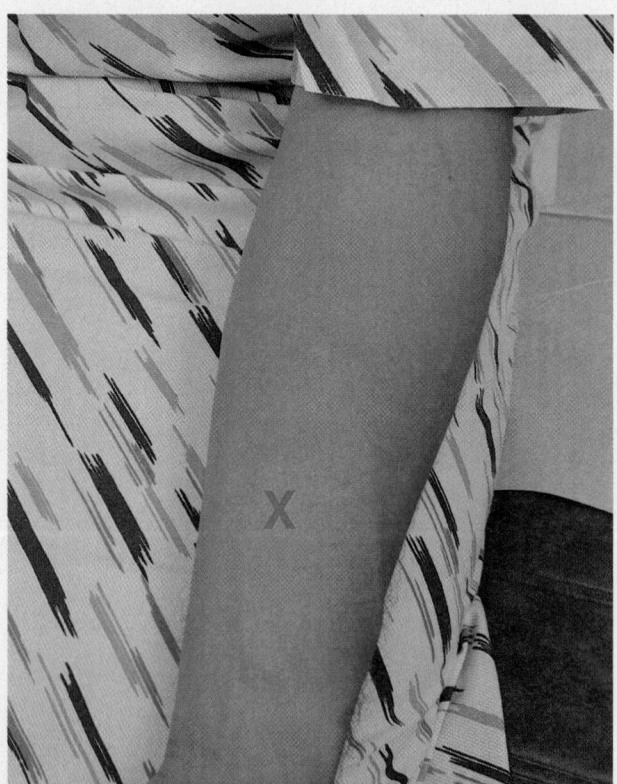

Figure 24-37A One site for administering an intradermal injection is near the center of the forearm.

Procedure 24-7 *(continued)*

25. Blot site. Do not massage. Dispose of equipment. Remove gloves.
26. Wash hands.
27. Observe the patient for signs of difficulty.
28. Provide for patient's safety.
29. Document the procedure. Example: 10/14/2001 10 AM 0.1 ml PPD I.D. (L) forearm. S. Jones, CMA.
30. The injected area should be read for the amount of induration (hardness) or reaction to the PPD to determine active or inactive tuberculosis exposure.
31. If injection area is hardened and elevated, make follow-up appointment for patient.

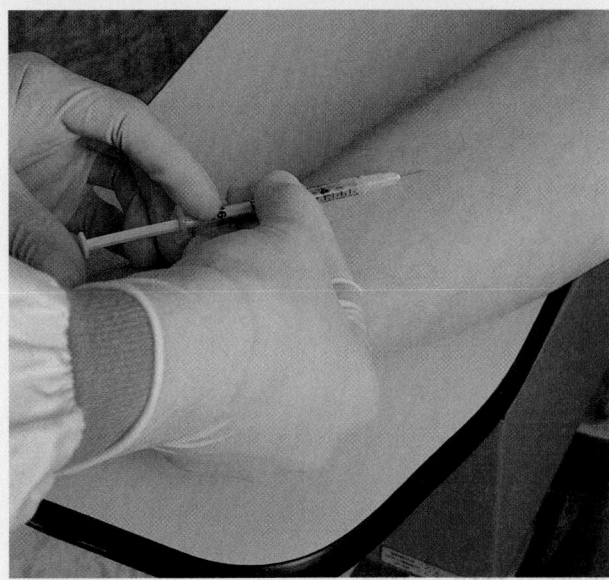

Figure 24-37B   Steadily inject the medicine.

Procedure 24-8 **Reconstituting a Powder Medication for Administration**

STANDARD PRECAUTIONS:

PURPOSE:
Drugs for injection may be supplied in a powdered (dry) form and must be reconstituted to a liquid for injection. A diluent (usually sterile water) is added to the powder, mixed well, and the appropriate dose is drawn up to be administered.

EQUIPMENT/SUPPLIES:
Medication as ordered by the physician and medicine card
Diluent
2 appropriately sized needles and syringe units
Alcohol wipes
Disposable gloves
Sharps container

PROCEDURE STEPS:
1. Medical assistant prepares the needle-syringe unit in preparation for reconstituting powder medication (Figure 24-38A).
2. Remove tops from diluent and powder medication containers and wipe with alcohol swabs (Figure 24-38B).
3. Insert the needle of a sterile needle-syringe unit through the rubber stopper on the vial of diluent that has been cleansed with an alcohol wipe. The needle-syringe unit should have an amount of air in it equal to the amount of diluent to be withdrawn (Figures 24-38C and D).
4. Withdraw the appropriate amount of diluent to be added to the powder medication (Figures 24-38E and F). Cover the sterile needle on the syringe containing appropriate amount of diluent.

(continues)

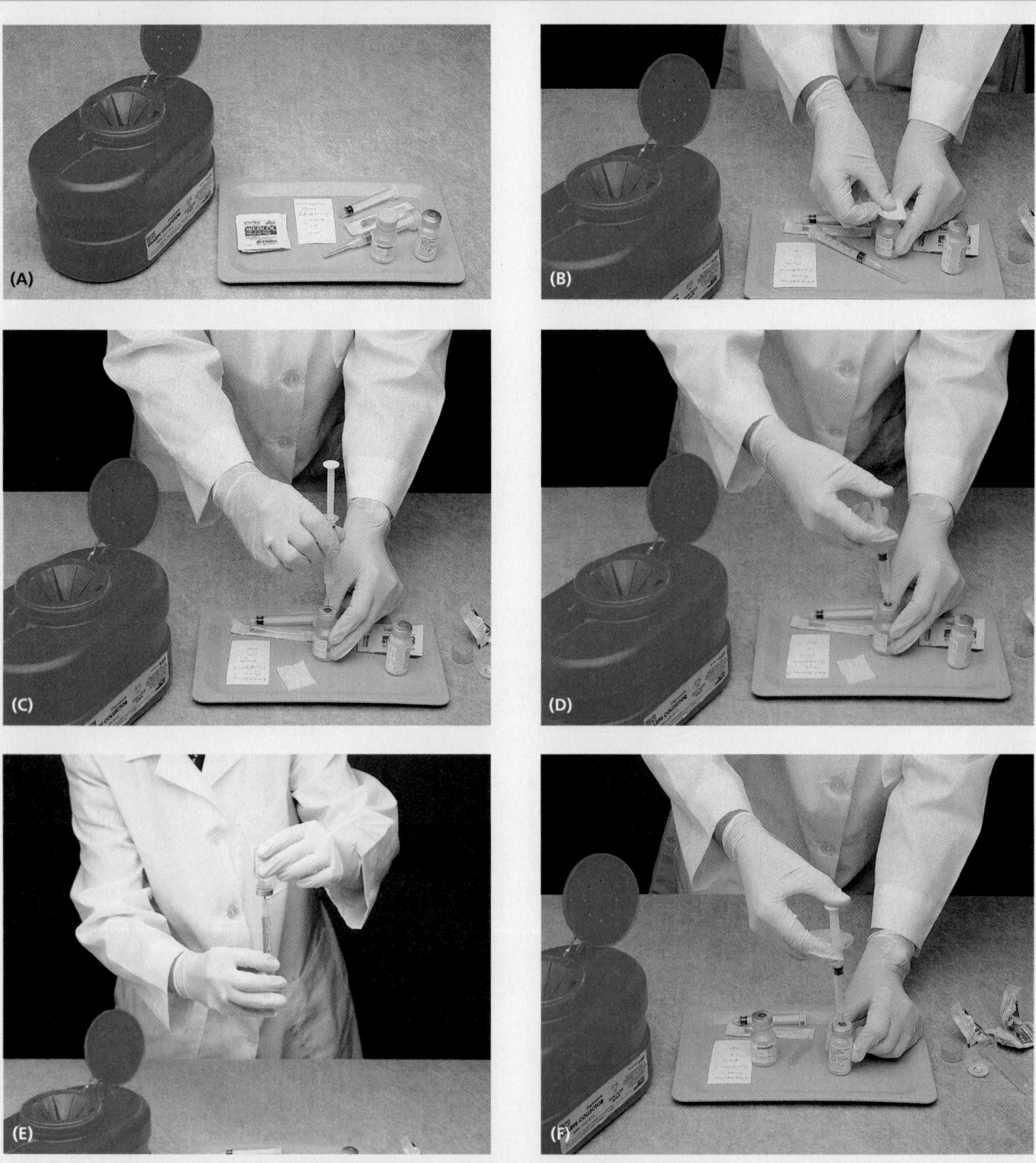

Figure 24-38 (A) Supplies for reconstituting powder medication. (B) Remove top from diluent and powdered medication. Wipe top of each with an alcohol wipe. (C) Prepare to inject air in an equal amount to diluent being removed from the vial. (D) Inject air into the vial. (E) Prepare to separate vial from needle-syringe unit after withdrawing diluent. (F) Inject diluent into vial containing powdered medication. Top of vial should be cleansed again with an alcohol wipe. *(continues)*

Procedure

24-8 (continued)

5. Add this liquid to the powder medication that has been cleansed with an alcohol wipe (Figure 24-38G).
6. Remove needle and syringe from vial with powder medication and diluent and discard into sharps container (Figure 24-38H).
7. Roll the vial between the palms of the hands to completely mix together the powder and diluent (Figure 24-38I). Label the multiple dose vial with the dilution or strength of the medication prepared, the date and time, your initials, and the expiration date.

8. With a second sterile needle and syringe, withdraw the desired amount of medication (Figure 24-38J).
9. Flick away any air bubbles that cling to side of syringe (Figure 24-38K).
10. The medicine tray with reconstituted medication is ready for transport to the patient (Figure 24-38L).
11. Proceed as in steps 11–32 of Procedure 24-6, Administering an Intramuscular Injection.

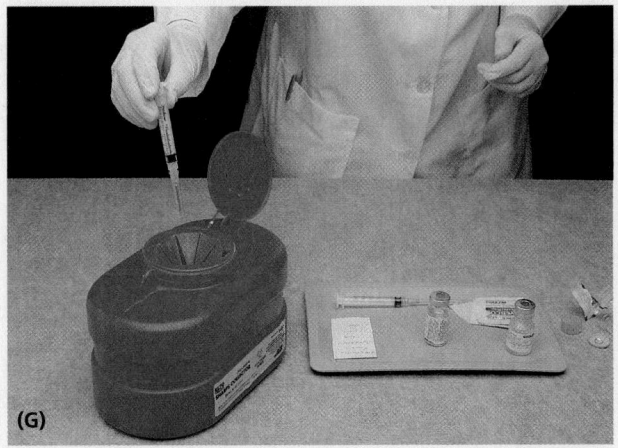
(G)

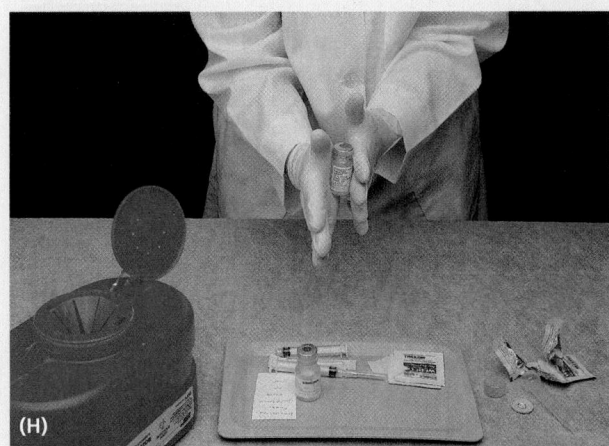
(H)

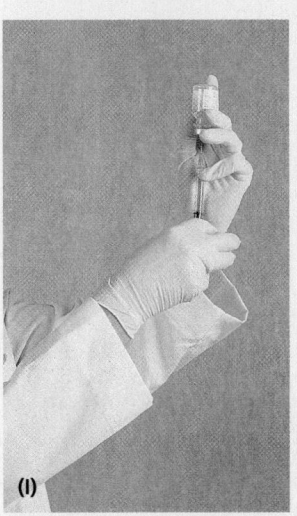
(I)

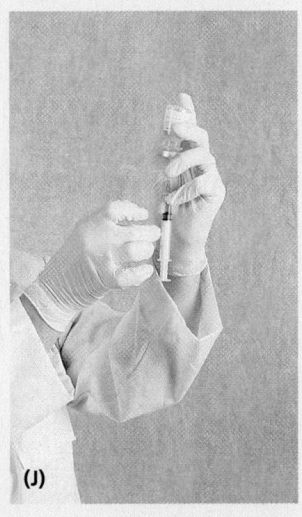
(J)

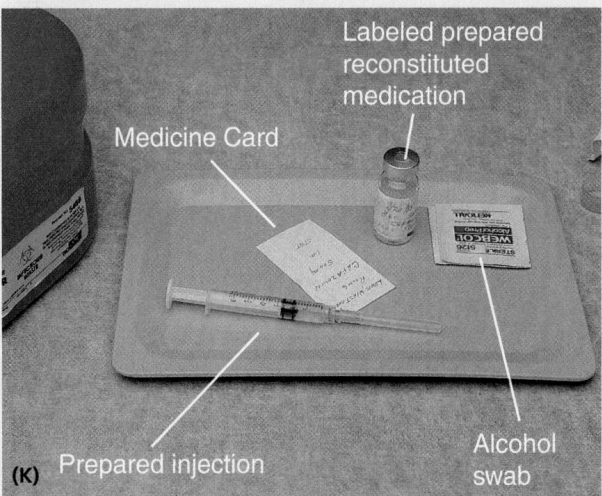
Labeled prepared reconstituted medication

Medicine Card

Prepared injection

Alcohol swab

(K)

Figure 24-38 *(continues)* (G) Discard recapped needle-syringe unit after mixing. (H) Roll vial of powdered medication between palms of hands with the diluent to mix well. Label vial with date, amount of diluent added, strength of dilution, time mixed, and your initials. (I) Use a second sterile needle-syringe unit to draw the prescribed dose of medication ordered by the physician. (J) Flick away any air bubbles that cling to the side of the syringe. (K) Medicine tray shows prepared injection ready for transport to patient. Labeled, reconstituted medication will be placed on the shelf or in the refrigerator according to the manufacturer's instructions.

Procedure 24-9

Z-Track Intramuscular Injection Technique

STANDARD PRECAUTIONS:

PURPOSE:

Correctly administer a Z-track intramuscular injection after receiving a physician's order and assembling the necessary equipment and supplies.

EQUIPMENT/SUPPLIES:

Medication ordered by physician and medicine card
Appropriately sized needle-syringe unit
Alcohol wipes
Disposable gloves
Sharps container

PROCEDURE STEPS:

1. Verify the physician's order. Make out a medicine card.
2. Follow the "Six Rights."
3. Perform medical asepsis handwash. Adhere to OSHA guidelines.
4. Work in a well-lighted, quiet, clean area.
5. Obtain the appropriate equipment and supplies.
6. Obtain the correct medication.
7. Compare the medication label with the medicine card (first time).
8. Check expiration date.
9. Calculate dosage, if necessary.
10. Correctly prepare the parenteral medication.
11. Compare medicine label with the medicine card (second time).
12. Replace medication on shelf and compare medication label with medicine card (third time).

13. Correctly transport the medicine to the patient.
14. Identify the patient. Explain the procedure.
15. Assess the patient. Put on gloves.
16. Prepare the patient for the injection (drape, position, allay apprehension).
17. Select an appropriate injection site.
18. Correctly cleanse the site using a circular motion and covering a 2-inch diameter. Allow the skin to dry.
19. Remove needle guard.
20. Pull the skin laterally 1½ inch away from the injection site.
21. Insert needle quickly, using a dart-like motion at a 90-degree angle. Maintain Z position (Figure 24-39).
22. Aspirate to check for blood.
23. Slowly inject medication.
24. Wait 10 seconds before removing needle to allow medication to begin to be absorbed.
25. Remove needle and syringe at same angle of insertion.
26. Release traction of the Z position in order to seal off the needle track. This prevents medication from reaching the subcutaneous tissues and the surface of the skin.
27. Immediately dispose of needle-syringe unit in a sharps container.
28. Cover site. Do not massage.
29. Remove gloves.
30. Wash hands.
31. Observe patient for signs of difficulty.
32. Provide for patient safety.
33. Document the procedure.

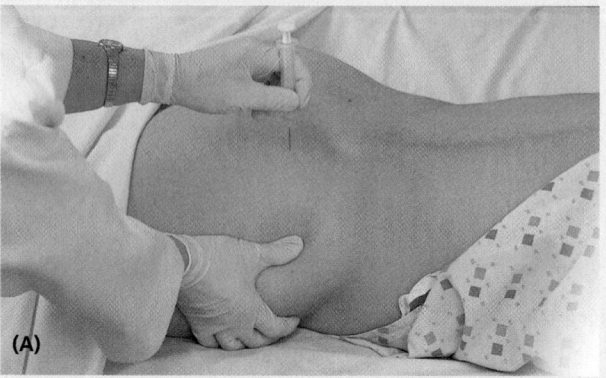

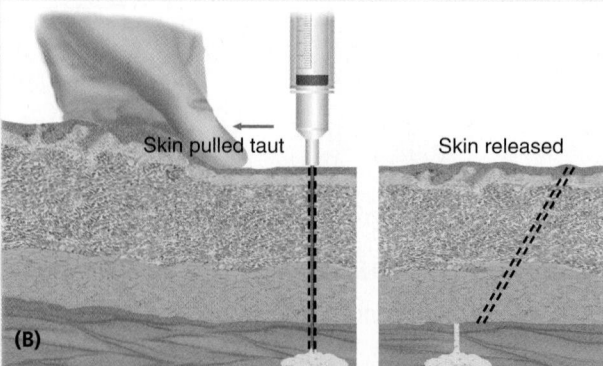

Skin pulled taut   Skin released

(A)   **(B)**

Figure 24-39 Z-track technique for IM injection: (A) With patient in prone position, grasp and pull the muscle laterally before injecting medication. (B) Inject medication. Keep skin pulled taut for 10 seconds. Quickly withdraw the needle and release the skin to seal the site.

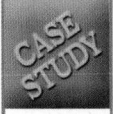

Abigail Johnson, a patient of Dr. Lewis, has been unable to keep her Type II noninsulin-dependent diabetes mellitus under control with oral hypoglycemics, and Dr. Lewis has decided that Abigail needs to begin to take insulin injections. Today in the clinic her fasting blood glucose level is 190 mg/mL. Dr. Lewis prescribes Humulin® insulin 10 units subcutaneously stat.

24-1

CASE STUDY REVIEW

1. What size insulin syringe should be used?
2. What does the medication label state are the number of units per milliliter? Show how to calculate the correct dosage.
3. Discuss the route of administration and the specifics about insulin administration that require it to be given slightly differently from other s.c. injections.
4. Describe several topics of discussion in which you would engage Abigail to help her learn how to better control her disease.

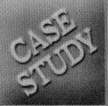

Alice Chambers weighs 28 pounds and is 33 inches tall. The adult dose is erythromycin 400 mg every 6 hours by mouth.

24-2

CASE STUDY REVIEW

1. Calculate the dose of erythromycin Alice needs.
2. If the physician ordered erythromycin by injection rather than by mouth, how would the dose be calculated if the erythromycin adult dose is 400 mg per milliliter?
3. What size needle and syringe is appropriate for giving Alice the injection?

SUMMARY

Administering medications is one of the most important and essential responsibilities that the medical assistant performs. In this chapter, a review of some of the fundamental elements of pharmacology, dosage calculations, and medication administration have been presented.

Each state has enacted laws governing the practice of medicine, nursing, and pharmacy. These laws vary from state to state; therefore, it is essential that one become familiar with the laws of the state in which one is employed before administering any medication.

Under the law, those administering medications are expected to be knowledgeable about the drugs that they administer and the effects the drug may and/or will have on the patient. They are responsible for their own actions.

REVIEW QUESTIONS

Multiple Choice

1. A written legal document that gives directions for compounding, dispensing, and administering medication to a patient is a:
   a. medicine card
   b. prescription
   c. medication order
   d. subscription

2. An abbreviation symbol that means nothing by mouth is:
   a. non rep
   b. NPO
   c. IM
   d. mm

3. Insulin-dependent diabetes mellitus is:
   a. Type I
   b. Type II

c. Type III
d. Type IV
4. Body surface area is used:
a. when calculating children's dosages
b. when calculating adult dosages
c. when determining an injection site
d. when selecting an appropriately sized needle
5. An injection given just below the surface of the skin is called a(n):
a. intramuscular injection
b. intradermal injection
c. subcutaneous injection
d. parenteral injection

Critical Thinking

1. Describe the process to follow to determine the state law regarding a medical assistant administering medications.
2. What is a medication order? Describe its purpose.
3. List nine parts of a prescription and define each part.
4. Name and describe factors that can affect medication dosage. Explain why and how the dosage is affected.
5. List the fundamental units of the metric system.
6. Name two methods used to calculate children's dosages of medication.
7. List and describe the "Six Rights."
8. A fellow student tells you that she accidentally gave a patient the incorrect dose of medication. Explain in detail what should be done.
9. You accidentally stick yourself with a used needle. What are the steps to take?
10. Discuss allergenic extracts. What are they? What safeguards are needed following administration?
11. List two reasons for the physician to prescribe oxygen for a patient. Describe how oxygen is administered and oxygen safety.

Calculation Problems

1. Calculate the following dosages according to body surface area (BSA):
    If the adult dose of E.E.S. tabs is 400 mg every 6 hours, what is the dosage for a child who is 35 inches tall and weighs 28 pounds (BSA 0.57)?
    If the adult dose of penicillin V potassium, USP, is 250 mg every 6 to 8 hours, what is the dosage for a child who is 24 inches tall and weighs 35 pounds (BSA 0.56)?

2. Calculate the following dosages according to kilogram of body weight:
    The physician orders Augmentin 20 mg/kg/day for Sally Whitney, who weighs 72 pounds. The dose is to be divided and given every 8 hours. What is the total dose? What is the amount to be given every 8 hours?
    The physician orders Cefadyl 40 mg/kg for George Kipperley, who weighs 78 pounds. The dose is to be divided into 4 equal doses. What is the total dose? What is the amount to be given in four equal doses?
    The physician orders Garamycin 2.0 mg/kg every 8 hours for a child who weighs 86 pounds. What is the correct dosage?

3. The physician ordered 64 units of U-100 Humulin insulin. Shade the correct dosage on the U-100 syringe pictured.

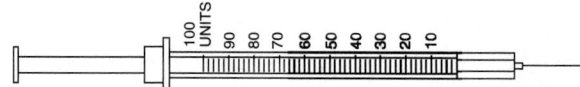

Using the proportional or formula method, calculate the following dosages.

4. The physician orders 125 mg of Diamox. On hand you have 250 mg tablets. You will give _____ tablets to your patient.
5. The physician orders 250 mg of Tagamet liquid. On hand you have 300 mg/5 mL. How many milliliters will you give?

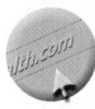

WEB ACTIVITIES

1. Search for a website to explore the various types of safety needles available for injection and venipuncture. What is the most recent ruling by OSHA in regard to these types of needles?

REFERENCES/BIBLIOGRAPHY

Pickar, G. D. (1999). *Dosage calculations* (6th ed.). Albany, NY: Delmar.

Rice, J. (1999). *Principles of pharmacology for medical assisting* (3rd ed.). Albany, NY: Delmar.

Taber's cyclopedic medical dictionary. (18th ed.). (1999). Philadelphia: F. A. Davis Company.

ELECTROCARDIOGRAPHY

KEY TERMS

Amplified
Amplitude
Angiogram
Arrhythmia
Artifact
Augment
Baseline
Bipolar
Bradycardia, Sinus
Calibration
Cardiac Catheterization
Cardiac Cycle
Cardioversion
Countershock
Defibrillation
Defibrillator
Deoxygenated
Depolarize
Diastole
Electrocardiogram
Electrocardiograph
Electrocardiography
Electrodes
Electrolyte
Galvanometer
Infarction
Ischemia
Isoelectric
Lead
Mounting
Noninvasive
Normal Sinus Rhythm
Oscilloscope

(continues)

OUTLINE

Anatomy of the Heart
**Electrical Conduction System of
  the Heart**
**The Cardiac Cycle and the ECG
  Cycle**
  Calculation of Heart Rate on
    ECG Graph Paper
Types of Electrocardiographs
  Single-Channel ECG
  Multichannel ECG
  Automatic ECG Machines
  ECG Telephone Transmissions
  Facsimile Electrocardiograph
  Interpretive Electrocardiograph
ECG Equipment
  Electrocardiograph Paper
  Electrolyte
  Sensors or Electrodes
  Care of Equipment
Lead Coding
**The Electrocardiograph and
  Lead Placement**
  Standard Limb or Bipolar Leads
  Augmented Leads
  Chest Leads or Precordial Leads

**Standardization of the Electro-
  cardiograph**
**Standard Resting Electro-
  cardiography**
Mounting the ECG Tracing
Interference or Artifacts
  Somatic Tremor Artifacts
  Alternating Current (AC)
    Interference
  Wandering Baseline Artifacts
  Interrupted Baseline Artifacts
Cardiac Conditions and Diseases
  Myocardial Infarctions
    (Heart Attacks)
Cardiac Arrhythmias
  Atrial Arrhythmias
  Ventricular Arrhythmias
Defibrillation
Other Cardiac Diagnostic Tests
  Holter Monitor (Portable
    Ambulatory Electro-
    cardiograph)
  Treadmill Stress Test or Exercise
    Tolerance ECG
  Echocardiography

OBJECTIVES

*The student should strive to meet the following performance objectives and demonstrate an
understanding of the facts and principles presented in this chapter through written and oral
communication.*

1. Define the key terms as presented in the glossary.
2. Follow the circulation of blood through the heart starting at the vena
   cave. *(continues)*

KEY TERMS
(*continued*)

Precordial
Repolarization
Rhythm Strip
Sonographer
Stylus
Syncope
Systole
Tachycardia, Sinus
Test Cable
Tracing
Transducer
Ultrasonography
Unipolar

OBJECTIVES (*continued*)

3. Describe the electrical conduction system of the heart.
4. State three reasons why patients may need an electrocardiogram.
5. Identify the various positive and negative deflections and describe what each represents in the cardiac cycle.
6. Explain the purpose of standardization of the electrocardiograph.
7. Identify the twelve leads of an ECG and describe what area of the heart each lead represents.
8. State the function of ECG graph paper, electrodes (sensors), and electrolyte.
9. Describe various types of ECGs and describe their capabilities.
10. Explain each type of artifact and explain how each can be eliminated.
11. Name and describe the purposes of the various cardiac diagnostic tests as outlined in this chapter.
12. Identify the placement of Holter monitor electrodes.
13. Describe the reason for a patient activity diary during ambulatory electrocardiography.
14. Identify six arrhythmias and explain the cause of each.
15. Explain how to calculate heart rates from an ECG tracing.
16. Identify a common coding system used to code each lead on an ECG tracing.
17. Describe the procedure for mounting and ECG tracing.

ROLE DELINEATION COMPONENTS

CLINICAL

Fundamental Principles

- **Apply principles of aseptic technique and infection control**
- **Comply with quality assurance practices**
- **Screen and follow up patient test results**

Diagnostic Orders

- **Perform diagnostic tests**

Patient Care

- **Obtain patient history and vital signs**
- **Prepare and maintain examination and treatment areas**

(continues)

SCENARIO

Wanda Slawson, CMA, clinical medical assistant at Inner City Health Care, recently had her own physical examination which included her first electrocardiogram. This is now Wanda's baseline ECG which provides a basis for future ECG readings to be compared. Since Wanda currently has no heart problems, future tests will indicate differences from her normal baseline ECG. It was very different for Wanda to be the patient versus the person performing the ECG. Having the test performed on her, Wanda can now relate to feelings many of her patients must have felt when having an ECG. These included feelings of fear that the test may be abnormal; a cold feeling because even though the room temperature was normal, she was uncovered and the electrolyte gel was cold when applied; and anxiousness because she found it difficult to stay completely still through the entire tracing. Wanda could empathize much more with her patients after she had the test than she did before her test. Wanda now makes a more concerted effort to allay patient fears and make patients comfortable during electrocardiograms.

INTRODUCTION

Many physicians include an **electrocardiogram** (ECG or EKG) as part of a complete physical examination, especially for patients who are 40 years or more of age, for patients with a family history of cardiac disease, or for patients who have experienced chest pain. It is a noninvasive, safe, and painless procedure that can provide the physician with valuable information about the health of the patient's heart. A graphic representation of the heart's electrical activity, an electrocardiogram measures the amount of the electrical activity produced by the heart and the time necessary for the electrical impulses to travel through the heart during each heartbeat.

Some reasons for **electrocardiography** are to: (1) detect myocardial **ischemia**, (2) estimate damage to the myocardium caused by a myocardial **infarction**, (3) detect and evaluate cardiac **arrhythmia**, (4) assess effects of cardiac medication on the heart, and (5) determine if electrolyte imbalance is present. The ECG is used in conjunction with other laboratory and diagnostic tests to assess total cardiac health.

In a medical office or ambulatory care setting, it is the medical assistant who records the ECG; therefore, special knowledge and skills are necessary and include these aspects of the correct electrocardiography procedures: patient preparation, operation of the **electrocardiograph**, elimination of **artifacts**, **mounting** and/or labeling the ECG, and maintenance and care of the instrument.

ANATOMY OF THE HEART

The heart has four chambers: two upper chambers known as atria, and two lower chambers known as ventricles. **Deoxygenated** blood enters the right atrium from the superior and inferior vena cavae and passes through the tricuspid valve into the right ventricle. In a healthy heart, the blood between right and left sides cannot mix together. It then travels to the lungs via the pulmonary arteries. The deoxygenated blood gives off the carbon dioxide and picks up oxygen in the capillary bed of the lungs. Oxygenated blood is pumped through the pulmonary vein into the left atrium, through the mitral valve, into the left ventricle. The oxygenated blood then passes through the aortic valve into the aorta and from the aorta to all cells, tissues, and organs of the body (Figure 25-1). The cycle begins with each heartbeat.

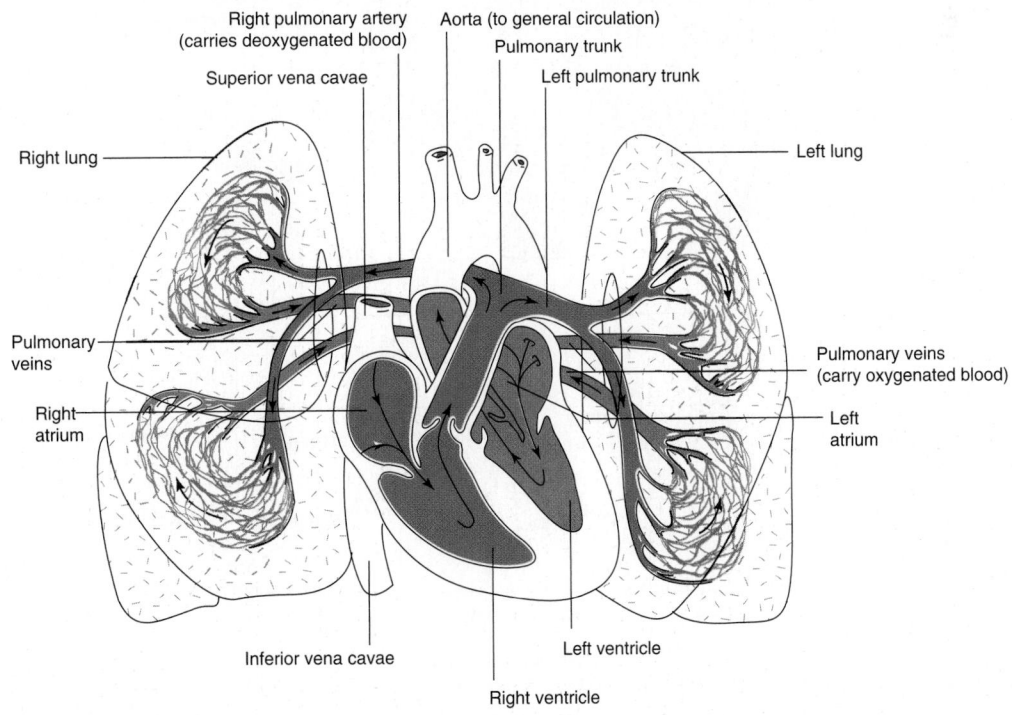

Figure 25-1 Oxygenated blood passing through the heart and onto the rest of the body.

On its external surface, the heart is surrounded by coronary arteries that supply the myocardium with its blood supply from which oxygen and nutrients are obtained. (See Chapter 18, Circulatory System.)

ELECTRICAL CONDUCTION SYSTEM OF THE HEART

The body's natural pacemaker, the sinoatrial (SA) node, is located in the upper part of the right atrium. It sends out an electrical impulse that begins and regulates the heartbeat. When the electrical impulses are dispersed through the atria, it causes them to **depolarize** or contract. From the atria, the electrical impulses travel toward the ventricles, to the atrioventricular (AV) node, located at the base of the right atrium. From here, the electrical impulses are transmitted to the bundles of His. The bundle of His divides into right and left bundle branches which continue the electrical impulses on to the Purkinje fibers. These fibers disperse the electrical impulses to the right and left ventricles causing them to contract. The heart relaxes very briefly (**repolarization**), then a new electrical impulse is begun by the SA node and the cycle begins again (Figure 25-2). This cycle is known as the **cardiac**

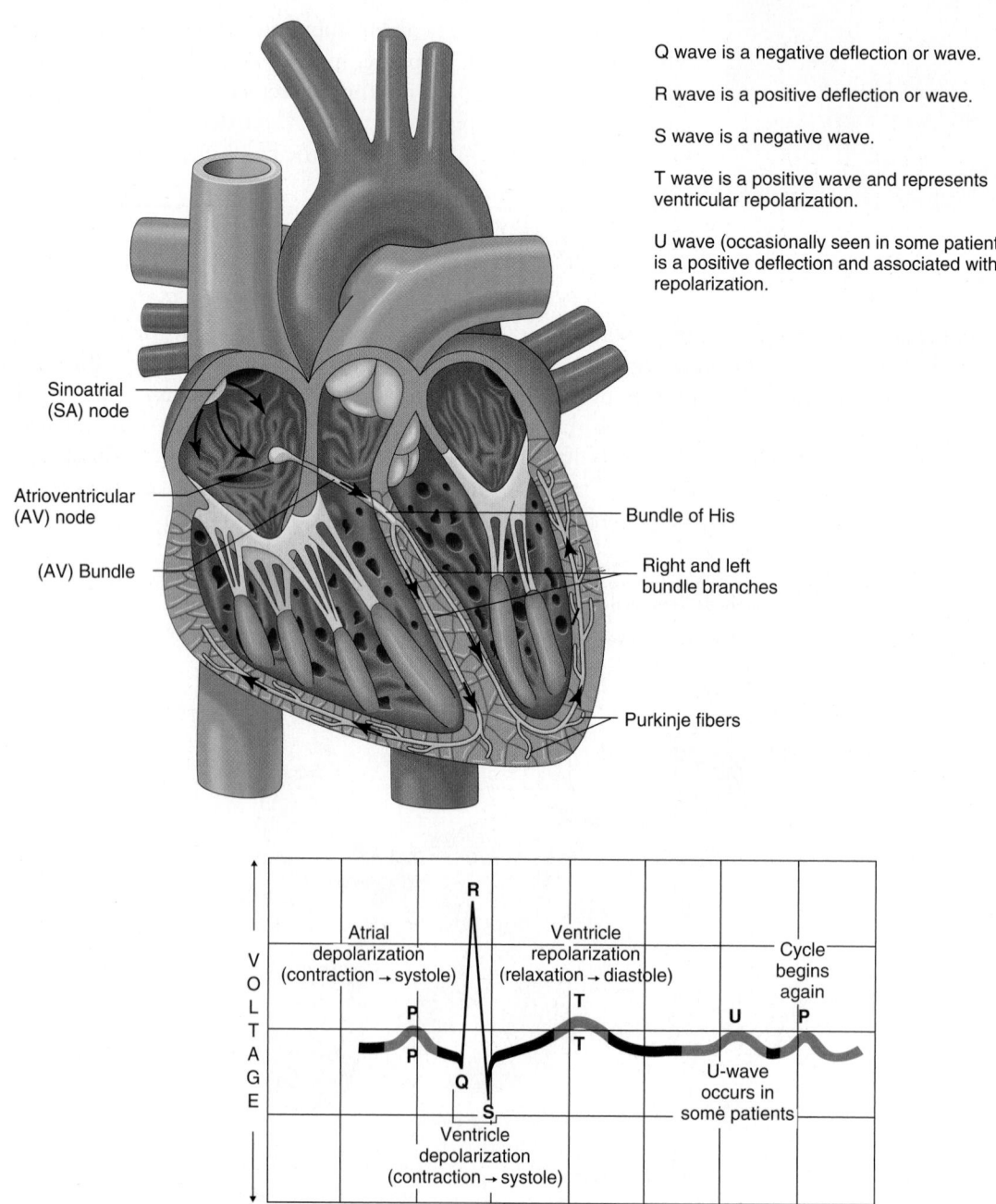

Q wave is a negative deflection or wave.

R wave is a positive deflection or wave.

S wave is a negative wave.

T wave is a positive wave and represents ventricular repolarization.

U wave (occasionally seen in some patients) is a positive deflection and associated with repolarization.

Figure 25-2 The heartbeat is controlled by electrical impulses which comprise the continuous cardiac cycle.

cycle and it represents one heartbeat. The electrocardiograph records the electrical activity that causes the contraction (**systole**) and the relaxation (**diastole**) of the atria and ventricles. The ECG cycle is the recording or the graphic representation of the cardiac cycle. These electrical impulses can be recorded on special ECG paper or displayed on an **oscilloscope**.

THE CARDIAC CYCLE AND THE ECG CYCLE

The **baseline**, or **isoelectric**, line is the flat line that separates the various waves. It is present when there is no current flowing in the heart. The waves are either deflecting upward, known as positive deflection, or deflecting downward, known as negative deflection from the baseline.

The P, QRS, and T waves, recorded during the ECG, represent the depolarization (contraction) and repolarization (relaxation) of the myocardial cells. The P wave represents atrial depolarization and is recorded as a positive deflection. The QRS complex represents ventricular depolarization and is measured from the beginning of the first wave of the QRS to the end of the last wave of the QRS (refer back to Figure 25-2).

Each complete cardiac cycle takes about 0.8 seconds with each wave taking an appropriate amount of time if the heart is healthy. By observing and measuring the size, shape, and location of each wave on an ECG recording, the physician can analyze and interpret the conduction of electricity through the cardiac cells, the heart's rhythm and rate, and the health of the heart in general.

Calculation of Heart Rate on ECG Graph Paper

ECG graph paper is divided into 1-mm squares (small squares) and 5-mm squares (large squares). Each large square is 25 small squares and is 5 mm high and 5 mm wide. On the horizontal line, one small square represents 0.04 second. On the vertical line, one small square represents 1 mm of voltage. Because a large square is five small squares wide and five deep, each small square represents 0.2 second horizontal and 5 mm vertical. **NOTE:** Every fifth line, both horizontally and vertically, is darker than the other lines, making squares that are 5 mm × 5 mm (Figure 25-3). These measurements are accepted worldwide and enable the physician to interpret the time of each deflection on the horizontal line and cardiac electrical

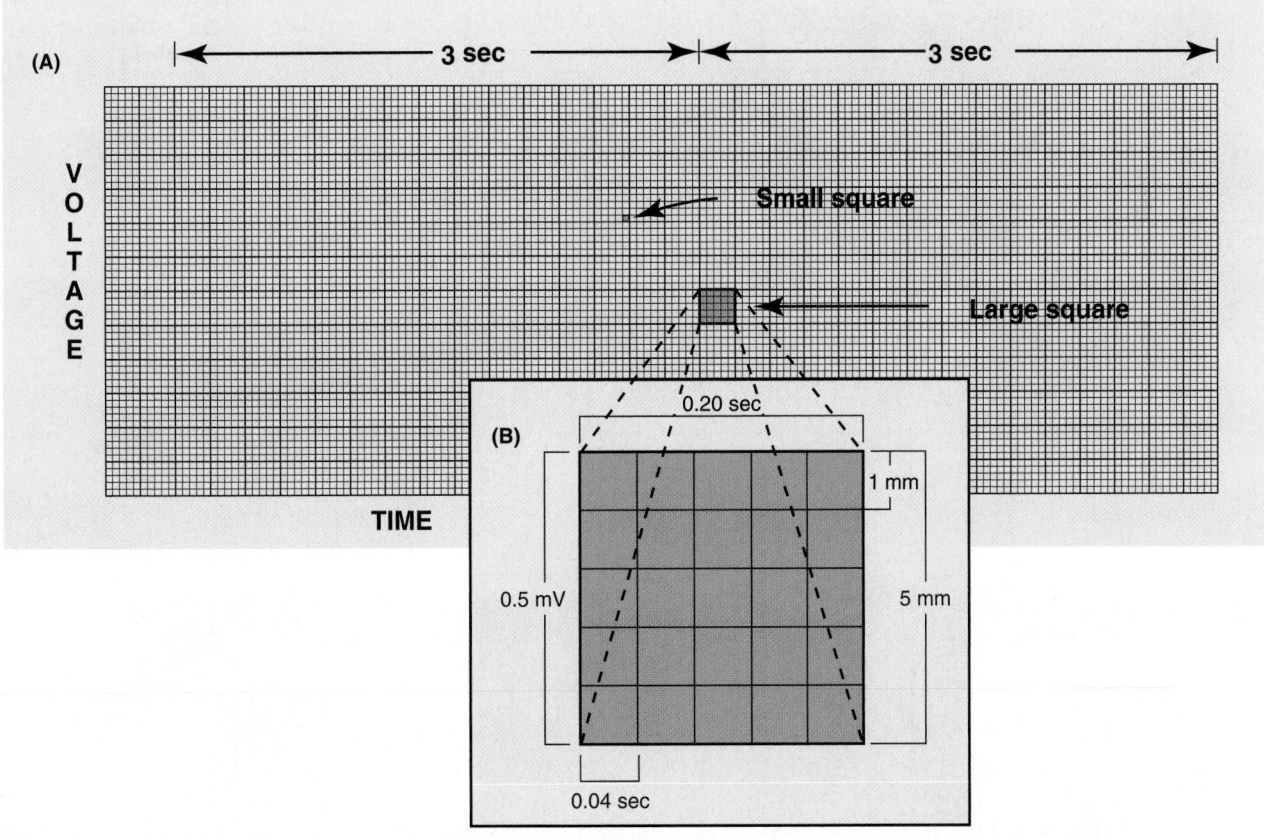

Figure 25-3 ECG graph paper measurements allow medical professionals to determine the time and voltage of heartbeats. (A) The small square is 1 mm wide and 1 mm high. One small square = 0.04 second. (B) The large square consists of 25 small squares and measures 5 mm wide and 5 mm high. One large square = 0.04 × 5 or 0.2 second.

activity (voltage) on the vertical line to help determine cardiac health.

Because all cardiac complexes consist of P, QRS, and T, and the electrocardiograph paper measures time on the horizontal line, it is possible to calculate heart rate. Count the number of 5-mm boxes (number within the dark lines) between two R waves. Divide this number into 300. The result will be the heart rate per minute.

Example: One small square (1 mm) = 0.04 second in time
One large square (5 mm) = 0.04 × 5 = 0.2 second
Divide 60 seconds (one minute) by 0.2 second
60 ÷ 0.2 = 300

Example: There are 3 large squares between two R waves.
300 ÷ 3 = 100
The heartbeat is 100 beats per minute.

TYPES OF ELECTROCARDIOGRAPHS

Single-Channel ECG

A conventional twelve-lead single channel electrocardiograph can be used in either manual mode or automatic mode. When using automatic mode, the twelve-lead ECG tracing is complete in less than 40 seconds. With a single channel machine, only one lead can be recorded at a time. If not automatic, the single-channel ECG requires manually turning the lead selector on and off between each of the twelve leads. It may also require the leads to be coded so that they can be identified later and properly mounted. Lead coding and mounting are explained more fully later in this chapter. The ECG tracing from a single-channel machine will need to be cut and mounted onto special forms, if available, or onto an 8½ × 11 inch plain piece of paper for filing into the patient record. See Figure 25-4 for a sample of a single-channel ECG machine and tracing.

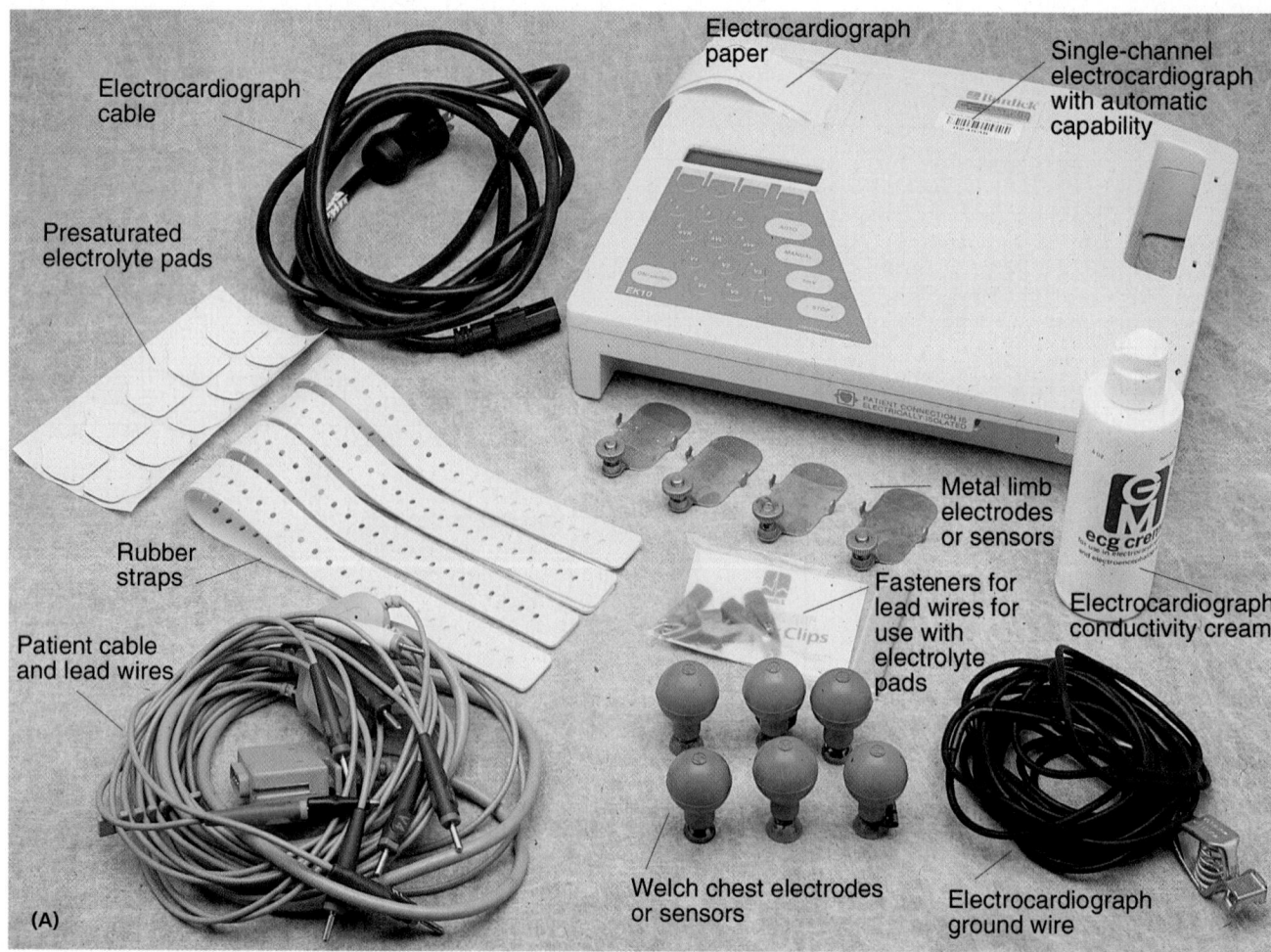

Figure 25-4 (A) Single-channel electrocardiograph and supplies needed for ECG.

(continues)

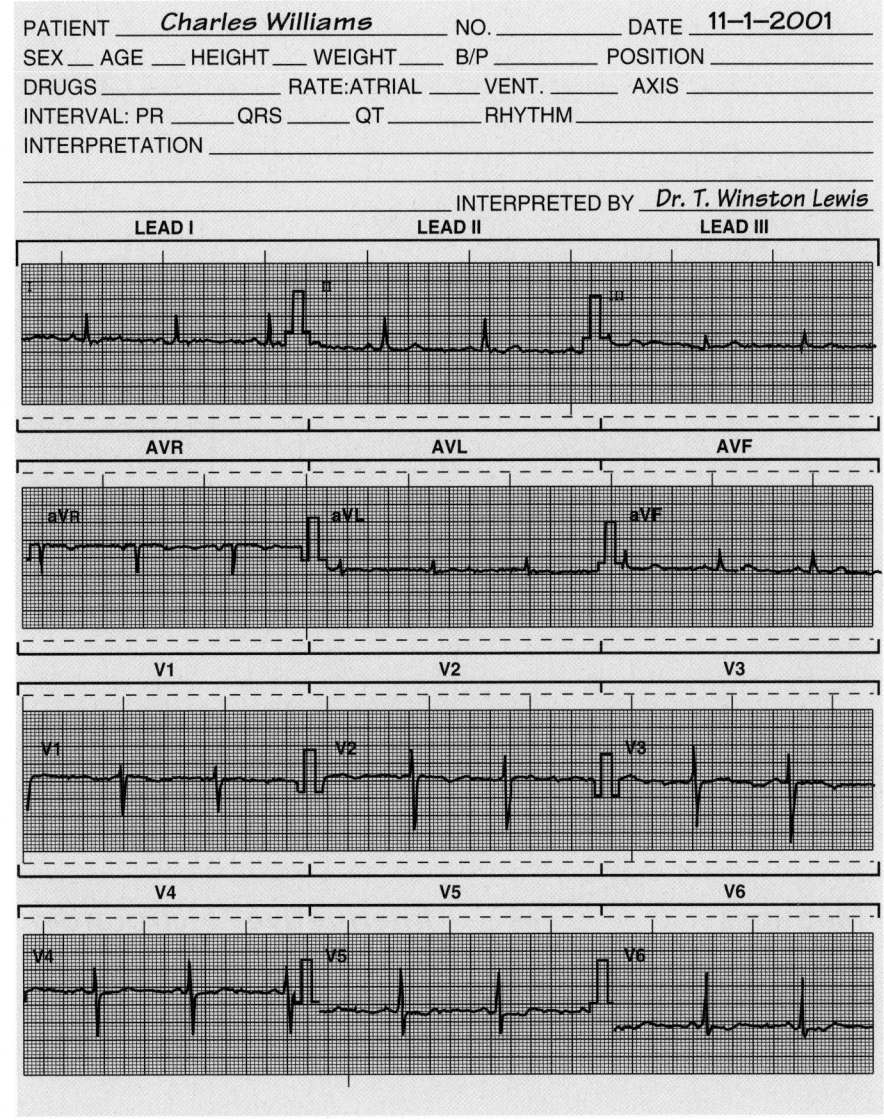

PATIENT _____ *Charles Williams* _____ NO. _____ DATE _11–1–2001_

SEX ___ AGE ___ HEIGHT ___ WEIGHT ____ B/P _____ POSITION _____

DRUGS _____ RATE:ATRIAL ____ VENT. _____ AXIS _____

INTERVAL: PR _____ QRS _____ QT _____ RHYTHM_____

INTERPRETATION _____

_____ INTERPRETED BY _Dr. T. Winston Lewis_

(B)

Figure 25-4 *(continued)* (B) Mounted single-channel ECG tracing or recording.

Multichannel ECG

An electrocardiograph that can simultaneously record several different leads is known as a multichannel electrocardiograph. The conventional electrocardiograph records one lead at a time. A three-channel machine, one type of multichannel ECG, records three channels at one time. It records Lead I, II, and III, followed by aVR, aVL, and aVF, followed by V_1, V_2, and V_3, followed by V_4, V_5, and V_6. The advantage of the multichannel machine is its speed. The most common multichannel machine used in the physician's office is the three-channel machine. This type of machine requires three-channel recording paper which is 8½ × 11 inches and fits into the patient record with no cutting or mounting. Refer to Figure 25-5 for an example of a multichannel machine and tracing.

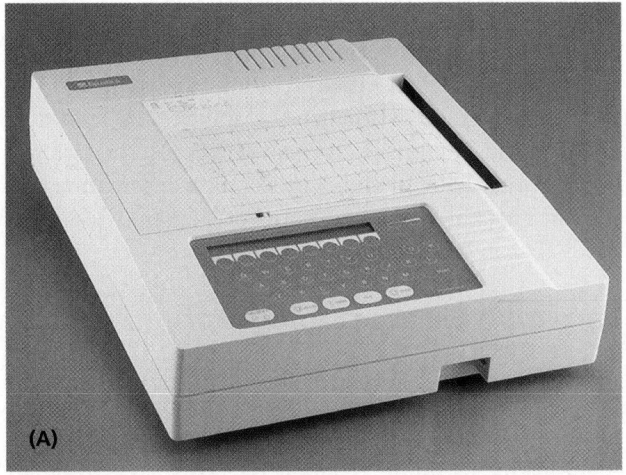

(A)

Figure 25-5 (A) Multichannel (three-channel) Burdick E350 ECG Machine.   *(continues)*

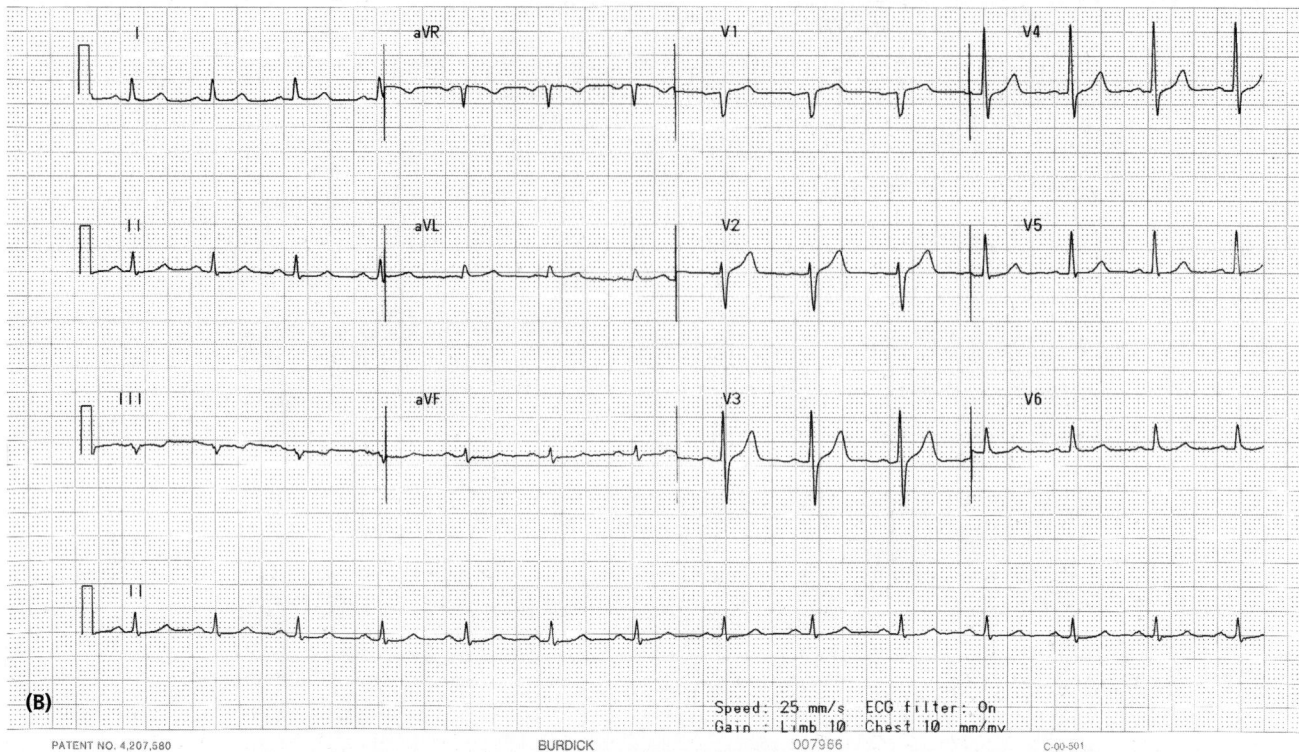

I aVR V1 V4
II aVL V2 V5
III aVF V3 V6
II

(B)

Speed: 25 mm/s   ECG filter: On
Gain : Limb 10 Chest 10 mm/mv
PATENT NO. 4,207,580   BURDICK   007966   C-00-S01

Figure 25-5 (*continued*) (B) Example of three-channel ECG recording where three leads are recorded simultaneously. (Courtesy of Siemens Burdick, Inc.)

Automatic ECG Machines

When using an automatic electrocardiograph, the lead length and switching of leads are done automatically by the electrocardiograph and there is no need to advance the control knob. For these reasons, both time and paper can be saved with the automatic instrument. The automatic instrument also comes equipped with a manual control that can be used if a longer tracing is necessary.

ECG Telephone Transmissions

An electrocardiogram can be transmitted via the telephone line to an ECG interpretation site when using an electrocardiograph with such capabilities. A recording printout and interpretation (many times interpretation is done by a cardiologist and/or by a computer) are transmitted automatically on the electrocardiograph. Results of the ECG can be verbally transmitted as well.

Facsimile Electrocardiograph

The physician may need a rapid, expert ECG interpretation from an off-site diagnostician. Direct ECG fax transmits from the electrocardiograph to a fax machine and a high-quality facsimile is produced. This saves time by eliminating the step of copying the report and sending it via the fax machine.

Interpretive Electrocardiograph

The interpretive electrocardiograph has a built-in computer program that interprets the ECG tracing while it is being recorded allowing for faster diagnosis and treatment. The physician in charge will review the tracing before a diagnosis is confirmed and treatment is begun.

ECG EQUIPMENT

Electrocardiograph Paper

ECG paper can be either black or dark blue and is wax or plastic coated with a white or pink background and color lines. The paper is heat and pressure sensitive so as the heated **stylus** of the electrocardiograph moves across the paper, the background coating is melted away revealing the black or blue color of the paper and the ECG cycles are recorded or traced. The heat of the stylus can be adjusted to obtain a sharp, clear recording, or **tracing**. Medical assistants should learn how to adjust the proper control using the specific manual or instructions that accompany the instrument in their facility.

Electrolyte

Because the skin is a poor conductor of electricity, there are various types of **electrolyte** applied with each elec-

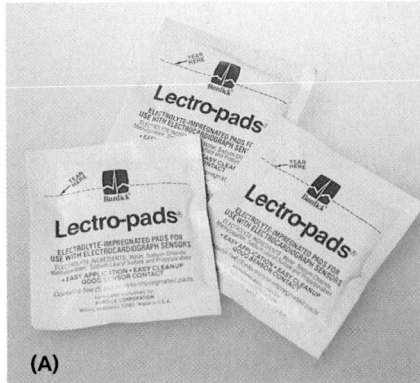 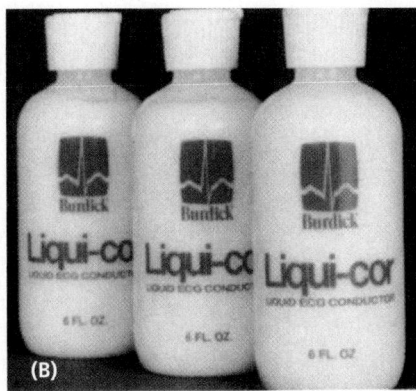 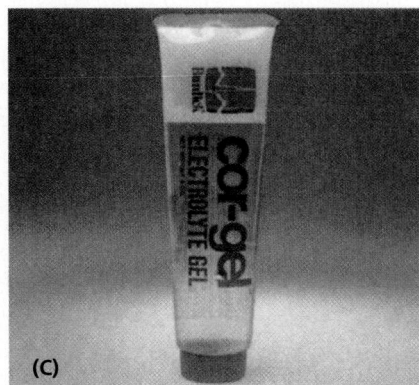

Figure 25-6 Various types of electrolyte: (A) Presaturated electrolyte pads. (B) Electrolyte lotion. (C) Electrolyte gel usually used with defibrillator. (Courtesy of Siemens Burdick, Inc.)

trode to help pick up the electrical current produced by the contraction and relaxation of the heart. The impulses are transmitted to the electrocardiograph by metal tips on the patient lead wires or cables that are attached to the electrodes. Electrolyte is manufactured in the form of a gel, lotion, or paste, or may be presaturated pads (Figure 25-6A-C).

Sensors or Electrodes

There are various types of sensors or **electrodes** made of metal or other conductive material used in taking an ECG. The sensors detect the electrical impulses on the body surface and relay them through cables, or leads, that are attached to the electrodes on one end to the ECG machine attached to the other end of the cables. Welch cups and metal sensors are found on some older model ECG machines and are still being used in some agencies. Other agencies have converted the Welch cups and metal sensors through the use of disposable electrodes and

reusable clips. The clips replace the metal sensors and are attached to the lead wires. The clips grasp hold of the disposable electrodes that have been applied to the limbs and chest.

Metal Sensors or Electrodes. Small metal sensors are secured to the fleshy parts of a patient's arms and legs using stretchable rubber straps. Electrolyte is applied to the side of the electrode touching the skin (Figure 25-7A).

Welch Sensors or Electrodes. A type of chest electrode, the Welch electrode consists of a rubber bulb with a metal suction cup. The electrolyte is placed onto the metal suction cup before it is applied to the chest wall (Figure 25-7B).

Disposable Electrodes. Disposable electrodes are permeated with electrolyte and can be used on both the limbs and chest (Figure 25-7C). They are made of a self-adhesive

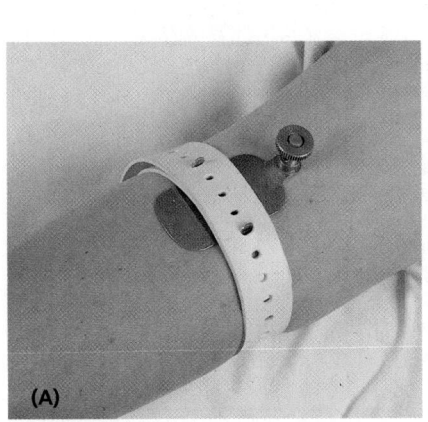 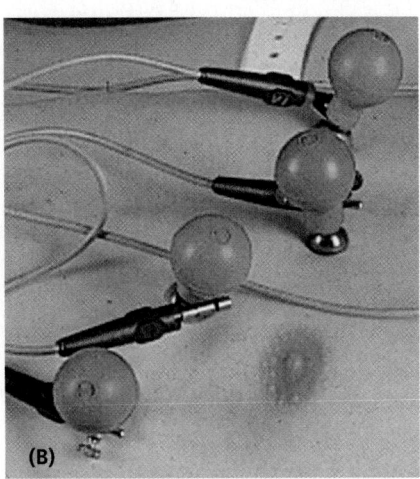 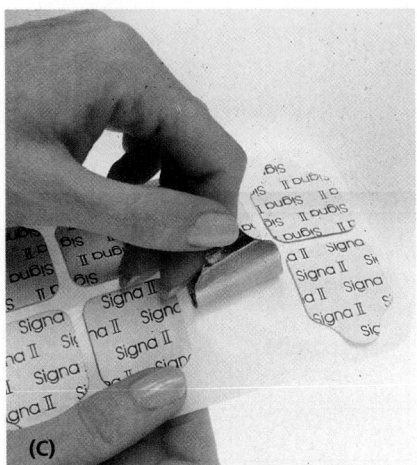

Figure 25-7 Various types of electrodes or sensors: (A) Metal limb electrode and strap. (B) Welch electrodes. (C) Signa II disposable sensors. (Courtesy of Siemens Burdick, Inc.)

conductive material that requires no additional electrolyte. These sensors are applied to the skin of the limbs
and chest and held in place by the adhesive backing. The
self-adhesive electrodes are discarded after use.

Care of Equipment

Many offices and ambulatory care areas use the standard
electrocardiograph with metal electrodes and rubber limb
straps. The newer computerized electrocardiographs require
disposable electrodes and presaturated electrolyte pads.

It is important to note that clean electrodes will
help ensure a good tracing. Metal electrodes should be
cleaned with a mild detergent and occasionally scrubbed
with a cleaner such as Soft Scrub®, rinsed, and dried. The
rubber straps used to attach the electrodes to the patient's
limbs should be washed in a mild detergent, rinsed, and
dried. Use a cotton-tipped applicator to clean the holes in
the rubber straps and inside the suction-type Welch chest
electrode.

LEAD CODING

There are a number of codes that are used to identify each
lead recorded on the ECG reading. These codes are necessary for later identification and for mounting purposes.
Newer electrocardiographs will automatically mark
(code) each lead in the upper margin of the ECG paper
during the recording. Older electrocardiographs must be
manually coded by depressing the lead marker button. See
Figure 25-8 for an example of a common coding system.

THE ELECTROCARDIOGRAPH AND LEAD PLACEMENT

The standard electrocardiogram consists of twelve leads
that record the heart's electrical activity from different
angles, allowing for a thorough three-dimensional interpretation of its activity. The electrical impulses given off
by the heart can be picked up by electrodes and then conducted into the instrument through **lead** wires. Electrodes
consist of materials that are good conductors of electricity.
Since the electrical activity that comes from the body is

Standard or bipolar limb leads	Electrodes connected	Marking code	Recommended positions for multiple chest leads (Line art illustration of chest positions)
Lead I	RA & LA	1 dot	
Lead II	RA & LL	2 dots	
Lead III	LA & LL	3 dots	
Augmented unipolar limb leads			V₁ Fourth intercostal space at right margin of sternum
aVR	RA & (LA-LL)	1 dash	V₂ Fourth intercostal space at left margin of sternum
aVL	LA & (RA-LL)	2 dashes	V₃ Midway between position 2 and position 4
aVF	LL & (RA-LA)	3 dashes	V₄ Fifth intercostal space at junction of left midclavicular line
Chest or precordial leads			V₅ At horizontal level of position 4 at left anterior axillary line
V	C & (LA-RA-LL)	(See data on right)	V₆ At horizontal level of position 4 at left midaxillary line

Figure 25-8   Example of a common coding system for ECG leads that must be manually coded on older electrocardiographs. Accurate coding is accomplished by pressing the lead marker button appropriately. (Courtesy of Siemens Burdick, Inc.)

small, it is made larger, or **amplified**, by the amplifier of the instrument. The voltage is changed into a mechanical motion by the **galvanometer** and recorded on the electrocardiograph by the stylus.

The electrodes are placed on the patient's four limbs and chest. The four limb leads are right arm (RA), left arm (LA), right leg (RL), and left leg (LL). The right leg electrode is not used as part of the recording. It is an electrical reference point only. The limb leads are placed on the fleshy area of upper arms and lower legs. The chest

leads are known as precordial leads, V leads, or C leads, and use an electrode for each of six areas on the chest wall or one electrode that is moved to six different positions on the chest wall. (This depends upon the type of electrocardiograph being used.)

Standard Limb or Bipolar Leads

The first three leads that are recorded on a standard ECG are called Lead I, Lead II, and Lead III (Figure 25-9A).

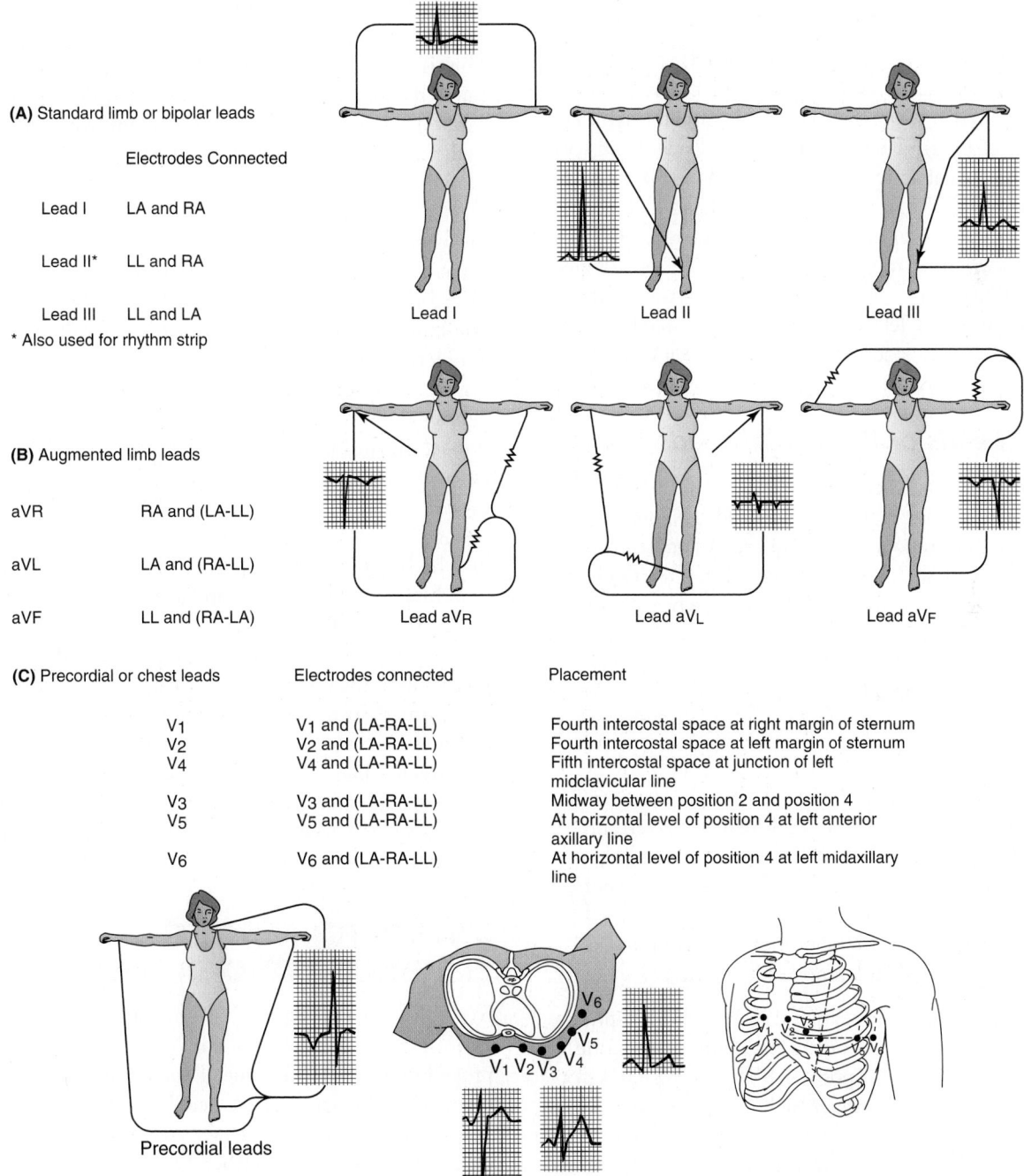

(A) Standard limb or bipolar leads

	Electrodes Connected
Lead I	LA and RA
Lead II*	LL and RA
Lead III	LL and LA

* Also used for rhythm strip

Lead I   Lead II   Lead III

(B) Augmented limb leads

aVR	RA and (LA-LL)
aVL	LA and (RA-LL)
aVF	LL and (RA-LA)

Lead aV$_R$ Lead aV$_L$ Lead aV$_F$

(C) Precordial or chest leads

	Electrodes connected	Placement
V$_1$	V$_1$ and (LA-RA-LL)	Fourth intercostal space at right margin of sternum
V$_2$	V$_2$ and (LA-RA-LL)	Fourth intercostal space at left margin of sternum
V$_4$	V$_4$ and (LA-RA-LL)	Fifth intercostal space at junction of left midclavicular line
V$_3$	V$_3$ and (LA-RA-LL)	Midway between position 2 and position 4
V$_5$	V$_5$ and (LA-RA-LL)	At horizontal level of position 4 at left anterior axillary line
V$_6$	V$_6$ and (LA-RA-LL)	At horizontal level of position 4 at left midaxillary line

Precordial leads

Figure 25-9 Lead types, connections, and placement: (A) Standard limb or bipolar leads. (B) Augmented limb leads. (C) Precordial or chest leads.

These are known as **bipolar** leads because each of them uses two limb electrodes that record simultaneously. Lead I records electrical activity between the right arm (RA) and left arm (LA); lead II records electrical activity between the right arm (RA) and left leg (LL); lead III records activity between the left arm (LA) and left leg (LL). Lead II is used as a **rhythm strip** because it portrays the heart's rhythm better than the other leads. The rhythm strip is usually a separate longer recording approximately 6 to 12 inches.

Augmented Leads

The next three leads are **augmented** leads and are designated aVR, aVL, and aVF (Figure 25-9B). The aV stands for augmented voltage; the R, L, and F stand for right, left, and foot (or leg). These are **unipolar** leads. Lead aVR records electrical activity from the midpoint between the left arm and left leg to the right arm. Lead aVL records electrical activity from the midpoint between the right arm and the left leg to the left arm. Lead aVF records electrical activity from the midpoint between the right arm and left arm to the left leg. Because these three leads produce such small electrical impulses, the ECG machine augments, or increases, their size in order to record them.

Chest Leads or Precordial Leads

The remaining six leads of the standard twelve-lead ECG are the chest leads or **precordial** leads (Figure 25-9C). These too are unipolar leads and are designated V_1, V_2, V_3, V_4, V_5, and V_6. These leads record the heart's electrical impulse from a central point within the heart to one of six predesignated positions on the chest wall where an electrode is attached. The correct position must be used for each lead recording.

The anatomical positions for placement of the chest or precordial leads are:

V_1—fourth intercostal space at right margin of sternum
V_2—fourth intercostal space at left margin of sternum
V_4—fifth intercostal space on left midclavicular line
V_3—midway between V_2 and V_4 (**NOTE:** This is correct order, V_3 after V_4.)
V_5—horizontal to V_4 at left anterior axillary line
V_6—horizontal to V_4 at left midaxillary line

When using a conventional electrocardiograph, the chest electrode must be moved manually one by one to each of the six chest lead positions. This necessitates stopping the instrument between each chest lead in order to move the electrode to the next appropriate position on the chest wall. Some electrocardiographs allow for all six chest leads to be applied at one time; therefore, there is no interruption between chest lead recordings. (See Figure 25-23 in Procedure 25-1).

STANDARDIZATION OF THE ELECTROCARDIOGRAPH

The value of an ECG recording depends on its being performed accurately. To ensure a precise and reliable recording, the ECG instrument must be standardized before an ECG is performed. The standardization of the instrument is a quality assurance check to determine if the machine is set and working properly. Standardization measurements have been adopted internationally as a means of accurate **calibration** according to universal measurements. The universal standard is that one millivolt of cardiac electrical activity will deflect the stylus exactly 10 mm high. This is the equivalent of 10 small squares on the ECG paper. Figure 25-10 shows an example of the 10-mm standardization and an electrocardiogram with all twelve leads recorded in minutes simultaneously with no interruption.

On occasion, R waves may be very large and go off the paper. Repositioning the stylus may not correct the situation. In such instances, the medical assistant can record the lead(s) in which the R wave is very large at one-half standard. This action will record all ECG cycles at half their normal **amplitude**.

Conversely, the waves of the ECG cycles may be very small, making it difficult to interpret. In this circumstance, the medical assistant can record the ECG cycles at twice the normal standard. This action will record ECG cycles at twice their normal amplitude. Whenever a change is made from a normal standardization mark (10 mm high) to either a one-half standardization mark (5 mm high) or a double standardization mark (20 mm high), the medical assistant must include the adjusted standardization mark with the particular lead to alert the physician to the change in standard. The instrument must be returned to normal standard to prevent accidentally running the next lead at a standard other than normal. The tracing paper is usually run at 25 mm per second. If cycles are too close together, speed can be adjusted to 50 mm per second. Make a note on the ECG paper if speed is changed.

STANDARD RESTING ELECTROCARDIOGRAPHY

Regardless of the type of electrocardiograph used, the basic components of the standard electrocardiography procedure remain the same. Patient preparation, placement of limb and chest leads, attachment of lead wires, and elimination of artifacts vary little from one electrocardiograph to another. Procedure 25-1 explains a twelve-lead ECG using a conventional single-channel electrocardiograph with reusable metal sensors for the limbs and six chest electrodes. Procedure 25-2 explains a

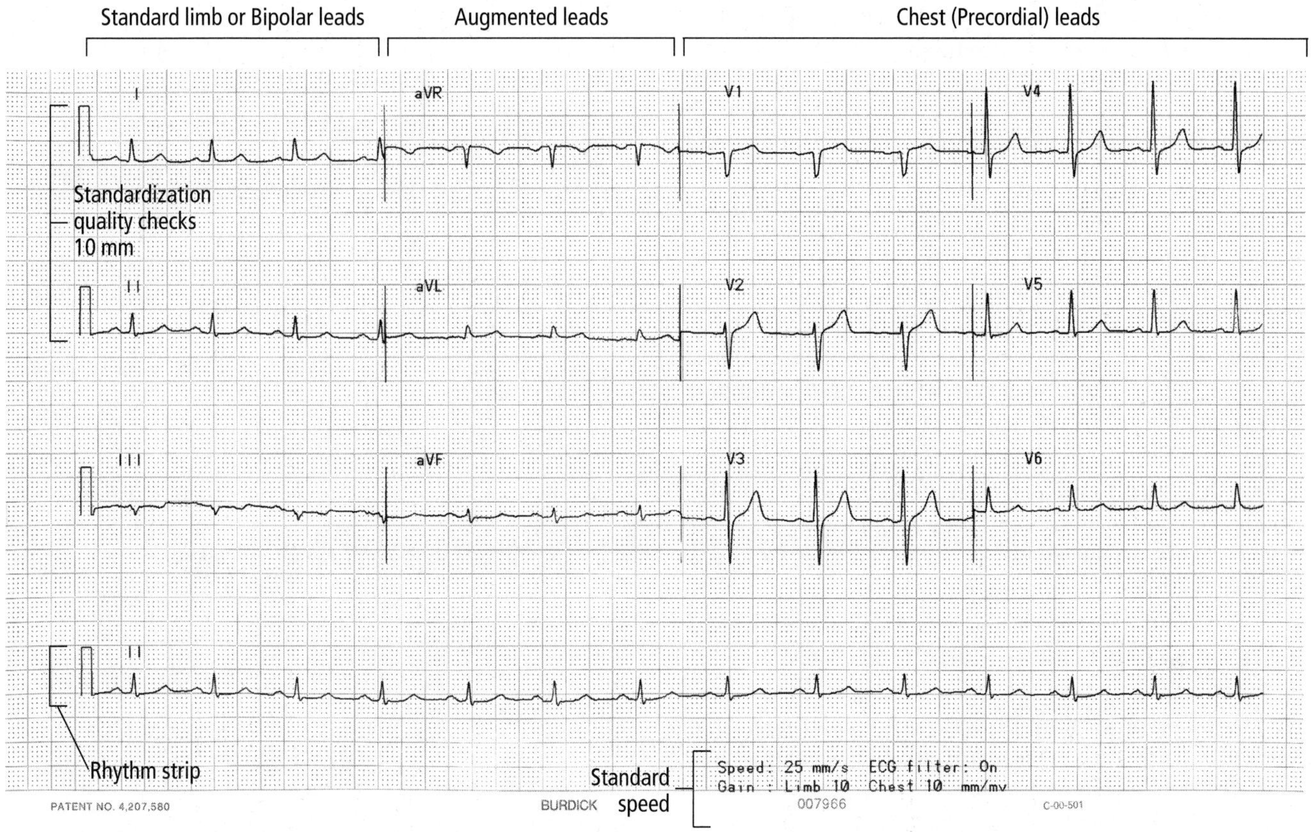

Standard limb or Bipolar leads	Augmented leads	Chest (Precordial) leads

Standardization quality checks 10 mm

Rhythm strip

PATENT NO. 4,207,580

BURDICK **Standard speed**

Speed: 25 mm/s ECG filter: On
Gain : Limb 10 Chest 10 mm/mv
007966   C-00-501

Figure 25-10 An electrocardiogram showing all twelve leads recorded in minutes at one time with no interruption.

twelve-lead ECG using a three-channel machine with disposable electrodes. Medical assistants must be familiar with the electrocardiograph machine in their facility and should thoroughly review the manufacturer's instruction manual that accompanies the machine prior to performing the procedure. Knowledge of the basic procedures included here can be adapted for all other electrocardiographs.

MOUNTING THE ECG TRACING

Commercially prepared mounting forms are available and the medical assistant should mount the completed tracing after the physician has reviewed the entire recording (Figure 25-11). It is important that each lead be individually cut, mounted, and identified. Include the patient's name, date, address, age, gender, blood pressure, height and weight, and cardiac medications on the mounting form.

INTERFERENCE OR ARTIFACTS

The ECG is a valuable diagnostic aid to the physician and must be performed accurately. The medical assistant is responsible for obtaining a recording that can be easily read and interpreted by the physician.

There can be unusual and unwanted activity in the tracing not caused by the electrical activity of the heart. These defects in the ECG tracing are known as artifacts and their appearance can make the ECG tracing difficult to read and interpret. Four of the more common artifacts are somatic tremor, alternating current interference, wandering baseline, and interrupted baseline. The medical

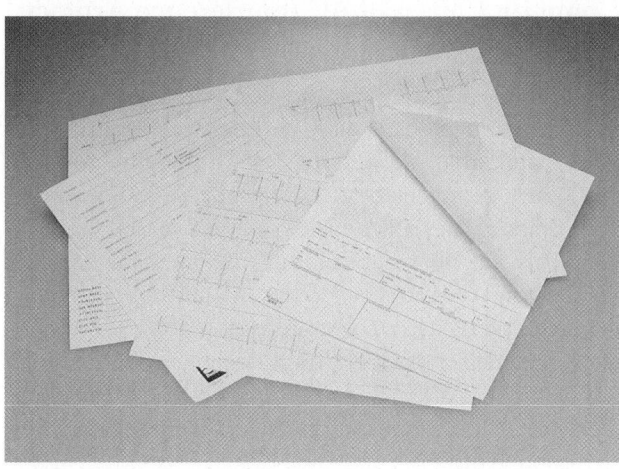

Figure 25-11 Various types of mounts for ECG tracing paper for patient's permanent record. (Courtesy of Siemens Burdick, Inc.)

assistant should understand the causes of each type of artifact and know how to eliminate them.

Somatic Tremor Artifacts

This type of artifact is also known as muscle tremor. It is characterized by unnatural baseline deflections such as jagged peaks or irregularity of spacing and height. The tracing appears fuzzy (Figure 25-12A). Somatic tremor occurs when the patient is apprehensive or uncomfortable and can result in involuntary muscle movement. Voluntary muscle movement occurs when the patient moves, talks, coughs, and so on. Parkinson's disease, a nervous system disorder, is an example of involuntary somatic tremor. It is not possible for the patient to control the muscle tremors. (Often, involuntary somatic tremor can be minimized somewhat by having the patient slide the hands under the buttocks during the recording.)

It is natural for the patient to feel apprehensive prior to and during the ECG tracing. Reassurance and an explanation of the procedure will allay apprehension and relax muscles. Be certain the patient is comfortable. Use pillows for the head and under the knees; be sure the temperature of the room is comfortable. These simple techniques will help to minimize somatic tremor.

Alternating Current (AC) Interference

This type of artifact is caused by electrical interference and appears as a series of small regular peaks (Figure 25-12B). Electricity present in medical equipment or wires in the area can leak a small amount of energy into the room in which the ECG is being recorded. The current can be picked up by the patient's body and it will be detected by the ECG tracing as an alternating current (AC) artifact.

Common Causes of AC Interference Artifacts.
Some common causes of AC interferences are:

1. Improper grounding of electrocardiograph. There are three-pronged plugs in the newer electrocardiographs that are inserted into a properly grounded three-receptacle outlet. This reduces AC interference. Older instruments may have only a two-pronged plug necessitating the use of a separate ground wire attached to the unit and connected to a ground such as a cold water pipe.
2. Presence of other electrical equipment in the room. Unplug other electrical equipment in the room (electrical examination tables, lamps, autoclaves, and so on).
3. Electrical wiring in the floor, ceiling, or walls. Move the ECG table away from walls.

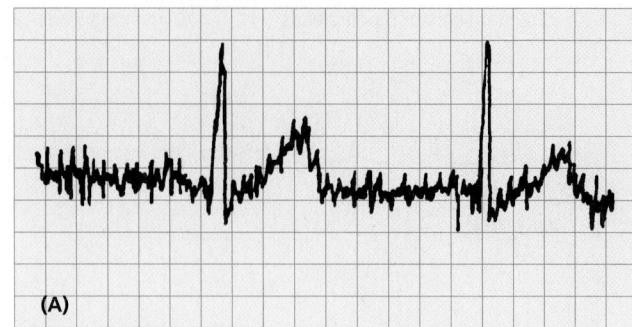

(A)

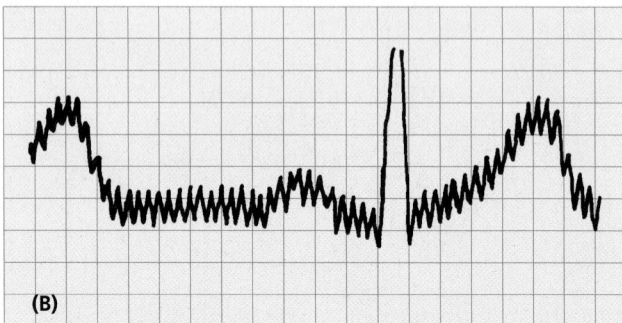

(B)

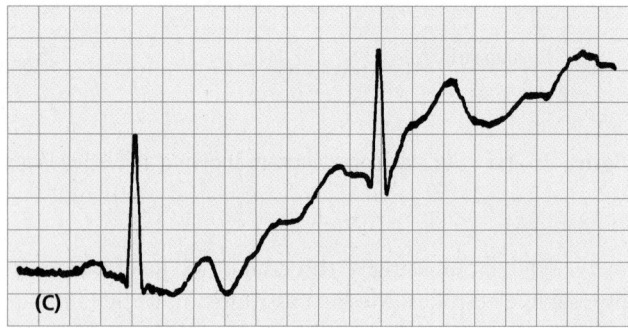

(C)

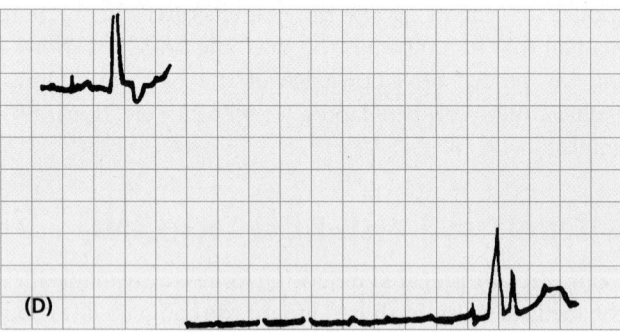

(D)

Figure 25-12 ECG artifacts. (A) Somatic tremor. (B) Alternating current (AC). (C) Wandering baseline. (D) Interrupted baseline. (Courtesy of Siemens Burdick, Inc.)

4. Crossed lead wires and lead wires not following body contour. Straighten lead wires and be sure they are positioned to follow the patient's body contour.
5. Corroded or dirty electrodes and/or metal tips of the lead wires. Reusable electrodes and tips of lead wires must be cleaned and rinsed completely after each use.

Wandering Baseline Artifacts

A wandering baseline occurs when the stylus suddenly moves from the center of the ECG paper resulting in the complexes "wandering" across the ECG paper; for example, from the top of the paper to the bottom, or bottom to top (Figure 25-12C). This makes it difficult to follow the complexes when the physician reads the recording and interprets it.

Common Causes of Wandering Baseline Artifacts. Wandering baseline artifacts can be caused by the following conditions:

1. Electrodes applied too loosely or too tightly. There should be equal tension on all four limb leads, metal tips should be firmly attached to the electrodes, and the patient cable should not have tension on it nor be dangling to cause pulling on the electrode.
2. Corroded or dirty electrodes and/or metal tips of the lead wires (refer to number 5 in AC interference).
3. Inappropriate amount or poor-quality electrolyte gel or paste. Each electrode should have the same amount of electrolyte gel or paste on it.
4. Lotions, oils, or creams on the patient's skin. Remove any of these substances before applying the electrode by vigorously rubbing the area with rubbing alcohol.

Interrupted Baseline Artifacts

On occasion, the baseline will become interrupted and there will be a break between complexes (Figure 25-12D). A probable cause could be a broken patient cable or a lead wire that may have become detached from an electrode.

CARDIAC CONDITIONS AND DISEASES

Myocardial Infarctions (Heart Attacks)

Myocardial infarctions (heart attacks) are the number one cause of death in the United States today. With the approval of your employer physician, medical assistants are in an excellent position to offer healthy tips and suggestions from which patients can benefit. For instance, they can offer patient health tips regarding diet and exercise while applying the ECG equipment (Table 25-1).

CARDIAC ARRHYTHMIAS

The medical assistant should recognize cardiac arrhythmias that occur during the ECG recording and make the physician aware of them as soon as they are noticed. The normal, healthy ECG cycle consists of P, QRS, and T in a regularly appearing sequence or pattern. The term **normal**

Patient Teaching Tip

Atherosclerosis is the build-up of fatty deposits on the lining of coronary arteries causing narrowing and obstruction of the arteries. Blood flow to the heart muscle is diminished particularly when the heart is called upon to work harder; e.g., during increased physical activity, emotional stress, exposure to cold temperatures, and after a heavy meal. The heart's muscle tissue responds to these conditions by symptoms of pain or discomfort beneath the sternum, into the neck, jaw, left arm and shoulder, and throat. Rest usually relieves the pain. This condition is known as angina pectoris.

Treatment for angina consists of rest and medication. Nitroglycerin may be prescribed in tablet or patch form. Change in lifestyle and other suggestions as noted in Table 25-1 may be recommended. Tests that the physician may order include a twelve-lead ECG, a stress ECG (stress test), blood tests, chest X ray, and coronary angiogram.

Pain that does not subside following rest may indicate a more serious condition: a complete obstruction of the coronary arteries and no blood flow to the heart muscle, a myocardial infarction, or heart attack. Seek immediate medical attention if pain persists.

sinus rhythm refers to an ECG that is within normal limits (WNL). The normal adult heart rate is 60 to 100 beats per minute. A rate less than 60 beats per minute is known as **sinus bradycardia** (Figure 25-13A); a rate greater than 100 beats per minute is known as **sinus tachycardia** (Figure 25-13B). These two heart rates, while regular in rhythm, are still considered to be cardiac arrhythmias.

TABLE 25-1 HEALTHY BEHAVIORS TO ADOPT FOR A HEALTHY HEART

The physician may want the medical assistant to remind patients of the following healthy behaviors:
1. Avoid tobacco.
2. Take medications as prescribed.
3. Report any unusual symptoms or problems to the physician.
4. Eat a low-fat, low-cholesterol, low-sodium diet.
5. Exercise regularly with physician's permission.
6. Get adequate rest.
7. Keep weight under control and at an acceptable level.
8. Practice stress reduction behaviors.

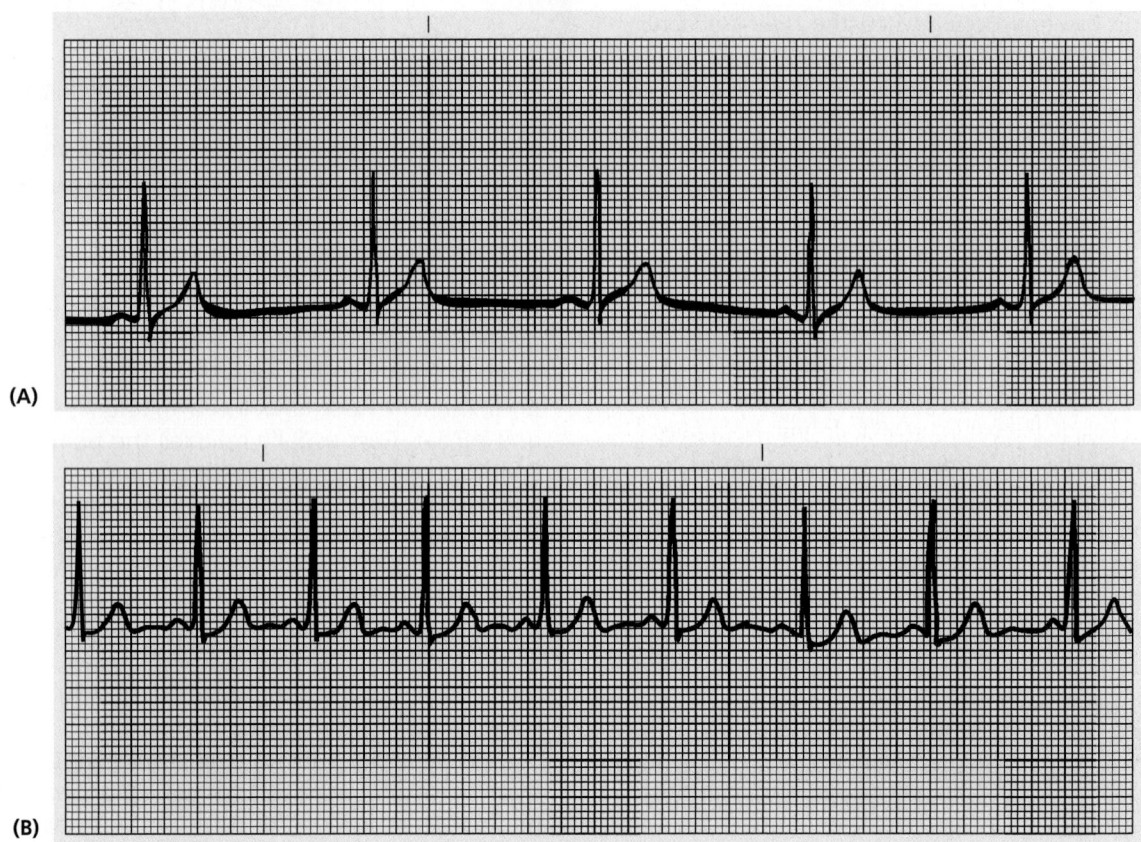

Figure 25-13   (A) Heart rate shown is 50 bpm, known as sinus bradycardia since it is less than 60 bpm. One large square = 0.2 second; one minute (60 seconds) ÷ 0.2 = 300. There are 6 large squares between R waves: 300 ÷ 6 = 50 bpm. (B) Sinus tachycardia is a heart rate faster than 100 bpm.

Atrial Arrhythmias

Premature Atrial Contractions (PAC). Healthy persons can experience premature atrial contractions. They are seen in patients who use tobacco and stimulants such as caffeine, but can forewarn of more serious cardiac problems. This type of arrhythmia is characterized by a cardiac cycle that occurs before the next cycle is due. The P wave is shaped differently from the P wave of the normal cycle (Figure 25-14A).

Paroxysmal Atrial Tachycardia (PAT). This arrhythmia also can be seen in healthy individuals; however, it can appear in persons with cardiac disease. PAT is characterized by its unprovoked sudden onset and abrupt termination. The heart rate is regular and ranges between 160 to 250 beats per minute. The episode usually lasts only a few seconds and the heart rate then returns to its original rate (Figure 25-14B). The patient may describe a fluttering in the chest, apprehension, shortness of breath, and on occasion, dizziness.

Atrial Fibrillation. This arrhythmia can be seen in healthy patients or those with cardiac disease. In younger patients, common causes can be congenital heart disease and mitral valve damage due to rheumatic heart disease. In older patients, the arrhythmia can be due to hypertension, coronary artery disease, or mitral valve prolapse. It is characterized by extremely rapid, incomplete contractions 400 to 500 bpm (beats per minute) resulting in small, irregular, and uncoordinated complexes that are difficult to measure accurately because the P waves cannot be distinguished (Figure 25-14C).

Ventricular Arrhythmias

Premature Ventricular Contractions (PVCs). This arrhythmia can be seen in healthy patients and patients with hypertension, coronary artery disease, and lung disease. In healthy patients, PVCs can be caused by tobacco, anxiety, alcohol, and medications that contain epinephrine (Figure 25-15A). PVCs are seen on ECG

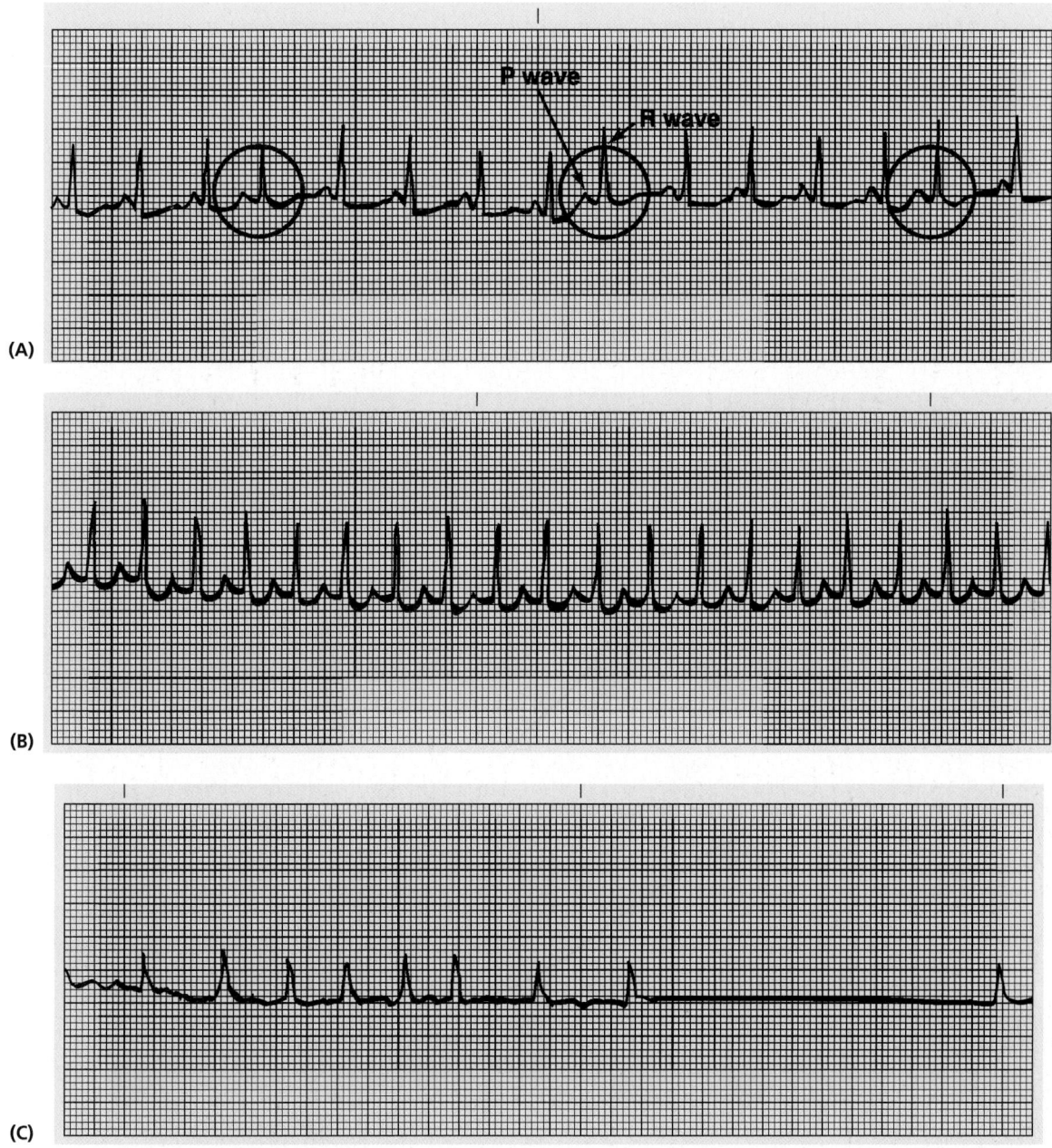

Figure 25-14   Atrial arrhythmias: (A) Premature atrial contractions (PAC). (B) Paroxysmal atrial tachycardia (PAT). (C) Atrial fibrillation.

tracings fairly frequently and are considered common disturbances in the rhythm. They are characterized by a beat that comes early in the cycle, has no P wave, a wide QRS complex, and a different T wave. The PVC is followed by a pause before the occurrence of the next normal cycle.

Ventricular Tachycardia. This arrhythmia is seen in patients with cardiac disease, both acute and chronic. It is common in coronary artery disease and frequently the patient experiencing a myocardial infarction will have ventricular tachycardia as a result of the infarction (Figure 25-15B). The arrhythmia is manifested by three or more

PVCs that occur at a rate ranging from 150 to 250 beats per minute. There are no P waves and the QRS complexes are distorted. Ventricular tachycardia is life threatening and can rapidly deteriorate into fibrillation and cardiac standstill.

Ventricular Fibrillation. This arrhythmia is seen in patients experiencing a myocardial infarction or in patients with existing cardiac disease. It may be preceded by PVCs or ventricular tachycardia or may begin as ventricular fibrillation. It is a life-threatening arrhythmia (Figure 25-15C).

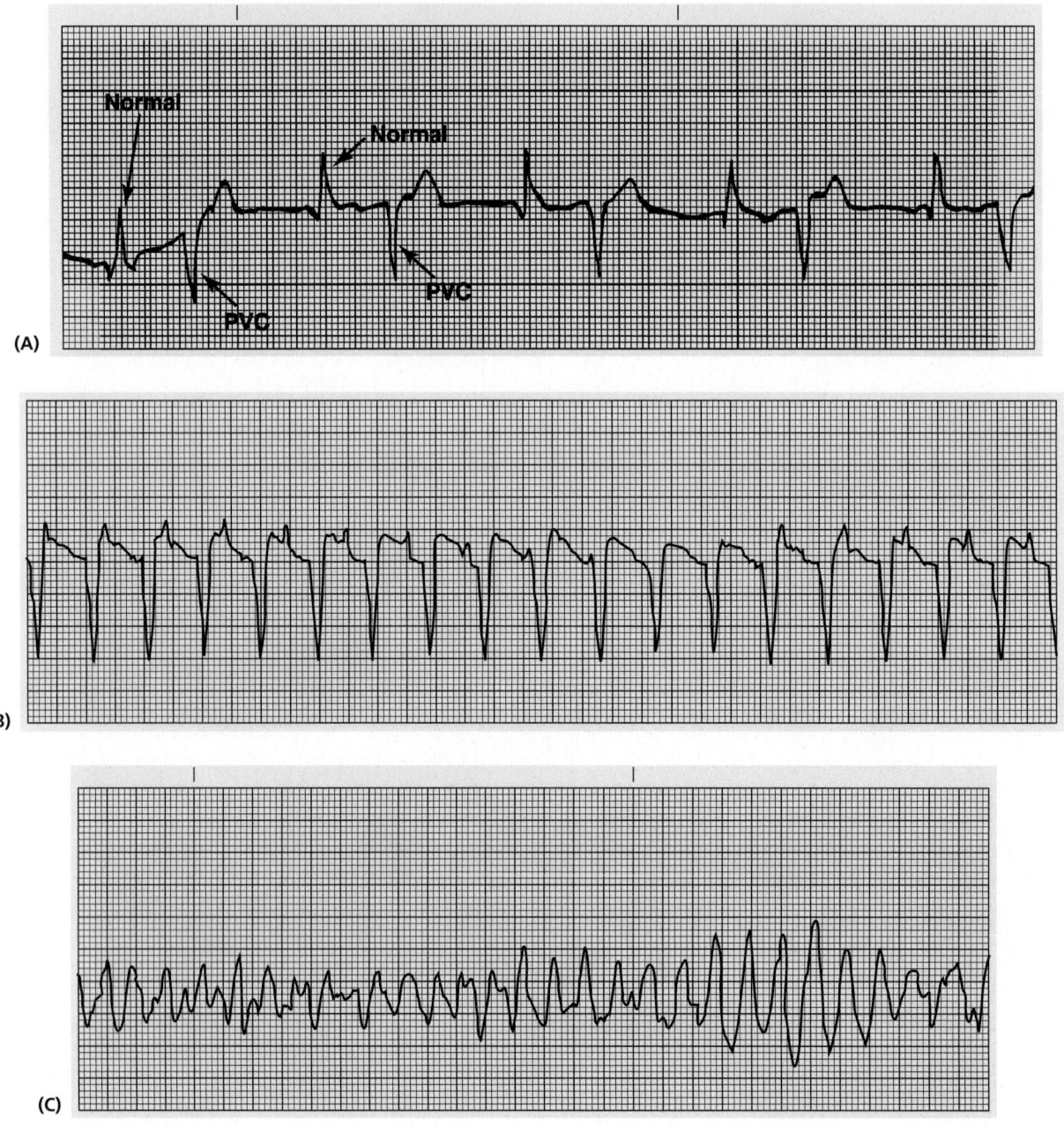

Figure 25-15 Ventricular arrhythmias: (A) Premature ventricular contractions (PVCs). (B) Ventricular tachycardia. (C) Ventricular fibrillation.

DEFIBRILLATION

A defibrillator is an electrical device that applies countershocks to the heart through electrodes or pads placed on the chest wall (Figure 25-16). The purpose is to convert cardiac arrhythmia into normal sinus rhythm. This is known as defibrillation or cardioversion. In some offices and clinics, a defibrillator is kept on a crash cart for quick access in emergency situations. The medical assistant should regularly check the equipment for proper operation and preparedness, and assist the physician as needed. See Chapter 9.

OTHER CARDIAC DIAGNOSTIC TESTS

Holter Monitor (Portable Ambulatory Electrocardiograph)

The Holter monitor is a portable continuous recording of cardiac activity for a 24-hour period (Figure 25-17). The patient is monitored while going about the usual daily activities with no restrictions. This noninvasive test helps to diagnose cardiac arrhythmias by correlating them

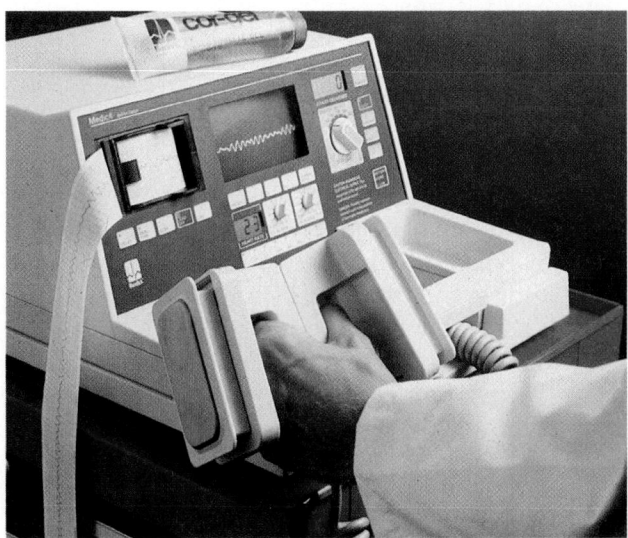

Figure 25-16 The Medic IV defibrillator. (Courtesy of Siemens Burdick, Inc.)

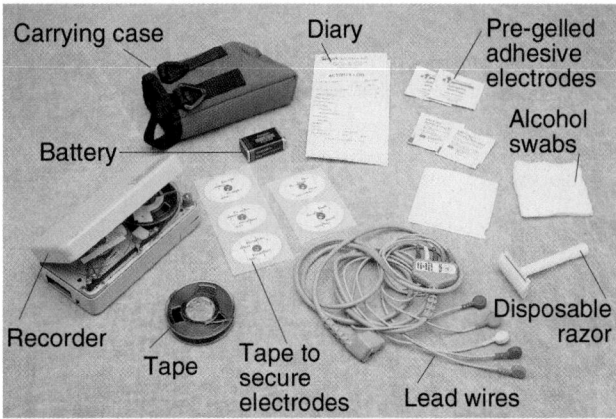

Figure 25-17 Holter monitor and supplies needed for application.

with the patient's symptoms. Some symptoms are syncope, fatigue, chest pain, and vertigo. This type of monitoring is useful for patients whose arrhythmias are sporadic in nature and whose arrhythmia is not able to be found on a twelve-lead ECG tracing. Also, ambulatory monitoring helps assess the function of an artificial pacemaker and the effectiveness of antiarrhythmic medications.

Special electrodes are placed in the appropriate areas of the patient's chest and lead wires are then attached to the electrodes. A special portable tape recorder, computer or magnetic, will continually record the heart's electrical activity for a 24-hour period. The monitor is a battery-operated recorder that is placed in a leather pouch or bag and is worn by the patient either on a belt around the waist or by a strap over the patient's shoulder.

Medical Assistant's Role. The medical assistant is responsible for preparing the patient, instructing the patient, and applying and removing the monitor.

Following are examples of some of the daily activities that should be recorded by the patient in the patient activity diary:

- Eating meals
- Ascending and descending stairs
- Sexual activity
- Medications taken
- Times of sleep
- Smoking
- Bowel movements
- Physical exercise

Holter Monitor Attachment. Once the Holter monitor has been attached to the patient, the monitor should be checked for effectiveness by attaching the **test cable** to the monitor and the other end to an ECG instrument. A baseline strip can be recorded to verify the correct wave activity and lack of artifact. If there are inaccurate readings, the monitor may not have been applied properly. The medical assistant can reconnect the leads to the electrodes or reposition the electrodes and reconnect the leads (see Procedure 25-3).

Holter Monitor Electrode Placement. Special disposable electrodes, which are round plastic and have an adhesive back, are available for the Holter monitor. These

Patient Teaching Tip

When preparing patients to wear a Holter monitor instruct them to:

1. Keep a diary of daily activities, symptoms, and emotions, and note the time of occurrence.
2. Do not shower, bathe, or swim while wearing the monitor because the recording could be interrupted or the monitor could be damaged.
3. Do not handle the electrodes. Doing so could cause artifacts.
4. Do not remove the recorder from its case.
5. Do not use an electric blanket. This can cause interference.
6. Depress the event marker only briefly and when experiencing a significant symptom. Overuse of the marker can mask the ECG tracing.

TABLE 25-2	HOLTER MONITOR ELECTRODE PLACEMENT	
Electrode	**Lead**	**Location**
A (black)	mV_1	Fourth intercostal space at right of the sternal edge
B (white)	mV_5	Right clavicle, just lateral to sternum
C (brown)	mV_1	Left clavicle, just lateral to the sternum
D (red)	mV_5	Fifth intercostal space at left axillary line
E (green)	Ground	Lower right chest wall

SPOTLIGHT ON AAMA ESSENTIALS THROUGH CAAHEP

● Take the time to talk with the patient when instructing him or her on keeping a daily activity record while wearing a Holter monitor. This will assist the patient to cut down on undue stresses and thus make the monitoring much more accurate and reliable.

● When preparing a patient for electrocardiography, it is important that the medical assistant be understanding and sensitive to the patient's fears and concerns about a possible heart problem.

● By explaining the electrocardiogram before performing the procedure, the medical assistant encourages the patient to be better informed and generally more cooperative and less anxious.

electrodes contain an electrolyte gel and are discarded once used. There may be either four or five electrodes depending on whether or not the monitor has a built-in ground. Notice that the leads for the Holter monitor are applied to different locations than the electrodes of a resting ECG. Table 25-2 explains the lead placement.

Patient Activity Diary. The patient activity diary is an important component of the monitoring procedures. As noted in the Patient Teaching Tip, all activities and emotional states, and the time of their occurrence, should be noted during the 24-hour monitoring time. Symptoms such as chest pain, shortness of breath, dizziness, palpitations, and so on, and the time the event occurred should also be noted. Patient symptoms recorded while being monitored can be compared to the patient's notations in the activity diary and correlated to the heart's activity. Symptoms can be further noted by the patient briefly depressing an event marker button located at one end of the monitor. This places an electronic "tag" on the tape. This signal can alert the person interpreting the ECG to look for a significant event or abnormality on the tape.

Holter Monitor Removal. The patient is instructed to return to the office or ambulatory care center 24 hours later to have the monitor removed. The tape is analyzed by a Holter monitor scanner or by a computer. This is usually done in the ECG department of a nearby hospital. The physician will receive a written report with samples of any abnormalities that were picked up during the monitoring period.

Treadmill Stress Test or Exercise Tolerance ECG

On occasion patients have symptoms of cardiac problems that do not appear as abnormalities on a resting ECG.

The physician may prescribe a treadmill stress test or exercise tolerance test to aid in the determination of the patient's diagnosis and prognosis. The test is done to diagnose heart disorders, to diagnose the probable cause of the patient's chest pain, and to assess the patient's cardiac ability following cardiac surgery. The treadmill stress test is a noninvasive ECG tracing taken under controlled conditions while the patient is closely monitored by the physician. Frequent blood pressure readings are done. The patient wears comfortable clothing and flat shoes such as sneakers with rubber soles and exercises on a treadmill at prescribed rates of speed (Figure 25-18). Electrodes are applied to the chest only.

The myocardium requires extra oxygen during exercise and in the presence of narrowed or obstructed coronary arteries. The additional workload on the myocardium will often be demonstrated as an abnormality on the ECG recording. There should be no pain, shortness of breath, or excess fatigue. If any of these or other unusual symptoms occur, the physician will terminate the test as this could indicate cardiac disease.

At the conclusion of the test, the patient is told to rest. Monitoring continues until the vital signs and heart rate return to normal. Prior to the patient leaving the office, the patient should be instructed to rest, refrain from a hot bath or shower, avoid stimulants such as caf-

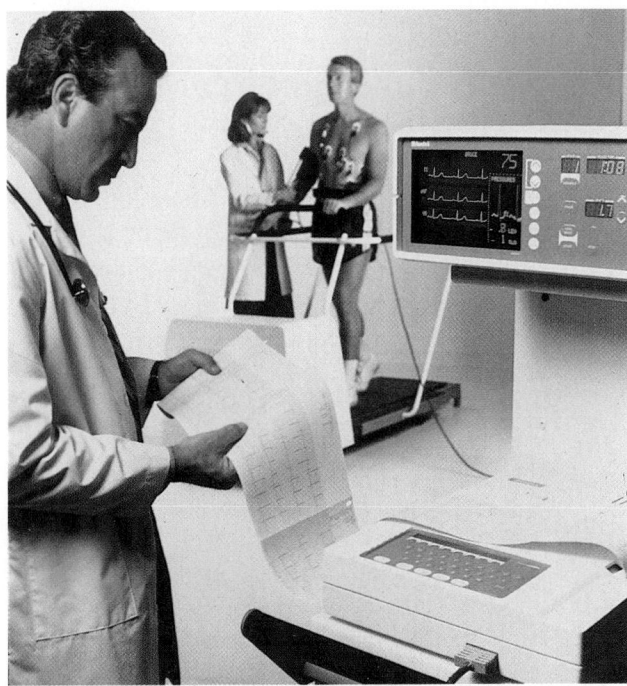

Figure 25-18 The EXTOL 350 ST Stress System. (Courtesy of Siemens Burdick, Inc.)

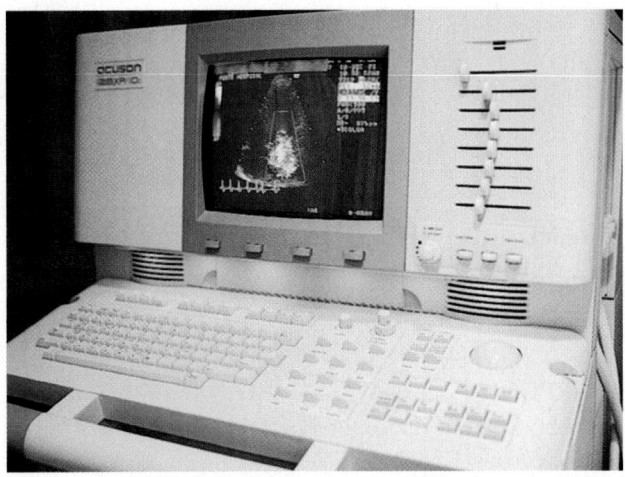

Figure 25-19 Echocardiograph. (Photo by Marcia Butterfield, Courtesy of W. A. Foote Memorial Hospital, Jackson, MI)

feine, and avoid extreme temperature changes for several hours.

Complications such as a myocardial infarction or a serious arrhythmia can occur during testing. While these events are unusual, appropriate emergency equipment must be readily available and checked frequently for proper functioning. Some equipment to have on hand for cardiac emergencies include oxygen, antiarrhythmic drugs, an Ambu-bag™, a defibrillator, an airway, an endotracheal tube, and a laryngoscope.

Further diagnostic tests such as **cardiac catheterization** may be necessary to diagnose the extent of the atheroscleratic buildup and obstruction of the coronary arteries.

Echocardiography

Echocardiography is a noninvasive, diagnostic test that uses ultrasound (ultrahigh-frequency sound waves) to image the internal structures of the heart (Figure 25-19). X rays are not used. General anatomy, myocardial function, valve function, and heart chamber size can be evaluated.

During **ultrasonography**, a handheld **transducer** acts as a transmitter and receiver of the high-frequency sound waves as it is held against the chest wall and moved over the heart area. As the sound waves go through the skin and hit internal structures, echoes are sent back to the transducer. A machine converts the images when the various structures provide different echoes. The images can then be examined by a computer and converted into photographs and films of structures and blood flow.

There is little patient preparation other than to have the patient lie on the examination table with the four-limb leads of a twelve-lead electrocardiograph attached. The test is usually performed by a **sonographer**.

Procedure 25-1

Perform Twelve-Lead Electrocardiogram, Single-Channel

STANDARD PRECAUTIONS:

PURPOSE:

To obtain an accurate, graphic, artifact-free reading of the electrical activity of the patient's heart to identify arrhythmias, estimate damage caused by MI, assess effects of cardiac medication, determine if electrolyte imbalance is present, identify cardiac ischemia, and determine the effects of hypertension or other disorders on the heart.

EQUIPMENT/SUPPLIES:

Examination or ECG table with pillow and sheet or blanket
Patient gown
Single-channel electrocardiograph with patient cable wires
Electrolyte (gel, lotion, paste, or presaturated pads)
ECG tracing paper
Metal electrodes (sensors)
Rubber straps
Gauze squares
Mounting form

PROCEDURE STEPS:

1. Perform tracing in a quiet, warm, and comfortable room away from electrical equipment that may cause artifacts. RATIONALE: Patient is less apprehensive in a quiet atmosphere. Alternating current (AC) interference is minimized when ECG is performed away from electrical equipment.

2. Wash hands, gather equipment, identify the patient, and explain the procedure to the patient. RATIONALE: Following these universal steps minimizes transmission of microorganisms and reassures patient.

3. Have the patient remove clothing from the waist up and uncover lower legs; Nylon stockings must be removed; socks can be worn. RATIONALE: Electrodes must be placed on bare skin for optimum conductivity of electricity. Provide a sheet or blanket for privacy and warmth. Place the patient in supine position on the examination table with arms and legs supported. Pillows may be used under the knees and head. RATIONALE: All four limbs and chest must be uncovered for proper electrode placement.

4. Explain that the procedure is painless and why it is necessary not to move or talk during the procedure. RATIONALE: Patient cooperation ensures good quality tracing.

5. Place the electrocardiograph with the power cord pointing away from the patient. Do not allow the cable to go underneath the table. RATIONALE: This helps reduce AC interference.

6. Apply the limb electrodes by first connecting the rubber straps to the tabs on the electrodes. Apply a pea-size dab of electrolyte to the electrode; either paste or gel can be used (Figure 25-20).

(continues)

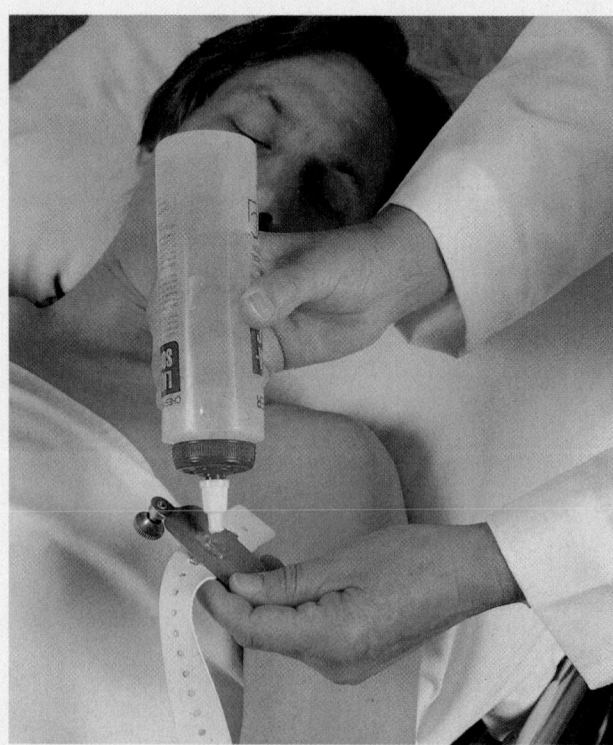

Figure 25-20   The rubber strap is attached to the metal electrode and a small amount of electrolyte gel is placed on the side of the electrode applied to the patient's skin.

Procedure 25-1 *(continued)*

Apply the electrodes to the fleshy parts of the four limbs. Rub the electrolyte into the patient's skin. Lead connectors of the electrodes should be pointing toward the feet. Pull the rubber strap around the limb until it just meets, then pull tighter one more hole and secure (Figures 25-21 and 25-22). RATIONALE: A more stable connection with the lead wires is possible when the lead connectors point to the feet. Electrolyte rubbed into the patient's skin helps ensure good contact between the electrode and the skin. Straps applied too tightly or too loosely can cause artifacts. By applying electrodes to the fleshy part of the limbs, artifacts are minimized.

7. If using a Welch cup chest electrode, apply electrolyte to chest position, rub the edge of each cup in the electrolyte, and secure it in position by squeezing the bulb end of the cup to create suction on the skin of the chest wall (Figure 25-23). When using the Welch cup electrode with a single channel non-automatic machine, only one chest lead can be recorded at a time because there is only one chest lead wire. Therefore, chest lead V_1 should be placed in position and be ready to be recorded. The first seven leads, I,

II, III, aVR, aVL, aVF, and V_1, can be recorded before it is necessary to temporarily stop recording while the Welch cup is moved to each successive chest lead. It is necessary to turn the machine to AMP OFF between each V lead because the medical assistant will manually remove the V lead and place it on the next

(continues)

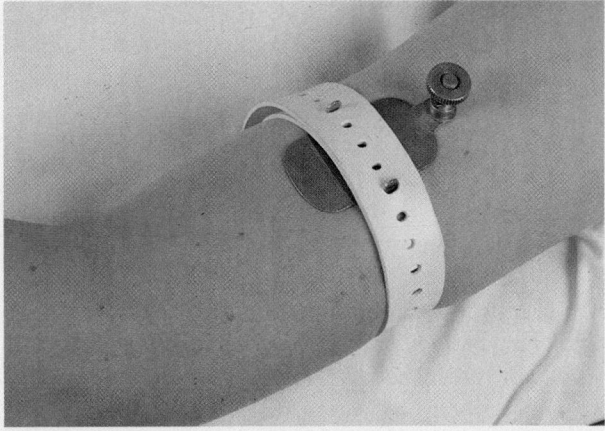

Figure 25-22 Electrode held in place on upper arm by rubber strap. Pull the rubber strap around until the holes line up with the protrusions on the electrode with no tension, then pull the strap one hole tighter and secure.

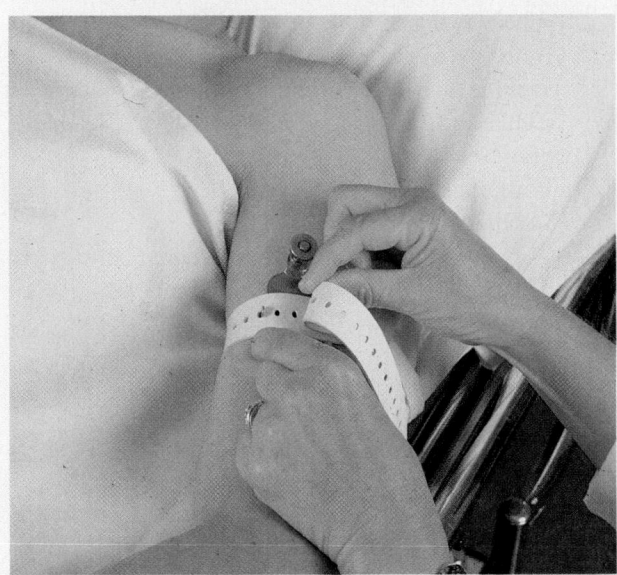

Figure 25-21 Application of rubber strap and electrode to patient's upper arm. Placing electrode on upper arm minimizes somatic tremor.

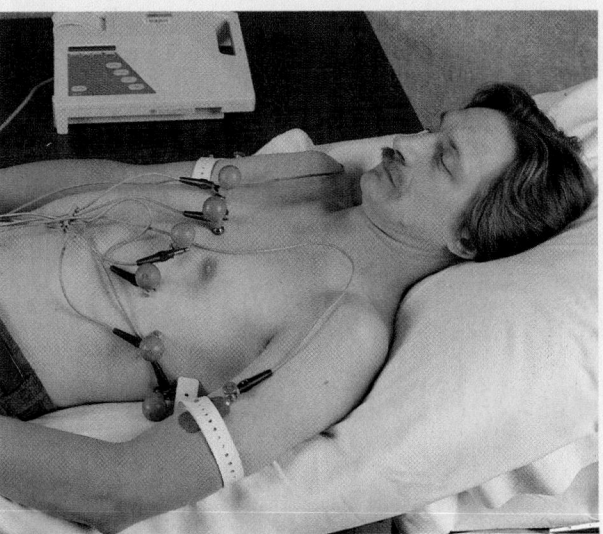

Figure 25-23 An automatic electrocardiograph with all six chest leads applied simultaneously using Welch electrodes allows all chest leads to be recorded at one time.

Procedure 25-1 (continued)

appropriate V lead position. If the machine were not turned to AMP OFF between each V lead as the medical assistant moves the Welch cup, this would interrupt the tracing, cause the stylus to become erratic, and distort the tracing. After the Welch cup has been moved to the next appropriate V lead, the stylus is adjusted, the machine is turned to AMP ON, and six to eight inches of the V lead is recorded.

8. Tightly connect the lead wires to the electrodes. Be sure to connect the correct lead wires to the correct electrodes. The lead wires are labeled with abbreviations (RA, LA, RL, LL, and V or C). The lead wires are color-coded as follows: RA=white, LA=black, RL=green, LL=red, V or chest=brown or multi-colored depending on model of machine. The lead wires should follow the patient's body contour. RATIONALE: Following body contour minimizes artifacts.

9. The patient cable is supported either on the table or the patient's abdomen. Plug the patient cable into the electrocardiograph.

10. Turn instrument to ON.

11. The lead selector switch should be on STD (standard). Center the stylus. The record switch should be on Run (25 mm/sec). Check the standardization for the instrument by quickly pressing the standardization button. The standardization mark should be 10 mm or 10 small squares high. If it is more or less than this, adjust the instrument appropriately. RATIONALE: Standardization ensures a dependable and accurate tracing.

12. Center the stylus and run about 4 to 5 complexes of each lead I, II, and III by placing the record switch on Run (25 mm/sec) and turning the lead selector switch appropriately.

    a. While recording, be sure the stylus and recording are near the center of the paper. If not, use the position control knob to move up or down to adjust as needed. None of the waves should fall off the graph paper.

    b. Watch for artifacts and correct if present.

    c. Determine if a change in standard or stylus position is needed by observing the amplitude of the R wave.

13. Continue with leads aVR, aVL, aVF, and record about 4 to 5 complexes of each lead by turning the lead selector to the appropriate position.

14. Record 6 to 8 complexes of each of the V leads by turning the lead selector control to the appropriate position.

15. Place another standardization at the end of the tracing by putting the lead selector on STD and depressing the button. Run the tracing through the instrument and turn the machine to OFF. Remove the tracing from the instrument and immediately label with patient's name, date, and time of day. Sign your initials. Unplug the power cord.

16. Disconnect the lead wires and remove the rubber straps and electrodes from the patient. Cleanse or wipe patient's skin to remove paste or gel electrolyte.

17. Assist patient as needed.

18. Provide physician with uncut tracing.

19. Clean and return equipment per OSHA guidelines.

20. Wash hands.

21. Document procedure.

22. Cut and mount the tracing, remembering to handle carefully. Label appropriately and place in patient's record.

Procedure 25-2: Perform Twelve-Lead Electrocardiogram, Three Channel

STANDARD PRECAUTIONS:

PURPOSE:

To obtain an accurate, graphic, artifact-free reading of the electrical activity of the patient's heart to identify arrhythmias, estimate damage caused by MI, assess effects of cardiac medication, determine if electrolyte imbalance is present, identify cardiac ischemia, and determine the effects of hypertension or other disorders on the heart.

EQUIPMENT/SUPPLIES:

Examination or ECG table with pillow and sheet or
blanket
Patient gown
Three-channel automatic electrocardiograph with
patient cable wires
Disposable electrodes
ECG tracing paper
Gauze squares
Mounting form

PROCEDURE STEPS:

1. Follow steps 1 through 5 of Procedure 25-1 for ECG with single-channel machine.
2. Prepare patient's skin for disposable electrode attachment. If patient's skin is oily, wipe electrode area with alcohol and let dry.
3. Apply electrodes firmly to fleshy parts of limbs. Point tabs of electrodes attached to arms in a downward position, place electrodes attached to legs in an upward position. RATIONALE: Tab position allows for better connection and keeps pulling on lead wires to a minimum.
4. Locate chest sites and apply electrodes with tabs pointing in a downward position.
5. Connect lead wires to the electrodes. An alligator clip (a special clip applied to the end of the lead wires) will grasp the tab on the electrode.
6. Plug patient cable into machine. Support patient cable to avoid pulling or tangling of it.
7. Turn on the ECG. Enter patient data by keying it into machine. Notice the data on the LCD screen (patient data includes: patient's name, age, height, weight, gender, ID number, and cardiac medications).
8. Press AUTO for automatic and run the ECG to obtain the tracing. The standardization is automatically inserted at the beginning and the twelve leads follow in the three-channel mode. Watch for artifacts and take the appropriate steps to eliminate them should they occur.
9. Disconnect the lead wires and remove the electrodes from the patient. Dispose of the electrodes.
10. Assist patient as needed.
11. Provide physician with uncut tracing.
12. Clean and return equipment per OSHA guidelines.
13. Wash hands.
14. Document procedure.
15. Cut and mount the tracing, remembering to handle carefully. Label appropriately and place in patient's record.

Procedure

25-3   **Perform Holter Monitor Application**

STANDARD PRECAUTIONS:

PURPOSE:
To detect sporadic cardiac arrhythmias, to determine correlation of symptoms with activity, to evaluate chest pain and cardiac status following pacemaker implantation or after acute myocardial infarction.

EQUIPMENT/SUPPLIES:

Holter monitor	Alcohol swabs
Patient activity diary	Gauze
Blank magnetic tape	Tape
Disposable electrodes	Carrying case
Razor	Belt or shoulder strap

PROCEDURE STEPS:

1. Wash hands and assemble equipment.
2. Prepare the equipment by removing old (used) battery from the monitor and replacing it with a new battery. Insert a blank magnetic tape into the monitor. RATIONALE: Installing a new battery each 24-hour period will ensure the monitor will function because it will have sufficient power.
3. Wash hands.
4. Identify the patient and explain the procedure. RATIONALE: Adherence to patient guidelines helps ensure an accurate tracing.
5. Have patient remove clothing from the waist up.
6. Have patient sit on the examination table or chair. RATIONALE: This allows for patient comfort and relaxation and for the medical assistant to place the electrodes appropriately.
7. Locate the correct electrode placement on the chest wall. The skin must be prepared in the following way:
   a. Dry shave patient's chest at each electrode site if chest is hairy.
   b. Rub the shaved area with an alcohol swab. Let area dry (Figure 25-24).
   c. Abrade the skin slightly with a dry 4 × 4 gauze. Areas should be red. RATIONALE: Shaved site and abraded skin help the electrodes to adhere better to the skin and facilitate easier removal.

8. Take the electrodes from the package and peel away the backing from one of them (electrode should be moist). Continue to remove electrodes one by one and attach as in step 9.
9. Apply adhesive-backed electrode to the appropriate sites by applying firm pressure at the center of the electrode and moving outward toward the edges. Starting at the center of the electrode, apply pressure firmly and move outward on the electrode. Run your fingers along the outer rim to ensure firm attachment. Avoid moving from one side of electrode to the other. Gel could be forced out and could cause interference. RATIONALE: Firmly attached electrodes ensure a good quality tracing.
10. Attach the lead wires to the electrodes. Connect them to the patient cable.
11. Secure each electrode with adhesive tape. RATIONALE: The tape secures the electrodes by reducing the tugging and pulling on them.

(continues)

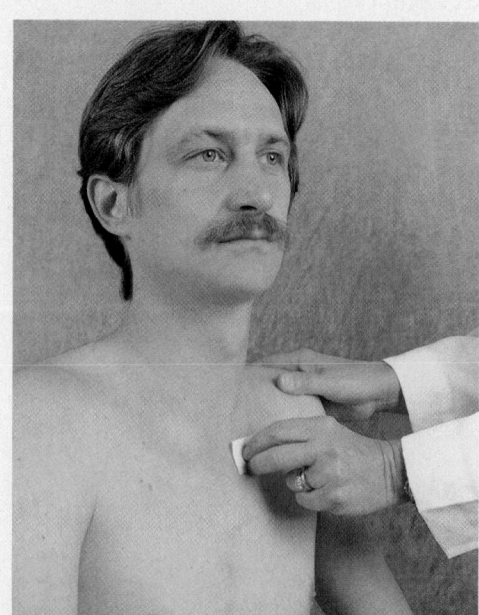

Figure 25-24   Preparation of patient skin with alcohol prior to placement of electrodes for Holter monitor.

Procedure

25-3   *(continued)*

12. Plug the monitor into an electrocardiograph with the test cable. Run a baseline tracing. RATIONALE: Running a baseline tracing will validate proper setup of electrodes and confirm there is no malfunction of the leads or cable.

13. Place the electrode cable so that it extends from between the buttons of the patient's shirt or from below the bottom of the shirt.

14. Place the recorder into its carrying case and either attach it to the patient's belt or over the patient's shoulder. Be certain there is no pulling on the lead wires (Figure 25-25). RATIONALE: Pulling on electrodes could cause them to become detached.

15. Plug the electrode cable into the monitor. Record the starting time in the patient activity log (diary). RATIONALE: The beginning time is noted in order to correlate cardiac activity with the patient activity log.

16. Give the activity log to the patient, being certain that the patient information is completed. RATIONALE: The activity log helps correlate cardiac activity with patient symptoms.

17. Inform patient what time the following day the monitor will be removed. Remind the patient to bring along the activity log.

18. Wash hands.

19. Document procedure in the patient's record.

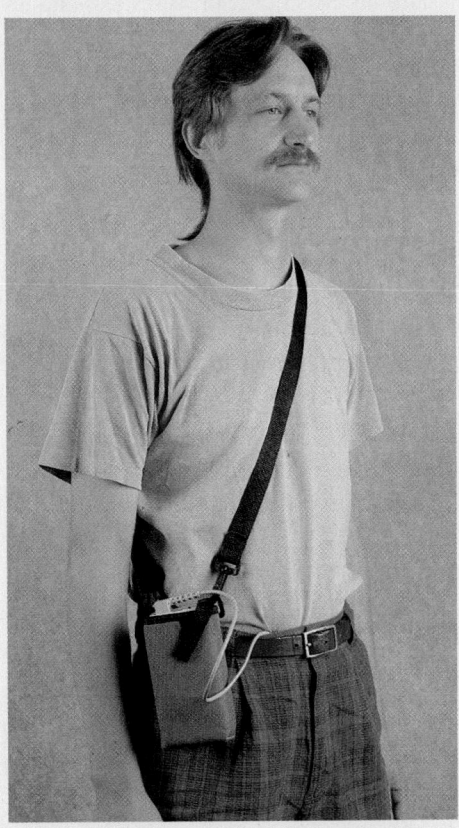

Figure 25-25   Holter monitor in its carrying case and secured by a shoulder strap. The monitor can also be applied on a belt and worn around the patient's waist.

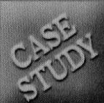

Abigail Johnson, in her mid-seventies, arrives at the urgent care center complaining of chest pains. She has been seen on two other occasions for similar pain and has a history of diabetes, hypertension, arteriosclerotic heart disease, and angina pectoris. Medical assistant Wanda Slawson immediately alerts Dr. Rice of Mrs. Johnson's chest pain and then takes her into the cardiac examination and treatment room. Dr. Rice tells Wanda to have Mrs. Johnson take one of her nitroglycerin tablets and to perform an ECG on her. Mrs. Johnson is restless and anxious as Wanda prepares for the ECG and while the tracing is in progress. There is significant somatic tremor. Wanda attempts to allay Mrs. Johnson's apprehension in order to obtain a good quality ECG. The patient's pain subsides within a few minutes and she begins to feel better.

CASE STUDY REVIEW

1. What immediate action could Wanda have taken if Mrs. Johnson's pain had not subsided?

2. Mrs. Johnson tells Wanda that Dr. Rice explained arteriosclerotic heart disease and angina pectoris to her, but that she was nervous and understood little and that she is embarrassed to admit that to Dr. Rice. How can Wanda explain, in language that the patient can comprehend, what causes arteriosclerotic heart disease and angina, and what Mrs. Johnson experiences during an attack of angina? What strategies can Wanda teach Mrs. Johnson to promote healthier habits and prevent more serious heart problems?

3. Research community resources that are available for persons with Mrs. Johnson's heart condition. Explain how Mrs. Johnson could benefit from them.

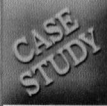

George Matthews, 79-year-old patient of Dr. Abbott, has a history of cardiovascular heart disease. He tells Dr. Abbott that today he has been experiencing "palpitations and slow and fast heartbeats and sometimes dizziness." Dr. Abbott orders a resting ECG that shows no evidence of arrhythmia and decides that a Holter monitor electrocardiograph for Mr. Matthews might be helpful in diagnosing a cardiac arrhythmia.

CASE STUDY REVIEW

1. Describe why Dr. Abbott ordered a Holter monitor electrocardiography for Mr. Matthews.

2. What instructions will you give to Mr. Matthews about wearing the monitor?

3. Mr. Matthews says he isn't certain what activities should be recorded in the patient activity diary. Explain what they are and the reason for their importance.

SUMMARY

Electrocardiography is a noninvasive painless procedure that is helpful in diagnosing heart disease. Cables with sensors are attached to the patient's arms, legs, and chest. The electrocardiograph amplifies the electrical currents generated when the myocardium contracts and relaxes with each heartbeat. A series of deflections (waves) is recorded on special ECG paper when a heated stylus on the electrocardiograph moves across the paper. The cardiac cycles that appear are then interpreted by the physician. The recording or tracing, known as an electrocardiogram, represents the heart's rate, rhythm, and other myocardial actions. Each of the twelve leads of the recording becomes part of the patient's permanent record.

In addition to a resting ECG, other types of electrocardiography can be done. Cardiac stress testing is done while the patient is physically challenged to perform increasingly strenuous exercises. The heart's tolerance to the increased demands placed on it during exercise can be observed and recorded while the patient is being closely monitored. This type of electrocardiography helps diagnose heart disease that would not be evident if a resting ECG were done.

Holter electrocardiography or ambulatory cardiac monitoring is an ECG test done as the patient goes about normal daily activities. The patient wears chest leads and carries a small recording device on a belt or on a strap over the shoulder for a period of 24 hours and documents activities in the patient activity diary. This type of electrocardiography helps diagnose cardiac arrhythmias that occur sporadically and may be difficult to capture on a resting ECG because of their unpredictability. Echocardiography is a diagnostic test that uses ultrasound to image the internal structures of the heart. Myocardial function, valvular function or defects, and chamber size can be determined.

In most instances, the medical assistant is responsible for patient preparation, patient education, operation of the electrocardiograph, elimination of artifacts, mounting, labeling, and placing ECG readings into the patient's file, and maintenance and care of the equipment. The diagnostic value of the test depends on the medical assistant's accuracy and skill.

REVIEW QUESTIONS

Multiple Choice

1. Which of the following is the most common type of artifact?
   a. somatic tremor
   b. AC interference
   c. wandering baseline
   d. interrupted baseline
2. Which of the following causes somatic tremor?
   a. too much electrolyte
   b. cable across patient's lap
   c. corroded sensors
   d. Parkinson's disease
3. One cardiac cycle (heartbeat) takes approximately how long?
   a. 0.2 second
   b. 0.4 second
   c. 0.6 second
   d. 0.8 second
4. Which of the following indicates ventricular depolarization?
   a. QRS complex
   b. P wave
   c. T wave
   d. S-T segment
5. Another name for V leads is:
   a. precordial
   b. augmented
   c. standard
   d. limb

Critical Thinking

1. The physician wants you to explain to Mrs. Johnson what behaviors she can adopt to have a healthy heart. With a partner, role-play medical assistant and patient and explain to the patient what she can do to improve her heart's health.
2. Mr. Williams has a diagnosis of Parkinson's disease. The physician requests an ECG. What strategies can you use to ensure an adequate tracing?
3. During the electrocardiogram, the equipment malfunctions. What options are available to the medical assistant?
4. Name four cardiac abnormalities that can be detected on an ECG.
5. Explain the significance of the small and large boxes on ECG paper. There are 2½ large boxes between each cardiac cycle. What is the heartbeat per minute?
6. Identify the placement of the twelve leads of the ECG.
7. The patient coughs and moves during the ECG. How can this affect the ECG tracing?
8. Explain standardization and why it is important.
9. What causes AC interference, wandering baseline, and interrupted baseline and how can they be eliminated?
10. State three purposes for a Holter monitor to be used and give the instructions that the patient will need to know while wearing the monitor.

WEB ACTIVITY

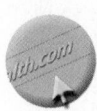

Search on the web for a national organization that focuses on heart and blood vessel disorders.

1. Print information about risk factors for cardiovascular heart disease.
2. What is the mortality rate for first-time myocardial infarctions for men versus women? Is there any difference in the mortality rate?
3. Are the symptoms identical in males and females when they are experiencing a myocardial infarction? Explain the similarities/differences between them.

REFERENCES/BIBLIOGRAPHY

Bonewit-West, K. (2000). *Clinical procedures for medical assistants* (5th ed.). Philadelphia: W. B. Saunders Company.

Keir, L., Wise, B., & Krebs, C. (1998). *Medical assisting. Administrative and clinical competencies* (8th ed.). Albany, NY: Delmar.

Krebs, C., & Heller, M. (1997). *Delmar's clinical handbook for healthcare professionals*. Albany, NY: Delmar.

Krebs, C., & Wise, B. (1998). *Medical assisting: Clinical competencies* (4th ed.). Albany, NY: Delmar.

Shea, D., & Carter-Ward, A. (1996). *Medical assisting: Clinical skills manual*. Albany, NY: Delmar.

Taber's cyclopedic medical dictionary. (18th ed.). (1999). Philadelphia: F. A. Davis Company.

Zakus, S. (1995). *Clinical procedures for medical assistants* (3rd ed.). St. Louis: Mosby-Year Book, Inc.

LABORATORY PROCEDURES

SAFETY AND REGULATORY GUIDELINES IN THE MEDICAL LABORATORY

26

KEY TERMS

Acetone
Aegis
Body Fluid
Calibration
Chemotherapeutic Agents
Communicable
Ethyl Alcohol
Excretion
Federal Register
Forensic
Formaldehyde
Fume Hood
Kit
Mandate
Medical Asepsis
Microscopy
Proficiency Testing
Pulmonary Edema
Quality Assurance
Quality Control
Reimbursement
Requisition
Secretion
Standard
Suppressed Immune System
Waived

OUTLINE

Clinical Laboratory Improvement Amendments of 1988 (CLIA '88)
The Intention of CLIA '88
General Program Description
Categories of Testing
Contents of the Law
CLIA '88 Regulation for Quality Control in Automated Hematology
Aftermath of CLIA '88
Impact of CLIA on Medical Assistants

Where to Find More Information Regarding CLIA '88
Occupational Safety and Health Administration (OSHA) Regulations
The Standard for Occupational Exposure to Hazardous Chemicals in the Laboratory
Chemical Hygiene Plan
OSHA Regulations and Students
Avoiding Exposure to Chemicals
Cumulative Trauma Disorders

OBJECTIVES

The student should strive to meet the following performance objectives and demonstrate an understanding of the facts and principles presented in this chapter through written and oral communication.

1. Define the key terms as presented in the glossary.
2. Identify the governmental agency that regulates procedures performed on patients and describe the agency's main concerns.
3. List the types of human specimens that CLIA regulates.
4. Name two performance requirements CLIA imposes on all laboratories.
5. Describe how CLIA '88 regulates the use of quality control in automated hematology instruments.
6. Recall the three categories of testing and list several from the waived category.
7. Discuss the importance of CLIA to the medical assistant.
8. Identify and discuss the contents of the law of CLIA '88.
9. Describe HCFA form 116 and explain its purpose.
10. Identify two OSHA standards that seek to safeguard employees.
11. Describe MSDS manuals and their purpose. Differentiate among the four colors and five numbers of the National Fire Protection Association.

CLINICAL

Fundamental Principles

- Apply principles of aseptic technique and infection control
- Comply with quality assurance practices

GENERAL (TRANSDISCIPLINARY)

Legal Concepts

- Follow federal, state, and local legal guidelines
- Maintain awareness of federal and state health care legislation and regulations
- Comply with established risk management and safety procedures

INTRODUCTION

Laboratory safety is a concern for all: management, staff, and patients. An unsafe work environment and/or work practices can threaten the emotional and physical health of the health care worker as well as the patient. Injuries are costly on many levels: personally to the injured individual, lost work days, workers' compensation, medical treatment, potential legal action, and potential fines from regulatory agencies. These situations have a direct effect on the individuals involved, but also have an indirect effect by lowering staff morale, ultimately resulting in less productivity. Management's response to safety is the key. Appropriate orientation, annual reviews, periodic drills, and consistent enforcement of staff adherence to policy are all part of a successful laboratory safety program.

All health care providers continually come into contact with patients who are ill. Some patients have **communicable** or contagious diseases; others may have a **suppressed immune system** that does not protect them from infection. In the course of performing your duties as a medical assistant, you will be in contact with blood and **body fluids** that may be highly infectious. It is of extreme importance that your health and safety as well as the health and safety of your patients be protected.

There are a number of infection control measures that can be used to reduce the transmission of bloodborne and other pathogens. **Medical asepsis**, also known as infection control, consists of procedures and practices that health care professionals use to prevent the spread of infection (see Chapter 10: Infection Control, Medical Asepsis, and Sterilization). State and federal

agencies also have established policies, procedures, and guidelines for health care providers and employers to follow in order to reduce the risk of transmission of infectious diseases. This chapter as well as Chapter 10 will examine the major guidelines.

The Centers for Disease Control and Prevention (CDC) in Atlanta, Georgia, a division of the United States Public Health Department, is an agency that investigates various diseases in an attempt to control them and makes recommendations on how to prevent the spread of disease. The CDC issued the system of seven isolation categories for patients with infectious diseases; it recommended the guidelines known as universal precautions; and, in 1996, it released standard precautions, which represent the most current and comprehensive approach to infection control.

The Clinical Laboratory Improvement Amendments of 1988 (CLIA '88) and the Occupational Safety and Health Administration (OSHA) also regulate the safety of patients and health care workers. CLIA '88 comes under the **aegis,** or protection, of the Health Care Financing Administration (HCFA) of the United States Department of Health and Human Services (HHS) of the federal government. OSHA comes under the United States Department of Labor. Both agencies require that health care settings, including clinical laboratories, adhere to the strict regulations that they set forth.

The purpose of CLIA '88 is to safeguard the public by regulating all testing of specimens taken from the human body. The purpose of OSHA is to require employers to ensure employee safety in regard to occupational exposure to potentially harmful substances.

CLIA '88 and OSHA guidelines will be examined independently. Table 26-1 summarizes both guidelines.

CLINICAL LABORATORY IMPROVEMENT AMENDMENTS OF 1988 (CLIA '88)

The Clinical Laboratory Improvement Amendments of 1988 (CLIA '88) were designed to set safety policies and procedures that protect patients.

In 1988 there was a public outcry as a result of articles published in the *Washington Post* and the *Wall Street Journal* and televised reports of deaths that were attributed to misread Pap smears. The public wanted action taken to ensure its safety, particularly in regard to laboratory testing. The outcry prompted the federal government to become more involved in regulating laboratories.

Although CLIA had been enacted into law in 1967, the issue of the misread Pap smears caused Congress to

TABLE 26-1   FEDERAL HEALTH AND SAFETY GUIDELINES

Guidelines	Issuing Agency	Purpose
Standard Precautions	Centers for Disease Control and Prevention (CDC), United States Public Health Department, Atlanta, Georgia	Issued in 1996 to augment and synthesize universal precautions and techniques known as body substance isolation (BSI). Standard precautions contain measures intended to protect all health care providers, patients, and visitors from infectious diseases.
Transmission-based Precautions	CDC	Designed to reduce the risk of airborne, droplet, and contact transmission of pathogens. These are used in addition to standard precautions and are intended for specific categories of patients.
Universal Blood and Body Fluid Precautions (Universal Precautions)	CDC	Released in 1985 to assist health care providers to greatly reduce the risk of contracting or transmitting infectious diseases, particularly AIDS and hepatitis B.
Clinical Laboratory Improvement Amendments of 1988 (CLIA '88)	Health Care Financing Administration (HCFA), United States Department of Health and Human Services (HHS)	Safeguards the public by regulating all testing of specimens taken from the body
Occupational Safety and Health Administration (OSHA) Guidelines	OSHA, United States Department of Labor	Requires employers to ensure employee safety in regard to occupational exposure to potentially harmful substances

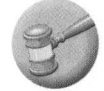

reexamine the regulations it had set forth in 1967. Thus, CLIA '88 was passed and included amendments to the original law. The amended regulations took effect on September 1, 1992.

States can seek exemptions from the CLIA standards if they have regulations that are comparable to those imposed by CLIA. If the federal government grants the state an exemption, laboratories in these states are under the control of state standards and applicable fees, not federal standards and fees. As of October, 1999, the states of California, New York, Oregon, and Washington have achieved state-exempt status.

Some accrediting bodies have revised their rules in an effort to meet HCFA's CLIA '88 requirements. HCFA can then give deemed status (equivalency) to these accrediting bodies. Laboratories accredited by these "deemed status" bodies are considered to meet HCFA's requirements. To date, HCFA has granted deemed status to the organizations listed in Table 26-2.

The Intention of CLIA '88

The intent of CLIA '88 is to protect the public by regulating all laboratory tests performed on specimens taken from the human body; i.e., blood and body **secretions** and **excretions.** The specimens are those used in the diagnosis, treatment, and prevention of disease. Previous regulations (Medicare, Medicaid, and CLIA '67) were based on the site and scope of the laboratory testing. CLIA '88 regulates laboratory testing irrespective of site, scope, volume, or frequency. As of July, 2000, registered CLIA laboratories total over 145,000 with physicians' office laboratories making up over 65 percent of the total. The regulations require that all laboratories in the

United States and its territories meet performance requirements that are based on how complex a test is and the risk factors that are associated with incorrect test results. Laboratories must comply with the requirements in order to be certified by the United States Department

TABLE 26-2   APPROVED ACCREDITING ORGANIZATIONS UNDER CLIA '88

American Association of Blood Banks
8101 Glenbrook Road
Bethesda, MD 20814-2749
Government Relations
(301) 907-6977

American Osteopathic Association
142 East Ontario Street
Chicago, IL 60611
(312) 202-8070

American Society of Histocompatibility and Immunogenetics
P.O. Box 15804
Lenexa, KS 66285-5804
(913) 541-0009

College of American Pathologists
325 Waukegan Road
Northfield, IL 60093-2750
Laboratory Accreditation Program
(800) 323-4040

Commission on Office Laboratory Accreditation
9881 Broken Land Parkway, Suite 200
Columbia, MD 21046-1158
(410) 381-6581

Joint Commission on Accreditation of Healthcare Organizations
One Renaissance Boulevard
Oakbrook Terrace, IL 60181
(630) 792-5783

of Health and Human Services (HHS). The following laboratories are exempt from the regulations: labs that perform only tests for **forensic**, or legal, purposes; research laboratories that do not produce results used in patient treatment; facilities certified by the National Institute on Drug Abuse to perform only urine drug testing; and states, territories, and municipalities with licensure. (Currently, California, Florida, Georgia, Hawaii, Nevada, North Dakota, Rhode Island, Tennessee, Virginia, the Commonwealth of Puerto Rico, and the municipality of New York City are licensed.)

It is necessary to understand what the CLIA '88 regulations encompass and how they impact medical assistants and other health care workers who participate in testing human specimens. It is important because all laboratories, including laboratories in ambulatory care physicians' office laboratories (POL), must abide by the CLIA law.

CLIA '88 regulations are based on the complexity of tests performed and they affect all aspects of the laboratory. They specify the type of test performed, personnel involved in testing, and **quality control.**

General Program Description

Congress passed CLIA in 1988, establishing quality standards for all laboratory testing to ensure the accuracy, reliability, and timeliness of patient test results regardless of where the test was performed. A laboratory is defined as any facility that performs laboratory testing on specimens derived from humans for the purpose of providing information for the diagnosis, prevention, or treatment of disease, or impairment or assessment of health. CLIA is user-fee funded; therefore, all costs of administering the program must be covered by the regulated facilities.

The final CLIA regulations were published on February 28, 1992 and are based on the complexity of the test method; thus, the more complicated the test, the more stringent the requirements. Three categories of tests have been established: waived complexity; moderate complexity, including the subcategory of provider-performed **microscopy** (PPM); and high complexity. CLIA specifies quality standards for proficiency testing (PT), patient test management, quality control, personnel qualifications, and quality assurance as applicable. Because problems in cytology laboratories were the impetus for CLIA, there are also specific cytology requirements.

The Health Care Financing Administration (HCFA) is charged with the implementation of CLIA, including laboratory registration, fee collection, surveys, surveyor guidelines and training, enforcement, approvals of PT providers, accrediting organizations, and exempt states. The Centers for Disease Control and Prevention (CDC) is responsible for test categorization and CLIA studies.

To enroll in the CLIA program, laboratories must first register by completing an application, pay fees, be surveyed if applicable, and become certified. CLIA fees are based on the certificate requested by the laboratory (i.e., waived, PPM, accreditation, or compliance) and the annual volume and types of testing performed. Waived and PPM laboratories may apply directly for their certificate because they are not subject to routine inspections. Those laboratories that must be surveyed routinely, i.e., those performing moderate and/or high complexity testing, can choose whether they wish to be surveyed by HCFA or by a private accrediting organization. The HCFA survey process is outcome-oriented and utilizes a quality assurance focus and an educational approach to assess compliance.

Data indicates that CLIA has helped to improve the quality of testing in the United States. The total number of quality deficiencies has decreased approximately 40 percent from the first laboratory survey to the second. Similar findings were demonstrated in the review of PT data. The educational value of PT in laboratories was known before CLIA existed. Initial PT failures are also addressed with an educational, rather than punitive, approach by CLIA.

Work is currently in progress with the CDC and HCFA to develop a final CLIA rule that will reflect all comments received and new technologies.

Categories of Testing

CLIA '88 is under the aegis of the Health Care Financing Administration (HCFA) of the HHS. HCFA has designated three categories of testing:

1. Waived tests
2. Moderate-complexity tests, including PPM
3. High-complexity tests

Each of these categories has different requirements for personnel and quality control.

Waived tests are simple, unvarying, and require a minimum of judgment and interpretation. Test error carries minimal hazard to the patient. Waived tests represent the lowest percentage of the total number of tests performed (Table 26-3).

Provider-performed microscopy tests are moderate-complexity tests but represent a subcategory which was added at the request of physicians.

To categorize moderate- and high-complexity tests, the following criteria are used:

- The degree of operator intervention needed

- The necessary knowledge and experience the operator possesses

- The degree of maintenance and troubleshooting needed to perform the tests

TABLE 26-3	LIST OF ANALYTES CURRENTLY ON THE CLIA '88 WAIVED LIST		
Amines	Gastric occult blood	Nicotine and/or metabolites	Urine qualitative dipstick glucose
Amphetamines	Glucose or glucose monitoring device	Opiates	Urine qualitative dipstick ketone
Bladder tumor-associated antigen	Glycosylated hemoglobin (HbA1C)	Ovulation test by visual color comparison	Urine qualitative dipstick leukocytes
Cannabinoids (THC)	hCG, urine	Phencyclidine (PCP)	
Catalase, urine	Helicobacter pylori antibodies	Prothrombin time	Urine qualitative dipstick nitrite
Cholesterol, HDL	Helicobacter pylori (bacteri-ology)	Spun microhematocrit	Urine qualitative dipstick pH
Cholesterol, total		Streptococcus group A	Urine qualitative dipstick protein
Cocaine metabolites	Hematocrit	Triglyceride	Urine qualitative dipstick specific gravity
Creatinine	Hemoglobin	Urine dipstick or tablet ana-lytes, nonautomated	
Erythrocyte sedimentation rate	Infectious mononucleosis antibodies	Urine qualitative dipstick bilirubin	Urine qualitative dipstick urobilinogen
Ethanol	Ketones, blood	Urine qualitative dipstick blood	Vaginal pH
Fecal occult blood	Methamphetamines		
Fructosamine	Microalbumin		

Source: Clara Sliva, Acting CLIA Coordinator

Note: Tests waived by FDA from January 31–July 26, 2000; CDC through March, 2000. There are over 500 Test Systems (products) approved for the analytes listed above. For an up-to-date list, visit the CDC website at www.phppo.cdc.gov.

Approximately 75 percent of all tests are of moderate complexity and 24 percent are of high complexity. Physicians' office laboratories are not restricted to tests in the waived category.

Thus far, over 5,000 tests have been categorized by CLIA '88 and, except those listed in Table 26-3, fall into either the moderate- or high-complexity category. It is important to realize that tests can be moved between or among categories and that revisions have been made since CLIA '88 went into effect in 1992. The best way to remain informed is by calling the manufacturer and asking whether your particular instrument or **kit** is in the moderate-complexity category. You can also obtain a list of categories as well as the complete CLIA '88 guidelines from the **Federal Register**. (Information on toll-free phone numbers, addresses, and order numbers are provided in the appendices.)

Contents of the Law

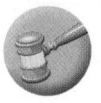

1. All laboratories are required to register with CLIA '88 even if just one test is performed and regardless of whether there is Medicare and Medicaid **reimbursement** and regardless in which of the categories the test is found.
2. The regulations apply to all laboratories. Previously unregulated laboratories could enroll until January 1, 1994.
3. The regulations are specific to the complexity of the test. Standards become more stringent as the complexity of the test increases.

4. A laboratory must obtain a certificate to perform tests. An initial filing for a certificate is made on form 116 with HCFA of the Department of Health and Human Services. One of five certificates can be obtained. (There can be a state exemption as previously mentioned.)
   a. *Certificate of Waiver.* This certificate is issued to a laboratory to perform only waived tests.
   b. *Certificate for Provider-Performed Microscopy (PPM) Procedures.* This certificate is issued to a laboratory in which a physician, midlevel practitioner, or dentist performs no tests other than the PPM procedures (Table 26-4). This certificate permits the laboratory to also perform waived tests.

TABLE 26-4	PROVIDER-PERFORMED MICROSCOPY (PPM) PROCEDURES

- All direct wet-mount preparations for the presence or absence of bacteria, fungi, parasites, and human cellular elements
- All potassium hydroxide (KOH) preparations
- Pinworm examinations
- Fern tests
- Postcoital direct, qualitative examinations of vaginal or cervical mucus
- Urine sediment examinations
- Nasal smears for granulocytes
- Fecal leukocyte examinations
- Qualitative semen analysis (limited to the presence or absence of sperm and detection of motility)

c. *Certificate of Registration.* This certificate enables the entity to conduct moderate and/or high complexity laboratory testing until the entity is determined by survey to be in compliance with the CLIA regulations.

d. *Certificate of Compliance.* This certificate is issued to a laboratory after an inspection finds the laboratory to be in compliance with all applicable CLIA requirements.

e. *Certificate of Accreditation.* This is a certificate that is issued to a laboratory on the basis of the laboratory's accreditation by an organization approved by HCFA.

As of July, 2000, over 145,000 CLIA certificates have been issued. Of certificates granted, 53 percent have been Certificates of Waiver, 22 percent have been Certificates for Provider-Performed Microscopy (PPM) Procedures, 15 percent have been Certificates of Registration or Compliance, and 10 percent have been Certificates of Accreditation.

All five certification categories must be renewed every two years and be accompanied by a fee ranging from $100 to $600.

HCFA Form 116

HCFA form 116 (Figures 26-1 and 26-2) for the clinical laboratory application for CLIA, HCFA-116 must be completed and returned to the Health Care Financing Administration of the United States Department of Health and Human Services within thirty days of receipt. The form collects information regarding a laboratory's operation and is needed to evaluate fees, to determine baseline data, to update existing data, and to fulfill legal requirements. The information obtained from the application will give the surveyor of the laboratory a perspective of the laboratory's operation and if it will be subject to an on-site inspection.

After a laboratory has been certified, it must notify HCFA within six months if it changes the types of tests it performs. This could alter the laboratory's classification.

5. Some examples of sanctions or penalties imposed by HCFA for noncompliance with the CLIA law follow:

DEPARTMENT OF HEALTH AND HUMAN SERVICES
HEALTH CARE FINANCING ADMINISTRATION

FORM APPROVED
OMB NO. 0938-0581

CLINICAL LABORATORY IMPROVEMENT AMENDMENTS OF 1988 (CLIA)
APPLICATION FOR CERTIFICATION

According to the Paperwork Reduction Act of 1995, no persons are required to respond to a collection of information unless it displays a valid OMB control number. The valid OMB control number for this information collection is 0938-0581. The time required to complete this information collection is estimated to average 30 minutes to 2 hours per response, including the time to review instructions, search existing data resources, gather the data needed, and complete and review the information collection. If you have any comments concerning the accuracy of the time estimate(s) or suggestions for improving this form, please write to: HCFA ,7500 Security Boulevard, N2-14-26, Baltimore, Maryland 21244-1850 and to the Office of the Information and Regulatory Affairs, Office of Management and Budget, Washington, D.C. 20503.

I. GENERAL INFORMATION

☐ Initial Application ☐ Change in Certification Type	CLIA IDENTIFICATION NUMBER _____D__________ *(If an initial application leave blank, a number will be assigned)*
Facility Name	Federal Tax Identification Number Telephone No. *(include area code)* Fax No.*(include area code)* ( ) ( )
Facility Address-*Physical Location of Laboratory (Building, Floor, Suite if applicable.)*	Mailing/Billing address *(If different from street address, include attention line and/or Building, Floor, Suite)*
Number, Street *(No. P.O. Boxes)*	Number, Street
City State Zip Code	City State Zip Code
Name of Director *last first middle initial*	

II. TYPE OF CERTIFICATE REQUESTED (Check One)

☐ Certificate of Waiver (*Complete Sections I - VI and VIII - X*)

☐ Certificate for Provider Performed Microscopy Procedures (PPMP) (*Complete Sections I - X*)

☐ Certificate of Compliance (*Complete Sections I- X*)

☐ Certificate of Accreditation (*Complete Sections I through X*) **and** indicate which of the following organization(s) your laboratory is accredited by for CLIA purposes, or for which you have applied for accreditation for CLIA purposes

☐ JCAHO ☐ AOA ☐ AABB
☐ CAP ☐ COLA ☐ ASHI

FORM HCFA-116 (11/98) Page 1 of 4

III. TYPE OF LABORATORY ***(check the one most descriptive of facility type)***

__ 01 Ambulatory Surgery Center	__ 09 Hospice	__ 17 School/Student Health Service
__ 02 Community Clinic	__ 10 Hospital	__ 18 Skilled Nursing Facility/Nursing Facility
__ 03 Comp. Outpatient Rehab. Facility	__ 11 Independent	__ 19 Physician Office
__ 04 Ancillary Testing Site in Health Care Facility	__ 12 Industrial	__ 20 Other Practitioner *(specify)*______
	__ 13 Insurance	__ 21 Tissue Bank/Repositories
__ 05 End Stage Renal Disease Dialysis Facility	__ 14 Intermediate Care Fac. for Mentally Retarded	__ 22 Blood Banks
__ 06 Health Fair		__ 23 Rural Health Clinic/Federally Qualified Health Center
__ 07 Health Main. Organization	__ 15 Mobile Laboratory	
__ 08 Home Health Agency	__ 16 Pharmacy	__ 24 Ambulance
Is this a Medicare/Medicaid certified facility? ☐ Yes ☐ No		__ 25 Other *(specify)*______

If yes, indicate Medicare provider number________ Medicaid number________

IV. HOURS OF LABORATORY TESTING (list times during which **laboratory testing** is performed)

	SUNDAY	MONDAY	TUESDAY	WEDNESDAY	THURSDAY	FRIDAY	SATURDAY
FROM: AM							
PM							
TO: AM							
PM							

(For multiple sites attach the additional information using the same format)

V. MULTIPLE SITES (Must meet one of the regulatory exceptions to apply for this provision)

Are you applying for the multiple site exception?

☐ No **If no,** go to section VI. ☐ Yes **If yes,** provide total number of sites under this certificate______ and complete remainder of this section .

Indicate which of the following regulatory exceptions applies to your facility's operation.

Is this a not-for-profit or Federal, State or local government laboratory engaged in limited (not more than a combination of 15 moderate complexity or waived tests per certificate) public health testing and filing for a single certificate for multiple sites? ☐ Yes ☐ No
If yes, list name, address and tests performed for each site below.

Is this a hospital with several laboratories located at contiguous buildings on the same campus within the same physical location or street address and under common direction that is filing for a single certificate for these locations? ☐ Yes ☐ No
If yes, list name or department, location within hospital and specialty/subspecialty areas performed at each site below.

If additional space is needed, check here ____ and attach the additional information using the same format.

NAME AND ADDRESS / LOCATION		TESTS PERFORMED / SPECIALTY / SUBSPECIALTY
Name of laboratory or hospital department		
Address/location (number, street, location if applicable)		
City, State, ZIP	Telephone No. ( )	
Name of laboratory or hospital department		
Address/location (number, street, location if applicable)		
City, State, ZIP	Telephone No. ( )	
Name of laboratory or hospital department		
Address/location (number, street, location if applicable)		
City, State, ZIP	Telephone No. ( )	

FORM HCFA-116 (11/98) Page 2 of 4

Figure 26-1 Form HCFA-116.

Infraction	*Penalty*
Failure to enroll with HCFA	Denial or revocation of certificate
Nonparticipation in proficiency testing	A score of zero (a score of 80 percent is required)
Failure to return the proficiency testing result	A score of zero

In addition, Medicare and Medicaid payments may be suspended or terminated and civil penalties of up to a $10,000 fine per violation or per day of noncompliance may be imposed.

For CLIA '88 conditions other than proficiency testing, newly regulated laboratories will not be subjected to penalties during the first inspection cycle unless it is determined that the laboratories' inadequacies pose immediate patient danger.

6. The law **mandates quality assurance** for nonwaived tests. Laboratories are required to establish policies and procedures through programs that assess test quality; identify problems and correct them; assure precise, dependable, and punctual reporting of test results; and guarantee sufficient competent staff. In addition, laboratories must assure that all quality control data are studied, and if there is a complaint, an investigation must be undertaken and appropriate action taken and recorded. It is a requirement that quality assurance records be maintained.
7. The law mandates quality control for nonwaived tests. Laboratories are required to have an adequate supply of equipment to perform the number and types of tests that they offer. A procedures manual must be available in the testing area and must include complete testing instructions. Documentation of maintenance programs for instruments, equipment, and test systems must be evident.
8. The law establishes requirements for the correct collection, transportation, and storage of specimens and the reporting of results. (See No. 14, Patient Test Management.)
9. The law mandates maintenance of records, equipment, and facilities of labs performing nonwaived tests. (See No. 15, Documentation.)
10. The law mandates personnel standards. There are requirements for personnel who perform nonwaived tests and they spell out the necessary qualifications and responsibilities required of them. Each person

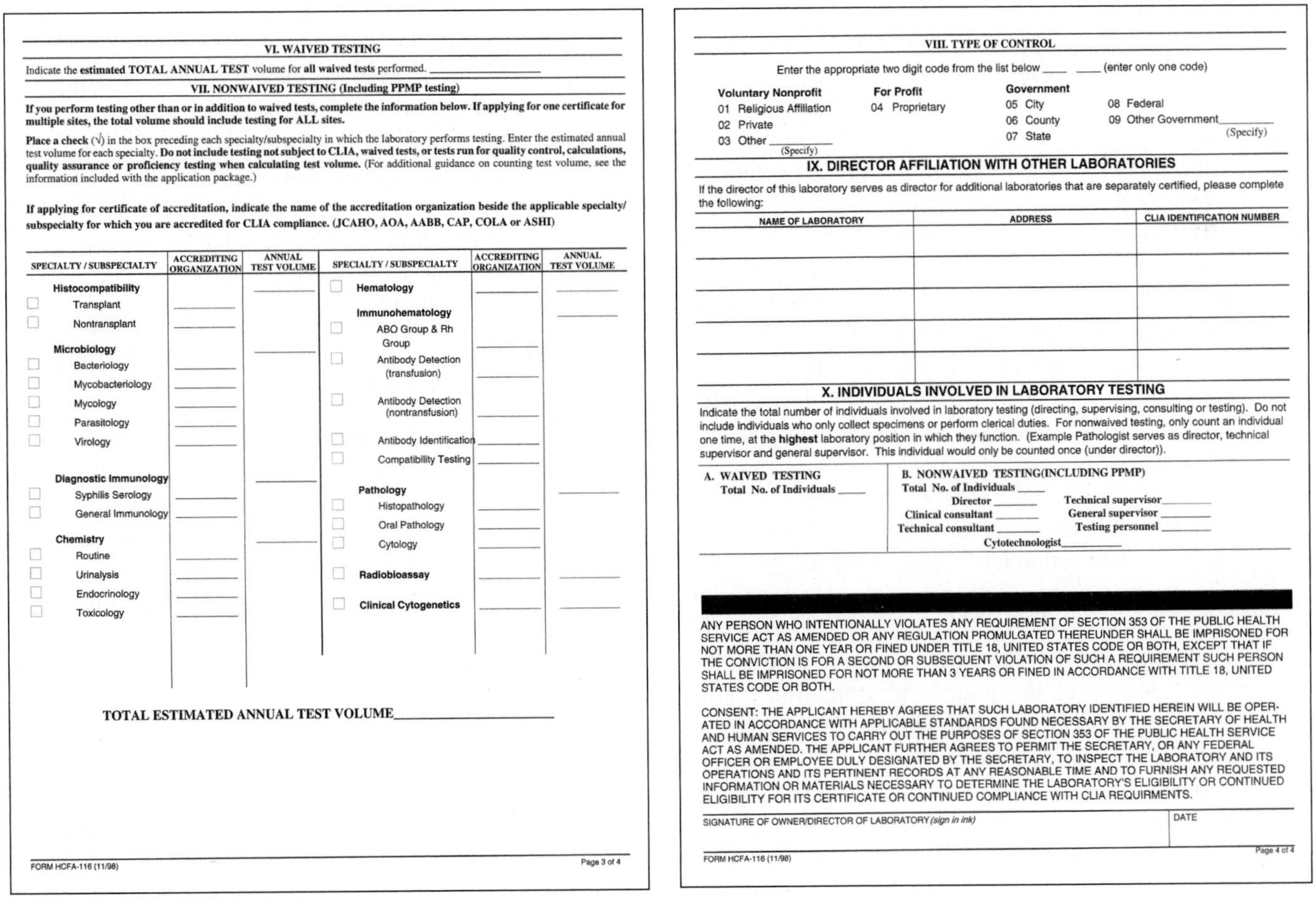

VI. WAIVED TESTING

Indicate the **estimated TOTAL ANNUAL TEST** volume for **all waived tests** performed. ____________

VII. NONWAIVED TESTING (Including PPMP testing)

If you perform testing other than or in addition to waived tests, complete the information below. If applying for one certificate for multiple sites, the total volume should include testing for ALL sites.

Place a check (√) in the box preceding each specialty/subspecialty in which the laboratory performs testing. Enter the estimated annual test volume for each specialty. **Do not include testing not subject to CLIA, waived tests, or tests run for quality control, calculations, quality assurance or proficiency testing when calculating test volume.** (For additional guidance on counting test volume, see the information included with the application package.)

If applying for certificate of accreditation, indicate the name of the accreditation organization beside the applicable specialty/subspecialty for which you are accredited for CLIA compliance. (JCAHO, AOA, AABB, CAP, COLA or ASHI)

SPECIALTY / SUBSPECIALTY	ACCREDITING ORGANIZATION	ANNUAL TEST VOLUME	SPECIALTY / SUBSPECIALTY	ACCREDITING ORGANIZATION	ANNUAL TEST VOLUME
Histocompatibility		______	☐ **Hematology**	______	______
☐ Transplant	______		**Immunohematology**		______
☐ Nontransplant	______		☐ ABO Group & Rh Group	______	
Microbiology		______	☐ Antibody Detection (transfusion)	______	
☐ Bacteriology	______		☐ Antibody Detection (nontransfusion)	______	
☐ Mycobacteriology	______		☐ Antibody Identification	______	
☐ Mycology	______		☐ Compatibility Testing	______	
☐ Parasitology	______		**Pathology**		______
☐ Virology	______		☐ Histopathology	______	
Diagnostic Immunology		______	☐ Oral Pathology	______	
☐ Syphilis Serology	______		☐ Cytology	______	
☐ General Immunology	______		☐ **Radiobioassay**	______	______
Chemistry		______	☐ **Clinical Cytogenetics**	______	______
☐ Routine	______				
☐ Urinalysis	______				
☐ Endocrinology	______				
☐ Toxicology	______				

TOTAL ESTIMATED ANNUAL TEST VOLUME____________

FORM HCFA-116 (11/98) Page 3 of 4

VIII. TYPE OF CONTROL

Enter the appropriate two digit code from the list below ____ ____ (enter only one code)

Voluntary Nonprofit	For Profit	Government	
01 Religious Affiliation	04 Proprietary	05 City	08 Federal
02 Private		06 County	09 Other Government ______ (Specify)
03 Other ______ (Specify)		07 State	

IX. DIRECTOR AFFILIATION WITH OTHER LABORATORIES

If the director of this laboratory serves as director for additional laboratories that are separately certified, please complete the following:

NAME OF LABORATORY	ADDRESS	CLIA IDENTIFICATION NUMBER

X. INDIVIDUALS INVOLVED IN LABORATORY TESTING

Indicate the total number of individuals involved in laboratory testing (directing, supervising, consulting or testing). Do not include individuals who only collect specimens or perform clerical duties. For nonwaived testing, only count an individual one time, at the **highest** laboratory position in which they function. (Example Pathologist serves as director, technical supervisor and general supervisor. This individual would only be counted once (under director)).

A. WAIVED TESTING
Total No. of Individuals ____

B. NONWAIVED TESTING(INCLUDING PPMP)
Total No. of Individuals ____
Director ______ Technical supervisor ______
Clinical consultant ______ General supervisor ______
Technical consultant ______ Testing personnel ______
Cytotechnologist ______

ANY PERSON WHO INTENTIONALLY VIOLATES ANY REQUIREMENT OF SECTION 353 OF THE PUBLIC HEALTH SERVICE ACT AS AMENDED OR ANY REGULATION PROMULGATED THEREUNDER SHALL BE IMPRISONED FOR NOT MORE THAN ONE YEAR OR FINED UNDER TITLE 18, UNITED STATES CODE OR BOTH, EXCEPT THAT IF THE CONVICTION IS FOR A SECOND OR SUBSEQUENT VIOLATION OF SUCH A REQUIREMENT SUCH PERSON SHALL BE IMPRISONED FOR NOT MORE THAN 3 YEARS OR FINED IN ACCORDANCE WITH TITLE 18, UNITED STATES CODE OR BOTH.

CONSENT: THE APPLICANT HEREBY AGREES THAT SUCH LABORATORY IDENTIFIED HEREIN WILL BE OPERATED IN ACCORDANCE WITH APPLICABLE STANDARDS FOUND NECESSARY BY THE SECRETARY OF HEALTH AND HUMAN SERVICES TO CARRY OUT THE PURPOSES OF SECTION 353 OF THE PUBLIC HEALTH SERVICE ACT AS AMENDED. THE APPLICANT FURTHER AGREES TO PERMIT THE SECRETARY, OR ANY FEDERAL OFFICER OR EMPLOYEE DULY DESIGNATED BY THE SECRETARY, TO INSPECT THE LABORATORY AND ITS OPERATIONS AND ITS PERTINENT RECORDS AT ANY REASONABLE TIME AND TO FURNISH ANY REQUESTED INFORMATION OR MATERIALS NECESSARY TO DETERMINE THE LABORATORY'S ELIGIBILITY OR CONTINUED ELIGIBILITY FOR ITS CERTIFICATE OR CONTINUED COMPLIANCE WITH CLIA REQUIRMENTS.

SIGNATURE OF OWNER/DIRECTOR OF LABORATORY *(sign in ink)* | DATE

FORM HCFA-116 (11/98) Page 4 of 4

Figure 26-2 Form HCFA-116.

who does the tests must be licensed by the state if required, have a high school diploma or equivalent, have adequate training, and be able to demonstrate an understanding of laboratory procedures, **calibration**, or standardization of instruments, specimen collection, and quality control. Personnel must report test results accurately and with dependability. All high-complexity tests must be done by technologists and technicians except for cytology, which requires more stringent qualifications.

11. The law mandates **proficiency testing** for non-waived tests. The procedures and tests found in the waived category are exempt from proficiency testing, regardless of the type of laboratory in which the tests are performed. Moderate- and high-complexity test laboratories must enroll in proficiency testing programs that are approved by the United States Department of Health and Human Services. The proficiency testing samples are checked in the same manner as patient specimens. Unsatisfactory performance on a proficiency testing check can result in various penalties ranging from termination of the laboratory's license to operate to the termination of reimbursement from Medicare and Medicaid. January, 1994 was the phase-in date for previously unregulated laboratories to enroll in proficiency testing, but proficiency testing will continue to be required for laboratories that were regulated by March 4, 1990.

12. The law mandates unannounced on-site inspection. All laboratories in the moderate- and high-complexity category are subject to unannounced inspections by HHS or an agency assigned to the task by HHS. Laboratories that perform only waived tests must prove that tests are being done according to the manufacturer's directions. Inspections can involve interviewing employees, observation of employees performing tests, analysis of data, and documentation of results. Violations of requirements by any laboratory can result in penalties. The cost of inspection will be billed to the laboratory.

13. The law mandates an annual listing of laboratories that have had action taken against them.

14. The law mandates patient test management. All laboratories must have a strategy for properly receiving and processing specimens and for the precise reporting of the results. Written instructions regarding collection, safeguarding of specimens, and labeling of specimens must be available for patients. There must be a specific procedure for the reporting of life-threatening results and a follow-through to the person requesting the test. Test records must be kept for two years following the reporting of results.

15. The law mandates documentation. The following documentation must be done and be available:
    - Specimen
      Patient preparation
      Specimen collection procedure
      Proper labeling technique
      Preservation of specimen if applicable
    - Proficiency testing
      Corrective action taken
    - Quality control and quality assurance
      Any corrective action taken
    - Problem and complaint log
    - **Requisitions** or written requests
      Patient name
      Name and address of laboratory
      Date and time of collection
      Name of test requested
      Diagnosis
    - Results
      Name and address of laboratory where test is done
      Test name
      Test results, including normal ranges listed on test results
      Disposition of unacceptable specimens must be released to authorized person
    - Log of Results
      Printouts from instruments report must be kept
      Identification of person performing test
      Patient identification number
      Specimen identification
      Date
      Time specimen is received in laboratory
      Specimen rejection log maintained
      Records and dates of all tests done

Criteria. To be categorized as a PPM procedure, the procedure must meet the following criteria:

1. The examination must be personally performed by one of the following practitioners:
   a. A physician during the patient's visit on a specimen obtained from his or her own patient or from a patient of a group medical practice of which the physician is a member or an employee
   b. A midlevel practitioner, under the supervision of a physician or in independent practice only if authorized by the state, during the patient's visit on a specimen obtained from his or her own patient or from a patient of a clinic, group medical practice, or other health care provider of which the midlevel practitioner is a member or an employee
   c. A dentist during the patient's visit on a specimen obtained from his or her own patient or from a

patient of a group dental practice of which the dentist is a member or an employee

2. The procedure must be categorized as moderately complex.
3. The primary instrument for performing the test is the microscope, limited to bright-field or phase-contrast microscopy.
4. The specimen is labile, or a delay in performing the test could compromise the accuracy of the test result.
5. Control materials are not available to monitor the entire testing process.
6. Limited specimen handling or processing is required.

CLIA '88 Regulation for Quality Control in Automated Hematology

CLIA '88 regulations require that three different procedures be performed in the quality control protocol for automated hematology instruments. The procedures include calibration, control samples, and proficiency testing. CLIA's regulations require that the automated hematology instrument be calibrated at regularly scheduled intervals with either a calibrator sample or a normal control sample. Many manufacturers of automated hematology instruments recommend or may require that the instrument be recalibrated at shorter intervals than are required by CLIA '88. CLIA '88 mandates that two levels of control samples be tested first each day on any parameter that will be performed on a patient's sample. These quality control checks must be performed before the patient's sample is tested. The results for quality control samples must fall within two standard deviations of the expected mean value for that sample. Standard deviations and Levy-Jennings charts were discussed in the quality control chapter. One of the two levels of control samples must be in the normal range; the other may be either an abnormal high or low sample.

In addition to calibrations and control sample testing, an ambulatory care setting that utilizes automated hematology instruments must enroll in a proficiency testing program with a reference laboratory that is CLIA '88 approved.

Aftermath of CLIA '88

There are many individuals who have serious concerns about whether CLIA has led to improved testing as was intended, or if the law has just produced an overload of paperwork and problems. Some question if the law will be fully implemented or even eliminated altogether.

 Important developments help to put the law into perspective. HCFA has postponed the date that Medicare payments would be cut off for fail-ure to register. The deadline has been postponed at least three times. The American Medical Association (AMA) complained that unannounced inspections of physicians' office laboratories (POL) would disrupt patient office visits. As a result, the Secretary of Health and Human Services declared that POL inspections would be announced.

The category of Provider-Performed Microscopy (PPM) was added as another certificate and testing category because physicians argued that the microscopic tests were essential to their practice. Already the PPM has expanded to include midlevel practitioners such as nurse practitioners, nurse midwives, and physician assistants.

The law states that CLIA must be self-supporting. There are far fewer laboratories registered than was originally anticipated, and the result is a significantly lower amount of revenue than had been expected.

It is interesting to note that the CDC has proposed easing CLIA regulations by adding another category of testing. It would fall between the waived tests and the moderately complex tests. The tests within this new category would be subject to minimal regulation. This proposal is under consideration. Many question whether CLIA will have any value if this event occurs.

Impact of CLIA on Medical Assistants

CLIA '88 requires every facility that tests human specimens for diagnosis, treatment, and prevention of disease to meet specific federal requirements. The law applies to any facility that performs tests for the preceding purposes. This includes any physicians' office laboratories and ambulatory care setting, two typical areas where medical assistants have found employment. The law covers all facilities even if only one test or a few basic tests are done and even if there is no charge for the testing.

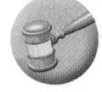 Medical assistants may be responsible not only for performing the tests, but also for maintaining personnel records including such information as workers' college diplomas, state licenses, national certifications, employees' continuing education, and re-credentialing. Employee hepatitis B status must also be on file. Medical assistants may be involved with compiling a procedures manual on how to perform every test done; these must be reviewed every year. An instrument log must be available on each piece of equipment. Systems must be in place for calibration, quality control, quality assurance test recording, and proficiency testing (if higher than waived category tests are performed). Documentation by medical assistants is of utmost importance; for instance, there may be a quality control plan in action, but it may not be written down in detail.

Due to the fact that HCFA has received only a fraction of the money that they expected to collect from application fees, there is very little money to carry the

CLIA '88 program forward. Medical assistants must realize that CLIA '88 is the law even though a number of laboratories have not seen inspectors nor felt any impact from the CLIA '88 regulations. Some laboratories are delaying concern about CLIA '88 rules and do not understand the law and, therefore, have not fully implemented the regulations. Medical assistants must know and comply with the law and be prepared for a CLIA inspection. Penalties are imposed on laboratories that are not in compliance with the law.

Medical assistants who perform clinical laboratory procedures need to be aware that they must keep up with government changes.

Where to Find More Information Regarding CLIA '88

The original CLIA '88 guidelines and updates are available from the Federal Register for a fee. See the appendices for ordering information or visit HCFA at www.HCFA.gov and click on the *Laboratory Testing* (CLIA) icon.

OCCUPATIONAL SAFETY AND HEALTH ADMINISTRATION (OSHA) REGULATIONS

The Occupational Safety and Health Administration (OSHA) regulations are intended to ascertain that employers have a safe and healthful work environment for their employees. They represent requirements that employers must follow to ensure employee safety and health.

There are two standards that comprise the regulations that have the primary impact on a clinical laboratory, *The Occupational Exposure to Hazardous Chemicals in the Laboratory*, an amended version of the original standard *The Hazard Communication Standard*, and *The Bloodborne Pathogen Standard*. Each **standard** will be described independently. See Chapter 10 for *The Bloodborne Pathogen Standard*.

The Standard for Occupational Exposure to Hazardous Chemicals in the Laboratory

In an effort to reduce the number of chemically related illnesses and injuries in the workplace, OSHA published its *Hazard Communications Standard* in 1983. This led many states to develop *right-to-know* laws. In 1992, OSHA expanded the *Hazard Communications Standard*, and published *The Occupational Exposure to Hazardous Chemicals in the Laboratory Standard* which specifically addressed clinical laboratories.

The intention of this law is to heighten employee awareness of risks linked with chemical dangers. It serves

SPOTLIGHT ON AAMA ESSENTIALS THROUGH CAAHEP

● When performing tests and procedures in the medical laboratory, it's important to remember to always maintain a safe environment, since unsafe working surroundings can often threaten the emotional and physical health of patients and health care workers.

● To avoid fear and the possibility of hurting oneself, if the medical assistant is required to work with hazardous chemicals, it's important that he or she learn about and understand the OSHA standards and comply with them.

● If caring for a patient diagnosed with an infectious disease such as AIDS or hepatitis B, instead of being fearful of working with these patients, the medical assistant should make every attempt to become educated on the regulations and guidelines set forth by the federal government, and then follow through by helping others implement them.

to improve work practices through employee training and identification of hazardous chemicals that exist in the workplace. The use of protective equipment is utilized to protect employees from harmful chemicals.

Chemical Hygiene Plan

The Chemical Hygiene Plan (CHP) on hazardous chemicals is the core of the OSHA safety standard on hazardous chemicals. A written plan must specify the training and information requirements of the standard. Certain specific control measures such as **fume hoods** and glove boxes must be included in the plan. A designated employee is the chemical hygiene or safety officer. Provisions for housekeeping and maintenance of the facility are included. OSHA standards are not optional and penalties are imposed for noncompliance with the standard. Employers must take the time to meet the requirements not only in order to be in compliance with the law, but to protect employees as well.

All laboratories and ambulatory care settings, including physicians' offices must comply with a chemical hygiene plan in order to meet the OSHA regulations. The only laboratories exempt from compliance are those that exclusively use methods that do not place employees at risk for exposure to chemicals that are hazardous. For example, there may be physicians' office laboratories (POLs) that perform only dipstick tests or use other commercially prepared kits in which reagents are not exposed and as a result they are exempt from compliance. The primary component of the OSHA standard is that a written chemical hygiene plan and program must be operational if chemicals are stored in a facility and handled by employees. Some examples of chemicals include, but are not limited to: stains, **ethyl alcohol**, sodium hypochlorite (household bleach), **formaldehyde**, fixatives, preservatives, injectables such as **chemotherapeutic agents**, **acetone**, and so on. Many laboratory accidents result in chemical-related illnesses ranging from eye irritations to **pulmonary edema**.

There are three primary goals that an employer must accomplish to be in compliance with the OSHA standard for chemical exposure. The first is that there must be an inventory undertaken and a list compiled of all chemicals considered hazardous. The following information must be documented (Figure 26-3): the quantity of chemical stored per month or year; whether the substance is gas, liquid, or solid; the manufacturer's name and address; and the chemical hazard classification.

Second, a material safety data sheet (MSDS) (Figure 26-4) manual must be assembled. MSDS manuals are often supplied by the manufacturer when the chemicals are ordered and will give information regarding whether or not a chemical is hazardous. All other MSDS information must be requested from the manufacturer. The MSDS sheets must be alphabetized and indexed and be reviewed on a regular basis and modifications made. The manual must be available to all employees. The various chemicals are labeled using the National Fire Protection Association's color and number method (Figure 26-5).

SAMPLE
CHEMICAL INVENTORY FORM

Office of _____

Date _____

Chemical Name	Catalog #	Quantity Stores L./gm. (monthly)	Physical State	Hazard Class				Manufacturer	Comments
				H	F	R	P		

(H) Health	(F) Fire Hazard	(R) Reactivity	(P) Protection
0 - Minimal	0 - Will not burn	0 - Stable is not reactive with water	A. - Goggles
1 - Slightly	1 - Slight		B. - Goggles/Gloves
2 - Moderate	2 - Moderate	1 - Slight	C. - Goggles/Gloves/Apron
3 - Serious	3 - Serious	2 - Moderate	D. - Face Shield/Gloves/Apron
4 - Extreme	4 - Extreme	3 - Serious	E. - Goggles/Gloves/Mask
		4 - Extreme	F. - Goggles/Gloves/Apron/Mask
			X. - Gloves

Figure 26-3 Sample chemical inventory form for listing chemicals on the premises, including quantity, physical state, hazard class, manufacturer, and comments. (Courtesy of POL Consultants)

MATERIAL SAFETY DATA SHEET

I – PRODUCT IDENTIFICATION

COMPANY NAME: We Wash Inc.

ADDRESS: 5035 Manchester Avenue
            Freedom, Texas 79430

Tel No: (314) 621-1818
Nights: (314) 621-1399
CHEMTREC: (800) 424-9343

PRODUCT NAME: Spotfree

Product No.: 2190

Synonyms: Warewashing Detergent

II – HAZARDOUS INGREDIENTS OF MIXTURES

MATERIAL:	(CAS#)	% By Wt.	TLV	PEL
According to the OSHA Hazard Communication Standard, 29CFR 1910.1200, this product contains no hazardous ingredients.		N/A	N/A	NA

III – PHYSICAL DATA

Vapor Pressure, mm Hg: N/A
Evaporation Rate (ether=1): N/A
Solubility in H_2O: Complete
Freezing Point F: N/A
Boiling Point F: N/A
Specific Gravity H_2O=1 @25C: N/A

Vapor Density (Air=1) 60–90F: N/A
% Volatile by wt N/A
pH @ 1%   Solution 9.3–9.8
pH as Distributed: N/A
Appearance: Off-White granular powder
Odor: Mild Chemical Odor

IV – FIRE AND EXPLOSION

Flash Point F: N/AV

Flammable Limits: N/A

Extinguishing Media: The product is not flammable or combustible. Use media appropriate for the primary source of fire.

Special Fire Fighting Procedures: Use caution when fighting any fire involving chemicals. A self-contained breathing apparatus is essential.

Unusual Fire and Explosion Hazards: None Known

V – REACTIVITY DATA

Stability - Conditions to avoid: None Known

Incompatibility: Contact of carbonates or bicarbonates with acids can release large quantities of carbon dioxide and heat.

Hazardous Decomposition Products: In fire situations heat decomposition may result in the release of sulfur oxides.

Conditions Contributing to Hazardous Polymerization: N/A

(continues)

Figure 26-4 Example of a Material Safety Data Sheet (MSDS) listing product name, hazardous ingredients, physical data, fire, explosion, reactivity, health hazard data, emergency and first aid procedures, spill or leak procedures, protection/control measures, and special precautions. (Courtesy of POL Consultants)

Spotfree
VI – HEALTH HAZARD DATA

EFFECTS OF OVEREXPOSURE (Medical Conditions Aggravated/Target Organ Effects)
A. ACUTE (Primary Route of Exposure)   EYES: Product granules may cause mechanical irritation to eyes.
   SKIN (Primary Route of Exposure): Prolonged repeated contact with skin may result in drying of skin.
   INGESTION: Not expected to be toxic if swallowed, however, gastrointestinal discomfort may occur.
B. SUBCHRONIC, CHRONIC, OTHER: None known.

VII – EMERGENCY AND FIRST AID PROCEDURES

EYES: In case of contact, flush thoroughly with water for 15 minutes. Get medical attention if irritation persists.
SKIN: Flush any dry Spotfree from skin with flowing water. Always wash hands after use.
INGESTION: If swallowed, drink large quantities of water and call a physician.

VIII – SPILL OR LEAK PROCEDURES

Spill Management: Sweep up material and repackage if possible.
   Spill residue may be flushed to the sewer with water.

Waste Disposal Methods: Dispose of in accordance with federal, state and local regulations.

IX – PROTECTION INFORMATION/CONTROL MEASURES

Respiratory: None needed   Eye: Safety   Glove: Not
                                                                  glasses   required

Other Clothing and Equipment: None required

Ventilation: Normal

X – SPECIAL PRECAUTIONS

Precautions to be taken in Handling and Storing: Avoid contact with eyes. Avoid prolonged or repeated contact with skin.
   Wash thoroughly after handling. Keep container closed when not in use.
Additional Information: Store away from acids.

Prepared by: D. Martinez   Revision Date: 04/11/_ _

Seller makes no warranty, expressed or implied, concerning the use of this product other than indicated on the label. Buyer assumes all risk of use and/or handling of this material when such use and/or handling is contrary to label instructions.

While Seller believes that the information contained herein is accurate, such information is offered solely for its customers' consideration and verification under their specific use conditions. This information is not to be deemed a warranty or representation of any kind for which Seller assumes legal responsibility.

Figure 26-4   *(continued)*

CHEMICAL WARNING LABEL DETERMINATION

The Hazard Communication Act contains specific labeling requirements. Labels must be on all hazardous chemicals that are shipped to and used in the workplace. Labels must not be removed. Material safety data sheets for all chemicals will be available to employees.

Manufacturer Requirements: Chemical manufacturers are required to evaluate chemicals, determine status as hazards, provide material safety data sheets (MSDS), and label all shipped chemicals properly. Manufacturer labels must never be removed. The best way to determine the hazards of the chemical is to read the MSDS, obtain an OSHA designated list or State Hazardous Substance list. For most mixed chemicals, it is necessary to contact the manufacturer for MSDS.

Office Chemicals: Search through your office and write down all chemicals you have in the office. Most pharmaceuticals and common household products do not come under this standard. Ingredients can then be compared to a list of regulated substances or MSDS sheets will provide necessary information.

Employer's Responsibility: Any hazardous chemical used in the workplace that is not in its original container *must* be labeled with the identity of the chemical and hazards. "Target Organ" chemical labels may be used. The label must include the chemical and common name, warnings about physical and health hazards, and the name and address of the manufacturer. The employer is to compile a chemical inventory list that is to be updated as needed. MSDS information should be located in a place where it is accessible to all employees. Label and MSDS information should be provided during the safety training program.

Identity: The term *identity* can refer to any chemical or common name designation for the individual chemical or mixture, as long as the term used is also used on the list of hazardous chemicals and the MSDS.

NOTE: If a chemical is poured into another container for immediate use, it does not need to be labeled.

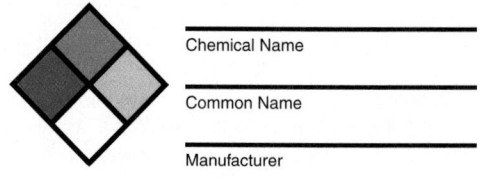

Chemical Name

Common Name

Manufacturer

Figure 26-5   Chemical warning label determination indicates necessary information for labels, including manufacturer's requirements, office chemicals, employer's responsibility, and identity of chemical or its common name. (Courtesy of POL Consultants)

There are four colors, each signifying a warning to the person handling the chemical(s). They are:

- Blue signifies a health hazard
- Red signifies a fire hazard
- Yellow signifies an instability hazard
- White signifies use of personal protective equipment (PPE)

The numbers 0–4 are used in conjunction with the colors to indicate the level of risk for each product and are assigned by the manufacturer using the rating system. The numbers can be found on the MSDS. See Figure 26-6.

Third, the employer is required to provide a hazard communication educational program to the employee

RED: FIRE HAZARD

4 = Danger: Flammable gas or extremely flammable liquid
3 = Warning: Flammable liquid
2 = Caution: Combustible liquid
1 = Caution: Combustible if heated
0 = Noncombustible

YELLOW: REACTIVITY

4 = Danger: Explosive at room temperature
3 = Danger: May be explosive if spark occurs or if heated under confinement
2 = Warning: Unstable or may react if mixed with water
1 = Caution: May react if heated or mixed with water
0 = Stable: Nonreactive when mixed with water

WHITE: PPE

A   Goggles
B   Goggles, gloves
C   Goggles, gloves, apron
D   Face shields, gloves, apron
E   Goggles, gloves, mask
F   Goggles, gloves, apron, mask
X   Gloves

BLUE: HEALTH HAZARD

4 = Danger: May be fatal
3 = Warning: Corrosive or toxic
2 = Warning: Harmful if inhaled
1 = Caution: May cause irritation
0 = No unusual hazard

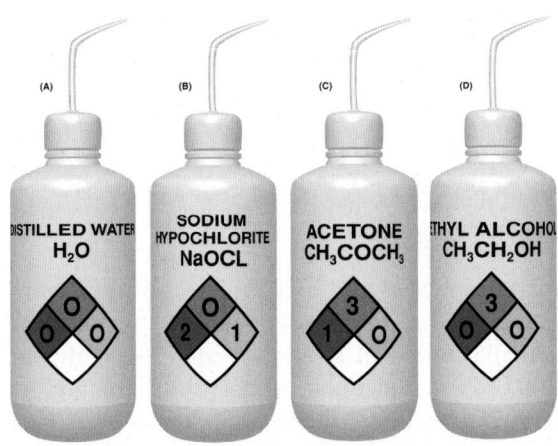

Figure 26-6 Four containers are marked using the National Fire Association's color and number method for identifying and warning of chemical hazards: (A) distilled water: presents no health, fire, or reactivity hazard and requires no PPE when used (all areas represented by zeros); (B) sodium hypochlorite: does not promote a fire hazard (red/0); is harmful if inhaled (blue/2); and it may react if heated or mixed with water (yellow/1); (C) acetone: a flammable liquid (red/3); may cause irritation (blue/1); stable and nonreactive when mixed with water (yellow/0); (D) ethyl alcohol: a flammable liquid (red/3); no unusual health hazard (blue/0); stable and nonreactive when mixed with water (yellow/0). (Courtesy of POL Consultants)

within thirty days of employment and before the employee handles any hazardous chemicals (Figure 26-7A). The training program should consist of the location and identification of hazardous chemicals, how to read and understand the labels on the chemicals, where the MSDS manual is kept, when to use personal protective equipment, and procedures to follow for chemical spills. The training sessions must be documented, signed by the employer, and permanently retained in the employee record (Figure 26-7B).

January, 1991 was the deadline for laboratories (including POLs) to have a chemical hygiene plan (CHP) in place.

Requirements of Chemical Hygiene Plan. The requirements for a CHP include:

- Employers must have an operational written plan (a manual) relevant to the safety and health of employees.

- Written instructions on the use of personal protection equipment must be available.

- Fume hoods or biohazard hoods must be checked regularly.

- Training sessions must be held for employees regarding their right to know what hazardous chemicals are in their work environment.

SAFETY TRAINING FORM

Safety training will be offered to all employees within 30 days of employment or before the employee assumes responsibilities that involve exposure to body fluids or chemicals.

Items to be covered in training session:

- General explanation of OSHA laws
- General explanation of the epidemiology and symptoms of HBV and HIV
- Who is at risk in office
- Modes of transmission of HBV and HIV
- Method of control in workplace
- Universal precautions
- Handwashing
- Personal protective equipment
- How to clean up spills
- What to do after a needlestick injury
- Medical follow-up after an exposure
- Cleaning protocol for office
- Hazardous Communication Standard
- Types of chemical labels
- How to read MSDS and NFPA signs
- Warning signs
- How to get MSDS
- Location of MSDS
- How to store chemicals
- How to record chemical inventory
- Hazardous Waste laws
- How to comply with laws
- How to use and label bio-bins and sharps containers
- How to keep records
- Who keeps the records
- Medical consent forms
- HBV forms
- Safety training certificate
- Engineering control records

Figure 26-7A Safety Training Form is an example of items to be covered by employer during training session regarding OSHA laws and exposure to chemicals, blood, body fluids, or OPIM. (Courtesy of POL Consultants)

- It is the employer's legal responsibility to provide medical attention for an employee should an accidental chemical spill occur.

- The responsibility for executing training sessions, keeping manuals current, and documentation is designated to an employer.

- Instruction must be provided regarding disposal of hazardous waste produced in the workplace.

SAMPLE

CERTIFICATE OF TRAINING

_____   _____   _____
First Name   Middle Initial   Last Name

has completed the

OSHA HAZARD COMMUNICATION
INFORMATION TRAINING PROGRAM

This certificate indicates your successful participation in a program instructing you of your rights as a worker and the proper handling of hazardous substances in the workplace.

_____   _____
Date   Employee Signature

                                              _____
                                              Instructor's Signature

                                              _____
                                              Employer's Signature

Figure 26-7B Sample Certificate of Training shows employee has completed OSHA hazard communication information training program. (Courtesy of POL Consultants)

(Usually a hazardous waste company is contracted by the employer.)

- Each employee's record must have a written statement, signed by the employer, stating the employer's responsibility to arrange for employee training and a safe work environment.

Importance of Chemical Standard to Medical Assistants. Meeting the requirements set forth by OSHA is not optional. All must comply or face penalties. All employees, including medical assistants, have the right to know and be given information and be educated regarding chemical hazards that they are exposed to in their place of employment. Medical assistants can be exposed to hazardous chemicals through skin contact, injection, or inhalation. Since many laboratory accidents result in chemical-related illnesses, it is important for medical assistants to understand how the law affects them, their place of employment, and

their employer. Medical assistants and other health care providers should know what hazards they face, and know the proper technique for handling, storing, and disposing of hazardous chemicals.

OSHA REGULATIONS AND STUDENTS

With the passage of the OSHA laws, all students with potential exposure to chemicals and bloodborne pathogens should follow all safety procedures as outlined by OSHA. Because students are not considered employees of a health care facility and are attending an educational institution, they do not fall under the OSHA guidelines. They should, however, take precautions to avoid contact with potentially infectious materials and toxic chemicals wherever learning is taking place.

Avoiding Exposure to Chemicals

Students may come into contact with harmful chemicals when doing procedures that can cause such problems as burns to the skin and eyes. Students will be made aware of these through information packaged with kits and the MSDS. As a general rule, if the chemical comes in contact with the skin, it must be flushed with water immediately and continued for five minutes. Chemicals that get into the eye must be flushed for fifteen minutes (unless contradicted on the label). Refer to the MSDS for specific post-exposure procotol. Eyewash stations and showers should be available in case of accidental exposure to hazardous chemicals with a follow-up in the emergency room.

Chemical spills should be carefully cleaned following the procedure for the particular chemical. Spill clean-up kits that consist of various items such as a shovel, cardboard, PPE, neutralizing agent, and/or absorbent material should be available.

Toxic fumes can occur with certain chemicals and certain tests can cause lung irritation and damage. This type of chemical should be handled under a fume hood that will take the fumes away by means of a ventilation mechanism.

A student safety laboratory manual outlining an exposure control plan with emphasis on standard precautions, PPE, work practice controls, lists of hazardous chemicals, and MSDS should be compiled and accessible. Students should be thoroughly familiar with its contents. Additionally, students should be educated as to the location and identification of hazardous chemicals just as employees are.

It is of utmost importance that students learn about and understand the OSHA standards and comply with them. In so doing, they will safeguard themselves from harmful chemicals and bloodborne pathogens.

CUMULATIVE TRAUMA DISORDERS

Recently OHSA has been focusing its attention on a new threat to the workplace, ergonomic hazards. Ergonomics is the study of the workplace. OSHA published its first standard, *Ergonomic Hazards*, in 1991. At the heart of these guidelines is the prevention of cumulative trauma disorders. Cumulative trauma disorders are injuries involving the musculoskeletal and/or nervous system, such as carpal tunnel syndrome and trigger finger. They are the result of long-term, repetitive work actions, such as gripping, keyboard use, pipetting, and microscopy. Limiting or preventing repetitive work actions is the key to minimizing cumulative trauma disorders. Use of ergonomically correct equipment and supplies, proper work site design, staff training, and job rotation are essential in creating an ergonomically sound workplace.

SUMMARY

Infectious diseases and accidents occur through lack of education and carelessness. Medical assistants must understand the importance of the regulations and guidelines set forth by the federal government and follow through by helping employers implement them. In doing so, the health and safety of patients and health care workers will be protected, the spread of infectious diseases can be kept under control, and the risk of contracting an infectious disease such as AIDS or hepatitis B will be greatly minimized.

Every medical office and ambulatory care setting must, by law, have clearly written and readily available manuals containing information about standard precautions, CLIA '88, and OSHA for the safe handling, storage, and disposal of blood, body fluids, and chemicals.

Through consistent use of standard precautions and adherence to the CLIA and OSHA laws, health care providers can acquire the behaviors and techniques needed to safeguard themselves and their patients.

Because of frequent changes in the laws, it is necessary for medical assistants and all other health care providers to keep abreast of the government mandates.

REVIEW QUESTIONS

Multiple Choice

1. Standard precautions were issued by:
   a. HHS
   b. CDC
   c. HCFA
   d. OSHA
2. CLIA '88 was made law in order to regulate:
   a. the disposal of infectious waste
   b. the use of chemicals in the workplace
   c. laboratory tests performed on specimens taken from the human body
   d. the transmission of the HIV virus
3. The core of the OSHA safety standard for chemical exposure is:
   a. the dipstick test
   b. the Chemical Hygiene Plan
   c. the quantity of chemical stored per month
   d. the MSDS manual
4. The agency that requires employers to ensure employee safety concerning occupational exposure to potentially harmful substances is:
   a. CDC
   b. United States Public Health Department
   c. HCFA
   d. OSHA
5. Successful laboratory safety programs include:
   a. threats to the emotional and physical health of health care workers
   b. lost work days and increased workers' compensation claims
   c. orientation, periodic drills, and consistent enforcement of policy
   d. potential fines from regulatory agencies
6. CLIA regulations specify all the following except:
   a. the type of test performed
   b. the personnel involved in testing
   c. quality control
   d. the methods used in testing
7. The agency charged with implementing CLIA is:
   a. CDC
   b. United States Public Health Department
   c. HCFA
   d. OSHA
8. Which is not an approved provider for PPM procedures?
   a. a physician
   b. a nurse practitioner

c. a dentist

d. a medical assistant

9. The standard published by OSHA to prevent cumulative trauma disorders is:

a. Workplace Standard

b. Standard for Prevention of Cumulative Trauma

c. Ergonomic Hazards

d. Ergonomic Standard

Match the chemical warning color with the hazard represented.

10. Blue   a. Reactivity or instability

11. Red   b. Use PPE

12. Yellow   c. Health

13. White   d. Fire

              e. Disaster

Critical Thinking

1. Explain the purpose of CLIA '88 and tell why the law was amended.
2. Name three categories of testing and explain each category.
3. Discuss the fifteen major components of CLIA '88.
4. Describe quality control and quality assurance. Why are they important?
5. What is HCFA form 116? Explain its use.

6. You have been asked to develop a manual for your physician/employer. The manual is to detail a Chemical Hygiene Plan (CHP) for all employees in the office. How would you proceed? What should be included in the plan? In the CHP include three major goals that will ensure the physician/employer's compliance with the hazard standard. You have been asked to compile a manual of the Material Safety Data Sheets. What must be included in the manual and from where does the information come?

WEB ACTIVITIES

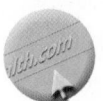

1. Search for CLIA on the web under the Department of Health and Human Services (HHS). Are there any recent updates or information on these guidelines?
2. What links can you find through OSHA's web site that are of specific relevance to medical assistants? To students?

REFERENCES/BIBLIOGRAPHY

Medical Economics Inc. (1993). *Medical laboratory observer.* Montvale, NJ: Medical Economics Inc.

Occupational Exposure to Hazardous Chemicals in Laboratories Federal Register 55:1450, 1990.

Occupational Safety and Health Administration Hazard Communication; final rule part III Federal Register 31852-31886, 1987.

U.S. Department of Health and Human Services, Health Care Financing Administration. (1992, February 28). *Clinical laboratory improvement amendments 1988.* (Federal Register No. 069-001-00042-4). Washington, DC: U.S. Government Printing Office.

INTRODUCTION TO THE MEDICAL LABORATORY

KEY TERMS

Assay
Asymptomatic
Baseline Values
Biopsy
Clinical Chemistry
Clinical Diagnosis
Condenser
Control Test
Cytology
Diagnosis
Diaphragm
Differential Diagnosis
Electrolyte
Glucose
Hematology
Histology
Hospital-Based Laboratories
Immunohematology
Immunology
Invasive
Microbiology
Mycology
Objective
Parasitology
Patient Service Centers
Physicians' Office Laboratories (POL)
Profile
Qualitative Test
Quantitative Test
Reagent
Reference Laboratories
Reference Values
Requisition
Serum
Urinalysis
Virology

OUTLINE

The Laboratory
  Purposes of Laboratory Testing
  Types of Laboratories
  Laboratory Personnel
  Laboratory Departments
Quality Controls/Assurances in the Laboratory
  Control Tests
  Proficiency Testing
  Preventative Maintenance
  Instrument Validations
  The Medical Assistant's Role

Laboratory Requisitions and Reports
Specimen Collection
  Proper Procurement, Storage, and Handling
  Processing and Sending Specimens to a Laboratory
Microscopes
  Types of Microscopes
  How to Use a Microscope
  How to Care for a Microscope

OBJECTIVES

The student should strive to meet the following performance objectives and demonstrate an understanding of the facts and principles presented in this chapter through written and oral communication.

1. Define the key terms as presented in the glossary.

2. Explain eight purposes of laboratory testing.

3. Describe the main similarities and differences between independent laboratories and physicians' office laboratories (POLs).

4. Explain the levels of laboratory personnel in relation to their education, skills, and duties.

5. List eight different departments within the medical laboratory and list at least two types of testing performed within each of those departments.

6. Name nine of the most common laboratory profiles and explain the body system or function being surveyed.

7. Explain the concepts of quality control and quality assurance in the medical laboratory.

8. Describe at least three methods of assuring quality in the medical laboratory.

(continues)

OBJECTIVES (*continued*)

9. Demonstrate how to correctly complete a laboratory requisition.
10. List ten pieces of information required on a written laboratory requisition.
11. Explain the rationale behind proper patient preparation prior to laboratory testing.
12. Explain where accurate and reliable information might be obtained about proper procurement, storage, and handling of laboratory specimens.
13. On a diagram, label the parts of a compound microscope.
14. Explain the function of a compound microscope.
15. Demonstrate the proper use of a compound microscope.
16. List six rules to assure proper care of a compound microscope.

ROLE DELINEATION COMPONENTS

CLINICAL
Diagnostic Orders
- Collect and process specimens
- Perform diagnostic tests

Patient Care
- Coordinate patient care information with other health care providers

GENERAL (TRANSDISCIPLINARY)
Legal Concepts
- Document accurately
- Comply with established risk management and safety procedures
- Participate in the development and maintenance of personnel, policy, and procedure manuals
- Develop and maintain personnel, policy, and procedure manuals (adv)

Instruction
- Instruct patients according to their needs

SCENARIO

At Inner City Health Care, Dr. Susan Rice has ordered urine tests for Annette Samuels, who came to the clinic complaining of stomach cramps. Certified medical assistant Wanda Slawson will obtain the necessary specimen and send it to an independent laboratory for testing. Wanda gives Annette specific instructions on how to prepare for the urine test and on how to collect the urine. She asks Annette if she has any questions and she has Annette repeat the instructions to be sure she understands them. When Annette returns with the specimen, Wanda immediately labels it and prepares it to be sent to the laboratory. With a reassuring smile, she tells Annette when to call the clinic for the results.

INTRODUCTION

Physicians use laboratory tests to diagnose illnesses, assess patients' health, and manage chronic diseases such as diabetes and arthritis. Medical assistants in physicians' offices, clinics, and laboratories may be responsible for patient preparation, obtaining specimens, and testing or sending specimens to an independent laboratory. It is important for medical assistants to be aware of laboratory procedures to ensure accurate testing.

THE LABORATORY

The current health care environment offers numerous options in the methods used to process laboratory tests. The specimen may be obtained and the test performed within the physician's office laboratory (POL) or the specimen may be procured and packaged for transport to a separate lab. Another option is to refer the patient to a separate laboratory for collection and testing of the specimen.

 Each laboratory setting has specific requirements for the training and qualifications of the health care personnel who work in that setting. The equipment, supplies, and paperwork as well as the instructions given to the patient are also determined by the type of laboratory. Whichever laboratory setting is selected, the focus should be on the safety of the public, the patient, and the health care personnel, while always maintaining quality testing to ensure accurate results.

Purposes of Laboratory Testing

Physicians (and other health care providers) depend on the ability of medical laboratories to help in determining a patient's state of health and/or disease in some of the following ways:

To Record an Individual's State of Health. Blood tests may be performed periodically, usually during a routine physical examination, to be assured of healthy normal ranges, also known as reference values. Then in the future, if illness occurs, the baseline values are available for comparison. Sometimes, places of employment or life insurance companies request laboratory tests to be assured that their employees or clients are free of illegal or dangerous drugs. Employment-required drug and alcohol testing is a classic example of this reason for testing.

To Detect Asymptomatic Conditions or Diseases. Occasionally a patient will have no complaints of illness and will be asymptomatic, exhibit no symptoms that might be associated with a disease process, but during routine screening or testing in another, perhaps unrelated, area, a disorder may be discovered. An example is a young man presenting at the office for an athletic physical. During routine urinalysis, it is discovered he is harboring a mild bladder infection.

To Confirm a Clinical Diagnosis. When a patient complains of specific symptoms and describes a particular condition (subjective information), and data is compiled through a clinical examination (objective information), the physician may be able to determine a diagnosis without the aid of laboratory tests. This is referred to as a clinical diagnosis. To confirm a clinical diagnosis, the physician will order laboratory tests. For example, a child has symptoms of a strep throat infection such as sudden onset of sore throat, fever, headache, and upset stomach. Upon visual examination, the physician discovers small abscesses on the child's tonsils. The physician is almost certain that the diagnosis will be strep throat, but a quick and simple strep test is performed to confirm the clinical diagnosis.

To Differentiate Between Two or More Diseases. Sometimes a patient presents with a combination of symptoms that can be related to more than one condition. In order for the physician to diagnose accurately, a laboratory test is performed. In situations like these, the physician chooses to perform the simplest and least invasive laboratory test in order to rule out a particular disease before requiring more extensive testing. This is known as a differential diagnosis. For example, if the child in the preceding case had a negative strep test but perhaps exhibited other more systemic symptoms, a blood test might confirm mononucleosis or another condition. The physician is then able to differentiate between the two diagnoses—strep throat and mononeucleosis.

To Diagnose. If symptoms are vague, thereby making the clinical diagnosis difficult for the physician, a series of laboratory tests may be required. Sometimes a profile, or group of related tests, is ordered. This helps narrow the field for diagnosis. An example is if a patient presents with complaints of severe fatigue, but preliminary testing does not reveal a diagnosis. Further testing will eventually either lead the physician in a specific direction or at least eliminate a wide variety of conditions.

To Determine the Effectiveness of Treatments. After a patient has been diagnosed and has begun treatment, the physician monitors the patient's health to be sure that the treatment is therapeutic. For example, a patient diagnosed with epilepsy must take an effective amount of antiseizure medication. A blood test is used to check the level of medication in the patient's system. A periodic blood test can also be used to determine the effectiveness of dietary and lifestyle changes in lowering blood cholesterol levels.

To Prevent Diseases/Disorders. Protection of the public, families, and coworkers can warrant laboratory tests. An example is protecting an unborn child from contracting genital herpes through the birthing process. A culture of the mother's cervical and vaginal mucosa helps to determine if the child is at risk. If the culture is positive, performing a caesarean section is the treatment of choice to protect the newborn from contracting herpes.

To Prevent the Exacerbation of Diseases. Patients with chronic conditions require regular blood tests to prevent exacerbation of the disease. When the results of the blood test are obtained, the physician or patient determines whether it is necessary to adjust the diet and/or medication. For example, a patient with diabetes tests her blood regularly to measure the blood sugar, or glucose, level. If the blood sugar level is too high or too low, the patient may adjust her insulin dosage or have something to eat to return her blood sugar level to normal.

Types of Laboratories

There are many different types and locations of medical laboratories. They are identified by their size, capabilities, and affiliations. Independent laboratories may be located within medical centers or large clinics. They often have small satellite **patient service centers** located near more isolated medical facilities or in areas of convenience to patients. Satellite laboratories facilitate patients' specimens being obtained closer to their neighborhoods and/or ambulatory care settings. The specimens are usually couriered back to the independent central laboratory for processing.

Hospital-based laboratories perform most of the tests required by that hospital area, but even large hospitals utilize reference laboratories for specialized testing. **Reference laboratories** are independent, regionally located laboratories that service larger areas. Reference laboratories are used by hospitals and physicians for complex, expensive, or specialized tests.

In a business sense, medical laboratories are quickly becoming more and more competitive. Growth and profitability depend on community relations and service, convenience, efficiency, cost, location, and even reputation. Competition often places the medical assistant and other medical personnel in a position of being asked to recommend a particular medical laboratory over another. Unless the physician-employer has a strong preference for utilizing a particular laboratory, or not referring to a particular laboratory, the patient should choose the laboratory. The patient's insurance plan may also be a factor in determining which laboratory is used. Many insurance plans require the patient to use a particular laboratory or to choose a laboratory from those participating in the plan in order to guarantee payment for the tests. The medical assistant is then a resource for options rather than a referral service. The law is very clear that a physician may not have a financial interest in the laboratory to which he or she refers patients.

Point-of-Care Testing (POCT). With the many changes in health care delivery and managed care, the clinical laboratory is also experiencing changes to improve clinical services in the laboratory area. On the forefront of change in the laboratory is point-of-care testing (POCT), also referred to as near-patient testing or bedside testing. Medical conditions, location of the patient, and treatment methods often require laboratory results as quickly as possible so proper medical care can be administered without delay. POCT uses small instruments that provide rapid, accurate results when used correctly.

Medical personnel can be trained to do laboratory tests of moderate complexity (as defined by CLIA '88) during POCT. The laboratory staff, because of their edu-

cation, knowledge, and experience in this area, are responsible for advice and management of the quality control and various aspects of this new area of testing. The extension of this laboratory service demands cooperation and cross-departmental efforts from all nontraditional personnel in the health care facility. POCT also has provided new career tracks for the laboratorian, along with multiple skills for several disciplines of health care providers.

Physicians' Office Laboratories. **Physicians' office laboratories (POLs)** are those laboratories physically set within the office. Some of the more commonly performed medical laboratory tests can easily and inexpensively be performed in the office by the medical assistant. With a simple fingerstick and a few readily available medical supplies, a patient's hematocrit and hemoglobin levels can be determined. Another commonly performed test in the ambulatory care setting is the **urinalysis** in which urine is physically, chemically, and microscopically examined for irregularities. With the availability of the many varieties of self-contained kits, tests for strep throat, pregnancy, blood sugar (serum glucose) levels, and hidden (occult) blood in stool can be performed quickly. Other kits are being developed daily. Patients may utilize a kit that can be purchased without a prescription at home. Some of the home kits available to the general public are "just as accurate" as the kits used in medical offices. The major difference is that the person performing the test may not be trained, which may affect the accuracy of the test results. More training, education, and credentialing are required as the complexity of the testing and equipment increases. If the results are not within normal limits (in some cases, positive), the physician needs to be consulted for confirmation and diagnosis/treatment. (See CLIA '88 in Chapter 26 for specific testing parameters.)

Laboratory Personnel

All independent medical laboratories must be managed by a pathologist, a physician who specializes in disease processes. Additional staffing consists of clinical laboratory scientists, technicians, clinical laboratory assistants, phlebotomists, and medical assistants. Many agencies certify laboratory personnel.

Clinical Laboratory Scientist. Certified clinical laboratory scientists are qualified to perform analysis testing in all departments of the laboratory. They often are department supervisors and have leadership roles within the laboratory personnel structure. Clinical laboratory scientists have earned a bachelor's degree and completed a minimum of one year of internship training. Certification is then obtained by passing a national certification examination issued by one of the following agencies:

MT (ASCP)—Medical Technologist
American Society of Clinical Pathologists
MT (AMT)—Medical Technologist
American Medical Technologists
CLS (NCA)—Clinical Laboratory Scientist
National Certification Agency for Medical
Laboratory Personnel
RMT (ISCLT)—Registered Medical Technologist
International Society for Clinical Laboratory
Technology
CLT (HHS)—Clinical Laboratory Technologist
Department of Health and Human Services

Clinical Laboratory Technician (CLT)/Medical Laboratory Technician (MLT).

Certified clinical laboratory technicians are qualified to perform qualitative and quantitative testing under supervision. Clinical laboratory technicians have completed two years of formal education and training. Certification is then obtained by passing a national certification examination issued by one of the following agencies:

MLT (ASCP)—Medical Laboratory Technician
American Society of Clinical Pathologists
MLT (AMT)—Medical Laboratory Technician
American Medical Technologists
CLT (NCA)—Clinical Laboratory Technician
National Certification Agency for Medical
Laboratory Personnel

RLT (ISCLT)—Registered Laboratory Technician
International Society for Clinical Laboratory
Technology

Medical Assistant. Medical assistants are multi-skilled professionals dedicated to assisting in patient-care management. Medical assistants work in medical offices, clinics, and ambulatory care centers. They perform administrative duties and clinical procedures, including basic waived laboratory tests. Formal education, training, and externship are obtained through community colleges, vocational-technical schools, and proprietary (private) institutions. Certification is obtained through a national certification examination issued by the following organizations (see Chapter 1 for additional information regarding certification):

CMA—Certified Medical Assistant
American Association of Medical Assistants and
the National Board of Medical Examiners
RMA—Registered Medical Assistant
American Medical Technologists

Laboratory Departments

Laboratories are usually divided into departments and may even be subdivided, depending on the size and specialties within the laboratory (Figure 27-1). The various departments perform special tests within their expertise (Table 27-1). Categorization becomes evident when test results are requested over the telephone or whenever

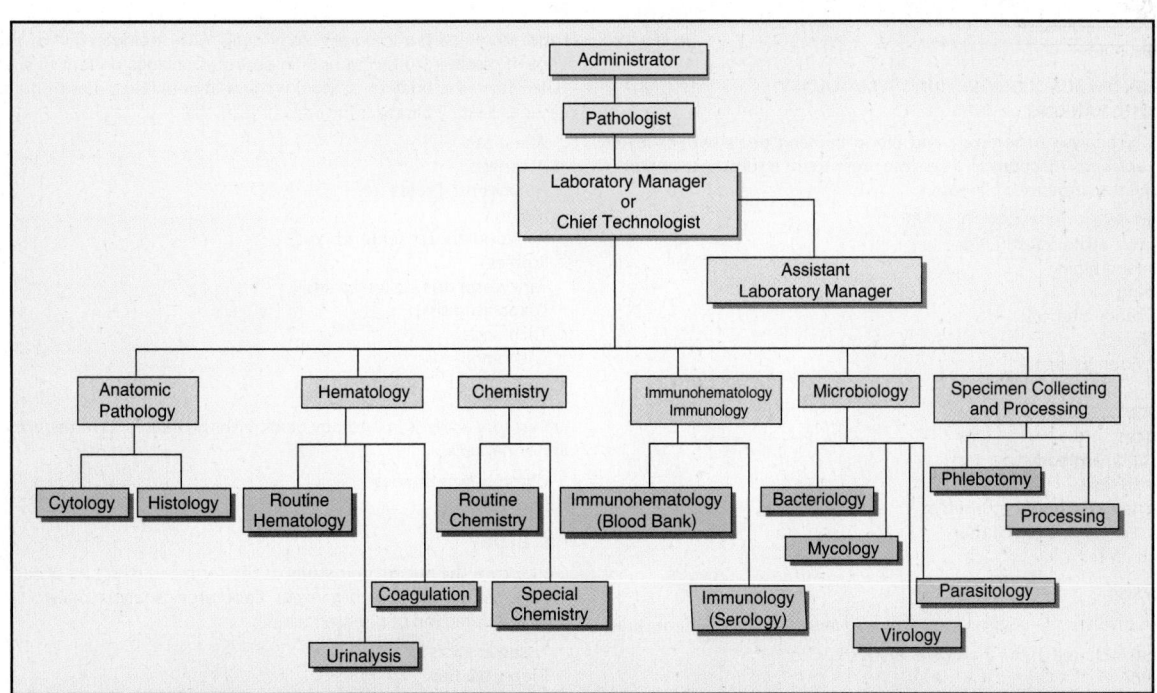

Figure 27-1 Departments in a typical medical laboratory.

TABLE 27-1   CATEGORIES OF LABORATORY TESTS

Categories of laboratory tests are listed, including the definition of each and commonly performed tests or pathologic condition in each category. Those tests that are commonly known by their abbreviations are listed as such.

HEMATOLOGY

Hematology is the science dealing with the study of blood and the blood-forming tissues. Laboratory analysis in hematology deals with the examination of blood for the detection of pathologic conditions and includes areas such as blood cell counts, cellular morphology, the clotting ability of the blood, and identification of cell types.

White blood cell count (WBC)
Red blood cell count (RBC)
Differential white blood cell count (Diff)
Hemoglobin (Hgb)
Hematocrit (Hct)
Prothrombin time (PT)
Erythrocyte sedimentation rate (ESR)
Platelet count

CLINICAL CHEMISTRY

Laboratory analysis in clinical chemistry involves detecting the presence of chemical substances or determining the amount of substances present in body fluids, excreta, and tissues (e.g., blood, urine, cerebrospinal fluid). The largest area in clinical chemistry is blood chemistry.

Glucose
Blood urea nitrogen (BUN)
Creatinine
Total protein
Albumin
Globulin
Calcium
Inorganic phosphorus
Chloride
Sodium
Potassium
Bilirubin
Cholesterol
Triglycerides
Uric acid
Lactate dehydrogenase, LD (LDH)
Aspartate aminotransferase, AST (SGOT)
Alanine aminotransferase, ALT (SGPT)
Alkaline phosphatase
Phospholipids

SEROLOGY (IMMUNOLOGY/IMMUNOHEMATOLOGY) AND BLOOD BANKING

Laboratory analysis in serology and blood banking deals with studying antigen-antibody reactions to assess the presence of a substance and/or to determine the presence of disease.

Syphilis detection tests (VDRL, RPR)
C-reactive protein test (CRP)
ABO blood typing
Rh typing
Rh antibody titer test
Cross-match
Direct Coombs' test
Cold agglutinins
Rheumatoid factor (RA factor)
Mono test
Heterophil antibody titer test
Hepatitis tests
HIV tests: ELISA and Western blot
Antistreptolysin O (ASO) titer
Pregnancy tests

URINALYSIS

Urinalysis involves the physical, chemical, and microscopic analysis of urine.

A. Tests included in the physical analysis of urine:
   Color
   Clarity
   Specific gravity

B. Tests included in the chemical analysis of urine:
   pH
   Glucose
   Protein
   Ketones
   Blood
   Bilirubin
   Urobilinogen
   Nitrite
   Leukocytes

C. Tests included in the microscopic analysis of urine:
   Red blood cells
   White blood cells
   Epithelial cells
   Casts
   Crystals

MICROBIOLOGY

Microbiology is the scientific study of microorganisms and their activities. Laboratory analysis in microbiology deals with the identification of pathogens present in specimens taken from the body (i.e., urine, blood, throat, sputum, wound, urethra and vagina, cerebrospinal fluid). Examples of infectious diseases diagnosed through identification of the pathogen present in the specimen include

Candidiasis
Chlamydia
Diphtheria
Gonorrhea
Meningitis
Pertussis
Pharyngitis
Pneumonia
Streptococcal sore throat
Tetanus
Tonsillitis
Tuberculosis
Urinary tract infection

PARASITOLOGY

Laboratory analysis in parasitology deals with the detection of the presence of disease-producing human parasites or eggs present in specimens taken from the body (e.g., stool, vagina, blood). Examples of human diseases caused by parasites include

Amebiasis
Ascariasis
Hookworm disease
Malaria
Pinworm disease (enterobiasis)
Scabies
Tapeworm disease (cestodiasis)
Toxoplasmosis
Trichinosis
Trichomoniasis

CYTOLOGY

Laboratory analysis in cytology deals with the detection of the presence of abnormal cells.

Chromosome studies
Pap test

HISTOLOGY

Histology is the microscopic study of the form and structure of the various tissues making up living organisms. Laboratory analysis in histology deals with the detection of diseased tissues.

Tissue analysis
Biopsy studies

(Adapted from *Clinical Procedures for Medical Assistants* (3rd ed.) by K. Bonewit-West, 1995, Philadelphia: W. B. Saunders Company. Adapted with permission.)

there is a need to converse with laboratory personnel. Through knowledge of the various departments within the laboratory, information can be more readily obtained.

Hematology Department. The **hematology** department tests the formed (cellular) elements of the blood. These tests may be quantitative or qualitative. The **quantitative tests** involve actual number counts such as counting the number of white blood cells (WBC), red blood cells (RBC), or platelets. The **qualitative tests** focus on the quality or characteristics of the components, such as the size, shape, and maturity of the cells. In addition, the hematology department tests the ability of the blood components to perform their individual tasks correctly. An example of this is testing the coagulation ability of clotting factors in blood.

Urinalysis Department. Urinalysis is the physical, chemical, and microscopic examination of urine. Required cultures are sent to the microbiology or bacteriology department (Figure 27-2).

Clinical Chemistry Department. The **clinical chemistry** department analyzes the chemical composition of blood, cerebrospinal fluid, and joint fluid. Some of the procedures within this department include **assay** of enzymes in the **serum**, serum glucose, or **electrolyte** levels. Toxicology, including therapeutic drug monitoring (TDM) and identification of drugs of abuse, is also performed in this department.

Immunohematology (Blood Bank) Department. **Immunohematology** is a special area that deals with blood typing procedures, cross-matching, and the separation and storage of blood components for transfusion as well as antibody-antigen reactions.

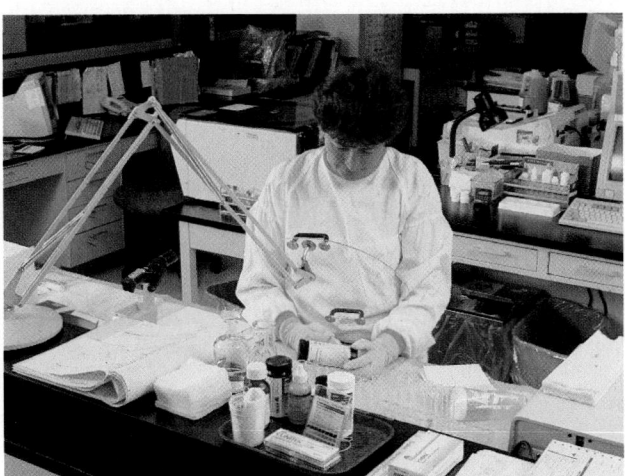

Figure 27-2 Clinical reference laboratories may have a separate urinalysis department where the laboratory professional tests urine for physical, chemical, or microbiological properties.

Serology (Immunology) Department. The serology (**immunology**) department is the area of the laboratory that performs tests to evaluate the body's immune response, both production of antibodies and the cellular immune response. Procedures in this area include the detection of antibodies to bacteria and viruses, as well as antibodies produced against one's own body (autoimmune), as in rheumatic diseases such as rheumatoid arthritis and lupus erythematosus. Diseases such as AIDS have helped move laboratory evaluation of the cellular immune system out of the research setting and into the diagnostic setting of the medical laboratory. Molecular biology and flow cytometry are becoming commonplace in today's medical laboratory. Traditionally serology has been an area within the microbiology department, but with the introduction of many new immunologic techniques, most medical laboratories now include a separate immunology department.

Microbiology Department. The **microbiology** department is the area in the laboratory where microorganisms such as bacteria and fungi are grown in an appropriate medium and then identified. Sensitivity tests are then performed to identify which antibiotics can effectively eradicate the pathogenic organisms. **Mycology** is an area within the microbiology department where fungi are studied. **Virology** is an area within the microbiology department where viruses are studied.

Parasitology Department. **Parasitology** is a subdivision of the microbiology department where ova and parasite (O & P) tests are performed on specimens such as feces. The specimens are examined for the presence of parasites and/or their eggs.

Cytology Department. The **cytology** department is the area in which microscopic examinations of cells are performed to detect early signs of cancer and other diseases. The Papanicolaou test, known as the pap smear, for irregular cervical cells is an example of a test performed in the cytology department.

Histology Department. **Histology** is the study of biopsied tissue samples for the determination of disease. Frozen samples or **biopsies** are sliced/stained and then microscopically examined for cancer and other anomalies.

Profiles of Laboratory Tests. Laboratory tests are often categorized into related groups to provide information about a particular body system or related bodily function. The groups are usually referred to as profiles (Figure 27-3). Additionally, laboratory tests are organized into panels for ease of ordering. For a current list of HCFA-approved organ- and disease-oriented panels, refer to Table 27-2.

TABLE 27-2 HCFA-APPROVED ORGAN- AND DISEASE-ORIENTED PANELS (WITH CPT CODES) EFFECTIVE APRIL 1, 2000

Basic Metabolic Panel (CPT code 80048)
BUN (84520)
Calcium, total (82310)
Carbon dioxide (82374)
Chloride (82435)
Creatinine (82565)
Glucose (82947)
Potassium (84132)
Sodium (84295)

General Health Panel (CPT code 80050)
Comprehensive metabolic panel (CPT code 80053)
CBC w/manual differential (80054) or CBC w/automated
   differential (85025)
TSH (84443)

Electrolyte Panel (CPT code 80051)
Carbon dioxide (82374)
Chloride (82435)
Potassium (84132)
Sodium (84295)

Comprehensive Metabolic Panel (CPT code 80053)
Albumin (82040)
Alkaline phosphatase (84075)
Bilirubin, total (82247)
BUN (84520)
Calcium, total (82310)
Carbon dioxide (82374)
Chloride (82435)
Creatinine (82565)
Glucose (82947)
Potassium (84132)
Protein, total (84155)
Sodium (84295)
SGOT (AST) (84450)
SGPT (ALT) (84460)

Obstetric Panel (CPT code 80055)
CBC w/manual differential (80054) or CBC w/automated
   differential (85025)
Hepatitis B surface antigen (87340)
Rubella antibody (86762)
Syphilis test, qualitative (e.g., VDRL, RPR) (86592)
Antibody screen, RBC (86850)
Blood typing, ABO (86900) and Rh (D) (86901)

Lipid Panel (CPT code 80061)
Cholesterol (82465)
HDL cholesterol (83718) and LDL cholesterol, calculated
Triglyceride (84478)

Renal Function Panel (CPT code 80069)
Albumin (82040)
BUN (84520)
Calcium, total (82310)
Carbon dioxide (82374)
Chloride (82435)
Creatinine (82565)
Glucose (82947)
Phosphorous (84100)
Potassium (84132)
Sodium (84295)

Arthritis Panel (CPT code 80072)
Uric acid (84550)
ESR, erythrocyte sedimentation rate (85651)
Fluorescent noninfectious agent, screen (86255)
Rheumatoid factor, qualitative (86430)

Acute Hepatitis Panel (CPT code 80074)
Hepatitis A antibody, IgM (86709)
Hepatitis B core antibody, IgM (86705)
Hepatitis B surface antigen (87340)
Hepatitis C antibody (86803)

Hepatic Function Panel (CPT code 80076)
Albumin (82040)
Alkaline phosphatase (84075)
Bilirubin, direct (82248)
Bilirubin, total (82247)
Protein, total (84155)
SGOT (AST) (84450)
SGPT (ALT) (84460)

TORCH Antibody Panel (CPT code 80090)
Cytomegalovirus antibody, IgG (86644)
Herpes simplex (1 & 2) antibody, IgG (86694/86695)
Rubella antibody, IgG (86762)
Toxoplasmosis antibody (86677)

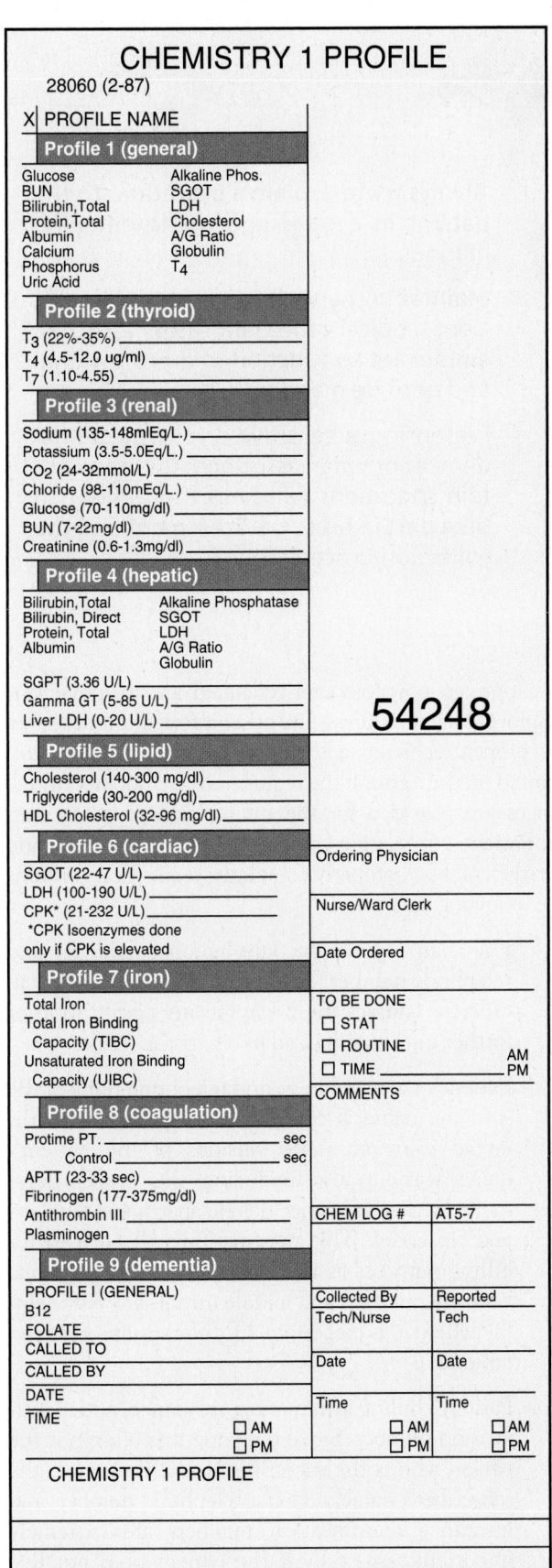

Figure 27-3 Example of a chemistry profile of laboratory tests.

QUALITY CONTROLS/ASSURANCES IN THE LABORATORY

The accuracy of any laboratory test result depends on all safeguards being followed. These standards ensure the quality of the testing equipment, supplies, personnel, and the accuracy of the test results. There are many factors that can compromise the accuracy of laboratory test results. Among these factors are collection of specimen, temperature, amount or age of specimen, time limits of test, and using chemicals or reagents past their expiration dates. Even when laboratory guidelines are strictly followed, inaccurate results may be obtained by using test kits that have been exposed to extreme heat or cold, or using chemicals or reagents after their expiration. It is important to follow all laboratory guidelines, but the medical assistant must also confirm that the specimen, chemicals, and test kits are handled and processed properly.

Control Tests

To further ensure accurate test results, **control test** samples are tested along with the patient's sample. The control samples have a known value, negative or positive result, or abnormal or normal result, which is compared with the results of the patient's test. One of the purposes of this control measure is to minimize human error. By being able to compare a sample of known value or positive (or negative) test result with the patient's test, the health care worker performing the test can accurately determine the result. An error in the testing method may be discovered if the control sample does not test accurately.

Another purpose of the control test is to check the **reagents** or chemicals. If the control sample is not showing accurate results, it may be determined that the chemicals (reagents) are faulty or have expired.

Proficiency Testing

CLIA '88 requires laboratories to participate in an accredited proficiency program for certain identified tests (see Chapter 26 for CLIA '88 requirements). Proficiency testing is similar to quality control in that "known" proficiency samples are tested the same as patient samples. The difference is an approved outside agency evaluates the accuracy of the testing and submits the performance records to HCFA for CLIA '88 compliance.

Preventative Maintenance

Preventative maintenance helps identify potential problems before they actually occur. Procedures include manufacturer-recommended maintenance on equipment; daily temperature checks on refrigerators, freezers, and incubators; daily checks on expiration dates of reagents and supplies; and instrument log and centrifuge checks.

Instrument Validations

The quality of test results can be ensured by consistently checking the calibration and linear range of the instruments and machines. If the equipment is not maintained or is functioning improperly, accurate test results cannot be assured.

The Medical Assistant's Role

Medical assistants are educated to perform administrative office duties, prepare patients, collect specimens, and perform tests in such a manner that patients and health care personnel are safe from contamination, the patient is not harmed, the sample is reliable, and the test is accurate. These four aspects of quality laboratory testing are critical for accuracy. When the patient is prepared properly, the specimen is obtained as expertly as possible, the reagents and equipment are in the best condition and calibration possible, and the test is performed by a trained professional, the test results will be accurate.

LABORATORY REQUISITIONS AND REPORTS

A written **requisition** for laboratory work must be sent to the laboratory with the patient or with the specimen (Figure 27-4). These forms are preprinted with the most commonly requested tests separated into logical categories. Additional space is provided for writing special requests. The laboratories that patients use will be happy to provide your medical agency with these forms. Laboratory requisi-

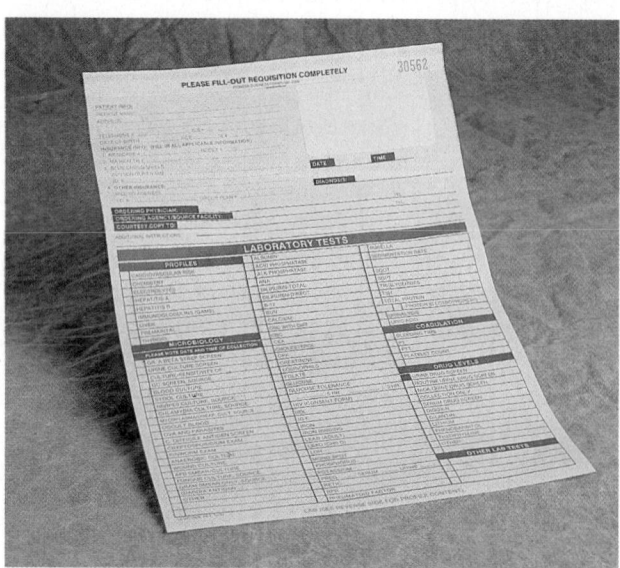

Figure 27-4 Sample laboratory requisition form.

tion forms are now computer-generated, and the physician-employer's name, address, and other information necessary for proper reporting and recordkeeping are often preprinted on the forms. If the requisitions are not preprinted, spaces are provided for the information to be written in. Patient information must be complete, accurate, and clearly legible. A properly completed requisition contains the following data:

● Physician's name, account number, address, and telephone number. This information is necessary in order to contact the office for any clarification or further information, and to report the results.

● Patient's name, address, and telephone number. Be sure the name is complete and spelled correctly. Avoid using alternate versions of the patient's name without also including the proper, legal name. Make certain to include apartment numbers and zip codes. This information will be used for billing purposes as well as medical records. Social Security numbers and middle initials are very helpful when it is necessary to differentiate between patients.

● Patient's billing information, insurance, and identification number. Since the patient is often not the person who is the subscriber to the insurance, the subscriber's name, address, telephone number, and insurance identification numbers are extremely important, especially if the patient does not live with the subscriber. Some patients have secondary insurance coverage. Be sure to include that data also. The laboratory would prefer to receive an additional sheet of information than to have incomplete insurance records in its business office.

- Unique patient identifier. This can be an identification number that is hospital- or laboratory-generated. In the outpatient setting this can be the patient's Social Security number or date of birth.

- Patient's age/date of birth and sex. Age and sex both influence the results of some tests and should not be assumed.

- Source of specimen. This information is especially important when dealing with tests such as cultures and biopsies. In the case of cultures, knowing the source of the specimen aids the laboratory in determining whether the specimen contains normal flora or is abnormal for that area of the body.

- Time and date of the specimen collection. Some tests require that the specimen be tested fairly quickly after leaving the body; other tests must be performed after a period of time has elapsed. The time and date of the specimen collection are important because accuracy can be compromised if the specimen is not sent to the laboratory in a reasonable amount of time.

- Test requested. This is usually a matter of putting a check mark in the appropriate box on the requisition, but it is surprising how often labs receive specimens with nicely completed requisitions and no indication of the test desired.

- Medications the patient is taking. Since medication can influence some test results, it is important that the laboratory be provided this information. Patients are often asked to refrain from taking certain medications prior to testing. Be sure to consult with the physician to verify orders.

- Clinical diagnosis. The physician's tentative diagnosis is very useful to the laboratory in helping to differentiate between diagnoses or confirm a diagnosis. The clinical diagnosis may also alert the laboratory personnel to any possible special considerations of which to be aware. For example, if diabetes is suspected, the laboratory will give special consideration to the glucose value. The diagnosis or preferably the ICD-9 code is also necessary for billing.

- Urgency of results. Sometimes the physician needs a test to be performed immediately (STAT) or would like a result as soon as possible (ASAP). The physician's orders need to be clearly stated on the requisition. Additional space is also provided for other special instructions if necessary.

- Special collection/patient instructions. Examples include fasting specimens, timed collections, and do not collect from a specific area.

The laboratory will send back a written report (Figure 27-5) that will contain the following information:

- Name, address, and telephone number of the laboratory

- Referring physician's name, address, and identification numbers

- Patient's name, identification number, age, and sex

- Date the specimen was received by the laboratory

- Date and time the specimen was collected

- Date the laboratory reported the results

- The test name, results, and normal reference ranges if applicable

When the results are received, the medical assistant should attach them to the patient's chart for the physician to review and initial before filing them. The physician should be alerted to any abnormal test results as soon as possible. Labs often send results via computer-generated reports directly to the physician's office or hospital (Figure 27-6).

Service Laboratories
734 Dunlap Street
Chicago, IL 60171
Telephone: 312-824-6925
Fax: 312-824-5829

Patient: Samuels, Annette (ID #ICH 041309)
            Female, Age 22

Referred by: Inner City Health Care
              Susan Rice
              #10004086

SAMP COLL: 04/24/__ 10:40 AM   SAMP RECD: 04/24/__ 12:10 PM

```
===============================================================
    TEST          RESULTS         REFERENCE RANGE      UNITS      *
===============================================================
CBC
Col: 04/26/  11:30                                              (1)
    WBC           5.3             5.0-16.0             X10-3
    RBC           4.5             3.9-5.3              X10-6
    HGB           12.8            11.5-13.5            G/DL
    HCT           37.2            34.0-40.0            %
    MCV           83              79-99                FL
    MCH           28              27-32                PG
    MCHC          34              32-37                G/DL
    RDW           13              11-15                %
    PLT           290             130-400              X10-3
    MPV           7               7-11                 FL

AUTO DIFF
Col: 04/26/  11:30                                              (1)

DIFFERENTIAL (MAN)
Col: 04/26/  11:30                                              (1)
    SEGS          34      L       41-85                %
    LYMPHS        56      H       15-48                %
    MONOS         9               2-15                 %
    EOS           1               0-55                 %
    RBC MORPH     RBC NORM

URINALYSIS (ROUTINE)
Col: 04/26/  11:31                                              (1)
    SP GRVTY      1.025           1.003-1.030
    PH            6.5             5.0-8.0
    PROTEIN       NEGATIVE        <= TRACE
    GLUCOSE       NEGATIVE        NEGATIVE
    KETONES       NEGATIVE        NEGATIVE
    BILIRUBIN     NEGATIVE        NEGATIVE
    UROBILINOGEN  0.2 E.U./dL     0.2-1.0
    BLOOD/HGB     NEGATIVE        NEGATIVE
    NITRITE       NEGATIVE        NEGATIVE
    LEUKOCYTES    NEGATIVE        NEGATIVE
```

Figure 27-5 Sample computerized laboratory report.

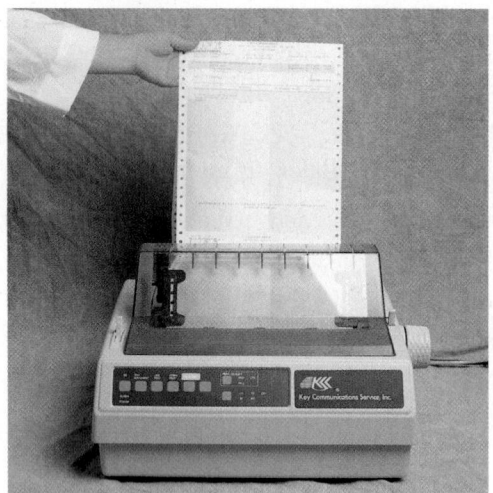

Figure 27-6 Computerized laboratory report transmitted directly from the reference lab to the physician's office.

SPECIMEN COLLECTION

Proper Procurement, Storage, and Handling

Instructions for procuring, storing, and handling and transporting laboratory specimens properly may be obtained from the independent laboratories. Most labs will provide the office/clinic with a step-by-step instruction manual (Figure 27-7) and will also be available to answer any additional questions by telephone.

Obtaining the specimen in the proper manner and using the right equipment will assure that a high-quality specimen is submitted to the laboratory. Some guidelines for specimen collection follow:

- Check the physician's orders and identify the patient.

PHLEBOTOMY GUIDELINES
(Labeling, Specimens, Patient ID, Etc.)

I. PRINCIPLE

The following sections concerning patient identification, patient information, venipuncture versus fingerstick, performing venipunctures and/or fingersticks, and potential problems are intended to establish basic guidelines. If any problems or unusual circumstances arise which are not covered, contact the main laboratory for assistance.

It must be stressed that the phlebotomists serve as laboratory representatives to the patients. A friendly, cooperative, cheerful attitude is mandatory. Please consult the Laboratory Manual, Compendium, or Central Laboratory before collecting the specimens for nonroutine procedures.

II. PHLEBOTOMY SAFETY

1. Smoking is prohibited in the patient drawing area and specimen processing area. Smoking is annoying to some patients, the burning cigarette is an ignition source to flammable liquids (such as alcohol), and the handling of cigarettes from bench to mouth is a route of exposure for potentially hazardous or infectious materials.
2. Laboratory coats are provided and must be worn when drawing or processing patient specimens.
3. Disposable laboratory gloves must be worn for patient contact or specimen handling. Gloves should be changed between patients or when they become soiled or damaged. They should be disposed of in the biohazard bag. If skin lesions are present on the hands (cuts, abrasions, punctures, burns, eczema, blisters, sores, etc.), the lesions should be covered with a bacteriostatic ointment such as Neosporin, and bandaged before putting on gloves.
4. Protective eye goggles/face shields should be worn when popping open specimen stoppers because of aerosols which may result. A piece of gauze wrapped over the specimen stopper as it is removed will also decrease aerosols. Standard eyeglasses do not provide the necessary protection and are not to be used in place of goggles/face shields.
5. Specimen spills are to be cleaned up immediately with a dilute bleach solution. If specimens spill on your lab coat, clean the area with soap and water, and then disinfect with bleach solution. If a spill soaks through to your street clothes, they should be removed and the area affected washed imme-

diately. Spills on countertops or centrifuges should be cleaned immediately with dilute bleach. All processing countertops should be wiped down routinely with dilute bleach at the end of each day.

A dilute bleach solution is prepared by adding one (1) part of household bleach (e.g., Clorox®) to nine (9) parts of water.

6. Needles should be used for phlebotomy only, and should never be recapped, cut, or bent. After use, they should be placed in a labeled, puncture-resistant container. When full, the container should be sealed and discarded into the biohazardous waste container. Never discard needles directly into the biohazardous waste container or empty full needle containers into the waste.
7. All contaminated waste (gloves, test tubes, bandages, cotton, towels, etc.) should be discarded in clearly labeled biohazard bags. When the bag becomes approximately two-thirds full, it should be securely tied to prevent spillage. All bags are picked up by a licensed waste disposal company for proper disposal. When the waste disposal company removes the waste, they will leave a paper called a "Hazardous Waste Manifest." All manifests must be kept on file at the drawstation.
8. Do not centrifuge uncapped tubes. Always make sure a centrifuge is on a level surface and properly balanced before turning it on.

III. PROCEDURE

A. *Patient Identification*
All patients must be identified on the test tube label.

B. *Patient Information*
It is the physician's responsibility to inform the patient of the necessity for the laboratory tests ordered. If questioned, the phlebotomist should refer any and all questions to the physician.

C. *Requisition Information*
A properly completed requisition should contain the following information:

a. Name of patient
b. Sex and age of patient
c. Requesting physician
d. Type of test(s) to be performed
e. Time and date of collection

Figure 27-7 Sample laboratory manual page. (Courtesy of Whatcom Pathology Laboratory, Bellingham, WA)

- Refer to the laboratory instruction manual or consult the laboratory for specific collection instructions.
- Instruct the patient in any necessary dietary restriction.
- Instruct the patient to ingest special food or take other substances if required.
- Select or provide to the patient appropriate containers with the proper preservatives in them, if required.
- Be certain to label the specimen with the patient's name, identification number, date, type of specimen, time of collection, and physician's name. Label the container, not the lid, since the lid will be removed during testing. Label the container, not the wrapping, since the wrapping will be separated from the container when testing is performed, e.g., throat swabs.
- Obtain the specimen or instruct the patient to provide the specimen according to the directions given by the laboratory.
- Follow applicable OSHA blood-borne pathogens guidelines (refer to Chapter 10) when packaging the specimen for transport so it will not leak or contaminate the courier or other office staff and so that it will safely arrive at the laboratory without being damaged or destroyed (Figure 27-8).

Processing and Sending Specimens to a Laboratory

Specimens collected by the medical assistant are often sent from the office to a laboratory many miles away or are picked up by a courier representing the outside laboratory. These are often large commercial laboratories that are not associated with a local hospital laboratory. The patient's

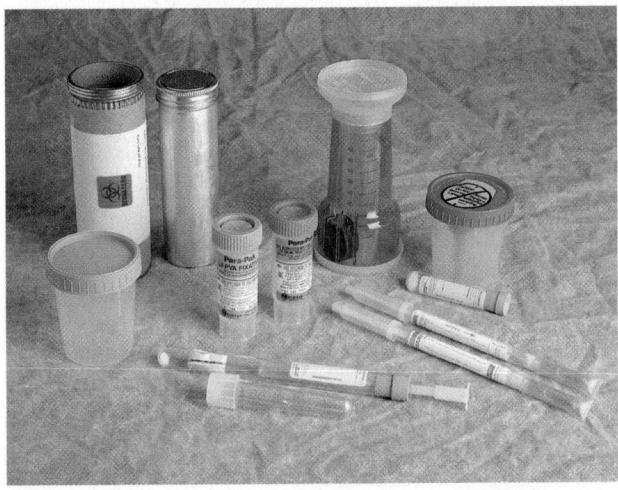

Figure 27-8 Various types of collection and transport containers used for laboratory specimens.

insurance often dictates the laboratory contracted to perform the patient's testing. It is not unusual for several different laboratories to pick up at one location. A situation could be that the blood work from patient Jones would go to laboratory A, the blood work from patient Smith would go to laboratory B, and a urine sample from patient Doe would be tested in the laboratory within the building. It sometimes can be confusing as to where to send the specimen.

All these laboratory test results are dependent on the quality of the specimen submitted. The quality of the specimen depends on the patient preparation, proper collection, correct patient identification, and transportation of the specimen. If there is any doubt or question regarding the type of specimen to be collected, it is imperative that the appropriate laboratory be called to clarify the specimen needed. There are often differences between laboratories; the type of specimen acceptable for one laboratory is not necessarily the acceptable specimen for another laboratory.

Serum Blood Collection. Most laboratory tests are performed on serum, plasma, or whole blood. Generally, when a serum sample is needed, a serum separator tube is used. There will be certain restrictions in some cases. When using a serum separator tube, several steps must be followed:

1. Perform venipuncture by the preferred method (refer to Chapter 28).
2. Invert the tube 5 times to activate the clotting.
3. Allow the tube to clot upright in a rack for at least 30 minutes but no longer than an hour.

4. Centrifuge the tube at 2,500 rpm for 15 minutes.
5. Store the tube upright or transfer the serum to a plastic transport vial for pickup by the laboratory. There will be different requirements for different laboratories.

NOTE: Do not use serum separator tubes for therapeutic drug monitoring or for toxicological studies. The gel has a tendency to lower the levels of constituents being tested. Collect the sample in a plain, red-top, evacuated tube. Remove the serum immediately after centrifugation and place the serum in a plastic transport vial.

Plasma and Whole Blood Collection.

Tubes containing an anticoagulant are used to collect plasma and whole blood samples. There are a variety of different anticoagulant tubes that can be used. The anticoagulant needed in the tube will be specified by the laboratory that will be testing the specimen. The anticoagulant is denoted by the color of the stopper of the tube. Preparing the plasma specimen for transport or testing is similar to specimen serum preparation.

1. Perform venipuncture by the preferred method (refer to Chapter 28).
2. Invert the tube 8–10 times to mix the blood with the anticoagulant.
3. Centrifuge the tube at 2,500 rpm for 10 minutes.
4. Transfer the plasma to a plastic transport vial for pickup by the laboratory. Do not allow any blood cells to mix with the plasma specimen. Indicate the specimen is a plasma specimen and what type of anticoagulant tube was used. There will be different requirements for different laboratories.

To prepare the whole blood specimen for transport or testing:

1. Perform venipuncture by the preferred method (refer to Chapter 28).
2. Invert the tube 8–10 times to mix the blood with the anticoagulant.
3. Maintain the tube at room temperature unless otherwise instructed. Never freeze a whole blood sample unless specifically instructed to do so.

Urine Collection.

For routine analysis and microscopic examination, a clean-catch midstream random urine is usually collected. The specimen is usually collected at the time of the patient's office visit.

1. With an antiseptic wipe, have the patient clean the glans (tip) of the penis for a male, or the labia for a female.
2. Following cleansing, rinse using a second antiseptic wipe to the area.
3. Void a small amount of urine in the toilet bowl.

4. Continue to void and collect the urine in a sterile urine collection cup. Instruct the patient not to touch the specimen cup on the inside or touch their body or clothing to the cup.
5. Carefully place the lid onto the specimen container. Screw the lid tightly to prevent leakage.
6. Give the urine to the medical assistant.

A 24-hour urine may also need to be collected. It is essential that the patient be thoroughly instructed in the proper method of collection to ensure the most accurate results. Some 24-hour urines require the addition of hydrochloric acid to the collection container before the start of the collection. Have the patient collect the urine in a smaller collection container and then pour the urine into the larger container to avoid acid burns to the patient. The collection procedure follows:

1. The patient should maintain the same amount of fluid intake as normal.
2. During collection, the urine should be kept in a refrigerator or a cool place.
3. At the start of the 24-hour collection, have the patient empty his or her bladder with the first morning void but do not include this urine in the 24-hour collection.
4. Collect the next voiding and all other urine voids for the next 24-hour period.
5. The last sample should be the following first morning void.
6. The total volume of urine is measured by the medical assistant. An aliquot of the urine is then poured into a transport container and sent to the laboratory with the total 24-hour volume noted. It is important to note the dates and times of collection. Some 24-hour urine tests require a corresponding blood test, e.g., creatinine clearance, to be collected during the collection period. Verify specific collection requirements with the testing laboratory.

Feces Collection.

Fecal specimens are required for a variety of laboratory tests. Various collection containers are provided by the laboratory depending on the specific test. Sterile urine collection cups can be used to collect random specimens for culture and examination for cells. Special collection cups containing formalin are used for ova and parasite testing. Mailing kits for the detection of occult blood are available to patients for ease of collection. As with all patient self-collections, detailed written instructions need to be reviewed with the patient. A special preweighed container is used for timed feces collection. As with the 24-hour urine collection, an aliquot of the feces is sent to the laboratory with the total weight recorded.

MICROSCOPES

One of the most used pieces of equipment in the medical laboratory is the microscope. Consisting of a light source, eyepieces, objectives, **condenser**, and **diaphragm**, the microscope enables us to see bacteria and other microorganisms that are much too small to be seen without magnification.

Types of Microscopes

The most commonly used microscope in the clinic is the compound microscope (Figure 27-9). As the name indicates, the image is compounded by the use of two different lenses. One lens compounds or increases the magnification produced by the other lens. The first lens system is located in the **objectives** and the second lens system is in the eyepiece (ocular). The light source is a bulb in the base. The light is directed up through the specimen on the slide and into the objective lenses. The light, or image, is then reflected by the condenser onto the specimen to the ocular lenses for visualization.

The eyepiece may have a single (monocular) lens, or there may be two (binocular) lenses. This lens is not adjustable or changeable. The magnification in the eyepiece is usually ten times (10X) the normal size of the object being viewed.

The objective lenses are adjustable between low power, high power, and oil immersion. The low-power objective lens allows the item being viewed to be magnified ten times larger than life. This magnification combined with the ten times magnification of the ocular lens allows us to see microscopically one hundred times the normal size (10X × 10X = 100X).

By combining the ten-power (10X) ocular lens with the high-power objective lens, which has the magnification power of forty-four times life (44X), we are able to increase our magnification vision to four hundred and forty times the normal size (10X × 44X = 440X). This is enough magnification to see large microorganisms, but it is still not enough to see smaller organisms, such as bacteria, clearly. An oil-immersion lens is needed to view bacteria closely.

The oil-immersion lens enables us to multiply the ocular lens magnification (10X) by one hundred (100X) to reach a possible total magnification of one thousand times normal life size (10X × 100X = 1,000X). Because more light is needed to actually see this amount of magnification, the lens is immersed in oil. This prevents the scattering and loss of light rays, which naturally occurs when light travels through air, consequently increasing the efficiency of the magnification.

Other types of microscopes have been developed especially for specific uses. One is the phase contrast microscope specifically designed for viewing specimens that are transparent and unstained. Some microscopic specimens must be stained with a fluorescent dye in order to be examined in detail (for example, when detecting specific bacteria). A fluorescent microscope is the instrument best suited for viewing those specimens. In dark-field microscopy, the light is reflected from an angle, which causes the specimen to appear as a bright object on a dark field.

Another type of microscope is the electron microscope (Figure 27-10). Special training is required to operate this very sophisticated instrument. The electron microscope is very large (several feet tall) and expensive; therefore, it is only found in larger regional and hospital laboratories. An electronic beam, rather than light, is passed through the specimen. The image is projected onto a fluorescent screen and may then be photographed and enlarged. Using the electron microscope enables us to view extremely small organisms, such as viruses, in great detail and in three dimensions. Figure 27-11 illustrates blood cells seen using an electron microscope.

How to Use a Microscope

Besides being able to adjust a microscope's magnification, it may be necessary to adjust focus. The microscope contains a coarse adjustment and a fine adjustment. The coarse adjustment is to be used with the low-power (short) objective only. The coarse adjustment is used to bring the object into view. The fine adjustment may then be used to sharpen the image. Depending on the individual microscope, the coarse and fine adjustments may raise and lower the nosepiece, which houses the objectives, or they may raise and lower the stage, or platform, on which the slide rests.

It is important always to remember to raise the platform of the lower objectives using the coarse adjustment and the low-power objective *while viewing the slide from the side*. This allows the lens to come close to the slide without

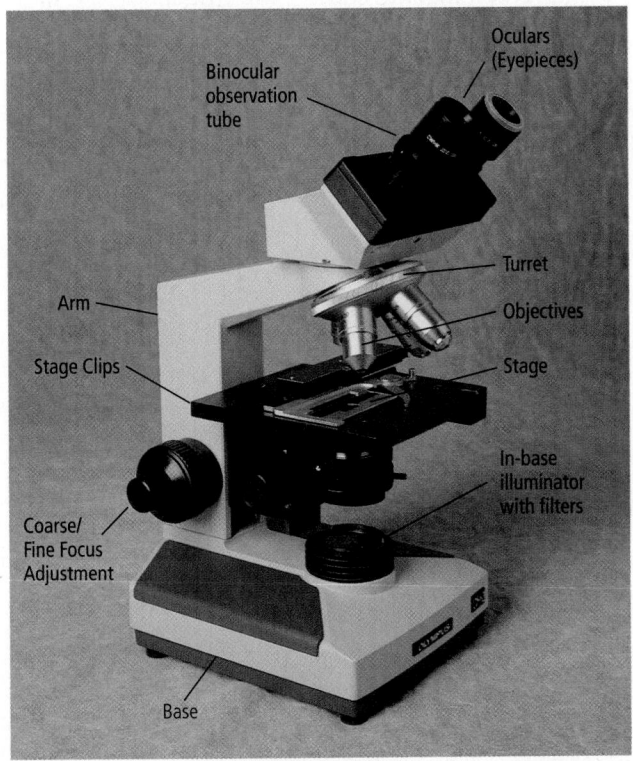

Binocular observation tube
Oculars (Eyepieces)
Arm
Stage Clips
Turret
Objectives
Stage
In-base illuminator with filters
Coarse/ Fine Focus Adjustment
Base

Figure 27-9 Compound microscope.

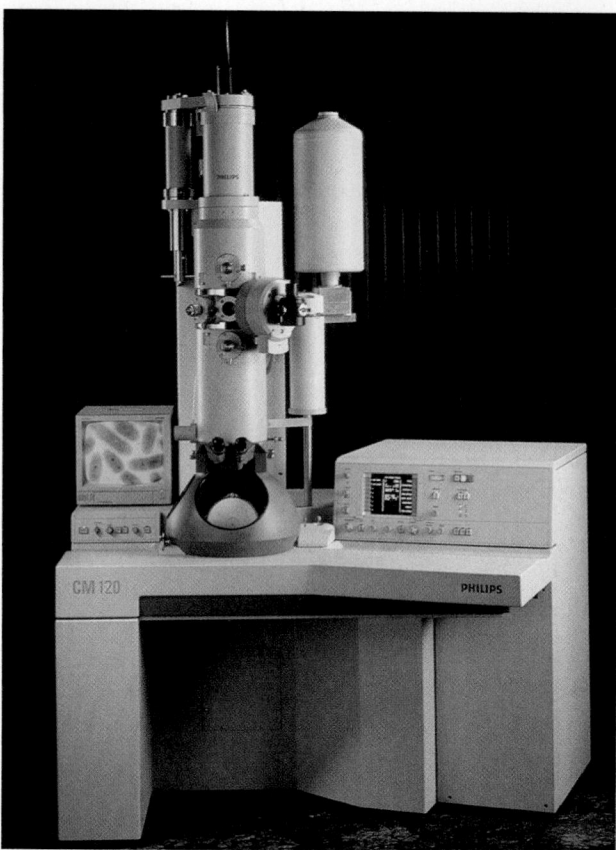

Figure 27-10 S440 scanning electron microscope. (Courtesy of Philips Electronic Instruments Co.)

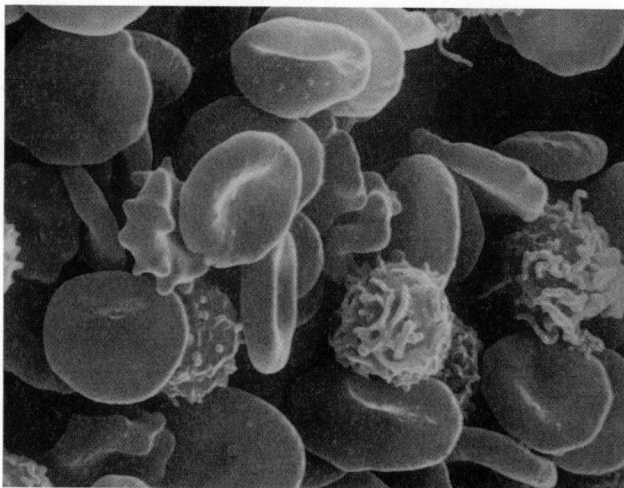

Figure 27-11 Blood cells as seen under an electron microscope. (Courtesy of Philips Electronic Instruments Co.)

- Always follow the manufacturer's and clinic's rules for the care and maintenance of the microscopes.
- Carry the microscope with one hand securely supporting the base and the other hand holding the arm (Figure 27-12).
- Keep the microscope covered when it is not being used.
- Clean the lenses with special lens paper and lens cleaner after each use. Using standard tissue can scratch the lenses.
- Always focus away from the lens to prevent the lens from coming into contact with the slide.
- Use oil only with the oil-immersion lens.

actually touching it. If the slide is not viewed from the side for the coarse adjustment, there is the possibility of running the objective through the slide and seriously damaging the lens and the microscope. After bringing the slide and objective together, the adjustments may be made through the ocular, always moving away from the slide. Once the item is in view, the fine adjustment may be used for clarity.

The bulb in the base, which directs light through the slide, first goes through a condenser and then through an iris diaphragm. The condenser is used to control the intensity of the light and the iris diaphragm may be adjusted to control the amount of light.

To use the oil-immersion lens, place a drop of cedar or mineral oil on top of the cover slip directly over the specimen on the slide. Then carefully lower the oil-immersion lens into the oil, making sure that the lens never actually touches the slide.

How to Care for a Microscope

Microscopes can be very expensive and, like any precision instrument, should be treated with care. Some practices that will extend the life of a microscope and maintain the quality of its performance are:

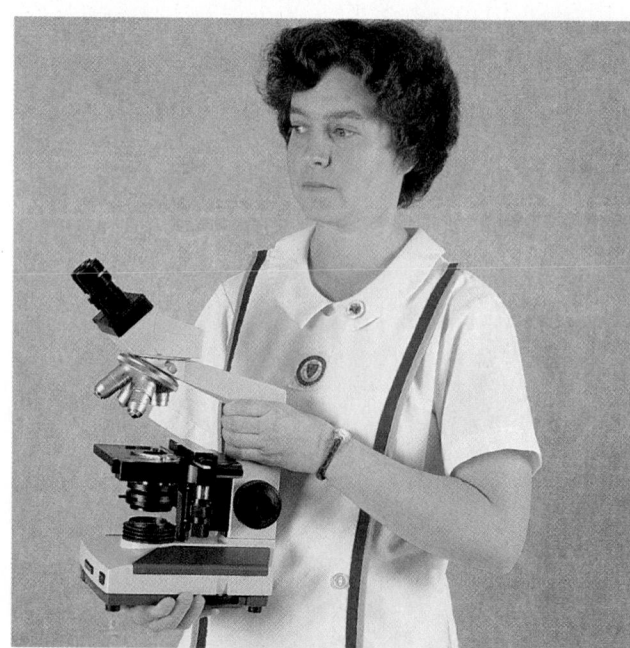

Figure 27-12 Proper way to carry a microscope.

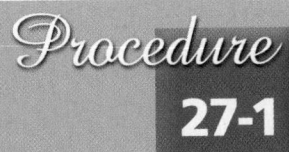

27-1 Using the Microscope

STANDARD PRECAUTIONS:

PURPOSE:

To properly use a microscope to view microscopic organisms using the coarse and fine adjustments as well as the low- and high-power objectives.

EQUIPMENT/SUPPLIES:

Hand disinfectant
Microscope (monocular or binocular)
Lens paper
Lens cleaner
Prepared slides (commercially available)
Immersion oil
Surface disinfectant
Note: Procedure will vary slightly according to microscope design. Consult the operating procedure in the microscope manual for specific instructions.

PROCEDURE STEPS:

1. Wash hands.
2. Assemble equipment and materials.
3. Clean the ocular(s) and objectives with lens paper.
4. Use the coarse adjustment to raise the nosepiece unit.
5. Raise the condenser as far as possible by turning the condenser knob.
6. Rotate the 10X, or low-power, objective into position, so that it is directly over the opening in the stage.
7. Turn on the microscope light.
8. Open the diaphragm until maximum light comes up through the condenser.
9. Place the slide on the stage (specimen side up) and secure with clips. The condenser should be positioned so that it is almost touching the bottom of the slide.
10. Locate the coarse adjustment.
11. Look directly at the stage and 10X objective and turn the coarse adjustment until the objective is as close to the slide as it will go. Stop turning when the objective no longer moves.
    Note: Do not lower any objective toward a slide while looking through the ocular(s).

12. Look into the ocular(s) and slowly turn the coarse adjustment in the opposite direction (as in step 11) to raise the objective (or lower the stage) until the object on the slide comes into view.
13. Locate the fine adjustment.
14. Turn the fine adjustment to sharpen the image.
    Note: If a binocular microscope is used, the oculars must be adjusted for each individual's eyes.
    a. Adjust the distance between the oculars so that one image is seen (as when using binoculars).
    b. Use the coarse and fine adjustments to bring the object into focus while looking through the right ocular with the right eye.
    c. Close the right eye, look into the left ocular with the left eye, and *use the knurled collar on the left ocular* to bring the object into sharp focus. (Do not turn the coarse or fine adjustment at this time.)
    d. Look into the oculars with both eyes to observe that the object is in clear focus. If it is not, repeat the procedure.
15. Scan the slide by either method:
    a. Use the stage knobs to move the slide left and right and backward and forward while looking through the ocular(s),
       or
    b. Move the slide with the fingers while looking through the ocular(s) (for microscope without movable stage).
16. Rotate the high-power (40X) objective into position while observing the objective and the slide to see that the objective does not strike the slide.
17. Look through the ocular(s) to view the object on the slide; it should be almost in focus.
18. Locate the fine adjustment.
19. Look through the ocular(s) and turn the fine adjustment until the object is in focus. Do not use the coarse adjustment.
20. Adjust the amount of light. This can be done by closing the diaphragm, lowering the condenser, or adjusting the light at the source.
21. Scan the slide as in step 15, using the fine adjustment if necessary to keep the object in focus.
22. Rotate the oil-immersion objective to the side slightly (so that no objective is in position).

(continues)

Procedure

27-1 *(continued)*

23. Place one drop of immersion oil on the portion of the slide that is directly over the condenser.
24. Rotate the oil-immersion objective into position, being careful not to rotate the 40X objective through the oil.
25. Look to see that the oil-immersion objective is touching the drop of oil.
26. Look through the ocular(s) and slowly turn the fine adjustment until the image is clear. Use only the fine adjustment to focus the oil-immersion objective.
27. Adjust the amount of light using the procedure in step 20.
28. Scan the slide using the procedure in step 15.
29. Rotate the 10X objective into position (do not allow the 40X objective to touch the oil).
30. Remove the slide from the microscope stage and gently clean the oil from the slide with lens paper.

A copeland jar containing a solvent cleaner, such as xylene, can be used to remove excess oil from the slide.

31. Clean the oculars, 10X objective, and 40X objective with clean lens paper and lens cleaner.
32. Clean the 100X objective with lens paper and lens cleaner to remove all oil.
33. Clean any oil from the microscope stage and condenser.
34. Turn off the microscope light and disconnect.
35. Position the nosepiece in the lowest position using the coarse adjustment.
36. Center the stage so that it does not project from either side of the microscope.
37. Cover the microscope and return it to storage.
38. Clean the work area; return slides to storage.
39. Wash hands.

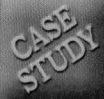

CASE STUDY 27-1

Edith Leonard came to Inner City Health Care because she was experiencing sight failure, constant thirst, and fainting spells. After examining Edith, Dr. Ray Reynolds ordered a glucose tolerance test. Certified medical assistant Wanda Slawson gave Edith a special diet that she was to follow for the three days preceding the test and instructions regarding fasting before the test.

Edith has returned to the clinic to have the test. "Did you follow the diet I gave you, Mrs. Leonard?" Wanda asks. "Yes, I did." "Did you have anything to eat this morning?" "No, but I did have a cup of coffee. I thought it would be all right because I drink it black. I can't start the day without my coffee."

CASE STUDY REVIEW

1. Should Wanda perform the test? Explain your answer.
2. How can Wanda emphasize the importance of following the diet, fasting, and test instructions?
3. What can Wanda do to try to ensure Edith's cooperation?

SUMMARY

If disease did not exist, we would have little need for clinical laboratories. If we were not susceptible to viral illnesses, if bacteria never infected our bodies, if our bodies always operated in their healthiest state regardless of what we did to them, and, perhaps most important of all, if we chose our parents wisely, there would be little that a clinical laboratory would be asked to do. The fact that our bodies are susceptible to disease necessitates the existence of clinical laboratories.

Along with clinical laboratory personnel, medical assistants play an important role in laboratory testing. They prepare patients for tests, obtain specimens, and perform simple, routine tests or send specimens to the appropriate laboratory. Medical assistants are educated to perform these tasks in a manner that ensures the accuracy of the test and safeguards the health of patients and health care personnel.

REVIEW QUESTIONS

Multiple Choice

1. All of the following statements concerning point-of-care testing (POCT) are true *except:*
   a. performed at the patient's bedside
   b. must be performed by certified laboratory professionals
   c. provides for rapid, accurate results
   d. the medical laboratory's role includes training and management of quality control
2. Independent medical laboratories must be managed by a:
   a. clinical laboratory technologist
   b. pathologist
   c. clinical laboratory technician
   d. medical assistant
3. The hematology department of a laboratory:
   a. studies microorganisms and their activities
   b. studies blood and blood-forming tissues
   c. detects the presence of disease-producing human parasites or eggs present in specimens taken from the body
   d. detects the presence of abnormal cells
4. The quality of patient test results is maintained by:
   a. instrument calibration procedures
   b. preventative maintenance procedures
   c. quality control testing
   d. all of the above
5. When a patient or specimen is sent to a laboratory for testing, the medical assistant also sends:
   a. a written requisition
   b. a report
   c. the patient's file
   d. an insurance form
6. The most commonly used microscope in the clinic is the:
   a. fluorescent microscope
   b. electron microscope
   c. phase contrast microscope
   d. compound microscope

Critical Thinking

1. A patient asks you to recommend a laboratory for the tests ordered by the physician. How will you respond to the request? What are some factors that will influence your response?
2. A patient performed a pregnancy test at home, but the physician has requested a pregnancy test in the office. Explain to the patient why the home test may not be as accurate as the test performed in the office.
3. Discuss the differences in education between a clinical laboratory technologist, a clinical laboratory technician, and a medical assistant.
4. The physician has ordered a chemistry profile for a patient. What is a profile and how will it help the physician to diagnose the patient's condition?
5. Explain why it is important to handle and process specimens, test kits, and chemicals properly.
6. Discuss the medical assistant's role in laboratory testing and how it affects the accuracy of test results.
7. The time and date of specimen collection were not included on the requisition form. Why is this data always important to the laboratory?
8. You have been asked to collect a plasma sample for testing at an independent laboratory. Describe how you will collect the sample. How will you determine which anticoagulant is needed in the tube?
9. Describe how to use a microscope to observe microscopic organisms.
10. Explain how a compound microscope is able to magnify.

WEB ACTIVITIES

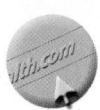

1. For each group of laboratory personnel discussed in this chapter, search the Internet for a web site that pertains to it. What kind of information does it offer?
2. Locate a local hospital's web site. Does it outline all the specialty departments described in this chapter? What unique services do they offer?
3. Visit your insurance company's web site. Does it specify which labs must be used?

REFERENCES/BIBLIOGRAPHY

Bonewit-West, K. (1995). *Clinical procedures for medical assistants* (4th ed.). Philadephia: W. B. Saunders Company.

Henry, J. B. (1996). *Clinical diagnosis and management by laboratory methods* (19th ed.). Philadelphia: W. B. Saunders Company.

Lane, K. (1993). *Saunders manual of medical assisting practice.* Philadelphia: W. B. Saunders Company.

Marshall, J. (1993). *Fundamental skills for the clinical laboratory professional.* Albany, NY: Delmar.

Walters, N. J., Estridge, B. H., & Reynolds, A. P. (2000). *Basic medical laboratory techniques* (4th ed.). Albany, NY: Delmar.

Wedding, M. E., & Toenjes, S. A. (1998). *Medical laboratory procedures* (2nd ed.). Philadelphia: F. A. Davis Company.

28

PHLEBOTOMY: VENIPUNCTURE AND CAPILLARY PUNCTURE

KEY TERMS

Additive
Aliquot
Anticoagulant
Buffy Coat
Cannula
Centrifuge
Constrict
Dilate
Edematous
Erythrocyte
Hematoma
Hemoconcentration
Hemolysis
Hypoglycemia
Integrity
Leukocyte
Luer
Lipemia
Oxygenated
Palpate
Phlebotomy
Plasma
Primary Container
Serum
Thixotrophic Separator Gel
Thrombocyte
Tourniquet
Venipuncture
Viscosity

OUTLINE

Why Collect Blood?
The Medical Assistant's Role in Phlebotomy
Anatomy and Physiology of the Circulatory System
Collection of Blood Specimens
Venipuncture Equipment
Syringes and Needles
Safety Needle
Evacuated Tube System
Anticoagulants
Tourniquets
Specimen Collection Trays
Venipuncture Technique
Approaching the Patient
Preparing Supplies and Greeting the Patient
Patient and Specimen Identification
Positioning the Patient

Selecting the Appropriate Venipuncture Site
Performing a Safe Venipuncture
Syringe Specimen Collection
Evacuated Tube Specimen Collection
Butterfly Collection System
Patient Reactions
The Unsuccessful Venipuncture
Criteria for Rejection of a Specimen
Factors Affecting Laboratory Values
Capillary Puncture
Composition of Capillary Blood
Capillary Puncture Sites
Preparing the Capillary Puncture Site
Performing the Puncture
Collecting the Blood Sample
Order of Draw

OBJECTIVES

The student should strive to meet the following performance objectives and demonstrate an understanding of the facts and principles presented in this chapter through written and oral communication.

1. Define the key terms as presented in the glossary.
2. Explain the medical assistant's responsibility to the patient in terms of quality of care and respect of the patient as a human being.
3. Explain why the medical assistant has a special responsibility to present a neat, pleasant, and competent demeanor.
4. Differentiate between serum and plasma. *(continues)*

OBJECTIVES (*continued*)

5. State the relationship between diameter and the gauge of the needle.
6. Explain the principle of the evacuated tube system.
7. State the manner in which anticoagulants prevent coagulation.
8. Name the anticoagulant associated with the various color-coded evacuated tubes.
9. State the purpose of additives to evacuated tubes.
10. Explain the three skills used in collecting blood specimen.
11. Explain the importance of correct patient identification, complete specimen labeling, and proper handling, storage and delivery.
12. Explain how a tourniquet makes the veins more prominent.
13. Describe the step-by-step procedure for drawing blood with a syringe, evacuated tube system, butterfly, or capillary puncture.
14. Explain how to handle the various reactions a patient might have to venipuncture.

ROLE DELINEATION COMPONENTS

CLINICAL

Fundamental Principles

- Apply principles of aseptic technique and infection control
- Comply with quality assurance practices
- Screen and follow up patient test results

Diagnostic Orders

- Collect and process specimens
- Perform diagnostic tests

GENERAL (TRANSDISCIPLINARY)

Legal Concepts

- Document accurately
- Comply with established risk management and safety procedures

SCENARIO

At Inner City Health Care, medical assistant Bruce Goldman often performs venipunctures. Bruce is personable and has an easy-going manner that makes patients feel comfortable with him. He takes time to talk to patients before performing a venipuncture to determine their feelings about the procedure and to learn about their previous experiences. Bruce is confident and professional in his interactions with patients. He is always well-groomed and he treats patients with respect. Using his social, technical, and administrative skills, Bruce is usually able to collect the necessary blood samples while providing a positive experience for patients.

INTRODUCTION

The task of collecting blood samples from patients for diagnostic testing is known as phlebotomy. The health care professional who performs this duty varies at each health care setting. The task of phlebotomy is not restricted to one individual. A variety of individuals are cross trained to do phlebotomy and other tasks. Many health care settings do not have enough patients to justify having a phlebotomist available at all times. Therefore, the medical assistant may be designated to perform phlebotomies.

WHY COLLECT BLOOD?

Phlebotomy is the process of collecting blood or bloodletting as a therapeutic measure. The history of bloodletting dates back to the early Egyptians and continues into modern times. Phlebotomy in the past was a method to cure individuals with "bad" blood. The blood was drained out of individuals as a treatment, thereby alleviating the patient's symptoms. Phlebotomy is now used to help determine the disease process taking place and to determine the method of treatment. Without the collection of blood samples, physicians would have few means available to assist them in making diagnoses.

THE MEDICAL ASSISTANT'S ROLE IN PHLEBOTOMY

A phlebotomist is a person trained to obtain blood specimens by venipuncture and capillary puncture techniques. The phlebotomist's primary role is to collect blood as efficiently as possible for accurate and reliable test results. How the medical assistant will be involved in phlebotomy will vary greatly from one health care environment to another. The medical assistant performing venipuncture will directly contact the patient, and perform tasks that are critical to the patient's diagnosis and care. During the direct contact with the patient, the medical assistant will leave an impression with the patient. It can be positive or negative depending on the skill with which the medical assistant performs the venipuncture.

It is the medical assistant's responsibility to provide high-quality care to patients. The medical assistant must act professionally when working with patients. Professionalism is displayed by performing tasks in an efficient, competent manner, wearing clean, neat attire, and showing concern for patients and their feelings.

Patients will not tell family and friends that their blood was run through expensive state-of-the-art instruments but rather that the person drawing their blood sample was friendly and skilled. A smile and a kind word can allay a patient's fear and do a lot to win a permanent customer and patient to the physician's office.

ANATOMY AND PHYSIOLOGY OF THE CIRCULATORY SYSTEM

To be prepared to collect blood, the medical assistant must understand the system that carries the blood and the composition of the blood. The system in which the blood is transported is the circulatory system. Blood forms in the organs of the body. The bone marrow is the primary factory for production of blood cells. The lymph nodes, thymus, and spleen are also sites for the production of blood cells. The function of blood is to carry oxygen to body tissues and to remove the waste product carbon dioxide. The blood also carries nutrients to all parts of the body and moves the waste products to the lungs, kidneys, liver, and skin for elimination.

The circulatory system consists of the heart, which pumps blood through the body by way of tubing called arteries, veins, and capillaries. When blood flows away from the heart, it flows in arteries. Blood flowing back to the heart flows through the veins. Connecting most of the arteries and veins are the capillaries (Figure 28-1).

ARTERIES VERSUS VEINS	
Arteries	**Veins**
1. Carry blood from the heart, carry oxygenated blood (except pulmonary artery)	1. Carry blood to the heart, carry deoxygenated blood (except pulmonary vein)
2. Normally bright red in color	2. Normally dark red in color
3. Elastic walls that expand with surge of blood	3. Thin walls/less elastic
4. No valves	4. Valves
5. Can feel a pulse	5. No pulse

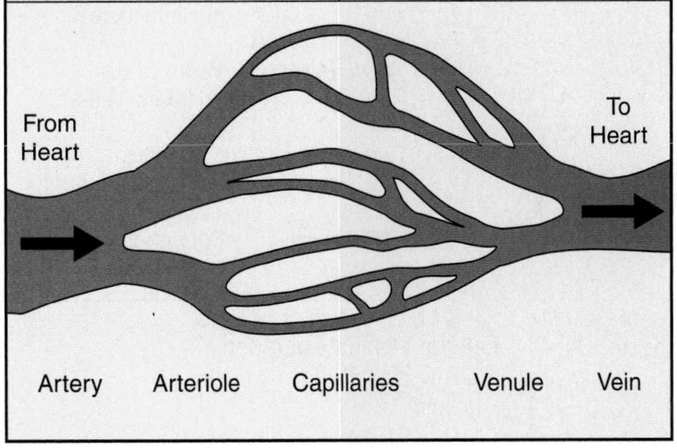

From Heart · Artery · Arteriole · Capillaries · Venule · Vein · To Heart

Figure 28-1 Blood flows from the heart through the arteries and back to the heart through the veins.

Arteries have a thick wall that helps them withstand the pressure of the pumping action of the heart. The arteries branch to form arterioles, which branch again to become capillaries. The capillaries then begin coming together to form venules and the venules then become veins. As blood flows through the body, it follows this path of artery-arteriole-capillary-venule-vein. **Oxygenated** arterial blood, which contains a high level of oxygen, leaves the heart and carries the oxygen to the tissue by releasing the oxygen through the cell walls of the capillaries. At the same time, carbon dioxide is being absorbed by the blood and then transported to the lungs to be exhaled as a waste product. The flow of the blood also regulates body temperature. When the body gets warm, the capillaries in the extremities **dilate** and let off heat. This process then cools the body. If the body becomes cold, the capillaries **constrict** and less blood flows through, thereby conserving heat for the rest of the body.

The body contains approximately 6 liters (l) of blood, 45 percent of which is formed elements. The formed cellular elements consist of **erythrocytes, leukocytes,** and **thrombocytes** (Figure 28-2). The remaining

	White Blood Cell (Leukocyte)	Red Blood Cells (Erythrocyte)	Platelet (Thrombocyte)
Function	Body defense (extravascular)	Transport of oxygen and carbon dioxide (intravascular)	Stoppage of bleeding
Formation	Bone marrow, lymphatic tissue	Bone marrow	Bone marrow
Size/shape	9–16 micrometers; different size, shape, color, nucleus (core)	6–7 micrometers; bioconcave disc. Normally no nucleus in circulatory blood	1–4 micrometers; fragments of megakaryocytes
Life cycle	Varies, 24 hours–years	100–120 days	9–12 days
Numbers	5–10,000/ cubic millimeter	4.5–5.5 million/ cubic millimeter	250–450,000/ cubic millimeter
Removal	Bone marrow, liver, spleen	Bone marrow, spleen	Spleen

Figure 28-2   Cellular elements of blood.

55 percent of the blood is liquid. Generally 2 milliliters (ml) of blood will yield about 1 milliliter of fluid. The liquid portion of uncoagulated blood is known as **plasma**. Blood flowing through the body contains a substance called fibrinogen. The clotting process converts the fibrinogen into fibrin. The fibrin is like a sticky spider web that traps the formed elements into the fibrin mass called a clot. The clot then contracts and the liquid (**serum**) portion is extracted. The serum is a clear straw-colored liquid that is used for many of the tests done in the laboratory. The main difference between serum and plasma is that plasma contains fibrinogen, serum does not.

The formed elements and the liquid portion of the blood are often separated for laboratory testing. To speed the removal of the serum from a tube of blood, an instrument called a **centrifuge** spins the blood. A carrier holds the tubes of blood and when the centrifuge is activated, the carrier spins. The spinning action of the carrier pushes the blood cells to the bottom of the tube. The blood separates according to weight. The clot goes to the bottom of the tube and the serum goes to the top.

To produce a plasma specimen, the blood must be prevented from clotting by the use of a chemical **anticoagulant**. Blood collected in a tube containing an anticoagulant can be centrifuged to separate the formed elements (cells) from the plasma. The bottom layer will contain the erythrocytes, then there will be a thin layer called the **buffy coat**. The buffy coat contains a mixture of leukocytes and thrombocytes. On top of all these layers is the plasma layer. The plasma will contain fibrinogen and usually is slightly hazy (Figure 28-3).

Collection of Blood Samples

The most commonly used method for blood collection is **venipuncture**. To obtain a blood sample, the medical

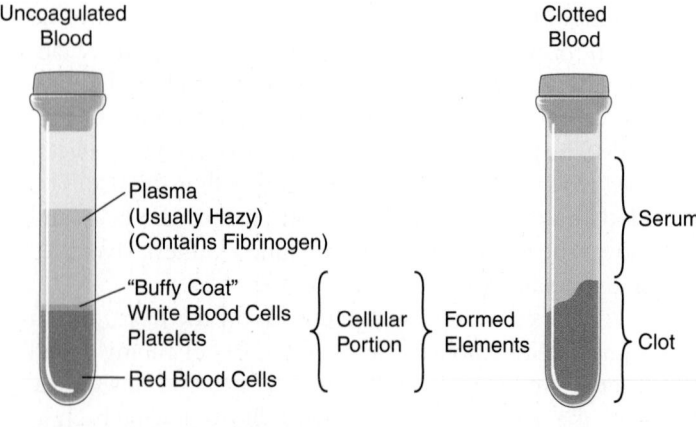

Figure 28-3   Blood tubes.

assistant must locate a vein that is acceptable for blood collection. The preferred site for venipuncture is the antecubital fossa, which is located anterior to the elbow on the inside of the arm. The veins are near the surface and are large enough to give access to the blood (Figure 28-4). The median cubital vein is the vein that is used the majority of the time. When this vein is not available, any of the other veins that can be felt may be used. These veins include the basilic, cephalic, and median veins. When necessary, veins on the dorsal surface of the hand or wrist may be used for venipuncture, but they are more painful for the patient and may require a smaller needle or the use of a butterfly apparatus.

The veins of the feet are an alternative when the arms are not available. A physician's permission is needed before drawing blood from the veins of the legs and feet.

The physician may not want the patient's leg or foot veins punctured because the act of drawing blood may cause clots to form. These clots then have the possibility of dislodging and causing a blockage elsewhere in the body. It would be extremely rare for a medical assistant to use this location. A phlebotomist or registered nurse in the physician's office should be consulted before a foot puncture is considered.

The arteries in the arm consist of the brachial artery in the brachial region of the arm and the radial and ulnar arteries in the wrist (Figure 28-5). Special techniques are necessary to puncture arteries to obtain a blood specimen for the examination of gases absorbed by the blood. Arterial punctures and the techniques used to draw blood from these locations for blood gas testing are not generally done by a medical assistant.

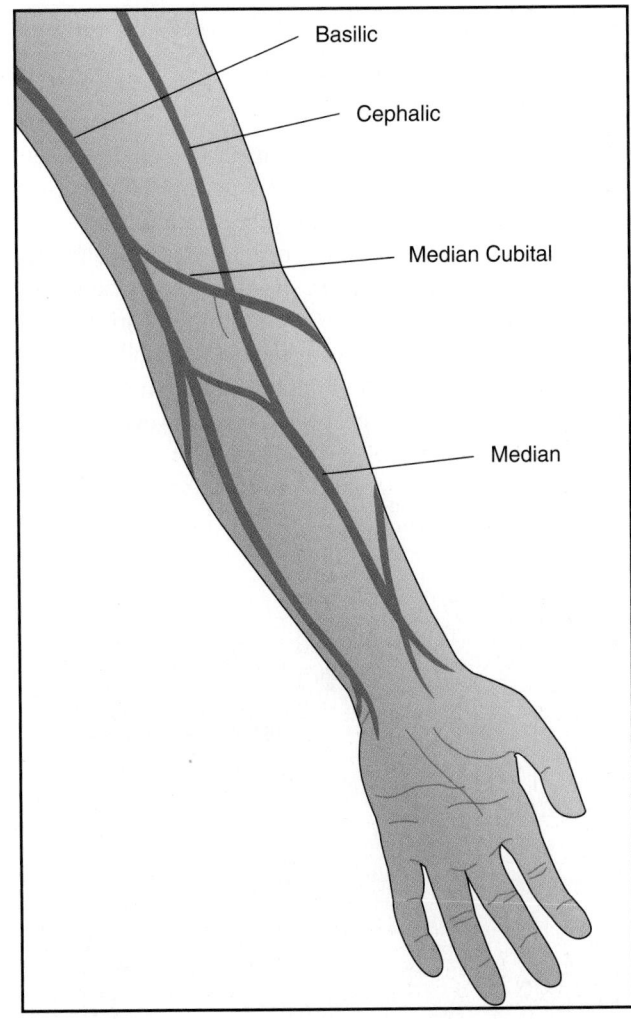

Figure 28-4 Superficial veins of the arm.

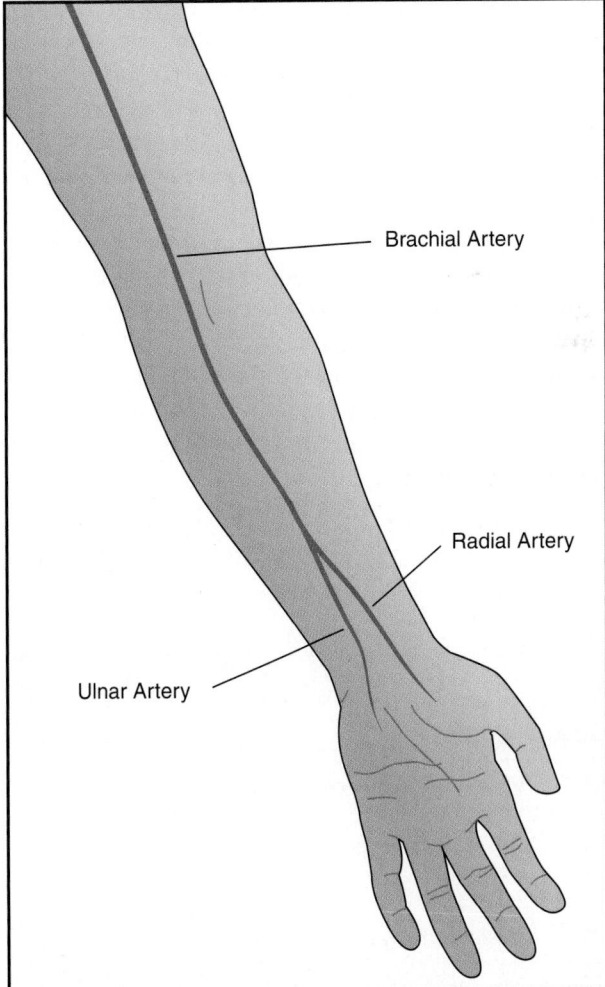

Figure 28-5 Arteries of the arm.

VENIPUNCTURE EQUIPMENT

All methods of venipuncture require the invasive procedure of opening a vein to obtain a blood sample.

Syringes and Needles

The syringe and needle method is one of the oldest methods known and does not destroy the **integrity** of the vein. Syringes are made of either glass or plastic. Most of the syringes currently being used are manufactured from plastic and are disposable (Figure 28-6). Syringes vary in volume from 1 milliliter to 50 milliliters.

Pulling on the plunger of a syringe creates a vacuum within the barrel. The larger the syringe, the greater the amount of vacuum that can be obtained. Too large a vacuum will have the tendency to pull too hard on the vein and may cause the vein to collapse. Vein collapse can be avoided by pulling the plunger slowly and by resting between pulls to allow the vein time to refill. Patients that have fragile, thin, or "rolling" veins that collapse when using an evacuated tube system are typical examples of patients that may be better venipunctured with a syringe. Pediatric or geriatric patients typically have these types of veins. The use of a syringe and needle is limited by the capacity of the syringe. The use of a syringe larger than 10–15 milliliters is not recommended. If a large amount of blood is needed, a butterfly collection set should be used. Syringes are also used in special procedures when the blood must be drawn and then transferred to a different container.

The recommended length of the needle is 1 to 1½ inches in length. The most common gauges of needles that are used in health care are 25, 23, 22, 21, 20, 18, and 16, with the smallest diameter needle being a 25 gauge and the largest being a 16 gauge (Table 28-1).

Safety Needle

 A new safety blood collection needle now available virtually eliminates risks associated with accidental needlesticks through an effective

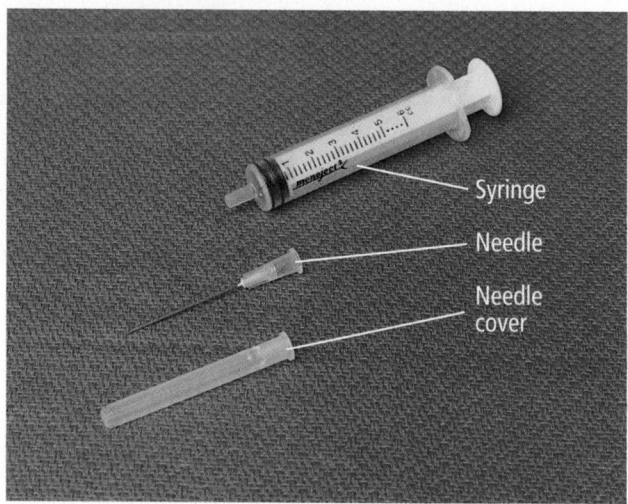

Figure 28-6 Needle and syringe components.

means of passive protection. The Bio-Plexus Punctur-Guard® needle is similar in appearance, size, performance, and general operation to the standard needles used in venipuncture. The unique feature of the needle assembly is a blunt **cannula**, called a blunting member, placed within an otherwise standard needle.

When the Punctur-Guard® needle assembly is inserted into the patient, the blunting member is in its retracted position. When the operator applies additional pressure to the blood collection tube, the blunting member locks into place beyond the needle's tip. The blunting member helps to prevent the needle from accidentally sticking anyone after it is removed from the patient (Figure 28-7). Since the blunting member is hollow, fluids flow normally through the Punctur-Guard® needle, similar to standard needles currently in use. However, because the Punctur-Guard® needle is blunted before it is removed from the patient, the danger of an accidental needlestick is virtually eliminated.

TABLE 28-1	NEEDLE GAUGES
Size	**Purpose**
25	Smallest gauge needle, often causes hemolysis of blood
23	Used with butterfly system, or syringes 0–5 ml in capacity
22	
21	Used with evacuated tube systems
20	
18	Large size, not often used for venipuncture
16	

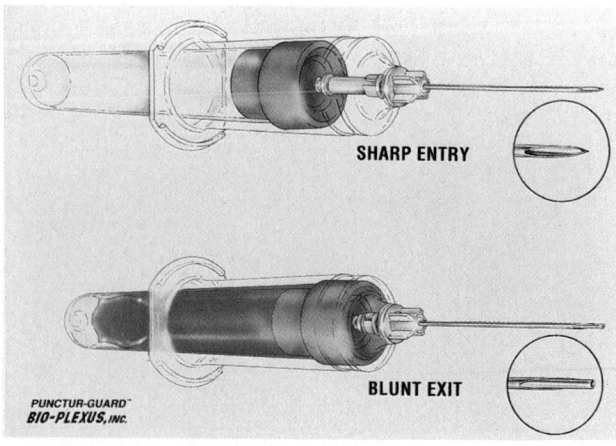

SHARP ENTRY

BLUNT EXIT

PUNCTUR-GUARD™
BIO-PLEXUS, INC.

Figure 28-7 Safety blood-collection needle. (Courtesy of Bio-Plexus, Inc., Tolland, CT.)

Evacuated Tube System

The evacuated tube system is often called the Vacutainer system. Vacutainer can be a misnomer because the term *Vacutainer*® is a brand name for the evacuated tube system manufactured by Becton Dickinson and Company, Rutherford, NJ. Medical assistants often say Vacutainer when they are using another company's product.

The principle of the evacuated tube blood collection system is the same principle as a syringe creating a vacuum when the plunger is pulled. A difference is the evacuated tube system is a closed system, adding an element of safety. In the evacuated tube system, a tube with a vacuum already in it attaches to the needle and the tube's vacuum is replaced by blood. The tubes can be glass or plastic. The total system consists of a double-pointed needle, a plastic holder or adapter, and a series of vacuum tubes with rubber stoppers (Figure 28-8).

The key to the evacuated tube system is the needle. The needle is a double-pointed needle with a different length needle on each end and a screw hub near the center. The longer needle has a bevel that enters the vein. The shorter needle pierces the rubber stopper in the blood collection tube. The needle that pierces the rubber stopper of the tube has a sleeve that functions as a valve to stop the flow of blood when the tube is removed (Figure 28-9). Pushing the tube into the holder compresses the sleeve and exposes the needle as it enters the tube. As the tube is removed, the sleeve slides back over the needle and stops the flow of blood.

The needle is thought of as a pipeline that is going to deliver blood from the patient to the tube. The blood is pulled out of the patient due to the vacuum inside the tube.

The patient will experience the least pain if the bevel of the needle is facing upward when the needle is inserted into the vein. The bevel of the needle is upward when the opening in the needle is visible when you look straight down on the needle as it is inserted into the skin. The needle should be inserted at a 15-degree angle to the surface of the skin (Figure 28-10). This technique allows the point of the needle to enter the skin first with little drag or bunching up of the skin, thereby reducing the pain of the puncture.

The holder for the needle makes the task of collecting the blood sample easier. The holder is held in the same manner as you would hold the barrel of a syringe. The holders come in two sizes, one size for adult venipuncture and one size for small diameter tubes used on pediatric patients (Figure 28-11). The holders have

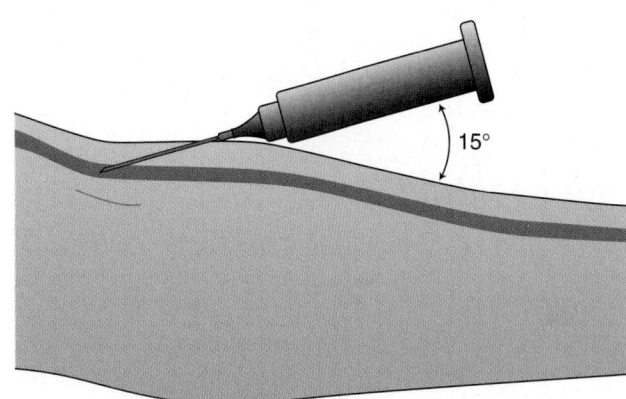

Figure 28-10 Proper angle of needle insertion for venipuncture.

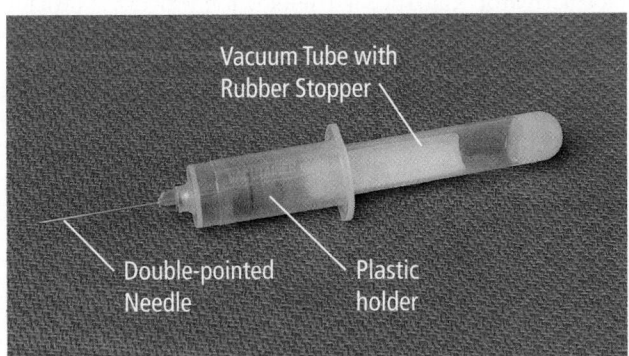

Figure 28-8 Evacuated tube blood-collection system.

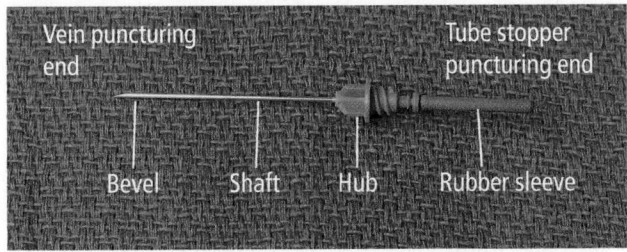

Figure 28-9 Needle for evacuated-tube system.

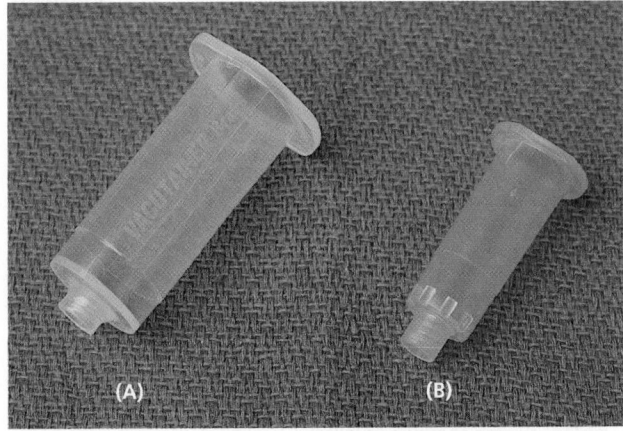

Figure 28-11 Holders for evacuated-tube system: (A) Adult holder. (B) Pediatric holder.

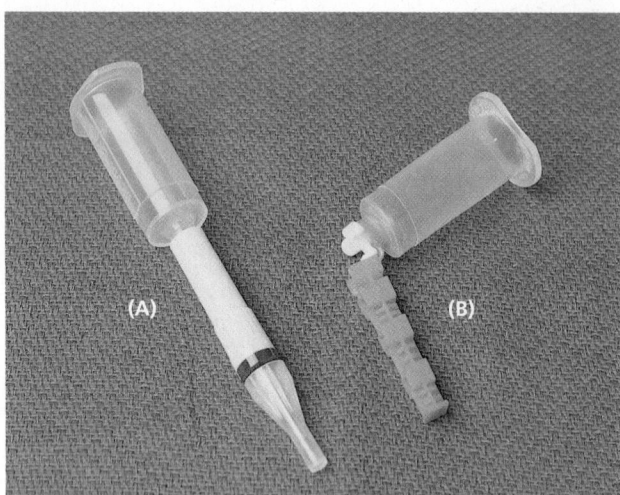

Figure 28-12 Safety tube holders: (A) Safety needle and holder. (B) Locking cover.

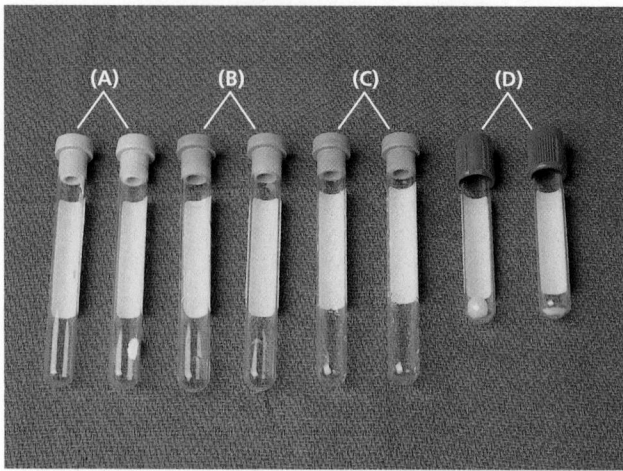

Figure 28-13 Basic anticoagulant tubes: (A) Gray: anti-glycocytic agent. (B) Light blue: citrate. (C) Lavender: EDTA. (D) Green: heparin. (A), (B), and (C) are B-D Vacutainer tubes with conventional stoppers. (D) is a B-D Vacutainer tube with Hemogard closure.

changed in recent years from the basic holders to include safety holders with outer sleeves that slide over the contaminated needle or covers that snap closed over the contaminated needle. The outer sleeve or locking cover protects the medical assistant from needlesticks until the needle and holder can be discarded into a puncture-proof container (Figure 28-12).

Anticoagulants

Different tests require different types of blood specimens. Some specimens require a serum sample and need to be drawn in a tube that allows the blood to clot. Others require a whole blood or plasma specimen and need to be drawn in a tube that does not allow the blood to clot. To prevent the clotting of the blood, the tube contains an anticoagulant. An anticoagulant is a chemical substance that prevents the clotting by removing calcium in the form of calcium salts or by inhibiting the conversion of prothrombin to thrombin. Coagulation occurs naturally according to the steps in Table 28-2. If a step is prevented, the blood does not clot.

The process of clotting can be prevented in the sample tube. A tube containing an anticoagulant removes one of the steps in the process, preventing the blood from clotting. The step removed depends on the anticoagulant

TABLE 28-2	STEPS TO BLOOD CLOTTING
1. Uncoagulated blood
2. Calcium utilized
3. Prothrombin converts to thrombin
4. Fibrinogen converts to fibrin
5. Clot forms

used. The basic anticoagulants used consist of oxalates, citrates, ethylenediaminetetraacetic acid (EDTA), or heparin (Figure 28-13). Anticoagulants are identified by tube color. It is important to use the correct anticoagulant for the test because the improper anticoagulant can alter test results (Table 28-3).

Various **additives** are used to improve the quality of the specimen. These additives are not anticoagulants or preservatives but are used to improve specimen quality or accelerate specimen processing. Some serum tubes have a clot activator that speeds the clotting process. The clot activator consists of silica (small glass) particles on the sides of the tubes that initiate the clotting process. The silica particles work as a catalyst for the clotting process by helping the clotting process to start.

A type of clot activator that is used for STAT (emergency) testing is thrombin. The thrombin is in the tube to chemically increase the speed of the clotting process and to hasten the complete formation of the clot.

Serum and plasma tubes can also be purchased with a **thixotrophic separator gel** (Figure 28-14). The gel is an inert material that undergoes a temporary change in **viscosity** during centrifugation. When centrifuged, the gel changes to a liquid and moves up the sides of the tube to engulf the cells or clot. The gel forms a solid plug and separates the cells/clot from the plasma/serum (Figure 28-15).

Tourniquets

The **tourniquet**, when applied to the arm, constricts the flow of blood in the arm and makes the veins more prominent. The tourniquet is a soft, pliable, rubber or elastic strip approximately 1 inch wide by 15 to 18 inches long.

TABLE 28-3   TUBE GUIDE

Tube stopper color*	Additive	Additive Action	Laboratory Use
Gray (1,2)	Potassium oxalate	Binds calcium	Glucose test/Alcohol levels
	Fluoride	Inhibits glycolysis	
	Iodoacetate	Inhibits glycolysis	
	Lithium heparin	Inhibits prothrombin to thrombin	
Light Blue (1,2)	Sodium citrate	Binds calcium	Used for coagulation studies. Tubes must be filled to the proper level
Lavender (1,2)	Ethylenediamine-tetraacetic acid (EDTA)	Binds calcium	Hematology testing—Complete blood count
Green (1,2)	Lithium heparin	Inhibits prothrombin to thrombin	Plasma determinations in chemistry
	Sodium heparin		
Royal Blue (1,2)	Sodium heparin	Inhibits prothrombin to thrombin	Plasma toxicology/Trace elements
	No additive	Clot forms	Serum toxicology/Trace elements
Yellow/Gray (1) Orange (2)	Thrombin	Fast clot formation	STAT serum determinations
Red (1,2)	No additive	Clot forms	Serum testing
Yellow (1,2)	SPS (sodium polyanetholesulfonate)	Binds calcium	Blood cultures
		Aids in recovery of microorganisms	
Red/gray (1) Gold (2)	Clot activator and thixotropic gel	Serum separator	Serum determination in chemistry
Brown (1,2)	Sodium heparin	Inhibits prothrombin to thrombin	Lead determination

*Tube stopper colors on Becton-Dickinson Vacutainer® brand tubes. (1) Color of conventional stopper, (2) Color of Hemogard closure.

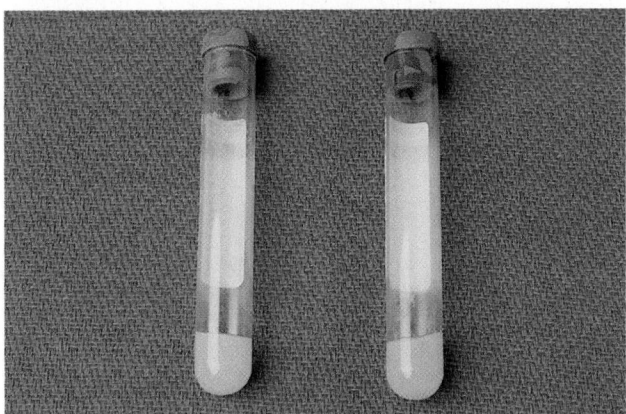

Figure 28-14   Thixotrophic gel tubes.

The rubber strip serves as the best tourniquet for all conditions. Velcro strips are also available. The Velcro strip cannot be cleaned easily and is too expensive to dispose of after each use. The rubber strip can easily be released with one hand. Being about 1 inch wide, it does not cut into the patient's arm but distributes the pressure. The tourniquet can easily be wiped off with alcohol to prevent spreading of infection and is inexpensive enough that it can be replaced often (Figure 28-16). If a patient has been identified as having a latex hypersensitivity, you must use a nonlatex tourniquet.

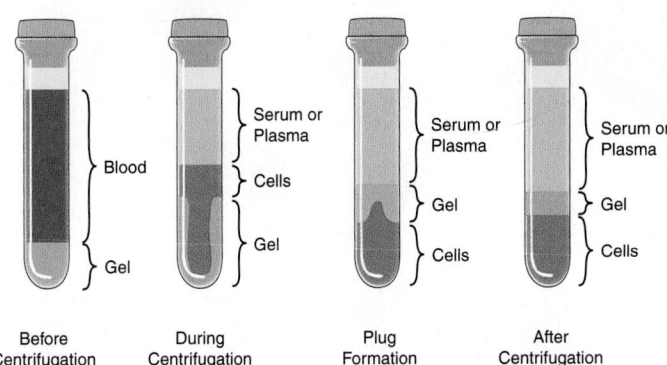

Figure 28-15   Separator gel tube: centrifugation process.

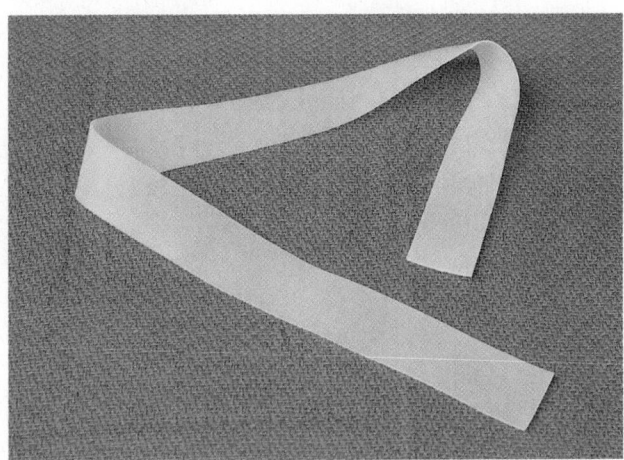

Figure 28-16   Soft rubber tourniquet.

A blood pressure cuff can also be used as a tourniquet. Its use is primarily for veins that are difficult to locate using a standard tourniquet. The blood pressure should be taken first and then the cuff should be maintained slightly below the diastolic pressure.

Specimen Collection Trays

The medical assistant may need a specimen collection tray to hold all the equipment necessary for proper specimen collection. The tray can be taken to the patient in the examination room so that whatever procedure is performed the phlebotomy can be conducted without searching for the proper equipment. The trays vary depending on the type of collections done. Since the tray is also used to transport blood specimens, the OSHA Bloodborne Pathogen Standard requires the tray be all red in color or prominently labeled with an approved biohazard symbol. In some cases, a tray will not be adequate and there will be the need for a stocked cart to roll from exam room to exam room. The tray is usually preferred because it is more portable and can easily be taken to the patient. The trays come in a variety of sizes and shapes to better fit the preference and needs of the individual collecting the blood sample (Figure 28-17). Most medical assistants will not need a tray or cart. The equipment will be in a special drawer for venipuncture equipment in each examination room or in a central lab area.

VENIPUNCTURE TECHNIQUE

Venipuncture is a detailed process that consists of many steps (Table 28-4).

TABLE 28-4 STEPS IN VENIPUNCTURE
1. Identify the patient.
2. Verify diet/drug restrictions; e.g., fasting vs. nonfasting.
3. Wash hands. Put on gloves, as well as safety glasses and mask if there is a potential for blood splatter.
4. Assemble supplies and inspect equipment.
5. Reassure the patient.
6. Position the patient.
7. Verify paperwork and tubes.
8. Perform venipuncture.
9. Fill the tubes (if syringe and needle are used).
10. Bandage the patient's arm.
11. Dispose of sharps in the proper container.
12. Label the tubes.
13. Remove gloves, safety glasses, and mask, and wash hands.
14. Chill specimen (only for certain tests).
15. Eliminate diet restrictions.
16. Process paperwork.
17. Send correctly labeled tubes to the office laboratory or prepare them to be sent to a reference laboratory.

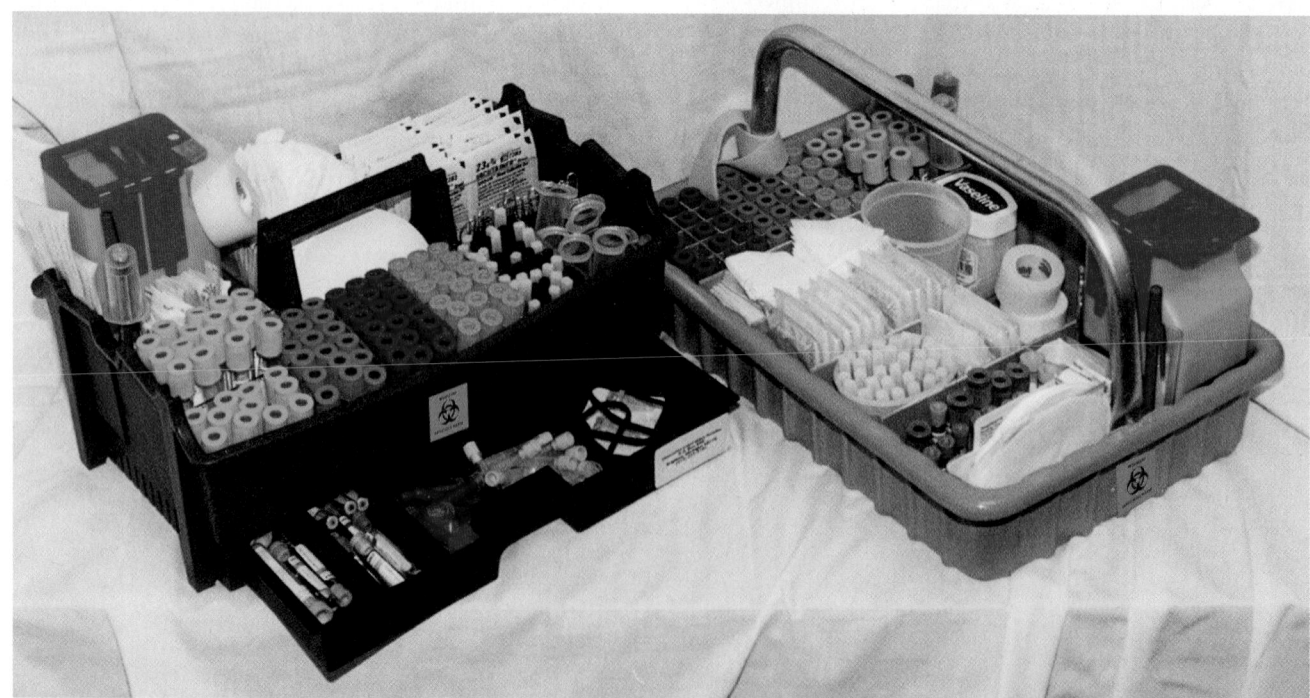

Figure 28-17 Two types of stocked phlebotomy trays.

Approaching the Patient

The medical assistant uses many skills when interacting with patients during phlebotomy. Three of the skills used are:

1. Social skills
2. Technical skills
3. Administrative skills

Social skills are used by the medical assistant to obtain cooperation from the patient. Some patients will be calm while others may be extremely frightened. The nicest patient may be irritable and may even become physically and/or emotionally abusive when placed in the unfamiliar health care setting. The medical assistant uses social skills to put the patient at ease, allay the patient's fears, and persuade the patient to allow blood to be drawn.

After calming the patient and explaining the procedure, the medical assistant uses technical skills to perform the phlebotomy with a minimum of pain to the patient. As important as it is to obtain a good specimen, it is equally important to treat the patient with empathy. Using social and technical skills, the medical assistant can provide a positive experience for the patient. A patient who has had a positive experience will talk with friends and neighbors about that experience, which could result in new patients for the physician's office, the clinic, or the laboratory.

For the medical assistant, administrative skills involve drawing the correct patient's blood and correctly labeling the specimen. Incorrect labeling constitutes the greatest number of errors in phlebotomy. All patient specimens must be positively identified on the **primary container**, the container that holds the specimen, to avoid any errors in reporting of results, thereby affecting patient diagnosis or treatment.

Preparing Supplies and Greeting the Patient

Prepare all supplies and equipment prior to the venipuncture. Place all tubes within easy reach in order to avoid crossing over the patient and possibly moving the needle after it is in the patient. Remember that occasionally a tube will not fill completely; therefore, it is best to keep a few spare tubes or have the phlebotomy tray within reach. The first step to a successful venipuncture is to put the patient at ease.

Patient and Specimen Identification

Proper patient and specimen identification is essential to accurate patient testing. The results of specimen testing will be incorrect if the specimen is not accurately identified. When entering the room, do not say, "Mr. Jones, I'm

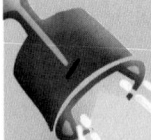

SPOTLIGHT ON AAMA ESSENTIALS THROUGH CAAHEP

- Maintaining a smile and offering a kind word can allay a patient's fear and do a lot toward winning a long-term patient for the physician's office.

- When performing a venipuncture, the medical assistant should be friendly, outgoing, and explain the procedure to the patient.

- Genuine concern for patients generally results in happier patients who choose the same physician for care in the future.

here to draw your blood," assuming if the patient says "Yes" this is Mr. Jones. The patient may not have been paying attention and may answer yes even if it is not his name. Ask the patient to state his full name. If the patient is in the hospital, a check of the patient's wristband is essential.

Greeting the Patient

1. Reassure the patient that the procedure is going to be simple and there will only be a slight inconvenience.
2. Be friendly, outgoing, and talk to the patient, explaining the procedure. Polite conversation with all patients gives them the feeling someone cares about them.
3. Do not tell the patient that the procedure will not be painful.
4. Exhibit concern for patients, as this will result in happier patients who will return in the future for care from the same physician.

Once the medical assistant has identified the patient and the blood is drawn, the specimen needs proper identification. The patient's first and last name, any assigned identification number, the date, the time, and the initials of the person collecting the specimen must be written on the tube immediately after drawing the patient's blood. Label the tubes before leaving the patient's presence. By doing so, if the tubes are taken to the physician's office laboratory or an outside reference laboratory, the specimens will be properly identified. Any paperwork or forms accompanying the specimens must be checked with the blood tubes to verify that names and numbers match.

Many offices are using various types of computer systems for test ordering and result reporting. The computer label has several advantages in that it lists the specific tests that are ordered and the required specimen and specimen requirements. The label can also be adhesive so it can be attached directly to the tube. Smaller labels can also be printed at the same time for smaller aliquot specimens. An **aliquot** specimen is a portion of a specimen that has been taken for use or storage. The computer has multiple advantages in timing the printing of orders, sorting lists of orders for one patient at one time, and speeding entry of draw times and test results. The computer labels print off in a roll with one label following the other. Two attached labels (Figure 28-18) require special attention. One label must be checked carefully with the other to assure that each label is for the same person, date, and time. Labels may also contain bar codes to assist in electronic patient and specimen identification. With computerized systems, the medical assistant will verify by entering information into the computer when the blood is drawn.

Positioning the Patient

The position of the patient is critical for proper patient blood collection. The best position is the position that is comfortable for the patient and the health care professional. Proper positioning of the patient will make the patient feel more at ease and facilitate the performance of the venipuncture.

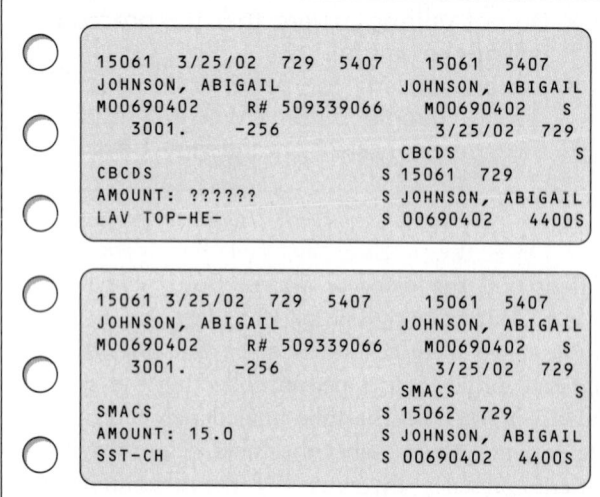

Figure 28-18 Adhesive computer labels for identifying specimen tubes from one patient.

Positioning the Patient

Before a patient's blood is drawn, discuss with the patient any previous problems with blood being taken. Usually one of two situations must be addressed:
1. Patient that does not have a problem with having blood drawn.
   a. The patient must be in a seated or reclining position before any attempt is made to draw blood.
   b. Do not allow the patient to sit on a tall stool or stand while drawing blood. There is always the possibility that the patient will faint (syncope) and be injured.
   c. The sitting position requires a chair with adequate arm supports that are adjustable for the best venipuncture position.
2. Patient who will faint (syncope).
   a. Apprehensive patients and patients who indicate they have fainted in the past when having blood drawn should be instructed to lie down.
   b. The reclining position is the ideal position from which to draw a blood sample from the patient.
   c. A pillow may be required to help support the patient's arm by keeping it straight for easier venous access.

Selecting the Appropriate Venipuncture Site

The appropriate venipuncture site can vary depending on the patient. The usual site that is first checked is the antecubital region of the arm. The primary vein used in the antecubital region of the arm is the median cubital vein. This is usually the prominent vein in the middle of the bend of the arm. Refer back to Figure 28-4. The basilic, cephalic, or median vein can be used as an alternative. These veins may not be accessible or may not be prominent enough to obtain a blood sample. The next step is to go to the back of the hand to determine other possibilities. The veins in the back of the hand have the tendency to "roll" more than the arm veins because they are not supported by as much tissue and are closer to the surface. To avoid this, the vein will have to be held in place by the index finger and the thumb while a smaller gauge needle or a butterfly is used. The hand veins are ideal for a 3–5 cc syringe with a 22 gauge needle. Careful, slow pulling on the syringe will obtain the blood sample without collapsing the vein or hemolyzing the blood. The veins at the back of the wrist are also an alternative, but they are generally much more painful than the other sites. The foot and ankle veins may also be used if the patient's physician gives permission to use them. The veins in the foot or ankle will also have the tendency to "roll." The medical assistant will in all likelihood never draw from the foot or ankle, but this is an area that will give an acceptable blood sample when all other attempts have failed.

The order for checking for the best available site is (1) antecubital region of the arm, (2) back of hand, (3) back of wrist, and (4) ankle or foot. The next alternative is to have a more experienced medical assistant check. If venous access is not possible, draw the sample by capillary puncture.

A tourniquet must be used to assist the medical assistant in feeling a vein. The tourniquet is applied 3–4 inches above the intended puncture site. It is applied tightly enough to stop the flow of blood in the veins but not so tightly as to prevent the flow of blood in the arteries (Figures 28-19A–D). This is similar to damming a small stream. When a stream is dammed, the water forms a pond in front of the dam. With the tourniquet applied, the veins fill with blood, pooling in the veins below the tourniquet. This pooling of blood makes the veins more prominent. The veins can then be **palpated** (examined with the fingertips) to determine their direction, depth, and size. The tourniquet should be on the arm no longer than one minute. A stream will become stagnant when it no longer flows. A tourniquet that is left on too long will cause **hemoconcentration** of the blood, an increased concentration of constituents in the blood sample that may lead to inaccurate test results. If the patient has very sensitive skin or a skin problem, the tourniquet should be applied over the patient's upper arm clothing or a piece of gauze pad. This will minimize the discomfort felt by the patient.

The tourniquet often causes greater discomfort for patients than the venipuncture itself. The tourniquet should ideally be removed as soon as blood flow is established. This is not practical for the novice medical assistant. The act of removing the tourniquet may move the needle and/or vein just enough so that no more blood can be obtained and a second venipuncture must be performed. It is recommended to wait until just before the needle is removed from the patient to remove the tourniquet. If the tourniquet is not removed before the needle is removed, the patient will bleed heavily. Blood will be forced out of the needle hole and into the surrounding tissue, resulting in a **hematoma** (an accumulation of blood around the venipuncture site).

Performing a Safe Venipuncture

The first step in collecting a venous blood specimen is to find the site that will give the best blood return. The vein

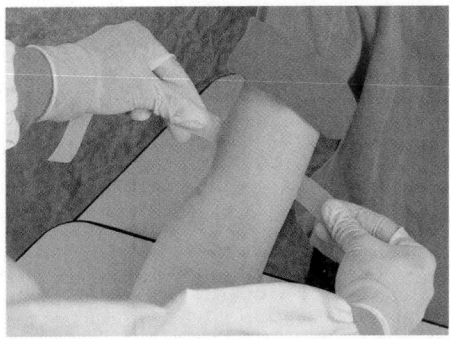

Figure 28-19A   Wrap the tourniquet around the arm 3 to 4 inches above the venipuncture site. Keeping the tourniquet flat to the skin will help minimize the discomfort felt by the patient.

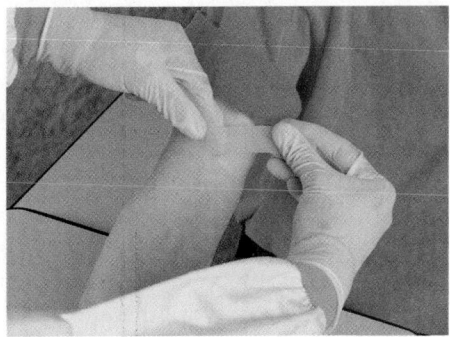

Figure 28-19B   Stretch the tourniquet tight and cross the ends.

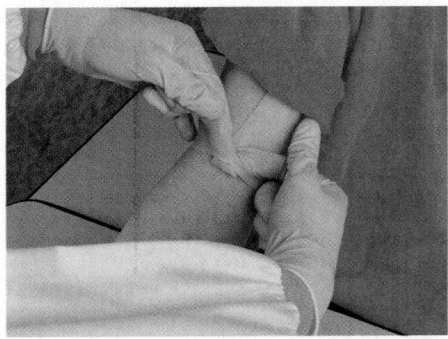

Figure 28-19C   While holding the ends tight, tuck one portion of the tourniquet under the other.

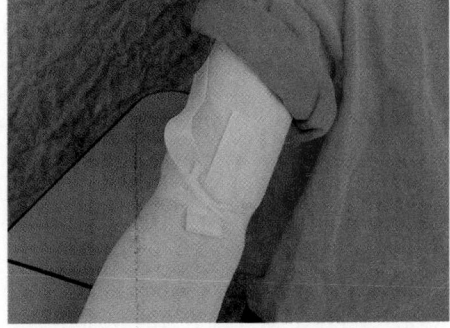

Figure 28-19D   Check that the tourniquet will not come loose. The ends of the tourniquet should be pointed upward and not hang into the intended venipuncture site.

must be palpated with the tip of the index finger. Feel for and trace the path of the vein several times. Avoid using the thumb because it has a pulse and is not as sensitive as the rest of the fingers. The vein will feel soft and bouncy to the touch. The roundness of the vein and the direction it follows may be determined. All veins are not straight up and down the arm. If no veins become prominent, retie the tourniquet tighter but not so tightly as to stop the flow of arterial blood into the arm. If the tourniquet is tied tightly enough to stop arterial blood flow, the patient will no longer have a pulse in the wrist. If this occurs, immediately remove the tourniquet as this indicates that blood has ceased flowing below the tourniquet.

If the "vein" that is felt has a pulsing action to it, it is an artery, not a vein, and the vessel should not be punctured. Tendons can be deceptive and give the appearance of veins. They do not have the soft, bouncy feel and will be hard to the touch. Puncturing a tendon will give no blood return and will be painful to the patient. Nerves also run the length of the arm. The nerves cannot be seen or felt, but by avoiding deep probing venipunctures, the chance of puncturing a nerve will be diminished. If the patient complains that the venipuncture is extremely painful, it is best to stop and try another site.

Veins of edematous arms, which are swollen due to fluid in the tissue, will not be prominent and the tourniquet will not be effective because of the swelling. Using the tourniquet in this instance may cause tissue damage. It leaves a temporary indentation in the arm. Areas of scarring should also be avoided due to possible injury or excessive pain to the patient. Specimens collected from an area of a hematoma may cause erroneous test results. If another vein site is not available, the specimen is collected distal from the hematoma. Because of the potential for harm to the patient due to lymphostasis (the stoppage of the flow of lymph), the arm on the side of a mastectomy should be avoided. If the patient has had a double mastectomy, a physician should be consulted prior to drawing the blood.

Syringe Specimen Collection

The patient has been identified, paperwork and tubes have been verified, equipment has been assembled, and the patient is in a comfortable position. Handwashing is the most critical step to preventing the spread of infection. Before touching the patient, medical assistants should wash their hands. It is good practice to wash your hands in view of the patient to give the patient confidence in your technique. The next step is to tie the tourniquet. Have the patient close the hand and then select a vein. If possible, place the patient's arm in a downward position. After locating an acceptable vein, mentally map the location. Set mental sites on the vein by visualizing the puncture site as the target for an accurate puncture. Cleanse the site with a gauze pad wet with 70 percent isopropyl alcohol solution. A commercially prepared alcohol pad or one with 0.5 percent chlorhexidine in alcohol may also be used. Clean the skin in a circular motion from the center of the intended puncture site to the outside. Allow the area to air dry to prevent hemolysis of the specimen and to prevent the patient from feeling a burning sensation from the puncture.

Some authorities suggest putting on gloves first and then palpating for the vein. This technique is required for the patient who is isolated due to a communicable disease and is good practice for all patients. Standard precautions require that personal protective equipment be worn when there is a chance of coming in contact with blood and body fluid. If the patient has veins that are difficult to palpate, the gloves may be put on after the site has been palpated and before the cleansing. To avoid forgetting where the collection site is, palpate the vein 1–2 inches above and below the intended puncture site. It helps the medical assistant feel that the vein is located in a straight line and these points can be used to "reset" the mental crosshairs without contaminating the venipuncture site. Safety glasses and a mask must be worn if there is a potential for blood spatter.

The syringe technique is used less often than the evacuated tube system. The techniques developed in the syringe method are building blocks for the evacuated tube technique and all other techniques that the medical assistant uses for obtaining a blood specimen.

The syringe is ideal for collecting small volumes of blood from fragile surface veins such as veins in the back

---

Correct Hand Position to Hold a Syringe

1. The needle is attached to the syringe.
2. Hold the syringe and needle system in your dominant hand, cradling it on your four fingers. A right-handed person would hold the syringe in the right hand, leaving the left hand to pull on the plunger. A left-handed person would do the opposite.
3. Place the thumb on top of the syringe (Figure 28-20).
4. With the syringe held in this position, turn it slightly so the bevel of the needle is facing up.
5. Hold the hand in such a position that by tilting the point of the needle down slightly the needle will enter the skin at a 15 degree angle and about 0.5 cm below the point where the vein was felt.

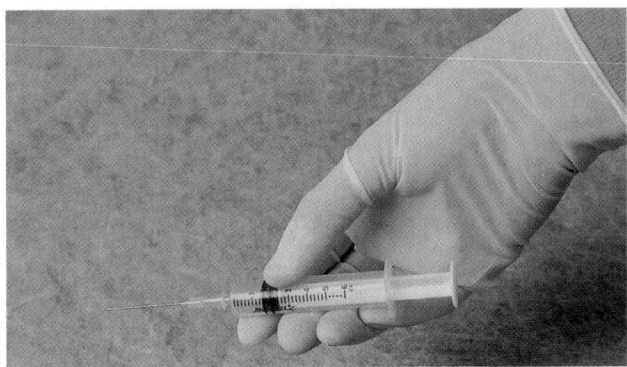

Figure 28-20   Proper hand position to hold a syringe.

of the hand. Procedure 28-2 gives detailed instructions for venipuncture with syringe.

When a syringe is used, the blood obtained must be placed in appropriate containers. To place the blood in empty evacuated tubes, puncture the stopper with the syringe needle and allow blood to enter the tube until the flow stops. Do not remove the rubber stoppers. Running blood down the side of the tube after removing the stopper is not recommended because aerosols and splattering of blood can occur. This is why masks and goggles are recommended for this type of venipuncture. Do not hold the tube in your hand as you puncture the stopper. There is the potential for missing the stopper or slipping off the stopper and puncturing yourself. The best method is to place the tubes in a test tube rack and then puncture the tubes using only one hand. The tube will fill itself; do not force the blood into the tube. This technique will maintain the proper ratio of blood to anticoagulant. Immediately upon filling, mix any tubes containing additives. The order of filling the tubes is important.

Fill sterile collection tubes first to prevent microorganism contamination. The additive tubes are filled before the nonadditive tubes to avoid contamination with microscopic clots. The blood that is last to come out of the syringe was the first blood to go in and has the poten-

tial to have started to clot. The empty syringe and needle are immediately placed into a sharps container without recapping the needle.

Evacuated Tube Specimen Collection

The evacuated tube system is an improvement over the syringe method yet maintains many similarities. When the syringe method is used, a vacuum is created as the medical assistant pulls on the syringe plunger. The evacuated tube method has the vacuum already in the tube. Another advantage of the evacuated tube system is that with multiple blood samples, syringes do not need to be changed; only the tubes need to be changed.

The similarity between the evacuated tube system and the syringe system is that the holder and needle are held in the same manner (Figure 28-21). The syringe is held in a manner that allows the medical assistant access to pull on the plunger. Access must be left in the evacuated tube system for one tube to be pulled out and another inserted. The hand that pulled on the plunger of the syringe is the hand that changes tubes with the evacuated tube system.

The procedure for venipuncture with the evacuated tube system follows the same steps as the syringe method with only slight variations.

With multiple tube draws, the order of drawing the tubes is important. Check with the tube manufacturer for the recommended order of draw. The National Committee for Clinical Laboratory Standards (NCCLS) recommends the following order of draw from a single venipuncture using the evacuated tube system.

Order of Filling Tubes from a Syringe

1. Blood culture tubes or bottles (sterile procedures)
2. Coagulation "citrate" tube (blue tube)
3. Heparin tube (green tube)
4. EDTA tube (lavender tube)
5. Oxalate/fluoride tube (gray tube)
6. Nonadditive "clot" tubes (red stoppered or gel tubes)

Evacuated Tube System Order of Draw

Purpose: Avoid possible test result error due to cross contamination from tube additives.

1. Blood culture tubes or bottles (for sterile procedures)
2. Tubes without additives (e.g., red stopper)
3. Tubes with additives:
   - Coagulation studies, citrate tube (e.g., light blue stopper)
   - Gel separator tube (red/gray or gold stopper)
   - Heparin (green stopper)
   - EDTA (lavendar stopper)
   - Other additives (gray stopper)

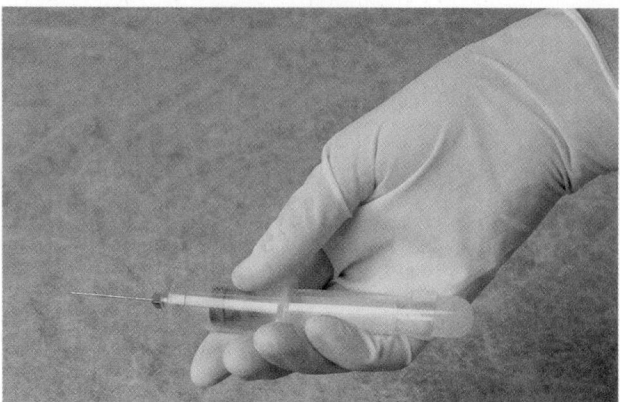

Figure 28-21 Proper hand position to hold an evacuated tube system.

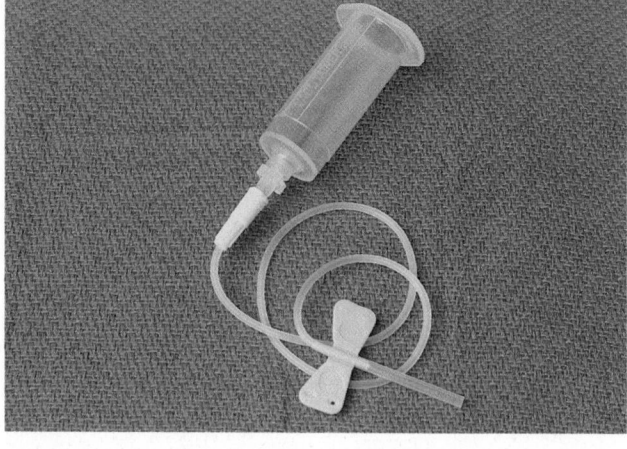

Figure 28-22 Butterfly needle assembly.

Butterfly Collection System

A system that combines benefits of the syringe system and the evacuated tube system is the butterfly collection system. The butterfly collection system has on one end a 21, 23, or 25 gauge needle with attached plastic wings. Six or twelve inches of tubing leads from the needle. On the other end of this tubing is a hub that can attach to a syringe. A needle covered by a rubber sleeve can also be attached to the tubing. The covered needle screws into an evacuated tube holder (Figure 28-22).

The butterfly system is used for small veins that are difficult to puncture with the evacuated tube system and standard evacuated tube system needle. The system also facilitates drawing from veins that have a tendency to collapse. The winged needle of the butterfly needle will slide into a small surface vein in the back of the hand, wrist, or foot. Instead of entering the vein at the usual 15 degree angle, the winged needle is inserted at approximately a 5 degree angle and then threaded into the vein. This procedure anchors the needle in the center of a small vein that is inaccessible by other methods. If the patient moves, the tubing gives flexibility so the needle will stay anchored and not pull out of the vein. The butterfly collection set works well on children who have small veins and the tendency to move while blood is being collected.

The system also gives the adaptability of initiating a draw with a syringe and then finishing it with the evacuated tube system. A syringe can be filled for procedures that require a syringe sample. It can then be removed, and the evacuated tube system can be attached for multiple tube collection. Although the butterfly collection system has many benefits, it is not used for all collections. It is much more expensive than the needle system. The additional expense is unnecessary for the majority of venipunctures.

Patient Reactions

Patients can have a variety of reactions to having their blood drawn. The medical assistant must anticipate these reactions and respond appropriately as quickly as possible. The most common patient reaction is pain. The patient will indicate that the venipuncture is painful. Slightly reposition the needle and then loosen the tourniquet. Loosening the tourniquet often helps because the tourniquet may be pinching the arm and causing discomfort rather than the needle. Avoid deep, probing venipunctures because they may go deeply into the arm and get too close to the nerves. If the pain persists, discontinue the venipuncture.

Other possible patient reactions and the medical assistant's appropriate responses are shown in Table 28-5.

The Unsuccessful Venipuncture

When a blood sample cannot be obtained, it may be necessary to change the position of the needle. Rotate the needle half a turn. The bevel of the needle may be against the wall of the vein. If the needle has not penetrated the vein far enough, advance it further into the vein. Advance it only slightly; a small change may mean the difference between a failed and a successful venipuncture. If the needle has penetrated too far into the vein, pull back a little. Always withdraw the needle slowly when the venipuncture has been unsuccessful. The blood often may start coming just as it seems the needle is ready to come out of the skin. The tube used may not have sufficient vacuum. Try another tube before withdrawing the needle. Methods of vein stimulation are shown in Table 28-6.

Probing the site is not recommended. Probing is painful to the patient and may cause a hematoma. Never attempt a venipuncture more than two times. If a blood

TABLE 28-5 PATIENT REACTIONS TO BLOOD DRAWS

Patient Reaction	Medical Assistant Response
1. Syncope (fainting)	Immediately remove the needle and stop the patient from falling. Lower the patient's head and arms. Wipe the patient's forehead and back of the neck with a cold compress if necessary. Pass an ammonia inhalant 4 to 5 inches away from the patient's nose (the patient will respond by coughing). If the patient still does not respond, notify a physician, move the patient to the floor, and place a pillow under the patient's legs.
2. Nausea	If a patient becomes nauseated, apply cold compresses to the patient's forehead. Give the patient an emesis basin, and have facial tissues ready if the nausea does not diminish. Deep slow breathing through the mouth may help.
3. Insulin shock/ hypoglycemia	The first signs of insulin shock are a cold sweat and pallor similar to the signs of syncope. The patient becomes weak and shaky, sudden mental confusion may follow, and it appears as though the patient's personality changes instantly. Call the physician if the patient loses consciousness.
4. Convulsions	The patient loses consciousness and exhibits violent or mild convulsive motions. Do not try to restrain the patient. Move objects or furniture out of the way to prevent the patient from striking objects and being hurt. Help the patient to the floor and into a reclining position. The patient usually recovers within a few minutes. Notify the physician about the patient's reaction. The physician will determine when to release the patient.
5. Cardiac arrest	The patient lapses into unconsciousness, has no pulse or respirations, the eyes are dilated, and there may be a blue or gray skin tone. Start cardiopulmonary resuscitation (CPR) immediately to avoid patient death. Only persons certified to do CPR can perform this procedure. Immediately notify the physician.

TABLE 28-6 METHODS OF VEIN STIMULATION

1. Position the patient's arm lower than the patient's heart.
2. Reapply the tourniquet.
3. Massage the arm from wrist to elbow.
4. Tap sharply at the venipuncture site with your fingers. This will cause the veins to dilate.
5. Use a blood pressure cuff in place of the tourniquet.
6. Warm the venipuncture site with a warming device or a warm washcloth (not hotter than 42°C).

diagnosis, the blood specimen may need to be redrawn to confirm the results. This is accomplished by either retesting the specimen or collecting another sample. This will either reconfirm that the correct patient was drawn and/or that the patient's test results changed significantly.

Factors Affecting Laboratory Values

There are numerous variables that can affect laboratory test results. The specimens are tested by analytical

sample cannot be obtained after two attempts, perform a microcollection (e.g., capillary puncture) if possible. Otherwise have another person attempt the draw. Notify the patient's physician if two medical assistants have been unsuccessful and a microcollection is not possible.

Criteria for Rejection of a Specimen

The primary goal of the medical assistant is to provide an acceptable specimen for laboratory testing as required by the physician. There are certain general criteria that must be met for a specimen to be acceptable. If the criteria are not met, the specimen is rejected and another venipuncture of the patient must be performed.

Table 28-7 lists quality assurance controls for specimen collection and processing. The list is not all inclusive. The type of specimen that is acceptable and the volume required are determined by the procedure ordered. The quality control checks done by the laboratory may indicate the results are valid. If the results do not agree with what the physician believes is the patient's

TABLE 28-7 QUALITY ASSURANCE FOR SPECIMEN COLLECTION AND PROCESSING

1. Each specimen must have its own label attached to the specimen's primary container.
2. Each specimen must have the test to be performed written on the label (CBC, Cholesterol, and so on).
3. Labels must have the patient's complete name and identification number.
4. Specimens in syringes with needles still attached are unacceptable.
5. All specimens must be in the appropriate anticoagulant.
6. Blood collection tubes with anticoagulant must be at least 75 percent full. All blood collection tubes for coagulation testing must be at least 90 percent full.
7. Uncoagulated blood specimens must be free of clots.
8. Certain tests require specimens to be free of hemolysis and lipemia, a milky appearance due to lipids.
9. The specimen may need to be recollected if the results do not agree with what the physician believes is the diagnosis of the patient.

instruments that give accurate and precise results. These results will accurately reflect what is wrong with the patient only if the specimen is collected correctly. A correctly collected specimen is the responsibility of the health care worker performing the collection procedure. Patient physiological factors may also contribute to inaccurate results. Other factors that can alter results are shown in Table 28-8.

Certain specimens must be chilled immediately after collection (Table 28-9). Place the blood tube into ice as it is withdrawn from the evacuated tube holder. Any delay in icing the specimen will alter test results. The longer the delay, the greater the change.

The medical assistant is not the only person who can affect test results. The patient can knowingly or unknow-

TABLE 28-9	EXAMPLES OF COMMON TESTS REQUIRING CHILLING OF THE SPECIMEN

Ammonia
Catecholamines
Gastrin
Lactic acid
Parathyroid hormone (PTH)
pH/blood gas

ingly alter the results by certain actions. An example of this occurs when a patient has had a cup of coffee but claims not to have had anything to eat or drink. The patient is often under the misconception that black coffee without sugar will not be a problem. Coffee and smoking affect the metabolism and can affect the test results.

CAPILLARY PUNCTURE

Venipuncture is the most frequently performed phlebotomy procedure, but it is not the procedure of choice in all circumstances. An alternative to venipuncture is capillary puncture, also known as dermal puncture or skin puncture.

Capillary puncture is the method of choice with two types of patients: when patient blood volume is a concern, such as with infants, and when vein access is difficult, such as with burned or scarred patients. Capillary puncture should not be used when a patient is edematous, dehydrated, or has poor peripheral circulation.

Composition of Capillary Blood

Blood obtained via capillary puncture is a mixture of blood from arterioles, venules, capillaries, and interstitial fluid. In most instances, a capillary puncture specimen most resembles arterial blood. Warming the site prior to puncture increases the blood flow as much as sevenfold. There may be significant differences between specimens obtained by capillary puncture and those collected by venipuncture. For example, the glucose level may be increased in capillary blood, while the potassium, calcium and total protein levels may be decreased. It is therefore important to always note on the specimen when capillary blood has been obtained.

Capillary Puncture Sites

The usual site for capillary puncture in adults and children is the fingertip (Figure 28-23). In adults, the ring finger is often selected because it usually is not callused. In infants, the lateral or medial plantar surface of the heel

TABLE 28-8	FACTORS AFFECTING LABORATORY RESULTS
Factor	**Effect**
Blood alcohol	When drawing a specimen for blood alcohol testing, a nonalcohol-based antiseptic should be used to clean the venipuncture site. The cleansing alcohol may falsely elevate the test result.
Diurnal rhythm	Some specimens must be drawn at timed intervals because of medication or diurnal (daily) rhythm. The exact time of collection must be noted on the specimen.
Exercise	Strenuous short-term exercise can make the heart work harder and increase the heart enzymes. Long-term exercise such as that performed by highly trained runners can cause erroneous results due to runner's anemia.
Fasting	Patient not in fasting state when fasting is required. Results of tests will not be accurate.
Hemolysis	Destruction of red blood cell membrane and release of intercellular contents into serum/plasma can be caused by: not allowing alcohol to air dry at venipuncture site, using a needle that is too small (less than 22 gauge), forcing the blood into a vacutainer tube from a syringe, or shaking the vacutainer tube instead of mixing by gentle inversion when mixing tubes with additives.
Heparin	Incorrect heparin used that interferes with tests being run on patient.
Stress	In children, violent crying before a specimen is collected can raise the WBC count.
Tourniquet on too long	Hemoconcentration, change in chemical concentration.
Volume	Not enough blood will cause a dilution factor, which can change the size of the cells and therefore produce a variation in test results.

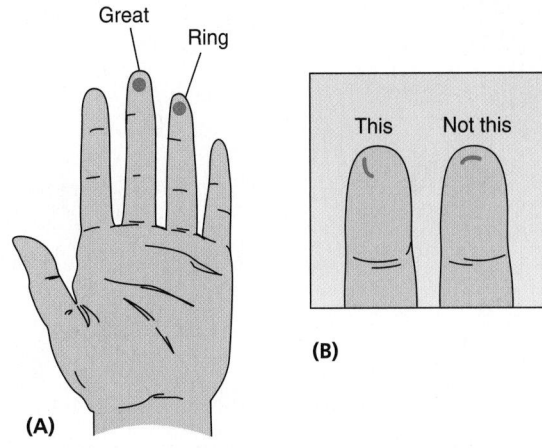

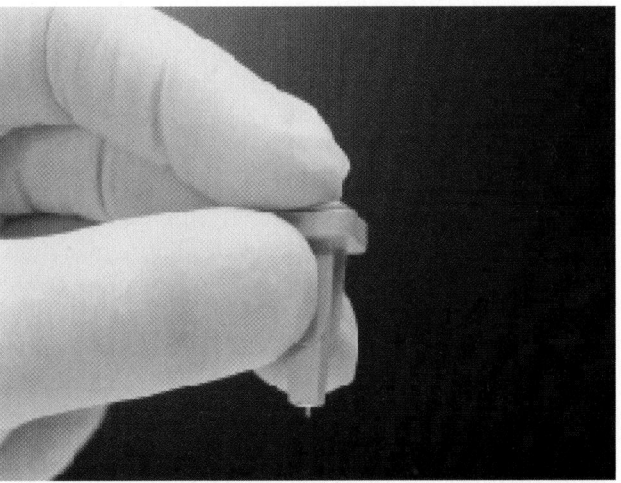

Figure 28-23 (A) Capillary blood collection sites. (B) Correct direction of capillary puncture.

pad is usually used, and the procedure is often called a heelstick. The heelstick is most often performed when testing for Phenylketonuria (PKU), which is covered in detail in Chapter 32, Specialty Laboratory Tests.

Preparing the Capillary Puncture Site

The area selected for a capillary puncture must be carefully prepared. The puncture site will be warm if blood circulation is adequate. Coolness of the skin indicates decreased circulation. To increase circulation, the site may be gently massaged or a warm, moist towel or face cloth at a temperature not higher than 42°C may be used to cover the site for three to five minutes.

Alcohol-soaked gauze or cotton should be used to cleanse and disinfect the puncture site. The site should then be allowed to air dry. Residual alcohol at the puncture site results in hemolysis of the specimen, which may affect test results as well as cause a burning sensation to the patient. Betadine (povidone iodine) should not be used to clean the puncture site. Blood contaminated with iodine may falsely elevate certain blood chemistries.

Performing the Puncture

Gloves must be worn by the medical assistant when performing the puncture. The patient's hand and finger should be held so the puncture site is readily accessible. The puncture is made at the tip of the fleshy pad and slightly to the side (Figure 28-23). The skin near the chosen site should be pulled taut. If the tips of the fingers are heavily callused or thickened, a special lancet with a longer point may be used. The puncture should be performed in one quick steady motion. Capillary punctures are performed using semiautomated devices such as the disposable MICROTAINER® Brand Safety Flow Lancet®

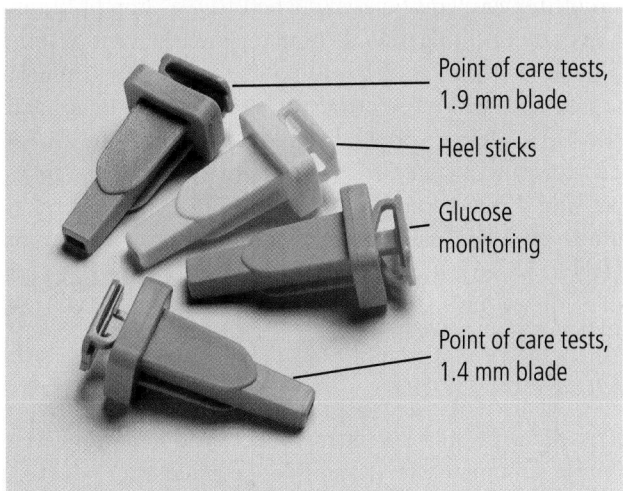

Figure 28-24 Microtainer® brand lancets are available in different types for various purposes. To use, hold lancet on skin and depress plunger with index finger to make puncture. Immediately release plunger while holding lancet on site. Discard lancet after use in biohazard container. (Courtesy of Becton-Dickinson Vacutainer Systems.)

(Figure 28-24). In the laboratory collection area, an acrylic safety shield can be placed between the patient and the medical assistant to protect the collector from blood splatters. Alternatively, safety glasses and a mask can be worn.

Collecting the Blood Sample

The first drop of blood is wiped away with dry, sterile gauze because it contains tissue fluid, which dilutes the blood drop and can also activate clotting. The second and following drops of blood are used for test samples. Depending on the tests to be performed, the blood may be collected in capillary tubes or other capillary collecting devices. Capillary tubes are glass or plastic tubes of small diameter.

It may be necessary to massage the finger to increase the blood flow. It is best to massage the whole hand, taking care not to apply direct pressure near the puncture site. Squeezing the fingertip should be avoided; this forces tissue fluid into the blood sample and dilutes it or may cause hemolysis. Do not use a scooping technique when collecting blood from the puncture site. Scooping can break the red blood cell membranes, leading to hemolysis. Allowing well-rounded drops of blood to form at the puncture site will aid in the collection process. If the flow of blood begins to slow, rewipe the puncture site with a sterile gauze pad (do not use alcohol). This will dislodge the platelet plug and cause the blood flow to increase.

The capillary tube should be held in an almost horizontal position, just tilted slightly downward. When the tip of the capillary tube is touched to the drop of blood, whether collecting directly from a patient's finger or from a collection tube, blood will enter the tube by capillary action because of the attraction between the liquid and the tube. Tubes should be filled two-thirds to three-quarters full (Figure 28-25). Usually, two to three tubes are filled from a capillary puncture. The capillary tubes are then sealed using either sealing clay or plastic caps (Figure 28-26). Manufacturer's instructions for the type of capillary tubes should be carefully followed.

Order of Draw

The order of draw for microcollection differs from that used in venipuncture. If multiple specimens are collected, EDTA specimens (lavendar caps) are collected first, then other additive specimens (green, gray caps) and lastly specimens that clot (red or gel caps).

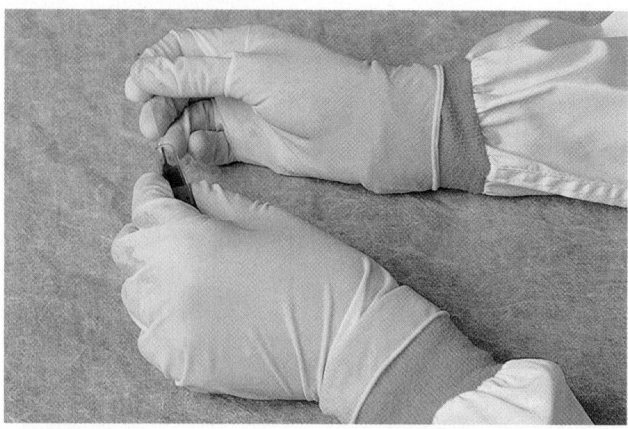

Figure 28-25   Filling a microhematocrit tube with blood by capillary action.

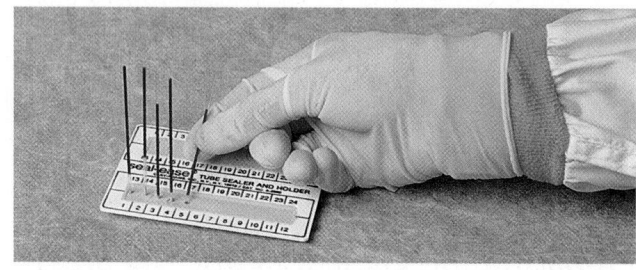

Figure 28-26   Sealing the microhematocrit tube with sealing clay.

In many ways the procedure for capillary puncture is similar to the other collection procedures discussed in this chapter, e.g., patient identification, safety precautions, specimen labeling. A detailed description of capillary puncture is found in Procedure 28-5.

Procedure

28-1   Finding a Vein in the Upper Arm

STANDARD PRECAUTIONS:

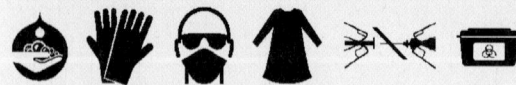

PURPOSE:
To obtain venous blood with limited discomfort to the patient.

EQUIPMENT/SUPPLIES:

Gloves	Gown or lab coat
Goggles and mask,	Tube holder
if necessary	Alcohol swab

Gauze	Tubes
Tourniquet	Bandage
Needle	Sharps container

PROCEDURE STEPS:
1. Identify the patient. Ask the patient's name and verify it with the computer label or identification number. If a fasting specimen is required, verify that the patient has not had anything to eat or drink.
2. Wash hands. Put on gloves, as well as safety glasses and mask if there is a potential for blood splatter.

(continues)

Procedure 28-1 (continued)

3. Apply tourniquet 3 to 4 inches above the venipuncture site. Apply tightly enough to stop blood flow but not so tight that blood flow in arteries is stopped. Refer to Figure 28-19.
4. Have the patient close the hand.
5. Place the patient's arm in a downward position.
6. Palpate the upper region of the arm, feeling for the median cubital, basilic, or cephalic vein with the tip of your index finger.
7. Feel for a soft bounce and a roundness to the vein. Follow the direction of the vein.
8. Feel the vein for its center and possibility of rolling.
9. After locating an acceptable vein, mentally map the location. Visualize the puncture site.
10. Clean the venipuncture site with a 70 percent isopropyl alcohol swab and complete the venous blood collection from the site.
11. If a vein cannot be found in the upper region of the arm, then the hand veins must be checked following the same procedure. The hand veins have a greater tendency to roll and venipuncture is more successful when a butterfly is used for hand vein collection.

Procedure 28-2 Venipuncture by Syringe Procedure

STANDARD PRECAUTIONS:

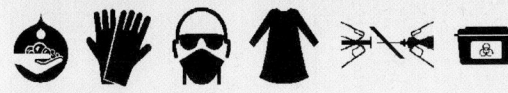

PURPOSE:

To obtain venous blood acceptable for laboratory testing as required by a physician.

SPECIMEN:

Venous blood collected to be aliquoted into evacuated tubes and/or special collection containers

EQUIPMENT/SUPPLIES:

Gloves
Safety glasses and mask, if necessary
Syringe, varies in size
Disposable needle for syringe, 21 or 22 gauge needle
Evacuated tube(s) or special collection tube(s)
Tourniquet
70% isopropyl alcohol swab
Gauze or cotton balls
Adhesive bandage or tape
Sharps container
Test tube rack

PROCEDURE STEPS:

1. Position and identify the patient. Ask the patient's name and verify it with the computer label or identification number.
2. If a fasting specimen is required, verify that the patient has not had anything to eat or drink.
3. Wash hands.
4. Put on gloves, as well as goggles and mask if there is a potential for blood splatter.
5. Open the sterile needle and syringe packages, attaching the needle if necessary.
6. Prevent the plunger from sticking by pulling it halfway out and pushing it all the way in one time.
7. Select the proper tube(s) to transfer the blood to after collection.
8. Select a site and apply the tourniquet (Figure 28-27A).
9. Ask the patient to close the hand. The patient must not be allowed to pump the hand. Pumping of the hand will change the values of the laboratory tests being collected. Place the patient's arm in a downward position if possible.

(continues)

Procedure

28-2   *(continued)*

10. Select a vein, noting the location and direction of the vein. The median cubital vein is most commonly used.
11. Clean the venipuncture site with a 70 percent isopropyl alcohol swab in a circular motion from the center outward (Figure 28-27B).
12. Do not touch the venipuncture site.
13. Draw the patient's skin taut with your thumb. Place the thumb 1 to 2 inches below or above the puncture site (Figure 28-27C). This will anchor the vein.
14. With the bevel up, line up the needle with the vein and perform the venipuncture (Figure 28-27D).
15. Do not enter at the exact location at which the vein is felt. Enter the vein approximately ¼ inch below the vein location. The bevel of the needle must enter the skin at the point where the vein was palpated. Push the needle into the skin. A sensation of resistance will be followed by easy penetration as the vein is entered. This is known as feeling the "pop." Once this point is reached, stop and do not move.
16. Take the opposite hand and pull on the plunger of the syringe. Pull gently and only as fast as the syringe will fill with blood. Pulling too hard or fast will cause temporary collapse of the vein. If the vein does collapse, stop pulling on the plunger and let the vein refill with blood (Figure 28-27E).
17. Pull the plunger back until the desired amount of blood has been obtained.
18. Ask the patient to open the hand.
19. Release the tourniquet (Figure 28-27F).
20. Lightly place a sterile gauze square or cotton ball above the venipuncture site.
21. Remove the needle from the arm (Figure 28-27G).
22. Apply pressure to the site for 3 to 5 minutes. The patient may assist if able by elevating the arm above heart level (Figure 28-27H). The arm should be held in a raised, outstretched position. Do not allow the patient to bend the arm at the elbow. Bending the arm at the elbow to apply pressure may lead to a hematoma.
23. Aliquot blood into appropriate tube(s). Tubes should be held in a test tube rack. Puncture the stopper of the evacuated tube with the syringe needle and allow the blood to enter the tube until the flow stops. Mix if any anticoagulant is present.

(continues)

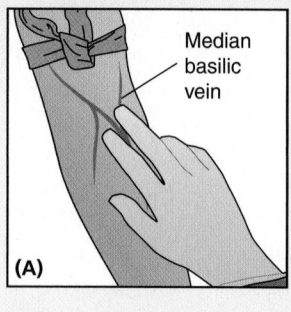
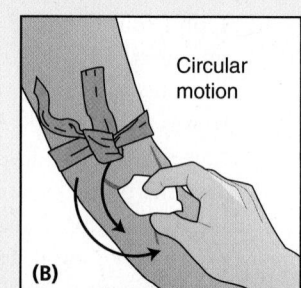
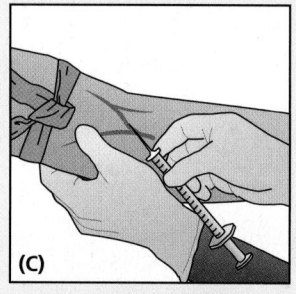
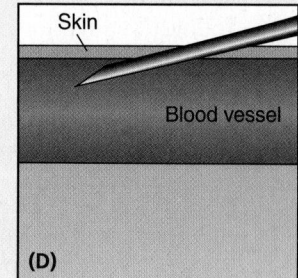
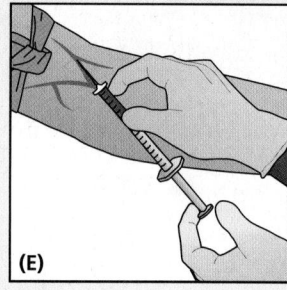
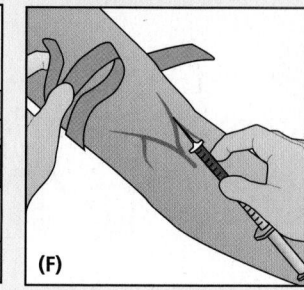
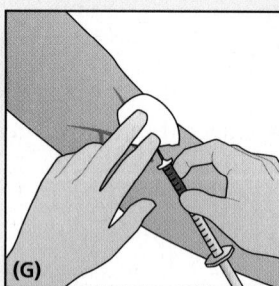
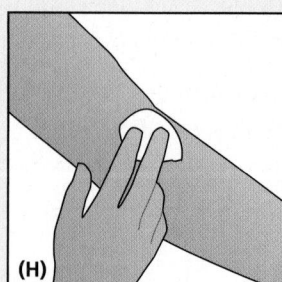

Figure 28-27   (A) Find vein and apply tourniquet.
(B) Apply alcohol and allow to air dry.
(C) Draw skin taut and insert needle.
(D) Needle entering the blood vessel.
(E) Withdraw blood slowly.
(F) Release tourniquet.
(G) Apply sterile pad before withdrawing needle.
(H) Have patient apply pressure to the site until clot forms.

Procedure 28-2 (continued)

24. Immediately discard the syringe and needle in the appropriate containers; e.g., needle to sharps container.
25. Discard the gauze and other waste in biohazard containers.
26. Label all tubes before leaving the examination room.
27. Apply an adhesive bandage (Figure 28-27I).
28. Remove and discard gloves and mask in a biohazard container.
29. Wash hands.
30. Thank the patient.
31. Document procedure.

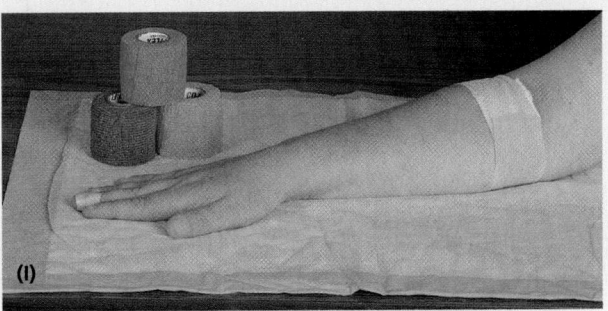

Figure 28-27 *(continued)* (I) Adhesive bandages for venipuncture are available in a variety of colors.

Procedure 28-3 Venipuncture by Evacuated Tube System

STANDARD PRECAUTIONS:

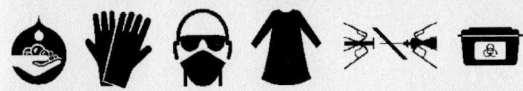

PURPOSE:
To obtain venous blood acceptable for laboratory testing as required by a physician.

SPECIMEN
Venous blood collected by evacuated tubes. Volume of blood dependent on size of tube and test requirements.

EQUIPMENT/SUPPLIES:

Gloves
Goggles and mask, if necessary
Evacuated tube holder
Disposable needle for evacuated tube system, 20, 21, or 22 gauge needle

Evacuated tube(s) or special collection tube(s)
Tourniquet
70% isopropyl alcohol swab
Gauze or cotton balls
Adhesive bandage or tape
Sharps container

PROCEDURE STEPS:
1. Position and identify the patient. Ask the patient's name and verify it with the computer label or identification number.
2. If a fasting specimen is required, verify that the patient has not had anything to eat or drink.
3. Wash hands.
4. Put on gloves, as well as goggles and mask if there is a potential for blood splatter.
5. Assemble equipment.
6. Break the needle seal. Thread the appropriate needle into the holder using the needle sheath as a wrench.
7. Before using, tap all tubes that contain additives to ensure that all the additive is dislodged from the stopper and wall of the tube.
8. Insert the tube into the holder until the needle slightly enters the stopper. Avoid pushing the needle beyond the recessed guideline, because a loss of vacuum may result. If the tube retracts slightly, leave it in the retracted position to avoid prematurely puncturing the rubber stopper.

(continues)

Procedure

28-3   (continued)

9. Apply the tourniquet.
10. Ask the patient to close the hand. The patient must not be allowed to pump the hand. Pumping of the hand will change the values of the laboratory tests being drawn. If possible, place the patient's arm in a downward position.
11. Select a vein, noting the location and direction of the vein.
12. Clean the venipuncture site with a 70 percent isopropyl alcohol swab.
13. Do not touch the venipuncture site.
14. Draw the patient's skin taut with your thumb. Place the thumb 1 to 2 inches below or above the puncture site (Figure 28-28). This will anchor the vein.
15. With the bevel up, line up the needle with the vein and puncture the vein. Remove your hand from drawing the skin taut. Grasp the flange of the evacuated tube holder and push the tube forward until the butt end of the needle punctures the stopper. Do not change hands while performing the venipuncture. The hand performing the venipuncture is the hand that holds the evacuated tube holder. The opposite hand manipulates the tubes.
16. Fill the tube until the vacuum is exhausted and blood flow into the tube ceases. This will assure the proper blood to anticoagulant ratio.
17. When the blood flow ceases, remove the tube from the holder. While securely grasping the evacuated tube holder with one hand, use the other hand to change the tubes. The rubber sleeve recovers the needle point, stopping the flow of blood until the next tube is inserted.
18. After drawing, immediately mix each tube that contains an additive. Gently inverting the tube 5 to 10 times provides adequate mixing without causing hemolysis.
19. Ask the patient to open the hand.
20. Release the tourniquet.
21. Lightly place a sterile gauze square or cotton ball above the venipuncture site.
22. Remove the needle from the arm. Be certain the last tube drawn has been removed from the holder before removing the needle. This prevents blood dripping from the tip of the needle.
23. Apply pressure to the site for 3 to 5 minutes. The patient may assist if able by elevating the arm above heart level to reduce blood flow. The arm should be held in a raised, outstretched position. Do not allow the patient to bend the arm at the elbow. Bending the arm at the elbow to apply pressure may lead to a hematoma.
24. Label all tubes at the patient's side before leaving the examination room.
25. Apply an adhesive bandage.
26. Remove and discard gloves and mask in a biohazard container.
27. Wash hands.
28. Thank the patient.
29. Document procedure.

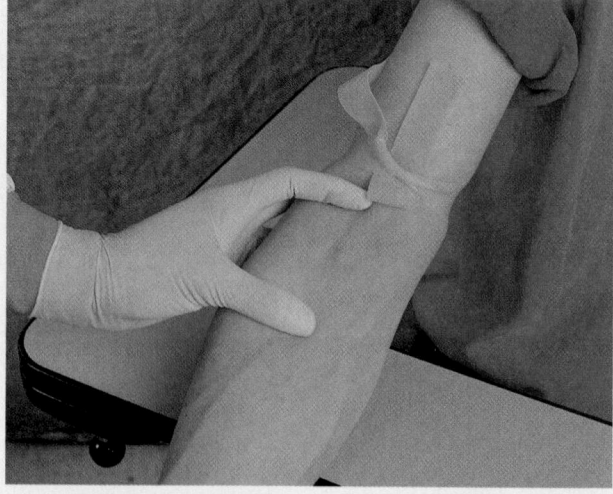

Figure 28-28   Pull the skin taut to prevent vein roll.

Procedure 28-4 — Venipuncture by Butterfly Needle System

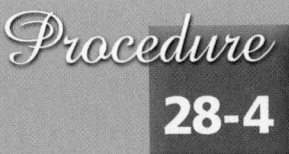

STANDARD PRECAUTIONS:

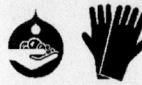   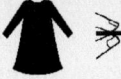 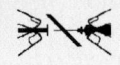

PURPOSE:
To obtain venous blood acceptable for laboratory testing as required by a physician.

SPECIMEN
Venous blood collected by butterfly needle system. Volume of blood dependent on size of tube and test requirements.

EQUIPMENT/SUPPLIES:

Gloves
Goggles and mask, if necessary
Evacuated tube holder
Butterfly needle system, 21, 23, or 25 gauge needle with or without luer adapter

Evacuated tube(s) or special collection tube(s)
Tourniquet
70% isopropyl alcohol swab
Gauze or cotton balls
Adhesive bandage or tape
Sharps container

PROCEDURE STEPS:

1. Position and identify the patient. Ask the patient's name and verify it with the computer label or identification number.
2. If a fasting specimen is required, verify that the patient has not had anything to eat or drink.
3. Wash hands.
4. Put on gloves, as well as safety glasses and mask if there is a potential for blood splatter.
5. Assemble equipment.
6. Open the package of butterfly needle system with evacuated tube luer adapter. The **luer** screws into the evacuated tube holder. The part inside the holder has a needle to puncture the tube top, the part outside the holder fits into a tubing port. Thread the luer needle into the holder.
7. Before using, tap all tubes that contain additives to ensure that all the additive is dislodged from the stopper and wall of the tube.
8. Insert the tube into the holder until the needle slightly enters the stopper. Avoid pushing the needle beyond the recessed guideline, because a loss of vacuum may result. If the tube retracts slightly, leave it in the retracted position.

9. Apply the tourniquet.
10. Ask the patient to close the hand. The patient must not be allowed to pump the hand. If possible, place the patient's arm in a downward position.
11. Select a vein, noting the location and direction of the vein.
12. Clean the venipuncture site with a 70 percent isopropyl alcohol swab.
13. Do not touch the venipuncture site.
14. Draw the patient's skin taut with your thumb and forefinger. Spread the thumb and forefinger 1 to 2 inches to each side of the puncture site.
15. Hold the wings of the butterfly with the bevel up. Line up the needle with the vein and perform the venipuncture. Remove your hand from drawing the skin taut. Grasp the flange of the evacuated tube holder and push the tube forward until the butt end of the needle punctures the stopper.
16. Fill the tube until the vacuum is exhausted and blood flow into the tube ceases. This will assure the proper blood to anticoagulant ratio. Due to air in the tubing, a loss of approximately 0.5 ml will result when collecting the initial evacuated tube.
17. When the blood flow ceases, remove the tube from the holder. While securely grasping the evacuated tube holder with one hand, use the other hand to change the tubes. The rubber sleeve recovers the point, stopping the flow of blood until the next tube of blood is inserted. Multiple draws require the same order of draw as an evacuated tube system draw.
18. After drawing, immediately mix each tube that contains an additive. Gently inverting the tube 5 to 10 times provides adequate mixing without causing **hemolysis**.
19. Ask the patient to open the hand.
20. Release the tourniquet.
21. Lightly place a sterile gauze square or cotton ball above the venipuncture site.
22. Remove the needle from the arm. Be certain the last tube drawn has been removed from the holder before removing the needle. This prevents blood dripping off the tip of the needle.
23. Apply pressure to the site for 3 to 5 minutes. The patient may assist if able by elevating the arm

(continues)

Procedure

28-4   *(continued)*

above heart level to reduce blood flow. The arm should be held in a raised, outstretched position. Do not allow the patient to bend the arm at the elbow. Bending the arm at the elbow to apply pressure may lead to a hematoma.

24. Label all tubes at the patient's side before leaving the examination room.
25. Apply an adhesive bandage.
26. Remove and discard gloves and mask in a biohazard container.
27. Wash hands.
28. Thank the patient.
29. Document procedure.

VARIATION TO THE PROCEDURE:
1. Draw with a butterfly system without a luer adapter.
2. Instead of threading the luer into the holder in step 6, attach a syringe.
3. Omit step 8.
4. In steps 15, 16, and 17, pull on the syringe instead of pushing the tube into the holder.
5. Aliquot blood into appropriate tubes as outlined in the syringe procedure.

Procedure

28-5   Capillary Puncture by Fingerstick

STANDARD PRECAUTIONS:

   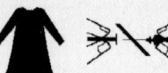

PURPOSE:
To obtain capillary blood acceptable for laboratory testing as required by a physician.

SPECIMEN:
Capillary blood collected by finger puncture. Volume of blood dependent on size of microcollection devices and test requirements.

EQUIPMENT/SUPPLIES:
Gloves
Goggles and mask, if necessary
70% isopropyl alcohol swab or pad
Microcollection tubes or capillary tubes
Lancet
Gauze
Adhesive bandage or tape
Sharps container

PROCEDURE STEPS:
1. Position and identify the patient. Ask the patient's name and verify it with the computer label or identification number.
2. If a fasting specimen is required, verify that the patient has not had anything to eat or drink.
3. Wash hands.
4. Put on gloves, as well as goggles and mask.
5. Assemble equipment.
6. Select puncture site on the palmar surface of the distal phalanx of the ring or middle finger. Do not use the side or tip of the finger. If necessary, warm site with a moist towel at a temperature not higher than 42°C for three to five minutes.
7. Clean the puncture site with a 70% isopropyl alcohol pad.
8. Allow the site to air dry.
9. Perform the puncture perpendicular to the fingerprint, holding the hand firmly to prevent sudden movement.
10. Using a clean gauze pad, wipe away the first drop

(continues)

Procedure **28-5** *(continued)*

of blood. Holding the finger in a downward position, apply gentle pressure to the finger. *Do not squeeze or milk the finger.*

11. Collect specimens using the proper order of draw.
12. Mix tubes with additives well.
13. Place a clean gauze pad on the puncture site and apply pressure until the bleeding stops.
14. Label all tubes at the patient's side before leaving the examination room.
15. Apply a bandage if necessary. Bandages are not recommended for children under the age of two. Parents or guardian must be instructed to monitor the child carefully as the potential for ingestion of the bandage exists.
16. Remove and discard gloves and mask in a biohazard container.
17. Wash hands.
18. Thank the patient.
19. Document procedure.

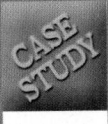

Inner City Health Care is short-staffed today and medical assistant Liz Corbin is feeling pressed for time. She has many tasks to complete, but first she must perform a venipuncture. She greets the patient, Wayne Elder, in a perfunctory manner, discouraging time-wasting conversation. Although Wayne appears apprehensive, he is not resistant, so Liz quickly assembles the necessary supplies, applies the tourniquet, and inserts the needle. While she is drawing his blood, Wayne faints.

CASE STUDY REVIEW

1. What should Liz do now?
2. What could Liz have done to prevent this situation from occurring?
3. In the future, what are some steps Liz can take to provide a positive experience for venipuncture patients?

SUMMARY

With a little practice, the medical assistant will become an expert at phlebotomy. The skills of phlebotomy cannot be learned primarily from a textbook; continuous practice will develop the skill to perfection. It may take months before the medical assistant feels comfortable and is able to obtain a sample without difficulty.

In all phlebotomy, safety is of the utmost consideration. Dispose of all sharps properly and separately from the noncontaminated trash. Proper handwashing between patients and wearing gloves, goggles, and masks with each phlebotomy will assure safety for both the patient and the medical assistant.

Proper specimen collection and handling of the specimen after collection by the medical assistant will assure that the patient obtains the most accurate result. The specimen must be treated in such a way that the integrity of the specimen is maintained. The quality of the sample must be the same when collected as when tested. Correct method of draw, order of draw, and the correct handling of the sample after collection will reduce the number of factors affecting the sample and give the most accurate result possible.

REVIEW QUESTIONS

Multiple Choice

1. Drawing blood with a 25 gauge needle increases the chance for:
   a. vein collapse
   b. hematomas
   c. hemoconcentration
   d. hemolysis

2. An anticoagulant is an additive placed in evacuated tubes in order to:
   a. dilute the blood prior to testing
   b. ensure the sterility of the tube
   c. make the blood clot faster
   d. prevent the blood from clotting

3. When collecting a blood sample with an evacuated tube system, the last tube drawn is withdrawn from the holder before removing the needle from the patient in order to:
   a. avoid hematoma at the venipuncture site
   b. avoid dripping blood out the end of the needle
   c. prevent clotting of the blood
   d. cause the blood to clot

4. Leaving the tourniquet on a patient's arm for an extended length of time before drawing blood may cause:
   a. hemoconcentration
   b. specimen hemolysis
   c. stress
   d. bruising

5. The single most important way to prevent the spread of infection from patient to patient is:
   a. gowning and gloving
   b. handwashing
   c. always wearing masks
   d. avoid breathing on clients

6. Under standard precautions, all used needles are to be disposed of in the following manner:
   a. recapped
   b. discarded intact in a sharps container
   c. bent
   d. broken or cut off

7. When drawing multiple specimens in evacuated tubes, it is important to fill which of the following color-stoppered tubes first?
   a. light blue
   b. green
   c. lavender
   d. red

8. The anticoagulant of choice when drawing coagulation studies such as PT and APTT is:
   a. (red) no anticoagulant
   b. (light blue) sodium citrate
   c. (lavender) EDTA
   d. (green) heparin

9. When the medical assistant cannot perform a venipuncture successfully after two attempts, the medical assistant should:
   a. try at least two more times
   b. notify the physician
   c. ask another medical assistant to try
   d. request the test for the next day

10. If the blood is drawn too quickly from a small vein, the vein has a tendency to:
    a. collapse
    b. bruise
    c. disintegrate
    d. roll

Critical Thinking

1. A frightened patient begins crying when you enter the room to perform a venipuncture. How will you handle the situation? What is your responsibility to the patient? Why are your demeanor and appearance important in this type of situation?

2. Explain the difference between serum and plasma. Describe how serum and plasma samples are collected.

3. You are preparing to perform a venipuncture on a geriatric patient who has fragile veins. Which system will you use—a syringe and needle or an evacuated tube system? Why? How can vein collapse be avoided?

4. Discuss how clots are formed and what can be done to stop the clotting process.

5. You've calmed the crying patient and successfully drawn the patient's blood. What will you do next? Why is this step important? Describe the skills you have used.

6. The patient cries out in pain when you insert the needle into the vein. What will you do to make the patient more comfortable? If you decide to try another site, how will you locate it?

WEB ACTIVITIES

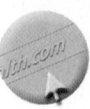

1. Visit the CDC and other government web sites for the most current information on Standard Precautions and proper protection during blood draws.

2. Search the keywords phlebotomy and puncture on the web. What organizations can you find that offer information for medical assistants?

REFERENCES/BIBLIOGRAPHY

Federal register, rules and regulations, 29 CFR part 1910.1030. (Vol. 56, 235). 1991, December 6.

Geller, S. J. (1992, March 3). *Effect of sample collection on laboratory test results.* ASCP Teleconference Series.

Hoeltke, L. B. (2000). *The complete textbook of phlebotomy* (2nd ed.). Albany, NY: Delmar.

National Committee for Clinical Laboratory Standards. (1991). *Protection of laboratory workers from infectious disease transmitted by blood, body fluids, and tissue* (2nd ed.). Approved Standard. NCCLS Document. M29-T2, Villanova, PA: National Committee for Clinical Laboratory Standards.

National Committee for Clinical Laboratory Standards. (1996). *Evacuated tubes and additives for blood specimen collection* (4th ed.). Approved Standard. NCCLS Document. H1-A4. Villanova, PA: Author.

National Committee for Clinical Laboratory Standards. (1998). *Collection, transport, and processing of blood specimen for coagulation testing and general performance of coagulation assays* (3rd ed.). Approved Guideline. NCCLS Document. H21-A3. Villanova, PA: Author.

National Committee for Clinical Laboratory Standards. (1998). *Procedures for the collection of diagnostic blood specimens by venipuncture* (4th ed.). Approved Standard. NCCLS document H3-A4. Villanova, PA: Author.

National Committee for Clinical Laboratory Standards. (1999). *Procedures and devices for the collection of diagnostic blood specimens by skin puncture* (4th ed.). Approved Guideline. NCCLS Document. H4-A4. Villanova, PA: Author.

Peek, G. J., Marsh, H., Keating, J., et al. (1990). The effects of swabbing the skin on apparent blood ethanol concentration. *Alcohol Alcoholism 25*, 639–640.

Tilton, R. C., Balows, A., Hohnadel, D. C., & Reiss, R. F. (1992). *Clinical laboratory medicine* (pp. 813–823). St. Louis: Mosby-Year Book.

Wedding, M. E., & Toenjes, S. A. (1992). *Medical laboratory procedures.* Philadelphia: F. A. Davis.

Chapter

29

HEMATOLOGY

KEY TERMS

Anisocytosis

Basophil

Centrifugal Hematology Analysis

Complete Blood Count (CBC)

Cyanmethemoglobin

Eosinophil

Erythrocyte

Erythrocyte Indices

Erythrocyte Sedimentation Rate

Erythropoietin

Hemacytometer (also spelled Hemocytometer)

Hematocrit

Hematology

Hematopoiesis

Hemoglobin

Hemoglobinopathy

Hypochromic

Impedance Principle

Leukocyte

Lymphocyte

Macrocytic

Microcytic

Monocyte

Neutrophil

Normochromic

Normocytic

Poikilocytosis

Polychromatic Stain

Thrombocyte

OUTLINE

Hematological Tests
   Hemoglobin and Hematocrit
      Determinations
   White and Red Blood Cell Counts
   White Blood Cell Differential
   Examination of a Blood Smear
Erythrocyte Indices
   Using Erythrocyte Indices to
      Diagnose
**Erythrocyte Sedimentation Rates
   (ESR)**
   Wintrobe Method

Westergren Method
Using the ESR to Diagnose
**Automated Hematology Instru-
   mentation and Quality Control**
   Hematology Instruments That
      Require Sample Dilutions
   Hematology Instruments That Do
      Not Require Sample Dilutions

OBJECTIVES

*The student should strive to meet the following performance objectives and demonstrate
an understanding of the facts and principles presented in this chapter through written and
oral communication.*

1. Define the key terms as presented in the glossary.

2. Describe the process of hematopoiesis.

3. Discuss how the clinical science of hematology and the CBC are used in
    the diagnosis and treatment of disease.

4. Compare the normal versus abnormal values of the CBC parameters.

5. Discuss how the hemoglobin and hematocrit are used to diagnose anemia.

6. Describe how the erythrocyte indices are used in the differential diag-
    nosis of anemias.

7. Perform the calculations necessary to derive the erythrocyte indices
    MCV, MCH, and MCHC.

8. List the steps required to prepare and stain a differential white blood cell
    smear.

9. List the five types of normal white blood cells that can be seen on a stained
    blood smear and give the identifying characteristics of each.   (*continues*)

10. Describe the differences in the procedures for the Wintrobe and Westergren erythrocyte sedimentation rates.

11. Recognize the physiological reasons why the erythrocyte sedimentation rate varies with different states of health and disease.

12. List the two general types of automated hematology instruments used in the ambulatory care setting and describe their technology.

13. Perform the laboratory procedures included in this chapter in a manner acceptable for entry-level employment.

ROLE DELINEATION COMPONENTS

CLINICAL

Fundamental Principles

- Apply principles of aseptic technique and infection control
- Comply with quality assurance practices
- Screen and follow up patient test results

Diagnostic Orders

- Collect and process specimens
- Perform diagnostic tests

GENERAL (TRANSDISCIPLINARY)

Legal Concepts

- Document accurately
- Comply with established risk management and safety procedures

SCENARIO

The physicians in the office of Doctors Lewis & King MD often order hematological tests to assist them in diagnosing and treating patients. As she performs the tests in the physician's office laboratory, clinical medical assistant Audrey Jones uses her knowledge of hematology every day. Audrey is comfortable using an automated hematology analyzer or performing tests manually because she understands the purposes and procedures of the tests. She always follows all safety and quality control guidelines to protect herself and others and to ensure the accuracy of test results.

INTRODUCTION

Hematology is the study of the blood cells and coagulation in both normal and diseased states. The two main components of the blood are plasma (the liquid portion) and cells. Cells of the blood are also known as the formed elements of the blood. The study of hematology is usually limited to the cellular components of the blood and does not include the chemistry of the blood.

The cellular components of blood include **erythrocytes** (red blood cells), **leukocytes** (white blood cells), and **thrombocytes** (platelets). Blood has many different functions. These include the process of supplying nutrients and oxygen to all cells as well as the removal of the end products of metabolism. Blood is also involved in fighting infection as well as producing antibodies which are used in our immune systems for defense against foreign antigens.

Hematopoiesis is defined as the formation of blood cells (Figure 29-1). The process of hematopoiesis, as well as the blood-forming tissues of the body, is included in the study of hematology. In the embryo, hematopoiesis occurs in the yolk sac, liver, and spleen. After we are born, the primary site for the production of erythrocytes, granulocytes, and platelets is the bone marrow. Lymphocytes are also produced in the bone marrow, as well as in the lymph nodes. At birth, most of the bone marrow in the body is capable of producing blood cells. This process is confined to the bone marrow of the ribs, vertebrae, sternum, and iliac crest by the age of 20. Bone marrow that is producing cells is known as red marrow. As the area for hematopoiesis is reduced, the red bone marrow is replaced by yellow marrow, which is stored fat. When a physician collects a bone marrow sample in an adult, the site chosen for sampling is the sternum or the iliac crest.

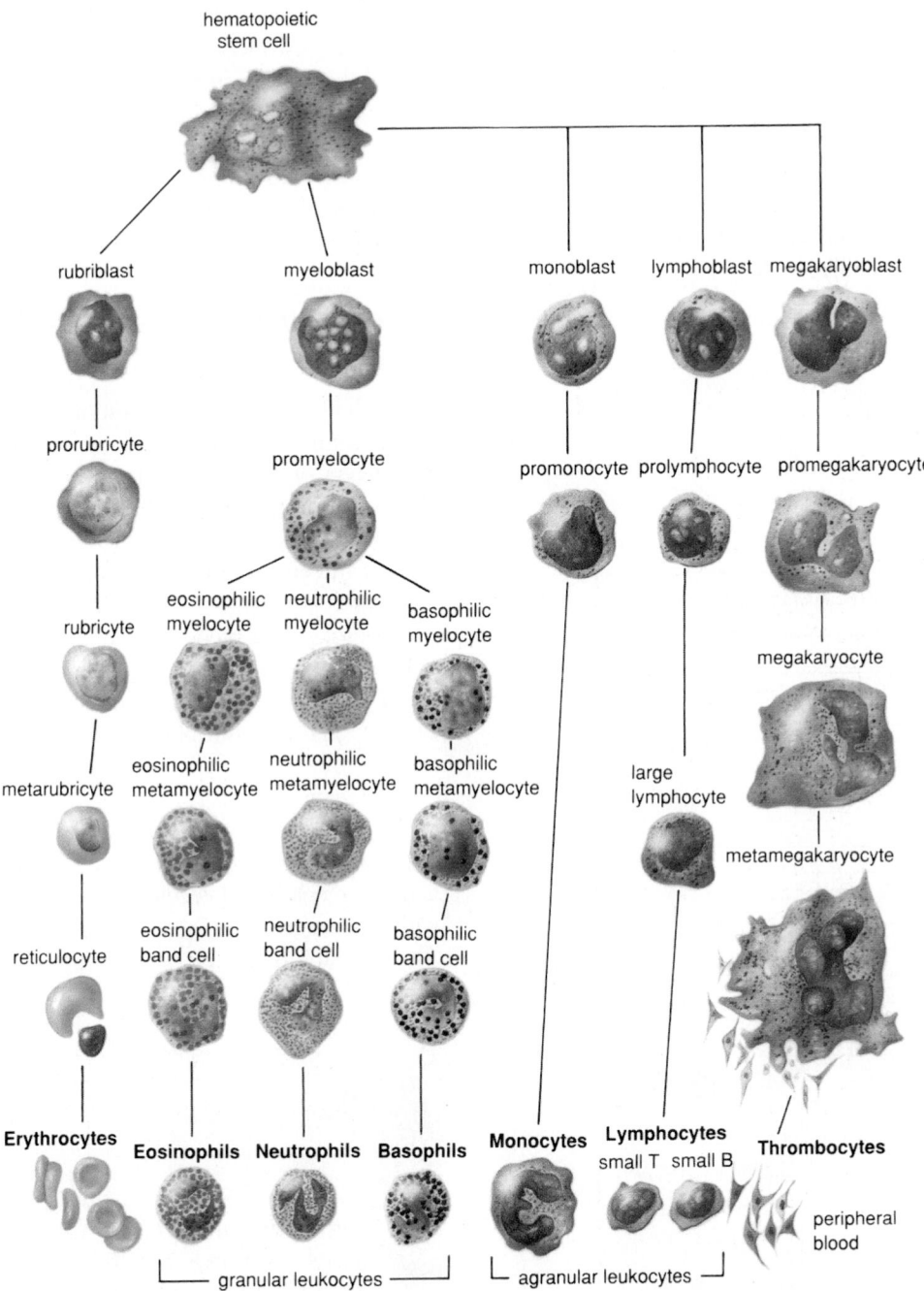

Figure 29-1   Hematopoiesis showing blood cells and platelet formation starting with hematopoietic stem cell.

HEMATOLOGICAL TESTS

Hematological tests are the second most common tests performed in the physician's office laboratory (POL). The most common test is the urinalysis. The cellular components of the blood may be affected by changes in either the blood-forming organs or in other tissues of the body. The study of these changes forms the basis of hematological tests performed in the POL.

Hematological tests performed in the clinical laboratory include:

- Hemoglobin
- Hematocrit
- White blood cell count (WBC)
- Red blood cell count (RBC)
- Platelet count
- Differential white blood cell count
- Erythrocyte sedimentation rate (ESR)
- Prothrombin time (PT)

The results of these hematological tests provide valuable information used by the physician in making a diagnosis, evaluating a patient's progress, and/or regulating further treatment.

The laboratory test ordered most frequently on blood in the ambulatory care setting is the **complete blood count (CBC)**. The exact number of parameters included in the CBC will vary from laboratory to laboratory (Figure 29-2). The CBC generally includes:

- Hemoglobin determination

- Hematocrit determination

- White blood cell count (WBC)

- Red blood cell count (RBC)

- Differential white blood cell count

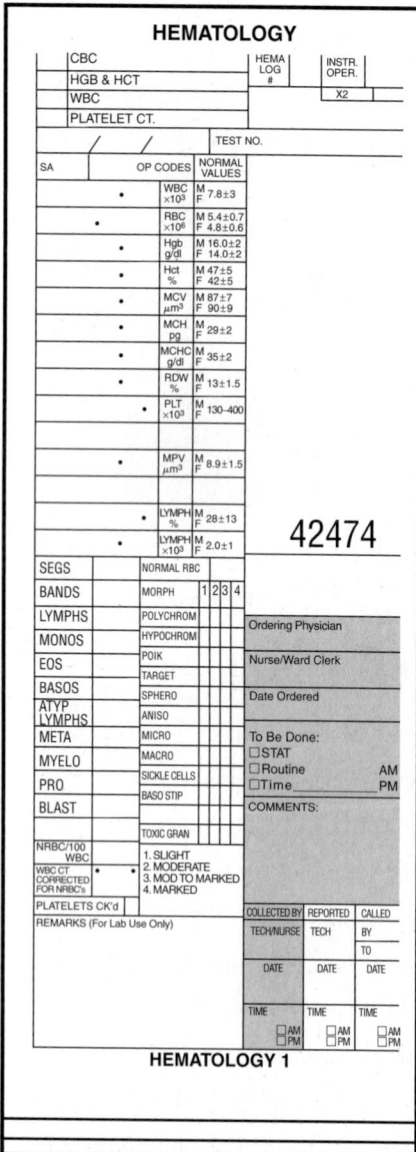

Figure 29-2 Hematology requisition form.

Erythrocyte indices are frequently included as a part of the complete blood count.

All of these tests can be performed by manual testing procedures or with an automated hematology analyzer. It is important to note that all automated hematology analyzers utilize a modification or adaptation of the manual methods. A complete understanding of each manual procedure will help you understand the automated methods.

Hemoglobin and Hematocrit Determinations

Hemoglobin and hematocrit tests are part of the complete blood count; however, they are frequently the only parameters of the CBC ordered by the physician. The abbreviations for hemoglobin and hematocrit are Hgb and Hct, respectively. **Hemoglobin** is the major component of the erythrocyte and serves as a transport vehicle for oxygen and carbon dioxide in the body. The **hematocrit** (packed red blood cell volume) is the ratio of the volume of packed red blood cells to that of the whole blood. Packed red blood cell volume is expressed as a percentage of the whole blood following centrifugation of the blood.

Hemoglobin is responsible for about 85 percent of the dry weight of the red blood cells. Hemoglobin is a conjugated protein composed of heme and globin. A single hemoglobin molecule consists of four globin chains with a heme group attached to each globin (Figure 29-3). The central ion of each heme group is an iron molecule.

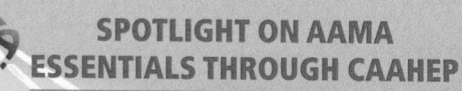

SPOTLIGHT ON AAMA ESSENTIALS THROUGH CAAHEP

- When required to perform hematology tests, the medical assistant should be knowledgeable in the skills necessary to perform the tests and sensitive to the patient's psychosocial needs and fears.

- By understanding methods used in hematology testing, the medical assistant will be better equipped to help the patient understand the procedures and to offer reassurance.

- It is important that the medical assistant remember to treat all patients with compassion and empathy when performing any type of hematology testing.

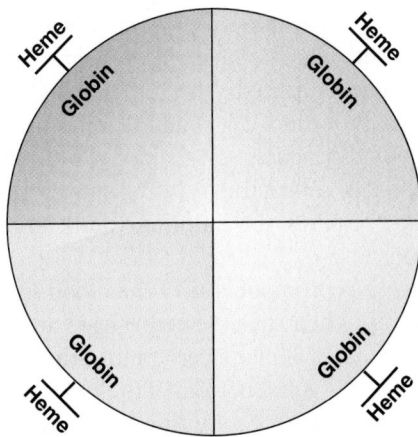

Figure 29-3 A normal hemoglobin molecule containing four globin chains with a heme group attached to each globin. One oxygen molecule can be transported by each heme group.

Synthesis of the heme portion of the hemoglobin molecule requires iron. The iron used in the synthesis of hemoglobin is normally absorbed in the duodenum of the small intestine following dietary intake. The daily iron requirement for an adult male is about 0.5 mg/day. A menstruating female requires about 2 mg/day.

As stated earlier, the major function of hemoglobin in the body is the transportation of oxygen to all the body cells. Hemoglobin carries 95 percent of all the oxygen to the cells and is responsible for transporting about 27 percent of the carbon dioxide produced by cellular metabolism back to the lungs where it is removed. The hemoglobin in the red blood cells also acts as a buffer system. This buffer system accounts for approximately 30 percent of the buffering capacity of whole blood.

The production of new red blood cells and consequently the formation of more hemoglobin is triggered by the hormone **erythropoietin**, which is produced in the kidney. This hematopoietic process is started when there is a decrease of available oxygen at the cellular level. Hgb A makes up the majority of normal hemoglobin found in the adult.

There are several forms of abnormal hemoglobin that are responsible for a group of diseases known as **hemoglobinopathies**. These abnormal forms of hemoglobin include hemoglobin S, hemoglobin C, and hemoglobin E. Hemoglobin S (Hgb S) is the most common abnormal form of hemoglobin observed in the laboratory. It is the form of hemoglobin that causes sickle cell anemia. When Hgb S molecules are subjected to certain conditions, they alter the physical structure of the red blood cells. The red blood cells assume a sickle shape, which makes it difficult, if not impossible, for the cell to pass through a capillary bed.

The most frequent hemoglobin disease seen in the ambulatory care setting is anemia, with iron deficiency anemia being the most common type. The laboratory findings of these individuals will be a normal or near normal hematocrit with a low hemoglobin value. The red blood cells of these individuals will be **hypochromic** because they lack hemoglobin. A decrease in available iron in the body is the most common cause of this type of anemia.

Hemoglobin values are determined by two methods: the specific gravity and **cyanmethemoglobin** methods. The specific gravity test is a procedure that utilizes different specific gravity solutions of copper sulfate. This is a screening technique used to determine the eligibility of blood donors; it is not an exact measurement method. The common way to measure hemoglobin levels in the ambulatory care setting is known as the cyanmethemoglobin method. This test is performed either by manual or automated methods. See Procedures 29-1 and 29-2.

The principle of the cyanmethemoglobin procedure is the same regardless of the method utilized. The red blood cells are lysed with a solution containing potassium ferricyanide and sodium cyanide which converts hemoglobin to cyanmethemoglobin. The cyanide solution is known as Drabkin's reagent and is sold under many brand names. Cyanmethemoglobin is a very stable compound, but it must be protected from light and excess heat. The pigmented solution of cyanmethemoglobin is read photometrically in a colorimeter or spectrophotometer at a wavelength of 540 nanometers (nm). The results are reported in grams per deciliter (g/dL). It is important to note that all forms of hemoglobin are converted to cyanmethemoglobin by this method except hemoglobin S.

 The Drabkin's solution is poisonous. Precautions to observe when working with any reagents includes wearing gloves, working in a well-ventilated area, properly disposing of used reagents, wiping up all spills, and handwashing.

The normal reference values for hemoglobin vary according to both the age and sex of the individual (Table 29-1).

The hematocrit (packed red blood cell volume) is the ratio of the volume of packed red blood cells to that of the whole blood. Packed red blood cell volume is expressed as a percentage of the whole blood. This is achieved by centrifuging a prepared blood sample. It

TABLE 29-1	NORMAL HEMOGLOBIN VALUES OR REFERENCE RANGES BY AGE AND/OR SEX
Newborn	15–20 g/dL
Age three months	9–14 g/dL
Age ten months	12–14.5 g/dL
Adult female	12–16 g/dL
Adult male	13–18 g/dL

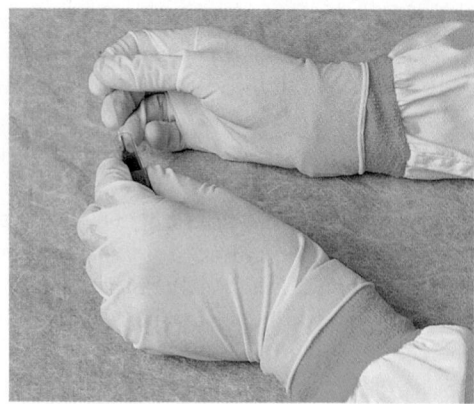

Figure 29-4   Filling a microhematocrit tube with blood by capillary action.

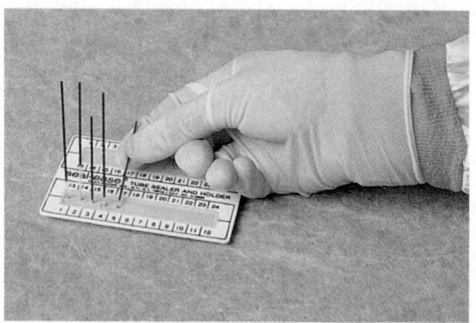

Figure 29-5   Sealing the microhematocrit tube with sealing clay.

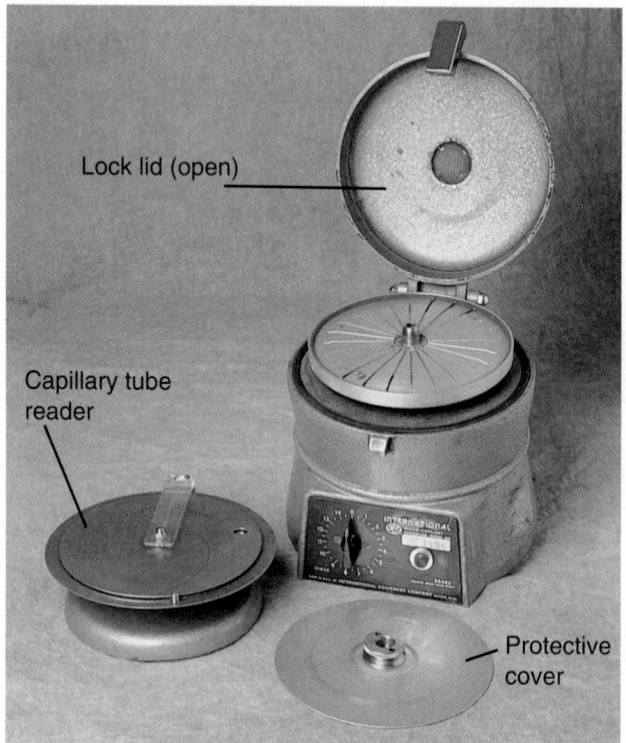

Figure 29-6   Microhematocrit centrifuge (right) with protective cover and lock lid (open) and a microhematocrit capillary tube reader (left).

can be performed using either a macrotechnique or a microtechnique. In the ambulatory care setting, the microtechnique is utilized. The test is called a microhematocrit (see Procedure 29-3) and requires only a couple drops of blood (Figures 29-4, 29-5, and 29-6). The macromethod is called the Wintrobe macrohematocrit. This method requires one milliliter (one cubic centimeter) of blood.

The cellular components of the blood sample separate into layers when they are centrifuged at high speeds (Figure 29-7). The cellular layers arrange themselves with the red blood cells at the bottom of the tube. White blood cells and platelets form a very thin layer called the buffy coat on top of the erythrocytes. The buffy coat has a whitish-tan appearance.

The white blood cell count of the sample can be estimated by measuring the buffy coat thickness. Each 0.1 mm of the buffy coat equals approximately 1,000 WBC/mm^3. Therefore, a buffy coat of 1 mm would equal a leukocyte count of approximately 10,000 WBCs/mm^3 and a 0.5 mm reading would equal 5,000 WBCs/mm^3. The cell counts may be reported in units of microliters (μL), which are equivalent to cubic millimeters.

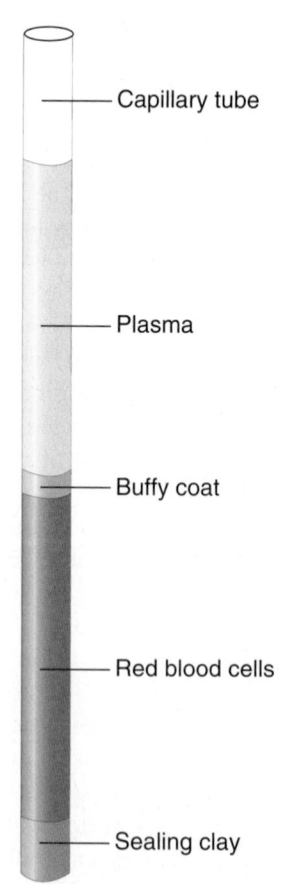

Capillary tube

Plasma

Buffy coat

Red blood cells

Sealing clay

Figure 29-7   Diagram of packed cell column in the hematocrit showing separation of cellular components after centrifugation.

TABLE 29-2	NORMAL HEMATOCRIT VALUES OR REFERENCE RANGES BY AGE AND/OR SEX	
Newborn	45–60%	
One year old	27–44%	
Adult female	36–46%	
Adult male	40–55%	

The normal values of hematocrit will vary according to the age and sex of the individual (Table 29-2).

Sources of error associated with the microhematocrit method include improper centrifugation, resulting in increased trapped plasma, and improper reading of the packed red cell volume, such as including the buffy coat layer.

 The microhematocrit capillary tubes are made of thin glass and are easily broken. Care must be observed when handling these tubes. Gloves must be worn. Hold the tube horizontally with your finger held over the clean end of the three-quarters blood-filled capillary tube. Remove excess blood by wiping off the outside of the filled capillary tube. While holding your finger over the wiped-off collection end, carefully insert the clean end into the sealing clay. Do not exert excessive pressure. Do not contaminate the clay with blood. Self-sealing plastic microhematocrit capillary tubes are now available.

White and Red Blood Cell Counts

White blood cell counts and red blood cell counts can be performed using either a manual or automated method (see Procedures 29-4 and 29-5). All white blood cell counts and red blood cell counts performed in the POL utilize an automated method. It is important to note that all automated testing methods are based on a modification or adaptation of the manual methods. Performing the manual methods gives the student an opportunity to observe what occurs in the automated hematology instrument. The knowledge gained gives students a better understanding of what is really happening and they become better laboratory workers. In the past, blood-diluting pipettes were utilized when a white or red blood cell count was performed. These have been replaced by the Unopette® systems (Figure 29-8) when a manual blood cell count is performed in the medical laboratory.

Both the manual white blood cell count and the red blood cell count can be performed using a Unopette® system. Unopette® systems require that an exact amount of blood sample be diluted with a known volume of diluting solution. The diluted sample is mixed and transferred to a hemacytometer, where the cells are counted with the aid of a microscope. The normal reference values for leukocyte (WBC) counts and erythrocyte (RBC) counts vary according to both age and sex of the individual (Tables 29-3 and 29-4).

White Blood Cell Count Manual Dilution. When a manual white blood cell count is performed using a Unopette® kit, the diluting solution is an acetic acid solution. The solution will lyse the red blood cells and leave only the white blood cells and platelets (thrombocytes) intact.

The Unopette® method for performing a manual WBC count employs the same principle as the classical procedure that was utilized by the WBC diluting pipette method. The disposable blood-diluting Unopette® kit includes a prefilled reservoir of 0.475 mL, 3 percent acetic acid, a 25 μL capacity capillary pipette, and a pipette shield (Figure 29-8). This Unopette® unit gives a dilution of 1:20. Unopette® units are also available that will produce a 1:100 dilution. The diluted sample should stand for ten minutes to allow time for all of the red blood cells to be hemolyzed. The sample is stable for three hours after dilution if it is kept at room temperature.

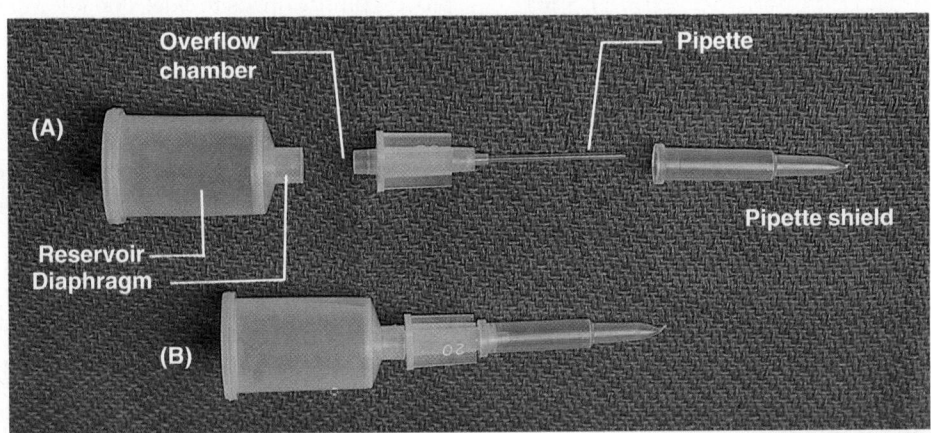

Figure 29-8 Parts of a disposable Unopette® blood-diluting unit: (A) Unassembled Unopette® unit. (B) Assembled unit.

Blood samples in either the white blood cell count or red blood cell count utilizing the Unopette® method may be collected directly from a capillary puncture. If a venipuncture sample is used, it should be collected in an EDTA (lavender) anticoagulant tube.

Red Blood Cell Count Manual Dilution. The manual red blood cell count is performed using the same procedure that was utilized with the white blood cell count. The method uses a pipette and a diluting solution. The diluting solution used with the RBC count is an isotonic salt solution also known as a Hayem and Gower, or Gower solution.

The Unopette® method for performing a manual RBC count employs the same principle as the classical procedure that was utilized by the RBC diluting pipette method. The disposable blood-diluting Unopette® unit includes a prefilled reservoir of 1.99 mL of diluent, a 10 μL pipette, and a pipette shield. The 10 μL pipette used with the 1.99 mL of diluent will give a dilution ratio of 1:200. It is best to perform the count immediately after the sample is diluted; however, the diluted specimen is stable for approximately six hours at room temperature.

The diluent used in the Unopette® RBC unit contains sodium azide which, if placed in an acid environment, can produce the extremely toxic compound hydrazoic acid. Care should be exercised when flooding or cleaning the hemacytometer and when discarding the diluent into the sink. Always dilute the solution with running water.

Both the WBC and the RBC manual counts are performed using a **hemacytometer** (Figure 29-9). The hemacytometer, also called a counting chamber, is a very precise piece of laboratory equipment which allows an exact volume of sample to be examined.

The hemacytometer utilizes a coverglass. Both the hemacytometer and coverglass must be completely clean, free of all dust, dirt, and grease. The process of filling the counting chamber is also known as flooding or charging.

Position the coverglass on the hemacytometer and be sure it covers both ruled areas on the counting cham-

When either a WBC or RBC count is performed using a hemacytometer, it is important that the sample be thoroughly mixed.

When a hemacytometer is filled with a Unopette®, the first two or three drops of diluted sample should be discarded before the counting chamber is flooded.

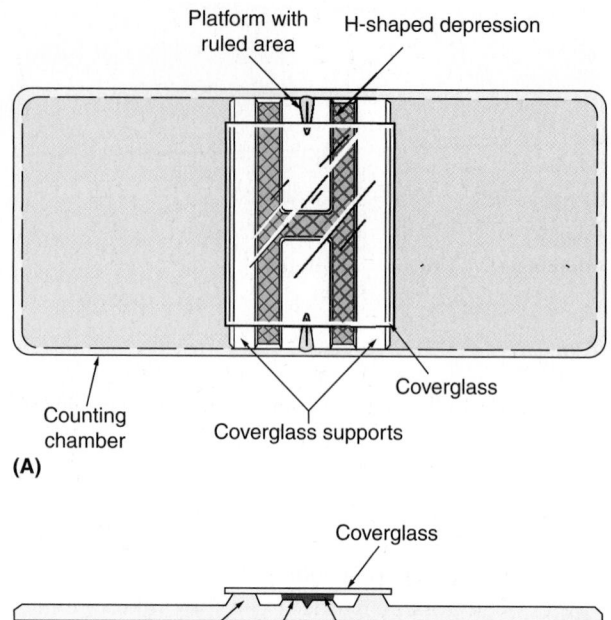

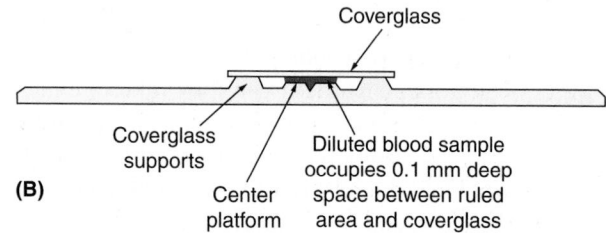

Figure 29-9   Hemacytometer: (A) Top view of hemacytometer with coverglass in place. (B) Side view with coverglass in place.

ber. Fill the chamber by letting the fluid from the Unopette® pipette flow evenly under the coverglass. The fluid should flow only on the platform of the hemacytometer. It *should not* flow into the H-shaped depressed areas (known as moats) that surround the platform. Most hemacytometers have a V-shaped trough to help in the flooding (charging) process. You will be able to see the fluid as it flows under the coverglass. If the hemacytometer is overflooded, it should be cleaned, dried, and the procedure should be repeated. After you have correctly flooded one side of the counting chamber, repeat the process on the opposite side. The filled counting chamber should stand for approximately two minutes to allow the cells to settle out of the fluid and stabilize before the count is performed (Figure 29-10).

Counting the WBC Sample Using Low-Power Magnification. The counting area on the hemacytometer when you are performing a WBC count is usually the four square millimeters indicated with the letter *W* (Figure 29-11). The count is performed using the low-power objective (10X). Remember that the total magnification observed when using the 10X objective is 100X. Magnification is the product of the power of both the objective and the eyepiece (ocular). The eyepiece on most microscopes is 10X; therefore, 10X × 10X = 100X.

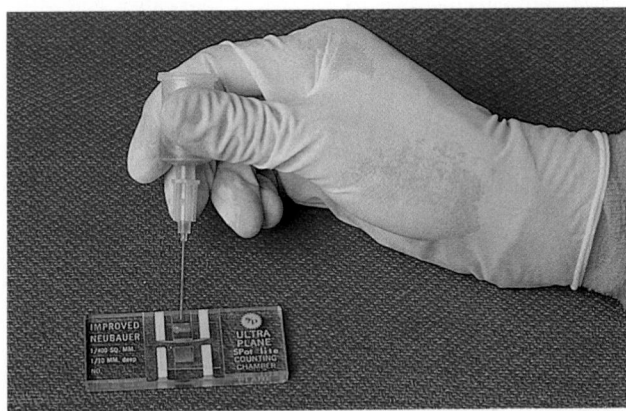

Figure 29-10 Filling the hemacytometer with a well-mixed diluted sample solution from a Unopette®.

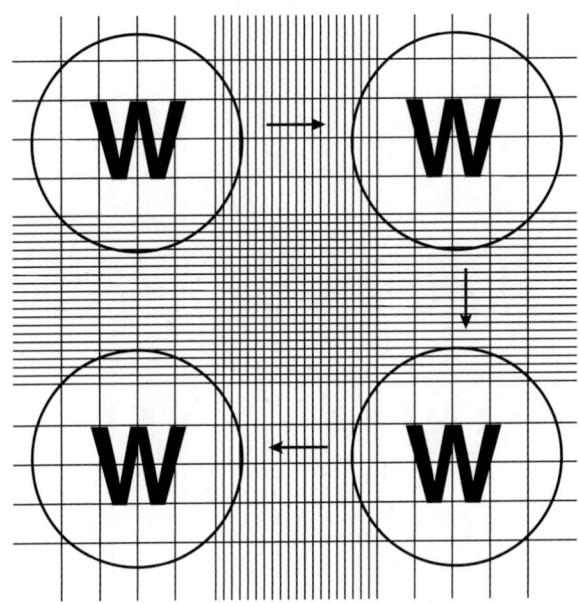

Figure 29-11 WBC counting areas marked with the letter *W*.

Each of the four areas counted in the WBC area contains sixteen squares. The order followed to count the four areas is not really important; however, it is customary to start in the upper left-hand corner and move in a clockwise direction (Figure 29-12). All the cells in each of the four squares marked *W* are counted using the following rule: Cells that touch the lines on two sides of the area should be counted; cells that touch the other two sides should not be counted (Figure 29-13). This same rule applies when you are performing an RBC count. If the number of cells counted in each of the four groups of sixteen small squares varies by more than plus or minus ten, the count should be discarded. The counting chamber should be cleaned, dried, and filled with a fresh drop of well-mixed sample. Uneven distribution of cells on the counting chamber usually occurs because of a dirty hemacytometer and/or coverglass.

NOTE: If the white blood cell count is very low (below 3,000 cells/cu mm), it would be more accurate to count all nine square millimeters on each side of the counting chamber (Figure 29-14). The total would then be divided by nine instead of four. Using the larger area should increase the accuracy of the count.

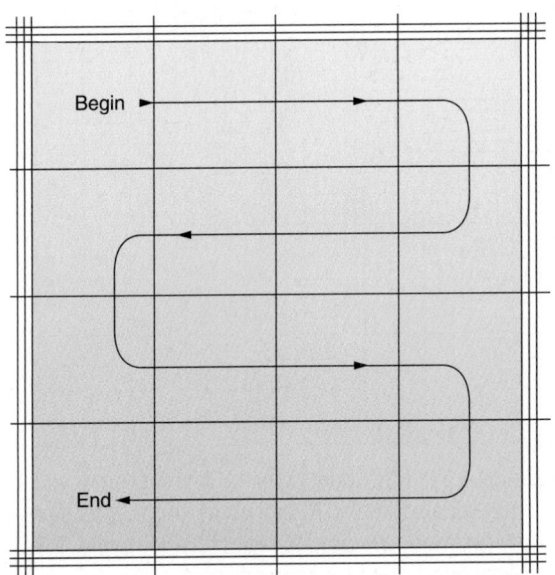

Figure 29-12 Counting pattern to follow when counting each of the one square millimeter areas of the hemacytometer.

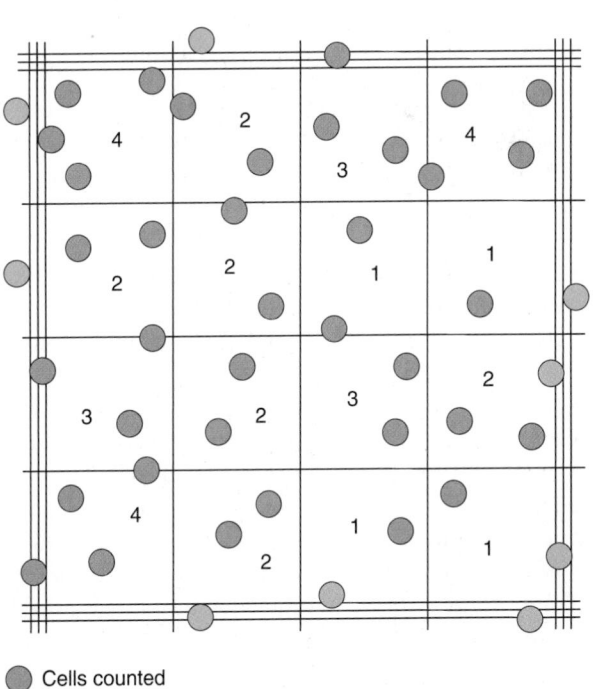

● Cells counted

● Cells not counted

Figure 29-13 Sample count in one square *W* area on one side of chamber. The purple cells and numbers shown denote the total number of cells counted in each square.

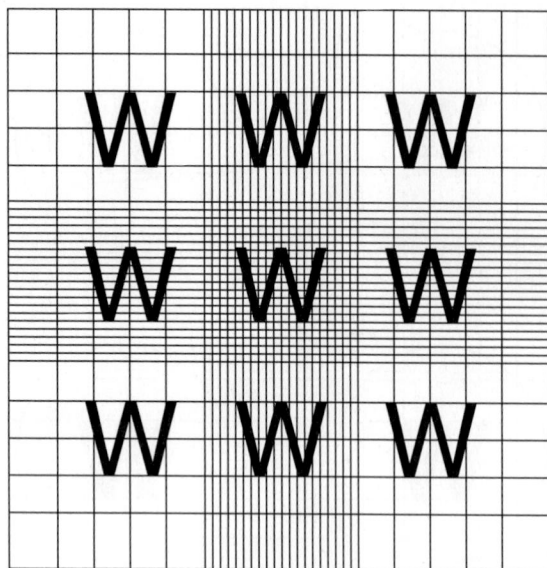

Figure 29-14   All nine large squares of the hemacytometer grid are used to count white blood cells when the count is low.

Calculating the White Blood Cell Count.

The total numbers of cells counted on both sides of the counting chamber are averaged. To calculate the number of white blood cells present in one cubic millimeter, the following formula is applied:

$$\text{WBC/mm}^3 = \frac{\substack{\text{average number cells counted}\\ \times \text{depth factor} \times \text{dilution factor}}}{\text{area counted (mm}^2)}$$

NOTE: The depth factor is always a value of 10 because the distance from the top of the platform of the hemacytometer to the bottom of the coverglass is 0.1 mm. To convert this value to 1 mm, it is multiplied by 10.

Counting the RBC Sample Using High-Power Magnification.

The area counted on the hemacytometer when performing a manual RBC count is usually one-fifth of a square millimeter. The procedure used to fill the hemacytometer for an RBC count is the same as that utilized in the WBC count. After the counting chamber is properly filled, it is allowed to settle for approximately two minutes. The RBC ruled area on the hemacytometer is first located using the low-power objective (10X). With the field in focus, change to the high-power objective (40X) and count the cells in the five RBC areas as indicated in Figure 29-15.

After counting the RBC area on one side of the counting chamber, repeat the procedure on the opposite side. The cells on the hemacytometer should be evenly distributed.

Example:

You perform a WBC count that has a dilution factor of 1:20 and you count the following number of cells. The cells are counted in the four *W* squares on the counting chamber.

1. Counting the cells:

Side 1		Side 2	
Square	Cells Counted	Square	Cells Counted
1	33	1	37
2	37	2	38
3	34	3	34
4	32	4	35
Total	136	Total	144

2. Calculating the average:
   a. 136 + 144 = 280
   b. 280 ÷ 2 = 140

3. Calculating the count:

$$\text{WBC mm}^3 = \frac{140 \times 10 \times 20}{4} = \frac{28,000}{4}$$
$$= \text{WBC mm}^3 = 7,000 \ (\text{or } 7.0 \times 10^3)/\text{mm}^3$$

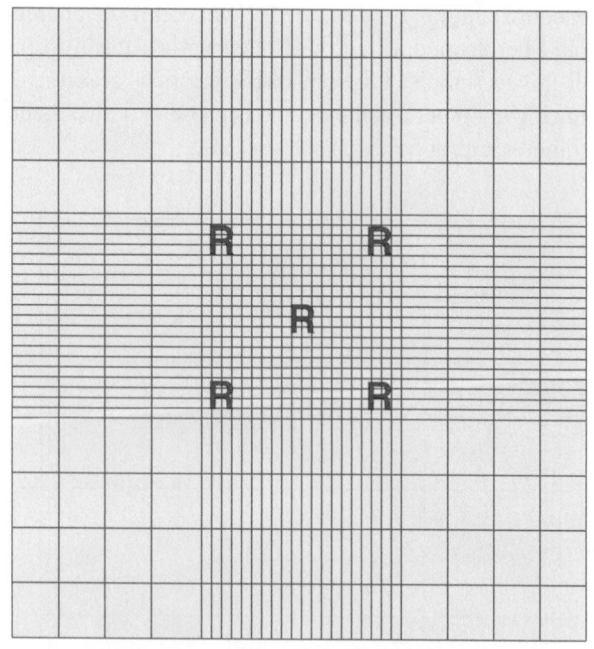

Figure 29-15   RBC counting area. The four corner squares and center square (labeled *R*) within the large center square on the hemacytometer are used to count red blood cells. These five areas equal one-fifth of a square millimeter.

TABLE 29-3 NORMAL LEUKOCYTE COUNTS

Leukocyte Count (Cells/mm³)

Age	Average	Reference Range
Newborn	18,000	9,000–30,000
One year	11,000	6,000–14,000
Six years	8,000	4,500–12,000
Adult	7,000	4,500–11,000

Example:

You perform an RBC count that has a dilution factor of 1:200 and you count the following number of cells. The cells are counted in the five *R* squares on the counting chamber.

1. Counting the cells:

Side 1		Side 2	
Square	Cells Counted	Square	Cells Counted
1	102	1	109
2	95	2	114
3	90	3	100
4	92	4	107
5	101	5	90
Total	480	Total	520

2. Compute the average:
   a. 480 + 520 = 1,000 cells
   b. 1,000 ÷ 2 = 500 average

3. Calculate the count:
   RBC mm³ = average number of cells × depth (mm) × dilution × area factor (mm)
   RBC mm³ = 500 × 10 (mm) × 200 × 5 (mm)²
   RBC mm³ = 500 × 10,000 (mm)³
   RBC mm³ = 5,000,000 or $5.0 \times 10^6/mm^3$

The number of cells in each of the five small areas should not vary by more than twenty-five. If the variation is greater than twenty-five, it indicates an uneven distribution of cells. This count should be discarded, the counting chamber should be cleaned and dried, and the process repeated.

Calculating the Red Blood Cell Count. The total number of cells counted on both sides of the counting chamber are averaged. To calculate the number of red blood cells present in one cubic millimeter, the following formula is applied:

$$RBC\ mm^3 = average\ number\ of\ cells \times depth_{(mm)}$$
$$\times dilution \times area\ factor_{(mm)}$$

The depth factor is always equal to 10 and the area factor in the RBC count is usually equal to 5. Remember that you usually count only one-fifth of a mm². To convert this to 1 mm², you must multiply by 5. The area factor in the formula can also be written as the denominator in the equation with a value of 0.20.

White Blood Cell Differential

The white blood cell (leukocyte) differential count is one of the most difficult tests to perform; it is also one of the most interesting. See Procedure 29-6. The reason it is so difficult is that there is no one way that a certain type of cell will always appear on a stained blood smear. The test is interesting because it provides the opportunity to visually examine all of the formed elements in the blood. It also enables the health care worker to see how the pathology of the patient is visible in the changes in the properties of

Some examples of blood cell changes associated with disease states are:

1. When a patient is experiencing an acute appendicitis, the white blood cell count will increase rapidly with a high percentage of neutrophils observed on the slide. There will also be an increase in the number of early or younger forms of these cells.
2. Patients who are suffering from a virus infection, especially adults, will frequently experience a reduction in white blood cells and the percentage of lymphocytes on the slide will increase. Patients with infectious mononucleosis will have increased numbers of lymphocytes, many of which will be atypical.
3. When patients have iron deficiency anemia, their differential slide will demonstrate red blood cells that show marked reduction in hemoglobin content. Their erythrocytes will appear hypochromic, lacking or low in color, because they lack the normal amount of hemoglobin in the red blood cell.

TABLE 29-4 NORMAL ERYTHROCYTE COUNTS

Age	Reference Range
Newborn	5.0 to $6.5 \times 10^6/mm^3$
One year	4.0 to $5.0 \times 10^6/mm^3$
Adult female	4.0 to $5.5 \times 10^6/mm^3$
Adult male	4.5 to $6.0 \times 10^6/mm^3$

the blood cells—both white cells and red cells—and how the types of cells will change with the pathology.

Making a Differential Blood Smear.

To perform a manual differential count, you must have a blood smear that has been stained. See Procedure 29-7. The most common way to make a differential blood smear is to use the two-slide or wedge method. The blood is spread out on the smear slide by using a second slide. This second slide is called the spreader slide.

The spreader slide should be held at a 30° to 35° angle. The greater the angle, the thicker the blood smear. If the angle is decreased during the end part of the spreading, the layer of cells on the smear slide will be very thin. A properly prepared blood smear has three distinct areas:

1. The heel of the smear, the area where the blood is too thick to examine properly
2. The feather edges of the slide where the smear is too thin and there are many holes or spaces between the cells
3. The body of the slide (between the thick area and the feather edge) where the cells are not overlaid and the smear does not have holes or large spaces between the cells

The smear slide should be allowed to air-dry and it should be stained as soon as it has dried. If the smear cannot be stained within a one-hour period after it is dried, it should be fixed to preserve the cells. Methyl alcohol is the fixative used to preserve blood smears.

Staining a Blood Smear.

Stains are applied to blood smears so that the formed elements may be more easily viewed and evaluated. A stained blood smear is evaluated in a procedure called the differential leukocyte count. This procedure is usually a part of the CBC (complete blood count). Stained smears may also be examined to detect and identify blood parasites such as those that cause malaria. A stained blood smear can provide important information regarding a patient's health. The evaluation of a blood smear often leads to the diagnosis or verification of disease.

Information gained during routine evaluation of blood smears may lead the physician to order special blood stains for further study. These special stains may be used to identify specific components of cells such as iron granules or nucleic acids. Bone marrow smears may be examined to evaluate blood cell production.

Types of Stains.

The stains most commonly used to stain a blood smear for routine microscopic examination are called **polychromatic stains**. Polychromatic blood stains contain methylene blue, a blue stain, and eosin, a red-orange stain. Polychromatic stains are also known as Wright's or Giemsa's stains.

The staining method utilized to stain the blood smear may be the two-step method or the three-step method. In most ambulatory care settings, the three-step method (also called the quick stain method) is utilized because it is easier and faster, and does not require the rigid control of the two-step method.

Two-step Method. In the two-step method, the methylene blue, eosin, and fixative are combined into one solution, which is placed on the dried smear slide first. The slide is allowed to stain for one to three minutes and then a buffer is added to the stain. The two solutions are mixed and allowed to stand. The slide is then rinsed gently with distilled water and allowed to air-dry. The two-step method requires four to six minutes.

Three-Step, or Quick Stain, Method. The quick stain method requires less than one minute to complete. It is called the three-step method because the slide is dipped first in a fixative solution then into two separate staining solutions (Figure 29-16).

 The fixative solution contains methyl alcohol in concentration greater than 99 percent. This solution can be fatal or cause blindness if swallowed. The methylene blue and eosin staining solutions are aqueous (water) solutions.

The slide is dipped into each of the three solutions approximately five times, allowing one second for each dip. The excess solution is allowed to drain away and at the end of each process, the excess solution is removed by touching the end of the vertical slide onto a paper towel. The process is repeated for each of the solutions and then the slide is gently rinsed with water and allowed to air-dry before it is examined microscopically.

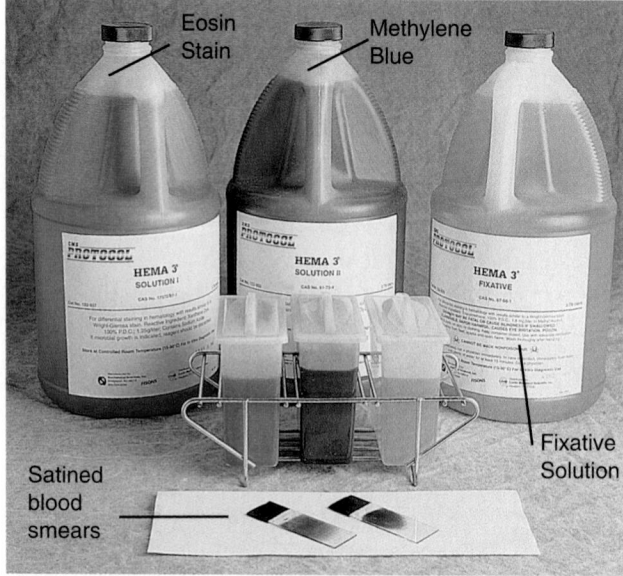

Figure 29-16   Hema-3 is a type of quick stain used in the ambulatory care setting.

Counting the Stained Differential Blood Smear. Cells are counted in the body area of the stained blood smear slides. The count usually consists of counting 100 white blood cells and determining the percentage of each of the five types. The characteristics of the white blood cells and the red blood cells are observed and noted. The relative number of platelets (thrombocytes) is noted on the lab report. When performing a differential leukocyte count, start in the thinnest area of the body portion of the slide and move in a serpentine pattern, making sure that cells are counted only once (Figure 29-17). The differential blood count is performed using the oil-immersion objective. Remember that this makes the total magnification 1,000X, because the oil-immersion objective is 100X and the eyepiece (ocular) is 10X.

The white blood cell features that must be studied to assist in the identification of the cell are: (1) the general size of the cell, (2) the nuclear characteristics, and (3) the cytoplasmic characteristics. The general size of the cell is determined by comparing it to the other types of cells on the slide as well as to the cells of the same type. Sometimes a single cell will be larger than the other cells of that type because it is younger. The characteristics of the nucleus that must be examined include shape, size, structure (such as dense or foamy), and color. The characteristics of the cytoplasm that must be examined and compared in the identification process include the amount, color, and types of inclusions.

It is very important that all of the preceding features of the cell be observed and studied during the identification and classification process. Probably the most common error made by beginners in white blood cell identification is that they let only one of these characteristics dominate their judgment when performing a differential count. The process of performing a correct differential leukocyte count requires a great deal of practice and study. It is imperative during the process to have access to a good blood cell atlas. *The Morphology of Human Blood Cells*, published by Abbott Laboratories, is an excellent reference.

Examination of a Blood Smear

The leukocytes on a stained blood smear can be divided into three groups: the myelocytic or granulocytic series (also called polymorphonuclear series), the lymphocytic, and the monocytic (Table 29-5; Figure 29-18). Mature cells in the granulocytic group have segmented nuclei and granules in the cytoplasm. The granulocytic group is further divided into three groups according to the types of granules in the cytoplasm. The three groups are the **neutrophil**, **eosinophil**, and **basophil**. The neutrophils are further indentified by the shape of the cell's nucleus. Mature cells have multiple nuclear lobes separated by a

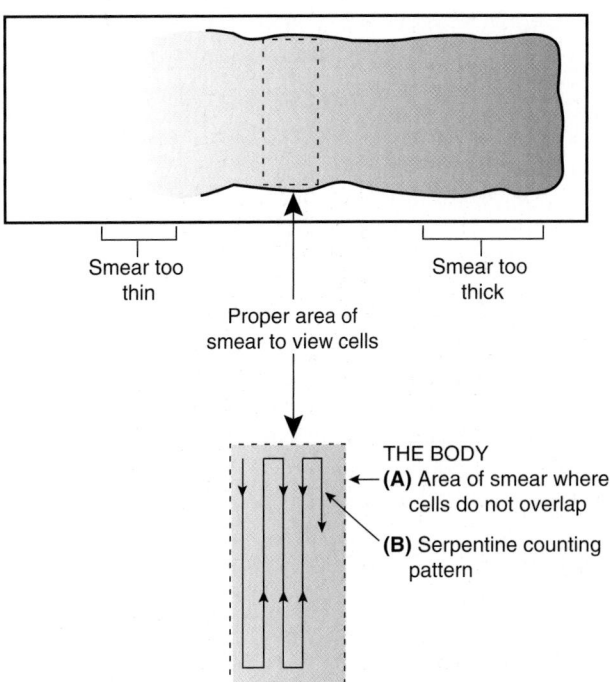

Figure 29-17 Proper area of slide to be viewed for differential count: (A) Close-up of proper body. (B) Counting pattern.

filament, hence the name segmented neutrophils (segs). Immature cells do not have distinct lobes, resulting in a nucleus that has a U shape. These cells are called band neutrophils (bands) (Figure 29-18 A and B). Eosinophils are easily recognized by the large red granules in the cell's cytoplasm (Figure 29-18E). Basophils are easily recognized by the large blue granules in the cell's cytoplasm (Figure 29-18F). The other two major divisions are the lymphocytic and monocytic divisions. Lymphocytes may be large or small in size. Table 29-6 and Figure 29-18 should be used in the process of identifying leukocytes on the stained blood smear.

After the leukocytes have been identified on the differential smear, the red blood cells and platelets (thrombocytes) are studied and evaluated. See Procedure 29-8. The average red blood cell is about 7.5 μm, which is slightly smaller than a small lymphocyte. Red blood cells that are about this size (7.5 μm) are called **normocytic**. Those

TABLE 29-5	LEUKOCYTE IDENTIFICATION GUIDE	
Divisions	**Cell Types**	**Polymorphonuclear Types**
I. Myelocytic, granulocytic, or polymorpho-nuclear	Neutrophil Eosinophil Basophil	Segmented cells Bands
II. Lymphocytic	Lymphocytes	
III. Monocytic	Monocytes	

TABLE 29-6 NORMAL VALUES FOR A DIFFERENTIAL LEUKOCYTE COUNT IN ADULTS

Neutrophil Bands: 3–5%
Neutrophil bands increase in appendicitis and many other diseases.

Neutrophil Segs: 54–62%
Segmented neutrophils increase in appendicitis and many other diseases. An elevation in neutrophils usually is indicative of an infectious disease.

Lymphocytes: 25–33%
Lymphocytes increase with infectious mononucleosis, lymphocytic leukemia, and many diseases of viral origin.

Monocytes: 3–7%
Monocytes increase in tuberculosis and monocytic leukemia.

Eosinophils: 1–3%
Eosinophils increase with allergic reactions, hay fever, and parasitic infections.

Basophils: 0–1%
Basophils increase in polycythemia vera, chicken pox, and ulcerative colitis.

that are larger are called **macrocytic** and those that are smaller are called **microcytic**. When the red blood cells on the differential slide show marked variation in size, this condition is called **anisocytosis**. The normal red blood cell has a round or slightly oval shape. If the shape of the red blood cells on the slide show marked variation, this is a condition known as **poikilocytosis**.

The red blood cell should contain hemoglobin that fills about one-half of the cell. The RBC is biconcave so most of the hemoglobin should be seen around the outer part of the cell. The central area of the RBC is pale. Red blood cells with the proper amount of hemoglobin are called **normochromic**. Those that do not have enough hemoglobin, that demonstrate too large of a pale central area, are called **hypochromic**.

The normal number of platelets observed on the differential smear averages about 10 per oil immersion field. The total platelet count can be estimated by counting the number of platelets in 10 fields and taking an average. The average number is then multiplied by 20,000. For example, if an average number of platelets is 15/oil immersion field, then the estimated total number of platelets is

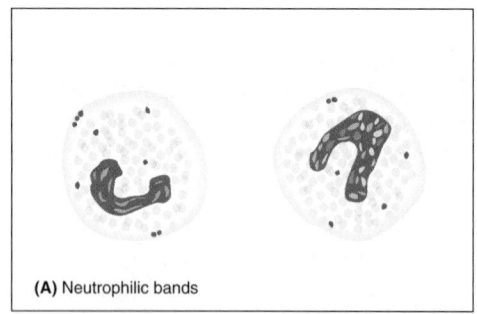

(A) Neutrophilic bands

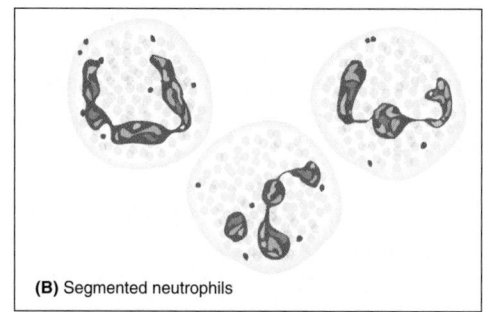

(B) Segmented neutrophils

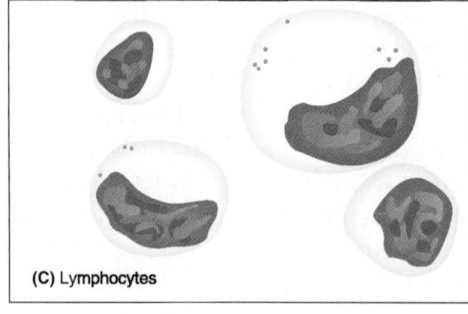

(C) Lymphocytes

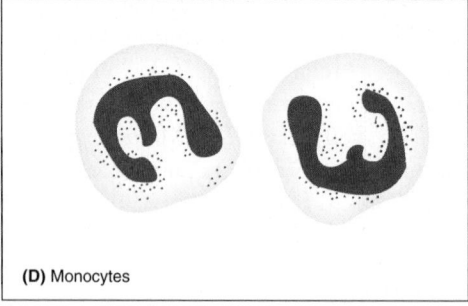

(D) Monocytes

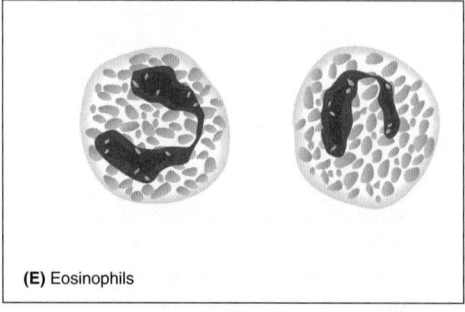

(E) Eosinophils

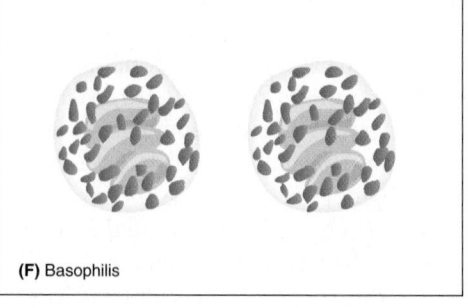

(F) Basophilis

Figure 29-18   Various divisions of leukocytes from a stained blood smear.

300,000/cm μL (15 × 20,000 = 300,000). The normal value for platelets (thrombocytes) is 140,000–400,000/cm μL. The differential count is performed automatically in most ambulatory care settings using an automated hematology instrument. This procedure is discussed later in this chapter.

> ## Clinical Laboratory Improvement Amendment, 1988 (CLIA '88) Regulation Regarding White Blood Cell Differential Counts
>
> - Laboratories that are certified for waiver-level testing only are not permitted to perform manual white blood cell differential counts.
> - Laboratories with a moderate-complexity certification can perform a manual differential white blood cell count but may only identify and report normal cells.
> - Laboratories certified to perform tests of high complexity can perform a manual differential white blood cell count and are permitted to identify and report both abnormal and normal cells.
>
> See Chapter 26 for details on CLIA '88 regulations.

ERYTHROCYTE INDICES

The **erythrocyte indices** include the mean corpuscular (cell) volume (MCV), the mean corpuscular hemoglobin (MCH), and the mean corpuscular hemoglobin concentration (MCHC). These indices (plural for index) are calculations that provide information about the size of the red blood cells and the hemoglobin content. The blood parameters needed to calculate all three indices are the red blood cell count, the hematocrit, and the hemoglobin. The erythrocyte indices values are important in the diagnosis or classification and treatment of different types of anemia. Table 29-7 shows normal values for the erythrocyte indices.

Before the automated hematology instrument became commonly used in the ambulatory care setting, the erythrocyte indices were not included as a part of the CBC because the red blood cell count was not an accurate measurement.

The following formulas are used to calculate the erythrocyte indices:

$$\text{Mean Corpuscular Volume (MCV)} = \frac{\text{Hematocrit}}{\text{RBC (in millions)}} \times 10$$

The result is reported in femtoliters (fL), a unit of volume 10^{-15} L, formerly reported in cubic microns (μm^3). This index gives the average volume of a red blood cell in the sample.

$$\text{Mean Corpuscular Hemoglobin (MCH)} = \frac{\text{Hemoglobin (in grams)}}{\text{RBC (in millions)}} \times 10$$

The result is expressed in picograms (pg), a micro microgram, or 1×10^{-12} g. This index estimates the weight of hemoglobin in a red blood cell of the sample.

$$\text{Mean Corpuscular Hemoglobin Concentration (MCHC)} = \frac{\text{Hemoglobin (in grams)}}{\text{Hematocrit}} \times 10$$

This result is expressed in grams/deciliter (g/dL). The MCHC is the average concentration of Hgb in a given volume of packed red blood cells (Hct).

Using Erythrocyte Indices to Diagnose

The MCH and MCV will be increased in megaloblastic anemias such as vitamin B_{12} and folate deficiency anemias. They will also be increased in acute blood loss anemia, chronic hemolytic anemias, aplastic anemias, hypothyroidism, and liver disease. The MCH and MCV will be decreased in hypochromic and microcytic anemias, including iron deficiency anemia, thalassemias, and occasionally in hyperthyroidism.

The MCHC will be increased in hereditary spherocytosis. It will be normal in macrocytosis. The MCHC will be decreased in iron deficiency anemia. The stained blood smear of a person with iron deficiency anemia will demonstrate red blood cells that are both hypochromic and microcytic.

ERYTHROCYTE SEDIMENTATION RATES (ESR)

The **erythrocyte sedimentation rate**, as the name implies, is a measurement of the rate at which the red blood cells in a well-mixed, anticoagulated blood sample will fall, or settle, toward the bottom when it is placed in a vertical tube. This test is commonly referred to in the

TABLE 29-7	NORMAL VALUES FOR THE ERYTHROCYTE INDICES
MCV	80–100 fL
MCH	27–33 pg
MCHC	32–36 g/dL

laboratory as a "sed rate." See Procedure 29-9. The ESR has been used for many years in the diagnosis and treatment of many disease states of the body. It is an inexpensive, accurate, and easy test to perform. Two factors that influence the sedimentation rate are the condition of the surface membrane of the red blood cell and changes in the level of fibrinogen in the plasma of the blood. During disease conditions in the body, the surface membrane of the red blood cell is altered, and this affects the rate at which the RBCs fall in the tube. Red blood cells will demonstrate this change even after the disease has subsided because RBCs have an average life of 120 days. For this reason, the ESR is a more accurate tool in diagnosing the onset of a disease than in checking the progress of treatment.

Fibrinogen is a plasma protein. The level, or concentration, of fibrinogen is altered during various disease states of the body.

Two ways to perform an ESR test are the Wintrobe method and the Westergren method. Both methods will provide the same information. Because of the simplicity in setting up the Westergren ESR, it has become the more widely used method in the ambulatory care setting.

Wintrobe Method

An EDTA venous blood sample is thoroughly mixed. With the use of a Pasteur pipette, the blood is transferred to a Wintrobe tube. The blood is added to the left zero mark at the top of the tube. It is important that no air bubbles are present in the blood column. The tube is placed exactly vertical in a rack and allowed to stand for exactly 60 minutes. The test is read by determining the number of millimeters (mm) the red cells have settled. The tube has a total capacity of 100 mm. The test is reported in mm/hr (Figure 29-19). Table 29-8 shows normal values for the Wintrobe method of ESR.

Westergren Method

The Westergren method differs from the Wintrobe method in that the blood sample is mixed with 3.8 percent sodium citrate solution before the tube is filled. The blood and sodium citrate are mixed and the tube is filled to the zero mark and placed exactly vertical in a rack. The tube is read after exactly 60 minutes, and the test is reported in mm/hr. Table 29-9 shows normal values for the Westergren method of ESR.

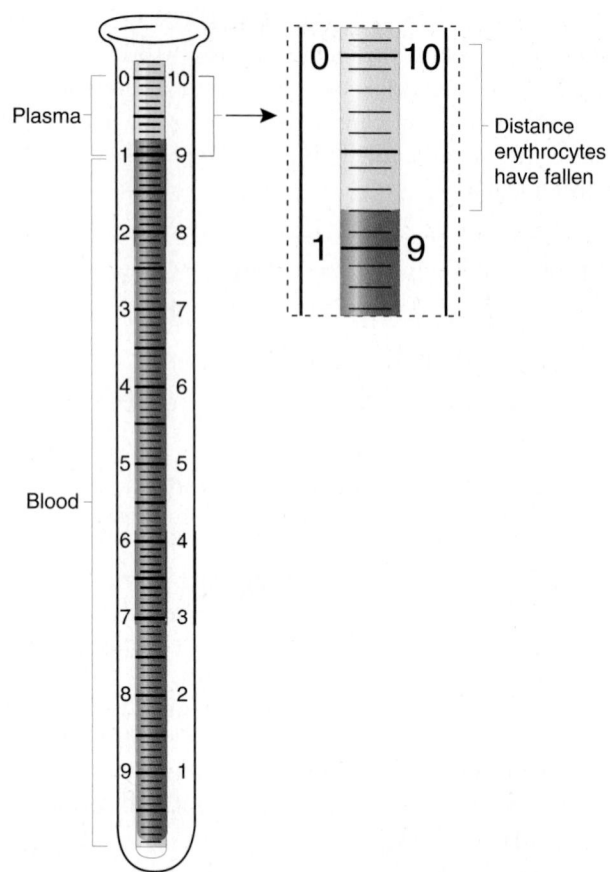

Figure 29-19   Wintrobe sedimentation tube showing settling of cells. The example shown illustrates a sedimentation of 8 mm.

The Polymedco company has produced a Sediplast® system to perform a Westergren ESR that is self-filling. It is a completely closed system that protects laboratory personnel from the risks associated with blood handling. The Sediplast® ESR System is shown in Figure 29-20.

The following guidelines should be followed when performing Wintrobe and Westergren ESR procedures to ensure accurate test results:

1. The tube must remain exactly vertical during the one-hour test time.
2. The test must be read at exactly 60 minutes (1 hour).
3. The counter on which the rack is placed must be free of vibrations.

TABLE 29-8	NORMAL VALUES FOR THE WINTROBE METHOD OF ESR
Males	0–9 mm/hr.
Females	0–20 mm/hr.

TABLE 29-9	NORMAL VALUES FOR THE WESTERGREN METHOD OF ESR
Males (under 50)	0–15 mm/hr.
Males (over 50)	0–20 mm/hr.
Females (under 50)	0–20 mm/hr.
Females (over 50)	0–30 mm/hr.

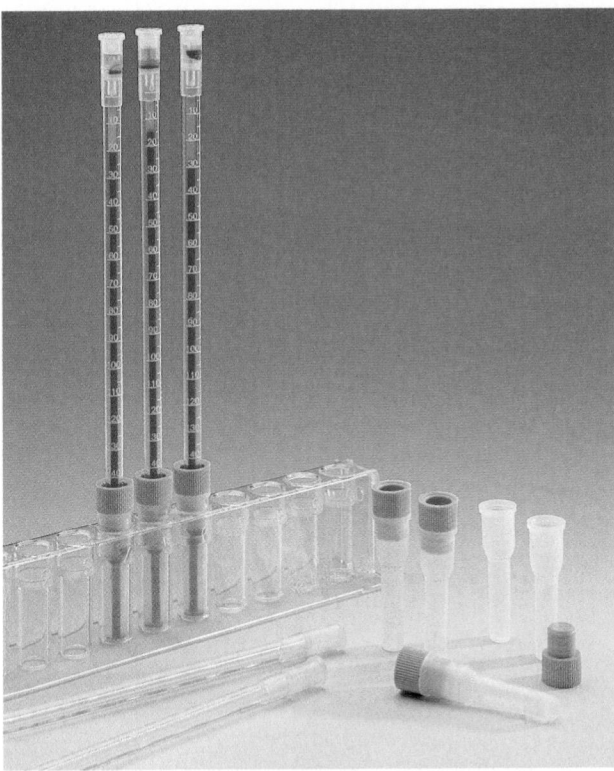

Figure 29-20 Sediplast® ESR System. The picture shows three filled tubes standing in the rack. Note the diluting vials with sodium citrate solution (right). (Courtesy of POLY-MEDCO Inc.)

4. The test should be set up within two hours after the blood is drawn.
5. The test should be conducted at room temperature.
6. The tube should not be placed in a draft, and it should not be exposed to direct sunlight.
7. The column of blood must be free of bubbles.

The erythrocytes in normal, nondiseased blood tend to remain suspended in the plasma. They do not aggregate (clump) together to form rouleaux. Rouleaux is a phenomenon where red blood cells form aggregates that look like rolls or stacks of coins (Figure 29-21).

This aggregate form causes the rate of sedimentation to increase. Red blood cells have membrane properties that tend to make them remain separated in the plasma. During certain diseased states, this repelling property is lost and the RBCs tend to aggregate.

Using the ESR to Diagnose

Erythrocyte sedimentation rates are increased in infections and inflammatory diseases, tissue destruction, and other conditions that lead to an increase in plasma fibrinogen. They are also increased with menstruation, pregnancy, malignant neoplasms, and multiple myeloma. With anemia, the ESR increases according to the severity of the condition.

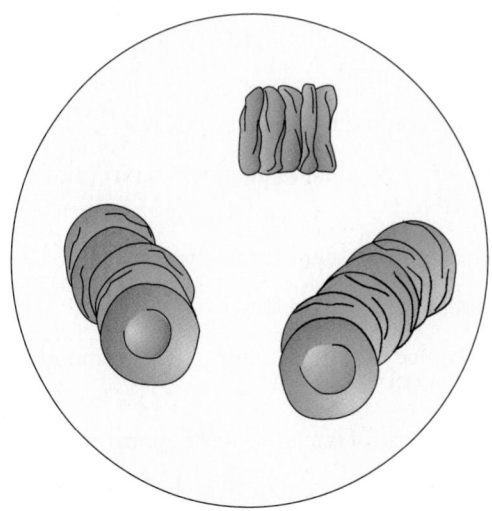

Figure 29-21 Erythrocytes forming rouleaux.

The ESR may be normal in osteoarthritis and in some cases of cirrhosis and malaria. The ESR values are decreased in polycythemia, spherocytosis, and sickle cell anemia.

AUTOMATED HEMATOLOGY INSTRUMENTATION AND QUALITY CONTROL

Most hematology tests performed in the ambulatory care setting today utilize some form of automated instrumentation. All procedures performed with automated instrumentation are modifications of manual methods. Automated hematology procedures have many advantages over the manual methods. They are faster, less expensive, simple to operate, and very accurate. The instruments can be calibrated and lend themselves to control testings. Most are equipped with printers that produce printed results. Many can store quality control results and print out quality control data summary sheets.

In addition to performing a wide variety of hematological tests, many automated hematology instruments also calculate part or all of the red blood cell indices and print the results. Some automated hematology instruments can be connected to other computers in the medical facility.

Semiautomated or completely automated hematology instruments can be purchased. The hematological parameters that are available on different automated office hematology instruments are:

- Red blood cell count
- White blood cell count
- Hemoglobin

- Hematocrit
- Platelet count
- Mean corpuscular volume (MCV)
- Mean corpuscular hemoglobin concentration (MCHC)
- Mean corpuscular hemoglobin (MCH)
- Percentage of granulocytes
- Granulocyte count (neutrophils, eosinophils, basophils)
- Percentage of lymphocytes/monocytes
- Nongranulocyte count (lymphocytes and monocytes)
- Mid-cell count (monocytes and band neutrophils)
- Percentage of mid-cells
- Lymphocyte count
- Percentage of lymphocytes
- Red blood cell distribution width (RDW)

The hematology instruments commonly utilized in the ambulatory care setting today employ two different principles of operation. One type takes the sample and makes appropriate dilutions before the sample is processed. The other type of instrument does not dilute the blood specimen but separates the sample into the different hematological values by centrifugation.

Hematology Instruments That Require Sample Dilutions

The type of technology utilized in the counting of particulate matter in the diluted sample is known as the **impedance principle** or resistance principle. A constant current is drawn across an electrolyte solution between two points. The blood sample is diluted with the same electrolyte solution. When the cells in the solution pass between these two points, they cause a change in the current flow at that point because they offer a resistance. The change in current flow produces an impulse which is counted as a cell. The various sizes of the cells can be interpreted by the instrument as different kinds of cells because they produce different amounts of resistance. Figure 29-22 shows an impedance hematology instrument that requires the operator to make manual dilutions. Fig-

ure 29-23 shows an impedance hematology instrument that is completely automatic. It pierces the rubber stopper of the blood sample, makes all of the necessary dilutions, reads the various parameters, and then self-cleans the instrument.

Hematology Instruments That Do Not Require Sample Dilutions

Centrifugal hematology analysis utilizes a nondiluted sample. Blood is drawn into a very precise capillary tube that has been treated on the inside with a special stain. This stain is picked up by the nuclei of the white blood cells. The tube is sealed and spun at very high speeds, causing the blood cells to separate into layers. These layers are read with the aid of a fluorescent microscope and a micrometer, which measures the thickness of the layer of each cell type.

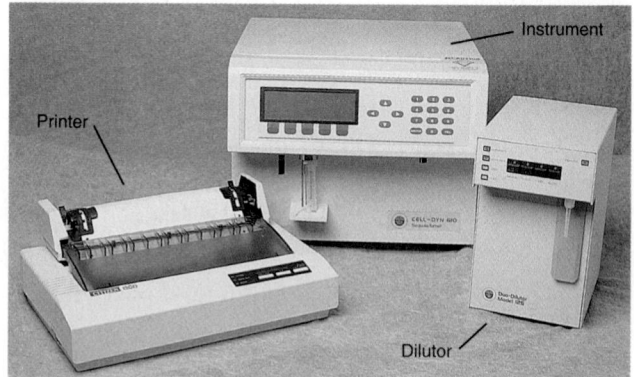

Figure 29-22   A semiautomated hematology instrument.

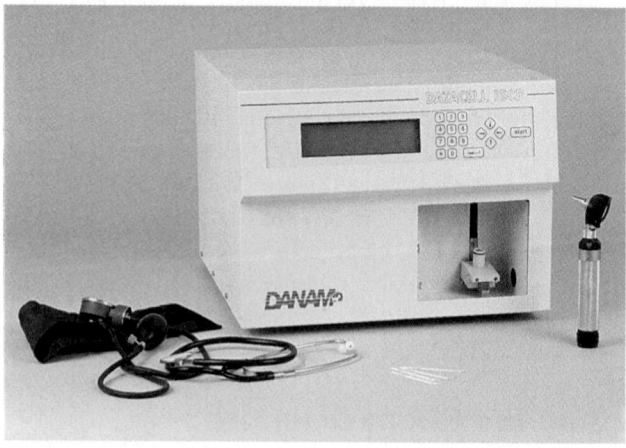

Figure 29-23   A completely automated hematology instrument.

Procedure 29-1 — Hemoglobin Determination (Manual Method Using a Spectrophotometer)

STANDARD PRECAUTIONS:

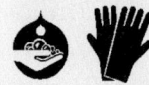   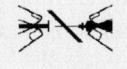

PURPOSE:

Properly and safely perform a manual hemoglobin determination using a spectrophotometer to evaluate the oxygen-carrying capacity of the blood.

EQUIPMENT/SUPPLIES:

Gloves
Hand disinfectant
EDTA blood sample(s) or supplies for a capillary puncture
Spectrophotometer (540 nm wavelength)
Hemoglobin standard solution
Cuvettes
Laboratory stretch film
10% chlorine bleach solution
UNOHEME® hemoglobin system *or* supplies for manual hemoglobin:
  Graduated pipette, 5 mL, with pipetting aid
  Drabkin's reagent
  Test tubes, 5 mL capacity
  Micropipettor to deliver 20 µL volume and tips
  Biohazard container
NOTE: Consult operating manual for specific instructions for spectrophotometer.

PROCEDURE STEPS:

1. Wash hands and put on gloves.
2. Assemble equipment and materials.
3. Turn on spectrophotometer.
4. Set wavelength at 540 nm.
5. For UNOHEME® method proceed with 5a–g. For manual method go to step 6.
   a. Draw 20 µL of well-mixed EDTA anticoagulated blood into the UNOHEME® capillary pipette.
   b. Insert the capillary pipette into the UNOHEME® reservoir and draw the blood into the reagent. Rinse the capillary pipette several times taking care not to overflow pipette.
   c. Mix contents by swirling. Let sit five minutes.
   d. Transfer contents of reservoir to a cuvette.
   e. Place diluting fluid from an unused UNOHEME® reservoir into a cuvette labeled "blank."
   f. Pipette 5 mL of a hemoglobin standard into cuvette labeled "Std."
   g. Proceed to step 7.
6. For manual method proceed with steps 6a–h.
   a. Label test tubes: blank, standard, and unknown (sample).
   b. Dispense 5.0 mL of Drabkin's reagent into blank and unknown tubes; dispense 5.0 mL of hemoglobin standard into standard tube.
   c. Mix blood sample for at least two minutes by hand or using mechanical mixer.
   d. Draw up 0.02 mL (20 µL) of blood with micropipette.
   e. Wipe excess blood from exterior of pipette with tissue.
   f. Dispense blood sample into the unknown (sample) tube.
   g. Mix contents of tube thoroughly and let stand for at least ten minutes (tubes can be mixed by inverting after placing laboratory stretch film over the top of the tube).
   h. Transfer contents of the tubes to cuvettes.
7. Place "blank" cuvette in the well of the spectrophotometer; set absorbance to zero following the manufacturer's instructions.
8. Place "standard" cuvette into the well of the spectrophotometer; read the absorbance and record the results.
9. Place "sample" cuvette (with UNOHEME® contents from step 5 or unknown from step 6) into the well of the spectrophotometer; read the absorbance and record the results.
10. Use the following formula to calculate hemoglobin concentration and record results:

$$\frac{A_{UNK}}{A_{STD}} \times Conc_{STD} = Conc_{UNK} \ (g/dL)$$

11. Discard all specimens and contaminated materials into biohazard container.
12. Disinfect and clean equipment and return to proper storage.
13. Clean work area with surface disinfectant.
14. Remove and discard gloves into biohazard container and wash hands with hand disinfectant.
15. Document the results.

Hemoglobin Determination (Hemoglobin Analyzer)

29-2

STANDARD PRECAUTIONS:

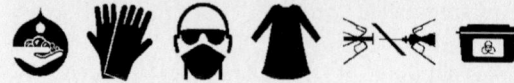

PURPOSE:

Properly and safely perform an automated hemoglobin determination to evaluate the oxygen capacity of the blood.

EQUIPMENT/SUPPLIES:

Gloves
Hand disinfectant
10% chlorine bleach solution
Capillary puncture equipment or blood samples collected in EDTA
Hb-Direct™ System, HemoCue® System, or other hemoglobin analyzer with supplies appropriate for the analyzer
Biohazard container
Puncture-proof biohazard container for sharps
NOTE: Consult manufacturer's instructions for specific procedure.

PROCEDURE STEPS:

1. Wash hands and put on gloves.
2. Assemble equipment and materials for analyzer method.
3. Turn on instrument to warm up. Calibrate or standardize the instrument according to the manufacturer's directions.
4. Perform a capillary puncture (see Chapter 28) observing the Bloodborne Pathogen Standard. Wipe away the first drop of blood with a tissue or sterile cotton ball.
5. Collect blood from the puncture using a capillary or cuvette appropriate for the analyzer to be used. Avoid trapping air bubbles in the collection device.
6. Wipe excess blood from the outside of the collection device (if appropriate) being careful not to touch the open end of the device.
7. For the Hb-Direct™, complete steps 7a–d. For HemoCue®, go to step 8.
   a. Insert the filled capillary tube into a cyanmethemoglobin vial. Place cap tightly on vial

and invert gently five to ten times until capillary tube is empty of blood. (The light red reaction color is stable for five days at room temperature.)
   b. Let vial stand at room temperature for five minutes.
   c. Insert vial into the Hemoglobin Analyzer, using the following procedure (these steps should be followed closely to ensure that the capillary tube does not obstruct the analyzer light path):
      (1) Invert the vial slowly, then hold it horizontally for three seconds. As the vial is *slowly* returned to its upright position, the capillary tube should adhere to the upper side of the vial.
      (2) Position the vial so that the capillary tube is at the *back* of the vial.
      (3) Wipe fingerprints from the sides of the vial with a tissue.
      (4) Check that the reagent vial is tightly capped.
      (5) Insert the vial into the Hemoglobin Analyzer with the capillary tube positioned to the back of the vial.
      (6) Wait five seconds. Read the analyzer display. Check to ensure that the capillary tube has remained in the upper half of the vial.
   d. Read the hemoglobin concentration from the display and record. Proceed to step 9.
8. For HemoCue®:
   a. Insert the filled cuvette into the HemoCue® photometer within ten minutes of filling the cuvette.
   b. Read the hemoglobin value from the display and record.
9. Discard all contaminated materials into biohazard containers.
10. Return all equipment to proper storage.
11. Wipe counters with surface disinfectant.
12. Remove and discard gloves into biohazard container.
13. Wash hands with hand disinfectant.
14. Document the results.

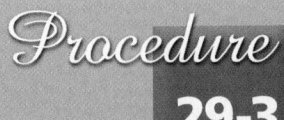

29-3 Microhematocrit

STANDARD PRECAUTIONS:

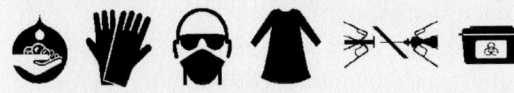

PURPOSE:
Properly and safely perform the microhematocrit procedure using a few microliters of blood in a capillary tube to separate the cellular elements of the blood from the plasma by centrifugation.

EQUIPMENT/SUPPLIES:
Gloves
Hand disinfectant
Capillary tubes, plain and with heparin
Acrylic safety shield
Precalibrated capillary tubes (optional)
Sealing clay or disposable plastic sealing caps (if not using self-sealing tubes)
Microhematocrit centrifuge and reader
Tube of anticoagulated venous blood (or commercially available simulated blood)
Paper towels or soft laboratory tissue
70% alcohol or alcohol swabs
Gauze or cotton balls, sterile
Blood lancets, sterile, disposable
Surface disinfectant or 10% chlorine bleach solution
Biohazard container
Puncture-proof biohazard container for sharps
NOTE: Consult the instruction manual for the centrifuge being used. Refer to the specific procedure being performed.

PROCEDURE STEPS:
1. Wash hands and put on gloves.
2. Assemble equipment and materials for capillary puncture and microhematocrit.

For direct specimen method, complete steps 3a–g. When utilizing a sample from a blood specimen tube, go to step 4.

3. Fill two capillary tubes from a capillary puncture.
   a. Perform a capillary puncture (see Chapter 28).
   b. Wipe away the first drop of blood.
   c. Touch one end of a heparinized capillary tube to the second drop of blood.
   d. Allow the tube to fill three-quarters full by capillary action. A slight downward angle of the tube may be necessary (if using precalibrated tubes, fill to the line).
   e. Fill a second tube in the same manner.
   f. Wipe the outside of the filled capillary tube with soft tissue, if necessary, to remove excess blood.
   g. Seal the capillary tube by placing the clean end into the tray of sealing clay (the sealing clay will stay cleaner if the dry/clean end of the capillary tube is sealed). Proceed to step 5.
4. Fill two capillary tubes using a tube of EDTA anticoagulated blood (if not available, proceed to step 5):
   a. Mix the tube of blood thoroughly by gently rocking the tube from end to end a minimum of two minutes by mechanical mixer or fifty to sixty times by hand.
   b. Remove cap from the tube (with an acrylic safety shield placed between worker and tube).
   c. Tilt the tube so that blood is very near the top edge of the tube.
   d. Insert the tip of a plain capillary tube into the blood and fill three-quarters full by capillary action (if using precalibrated tubes, fill to the line). NOTE: Wipe the outside of the filled capillary tube with tissue, if necessary, to remove excess blood.
   e. Seal the tube by placing the clean end into the tray of sealing clay or by using a plastic sealing cap. If using self-sealing tubes, check to see that the plug expanded.
   f. Fill a second tube in the same manner.
5. Check to see if the interior sealing clay edge appears level in the tubes.
6. Place tubes into the microhematocrit centrifuge with *sealed* ends securely against the gasket (balance the centrifuge by placing the tubes opposite each other).
7. Fasten both lids securely.
8. Set the timer and adjust the speed if necessary.
9. Centrifuge for the prescribed time.
10. Allow the centrifuge to come to a complete stop and unlock the lid(s).
11. Determine the microhematocrit values using one of the following methods:
    a. A centrifuge that requires calibrated tubes and has a built-in scale:

(continues)

Procedure 29-3 (continued)

(1) Position the tubes as directed by the manufacturer's instructions.

(2) Read the microhematocrit value.

b. A centrifuge without a built-in reader:

(1) Carefully remove capillary tubes from centrifuge.

(2) Place tube on the microhematocrit reader provided.

(3) Follow instructions on the reader to obtain the microhematocrit value.

12. Average the values from the two tubes and record the microhematocrit.

13. Discard the capillary tubes and used lancets into a puncture-proof biohazard container for sharps.

14. Clean and return equipment to proper storage.

15. Clean the work area with surface disinfectant.

16. Remove and discard gloves into biohazard container and wash hands with hand disinfectant.

17. Wash hands with hand disinfectant.

18. Document the results.

Procedure 29-4 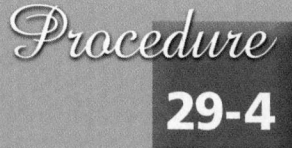 White Blood Cell Count (Unopette® Method)

STANDARD PRECAUTIONS:

    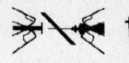

PURPOSE:
Properly and safely perform the white blood cell count using a self-contained system to determine the total number of white blood cells per cubic millimeter of blood.

EQUIPMENT/SUPPLIES:
Gloves
Surface disinfectant (10% chlorine bleach solution)
Tube of EDTA blood or supplies for a capillary puncture
Hand disinfectant
Unopette® WBC or WBC/Platelet system
Hemacytometer with coverglass
Hand tally counter
70% alcohol
Microscope
Lens paper
Acrylic safety shield or goggles and mask
Biohazard container
Biohazard container for sharps
NOTE: Following is a general procedure for the use of the Unopette® system. Consult the manufacturer's package insert for specific instructions.

PROCEDURE STEPS:
1. Assemble equipment and materials; obtain a Unopette® system for WBC or WBC/Platelet count.

2. Place a clean hemacytometer coverglass on a clean hemacytometer.

3. Pierce the diaphragm of the Unopette® reservoir with the pipette shield.

4. Set up acrylic safety shield or wear goggles and mask.

5. Wash hands and put on gloves.

6. Remove the shield from the pipette assembly. (Perform steps 7–14 with safety shield between you and the blood or blood solution.)

7. Fill the capillary pipette from a capillary puncture or from a tube of well-mixed EDTA blood.

8. Allow the blood to rise in the capillary until it automatically stops.

9. Wipe any excess blood from the outside of the pipette, being careful not to touch the tip with the tissue.

10. Squeeze the reservoir slightly, being careful not to expel any of the liquid.

11. Maintain pressure on the reservoir and insert the capillary pipette into the reservoir, seating the pipette firmly into the neck of the reservoir. Do not expel any of the liquid.

(continues)

Procedure 29-4 (continued)

12. Release the pressure on the reservoir, drawing the blood out of the capillary pipette and into the diluent.
13. Squeeze the reservoir gently three to four times to rinse the remaining blood from the capillary pipette. NOTE: Do not allow the blood-diluent mixture to flow out the top.
14. Swirl or turn the reservoir from side to side to gently mix the contents.
15. Let the reservoir sit for ten minutes (but no longer than an hour) to destroy the red blood cells.
16. Remove the pipette from the reservoir and insert it into the neck of the reservoir so that the pipette tip extends *upward* from the reservoir.
17. Thoroughly mix the contents of the reservoir. Invert the reservoir and gently squeeze to discard four or five drops onto paper towel or gauze.
18. Touch the tip of the pipette to the edge of the coverglass and counting chamber. Fill both chambers.
19. Place the filled hemacytometer into a Petri dish beside a damp cotton ball. Cover and let stand for ten minutes.
20. Carefully place the hemacytometer on the microscope stage and secure it.
21. Use the low-power (10X) objective to bring the ruled area into focus. Identify the nine white

blood cell squares.
22. Count the white blood cells lying within all nine squares, using the boundary rule.
23. Record the results.
24. Repeat the count, using the other side of the hemacytometer, and record the results.
25. Obtain the average count by adding the results from the two sides and dividing by two.
26. Calculate 10 percent of the average and add that to the average. Then multiply that total by 100 to get the number of white blood cells per cubic millimeter.
27. Place the hemacytometer and coverglass into the bleach solution for ten minutes, then rinse with water. Dry carefully with lens paper.
28. Discard any sharps into a puncture-proof biohazard container.
29. Return the tube of blood to the storage area or discard into biohazard waste. Discard the Unopette® assembly in the biohazard sharps container.
30. Return equipment to proper storage.
31. Clean the work area with surface disinfectant.
32. Remove and discard gloves into biohazard container.
33. Wash hands with hand disinfectant.

Procedure 29-5 — Red Blood Cell Count (Unopette® Method)

STANDARD PRECAUTIONS:

   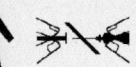

PURPOSE:
To count red blood cells.

EQUIPMENT/SUPPLIES:
Gloves
Hand disinfectant

Materials for capillary puncture, or blood sample, anticoagulated with EDTA
Hemacytometer with coverglass
Test tube rack or beaker to hold blood sample
Unopette® for RBC count (reservoir and pipette assembly)
Microscope
Lens paper
Alcohol (70% ethanol)

(continues)

Procedure

29-5   *(continued)*

Hand tally counter
Surface disinfectant or 10% chlorine bleach solution
Biohazard container
Biohazard container for sharps
Acrylic safety shield or goggles and mask
NOTE: Following is a general procedure for the use of the Unopette® system. Consult the package insert for specific instructions.

PROCEDURE STEPS:

1. Assemble equipment and materials. Set up acrylic safety shield or put on goggles and mask.
2. Place a clean hemacytometer coverglass over a clean hemacytometer.
3. Wash hands and put on gloves.
4. Puncture the diaphragm of the Unopette® reservoir. Hold the reservoir firmly on a flat surface with one hand and use the tip of the pipette shield to puncture the diaphragm. NOTE: The opening must be made large enough to easily accommodate the pipette.
5. Remove the shield from the pipette assembly.
6. Fill the capillary pipette from a capillary puncture or from a tube of well-mixed EDTA anticoagulated blood. The pipette will fill by capillary action and will stop filling automatically. NOTE: Keep pipette horizontal or at a slight (5°) upward angle to avoid overfilling.
7. Wipe excess blood from the outside of the capillary pipette with soft laboratory tissue. NOTE: Do not allow tissue to touch pipette tip.
8. Squeeze the reservoir slightly, being careful not to expel any of the liquid.
9. Maintain the pressure on the reservoir and insert the capillary pipette into the reservoir, seating the pipette firmly into the neck of the reservoir. Do not expel any of the liquid.
10. Release the pressure on the reservoir, drawing the blood out of the capillary pipette into the diluent.
11. Squeeze the reservoir gently three to four times to rinse the remaining blood from the capillary pipette. NOTE: Do not allow the blood-diluent mixture to flow out the top.
12. Thoroughly mix the contents of the reservoir by gently swirling the reservoir and/or turning it side to side.
13. Withdraw the capillary pipette from the reservoir and insert it into the neck of the reservoir in reverse position (the pipette tip should now project upward from the reservoir).
14. Thoroughly mix the contents of the reservoir. Invert the reservoir and gently squeeze to discard four to five drops onto gauze or paper towel.
15. Fill both sides of the hemacytometer.
16. Carefully place the hemacytometer on the microscope stage and secure.
17. Use the low-power (10X) objective to bring the ruled area into focus.
18. Locate the large central square.
19. Carefully rotate the high-power (40X) objective into position and focus with the fine adjustment knob until lines are clear.
20. Adjust the light and/or condenser so that red blood cells are visible.
21. Count the cells in the four corner squares and one center square within the larger center square of the counting area, using the left-to-right, right-to-left counting pattern.
22. Record the results for each of the five squares (four corner and one center).
23. Repeat the count using the other side of the hemacytometer.
24. Use the worksheet to calculate the RBC count.
25. Record the result.
26. Disinfect the hemacytometer and coverglass.
27. Discard the specimen and disposable materials appropriately.
28. Return equipment to proper storage.
29. Clean work area with surface disinfectant.
30. Remove and discard gloves into biohazard container and wash hands with hand disinfectant.

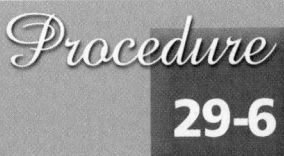

Preparation of a Differential Blood Smear Slide

STANDARD PRECAUTIONS:

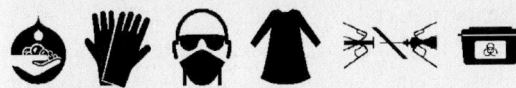

PURPOSE:
Properly and safely prepare an anticoagulated blood smear and a capillary blood smear by spreading blood on a microscopic slide, altering the form, structure, and distribution of cells (morphology) as little as possible, to microscopically view the cellular components.

EQUIPMENT/SUPPLIES:
Gloves
Hand disinfectant
Pencil
Microscope slides (1″ × 3″), frosted end optional
95% ethyl alcohol
Laboratory tissue
Capillary tubes (plain and heparinized)
Slide drying rack
Hot water
Detergent
Distilled water
Methanol in covered staining (Coplin) jar
EDTA anticoagulated blood specimen (fresh)
Materials for capillary puncture
Surface disinfectant or 10% chlorine bleach solution
Biohazard container
Puncture-proof container for sharp objects

PROCEDURE STEPS:
1. Assemble equipment and materials.
2. Place a clean slide on a flat surface (be sure to touch only the edges of the slide with fingers). Write patient identification on the frosted area with a pencil.
3. Wash hands and put on gloves.
4. Obtain an EDTA anticoagulated blood sample (provided by the instructor).
5. Mix blood well and fill a plain capillary tube with blood.
6. Dispense a small drop of blood from the capillary tube onto the slide about one-half to three-fourths inch from the right end (if left-handed, reverse instructions) (Figure 29-24A).
7. Place the end of a clean, polished, unchipped spreader slide in front of the drop of blood at a 30°–35° angle. Spreader should be lightly balanced with fingertips (Figure 29-24B).
8. Pull the spreader slide back into the drop of blood by sliding gently along the slide until the blood spreads along three-fourths of the width of the spreader (Figure 29-24C).
9. Push the spreader slide forward with a quick steady motion (use other hand to keep slide from moving while spreader is pushed) (Figure 29-24D).
10. Examine the smear to see if it is satisfactory (Figure 29-24E).

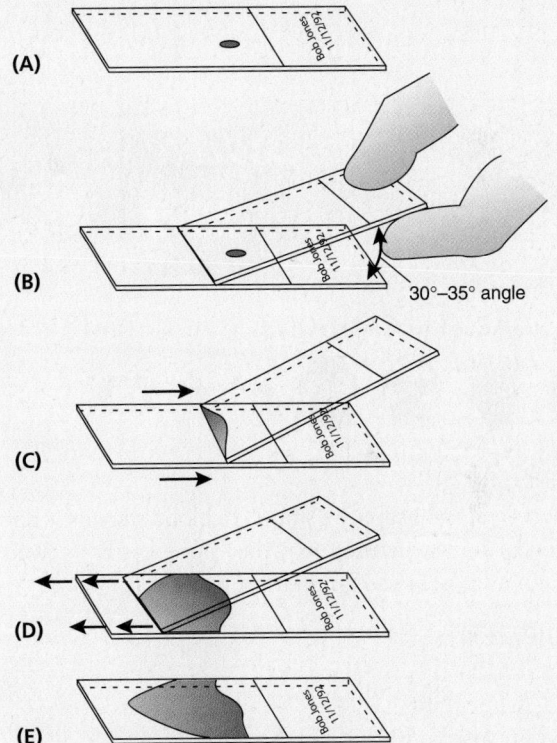

Figure 29-24 Making a blood smear for a differential white blood cell count using a spreader slide.
A. Position labeled end to right if you are right-handed, or to left if you are left-handed.
   Place a small drop of blood on the slide.
B. Grasp the slide with your left hand to steady it.
C. Pull the spreader slide back into the drop of blood.
   Let the blood spread along the back side of the spreader slide.
D. Quickly, without jerks, push the spreader slide to the left.
E. Allow the blood smear to air-dry before it is stained.

(continues)

Procedure 29-6 *(continued)*

11. Repeat the procedure until two satisfactory smears are obtained.
12. Allow the smear to air-dry quickly (stand slide on end in slide drying rack).
13. Place the dried smear in absolute methanol for thirty to sixty seconds to preserve the smear.
14. Remove the slide from methanol and allow to air-dry.
15. Store slide for staining.
16. Perform a capillary puncture, wipe away the first drop of blood, and fill one or two EDTA anticoagulated capillary tubes.

17. Prepare two blood smears from capillary blood, repeating steps 6–15.
18. Discard blood specimens appropriately or store for later use. Place contaminated materials into biohazard or sharps container.
19. Clean equipment and return to proper storage.
20. Clean work area with surface disinfectant.
21. Remove and discard gloves into biohazard container and wash hands with hand disinfectant.

Procedure 29-7   **Staining a Differential Blood Smear Slide**

STANDARD PRECAUTIONS:

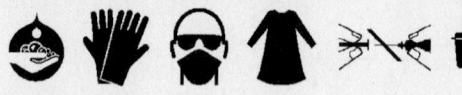

PURPOSE:
Properly and safely apply a stain to a blood smear so that the cells and structures may be more easily viewed through microscopic examination.

EQUIPMENT/SUPPLIES:
Gloves
Hand disinfectant
Blood smears, freshly prepared or preserved
Blood stain reagents:
  Wright's stain and buffer and/or
  commercial blood stain kit (quick stain)
Tube of EDTA anticoagulated blood (optional)
Staining rack
Immersion oil
Microscope
Lens paper
Forceps
Laboratory tissue
Lab apron or lab coat
Staining jars for quick stains

Surface disinfectant or 10% chlorine bleach solution
Biohazard container
Puncture-proof container for sharp objects
Slide storage box
NOTE: Stain characteristics may vary with stain lot. Follow the manufacturer's instructions for best results.

PROCEDURE STEPS:
1. Wash hands and put on gloves.
2. Assemble equipment and materials.
3. Prepare a blood smear (as in Procedure 29-6) or obtain a previously prepared, fixed smear.
4. Stain a blood smear by one of the following methods:
   a. Two-step method
      (1) Place the dried smear on the staining rack or on a flat surface, blood side up.
      (2) Flood the smear with Wright's stain but do not let stain overflow the sides of the slide.
      (3) Leave stain on slide one to three minutes (get exact time from instructor).
      (4) Add buffer, dropwise, to the stain until the buffer volume is about equal to the stain.

(continues)

Procedure 29-7 *(continued)*

(5) Blow gently on the surface of the fluid to mix the solutions. A green metallic sheen should appear on the surface.

(6) Allow buffer to remain on slide for two to four minutes (do not allow mixture to run off slide); get exact time from instructor.

(7) Rinse thoroughly and continuously with a gentle stream of tap or distilled water.

(8) Drain water from slide.

(9) Wipe the *back* of the slide with a wet gauze to remove excess stain.

(10) Stand smear on end to dry.

b. Three-step method (quick stain)

(1) Dip dry smear into solutions as directed by manufacturer's instructions (do not allow slide to dry between solutions).

(2) Rinse slide (if instructed to do so).

(3) Remove excess stain from the *back* of the slide with wet gauze.

(4) Allow slide to air-dry by standing on end.

5. Place thoroughly dried slide on microscope stage, stain side up.

6. Focus with low-power (10X) objective.

7. Scan slide to find area where cells are barely touching each other (in feathered edge of smear).

8. Place a drop of immersion oil on the slide.

9. Rotate oil-immersion lens carefully into position.

10. Focus with fine adjustment knob only.

11. Observe erythrocytes; color should be pink-tan.

12. Observe leukocytes; nuclei should be purple; neutrophil granules should be pink-lavender.

13. Observe platelets; they should appear purple and granular.

14. Rotate the low-power (10X) objective into position.

15. Remove slide from microscope stage.

16. Clean oil objective thoroughly with lens paper.

17. Gently wipe oil from slide with soft tissue.

18. Clean equipment and return to proper storage.

19. Discard slides as instructed or store in slide box for use in Procedure 29-8.

20. Clean work area with surface disinfectant.

21. Remove and discard gloves into biohazard container and wash hands with hand disinfectant.

Procedure 29-8 Differential Leukocyte Count

STANDARD PRECAUTIONS:

PURPOSE:

Properly and safely examine a stained blood smear to observe, identify, and record 100 leukocytes and "differentiate" the five types of leukocytes by size, nuclear characteristics, and cytoplasmic characteristics.

EQUIPMENT/SUPPLIES:

Gloves
Hand disinfectant
Stained normal blood smears
Microscope with oil-immersion objective
Immersion oil
Lens paper
Soft tissue or soft paper towels
Blood cell atlas; drawings or photographs and descriptions of stained blood cells
Tally counter or differential counter
Worksheet
Puncture-proof container for contaminated sharps
Surface disinfectant or 10% chlorine bleach solution

(continues)

Procedure

29-8   *(continued)*

PROCEDURE STEPS:

1. Wash hands and put on gloves.
2. Assemble equipment and materials.
3. Place stained smear on microscope stage and secure with clips.
4. Use the low-power (10X) objective to locate the feathered edge of the smear.
5. Bring the cells into focus using the 10X objective and coarse adjustment.
6. Scan the smear to find an area where the red blood cells are barely touching.
7. Place one drop of immersion oil on the smear.
8. Rotate the oil-immersion objective (97X or 100X) carefully into position.
9. Using the fine adjustment, focus until cells can be seen clearly.
10. Raise the condenser and open the diaphragm to allow maximum light into the objective.
11. Scan the slide to observe the leukocytes.
12. Study the smear; try to find and identify all five types of leukocytes.
13. Scan the smear to find platelets.
14. Scan the smear to observe red cells.
15. Repeat steps 3–14 until cells can readily be identified.
16. Repeat steps 1–10 using the same smear or a different one.
17. Count 100 consecutive leukocytes moving the slide or the movable stage so that consecutive microscopic fields are viewed; use the counting pattern illustrated in Figure 29-17.

18. Record on the worksheet how many of each type of leukocyte are seen.
19. Observe the red blood cells in at least ten fields. Note the hemoglobin content; record as normochromic or hypochromic. Look for any variation in shape.
20. Observe the red blood cell size. Record as normocytic, microcytic, or macrocytic. An approximation of the number of cells affected can be made by using a system of 1+ to 4+, or using small, medium, or large amount.
21. Observe platelets in at least ten fields:
    a. Note morphology.
    b. Estimate the number of platelets per oil immersion field: record as adequate, decreased, or increased, using the guide on the worksheet.
22. Rotate the low-power (10X) objective into place.
23. Remove the slide from the stage.
24. Using lens paper, clean the oil-immersion objective thoroughly.
25. Check the microscope stage and condenser for oil and clean with soft tissue if necessary.
26. Place the slide on its edge in a plastic slide box so oil can drain, or discard slide as instructed.
27. Clean remaining equipment and return it to proper storage.
28. Wipe work counter with surface disinfectant.
29. Remove and discard gloves into biohazard container and wash hands with hand disinfectant.

Procedure

29-9   **Erythrocyte Sedimentation Rate**

STANDARD PRECAUTIONS:

    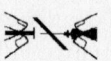

PURPOSE:
Properly and safely examine a blood sample by using either the Sediplast® (Westergren) or Wintrobe method to record the erythrocyte sedimentation rate.

(continues)

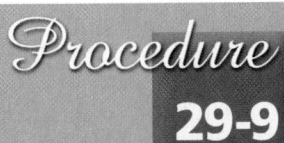

Procedure

29-9   *(continued)*

EQUIPMENT/SUPPLIES:

Gloves
Hand disinfectant
Sample of venous blood collected in EDTA
Sediplast® kit (or other ESR kit):
  sedivial and sedirack
  Sediplast® autozeroing pipette
  Pipette capable of delivering up to 1.0 mL
Wintrobe method:
  Wintrobe sedimentation tube (disposable or
    reusable)
  Wintrobe sedimentation rack
  Long-stem Pasteur-type pipette with rubber bulb
Timer
10% chlorine bleach solution
Biohazard disposal container
Acrylic safety shield or goggles and mask
Puncture-proof biohazard container for sharps
NOTE: Consult the manufacturer's package insert for
  specific instructions for the ESR kit being used.

PROCEDURE STEPS:

1. Wash hands and put on gloves.
2. Assemble equipment and materials.
3. Gently mix blood sample for two minutes.
4. Perform either method a (Sediplast® ESR) or
   method b (Wintrobe):
   a. Sediplast® ESR (modified Westergren)
      (1) Remove stopper on sedivial and fill to the
          indicated mark with 0.8 mL blood. Re-
          place stopper and invert vial several times
          to mix (or mix using pipette).
      (2) Place sedivial in Sediplast® rack on a level
          surface.
      (3) Gently insert the disposable Sediplast®
          pipette through the pierceable stopper
          with a twisting motion and push down
          until the pipette rests on the bottom of the
          vial. The pipette will autozero the blood
          and any excess will flow into the sealed
          reservoir compartment.
      (4) Set timer for one hour.
      (5) Return blood sample to proper storage. (If
          no laboratory work will be performed dur-

ing the incubation, remove gloves, discard
appropriately, and wash hands. Reglove
before handling test materials.)
      (6) Let the pipette stand undisturbed for
          exactly one hour and then read the results
          of the ESR: Use the scale on the tube to
          measure the distance from the top of the
          plasma to the top of the red blood cells.
      (7) Record the sedimentation rate:
          ESR (Mod. Westergren, 1 hr) = ___ mm
      (8) Dispose of tube and vial in appropriate
          biohazard container.
   b. Wintrobe method:
      (1) Place tube in Wintrobe sedimentation
          rack.
      (2) Check the leveling bubble to ensure that
          the Wintrobe rack is level.
      (3) Fill Wintrobe tube to the zero mark with
          well-mixed blood using the Pasteur pipette
          and being careful not to overfill.
          NOTE: Tube must be filled from the bottom
          to avoid getting air bubbles in the tube.
      (4) Set timer for one hour. Be certain the tube
          is vertical.
      (5) Return blood sample to proper storage. (If
          no other laboratory work is scheduled, re-
          move gloves, discard appropriately, and
          wash hands. Reglove before handling test
          materials.)
      (6) Measure the distance the erythrocytes
          have fallen (in mm): after exactly one
          hour, use the scale on the tube to measure
          the distance from the top of the plasma to
          the top of the red blood cells.
      (7) Record the sedimentation rate:
          ESR (Wintrobe, 1 hr) = ___ mm
      (8) Disinfect and clean equipment and return
          to storage.
      NOTE: If disposable equipment is used, dispose
      of in biohazard container.
5. Clean work area with surface disinfectant.
6. Remove gloves and discard into biohazard container.
7. Wash hands with hand disinfectant.

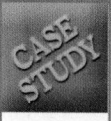

CASE STUDY 29.1

Today is busier than usual at Doctors Lewis & King. While she is performing an erythrocyte sedimentation rate for Jim Marshal, a patient in his late thirties, medical assistant Audrey Jones is called upon to help with another patient. She hurriedly places the sedimentation rack on top of an incubator in the sunlight by an open window and leaves to assist Dr. King.

CASE STUDY REVIEW

1. List two ways in which the test results may be affected.
2. What are the normal Westergren ESR values for males and females under 50 years of age?
3. What are the best conditions for an accurate test?

SUMMARY

Hematology tests are the second most frequently performed tests in the ambulatory care setting. Only the urinalysis is performed more frequently. Medical assistants must have a knowledge of hematology to accurately and efficiently perform the tests. The study of hematology includes hematopoiesis, which is the formation of the blood elements, as well as the hematological tests and their relationship to the pathology of the body.

This chapter has introduced the more common hematological tests that are performed in the ambulatory care setting, including all the parts of the complete blood count (CBC), the erythrocyte sedimentation rates methods, and the erythrocyte indices. All of these tests are utilized by the physician in the diagnosis and treatment of disease.

Most of the hematology procedures performed in today's ambulatory care setting utilize some type of automated instrumentation. Some automated hematology instruments require a diluted blood sample while others do not require a diluted sample. Both methods of automated instrumentation are discussed in the chapter.

Blood specimens used in the sampling of hematological procedures are biohazardous material. Be sure to follow Universal and Standard Precautions when you work with these specimens. Refer back to Chapter 10.

REVIEW QUESTIONS

Multiple Choice

1. Which of the following is *not* a cellular component of blood?
   a. erythrocytes
   b. leukocytes
   c. thrombocytes
   d. erythropoietin
2. The formation of blood is defined as:
   a. erythropoietin
   b. hematopoiesis
   c. mean corpuscular volume
   d. hemoglobinopathy
3. Sickle cell anemia, a hereditary disease, has which type of hemoglobin?
   a. hemoglobin S
   b. hemoglobin A
   c. hemoglobin E
   d. hemoglobin C
4. The volume of packed red cells compared to the total volume of the sample is calculated from which test?
   a. hematocrit
   b. hemoglobin
   c. MCH
   d. MCV
5. Manual blood cell counts are made using the:
   a. hemacytometer
   b. QBC
   c. nanometer
   d. spectrophotometer
6. The most common white cell type found in the granulocytic series is the:
   a. lymphocyte
   b. monocyte
   c. neutrophil
   d. basophil

7. The erythrocyte indices are used for the diagnosis, classification, and treatment of different:
   a. infections
   b. anemias
   c. inflammatory diseases
   d. neoplasms
8. Which hematological test result shows an increase with infections, inflammatory disease, pregnancy, and tissue destruction?
   a. hemoglobin
   b. MCV
   c. hematocrit
   d. ESR
9. The most frequent hemoglobin disease seen in the ambulatory care setting is:
   a. iron deficiency anemia
   b. sickle cell anemia
   c. leukemia
   d. anisocytosis

Critical Thinking

1. Describe three changes from normal, and their causes, that can be observed on a stained blood smear.
2. What hematological factors do the erythrocyte indices provide information about? List one example for each index in which a disease causes an elevation or decrease.

3. You are serving your externship in a local clinic. A physician has made a tentative diagnosis of appendicitis for a patient. In addition to the urinalysis, what single hematological test is most likely to confirm the diagnosis?
4. List the guidelines that must be followed in order to assure accurate sed rate results.
5. How is quality control maintained with automated hematology instruments? Refer to Chapter 26.

WEB ACTIVITIES

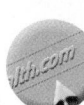

1. Visit the CDC's web site to review Standard Precautions required during blood collection.
2. Does the American Heart Association's web site offer parameters for different blood counts and hematology values? Are guidelines and tips on specimen collection outlined?

REFERENCES/BIBLIOGRAPHY

Henry, J. B. H. (Ed.). (1996). *Clinical diagnosis and management by laboratory methods* (19th ed.). Philadelphia: W. B. Saunders Company.

Palko, T., & Palko, H. (1996). *Laboratory procedures for the medical office*. Columbus, OH: Glencoe/McGraw-Hill.

Walters, N. J., Estridge, B. H., & Reynolds, A. P. (2000). *Basic medical laboratory techniques* (4th ed.). Albany, NY: Delmar.

URINALYSIS

KEY TERMS

Acetest®
Acid/Base Balance
Amorphous
Bilirubin
Casts
Circadian Rhythm
Clinitest®
Creatinine
Critical Values
Crystals
Cultures
Glucose
Hematuria
Hyaline
Ictotest®
Ketoacidosis
Ketone
Leukocyte Esterase
Meniscus
Midstream Collection
pH
Quality Control
Reagents
Reagent Test Strip
Refractometer
Screening
Sediment
Specific Gravity
Supernatant
Tamm-Horsfall
Turbid
Urea
Urinalysis
Urinometer
Urobilinogen
Urochrome

OUTLINE

Urine Formation
    Filtration
    Reabsorption
    Secretion
Urine Composition
Safety
Quality Control
CLIA '88
Urine Containers

Urine Collection
    Urine Specimen Types
    Collection Methods
Examination of Urine
    Physical Examination of Urine
    Chemical Examination of Urine
    Microscopic Examination of Urine
        Sediment

OBJECTIVES

The student should strive to meet the following performance objectives and demonstrate an understanding of the facts and principles presented in this chapter through written and oral communication.

1. Define the key terms as presented in the glossary.

2. Explain the process of urine formation.

3. Discuss the importance of safety procedures and quality control when working with urine.

4. Describe the importance of proper collection and preservation of the random, midstream, clean-catch, and 24-hour urine specimens.

5. Identify the proper technique for examining the physical characteristics of a urine specimen.

6. Explain causes of abnormal physical characteristics of urine.

7. Describe methods for chemical examination of a urine specimen.

8. Explain the need to confirm abnormal results.

9. Describe the confirmatory tests for ketones, glucose, protein, and bilirubin.

10. Identify the proper method of preparing urine sediment for microscopic examination.

11. Identify normal and abnormal structures found during the microscopic examination of urine sediment.

CLINICAL

Fundamental Principles

- Apply principles of aseptic technique and infection control
- Comply with quality assurance practices
- Screen and follow up patient test results

Diagnostic Orders

- Collect and process specimens
- Perform diagnostic tests

GENERAL (TRANSDISCIPLINARY)

Legal Concepts

- Document accurately
- Comply with established risk management and safety procedures

Instruction

- Instruct individuals according to their needs

At Inner City Health Care, clinical medical assistant Wanda Slawson performs many urinalyses. Although urinalysis is a routine procedure, Wanda recognizes its importance as a diagnostic tool and she performs each test carefully to ensure accurate results. Wanda takes time to instruct patients in the proper collection procedures. She encourages patients to ask questions before collecting the urine sample and she provides written instructions for easy reference. When she performs the urinalysis, Wanda follows safety and quality control guidelines. By paying attention to the details of the procedure, Wanda does her best to ensure the quality of the urinalysis results.

INTRODUCTION

Examination of the urine (**urinalysis**) as a diagnostic tool for many diseases has been performed for centuries by medical practitioners. Urinalysis refers to the study of urine as an aid in patient diagnosis or to follow the course of disease. The urine examination is a routine part of most physical examinations.

The routine urinalysis is one of the most frequently performed procedures in the medical office laboratory. Many tests can be performed on one urine sample. This procedure is often ordered because urine is easily obtained, and much information about the body's metabolism may be gained from the results of this testing.

When physicians order a "routine urinalysis," they expect timely and accurate results. Results can indicate a systemic disease process and/or renal (kidney) or urinary tract disease.

Practice, experience, and attention to detail are the most important tools in achieving quality results. Following standard precautions when working with any body fluid is mandatory.

URINE FORMATION

Before discussing the analysis of urine, it is helpful to understand how urine is formed in the human body. The formation and excretion of urine is the principal way the body excretes water and gets rid of waste. These waste products, if not removed, rapidly can become toxic.

The kidney is a highly specialized organ that eliminates soluble (dissolved in water) waste products of metabolism. Urine is formed in the kidney and is excreted from the body by way of the urinary tract system (Figure 30-1). The kidney also regulates the fluid outside the cells of the body by eliminating certain fluids and returning other fluids, maintaining a careful balance (homeostasis). In this manner, the body is protected from dramatic changes in fluid volume, acidity and alkalinity (**acid/base balance**), composition, and pressure.

There are two kidneys, one on each side of the body. They are about 11 to 12 centimeters long and 5 to 6 centimeters wide. Kidneys are shaped like a lima bean with their concave border directed toward the midline of the body. The left kidney is slightly higher than the right.

Filtration

The kidney filters waste products, salts, and excess fluid from the blood. The filtering unit of the kidney is called the glomerulus. The part of the kidney that concentrates the filtered material is called the tubule. Together, the glomerulus and the tubule combine to form the nephron (Figure 30-2).

Most of the work of the kidney is done by the nephrons. There are approximately one million nephrons in each kidney. Each minute, more than 1,000 milliliters of blood flow through the kidney to be cleansed. In the glomerulus, certain substances are filtered out of the blood. The remaining filtrate then passes into the tubule where various changes occur. Substances filtered out from the body can include water, ammonia, electrolytes, **glu-**

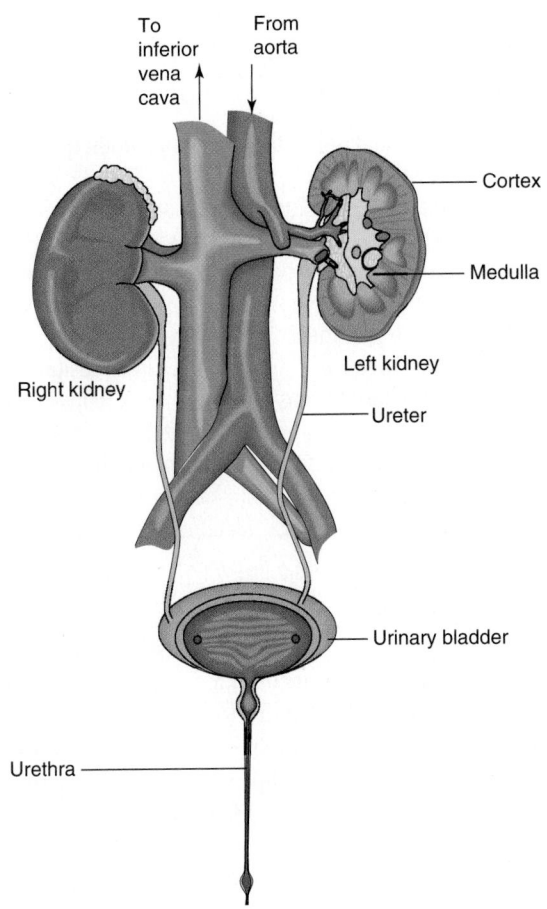

Figure 30-1 The urinary system.

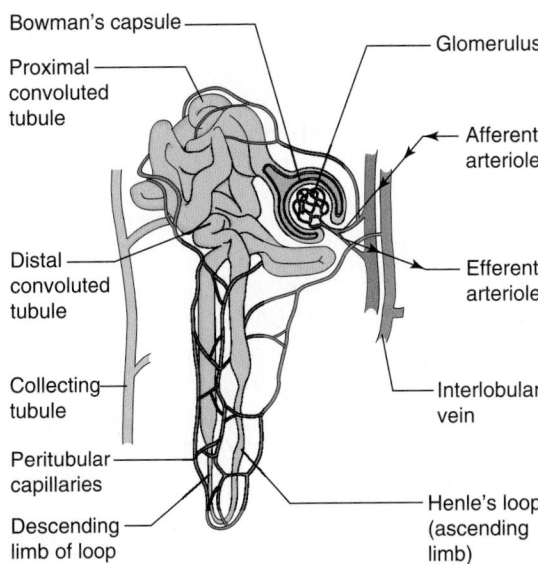

Figure 30-2 Parts of the nephron unit.

cose, amino acids, **creatinine**, and **urea**. These wastes leave the body in the eliminated urine.

For example, when diabetics have excess sugar in their blood, the body attempts to eliminate the excess glucose through the urine. Routine urinalysis testing will reveal the excess glucose, alerting the physician to the presence of too much glucose. Diabetes can be diagnosed in this manner, as well as determining that a diabetic is not taking enough insulin to control the glucose in the blood.

Reabsorption

While passing through the kidney, some substances may need to be reabsorbed by the blood. Approximately 180 liters of filtrate are produced daily by the body, but only 1 to 2 liters of urine are eliminated from the normally functioning human body. Therefore, much of the filtrate, including water, sodium, chloride, potassium, bicarbonate, glucose, calcium, and amino acids, is reabsorbed into the body.

Under normal conditions, blood cells and most proteins stay in the blood plasma because they are too large to pass through the walls of the capillaries of the glomerulus.

If blood cells and excess protein are found in the urine, the physician is alerted that the kidney is not filtering properly due to an irregular condition affecting the urinary tract.

As long as the concentration of glucose in the blood is below 180 mg/dL (milligrams per deciliter), the glucose will be completely reabsorbed. If the level increases above 180 mg/dL, the glucose is not reabsorbed. Substances such as glucose that are reabsorbed in relationship to their concentration in the blood are known as threshold substances. The needs of homeostasis call for sugar and protein to be almost completely reabsorbed, while other threshold substances such as creatinine, amino acids, potassium, sodium, and chloride are only partially reabsorbed.

Secretion

Near the end of the blood's journey through the kidney, specifically in the distal convoluted tubule, other substances that have not already been filtered are secreted into the urine. Such substances as hydrogen and ammonium ions may be secreted into the urine in exchange for sodium. Certain drugs in the blood at this point may also be secreted into the urine.

URINE COMPOSITION

After urine progresses through a healthy kidney, it is approximately 96 percent water and 4 percent dissolved substances, most of which come from either dietary intake or metabolic waste products. These substances are primarily urea, salt, sulfates, and phosphates. Abnormal constituents of urine include red and white blood cells, fat, glucose, casts, bile, acetone, and hemoglobin (Table 30-1).

TABLE 30-1	NORMAL AND ABNORMAL SUBSTANCES IN URINE
Normal	**Abnormal**
Urea	Bile
Uric acid	Blood
Creatinine	Fat
Sodium	Glucose
Potassium	Protein
Ammonium	White blood cells
Sulfate	Urobilinogen
Chloride	Microorganisms (bacteria and/or parasites)

Precautions To Use When Handling Urine Specimens

- Treat all specimens as if they were infectious, handling them with gloved hands.
- Avoid splashes or creation of aerosols when handling or disposing of urine specimens. Wearing face shields will prevent splashes from getting into the eyes, nose, or mouth.
- Process urine specimens as soon as possible.
- Store urine specimens appropriately in a designated refrigerator that contains no food or drink items.
- Dispose of urine appropriately, possibly in a special sink (run water to wash the specimen into the drain) or toilet.

When certain disease processes occur in the human body, the following changes in urine production and composition can occur:

- The amount of urine excreted can rise or fall
- Urine color can change
- Urine appearance can vary
- Urine odor can change
- Cells can be present in urine
- Chemical constituents in urine can change
- Urine concentration (specific gravity) may vary

SAFETY

Chapter 26 of this textbook covers the guidelines set up by government agencies to ensure the safety of everyone working in the health care field and for the protection of our environment. These guidelines are now referred to as standard precautions. Other terms used to describe care when handling infectious materials are transmission-based precautions and biohazard precautions.

QUALITY CONTROL

As in every area of the laboratory, every effort must be made by health care professionals to produce test results free from error. Much pressure is placed by regulatory agencies on facilities that perform laboratory tests such as urinalysis to maintain standards that will ensure reliable results. **Quality control** (QC) programs are an important part of urine testing to ensure accurate and reliable results for the patient. Quality control programs must be incorporated into every urine testing procedure. Because many of the tests are interpreted by visual examination, the quality control procedures are dependent on the expertise of the person performing the examination.

Testing protocols must be written out and available to personnel. Records of testing must be maintained. Equipment and instruments used for urine testing must be maintained and checked daily for proper calibration. If the instrument should require recalibration, the manufacturer's instructions are provided with the instrument.

Always be careful to perform the quality control procedures *exactly* as you perform the procedures on actual patient samples. Documentation of the performance of daily control testing must be kept for at least three years. With the advent of computer storage, the data can now be stored indefinitely. Commercially available urine control samples can be purchased from a number of manufacturers. Positive and negative controls should be run each day on all tests to be performed. Control results should be recorded on a daily log for easy access. The control samples should be stored as directed by the manufacturer.

CLIA '88

The regulations under the new Clinical Laboratory Improvement Amendments (CLIA) are discussed in Chapter 26. Several CLIA '88 regulations apply to the medical assistant performing urine testing. They include:

- Appropriate training in the methodology of the test being performed
- Understanding of urine-testing quality control procedures
- Proficiency in the use of instrumentation, being able to troubleshoot problems
- Knowledge of the stability and proper storage of **reagents** (substances involved in urine testing)
- Awareness of factors that influence test results
- Knowledge of how to verify test results

URINE CONTAINERS

The first step toward achieving proper results during laboratory testing is proper collection of the specimen to be tested. There are a variety of containers (Figure 30-3) used for urine collection, including nonsterile containers for random specimens (urinalysis), sterile containers for **cultures** (testing specimens for growth of bacteria), and 24-hour collection containers with added preservatives.

After specimen collection, the container must be labeled immediately with all the following information: patient's name, age, sex, identifying number, date, time of collection, and physician's name. These requirements may differ in various facilities. To prevent specimen mislabeling, the following procedures should always be followed. Specimen labeling should be done immediately following specimen collection. Never prelabel a specimen collection container. The only exception is when a patient is asked to collect a specimen on his or her own. Before the container is given to the patient, it should be labeled properly. If the patient cannot void, the container must be discarded immediately. This will prevent the container being used for some future patient collection. Always place the specimen label on the specimen collection container, never on the lid.

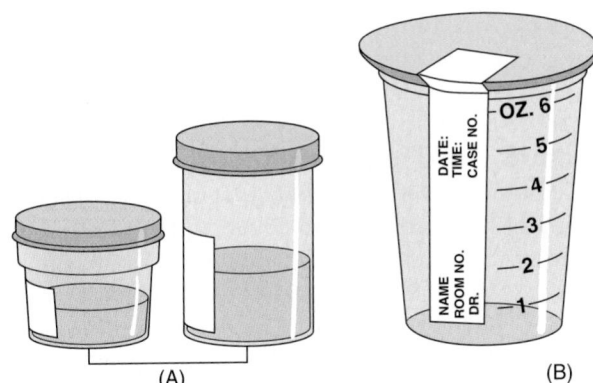

Figure 30-3 Urine collection containers: (A) Sterile. (B) Random.

Patients may have questions about how a specimen should be collected. The medical assistant must be able to give proper instructions using common terms that the patient will be able to understand. Most laboratories have containers made specifically for urine collection, but any container can be used for urinalysis testing as long as it is clean and dry. However, if the sample is to be cultured (tested for microorganisms), it must be collected in a sterile container. In some cases, catheterization, which is discussed later in this chapter, also is used.

URINE COLLECTION

Urine Specimen Types

Following are common types of urine specimens that might be ordered frequently by physicians.

Random (Spot) Specimen. Random (spot) urine samples are specimens that can be obtained at any time and are the most commonly collected specimens. Any random urine specimen can be used for routine urinalysis. However, a concentrated specimen is preferable to one that is dilute. The first morning void is typically the most concentrated specimen and is usually the specimen of choice for many urine tests.

Fasting/Timed Specimens. A fasting (going without food and drink) urine specimen is ordered less often than a random specimen. The physician may want to measure a urinary substance without interference from food intake. Some physicians may require an overnight fast. Others may ask the patient to have a meal and then urinate four hours later (that urine is not collected as the next voided specimen but is considered a *timed* specimen).

It is up to the medical assistant to give the patient proper instruction as to how to collect a fasting, or timed, specimen. Written directions given to the patient in addition to oral instructions are best. A regular urinalysis container can be used for a fasting specimen. It does not require a sterile container.

Twenty-Four-Hour Specimen. Urine varies in its concentration of certain substances at different times during any 24-hour period due to **circadian rhythm** and the intake of food and water. For instance, the amount of water excreted is highest from 10 A.M. to noon and 4 to 6 P.M. Chloride is in its highest concentration from noon to 2 P.M. Therefore, a 24-hour specimen is sometimes requested when quantitative tests (measuring the amount) for different substances are desired. The results of this type of collection then will be expressed in *units per 24 hours*. Some commonly tested substances include sodium, potassium, calcium, and creatinine.

The container used to collect this amount of urine should be of adequate size. Usually a one-gallon, dark-colored plastic bottle is used. For measuring some urine constituents, preservatives need to be added to the bottle before the collection begins. Without the preservative, these substances may break down and be impossible to quantify. Preservatives include thymol, toluene, and certain acids.

Urine collected over a 24-hour period of time is refrigerated between collections. After the collection is complete, it must be returned to the medical laboratory as soon as possible.

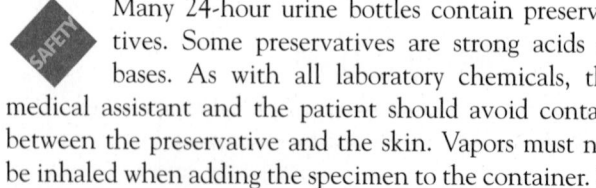 Many 24-hour urine bottles contain preservatives. Some preservatives are strong acids or bases. As with all laboratory chemicals, the medical assistant and the patient should avoid contact between the preservative and the skin. Vapors must not be inhaled when adding the specimen to the container. In the patient's written instructions, there should be a warning about avoiding contact with preservatives.

Physicians sometimes choose to have a 2-hour or a 12-hour specimen instead of the usual 24-hour collection. All of the collection steps for a 24-hour specimen apply. Recording the time of day is very important (a 2-hour specimen is usually collected in the afternoon).

Collection Methods

In addition to ordering what type of urine specimen is desired (random, fasting, 24-hour), the physician might also order a certain type of collection method to collect the specific sample. These methods include random, clean-catch, midstream, and catheterization.

Random Collection. The patient simply urinates into a cup until the cup is fairly full. Patients often find collecting urine very awkward. In the process of collection, the specimen can become contaminated from such

1. When giving a patient any type of instructions, make sure that the patient understands the importance of each step. Always provide written instructions as well. Emphasize that failing to follow the instructions will cause the results to be invalid, requiring another collection.
2. The patient begins a 24-hour collection by emptying the bladder and not keeping the specimen. The container is then labeled with the time of bladder emptying. Patients generally start the collection between 6 and 8 P.M., but any 24-hour period is acceptable.
3. Explain that each time the patient urinates within the 24-hour period, the urine is placed into the collection bottle.
4. Instruct the patient to refrigerate the bottle between urinations.
5. Explain to the patient that at the end of the 24-hour period, the patient should urinate and place the urine in the bottle. The exact time should be written on the label as the "ended" or "completed" time.
6. The most common errors in the 24-hour urine specimen collection are the inclusion of the first voided specimen and the discarding of one or more of the voided specimens during the 24-hour period. Be sure the patient understands these steps.

sources as epithelial cells (skin cells) around the genital area, bacterial contamination from the skin, excess mucus, or fecal contamination from the rectal area.

Clean-Catch Method. To avoid as much contamination as possible when collecting a specimen, physicians prefer that the patient cleanse the genital area before collection. The clean-catch order means that an antiseptic towelette is provided in addition to a urine container. Men cleanse the urethral opening with a single stroke of an antiseptic towelette. The stroke should be directed from the tip of the penis toward the ring of the glans. This should be repeated with another towelette.

Female patients should spread the outer vulval folds and cleanse the inner side of both folds with a single stroke from front to back. A second towelette is used to cleanse the urethral opening with a single front-to-back stroke. Female patients should also be instructed to notify the medical assistant if they are menstruating during the collection.

Midstream Collection. Sometimes a physician will order a **midstream collection**. After cleansing, the patient should begin to urinate into the toilet. The patient then stops the stream of urine and collects the next portion into a collection cup, voiding the final stream into the toilet. By this method, the initial urine stream will carry away any contamination left after cleansing. The midstream urine should be as free of contamination as possible.

Catheterized Collection. At times it is necessary to catheterize a patient. This procedure is performed by a physician or a health care worker specifically trained to do catheterizations.

A catheterization involves inserting a sterile tube directly into the bladder through the urethra. Samples obtained in this way are suitable for all urinalysis and microbiological procedures because they are not contaminated by the outside environment.

Due to the invasive action, this procedure can cause infection in the patient if not done correctly. Physicians order this method of collection only when other methods are contraindicated. A catheterization may be necessary when urine specimens collected by other methods continually test positive for bacteria.

EXAMINATION OF URINE

Urine should be examined in a fresh state, preferably while still warm if possible. However, urine usually cannot be tested immediately. If immediate testing is not possible, the urine should be refrigerated at about 4°C or stored on ice. The urinalysis should be performed as soon as possible, preferably within 2 hours. **Crystals** and **casts** begin to break down after 2 hours. Any time delay allows bacteria to multiply and can lead to inaccurate microbiology results.

The routine urinalysis procedure is composed of three parts:

- *Physical* examination of the urine
- *Chemical* examination of the urine
- *Microscopic* examination of urine sediment

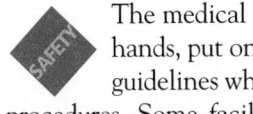 The medical assistant should remember to wash hands, put on gloves, and follow all of the safety guidelines when performing any of the following procedures. Some facilities require eye protection when pouring urine or any procedure where splashing urine into the eye could occur.

Physical Examination of Urine

When the medical assistant begins the process of performing a urinalysis, the first step is performing the physical examination. This examination consists of:

Patient Teaching Tip

When instructing the patient in collecting a clean-catch, midstream urine specimen for laboratory analysis:

1. Instruct the patient in proper cleansing of the genital area. It is best to give the patient written instructions as well. Men and women should have separate instructions.
   - *Men:* After thoroughly washing his hands, the male patient should retract the foreskin on the penis (if not circumcised) using a sterile towelette. A second towelette should be used to cleanse the urethral opening with a single stroke directed from the tip of the penis toward the ring of the glans. The cleansing procedure should be repeated again using a new towelette.
   - *Women:* After thoroughly washing her hands, the female patient should position herself comfortably on the toilet seat and should swing one knee to the side as far as she can. She should spread the outer vulval folds using a sterile towelette. The inner folds should be cleansed using the towelette with a single stroke from front to back (some instructions may call for cleansing one side, discarding the towelette, and then cleansing the other side with a fresh towelette). Another towelette is used to cleanse the urethral opening with a single front-to-back stroke.

2. Instruct the patient also about the midstream collection technique. Explain why it is necessary. These instructions should also be written and included with the clean-catch written directions.
   - After cleansing the area using the clean-catch directions, the patient should begin to void into the toilet. The urine stream should be interrupted to collect the urine into the supplied container. Only the middle portion of the urine flow is included in the sample. After the specimen has been collected, the container should be closed. The patient should always avoid touching the inside of both the container and the lid.

3. Before the container is given to the patient, it should be labeled properly. After collection, the container should be given promptly to the medical assistant or placed in a proper collection area.

CAUTION: The medical assistant should always wear gloves when handling urine specimens or body fluid specimens.

● Assessing the volume of the urine specimen, making sure that the specimen is sufficient for testing

● Observing and recording the color and transparency of the specimen

● Noting any unusual urine odor

● Measuring the specific gravity of the specimen

Specimen Volume. The first step in performing a urinalysis is to determine if the sample's volume is adequate for testing. Procedure 30-1 illustrates how initially to assess the volume of the urine specimen.

Urine Color. There is a wide range of color in normal urine, usually ranging from a pale yellow to a dark yellow or amber. The range of color usually is due to the concentration of the urine. A darker color generally indicates a more concentrated urine. The color (urochrome) comes from normal metabolic processes, the end products of which are deposited in the urine.

After assessing the adequacy of the urine volume, the medical assistant then observes and records the color of the urine, as in Procedure 30-2.

The diet and certain drugs can add substances to the urine that give it a specific color. The medical assistant should be familiar with some reasons for abnormally colored urine. For example, the most common cause of red urine is red blood cells, known as hematuria. Blood cells in urine may indicate bleeding in the urinary tract. The medication Pyridium is commonly used for bladder infections and gives urine a bright orange color. Table 30-2 lists several urine color variations and possible causes.

Urine Transparency. Urine transparency normally is not significant by itself. However, it may be helpful when included with the rest of the urinalysis information.

TABLE 30-2	URINE COLORS AND POSSIBLE CAUSES
Color	**Possible Cause**
Straw to yellow	Normal
Orange to amber	Concentrated urine
Colorless	Dilute urine
Deep yellow	Vitamin intake
Bright orange	Drugs, usually Pyridium
Orange-brown	Urobilin
Greenish-orange	Bilirubin
Smokey	Red blood cells
Wine red/reddish brown	Hemoglobin pigments
Green or blue	Methylene blue

Transparency of urine usually is recorded as clear, cloudy, hazy, or turbid (opaque), as in Procedure 30-3. These descriptive terms may vary in different facilities.

There are many causes of cloudy urine, most of which are considered normal. Cloudiness could be contributed to contamination from vaginal discharges, white blood cells, bacteria, or yeast. As urine cools, sometimes crystals form that also may give urine a cloudy appearance.

Urine Odor. With experience, the medical assistant will recognize certain odors in the urine that can indicate specific conditions. Odors, though not recorded on the final laboratory urinalysis report, should not be disregarded. For example, the urine of a diabetic who may have a condition known as ketoacidosis may have a sweet odor. Urine full of bacteria will have a foul odor that is easily recognized.

Urine Specific Gravity. Specific gravity is defined as the ratio of the weight of a given volume of a substance to the weight of the same volume of distilled water at the same temperature. Distilled water used as the reference point has been given the specific gravity value of 1.000. The specific gravity of urine indicates the concentrations of solids such as phosphates, chlorides, proteins, sugars, and urea that are dissolved in urine.

Variations in urine specific gravity can give the physician diagnostic information. In diabetes mellitus, glucose molecules will be very dense and give the urine a high specific gravity. The normal range of specific gravity for urine is from 1.003 to 1.035. Specific gravity is highest in the first morning samples because the urine is more concentrated.

Specific gravity is often tested by using either a urinometer or a refractometer. A urinometer is a calibrated, floating device. A refractometer measures the amount of light that is bent by particles suspended in a liquid. The two methods do not give exactly the same results but are close enough for most clinical applications. A specific gravity reading is also available in conjunction with chemical testing on some reagent strips.

Urinometer. A urinometer (Figures 30-4A and B) is made from a small glass tube weighted to float in a sample of urine (usually 15 mL). The glass tube has been calibrated, and the stem of the tube has been marked accordingly to read 1.000 at the bottom of the meniscus in distilled water at room temperature. The meniscus is the curvature that appears in a liquid's upper surface when the liquid is placed in a container. The medical assistant reads the specific gravity of the urine from the stem at the meniscus (Figure 30-4C). However, the temperature of the urine must be taken into account if it differs from 20

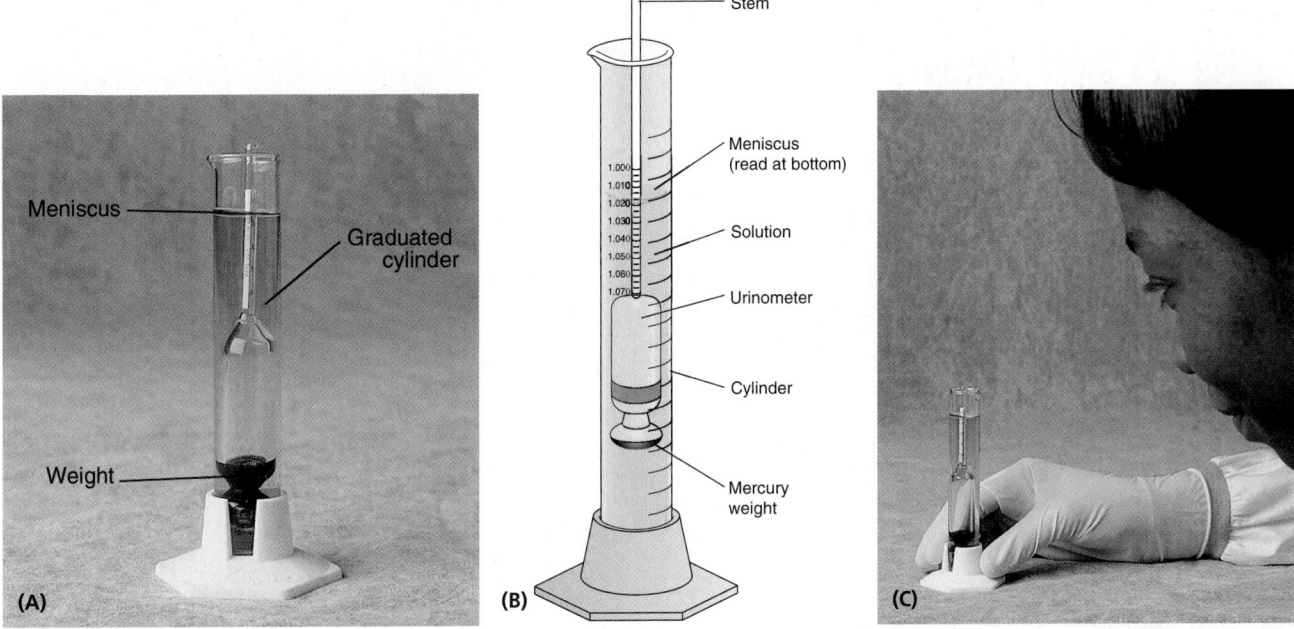

Figure 30-4 (A) Urinometer. (B) Urinometer parts. (C) The medical assistant reads the specific gravity of the urine from the urinometer stem at the meniscus.

degrees centigrade, which is normal room temperature. Add 0.001 to the reading for every 3 degrees above 20 degrees centigrade, and subtract 0.001 for every 3 degrees below 20 degrees centigrade. The buoyancy of a liquid changes with the temperature. The need for temperature correction can be avoided by allowing the sample of urine to come to room temperature.

Refractometer. The most common tool for determining the specific gravity of liquids is the refractometer (Figure 30-5). This instrument measures the refractive index of urine, which is the speed at which light travels through the air as compared to the speed at which it passes through urine. Light is slowed and therefore bent as it encounters particles—the more particles, the more bend. The bend can be used to determine the total number of particles and is not affected by the weight of the particles.

The refractometer reading is about 0.002 below that of the true specific gravity. This slight difference is more than made up for by the ease of using the instrument and the instrument's reliability. This instrument only needs a drop or two of urine, and the result does not have to be adjusted for temperature as long as the temperature is between 60° and 100°F. See Procedure 30-4.

Chemical Examination of Urine

After the physical testing of a urine specimen, the next step in urinalysis testing is chemical testing. This procedure once was complex, but today many manufacturers have made the task simple through a wide range of ready-to-use reagents and the reagent test strip, or dipstick (Figure 30-6) as it is more commonly known.

A **reagent test strip**, or dipstick, is a narrow strip of plastic on which pads containing reagents for different reactions are attached. The pads have reagents to test for many metabolic processes, including kidney and liver functions, urinary tract infection, and pH balance. The reagent test strip is the primary tool used for chemical

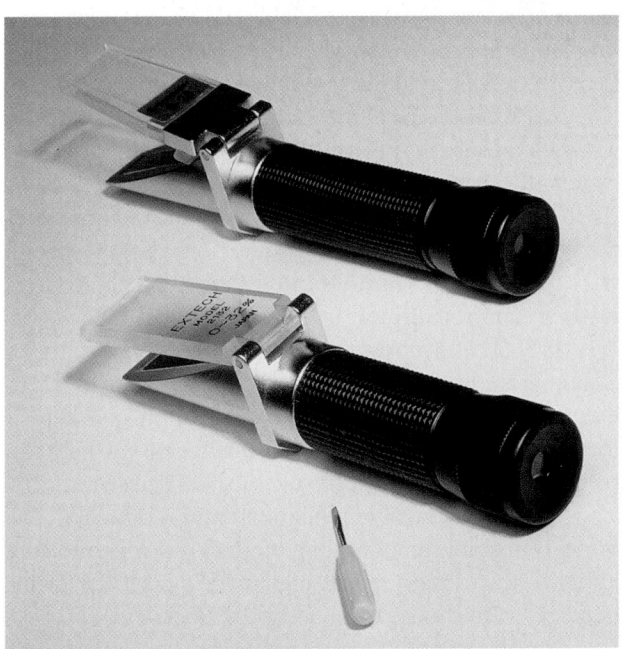

Figure 30-5 Refractometers.

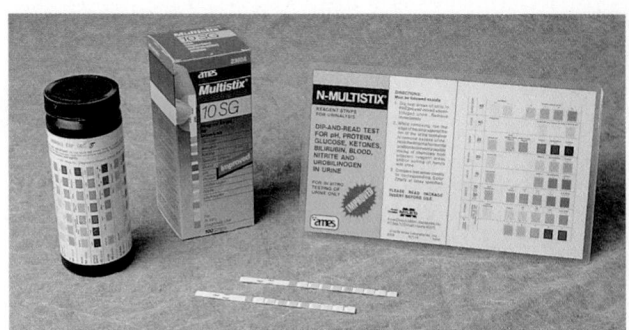

Figure 30-6 Multistix reagent strips with color-coded chart are used for chemical analysis of urine.

examination of urine. Specific confirmatory tests or methods may be necessary based on the result of the reagent test strip. Table 30-3 lists some tests available on urine reagent strips.

Specific Reagent Test Strip Tests.
Bilirubin. **Bilirubin** is a product of the breakdown of hemoglobin. Bilirubin in urine can indicate problems such as liver disease, hepatitis, and bile duct destruction. Bilirubin can break down in sunlight, so a urine sample should be protected from sunlight prior to testing for bilirubin.

Blood. Small amounts of blood (from blood cells or hemoglobin) can be detected by reagent strips. Urinary blood can indicate infection, urinary tract trauma, kidney bleeding, menses, and other conditions.

Glucose. A glucose test is added to a reagent strip to detect unsuspected diabetes or to check efficiency of insulin therapy in diabetics.

Ketones. **Ketone** bodies appear when excessive amounts of fatty acids are catabolized (broken down into simpler compounds) and when glucose availability is limited. Ketones occur during prolonged fasting.

Leukocyte. The **leukocyte esterase** test indicates white blood cells in the urinary tract, presumably attracted by invading bacteria.

Nitrites. The presence of urinary nitrites indicates the possibility of a urinary tract infection. Certain species of bacteria convert nitrates into nitrites, which are normally absent from urine.

pH. The **pH** test indicates the relative acidity or alkalinity of the urine. The urine has a pH range of 4.6 to 8.0, with a mean reading of 6.0. Starvation and ketosis increase urine acidity (pH reading goes below 7.0). Bacteria can make the pH alkaline (over 7.0), as can some drugs.

Protein. A small amount of protein is normal in the urine. Detectable amounts of protein in the urine indicate injury to the kidney, specifically to the glomerular membrane. Protein can increase during a high fever.

Specific gravity. Some reagent strips contain an indicator that turns various colors depending on the ion con-

TABLE 30-3	CHEMICAL TESTING AVAILABLE ON URINE REAGENT TEST STRIPS
• Bilirubin	• Nitrites
• Blood	• pH
• Glucose	• Protein
• Ketones	• Specific gravity
• Leukocyte esterase	• Urobilinogen

centration of the urine. This test reads up to a 1.030 result.

Urobilinogen. **Urobilinogen** is a degradation product of bilirubin formed by intestinal bacteria. Increased levels of this substance suggest liver disease or bleeding disorders.

Reagent Test Strip Quality Control. Reagent test strips are easy to use, but the complexity of the chemical testing should not be overlooked. As with any chemical reaction, each test involves multiple steps that are sensitive to temperature, time, dilution, and other factors. Outdated strips or reagents should never be used. To get optimum results, a certain amount of care must be taken when handling and storing the reagent strips. They must not be exposed to moisture, volatile substances, direct sunlight, or excess heat. The strips should not be removed from their original container except at the time of use. Always follow the manufacturer's instructions for storage. Test results are represented by a color change. The test result is compared to a color chart on the label of the reagent test strip container. Employees performing this test should be tested for color blindness as many of the color changes are subtle.

Reagent test strips are ready to use directly from their container. Correct quality control procedures should be followed as required by CLIA '88 and the facility where the testing is performed. This usually includes using a quality control urine sample (with predetermined results). All that is needed for this testing are the strips, quality control specimen, and patient specimens. Procedure 30-5 explains how to perform a urinalysis chemical examination.

There are also automated urine analyzers (Figure 30-7A and B) capable of timing and reading the test strip. These instruments can be quite expensive and are not available in every laboratory. Today, automated urine analyzers are used more frequently as they are more accurate and cut down on human error.

When reporting results, it is important to use the proper units and terms as directed by your laboratory. An example of the sensitivity of the reagent strips is shown in Table 30-4 (there is variation in sensitivity among manufacturers).

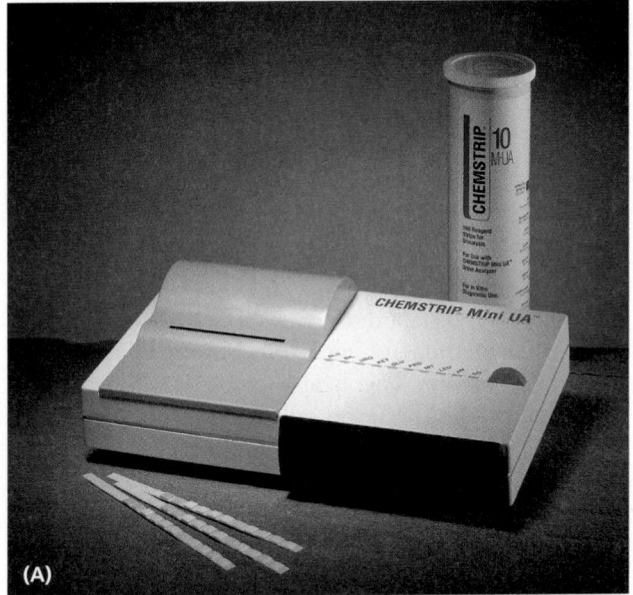

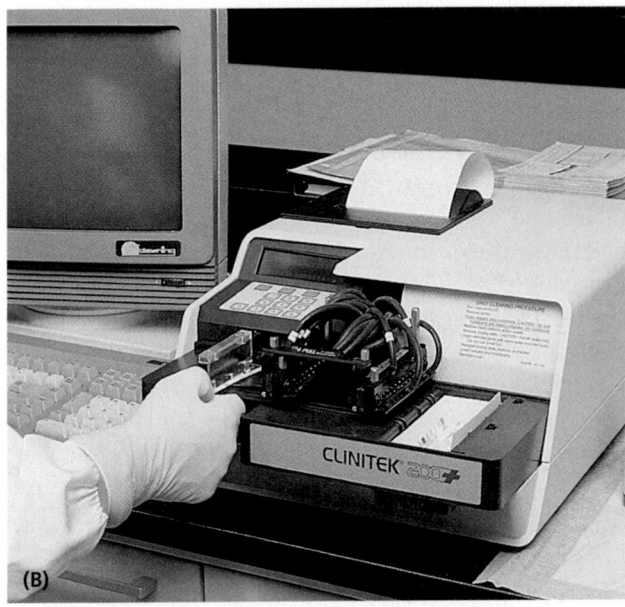

Figure 30-7 (A) The Chemstrip Mini UA Urine Analyzer is a semiautomated analyzer that provides accuracy and consistency of results when properly used. It is often used in laboratories where the volume of tests analyzed is less than forty strips per hour. (Courtesy of Boehringer Mannheim) (B) The Clinitek 200 semiautomated urine analyzer may be used in larger laboratories where there is a moderate to high volume of tests. Results are printed on a paper printout.

Confirmatory Testing. Since the reagent test strips are actually **screening** tests, some positive results must be confirmed with more sensitive and/or specific methods. The results of the dipstick test cannot be reported until positive results on the following tests are confirmed by the following methods. These tests include but are not limited to protein, ketones, bilirubin, and reducing sugars (to use when the glucose result is positive). Each laboratory will have a specific procedure for performing these confirmatory tests.

Protein. The most common confirmatory test for protein is the sulfosalicylic acid (SSA) test. It relies on

the precipitation of protein, causing turbidity (cloudiness) in the test tube when added to a sample of urine. Urine samples should be centrifuged and a clear supernatant used. The amount of precipitate found is roughly proportional to the protein concentration present. A negative test has no cloudiness; a trace amount is barely perceptible; a 1+ result is cloudy but not granular; a 2+ result is cloudy and granular; a 3+ result is heavy cloudiness with clumping; and a 4+ result is dense with large clumps. This is a qualitative method. A semiquantitative method is available by using a set of commercially available standards and comparing the turbidity of the patient sample to that of the standards.

Ketones. The **Acetest®** is a test for ketones that is available in tablet form. Ketones are produced during increased metabolism of fat. If ketones are present in urine, a drop of urine added to the tablet will produce a purple color (Figure 30-8).

TABLE 30-4	REAGENT STRIP SENSITIVITY	
Test	**Range**	**Normal Value**
pH	5–9	5–8
Protein	Negative to positive*	Negative
Glucose	Negative to >1,000 mg/dl	Negative
Ketone	Negative to >80 mg/dl	Negative
Bilirubin	Negative to large	Negative
Blood	Negative to large	Negative
Leukocyte Esterase	Negative to large	Negative
Nitrites	Negative to positive	Negative
Urobilinogen	0.2 to 8.0 mg/dl	2.0 mg/dl

*Note that positive results in a newborn for glucose, ketone, and protein are considered critical values and should be reported to the physician immediately.

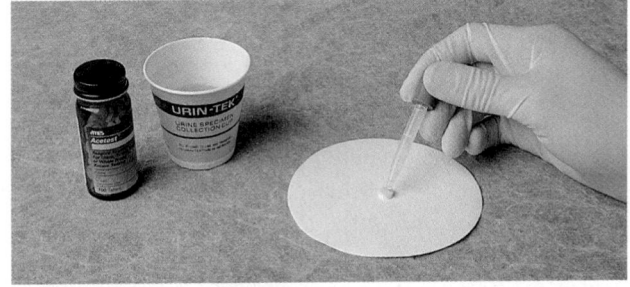

Figure 30-8 The Acetest® is a common test used to confirm the presence of ketones in urine.

Bilirubin. The Ictotest® is a specific test for bilirubin. It is approximately four times as sensitive as the reagent strip method. The test includes a tablet and an absorbent mat. If bilirubin is present, a purple color will develop when a urine drop is placed on the tablet.

Reducing sugars. The Clinitest® uses a prepared tablet and a color reaction comparison chart to help determine the quantity of sugar in the urine, as shown in Procedure 30-6. This test is used to detect reducing sugars (called reducing because these sugars give up electrons easily in chemical reactions) such as lactose and galactose, which are not detected by the glucose test on the reagent test strip. Screening for reducing substances is especially important in pediatric populations. The tablet used in the test contains copper sulfate, citric acid, sodium hydroxide, and sodium carbonate. The test is based on a copper reduction reaction known as the Benedict's test.

Microscopic Examination of Urine Sediment

In addition to the physical and chemical examination of urine, the medical assistant may also be required to perform a microscopic examination of a sample of urine after it has been centrifuged. The sediment (insoluble material) at the bottom of the centrifuge tube is used for the microscopic examination (see Chapter 27 for proper use of the microscope). The microscopic examination is helpful in determining kidney disease, disorders of the urinary tract, and systemic disease. It is particularly important that urine be freshly voided and examined as soon as possible to prevent deterioration of sediment components.

One of the most important items to have on hand when performing a microscopic urine examination is a urine color atlas. It takes years to be able to correctly identify abnormal components of urine. A color atlas should always be available to the medical assistant to help with identification.

Some laboratories make use of urine stains to add color to certain structures in the urine sediment. Sedistain® is an example of such a stain.

Sediment Components.
Sediment is obtained by centrifugation of 10 to 15 mL of urine. The supernatant urine is carefully poured off, and the sediment in the tube is resuspended by shaking. A drop of sediment is then placed on a slide and examined microscopically.

When viewing a normal urine specimen, the medical assistant may see very little under the microscope. Squamous epithelial cells (Figure 30-9) may be seen, especially in women. These cells have no medical significance as they are skin cells continuously sloughed off into the urine.

They are generally reported as few, moderate, or many. If the physician sees many epithelial cells in the urine specimen, it is indicative that the specimen is contaminated.

Normal urine sediment can also contain a few red or white blood cells and a few bacteria resulting from external contamination. Clean-catch urine collecting techniques are designed to eliminate as much of this contamination as possible.

Abnormal Urine Sediment Cells and Microorganisms. The methods of reporting abnormal urine sediment may vary among health facilities. The medical assistant looks at the urine sediment microscopically to see if the specimen has one or more of the following components:

Red blood cells. Red blood cells appear as pale, light-refractive disks when seen under high power. Large amounts of red blood cells in urine (hematuria) indicate disease or trauma. These cells are counted in a microscopic field (high-power field or HPF) and reported as cells counted per HPF (e.g., 10/HPF).

White blood cells. A few white blood cells can appear in normal urine. More than a few white blood cells in urine often indicate a urinary tract infection. White blood cells are slightly larger than red blood cells, may appear granular, and have a visible nucleus (the red blood cell has no nucleus). Figure 30-10 shows both red and white blood cells in urine. White blood cells are reported in the same manner as red blood cells.

Renal epithelial cells. Renal epithelial cells (Figure 30-11) can indicate kidney disease if they are present in large numbers. They can be confused with both white blood cells and other epithelial cells. If these cells are suspected, they should be reviewed by a physician before reporting them. They are also reported in the same manner as white and red blood cells.

Bacteria. Bacteria can appear as tiny round or rod-shaped objects (Figure 30-12). Rod-shaped bacteria are generally easier to see as round bacteria may appear as amorphous, or shapeless, material. Bacteria can be reported as few, moderate, many, and loaded.

Yeast. Yeast cells (Figure 30-13) may be present in urine, possibly indicating a yeast infection in the urinary tract. Yeast cells are smaller than red blood cells but may appear similar to them. Yeasts are round and can be observed budding. To distinguish between yeast and red blood cells if there is a question, a drop of dilute acetic acid is added to the urine sediment. The red blood cells will lyse, but the yeast will not. The most common yeast found is *Candida albicans.* Yeasts are reported as the amount per high-power field.

Parasites. The most frequently seen parasite in urine is *Trichomonas vaginalis* (Figure 30-14). *Trichomonas*

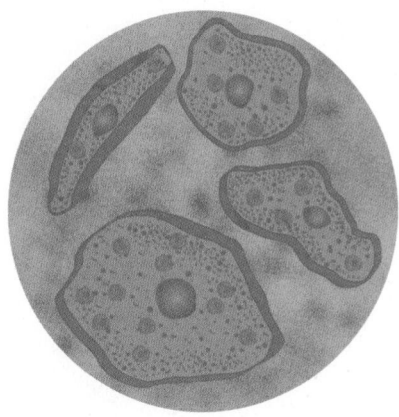

Figure 30-9   Squamous epithelial cells.

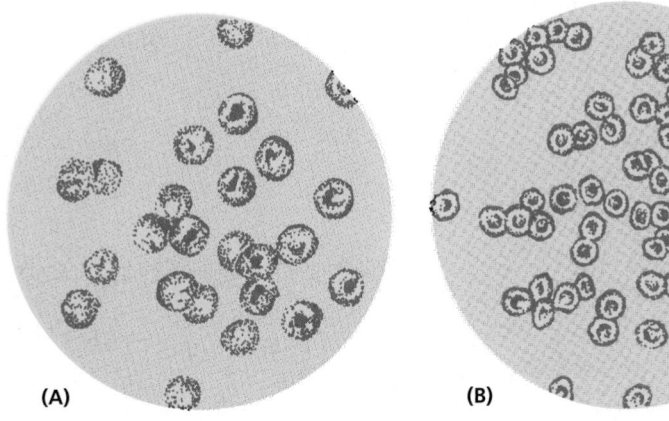

(A)   **(B)**

Figure 30-10   (A) White blood cells in urine. (B) Red blood cells in urine.

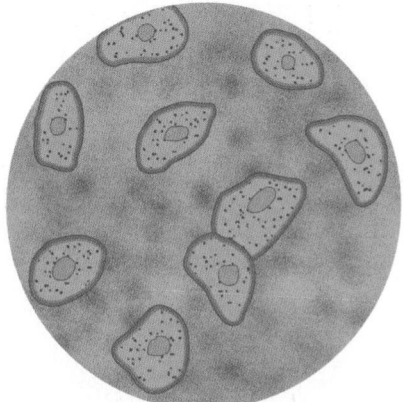

Figure 30-11   Renal epithelial cells.

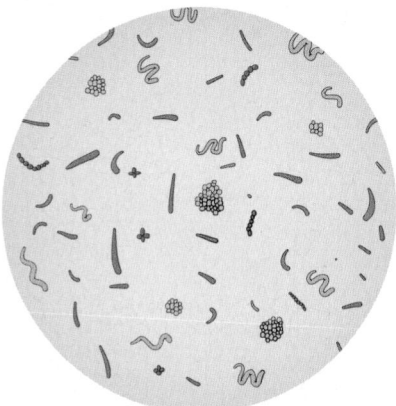

Figure 30-12   Bacteria in urine sediment.

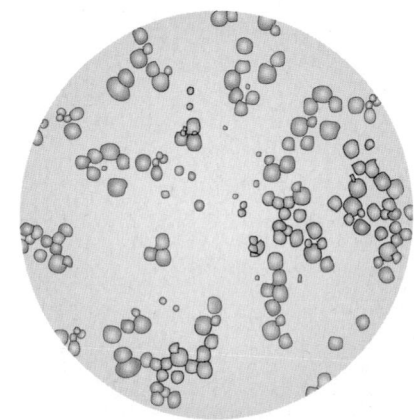

Figure 30-13   Yeast in urine sediment.

is a parasite that can infect the urinary tract. It is often recognized by the movement of its tail (flagella). Always check with a physician or someone more familiar with these organisms before reporting this organism.

Sperm. Sperm is reported only when seen in male urine unless specifically requested by a physician. Sperm have oval bodies with one long, thin flagella (Figure 30-15A).

Artifacts. Hair, fibers, baby powder, and oil are among the substances that may appear in urine sediment as a result of contamination during collection or later. If a structure cannot be identified using a good urine atlas, it probably is an artifact. A urine atlas will also show illustrations of artifacts. If in doubt, get an expert opinion (Figure 30-15B).

Crystals in Urinary Sediment. Crystals make up unorganized urine sediment. Since crystals are big, the tendency of the medical assistant is to pay attention to them. However, they are the most insignificant part of the urinary sediment; thus, they require little attention. These crystals include calcium phosphate, triple phosphate,

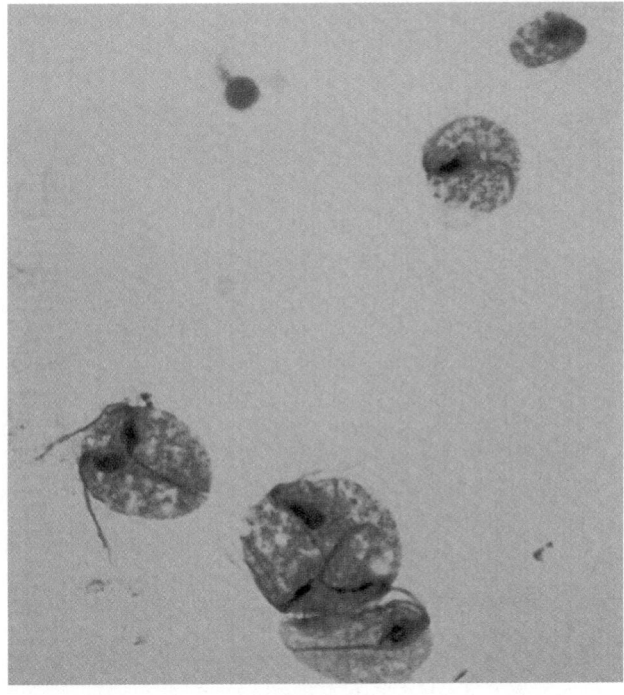

Figure 30-14   *Trichomonas* in stained urine sediment.

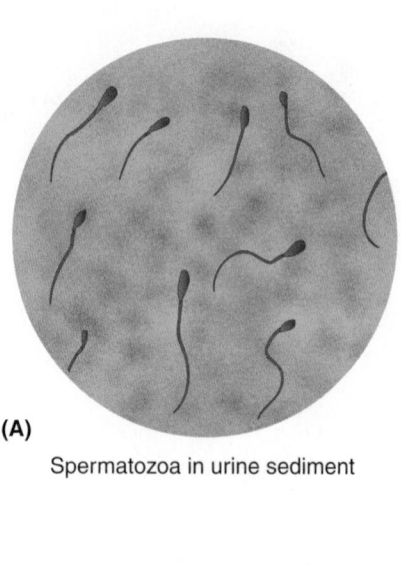

(A)

Spermatozoa in urine sediment

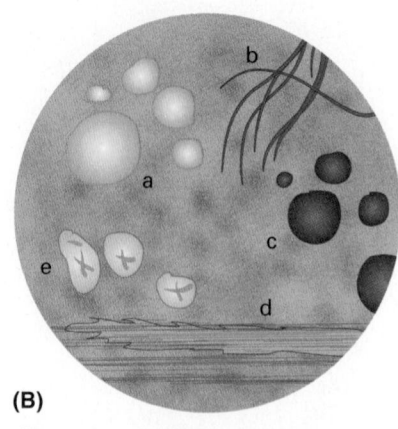

(B)

Examples of artifacts which may be
seen in urine sediment: (a) air bubbles,
(b) fibers, (c) oil droplets, (d) hair,
(e) starch or talc granules

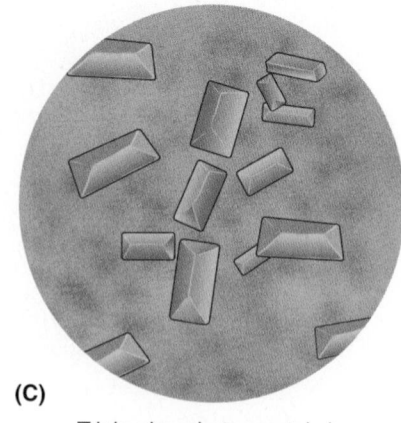

(C)

Triple phosphate crystals in
urine sediment

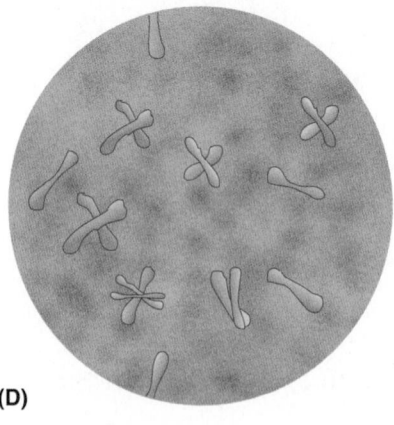

(D)

Calcium carbonate crystals in
urine sediment

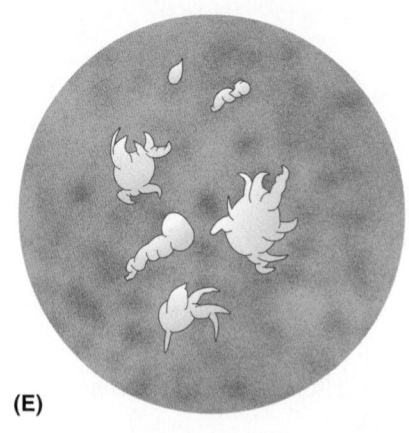

(E)

Ammonium biurate in
urine sediment

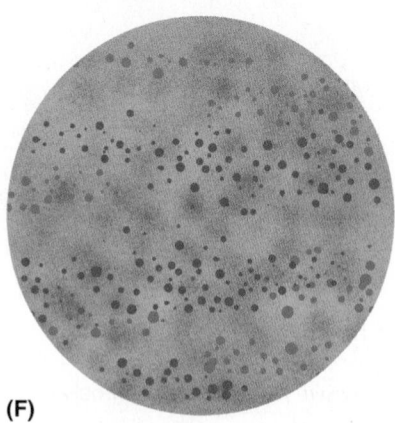

(F)

Amorphous phosphates in
urine sediment

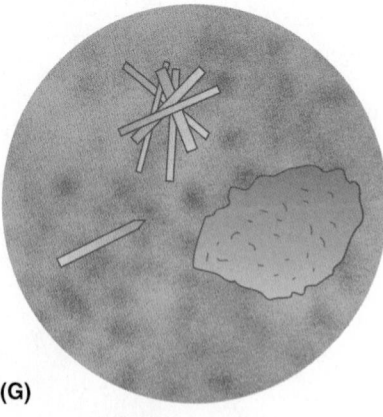

(G)

Calcium phosphate in urine sediment

Figure 30-15   Crystals and miscellaneous structures that can appear in urine.

calcium oxalate, amorphous phosphates and urates, and calcium carbonate. These crystals generally form as urine specimens stand, especially when refrigerated. Many laboratories do report these crystals. Refer to a urine color atlas to identify crystals. Figure 30-15 (C–G) illustrates several kinds of crystals that can be found in urine.

A few crystals in urine should be particularly noted if seen as they may indicate disease states. Uric acid, cystine, and sulfa drug crystals can indicate disease states. Refer to a urine atlas to observe the shape of these crystals.

Casts in Urinary Sediment. Casts are very important to see and identify in urine sediment. It takes a great deal of experience and expertise to recognize the many different kinds of casts that can be in sediment. When casts are suspected, the medical assistant should get an expert opinion before reporting their presence.

Casts are formed when protein accumulates and precipitates in the kidney tubules. The casts are then washed into the urine. Most casts are made from a particular type of protein called **Tamm-Horsfall** mucoprotein. Other proteins can also form casts. Serum proteins can form waxy casts. The presence of casts in the urine may indicate kidney disease.

Casts are cylindrical with rounded or flat ends. They are classified according to the substances observed inside them. Some casts may include debris as they are forming and may appear cellular or granular.

The most common cast seen in urine sediment is the **hyaline** cast. Rare hyaline casts can be seen in normal urine but increase with any kidney disease. They can also be seen as a result of fever, emotional stress, or strenuous exercise. Hyaline casts are nearly transparent and can be difficult to see under the microscope without some light adjustment.

Other types of casts include granular casts, containing remnants of disintegrated cells that appear as fine or coarse granules. Cellular casts may contain epithelial cells, red blood cells, or white blood cells. Figure 30-16 illustrates hyaline, granular, and cellular casts.

As mentioned before, identification of casts in urine takes an experienced eye. The medical assistant should always ask for assistance when identifying casts in urine sediment. See Procedures 30-7 and 30-8.

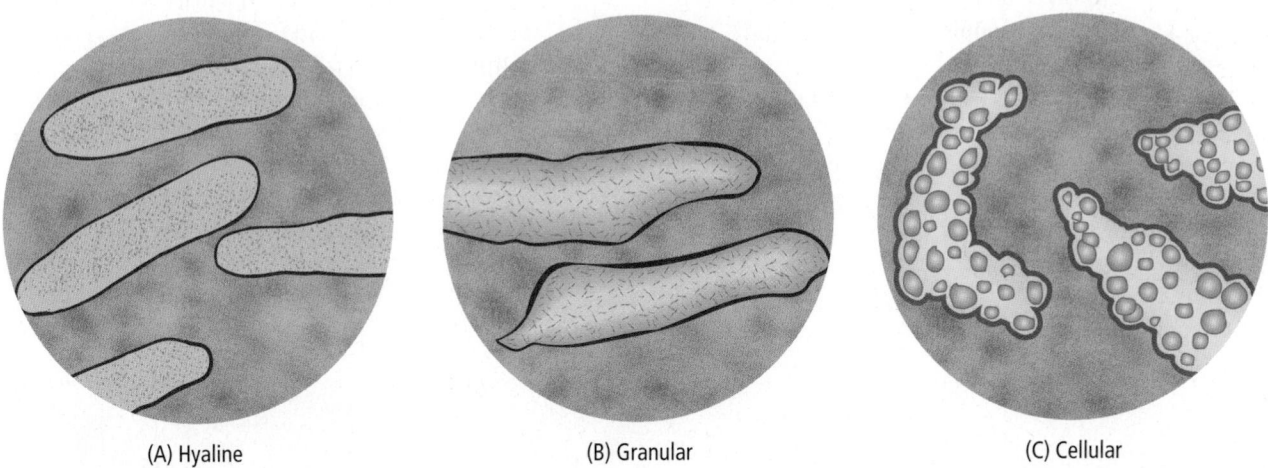

(A) Hyaline   (B) Granular   (C) Cellular

Figure 30-16 Casts in urine sediment.

Procedure 30-1　Assessing Urine Volume

STANDARD PRECAUTIONS:

   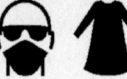 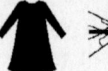 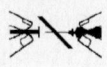

PURPOSE:

Determine and document the volume of a urine sample.

EQUIPMENT/SUPPLIES:

Gloves	Biohazard container
Graduated urine container	Antiseptic cleaner
Graduated cylinder	Laboratory report form

PROCEDURE STEPS:

1. Wash hands.
2. Put on gloves.
3. Assemble equipment and materials.
4. Follow all safety guidelines, being careful not to splash the urine sample. Wipe up all spills with antiseptic cleaner.
5. The sample must first be observed for proper labeling. Any unlabeled specimen is not tested. The medical assistant is required to determine whose urine is unlabeled. Then the patient is notified, and a new specimen is ordered. Guessing what urine belongs to which patient is not permissible.
6. After making sure that the urine container lid is tightly closed, mix the urine thoroughly.
7. If the container is not graduated, pour the urine into a suitable measuring device, such as a graduated cylinder.
8. The volume of the urine should be recorded in milliliters (mL); 10 to 12 mL is considered an adequate specimen. Some facilities do not require the recording of volume unless the quantity is insufficient.
9. In samples from 4 to 10 mL, the medical assistant should record the following comment on the results report: *"Interpret with caution. Quantity not sufficient for accurate quantitative analysis."* Some laboratories may not require this warning.
10. Samples of less than 4 mL (except for newborns) should be marked "QNS" (quantity not sufficient) and should not be tested. This policy also may differ from facility to facility.
11. After the volume is recorded on the laboratory report form, an aliquot (a smaller portion of the sample) may be used to continue the urinalysis. This aliquot should be placed in a standard urinalysis centrifuge tube.

Procedure 30-2　Observing Urine Color

STANDARD PRECAUTIONS:

    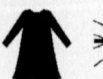

PURPOSE:

Observe and record the color of a urine specimen.

EQUIPMENT/SUPPLIES:

Gloves	Biohazard container
Urine specimen	Antiseptic cleaner
White card	Laboratory report form

PROCEDURE STEPS:

1. Wash hands.
2. Put on gloves.
3. Assemble equipment and materials.
4. Follow all safety guidelines, being careful not to splash the urine sample. Wipe up all spills with antiseptic cleaner.
5. Mix the urine specimen thoroughly.
6. Observe the color of the urine in a clear centrifuge tube. Use good light against a white background (a white card or sheet of paper will do).
7. Record the results on the laboratory report form.

Procedure 30-3 Observing Urine Clarity

STANDARD PRECAUTIONS:

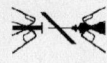

PURPOSE:
Observe and record the clarity of the urine specimen.

EQUIPMENT/SUPPLIES:

Gloves
Urine specimen in a
   centrifuge tube
White sheet of paper
   with print

Biohazard container
Antiseptic cleaner
Laboratory report form

PROCEDURE STEPS:
1. Wash hands.
2. Put on gloves.
3. Assemble equipment and materials.

4. Follow all safety guidelines, being careful not to splash the urine sample. Wipe up all spills with antiseptic cleaner.
5. Hold the centrifuge tube close to a printed sheet of white paper.
6. If you can clearly see the print on the paper, the specimen should be described as clear.
7. If the urine is slightly blurry, it might be described as hazy.
8. If the urine has cloudy material in it, describe it as cloudy.
9. If the urine is impossible to see through, it might be described as turbid.
10. Record the results on the laboratory report form.
11. Dispose of all biohazardous wastes in the biohazard container.

Procedure 30-4 Using the Refractometer to Measure Specific Gravity

STANDARD PRECAUTIONS:

PURPOSE:
Measure and record the specific gravity of a urine specimen.

EQUIPMENT/SUPPLIES:

Refractometer
Urine sample
Gloves
Pipettes
Distilled water
5% saline solution

Lint-free tissues
Quality control
   urine sample
Biohazard container
Antiseptic cleaners
Laboratory report form

PROCEDURE STEPS:
1. Wash hands.
2. Put on gloves.
3. Assemble equipment and materials.
4. Follow all safety guidelines, being careful not to splash the urine sample. Wipe up all spills with antiseptic cleaner.
5. Quality control must be done on the refractometer before working with a urine specimen. This is done by checking the value of distilled water, which should read 1.000.
6. Clean the surface of the cover and the prism with a lint-free tissue moistened with distilled water. Wipe them dry.
7. Close the cover. Apply a drop of distilled water to the notched portion of the cover so that it flows over the prism (Figure 30-17).

(continues)

Procedure 30-4 (continued)

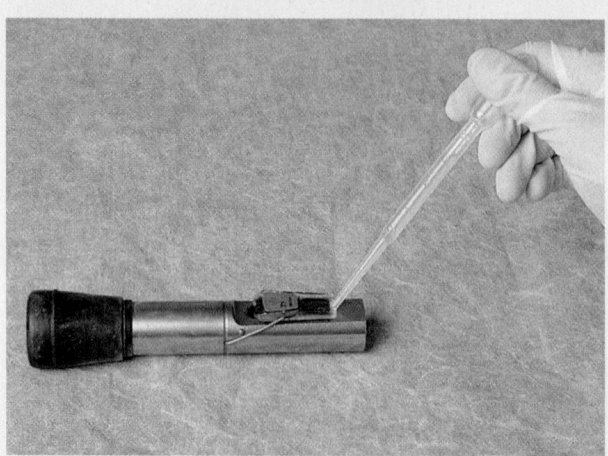

Figure 30-17   A pipette or dropper may be used to fill the refractometer with the urine sample.

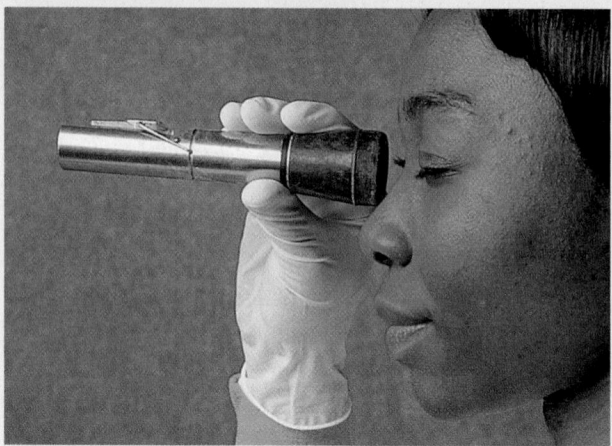

Figure 30-18   The medical assistant reads the refractometer to determine the specific gravity of the urine sample.

8. Tilt the instrument to allow light to enter. Read the specific gravity scale, which is the sharp dividing line between the dark and light areas (Figure 30-18). This reading should be at 1.000. If the reading is not 1.000, use a fresh sample of distilled water from another source.
9. Wipe the cover and prism between samples.
10. Next, test a sample of 5% saline solution, which should read 1.023 +/– 0.001. The instrument is now standardized. You are now ready to analyze quality control samples and patient samples. Use

the same method as in steps 1–9 and record your results on your quality control sheet.
11. Use the same procedure for each urine sample and record the result on the patient requisition.
12. Be sure to clean the area after finishing the procedure. Make sure any spills are cleaned with antiseptic solution. Make sure the refractometer is thoroughly cleaned with distilled water and a lint-free tissue. Dispose of all biohazardous waste in the biohazard container.

Procedure 30-5   Performing a Urinalysis Chemical Examination

STANDARD PRECAUTIONS:

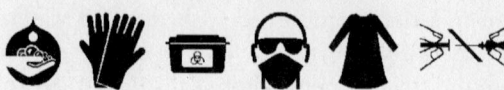

PURPOSE:
Detect any abnormal chemical constituents of a urine specimen.

EQUIPMENT/SUPPLIES:
Gloves
Dipsticks
Urine specimen
Biohazard container
Antiseptic cleaner
Laboratory report form

(continues)

Procedure

30-5 *(continued)*

PROCEDURE STEPS:

1. Wash hands.
2. Put on gloves.
3. Assemble equipment and materials.
4. Follow all safety guidelines, being careful not to splash the urine sample. Wipe up all spills with antiseptic cleaner.
5. Mix the urine specimen thoroughly.
6. Remove a test strip from the container and replace the cap tightly (strips are adversely affected if the bottle is left open for long periods).
7. Immerse the strip completely in the uncentrifuged urine and remove it immediately (Figure 30-19A).
8. While removing the strip from the urine, run the edge of the strip against the rim of the container, tapping it lightly on the container to remove any excess urine (Figure 30-19B). RATIONALE: Excess urine can bridge the gap between reagent pads, causing inaccurate results.

9. Proper timing is essential for correct results. The proper time for each pad will be listed on the dipstick container.
10. Hold the dipstick close to the container, but do not touch it against the container. Compare the test areas to the proper area on the container and record the results (Figure 30-19C).
11. Record the results on the laboratory report form.
12. Discard the used reagent strips and other disposable items in the proper receptacles.

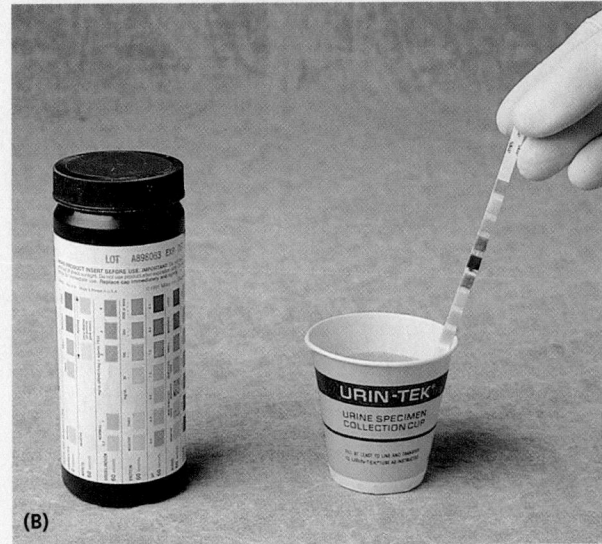

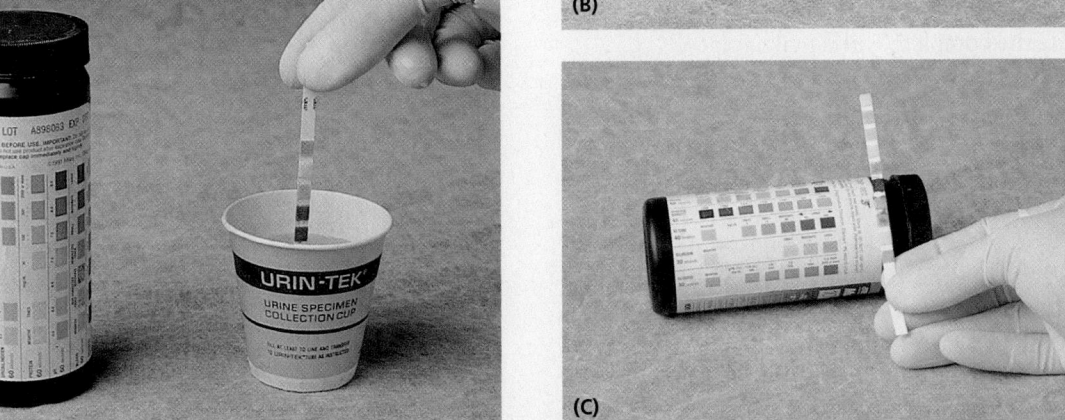

Figure 30-19 (A) Immerse the reagent strip in the urine sample. (B) After immersing the reagent strip, tap it lightly to remove excess urine. (C) Read the reagent strip by matching the color on the strip to a color on the container.

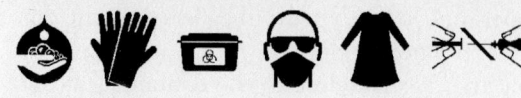

30-6   Testing for Sugar in the Urine

STANDARD PRECAUTIONS:

PURPOSE:
Perform a Clinitest on a urine specimen to detect reducing sugars.

EQUIPMENT/SUPPLIES:

Gloves	Disposable pipettes
Clinitest tablets	Biohazard container
Urine specimen	Antiseptic cleaner
Clean glass test tube	Laboratory report form
Distilled water	

PROCEDURE STEPS:
1. Wash hands.
2. Put on gloves.
3. Assemble equipment and materials.
4. Follow all safety guidelines, being careful not to splash the urine sample. Wipe up all spills with antiseptic cleaner.
5. Transfer 5 drops (0.3 mL) of urine into a clean glass test tube.
6. Add 10 drops (0.6 mL) of distilled water. Mix well, being careful not to splash the contents of the tube (Figure 30-20).
7. Drop one tablet into the tube. Watch the mixture while the complete boiling takes place.
   CAUTION: Do not touch the bottom of the tube. The bottom becomes very hot during the test reaction and can cause serious burns.
8. Do not shake the tube after adding the tablet until at least 15 seconds after the boiling stops.
9. At the end of the 15-second waiting period, gently shake the tube to mix. Do not touch the bottom of the tube as the heat of reaction is still present.
10. Compare the color of the liquid to the proper color chart. Ignore any color changes that occur after the waiting period.

11. There are two methods of reporting. One method is by percentage, and the other uses trace through 4+:

¼% or trace; ½% or 1+; ¾% or 2+; 1% or 3+; 2% or 4+

12. Urine containing more than 5% sugar will cause a rapid color change during the boiling. Observe closely during this time to detect a "pass-through" phenomenon in which the color changes from green to tan to orange to black or dark brown. If this happens, report as greater than 2% or 4+.
13. Record the results on the laboratory report form.
14. Dispose of all biohazardous waste in the biohazard container.
    NOTE: If a reducing sugar is present in the urine, the color changes from blue to green and then orange, depending on the amount of sugar present. This test is not specific for glucose, and many drugs may cause positive results. The Clinitest is not used for insulin monitoring.

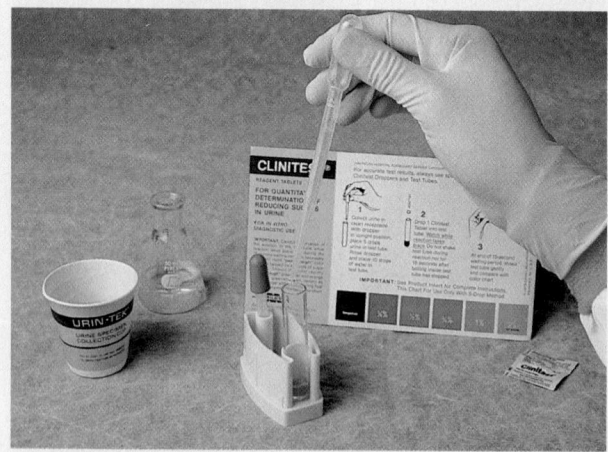

Figure 30-20   The Clinitest® confirmatory test.

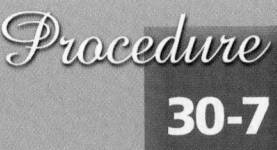 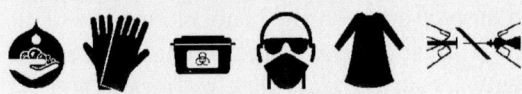

Microscopic Examination of Urine Sediment

STANDARD PRECAUTIONS:

PURPOSE:
Perform a microscopic examination of urine sediment.

EQUIPMENT/SUPPLIES:

Gloves	Centrifuge tube
Microscope	Urine sediment
Centrifuge	containing casts
Microscope slides	Urine atlas
Cover slips	Antiseptic cleaner
Disposable pipettes	Biohazard container

PROCEDURE STEPS:

1. Wash hands.
2. Put on gloves.
3. Assemble equipment and materials.
4. Follow all safety guidelines, being careful not to splash the urine sample. Wipe up all spills with antiseptic cleaner.
5. Obtain a urine specimen. The first morning specimen is preferred due to its concentration and pH, which tend to preserve the formed elements. The urine should be examined as soon as possible but may be refrigerated for a short time.
6. Mix the entire specimen well, then centrifuge a 10–15 mL aliquot (portion) at 1,500 revolutions per minute for 5 minutes.
7. After centrifugation, pour off the supernatant, leaving about 1 mL in the bottom of the centrifuge tube.
8. Tap or "flick" the bottom of the tube to resuspend the sediment in the remaining fluid.
9. Place a drop of the sediment on a microscope slide, carefully placing a coverglass over the drop of sediment.
10. Place the slide on the microscope stage and examine immediately. When examining urine sediment, it is important to keep the light subdued by lowering the condenser and to constantly vary the fine focus adjustment in order to view structures that are very faint. Again, proper light and focus adjustments take a great deal of practice.
11. Scan the sediment using a 100X (low power) magnification.
    NOTE: A 100X magnification is achieved by using the 10X objective lens, remembering that the ocular also is a 10X lens. 10X × 10X = 100X.
12. View 10 to 15 fields and around the edges of the drop for casts.
    NOTE: When using a cover slip, the casts can be forced to the edges.
13. Record the average number of each type of cast viewed per LPF (low-power field). It may be necessary to use the 40X objective (high power) to identify some of the casts. For example: If a type of cast is seen from two to four times in each field, report as 2–4 casts/LPF.
14. Scan the drop using a 400X (high power) magnification. Count and average the numbers of other formed elements in 10 to 15 fields.
15. Record the results on the laboratory report form.
16. Dispose of all biohazardous waste in the biohazard container. Be sure to clean off the microscopic lenses with lens paper. Wipe up all spills with antiseptic cleaner.

30-8 Performing a Urinalysis

STANDARD PRECAUTIONS:

PURPOSE:
Perform a complete urinalysis, including the physical, chemical, and microscopic examination.

EQUIPMENT/SUPPLIES:

Gloves
Urine specimen
Measuring cylinder
Test tubes
Pipettes
Centrifuge tube
Centrifuge
Microscope
Microscope slides
Coverglasses

Reagent strips (dipsticks)
Control urine sample
Urine atlas
Refractometer
  (or urinometer)
Distilled water
Lint-free tissues
Biohazard container
Antiseptic cleaner
Laboratory report form

PROCEDURE STEPS:
1. Wash hands.
2. Put on gloves.
3. Assemble equipment and materials.
4. Follow all safety guidelines, being careful not to splash the urine sample. Wipe up all spills with antiseptic cleaner.

PHYSICAL EXAMINATION:
5. Obtain a urine specimen. Measure the amount of the specimen in a measuring cylinder if there are no measurement markings on the specimen container. Make sure there is more than 12 mL of urine.
6. Mix gently and pour approximately 5 mL of urine into a test tube.
7. Observe and record the color of urine (straw, yellow, amber, red).
8. Observe and record the transparency of urine (clear, slightly cloudy, turbid).
9. Note unusual odors of the urine (not recorded).
10. Measure the specific gravity using either a refractometer or a urinometer.
   Refractometer: Place one drop distilled water on the glass plate and close. Look through the ocular and read the specific gravity from the scale. The reading should be 1.000. Then wipe the water from the glass plate using lint-free tissues. Place one drop of urine on the plate, closing the plate. Look through the ocular, reading the specific gravity. Clean the glass plate with water and dry with a tissue. Record the results.
   Urinometer: Pour 40 to 50 mL of distilled water into the glass cylinder (about three-fourths full). Insert the urinometer with a spinning motion. Read the specific gravity from the scale on the stem of the urinometer as it stops spinning. The reading should be 1.000. Rinse the equipment with distilled water. Repeat the procedure using a urine specimen. Clean the equipment carefully using detergent, rinsing thoroughly with distilled water, and drying carefully. Record the results.

CHEMICAL EXAMINATION:
1. Continue to wear gloves and use the same specimen as in the physical examination.
2. Test the urine control sample with a reagent strip. Dip the strip into the urine sample, moistening all pads.
3. Immediately remove the strip from the urine and tap it to remove excess urine.
4. Observe the reagent pads and compare colors to the color chart at appropriate intervals.
5. Record the results on a laboratory report form after properly disposing of the reagent strip.
6. If any tests are positive that need confirmation (protein, glucose, bilirubin, acetone), perform that test following the manufacturer's directions. Follow all safety precautions necessary.
7. Dispose of all biohazardous materials in a biohazard container.

MICROSCOPIC EXAMINATION:
1. Continue to wear gloves. Use the same urine sample. Follow all safety precautions necessary for this procedure.
2. Carefully pour 12 mL of specimen into a centrifuge tube. Centrifuge the specimen at 1,500 to 2,500 rpm for 5 minutes.
3. Carefully decant the supernatant and resuspend the sediment.
4. Pipette one drop resuspended urine sediment on a clean glass slide.

(continues)

Procedure 30-8 (continued)

5. Place a coverglass over the drop of urine.
6. Carefully place the slide under the microscope.
7. Under low power (10X), scan the slide with reduced light for casts. Refer to a urine atlas to refresh your memory about cast appearances.
8. Rotate to high power (40X and 45X objective).
9. Scan the slide and identify any blood cells, bacteria, yeast, parasites, and epithelial cells that may be seen.
10. Identify any crystals or amorphous deposits seen.

11. Record all the results on the laboratory report form.
12. Discard all biohazardous materials in the biohazard container.
13. Clean and return the equipment to proper storage, if necessary.
14. Clean the work area with disinfectant.
15. Discard gloves in the biohazard container.
16. Thoroughly wash hands with disinfectant soap.

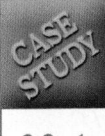

CASE STUDY

30-1

Annette Samuels came to Inner City Health Care today because she is experiencing frequent urination, itching, and burning when urinating. Dr. Rice ordered a urinalysis, which clinical medical assistant Wanda Slawson is performing. Wanda notes that the urine has a cloudy appearance and the dipstick tests positive for nitrites. Wanda confers with Dr. Rice, who instructs her to perform a microscopic examination of the specimen.

CASE STUDY REVIEW

1. Why does Dr. Rice want this specimen examined microscopically?
2. What should Wanda look for when she examines the specimen?
3. How should she report her findings?

SUMMARY

This chapter summarizes the basics of the urinalysis. Physicians order a variety of tests on urine to help them determine or rule out certain abnormalities in order to make a correct diagnosis and prescribe treatment.

Urine is formed as blood is filtered through the kidney. Substances such as by-products of metabolism, mineral excesses, cells, bacteria, parasites, crystals, and casts can be found in the urine during examination.

It is important for the medical assistant to:

- Understand the proper collection techniques for urine specimens. Medical assistants are often called upon to instruct patients in the proper collection procedures.

- Understand the safety guidelines involved with collecting and handling specimens, preservatives, and reagents. These guidelines must *always* be observed.
- Understand the importance of and the procedures for maintaining a consistent quality control program.
- Understand how to properly perform the urinalysis, following up with proper confirmatory tests when necessary.
- Understand and be constantly aware of factors that may interfere with the accuracy of a urinalysis.

REVIEW QUESTIONS

Multiple Choice

1. What safety guideline is important to follow during a routine urinalysis?
   a. use the same pipette for all patients' urine samples
   b. allow urine to sit at room temperature to ferment the urine properties
   c. once tested, urine can be disposed of by the janitorial service
   d. treat all specimens as if they were infectious

2. What are the three basic parts of a typical urine examination?
   a. volumetric, chemical, and macroscopic
   b. pathological, chemical, and confirmatory
   c. physical, chemical, and microscopic
   d. random, 24-hour, and catheterized

3. What is the specimen of choice for routine urinalysis?
   a. random
   b. clean-catch
   c. catheterized
   d. timed

4. A diabetic patient will normally have an excess of what substance in the urine?
   a. hemoglobin
   b. glucose
   c. insulin
   d. sodium

5. What is the most common way of doing a chemical analysis of urine in a physician's office?
   a. reagent strip test
   b. Clinitest®
   c. culture test
   d. Acetest®

6. Positive results for the following during chemical testing of newborn urine should be immediately reported to the physician:
   a. blood, pH, nitrates
   b. bilirubin, blood, leukocyte esterase
   c. pH, urobilinogen, specific gravity
   d. glucose, ketone, and protein

7. Confirmatory tests are done to:
   a. confirm negative results from initial testing
   b. confirm positive results from initial testing
   c. confirm urine volume
   d. confirm urine turbidity

8. What confirmatory urine test is done to test for evidence of incomplete fat metabolism?
   a. Clinitest®
   b. sulfosalicylic acid test
   c. Ictotest®
   d. Acetest®

9. Which substance or structure is automatically considered abnormal when found in urine?
   a. phosphates
   b. urea
   c. blood
   d. salt

Critical Thinking

1. What is the importance of proper urine collection?
2. How is a clean-catch urine sample collected?
3. What is a midstream urine specimen?
4. When is a urine preservative necessary?
5. Why is the first morning specimen preferred for routine urinalysis?
6. What would give a urine sample a cloudy appearance?
7. What is the normal specific gravity of urine?
8. If urine was kept at a temperature of 16° centigrade and specific gravity was performed, what adjustment, if any, would have to be made to the results?

WEB ACTIVITIES

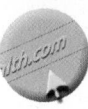

1. Search for CLIA information on the Internet. Are guidelines posted for specimen collection? When were these guidelines last updated?
2. Visit the CDC's web site and review the Standard Precautions that apply to urine collection and analysis.

REFERENCES/BIBLIOGRAPHY

Akron City Hospital Procedure Manual. (1996). Akron, OH: Author.

Flynn, J., & Whitlock, S. (1997). *Delmar's clinical lab manual series: Urinalysis* (1st ed.). Albany, NY: Delmar.

Henry, J. B. (1996). *Clinical diagnosis and management by laboratory methods* (19th ed.). Philadelphia: W. B. Saunders.

Walters, N. J., Estridge, B. H., & Reynolds, A. P. (2000). *Basic medical laboratory techniques* (4th ed.). Albany, NY: Delmar.

KEY TERMS

Aerobic
Aerosols
Anaerobic
Biochemical Tests
Broth Tubes
Check Cell Slides
Concentration Method
Counterstain
Culture
Decolorizer
Dermatophytes
DNA
Enterobacteriaceae
Expectorate
Fastidious Bacteria
Genus
Gram Stain
Holding Media
Immunosuppressed
Inoculate
Kirby Bauer
Lumbar Puncture
Microbiology
Mordant
Morphology
Mycobacteria
Mycology
Nematode
Normal Flora
Nosocomial
Ova
Parasitology
Pathogen

(continues)

OUTLINE

The Medical Assistant's Role in the Microbiology Laboratory
Microbiology
  Classification
  Nomenclature
  Cell Structure
Equipment
  Autoclave
  Microscope
  Safety Hood
  Incubator
  Anaerobic Equipment
  Inoculating Equipment
  Incinerator
  Media
  Refrigerator
Safety When Handling Microbiology Specimens
  Personal Protective Equipment
  Work Area
  Specimen Handling
  Disposal of Waste and Spills
Quality Control
Collection Procedures
  Specific Collection Requirements
Microscopic Examination of Bacteria
  Bacterial Shapes
  Dyes (Stains)

Simple Stain
Differential Stain
Acid-Fast Stain
Special Techniques
Potassium Hydroxide (KOH)
  Preparation
Culture Media
  Media Classification
Microbiology Culture
  Inoculating the Media
  Other Types of Streaking
  Primary Culture
  Subculture
Biochemical Tests
  Direct Tests
  Biochemical Tube Testing
Identification Systems
  Streptococcus Screening
    (Rapid Strep Testing)
  Packaged Systems
  Semiautomated and Automated
    Instruments
Sensitivity Testing
Parasitology
  Examination Methods
  Specimen Collection
  Common Parasites
Mycology

OBJECTIVES

The student should strive to meet the following performance objectives and demonstrate an understanding of the facts and principles presented in this chapter through written and oral communication.

1. Define the key terms as presented in the glossary.
2. Define microbiology, discussing classifications, and nomenclature relevant to the microbiology laboratory. *(continues)*

KEY TERMS (*continued*)

Petri Dish
Protozoa
Quality Control
Reagents
Sensitivity
Species
Stab Culture
Taxonomy
Tetrads
Virology
Wood's Lamp

OBJECTIVES (*continued*)

3. Describe bacterial cell structure.
4. List and describe the equipment used in the microbiology laboratory.
5. Explain how to safely handle microbiology specimens.
6. Describe the importance of and steps involved in quality control in the microbiology laboratory.
7. Explain the types of specimens collected for the microbiology laboratory and how they are collected.
8. List different types of stains used to microscopically observe microorganisms.
9. Perform a Gram stain.
10. List the different classifications of media used in the microbiology laboratory.
11. Describe how organisms are cultured onto various media.
12. Explain how biochemical testing is used to identify microorganisms.
13. Discuss identification systems used to identify bacteria.
14. Describe the significance of sensitivity testing.
15. List two parasites and two fungi that can be observed in the microbiology laboratory.

ROLE DELINEATION COMPONENTS

CLINICAL

Fundamental Principles

- Apply principles of aseptic technique and infection control
- Comply with quality assurance practices
- Screen and follow up patient test results

Diagnostic Orders

- Collect and process specimens
- Perform diagnostic tests

GENERAL (TRANSDISCIPLINARY)

Legal Concepts

- Document accurately
- Comply with established risk management and safety procedures

SCENARIO

To aid in diagnosing and treating patients, the physicians at Lewis and King MD order tests to identify disease-causing bacteria, fungi, viruses, and parasites. Some of these tests, such as the latex agglutination test for Group A Streptococcus, are performed in the office laboratory, while other tests are sent to a reference laboratory. Regardless of where the test will be performed, medical assistant Joe Guerrero follows all safety precautions when handling specimens. He checks the test manufacturer's or laboratory's procedures and carefully completes each step. By following all safety guidelines and test procedures, Joe ensures his and others' safety. He obtains a high-quality specimen for testing.

INTRODUCTION

The field of **microbiology** encompasses the study of all microorganisms, living structures that can be seen only with the powerful magnification of a microscope. The word *microbiology* comes from the Greek words *micro* (small) and *bios* (living). The field of microbiology includes the study of such organisms as bacteria, fungi, viruses, parasites, and algae (Table 31-1).

Many medical textbooks in microbiology include extensive study of all of the preceding organisms, including lesser known species in each category. It is the goal of this chapter to introduce the student to the field of microbiology with emphasis on bacteria, fungi, and parasites. Safety while working with microorganisms in the laboratory is emphasized. The relationship of bacteria to diseases also is explored.

TABLE 31-1   BIOLOGICAL SCIENCES

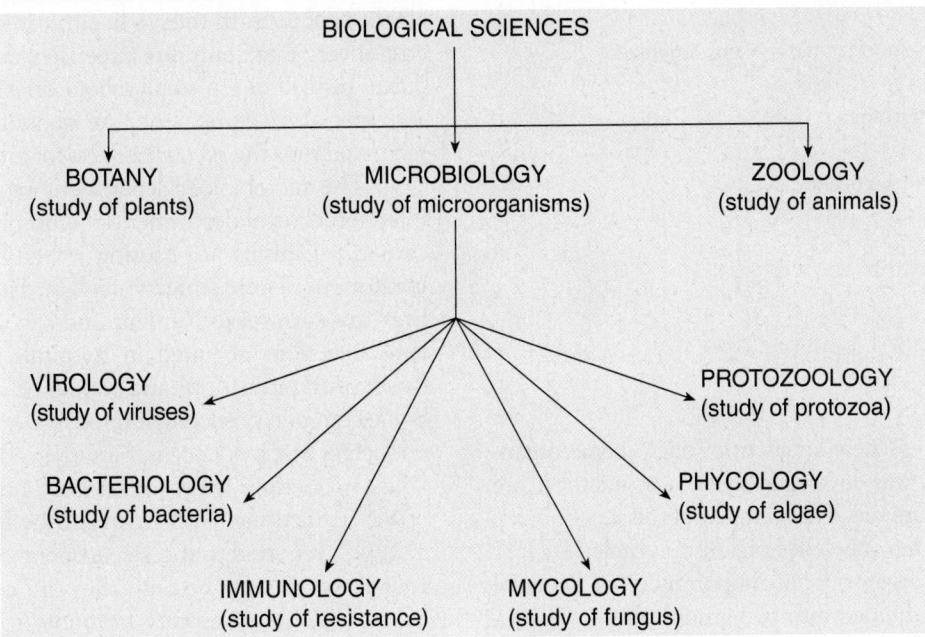

THE MEDICAL ASSISTANT'S ROLE IN THE MICROBIOLOGY LABORATORY

The role of the medical assistant in the microbiology laboratory may be to assist in isolating and identifying microorganisms that can cause harm and disease. A medical assistant might be asked to carefully smear a microscopic slide with body material that is suspected of being contaminated with bacteria. This slide is then stained in a special manner (described later in the chapter) and read under a microscope. The medical assistant may also place a sample of body secretions or excretions (urine, material from a sore throat, blood, sputum coughed up from the lungs, and so on) on special media to allow bacteria to grow. This is called a **culture**. The bacteria is usually allowed to grow at least twelve hours before the culture can be examined to identify the offending organism. In certain situations, a physician may request a **sensitivity** in addition to the culture. This is a test that will identify which antibiotic or antibiotics will effectively kill the microorganism identified as causing the infection.

In healthy individuals, several types of bacteria are found in various parts of the body. For instance, the throat has bacteria in it, called **normal flora**. These organisms are always present and help with the body's immune system. In disease, the causative microorganism is called a **pathogen** because it causes harm to the body.

The medical assistant's technique must be exact to avoid laboratory error. The medical assistant also must be assured the specimen for culture was taken with sterile

supplies and brought to the laboratory in a reasonable amount of time. Delivery time of the specimen or culture may vary due to the type of specimen collected for culture. Some specimens may be refrigerated without harm. Some may be kept in **holding media**, media that will keep a specimen on a swab moist until it is cultured. These variations will be discussed later in specimen processing.

By doing the smear, culture, and identification through biochemical tests, the microbiologist can identify the organism and aid the physician in diagnosing and treating the patient. Most identification of organisms can be done successfully within 24 to 72 hours. Some organisms may take longer to grow. The acid-fast bacterium *Mycobacterium tuberculosis*, the causative organism of tuberculosis, may take longer; however, modern techniques are making it possible to identify this microorganism more rapidly.

MICROBIOLOGY

Classification

Taxonomy deals with the classification of living organisms. The scheme of naming organisms is based on similarities of structures. The current classification is based on a system devised by Carolus von Linne, a Swedish biologist. Although there are a number of classifications, there is no universal agreement on one particular system.

A common system divides living organisms into kingdoms. Prior to the discovery of the microscope in the sixteenth century, there were two known kingdoms,

TABLE 31-2   KINGDOM PROTISTA

I. Lower protists
   1. Prokaryotic—nuclear material not organized
      A. Bacteria
      B. Blue-green algae
II. Higher protists
   1. Eukaryotic—true nucleus
      A. Algae
      B. Slime molds
      C. Fungus
      D. Protozoa

animal and plant. A new kingdom of microscopic organisms, the *Protista,* was developed since most microbes are neither plant nor animal. The members of this kingdom are called *protists* and are one-celled organisms (Table 31-2).

The microorganisms of importance in medical microbiology are divided into two groups: the lower protists or *prokaryotes* (including blue-green algae and bacteria) and the higher protists or *eukaryotes* (including protozoa, algae, and fungi).

Nomenclature

The system used for naming bacteria is the binomial (two) nomenclature (system of names). Two Greek or Latin names are used, the first name being a genus, which is capitalized. The second name is the species name, which is not capitalized. These names may reflect a characteristic of a bacterium and/or names of places or persons associated with the discovery of the microorganism. For example, *Salmonella typhi* was discovered by an American microbiologist named Salmon. The bacterium causes typhoid fever.

Individuals who study bacteria are referred to as bacteriologists or microbiologists. These individuals have taken extensive courses in the field of microbiology. In most laboratories, clinical laboratory scientists or assistants help perform microbiology procedures. The job of these individuals is to quickly and efficiently identify the organism in a given culture that has been properly obtained and brought to the laboratory within a reasonable time frame.

Along with routine bacteriological cultures, many microbiology departments, especially in larger health care facilities, perform parasitology procedures for the identification of parasites; virology procedures for the identification of viruses; and mycology procedures for the identification of fungi. If an institution such as a clinic or physician's office laboratory is too small to properly identify many microorganisms, cultures often are sent to a reference laboratory. These laboratories are specialized laboratories set up with up-to-date equipment to handle large amounts of tests. In today's health care environment, it is cost-effective to centralize expensive and complex procedures. Instead of ten small laboratories each having their own specialized equipment, one laboratory buys the equipment and runs the specialized test for all ten laboratories.

The microbiology department works closely with the infection control department of a hospital to determine if certain organisms are causing infections throughout an institution. These infections can be acquired by an immunosuppressed patient and become a serious problem. Infections acquired in hospitals are referred to as nosocomial infections and should be closely monitored. Some common nosocomial infections are caused by bacteria such as Staphylococcus, Serratia, and monilia (a yeast).

Certain types of bacteria and yeasts that are identified and grown in the laboratory must be reported to the Department of Public Health in your town or state because they are communicable diseases. These diseases vary from city to city and state to state. Some of the common bacteria that are reported are Salmonella, Shigella, and those organisms that cause sexually transmitted diseases (STDs), such as gonorrhea, syphilis, chlamydia, and herpes. The state and town you work in will have a list of reportable diseases that the clinic or physician's office laboratory will have posted.

Cell Structure

All living forms are alike in that their cells contain a nuclear material referred to as DNA (deoxyribonucleic acid, which carries special genetic information). The main structural difference of eukaryotes and prokaryotes is the arrangement of the nucleus. A eukaryote has a well-defined or true nucleus and is a higher form of microorganism. The prokaryote is a lower form of microorganism and has a simple nucleus that is not well-defined.

The bacterial cell, classified as a lower protist, is a single-celled organism with a cytoplasmic cell membrane, cell wall, and nucleus. The nucleus is not well-defined. The cell grows by taking in materials from the environment. After a certain amount of growth, the bacteria reproduce by division of the cell. Certain conditions are required for this reproduction to take place.

Figure 31-1 illustrates a basic bacterial cell. Not all bacteria possess flagella for motility, as some are not motile. Some bacteria can produce capsules around the outside of the cell, providing protection from antibiotic penetration and white blood cell attack. Some bacteria produce spores, an inactive state that can help bacteria resist chemicals, freezing, drying, radiation, and heating. Bacterial spores are so resistant they can live 150,000 years and can survive in dust.

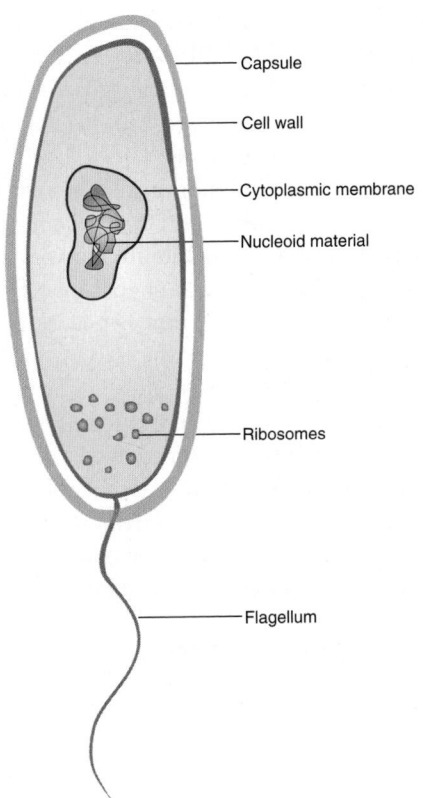

Figure 31-1   Basic bacterial cell.

Labels: Capsule, Cell wall, Cytoplasmic membrane, Nucleoid material, Ribosomes, Flagellum

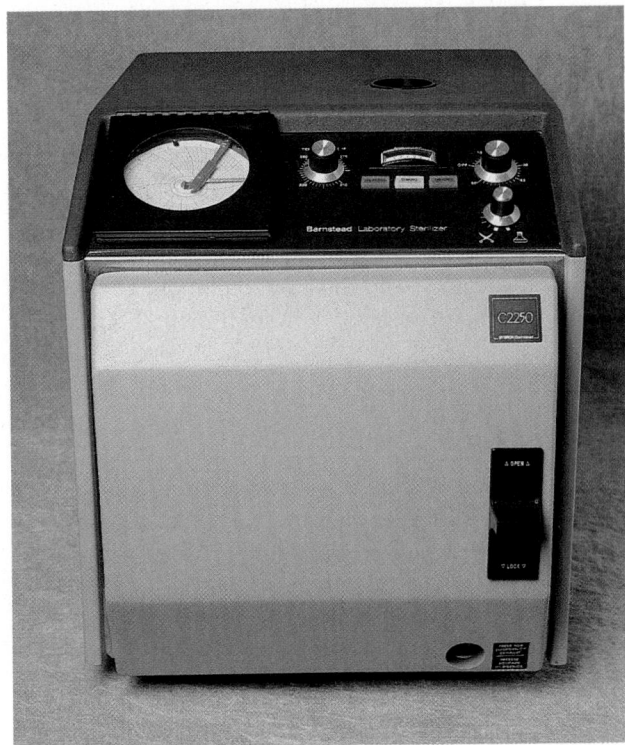

Figure 31-2   Small laboratory autoclave.

EQUIPMENT

Basic equipment needed in a microbiology department of a clinic or a physician's office laboratory varies depending on the size of the facility. Most laboratories have some of the following equipment.

Autoclave

An autoclave (Figure 31-2) is used in the laboratory to sterilize equipment that may have been contaminated while processing specimens. It can be used to sterilize contaminated materials as well. The setting of 15 lb./sq. in. and a temperature of 121°C for 15 to 20 minutes is sufficient to kill infectious agents, spores, viruses, and contaminants. Small microbiology departments use a bench-top autoclave, and larger departments have a separate room with a large autoclave. Many laboratories no longer use autoclaves because of the use of presterilized and disposable equipment. Waste products are put into biohazardous bags and are disposed of by a service outside the health care facility.

Microscope

An important piece of equipment for the physician's office laboratory or clinic is the microscope. This instrument is used to view organisms that cannot be seen with the naked eye on a prepared slide. Skill in using the microscope is necessary to gain information from studying the slide. The microscope is a delicate instrument and should be cared for properly as stated by the manufacturer. (Refer to Chapter 27, Introduction to the Medical Laboratory, for more information on the microscope.)

Safety Hood

Some laboratories, especially if they are culturing specimens with aerosols, will have a safety hood (Figure 31-3).

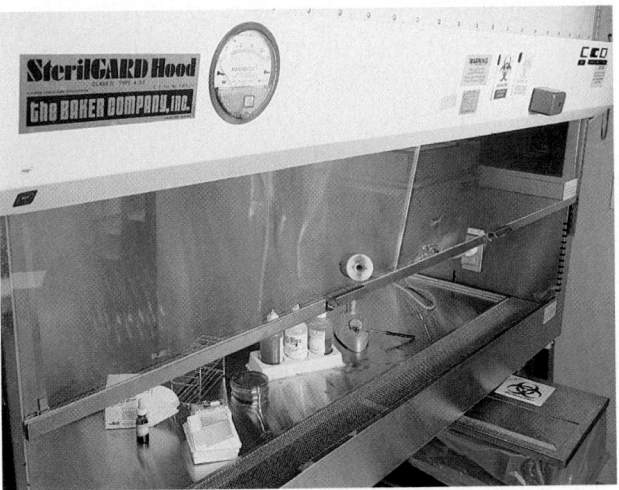

Figure 31-3   Laboratory safety hood.

Aerosols are airborne particles that can be released into the air when culturing. They are potentially dangerous if inhaled. By using the safety hood, the health care worker is separated from the specimen by a glass in front of the face, with fumes and aerosols suctioned into the hood. The use of a safety hood is mandatory when performing a culture on a specimen with a potential aerosol. Aerosols are particularly dangerous in fungus and mycobacterium cultures. It is a good idea to use the safety hood with foul-smelling specimens to minimize odors.

Incubator

The incubator is a cabinet that has a constant temperature of 35 to 37°C. Most organisms, whether **aerobic** (grow well in oxygen) or **anaerobic** (will not grow well or at all in oxygen), grow at these temperatures. Some bacteria, such as Yersina, grow at a lower temperature (26°C). A bacterium called Campylobacter requires a higher temperature (42°C). When working with these organisms, temperature requirements must be met for adequate growth.

Anaerobic Equipment

Certain types of cultures, such as deep wound cultures, could contain anaerobic pathogens. At the time of culturing, the medical assistant sets up some cultures in an oxygenated environment as well as an oxygen-reduced environment. Most laboratories post lists of cultures that need an anaerobic setup.

To grow anaerobic bacteria, the absence of oxygen is achieved by using something as simple as a candle jar (Figure 31-4) containing a lighted candle into which the inoc-

ulated petri dish is placed. When the cover is put on the jar the burning of the candle will use up the available oxygen and generate carbon dioxide. Organisms, such as *Neisseria gonorrhoeae,* which causes gonorrhea, need a high carbon dioxide atmosphere to survive. The use of a candle jar allows an easy collection and transport system that maximizes the recovery rate of certain microorganisms.

Another method of maintaining an anaerobic condition is a specialized jar called a gas pack jar (Figure 31-5). This jar contains a foil pack that, when activated, gives off carbon dioxide, decreasing the oxygen in the jar. Extensive culturing of anaerobes often is not performed by smaller laboratories. Anaerobic specimens are sent to reference laboratories better equipped to process them. Some small laboratories will perform a Gram stain on the suspected anaerobic cultures. The **Gram stain** is the most common stain used to observe the gross morphological features of bacteria and will be discussed later in this chapter.

Inoculating Equipment

An *inoculating loop* (Figure 31-6) is a piece of wire with a rounded end and a handle at the other end. The loop is used to **inoculate** organisms onto a culture medium in a plate or broth. If it is made of wire, the loop can be flamed to sterilize it before and after use. As an alternative, sterile plastic disposable loops can be used. These are one-time use and are disposed of in the biohazardous waste.

An *inoculating needle* (Figure 31-7) is similar to the loop but has a straight end. The needle is used when performing a **stab culture**. The needle is flamed, and the culture material is "stabbed" on the needle into medium in a tube. This technique is used for certain **biochemical tests** used for identification.

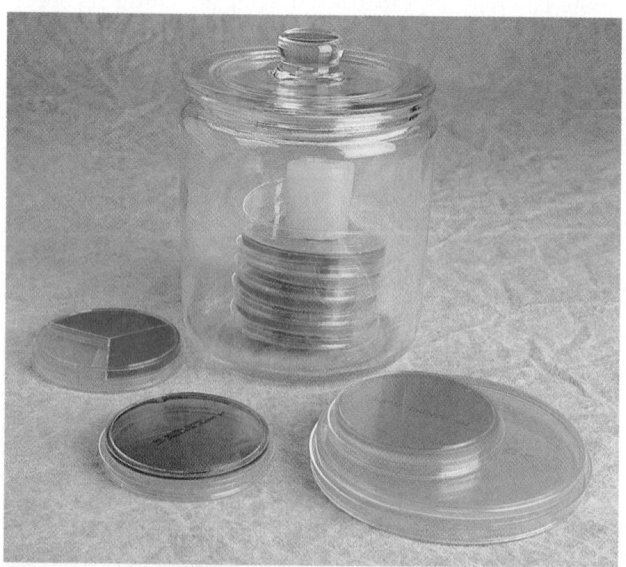

Figure 31-4   Candle jar with media for high CO_2 conditions.

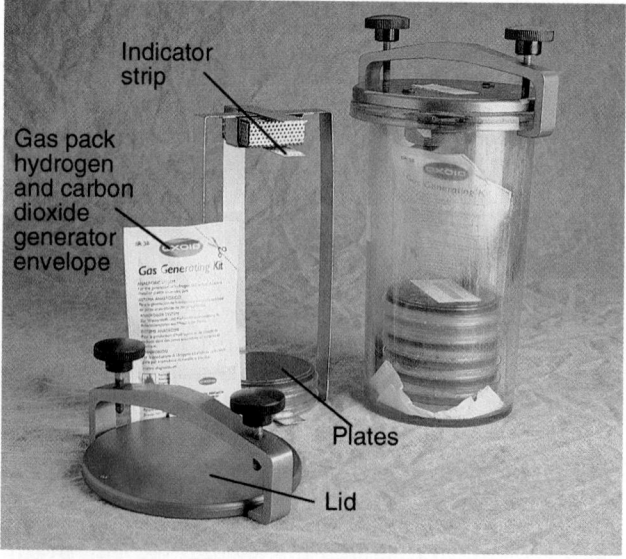

Figure 31-5   Gas pack anaerobic system.

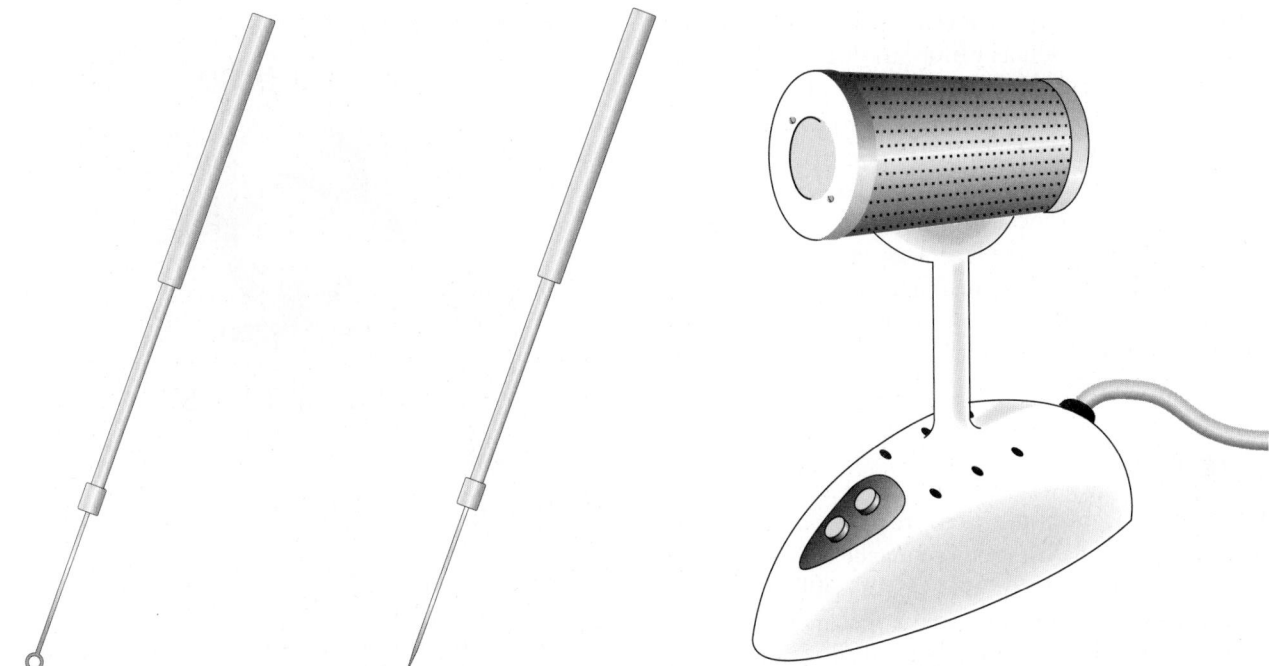

Figure 31-6   Inoculating loop.   **Figure 31-7**   Inoculating needle.   **Figure 31-8**   Electrical incinerator.

Incinerator

Incineration is the quickest method of sterilization. This can be accomplished by using an electrical incinerator (Figure 31-8) or a Bunsen burner (less popular today because of the open flame danger). When doing cultures, the inoculating needle or loop must be sterilized before and after it is used. This is done by placing the loop in the incinerator or passing through the flame of the Bunsen burner.

Media

Media in the microbiology laboratory refers to a host of substances used to foster the growth of bacteria. It is listed in this section of basic equipment (Figure 31-9), but will be explained in detail in the section about media.

Refrigerator

A refrigerator is needed to store certain materials, such as media and testing kits that need a temperature of 2 to 8°C. Food or drink should never be stored in the refrigerator with any specimens, kits, or media.

SAFETY WHEN HANDLING MICROBIOLOGY SPECIMENS

Safety should be practiced in every area of the clinical laboratory at all times. Microbiology specimens can be dangerous because of potential pathogens. Following safety rules will reduce danger to all personnel concerned. Some important safety measures follow. A detailed discussion can be found in Chapters 10 and 26.

Personal Protective Equipment

Personal protective equipment should be worn at all times when processing microbiology specimens. It should be removed when leaving the work area. When processing microbiology specimens, the medical assistant wears a

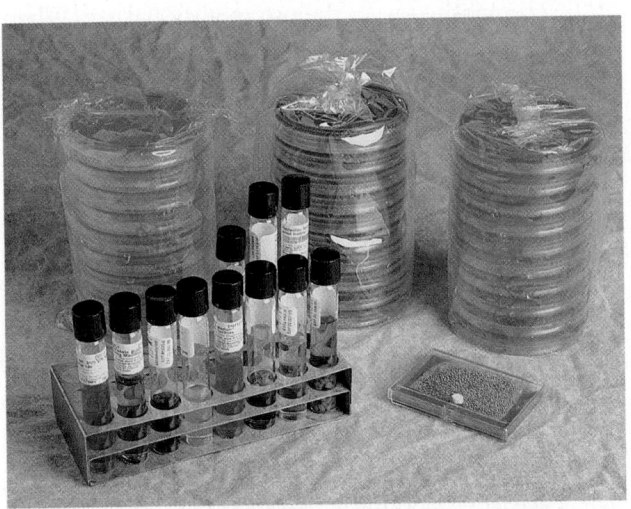

Figure 31-9   Various types of media tubes and plates.

buttoned laboratory coat or apron, safety goggles, and gloves. At times, personnel performing microbiology testing will work behind a shield or use a safety hood to avoid inhalation of aerosol pathogens and to avoid splashes and spatters of blood and/or body fluids.

There is never any eating, smoking, drinking, or putting objects into the mouth while working with microbiology specimens or in the laboratory area itself. Contact lenses should not be touched nor should makeup be applied. The practice of washing hands several times should be a habit. Washing hands after glove removal is important.

Work Area

The bench area where specimens are processed and set up should be cleaned with a strong germicide before and after daily use or immediately following a spill. Pathogens could be present where microbiology specimens are cultivated. This area should be dust-free and clean at all times.

Care should be taken not to have a cluttered work area. If using burners or incinerators, caution should be practiced to avoid body burns or fires.

Specimen Handling

Microbiology specimens will be brought to the physician's office laboratory or clinic to be processed, so the medical assistant should look for leaks and contamination on the outside of the transporting containers. It is a good practice always to wear gloves when receiving specimens. Most specimens will arrive in an "outside" plastic bag to avoid danger to laboratory personnel. When sending specimens to an outside laboratory to be cultured, it is important to use the appropriate container to avoid contamination of others. If there is a possibility of an aerosol specimen, the specimen must be cultured under a safety hood. All specimens should be handled as if they were contaminated. (Refer to Chapters 10 and 26 concerning standard precautions.)

Disposal of Waste and Spills

Most facilities will have a plan for disposal of dangerous biohazardous waste that should be strictly followed. Biohazardous waste generally is placed in red biohazard-marked bags (Figure 31-10). Most clinics or physician's office laboratories employ an outside agency to dispose of waste. It is extremely important that biohazardous waste is not placed with the regular waste and disposal guidelines are followed.

If a spill should occur, follow the agency's or employer's rules. Remember to disinfect with a 5 percent phenol or a 10 percent bleach solution.

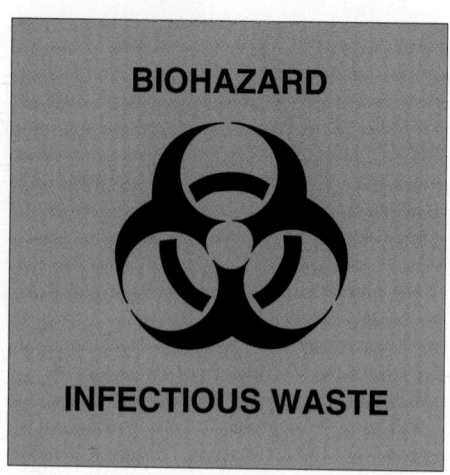

Figure 31-10   Biohazard symbol.

QUALITY CONTROL

Quality control is practiced in all areas of the clinical laboratory. The microbiology department has equipment, media, and reagents that need quality control checks periodically. Employees in the microbiology laboratory are also checked for accuracy by quality control programs. The following list details some measures that are a part of a quality control program in the microbiology laboratory:

- All equipment with temperature controls should be monitored daily.

- The microscopes should be cleaned and kept dust-free.

- All staining reagents should be checked with known check cell slides, which are preinoculated with known organisms, to determine the accuracy. This check is done when a new kit is received or a new batch of dyes are made.

- Testing for microorganism identification is often accomplished with the use of a special kit. When using kits for different tests, the positive and negative controls must be run at all times. Before use, the expiration date should be checked.

- Media of all types should not be used past the shelf life and should be stored at the proper temperatures and checked for growth with known organisms for quality control. All laboratories should have a specific list of bacteria to use on various media to test for growth.

- A procedure manual with all standard operating procedures written down should be updated periodically. All chemicals or reagents with material safety data sheets (MSDSs) should be available to reference when working with something with which one is not familiar.

• Many microbiology laboratories subscribe to associations that periodically send unknown samples to be set up and identified. This is known as proficiency testing. The laboratory is then graded on its performance, to make sure technique is correct.

COLLECTION PROCEDURES

When a physician needs an identification of an organism that is causing infection, he or she orders a culture from that site. Before a culture is processed, it first should be checked to see if it was collected properly, delivered within a reasonable period of time, and collected in sufficient quantity. The results of the culture will depend on the quality of the original specimen. All specimens obtained for identification of infectious organisms must be taken from the site of the infection, not the surrounding area. Figure 31-11 lists methods of transmission for many common communicable diseases.

Once the specimen is collected correctly, it should be placed in the appropriate container and brought to the laboratory soon after collection. Many organisms, if not

Disease	How Agent Leaves the Bodies of the Sick	How Organisms May Be Transmitted	Method of Entry into the Body
Acquired immuno-deficiency syndrome (AIDS)	Blood, semen, or other body fluids, including breast milk	Inoculation by use of contaminated needles or by direct contact so that infected body fluids can enter the body	Transplacentally to embryo or fetus Nursing at breast
Cholera	Excreta from intestinal tract	As in typhoid fever	As in typhoid fever
Diphtheria	Sputum and discharges from nose and throat Skin lesions	Direct contact Droplet infection from patient coughing Hands of nurse Articles used by and about patient	Through mouth to throat or nose to throat
Gonococcal disease	Lesions Discharges from infected mucous membranes	Direct contact as in sexual intercourse Towels, bathtubs, toilets, etc. Hands of infected persons soiled with their own discharges Hands of attendant	Directly onto mucous membrane Through breaks in membrane
Hepatitis A, viral	Feces	As in typhoid fever	As in typhoid fever, rarely by blood transfusion
Hepatitis B, viral and delta hepatitis	Blood and serum-derived fluids, including semen and vaginal fluids	Contact with blood and body fluids	Transfusion Exposure to body fluids including during hetero- or homosexual intercourse
Hepatitis C	Blood	Transfusion Parenteral drug use Laboratory exposure to blood	Infected blood Contaminated needles

(continues)

Figure 31-11 Methods of transmission of some common communicable diseases. (From *Taber's Cyclopedic Medical Dictionary* [17th ed.], by C. L. Thomas [Ed.], 1993, Philadelphia: F. A. Davis Company. Reprinted with permission.)

Disease	How Agent Leaves the Bodies of the Sick	How Organisms May Be Transmitted	Method of Entry into the Body
Hookworm	Feces	Health care workers exposed to blood, i.e., dentists and their assistants, and clinical and laboratory staff Direct contact with soil polluted with feces Eggs in feces hatch in sandy soil Feces may also contaminate food	Larvae enter through breaks in skin, especially skin of feet, and after devious passage through the body settle in the intestine
Influenza	As in pneumonia	As in pneumonia	As in pneumonia
Leprosy	Uncertain, may be from lesions Bacilli found in nodules that may break down, forming lesions	Uncertain, probably nasal discharges of untreated patients	Uncertain, probably via upper respiratory tract and broken skin
Measles (rubella)	As in streptococcal sore throat	As in streptococcal sore throat	As in streptococcal sore throat
Meningitis, meningococcal	Discharges from nose and throat	Direct contact Hands of nurse or attendant Articles used by and about patient Flies	Mouth and nose
Mumps	Discharges from infected glands and mouth	Direct contact with persons affected	Mouth and nose
Ophthalmia neonatorum (gonococcal infection of eyes of newborn)	Purulent discharges from the eye	Direct contact with infected areas as vagina or infected mother during birth Other infected babies Hands of doctor or nurse Linens	Directly on the conjunctiva
Pneumonia	Sputum and discharges from nose and throat	Direct contact Hands of caretaker Articles used by and about patient	Through mouth and nose to lungs
Poliomyelitis	Discharges from nose and throat, and via feces	Direct contact Hands of caretaker or attendant Rarely in milk	Through mouth and nose

(continues)

Figure 31-11   *(continued)*

Disease	How Agent Leaves the Bodies of the Sick	How Organisms May Be Transmitted	Method of Entry into the Body
Rubeola	Secretions from nose and throat	Droplet spread from nose or throat by direct contact with nasal or throat secretions Airborne spread is possible	Through mouth and nose
Streptococcal sore throat	Discharges from nose and throat Skin lesions	Direct contact Hands of caretaker Articles used by and about patient	Through mouth and nose
Syphilis	Infected tissues Lesions Blood Transfer through placenta to fetus	Direct contact Kissing or sexual intercourse Contaminated needles and syringes	Directly into blood and tissues through breaks in skin or membrane Contaminated needles and syringes
Tetanus	Excreta from infected herbivorous animals and man	Soil, especially that with manure or feces in it Dust, etc. Articles used about stables	Directly into bloodstream through wounds (organism is an anaerobe and prefers deep, incised wound)
Trachoma	Discharges from infected eyes	Direct contact Hands, towels, handkerchiefs	Directly on conjunctiva
Tuberculosis, bovine		Milk from infected cow	As in tuberculosis, human
Tuberculosis, human	Sputum Lesions Feces	Direct contact such as kissing Droplet infection from person coughing with mouth uncovered Sputum from mouth to fingers, thence to food and other things Soiled dressings	Through mouth to lungs and intestines From intestines via lymph channels to lymph vessels and to tissues
Typhoid fever	Feces and urine	Direct contact with food, water, articles, or insects contaminated with feces, or urine from patients	Through mouth via infected food or water and thence to intestinal tract
Whooping cough	Discharges from respiratory tract	Direct contact with person affected	Mouth and nose

Figure 31-11   (*continued*)

placed in a holding or transport medium to keep them viable (alive), will die if not kept moist. Transport media can have a moistening agent to keep the specimen from drying out. This media is then disposed of and not reused.

If a specimen comes into the laboratory in an improper container or has not been brought in within a reasonable period of time soon after collection, it should be rejected and another specimen obtained. The container in which the specimen has been placed should be sterile, and the right type should be used for a specific culture (Figure 31-12). Sterile containers are used for most collections, with the exception of stool collection containers, which do not have to be sterile. Culturette cultures are from swabs and should be kept moist. This system is a plastic tube that has a sterile swab used to collect the specimen and then placed back into the tube. Once in the tube, an ampule containing Stuart medium or another medium is squeezed, releasing the fluid to keep the swab moist.

The laboratory's success in isolating the causative pathogens depends on the following factors:

1. Proper collection from infection site
2. Collection of specimen during infection period
3. Sufficient amount of specimen
4. Appropriate specimen container
5. Appropriate transport medium
6. Specimen labeled properly
7. Specimen brought to the laboratory in a minimal amount of time

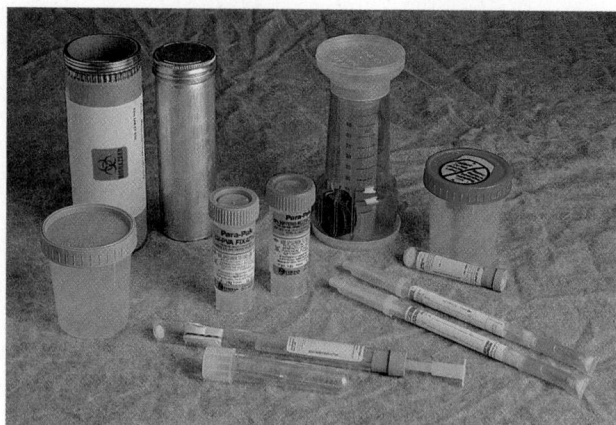

Figure 31-12 Various collection and transport containers for bacteriological specimens.

8. Specimen collected before the administration of antibiotics
9. Specimen inoculated onto proper media and placed in correct atmosphere to ensure growth

When collecting specimens, it is important that the medical assistant carefully follow procedures designated by the health care facility. Everyone handling specimens should wear gloves to protect themselves from leakage of the container and contamination with a pathogenic organism.

Specific Collection Requirements

Urine. Patients should be instructed to obtain a clean-catch urine in a sterile container. A clean-catch midstream specimen is obtained by first cleaning the genital area and then urinating midstream into a specimen container. Details of this procedure are found in Chapter 30. Patients should be given strict instructions so that a quality specimen for culturing can be obtained.

Sometimes a catheterization is done to collect the urine for culture. The urine must be collected into a sterile container if obtained by this method.

Throat. A specimen for throat culture is obtained by using a sterile tongue depressor to hold the patient's tongue down. With a sterile swab, have the patient say "ah." Gently swab the back portion of the throat and tonsils (if present). Avoid swabbing the sides of the mouth and tongue. Place the specimen swab in a sterile tube for delivery to the laboratory.

Taking a Throat Culture. Explain to the patient that a throat culture is necessary to identify certain organisms. Be sure to tell the patient that there might be some momentary discomfort in obtaining the specimen, and answer all questions about the process of obtaining the specimen. See Procedure 31-1.

SPOTLIGHT ON AAMA ESSENTIALS THROUGH CAAHEP

- A medical assistant taking a specimen or a secretion from a patient needs to be sensitive to the potential embarrassment the patient may experience from submitting to the collection process.

- By explaining the purpose and value of a specimen collection, the medical assistant can do much to allay the patient's fears.

- A calm and professional attitude displayed by a medical assistant while explaining the collection of such specimens as sputum and stool can often mean the difference between obtaining a useful specimen and a contaminated one.

The specimen is taken directly from the affected area with a sterile swab and distributed over the agar in a petri dish of clear plastic. Many physicians obtain, incu-bate, and read their own cultures for the patient's conven-ience and to maintain efficiency in the ambulatory care setting (Figures 31-13 and 31-14).

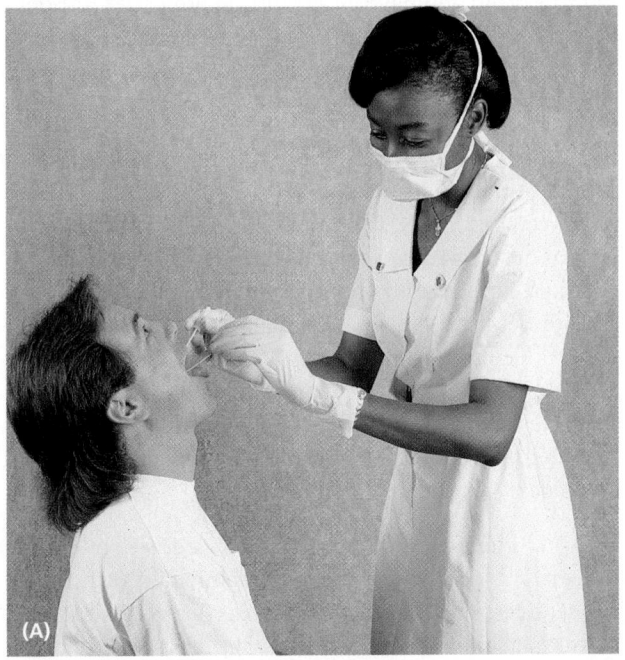

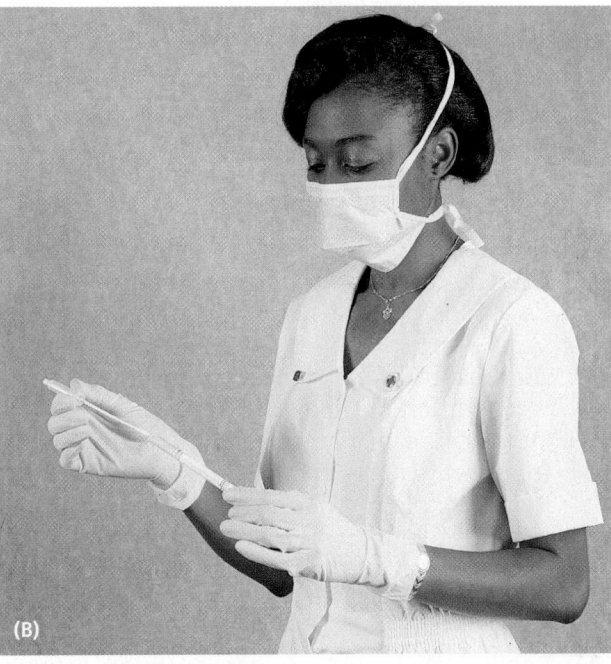

Figure 31-13   (A) The medical assistant obtains a throat culture using a commercially available sterile swab and culture tube with growth medium. Note the medical assistant wears gloves and mask. (B) After swabbing patient's throat for a culture, the medical assistant replaces swab into culture tube. A laboratory requisition form will be attached to the labeled tube and sent to the laboratory.

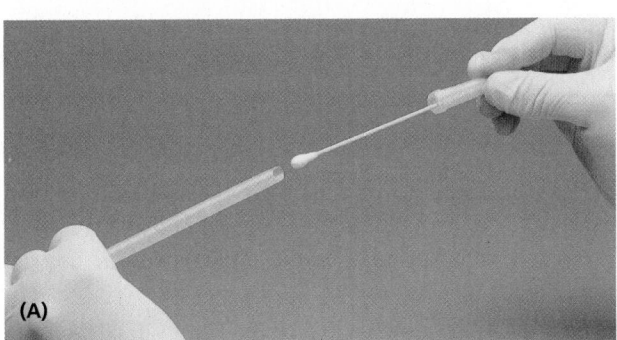

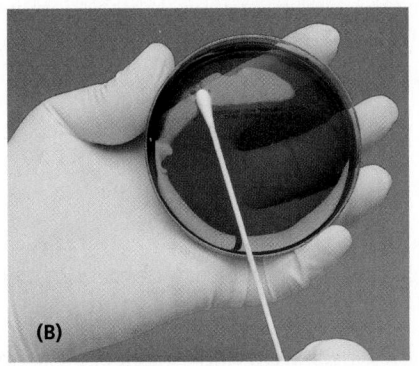

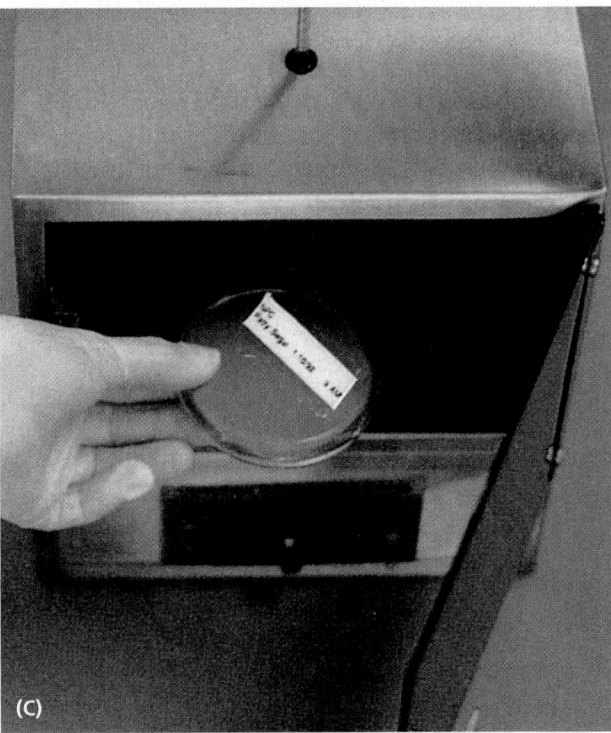

Figure 31-14   (A) The swab with specimen is put into transport container with culture media for laboratory analysis. (B) The med-ical assistant smears the culture plate with specimen from the swab; it is then streaked as shown in Procedure 31-6. (C) The culture plate is placed in an incubator with agar side up.

Patient Teaching Tip

As you obtain throat cultures from patients, you may want to give them some helpful advice concerning their condition. Generally when a person has a sore throat, it is associated with other respiratory symptoms as well. The following suggestions may provide some relief from discomfort and help them toward better health.

1. Advise patients to drink plenty of liquids (fruit juices) and to eat sensibly from the basic food groups.
2. Urge patients to get extra rest and dress comfortably (according to the weather/temperature outside).
3. Suggest use of gargles or throat lozenges (or both) to relieve painful sore throat.
4. Remind them to avoid tobacco/smoking.
5. Instruct them to cough/sneeze into tissue and discard into proper waste container wherever they are to prevent the spread of microorganisms.
6. Remind them not to eat or drink from another person's plate or glass and to use disposables at home when there is illness.

Nose. A nasal-pharyngeal swab may be requested with a throat culture. This is collected with a swab on a thin wire. A separate swab may be used for each nostril. The patient tilts back the head, and each swab is gently inserted into each of the nostrils. The swab is then placed into a sterile tube for transport to the laboratory.

Wound. When culturing a wound, a sterile needle might be used to aspirate pus-filled fluid from the wound, or a swab is used. It is important to get the swab deep into the wound without touching the surrounding skin. Specimens for wound cultures often are placed in anaerobic transport medium, especially if the wound is not superficial.

Sputum. To collect this specimen correctly, the patient should cough deeply and **expectorate** into the sterile container. The specimen should be a morning specimen and placed into a special container designed to protect all who handle the specimen from contamination. (Refer to Procedure 18-18.)

Stool. Stool specimens are brought to the laboratory for various tests. If the stool is to be examined for **ova** or parasites, the specimen should be as fresh as possible. Special containers often are used for ova and parasites.

For bacterial cultures of stool material (as well as for ova and parasites), several different specimens may be sent for testing at different times. The collection containers for stool cultures do not have to be sterile, but they must be clean and have a tight-fitting lid. Patients should be instructed to be careful not to contaminate the specimen with urine since urine may alter the results of the stool culture.

Cerebrospinal Fluid (CSF). The physician obtains cerebrospinal fluid by doing a **lumbar puncture**. (Refer to Procedure 18-24.) The fluid generally is dispersed in several departments of the clinical laboratory. Generally, the fluid goes first to the microbiology laboratory for a culture before it becomes contaminated by doing other tests. If a culture cannot be set up immediately, the tube should be placed in an incubator or left at room temperature. Refrigeration of spinal fluid can kill two common meningitis-causing bacteria, *Haemophilus influenzae* and *Neisseria meningitidis*.

Blood. Human blood is free from bacteria in a healthy human. If blood does become contaminated with bacteria, septicemia (septic blood infection) can result. Blood cultures are collected by the same means as regular blood collection, with special considerations to avoid any contamination of the blood. A variety of collection devices are available for collecting blood cultures, all requiring careful sterile techniques.

MICROSCOPIC EXAMINATION OF BACTERIA

There are usually two procedures involved in properly identifying bacteria: the microscopic examination and the culture. The microscopic examination involves viewing stained or unstained bacteria through the microscope. (See Procedure 31-2.)

Culturing is a means of isolating a disease-causing microorganism for identification. A specimen is obtained and placed in a culture medium, which contains nutrients comparable to human tissue to encourage growth of microorganisms. The medium is agar, a gelatinlike substance, mixed with nutrients.

Bacterial Shapes

Each genus of bacteria has a characteristic shape. A knowledge of the shapes of bacteria helps in identification (Figure 31-15). Bacteria have three basic shapes:

1. *Cocci.* Cocci are round in shape, occurring in clusters, pairs, singles, and **tetrads**. They are nonmotile microorganisms. (They do not move on their own accord.)

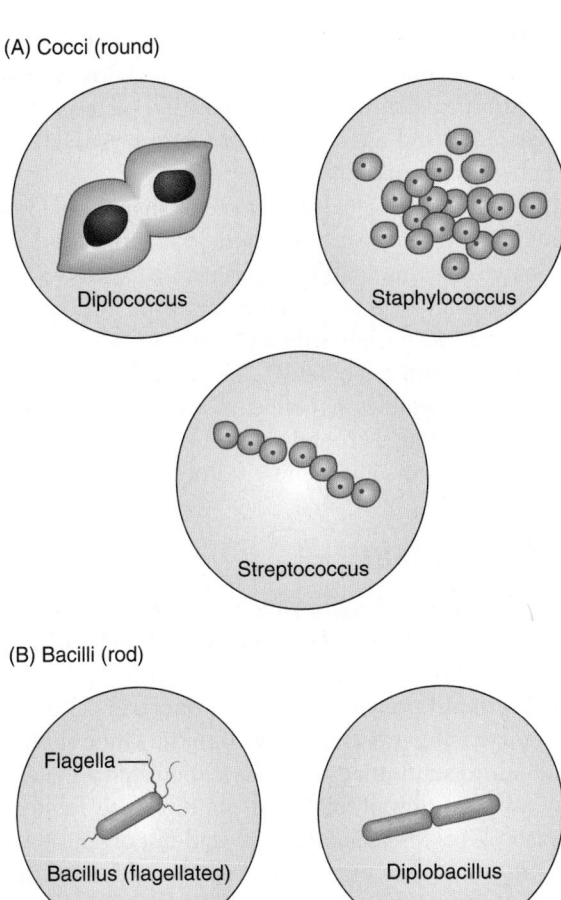

(A) Cocci (round)

Diplococcus

Staphylococcus

Streptococcus

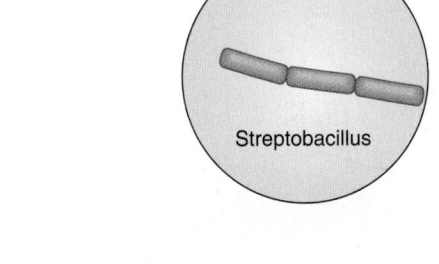

(B) Bacilli (rod)

Flagella

Bacillus (flagellated)

Diplobacillus

Streptobacillus

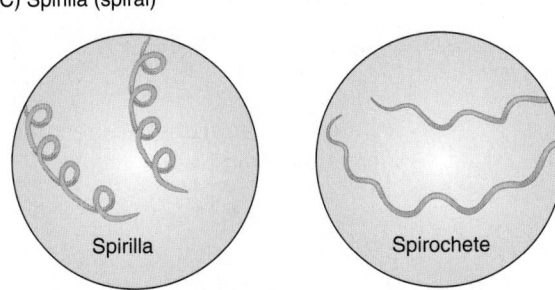

(C) Spirilla (spiral)

Spirilla

Spirochete

Figure 31-15 Three types of bacteria.

2. *Bacilli.* Bacilli are rod-shaped and can have rounded, straight, or pointed ends. Some bacilli have flagella that give bacteria motility (movement). Most bacteria are the shape of bacilli.
3. *Spirilla.* Spirilla are spiral-shaped bacteria that have one too many turns. Most spirilla are motile.

The microscopic examination produces information that is often needed to identify bacteria. However, biochemical reactions and the sensitivity pattern (how the organisms respond to antibiotics) are also needed to make the full identification.

Dyes (Stains)

The dyes used in microbiology are derived from coal tar. These dyes are acidic or basic and impart a color to the microorganism. Basic dyes carry a positive ion and stain structures that are acidic in nature. Methylene blue, a common stain, is a basic dye and binds to the DNA and RNA of the cell. An acid dye carries a negative ion and stains structures that are basic in nature such as cytoplasmic structures. An example of an acidic dye is safranin. Several different types of stains are used depending upon what test is ordered (Table 31-3).

Simple Stain

A simple stain uses a single stain on a fixed slide for a given period of time. A simple stain will show the arrangement and structure of the bacterial cell. It is fast, taking no more than three minutes to stain, but does not give much information.

Differential Stain

A differential stain is more complex than a simple stain. It is known as a differential stain because the stain result varies. A common differential stain is the Gram stain.

TABLE 31-3   STAINS AND THEIR USE

Stain	Example
Simple	Carbolfuchsin
	Gentian violet
	Methylene blue
	Safranin
Differential	Gram
	Acid-fast (Ziehl-Neelsen, Kinyoun)
Special	Capsule (Welch negative)
	Flagella (Leifson)
	Nuclei (Feulgen)
	Spore (Doerner)

The Gram stain uses a primary stain, a **decolorizer**, and a **counterstain**.

The Gram stain was developed in 1884 by Dr. Hans Christian Gram. More than 100 years later, this famous stain is still in use with little variation. This staining procedure differentiates bacteria by their Gram stain ability of being either negative or positive. A bacterium is Gram negative or positive by the nature of the cell wall and the ability of it either to retain or lose color through decolorization. This identification of Gram-positive or Gram-negative aids in identification of an organism. Gram-positive bacteria have a lower lipid (fat) content and are not decolorized as compared to Gram-negative bacteria, which have a higher lipid content and are readily decolorized.

The **reagents** used in the Gram stain are gentian or crystal violet, a purple stain that is the primary stain. Iodine, which acts as a **mordant**, holds the purple stain. Alcohol-acetone is the decolorizer that removes the purple color. Safranin is the red counterstain. When stained according to the manufacturer's directions, the Gram-positive bacteria stain purple, and the Gram-negative bacteria stain pink. Sometimes an organism will appear Gram-variable. This is found with Gram-positive organisms that have been exposed to acidic media, that are often old and lose their ability to retain the gentian violet, or the proper procedure has not been followed. See Procedure 31-3 and Figure 31-16.

The Gram stain is one of the most important procedures in the microbiology laboratory, giving valuable information by identifying Gram-positive bacteria such as *Staphylococcus* and *Streptococcus* or Gram-negative bacteria such as *E. coli* and Proteus.

The morphological arrangement, shape, and Gram-stain characteristic will begin to help identify the bacteria. Sometimes this is all the physician needs to know to start treatment for a pathogenic organism. For example, the bacteria causing gonorrhea (*Neisseria gonorrhoeae*) is a distinctive organism, having a characteristic diplococci shape that resembles a coffee or kidney bean. These organisms are found in and outside of white blood cells and can be identified by a Gram stain.

Acid-Fast Stain

Another differential stain, which is often referred to as a specific stain, is the acid-fast stain. This stain is either differential or specific in that it allows microscopic examination of acid-fast organisms, or **mycobacteria**. This group of organisms does not respond well to the Gram stain and is difficult to stain under ordinary circumstances due to a waxy capsule cell wall that resists staining. See Table 31-4 for examples of diseases caused by acid-fast organisms.

To stain these organisms, heat or a powerful dye is used in the procedure to stain the bacteria. The bacteria, once stained, resist decolorization with an acid alcohol,

Step	Time	Procedure	Result
1	one minute	Primary stain: Apply crystal violet stain (purple) ↓ Rinse slide	All bacteria stain purple 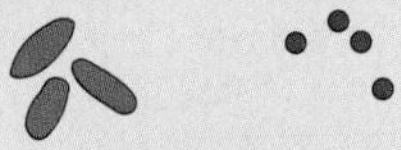
2	one minute	Mordant: Apply Gram's iodine ↓ Rinse slide	All bacteria remain purple 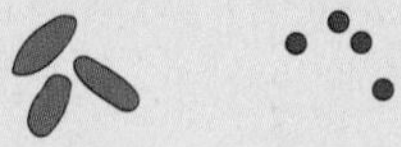
3	three to five seconds	Decolorize: Apply alcohol ↓ Rinse slide	Purple stain is removed from Gram-negative cells 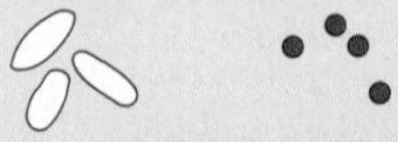
4	one minute	Counterstain: Apply safranin stain (red) ↓ Rinse slide	Gram-negative cells appear pink-red; Gram-positive cells appear purple 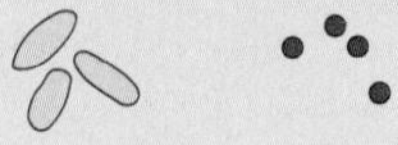

Figure 31-16   Steps in the Gram stain procedure.

TABLE 31-4	SOME ACID-FAST ORGANISMS	
Genus	**Species**	**Disease**
Mycobacterium	Tuberculosis	Tuberculosis (TB)
Mycobacterium	Leprae	Hansen's disease (leprosy)
Mycobacterium	Kansasii	Pulmonary disease
Mycobacterium	Avium-intracellulare complex	AIDS-related pulmonary disease

giving them the acid-fast name. The bacteria that causes tuberculosis is an acid-fast organism.

Two methods commonly used to stain acid-fast organisms are the Ziehl-Neelsen stain, shown in Procedure 31-4, which uses heat, and the Kinyoun stain, a cold method that does not include a heating process. Either of these stains is satisfactory.

Special Techniques

There are several special situations when more than the Gram stain or the shape and arrangement of an organism is needed to aid in the identification. Such situations would be the demonstration of the presence of flagella, spore, capsule, or nuclei of cells. The technique of these stains can be found in a detailed microbiology text.

There also are microscopic examinations of organisms in a living state, without staining. Characteristics that can be studied by this method include motility, shape, and arrangement of organisms. This technique requires the microorganisms to be in a liquid suspension.

For vaginal secretions, a swab of the vaginal discharge is placed in a sterile tube containing 1 mL of normal saline and mixed. Then the suspension is viewed under a microscope. For stool or other bacterial specimens, a small amount of specimen is mixed with a drop of normal saline, then viewed under a microscope. These methods are known as the wet mount preparation and the hanging drop preparation. Refer to Procedure 31-5.

The wet mount preparation is a valuable diagnostic tool in determining the cause of vaginosis. Bacterial vaginosis is identified by the presence of "clue cells," epithelial cells covered by coccobacillary bacteria. Motile trichomonads are seen in case of *Trichomonas vaginalis*. The presence of pseudohyphae indicates a yeast infection. In many cases an accurate diagnosis can be made from the wet mount preparation, thus making more complex techniques unnecessary.

Potassium Hydroxide (KOH) Preparation

Another type of wet preparation is using 10 percent solution of potassium hydroxide in a wet preparation for the study of fungi and spores. The slide is prepared by using fragments of human hair, skin, or nails that could have fungus. These fragments are placed on a slide with a drop of 10 percent KOH and a coverslip on top. The KOH will clear debris. The slide should sit at room temperature for about one-half hour before examination for debris settlement.

The direct examination of specimens is best viewed with a phase or dark-field microscope rather than a bright-field microscope due to reduced illumination. If using a bright-field microscope, lower the condenser to reduce transmitted light. Proper disposal of these specimens is important as the organisms are alive and possibly pathogenic.

Table 31-5 is a listing of microscopic findings for several pathogens under direct microscopic examination.

TABLE 31-5	DIRECT MICROSCOPIC EXAMINATION OF CULTURE AND INFECTIOUS BACTERIA		
Specimen	**Procedure**		**Microscopic Findings**
Cerebrospinal fluid	Gram stain	Haemophilus	Small Gram-negative pleomorphic bacteria
		Neisseria meningitides	Gram-negative diplococci
		Streptococcus pneumoniae	Gram-positive diplococci
	Gram stain Hanging drop	Listeriosis	Gram-positive nonsporing bacillus
Eye	Gram stain	Various Gram-positive and Gram-negative organisms	
Feces	Gram stain	WBCs	Gram-positive bacteria
	Direct mount		Motility
	Iodine		Ova and parasite *(continues)*

TABLE 31-5   (continued)

Specimen	Procedure	Microscopic Findings	
Genital	Gram stain	Neisseria gonorrhoeae	Gram-negative Intracellular diplococci
		Gordnerella vaginalis	Clue cells
		Chancroids	Small Gram-negative bacilli
	Darkfield Microscope	Syphilis	Coiled spirochetes
	Direct mount	Trichomonas	Darting Flagellates
	Direct 10% KOH	Yeast	Budding yeast forms
Skin	Direct 10% KOH	Fungus infection	Hyphae, mycellium, and spores
Sputum	Gram stain	Various Gram-negative and Gram-positive organisms	
	Acid-fast test	Acid-fast bacilli	
	Direct	Fungal infections	Hyphae, mycellium, and spores
Throat	Fluorescent Microscope	Strep infection	Fluorescent cocci in chains
Urine	Gram stain	Various bacterial organisms and yeast	
Wound	Gram stain	Gas gangrene	Gram-positive bacillus with spores
		Cellulitis	Various Gram-negative and Gram-positive organisms
	Direct mount	Fungal infections	Hyphae, mycellium, and spores

CULTURE MEDIA

After the proper collection of the specimen, the material collected must be inoculated on a proper culture medium. This is necessary for growth and eventual identification of an organism.

The results of culture, the growing of an organism on special media in the laboratory, are only as reliable as the method used in collecting the specimen. In addition, growth requirements of different organisms must be considered, such as moisture, temperature, oxygen, carbon dioxide, and essential nutrients. Organisms that are sensitive to drying must be put into transport medium immediately after collection to prevent loss of viability. Some bacteria require a specialized medium to grow and multiply. These are called fastidious bacteria. Aerobic bacteria grow only in the presence of oxygen. Anaerobic bacteria live and grow in the absence of oxygen. Examples

of some common bacteria and their growth requirements are illustrated in Table 31-6.

When specimens are collected for the laboratory, the microorganism's growth requirements must be considered. No matter how good the specimen, if an anaerobic organism is kept in an aerobic atmosphere while being transported to the reference laboratory, it will probably not survive. Special anaerobic transport systems must be used.

Neisseria gonorrhoeae, the causative agent of the sexually transmitted disease (STD) gonorrhea, requires special media and an atmosphere of reduced oxygen and increased carbon dioxide. Therefore, the specimen must be collected from the patient and immediately placed on a special media in a reduced oxygen atmosphere.

Laboratory personnel who send bacterial specimens to a reference laboratory must be familiar with the trans-

TABLE 31-6   SOME COMMON BACTERIA AND THEIR GROWTH REQUIREMENTS

Organism	Disease	Medium	Oxygen Requirements
Streptococcus	Strep Throat	Blood agar	$\downarrow O_2$, $\uparrow CO_2$
Neisseria gonorrhoeae	Gonorrhea	Chocolate agar, modified Thayer-Martin (MTM)	$\downarrow O_2$, $\uparrow CO_2$
Staphylococcus	Infections, boils	Blood agar	O_2
Escherichia coli	Urinary tract infections	Blood agar, eosin methylene blue (EMB), MacConkey's	O_2

port media the reference laboratory provides. The reference laboratory should provide a procedure manual that explains how and when to use the various microbiology transport systems.

Media can be a solid, liquid, or semisolid substance that has the required nutrients to support the growth of bacteria. Such ingredients include vitamins, sugar, salt, minerals, and amino acids. Some media have the addition of special products like egg, potato, meat, milk, blood, and dyes.

The solid form of media is called agar. Agar has an appearance similar to gelatin. When heated, agar is a liquid; when cooled, it solidifies. Agar is poured into a **petri dish** (a plastic dish used to grow bacteria) so the bacteria can be studied for gross **morphology** (form and structure). Agar can also be placed in tubes.

Semi-solid media is made by adding less agar. Media in a liquid broth form is stored in tubes called **broth tubes** and allows for the observation of gas production, change in pH, and odor. Figure 31-7 shows many different types of media that can be used to identify bacteria. Media can be purchased already prepared, or it can be produced from ingredients in the laboratory. Charts listing the proper media to set up for specific types of cultures generally are prominently displayed in the set-up area of most microbiology laboratories.

Media Classification

There are several classifications of media, including:

- *Basic*. Basic media is used for general purposes and does not contain added nutrients. It will support the growth of many Gram-negative and Gram-positive organisms.

- *Differential*. Differential media contains substances that alter the appearance of some types of organisms and not other types. An eosin methylene blue (EMB) plate for lactose and nonlactose fermenters is an example of differential media. The lactose fermenter can use lactose and looks different on the agar.

- *Selective*. Selective media supports the growth of one type of organism, while inhibiting the growth of another. This is done by the addition of either a salt, dye, chemical, or antibiotic. A hektoen enteric (HE) plate for the growth of salmonella and shigella is a selective type of media.

- *Enriched*. This type of media contains substances that inhibit certain bacteria from growing. This media works well with cultures from sites that possess normal flora, like the throat. The normal flora is inhibited and pathogenic bacteria are encouraged to grow. Blood agar and chocolate agar are examples of enriched media.

All media that is used should first be checked with known organisms for quality control and for contaminants. The manufacturer will usually suggest a list of organisms for a quality control check. A check for contaminants involves a thorough visual check of the plate before using it. It is also important to store media according to the manufacturer's direction. *Never use outdated media.*

Table 31-7 lists common media by classification and use and Table 31-8 is a listing of media that might be selected for specific sources. All laboratories vary slightly in their recommendations of media to set up on specimens.

TABLE 31-7	COMMON MICROBIOLOGY MEDIA BY CLASSIFICATION AND USE	
Type	**Name**	**Use**
Basic	Trypticase agar	Supports the growth of most organisms
	Trypticase broth	
Differential	Blood agar	Supports the growth of Streptococcus and Staphylococcus; demonstrates hemolysis
	MacConkey	Certain Gram-negative organisms
	Eosin methylene blue (EMB)	Escherichia coli
Selective	Salmonella and Shigella (SS)	Gram-negative Salmonella and Shigella
	Hektoen	Enteric organisms
	Phenylethyl alcohol	Inhibits Gram-negative growth
	Mannitol salt	Promotes growth of Staphylococcus
	Selenite (GN) broth	Promotes growth of enteric organisms
	Thayer Martin	Promotes growth of Neisseria species
	Thioglycollate broth	Promotes growth of anaerobes
Enriched	Loefflers	Promotes growth of Corynebacterium
	Chocolate	Promotes growth of Haemophilus species
	Lowenstein Jensen	Promotes growth of mycobacteria

TABLE 31-8   COMMON SPECIMENS, SUSPECTED PATHOGENS, MEDIA RECOMMENDATIONS

Specimen Source	Potential Pathogens	Blood agar	Choc.	EMB	MacConkey	SSHE	Selenite	Thayer Martin	Thio.	CO_2
Eye/Ear	Neisseria gonorrhoeae Haemophilus species Staph. aureus Strep. pyogenes Pseudomonas aeruginosa Moraxella species	x	x	x	x			x	x	x
CSF	Neisseria meningitidis Strep. pneumoniae Haemophilus influenzae	x	x						x	x
Throat	Strep. pyogenes	x								x
Sputum	Strep. pneumoniae	x								
Urine	E. coli Klebsiella Proteus Pseudomonas aeruginosa Enterococcus	x		x	x					
Wounds	Staphylococcus Streptococcus Enterobactericae Anaerobic bacteria	x	x	x	x				x	x
Stool	Salmonella Shigella			x	x	x	x			
Stool	Pathogenic E. coli Yersinia species									
Vaginal	Neisseria gonorrhoeae	x	x					x		x

MICROBIOLOGY CULTURE

Inoculating the Media

After selecting the right medium for the culture and observing the specimen to make sure it is properly collected, the specimen is then inoculated onto the medium. If the specimen is on a swab, the swab is rolled directly onto the upper quadrant of the agar plate. If the specimen is a sputum or liquid, it is inoculated onto the plate with a loop.

The inoculum is spread back and forth in a sweeping motion with a flamed loop or needle. This is done to dilute the bacteria to obtain isolated colonies. The loop or needle should be cooled before streaking the bacteria. A hot loop will damage the agar, kill bacteria, and cause aerosols to form. To cool, touch it to the inside lid of the petri dish or stab into part of the media that is not inoculated. Never wave the loop or needle in the air to cool as this will contaminate it.

After the agar plate has been inoculated and properly labeled, it should be turned upside down and placed in the proper environment for growth. By turning the agar upside down, any condensation that forms from bacterial growth will be on the inside lid.

Liquid broths and agar slant tubes have screw caps. These caps must not be screwed on too tightly due to gas production by some organisms that can break the tube. See Procedures 31-6, 31-7, and 31-8.

Other Types of Streaking

Other types of streaking include the lawn streak. This streaking technique is used to place an organism over an entire area of an agar plate for sensitivity testing. The bacteria is spread over the entire plate using a swab (Figure 31-17), streaking over the entire area several times from different angles. After the streaking has been completed, disks saturated with different antibiotics are placed equidistant throughout the streaked area.

The colony count is a streaking technique much like the lawn technique. This technique is used to plate urine cultures. A special calibrated urine loop is used to make the first streak, followed by a second streak that goes across the entire length of the initial streak. Then another

Figure 31-17 Lawn or spread streak.

complete streaking is placed over the original streaks after rotating the plate (Figure 31-18). This method of using a calibrated loop to get a more accurate inoculation gives the physician an idea of how many colonies of bacteria are present.

Every laboratory will use slightly different ways of performing the basic streaks. The important factor is to use good aseptic techniques so there is no contamination from outside organisms, and all organisms that are streaked out are isolated enough to further test if necessary.

Primary Culture

After the media has been incubated for 24 to 48 hours, the initial or primary culture is read. The agar is observed for gross colony characteristics on the agar surface. In identifying the characteristics, the following aspects of the bacterial colonies are observed: size, shape, color, elevation, density, consistency, hemolytic versus nonhemolytic (if grown on blood agar), odor, and pigment production. Colonies that are hemolytic will utilize blood on a blood agar plate, while nonhemolytic colonies will not. By assessing the various characteristics, the microbiologist is able to make an initial identification of what bacteria are present. These characteristics are useful in the selection of various biochemical tests and differential media to make a final identification.

Specialized skill is required to examine an agar plate for colony characteristics. In many laboratories, these tasks are left to the microbiology professional staff. The medical assistant in these instances may be asked to set up and incubate the cultures, but not read the results.

The observation of the growing bacteria is made under a bright direct light by tilting the plate at various angles to see all characteristics. Often, a dissecting microscope or hand lens is used for better observation. On the

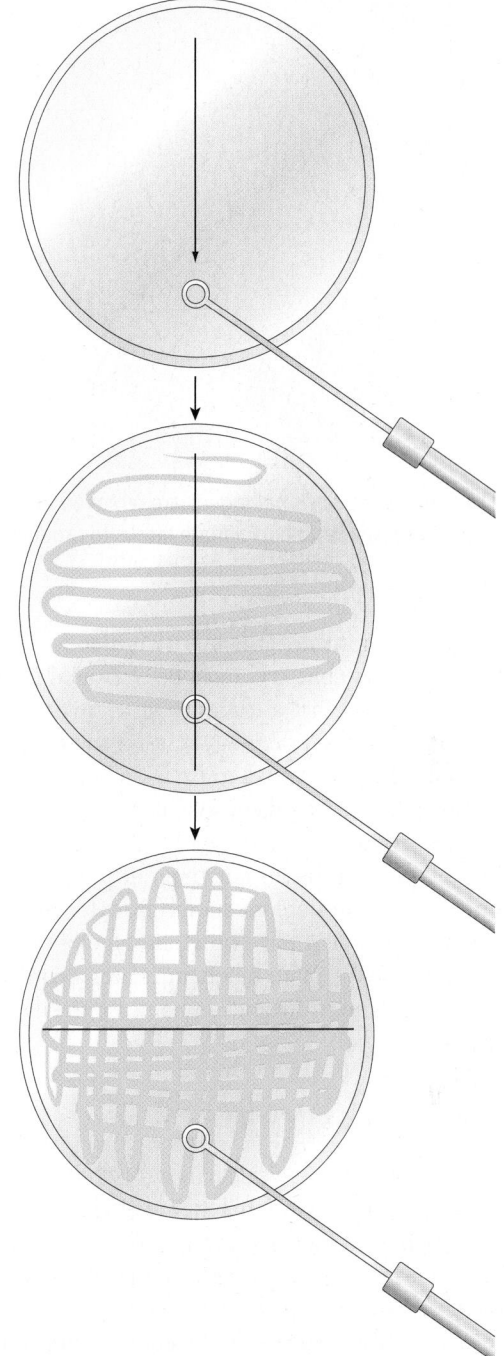

Figure 31-18 Colony count streak.

initial culture, the pathogens are mixed in with the normal flora in the first quadrant streaks, and it takes a trained eye to separate them.

Subculture

When working with bacterial cultures, there can be more than one pathogen growing in the culture. For instance, a wound culture may have both Gram-positive and

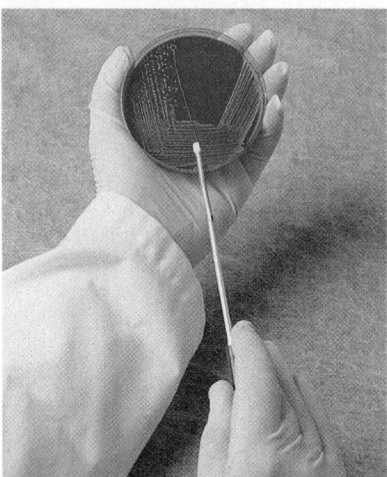

Figure 31-19   Suspicious pathogens are removed from one plate and streaked onto appropriate media to produce subcultures.

Gram-negative organisms growing. In order to identify each organism, these bacteria must be separated to other media. It is also necessary at times to separate the pathogenic bacteria from the normal flora, as in the throat and sputum cultures. Some initial cultures do achieve excellent isolation without having to subculture.

A pure culture is set up by using an inoculation loop or needle and picking the suspicious pathogen and streaking it onto the appropriate media for growth (Figure 31-19). This new plate will have only one type of organism present and from this plate biochemical tests can be set up. This step takes an additional 24 hours for the new subcultures to grow.

BIOCHEMICAL TESTS

In order to report to the physician exactly what organisms are causing patient infection, further testing may be necessary. Through the Gram stain, it is determined that the organism is either Gram-positive or Gram-negative. Initial growth on plates gives the microbiologist an impression of the colonies of the bacteria, and sometimes this is enough for identification if the bacteria has distinctive colonies. But most bacteria have similar characteristics on the initial plates. Further testing is needed to determine both the genus and species of the organisms. Table 31-9 illustrates a flowchart with biochemical testing as one of the final identification steps in this process.

Usually, laboratories will have a set procedure of tests to run when identifying certain genuses and species. Some organisms are much easier to identify than others. For example, the organism that causes strep throat will be obvious on blood agar. The *Beta Streptococcus, Group A* organism will use the red blood cells in the agar and produce a clear colony. Confirmation of this organism can be

TABLE 31-9   FLOWCHART OF SPECIMEN FOR IDENTIFICATION

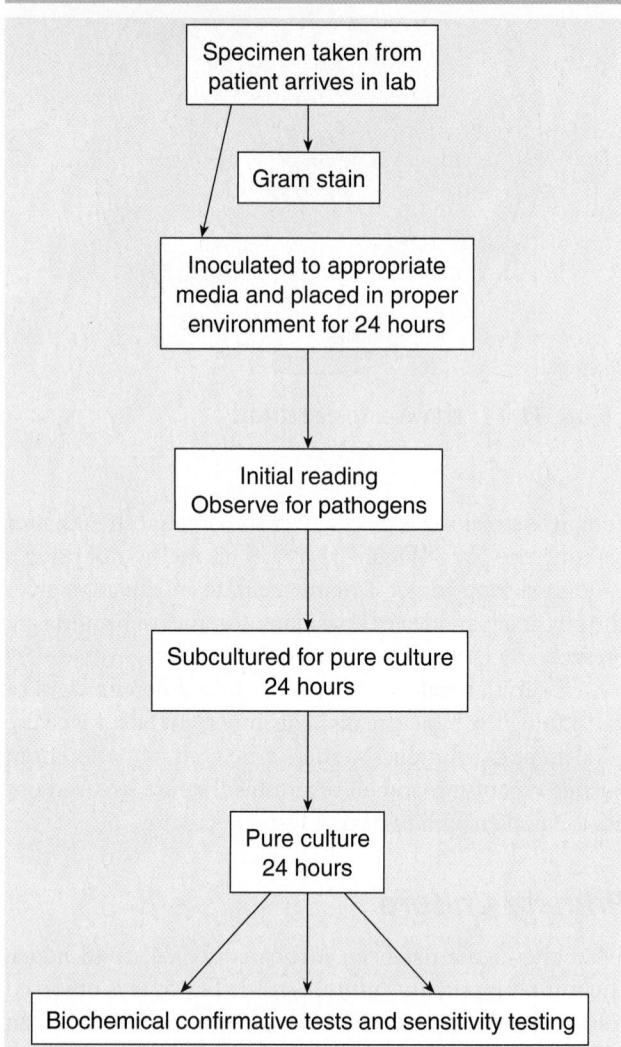

done rapidly with a specialized kit. Direct testing on isolated colonies has become very popular in today's health care environment due to the demand for immediate results.

Direct Tests

The following tests are done with immediate results. The directions included with the product by the manufacturer must be followed carefully.

- *Bile solubility.* *Streptococcus pneumoniae* is a Gram-positive coccus that can cause serious pneumonia. When a few drops of sodium desoxycholate are placed on these colonies, the colonies will lyse and disappear.

- *Catalase.* Colonies of Staphylococcus will foam (effervesce) when placed on a slide with a drop or two of hydrogen peroxide (catalase). This indicates hydrogen gas and is a positive test for staphylococcus species. Streptococcus organisms do not effervesce with catalase, although their colonies may look like Staphylococcus.

- *Coagulase*. Staphylococcus colonies that are coagulase-positive will clump when placed on a slide with rabbit plasma. Some Staphylococcus colonies are coagulase-negative. Different antibiotics may be used for coagulase-positive and coagulase-negative Staphylococci.

- *Indole*. Bacteria that possess the substance tryptophanase will react with Kovac's reagent to produce a red color (positive test). This test is also called the spot indole test.

- *Cytochrome Oxidase*. Certain bacteria will produce a blue-purple color when colonies are placed on a strip saturated with cytochrome oxidase.

- *Motility*. Some bacteria have motility and some do not. A direct microscopic examination can result in the observation of organized movement and the determination that the organism is motile.

These direct simple tests can be performed to make a final identification on some organisms or to give an indication as to what additional tests should be performed. Some highly sophisticated microbiology laboratories are now using high-tech systems that produce rapid identification results for many bacteria. (See Identification Systems section later in this chapter.) The identification techniques that follow will eventually be outdated with the increased demand for immediate results.

Biochemical Tube Testing

Identification of many bacteria can be facilitated by placing isolated colonies in a variety of tube media to determine how the bacteria will react. **Enterobacteriaceae**, a large group of Gram-negative bacteria, grow readily on many types of media. Many of these bacteria colonize the human intestinal tract and cause no problems. However, colonizing bacteria can cause problems if introduced into a susceptible site (the lung, spinal fluid, and so on) of a compromised host. Tube media often is used to help in the identification of Enterobacteriaceae, as well as other types of bacteria. Listed below are a few of the many tube media options available for bacterial identification. A larger, more complete list can be found in medical microbiology reference textbooks.

- *Triple Sugar Iron Agar (TSI); Kligler Iron Agar (KIA).* These complex carbohydrate media test the characteristic reactions of specific bacteria to various chemicals, especially the enterobacteriaceae. TSI contains lactose, glucose, sucrose, an iron salt, and indicators. KIA contains lactose, glucose, an iron salt, and indicators. The tubes are allowed to solidify on a slant. Several reactions can be observed in the bottom (butt) of the slant, as well as on the slant surface itself. The carbohydrate reaction in the butt and slant, the gas production of hydrogen and hydrogen sulfide, and pH change can be observed (Figure 31-20).

- *Citrate*. Only organisms that can utilize citrate as the sole source of carbon will react in this media.

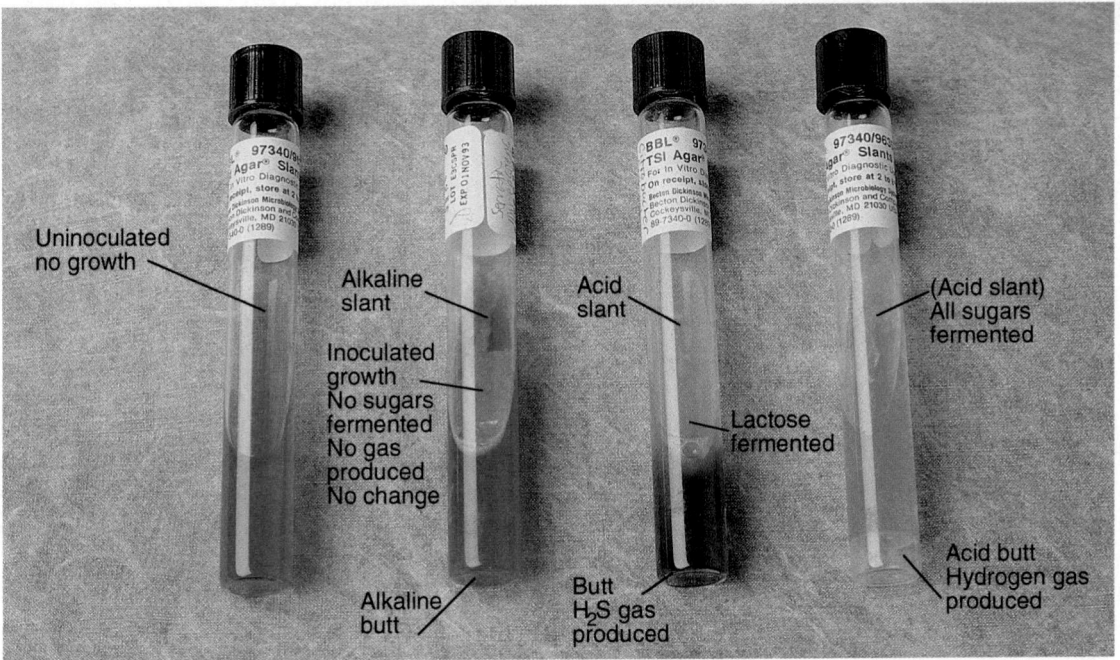

Figure 31-20 Triple sugar iron (TSI) agar.

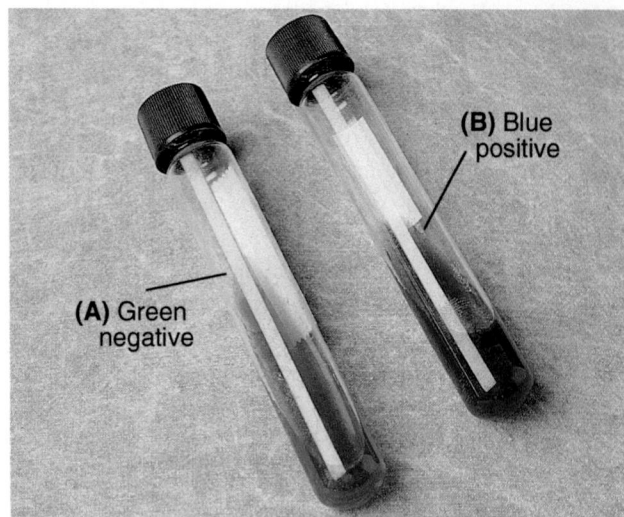

(B) Blue positive

(A) Green negative

Figure 31-21   Citrate tubes: (A) E. coli. (B) Citrobacter Klebsiella.

The media is Simmons citrate agar with bromthymol blue as an indicator. The agar is made as a slant. When an organism has utilized citrate, the media turns from green to blue (Figure 31-21).

● *Urease Production.* Organisms that have the enzyme urease will break down the substance urea, producing ammonia and a pink-red color in the medium.

● *Bile Esculin.* This test is based on an organism's ability to break down the substance esculin in the presence of 1 percent to 4 percent bile. Some Streptococci organisms give a positive bile esculin reaction, seen as a blackened color on the media.

Table 31-10 is a listing of common pathogens and biochemical tests that might be used to help in their identification. Some tests are listed that are not explained in this text. Refer to a medical microbiology reference textbook for information on such tests.

IDENTIFICATION SYSTEMS

The age of high technology and computerized equipment has also made inroads into microbiology laboratories, clinics, and physician's office laboratories. Every day, traditional methods of identifying bacteria are being replaced by rapid identification tests, packaged systems (kits), and automated systems.

Rapid test systems give a quick identification, are economical, and allow physicians to start treatment sooner. A system is considered rapid if the physician can receive an answer while the patient is still in the physician's office.

TABLE 31-10   RECOMMENDED DIFFERENTIAL CHARACTERISTICS OF VARIOUS BACTERIA FOR IDENTIFICATION

Pathogen	Biochemical Test
Staphylococcus	Coagulase Mannitol Catalase
Streptococci	Catalase
Strep. pneumoniae	Bacitracin disk Bile esculin Quelling Bile solubility Camp test
Neisseria Moraxella	Oxidase activity CTA carbohydrate (maltose, sucrose, glucose, lactose)
Enterobacteriaceae	Lactose fermentation Oxidase activity H_2S production Decarboxylase activity Motility IMVIC reaction Urease
Nonfermentative Gram-negative bacilli	Oxidase activity Motility Indole Urease Growth on Mac Pigment production
Haemophilus	Enriched media with X and V factor Catalase Required CO_2 for growth Oxidase

Streptococcus Screening (Rapid Strep Testing)

There are a number of instant or rapid test kits on the market to identify Group A Streptococcus (also known as Beta Hemolytic Streptococcus Group A), the causative agent of a serious sore (strep) throat. It is very important to identify this Gram-positive Streptococcus as soon as possible because the bacteria can do serious damage (i.e., kidney and heart valve damage) if not treated with antibiotics immediately.

One test kit out today is based on the principle of enzyme immunoassay (EIA). This test is very sensitive and eliminates false positive tests. The directions should be strictly followed to produce an accurate test result. The results are based on color development of a spot on the test filter. Test results are available in minutes.

A latex agglutination test for Group A Streptococcus is based on an antigen and antibody agglutination. A throat swab is placed directly on the antibody coated slide, and the presence of a positive test is seen by the appearance of agglutination (clumping). Although these tests are quick and convenient, the following rules should be strictly followed:

1. Use the correct swab in taking the throat cultures. Some cottons and chemicals on the swab will interfere with test reagents.
2. Always run positive and negative control along with the actual test.
3. Read and understand directions before starting the test.
4. Never use outdated kits and materials.
5. Observe all safety guidelines.

If a patient has symptoms of an infected throat and the slide test is negative, the physician will also order a regular throat culture to make sure there is no infection present. Latex kits can give false readings, and it is best to follow up with the throat culture. Table 31-11 lists "Rapid Strep" kits approved for CLIA '88 waived testing.

Packaged Systems

Packaged systems are identification systems that have multiple tests within the container. These systems are used for identification of such microorganisms as anaerobic bacteria, enterobacteriaceae, and yeasts. These systems have replaced the many test tubes filled with various biochemicals.

Multitest media systems that will identify the Enterobacteriaceae bacteria include:

- *Enterotube®*. The Enterotube is a pencil-shaped chamber with eight compartments from which eleven reactions can be determined. To inoculate,

unscrew each end of the tube. One end will have a wire needle for inoculation and the other end a small handle. To inoculate, touch the needle end to an isolated colony. With a slow rotary motion, pull the handle of the wire back through the chambers and out of the tube. Reinsert the wire into the first four compartments for anaerobic conditions. Also pull the plastic sleeve over these compartments. Incubate horizontally for 18 to 24 hours at 37°C. Add Kovac's reagent to the indole chamber of the tube and 10% ferric chloride to the phenylalanine chamber. This is best done with a hypodermic needle directly into the chamber. Read the reactions according to the manufacturer's directions, convert to a four-digit number, and compare the number to the organism in the code book (Figure 31-22).

- *API® System.* The API System consists of a plastic strip with twenty small cupules that are filled with a bacterial suspension for inoculation. The cupules contain dehydrated substrates for specific tests. There is an incubation tray to put the strip in with

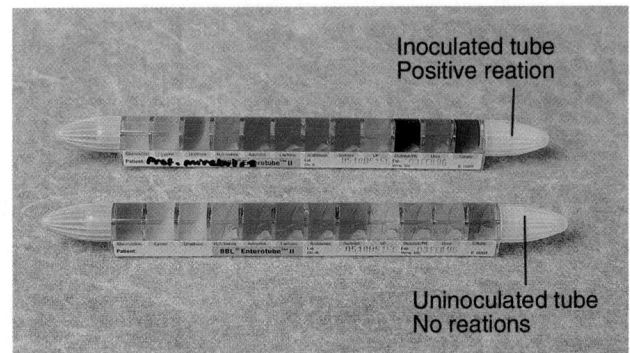

Figure 31-22 Enterotube.

TABLE 31-11	LIST OF WAIVED TESTS FOR *STREPTOCOCCUS, GROUP A (STREP A)*	
Manufacture	**Kit Name**	**Specimen**
Abbott	Signify Strep A Test	Direct from throat swab
Applied Biotech	SureStep Strep A	Direct from throat swab
Becton Dickinson	LINK 2 Strep A (II)	Direct from throat swab
Bianax	NOW Strep A Test	Direct from throat swab
BioStar Acceava	Strep A Test	Direct from throat swab
Genzyme	Contrast Strep A	Direct from throat swab
Jant Pharmacal	AccuStrip Strep A	Direct from throat swab
Mainline Technology	Mainline Confirms Strep A Dots Test	Direct from throat swab
Meridian Diagnostics	ImmunoCard STAT Strep A	Direct from throat swab
Quidel	QuickVue In-Line One-Step Strep A Test	Direct from throat swab
SmithKline	ICON Fx Strep A Test	Direct from throat swab
Wyntek Diagnostics	OSOM Strep A Test	Direct from throat swab

Reference: CLIA '88 Test Categorization List as of April 26, 1999. This list changes rapidly. For the most current listing, refer to the CDC website at www.cdc.gov.

a loose-fitting lid. Some cupules are overlaid with oil to reduce oxygen. The tray is incubated for 5 to 6 hours for the rapid test or 18 to 24 hours at 37°C. The tests are read visually as positive or negative and converted to a seven-digit number that corresponds to a bacterial organism in the code book. There are also API strips for the identification of yeasts, anaerobic organisms, and nonfermentative Gram-negative bacilli (Figure 31-23).

- *r/b System*®. This system consists of four constricted tubes called Beckford tubes. These four tubes contain eight types of biochemicals in media that will determine fourteen characteristic reactions. The medium above the constriction is a slant for aerobic reactions and the medium below the constriction is for anaerobic conditions. The tubes are inoculated with an inoculating needle for stabbing to the bottom and streaking to the top. They are incubated in an upright position at 37°C for 18 to 24 hours. The color changes in the tubes are compared to the color chart provided by the manufacturer.

There are several other packaged systems on the market. Selection of specific systems depends on the volume of work and cost for the particular size laboratory.

Semiautomated and Automated Instruments

The microbiology department of the clinical laboratory has been among the last departments to become automated. The nature of reading cultures has not lent itself well to automation until the past few years. Now systems such as ALADIN® and Vitek® are known as "walk-away" systems, where the microbiologist sets up the machine, and the work is done automatically. Semiautomated systems such as Biolog® and MicroScan® require more interaction between the microbiologist and the instrument. These automated and semiautomated systems are expensive and are used in high-volume laboratories.

SENSITIVITY TESTING

Antibiotic sensitivity testing often is ordered on the pathogenic organisms recovered from the culturing process. By setting up an antibiotic sensitivity test, the laboratory can identify which antibiotics destroy the pathogen, and the physician will be able to set up antibiotic treatment for the patient. Today's health care environment demands that this information be made available to the physician as soon as possible. Automated systems mentioned in the previous section are designed to produce this information as rapidly as possible.

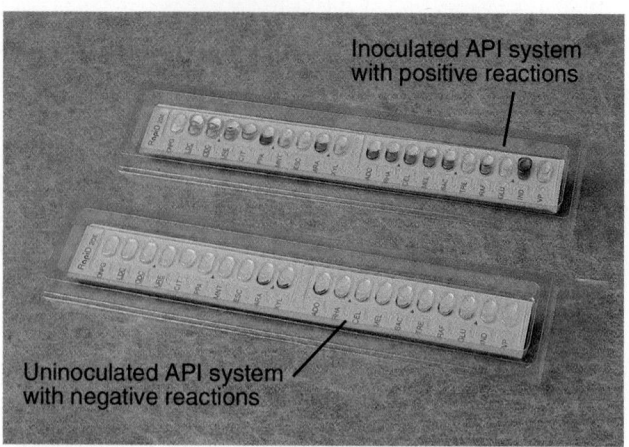

Figure 31-23 The API System identifies Gram-negative bacilli.

A traditional manual method of performing sensitivity testing is the **Kirby Bauer** method. It involves placing antibiotic disks on top of an inoculated plate. The plate is incubated for up to 24 hours. The pathogen will grow closely around a disk if the antibiotic is not destroying the organism. However, if an antibiotic will destroy the pathogen, there will be no growth at all around the disk. An obvious zone will be apparent.

To set up the Kirby Bauer test, a bacterial suspension of the isolated organism is compared to a barium sulfate standard to be sure that it is not too concentrated. A large Mueller Hinton plate is lawn streaked with a swab. The antibiotic disks are placed on the agar and gently pressed down for contact.

After 18 to 24 hours of incubation, the disk zones are measured with a metric ruler. Zones are measured for (R) resistant organisms (those the antibiotic cannot destroy), (I) intermediate (the organism is partially destroyed), and (S) sensitive (the organism is destroyed by the antibiotic).

The type of antibiotics used will vary depending on the organism that is grown. Zone sizes for R, S, and I will vary and the manufacturer's guidelines should be followed (Figure 31-24). As related to antimicrobial agents, bacteria are categorized as susceptible, moderately susceptible, or resistant to the antimicrobial agent. Definitions of these categories for various bacteria are published by the National Committee for Clinical Laboratory Standards. Refer to M2-A7, *Performance Standards for Antimicrobial Disc Susceptibility Tests*, 7th edition (2000); M7-A5, *Methods for Dilution Antimicrobial Susceptibility Tests for Bacteria That Grow Aerobically*, 5th edition (2000); M100-S10, Supplemental tables for M2-A7 and M7-A5; M11-A4, *Methods for Antimicrobial Susceptibility Tests for Anaerobic Bacteria*, 4th edition (1997).

There are several automated and semiautomated systems that utilize the antibiotic in several concentra-

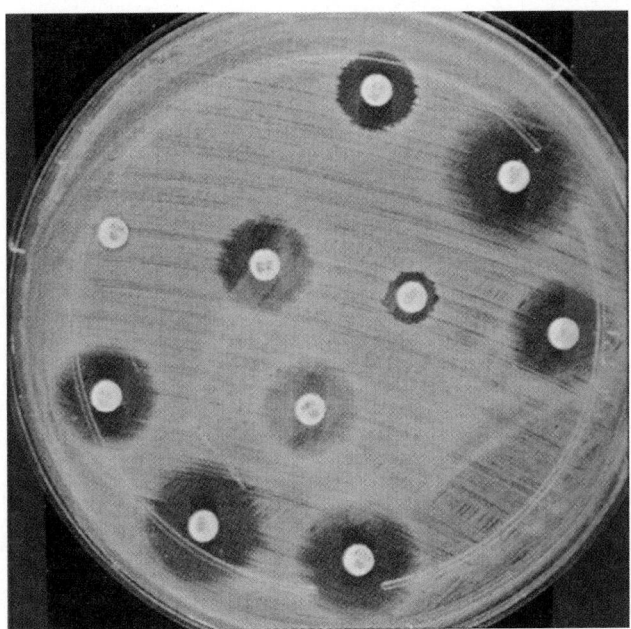

Figure 31-24 Zones of inhibition in an agar diffusion method of sensitivity testing.

tions against the isolated pathogen. The instrument prints out the most effective antibiotics. These systems are efficient and give results in a shorter period of time, but they are costly.

PARASITOLOGY

With the age of travel and more public awareness, we are beginning to see more parasitic infections. The field of parasitology is a vast one with many different types of parasites. They range from extremely small microscopic ones to those that are large and macroscopic in size. Parasites have varying life cycles. The degree of severity of illness depends on which parasite enters the human body and infects it. Parasites can be found in the blood, urine, or feces. The more common ones are found in the feces.

The study of parasitology in the clinic or physician's office laboratory is usually limited. Different geographical areas have different types of parasites that are seen. Resettled immigrant populations may be infected with a parasite previously unseen in a geographic area. World travelers can also bring back rare parasitic infections from their adventures.

Examination Methods

There are several methods used to examine parasites. They can be examined in permanent stained slides. (Refer to Procedures 31-2 and 31-3.) This type stains the parasite and provides a permanent record of the parasite seen. Another microscopic method is the direct wet mount.

(Refer to Procedure 31-5.) It is the examination of the feces in a suspension of saline or formalin applied in a thin layer on the slide.

The **concentration method**, either by flotation or sedimentation, is a procedure done to have a better view of the protozoa or ova in a specimen. In the sedimentation method, the parasites are found in the bottom layer of the test tube. In the flotation method, the parasites are found on the top layer. These procedures are not commonly performed in a physician's office laboratory. More detailed information can be found in a medical microbiology reference textbook.

One of the most common methods of fecal specimen examination for parasitic identification in a clinic or physician's office laboratory is the direct wet mount slide. The permanent stained slide and fecal concentration take more time and are done in the microbiology department of a hospital or reference laboratory.

Specimen Collection

Fecal specimens for identification of ova and parasites should be collected in wide-mouth containers with a tight lid to prevent leakage. The container should be put in a biohazard transport bag to avoid contamination and sent for examination immediately. The patient should be instructed not to contaminate the specimen with urine because it could interfere with testing. Special vials containing formalin are also available for ova and parasite testing that are preferred by some laboratories.

The laboratory procedure for collection and processing of the parasite specimen should be strictly followed to provide an accurate testing of the specimen. The collection time of the specimen should be followed as directed by the physician. Three specimens may be ordered over a specified period of time. Physician's offices will have specific instructions and containers with a preservative in them when an ova and parasite examination is requested.

When the specimen is sent for testing, it should be labeled correctly with the patient's name, date, and time of the specimen. It is important to know if the patient has been traveling, to what area of the world, and what is suspected by the physician to help aid in identification.

Before the microscopic examination is done, a description of the gross appearance of the stool should be recorded. The specimen should be checked for color, consistency, blood, and mucous. When working with the fecal specimens, all safety procedures should be followed and gloves should be worn at all times. The specimen should be disposed of by the procedures set forth by the clinic or physician's office laboratory using standard precautions and OSHA guidelines.

Common Parasites

Some of the more common parasites identified in the physician's office laboratory are *Enterobius vermicularis,* the causative organism of pinworm infection, and *Trichomonas vaginalis,* a parasite that infects the urogenital tracts of men and women.

Enterobius vermicularis. This **nematode** (round worm) is found worldwide, predominantly in children. The adult worm is shaped like a pin, wide at one end and pointed at the other end. The female worm is larger than the male. Infection with pinworm can cause severe itching, irritability, and insomnia, depending upon the severity of the infection. The adult female worm migrates to the anus at night, depositing ova (eggs) that cause itching during hatching. At times, the adult worm can be found around the anus and on the stool. The adult worm measures approximately 7 to 12 mm long (Figure 31-25A). The egg is the infectious stage of the parasite (Figure 31-25B).

To diagnose the presence of the parasite, either the adult worm or ova has to be located in the specimen. A negative test should be confirmed by as many as six negative tests performed. The test is performed by taking a cellophane tape swab and placing the sticky side down to the skin around the anal area. The tape is placed on a slide and brought to the laboratory for examination (Figure 31-26).

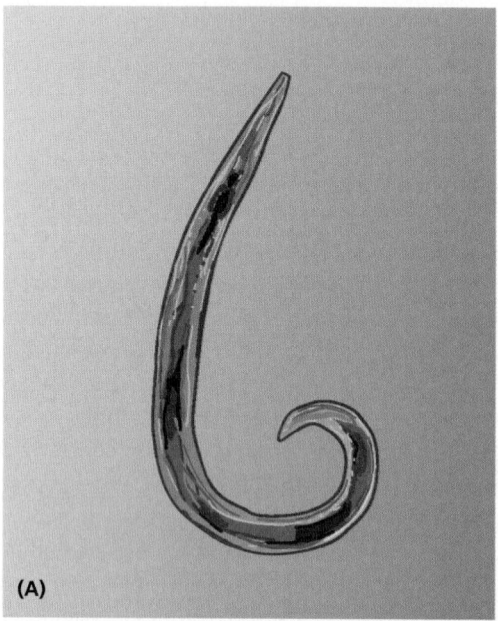

(A)

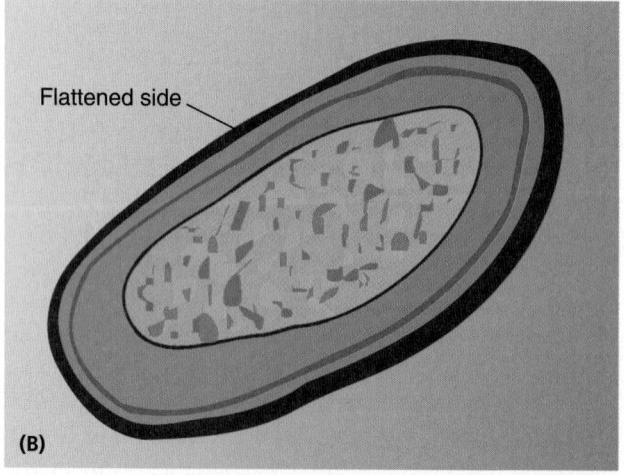

Flattened side

(B)

Figure 31-25   (A) Adult pinworm, *Enterobius vermicularis.* (B) *Enterobius vermicularis* egg (pinworm egg) at the infectious stage.

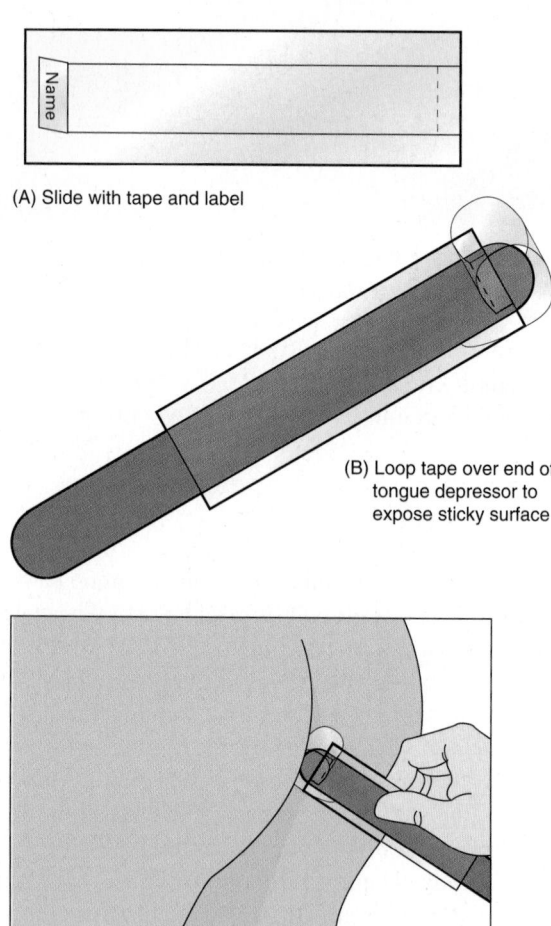

(A) Slide with tape and label

(B) Loop tape over end of tongue depressor to expose sticky surface

(C) Press sticky surfaces against perianal areas

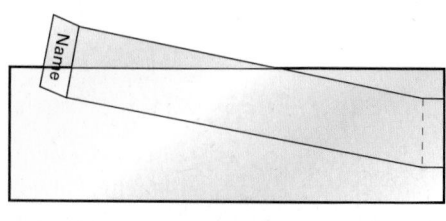

(D) Replace tape

Figure 31-26   Technique for preparing and using a cellophane tape swab.

Trichomonas vaginalis. This parasite is found in both men and women, but its presence is five times higher in women (men can harbor the organism for years without symptoms). The organism belongs to the flagellate (possesses flagella) class and is extremely motile. Infection with this flagellate causes a purulent yellowish-green discharge and dysuria. The organism is recovered from the discharge or urine and is transmitted sexually.

The trichomonad is recovered in a wet preparation slide of spun urine or vaginal secretion mixed with a drop of saline. (Refer to Procedure 31-5.) The specimen should not be contaminated with fecal material that could contain *Trichomonas hominis,* another flagellate. The prepared slide is examined under the low and high objectives of the microscope to observe the motility and morphology of the parasite (see Figure 30-14). There are also test kits and fluorescent stains used to diagnose this parasite.

MYCOLOGY

The field of mycology and the infections that cause fungi are extensive. Most identification and sensitivities testing for fungal organisms take place in larger laboratories and specific reference laboratories. Identification of two of the common fungal infections can be made quickly in the clinic or physician's office laboratory.

The genus Candida has several species that cause yeast infections in the body. Candida species are also present in the environment around us. They present a particular problem in the health care setting where they can cause serious nosocomial infections. Equipment can be easily contaminated with Candida organisms.

Yeast infections commonly are found on the moist areas of the body and in the subcutaneous tissue. An infection with yeast can range from mild to serious. *Candida albicans* is the causative agent of vaginal yeast infections. The specimen is examined microscopically for the characteristic budding yeast forms. (Refer to Procedure 31-5.) If the specimen is fluid and clear, it is placed on a slide with a drop of saline. If the specimen is thick, it should be mixed with 10 percent potassium hydroxide (one drop) on the slide to clear away debris. Once the specimen is prepared, it is microscopically examined.

Another group of significant fungi that sometimes can be generally identified are the **dermatophytes**. These fungi cause infections on the hair, skin, and nails. The microscopic structure of these fungi is very detailed. Some of the fungi that cause dermatophytic infections can be diagnosed using a **Wood's lamp**. This is a lamp with an ultraviolet light. Some dermatophytes will fluoresce (glow brightly) under this light.

Mycotic infections can also be identified through culture and kit identification systems. Fungi can produce heavy aerosols and should be processed and observed under the safety hood.

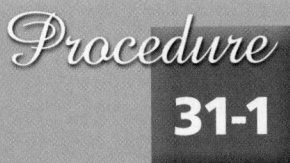

Procedure 31-1
Procedure for Obtaining a Throat Culture

STANDARD PRECAUTIONS:

PURPOSE:
To obtain secretions from the nasopharynx and tonsillar area in order to incubate for means of identifying a pathogenic microorganism.

EQUIPMENT/SUPPLIES:
Tongue depressor
Culture tube with applicator stick or commercially prepared culture collection system
Label and requisition form
Gloves and mask

PROCEDURE STEPS:
1. Explain procedure to patient.
2. Have patient in sitting position. Adjust good light source.
3. Wash hands. Gather equipment.
4. Apply mask and gloves.
5. Remove sterile applicator from culture tube.
6. Ask patient to open mouth widely.
7. Depress tongue with tongue depressor.
8. Swab the back of throat and the tonsillar area. RATIONALE: Be certain to obtain a good sample of secretions or exudate from the very back of the throat paying special attention to red, raw, or with pustules.

(continues)

Procedure

31-1 (*continued*)

NOTE: On occasion separate cultures from each side of the throat may be taken per the physician's direction.

9. Remove applicator stick and place in culture tube(s).
10. Remove tongue blade and discard in biohazard waste container.
11. Push the applicator stick into the culture medium until the medium compartment is punctured and

medium is released. RATIONALE: This keeps sample alive because medium contains nutrients similar to human tissue.

12. Ensure patient comfort.
13. Label culture tube(s) and send to outside laboratory or process the specimen according to agency policy.
14. Remove gloves and mask.
15. Wash hands.

Procedure

31-2 Preparing a Bacteriological Smear

STANDARD PRECAUTIONS:

PURPOSE:
Prepare a bacterial suspension for staining to examine bacteria microscopically.

EQUIPMENT/SUPPLIES:

Gloves	Loop or swab
Laboratory coat	Organism to be examined
Goggles (barrier shield	Heat
or face shield can also	Stain rack
be used)	Tray
Clean glass slide	Stains
Distilled water	

PROCEDURE STEPS:
1. Wash hands.
2. Put on personal protective equipment.
3. Assemble equipment and materials.

4. Apply a thin film of bacteria using a sterile or flamed loop or rolling a swab onto the surface of the slide, making a smear about the size of a nickel. If the bacteria is in a liquid suspension, apply directly to the slide; if not, add a drop of sterile water to the slide first.
5. Allow the bacteria to air-dry completely.
6. After the slide air dries, it is ready to be heat fixed. To heat fix the slide, pass it through the flame two or three times. This step is an important one. RATIONALE: If heat fixing is omitted, the bacteria will wash off in the staining process when water is applied. Avoid too much heat fixing because it can distort cells.
7. Allow the slide to cool before staining.

CAUTION: Use all safety precautions and make sure the suspension is air-dried before applying heat so that bacteria does not splatter.

Procedure

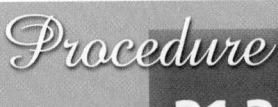

31-3 Gram Stain

STANDARD PRECAUTIONS:

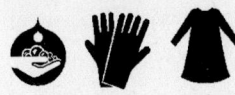

PURPOSE:
View organism microscopically to differentiate Gram-negative or Gram-positive bacteria through staining technique.

EQUIPMENT/SUPPLIES:

Gloves
Laboratory coat
Goggles (barrier shield or face shield can also be used)
Distilled water in beaker or plastic squeeze bottle
Loop or swab

Paper towels
Bibulous paper
Prepared bacteriological smear
Heat
Gram stain kit or individual Gram stain reagents
Staining tray and rack

PROCEDURE STEPS:
1. Wash hands.
2. Put on personal protective equipment.
3. Assemble equipment and materials.
4. Flood the fixed smear with crystal violet for the manufacturer's recommended time period, usually one minute.
   NOTE: All bacteria cells will be purple.

5. Rinse the stain off the smear with a gentle stream of water from a beaker or plastic squeeze bottle.
6. Tilt the smear to remove excess water.
7. Flood the smear with Gram's iodine for the recommended time. RATIONALE: The iodine is a mordant that will hold the crystal violet to the Gram-positive bacteria.
   NOTE: All bacteria cells are still purple.
8. Rinse the smear as in steps 2 and 3.
9. Hold the smear by the short edge using forceps. Add the acetone-alcohol decolorizer by squeeze bottle or pasteur pipette until purple no longer runs off the slide.
   CAUTION: It is important to decolorize no longer than a few seconds to prevent over-decolorization.
   NOTE: Gram-positive bacteria remain purple; Gram-negative cells have no color.
10. Rinse the smear immediately to remove the decolorizer; tilt the slides to remove excess water.
11. Counterstain the smear by flooding the smear with safranin for the recommended time.
    NOTE: Gram-negative bacteria cells now have pink color.
12. Rinse the smear, tilt to remove excess water; wipe the back of the smear with paper towel to remove stain; stand smear on end or blot between sheets of bibulous paper to dry.

Procedure

31-4 Ziehl-Neelsen Stain

STANDARD PRECAUTIONS:

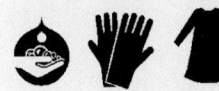

PURPOSE:
Identify acid-fast and non-acid-fast organisms.

EQUIPMENT/SUPPLIES:

Gloves
Laboratory coat
Safety hood
Barrier shield
Face shield or goggles
Glass slide
Organism
Distilled water

Loop or swab
Heat
Ziehl-Neelsen stain reagents (carbolfuchsin, acid alcohol and methylene blue or malachite green)
Staining rack and tray

(continues)

Procedure

31-4 (continued)

PROCEDURE STEPS:

1. Wash hands.
2. Put on personal protective equipment.
3. Assemble equipment and materials.
4. Place a prepared smear on a staining rack and apply heat, staining with carbolfuchsin. Apply heat under the smear until steaming. *Do not let the stain dry on the smear*; generously apply the carbolfuchsin.
5. Wash off the carbolfuchsin with *distilled* water. **CAUTION:** Do not flood with water when the smear is still very hot as it will crack.
6. Decolorize with acid alcohol about two minutes until no more stain is in the washing. All acid-fast organisms will retain the carbolfuchsin, which is red.
7. Wash off with distilled water.
8. Apply a counterstain of methylene blue or malachite green for 30 seconds. The counterstain will stain all the non-acid-fast material that did not retain the carbolfuchsin. These organisms will appear green or blue (Figure 31-27).
9. Wash off the smear with distilled water and air-dry completely. The smear can also be dried for several hours on a heat block.

CAUTION: All safety precautions for the microbiology laboratory should be followed. This smear should be prepared under a safety hood.

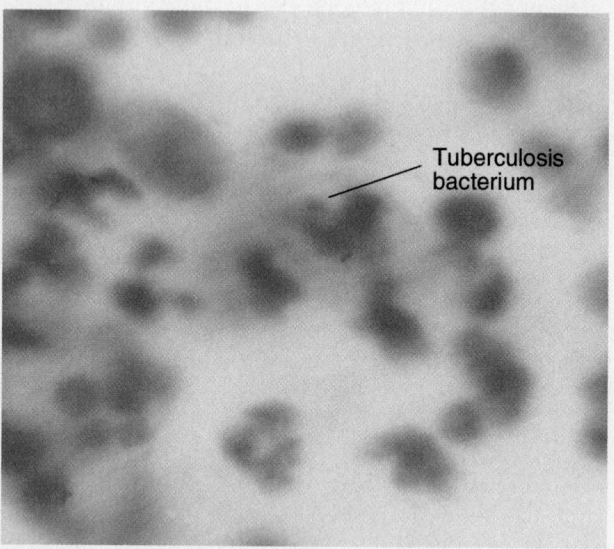

Tuberculosis bacterium

Figure 31-27 These non-acid-fast organisms have turned blue after the Ziehl-Neelsen stain.

Procedure

31-5 Wet Mount and Hanging Drop Slide Preparations

STANDARD PRECAUTIONS:

PURPOSE:

Prepare a slide for viewing live organisms for motility and identifying characteristics.

EQUIPMENT/SUPPLIES:

Gloves	Coverslips
Laboratory coat	Petroleum jelly
Clean glass slide	Dropper

Glass slide with concave well   Bacterial suspension

PROCEDURE STEPS:

1. Wash hands.
2. Put on personal protective equipment.
3. Assemble equipment and materials.

Wet Mount Preparation

4. Place a drop of the bacterial suspension on a clean glass slide (Figure 31-28A).
5. Place petroleum jelly around the edges of the coverslip (Figure 31-28B).

(continues)

Procedure
31-5 *(continued)*

6. Place a coverslip with the petroleum jelly on top of the bacterial suspension. RATIONALE: This cuts down on air currents and keeps the slide from drying out.

7. After the smear is prepared properly, it can be observed microscopically at any power (Figure 31-28C).

Hanging Drop Slide Preparation

8. The bacterial specimen is placed in the center of the coverslip with petroleum jelly around the edges of the coverslip (Figure 31-29A).

9. The slide is inverted and the concave well of the slide is placed over the coverslip (Figure 31-29B).

10. The slide is carefully turned right side up for examination (Figure 31-29C).

CAUTION: All laboratory safety precautions should be followed. Extreme caution should be followed. The organisms involved in this procedure are alive, not having been killed by heat fixation.

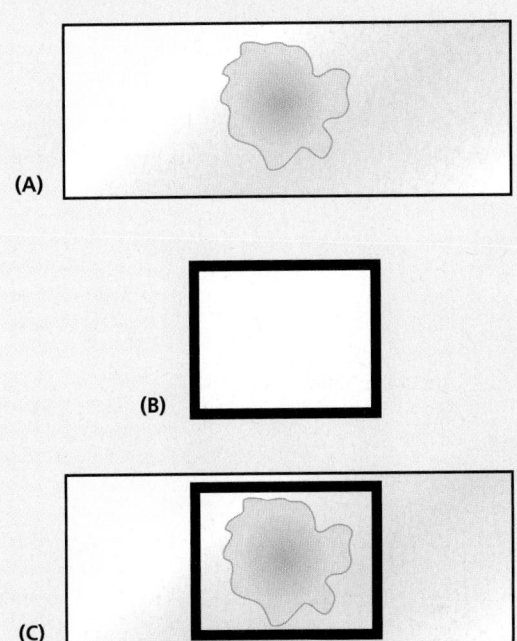

(A)

(B)

(C)

Figure 31-28 (A) Specimen placed on a glass slide. (B) Coverslip with petroleum jelly on edges. (C) Coverslip placed directly on top of slide with specimen.

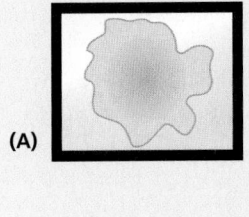

(A)

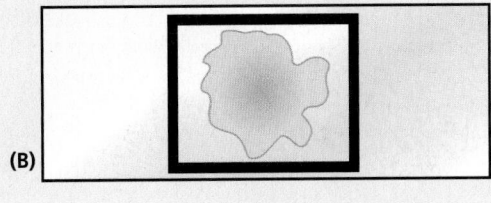

(B)

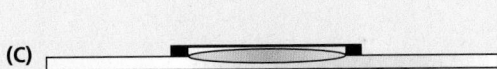

(C)

Figure 31-29 (A) Specimen placed on coverslip. (B) Slide placed over coverslip. (C) Slide turned right side up for examination.

Procedure 31-6

Specimen Inoculation and Dilution Streaking

STANDARD PRECAUTIONS:

PURPOSE:

Inoculate solid media to study bacterial growth on agar.

EQUIPMENT/SUPPLIES:

Gloves
Laboratory coat
Plates
Barrier shield
Face shield or safety glasses
Heat
Blood agar
Inoculating loop
Bacterial specimen

PROCEDURE STEPS:

1. Wash hands.
2. Put on personal protective equipment.
3. Assemble equipment and materials.
4. Flame the loop (if a metal loop is used) and allow to cool. Apply the specimen to the plate with the sterile flamed loop or the specimen's swab. Once the specimen is applied, flame the loop again (Figure 31-30).
5. Use the loop to spread through the first streak and streak, turning the plate. Flame the loop.
6. Use the loop to spread through the second streak and streak, turning the plate.
7. Use the loop to spread through the third streak. Flame the loop.

CAUTION: All safety precautions for the microbiology laboratory should be followed. All cultures should be plated under a safety hood.

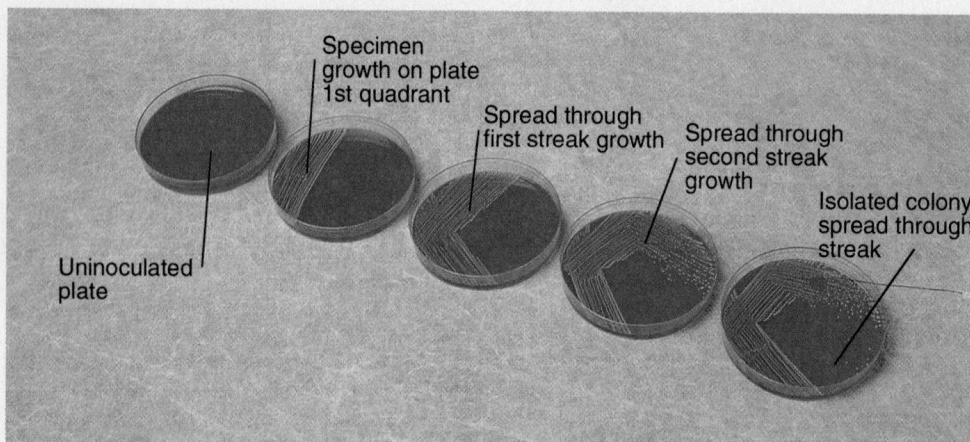

Figure 31-30   Stages of dilution streak.

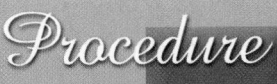

31-7   Broth Tube Inoculation

STANDARD PRECAUTIONS:

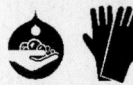

PURPOSE:
Inoculate liquid media to observe bacterial growth.

EQUIPMENT/SUPPLIES:
Gloves   Broth
Laboratory coat   Inoculating loop
Barrier shield   Liquid specimen
Face shield or goggles   Heat

PROCEDURE STEPS:
1. Wash hands.
2. Put on personal protective equipment.
3. Assemble equipment and materials.
4. Flame the loop. If disposable loop, do not flame!
5. Pick up the specimen carefully with the inoculating loop.
6. Slant the tube at a 30 to 40 degree angle and touch a loop to the inside of the tube just above the agar. When the tube is placed in an upright position, the inoculation will be submerged (Figure 31-31).
7. Then gently mix the tube. RATIONALE: To inoculate liquid media for bacterial growth.

CAUTION: All safety precautions for the microbiology laboratory should be followed. Certain cultures should be plated under a safety hood.

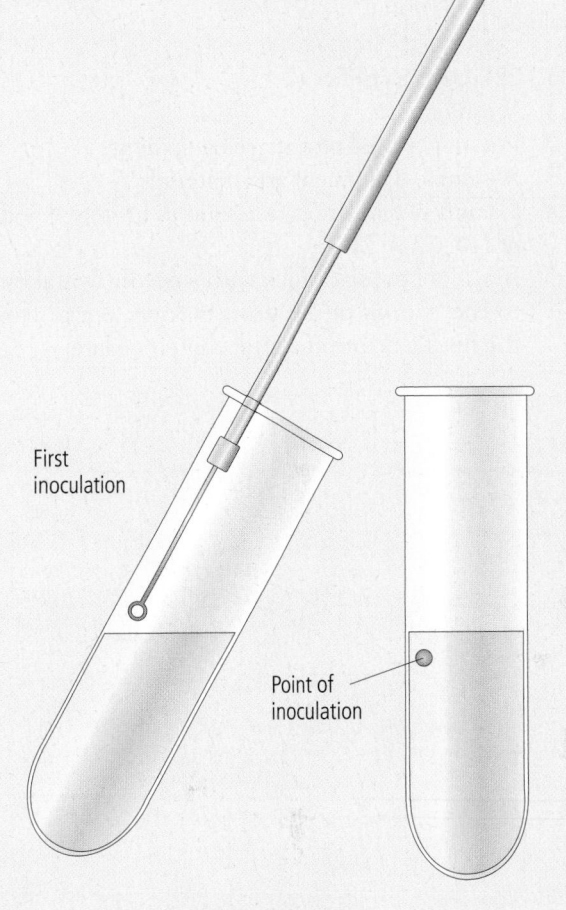

First inoculation

Point of inoculation

Figure 31-31   Broth tube inoculation.

31-8   Deep Inoculation/Slant

STANDARD PRECAUTIONS:

PURPOSE:
To study motility and biochemical reactions in slant media.

EQUIPMENT/SUPPLIES:
Gloves
Laboratory coat
Barrier shield
Face shield or goggles
Inoculating needle

(continues)

Procedure

31-8   *(continued)*

Deep agar or slant
Heat
Isolated bacteria

PROCEDURE STEPS:

1. Wash hands.
2. Put on personal protective equipment.
3. Assemble equipment and materials.
4. Using a needle, inoculate slant as in steps 4 and 5 of Procedure 31-7.
5. Inoculate the slant tube with a needle by stabbing to the bottom of the tube, making sure to flame the needle before and after this procedure.
6. For the slanted portion of the agar, use a needle to streak an "S" motion up the slant (Figure 31-32A).
7. The stab made deep in the agar can show whether or not the organism can move through the agar (motile) or just grow right around the stab (non-motile). The streak on the slant gives the bacteria a surface on which to grow. Some slants and deeps have biochemicals in them that change colors with different chemical reactions with the growing bacterial colonies (Figure 31-32B).

CAUTION: All safety precautions for the microbiology laboratory should be followed. Certain cultures should be plated under a safety hood.

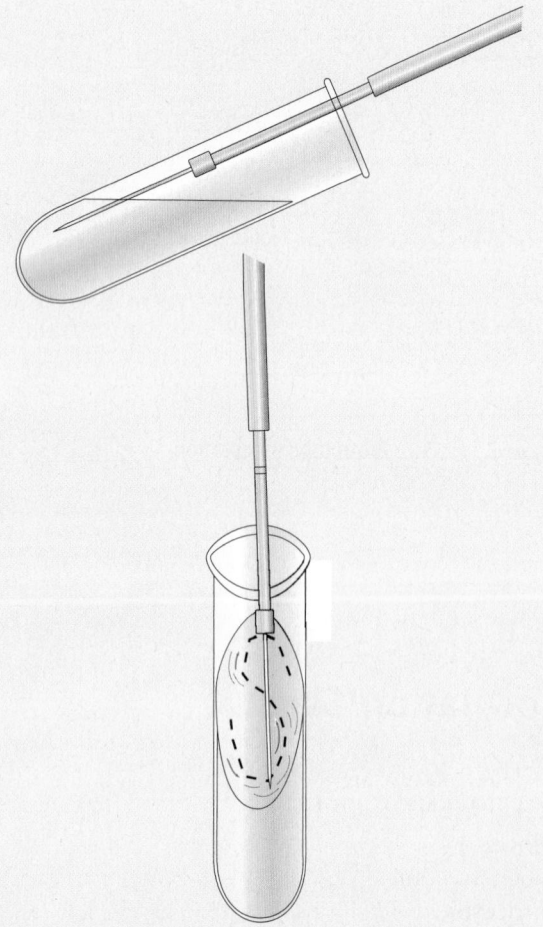

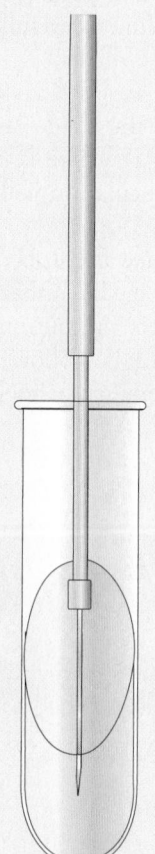

(A)   **(B)**

Figure 31-32   (A) Slant inoculation. (B) Deep inoculation.

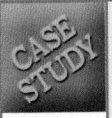

31·1

Mary O'Keefe has brought her three-year-old son Chris to the office of Doctors Lewis and King with a temperature of 102°F and an extremely sore and red throat. He is irritable and crying. After examining Chris, Dr. King orders a STAT latex agglutination test for Group A Streptococcus. Medical assistant Joe Guerrero has a difficult time acquiring the throat swab for the test due to Chris's condition. The test is run, and the results are negative.

CASE STUDY REVIEW

1. What are some reasons the test is negative?
2. What other procedure can be done to diagnose strep throat?
3. How would the test in question 2 be set up?

SUMMARY

The field of microbiology is vast. There are many microorganisms that are pathogenic and can cause serious infection in patients. The successful culturing and identification of such organisms is an important aspect of the successful treatment of patients. All specimens that are processed in the physician's office laboratory should be handled carefully, and all safety guidelines should be followed.

In order for the pathogen to be identified correctly, the utmost care must be taken in obtaining the culture. Sterile equipment must be used by the health care worker. When the culture is processed, the correct microscopic examination, media, incubation, and confirmatory tests must be used correctly to identify the pathogen.

Often a sensitivity test will be requested along with the culture. The information from this test will guide the physician in selecting the appropriate treatment for the patient.

Physicians' office laboratories vary in the type and number of cultures that are performed on the premises and those that are sent out to be performed in a reference laboratory. It is important to provide the best care for the patient by doing only those tests that a laboratory can reasonably handle given equipment and personnel limitations.

In addition to performing bacterial identification, some physician's office laboratories perform parasitology and mycology tests on a limited basis. When performing parasitology tests, it is important to obtain the proper specimen in the correct manner. When performing mycology tests, it is important to work under a safety hood to minimize the risk of exposure to spores from the fungal specimens.

Of utmost importance is the careful following of safety and quality control guidelines. These procedures help ensure patient and health care worker safety, as well as the integrity of test results.

REVIEW QUESTIONS

Multiple Choice

1. A structure that is *not* found on bacterial cells is the:
   a. nucleus
   b. ribosome
   c. spore
   d. cell wall
2. The proper sequence of staining in the Gram stain is:
   a. crystal violet, alcohol, Gram's iodine, safranin
   b. crystal violet, safranin, alcohol, Gram's iodine
   c. crystal violet, Gram's iodine, alcohol, safranin
   d. safranin, iodine, alcohol, Gram's iodine

3. An example of a nonselective media would be media that:
   a. contains a substance that alters the appearance of some organisms
   b. will support the growth of all organisms and does not alter their appearance
   c. supports the growth of one type of organism and inhibits the growth of other types of organisms
   d. identifies the biochemical activity of some organisms

4. When a CSF culture cannot be set up immediately, it should be placed in the incubator or remain at room temperature as opposed to being placed in the refrigerator because some organisms are affected by a low temperature. An example of this type of organism would be:
   a. *Beta streptococci*
   b. *Neisseria meningitidis*
   c. *Streptococcus pneumoniae*
   d. *Staphylococcus aureus*

5. The enterobacteriaceae are:
   a. Gram-positive organisms that include staphylococcus and streptococcus species
   b. fungal organisms that are easily identified in the laboratory
   c. Gram-negative organisms that commonly reside as normal flora in the intestinal tract but can cause infection
   d. common agents of sore throats

6. A culture from a knee wound on a young child showed a yellow creamy colony on blood agar. Given the following results, what is the most likely organism?

   Catalase—positive   Mannitol—positive
   Taxo A—negative   Coagulase—positive
   a. *Streptococcus pneumoniae*
   b. *Beta streptococcus*
   c. *Staphylococcus aureus*
   d. *Alpha streptococcus*

7. The best method of taking a specimen for the recovery of anaerobic organisms is to:
   a. swab deep and place into an anaerobic container
   b. aspirate purulent fluid and place into a test tube
   c. swab around the wound and place into an anaerobic container
   d. take as any other specimen for culture

Critical Thinking

1. Name two ways to identify whether an organism is motile.
2. If the iodine step was forgotten in a Gram stain, what color would the colonies appear?

3. Define an aerosol and explain how protection is provided when working with an aerosol.
4. What color is an acid-fast organism on a Ziehl-Neelsen stain?
5. Identify one potential pathogen and list the specimen source, media for culture, microscopic appearance, and the disease it causes.
6. A patient is given a requisition slip for a stool culture, ova and parasite examination. How would you instruct this patient to collect the specimen?
7. Explain why pinworm specimens are collected at a certain time of the day.

WEB ACTIVITIES

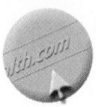

1. Visit the Centers for Disease Control and Prevention's website and other websites to review guidelines on Standard Precautions and use of personal protective equipment.

REFERENCES/BIBLIOGRAPHY

Barnett, M. (1992). *Microbiology laboratory exercises short version* (1st ed.). Dubuque, IA: Wm. C. Brown.

Baron, E. J., & Finegold, S. M. (1990). *Bailey and Scott's diagnostic microbiology* (8th ed.). St. Louis, MO: Mosby-Year Book Inc.

Garcia, L. S., & Bruckner, D. A. (1988). *Diagnostic medical parasitology* (1st ed.). New York: Elsevier.

Grover-Lakomia, L., & Fong, E. (1999). *Microbiology for health careers* (6th ed.). Albany, NY: Delmar.

Howard, B. J., Keiser, J. F., Smith, T. F., Weissfeld, A. S., & Tilton, R. C. (1994). *Clinical and pathogenic microbiology* (2nd ed.). St. Louis, MO: Mosby-Year Book Inc.

Koneman, E. W., Allen, S. D., Janda, W. M., Schreckenberger, P. C., & Winn, Jr., W. C. (1992). *Color atlas and textbook of diagnostic microbiology* (4th ed.). Philadelphia: J.B. Lippincott.

Morello, J. A., Mizer, H. E., & Wilson, M. E. (1991). *Laboratory manual and workbook in microbiology applications to patient care* (4th ed.). Dubuque, IA: Wm. C. Brown.

Walters, N. J., Estridge, B. H., & Reynolds, A. P. (2000). *Basic medical laboratory techniques* (4th ed.). Albany, NY: Delmar.

SPECIALTY LABORATORY TESTS

KEY TERMS

ABO Blood Group

Agglutination

Antibody

Antigen

Antiserum

Bilirubin

Blood Urea Nitrogen

Cholesterol

Choriocarcinoma

Cushing's Syndrome

Diabetes Mellitus

Ectopic Pregnancy

Enzyme Immunoassay

Epstein-Barr Virus (EBV)

Guthrie Screening Test

Hemolytic Anemia

Heterophile Antibodies

High-Density Lipoprotein (HDL)

Human Chorionic Gonadotropin (hCG)

Hydatidiform Mole

Hyperglycemia

Hypoglycemia

Infectious Mononucleosis

Insulin

Latex Beads

Low-Density Lipoprotein (LDL)

Mantoux Test

Phenylketonuria (PKU)

Purified Protein Derivative (PPD)

Rh Factor

Semen

Tine Test

Triglycerides

Tuberculosis

Wheal

OUTLINE

Pregnancy Tests

Commercial/Home Pregnancy Tests

Testing Methods

Slide Test or Agglutination Inhibition Test

Enzyme Immunoassay (EIA) Test

Infectious Mononucleosis

Transmission of EBV

Symptoms of Mononucleosis

Treatment of Mononucleosis

Diagnosis of Infectious Mononucleosis

Slide Test for Infectious Mononucleosis

Blood Typing: ABO Blood Groups and Rh Factor

ABO Blood Typing

Rh Blood Typing

Semen Analysis

Semen Composition

Altering Factors in Semen Analysis

Phenylketonuria (PKU) Test

Blood Testing for PKU

Urine Testing for PKU

Tuberculosis: *Mycobacterium* and TB Testing

Cause of Tuberculosis

Resistance in Mycobacteria

Transmission of Infectious Tuberculosis

Diagnosis of Tuberculosis

Screening for Tuberculosis: Skin Testing

The Mantoux Test

Blood Glucose

Fasting Blood Glucose

Two-Hour Postprandial Blood Glucose

Glucose Tolerance Test

Automated Methods of Glucose Analysis

Testing Profiles

Glycosylated Hemoglobin

Cholesterol

The Chemistry of Cholesterol

Functions of Cholesterol

Lipoproteins and Cholesterol Transport

Triglycerides

Blood Urea Nitrogen (BUN) Test

OBJECTIVES

The student should strive to meet the following performance objectives and demonstrate an understanding of the facts and principles presented in this chapter through written and oral communication.

1. Define the key terms as presented in the glossary.

2. List the three main precautions to be observed during all tests and the collection of samples included in this chapter. *(continues)*

OBJECTIVES (*continued*)

3. Collect samples and perform and interpret all tests included in this chapter.

4. Discuss factors to be considered when evaluating test results.

5. Discuss transmission, incubation period, and symptoms of EBV infectious mononucleosis.

6. List the blood group antigens and antibodies found in each of the four ABO groups and the Rh factor.

7. Explain the cause of PKU and the symptoms caused by untreated PKU.

8. Indicate normal and elevated levels of phenylalanine and the dietary restrictions to be observed by PKU patients.

9. Discuss the cause of tuberculosis and some major characteristics of *Mycobacterium tuberculosis*.

10. Discuss the role of insulin in the regulation of blood glucose levels.

11. List and discuss differences between the normal values for fasting blood glucose, two-hour postprandial glucose, and the glucose tolerance test.

12. Explain the importance of cholesterol and triglyceride testing to identify patients at high risk for coronary heart disease.

13. Give the average values of cholesterol for adults, children, infants, and newborns.

14. Give the acceptable level of LDL in persons with or without coronary heart disease and discuss the role of HDL and LDL in coronary heart disease.

15. Give the normal values of urea nitrogen for adults, children, infants, and newborns and discuss the significance of elevated blood urea levels.

ROLE DELINEATION COMPONENTS

CLINICAL

Fundamental Principles

- Apply principles of aseptic technique and infection control
- Comply with quality assurance practices
- Screen and follow up patient test results

Diagnostic Orders

- Collect and process specimens
- Perform diagnostic tests

(*continues*)

SCENARIO

Audrey Jones, CMA, has worked at Doctors Lewis and King for over five years. In that time, Audrey has become proficient in obtaining specimens from patients for various laboratory tests. Audrey enjoys the work and finds it extremely challenging. She also realizes that communicating with patients to help them understand why their specimens are necessary for testing is just as important as being skillful in collecting and testing the specimens. Audrey has found that when she explains the reason the specimen is needed in terms patients can understand, they are often less fearful, which helps them relax. This can be especially helpful when collecting blood specimens.

INTRODUCTION

An increasing number of tests are performed in the ambulatory care setting, many of them by the medical assistant. In order to meet these new demands, the medical assistant must have a strong background in a variety of areas including medical terminology, laboratory safety procedures, and specimen collection. Because many procedures require collection of a blood specimen, the medical assistant must also be an excellent phlebotomist. Good record-keeping and communications skills round out the requirements. A quality control program is necessary to assure that the results are accurate and reliable. This will require a commitment on the part of the medical assistant to maintain the highest standards throughout the process.

A variety of specialty tests are covered in this chapter, including testing for pregnancy, infectious mononucleosis, blood types, semen analysis, phenylketonuria (PKU), tuberculosis, blood glucose, cholesterol, triglycerides, and blood urea nitrogen (BUN).

PREGNANCY TESTS

Pregnancy tests are used when pregnancy is suspected. Pregnancy tests may also be used to rule out pregnancy before prescribing birth control pills, X-ray studies, certain antibiotics or other drugs, and for females who are to undergo surgery.

Pregnancy testing is based on detection of **human chorionic gonadotropin (hCG)**, a hormone secreted by the placenta that can be detected in the serum or urine of pregnant women as early as five days after conception. During pregnancy, hCG levels peak at about eight weeks, then drop to lower but detectable levels for the remainder of the pregnancy.

Commercial/Home Pregnancy Tests

A variety of accurate and easy-to-use commercial tests are available for use in the medical office. Manufacturers of pregnancy test kits have designed them to be sensitive, easy to perform and interpret, and to give rapid results. Pregnancy tests are one of the few tests available for purchase as an over-the-counter product. However, results of tests performed at home should be confirmed by a laboratory test using appropriate controls.

Testing Methods

Two testing methods using urine are discussed in this section: the slide test or agglutination inhibition test and the modified enzyme immunoassay (EIA). Diagnosis of pregnancy is made using these test results in conjunction with a physical examination including a pelvic exam by a physician. Serum pregnancy testing requires special equipment and is not usually performed in the medical office.

A positive reaction to any pregnancy test does not necessarily indicate a normal pregnancy. Detection of hCG can also indicate such abnormal conditions as an **ectopic pregnancy**, a developing **hydatidiform mole** of the uterus, **choriocarcinoma**, or cancer of the lung, stomach, pancreas, colon, or breast.

Quality Control. Kits must be stored and used at the temperature directed by the manufacturer. Most kits contain a built-in control; however, appropriate positive and negative urine controls must always be run with patient specimens. Kits and/or reagents must not be used after the expiration date. Manufacturer's instructions must be rigorously followed for the particular test used.

Slide Test or Agglutination Inhibition Test

The slide test is based on inhibition of **agglutination** (clumping) of hCG-coated **latex beads**. The hCG

Precautions for Pregnancy Testing

1. Use a clean container for collection of the urine specimen. Disposable containers are preferred. Detergent residue on nondisposable containers may interfere with test results.

2. The first-voided morning urine has the highest concentration of hCG and is the preferred specimen. If this is not available, a urine specimen with a specific gravity of at least 1.010 is acceptable.

3. If the specimen cannot be tested immediately, it may be stored at 4°C for up to twenty-four hours. Both urine and serum specimens may be used with some test kits; other kits use only one or the other.

4. Allow refrigerated urine specimens and test reagents to come to room temperature.

5. If using the slide test procedure:
   A. Avoid cross contamination with other urine specimens.
   B. Use a new stirrer for each test.

antiserum (antibody against hCG) is added to urine on a microscope slide. If hCG is present in the urine, an hCG/anti-hCG complex forms between the antiserum and the patient's hCG. Next, an antigen reagent containing latex beads coated with hCG is added to the mixture. If the hcG/anti-hCG complex formed, then there is no hCG antiserum available to react with the latex beads, and agglutination will *not* occur. Negative agglutination indicates positive pregnancy. Positive agglutination of the latex beads indicates negative pregnancy (Figure 32-1).

Enzyme Immunoassay (EIA) Test

The enzyme immunoassay (EIA) is a more complex procedure than precipitation or agglutination. The test can be designed in several different ways, but it always involves an antigen, an antibody specific for the antigen, and a second antibody conjugated to an enzyme. The test may be designed to detect a particular antibody in a patient's serum or to detect an antigen in a patient specimen.

Numerous tests are based on variations of the EIA. New technologies have been developed called membrane

EIAs. In these tests, most of the reagents are incorporated into an absorbent membrane, which is enclosed in plastic. When the sample (serum or urine) is added, it migrates through the membrane, reacting with the reagents and forming a color. Many of these tests are simple to set up and interpret even though the technology is complex. Examples of membrane EIAs include over-the-counter pregnancy test kits and tests for group A *Streptococcus*.

Enzyme immunoassays for hCG vary in design, but have some features in common. Most have the reagents incorporated into an absorbent membrane within a self-contained test unit, which may look like a plastic slide, a reagent strip, or a test cylinder. Tests may require the addition of the sample only or the addition of the sample and reagents to the test unit (Figure 32-2). Procedure 32-1 shows how to perform the enzyme immunoassay or agglutination inhibition test for pregnancy.

INFECTIOUS MONONUCLEOSIS

Infectious mononucleosis (IM) is a contagious disease that may have vague clinical symptoms and can mimic

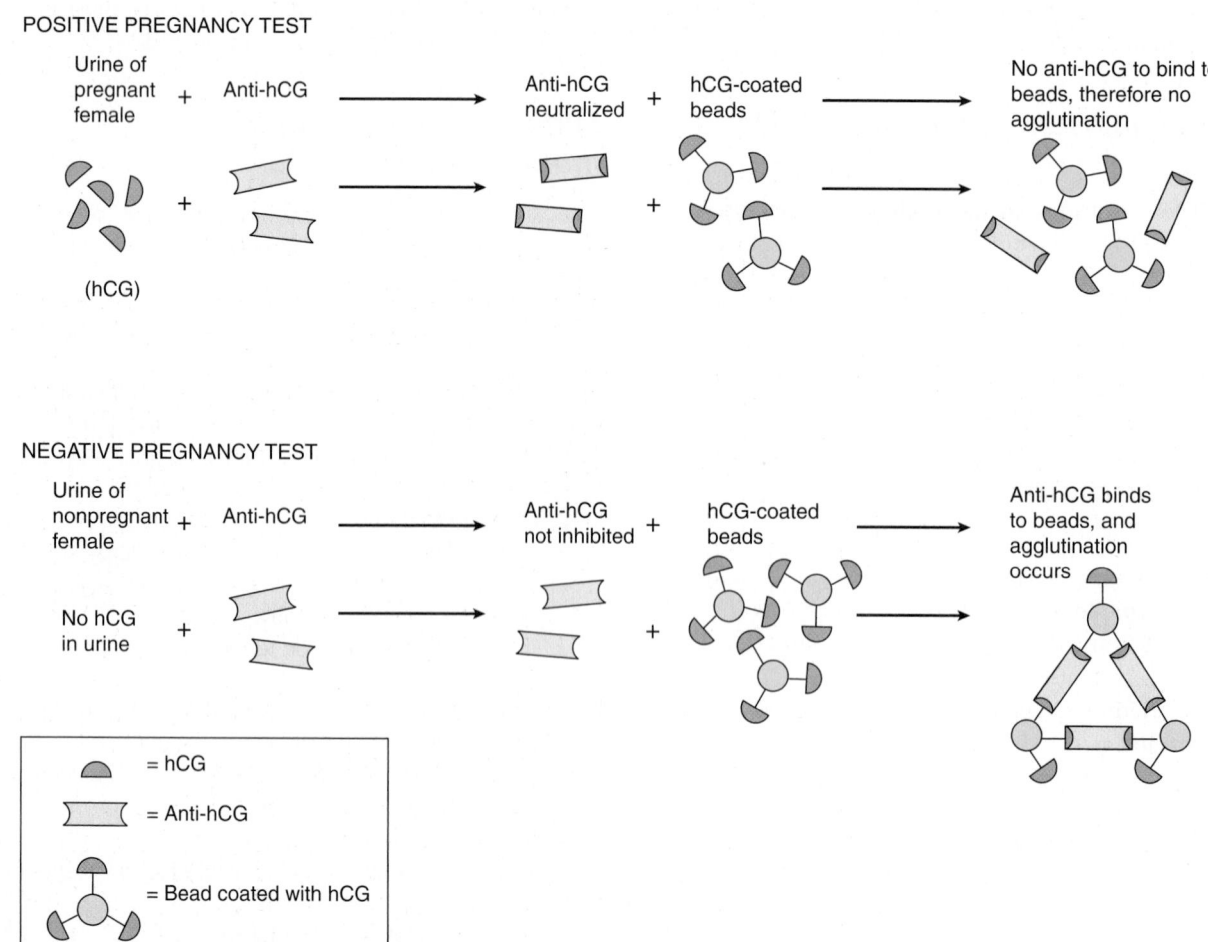

Figure 32-1   Principles of agglutination inhibition test for hCG.

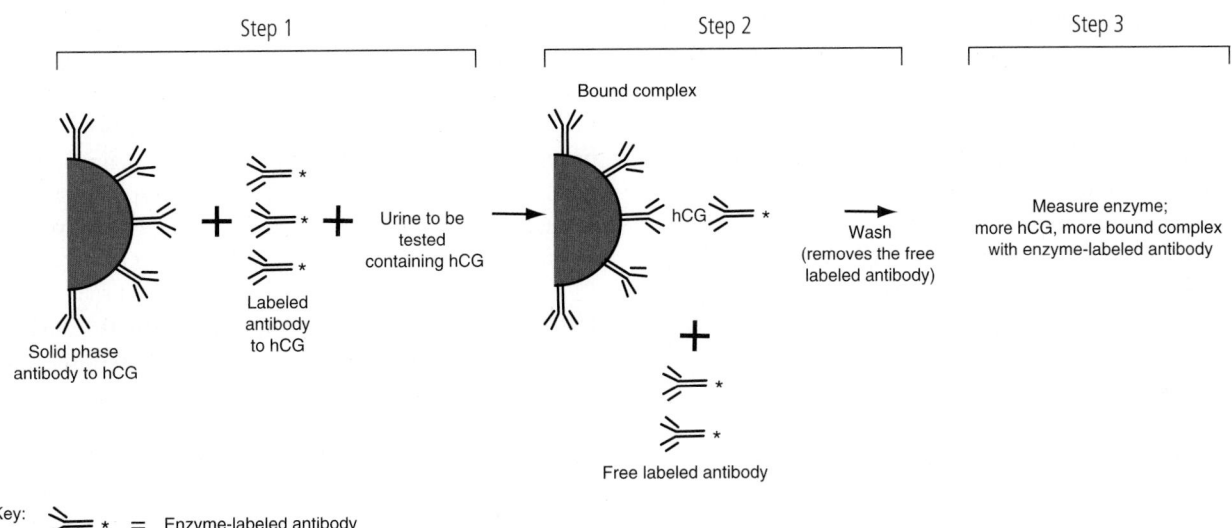

Figure 32-2   EIA test for hCG.

other diseases. Serological tests are often the basis for an early diagnosis of the disease and may also be used to follow the course of the disease.

Infectious mononucleosis is commonly called "mono" or "kissing disease." The disease is a result of infection of the lymphocytes by the **Epstein-Barr virus (EBV)**. EBV is common in our population. By five years of age approximately 50 percent of the population are infected, increasing to 90 to 95 percent in adults. After the primary infection, the virus establishes a lifelong latency. The infectious virus may be isolated from saliva for several months, while antigens may be detected for life. In addition to causing infectious mononucleosis, EBV has been implicated in other diseases such as African Burkitt's lymphoma (a lymphoma of the lower jaw), nasopharyngeal carcinoma (NPC), and chronic fatigue syndrome.

Transmission of EBV

Transmission of EBV infectious mononucleosis is primarily by saliva which is why it is often referred to as "the kissing disease." EBV may also be spread by the sharing of drinking glasses and less often by blood transfusion. The disease is moderately contagious and is transmitted approximately 10 to 38 percent of the time in close social groups. In the home or in the hospital, careful handwashing will help prevent transmission of the virus.

Symptoms of Mononucleosis

Mononucleosis is seen most often in children and young adults. Incubation may vary from 4 to 50 days, however 7 to 14 days is the average. Infection in younger children is usually asymptomatic or manifests minor symptoms such as pharyngitis, otitis media, bronchitis, and other upper respiratory discomforts.

Classic symptoms usually occur when the primary infection is delayed until the second decade of life. It is the 15- to 25-year-old age group in which infectious mononucleosis is most often observed. Symptoms usually begin with a fever and swollen glands lasting for 3 to 5 days. Over the next 7 to 20 days the patient may develop a headache, malaise, chest pain, a cough, tonsillitis, a rash, soft, swollen lymph nodes, and a swollen spleen. Symptoms usually persist for 2 to 4 weeks and in more serious cases may last for more than a month.

Treatment of Mononucleosis

Because there are currently no effective drugs available for EBV infectious mononucleosis, treatment is primarily supportive. Although a vaccine is not yet available, some important work in that direction is ongoing.

Diagnosis of Infectious Mononucleosis

In order to properly diagnose IM, hematological and serological test results must be considered along with the clinical symptoms.

Hematological Test for Infectious Mononucleosis. The hematological test for IM includes a white blood cell count and evaluation of the patient's lymphocytes. In IM, a lymphocytosis, or increase in lymphocytes, usually occurs and large numbers of lymphocytes (greater than 20 percent) have an unusual or atypical appearance. Atypical lymphocytosis has a 95 percent specificity for patients with EBV mononucleosis, but is relatively insensitive for diagnosis. Because of this, serological testing is the method of choice for diagnosis of IM.

Serological Test for Infectious Mononucleosis. Persons with IM produce antibodies called heterophile antibodies by the sixth to tenth day of the illness. Heterophile antibodies are antibodies that react with similar antigens in more than one species. They are usually of the IgM class.

Detection of heterophile antibodies combined with the hematological and clinical findings provide the basis for the diagnosis of IM. The serological test is usually positive after the first week of illness. However, if test results are negative, the test should be repeated after a week if clinical symptoms are still present.

Slide Test for Infectious Mononucleosis

The most common serological test used for IM is a rapid slide test, which tests patients' serum for the presence of heterophile antibodies. The slide test gives quick, reliable results and is simple to perform. Tests are also available that detect antibodies to Epstein-Barr virus, the cause of IM.

Several commercial kits are available to test for IM. Most kits are based on agglutination principles and are adaptations of the Davidsohn differential test for heterophile antibodies, a cumbersome, time-consuming test. Colorimetric immunoassay kits for IM are also available from several manufacturers. Examples of IM kits include Color Slide® II Mononucleosis Test by Seradyn, BBL®

Monoslide™ Test by Becton Dickinson, Monospot® Slide Test by Meridian Diagnostics, and Monosticon Dri-Dot® by Organon Teknika Corporation.

Serological kits for infectious mononucleosis usually provide all the necessary reagents, materials, and controls. The laboratory must provide only the specimen to be tested, which is usually a small sample of the patient's plasma or serum, or a drop of capillary blood.

Performing the Slide Agglutination Test for IM. The principles for each manufacturer's test are the same; however, the instructions for the specific kit used should be strictly followed. The procedure for detecting the heterophile antibodies of IM described in this example is based on the Monospot® test by Meridian Diagnostics.

The test is performed using a glass slide that has two squares (I and II) etched on the slide. The reagent and patient sample are mixed thoroughly and a drop of indicator cells (horse erythrocytes) is added to a corner of each square using the capillary pipette provided in the kit (Figure 32-3).

The serum and reagent I are mixed using at least ten stirring motions with a clean wooden applicator stick. The indicator cells are then blended in so that the entire surface of the square is covered. The contents of square II are mixed in the same manner as square I (Figure 32-4).

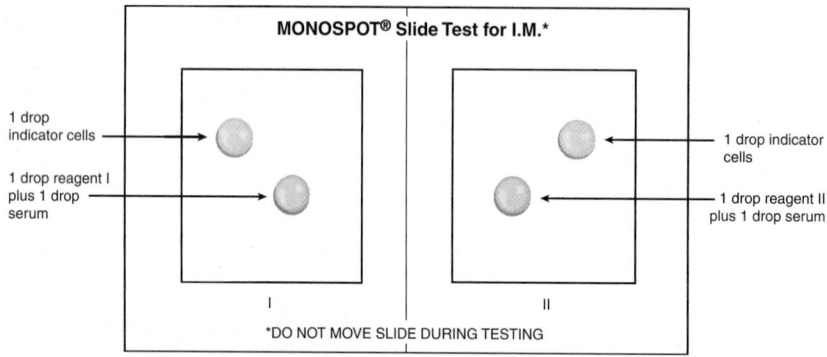

Figure 32-3   Monospot® slide with reagents added.

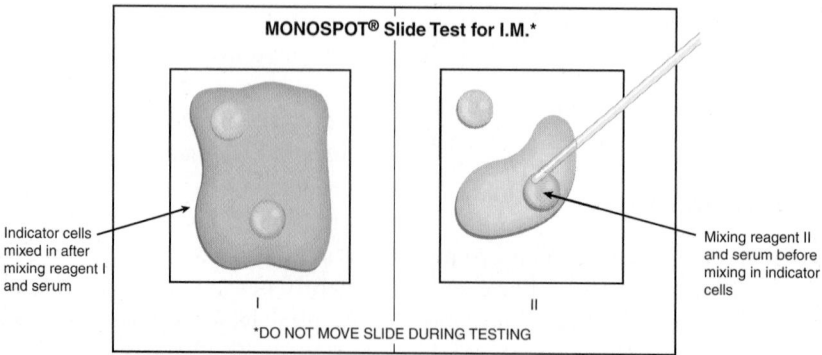

Figure 32-4   Mixing reagents on Monospot® slide using wooden applicator.

Do not use the contaminated applicator stick used to mix reagent I.

A timer is started as soon as mixing is completed and the slide is observed for one minute for agglutination of the horse cells. During this time, the slide should not be moved or picked up. At the end of one minute, the results are recorded and interpreted. Positive and negative serum controls provided with the kit should be tested in the same manner to ensure that all reagents are reacting properly.

Interpreting Results of Slide Test for IM. The presence or absence of heterophile antibodies of infectious mononucleosis will be indicated by the presence or absence of agglutination, as indicated in Table 32-1. See Procedure 32-2 for the steps involved in performing a slide test for infectious mononucleosis.

BLOOD TYPING: ABO BLOOD GROUPS AND RH FACTOR

Blood typing is based on the presence or absence of certain antigens on the surface of red blood cells (RBC). These antigens are carbohydrate molecules that react with antibodies specific to them to cause agglutination of the RBCs. Antibodies are protein molecules that are found in serum; they are also referred to as immunoglobulins (Ig). When RBC antigens and antibodies react, they cause the RBCs to agglutinate. This process is called hemagglutination. Hemagglutination reactions are used in the typing of blood. The two major categories of blood typing are for the **ABO blood group** and the **Rh factor**. Figure 32-5 illustrates how red blood cells are tested for blood type.

The ABO and Rh systems place certain restrictions on how blood may be transfused from one individual to another. Depending on their blood type, persons with a particular RBC antigen may have antibodies against the other type or types (Table 32-2). An incompatible blood transfusion results when the antigens of the donor RBCs react with the antibodies of the recipient RBCs. This is a potentially life-threatening situation, varying in severity from mild fever to anaphylaxis with severe intravascular hemolysis. Although ABO and Rh typing does not completely rule out the possibility of reaction, it greatly reduces the chances.

ABO Blood Typing

ABO blood typing is determined by the presence or absence of two major antigens, A and B. All people have one of the four blood group categories: A, B, AB, or O. People with group A RBCs have A antigens, group B RBCs have B antigens, group AB RBCs have antigens for

TABLE 32-1	INTERPRETATION OF MONOSPOT® TEST RESULTS
Positive Test	**Negative Test**
Agglutination pattern is stronger on the left side of the slide (square I) than on the right side of the slide (square II).	A. Agglutination pattern is stronger on the right side of the slide (square II) than on square I. *or* B. No agglutination appears in either square. *or* C. Agglutination is equal in both squares of the slide.

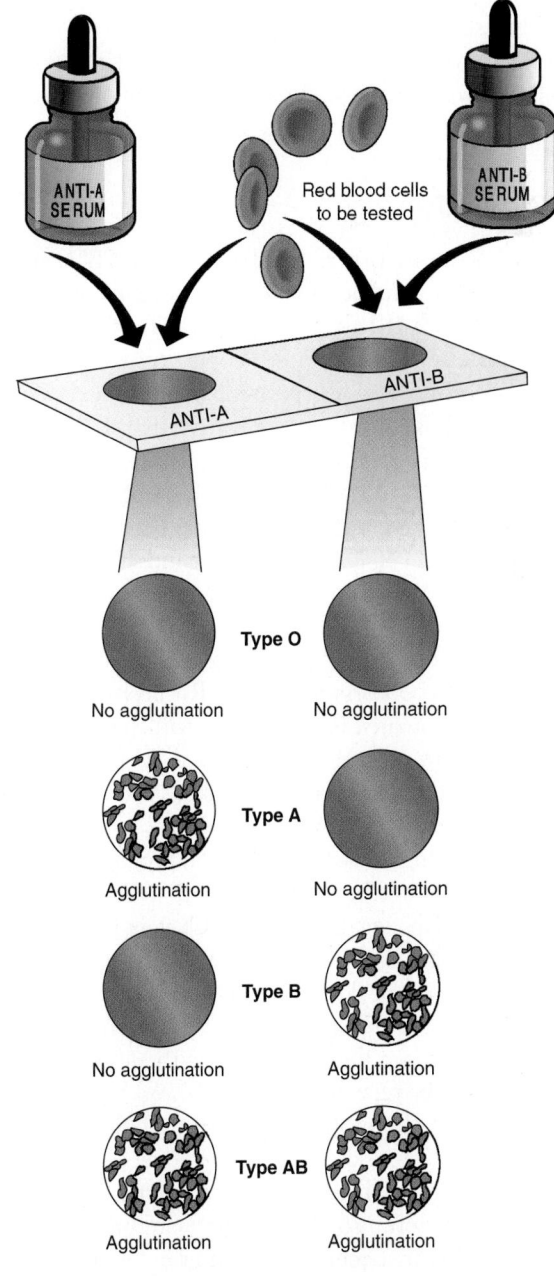

Figure 32-5 Blood typing ABO groups.

TABLE 32-2	ANTIGENS AND ANTIBODIES IN ABO AND RH BLOOD SYSTEMS	
Blood Group/Type	**Antigen on RBC**	**Serum Antibodies**
O (Universal donor)	None	Anti-A and Anti-B
A	A	Anti-B
B	B	Anti-A
AB	A and B	None
Rh+	D	No anti-D*
Rh–	D	No anti-D*

*There are no naturally occurring antibodies to the Rh system.

both A and B, and group O RBCs lack both A and B antigens. Naturally occurring antibodies to the other antigen types are found in the serum.

ABO type may be determined by the slide or tube method. The tube method is now most often used for blood typing.

Rh Blood Typing

Rh typing is routinely performed along with ABO typing. The Rh system is named for the rhesus monkey used in experiments that led to its discovery. The Rh factor is found on the surface of RBCs. People possessing the Rh factor are said to have Rh positive (Rh+) blood. Those without the Rh factor have Rh negative (Rh–) blood.

About 85 percent of North Americans are Rh positive, 15 percent Rh negative. Neither Rh negative nor Rh positive people have naturally occuring Rh antibodies in their blood. However, if an Rh negative individual receives a transfusion of Rh positive blood, he or she will develop antibodies to it. The antibodies take two weeks to develop. Generally, there is no problem with the first transfusion. However, if a second transfusion of Rh positive blood is given, the accumulated Rh antibodies will clump with the Rh antigen of the blood being received. Therefore, both blood type and Rh factor must be taken into account for safe and successful transfusions.

Blood typing is also performed on pregnant patients to determine the mother's blood type. In situations where the mother is Rh negative or type O, it is necessary to determine the father's blood type as well. If his blood is Rh positive or types A or B or AB, the mother's blood should be further tested for the presence of Rh antibodies. If the test is negative, then there is no risk to the fetus. A negative test should be repeated at weeks 30 and 36. If the test is positive, then the mother has been immunized by the Rh factor of the fetus and has produced antibodies referred to as anti-D (D is a major factor in the Rh group). A positive reaction also means that maternal hemolysis of fetal RBCs can occur. This condition is also called hemolytic disease of the newborn (HDN). The severity of

hemolytic anemia can be determined by evaluation of the quantity of bilirubin in the amniotic fluid. Fortunately, most cases of HDN can be prevented by administering RhoGAM to the Rh negative mother. RhoGAM is a concentrated solution of anti-D. When injected into the mother, RhoGAM will prevent her from producing the anti-D antibody. The injection must be administered within 72 hours after delivery of an Rh-positive baby or termination of pregnancy.

SEMEN ANALYSIS

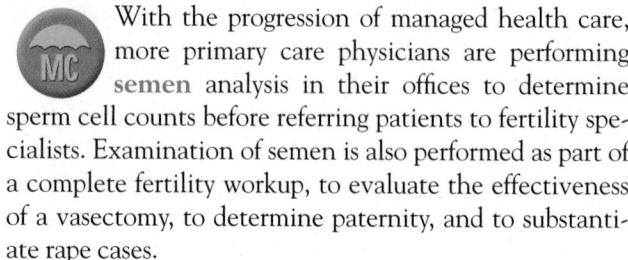

With the progression of managed health care, more primary care physicians are performing semen analysis in their offices to determine sperm cell counts before referring patients to fertility specialists. Examination of semen is also performed as part of a complete fertility workup, to evaluate the effectiveness of a vasectomy, to determine paternity, and to substantiate rape cases.

When semen analysis is performed as part of a fertility workup, the procedure involves macroscopic and microscopic analysis of seminal fluid for determination of total sperm count, percent of motility, presence of agglutination, and percent of normally formed sperm cells (Table 32-3). All individuals will have variable sperm counts; therefore a single analysis is insufficient. To achieve a reasonable estimate of these factors, the seminal analysis should be repeated at least three times over a two-month

TABLE 32-3	REFERENCE VALUES FOR SEMEN ANALYSIS
Parameter	**Normal Range**
Appearance	White, viscid, opaque
Volume	1.5–5 mL
pH	7.12–8.00
Total count	50–200 million
% normal sperm	At least 80%
% motility	At least 60%

period. A complete analysis will also include an evaluation of the partner's cervical secretions and sperm survival. This involves determining the ability of sperm to penetrate the mucus and maintain motility.

Vasectomies are evaluated about six weeks after surgery. If sperm are seen at that time, then the effectiveness of the procedure is questionable and a follow-up analysis is required.

Semen Composition

Semen is a composite solution produced by the testes and the accessory male reproductive organs. It consists primarily of spermatozoa suspended in seminal plasma. Because there is considerable variation in composition between different portions of the fluid as ejaculated, it is important to collect the entire sample.

Altering Factors in Semen Analysis

Many factors can alter the results of semen analysis. Several drugs such as Cytoxan (cyclophosphamide) and nitrogen mustard lower sperm count. So may orchitis (inflammation of the testes), testicular atrophy, testicular failure, and obstruction of the vas deferens. Cigarette

---

Patient Teaching Tip

The following instructions should be given to male patients when a semen sample is required for analysis:

1. Advise the patient to avoid consumption of alcohol for several days prior to the test. He should also avoid ejaculation for three days prior to collection of the semen sample.
2. Provide the patient with instructions and a container. The entire sample should be collected in a clean, dry, glass bottle that has been labeled, dated, and timed. The sample is collected by masturbation or interrupted coitus at home or may be collected at the medical office of the laboratory. Never collect the specimen into a condom.
3. Specimens for complete fertility analysis collected outside the laboratory must be brought to the laboratory within 30 minutes. Postvasectomy specimens should be brought to the laboratory within one hour of collection.
4. The sample must be transported to the laboratory at 37°C (98.6°F). Low temperature during transport will decrease the motility of sperm.

---

smoking is associated with a decrease in the volume of semen, while coffee drinking results in increased sperm density and an increase in the percentage of cells with abnormal morphology. Fever may temporarily suppress the count. Although research suggests that consumption of alcohol does not affect sperm function as measured by semen analysis, the patient is instructed to avoid alcohol for several days prior to testing as a precaution.

Although research suggests that fertility is most closely correlated with motility and morphology, men with very high (> 200 million/mL) or very low (≤ 20 million/mL) counts are likely to be infertile. Patients with aspermia (no sperm) or oligospermia (low sperm count, ≤ 20 million/mL) should be endocrinologically evaluated for pituitary, testicular, adrenal, or thyroid abnormalities.

Procedure 32-3 gives the steps for analyzing semen.

PHENYLKETONURIA (PKU) TEST

Phenylketonuria (PKU) is an inherited condition in which the amino acid phenylalanine is not metabolized, causing urine to have a mousy or musty odor. It is important that all newborns be tested for PKU because progressive mental retardation, tremors, and loss of muscle coordination can result if the condition is allowed to go untreated. Diagnosis must be made early so that a low-phenylalanine diet can begin immediately. Although the phenylalanine-restricted diet will prevent mental retardation, it will not cure the underlying condition. Routine screening of newborns for PKU is mandatory in most states and may be performed in the hospital or the medical office. The medical assistant's role is to properly explain the procedure to the infant's parents and collect the blood specimen for analysis.

Excess phenylalanine can be detected in blood or in urine. Normal levels of phenylalanine are less than 2 mg/deciliter (dL); more than 4 mg/dL is considered elevated. The **Guthrie screening test** is used to evaluate blood and is considered more accurate than urine tests. Phenylalanine can be detected in the blood of infants with PKU after three to four days on a breast milk or formula milk diet. Testing of breast-fed infants is delayed a few days due to the lack of phenylalanine in colostrum, the first breast milk. Colostrum is produced for the first two to three days after birth and is rich in antibodies, protein, and calories. True breast milk production begins after this time. Urine testing can detect PKU in infants who are at least 6 weeks of age and is usually done at the first checkup. A positive urine test is followed up with a blood test. Positive results from either blood or urine testing are confirmed by measuring serum phenylalanine and tyrosine levels. Infants with PKU have increasing phenylalanine levels (> 4 mg/dL) and decreasing tyrosine levels (< 0.6 mg/dL).

Patient Teaching Tip

Infants who test positive for PKU require a restricted-phenylalanine diet for normal development to occur. Instruct the mother to provide a low-phenylalanine diet. This will include a suitable milk substitute such as Lofenalac™, and later the addition of strained, low-protein foods. Blood and urine testing will continue to monitor the special diet.

Women of reproductive age who have PKU and want to have children must be instructed to begin a restricted-phenylalanine diet prior to conception to reduce the risk of damage to the fetus. Remaining on a general diet poses a high risk of producing a mentally retarded infant.

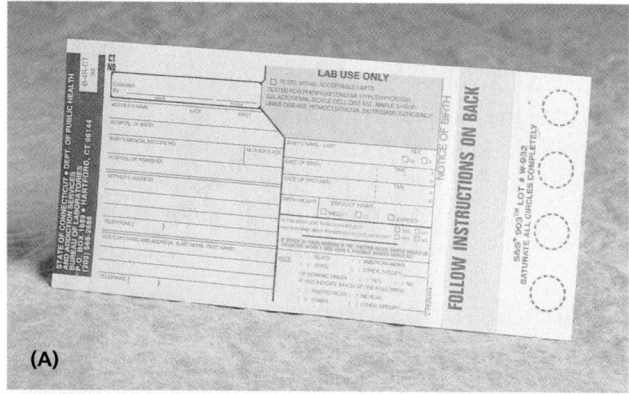

(A)

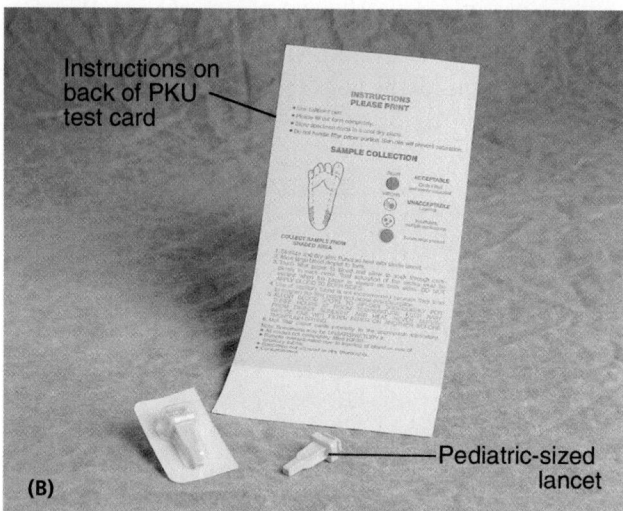

Instructions on back of PKU test card

Pediatric-sized lancet

(B)

Figure 32-6   (A) A filter paper test card is used to collect samples of infant's blood to screen for PKU. (B) Pediatric-sized lancets are available to limit the depth of the puncture when obtaining the blood sample from the infant. The back of the filter paper test card provides detailed instructions on performing the test and completing the card for testing.

Blood Testing for PKU

The Guthrie test was developed to screen for phenylalanine in the blood and is usually performed prior to the discharge of infants from the hospital. However, with managed care and the trend toward very short hospital stays for newborns, many pediatrician offices are now performing this test. Capillary blood is collected from a heel stick onto a "filter paper" test card and sent to the laboratory for testing. Patient, physician, and test information along with the blood samples are placed directly on the lab test card which is typically provided by most State Departments of Health (Figure 32-6). See Procedure 32-4, Obtaining Blood Sample for Phenylketonuria (PKU) test. Refer to Chapter 28 for proper capillary puncture technique.

Factors that May Influence the Guthrie Test

1. Feeding problems such as vomiting may result in a false negative reaction.
2. Failure to ingest sufficient phenylalanine—testing prior to three to four days of the beginning of a milk diet—will result in a false negative reaction.
3. Premature infants may give false positive test results due to a delay in the development of certain liver enzymes.
4. If either the mother (if breastfeeding) or the child is taking drugs such as salicylates, aspirin, or antibiotics, they may interfere with the test results.

Urine Testing for PKU

Urine testing can detect PKU in infants who are at least 6 weeks of age and is usually done at the first checkup and on infants who are on low-phenylalanine diets due to a previous positive test for PKU. Procedure 32-5 gives the steps to obtain a urine sample for the PKU test.

A positive urine test should be followed up with a blood test for PKU.

TUBERCULOSIS: MYCOBACTERIUM AND TB TESTING

Despite efforts to control its spread, **tuberculosis** infections are on the increase in the United States and around the world. Latent infection with tuberculosis is estimated in approximately 10 million United States residents and 2 billion persons worldwide. Because tuberculosis morbidity is on the rise, increasing 14 percent from 1985 to 1993 (*Nursing*, 1995) more patients are screened for the disease now than ever before. The Advisory Council for Elimination of Tuberculosis, an independent group of TB-control experts, recommends screening all patients who fall into high-risk groups. High-risk patients include those infected with the HIV virus, those who have had close contact with someone who has active TB, and those living or working in high-risk gathered settings (such as health care facilities, correctional facilities, and homeless shelters).

Cause of Tuberculosis

Infectious tuberculosis is caused by the small, rod-shaped bacterium, *Mycobacterium tuberculosis*. This aerobic bacterium is nonmotile and has a high content of lipid in its cell wall making it difficult to stain using basic aniline dyes. For this reason, the Ziehl-Neelsen method was developed and is used as a tool for identification of mycobacteria. Mycobacteria will retain the red stain in the presence of acid alcohol and are therefore referred to as "acid-fast." Other bacterial species stain blue. Refer back to Chapter 31 for additional information on the Ziehl-Neelsen stain.

Resistance in Mycobacteria

Mycobacteria exhibit an unusual degree of resistance on many fronts. They are able to tolerate drying and the effects of many disinfectants. Mycobacteria also show resistance to most antibiotics, making these infections very difficult to treat. To help overcome bacterial resistance to antimicrobial agents, patients take two or three drugs for a period of six to nine months. Mycobacteria are, however, susceptible to heat and are killed in milk by pasteurization (62°C for 30 minutes).

Transmission of Infectious Tuberculosis

Infectious tuberculosis is highly contagious. Seventy-five percent of new cases occur by inhalation of cough-produced airborne droplets from symptomatic or asymptomatic persons. Crowded conditions contribute to this transmission. Tuberculosis is often associated with poverty and is often seen in prisons and mental health hospitals. Occasionally, transmission through the skin or the GI tract may occur. A recent increase in tuberculosis is related to the rise in AIDS.

Diagnosis of Tuberculosis

One factor that complicates the diagnosis of tuberculosis is the fact that Mycobacteria are slow growers in the laboratory taking anywhere from 30 to 60 days. The average for *Mycobacterium tuberculosis* is 14 to 21 days with best growth in the laboratory on Lowenstein-Jensen agar. This means that isolation, identification, and diagnosis may take up to eight weeks. Recently, DNA probe technology for the identification of *Mycobacterium* species has been developed for the medical laboratory. The major advantage of these probes is rapid identification, within 1 to 2 hours.

Patients exhibiting a positive or questionable **purified protein derivative (PPD)** reaction should have a chest X ray to examine for tubercles, and a sputum sample should be stained to search for acid-fast rods. The presence of acid-fast rods in the sputum confirms active tuberculosis. Reasons for a positive reaction to PPD are varied. First and most obvious is that the patient has an active case of tuberculosis. Persons with an old, inactive case will also give a positive skin test as will persons who have been vaccinated with BCG. BCG (the bacille of Calmette and Guerin) is a vaccine made from live, avirulent M. *bovis*. The vaccine is used in Europe to help prevent childhood cases of tuberculosis. Persons who receive BCG will give a positive skin reaction for a minimum of four years, much longer in many cases.

Screening for Tuberculosis: Skin Testing

Screening for tuberculosis may be performed as part of a routine medical examination or as a prerequisite for school or employment. In states where medical assistants can legally perform injections, they may be responsible for administration and interpretation of the skin test. The most accurate method used is the **Mantoux test**. The **tine test**, which is a multiple-puncture test, may still be used in some areas but is no longer recommended by the American Academy of Pediatrics. Both the Mantoux and the tine methods use tuberculin, which is also referred to as PPD. PPD stands for purified protein derivative, and is a filtrate of tuberculin cultures that are used for skin testing. Persons who have been exposed to tuberculosis will develop a hypersensitive response to PPD resulting in the formation of an induration. An induration is a hard, red spot on the skin that is the result of sensitized lymphocytes migrating to the site of the injection. It is important to keep in mind that a positive skin test does not distinguish between active or inactive cases of tuberculosis. Again, a positive skin test will require further diagnostic testing including an X ray for lung lesions and an acid-fast stain of sputum to examine for the presence of *Mycobacterium tuberculosis*. Because of the severity of the reaction, do not administer the skin test to persons who have had a positive reaction in the past.

The Mantoux Test

In the Mantoux test, 0.1 mL of 5 TU (toxin unit) strength PPD is injected intradermally using a 1.0 mL tuberculin

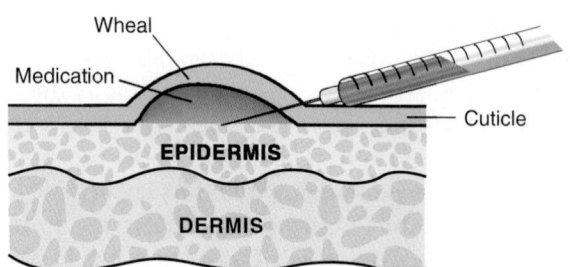

Figure 32-7   A raised wheal will form when the PPD is properly administered with an intradermal injection.

syringe. A short (⅜–½″), 26 or 27 gauge needle is used. Care must be taken to inject the PPD so that a **wheal** forms (Figure 32-7). If the injection is too deep, it will be impossible to read the wheal. If the injection is too shallow, the PPD may leak onto the skin. Either of these two errors would invalidate the test results. It is also very important to draw exactly 0.1 mL of the PPD as too much or too little would also lead to erroneous test results.

Choosing a Site to Administer the Mantoux Test. To select a site for the Mantoux test, locate a site approximately 3 to 4 inches down from the bend of the arm on the anterior side. Avoid areas with excess hair, visible blood vessels, or scar tissue. The chosen site should be cleaned with alcohol and allowed to dry prior to administering the PPD.

SPOTLIGHT ON AAMA ESSENTIALS THROUGH CAAHEP

● When assisting pediatric patients, one way the medical assistant can gain the patient's trust and put him or her at ease is to make a game out of the procedure.

● Being aware of a patient's modesty and sensitivity while he or she is being examined will help to establish a positive rapport and help the patient to get through the examination in an expeditious manner.

● Often, taking a few moments to hold a patient's hand or talk to him or her before an examination will help to alleviate excessive fears and undue stress the patient may be experiencing.

BLOOD GLUCOSE

Glucose is the principal and almost exclusive carbohydrate found circulating in blood. It may also be detected in urine, cerebral spinal fluid, and semen. Glucose serves as an energy source for the body. Excess glucose is converted into glycogen for short-term storage in the liver and muscle cells, and as adipose tissue for long-term storage. Tests for blood glucose levels are commonly performed in the medical office. The results are used to screen for carbohydrate disorders such as **hypoglycemia** (low blood glucose level), **hyperglycemia** (high blood glucose level which occurs in **diabetes mellitus**), and liver dysfunction. A variety of testing methods have been developed to diagnose, evaluate, and monitor abnormalities in carbohydrate metabolism. They include the fasting blood sugar, the two-hour postprandial blood sugar, and the glucose tolerance test. All are briefly discussed here.

Blood glucose concentrations rise after a meal and are regulated by the action of several hormones including **insulin** and glucagon. Both insulin and glucagon are produced by the pancreas. Insulin is secreted by pancreatic cells in response to increased glucose levels and aids with the entry of glucose into cells for conversion into energy. Insulin is also required for proper storage of glucose (which is first converted into glycogen) in the liver and in muscle cells. Glucagon is secreted by the pancreas when blood sugar levels drop and triggers the breakdown of glycogen to help raise and regulate blood sugar levels.

Fasting Blood Glucose

Evaluation of fasting blood glucose levels is commonly used to screen for diabetes mellitus. Diabetes mellitus is a type of carbohydrate disorder characterized by insulin deficiency (or no insulin) and a state of hyperglycemia.

The normal fasting value of glucose ranges from 70–110 mg/100 mL (mg/dL). Refer to Table 32-4 for reference glucose values. 120 mg/dL of glucose is the dividing point between normal and hyperglycemic individuals.

Patient Teaching Tip

In preparation for the test, the patient should be instructed to fast for 12 hours (except for water). A fasting blood sample is usually collected in the morning to minimize inconvenience to the patient. Certain drugs such as oral contraceptives, salicylates, diuretics, and steroids may alter the results so the physician may restrict their use for two to three days prior to the test.

TABLE 32-4	REFERENCE VALUES FOR BLOOD GLUCOSE LEVELS
Test	**Glucose Concentration (mg/dL)**
Fasting	
Serum	70–110
Whole blood	60–100
2-hour postprandial	≤ 110
Glucose Tolerance (oral, serum)	
Fasting	70–110
1 hour	20–50 above fasting
2 hour	5–15 above fasting
3 hour	fasting level or below
Values vary slightly between laboratories depending on testing method used.	

Generally, truly elevated glucose levels indicate diabetes mellitus. Other causes of hyperglycemia include **Cushing's syndrome** and acute stress response. Elevated blood glucose levels should be further evaluated using the glucose tolerance test.

Two-Hour Postprandial Blood Glucose

The two-hour postprandial (after eating) evaluation of blood glucose levels is used to screen for diabetes and to monitor insulin dosage. After fasting from midnight the night before, the patient eats a prescribed meal containing 100 grams of carbohydrate or consumes a 100-gram glucose test load solution such as Glucola®. Two hours later a blood specimen is collected and tested for glucose concentration. Glucose levels will return to or fall below the fasting level within two hours in nondiabetic individuals. Diabetic patients will have glucose levels of 140 mg/dL or higher. Elevated glucose levels should be further examined using the glucose tolerance test.

Glucose Tolerance Test

The glucose tolerance test provides more detailed information used to assess insulin response to glucose and to diagnose diabetes.

Patient Teaching Tip

The patient should be instructed to eat a high carbohydrate diet (300 g/day) for three days prior to the glucose tolerance test and to fast for 12 hours prior to collection of the blood specimen.

Fasting blood and urine specimens are drawn and evaluated for glucose level. If the results indicate hyperglycemia, the physician should be notified immediately. Hyperglycemia after fasting is abnormal and not an appropriate condition for further loading with additional glucose and may be dangerous to the patient. If glucose levels fall within the normal reference values, then the test may continue.

After providing the fasting urine and blood specimens, the patient consumes a glucose test solution containing 1.75 grams of glucose/kilogram of body weight, or the standard adult dose of 100 grams. Blood and urine specimens are typically collected at thirty minutes, one hour, two hours, three hours (and sometimes six hours) after ingestion of the glucose solution and are tested for glucose level. These measurements help determine the patient's ability to deal with increased glucose. During the test, the patient must not ingest anything except water. The patient must also abstain from smoking, as smoking acts as a stimulant and increases blood glucose levels.

During the second and third hours of the test, the patient may experience weakness, slight faintness, and perspire. These are all normal symptoms. If, however, the patient develops a headache, faints, or displays irrational speech or behavior, she may be experiencing hypoglycemic shock and the physician should be notified immediately.

The blood glucose level of nondiabetic patients usually peaks thirty to sixty minutes after consumption of the test load at 160–180 mg/dL and returns to the fasting level after two to three hours. Diabetic patients will still have elevated glucose levels at the end of the test.

Automated Methods of Glucose Analysis

Several types of glucose analyzers are available that are suitable for physician's office laboratories (POLs) or small clinical laboratories. Many of these operate on the principle of reflectance photometry and use adaptations of the enzymatic methods of glucose analysis. One example of an instrument suitable for small laboratories is the HemoCue® blood glucose analyzer.

Several small, inexpensive, handheld glucose meters are also made and are designed for home use by diabetics. Most of these are suitable for use in point-of-care (POC) testing or in physician's offices (Figure 32-8).

Glucose controls may be purchased from the instrument manufacturers to check instrument performance. It is always necessary to use test materials that are made for a particular instrument only with that instrument.

All of these analyzers are designed to be easy to use and to give rapid results. In general, better accuracy and precision (reproducibility) is obtained with the analyzers

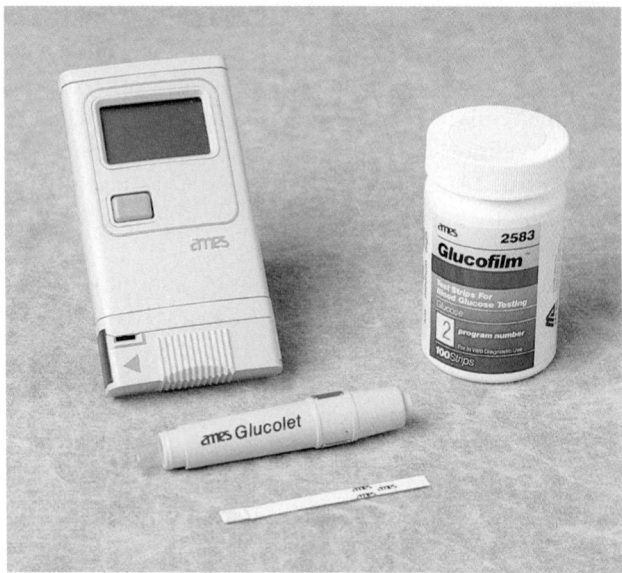

Figure 32-8 A variety of handheld glucose analyzers are now available for home and office use. These analyzers have become less expensive; however, the cost of the strips needed for the tests used can be expensive especially if used three times a day as recommended by most manufacturers. These analyzers do allow diabetics to safely test and track their blood glucose levels to help control diabetes.

designed for laboratory use than with the handheld photometers. With all instruments, it is necessary to use consistent proper specimen collection and testing technique to avoid variations in results.

Photometry Analyzers. The HemoCue® Blood-Glucose system is a compact glucose analyzer based on the principle of photometry. The system consists of a compact photometer and disposable microcuvettes. The self-filling microcuvette automatically draws up 5 μL of blood from a capillary puncture into its reaction chamber. The micro-

cuvette is then placed into the holder and pushed into the photometer. The glucose concentration in mg/dL is displayed within 45 to 240 seconds (Figure 32-9). This system is ideal for POLs and POC testing because of the stability of calibration and the minimum operator training required.

Reflectance Photometry Analyzers. Several glucose analyzers are available that are based on reflectance photometry. Blood from a fingerstick, serum, or plasma is applied to the reagent area of a test strip. The glucose in the sample reacts with the reagents in the pad(s) causing a color to form. The more glucose present in the sample, the darker or more intense the color. At the appropriate time, the strip is inserted into the test chamber and light is directed onto the test area. The amount of light reflected from the colored test area is measured by the photometer and converted to a digital readout showing the glucose concentration in mg/dL or mmol/L. Most instruments give results in one to three minutes. Instructions included with the test strips must be followed carefully for reliable test results. See Procedure 32-7, Measurement of Blood Glucose Using an Automated Analyzer.

Testing Profiles

Glucose testing may be part of a general profile chemistry test which can be useful in giving an overall view of an individual's state of health, especially when used in conjunction with other tests. Glucose testing may also be performed as part of a specific chemistry profile (renal profile) to determine the function of a particular biological system (Figure 32-10). The renal profile helps determine normal or abnormal function of the kidney. Another test in the renal profile of tests is the BUN, which is discussed later in this chapter.

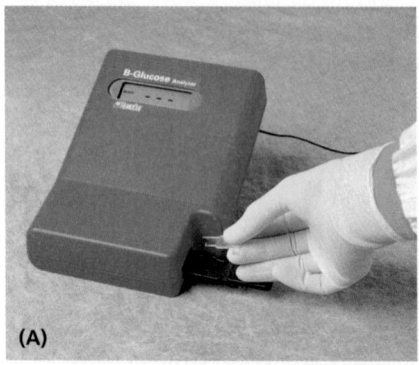
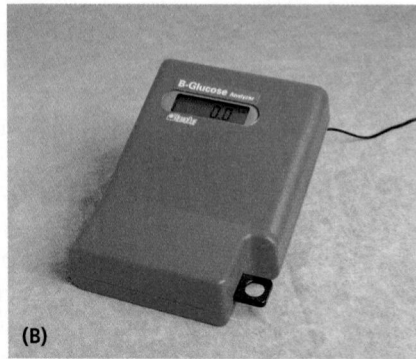
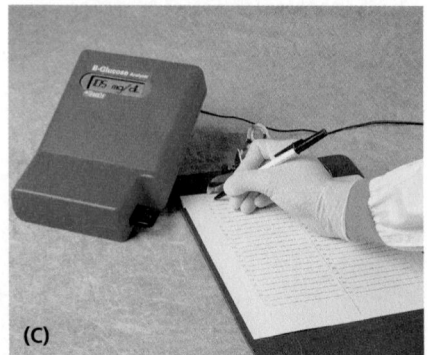

(A) **(B)** **(C)**

Figure 32-9 HemoCue® Blood-Glucose System: (A) A blood specimen is placed on the microcuvette, inserted into its holder, and pushed into the photometer. (B) Specimen is allowed to remain in analyzer until test is complete. (C) Glucose concentration is displayed in mg/dL after 45 to 240 seconds.

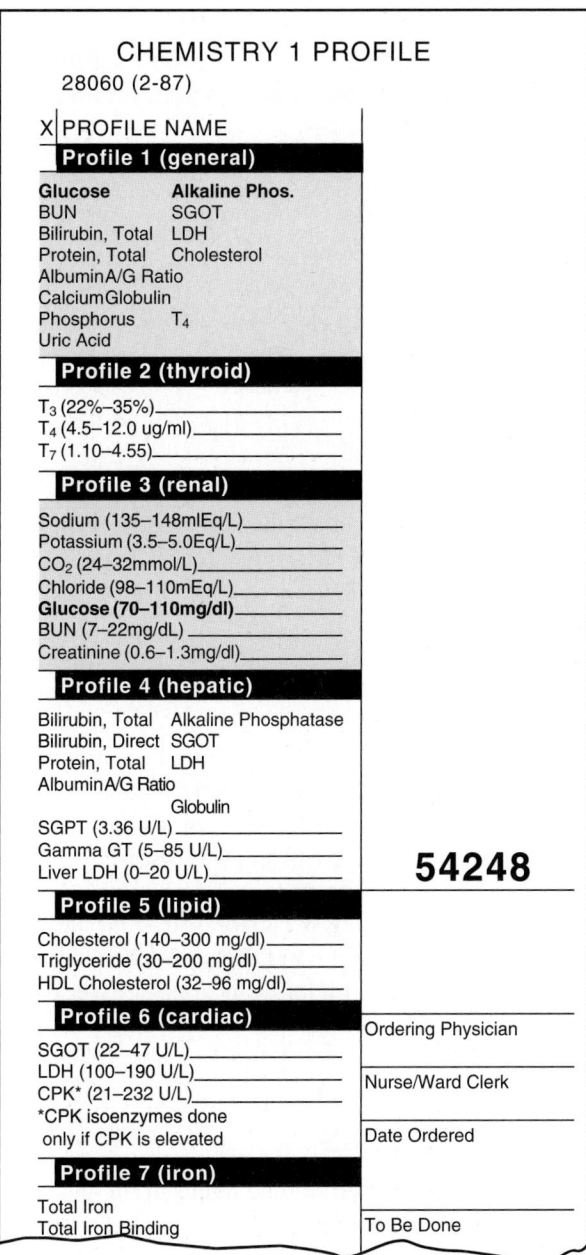

CHEMISTRY 1 PROFILE
28060 (2-87)

X | PROFILE NAME

Profile 1 (general)

Glucose	Alkaline Phos.
BUN	SGOT
Bilirubin, Total	LDH
Protein, Total	Cholesterol
Albumin	A/G Ratio
Calcium	Globulin
Phosphorus	T₄
Uric Acid	

Profile 2 (thyroid)

T₃ (22%–35%)_____
T₄ (4.5–12.0 ug/ml)_____
T₇ (1.10–4.55)_____

Profile 3 (renal)

Sodium (135–148mlEq/L)_____
Potassium (3.5–5.0Eq/L)_____
CO₂ (24–32mmol/L)_____
Chloride (98–110mEq/L)_____
Glucose (70–110mg/dl)_____
BUN (7–22mg/dL)_____
Creatinine (0.6–1.3mg/dl)_____

Profile 4 (hepatic)

Bilirubin, Total	Alkaline Phosphatase
Bilirubin, Direct	SGOT
Protein, Total	LDH
Albumin	A/G Ratio
	Globulin

SGPT (3.36 U/L)_____
Gamma GT (5–85 U/L)_____
Liver LDH (0–20 U/L)_____

54248

Profile 5 (lipid)

Cholesterol (140–300 mg/dl)_____
Triglyceride (30–200 mg/dl)_____
HDL Cholesterol (32–96 mg/dl)_____

Profile 6 (cardiac)

SGOT (22–47 U/L)_____
LDH (100–190 U/L)_____
CPK* (21–232 U/L)_____
*CPK isoenzymes done
  only if CPK is elevated

Profile 7 (iron)

Total Iron
Total Iron Binding

Ordering Physician

Nurse/Ward Clerk

Date Ordered

To Be Done

Figure 32-10 Example of a laboratory requisition form for chemistry profile tests. On this sample lab form, glucose testing is part of the general chemistry tests (Profile 1) and the renal tests (Profile 3).

Glycosylated Hemoglobin

Glycosylated hemoglobin (Hb A₁c) determination is a blood test that measures how well the glucose level has been controlled over the past four to six weeks versus the conventional blood test which shows only current day status. Physicians can use this test to determine if diabetics are consistently adhering to their diet and health guidelines or are adhering to their diet only for a day prior to their office visit.

Glycosylated hemoglobin is a stable molecule formed when sugar and hemoglobin bind together on the RBC. An elevated finding of glycosylated hemoglobin indicates poor glucose control in the assessment of glucose in the diabetic patient.

CHOLESTEROL

Cholesterol is a fatty compound that is essential for many vital life functions and is a normal constituent of blood. It is a steroid alcohol and a saturated fatty acid. Although it is required for life, cholesterol is not a necessary part of the diet. Sufficient quantities are manufactured by the body from carbohydrates and other fats. Because cholesterol has been linked to coronary artery disease, an increased interest in cholesterol levels and diet has developed. Typical cholesterol values for various age groups are shown in Table 32-5. To help reduce the risk of coronary artery disease, nutritionists and agencies such as the American Heart Association and the National Cholesterol Education Program advise that fats make up no more than 30 percent of the total intake of calories daily, and that the concentration of cholesterol in blood not exceed 200 mg/dL. Cholesterol of 240 mg/dL or above is considered to present a high risk of heart disease. Cholesterol levels between 200 and 239 mg/dL are considered borderline.

The Chemistry of Cholesterol

The cholesterol molecule consists of carbon, hydrogen, and oxygen. Most of the carbon atoms in the molecule are arranged into rings, rather than into long hydrocarbon chains as in most other lipids. A hydroxyl group (OH) attached to one of the carbon rings is what makes cholesterol an alcohol. Cholesterol is also a saturated, fatty acid. Saturated refers to the number of hydrogen atoms attached to the molecule. The more saturated the fat, the harder it is at room temperature. Fats of animal origin, for example, butter and animal fat, are saturated and are solid

TABLE 32-5	REFERENCE VALUES FOR TOTAL BLOOD CHOLESTEROL		
Age (years)	Range* mg/dL	Males mg/dL	Females mg/dL
0–19	120–230	—	—
20–29	120–240	235	220
30–39	140–270	265	240
40–49	150–310	280	265
50–59	160–330	300	320

*The upper limits of ranges are not necessarily the desired levels, but represent levels found in the U.S. population.

at room temperature. Monounsaturated and polyunsaturated fats are liquid at room temperature. Research into coronary artery disease has shown that saturated fats tend to raise levels of blood cholesterol. Monounsaturated fats (olive and peanut oils) do not change blood cholesterol levels and polyunsaturated fats (corn, safflower, sunflower, and many fish oils) tend to lower those levels.

Functions of Cholesterol

The human body is efficient at manufacturing cholesterol. Most cells are capable of doing so, especially the liver, the adrenal cortex, the testes, and the ovaries. All of the preceding cells, with the exception of the liver, use cholesterol to manufacture steroid hormones. Additionally, cholesterol is an important component of bile and cellular membranes. Although the body is very efficient at making cholesterol, it is not as easily degraded and may accumulate in the body and reach dangerous levels.

In addition to what the body produces, humans take in additional cholesterol through the ingestion of meat, eggs, and dairy products. The liver metabolizes cholesterol to its free form, which is then bound to lipoprotein and transported through the blood. Over time, excess cholesterol in the diet can result in a gradual increase of cholesterol concentration in the plasma. Increased concentrations of cholesterol in the plasma can rise to pathogenic levels. Some of the excess is stored in the liver while some is deposited on the walls of blood vessels (atherosclerosis) Atherosclerosis of the coronary arteries is the most common cause of acute myocardial infarction (heart attack).

Lipoproteins and Cholesterol Transport

Two kinds of lipoprotein are involved in the transport of cholesterol: **high-density lipoprotein (HDL)** and **low-density lipoprotein (LDL)**. Cholesterol bound to HDL is transported to the liver where it is excreted in the form of bile. HDL is sometimes referred to as good cholesterol. LDL cholesterol is deposited in the tissues as fat and inside the walls of blood vessels, and is referred to as bad cholesterol. High levels of LDL are associated with an increased risk of coronary artery disease. Persons with coronary artery disease should have levels of less than 160 mg/dL

Patient Teaching Tip

The patient is instructed to eat a low-fat diet for two weeks before the test, ending with a twelve- to fourteen-hour fast prior to collection of the blood sample.

TABLE 32-6 REFERENCE RANGES FOR HDL AND LDL CHOLESTEROL

Age (years)	HDL Male Range mg/dL	HDL Female Range mg/dL	LDL Male and Female mg/dL
0–19	30–65	30–70	50–170
20–29	30–65	36–78	60–170
30–39	30–59	33–77	70–190
40–49	25–61	40–81	80–190
50–75	29–72	38–91	80–210

LDL while those without the disease should have levels of less than 180 mg/dL. Typical values for HDL and LDL are shown in Table 32-6. Levels of HDL and LDL are influenced by many factors, both genetic and environmental. It is possible to raise HDL levels through a combination of weight loss, a diet low in saturated fats, exercise, and cessation of smoking.

Blood cholesterol may be reported as total cholesterol or as total cholesterol and the HDL and LDL fractions. Cholesterol screening is used to help identify patients that are at a high risk for heart disease. See Procedure 32-8, Cholesterol Testing.

Cholesterol testing is part of a lipid profile which also evaluates lipoproteins and triglycerides to help identify patients at a high risk for heart disease. Refer back to Figure 32-10, which shows tests performed for lipid profiles on the lab form.

TRIGLYCERIDES

Triglycerides are a type of lipid found in the blood that serve as a source of energy. Fatty acids and glycerol from the diet are converted into triglycerides by the liver. When triglyceride levels in the blood are excessive, they are deposited in tissues as adipose tissue (Table 32-7). Triglycerides are transported within the bloodstream by low-density lipoproteins (LDL) and very low-density lipoproteins (VLDL).

Many factors influence serum triglyceride levels; several of these are listed in Table 32-8. Serum triglyceride

TABLE 32-7 REFERENCE VALUES FOR TRIGLYCERIDES

Age	Male	Female
Adults/Elderly	40–160 mg/dL	35–135 mg/dL
0–11 years	30–108 mg/dL	32–114 mg/dL
12–19 years	36–163 mg/dL	41–128 mg/dL

TABLE 32-8	FACTORS THAT INFLUENCE SERUM TRIGLYCERIDE LEVELS	
Factors that Increase Concentration	**Factors that Decrease Concentration**
Pregnancy	Fasting
Estrogens, oral contraceptives	Ascorbic acid, clofibrate
Ingestion of fatty food	Uncontrolled diabetes mellitus
Ingestion of alcohol	Hyperthyroidism
Gout	Malnutrition

Patient Teaching Tip

Instruct the patient to remain on a stable diet for two weeks prior to collection of a blood specimen for triglyceride testing. The patient must also fast for the last 12 to 16 hours and avoid consumption of alcohol for 48 hours prior to the test.

concentration will rise moderately after ingesting a meal containing fat, peaking 4 to 5 hours later. Elevated concentrations of triglycerides are associated with an increased risk of coronary and vascular disease.

BLOOD UREA NITROGEN (BUN) TEST

The **blood urea nitrogen** (BUN) test measures the concentration of urea in blood. The amount of urea in blood reflects the metabolic function of the liver and the excretory function of the kidneys. Most renal diseases result in inadequate excretion of urea from the body; therefore, elevated concentrations of urea appear in the blood. BUN is one of several tests that are used to screen for renal disease and is especially useful for evaluating glomerular function.

Excess protein in the diet is not stored in the body but is metabolized (catalyzed) for energy production. Urea is the nitrogenous end-product of protein catabolism and is produced in the liver. It is deposited in the blood and carried to the kidneys for excretion. Surplus urea is measured as blood urea nitrogen, or BUN. Normal values of urea vary but in adults range between 8–25 mg/dL (see Table 32-9); concentrations above 100 mg/dL indicate serious impairment of renal function. Many factors other than renal disease may cause changes in urea concentration and should be considered in the process of diagnosis (Tables 32-10 and 32-11). Automated equipment is available to measure serum urea nitrogen.

TABLE 32-10	FACTORS THAT INFLUENCE SERUM UREA NITROGEN CONCENTRATION	
Factors that Increase Urea	**Factors that Decrease Urea**
Kidney disease	Pregnancy
High-protein diet	Low-protein diet
Steroid use	Poor hepatic function
Urinary obstruction	Malnutrition
Dehydration	Overhydration
Gastrointestinal bleeding	
Enlarged prostate	
Diabetes	
Heart failure	
Shock	
High fever	
Infection	

TABLE 32-11	DRUGS THAT INFLUENCE SERUM UREA NITROGEN CONCENTRATION	
Drugs that Increase Urea Concentration	**Drugs that Decrease Urea Concentration**
Tetracyclines	Streptomycin
Thiazide diuretics	Chloramphenicol
Allopurinol	
Aminoglycosides	
Cephalosporins	
Chloral hydrate	
Cisplatin	
Furosemide	
Guanethidine	
Indomethacin	
Nephrotoxic drugs: aspirin, methicillin, vancomycin, etc.	
Methotrexate	
Methyldopa	
Rifampin	
Spironolactone	

TABLE 32-9	UREA NITROGEN REFERENCE VALUES	
	Concentration of Urea in mg/dL
Adults (slightly higher in elderly)	10–20
Infants and children	5–18
Newborns	3–12

Procedure

32-1 Pregnancy Tests

STANDARD PRECAUTIONS:

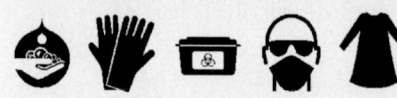

PURPOSE:

To perform the enzyme immunoassay or agglutination inhibition test to detect hCG in urine to determine positive or negative pregnancy results.

EQUIPMENT/SUPPLIES:

Gloves

Hand disinfectant

Urine specimen

Stopwatch

Surface disinfectant (10% chlorine bleach solution)

Biohazard container

hCG negative urine control

hCG positive urine control

Pregnancy test kit for enzyme immunoassay (EIA) and/or the agglutination inhibition pregnancy test. Kits should include slide or test unit, dispensers, reagents, and so on.

PROCEDURE STEPS:

1. Wash hands and put on gloves.
2. Assemble all equipment and supplies.
3. Perform a modified enzyme immunoassay test for hCG following the manufacturer's instructions (if not available, skip to step 4).

   a. Obtain test kit materials, reagents, and urine specimen. Allow all materials to reach room temperature.

   b. Apply urine to the test unit using dispenser provided (Figure 32-11).

   c. Wait appropriate time interval (use stopwatch to time test).

   d. Apply first reagent/antibody to test unit using dispenser provided.

   e. Rinse unreacted reagent from unit after appropriate time.

   f. Apply color reagent/substrate to test unit.

   g. Observe color development after appropriate time interval.

   h. Stop reaction.

   i. Record results. Consult manufacturer's package insert to interpret test results (Figure 32-12).

   j. Repeat steps 3a–i using both positive and negative urine controls.

   k. Proceed to step 5.

4. Perform an agglutination inhibition test for hCG following the manufacturer's instructions.

   a. Obtain slide test kit, reagents, and urine specimen.

   b. Place one drop of antiserum in the center of the circled area of slide.

(continues)

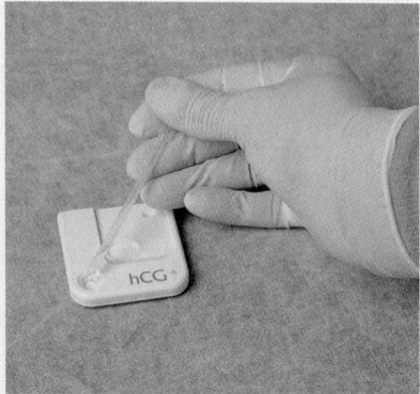

Figure 32-11 A drop of urine is placed in the urine test unit.

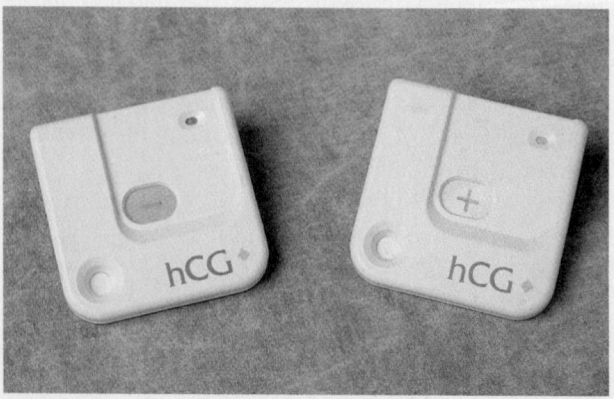

Figure 32-12 The package instructions will specify how the test is to be interpreted. The most common interpretation is with a negative sign (left) and positive sign (right).

Procedure

32-1 *(continued)*

c. Dispense one drop of urine beside the drop of antiserum.

d. Mix urine and antiserum with stirrer provided.

e. Rock the slide in a figure-eight motion for the appropriate time, usually one to two minutes (use stopwatch to measure time).

f. Apply one drop of well-mixed indicator particles to mixture on slide.

g. Mix indicator particles with antiserum-urine mixture and spread the mixture over the entire circled area of the slide using a stirrer.

h. Rock slide slowly in a figure-eight motion for the appropriate time, usually one to two minutes.

i. Observe slide for agglutination at the end of the time interval and record the results (no agglutination = positive; agglutination = negative). Refer to Figure 32-13.

j. Repeat steps 4a–i using positive and negative urine controls.

5. Disinfect reusable equipment by soaking in 10% chlorine bleach solution a minimum of ten minutes. Wash and rinse thoroughly.

6. Discard disposable supplies into biohazard container.

7. Dispose of specimen as instructed.

8. Clean work area with surface disinfectant.

9. Remove gloves and discard into biohazard container.

10. Wash hands with hand disinfectant.

11. Document procedure.

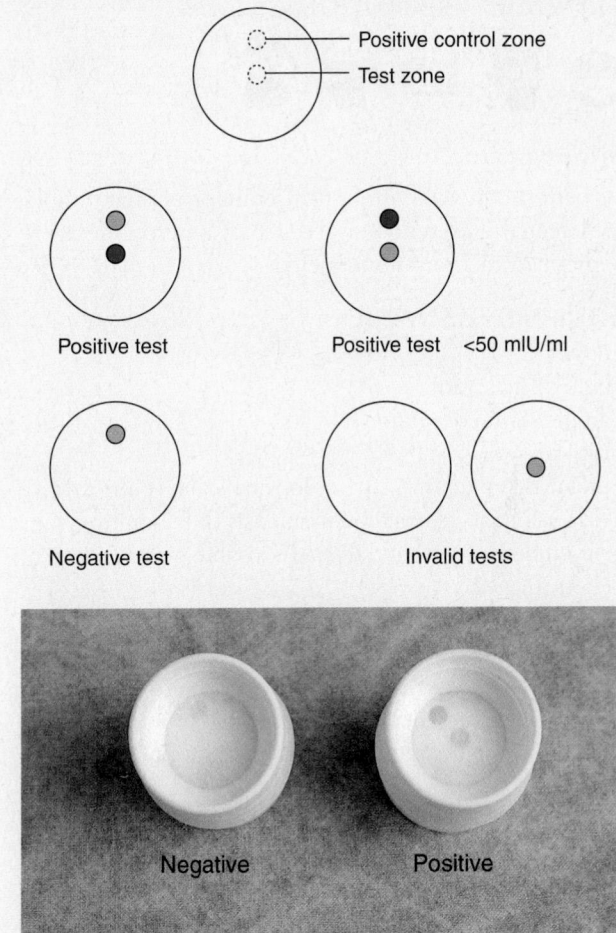

Figure 32-13   Illustration and photograph of positive and negative results with ICON II® hCG test.

Slide Test for Infectious Mononucleosis

Procedure 32-2

STANDARD PRECAUTIONS:

PURPOSE:
To perform an accurate test of serum or plasma sample to detect the presence or absence of heterophile antibodies of infectious mononucleosis.

EQUIPMENT/SUPPLIES:
Gloves
Hand disinfectant
Sample serum or plasma
Stopwatch
Surface disinfectant (10% chlorine bleach solution)
Test kit for infectious mononucleosis (kit should include instructions, slide, disposable pipettes, stirrers, reagents)
Biohazard container
NOTE: The procedure given is for Monospot® test by Meridian Diagnostics. Package insert should be consulted before the test is performed. If another kit is used, the specific manufacturer's instructions should be followed.

PROCEDURE STEPS:
1. Wash hands and put on gloves.
2. Assemble all equipment and supplies. Allow all materials to come to room temperature.
3. Place the Monospot® slide on a flat work surface.
4. Mix the reagent vials several times by inversion.
5. Fill the capillary pipette to the top mark:
   a. Place the rubber bulb on the end of the capillary pipette with the heavy black line.
   b. Insert the pipette into the vial of indicator cells.
   c. Allow the pipette to fill by capillary action to the top mark.
6. Place the index finger over the hole in the bulb and squeeze gently to dispense half the cells (10 µL) on a corner of square I of the slide (the level of the cells should now be at the lower mark on the pipette).

7. Deliver the remaining cells (10 µL) to a corner of square II.
8. Place one drop of thoroughly mixed reagent I in the center of square I.
9. Place one drop of thoroughly mixed reagent II in the center of square II.
10. Add one drop of serum to the center of each square using the disposable plastic pipette provided.
11. Use a clean applicator stick to mix reagent I with the serum using at least ten stirring motions and avoiding touching the indicator cells.
12. Blend in the indicator cells in square I with the applicator stick using no more than ten stirring motions and spread the mixture over the entire surface of the square.
13. Repeat steps 11 and 12 using reagent II in square II, using a clean applicator stick.
14. Start the stopwatch upon completion of the mixing of both squares.
15. Do not pick up or move the slide.
16. Observe for agglutination at the end of one minute (no longer) without moving the slide or picking it up.
17. Record the agglutination in each square and interpret the results. If the agglutination pattern is stronger in square I than in square II, the test is positive for the heterophile antibody of infectious mononucleosis. Any other combination of reactions is negative.
18. Record test results as positive or negative.
19. Repeat the test procedure (steps 3–18) using positive and negative control sera.
20. Discard contaminated materials into biohazard container.
21. Dispose of specimen appropriately and disinfect reusable materials by soaking in 10 percent chlorine bleach solution for at least ten minutes. Wash and rinse thoroughly.
22. Clean work area with surface disinfectant.
23. Remove gloves and discard into biohazard container.
24. Wash hands with hand disinfectant.
25. Document results.

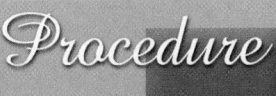

32-3 Analyzing Semen

STANDARD PRECAUTIONS:

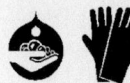

PURPOSE:
To analyze semen to determine total sperm count, percent of motility, and percent of normally formed sperm cells.

EQUIPMENT/SUPPLIES:
Gloves
10 mL graduated cylinder
pH test paper (approximate range: 6.1–10.0)
Automatic pipette
Hemacytometer
Diluting fluid
Sodium bicarbonate
Distilled water
Slides and coverslips
Petri dishes
Microscope
Coplin jar

PROCEDURE STEPS:
Macroscopic Examination

1. Wash hands and apply gloves.
2. Assemble all equipment and supplies.
3. Measure the specimen volume in a graduated cylinder.
4. Measure the pH using pH test paper.
5. Evaluate the viscosity:
   a. Upon collection, the gel-like specimen liquifies within 30 minutes and forms a translucent but viscous fluid. This is the result of the action of various enzymes contained in seminal fluid.
   b. As the specimen is poured into the cylinder, viscosity can be determined. A normal specimen will not appear watery or clumped and will pour in droplets. Some laboratories give a 0 to 4 rating to viscosity: 0 (watery) to 4 (clumped).
6. Remove gloves and wash hands.
7. Document results.

Microscopic Examination

1. Wash hands and apply gloves.
2. Assemble all equipment and supplies.
3. Mix semen specimen.
4. NOTE: Motility should be observed within 3 hours of collection.
   Place one drop of liquified specimen on a glass slide and cover with a coverslip. Examine for motility. Initially, 70–80% of the spermatozoa should be actively motile. Agglutination of sperm should be noted. Agglutination should be described by the orientation of the sperm sticking to each other: head to head, tail to tail, or other combinations.
5. Sperm count:
   a. Using automatic pipettes, make a 1:20 dilution of sample with sodium bicarbonate solution. Mix well.
   b. Fill both sides of the hemocytometer (also used for red and white cell counts) and allow the sperm to settle for 5–10 minutes.
   c. Count the sperm in 2 large WBC squares or 5 RBC squares. To calculate:
      If 5 RBC squares used:
      Count number of sperm × 1 million = sperm per milliliter
      If 2 WBC squares used:
      Count number of sperm × 100,000 = sperm per milliliter
6. Morphology: sperm are evaluated on the appearance of their tail and head in a stained preparation by a pathologist or trained technologist.
   a. Prepare two slides using the technique to make a blood smear. Do not allow the slides to air dry. Immediately immerse both slides into a coplin jar containing 95% alcohol.
   b. Deliver the slides to the pathologist to view for morphology.
7. Remove gloves and wash hands.
8. Document results.

Procedure
32-4   Obtaining Blood Specimen for Phenylketonuria (PKU) Test

STANDARD PRECAUTIONS:

PURPOSE:
To obtain a blood specimen using a PKU test card or "filter paper" to determine phenylalanine levels in newborns who are at least 3 to 4 days old.

EQUIPMENT/SUPPLIES:
Gloves
PKU filter paper test card and mailing envelope
Alcohol swabs
Cotton balls
Sterile pediatric-sized lancet
Biohazard waste container

PROCEDURE STEPS:
1. Wash hands and put on gloves.
2. Identify the infant. Explain the purpose of the test and the procedure to the parents. Discuss the feeding pattern of the infant prior to beginning the procedure. RATIONALE: Certain antibiotics, aspirin, or vomiting problems may cause false results.
3. Select and clean an appropriate puncture site (Figure 32-14).
4. Grasp the infant's foot taking care not to touch the cleansed area. Make a puncture approximately 2–3 mm deep in the infant's heel making sure the infant's lateral, or side, portion of the heel pad is used. A pediatric-sized lancet, which limits the depth of puncture, should be used (Figure 32-15). If possible, recent puncture sites should always be

avoided. Refer to Chapter 28, Phlebotomy: Venipuncture and Capillary Puncture.
5. Wipe away the first drop of blood with a cotton ball. RATIONALE: The first drop is diluted with alcohol and should not be collected for the test.
6. To collect blood for the test, press the back side of the filter paper test card against the infant's heel while exerting gentle pressure on the heel (Figure 32-16). The drop of blood should be large enough

(continues)

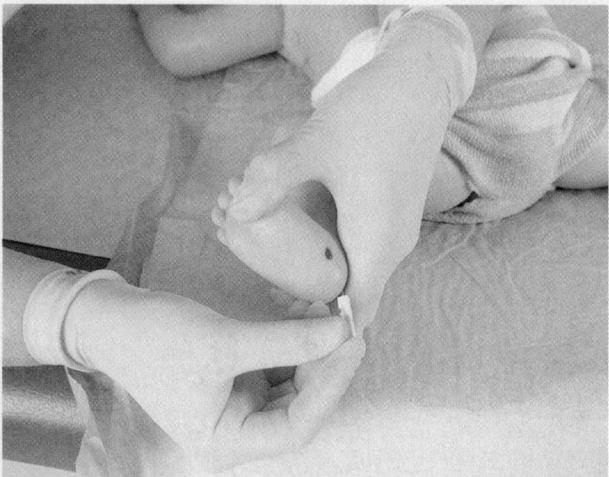

Figure 32-15   The infant's leg should be held securely with the nondominant hand and arm, while the dominant hand uses a pediatric lancet to perform a capillary heel stick.

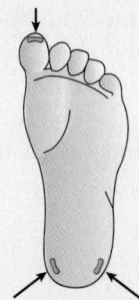

Figure 32-14   Capillary blood collection sites on an infant's foot. The most common site is the side of the infant's heel pad.

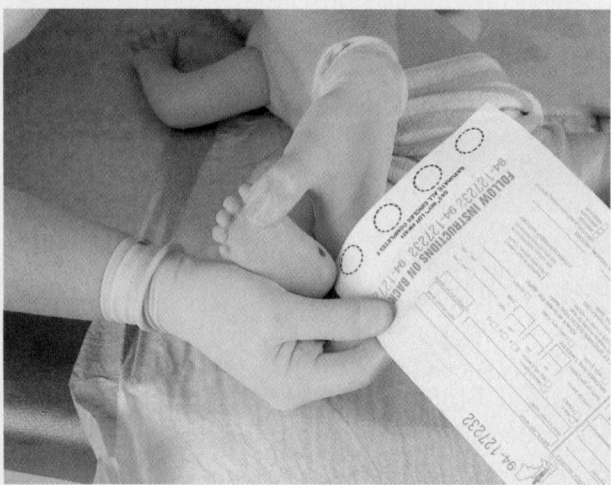

Figure 32-16   Drops of blood are transferred from the capillary puncture to all circles on the filter paper test card.

Procedure 32-4 *(continued)*

to completely fill and soak through the circle. *Do not* layer the multiple blood drops within a single circle. Completely fill all of the circles on the test card. RATIONALE: Failure to do so will require a retest.

7. Hold a cotton ball or gauze pad over the puncture and apply gentle pressure until the bleeding stops.
8. Properly dispose of all waste in biohazard container.
9. Remove the gloves and wash hands.
10. Allow the PKU test card to completely dry on a nonabsorbent surface at room temperature. This will take about two hours. If collecting more than

one card, *do not* lay one card on another when drying. This could cause cross-contamination of blood between the cards.

11. After the test card is dry, put on gloves and complete the PKU test card with all patient and physician information.
12. Place the test card in the mailer envelope and send it to the laboratory within two days.
13. Remove gloves and wash hands.
14. Document the procedure in the patient's medical record. When test results are returned, these should also be placed in the patient's medical record.

Procedure 32-5 Obtaining Urine Specimen for Phenylketonuria (PKU) Test

STANDARD PRECAUTIONS:

PURPOSE:
To obtain a urine specimen using the diaper test or the Phenistik test to determine phenylalanine levels in newborns who are at least 6 weeks old.

EQUIPMENT/SUPPLIES:
Gloves
10% ferric chloride for the diaper test
or
Phenistik for the Phenistik Method Test
Biohazard waste container

PROCEDURE STEPS:
1. Identify the infant. Verify that the infant is at least 6 weeks of age. Explain the purpose of the test and the procedure to the parents.

2. Wash hands and apply gloves.
3. Follow one of the two following procedures:
   Diaper Test:
   Apply several drops of 10% ferric chloride to a diaper that contains fresh urine. Development of a green color indicates a positive test.
   Phenistik Test:
   Dip the Phenistik test strip into fresh urine or press it against a diaper containing fresh urine. Development of a green color indicates a positive test.
4. A positive urine test should be followed up with a blood test.
5. Properly dispose of all waste in a biohazard waste container.
6. Remove gloves and wash hands.
7. Document the procedure and results in the patient's medical record.

Procedure

32-6   Mantoux Test

STANDARD PRECAUTIONS:

   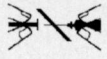

PURPOSE:
To safely and accurately inject 0.1 mL of intermediate strength (5 TU) purified protein derivative (PPD) intradermally to present an indurated wheal to determine if an active or inactive tuberculous infection is present.

EQUIPMENT/SUPPLIES:
Gloves
Goggles
Tuberculin syringe
Short (⅜–½″) 26 or 27 gauge needle
PPD (5 TU strength)
Alcohol
Cotton balls or gauze
Sharps container
Biohazard waste container

PROCEDURE STEPS:
1. Wash hands and put on gloves and goggles.
2. Identify the patient and explain the procedure.
3. Select the site approximately 3 to 4 inches from the bend of arm on the anterior side.
4. Clean the site with alcohol and allow surface to dry. Do *not* touch the site after cleaning. If the site is touched, recleaning will be necessary.
5. Use a 1.0 mL tuberculin syringe fitted with a ⅜–½″, 26 or 27 gauge needle. Draw 0.1 mL of 5 TU strength PPD into the syringe.
   CAUTION: Be careful to draw the correct amount of PPD into the syringe.
   RATIONALE: Too much or too little PPD will cause erroneous results.
6. Hold the patient's forearm just under the chosen site to prevent movement during the injection (Figure 32-17A).
7. Slowly inject the PPD intradermally into the skin of the anterior portion of the arm to form a wheal approximately 6–10 mm (Figure 32-17B). A small amount of blood at the puncture site will not interfere with the test results. Do not rub the injection site.

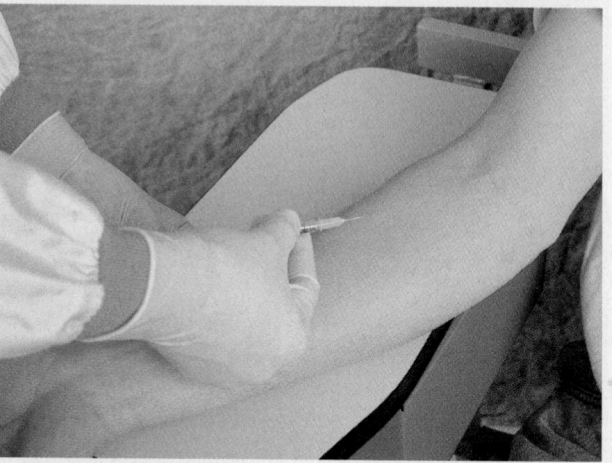

Figure 32-17A   The syringe should be at a 10 to 15 degree angle to allow the needle to penetrate the dermal layer of skin. If the injection is too deep, it will be impossible to read the wheal.

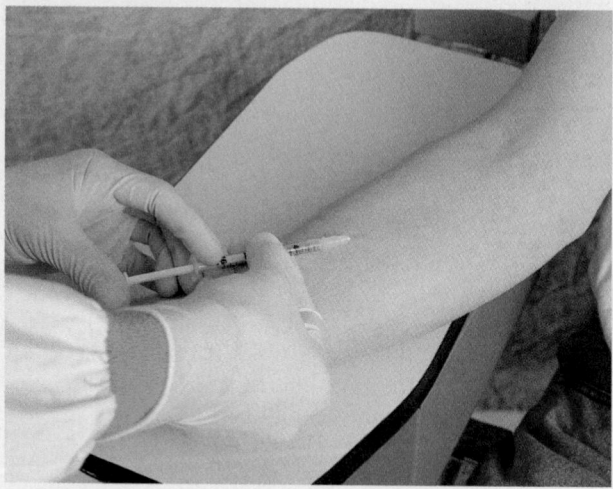

Figure 32-17B   It is important to inject the PPD slowly since absorption in this area is slow. If the medication is injected too fast, it may leak onto the skin and invalidate the test.

8. Dispose of the syringe and needle in a sharps container.
9. Watch the patient carefully and notify the physician immediately of any adverse reactions to the medication.

(continues)

Procedure
32-6 *(continued)*

10. Instruct the patient to return within 48–72 hours of the injection for test interpretation.
11. Remove gloves and wash hands.
12. Document procedure in the patient's medical record.

When patient returns for test interpretation:

13. Wash your hands and bend the patient's arm at the elbow. Inspect the injection site. Gently rub a

finger across the induration to evaluate its size, then measure in millimeters (Figure 32-18).
14. Read the test according to Figure 32-19. Questionable results will require retesting. Document the test results in the patient's medical record.

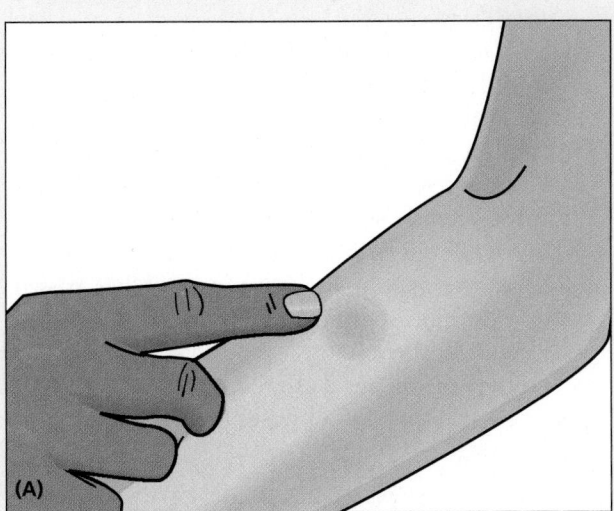 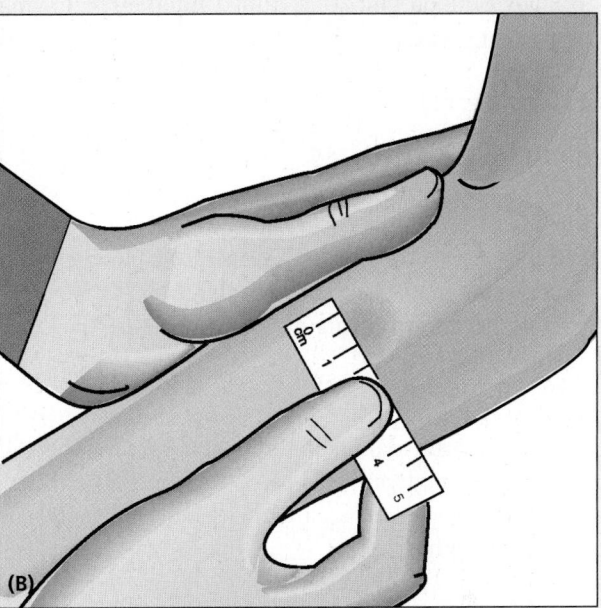

Figure 32-18 Gently inspect and measure the size of induration in response to tuberculin test 48 to 72 hours after administration.

Induration

(A) **Positive reaction** for past or present infection: 10 mm or more of induration

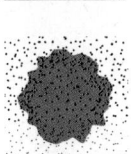

(B) **Doubtful reaction:** 5–9 mm
(In persons who are suspected to have been exposed to TB an induration of 5–9 mm is considered suspicious. Further diagnostic testing should follow.)

(C) **Negative reaction:** without induration or less than 5 mm.

Figure 32-19 The results of an induration are read as shown. A positive result should be communicated immediately to the physician.

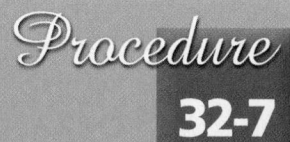

Measurement of Blood Glucose Using an Automated Analyzer

STANDARD PRECAUTIONS:

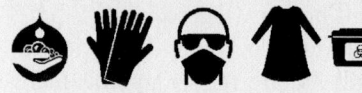

PURPOSE:

To analyze blood glucose at timed intervals following the patient's ingestion of a standard glucose dose to aid in the diagnosis and management of diabetes or in the management of hypoglycemia.

EQUIPMENT/SUPPLIES:

Gloves
Goggles
Sterile lancet
Alcohol swabs or 70%
   alcohol and cotton balls
Glucose analyzer
Control solutions for
   glucose analyzer
Test strips for glucose
   analyzer
Laboratory tissue

PROCEDURE STEPS:

1. Review the manufacturer's manual for the specific glucose analyzer being used. Turn on the analyzer.
2. Clean the work area and assemble all materials and supplies.
3. Wash hands.
4. Put on gloves and goggles.
5. Record the control ranges, control lot number, and test strip lot number.
6. Perform the check test and the control test according to the manufacturer's instructions. If both tests are within range, proceed to the glucose test. Repeat both tests if either is out of acceptable range.

To perform the glucose test:

1. Remove a test strip from the bottle and replace the lid.
2. Perform a capillary puncture (refer to Chapter 28).
3. Apply a large drop of blood to the test strip.
4. Blot the test strip with tissue after the time interval recommended by the manufacturer.
5. Insert the test strip into the test chamber.
6. After the appropriate time interval has passed, read the glucose concentration.
7. Document the results.
8. Remove gloves and wash hands.
9. Properly dispose of all waste in a biohazard waste container.

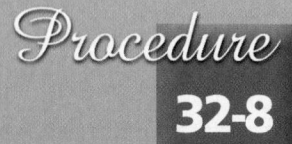

Cholesterol Testing

STANDARD PRECAUTIONS:

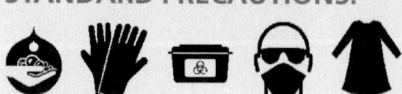

PURPOSE:

To determine the total cholesterol level to aid in diagnosis of coronary artery disease.

EQUIPMENT/SUPPLIES:

Gloves
Blood collecting equipment
Pipettes with disposable tips
Chlorine bleach
Commercial kit for manual determination of cholesterol
Controls and standards
Marking pen
Biohazard container

PROCEDURE STEPS:

1. Assemble all necessary equipment and materials.
2. Wash hands; apply gloves and goggles.
3. Obtain a blood sample from the patient, either by fingerstick or venipuncture, depending on the manufacturer's instructions (refer to Chapter 28).
4. Follow the manufacturer's instructions to perform the cholesterol test.
5. Properly dispose of all waste in biohazard container.
6. Document results.

CASE STUDY 32-1

Anna Preciado, CMA, a clinical medical assistant at Doctors Lewis and King, has performed many venipunctures during her training at college, throughout her internship, and since her employment with Lewis and King. She has not, however, drawn a heelstick specimen from an infant since she was in college and even then she typically practiced on a doll. With more mothers and infants leaving the hospital so soon after the birth of the baby, she noticed that the practice is now scheduling infants for PKU tests. Anna is concerned and somewhat nervous about obtaining a PKU blood specimen from an infant.

CASE STUDY REVIEW

1. What course of action should Anna take to prepare herself for performing a procedure that she has not done in several years?

2. Should Anna simply tell the office manager or one of the physicians that she is not capable of obtaining the blood specimen?

3. Once Anna feels she is technically ready to perform the PKU blood test, what should she do to assure that the procedure goes well?

SUMMARY

A number of rapid test kits and automated methods are available for use in the ambulatory care setting by the medical assistant. For all of the tests discussed in this chapter, it is important for the medical assistant to have a basic understanding of the principles involved and the proper sampling procedures required. Safety procedures and standard precautions must be observed at all times and include the proper disposal of infectious materials and reagents. Gloves and goggles are always used when obtaining samples and while performing the actual test. Careful documentation by the medical assistant will help the physician in the diagnosis of the patient.

REVIEW QUESTIONS

Multiple Choice

1. The slide test for pregnancy and the detection of the hormone hCG is the same as the test method based on:
   a. agglutination inhibition test
   b. modified enzyme immunoassay
   c. antigen-antibody reaction
   d. color reaction

2. In addition to pregnancy, a positive hCG test can be found in the following pathological conditions *except:*
   a. ectopic pregnancy
   b. hydatidiform mole of the uterus
   c. pelvic inflammatory disease
   d. cancer of the lung

3. If a urine sample for a pregnancy test cannot be tested immediately, it may be stored in the following way for 24 hours:
   a. room temperature 25°C
   b. body temperature 37°C
   c. frozen
   d. refrigerated at 4°C

4. The kissing disease is synonymous with the disease:
   a. tuberculosis
   b. infectious mononucleosis
   c. hemolytic anemia
   d. hypoglycemia

5. Serum or blood would be the *specimen of choice* for all but the following test:
   a. ABO typing
   b. testing for the Epstein-Barr virus
   c. cholesterol
   d. hCG hormone

6. All but one of the following are correct statements about blood type:
   a. type A RBCs have A antigens on the cell
   b. type B RBCs have B antigens on the cell
   c. type O RBCs have A and B antigens on the cell
   d. type AB RBCs have both A and B antigens on the cell

7. Which of the following is a *true* statement about the Rh factor?
   a. Rh factor is a rare blood type
   b. Rh factor is present on all red blood cells
   c. Rh factor was discovered from rhesus monkeys
   d. People without the Rh factor on their RBCs have naturally occurring antibodies called anti-D in their plasma.

8. When instructing a patient in the correct collection of a specimen for semen analysis, all of the following should be considered *except*:
   a. avoid the consumption of alcohol several days before the test
   b. collection of semen into a condom is unacceptable
   c. specimen should be transported to the laboratory at 37°C within 30 minutes of collection
   d. avoid the consumption of fats several days before the test

9. Testing for phenylketonuria (PKU) is done on:
   a. newborns
   b. children 1 to 3 years of age
   c. teenagers
   d. adults over 40

10. The best site location for a tuberculin Mantoux test is:
    a. back of the hand
    b. forearm 3 to 4 inches from bend of arm
    c. ½″ above the back of the knee
    d. upper part of the arm in the deltoid muscle

11. A patient with hypoglycemia would have a blood glucose level of:
    a. 50–70 mg/dL
    b. 70–110 mg/dL
    c. 110–150 mg/dL
    d. 150–200 mg/dL

Critical Thinking

1. Why is the first-voided morning urine the preferred specimen for a pregnancy test?
2. In addition to causing infectious mononucleosis, in what other diseases has EBV been implicated?
3. Why is it necessary to repeat the seminal analysis three times over a two-month period?
4. List three reasons for a positive skin test for tuberculosis.
5. What factors may alter the results of a blood glucose measurement?

6. How can you distinguish between the diabetic and nondiabetic patient based on the results of the two-hour postprandial glucose evaluation?
7. Discuss the relationship between saturated fats and coronary artery disease.
8. What is the function of triglycerides in the body?
9. What instructions should the patient be given in preparation for a triglyceride evaluation?
10. What is the source of urea in the blood?

WEB ACTIVITIES

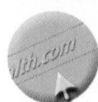

1. Search the CDC's and other government websites for information on infectious diseases such as mononucleosis.
2. Use search engines to research some of the conditions discussed in this chapter, such as phenylketonuria and tuberculosis.

REFERENCES/BIBLIOGRAPHY

Avey, A. M. (1993). TB skin testing: How to do it right. *American Journal of Nursing, 93,* 42–45.

Braun, M. M., Cote, T. R., et al. (1993). Trends in death with *tuberculosis* during the AIDS era. *Journal of the American Medical Association, 269,* 2865–2869.

Kaiser Permanente, Southern California Region. (1993). *Guide to laboratory services.* [Brochure].

Marshall, J. (1993). *Fundamental skills for the clinical laboratory professional.* Albany, NY: Delmar.

Meyers, R. (1989). *Immunology: A laboratory manual.* Dubuque, IA: Wm. C. Brown Publishers.

Pagana, K., & Pagana, T. (1992). *Mosby's diagnostic and laboratory test reference.* St. Louis: Mosby-Year Book, Inc.

Reese, R., & Betts, R. (Eds.). (1991). *A practical approach to infectious disease* (3rd ed.). Boston: Little, Brown and Co.

Reiss, B., & Evans, M. (1996). *Pharmacological aspects of nursing care* (5th ed.). Albany, NY: Delmar.

Sherris, J. C. (Ed.). (1990). *Medical microbiology: An introduction to infectious disease* (2nd ed.). New York: Elsevier Science Publishing Co.

Walters, N. J., Estridge, B. H., & Reynolds, A. P. (2000). *Basic medical laboratory techniques* (4th ed.). Albany, NY: Delmar.

Wedding, M. E., & Toenjes, S. A. (1992). *Medical laboratory procedures.* Philadelphia: F. A. Davis Company.

Wyngaarden, J. B., Smith Jr., L. H., & Bennett, J. C. (Eds.). (1992). *Cecil textbook of medicine* (19th ed.). 2 vols. Philadelphia: W. B. Saunders.

III

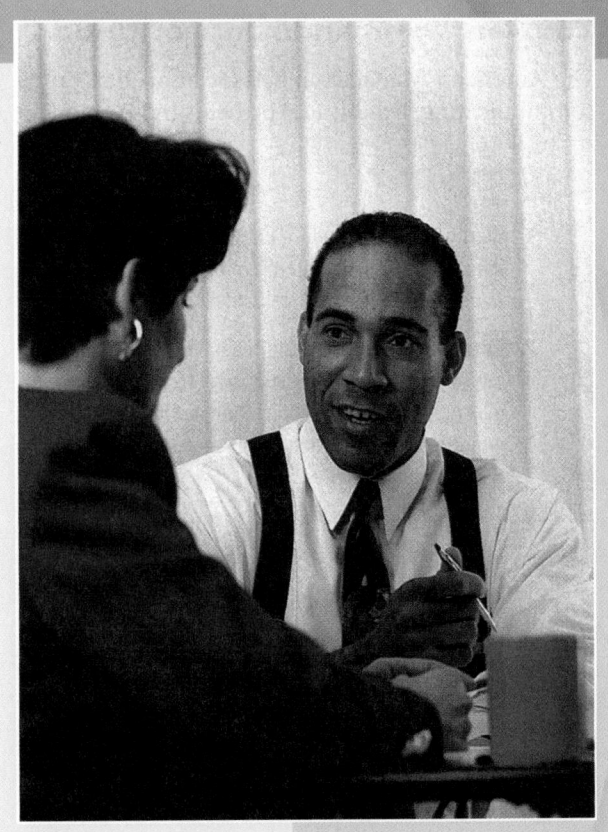

PROFESSIONAL
PROCEDURES

Unit

8

OFFICE AND HUMAN RESOURCE MANAGEMENT

Chapter 33

THE MEDICAL ASSISTANT AS OFFICE MANAGER

KEY TERMS

Agenda
Ancillary Services
Benchmark
Benefit
Bond
Brainstorming
Charisma
Embezzle
Emulate
Externship
Fringe Benefit
"Going Bare"
Hierarchy
Internet
Itinerary
Liability
Malpractice
Marketing
Minutes
Negligence
Paradigm
Practicum
Procedures Manual
Professional Liability Insurance
Profit Sharing
Risk Management
Search Engine
Self-actualization
Shadow
Subordinate
Teamwork
Web Site
Work Statement

OUTLINE

The Medical Assistant as Manager
Qualities of a Manager
Management Styles
 People-oriented Personality
 Things-oriented Personality
 Idea-oriented Personality
 Other Management Styles
 Changing Styles for the Twenty-
  first Century
The Importance of Teamwork
 Getting the Team Started
 Using a Team to Solve a Problem
 Planning and Implementing a
  Solution
 Recognition
Supervising Personnel
 Staff Meetings
 Supporting Staff Members
Travel Arrangements
 Itinerary
Supervising Student Practicums
Time Management

Procedures Manual
 Organization of the Procedures
  Manual
 Updating and Reviewing the
  Procedures Manual
Marketing Functions
 Seminars
 Brochures
 Newsletters
 Press Releases
 Special Events
Record and Financial
 Management
 Payroll Processing
Facility and Equipment
 Management
 Inventories
 Equipment and Supplies
  Maintenance
Risk Management
Liability Coverage and Bonding

OBJECTIVES

The student should strive to meet the following performance objectives and demonstrate an understanding of the facts and principles presented in this chapter through written and oral communication.

1. Define the key terms as presented in the glossary.
2. Describe the qualities of a manager.
3. Identify three types of personalities and their management styles.
4. Differentiate between authoritarian and democratic management styles.
5. Discuss characteristics of managers and leaders.

(continues)

OBJECTIVES (*continued*)

6. Recall a minimum of four descriptions of managers/leaders for the new millennium.
7. List three benefits of a teamwork approach.
8. Discuss the importance of a meeting agenda.
9. List pieces of information that should be included in meeting minutes.
10. Identify the steps required to make travel arrangements.
11. Define the term itinerary and list important information the itinerary should contain.
12. List three methods of increasing productivity and efficient time management.
13. Describe the purpose of a procedures manual.
14. Describe the general concept of marketing and recall at least three marketing tools.
15. Describe the purpose and benefit of marketing.
16. Define records management, financial management, facility and equipment management, and risk management.
17. Describe the steps involved in payroll processing.
18. Describe liability coverage and what bonding means.

ROLE DELINEATION COMPONENTS

ADMINISTRATIVE

Practice Finances

- **Process Payroll**
- **Manage renewals of business and professional insurance policies (adv)**

GENERAL (TRANSDISCIPLINARY)

Professionalism

- **Work as a team member**
- **Manage time effectively**
- **Prioritize and perform multiple tasks**
- **Facility planning (adv)**
- **Lead/motivate employees (adv)**
- **Plan and conduct staff meetings (adv)**
- **Train/orient employees (adv)**

(continues)

SCENARIO

Marilyn Johnson has been employed by Doctors Lewis & King for the past eight years. Three years ago, she was promoted to the position of office manager when the facility added the second office for its associates in the next suburb. Marilyn has a baccalaureate degree in business administration. Her responsibilities at Doctors Lewis & King include various duties involving personnel, finances, and office efficiency.

INTRODUCTION

The skills and growing complexity of medical specialization have broadened the scope of employment options for the medical assistant. Many ambulatory health care facilities are turning to managed care as a means of ensuring consumer use of the appropriate level of care and to facilitate cost containment. This approach has created opportunity for medical assistants to advance to the office manager (OM) position based on individual facility needs.

In general, the office manager should have a minimum of an associate's degree. Large corporate settings may employ an OM and a human resource (HR) person with some crossover of responsibilities depending on the needs and organizational structure of the facility. Most HR positions require a minimum of a bachelor's degree with validation that the person has been accepted to an accredited master's program. The role of the medical assistant as a human resources manager is covered in Chapter 34.

ROLE DELINEATION COMPONENTS (continued)

Communication Skills

- Promote the practice through positive public relations
- Serve as liaison (adv)

Legal Concepts

- Comply with established risk management and safety procedures
- Follow employer's established policies dealing with the health care contract
- Follow federal, state, and local legal guidelines
- Maintain awareness of federal and state health care legislation and regulations
- Participate in the development and maintenance of personnel, policy, and procedure manuals
- Develop and maintain personnel, policy, and procedure manuals (adv)

Instruction

- Locate community resources and disseminate information
- Develop educational materials (adv)

Operational Functions

- Maintain supply inventory
- Evaluate and recommend equipment and supplies
- Supervise personnel (adv)
- Negotiate leases and prices for equipment and supply contracts (adv)
- Negotiate managed care contracts (adv)
- Create spreadsheets and input data (adv)
- Create databases and input data (adv)
- Perform computer searches (adv)
- Transmit and receive data and messages by Internet, e-mail, and web site (adv)

THE MEDICAL ASSISTANT AS MANAGER

The office manager of a medical office or ambulatory care facility is a role that can have vast and diverse responsibilities. In some offices, there may be one office manager and a separate human resources manager. In others, one person may be responsible for all duties that can fall under the role of office manager and human resources manager. This chapter covers the following office manager duties:

1. Create and update the office procedures manual
2. Supervise office personnel
3. Assist in improving work flow and office efficiencies (time management)
4. Prepare staff meeting agenda, conduct the meeting, and record minutes
5. Supervise the purchase, repair, and maintenance of office equipment
6. Supervise the purchase and storage of office supplies
7. Supervise the purchase and storage of controlled substances
8. Approve financial transactions and account disposition; generate financial reports as needed
9. Make travel arrangements and prepare an itinerary
10. Prepare patient education materials and arrange patient/community education workshops as needed
11. Arrange and maintain practice insurance and develop risk management strategies

QUALITIES OF A MANAGER

Qualifications of the manager will vary from office to office, however, some general requirements are common to any office setting. Attributes needed to perform as a high quality manager include but are not limited to the following:

- *People Skills.* The office manager must like people in general and enjoy working with them. Building confidence and self-esteem in others and being interested in promoting constructive relationships are essential qualities of the office manager. The ability to function as an effective team leader provides a role model for other staff members to **emulate**.

- *Truthfulness.* Lead by example! If an honest mistake is made, be the first to admit to the error and seek the best solution for preventing it from happening again. Respond honestly to requests. For example, two staff members ask for the same day off. The office manager will make the decision that only one member may have the day off and will review the policy manual to determine the appropriate criteria for designating who will have the request granted.

- *Fairmindedness.* It is important to always be fair with co-workers. Decisions that impact one fellow employee create a ripple effect. That is, you may have to make the same decision for another employee at another time. Decisions should be based, as much as possible, on the assumption that what is granted to one employee will be granted to others in similar situations. This approach will decrease the risk of being accused of playing favorites or being unfair.

- *Effective Communication Skills.* Communication skills include written and oral methods. The manager must communicate clearly, diplomatically, tactfully, and with respect for the feelings of others.

Organizational Skills. Being organized includes being able to prioritize tasks, working efficiently and methodically. Know when and be willing to delegate tasks when others have the expertise and time to complete the task within the time lines.

Objectivity. The manager must be able to view challenges without bias or prejudice. For example, when promotions are made, the office manager must be able to focus on the job description criteria and individual qualifications without introducing personal preference.

Problem-solving Skills. The office manager must be a problem solver. This may include being creative and doing away with old **paradigms** and traditional approaches to solving a problem. When difficult issues arise, focus on the situation, issue, or behavior, not on the person. A discussion about solving the problem without laying blame is much more productive. Positive solutions may be more readily attained when discussing what was observed rather than what was told by someone else.

Technical Expertise. The office manager should have a working knowledge of each procedure performed in the office, although it is not necessary to be the acknowledged technical expert. A good office manager is continually learning and encourages **subordinates** to seek opportunities to continue their education and advance their technical skills.

MANAGEMENT STYLES

There is a direct correlation between a person's personality and his or her management style. Three types of personalities and their management styles are discussed here (Institute for Management Excellence, 1998; Pyzdek, 1996).

People-oriented Personality

A team-oriented management style is most often used by people-oriented personalities. This personality is comfortable teaching, coaching, helping, communicating, advising, motivating, guiding, leading, and inspiring others. People-oriented managers tend to use the participatory management style by establishing and communicating the purpose and direction of the task and soliciting the participation of employees. These managers are leaders who use actions and words to show the way and inspire employees. They tend to coach by evaluating and advising, motivating and guiding.

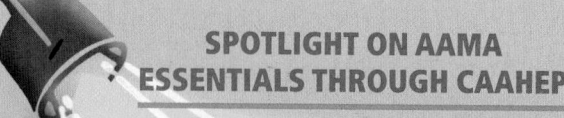

Things-oriented Personality

Things-oriented personalities tend to have more process-oriented management styles. They are most comfortable with physical dexterity, building, constructing, modeling, remodeling, and working with tools or instruments. The autocratic management style is often used by this personality. Autocratic managers function on the premise that in most cases employees cannot make a contribution to their own work, and that even if they could, they wouldn't. Autocratic managers deal with this perception by using "carrots" and "sticks." The "carrot," in most cases, is a monetary incentive and the "stick" is docked pay for poor quality work.

Idea-oriented Personality

The innovation-oriented management style is most often employed by idea-oriented personalities. These managers are most comfortable working with ideas and information. Management by wandering around (MBWA) is often used by them to collect information that can then be used to generate new ideas and approaches to doing the job. MBWA users are observant and ask questions to get at the problem. Once the problem has been clearly identified they enjoy research, data collection, and then brainstorming sessions to arrive at solutions.

Other Management Styles

In some organizations the **hierarchy** is viewed as a "chain-of-command." The person in the topmost position on the organizational chart is the ultimate authority. This person may delegate authority to a subordinate who may, in turn, delegate authority to positions further down in the hierarchy. But these managers must possess complete knowledge of the work being done by their subordinates. This management style is often referred to as the authoritarian style. The manager holds all authority and responsibility and communicates from the top of the hierarchy down.

In the democratic management style, the person at the top of the organization holds final responsibility but also delegates authority to others by developing a shared vision of the goals and objectives of the organization. Communication is very active, flowing upward to higher authorities and downward to subordinates.

Changing Styles for the Twenty-first Century

Today, managers are often seen as administrators rather than leaders. An administrator is one who executes, directs, or manages affairs. A leader, on the other hand, is a person who shows the way or guides. As we move into the twenty-first century, office managers will be called upon to be leaders and possess leadership qualities.

A good leader is one who can inspire others by example. In the medical office setting, a leader has the ability to inspire employees in a direction that benefits the entire facility. A leader excels in achieving goals and therefore influences others to be goal setters and achievers as well. Managers become leaders by demonstrating on a daily basis that they believe in their vision for the organization. Leaders have **charisma**, that is, they motivate others and inspire allegiance and devotion. Table 33-1 contrasts some management and leadership characteristics. Table 33-2 contains suggested management techniques and a brief description of the managers and leaders of the new millennium. Notice the importance of leadership characteristics as opposed to management characteristics in these descriptions.

TABLE 33-1 MANAGEMENT AND LEADERSHIP CHARACTERISTICS	
Management Characteristics	**Leadership Characteristics**
Punishment	Reward
Demands respect	Invites speaking out
Drill sergeant	Motivator
Limits and defines	Empowers
Imposes discipline	Values creativity
Bottom line	Vision
Control	Change
Hierarchy	Network
Rigid	Flexible
Automatic annual raises	Pay for performance
Dominates	Facilitates
Issues orders	Acts as role model
Demands unquestioning obedience	Coaches and mentors others
Knows all the answers	Asks the right questions
Not interested in new answers	Seeks to learn and draw out new ideas

Source: The Institute for Management Excellence. (1996, October). Managers vs. leaders. *Management vs. Leadership* [On-line]. Available: www.itstime.com/oct96b.htm.

THE IMPORTANCE OF TEAMWORK

The use of **teamwork** to improve the efficiency of the office may at first seem incongruent to your desire to improve office efficiency, since it seems that several people are now involved in solving a problem that you the manager should solve and explain. Teamwork builds morale and actually results in getting more accomplished with the resources you have because the team members

TABLE 33-2 DESCRIPTIONS OF MANAGERS AND LEADERS	
Management by Coaching and Development (MBCD)	Managers see themselves primarily as employee trainers.
Management by Competitive Edge (MBCE)	Individuals and groups within the organization compete against one another to see who can achieve the best results.
Management by Decision Models (MBDM)	Decisions are based on projections generated by artificially constructed situations.
Management by Exception (MBE)	Managers delegate as much responsibility and activity as possible to those below them, stepping in only when absolutely necessary.
Management by Performance (MBP)	Managers seek quality levels of performance through motivation and employee relations.
Management by Styles (MBS)	Managers adjust their approaches to meet situational needs.
Management by Walking Around (MBWA)	Managers walk around the company, getting a "feel" for people and operations; stopping to talk and to listen.
Management by Work Simplification (MBWS)	Managers constantly seek ways to simplify processes and reduce expenses.

Source: The Institute for Management Excellence. (1996, October). Management styles. *Management vs. Leadership* [On-line]. Available: www.itstime.com/oct96.htm.

develop ownership of the solution to a problem and want to make it work. When it works, it flatters them and builds their esteem.

Efficiency of a team results from the collective working together to plan how to "work smarter" and how to dovetail tasks and support each other so that wasted effort is avoided. In order to achieve all of these things, a team must not only be given the responsibility and the authority to plan and execute their plan to solve a problem, but they must know your expectations for them. Sometimes this means that you, the office manager, must stick your neck out for them. They will reward you handsomely for doing so.

Getting the Team Started

A successful teamwork approach is not a mysterious event that just happens, it is the result of clear vision, specific goals, and a well-planned strategy on the part of the team leader. For teamwork to be successful, individual team members must understand and support the specifics of the problem they are being asked to solve. This is probably the most significant task of the team leader or the office manager. It is helpful in taking this important step to let the team develop its own **work statement**, for in this way they assume ownership of the goals and objectives you want them to achieve. The work statement frequently outlines specific tasks and their sequential order of accomplishment. Its purpose is to ensure that everyone is working toward the team goals and objectives.

A major pitfall at this stage may be diverse opinions which can lead to a work statement that does not meet the manager's goals and objectives for the team. It is your job as office manager to try to direct the team back to what you want them to work on without undermining their team spirit. Take care at this stage not to begin making assignments or to let team members start solving the problem until the work statement is complete. Under some circumstances it may be necessary for you, the office manager, to exercise your authority in defining the work statement, but be careful, as this approach could harm the team's collective spirit.

The next step in team development is to establish a timetable for achieving results and identifying the standards that must be maintained. Without a timetable a team feels no sense of urgency and tends to lose direction. You also have to paint a clear picture of the standards that must be maintained as you attempt to solve the problem. You should let the team develop both the standards as well as the timetable, but with your leadership and support.

Using a Team to Solve a Problem

Problem solution is the next step in team development. Some people call this stage **brainstorming** a solution.

Brainstorming is fun, but unless it is controlled by the leader, it will bog down into needless arguments and hurt feelings. In a successful brainstorming session everyone should feel free to contribute solutions to the problem without any consideration for practicality or flaws in the proposal. Only after everyone has had a chance to speak are the solutions looked at in terms of practicality and for technical correctness. At this point the team should not look at what is wrong with the solution, but what needs to be done to make it a workable solution.

Prioritization of the solutions comes next. In order to do this it is helpful to assign scores for impact on solving the problem and for changeability, or the difficulty in implementing a particular solution in your office environment. The result will be a list of solutions to the problem in descending order from the greatest impact on the problem with the least cost or difficulty in implementation. Do a needs assessment, remove oneself from the issue, and look at it from a different perspective. **Benchmark** (compare) your facility to other facilities and organizations to see how they accomplish tasks, compensate employees, and so on.

Planning and Implementing a Solution

The team should work out a detailed plan for implementation of the solution selected, including a schedule. Assignments should be made, resources of equipment and funds available to the team should be defined, and any remaining problems assigned to subteams that will function just as the primary team did in solving them. The team should continue to meet to discuss progress and to resolve additional problems that may occur.

Recognition

A successful team should not be disbanded until it is acknowledged for its efforts and physical recognition is given in the case of an important problem that was solved. In some cases, a dinner or luncheon is in order. This is the most important phase of team development, as it is responsible for developing a team spirit or sense of **self-actualization** within the organization. Once this spirit is implanted into an organization, it becomes infectious.

SUPERVISING PERSONNEL

Creating an atmosphere in which open and honest communication can take place is critical to supervising personnel. This type of communication may be encouraged through the establishment of regular staff meetings, with each staff member sharing ideas for improvement and areas of concern. Eliciting the help of others in problem-solving strategies will promote harmony (Figure 33-1).

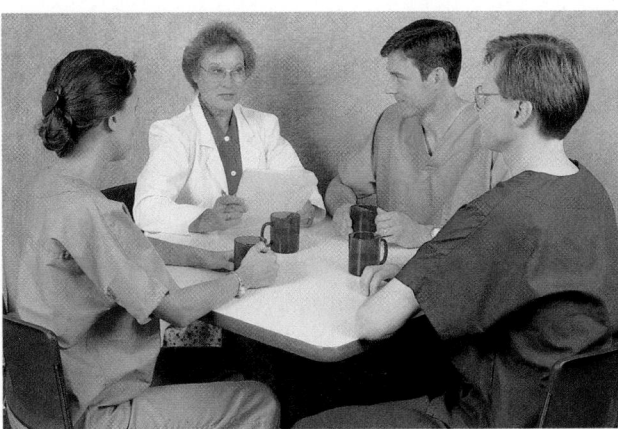

Figure 33-1 Consistently scheduled staff meetings can help office managers understand staff concerns as well as allow managers to communicate with the staff. This personal communication can help promote harmony among the health care team.

Staff Meetings

The office manager usually initiates the staff meeting idea and should officiate at such meetings. Failure of the office manager to be present may convey a message that the meeting is an event not worthy of attention. It is important that the office manager be familiar with basic parliamentary procedures. The purchase of books such as *Robert's Rules of Order* or *Parliamentary Procedure at a Glance* is an excellent investment.

Successful staff meetings are announced well in advance or on established time lines to enable the majority of the office personnel to attend. An **agenda** identifying the subjects to be covered during a given meeting should be issued prior to the meeting so that each attendee arrives prepared with input and/or questions relevant to the topics. Procedure 33-1 outlines the procedural steps for creating a meeting agenda. Figure 33-2 is a sample agenda. Each meeting should end with opportunity for nonagenda items to be discussed or suggested for inclusion in the next meeting. The meeting should have a fixed time to end.

A written record in the form of **minutes** should be maintained and sent to all team members regardless of whether they attended the meeting. This policy will keep all members informed about policy changes and decisions that impact the office operations. The minutes also trigger a reminder for any new procedures or revisions to be made in the procedures manual.

The first paragraph of the minutes should contain the following pieces of information:

- Kind of meeting (scheduled staff meeting, special meeting)

AGENDA

STAFF MEETING Wednesday, February 16, 2002
2:00 PM — Conference Room

1. Read and approve minutes of last meeting

2. Reports

   A. Satellite facility — Marilyn Johnson

   B. Patient flow — Joe Guerrero

   C.

3. Discussion of new telephone system

4. Unfinished Business

   A. Review new procedure manual pages

   B.

5. New Business

   A. Appoint committee for design of new marketing brochure

   B.

6. Open discussion and/or topics for next meeting's agenda

7. Set next meeting time

8. Adjourn

Figure 33-2 Sample meeting agenda.

- Name of the organization (Doctors Lewis & King)
- Date, time, and place of the meeting
- Names of those attending and who was the chair of the meeting
- Approval of previous minutes

The following paragraphs should address each of the agenda topics and include a brief summary of discussions, actions taken, name of person making any motions, the exact wording of the motion, and whether the motion was approved.

In addition to recording action plans under each agenda topic, it is desirable to summarize all action items agreed to in the meeting in one section of the minutes. This will facilitate easy access to information at a later date should it be required.

The last paragraph should include the date, time, and place of the next meeting and the hour of adjournment for this meeting. The person preparing the minutes should always sign them. A copy of the minutes should always be maintained in a book for easy reference.

Supporting Staff Members

The office manager may also be responsible for the following roles related to supporting staff employees. In large offices or clinics some of these responsibilities may be delegated to the human resources manager and are more fully covered in Chapter 34.

- Interview, hire, and terminate employees as delegated by the physician(s)/employer.

- Supervise or personally train employees. These responsibilities apply to new staff members as well as to updating current staff.

- Make weekly work schedules, vacation schedules, and determine how sick days will be covered effectively.

- Provide adequate staffing for employee absences.

- Establish probation periods within the legal boundaries of the employer and conduct performance evaluations as delegated by the physician(s)/employer.

- Establish increases and changes in the benefit package. These responsibilities should always be discussed with the physician(s)/employer first to be sure that the office manager is acting within the guidelines and scope of tasks delegated to that position.

TRAVEL ARRANGEMENTS

The office manager may be asked to make travel arrangements for physicians going on vacation or to conventions, symposiums, or out-of-town seminars and continuing medical education (CME) courses. If the physicians do a fair amount of travel or if they live in a metropolitan area, they may utilize the services of a travel agent. Attention to detail is extremely important in preventing travel disruptions.

Read carefully the instructions for completing registration forms, complete them, and mail them as quickly as possible to secure reservations to conventions, etc. Next make hotel and travel arrangements. General information regarding the physician's travel preferences should be maintained in a file folder and be referred to when making travel arrangements. Helpful information to maintain in this file includes:

- Name of travel agents used in the past (ranked by reputation and recommendation)

- Physician's or office credit card numbers

- Car rental preference

- Preferred airline, class of travel, seating choice

- Hotel/motel accommodations (bed size, suite, studio, connecting rooms, price range, amenities)

- Shuttle service

Next, contact the travel agent and identify the destination, date and time for departure and return, number traveling in party, and seating preference. A travel agent can also assist with rental car and hotel accommodations if needed. Take your time and pay attention to detail. When tickets are received, always check to see that all departure and arrival times match what is needed and that a confirmation number has been provided for car rentals and hotel arrangements. Procedure 33-2 outlines the procedural steps involved in making travel arrangements through a travel agent.

The Internet may be used to search for the lowest cost air, auto, and lodging reservations. The procedures do not require extensive knowledge of travel and airline reservation protocols. Searching for information on the **Internet** requires the use of a search engine if you do not already have a list of favorite travel **web sites**. A **search engine** is a special computer program available through your Internet service provider. With a search engine, you enter only the subject of your search and the engine will provide a list of web sites related to your subject. For example, if you are making travel arrangements you might access a search engine such as Lycos and key in the subject "air fares." The engine will return either a list of web sites or ask you to further refine your subject with suggestions such as cheap air fares, international travel, etc. Once you have refined your search, you may have choices such as Only-Travel.com, Expedia.com, or Priceline.com. Select the appropriate web site and follow its instructions.

Priceline.com and similar web sites are services that allow you to name the price you want to pay; Priceline finds a major airline willing to release seats on flights where they have unsold space. You need to have a reasonable idea of the price of the service you are trying to purchase; unreasonably low bids will just waste your time and effort. Procedure 33-3 outlines the steps for making travel arrangements via the Internet.

Itinerary

If you have utilized a travel agent in making the travel arrangements the agency will most likely provide several copies of the **itinerary**. An itinerary is a detailed plan for a proposed trip. The office should maintain one copy of the itinerary in case the physician must be reached for emergencies. The physician should have one copy to carry with him or her and a copy to leave with family members.

TRAVEL ITINERARY

James Whitney, MD
Inner City Health Care
400 Inner City Way
Seattle, WA 98400

Sept 15, 20--   INVOICE: 880133795

29 Sept 20-Friday
USAIR   6:30   Coach Class   Equip-Boeing 757 Jet
LV: Seattle   11:55P   Nonstop   Miles-2125   Confirmed
AR: Pittsburgh   7:23A   Elapsed time-4:28   Arrival Date-30Sept
                                        Seat-31C

30 Sept-Saturday
Alamo   1 Compact 2/4 DR   Drop-101CT   Confirmed
Pickup-Pittsburgh   Pittsburgh Airport   Chg-USD .00
Rate-   59.98   Baserate   Guaranteed   Extra Hr 10.00-UN
Phone-412-472-5060
                        Confirmation-1870649

01 Oct 20-Sunday
USAIR   1419 Coach Class   Equip-Boeing 737 Jet
LV: Pittsburgh   3:05P   Nonstop   Miles-2125   Confirmed
AR: Seattle   5:27P   Elapsed time-5:22
Lunch   Seat-20A

Ticket Number/s:
Whitney/James   35709334923   BA Card   461.00
    Air Transportation   416.36   Tax   44.64   TOTAL   461.00
                                       Sub Total   461.00
                                       Credit Card Payment   461.00-
                                       Amount Due   0.00

TICKET IS NON REFUNDABLE. TRIP INSURANCE IS AVAILABLE. RECONFIRM ALL FLTS 24 HRS PRIOR TO DEPARTURE

Figure 33-3   Sample travel itinerary.

You may need to develop the itinerary if you have made the travel arrangements via computer. Figure 33-3 shows a sample travel itinerary.

Important information to be included on any itinerary includes:

- Air travel: departure and arrival date and time, meals, airline name and telephone number, airport
- Car rental: name of provider, telephone number, confirmation number
- Hotel/motel: name, confirmation number, dates, telephone number

- Meeting location: name, address, room number, telephone number

SUPERVISING STUDENT PRACTICUMS

The student **practicum** is a transitional stage that provides opportunity for the student to apply theory learned in the classroom to a health care setting through practical, hands-on experience. Institutions accredited by the Committee on Accreditation of Allied Health Education Programs (CAAHEP) call this period **externship**. Some institutions may use the term *internship* and still others may operate through a co-operative education program. The number of hours for the practicum are predetermined along with criteria for site selection and tasks performed by the student.

The office manager should schedule an information interview with the extern student before the practicum begins. During this time a discussion of the expectations of the office manager and the extern may be established. A tour of the facility and introductions to key personnel aids the extern in feeling more comfortable the first day of "work."

Since the extern will be writing in medical records where correct spelling is mandatory or may be scheduling appointments and must write telephone numbers without transposition, some pretesting may be offered. By giving a spelling test of ten commonly used medical terms or verbally stating five telephone numbers for the extern to write down, an immediate evaluation is attained.

The office manager should directly supervise or identify someone else to supervise the extern. During the first few days of the practicum, the extern may simply shadow the supervisor, learning the routine, physician preference, and protocols for that particular office. As the extern begins to feel comfortable in the new environment, minimal tasks should be assigned. Based on the extern's ability to follow directions and perform tasks, increased skill-level tasks may be added.

The supervisor will supervise and evaluate the extern's progress; schedule activities that will provide experience in all aspects of medical assisting, including administrative, clinical, and laboratory procedures; maintain accurate records of attendance and hours "worked"; and communicate the extern's progress to the medical assisting supervisor from the educational institution. Procedure 33-4 provides steps for supervising a student practicum.

When working with externs, it is important to remember that they still have much to learn. When you take time to explain each step and to provide the rationale for each, students will learn more quickly. Demonstrating new and/or different techniques and approaches helps students by providing them with options that they may find more comfortable.

Remember that this type of learning is very stressful. The extern is not yet accustomed to communication with a "real" patient, let alone working with a physician. Your role as office manager is to reduce as much stress as possible for everyone concerned. Introduce the extern to the patient and ask the patient's permission to allow the student to perform a procedure. Many patients will be very tolerant when they realize the circumstances and will be quite cooperative.

TIME MANAGEMENT

Because medical office managers are responsible for numerous tasks and may experience many interruptions during the course of the day, it is important that they become disciplined and work well independently as well as with others. By focusing and pinpointing specific goals, which in turn may be translated into tasks to be completed during the workday, much can be accomplished.

Many office managers find it helpful to develop a "To Do" list on which tasks to be accomplished are listed. These tasks may be prioritized or simply listed as they come to mind or occur during the day. As each task is completed, it is crossed off. At the end of the day a sense of accomplishment is the reward for a clean list. Any tasks not yet completed may be prioritized and transferred to the next day's "To Do" list.

As much as possible, try to handle a paper only once. Read it, decide what action needs to be taken, and complete it. When responding to telephone calls, try also to bring closure to the call so that it is not necessary to make another call.

Do not procrastinate. Complete tasks as they arise whenever possible. Sometimes it takes longer to list a task on the "To Do" list and then have to rethink the solution than to just do it.

PROCEDURES MANUAL

The **procedures manual** provides detailed information relative to the performance of tasks within the facility in which one is employed. Each procedures manual should be designed for that specific office setting and should satisfy its requirements.

The procedures manual serves as a guide to the employee assigned a specific task and may also be useful in evaluating the employee's performance. If a temporary employee is assigned the task, the procedures manual will be invaluable in assuring that each procedure is completed as outlined.

The physician(s) and the office manager should have copies of the procedures manual and it should also be accessible to all employees. Copies of individual sections may be given to the employee responsible for the task; the employee should be instructed to follow these guidelines and told that they may be used as employee evaluation tools.

Organization of the Procedures Manual

It is best to use a loose-leaf binder with separator pages denoting each procedure. Many office managers find it helpful to divide the binder into administrative and clini-

Administrative Section	Clinical Section
Personnel Management	Physical Examinations
Communication	Infection Control
(oral and written)	Collecting Specimens
Patient Scheduling	Laboratory Procedures
Records Management	Surgical Asepsis
Financial Management	Emergencies
Facility and Equipment	
Management	

Figure 33-4 Many offices find that dividing the procedures manual into tabbed sections helps organize the material. A table of contents for the manual can also help locate information easily.

cal sections with subdivisions for each primary task performed (Figure 33-4).

To facilitate using the procedures manual, a consistent format should be developed and used throughout the manual. Each procedure should be a step-by-step outline or list of steps to be taken to complete a task as desired in that facility. Providing the rationale for a step, when appropriate, enhances the learning process, especially for new staff members. Procedure 33-5 provides steps for developing and maintaining a procedures manual.

Updating and Reviewing the Procedures Manual

When new procedures are added to the office routine, a new procedure page should be developed immediately. The new page is then useful as an educational tool or job aid while team members are learning new techniques.

An annual page-by-page review should be done to ascertain if each procedure is still being used and assure that each page is correct in each detail and satisfies all criteria established by the staff personnel. This contributes to an efficient office and gives all employees a sense of pride and satisfaction that they are performing within the scope of their training and to their greatest potential. The procedures manual should be reviewed by personnel performing the various tasks and their suggestions should be evaluated and incorporated into the revisions when appropriate. All new procedure pages and revisions should be dated (Rev. 02/15/02).

MARKETING FUNCTIONS

Effective communication skills are essential in the management of the ambulatory care setting. These skills are used by the office manager inside the ambulatory care setting to establish friendly, professional relationships with colleagues and patients. Communication is just as critical when relating to external audiences: other organizations, potential new patients, and community members. Developing relationships outside the office is often called marketing, a concept that office managers may utilize to enhance the image and visibility of an ambulatory care setting while also providing benefits to patients, potential patients, and the neighboring community.

In its broadest sense, **marketing** can be defined as the process by which the provider of services makes the consumer aware of the scope and quality of these services. While marketing is a tool traditionally used by for-profit organizations to promote and sell products and services, it has become increasingly acceptable among health care organizations, whether they are for- or not-for-profit.

Marketing functions and materials are diverse and can include seminars and workshops, patient education brochures, brochures that describe the ambulatory care setting and its scope of services, newsletters, press releases, and special events such as open houses or participation in community health care events. Depending on the size and resources of the medical office, the manager may choose to use all or some of these tools (Figure 33-5).

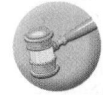 When producing written material and organizing events, it is essential that ethical guidelines be respected at all times. Marketing tools should be appropriate, in good taste, and designed to quietly enhance the reputation of the office. Cultural issues should always be considered. For example, patient education brochures for a practice with many Spanish-speaking patients should be produced in bilingual editions, with English on one side and Spanish on the other. Legal issues are important as well; when presenting material of a medical nature, it is extremely important that information be accurate and up-to-date.

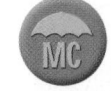 Effective marketing is a valuable tool for the office manager, especially as managed care calls on all health care professionals to become more competitive in order to survive. Marketing can increase visibility and credibility. The effective manager will enlist the talents and skills of the entire team in developing a marketing plan.

Seminars

As consumers become increasingly aware of lifestyle choices, they look to health care professionals for information and guidance. Seminars and workshops are useful vehicles for presenting health-related information; while expert advice can be given, there is also the opportunity for patients and health care professionals to interact.

Marketing Tool	Potential Uses and Value
Seminars	Can educate patients and provide good will in the community. All staff—administrative and clinical—can work as a team to organize, publicize, and deliver the seminars.
Brochures	Brochures are typically of two types: patient education brochures and brochures on office services. Can be simple 8 1/2" x 11" fact sheets, with text only, or more elaborate brochures folded to 4" x 9" that incorporate both text and graphics or photos. Both types of brochures are informative for patients and present a professional image of the ambulatory care setting.
Newsletters	Newsletters can be produced on a biannual or quarterly basis and can form the nucleus of a marketing program. Because they are versatile tools, they can include a wide range of information from health-related articles to staff introductions to insurance updates. They should be sent to individuals on the office's mailing list and be available in the reception area.
Press Releases	Periodic press releases on new equipment, new staff, and expanded or remodeled office space can be a vital link to the local community.
Special Events	Special events are an effective way to join with other community organizations to promote wellness. They can include participation in health fairs, cosponsorship of a charity event, or an open house on the premises to acquaint the community with new services or equipment.

Figure 33-5 Marketing tools and their use in a medical environment.

Seminars can be organized to meet patient and community needs. Some popular seminar topics include hypertension, diabetes, eating disorders, and exercise and weight management programs.

No matter what the topic area, the content should be oriented to the lay person's level of understanding, with a focused message and a delivery designed to maintain attention. Interactive seminars, which encourage audience participation, can be productive and enjoyable. Audiovisuals, such as projected slides, will provide visual reinforcement. Handouts, either from professional organizations or those produced by office staff, can elaborate on seminar content and help the participant review and remember what was said.

Brochures

Despite the promise of a paperless society, brochures continue to be valuable sources of information. In the health care setting, patients welcome a rack of brochures as a source of current, accurate background on medical issues. New patients also find that a brochure on office services will answer many questions about the practice, its philosophy, and its scope of services, and provide physician profiles.

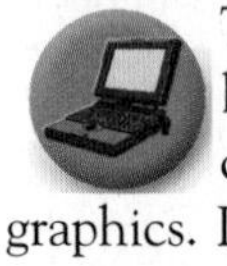

Today, it is possible to produce a professional-looking brochure in the office using one of the computer programs that integrate text and graphics. If a brochure is produced in-house, it is important to consider writing, design, and production. Writing should be clear, to the point, and grammatically correct. Always proofread carefully before printing. Design should be kept simple; while computer programs offer sophisticated options, these are best left to experienced designers. Avoid the use of too many typefaces; choose a typeface and size for readability, and, if using artwork or photography, consider its reproduction qualities. Typically, brochures will be printed in one or two colors. Black or another dark ink is best for readability.

Often, a local printer will be able to advise the office manager on how to prepare a brochure or handout for printing. The simplest handouts can be quick-copied (a high-speed photocopy) on a white or lightly colored or textured stock. After printing, brochures should be made accessible to patients and other visitors in a rack or neatly arranged in piles (Figure 33-6). Occasionally, a brochure will be mailed; one that folds to 4″ × 9″ will fit into a standard #10 business envelope.

Patient Education Brochures. Like seminars, patient education brochures can address a variety of topics, including hypertension, diabetes, eating disorders, and exercise and weight management programs. When writing these brochures, always research material carefully, request permission for copyrighted materials, and present the information in a manner that is accessible to your patient population.

Office Brochures. A brochure on the practice can provide a wide range of information and will orient the new patient to the practice. One way to determine what information to include is to develop a list of frequently asked patient questions. Once this list is compiled, it can serve as the beginning of the brochure outline. Issues to consider might include:

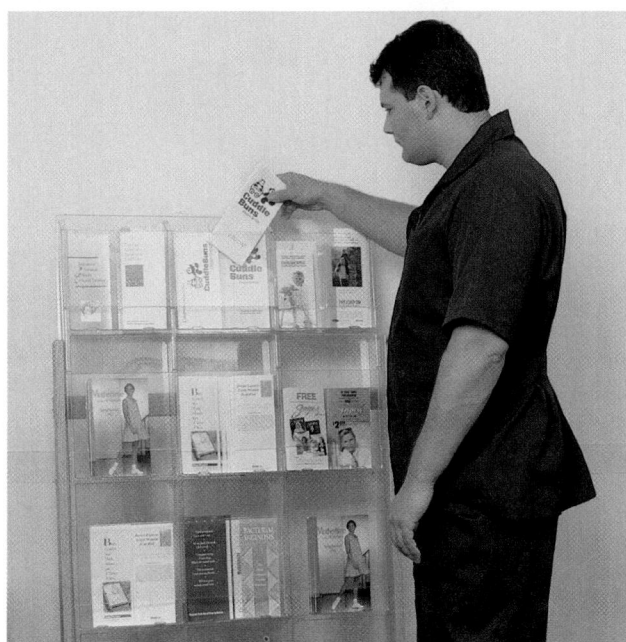

Figure 33-6 Brochures and handouts should be accessible and inviting to patients and office visitors.

- Brief history of the practice
- Brief resumes or credentials of physicians
- Philosophy of the practice
- Scope of services
- How to reach the practice in case of emergency
- Insurances accepted
- Rights of patients
- Policies regarding the release of information
- Scheduling information: How to schedule an appointment, cancellation policies
- Amenities on the premises such as parking, pharmacy, lab
- Location, map if necessary, and location of satellite offices

Newsletters

Newsletters are effective communication tools because they encourage regular contact with patients and other readers. Newsletters are a versatile medium, too; they can contain patient education articles, updates on staff changes, awards, information on insurance carriers, calendars of events, even recipes that are consistent with a healthful lifestyle.

Most newsletters can be written and produced in the office. Like brochures, they should be simple in design

and format. An additional factor in newsletter production is mailing; an up-to-date database must be maintained, postal regulations must be followed, and the costs of mailing considered.

Press Releases

Press releases are simple, inexpensive marketing tools. Use them to announce new staff, promote a new service, or publicize a series of seminars. If a professional, courteous relationship is developed with the local press, most will be happy to receive and publish releases. When writing releases, always follow proper format, which includes a date of release, a contact person's name and telephone number, and a short headline. Releases are best kept to one double-spaced typed page. At the end of the release, type "30" or a number sign (#). Maintain an active list of local newspapers and editors' names so that you can mail or fax the release to the appropriate editor.

Special Events

While they can be time-consuming to organize and participate in, special events are rewarding, for they present an opportunity to interact with the community. They have high visibility, for often a group of community organizations will collaborate to cosponsor an event such as a walk-a-thon, blood pressure clinic, health fair for seniors, or wellness day for children and families. Sponsorship can be as simple as a donation to the cause; other times, staffing a booth or offering a service such as blood pressure checks is appropriate.

Like all marketing efforts, special events require organizational skills and teamwork, but they often result in heightened communication with the community and provide an educational service to patients and their families.

RECORD AND FINANCIAL MANAGEMENT

Physicians entrust a great deal of responsibility to their medical office managers. The daily payments received through the mail and office visits must be processed and prepared for banking. Office expenses must be processed and paid in a timely fashion to capitalize on any discounts available. Employee requirements and records such as Social Security records, Withholding Allowance Certificates (W-4 forms) (Figure 33-7) indicating the number of exemptions claimed, and Employment Eligibility Verification Forms (I-9) ensuring that all persons employed are either United States citizens, lawfully admitted aliens, or aliens authorized to work in the United States must be completed and filed with the appropriate federal agencies. Also, state and local tax records must be filed and maintained for each employee.

Form W-4 (2000)

Purpose. Complete Form W-4 so your employer can withhold the correct Federal income tax from your pay. Because your tax situation may change, you may want to refigure your withholding each year.

Exemption from withholding. If you are exempt, complete only lines 1, 2, 3, 4, and 7, and sign the form to validate it. Your exemption for 2000 expires February 16, 2001.

Note: *You cannot claim exemption from withholding if (1) your income exceeds $700 and includes more than $250 of unearned income (e.g., interest and dividends) and (2) another person can claim you as a dependent on their tax return.*

Basic instructions. If you are not exempt, complete the **Personal Allowances Worksheet** below. The worksheets on page 2 adjust your withholding allowances based on itemized deductions, adjustments to income, or two-earner/two-job situations. Complete all worksheets that apply. They will help you figure the number of withholding allowances you are entitled to claim. **However, you may claim fewer (or zero) allowances.**

Child tax and higher education credits. For details on adjusting withholding for these and other credits, see **Pub. 919,** How Do I Adjust My Tax Withholding?

Head of household. Generally, you may claim head of household filing status on your tax return only if you are unmarried and pay more than 50% of the costs of keeping up a home for yourself and your dependent(s) or other qualifying individuals. See line E below.

Nonwage income. If you have a large amount of nonwage income, such as interest or dividends, you should consider making estimated tax payments using **Form 1040-ES,** Estimated Tax for Individuals. Otherwise, you may owe additional tax.

Two earners/two jobs. If you have a working spouse or more than one job, figure the total number of allowances you are entitled to claim on all jobs using worksheets from only one Form W-4. Your withholding usually will be most accurate when all allowances are claimed on the Form W-4 prepared for the highest paying job and zero allowances are claimed for the others.

Check your withholding. After your Form W-4 takes effect, use Pub. 919 to see how the dollar amount you are having withheld compares to your projected total tax for 2000. Get Pub. 919 especially if you used the **Two-Earner/Two-Job Worksheet** on page 2 and your earnings exceed $150,000 (Single) or $200,000 (Married).

Recent name change? If your name on line 1 differs from that shown on your social security card, call 1-800-772-1213 for a new social security card.

Personal Allowances Worksheet (Keep for your records.)

A Enter "1" for **yourself** if no one else can claim you as a dependent . . . . . A ____

B Enter "1" if: { • You are single and have only one job; or • You are married, have only one job, and your spouse does not work; or • Your wages from a second job or your spouse's wages (or the total of both) are $1,000 or less. } . . B ____

C Enter "1" for your **spouse.** But, you may choose to enter -0- if you are married and have either a working spouse or more than one job. (Entering -0- may help you avoid having too little tax withheld.) . . . C ____

D Enter number of **dependents** (other than your spouse or yourself) you will claim on your tax return . . . D ____

E Enter "1" if you will file as **head of household** on your tax return (see conditions under **Head of household** above) . E ____

F Enter "1" if you have at least $1,500 of **child or dependent care expenses** for which you plan to claim a credit . . F ____

G **Child Tax Credit:**

- If your total income will be between $18,000 and $50,000 ($23,000 and $63,000 if married), enter "1" for each eligible child.
- If your total income will be between $50,000 and $80,000 ($63,000 and $115,000 if married), enter "1" if you have two eligible children, enter "2" if you have three or four eligible children, or enter "3" if you have five or more eligible children . G ____

H Add lines A through G and enter total here. **Note:** *This may be different from the number of exemptions you claim on your tax return.* ► H ____

For accuracy, complete all worksheets that apply.

- If you plan to **itemize or claim adjustments to income** and want to reduce your withholding, see the **Deductions and Adjustments Worksheet** on page 2.
- If you are **single,** have **more than one job** and your combined earnings from all jobs exceed $34,000, OR if you are **married** and have a **working spouse or more than one job** and the combined earnings from all jobs exceed $60,000, see the **Two-Earner/Two-Job Worksheet** on page 2 to avoid having too little tax withheld.
- If **neither** of the above situations applies, **stop here** and enter the number from line H on line 5 of Form W-4 below.

Cut here and give Form W-4 to your employer. Keep the top part for your records.

Form **W-4** — Department of the Treasury, Internal Revenue Service

Employee's Withholding Allowance Certificate

► For Privacy Act and Paperwork Reduction Act Notice, see page 2.

OMB No. 1545-0010 **2000**

1 Type or print your first name and middle initial | Last name | 2 Your social security number

Home address (number and street or rural route) | 3 ☐ Single ☐ Married ☐ Married, but withhold at higher Single rate.
Note: *If married, but legally separated, or spouse is a nonresident alien, check the Single box.*

City or town, state, and ZIP code | 4 If your last name differs from that on your social security card, check here. **You must call 1-800-772-1213 for a new card** . . . ► ☐

5 Total number of allowances you are claiming (from line H above **OR** from the applicable worksheet on page 2) | 5 |

6 Additional amount, if any, you want withheld from each paycheck . . . | 6 | $

7 I claim exemption from withholding for 2000, and I certify that I meet **BOTH** of the following conditions for exemption:
- Last year I had a right to a refund of **ALL** Federal income tax withheld because I had **NO tax liability AND**
- This year I expect a refund of **ALL** Federal income tax withheld because I expect to have **NO tax liability.**

If you meet both conditions, write "EXEMPT" here . . . ► | 7 |

Under penalties of perjury, I certify that I am entitled to the number of withholding allowances claimed on this certificate, or I am entitled to claim exempt status.

Employee's signature (Form is not valid unless you sign it) ► Date ►

8 Employer's name and address (Employer: Complete lines 8 and 10 only if sending to the IRS.) | 9 Office code (optional) | 10 Employer identification number

Cat. No. 10220Q

Form W-4 (2000) Page **2**

Deductions and Adjustments Worksheet

Note: *Use this worksheet only if you plan to itemize deductions or claim adjustments to income on your 2000 tax return.*

1 Enter an estimate of your 2000 itemized deductions. These include qualifying home mortgage interest, charitable contributions, state and local taxes, medical expenses in excess of 7.5% of your income, and miscellaneous deductions. (For 2000, you may have to reduce your itemized deductions if your income is over $128,950 ($64,475 if married filing separately). See **Worksheet 3** in Pub. 919 for details.) . . . 1 $____

2 Enter: { $7,350 if married filing jointly or qualifying widow(er); $6,450 if head of household; $4,400 if single; $3,675 if married filing separately } . . . 2 $____

3 **Subtract** line 2 from line 1. If line 2 is greater than line 1, enter -0- . . . 3 $____

4 Enter an estimate of your 2000 adjustments to income, including alimony, deductible IRA contributions, and student loan interest 4 $____

5 **Add** lines 3 and 4 and enter the total (Include any amount for credits from **Worksheet 7** in Pub. 919.) . 5 $____

6 Enter an estimate of your 2000 nonwage income (such as dividends or interest) . . . 6 $____

7 **Subtract** line 6 from line 5. Enter the result, but not less than -0- . . . 7 $____

8 **Divide** the amount on line 7 by $3,000 and enter the result here. Drop any fraction . . . 8 ____

9 Enter the number from the **Personal Allowances Worksheet,** line H, page 1 . . . 9 ____

10 **Add** lines 8 and 9 and enter the total here. If you plan to use the **Two-Earner/Two-Job Worksheet,** also enter this total on line 1 below. Otherwise, **stop here** and enter this total on Form W-4, line 5, page 1 . 10 ____

Two-Earner/Two-Job Worksheet

Note: *Use this worksheet only if the instructions under line H on page 1 direct you here.*

1 Enter the number from line H, page 1 (or from line 10 above if you used the **Deductions and Adjustments Worksheet**) 1 ____

2 Find the number in **Table 1** below that applies to the **LOWEST** paying job and enter it here . . . 2 ____

3 If line 1 is **MORE THAN OR EQUAL TO** line 2, subtract line 2 from line 1. Enter the result here (if zero, enter -0-) and on Form W-4, line 5, page 1. **Do not** use the rest of this worksheet . . . 3 ____

Note: *If line 1 is **LESS THAN** line 2, enter -0- on Form W-4, line 5, page 1. Complete lines 4–9 below to calculate the additional withholding amount necessary to avoid a year end tax bill.*

4 Enter the number from line 2 of this worksheet . . . 4 ____

5 Enter the number from line 1 of this worksheet . . . 5 ____

6 **Subtract** line 5 from line 4 . . . 6 ____

7 Find the amount in **Table 2** below that applies to the **HIGHEST** paying job and enter it here . . . 7 $____

8 **Multiply** line 7 by line 6 and enter the result here. This is the additional annual withholding needed . . 8 $____

9 Divide line 8 by the number of pay periods remaining in 2000. For example, divide by 26 if you are paid every other week and you complete this form in December 1999. Enter the result here and on Form W-4, line 6, page 1. This is the additional amount to be withheld from each paycheck . . . 9 $

Table 1: Two-Earner/Two-Job Worksheet

Married Filing Jointly				All Others			
If wages from LOWEST paying job are—	Enter on line 2 above	If wages from LOWEST paying job are—	Enter on line 2 above	If wages from LOWEST paying job are—	Enter on line 2 above	If wages from LOWEST paying job are—	Enter on line 2 above
$0 - $4,000	0	41,001 - 45,000	8	$0 - $5,000	0	65,001 - 80,000	8
4,001 - 7,000	1	45,001 - 55,000	9	5,001 - 11,000	1	80,001 - 100,000	9
7,001 - 13,000	2	55,001 - 63,000	10	11,001 - 17,000	2	100,001 and over	10
13,001 - 19,000	3	63,001 - 70,000	11	17,001 - 22,000	3		
19,001 - 25,000	4	70,001 - 85,000	12	22,001 - 27,000	4		
25,001 - 31,000	5	85,001 - 100,000	13	27,001 - 40,000	5		
31,001 - 37,000	6	100,001 - 110,000	14	40,001 - 50,000	6		
37,001 - 41,000	7	110,001 and over	15	50,001 - 65,000	7		

Table 2: Two-Earner/Two-Job Worksheet

Married Filing Jointly		All Others	
If wages from HIGHEST paying job are —	Enter on line 7 above	If wages from HIGHEST paying job are —	Enter on line 7 above
$0 - $50,000	$420	$0 - $30,000	$420
50,001 - 100,000	780	30,001 - 60,000	780
100,001 - 130,000	870	60,001 - 120,000	870
130,001 - 250,000	1,000	120,001 - 270,000	1,000
250,001 and over	1,100	270,001 and over	1,100

Privacy Act and Paperwork Reduction Act Notice. We ask for the information on this form to carry out the Internal Revenue laws of the United States. The Internal Revenue Code requires this information under sections 3402(f)(2)(A) and 6109 and their regulations. Failure to provide a **properly** completed form will result in your being treated as a single person who claims no withholding allowances; **providing fraudulent information may also subject you to penalties.** Routine uses of this information include giving it to the Department of Justice for civil and criminal litigation, to cities, states, and the District of Columbia for use in administering their tax laws, and for use in the National Directory of New Hires.

You are not required to provide the information requested on a form that is subject to the Paperwork Reduction Act unless the form displays a valid OMB control number. Books or records relating to a form or its instructions must be retained as long as their contents may become material in the administration of any Internal Revenue law. Generally, tax returns and return information are confidential, as required by Code section 6103.

The time needed to complete this form will vary depending on individual circumstances. The estimated average time is: **Recordkeeping** 46 min., **Learning about the law or the form** 13 min., **Preparing the form** 59 min. If you have comments concerning the accuracy of these time estimates or suggestions for making this form simpler, we would be happy to hear from you. You can write to the Tax Forms Committee, Western Area Distribution Center, Rancho Cordova, CA 95743-0001. **DO NOT** send the tax form to this address. Instead, give it to your employer.

Figure 33-7 The Form W-4 indicates the number of exemptions claimed by the employee for income tax purposes.

Payroll Processing

In some cases it is the office manager's responsibility to prepare payroll checks for each employee and record all deductions withheld. A W-2 form (Figure 33-8) summarizing all earnings and deductions for the year must be prepared for each employee by January 31 of each year. The Social Security Administration must receive a report of W-2 forms each year.

To comply with all governmental regulations, federal, state, and local, it is important that the office manager who processes payroll maintain complete, up-to-date records on every employee. This information should be gathered from new employees and updated every year and upon any change in employee status. Every employee file should contain social security number, number of exemptions claimed on the W-4 Form, the employee's gross salary, and all deductions withheld for all taxes including Social Security, federal, state, local, plus unemploy-

ment tax (where applicable), and disability insurance (where applicable).

In order to process payroll, the physician's office must have a federal tax reporting number, obtained from the Internal Revenue Service. In some states, a state employer number also is needed.

Preparing Payroll Checks. When preparing payroll checks, it is important to keep a record of all tax and insurance amounts deducted from an employee's earnings. Many ambulatory care settings that operate on a manual bookkeeping system find that the write-it-once system is the most efficient way to accurately maintain these records. Payroll records should include:

- Employee name, address, and telephone number
- Social security number
- Date of employment

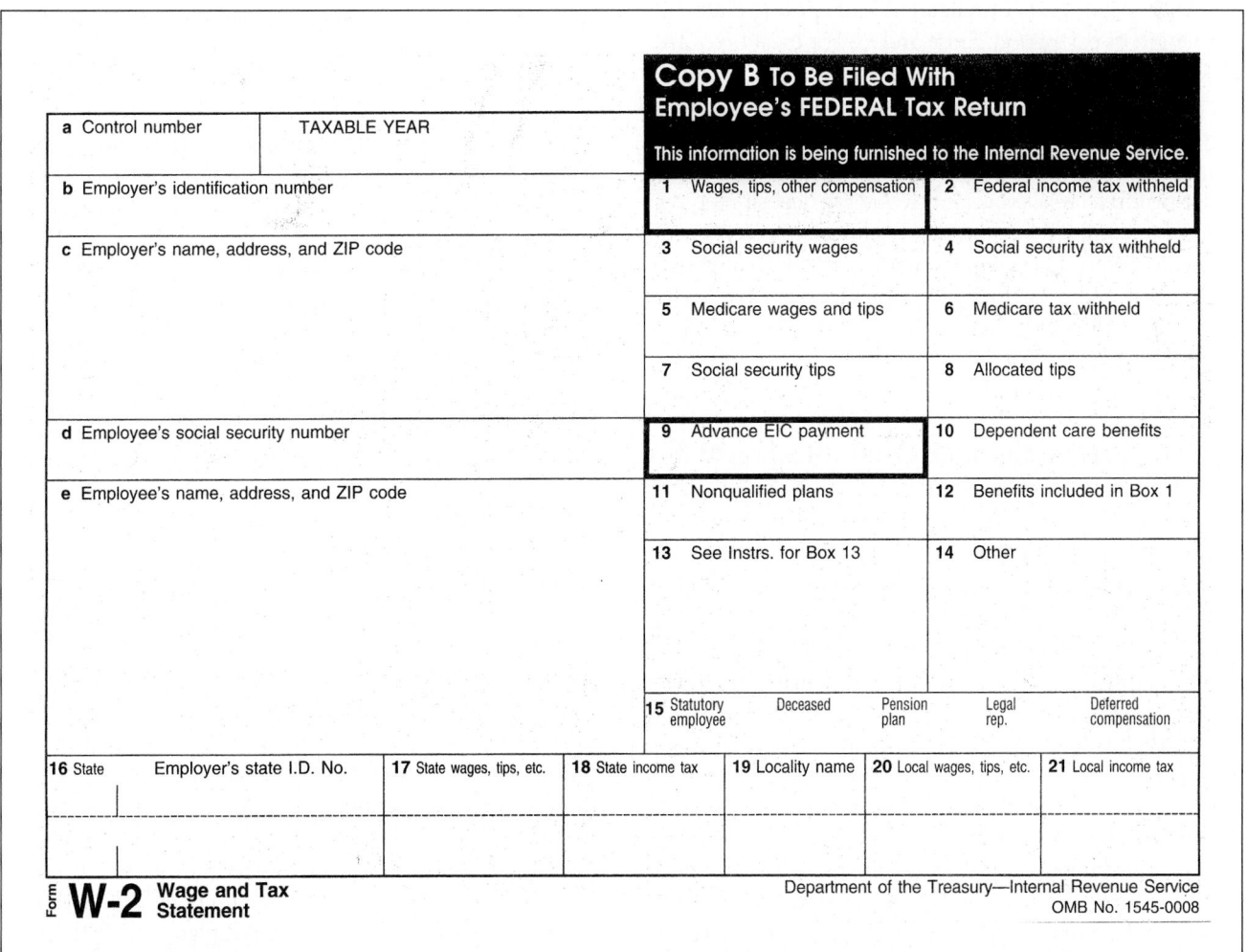

Figure 33-8 The Form W-2 summarizes all earnings and deductions for the year and must be prepared for each employee by January 31.

Each paycheck stub should contain:

- Number of hours worked, including regular and overtime (if hourly)
- Date of pay periods
- Date of check
- Gross salary
- Itemized deductions for federal income tax, social security (FICA) tax, state taxes, city or local taxes
- Itemized deductions for health insurance, disability insurance
- Other deductions such as uniforms, loan payments, and so on
- Net salary (gross earnings minus taxes and deductions)

Figuring Taxes. When figuring federal income taxes and social security taxes, use the charts provided by the Internal Revenue Service. Federal tax is based on amount earned, marital status, number of exemptions claimed, and length of pay period. State and city or local taxes are typically a percentage of the gross earnings.

All federal and state taxes withheld must be paid on a quarterly basis to the appropriate government offices. These monies should be accompanied by the required reporting forms. It is important to observe deposit requirements for withheld income tax and social security and Medicare taxes. These requirements, which change frequently, are listed in the Federal Employer's Tax Guide, available from the U.S. Government Printing Office, Internal Revenue Service, or on-line at ftp://ftp.fedworld.gov/pub/irs-pdf/p15.pdf.

Managing Benefits and Other Responsibilities. Benefits, or additional remuneration to the salary earned by full-time employees, must also be managed and records maintained for each employee. Examples of benefits may include paid vacation, paid holidays, health/dental insurance, disability, profit-sharing options, and complimentary health care. Some ambulatory care settings may refer to all or some of these benefits as fringe benefits.

Other responsibilities of the office manager may include maintaining a personal file for each employee providing their history with the facility, application for their current position, evaluations, promotions, problems, awards, entitlements, legal forms required by state and federal agencies, and so on. All Occupational Safety and Health Administration (OSHA) data, hazard material training and documentation, cardiopulmonary resuscita-

tion (CPR) certifications, and continued education units (CEUs) must be recorded and maintained.

FACILITY AND EQUIPMENT MANAGEMENT

The physical plant or building must be observed and maintained with safety being a key ingredient. It should be the responsibility of each staff member to report to the office manager any facility repairs that require attention and suggest replacement or recommend new pieces of equipment as required by the practice to support the health care needs of its population.

The office manager is usually responsible for the maintenance of the office and may hire ancillary services to provide janitorial and laundry services, dispose of hazardous materials, and maintain aquariums or plants that may enhance the environment of the facility. The office manager must stress the importance of patient confidentiality at the close of each day. Ancillary services must not have access to confidential material.

Magazine subscriptions and health-related literature for the reception area are the responsibility of the office manager. Selections should be made carefully, keeping in mind the interests of the patients and their cultures. These materials should not be kept once they become dog-eared, torn, and outdated. The use of plastic protectors and appropriate storage shelving aid in keeping the area and materials tidy.

The office manager is also responsible for facility improvements including any necessary repairs, decorating and color scheme, and floor plan suggestions. The wise office manager does not make these decisions independently, but asks for suggestions from the physician(s) and staff members. Remember, the team-building approach adds a cohesive element to any office environment.

Inventories

All equipment in the facility must be inventoried and maintained. Documented files should be maintained for each piece of equipment. These files are maintained in a separate reference loose-leaf binder and may be divided into administrative and clinical categories. The binder may contain pocket pages in which copies of any warranties, service agreements/contracts, and instructions for use and maintenance may be placed. This binder should be accessible to anyone who may need to refer to its pages. It is also important that as new items or updated service agreements/contracts are purchased, the old ones are removed from the binder and replaced with the new items.

Equipment and Supplies Maintenance

The office storage areas should be well maintained, and each item should always be put back in its place with lids replaced properly to prevent any accidents. Medication storage requires special attention. Many medications must be stored at certain temperatures, kept dry, or stored in dark, airtight containers. Narcotics should always be stored in a locked cabinet. Require two individuals to sign off when narcotic supplies are used and maintain a daily inventory.

Laboratory equipment must be maintained and quality control measures utilized. Calibration checks are required for a number of pieces of equipment: sphygmomanometers and centrifuges to name two. Microscopes and various types of scopes used during physical examinations and specialty procedures contain light sources that must be checked before each use. A replacement supply of bulbs should be available. Refer to Safety and Regulatory Guidelines in the Medical Laboratory, Chapter 26, for more information on quality control and safety in the medical laboratory.

RISK MANAGEMENT

The office manager must practice **risk management**. The risk management process includes the identification, analysis, and treatment of risks within the medical office. The office manager should evaluate the practice to determine when potential risks are present and act to eliminate the risks or to prevent injuries from the risks.

A comprehensive safety program is essential to risk management. This safety program is responsible for meeting the basic safety needs of patients, employees, and visitors. The manager will make sure that all safety guidelines and practices are followed throughout the office and that all staff members work within the scope of their training and qualifications.

The primary principle behind the risk management role is loss prevention. With the increased number of legal actions occurring in the health care field, the risk management program is even more vital for the protection of the facility's assets. Maintenance of practice liability coverage is essential to protect the facility from risk that cannot be avoided.

LIABILITY COVERAGE AND BONDING

Negligence is performing an act that a reasonable and prudent physician would not perform or failure to perform an act that a reasonable and prudent physician would perform. The common term used to describe professional **liability**, or legal responsibility, today is **malpractice**, a term that has negative connotations. It is much easier to prevent malpractice than to defend it in litigation so every effort should be taken to prevent negligence.

Insurance policies specifically designed to protect the physician's assets in the event a liability claim is filed and awarded in the patient's favor are available. Any physician not carrying such insurance is said to be **"going bare"** and would personally be responsible for any court costs, damages, and attorney fees if a malpractice suit were lost.

Practicing medical assistants should carry **professional liability insurance** for protection. Medical assistants who are members of the American Association of Medical Assistants (AAMA) have the option of purchasing personal and professional insurance through the organization at corporate rates.

Some physicians will carry the names of their employees on their policies. If this is the case, always ask to see the policy and verify that your name is printed on the policy—no name indicates no coverage. The manager may need to see that professional liability insurance has been purchased, all appropriate names are listed, and the premiums are paid in a timely fashion.

Professional liability insurance is important if the physician/employer is sued. In this event, the physician and the medical assistant could be named in the suit. If the case were lost, both the physician and the medical assistant could be liable.

Individuals who are responsible for handling financial records and money in the medical office may be bonded. A **bond** is purchased for a cash value in an employee's name which insures that the physician will recover the amount of loss in the event that an employee **embezzles** funds. It is the office manager or the human resources manager's responsibility to ask prospective employees if they are bondable. Individuals who are not bondable may not be the best candidates for the position.

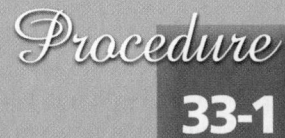

33-1   Preparing a Meeting Agenda

PURPOSE:
To prepare a meeting agenda, a list of specific items to be discussed and/or acted upon, in order to maintain the focus of the group and allow business to be transacted in a timely fashion.

EQUIPMENT/SUPPLIES:
List of participants
Order of business
Names of individuals giving reports
Names of any guest speakers
Computer and paper to print agendas

PROCEDURE STEPS:
1. Reserve proposed date, time, and place of meeting. RATIONALE: Ensure that the facilities are available for the meeting.

2. Collect information for meeting agenda by previewing the previous meeting's minutes for old business items, checking with others for report items, determining any new business items. RATIONALE: Ensure that all old and new business items have been identified.
3. Prepare a hard copy of the agenda and have it approved by chair of the meeting. RATIONALE: Confirmation by the chair of the agenda content ensures that agenda is correct and complete.
4. Send agenda to meeting participants two weeks in advance of the meeting. RATIONALE: Permits participants to prepare for the meeting by completing any tasks required and preparing any necessary documentation.

33-2   Making Travel Arrangements

PURPOSE:
To make travel arrangements for the physician.

EQUIPMENT/SUPPLIES:
Travel plan
Telephone and telephone directory
Computer
Physician's or office credit card to pay for reservations

PROCEDURE STEPS:
1. Confirm the details of the planned trip: dates, time, and place for departure and arrival; preferred mode of transportation (plane, train, bus, car); number of travelers; preferred lodging type and price range; and whether travelers checks are required. RATIONALE: Confirming pertinent travel details ensure that correct arrangements will be made.
2. Make travel and lodging reservations by calling travel agent or using the computer for on-line ticket services. RATIONALE: Ensure that space for physician is reserved at desired times.

3. Pick up tickets or arrange for their delivery.
4. Check to see that ticket arrangements are accurate (dates, times, places).
5. Check to see that car rental and lodging accommodations are accurate and confirmed. RATIONALE: Avoid inaccuracies and confusion with schedule.
6. Make additional copies of the itinerary or create the itinerary if making arrangements via computer. The itinerary should list date and time of departures and arrivals, including flight numbers and seat assignments. Note mode of transportation to lodging (shuttle, bus, car, taxi). Include name, address, and telephone number of lodgings and meeting places.
7. Maintain one copy of the itinerary in the office file.
8. Give several copies of the itinerary to the physician. RATIONALE: Ensure that a copy is on file with the office and that there are sufficient copies for the traveler(s) and their families.

Procedure 33-3 — Making Travel Arrangements Via Internet

PURPOSE:
To make travel arrangements for the physician using the Internet.

EQUIPMENT/SUPPLIES:
Travel plan
Computer
Physician's or office credit card to pay for reservations.

PROCEDURE STEPS:
1. Confirm the details of the planned trip: dates, time, and place for departure and arrival; preferred mode of transportation (plane, train, bus, car); number of travelers; preferred lodging type and price range; and whether travelers checks are required. RATIONALE: Confirming pertinent travel details ensures that correct arrangements will be made.
2. Go to the computer and access the Internet.
3. Select a search engine to locate web pages under the subject "air fares." Web pages may provide links to air fares, auto reservations, and hotel/motel reservations. Follow web page instructions for making arrangements. Review and copy confirmation of your transaction. RATIONALE: The Internet can be a time saver and cost-effective way of securing travel arrangements.
4. Pick up tickets or arrange for their delivery, if necessary. Tickets purchased on the Internet may be mailed or picked up at an airport, or they may be electronic tickets.
5. Make additional copies of the itinerary or create the itinerary. The itinerary should list date and time of departures and arrivals, including flight numbers and seat assignments. Note the mode of transportation to lodging (shuttle, bus, car, taxi). Include name, address, and telephone number of lodgings and meeting places.
6. Maintain one copy of the itinerary in the office file.
7. Give several copies of the itinerary to the physician. RATIONALE: Ensure that a copy is on file with the office and that there are sufficient copies for the traveler(s) and their families.

Procedure 33-4 — Supervising a Student Practicum

PURPOSE:
To prepare a training path for a student extern being assigned to the office. To make the involved office personnel aware of their responsibilities. To preplan which jobs the student extern performs and in what sequence they will be assigned. To make the externship successful by providing as much supervision and assistance as necessary.

EQUIPMENT/SUPPLIES:
None needed

PROCEDURE STEPS:
1. Review the clinical externship contract or agreement between your agency and the educational institution. RATIONALE: Guidelines and procedures are reviewed and refreshed in your mind.
2. Determine the amount of supervision the extern will require. RATIONALE: Prepares you to speak with the student and site supervisor regarding supervision.
3. Identify the supervisor who will be immediately responsible for the extern. RATIONALE: Establishes a person who knows he or she is to supervise the student and be responsible for the externship procedures.
4. Plan what tasks the extern will be allowed or encouraged to perform. RATIONALE: The office may or may not permit the student to perform

(continues)

Procedure 33-4 *(continued)*

invasive procedures. Determining tasks the student can and can not perform beforehand promotes a better relationship.

5. Create a schedule outlining the time the extern will be assigned to each unit. RATIONALE: Establishing a schedule keeps everyone appraised of what is happening and when.

6. Begin orientation for the extern as soon as he or she arrives at the office. Include a tour of the office and introduction to the staff. RATIONALE: Orients student and staff to each other and establishes guidelines for procedures.

7. Give the extern a copy of the Office Policy Manual and the work schedule for the entire externship. Answer any questions the extern might have. RATIONALE: Orients student and staff to each other and establishes guidelines for procedures.

8. Maintain an accurate record of the hours the extern works. Also log the date and reason for any missed days, late arrivals, or early dismissals. RATIONALE: Provides necessary documentation for the hours completed by the student.

9. Check with the extern frequently to be sure the extern is receiving meaningful training from the work experience. RATIONALE: Verifies that necessary training is being provided.

10. Consult physicians and staff members with whom the extern has worked for their opinion of the student's capabilities. Follow up on any problems that might be identified. RATIONALE: Verifies that necessary training is being provided.

11. Report the extern's progress to the medical assisting supervisor from the educational institution. This person usually visits once or twice each rotation. RATIONALE: Verifies that necessary training is being provided.

12. Prepare the student extern evaluation report from comments provided by the supervisor assigned and each employee who worked with the extern. RATIONALE: Provides necessary documentation for the externship experience.

Procedure 33-5 **Developing and Maintaining a Procedures Manual**

PURPOSE:

To develop and maintain a comprehensive, up-to-date procedures manual covering each medical, technical, and administrative procedure in the office, with step-by-step directions and rationale for performing each task.

EQUIPMENT/SUPPLIES:

Computer or electronic typewriter (electronic storage allows changes and revisions to be made easily)
Binder, such as a three-ring binder
Paper
Standard procedures manual format

PROCEDURE STEPS:

1. Write detailed, step-by-step procedures and rationales for each medical, technical, and administrative function. Each procedure is written by experienced employees close to the function and then reviewed by a supervisor and/or office manager. Rationales help employees understand *why* something is done. RATIONALE: Establishes consistent guidelines to be followed.

2. Collect the procedures into the Office Procedures Manual. RATIONALE: Provides a reference

(continues)

Procedure

33-5 (*continued*)

guide with step-by-step instruction and examples where appropriate.

3. Store one complete manual in a common library area. Provide a completed copy to the physician/employer and the office manager. Distribute appropriate sections to the various departments. RATIONALE: Provides a reference guide with step-by-step instruction and examples where appropriate.

4. Review the procedures manual annually and add any new procedures, delete or modify as necessary, and indicate the revision date (Rev. 10/12/02). RATIONALE: Maintains current office protocols.

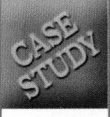

33-1

Dr. Lewis and Dr. King have requested sigmoidoscopy procedures to be scheduled for two different patients. The patients are scheduled. Both patients are put on a strict diet and pretest protocol for several days to prepare for the procedures. The day of the appointments, it is discovered that the two sigmoidoscopy procedures have been scheduled at the same time. The problem is that the office has only one sigmoidoscope available.

CASE STUDY REVIEW

1. Divide the class into two groups to discuss problem-solving solutions. Assume that rescheduling a patient is not an acceptable solution because of the patient's pretest protocol. The patients would be very upset if the procedure could not be performed due to a scheduling problem.

2. How could this problem have been avoided?

3. Both patients have been told about the scheduling problem and one is very upset and argumentative. What role should the office manager assume in this predicament?

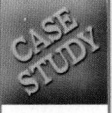

33-2

The office manager for Doctors Lewis and King has many leadership qualities and utilizes them effectively in her management style. She sets realistic goals and becomes a role model for subordinates to emulate. She empowers her subordinates and encourages creativity.

CASE STUDY REVIEW

1. Divide the class into small groups and ask them to brainstorm the pros and cons of this management style.

2. Discuss with your small group other management styles and your comfort level working under these management styles.

3. Within your group, develop a set of questions that might be asked at an interview to determine the management style of this manager prior to accepting employment.

SUMMARY

The office manager is the glue that holds the office together and keeps it running smoothly. When the manager sets a positive example for others, is considerate and aware of the diversity of others, a positive environment is created for teamwork. A teamwork approach enables the entire office to be more productive, provide the best health care, and foster an enjoyable work relationship.

The role of office manager varies greatly depending upon the size of the medical practice, the physician's trust in the manager's competency level, and the physician's comfort in delegating authority to others. An effective office manager is a tremendous asset to physicians. The personal and financial rewards are worthwhile to the medical assistant who desires a new dimension to explore and enjoys a challenge.

REVIEW QUESTIONS

Multiple Choice

1. The office manager should have a minimum of a (an):
   a. associate's degree
   b. bachelor's degree
   c. master's degree
   d. doctoral degree
2. When the office manager is too busy to perform a task, he or she should:
   a. refuse to do it
   b. delegate the task to someone who is knowledgeable
   c. put it off and do it when there is time later
   d. hope that no one will notice it did not get done
3. For teamwork to be successful, individual team members must:
   a. do as they are told by the office manager
   b. not ask why they are doing something a certain way
   c. understand and support the task
   d. think independently and solve the problem on their own
4. People-oriented personalities:
   a. are most comfortable with physical dexterity, building, construction, and working with tools or instruments
   b. are most comfortable working with ideas, information, and data
   c. are most comfortable teaching, coaching, helping, leading, and inspiring others
   d. use "carrots" and "sticks"
5. Meeting minutes:
   a. should address each agenda topic and include a brief summary of discussions, actions taken, name of each person making a motion, the exact wording of motions, and motion approval or defeat
   b. are a detailed plan for a proposed trip
   c. include information regarding mode of transportation and lodging reservations
   d. must follow parliamentary procedures

6. When working with externs, it is important to remember that:
   a. they should have expert knowledge about their field
   b. they do not need supervision when working with a patient
   c. they are very experienced with working on real patients
   d. they have much to learn
7. The procedures manual:
   a. is a detailed plan for a proposed trip
   b. provides detailed information regarding mode of transportation and lodging reservations
   c. provides detailed information relative to the performance of tasks within the health care facility
   d. summarizes action details of staff meetings
8. Which of the following statements is *not* correct regarding a student practicum?
   a. It is a transitional stage that provides opportunity for students to apply theory learned in the classroom to a health care setting through hands-on experience.
   b. It assumes that the student is an employee who does not need to be introduced to patients.
   c. It may require the student to shadow another medical assistant for a few days.
   d. It involves an evaluation of the student's progress.
9. Developing relationships outside the office is often called:
   a. marketing
   b. benchmarking
   c. advertising
   d. sales
10. Record and financial management involves all of the following *except*:
    a. payroll processing
    b. preparing payroll checks
    c. figuring taxes
    d. equipment and supplies maintenance

Critical Thinking

1. How would you, as the office manager, handle someone who is spreading a harmful rumor about another employee in the office?
2. Discuss teamwork and the benefits of the teamwork approach.
3. How can the office manager promote open and honest communication?
4. This chapter identifies various management styles. Under which management style would you feel most comfortable working and why? Does this management style promote a teamwork atmosphere? Why or why not?
5. The student practicum can be a very stressful time for the extern. As an office manager, how can you help the extern feel more at ease the first day of "work"?
6. This chapter describes various tactics you can use to keep yourself organized, such as making a "To Do" list, handling a paper only once, and avoiding procrastination. Describe things that you do to keep yourself organized.
7. Describe how a procedures manual for a single-physician practice would differ from a procedures manual for a multi-physician practice.
8. Describe how a procedures manual could become outdated and need revision.
9. In what cases would a press release be used?
10. Explain why the primary principle behind the risk management role is loss prevention.

WEB ACTIVITIES

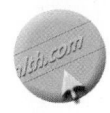

Use the web sites described in the text, or alternative sites you know about, to plan a trip between two cities within the United States. Compare the fares for Sunday departure and Friday return dates with the fares for low volume days as obtained from the Priceline.com site. Also compare fares on flights purchased within one week of departure with fares on flights purchased a month prior to departure. Follow the instructor's instructions on completing and turning in your results.

REFERENCES/BIBLIOGRAPHY

Colbert, B. J. (2000). *Workplace readiness for health occupations.* Albany, NY: Delmar.

Frew, M. A., Lane, K., & Frew, D. R. (1995). *Comprehensive medical assisting: Competencies for administrative and clinical practice* (3rd ed.). Philadelphia: F. A. Davis.

Institute for Management Excellence (June 1998). Linking personality with management style. [On-line]. Available: http://itstime.com/jun98.htm.

Lewis, M. A., & Tamparo, C. D. (1998). *Medical law, ethics, and bioethics for ambulatory care* (4th ed.). Philadelphia: F. A. Davis.

McConnell, C. R. (1998). *Case studies in health care supervision.* Gaithersburg, MD: Aspen Publishers.

Pyzdek, T. (1996). Management styles: Participatory management style. [On-line]. Available: http://www.qualityamerica.com/knowledgecente/articles/CQMStyle2.html.

THE MEDICAL ASSISTANT AS HUMAN RESOURCES MANAGER

KEY TERMS

Conflict Resolution
Educational History
Evaluation
Exit Interview
Involuntary Dismissal
Job Description
Letter of Reference
Letter of Resignation
Mentor
Networking
Overtime
Probation
Resumes
Salary Review
Work History

OUTLINE

Tasks Performed by the Human Resources Manager
The Office Policy Manual
Recruiting and Hiring Office Personnel
  Job Descriptions
  Recruiting
  Preparing to Interview Applicants
  The Interview
  Selecting the Finalists
Orienting and Training New Personnel
Evaluating Employees and Planning Salary Review
  Performance Evaluation
  Salary Review

Dismissing Employees
  Involuntary Dismissal
  Voluntary Dismissal
  Exit Interview
Maintaining Personnel Records
Complying with Personnel Laws
Special Policy Considerations
  Temporary Employees
  Smoking Policy
  Discrimination
  Employees with Chemical
    Dependencies or Emotional
    Problems
Providing/Planning Employee Training and Education
Conflict Resolution

OBJECTIVES

The student should strive to meet the following performance objectives and demonstrate an understanding of the facts and principles presented in this chapter through written and oral communication.

1. Define the key terms as presented in the glossary.

2. Describe the role of the human resources manager.

3. Explain the function of the office policy manual.

4. Identify methods of recruiting employees for a medical practice.

5. Discuss the interview process.

6. Describe appropriate evaluation tools for employees.

7. Recall procedures to follow when dismissing employees.

8. Identify items to keep in an employee's personnel record.

9. List and define a minimum of four laws related to personnel management.

10. Recall effective methods of resolving conflicts.

ADMINISTRATIVE

Practice Finances

- Manage personnel benefits and maintain records (adv)

GENERAL
(TRANSDISCIPLINARY)

Legal Concepts

- Follow federal, state and local legal guidelines
- Participate in the development and maintenance of personnel, policy and procedure manuals
- Develop and maintain personnel, policy and procedures manuals (adv)

Instruction

- Train and orient personnel (adv)
- Conduct continuing education activities (adv)

Operational Functions

- Supervise personnel (adv)
- Interview and recommend job applicants (adv)

SCENARIO

Jane O'Hara, CMA, is the officer manager at Inner City Health Care. She also functions in the role of the human resources manager. Part of her responsibilities includes recruiting, hiring, training, and dismissing employees.

In one day Jane may meet with Dr. Rice to update the policy manual, place an advertisement in the local newspaper for a new medical assistant, welcome a new physician to the practice, being sure she completes all of the necessary forms, and meet with Karen Ritter to evaluate her salary.

INTRODUCTION

The medical assistant, while performing the tasks and assuming the responsibility of an office manager, also may function in the role of the human resources manager.

The title human resources manager is often reserved for an individual who manages a human resources department in a large, corporate setting. Many of the duties performed by this individual, however, may be performed in a sole proprietor's medical practice with only one or two employees.

TASKS PERFORMED BY THE HUMAN RESOURCES MANAGER

Tasks usually assigned to the human resources manager include determining job descriptions, hiring, training, and dismissing employees, and maintaining employee personnel records. But with today's quest for greater office efficiency and the tremendous increase in federal and state regulatory requirements, the skills required of a human resources manager have greatly broadened. Former responsibilities have been expanded to include writing the policy manual, planning employee evaluation, preventing and investigating discrimination

and harassment claims, and complying with regulatory agencies. The human resources manager also assists in providing training and educational opportunities for employees so they are up to date in all aspects of quality patient care.

Increasingly, human resource managers are expected to be able to support the organization's efforts that focus on productivity, service, and quality. In a climate in which there are too few persons for the positions to be filled, and the delivery methods for health care are changing almost daily, productivity, service, and quality are essential to a successful practice. It becomes the responsibility of the human resource manager to see that every employee's productivity level is high, that the service is A+, and that quality is at the highest level. Today's customers, the patients, will often choose their health care provider on the basis of service and quality.

The position of human resources manager now requires a higher level of education and experience to better grasp the legal and regulatory aspects of personnel management. The human resources manager also must have excellent people skills, a strong sense of fairness, and the ability to resolve conflicts. None of this is accomplished in a vacuum. It requires working in close cooperation with the office manager and the physician-employer(s).

This chapter discusses these responsibilities in groups of eight separate but overlapping functions:

1. Creating and updating the office policy manual
2. Recruiting and hiring office personnel
3. Orienting and training new personnel
4. Evaluating and planning salary review
5. Dismissing employees

6. Maintaining personnel records
7. Complying with all state and federal regulations regarding personnel
8. Planning/providing employee training and education

THE OFFICE POLICY MANUAL

The procedures manual described in Chapter 33 identifies specific methods of performing tasks. The policy manual provides more general guidelines for office practices.

Possible content of policy and procedure manual

Policy Manual	Procedure Manual
General practices and policies of an office	Daily guide; step-by-step instructions for procedures

---

The policy manual will identify clear guidelines and directions required of all employees as well as define appropriate expectations and boundaries of the employment relationship. Having written policies means not having to determine a policy on a case-by-case basis. Policy manuals will vary by the size of the practice or problems to be addressed, but some topics include the mission statement of the practice, biographical data on each physician, employment policies, wage and salary policies, benefits to be awarded, and employee conduct expectations.

Establishing and stating the mission of the practice clearly identifies for employees the goals and objectives to be sought by each employee. Having biographical data of each physician helps employees to respond to queries from patients about a physician's training, education, and interests.

Employment policies might include statements on equal employment opportunity, job requirements for particular positions and to whom the person reports, recruitment and selection procedures, orientation of new employees, probation, and dismissal. Wage and salary policies should be in writing. How are employees classified, what are the working hours, how is overtime compensated, how are salary increases determined, what benefits (medical, retirement, vacation, holidays, sick leave) does the practice have? The answers to such questions are part of the policy manual. Employee conduct is another piece of the policy manual. Guidelines should be established about uniforms and appearance. Can an employee hold a second job outside the practice? Is smoking allowed? Are staff members responsible for housekeeping duties? A statement regarding the confidentiality of all information received in the practice is essential in this area of the policy manual.

Having a policy manual with clearly written directives helps employees understand the expectations and boundaries of the employment relationship. The policy manual should be reviewed with each new employee and updated on a regular basis. See Procedure 34-1 for details on developing and maintaining a policy manual.

RECRUITING AND HIRING OFFICE PERSONNEL

Before recruiting and hiring personnel to fill positions within the medical office, the human resources manager and physician-employer must know exactly what the role and responsibilities of the position are by having a job description for the position and follow a recruiting policy that is effective, fair, and observes all appropriate laws and regulations.

Job Descriptions

Before any position is filled, a **job description** must be in place. This is done cooperatively with the office manager and the physician-employer. Once the job qualifications are defined, the human resources manager can begin efforts to fill the position.

In daily operations most job descriptions are on file, but if the situation involves a new or greatly expanded office, a complete set of job descriptions is needed before recruiting can begin. Even when a written description is on file, it should be reviewed when a new employee is to be hired. The person who is leaving the position is often an excellent resource for the accuracy of the current job description and any changes that should be made.

The job description must include basic qualifications for the position and have enough information to provide both the supervisor and the employee with a clear outline of what the job entails (Figure 34-1). Necessary work experience, skills, education, and any special certification or licensure that is expected is to be identified in the job description. See Procedure 34-2 for details on preparing job descriptions.

Another important point with respect to the job description is that a review and update of the description should be done every year. Most jobs change constantly whether from a minor shifting of duties or the addition

JOB DESCRIPTION FORMAT

JOB TITLE:
Describes the job in one to three words; should be a title an employee can identify with and be proud of.

REPORTS TO:
Identifies position or person to whom the employee reports.

PURPOSE/OBJECTIVE:
A short statement outlining the purpose or mission of the job, explaining basically why this job exists; should make the person feel like an integral part of the whole organization.

RESPONSIBILITIES AND DUTIES:
Duties are statements that outline a particular function or task and identify what is being done; all statements are related to the work to be performed. Duties should identify the most predominant and significant tasks and convey a measure of frequency of occurrence. *Responsibilities* are simply names or titles for types of work areas. Duties are subsets of responsibilities.

WORK RELATIONSHIPS AND AUTHORITY BOUNDARIES:
When significant to the job, a statement describing the relationships and degree of interface of the job with internal and external groups.

POSITION REQUIREMENTS:
Education and experience that are required for the person to function in this capacity.

Figure 34-1   This sample format describes the main features of a job description with definitions for each feature. (From *Personnel Management Handbook*, 2nd ed., by Maryann Ricardo, The McGraw-Hill Companies, Inc. Copyright 1992. Reprinted with permission.)

of some new technical procedure or device. Without updating a job description, the wrong person may be recruited to fill a vacancy.

Recruiting

A major challenge facing the human resource manager today is recruitment. Medical assistants are listed in the top ten occupations with the fastest employment growth through 2006 according to the U.S. Department of Labor, Bureau of Labor Statistics. One reason for this demand is the aging of the U.S. population. It is estimated that over 80% of jobs are in the service industry, and all health care positions fit into that category. When physician-employers have been unsuccessful in recruiting qualified medical assistants, they have turned to contracting out some work, such as transcription and billing.

The human resources manager begins the recruitment process. Often a process called networking is a highly effective method of finding employees. **Networking** is a process in which people of similar interests exchange information in social, business, or professional relationships. For instance, the human resources manager may network with members of the American Association of Medical Assistants and express an interest in a new employee for a position that is open. Current employees are often an excellent resource because they may know of a qualified person who is looking for a position.

Checking with nearby universities, community, and technical colleges' medical assistant departments is another good resource. Employing a private or state placement agency is another possibility. While newspaper advertisements may generate many **resumes**, they are only marginally effective as a search tool. It is often far too time consuming to review the large volume of applications generated by this approach.

Preparing to Interview Applicants

Once several applicants have expressed interest in the position, preparation for the interview begins. The human resources manager should have a number of resumes to consider. Some may have already filled out a job application when they dropped off a resume. The resumes and applications can be reviewed together. Some important points to remember in reading resumes and applications follow.

Under **educational history**, look beyond the degree earned. Look for a good performance record at school and the kinds of supplemental education achieved. Does attendance at seminars and short-course training programs relate to your position needs? When reading a person's **work history**, make note of unexplained gaps in employment. You may want to ask specific questions in the interview. Has advancement been gained in each new position? Are the responsibilities and duties of the applicant's positions explained or will questions need to be asked of the prospective employee?

Look for information that indicates if this candidate really enjoys the kind of work setting you have. Is the applicant comfortable serving the infirm? Can you truly identify the level of skill from the descriptions or are the skills vague? The cover letter, if one is included, should address the specifics required of your position. Does the person display a negative or a positive attitude? Do not excuse any errors or unprofessional appearance in the job application or the resume. Each should be letter perfect. An individual who is careless in this respect is likely to be careless on the job.

Some applications will be set aside after using the preceding guidelines. With the remaining candidates, determine who is to be interviewed and make telephone calls to establish interviews. You may make note of the quality of speaking skills, especially if this person will be using the telephone on the job. Make an interview appointment date with only those who seem truly interested in the position during your telephone conversation.

The Interview

The interview is usually conducted by only one person if second interviews are anticipated. The physician-employer, office manager, or another employee may be present in either the first or the second interview, however. This is a decision made by the human resources manager and the physician-employer (Figure 34-2). The interviewer(s) will want to review the application and resume prior to the interview for particular points to ask the candidate. An interview worksheet is an excellent tool to use to make certain that you are fair and equitable with each candidate. The worksheet should provide enough room for notes taken during the interview.

Suggested items for the interview worksheet are:

- Applicant's name
- Telephone number
- Education and training

- Work experience
- Special skills
- Professional demeanor
- Voice and mannerisms specific to position
- Responses to questions
- Ability to problem solve when given a scenario
- Any health-related or work-related problems applicant discloses
- Interviewer's personal impressions and recommendations

Conduct interviews in a quiet and private setting. Do not schedule interviews back to back without time to collect your thoughts or to allow you to compare notes with others participating in the interview. Ask job-related questions such as Describe your last job. What did you like best about it? What did you like least? What is most important to you about a job? Describe your administrative and clinical skills. Figure 34-3 shows some sample questions. Let the applicant do the most of the talking.

Any questions related to age, sex, race, religion, or national origin are inappropriate. Inquiries about medical

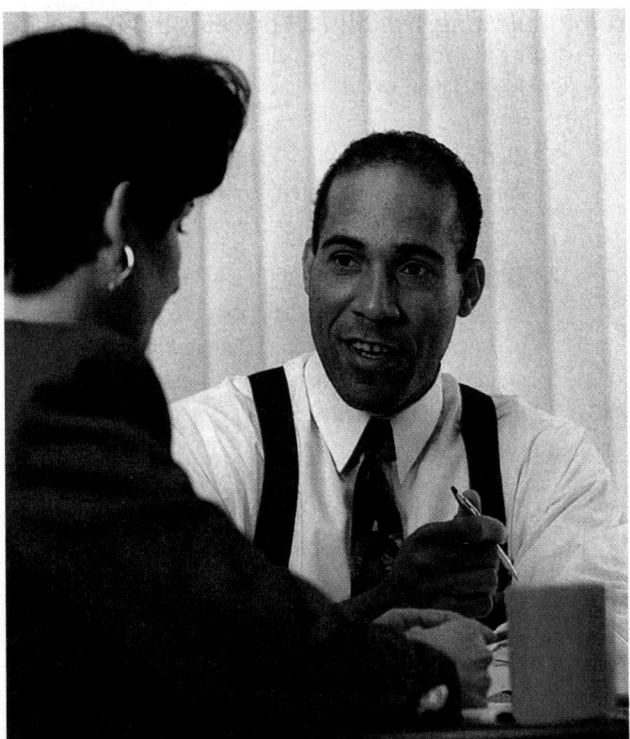

Figure 34-2 The interview can be conducted on a one-to-one basis with only the applicant and one staff member or with several staff members meeting with the applicant at once.

General Questions

- What are your strengths and weaknesses?
- Why did you leave your last job?
- Identify what is most important to you in a job.

Questions Related to Work Relationships

- Describe an individual you have enjoyed working with.
- Explain how a conflict with a coworker was resolved.
- How would a coworker describe you?

Questions Related to Problem Solving

- Describe a work-related decision that made you very proud.
- Identify a task/procedure/assignment you could not do, and explain why.
- How do you approach a task when it seems mundane or boring?

Questions Related to Integrity

- If asked to do something illegal or unethical, what would you do?
- Tell us about a time when you broke a confidence.
- If you saw a coworker put a patient at risk, what would you do?

Figure 34-3 Common interview questions.

history, drug use, or arrest records may not be made. Keep your questions related to performance on the job. If you may want to bond this employee, you may ask candidates if they have been bonded before or are willing to be bonded. It may be best to leave salary discussions for a second interview, but it can also be helpful to determine if applicants' salary expectations are in line with what you can offer. A question such as What salary are you expecting? is appropriate. Do not make a job offer until all the candidates selected for interview have been interviewed, and do not prejudge someone on appearance or any other physical factor during or following the interview. Only the person's qualifications are to be considered.

At the close of the interview, let the applicant know when a decision will be made or whether a second interview will be conducted. A tour of the facility and introduction to key staff members may be offered, but are not necessary at the time of the first interview. Finally, thank the applicant for participating in the interview and being interested in the position.

Selecting the Finalists

Shortly after the final interview is complete, the human resources manager should compare notes with all the others involved in the interview to select the top candidates. This is done by comparing notes and impressions from the interviews and by taking into consideration the ability of a candidate to work with patients and colleagues having a variety of problems and cultural backgrounds. The next step is to check references of former employers, supervisors, coworkers, and teachers. A large corporate medical practice may even have a consent form each candidate is asked to sign that gives permission to check references and call former employers. You may need to recognize, however, that even with a release from a potential new hire, many organizations and businesses restrict the release of reference information to only name, dates of employment, and title of position served. Telephone checks for references are an excellent strategy since you receive an immediate response. If you stress confidentiality when you make the contact, it will be easier for the person to respond to your questions. Always check with more than one reference and former employer to get an accurate assessment of the candidate. A sample telephone reference check form is shown in Figure 34-4.

A checklist of questions to ask might include:

1. What were the dates of employment of (name of applicant) in your firm?
2. Describe the job performed.
3. Reason for leaving the job?
4. Strong points of the employee?
5. Limitations of the employee?

TELEPHONE REFERENCE CHECK FORM

Name of Applicant _____

Person Contacted _____

Position _____

Telephone Number _____

Relation to Applicant _____

1. I would like to verify some information given to us by (applicant's name) who is applying for a position with our organization. What are the dates of his employment with you?

   _____, 20___ to _____, 20___

2. What was the nature of his job?
3. What did you think of his work?
4. How did he get along with the other employees?
5. Did you see any difference in his job performance during the employment period?
6. What was his salary?
7. Why did he leave the job?
8. What are his strong points?
9. What are his limitations?
10. Please describe his attitude.
11. What degree of supervision did he need?
12. Could you comment on his attendance and dependability?
13. Were there any personal difficulties that you know of that may have interfered with his work?
14. Given the right opportunity, would you rehire him?
15. Is there anything else that we should know?

Reference call made by _____ Date _____

Figure 34-4 A telephone reference check form such as this one can help the interviewer ask consistent questions of several references. (From *Personnel Management Handbook*, 2nd ed., by Maryann Ricardo, The McGraw-Hill Companies, Inc. Copyright 1992. Reprinted with permission.)

6. Can you comment on attendance and dependability?
7. Any personal difficulties you were aware of that interfered with the work?
8. Would you rehire?
9. Anything else we should know about this candidate?

Offer the position when a first-choice candidate has been determined and indicate when a response is needed. Be prepared with a second-choice candidate should the preferred candidate respond negatively. At the time of the offer, the candidate should understand the salary offered, the starting date, the practice policies, and the benefits. When a candidate has accepted the position, a confirmation letter should be written that clearly spells out details discussed earlier. Give specific instructions on when and where the new employee should report the first day on the job. If practical, the employee should be given the policy and procedures manuals to read.

For the unsuccessful applicants, send a letter explaining that they are no longer being considered for the position and thank them for applying. Copies of these letters as well as the interview checklists should be kept for a minimum of six months should any questions arise regarding your choice of candidates. See Procedure 34-3 for details on interviewing.

ORIENTING AND TRAINING NEW PERSONNEL

Orienting and training new employees is the responsibility of both the human resources manager and the office manager who is most likely to work the closest with the new employee. It is common for a new employee to be placed on **probation** for sixty to ninety days during which time both the employee as well as supervisory personnel may determine if the environment and the position are satisfactory for the employee. Procedure 34-4 outlines how to orient and train personnel.

Important elements to orientation include the introduction of the new employee to other staff members, assigning a **mentor** who can respond to questions, and making the employee aware of the procedures to be performed in this new position. If the procedure's manual is detailed and accurate, this manual now becomes the daily "guide" for the new employee. Sometimes the individual leaving a position may still be present and is asked to assist in the orientation process. This is especially beneficial if there is a good working relationship between the employee who is leaving and the management of the practice. Depending upon the responsibilities of the new employee, a supervisor may be asked to monitor all procedures for a period of time for accuracy, safety, and patient protection. During the probation period, the employee should be officially evaluated by the human resources manager (see sample form in Figure 34-5). This **evaluation** becomes part of the employee's personnel record.

EVALUATING EMPLOYEES AND PLANNING SALARY REVIEW

It is very important that all employees know whether they are performing their job as expected and know how they can improve their performance if necessary.

PROBATIONARY EMPLOYEE EVALUATION FORM

Name _____

Hire Date _____

Job Title _____

Pay Rate_____ Supervisor _____

Do you recommend the employee continue in employment?
_____ Yes _____ No

Please state your reasons for whatever action you recommend. Use the guidelines below to make your decision.

1. Has the employee required more training than is normally needed for the job?

2. Has the employee grasped this job with very little training?

3. Is the employee performing at, above, or below (circle one) the standard for this job?

4. If below, when do you expect the employee to reach the standard?

5. Does the employee get along well with all staff members?

6. Has the employee maintained a good attendance record and a good work attitude?

7. Has the employee expressed any dissatisfactions?

_____ _____
Supervisor's Signature   Date

Figure 34-5 Sample probationary employee evaluation form. (From *Personnel Management Handbook*, 2nd ed., by Maryann Ricardo, The McGraw-Hill Companies, Inc. Copyright 1992. Reprinted with permission.)

Performance Evaluation

Not only is evaluation of employees necessary during the probation period, it is necessary for current employees as well. Evaluations should be performed no less than once a year on the anniversary of the hire date. Some human resources managers may wish to evaluate an employee more often, especially if a problem has surfaced in an evaluation.

The evaluation may take many forms; it can be formal or informal; it may involve more than one person. The results of the evaluation, however, must be a part of the employee's personnel record. For that reason, a formal evaluation is preferred. Many practices use a written evaluation that requires that the employee evaluate himself prior to meeting with the human resources manager (Figure 34-6). The human resources manager uses the same form for evaluation. During the meeting, notes are compared as the evaluation is conducted.

PERFORMANCE REVIEW FORM

_____   _____
Employee Name   Title

_____   _____
Supervisor   Department

TYPE OF REVIEW (Check One)
_____ Quarterly
_____ Annual
_____ Probation
_____ Other _____

Review Period Covered _____ to _____

PERFORMANCE DEFINITIONS

5 = Outstanding	Performance that is clearly superior, beyond the call of duty, or substantially above standard level. Seldom attained level of performance but achievable.
4 = Above Standard	Very commendable performance; exceeds the norm for the job.
3 = Standard	Competent and consistent performance; expected level of activity and performance for the job. Most often rating received.
2 = Below Standard	Performance needs improvement. This level of performance is unacceptable; needs improvement to meet the standards for the job. **Employee new to the job:** Performance might receive below standard rating due to lack of job knowledge and is expected to improve with experience. **Experienced Employee:** Performance is below acceptable level and requires direction and/or counsel.
1 = Unsatisfactory	Performance is unacceptable. Job activity is clearly and substantially lacking in quality, quantity, or timeliness. May also not be meeting cost or budget constraints. Needs much improvement to meet the standards for the job.

(office use only) EVALUATION SUMMARY Total I _____ + Total II _____	FINAL RATING: CHECK ONE (office use only) _____ Merit Increase Recommended _____ No Merit Increase—Satisfactory Performance/No Growth _____ No Merit Increase (Probationary/Special Evaluation) _____ No Merit Increase (Performance Probation) Re-evaluate in 90 Days for Unsatisfactory or in 180 Days for Needed Improvement

GENERAL PERFORMANCE RATING (PART I)

General Criteria	Rating	Comments Supporting Rating
1. **Patient Relations:** How well does the employee communicate a "we care" image to the patients, visitors, physicians, and fellow employees?		
2. **Work Responsibilities:** What is the quality of the employee's work relative to quality, quantity, and timeliness?		
3. **Teamwork:** Does the employee have a team spirit? Does the employee interact well with co-workers/supervisor/manager?		*(continues)*

Figure 34-6 Sample performance review form. (Adapted from *Personnel Management Handbook*, 2nd ed., by Maryann Ricardo, The McGraw-Hill Companies, Inc. Copyright 1992. Reprinted with permission.)

General Criteria	Rating	Comments Supporting Rating
4. **Adaptability:** Is the employee open to change and new ideas? Does the employee remain flexible to changes in routine, work-load, and assignments?		
5. **Personal Appearance:** How well does the employee maintain appropriate personal appearance, including proper attire, hygiene?		
6. **Communication:** Does the employee communicate well? Is information given and received clearly? Does he/she have good verbal and written skills?		
7. **Dependability:** Can the employee be relied upon for good attendance? Does the employee perform and follow through on work without supervisory intervention or assistance?		

Subtotal I _____ + 7 General Criteria = _____

JOB-SPECIFIC CRITERIA RATING (PART II) (To be used with Job Description attached)

Responsibility and Standard	Rating	Comments Supporting Rating
Complete a section for each responsibility listed on the employee's job description.		

Subtotal II _____ + _____ = _____
job duties

Contributions made since last review:

_____

_____

_____

Education or training received since last review:

_____

_____

_____

Action to be taken based on performance:

_____

_____

_____

Comments:

_____

_____

_____

_____	_____
Employee Signature	Date
_____	_____
Supervisor Signature	Date
_____	_____
Physician Signature	Date

Figure 34-6 (*continued*)

The climate of the performance evaluation should be comfortable and provide privacy (Figure 34-7). The meeting should be friendly, but the employee must sense the importance of the evaluation. Do not allow any disagreements to escalate into arguments during the evaluation. Without reading the employee's self-evaluation, ask the employee to tell about the self-assessment. Acknowledge the employee's point of view and identify when you agree or differ from the self-assessment. Be prepared to describe specific examples of positive performance and/or negative performance.

When negative performance is identified, ask the employee for possible solutions. Then a plan can be determined to alter the negative performance. In this way, a trusting atmosphere is established in that both of you are working together for a solution that will benefit the medical practice. Always look for and seek a win-win situation whenever possible. The action plan determined should then be evaluated at the next performance evaluation.

At the close of the evaluation, always express your confidence in the individual to make any changes necessary, offer assistance where needed, and thank the employee for participating. End any evaluation with a positive statement about some portion of the employee's performance.

There are occasions when reviews are performed more frequently than annually. A review would occur two to three months after a significant promotion to measure how things are progressing. Reviews occur more often when general performance falls well short of past efforts or a serious error in judgment has been made. This type of review may end with a reprimand, a warning to correct the problem by a given date, or possibly, immediate dismissal. Document any steps to be taken to correct a problem and any reason that is cause for dismissal.

Salary Review

Although the practice is common in some areas, it may be better not to tie salary increases or bonuses with the annual performance evaluation. Conduct the **salary review** at the beginning of the new year separate from performance evaluations.

Salary review is important. Unfortunately, in smaller medical offices and ambulatory care settings, the review of salary may have to be raised by the employee. Physician-employers tend to forget that their employees have been with them for over a year without a raise or a discussion of financial reimbursement. If such is the case, it is perfectly acceptable for the employee to raise the issue on a yearly basis. However, the best approach is for the human resources manager to conduct salary reviews at the beginning or end of each calendar year.

Data should be collected prior to a salary review. The human resources manager should network with other

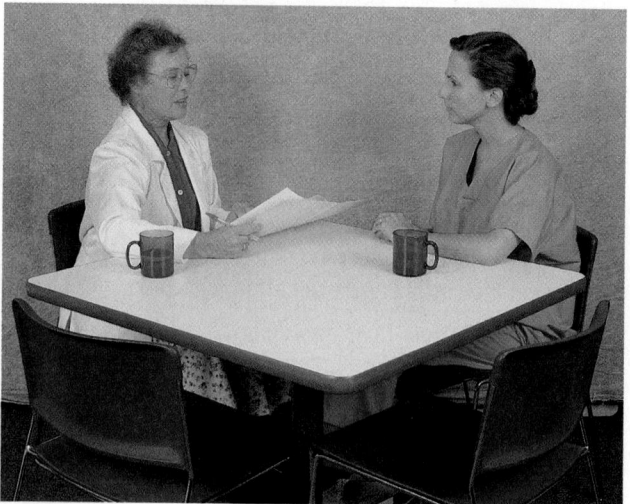

Figure 34-7 A comfortable, private setting encourages discussion during an employee evaluation.

human resources managers to determine wages and salaries for comparable individuals with comparable skills. Remember, also, that it is far more cost-effective to reward good employees with a salary increase than it is to train a new employee who commands a lesser salary than current employees. Reward employees well and provide benefits that encourage them to stay with the practice. Employees who stay with the practice for a long time not only fully understand how best to serve their physician-employers, they have established a relationship with patients that is very beneficial.

How much of a raise is to be awarded at the time of salary review is difficult to determine and will depend upon many factors which might include the profits of the year, the patient load, the workload, and the current cost of living.

The critical shortage of health care employees today is reflected in the shortage of medical assistants across the country. Newspapers advertising for individuals to work in the ambulatory care setting tell the story. A consideration worth mentioning is that often the salary does not match the education, experience, and special training required of someone working in the health care field. Educators often hear, "Why would I spend a year or more in education to be paid what I would make working in a fast food restaurant?" Because it is costly in time and resources to replace employees, it is best to invest that cost into a fair and just salary increase for valued employees.

DISMISSING EMPLOYEES

Most human resources managers do not enjoy rating the performance of other employees particularly when difficult topics are involved and it may be necessary to dismiss an employee. However, the written performance evaluation actually establishes the format for such a dismissal when necessary and is more likely to remove the emotion from the situation. **Involuntary dismissal** is still difficult when it is necessary.

Involuntary Dismissal

Involuntary dismissal results from two primary causes: poor performance or serious violation of office policies or job descriptions. When it becomes apparent to the human resources manager that the effectiveness of an employee is dropping well below expectations, it will be known in the review or a performance review may be called. The review allows the employee to be informed of the shortcomings, to explain any reasons for the present situation, and to determine a plan to alleviate the problem. If the problem is a serious one, probation is usually invoked and any lack of significant improvement in the time provided results in immediate dismissal.

When the problem is a violation of either office policy or procedures, both a verbal and a written warning are given to the employee. Involuntary dismissal follows if the situation persists. Dismissal may be immediate if the action is a serious violation of policy. Serious violations will depend upon the office practice, but some causes for immediate dismissal include theft, making fraudulent claims against insurance, placing the patient in jeopardy by not practicing safe techniques, and breach of patient confidentiality.

Some key points to keep in mind when dismissal is necessary are:

1. The dismissal should be made in privacy.
2. Take no longer than 10 minutes for the dismissal.
3. Be direct, firm, and to the point in identifying reasons.
4. Do not engage in an in-depth discussion of performance.
5. Explain terms of dismissal (keys, clearing out area, final paperwork).
6. Listen to employee's opinion and emotions; it is not necessary to agree.
7. Accompany the employee to their desk to pack their belongings.
8. Escort the employee out of the facility; do not allow to finish the work of the day.

Voluntary Dismissal

Other reasons for dismissal may be more pleasant. Changes in personnel occur for many good reasons and people voluntarily leave their jobs. They may relocate, seek advancement in another facility, or simply have personal reasons for leaving. These employees will give their manager proper notice and be able to turn their current projects and duties over to their replacements. They have time to say good-bye to their friends and leave with a good feeling about their employment.

Exit Interview

An **exit interview** is an excellent opportunity for the employee who voluntarily leaves a practice and the human resources manager to discuss the positive and negative aspects of the job and what changes might be made for a new person coming into the facility. A sample exit interview form is shown in Figure 34-8. It also allows the opportunity for the employee to ask for a **letter of reference** or to view the personnel file before leaving. In a voluntary dismissal, request a **letter of resignation** for the personnel file.

Any dismissal process, voluntary or involuntary, must include a statement in the personnel file. For involuntary dismissal, be certain that the reasons for the dismissal are well documented. Be honest, nonjudgmental, and do not allow emotions to escalate into hostility and anger. State only the facts in the personnel file; do not

---

EXIT INTERVIEW FORM

1. What did you like and dislike about the work you have been doing?
   (Including: support on the job; opportunity for personal growth; recognition and rewards)

2. What kind of people have you found the doctors, your immediate supervisor, and co-workers to be?
   (Including: attitude; fairness; scheduling and assignment of work; work expectations; technical competence; assistance and guidance available; team spirit)

3. What is your view of our management practices and policies?
   (Including: clarity and fairness of practice policies; communications; management and staff)

4. How have you felt about performance appraisals, your salary and benefits?
   (Including: adequacy of salary; regularity and fairness of appraisals)

5. What are your principal reasons for leaving the practice?
   (Including: primary dissatisfactions; job or personal changes)

6. In what areas do you feel we need to improve?

Interviewer signature: _____ Date _____

Employee signature: _____ Date _____

Figure 34-8 Sample exit interview form. (From *Personnel Management Handbook*, 2nd ed., by Maryann Ricardo, The McGraw-Hill Companies, Inc. Copyright 1992. Reprinted with permission.)

state opinion. Remember that employees have the right to view their personnel file at any time.

The physician-employer should always be informed of any dismissal as quickly as possible. Some will be involved in the actual dismissal process. A physician-employer is most likely going to be concerned about ongoing assistance in the practice and that a break not occur in quality care given to patients.

MAINTAINING PERSONNEL RECORDS

An important aspect of the responsibilities of the human resources manager is maintaining personnel records. All documentation and correspondence related to each employee from application to dismissal, from awards to reprimands including the formal reviews, must be kept in the confidential personnel file. Access to this file is limited to certain management personnel and the employee. Not all of these people are allowed to see the entire file. These files are usually kept for a period of three to five years.

This file also includes the kind of information normally maintained for payroll and business practices. That information includes name, address, and sex of employee. The position title, date of beginning employment, rate of pay (hourly or otherwise), total overtime pay, deductions or additions to wages, wages paid each pay period, and date of dismissal.

COMPLYING WITH PERSONNEL LAWS

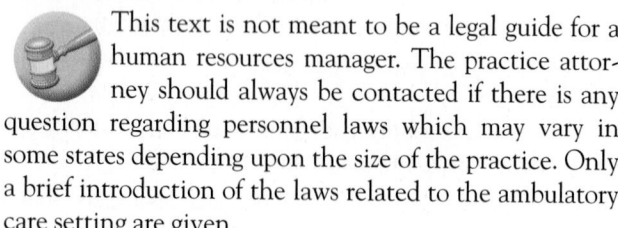 This text is not meant to be a legal guide for a human resources manager. The practice attorney should always be contacted if there is any question regarding personnel laws which may vary in some states depending upon the size of the practice. Only a brief introduction of the laws related to the ambulatory care setting are given.

Overtime must be addressed in each practice. Who is reimbursed for overtime and how is that reimbursement determined? Typically, medical receptionists and secretaries, insurance billers, medical transcriptionists, and medical assistants are likely to be paid overtime. Overtime pay at a rate of not less than one and one-half times the regular rate of pay after a forty-hour work week is standard. Each week stands alone and one week cannot compensate for another. If the practice does not want to be involved in overtime situations, require that any overtime be preauthorized in advance.

The Equal Pay Act of 1963 prevents wage discrimination for jobs that require equal skill, effort, and responsibility. The Civil Rights Act of 1964 prevents employers from discriminating against individuals on the basis of race, color, religion, sex, age, or national origin.

Sexual harassment violates Title VII of the Civil Rights Act. Steps must be taken to ensure that all employees are working in an atmosphere that is not hostile, where sexual gestures, the presence of pornographic or offensive materials, or obscene language are not allowed.

Employees have a right to expect safe working conditions. The Occupational Safety and Health Act (OSHA) was established to prevent injuries and illnesses resulting from unsafe or unhealthy working conditions. (Refer to Chapter 10 for detailed discussion of the standards and requirements, especially the section on bloodborne pathogens which went into effect in 1992.) Compliance with this law requires that each employee be aware of possible risks associated with chemical hazards and how to protect themselves. Since there are many of these hazards in a medical practice, compliance and protection for employees are extremely important, and training sessions should be held in this area.

The Immigration Reform Act requires employers to verify the right of employees to work in the United States. Documentation acceptable for verification is a Social Security card or birth certificate. The United States Department of Justice Immigration and Naturalization Service will provide instructions and a form for employees and employers to complete (Figure 34-9).

Employers cannot discriminate or condemn any full-time employee for jury duty. While the employer does not have to continue pay during jury duty, the employee cannot lose seniority, insurance, or other benefits. Many employers continue an employee's full pay during the time of service on a jury since the reimbursement for jury service is so small. This is a way to benefit your employees and encourage good citizenship.

This list is by no means comprehensive, but does include personnel regulations most likely to affect the medical practice. Any concerns should be directed to the practice's attorney.

SPECIAL POLICY CONSIDERATIONS

There are several other managerial issues that may arise in a medical office for which the office manager will have to plan. These can include policies for temporary employees, smoking, avoiding discrimination, and having a support system in place for employees who need physical or emotional help.

Temporary Employees

Temporary employees who may be employed for ninety days or less include students who are serving an internship

U.S. Department of Justice
Immigration and Naturalization Service

OMB No. 1115-0136
Employment Eligibility Verification

Please read instructions carefully before completing this form. The instructions must be available during completion of this form. ANTI-DISCRIMINATION NOTICE. It is illegal to discriminate against work eligible individuals. Employers CANNOT specify which document(s) they will accept from an employee. The refusal to hire an individual because of a future expiration date may also constitute illegal discrimination.

Section 1. Employee Information and Verification. To be completed and signed by employee at the time employment begins

Print Name: Last	First	Middle Initial	Maiden Name

Address *(Street Name and Number)* | Apt. # | Date of Birth *(month/day/year)*

City | State | Zip Code | Social Security #

I am aware that federal law provides for imprisonment and/or fines for false statements or use of false documents in connection with the completion of this form.

I attest, under penalty of perjury, that I am (check one of the following):
- ☐ A citizen or national of the United States
- ☐ A Lawful Permanent Resident (Alien # A_____)
- ☐ An alien authorized to work until ____/____/____
  (Alien # or Admission #_____)

Employee's Signature | Date *(month/day/year)*

Preparer and/or Translator Certification. *(To be completed and signed if Section 1 is prepared by a person other than the employee.) I attest, under penalty of perjury, that I have assisted in the completion of this form and that to the best of my knowledge the information is true and correct.*

Preparer's/Translator's Signature | Print Name

Address *(Street Name and Number, City, State, Zip Code)* | Date *(month/day/year)*

Section 2. Employer Review and Verification. To be completed and signed by employer. Examine one document from List A OR examine one document from List B **and** one from List C as listed on the reverse of this form and record the title, number and expiration date, if any, of the document(s)

List A	OR	List B	AND	List C
Document title: _____		_____		_____
Issuing authority: _____		_____		_____
Document #: _____		_____		_____
Expiration Date *(if any):* ___/___/___		___/___/___		___/___/___
Document #: _____				
Expiration Date *(if any):* ___/___/___				

CERTIFICATION - I attest, under penalty of perjury, that I have examined the document(s) presented by the above-named employee, that the above-listed document(s) appear to be genuine and to relate to the employee named, that the employee began employment on *(month/day/year)* ____/____/____ and that to the best of my knowledge the employee is eligible to work in the United States. (State employment agencies may omit the date the employee began employment).

Signature of Employer or Authorized Representative | Print Name | Title

Business or Organization Name | Address *(Street Name and Number, City, State, Zip Code)* | Date *(month/day/year)*

Section 3. Updating and Reverification. To be completed and signed by employer

A. New Name *(if applicable)* | B. Date of rehire *(month/day/year)* *(if applicable)*

C. If employee's previous grant of work authorization has expired, provide the information below for the document that establishes current employment eligibility.

Document Title:_____ | Document #:_____ | Expiration Date (if any):___/___/___

I attest, under penalty of perjury, that to the best of my knowledge, this employee is eligible to work in the United States, and if the employee presented document(s), the document(s) I have examined appear to be genuine and to relate to the individual.

Signature of Employer or Authorized Representative | Date *(month/day/year)*

Form I-9 (Rev. 11-21-91) N

Figure 34-9 Employment Eligibility Verification, Form I-9.

from a local college practicing their skills for when they will be on the job. They should be reviewed every two to three weeks in cooperation with their college supervisor. Give them as much actual hands-on experience as possible; they are your future employees and the employees of your colleagues.

Smoking Policy

Smoking on the premises has become a greater concern in the past ten years. Many places of employment do not allow smoking at all. Some states and cities have laws that may govern this issue for you. When a policy is established, it should cover everyone—employers, employees, and patients. The objective is to have a policy that is workable and enforceable, promotes health, encourages employee morale and productivity, and sets examples for patients. A designated place for smoking may be necessary.

Discrimination

The Americans with Disabilities Act (ADA) establishes guidelines prohibiting discrimination against a "qualified individual with a disability" in regard to employment. Someone with a disability who satisfies the skills necessary for the job, has the experience, education, and any other job requirements, and who, with reasonable accommodation, can perform the job cannot be discriminated against. Employers often find that persons with disabilities are their finest employees. Of particular note for medical personnel is that persons with AIDS are included in the guidelines set forth by the ADA. Persons with AIDS cannot be discriminated against. It can be assumed that if you are providing a safe working environment and all employees follow the rules for standard precautions (see Chapter 10), that reasonable accommodation has been made for the person with AIDS.

Employees with Chemical Dependencies or Emotional Problems

Employees with chemical dependency or emotional problems are ill and are to be treated as such. The situation should be approached constructively rather than punitively. Make a commitment to the employee to assure that the employee is fit for and capable of quality patient care. The human resources manager and physician-employer must be able to recognize the problem when it exists and deal openly and honestly with the issue. If drug or alcohol treatment becomes necessary and an employee is temporarily suspended from employment, do not allow the employee to return unless it is made certain the employee will not endanger herself or anyone else.

PROVIDING/PLANNING EMPLOYEE TRAINING AND EDUCATION

Health care changes daily; new procedures are established, a better technique is discovered for performing a particular task. Major changes regularly occur in medical insurance. Computer systems are updated or new software is added. A more sophisticated telephone system is installed to make certain patients are responded to promptly. New state or federal regulations demand additional training or compliance to safety regulations not previously necessary. New medications become available which physicians may prescribe and employees must understand. All this demands that employees receive a continuing and constant update in their area of employment.

Training and education may be done within the practice or outside the practice. When an employee is a member of a professional organization such as the American Association of Medical Assistants or the American Association of Medical Transcriptionists, many monthly meetings will include continuing education opportunities. Numerous seminars and conferences held throughout the country may be beneficial to employees. Local hospitals often have continuing education opportunities that might be beneficial. The human resources manager will keep abreast of these opportunities and encourage employees to attend. Any continuing education opportunity that may benefit the employee on the job and the medical practice itself should ideally be paid for by the physician-employer(s).

It is often best to provide training and education within the facility when the training necessary is very specific to the medical practice. For instance, training on new computer software is apt to be very specific to the particular setting. When sophisticated new equipment is purchased, companies often provide in-house training for the individuals who will be using the equipment. Take advantage of as many of those opportunities as are available and for as many of your employees as possible. When the training is quite expensive or time consuming, make certain one person receives the training. Then have that individual train others. Whenever possible, provide training outside of regular hours when patients are not being seen—before or after the office closes or during a lunch period. Always pay employees for any time served over their regular working hours.

Careful attention to continuing education and training for employees will pay for itself many times over

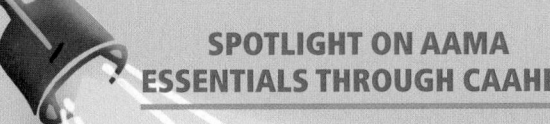

SPOTLIGHT ON AAMA ESSENTIALS THROUGH CAAHEP

● Conducting an exit interview with an employee who voluntarily leaves his or her position provides an atmosphere where the positive and the negative aspects of the position can be discussed. It can also identify what changes might be necessary when a new person fills the position.

● Part of being a good human resources manager is being able to solve conflicts between other employees, coworkers, supervisors, and physician-employers.

● Being able to acknowledge what stresses employees on the job will help to generate new ways or tasks to decrease or prevent stress.

again. The more confident and secure employees feel in the skills they are expected to perform, the more satisfied the practice's patients will be.

CONFLICT RESOLUTION

A good human resources manager will be a master at **conflict resolution**, solving problems between any two parties. The most difficult task is to prevent or solve conflicts that occur between employees or between employees and supervisors or physician-employers. Most conflict occurs because of poor communication or a misunderstanding, so effective communication is a goal for any manager.

Volumes of materials have been written about successful conflict management. One can probably never get enough material on the subject. Some guidelines that may be helpful in preventing and resolving conflicts follow:

● Listen to your employees. What do they say? What do they communicate nonverbally?

● Be prepared to temporarily assist an employee having a difficult time.

● Create a safe environment for an employee to admit a mistake.

● Manage by walking around and talking to your employees.

● Acknowledge the stressors of the job and compensate employees.

● Give ample verbal positive comments and pats on the back.

● Be honest with employees at all times.

● Provide office staff meetings in which employees can express their concerns.

● Treat employees fairly.

● Do not tolerate negative comments or actions among employees.

● Remember birthdays and special occasions with cards or small gifts.

● Provide small rewards when possible.

● Expect to work longer and harder than any employee.

● Have the physician-employer host a social lunch every 60 days.

● Keep employees informed of changes impacting them.

● Encourage an open door policy for concerns and complaints.

● Be a role model for all employees.

● Keep confidences.

● Encourage continuing education through workshops and seminars.

There is no end to such a list. A human resources manager who cares about each employee, who "carries water for the workers in the trenches," who administers fairly and honestly creates an environment where conflict will be at a minimum.

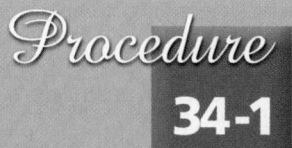

Develop and Maintain a Policy Manual

34-1

PURPOSE:
To develop and maintain a comprehensive, up-to-date policy manual of all office policies relating to employee practices, benefits, office conduct, and so on.

EQUIPMENT/SUPPLIES:
Computer
Binder, such as a three-ring binder
Paper
Standard policy manual format

PROCEDURE STEPS:
1. Following office format, develop precise, written office policies detailing all necessary information pertaining to the staff and their positions. The information should include benefits, vacation, sick leave, hours, dress codes, evaluations, rules of conduct, and grounds for dismissal. RATIO-NALE: Well-defined policies clearly outlined for each employee are necessary for efficient and effective staff operations.
2. Identify procedures for reimbursing overtime, preventing discrimination and harassment, creating a safe working environment, and allowing for jury duty.
3. Include a policy statement related to smoking.
4. Identify steps to follow should an employee become disabled during employment.
5. Determine what employee opportunities for continuing education, if any, will be reimbursed; include requirements for recertification or licensure.
6. Provide a copy of the policy manual for each employee.
7. Review and update the policy manual regularly. Add or delete items as necessary, dating each revised page.

Preparing a Job Description

34-2

PURPOSE:
To provide a precise definition of the tasks assigned to a job, to determine the expectations and level of competency required, and to specify the experience, training, and education needed to perform the job for purposes of recruiting and performance evaluation.

EQUIPMENT/SUPPLIES:
Computer
Paper
Standard job description format

PROCEDURE STEPS:
1. Detail each task that creates the job. RATIO-NALE: A detailed job description identifies clear expectations for each employee.
2. List special medical, technical, or clerical skills required.
3. Determine the level of education, training, and experience required for the position.
4. Determine where the job fits in the overall structure of the office.
5. Specify any unusual working conditions (hours, locations, and so on) that may apply.
6. Describe career path opportunities.

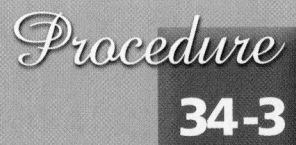

34-3   Interviewing

PURPOSE:
To screen applicants for training, experience, and characteristics to select the best candidate to fill the position vacancy.

PROCEDURE STEPS:
1. Review resumes and applications received.
2. Select candidates who most closely match the education and experience being sought.
3. Create an interview worksheet for each candidate listing points to cover.
4. Select an interview team; this team should always include the human resources or office manager and the immediate supervisor to whom the candidate will report.
5. Call personally to schedule interviews; this allows you to judge the applicant's telephone manners and voice.
6. Remind the interviewers of various legal restrictions concerning questions to be asked.
7. Conduct interviews in a private, quiet setting. RATIONALE: Careful interviewing of potential employees is an important step in hiring the best candidate for the position.
8. Put the applicant at ease by beginning with an overview about the practice and staff, briefly describing the job, and answering preliminary questions.
9. Ask questions about the applicant's work experience and educational background using the resume and interview worksheet as a guide.
10. Provide the most promising applicants additional information on benefits and a tour of the office if practical.
11. Applicant's general salary requirements may be discussed, but avoid discussion of a specific salary until a formal offer is tendered.
12. Inform the applicants when a decision will be made and thank each for participating in the interview.
13. Do not make a job offer until all the candidates have been interviewed.
14. Check references of all prospective employees.
15. Establish a second interview between the physician-employer(s) and the qualified candidate if necessary.
16. Confirm accepted job offers in writing, specifying details of the offer and acceptance.
17. Notify all unsuccessful applicants by letter when the position has been filled.

34-4   Orient and Train Personnel

PURPOSE:
To acquaint new employees with office policies, staff, what the job encompasses, procedures to be performed, and job performance expectations.

PROCEDURE STEPS:
1. Tour the facilities and introduce the office staff.
2. Complete employee-related documents and explain their purpose.
3. Explain the benefits programs.
4. Present the office policy manual and discuss its key elements.
5. Review federal and state regulatory precautions for medical facilities.
6. Review the job description.
7. Explain and demonstrate procedures to be performed and the use of procedure manuals supporting these procedures.
8. Demonstrate the use of any specialized equipment.
9. Assign a mentor from the staff to help with the orientation. RATIONALE: Without proper orientation and training, the best new employee can fail.

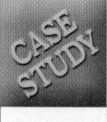

CASE STUDY

34·1

Bruce Goldman, CMA, has been with Inner City Health Care for one year. It is time for his first annual evaluation. The office manager, Jane O'Hara, gives Bruce a performance review form to complete before the formal evaluation. The following day, Bruce has an appointment to meet with Jane to discuss the evaluation. During the meeting, they discover they agree on most points.

CASE STUDY REVIEW

1. How should Jane handle discussing Bruce's frequent long lunches that extend beyond his scheduled lunch break time?
2. Would it be appropriate for Jane to ask a fellow CMA who works with Bruce to sit in to help her to evaluate him?
3. How should Jane end the formal evaluation?

SUMMARY

As you have seen from this discussion, human resources management is a challenge. It is, however, a rewarding one. While physician-employers are responsible for patients' physical care, the human resources manager is responsible for the employees in the organization. The human resources manager who is successful will manage these employees in a way that enables and encourages them to give the very best patient care possible. The medical assistant who has good communication skills and acquires additional training in human resources management will always have variety on the job and will have the satisfaction of watching a health care team run smoothly and efficiently.

REVIEW QUESTIONS

Multiple Choice

1. Human resources managers:
   a. need no special training for the job
   b. are responsible for hiring, training, and managing personnel
   c. usually work harder and longer hours than employees
   d. both b and c
2. The following questions may be asked in an interview:
   a. How old are you?
   b. Have you ever been arrested?
   c. Can you supply a birth certificate or a Social Security card?
   d. Do you plan to start a family soon?
3. Causes for immediate dismissal of an employee include:
   a. being late for work three times within a month
   b. theft, making fraudulent insurance claims
   c. placing a patient in jeopardy and breaching confidentiality
   d. both b and c

4. The most difficult tasks of the human resources manager may be:
   a. resolving conflicts between personnel and dismissing an employee
   b. evaluating employees and planning salary review
   c. planning for continuing education
   d. communicating with the physician-employer
5. The human resources manager will work closely with:
   a. the physician-employer
   b. the office manager
   c. all employees
   d. all the above
6. OSHA:
   a. requires employers to verify an employee's right to work in the United States
   b. protects employees who have disabilities from employment discrimination
   c. protects employees with chemical dependencies or emotional problems
   d. protects employees from unsafe or unhealthy working conditions

7. Conflict between employees:
   a. usually is the result of personality differences
   b. results when the manager is dictatorial
   c. usually is the result of poor communication or a misunderstanding
   d. is better ignored to allow employees to work it out
8. Employees receiving training or education necessary to the job:
   a. will seek that training after hours and not expect reimbursement
   b. will be continuous and constant in the health care field
   c. should always be paid for any time served over regular working hours
   d. both b and c
9. Personnel records:
   a. are usually kept for three to five years and may include payroll data
   b. are not available for everyone to view and must be kept confidential
   c. include all papers related to employment and personal data
   d. all the above
10. Dismissal:
    a. may be voluntary or involuntary
    b. should always be documented
    c. is a good time for an exit interview
    d. all the above

Critical Thinking

1. Discuss the importance of having employees participate in providing input to the job description.
2. How are references checked for prospective employees?
3. Discuss the advantages of having established policies and procedures for performance reviews.
4. How and when might physician-employers be directly involved in personnel matters?
5. You have an employee who gossips about other employees and is negative to everyone. She is otherwise an excellent employee. Plan a strategy to correct the situation.
6. You have just accepted a position to work in a larger more specialized clinic where you will be able to use skills you are not currently able to exercise. Identify two or three main points for a letter of resignation you will prepare.

7. An employee approaches you, the human resource manager, identifying that he/she has just become responsible for the care of an aging parent that may require occasional time away from work. You have no policy about how this absence should be treated. What kind of policy might be helpful? Where would you look for suggestions?
8. An exit interview form has been introduced in this chapter. Another simple form for an exit interview is to use the ABCs. *A* stands for "awesome." What do we do that is really good? *B* stands for "better." What could we do better in our organization? *C* stands for "change." What would you recommend we change? Discuss the merits of both forms for an exit interview.
9. Do a simple comparison of salaries in your community. Compare the hourly wages of a secretary, a medical assistant, a plumber, your automobile mechanic, and a person working in a fast-food restaurant. What conclusions can you make, if any?
10. What might physician-employers and human resource managers do to make certain they keep valued employees? Is salary really the most important issue?

WEB ACTIVITIES

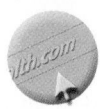 Research the World Wide Web for information about how to hire individuals. Consider http://www.ruf.rice.edu/~humres/Training/HowToHire as one resource for your search. Are there any differences in hiring for the medical profession as opposed to other types of businesses? What tips do you *not* find mentioned in the text?

REFERENCES/BIBLIOGRAPHY

Andress, A. A. (1996). *Manual of medical office management.* Philadelphia: W. B. Saunders Company.

Kinn, M. E., & Woods, M. A. (1999). *The medical assistant: Administrative and clinical* (8th ed.). Philadelphia: W. B. Saunders Co.

Mathis, R. L., & Jackson, J. H. (2000). *Human resource management* (9th ed.). Cincinnati, OH: South-Western College Publishing.

Ricardo, M. (1992). *Personnel management handbook* (2nd ed.). New York: McGraw-Hill, Inc.

Sullivan, D. (1992). *Effective management in nursing.* New York: Addison-Wesley.

ENTRY INTO THE PROFESSION

Chapter

35

PREPARING FOR MEDICAL ASSISTING CREDENTIALS

KEY TERMS

Accrediting Bureau of Health
    Education Schools (ABHES)
American Association of Medical
    Assistants (AAMA)
Certification Examination
Certified Medical Assistant (CMA)
Continuing Education Units (CEUs)
National Board of Medical Examiners
    (NBME)
Not current status
Recertification
Registered Medical Assistant (RMA)
Revalidation
Task Force for Test Construction

OUTLINE

Purpose of Certification
Preparing for the Examination
Registered Medical Assistant
    (RMA)
    Examination Format and Content
    Application Process
    Application Completion and Test
        Administration Scheduling

Certified Medical Assistant
    (CMA)
    Examination Format and Content
    Application Process
    Eligibility Categories and
        Requirements
    Grounds for Denial of Eligibility
    How to Recertify

OBJECTIVES

*The student should strive to meet the following performance objectives and demonstrate
an understanding of the facts and principles presented in this chapter through written and
oral communication.*

1. Define the key terms as presented in the glossary.
2. Differentiate between being certified and being registered.
3. Identify the benefits of certification and registration.
4. List the necessary qualifications to sit for the CMA certification
    examination.
5. List the necessary qualifications to sit for the RMA examination.
6. State when the CMA certification examination is offered and the
    registration deadlines.
7. State when the RMA examination is offered and the registration
    protocols.
8. Describe several methods for continuing education opportunities.
9. Explain when recertification/revalidation must take place.
10. Describe the procedure for recertification/revalidation.

**GENERAL
(TRANSDISCIPLINARY)**

Professionalism

- Enhance skills through
  continuing education

Legal Skills

- Recognize professional
  credentialing criteria

Dr. Ray Reynolds currently is the senior physician at Inner City Health
Care, a multi-physician urgent care center. When he began his practice
thirty-two years ago, however, he had a private practice and employed one
full-time and two part-time medical assistants. Dr. Reynolds felt the office
ran smoothly, except when an assistant had to be replaced. Retraining a new
person consumed a great deal of valuable time. Even if the new employee
came with experience from another medical office, the procedures still
required retraining.

Dr. Reynolds finds that when he needs to replace a medical assistant
now, he looks at the applicants' resumes and interviews only those
candidates who are certified medical assistants (CMAs) or registered medical
assistants (RMAs). The office is too busy to spend time training and
retraining new people.

INTRODUCTION

Thirty years ago medical assistants were trained on the job
by the practitioner for whom they were employed. Quality
control of training varied since there were no established
criteria for evaluating such training.

Hence, the certification examination was developed
by AAMA and the RMA examination was developed by

the AMT. Both examinations, along with methods of
continuing education and recertification, or revalidation,
establish criteria for evaluating training.

PURPOSE OF CERTIFICATION

Certification is intended to set a consistent minimum
standard for evaluating an individual's professional competence as a medical assistant. The **certification examination** is offered by the **American Association of
Medical Assistants (AAMA)**. Hiring physicians view
the credential as professional and an indication of entry-
level skills. Maintaining the credential demonstrates a
lifelong commitment to continuing education. The graduate medical assistant has a goal and challenge to which
to aspire, first by earning the credential, and second by
maintaining the credential through recertification.

Formal medical assistant education programs are
offered throughout the country in vocation-technical
high schools and colleges, proprietary schools, postsecondary vocational schools, community and junior colleges, and four-year colleges and universities. Medical
assistants may be trained on the job; however, physicians
recognize that their offices operate more efficiently with
professionally educated personnel.

PREPARING FOR THE EXAMINATION

Preparation for the examination requires forethought,
scheduling, and discipline. It is important to plan well in
advance to ensure confidence and a positive test result,
earning your credential. If you are sitting for the examination immediately upon graduation, your preparation
time for the examination may only require two to three
months. If you have been out of school for some time or
your work experience has been very specialized, you may
need six to eight months to prepare for the examination.

During the forethought stage, determine the date
you want to sit for the examination. Check with the
appropriate Web site or make a telephone call to the
examination department to obtain the current application
form. The application form will contain information such
as dates, times, and locations of test sites, policies regarding
deadlines, incomplete applications, examination verification information, and information regarding study guides.

It is also important to consider looking for a study group or partner. The right study environment can be invaluable to your success for several reasons. First, it is important to select a study partner or group who shares your commitment to a successful outcome and who plans to sit for the examination near the same date you have selected. A study partner can also give you some accountability for keeping to the planned schedule.

Once it has been determined when and where you will sit for the examination and who your study partner, if any, will be, a meeting should be scheduled to discuss the review/study approach. It may be that your group will decide to review/study each subject provided in the Curriculum Content Outline accompanying the application. Other groups review/study only those areas in which they feel less confident. A plan that meets the needs of each group member and that all can agree to works best.

Meeting once or twice a week helps the group stay focused and on task. Independent study should be done throughout the week. During the independent study time, each group member may be asked to write 10 multiple choice questions relevant to the weeks' study topic. Answers to these questions should be on a separate page. Some find it helpful to also provide the rationale or textbook page number that supports their answer. When the group meets, a discussion of the study topic could take place and copies of the questions distributed for answering. The questions could then be corrected and discussion of any questionable or missed answers could take place.

Once a schedule has been established and agreed upon, discipline is required. It is critical that each group member spend time individually preparing for the next group meeting. Someone should be put in charge of each group meeting to keep the event from turning into a social time. To help with this, it is a good idea to set a specific time limit for the study/review session. If individuals want to visit after the session, they are free to do that without disrupting the purpose of the session. All members should be committed to being prepared and attending each scheduled review/study session.

REGISTERED MEDICAL ASSISTANT (RMA)

The American Medical Technologists (AMT), a national certifying body for health professionals, established the **Registered Medical Assistant (RMA)** credential in 1972. The RMA/AMT has its own bylaws, officers, local, state, and national organizations. Applicants for the RMA examination are graduates of schools accredited by the **Accrediting Bureau of Health Education Schools (ABHES)**, a regional accrediting commission, or other acceptable agency. Currently, there are over 52,000 RMAs certified by AMT. Registered medical assistants

SPOTLIGHT ON AAMA ESSENTIALS THROUGH CAAHEP

● Joining professional organizations, such as AAMA and AMT, and participating in the activities they afford, such as becoming certified or registered, helps a medical assistant to grow both personally and professionally.

● Obtaining certification or registration as a medical assistant requires a professional attitude, a high degree of understanding of medical assistant skills, and a positive approach to working with all types of patients and coworkers.

● A skilled and credentialed medical assistant should possess the ability to see beyond the complaining patient who may not be feeling well, and project a positive and professional caring attitude toward that patient.

and members of the AMT Registry are entitled to wear the RMA insignia.

AMT certification examinations are intended to evaluate the competence of entry-level practitioners. Content areas defined and validated by subject-matter experts, educators, and individuals working in their respective fields make up the test. Registration is granted in conjunction with other indicators of training and experience, since the tests provide only one source of information regarding examinee competence.

Examination Format and Content

The AMT registration examination consists of 200 to 210 multiple-choice questions. Examinees are required to select the single best answer; multiple answers for a single item are scored as incorrect. Test questions may require examinees to recall facts, interpret graphic illustrations, interpret information presented in case studies, analyze situations, or solve problems. The approximate percentages of questions in content areas are as follows:

1. General Medical Assisting Knowledge—42.5%
   - anatomy and physiology
   - medical terminology
   - medical law
   - medical ethics
   - human relations
   - patient education

2. Administrative Medical Assisting—22.5%
   - insurance
   - financial bookkeeping
   - medical secretarial-receptionist

3. Clinical Medical Assisting—35.0%
   - asepsis
   - sterilization
   - instruments
   - vital signs
   - physical examinations
   - clinical pharmacology
   - minor surgery
   - therapeutic modalities
   - laboratory procedures
   - electrocardiography
   - first aid

Application Process

The following criteria have been established for applicants sitting for the RMA Examination:

1. Applicant shall be of good moral character.
2. Applicant shall be a graduate of an accredited high school or acceptable equivalent.
3. Applicant must meet one of the following requirements:
   A. Applicant shall be a graduate of a
      - medical assistant program or institution accredited by an organization approved by the United States Department of Education
      - medical assistant program accredited by a Regional Accrediting Commission or by a national accrediting organization approved by the United States Department of Education
      - formal medical services training program of the United States Armed Forces
   B. Applicant shall have been employed in the profession of medical assisting for a minimum of five years, no more than two years of which may have been as an instructor in a postsecondary medical assistant program.
4. All applicants taking the AMT examination must pass to receive the Registered Medical Assistant (RMA) credential.

Application Completion and Test Administration Scheduling

The candidate should allow ample time for documentation to be completed before considering the scheduling of a test when submitting an application. It is the candidate's responsibility to keep abreast of the progress of the application and to aid in the timely response of references and employers. Tests may be scheduled *only* after applications are completed.

Examinations are administered throughout the year at testing center locations. Although most centers offer tests every week of the year, several locations administer tests only on specific days of the year. A complete and up-to-date list of sites will be forwarded when the candidate's application is approved. Most examinations may be scheduled within three days of application completion.

CERTIFIED MEDICAL ASSISTANT (CMA)

The American Association of Medical Assistants (AAMA) offers the certification examination. After successfully passing the certification examination, the **Certified Medical Assistant (CMA)** credential is awarded by the Certifying Board of the AAMA. The credential appears after your name and distinguishes you as a professional signifying achievement in a demanding career field.

CMAs are recognized by peers for their commitment to continued professional development. Survey results indicate that employers recognize the value of the credential by paying higher salaries and offering more benefits to CMAs. Broader career advancement opportunities and enhanced job security represent other benefits of certification. The CMA credential is a national credential and therefore is valid wherever the practitioner is employed within the United States.

Examination Format and Content

The CMA certification examination is a comprehensive test of the knowledge actually utilized in today's medical office. The content is drawn from an in-depth analysis of the numerous tasks medical assistants perform on a daily basis. The consultant for the examination is the **National Board of Medical Examiners (NBME)**, the same organization that develops licensure and specialty board examinations for physicians nationwide.

Examination questions are formulated by the Certifying Board's **Task Force for Test Construction**. This group is comprised of practicing medical assistants, physicians, and medical assisting educators from across the United States. Working with NBME, the Task Force updates the CMA examination annually to reflect changes in medical assistants' day-to-day responsibilities, as well as the latest developments in medical knowledge and technology.

The three major areas tested include:

1. *General medical knowledge:* terminology, anatomy, physiology, professionalism, communication, medicolegal guidelines/requirements
2. *Administrative knowledge:* typing and data entry, equipment, records management, screening and processing mail, scheduling and monitoring appointments, resource information/community services, managing physician's professional schedule and travel, managing the office, office policies and procedures, managing practice finances
3. *Clinical knowledge:* principles of infection control, treatment area, patient preparation and assisting the physician, patient history interview, collecting and processing specimens, preparing and administering medications, emergencies, first aid

Students must enroll as an AAMA member before their graduation date to be eligible for the reduced student rate. Once they are a student member they may stay at the student rate for one year after graduation if they don't choose to be an active or associate member and pay the higher dues amount. The additional year of membership at the reduced rate helps the recent graduate maintain membership while finding a job and getting established in a career.

Application Process

Candidates will want to read all instructions carefully before completing the application form. Incomplete or incorrect applications will not be processed and will be returned to the candidate. Postmark deadlines for applications, cancellations, and examination location changes are strictly enforced.

The examination is offered at over 250 test sites nationwide. A complete listing of the locations is included in the application. Applications are available from the AAMA Certification Department, 20 North Wacker Drive, Suite 1575, Chicago, IL 60606-2903 or telephone 312-424-3100 or e-Mail: certification@aama.ntl.org.

The appropriate application form must be completed and postmarked by October 1 for the January exam and by March 1 for the June exam.

The certification examination is scheduled from 9:00 AM to 1:00 PM the last Friday of January and the last Saturday in June.

It is recommended that the application be sent by certified mail, return receipt requested to verify delivery. The application must be typewritten or printed using black ink only. Be sure the application is signed and dated properly and the eligibility category section is completed appropriately.

Tear off the application page from the instruction pamphlet. Do not mail the instructions back with the application. Keep this information for future reference along with a copy of everything submitted, including a copy of your completed payment check or money order. If you are paying by VISA or MasterCard, provide the requested information at the top of the application.

A guide for the certification examination entitled *A Candidate's Guide to the AAMA Certification Examination* provides explanations of how to approach the types of questions used on the examination and tips on how to study for the content that will be tested. A sample 120-question examination is included.

Eligibility Categories and Requirements

You must fulfill one of the four eligibility categories to apply for the CMA examination. Figure 35-1 describes these requirements.

Grounds for Denial of Eligibillity

The following are grounds for denial of eligibility for the Certified Medical Assistant (CMA) credential, or for discipline of Certified Medical Assistants (CMAs):

- obtaining or attempting to obtain certification, or recertification of the CMA credential, by fraud or deception

- knowingly assisting another to obtain or attempt to obtain certification or recertification by fraud or deception

- misstatement of material fact or failure to make a statement of material fact in application for certification or recertification

- falsifying information required for admission to the CMA examination, inpersonating another examinee, or falsifying education or credentials

- copying answers, permitting another to copy answers, or providing or receiving unauthorized advice about examination content during the CMA examination

- unauthorized possession or distribution of examination materials, including copying and reproducing examination questions and problems.

Individuals who have been found guilty of a felon, or pleaded guilty to a felon, are not eligible to take the CMA Exam. However, the Certifying Board may grant a waiver based upon mitigating circumstances, which may include, but need not be limited to the following:

CATEGORY 1—CAAHEP GRADUATING STUDENT OR RECENT GRADUATE

Graduating students must have completed, by January 31 for the January test and by June 30 for the June test, formal training, including an externship, in a medical assisting program accredited by CAAHEP. If the student fails to complete the program by the required date, the exam will be considered invalid. Scores will not be released, and refunds will not be provided.

Requirement: Applications must be signed by the program director and an official transcript must accompany the application.

Recent graduates must take the exam within 12 months of graduation to qualify for the discounted fee.

Requirement: An official transcript must accompany the application to verify graduation from the program.

CATEGORY 2—CAAHEP GRADUATE

The candidate must be a graduate of a medical assisting program accredited by CAAHEP.

Requirement: An official transcript must accompany the application to verify graduation from the program.

CATEGORY 3—ABHES GRADUATE

The candidate must have graduated from an ABHES accredited medical assisting program that was ABHES accredited at the time of graduation.

Requirements: An official transcript must accompany the application to verify graduation from the program.

CATEGORY 4—RECERTIFICANT

The candidate must be a Certified Medical Assistant applying for the CMA Examination to recertify his or her credential.

Requirement: A copy of the candidate's CMA certificate should accompany the application. (Contact the AAMA Certification Department if you are unable to locate your certificate. The month and year that you passed the CMA Examination will be required to research your records.)

Figure 35-1   CMA Eligibility Categories and Requirements through June 2002. (Source: *AAMA's CMA Examination.* AAMA Certification Department, Dept. 79-7999, Chicago, IL 60678-7999.)

- the age at which the crime was committed
- the circumstances surrounding the crime
- the nature of the crime committed
- the length of time since the conviction
- the individual's criminal history since the conviction
- the individual's current employment references
- the individual's character references
- other evidence demonstrating the ability of the individual to perform the professional responsibilities competently, and evidence that the individual does not pose a threat to the health or safety of patients

How to Recertify

Recertification of the CMA credential may be achieved by either reexamination or by the continuing education method. Recertification credits are evaluated on supportive documentation, and on their relevancy to medical assisting as defined by the AAMA Medical Assistant Role Delineation Study or the Content Outline for the Certification/Recertification Examination.

A total of 60 points is necessary to recertify the CMA credential. At least 20 points must be from AAMA **continuing education units (CEUs)**. The remaining 40 points may be any formal credit (e.g., non-AAMA CEUs, contact hours, college credit) that has relevancy to medical assisting as defined by the AAMA Medical Assistant Role Delineation Study (shown in the appendices) or the Content Outline for the Certification/Recertification Examination. All 60 points may be from AAMA CEUs, but 20 *must be* from AAMA CEUs.

Continuing education courses are offered by local, state, and national AAMA groups. Guided study programs are also available through AAMA's "Quest for Excellence" program. *The Professional Medical Assistant,* the official bimonthly publication of AAMA, provides articles designated for continuing education units.

The CMA credentials must be recertified every five years. Certificates are current through December 31 of the fifth year following certification or recertification. For example, if you certified or recertified in 1996, your credential would hold current status through December 31, 2001. Failure to recertify will result in a **not current status**.

A CMA need not be a member of the AAMA, nor currently employed, in order to recertify. Figure 35-2 illustrates the Continuing Education Verification Form used to submit CEUs to AAMA for recertification. The entire recertification by continuing education instructions and application can be downloaded from AAMA's website (www.aama-ntl.org). Review of recertification applications can take up to 90 days. If all criteria are met, recertification is granted. The date that the application is postmarked to the AAMA Executive Office will be the date of recertification.

Upon meeting recertification requirements, the applicant receives a seal to affix to the original certificate. A Recertification Certificate is also available for purchase. AMT promotes continued education and **revalidation** of the RMA credential. Revalidation is processed through the American Medical Technologists Institute for Education (AMTIE) and is required on a five-year cycle. *Vital Signs*, a quarterly publication by AMT, is designed for registered medical assistants and students of ABHES schools.

The American Medical Technologists Institute for Education (AMTIE) offers STEP, a continuing education home-study program for healthcare practitioners. STEP is published in AMT's *Journal of Continuing Education Topics & Issues*. Health care practitioners may earn continuing education credit for reading articles, answering self-study questions, and returning answer sheets to the AMT office for scoring. AMT records credit earned and issues annual reports of STEP activities to program participants.

AAMA's CMA Recertification by Continuing Education
Continuing Education Verification Form

Name: Jane Doe   **Social Security Number:** 000-00-0000   **Page Number:** 1

Read the application instructions before completing this sheet. If additional space is needed, this form may be photocopied. You may use computer-formatted facsimiles of any part of this application. TYPE or neatly PRINT the information. This form is also available in a Word or WordPerfect format. You may call the AAMA to request it be sent to you by email or on disk. On each page you use, enter your name, Social Security number, and the page number above. To convert credits to points, see How to Convert Credit to Recertification Points in the instructions. For information on how to determine the content category, refer to the section Content Areas Defined. Supportive documents must be attached to this form. Also attach a photocopy of your original certificate. Do *not* send your original certificate.

1	2	3	4	5	6	7	8	9
Date of activity (m/d/y)	Sponsor (group or organization issuing the credit for the continuing education activity)	Program title	Amount and type of credit earned (eg, CEU, CME, contact hour or college credit)	Recertification points — AAMA CEUs	Recertification points — Other credit	Points per content area — Gen.	Adm.	Clin.
	If using more than one page, copy the cumulative total for each column (5–9) from the previous page ☞							
7/3/00	AAMA 10259	Managing the Medical Office	.4 CEU	4			4	
8/24/00	Trident Chapter of Medical Assistants	Medical Nutritional Needs	.6 CEU	6		6		
9/2/98	Eli Lily Co.	Aspects of Diabetes	.2 CEU		2			2
10/11/00	Tri-City Chapter of Medical Assistants	Improving Your Coding Skills	.4 CEU	4			4	
11/17/00	28784	Quality Urinalysis Testing	.2 CEU	2				2
1/9/01	Administrative Seminars Inc.	Personnel Management	.8 CEU		8		8	
3/19/01	Riverside Hospital	Hepatitis In-service	1 Contact Hr.		1			1
4/24/99	South Carolina AAMA St. Soc.	Child Abuse	.4 CEU	4		2	1	1
6/21/01	U. of South Carolina	AIDS Awareness	2 Semester Hrs.		30	15		15
9/8/01	American Heart Association	CPR	4 Contact Hrs.		4	1		3
		Total points in each column (5–9): (If using more than one page, copy the cumulative total for each column (5–9) to the top of the next page.)		20	45	24	17	24

SAMPLE

Figure 35-2   Sample Continuing Education Verification Form for AAMA. (Source: *AAMA's CMA Examination.* AAMA Certification Department, Dept. 79-7999, Chicago, IL 60678-7999.)

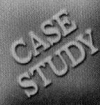

It is February, and Juan Estaban is beginning to research the procedures and requirements for taking the medical assisting certification examination. Juan is enrolled in a CAAHEP-accredited program.

35-1

CASE STUDY REVIEW

1. If Juan wants to take the examination in June, what is the procedure for applying?

2. Juan is setting up a study schedule. He plans to review course textbooks and tests, purchase a certification review study guide, and set up a study group. Set up a sample study schedule.

3. What criteria should Juan use when asking people to join his study group?

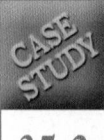

It is May, and Nancy McFarland, who graduated from an ABHES-accredited program four and a half years ago, is beginning to research the procedures and requirements for taking the medical assistant examination. Nancy completed her internship at Inner City Health Care and was hired to work there full-time (35 hours per week) when she graduated.

35-2

CASE STUDY REVIEW

1. If Nancy wants to take the exam in January, what is the procedure for applying?

2. Nancy is setting up a study schedule. She plans to review course textbooks and tests, purchase a study guide, and set up a study group. Develop a simple study schedule.

3. What criteria should Nancy use when asking people to join her study group?

SUMMARY

Many advantages for certification/recertification and registration have been discussed in this chapter. Although certification examinations are not legally required for practicing medical assistants, it is the goal of CAAHEP-accredited and ABHES-accredited institutions to encourage graduates to sit for and maintain their credentials.

Membership in the AAMA or in the AMT is also encouraged. In addition to the previously mentioned advantages of AAMA, other benefits such as receiving quarterly newsletters, *The Professional Medical Assistant* journal, credit card privileges, group insurance plans, legal advice, a loan program, and a discounted car rental program are available.

With nearly 400 local AAMA chapters and 51 affiliate state societies, there is the benefit of networking with others in the profession. As an information source for both professional and association issues, the executive staff at the AAMA's national headquarters is available to answer questions at a toll-free number (1-800-228-2262).

AMT currently has 37 chapters which meet regularly and allow networking with other Registered Medical Assistants plus other allied health professionals registered through the AMT, including phlebotomists, medical laboratory technicians, and dental assistants.

REVIEW QUESTIONS

Multiple Choice

1. The goal and challenge of each graduating medical assistant should be to:
   a. find employment
   b. have a good benefit package
   c. possess entry-level skills
   d. earn the CMA credential and maintain it

2. The certification examination is:
   a. a comprehensive test based on tasks medical assistants perform daily
   b. all true/false questions
   c. developed by the AMTIE
   d. developed by the NBME

3. Benefits from membership in a professional organization such as AAMA or AMT include all of the following *except:*
   a. discounted rates on legal representation
   b. legal advice
   c. nationwide networking opportunities
   d. professional journal publications
4. Recertification of the CMA credential options include:
   a. submit work experience
   b. reexamination or CEU method
   c. submit on-the-job training
   d. submit military training
5. Applications for the CMA exam must be postmarked by:
   a. October 1 for January exam and March 1 for June exam
   b. October 31 for January exam and March 31 for June exam
   c. September 30 for January exam and April 30 for June exam
   d. September 1 for January exam and April 1 for June exam
6. The RMA was established by the:
   a. ABHES
   b. CAAHEP
   c. AMT
   d. AAMA
7. Candidates who graduate from a medical assisting program that is not CAAHEP-accredited on the date of graduation, but is accredited by CAAHEP within 36 months of that date, are eligible to apply for the CMA exam under which category(ies)?
   a. Category 1
   b. Category 4
   c. Categories 3 or 4
   d. Categories 1 or 2
8. RMA examinations:
   a. are offered at Cogent testing center locations
   b. are offered twice a year
   c. are offered three times a year
   d. are offered six times a year

Critical Thinking

1. Describe the purpose and benefits of certification.
2. Identify the necessary qualifications for maintaining current CMA status
3. Identify the necessary qualifications for the certification examination as an RMA.

4. Differentiate between the methods of recertification for the CMA.
5. Identify several approaches to collecting CEUs.
6. List advantages of membership in a professional organization for medical assistants.

WEB ACTIVITIES

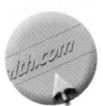

Using the World Wide Web, search your local and state AAMA or AMT web sites. Print and turn in to your instructor the location, meeting schedules, and any upcoming events planned for your state.

DOCUMENTATION

Upon successfully passing the Certification Examination and earning the CMA credential, one should begin to document all CEUs earned. Copies of the form illustrated in Figure 35-2 may be obtained from the AAMA for this purpose. It is important to have the following information for CEU documentation:

- complete date of the activity
- sponsor (group or organization issuing the credit for the CE activity)
- program title
- amount and type of credit earned (e.g., CEU, CME, contact hour or college credit)
- recertification points (AAMA CEUs or other credit)
- points per content area (general, administrative, clinical)

REFERENCES/BIBLIOGRAPHY

AAMA. (1997–1998). AAMA *certification/recertification examination for medical assistants;* January and June 2000 Application Instructions. Chicago: AAMA.

American Medical Technologists. [On-line]. Available: http://www.amt1.com.

Frew, M. A., Lane, K., & Frew, D. R. (1995). *Comprehensive medical assisting: Competencies for administrative and clinical practice.* Philadelphia: F. A. Davis Company.

Chapter

36

EMPLOYMENT STRATEGIES

KEY TERMS

Accomplishment Statements
Application/Cover Letter
Application Form
Bullet Point
Career Objective
Chronological Resume
Contact Tracker
Functional Resume
Interview
Power Verbs
References
Resume
Targeted Resume

OUTLINE

Developing a Strategy
  Self-Assessment
Job Analysis and Research
Budgetary Needs Analysis
Resume Preparation
  Resume Specifications
  Clear and Concise Resumes
  Accomplishments
  References
  Accuracy
  Resume Styles
  Vital Resume Information

Application/Cover Letters
Completing the Application Form
The Look of Success
  Personal and Professional Poise
The Interview Process
  Preparing for the Interview
  The Actual Interview
  Closing the Interview
Interview Follow-Up
  Follow-Up Letter
  Follow Up by Telephone

OBJECTIVES

The student should strive to meet the following performance objectives and demonstrate an understanding of the facts and principles presented in this chapter through written and oral communication.

1. Define the key terms as presented in the glossary.
2. List the steps involved in job analysis and research.
3. Describe a contact tracker and its usefulness.
4. Give three examples of accomplishment statements.
5. Differentiate chronological, functional, and targeted resumes.
6. Identify the purpose and content of a cover letter.
7. Demonstrate effective ways to anticipate and respond to an interviewer's questions.
8. Describe appropriate overall appearance and dress for an interview.
9. Identify the benefits of writing a follow-up letter.

**GENERAL
(TRANSDISCIPLINARY)**

Professionalism

- Project a professional manner and image
- Demonstrate initiative and responsibility
- Adhere to ethical principles

Communication Skills

- Use effective and correct verbal and written communications
- Recognize and respond to verbal and nonverbal communications

Eun Mee Soo is a graduate of a CAAHEP-accredited medical assisting program and recently passed the certification examination. She is now preparing her resume and beginning her job search. Eun Mee plans to move out of state (she always dreamed of moving north), so she will also be looking for a new apartment. All of these changes are a bit unsettling for Eun Mee. She is beginning to wonder if she should not relocate at this time but stay close to home until she feels more secure.

INTRODUCTION

So you are about to graduate from the medical assistant program! This time is often unsettling since many changes are occurring; the loss of security the classroom environment provided, loss of contact with fellow classmates, and loss of a structured schedule are just a few changes. Questions such as: Am I ready for my first job? How do I find a job? What do I say at the interview? begin to surface.

The focus on employment may represent apprehension and doubt or be sparked with anticipation and a sense of fulfillment. This chapter has been included to provide direction and to help answer some of the questions related to the job search.

DEVELOPING A STRATEGY

Positive thinking is one of the primary keys to success in planning your career and job search. Positive thinking leads to positive attitudes, positive feelings about yourself and others, and positive words and actions.

There is a job out there for you! Those individuals who are successful at finding that first job devote a minimum of forty hours per week at job strategy tactics. In other words, finding their first job is their first job. These individuals do not become discouraged by rejection, rather they learn from it and work harder for the next opportunity.

Self-Assessment

Perhaps the first place to begin the job campaign is with a self-assessment exercise. This exercise should stimulate your thought process related to the type of employment upon which you want to focus. Take a moment now to complete the exercise, Self-Evaluation Work Sheet (Figure 36-1).

JOB ANALYSIS AND RESEARCH

Begin to compile a list of potential employers in your immediate area or the geographical area in which you want to work. This may be accomplished by looking through the yellow pages of the telephone directory and/or the business listings. Select facilities that are within your geographic boundaries, provide the work setting and/or specialty you have selected, and appear to offer the basic guidelines you have established.

Now begin your research. Many offices have brochures available that describe their services, appointment scheduling, telephone policy, fees and insurance protocol, confidentiality issues, after-hours medical coverage, and mission statement or philosophy of practice criteria. Most of the larger medical centers offer community education series and prepare a calendar of events publication. Also found in these publications are articles on wellness issues, safety precautions, financial reports, and introductions of new procedures, equipment, and staff members. These documents are an excellent resource tool for learning more about a particular facility and should be studied carefully.

The computer can be of great value in your job search. There are multitudes of employment sites on the Internet and it is possible to search newspaper want ads for almost any large city you desire. The yellow pages are also on-line for most cities, permitting you to easily search for medical facilities that are in line with your goals and objectives.

It may also be helpful to develop your own list of "Hot Line" telephone numbers. Television and radio sta-

---

SELF-EVALUATION WORK SHEET

Respond to the following questions honestly and sincerely. They are meant to assist you in self-assessment.

1. List your three strongest attributes as related to people, data, or things.
   i.e.; Interpersonal skills related to people
      Accuracy related to data
      Mechanical ability related to things

   _____ related to _____
   _____ related to _____
   _____ related to _____

2. List your three weakest attributes as related to people, data, or things.
   _____ related to _____
   _____ related to _____
   _____ related to _____

3. How do you express yourself? excellent, good, fair, poor
   Orally _____ In writing _____

4. Do you work well as a leader of a group or team? Yes _____ No _____

5. Do you prefer to work alone and on your own? Yes _____ No _____

6. Can you work under stress/pressure? Yes _____ No _____

7. Do you enjoy new ideas and situations? Yes _____ No _____

8. Are you comfortable with routines/schedules? Yes _____ No _____

9. Which work setting do you prefer?
   Single-physician setting _____ Multiple-physician setting _____
   Small clinic setting _____ Large clinic setting _____
   Single specialty setting _____ Multi-specialty setting _____

10. Are you willing to relocate? _____ Willing to travel? _____

Figure 36-1   Self-evaluation work sheets can help determine a person's strengths, weaknesses, and preferences before the job search begins.

---

tions often share these numbers. By compiling these numbers into a list, you can efficiently make calls to determine if positions are open and the correct name and spelling of the person to whom the application should be addressed. A visit to your local employment agency may also provide additional resources. Remember to check for job openings on bulletin boards in laundromats, churches, health clubs, and any variety of locations. The Chamber of Commerce in your community may be another resource to consider. Journals and publications such as *The Professional Medical Assistant* (PMA) and your local AAMA chapter will be valuable resources to utilize. Network with professionals at every opportunity. Employers will often report employment opportunities to the Job Placement Center in the college campus or to your medical assistant instructors.

Competition in today's employment arena is very keen. Solicit all help possible as you search for that first job. Friends, relatives, and acquaintances provide the most successful leads to potential employment opportunities. Tell everyone you are looking for a job, the type of position, and the setting in which you would most like to work. Do not forget to tell your personal physician, ophthalmologist, and dentist about your employment goals. They have contact with other professionals who may need help and want to hire a medical assistant.

Direct contact with employers is the second most successful means of finding employment. It takes a lot of nerve and self-confidence to call on prospective employers unannounced or to pick up the telephone to call and ask if they are likely to be hiring medical assistants in the near future. This is an effective approach, however.

The third most effective way to gain employment is a combination of the methods previously discussed. For example, you are visiting the physician's office for an allergy injection. The medical assistant administering the injection asks how your classes are progressing and you share that you are about to graduate and are looking for an entry-level position. The medical assistant tells you that the office next door has a position open. After the injection, if you are dressed appropriately, you could stop in to inquire about the position and ask for an application form.

Don't overlook your externship facility if you participated in an externship program. Very frequently new MAs entering the job market are hired by the site where they did their externship. The site has had time to come to know them, their work ethic, and their knowledge. In addition the site has already invested time in some training so former externs are knowledgeable of the policies and procedures of the facility. Even if the site decides to advertise for the position and interview candidates, you will have an advantage over the other applicants provided your performance was good during your work there.

Review the reasons for employers not hiring shown in Figure 36-2. This figure lists the qualities employers want and do not want in an employee.

When you are serious about the job search and are giving forty hours per week to the process, you will contact numerous individuals. By devising some means of recording these contacts, their responses, and your action, you will not become confused or forget valuable information. A **contact tracker** such as the one suggested in Figure 36-3 may be helpful.

BUDGETARY NEEDS ANALYSIS

It is critical that you know just how much income is required to meet your living expenses. To accomplish this, begin to keep a diary of all purchases and payments. By

reviewing your checkbook register you should be able to itemize basic expenditures; i.e., rent, utilities, payments (car, credit card), food, clothing, insurance, taxes, and so on. Once a monthly expenditure record is established, an estimate of the money required to live on may be calculated.

REASONS FOR EMPLOYERS NOT HIRING

Employers in business were asked to list reasons for not hiring a job seeker. Given in rank order (from most unwanted to least unwanted), the 15 biggest gripes are as follows:

1. Poor appearance (not dressed properly, poorly groomed).
2. Acting like a know-it-all.
3. Cannot express self clearly; poor voice, diction, grammar.
4. Lack of planning for work—no purpose or goals.
5. Lack of confidence or poise.
6. No interest in or enthusiasm for the job.
7. Not active in school extracurricular programs.
8. Interested only in the best dollar offer.
9. Poor school record (academic, attendance).
10. Unwilling to start at the bottom.
11. Making excuses, hedges on unfavorable record.
12. No tact.
13. Not mature.
14. No curiosity about the job.
15. Critical of past employers.

Figure 36-2   Reasons for employers not hiring. (Courtesy of Highline Community College, Counseling/Career Center, Des Moines, WA)

CONTACT TRACKER

	Company Name/Address	Telephone Number	Contact's Name	Resume Sent	Application/ Cover Letter	Application Form Sent	Follow-Up Phone	Follow-Up Letter	Result
1.									
2.									
3.									
4.									
5.									
6.									

Figure 36-3   A simple contact tracker such as this can help organize all communication you may have with potential employers.

RESUME PREPARATION

A **resume** is a summary data sheet or a brief account of your qualifications and progress in the career you have chosen. It is a useful tool for selling yourself and provides opportunity to describe your education, what you have done, and what you can do, and lists those who can vouch for your integrity and experience. A resume that is well thought out and written in such a way as to create interest in what you have to contribute to the employer may reward you with many interviews. During the interview your resume serves as a reference from which the interviewer may be prompted to ask questions.

Resume Specifications

The resume should be limited to one page in length. Keep a 1 to 1½ inch margin on all four sides of the page to create a picture-like frame. Capitalize major headings and single space between lines. Double space between sections. The use of **bullet point** lists instead of paragraphs aids the interviewer in gleaning key points quickly.

Select a high-quality bond stationery that is standard 8½ × 11 inches with a weight of between 16 and 25 pounds. This paper weight provides aesthetic benefit and will also accept the ink better resulting in a clean, sharp print resolution. Buff or ivory paper with matching envelope has the greatest eye appeal and distinguishes your resume from others.

Use a computer or word processor to produce your resume. It allows you the freedom to experiment with placement to create a picture-perfect resume or to individualize the resume for a particular position or facility.

Clear and Concise Resumes

Your resume must be short and easy to read and understand. Use statements that are positive and reflect confidence and portray you as a problem solver. Be sure that any information given within your resume or application form is not misleading or exaggerated. Leave out the word *I* when writing your resume. This is your personal resume and it is understood that you are referring to yourself.

Accomplishments

Use **accomplishment statements** if you have them from your externship or work experience. Accomplishment statements begin with **power verbs**, give a brief description of what you did, and the demonstrable results that were produced. Figure 36-4 provides a list of sample power verbs. Some accomplishment statement examples are: "Utilized computer skills to schedule and reschedule patient appointments" and "Demonstrated skills in setting up sterile trays and assisting with sterile procedures."

Accompanied	Billed	Computed	Demonstrated	Enumerated	Graded
Accumulated	Bought	Conducted	Deposited	Established	Graphed
Achieved	Budgeted	Conferred	Described	Estimated	Greeted
Acquired	Built	Constructed	Detailed	Evaluated	Headed
Administered	Calculated	Consulted	Determined	Examined	Hired
Admitted	Cashed	Contacted	Developed	Exchanged	Identified
Advised	Catalogued	Contracted	Devised	Exhibited	Implemented
Allowed	Changed	Contrasted	Diagnosed	Expanded	Improved
Analyzed	Charged	Contributed	Directed	Expedited	Improvised
Answered	Charted	Controlled	Discovered	Experienced	Increased
Applied	Classified	Converted	Dismantled	Fabricated	Indexed
Appointed	Cleaned	Convinced	Dispatched	Facilitated	Indicated
Appraised	Cleared	Coordinated	Distributed	Figured	Influenced
Arranged	Closed	Copied	Documented	Filled	Informed
Assembled	Coded	Corrected	Drew	Financed	Initiated
Assessed	Collated	Corresponded	Drove	Finished	Inspected
Assigned	Collected	Counseled	Earned	Fitted	Installed
Attached	Commanded	Created	Educated	Fixed	Instructed
Attained	Communicated	Debated	Employed	Formalized	Insured
Attended	Compiled	Decided	Encouraged	Formulated	Integrated
Authorized	Completed	Delegated	Engineered	Fulfilled	
Balanced	Composed	Delivered	Entertained	Generated	*(continues)*

Figure 36-4 These sample power verbs may help you define your previous job responsibilities.

Interpreted	Maintained	Overcame	Prompted	Related	Showed
Interviewed	Managed	Packaged	Proofread	Relayed	Sold
Introduced	Manufactured	Packed	Proposed	Renewed	Solicited
Inspected	Marked	Paid	Proved	Reorganized	Sorted
Inventoried	Marketed	Participated	Provided	Repaired	Stocked
Investigated	Measured	Patrolled	Published	Replaced	Stored
Invoiced	Met	Perfected	Purchased	Reported	Straightened
Issued	Modified	Piloted	Ran	Requested	Summarized
Judged	Monitored	Placed	Rated	Researched	Supervised
Justified	Motivated	Planned	Read	Responsible for	Supplied
Kept	Negotiated	Posted	Rearranged	Retrieved	Taught
Learned	Nominated	Prepared	Rebuilt	Revised	Telephoned
Lectured	Noted	Prescribed	Recalled	Routed	Tested
Led	Notified	Presented	Received	Scheduled	Trained
Licensed	Observed	Priced	Recommended	Secured	Transferred
Listed	Obtained	Printed	Reconciled	Selected	Transported
Listened	Opened	Processed	Recorded	Sent	Typed
Loaded	Operated	Procured	Reduced	Separated	Verified
Located	Ordered	Produced	Referred	Served as	
Logged	Organized	Programmed	Registered	Serviced	
Mailed	Outlined	Promoted	Regulated	Set up	

Figure 36-4 *(continued)*

References

Select a variety of **references** to be included on or with your resume. References may be listed on a separate sheet of paper that matches your resume. An individual who knows you or has worked with you long enough to make an honest assessment and recommendation regarding your background history is an excellent reference person. Use only nonrelated persons as references unless the work relationship has been formalized.

Choose references who are well-respected and are clear speakers and writers. No matter how much someone likes you and your work, it can hurt you if they cannot convey the information in a business-like manner. Professional references such as a former instructor, physician, externship supervisor, or fellow coworkers are excellent reference choices.

Always ask permission to use someone as a reference *before* the name is printed on the resume or reference list. You will want to verify the correct spelling of the reference's name, title, place of employment and position, and telephone number for prospective employers.

Help your references aid you in obtaining an interview and employment. A personal visit or telephone call to discuss your career objectives and how you plan to conduct your job search will be helpful. Ask for any suggestions they may have to offer. Provide them with a copy of your resume and cover letter. This helps them visualize the position for which you are applying and picture how you may benefit that employer.

Keep in touch with references. Check back to see who has called and how things went. Knowing what employers ask may produce some valuable pointers for your next letter, resume, or interview.

Finally, thank your references. They will appreciate knowing how you are doing and that you value their assistance.

Leave out "References Upon Request" if necessary to shorten your resume to save space. Employers know they can ask for references at a later date.

Accuracy

Proofread, proofread, and proofread your resume. Ask someone who is a good speller or your references to edit your resume. Then proofread it again yourself. Do not rely on your computer spell check; it does not differentiate between words such as to, too, two or here and hear. Eliminate repetition of information such as task descriptions. Summarize employment prior to ten years ago or leave it off if not relevant to the position you are seeking.

Resume Styles

Various resume styles have been developed, each having specific advantages and disadvantages. You will want to choose the style or combination of styles that best describes your strengths and ability to do the job. It may be to your advantage to check with the human resources department of the facility to which you are applying to see if there is a resume style preference.

Chronological Resume. The **chronological resume** is used by individuals who have job experience. The job history begins with the most recent experience first and concludes with the earliest experience at the bottom.

The chronological resume is advantageous when:

- The position is in a highly traditional field, such as teaching, law, or health care, where specific employers are of paramount interest

- You are staying in the same field as prior jobs

- Job history shows real growth and development

- Prior titles are impressive

The chronological resume is *not* advantageous when:

- Your work history is spotty

- You are changing career goals

- You have been in the same job for many years

- You are looking for your first job

Figure 36-5 is an illustration of a chronological resume.

Ashley Jackson
2031 Craig Street
Renton, Washington 98055
(206) 255-1365

WORK EXPERIENCE

September, 1996–Present   GROUP HEALTH COOPERATIVE
Direct support for a dermatology/surgery practice.
Patient preparation.
Medical and surgical asepsis.
Assist with sterile procedures.
Patient follow-up.

June, 1994–August, 1996   VALLEY INTERNAL MEDICINE
Clinical responsibilities.
Assisted with surgeries in ambulatory care setting.
Patient preparation.
Medical and surgical asepsis.
Assisted with sterile procedures.

March, 1994–June, 1994   VALLEY INTERNAL MEDICINE
Medical Assistant Externship
Administrative duties and clinical responsibilities utilizing all medical assisting skills, including patient induction, chief complaint, vital signs, patient preparation, EKGs, medical and surgical asepsis, and sterile procedures.

EDUCATION/CERTIFICATION

Associate in Applied Science degree, June, 1994, Highline Community College, Des Moines, Washington, 98198-9800.

Certified Medical Assistant, June, 1994.

Figure 36-5 Sample chronological resume.

Functional Resume. The **functional resume** highlights specialty areas of accomplishment and strengths. It allows you to organize these in an order that supports your work objective.

The functional resume is advantageous when:

- Your experience can be sorted into areas of function; i.e., administrative, clinical, supervisory
- You are changing careers
- You are reentering the job market after an absence
- Your career path or growth is not clear from a chronological listing
- You have had a variety of different, apparently unconnected work experiences

- Much of your work has been volunteer, freelance, or temporary
- You want to eliminate repetition of descriptions of job duties
- You have extensive specialized experience

The functional resume is *not* advantageous when:

- You want to emphasize a management growth pattern
- Your most recent employers have been highly prestigious and the specific employers are of paramount interest

A sample of a functional resume for a person reentering the job market is shown in Figure 36-6.

Joan Bishop
4320 Spraig Street
Renton, Washington 98055
(206) 255-2620

TEACHING:

Instructed community groups on issues related to child abuse.

Taught volunteers how to set up community program for victims of domestic violence.

Ran workshops for parents of abused children.

Instructed public school teachers on signs and symptoms of potential and actual child abuse.

COUNSELING:

Consulted with parents for probable child abuse and suggested courses of action.

Worked with social workers on individual cases, in both urban and suburban settings.

Counseled single parents on appropriate coping behaviors.

Handled pre-take interviewing of many individual abused children.

ORGANIZATION/COORDINATION:

Coordinated transition of children between original home and foster home.

Served as liaison between community health agencies and schools.

Wrote proposal to state for county funds to educate single parents and teachers.

WORK HISTORY:

1986–1990   Community Mental Health Center, Tacoma, Washington
            Volunteer Coordinator—Child Abuse Program
1990–1994   C.A.R.E.—Child-Abuse Rescue-Education, Trenton, New Jersey
            County Representative

EDUCATION:

1970   B.S. Sociology, Douglass College, New Brunswick, New Jersey

---

Figure 36-6   Sample functional resume; this style is useful for a person reentering the job market.

Targeted Resume. The **targeted resume** is best for focusing on a clear, specific job target. It should contain a **career objective**, and list your skills, capabilities, and any supporting accomplishments related to that objective. Graduating students will find this resume style enables them to list classes related to their career objective, grade point average, student awards, and achievements. This information adds substance to a resume when work experience is minimal and should be at the beginning of the resume since it is your most significant asset.

The targeted resume is advantageous when:

- You are very clear about your job target
- You have had a variety of experiences that appear unrelated to each other, but that include skills that you can use in a skills list related to your job target

- You can go in several directions and want a different resume for each
- You are just starting your career and have little experience, but know what you want and are clear about your capabilities
- You are able to keep your resume on a computer disk

The targeted resume is *not* advantageous when:

- You want to use one resume for several different applications
- You are not clear about your abilities and accomplishments

Figure 36-7 provides a sample of a targeted resume.

Ashley Jackson
2031 Craig Street
Renton, Washington 98055
(206) 255-1365

CAREER OBJECTIVE: To obtain a challenging position as a medical assistant in an ambulatory care/surgery facility.

ACHIEVEMENTS:
Certified Medical Assistant.
Graduate of an Accredited Medical Assistant Program.
Experienced in providing assistance with surgeries in an ambulatory care setting.
Excellent communication and interpersonal skills.

SKILLS AND CAPABILITIES:
Post-surgery patient follow-up.
Patient induction.
Vital signs.
Patient preparation.
EKGs.
Medical and surgical asepsis.
Sterile procedures.

WORK HISTORY:
September, 1996–Present	Group Health Cooperative, Seattle, WA, Surgical Medical Assistant.
June, 1994–August, 1996	Valley Internal Medicine, Renton, WA, Clinical Medical Assistant.
March, 1994–June, 1994	Valley Internal Medicine, Renton, WA, Externship Student/Trainee.

EDUCATION/CERTIFICATION:
Associate in Applied Science Degree, Highline Community College.
Certified Medical Assistant.

AFFILIATIONS:
American Association of Medical Assistants

Figure 36-7 Sample targeted resume; this style is useful when focusing on a specific job target.

Vital Resume Information

All resume styles must contain certain vital information about the job applicant. Essential information includes:

- Your full name, address including street number, city, state, and zip code.
- Your telephone number or a number where a message may be left. Always include the area code with the number.
- Your education. Begin with the most recent school attended and include the name, address, and graduation date with the diploma, certificate, or degree earned.
- Work experience. List company name and address. Do not underestimate the value of any job; relate transferable skills to your career objective.

APPLICATION/COVER LETTERS

The application/cover letter is a means of introducing yourself and submitting your resume to a potential employer with the goal of obtaining an interview. A well-written cover letter will highlight your qualifications and experience for employment and will enhance the information contained within your resume. The letter should follow a standard business style and should never be more than one page in length. It should be printed on the same paper as the resume.

Since this may be your first contact with a potential employer, the letter should sell you and describe your intentions regarding employment, display your personality, and create an interest in reading your enclosed resume.

Some guidelines to follow in writing the application/cover letter include:

1. Address your letter to a specific individual whenever possible. You may need to make a telephone call to obtain the name and correct spelling.
2. Keep the letter short, use correct grammar and spelling, and follow standard business letter format.
3. The first paragraph should state your reason for writing and focus the reader's attention.
4. The second paragraph should identify how your education, experience, and qualifications relate to the job and refer to the enclosed resume.
5. The last paragraph should close with a request for an interview.
6. Do not reproduce cover letters. An original letter should be sent to each individual.
7. The cover letter and resume should be mailed in a business size envelope that matches its contents or in an 8½ × 11 manila envelope containing your return address.

A sample of an application/cover letter is shown in Figure 36-8A.

An alternate example of an application/cover letter using Information Mapping® to highlight and draw attention to specific information in your letter is shown in Figure 36-8B. This format is considered easier to read because the focus is on specific blocks of information. In addition, its uniqueness draws attention to your letter and resume and may result in your being selected when competition is keen.

COMPLETING THE APPLICATION FORM

Sooner or later during the job search you will be asked to complete an application form. How well you complete this task may be a key factor in obtaining an interview and/or that first job.

Reading through the application form questions, you may be tempted to write in "See resume" rather than repeat pertinent information already contained within your resume. Do not fall into this pitfall. Answer every item completely. Read all the directions carefully. Look for seemingly insignificant directions placed at the top or bottom of the page that state "Print Carefully," "Complete in Your Own Handwriting," or "Please Type." Employers may use this to assess your ability to read and follow directions.

If the application is to be handwritten, use black ink to complete the form. Black ink is considered legal and often is an indelible (permanent) ink and is more legible if the form must be duplicated. Concentrate when completing the form and be sure to print clearly and make no errors.

The current trend is toward on-line application forms. These forms are prepared by keying information into the appropriate spaces or blocks by using a computer. The completed forms may then be printed and mailed to the perspective employer or sent electronically. Sending electronically is increasingly the preferred method. All of the concerns relative to care in following instructions, providing complete and accurate information, and proofing the application for any errors before sending are applicable.

If you are asked to list experience but the application does not specify "paid experience," be sure to list any volunteer or externship experience that relates to the position you are seeking. Part-time employment can be important as an indicator of your willingness to work, your ability to serve the public, and your organizational skills.

You may be asked to complete the application form "on the spot." Plan ahead for this event and carry a completed copy of your resume, reference list, and

2031 Craig Street
Renton, Washington 98055
August 22, 20___

Sarah Molles, Manager
Seattle Group Health Cooperative
304 Fourth Avenue
Seattle, Washington 98124-1716

SUBJECT: SURGICAL MEDICAL ASSISTANT POSITION

Background	I read your advertisement in the *Seattle Times* for a medical assistant to assist in a dermatology surgery practice. I meet the qualifications listed and would like to be considered for the position.
Qualifications	I am a certified medical assistant graduated from a two-year accredited program. I have experience as a clinical assistant in an internal medicine clinic and have excellent communication and interpersonal skills.
Requested Action	I would like to request an interview to discuss how I could be of value to your organization in the subject position.

Yours truly,

Ashley Jackson

Ashley Jackson

Enclosure, Resume

Figure 36-8(B)   Sample information mapped letter.

2031 Craig Street
Renton, Washington 98055
August 22, 20___

Sarah Molles, Manager
Seattle Group Health Cooperative
304 Fourth Avenue
Seattle, Washington 98124-1716

Dear Ms. Molles:

I read your advertisement in the *Seattle Times* for a medical assistant to assist in a dermatology surgery practice. I meet the qualifications listed and would like to be considered for the position.

I am currently a certified medical assistant graduated from a two-year accredited program. I have experience as a clinical assistant in an internal medicine clinic and have excellent communication and interpersonal skills.

I would like to request an interview to discuss how I could be of value to your organization in the subject position.

Yours truly,

Ashley Jackson

Ashley Jackson

Enclosure, Resume

Figure 36-8(A)   Sample application/cover letter.

application/cover letter with you. Information not included in your resume, such as which years you attended high school and your salary history, should also be carried with you. These documents should provide all the information needed to complete the application form and may be submitted with the application form. This demonstrates to the potential employer your seriousness and preparedness for finding a job.

THE LOOK OF SUCCESS

The look of success begins with the outward appearance. First impressions are lasting, so strive for a favorable, professional look from head to toe.

Hair should be clean, shiny, and healthy looking, and worn in an appropriate style for the ambulatory care setting. Long hair should be worn off the collar in perhaps a French braid or twist. Long hair that is worn on the shoulders or down the back has the potential for being caught in equipment. It also serves as a host for many airborne pathogens.

The skin should have a healthy glow. Consultation with a cosmetician may prove helpful in solving skin problems or provide opportunity for trying new products. A basic understanding of your personal skin type and selection of cosmetics that complement your skin tone aid in the presentation of a professional appearance. The natural look is most appropriate for the medical office.

Daily bathing, whether by soaking in a tub and using a loofah sponge or using a pulsating shower, cleanse and relax the body. If your skin tends to be dry, apply lotion or emollient cream to replace the natural oils depleted by the water. Many lotions, talcum powders, and deodorants are scented. Remember to use caution where perfumes and scents are concerned since many magnify when the body is under stress and the scent may be offensive or cause allergic reactions in others.

Bathe the feet, carefully washing between each toe, and take care to dry the feet completely. This aids in the prevention of fungal growth. To prevent ingrown toenails, trim the nails straight across rather than rounding the nails as you do the fingernails.

Fingernails should be manicured on a weekly basis. Nails should be short and oval shaped or have rounded corners. Cuticles should be softened by soaking the fingertips in warm water. Gently use an orange stick or a cotton-tipped swab and push the cuticle back. To prevent hangnails, apply cuticle oil as you gently push the cuticle back. Only clear nail polish should be worn in the ambulatory care setting. Nail polish that is chipped or cracked must be removed or replaced immediately as it creates crevices in which pathogens may hide, multiply, and be spread.

First impressions are lasting so make yours professional in all respects. Conservative business attire is appropriate. A tailored suit or a classic dress are effective in portraying a professional image. Pay attention to details such as your jewelry and shoe selection. Shoes should be polished and in good repair. They should fit properly and be comfortable and easy to walk in (Figure 36-9).

Personal and Professional Poise

When you feel well and know that you look good, you project a confident and professional appearance. In other words, you are professionally poised. Webster's dictionary defines poise as balance and stability; ease and dignity of manner. Personal poise combines all of the previously mentioned body appearances plus smoothness of movement and physical flexibility.

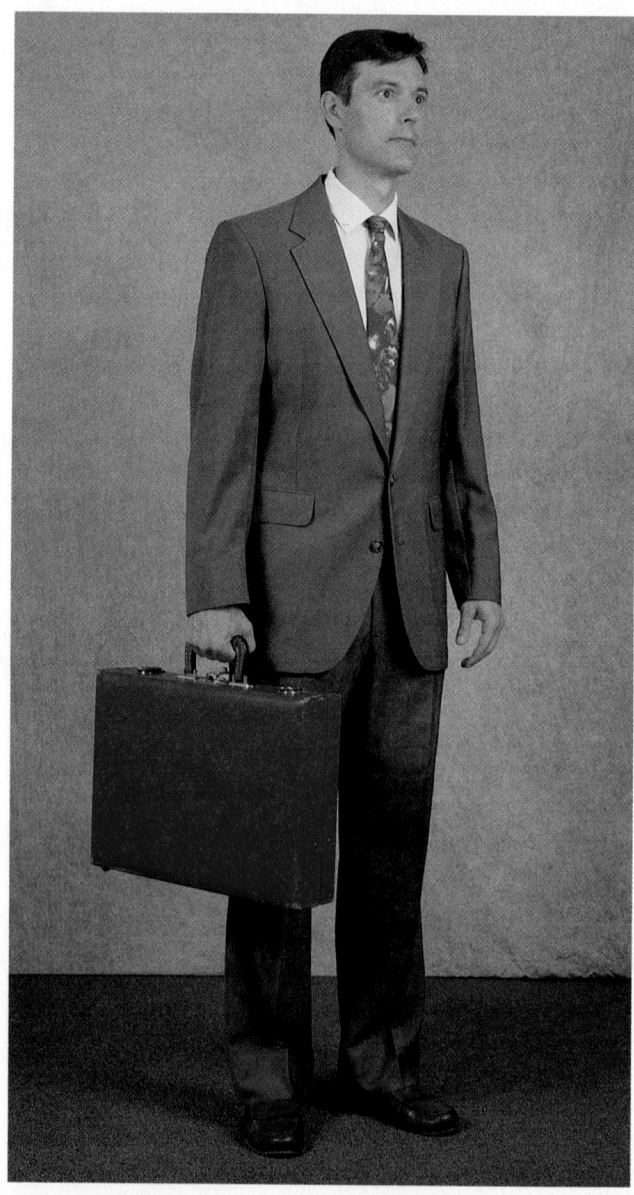

Figure 36-9 Medical assistant appropriately dressed and prepared for the interview.

SPOTLIGHT ON AAMA ESSENTIALS THROUGH CAAHEP

- Positive thinking is one of the primary keys to success in planning a career and conducting a job search.

- A person's outward appearance and first impression are lasting; they can make the difference between a positive and a negative job interview.

- Feeling well and dressing in an appropriate manner will help you to project the image of a confident and poised professional member of the health care team.

THE INTERVIEW PROCESS

If your application/cover letter and resume have made a favorable impression with the organization, you may be invited for an interview. An **interview** is a meeting in which you and the interviewer discuss the employment opportunities within that particular organization. It will be the interviewer's responsibility to determine if you have the personality, education, and skills to perform the job. You, on the other hand, will be selling your qualifications and assessing if this is an organization in which you want to be employed.

Being well prepared for the interview will increase your self-confidence and ability to focus during the actual interview. Knowing that your application/cover letter, resume, and references all support your career goal and objectives allows you time to concentrate on interview preparation and presentation.

Preparing for the Interview

Before the interview takes place, you will want to study carefully the organization for which you are interviewing. Be prepared to relate your skills and interests to the needs of this organization. In other words, what can you contribute and why should they hire you? The interview is your opportunity to sell yourself and identify ways in which you can benefit the employer.

A copy of your resume and cover letter should be brought along to the interview just in case the interviewer can not locate the original or wants another copy. You should also have copies of letters of recommendation, a list of references, a copy of your transcript from the schools you attended, and copies of any certificates such as

AIDS training, First Aid, and CPR. These items should not be presented unless dictated by events that take place during the interview. You might also have with you the name of the interviewer and a copy of any questions you plan to ask the interviewer. A last minute review will refocus your thoughts before you go into the interview. You could also keep your list available for quick reference in the event that your mind goes blank when you are asked if you have questions.

In order to arrive five to ten minutes early, you may need to check a map for directions or make a trip the day before your interview. Try to travel about the same time as you would for the interview so you have an idea of the time it takes, traffic flow, construction areas encountered, and parking availability.

Introduce yourself confidently to the receptionist and identify by name the person you wish to see and the time of your appointment. Always arrive alone. The employer wants to see you and sense your self-reliance and responsibility. While you wait, try to relax and observe the office setting, other employees, what they are wearing, and their manner of conducting business. This may be helpful to you during the interview and in making a decision to work here.

The Actual Interview

When you enter an interviewer's office, think of yourself as a guest and take your cues from him or her. Most interviewers will introduce themselves and extend their hand. A firm handshake, responding by introducing yourself and smiling confidently convey a positive professional image. Remain standing until you are invited to be seated. Keep your personal items on your lap or place them on the floor near your chair. Do not invade the interviewer's territory by placing your things on the desk.

Sit erect in the chair with your feet flat on the floor or crossing only your ankles. Avoid nervous mannerisms while you speak and maintain good eye contact. Be natural and positive about the position, organization, and yourself. Present a professional image by using medical terminology when responding to questions or providing information. Observe the interviewer carefully for cues. Respond to questions completely, trying not to repeat yourself or give more information than was requested.

Be prepared for the kinds of questions that may be asked during the interview process. Ask yourself, "If I were the employer, what would I want to know about the applicant?" Figure 36-10 contains examples of standard questions asked by most employers. Consider how you would respond to each question.

Remember that the interviewer is asking questions to determine if you are qualified for the position and if you are the kind of person that will fit into the organization.

TYPICAL QUESTIONS ASKED DURING AN INTERVIEW

1. I see from your resume you graduated from _____ college. What did that college have to offer that others didn't?
2. What subjects did you enjoy the most and why?
3. What do you see yourself doing five years from now?
4. Tell me about yourself.
5. What do you consider to be your greatest strengths and weaknesses?
6. How do you think a friend or professor who knows you well would describe you?
7. What qualifications do you have that make you think you would be successful in this position?
8. In what ways do you think you can make a contribution to our organization?
9. What two or three accomplishments have given you the most satisfaction?
10. How well do you work under pressure?
11. Will you be able to work overtime occasionally?
12. Do you have any questions you would like to ask?

Figure 36-10   Knowing how you would answer some of these typical questions can prepare you for your interview.

Think before answering questions; try to provide the information requested in a positive and professional manner. *Listen* carefully so that you understand what information the question is requesting. *Ask* for clarification if you are uncertain. This demonstrates your ability to be open enough to ask questions when in doubt.

Closing the Interview

By observing the interviewer and listening carefully, you will be able to determine when the interviewer feels he or she has enough information about you to make a decision. Usually during the closing the interviewer will ask if you have any additional questions. This is your opportunity to collect information helpful in making a decision to accept or decline an offer. Your questions provide another opportunity to sell yourself, show that you have done your homework about the organization, and have listened carefully during the interview. Select three or four questions that will help you the most.

Questions about the organization are excellent choices. Examples might be:

- "What are the opportunities for advancement with this organization?"
- "I read that your organization has educational benefits. Could you explain briefly how that program works?"
- "You mentioned in-house training programs for employees. Could you give one or two examples?"

You may also have some questions about the job itself. Examples of these types of questions are:

- "Is this a newly created position? If so, what results are you hoping to see?"
- "Was the last person in this position promoted? What contributed to their advancement?"
- "What do you consider the most difficult task on this job?"
- "What are the lines of authority for this position?"

Do not use this question time to ask about salary, sick leave, vacations, or retirement benefits. At this point, your focus should be on the value and skills you can contribute to the organization. These questions may be asked during a second interview or when a position is offered.

Before you leave, thank the interviewer for taking time to discuss the position with you. If you definitely are interested in the position, ask to be considered as a candidate for the position. If follow-up procedures have not been explained, now is the time to ask when the final selection will be made and how you will be notified. A firm handshake as you leave, a pleasant smile, and confidence as you exit will leave a professional picture in the interviewer's mind.

INTERVIEW FOLLOW-UP

Following up after the interview is essential. This is the time to telephone your references to let them know the name of the organization and the person's name with whom you interviewed, something about the position, and your qualifications. Share any information that will help your references support you in obtaining the position.

Follow-Up Letter

Take time to write a follow-up letter to the interviewer a day or two after your interview. The letter should be written in standard business format and printed on the same paper as your application/cover letter and resume. Be sure that all spelling and grammar are correct.

The follow-up letter provides another opportunity to express your interest in the organization and the position. You can briefly emphasize the experience and skills you have to offer and again request being considered a candidate for the position.

Record the mailing date on your contact tracker and keep a copy of the letter in a file with other information about the organization. Figure 36-11 is a sample follow-up letter.

Follow Up by Telephone

Allow a few days for your follow-up letter to reach the interviewer. If you do not hear from the interviewer within a week or by the designated time established during the interview, you may telephone to ask if you are still being considered for the position or if a decision has been made.

Speak directly into the mouthpiece of the telephone using good diction and voice volume. Identify yourself and provide some information to aid the interviewer in recalling who you are. Perhaps mentioning the date you interviewed will suffice. Be polite and professional and remember to thank the individual for speaking with you. At the end of the conversation say good-bye and wait until they hang up before you break the connection. Log the telephone call and its response on your contact tracker for future reference.

2031 Craig Street
Renton, Washington 98055
August 28, 20--

Sarah Molles, Manager
Seattle Group Health Cooperative
304 Fourth Avenue
Seattle, Washington 98124-1716

Dear Ms. Molles,

Thank you for scheduling a personal interview with me last Wednesday, August 26, at 9:45 AM. I enjoyed discussing the medical assistant position open in one of your dermatology surgery practices. I would like to be considered for the position.

After talking with you, I feel my qualifications match closely with those you requested. My communication and interpersonal skills are excellent and a necessary ingredient for any medical assistant.

I look forward to hearing from you September 5 as you mentioned during the interview. If there are any questions I may answer, please telephone me.

Sincerely,

Ashley Jackson

Ashley Jackson
(206) 255-1365

Figure 36-11   Sample follow-up letter.

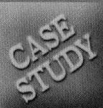

Eun Mee Soo is a recent graduate of an accredited medical assisting program and has no medical work experience except her externship at Inner City Health Care. Eun Mee has been employed part-time as a sales representative (clerk) in one of the city's prestigious clothing stores while she attended school.

36-1

CASE STUDY REVIEW

1. Which resume style would represent Eun Mee best and why?

2. What information should Eun Mee provide in the vital information section of the resume?

3. What is the purpose of an accomplishment statement? Provide an example of one that Eun Mee might use.

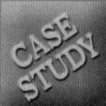

Doctors Lewis and King maintain a two-doctor family physicians' office. They are in need of a new medical assistant to take the place of one who will be leaving at the end of the month. They have established interviews with five applicants. Eun Mee Soo is the first candidate to be interviewed.

36-2

CASE STUDY REVIEW

1. Eun Mee enters the interview with some papers in her hand. What paperwork should she have brought with her?

2. Why should Eun Mee arrive five to ten minutes early for the interview?

3. How should Eun Mee enter the room?

SUMMARY

Finding your first job is your first job. How well you research, plan, prepare, and implement your tasks will make the difference between being hired or not being hired. Learn from each interview session. Listen to the questions that were asked and formulate answers that you feel would be appropriate for your next interview. Tell everyone you are looking for a job and solicit their help. Follow up on all leads and do not become discouraged.

Once you have been hired at that first job, continue your learning experience. Ask appropriate questions and try not to ask the same question a second or third time. Pay attention to details and learn individual preferences. Become a team player and look for ways you can help others. Carry your share of responsibility and do not be afraid to admit you are unfamiliar with certain aspects of the office. Employers need to know you can be trusted to work within the scope of your education and not beyond. Practice being an asset to your employer.

REVIEW QUESTIONS

Multiple Choice

1. The resume:
   a. is a summary data sheet or brief account of your qualifications and progress in your career
   b. is also known as a contact tracker
   c. always includes references
   d. is used to introduce yourself and identify qualifications

2. References:
   a. must always be listed on the resume
   b. should be a relative
   c. should be someone who likes you and your work but may not be a good communicator
   d. should be someone who knows you or has worked with you long enough to make an honest assessment of your capabilities and integrity

3. The targeted resume is advantageous:
   a. when prior titles are impressive
   b. when reentering the job market after an absence
   c. when you are just starting your career and have little experience
   d. when you have extensive specialized experience

4. The application/cover letter is:
   a. a detailed data sheet describing your vital information, education, and experience
   b. introduces you to a prospective employer and captures their interest in you as a candidate for the position
   c. lists individuals who can vouch for you
   d. should be lengthy and detailed

5. The interview:
   a. does not require much thought or preparation
   b. requires you to think before answering questions, listen carefully, and ask for clarification if uncertain of the question
   c. provides time to ask questions about salary, vacation, and benefits
   d. does not require any follow-up

6. Preparing for the interview:
   a. bathe yourself, groom your hair and fingernails, and wear clean and pressed conservative business attire
   b. allow adequate time to get to the interview
   c. prepare a packet to give the interviewer containing certificates, letters of recommendation, a list of references, and your list of questions
   d. a, b, and c

7. Job analysis should include:
   a. compiling a list of potential employers
   b. gathering information about employers in whom you have interest
   c. preparing a budgetary needs analysis
   d. all of the above

8. The best source for job search data is:
   a. the Internet
   b. friends and acquaintances
   c. the yellow pages and classified ads
   d. all the above

9. A frequently overlooked potential employer is:
   a. your personal health care provider
   b. your externship site
   c. the local hospital
   d. all of the above

10. You can impress the interviewer by:
    a. acting like you know it all
    b. having poise and good appearance
    c. showing flexibility by having no specific goals
    d. all of the above

Critical Thinking

1. Discuss the various resume styles and determine which style would be most suitable for you.
2. Discuss methods of researching a prospective employer.
3. Review Figure 36-2 and discuss the rationale behind each reason for employers not hiring.
4. Prepare a budget and discuss it with a classmate.
5. Collect and review numerous application forms.

WEB ACTIVITIES

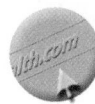

Select a location in the United States and use the Internet to research potential openings for medical assistants. Go to the Internet site Yahoo! [http://www.yahoo.com/] and research positions available at the location you have selected. Then research salaries for medical assistants in that area. If you have trouble working through the menu, select the site careers.yahoo.com and use the sections on job search and researching salaries to obtain the information. After you have completed these tasks, prepare an information packet on one of the facilities with a job opening for medical assistant. Include address, phone number, person to contact, and type of procedures performed at the location. You may need to do further Internet research to obtain some of this information. Follow the instructor's instructions on completing and turning in your results.

DOCUMENTATION

Copy or design your own contact tracker form and document all pertinent information regarding your job search contacts.

REFERENCES/BIBLIOGRAPHY

Yate, M. (1994). *Knock 'em dead the ultimate job seeker's handbook*. Holbrook, MA: Bob Adams, Inc.

Yate, M. (1993). *Resumes that knock 'em dead*. Holbrook, MA: Bob Adams, Inc.

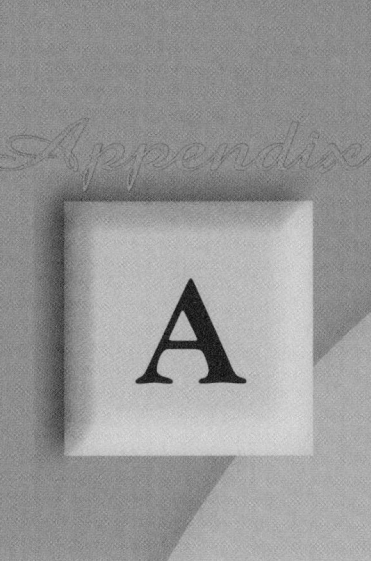

a̅a̅	of each	aq	water	BW	below waist
AAMA	American Association of Medical Assistants	A/R	accounts receivable		birth weight
		ARU	automated routing unit		body weight
AAMT	American Association of Medical Transcription	AS	left ear (auris sinistra)	Bx	biopsy
		ASA	acetylsalicylic acid		
ab	abortion	ASAP	as soon as possible	C	Celsius
abd	abdomen	ASCAD	arteriosclerotic coronary artery disease		centigrade
ABE	acute bacterial endocarditis			c̄	with
ABG	arterial blood gases	ASCVD	arteriosclerotic cardiovascular disease	C1	first cervical vertebra
ABHS	Accrediting Bureau of Health Education Schools			CA	cancer
			atherosclerotic cardiovascular disease		carcinoma
ABO	blood groups	AU	each ear (aures unitas)	Ca	calcium
abs	absent	A&W	alive and well	CAAHEP	Commission on Accreditation of Allied Health Education Programs
ac	before meals (ante cibum)				
ac	acute	Ba	barium		
ACTH	adrenocorticotropic hormone	BaE	barium enema	CAD	coronary artery disease
AD	right ear (auris dexter)	BBB	bundle branch block	CAHD	coronary arteriosclerotic heart disease
ADA	Americans with Disabilities Act	BC	birth control		
		BC/BS	Blue Cross/Blue Shield	caps	capsules
ADL	activities of daily living	BE	bacterial endocarditis	CAT	computerized axial tomography
ad lib	as desired		barium enema		
adm	admission	bid	twice a day	CBC	complete blood count
AFP	alpha fetal protein	bil	bilateral	CC	chief complaint
AHD	arteriosclerotic heart disease	BM	basal metabolism	cc	cubic centimeter
	atherosclerotic heart disease		bowel movement	CCU	coronary care unit
AIDS	acquired immunodeficiency syndrome	BMR	basal metabolism rate	C&D	cystoscopy and dilation
		BP	blood pressure	CDC	U.S. Centers for Disease Control and Prevention
AL	left ear (auris laevus)	BPH	benign prostatic hypertrophy		
alb	albumin	BS	blood sugar	CE	continuing education
AM	before noon (ante meridiem)		bowel sounds	cerv	cervical
AMA	against medical advice		breath sounds		cervix
	American Medical Association	BSA	body surface area	CEU	continuing education unit
		BSI	body substance isolation	CHAMPUS	Civilian Health and Medical Program of the Uniformed Services
AMI	acute myocardial infarction	BSL	blood sugar level		
amt	amount	BSN	bowel sounds normal		
ant	anterior	BSO	bilateral salpingo-oophorectomy	CHAMPVA	Civilian Health and Medical Program of the Veterans Administration
ante	before				
A&P	anterior and posterior	BSR	blood sedimentation rate		
	auscultation and palpation	BUN	blood urea nitrogen	CHD	childhood disease
	auscultation and percussion				congenital heart disease

CHD	congestive heart disease	DOB	date of birth	fl	fluid
	coronary heart disease	DOD	date of death	fl dr	fluid dram
CHF	congestive heart failure	DOE	dyspnea on exertion	fl oz	fluid ounce
CHO	carbohydrate	dos	dosage	FMP	first menstrual period
CIN	cervical intraepithelial	DPM	doctor of podiatric medicine	FP	family practice
	neoplasia	DPT	diphtheria, pertussis, and	freq	frequent
ck	check		tetanus	FSH	follicle-stimulating hormone
Cl	chlorine	DR	delivery room	ft	foot
cldy	cloudy	Dr	doctor	FTP	file transfer protocol
CLIA	Clinical Laboratory	dr	dram	fx	fracture
	Improvement	DRGs	diagnosis-related groups		
	Amendments	DSD	dry sterile dressing	G	gravida
cm	centimeter	dsg	dressing	g	gram
CMA	certified medical assistant	DT	delirium tremens	GB	gallbladder
CME	continuing medical education	DTR	deep tendon reflex	GC	gonococcus
CNS	central nervous system	D&V	diarrhea and vomiting		gonorrhea
C/O	complains of	DW	distilled water	GI	gastrointestinal
CO₂	carbon dioxide	D/W	dextrose in water	gm	gram
COB	coordination of benefits	dx	diagnosis	GP	general practice
COPD	chronic obstructive			gr	grain
	pulmonary disease	ea	each	grav	pregnancy
CPR	cardiopulmonary resuscitation	EBV	Epstein-Barr virus	GTH	gonadotropic hormone
CPT	Current Procedural Code	ECG	electrocardiogram	GTT	glucose tolerance test
CPU	central processing unit	Echo	echocardiogram	gtt(s)	drop (drops)
crit	hematocrit		echoencephalogram	GU	genitourinary
CS	cerebrospinal	*E. coli*	*Escherichia coli*	GYN	gynecology
CS	cesarean section	ECT	electroconvulsive therapy		
C&S	culture and sensitivity	EDC	estimated date of confinement	h	hour
CSF	cerebrospinal fluid		or expected date of	HBP	high blood pressure
CSR	continuous speech		confinement	HCFA	U.S. Health Care Financing
	recognition	EDD	estimated date of delivery or		Administration
CT	computerized tomography		expected date of delivery	hCG	human chorionic
CVA	cerebrovascular accident	EEG	electroencephalogram		gonadotropin
CVP	central venous pressure	EENT	eyes, ears, nose, and throat	HCL	hydrochloric acid
CVS	chorionic villus sampling	eg	for example	HCPCS	HCFA Common Procedure
cx	cervix	EKG	electrocardiogram		Coding System
CXR	chest x-ray	elix	elixir	Hct	hematocrit
cysto	cystoscopic examination	EMG	electromyography	HCVD	hypertensive cardiovascular
	cystoscopy	EMS	emergency medical service		disease
		ENT	ear, nose, and throat	HEENT	head, eyes, ears, nose, and
DACUM	developing a curriculum	EOB	explanation of benefits		throat
DC	doctor of chiropracty	eos	eosinophil	Hgb	hemoglobin
D&C	dilation and curettage	EPO	exclusive provider	H&H	hemoglobin and hematocrit
DDS	doctor of dentistry		organization	HHS	U.S. Department of Health
DEA	U.S. Drug Enforcement	eq	equivalent		and Human Services
	Agency	ER	emergency room	HMO	health maintenance
dec	decrease	ERT	estrogen replacement therapy		organization
del	delivery	ESR	erythrocyte sedimentation rate	H/O	history of
diab	diabetic	EST	electroshock therapy	H₂O	water
diag	diagnosis	exam	examination	H&P	history and physical
diff	differential white blood cell	ext	extract	HPI	history of present illness
	count			HPV	human papilloma virus
dil	dilute	F	Fahrenheit	HR	human resource
disc	discontinue		female	hs	at bedtime
disp	dispense	fax	facsimile		hour of sleep
DM	diabetes mellitus	FBS	fasting blood sugar	ht	height
DNA	deoxyribonucleic acid	FDA	U.S. Food and Drug	hx	history
	does not apply		Administration	Hz	hertz
DNR	do not resuscitate	FH	family history		
DO	doctor of osteopathy	FHR	fetal heart rate	ICCU	intensive coronary care unit
DOA	dead on arrival	FHS	fetal heart sound	ICD	International Classification of
					Diseases, Adapted

ICD-9-CM	International Classification of Diseases, 9th revision, Clinical Modification	MBCE	management by competitive edge	noct	at night
ICU	intensive care unit	MBDM	management by decision models	non rep	do not repeat
ID	intradermal	MBP	management by performance	NOS	not otherwise specified
I&D	incision and drainage	MBS	management by styles	NPO	nothing by mouth
IM	internal medicine	MBWA	management by wandering around	NR	nonreactive
	intramuscular				no refill
imp	impression	MBWS	management by work simplification		normal range
inf	infusion			NS	nonspecific
inj	injection	MCHC	mean corpuscular hemoglobin and red cell indices		normal saline
I&O	intake and output				not significant
IPPB	intermittent positive pressure breathing	MCO	managed care organization		not sufficient
		MCV	mean corpuscular volume and red cell indices	N&T	nose and throat
IUD	intrauterine device			N&V	nausea and vomiting
IV	intravenous	MD	muscular dystrophy	NVD	nausea, vomiting, and diarrhea
IVP	intravenous pyelogram		doctor of medicine		
		MDR	minimum daily requirement	O	oral
JAAMT	*Journal of the American Association for Medical Transcription*	med	medicine		oxygen
		mEq/L	milliequivalents per liter		pint
		mg	miligram	O_2	oxygen
JAMA	*Journal of the American Medical Association*	MH	marital history	OB	obstetrics
			medical history	OB-GYN	obstetrics-gynecology
JCAHO	Joint Commission on Accreditation of Healthcare Organizations		menstrual history	OC	office call
		MHx	medical history		on call
		MI	maturation index		oral contraceptive
jt	joint		myocardial infarction	occ	occasionally
		ml	milliliter	OD	drug overdose
K	potassium	mm	millimeter		right eye (oculus dexter)
kg	kilogram	mm^3	cubic millimeter		doctor of optometry
KOH	potassium hydroxide	mmHg	millimeters of mercury	OGTT	oral glucose tolerance test
KUB	kidney, ureter, and bladder	MMR	measles, mumps, and rubella	OM	office manager
KV	kilovolt	MOM	milk of magnesia	OOB	out of bed
		mono	mononucleosis	OP	outpatient
L	liter	MP	menstrual period	O&P	ova and parasites
	left	MRI	magnetic resonance imaging	OPIM	other potentially infected material
l	length				
LA	left atrium	MS	mitral stenosis	OPV	oral poliovaccine
	lactic acid		morphine sulfate	OR	operating room
L&A	light and accommodation		multiple sclerosis	ortho	orthopedics
lab	laboratory	MT	medical technologist	OS	left eye (oculus sinister)
lac	laceration		medical transcriptionist	os	mouth
lap	laparotomy	MTCP	Medical Transcriptionist Certification Program	OSHA	U.S. Occupational Safety and Health Administration
lat	lateral				
lb	pound	multip	multipara	OT	occupational therapist
LBBB	left bundle branch block	MVP	mitral valve prolapse		occupational therapy
LDL	low-density lipoprotein			OTC	over the counter
LE	lupus erythematosus	NA	not applicable	OU	both eyes (oculus unitas)
liq	liquid	NaCl	sodium chloride	OURQ	outer upper right quadrant
LLQ	lower left quadrant	narc	narcotic	OV	office visit
LMP	last menstrual period	NB	newborn	oz	ounce
LP	lumbar puncture	NBME	National Board of Medical Examiners		
LRQ	lower right quadrant			P	phosphorus
LUQ	left upper quadrant	N/C	no complaints		pulse
L&W	living and well	ND	doctor of naturopathy	PA	posteroanterior
lymphs	lymphocytes	NEC	not elsewhere classified	P&A	percussion and auscultation
		neg	negative	PA	physician's assistant
M	male	NG	nasogastric	PAC	phenacetin, aspirin, and codeine
m	meter	NGU	nongonococcal urethritis		
℥	minim	NL	normal limits		premature atrial contraction
MBCD	management by coaching and development	NMP	normal menstrual period	Pap	Papanicolaou (smear, test)
				para	number of pregnancies

para I	primipara
PAT	paroxysmal atrial tachycardia
path	pathology
PBI	protein-bound iodine
pc	after meals
PCC	Poison Control Center
PCN	penicillin
PCP	primary care physician
PCV	packed cell volume
PDR	*Physician's Desk Reference*
PE	physical examination
peds	pediatrics
PEG	pneumoencephalography
PERRLA	pupils equal, round, regular, react to light, and accommodation
PET	positron emission transmission or tomography
PH	past history
	personal history
	public health
pH	hydrogen in concentration
PHO	physician-hospital organization
PI	present illness
	pulmonary infarction
PID	pelvic inflammatory disease
PKU	phenylketonuria
PM	after noon (post meridiem)
	post mortem (after death)
PMN	polymorphonuclear neutrophils
PMP	past menstrual period
PMS	premenstrual syndrome
PNC	penicillin
PO	postoperative
po	by mouth
POB	place of birth
POMR	problem-oriented medical record
POS	point-of-service plan
pos	positive
poss	possible
postop	postoperative
PP	postprandial
PPB	positive pressure breathing
PPBS	postprandial blood sugar
PPD	purified protein derivative
PPO	preferred provider organization
PPT	partial prothrombin time
preop	preoperative
PRERLA	pupils round, equal, react to light and accommodation
primip	woman bearing first child
prn	as the occasion arises, as necessary
procto	proctoscopy
prog	prognosis
PROM	premature rupture of membranes

pro-time	prothrombin time
PSA	prostate-specific antigen
PSRO	Professional Standards Review Organization
PT	physical therapy
	prothrombin time
pt	patient
PTA	prior to admission
pulv	powder
PVC	premature ventricular concentration
px	physical examination
	prognosis
q	each; every
q AM	every morning
QA	quality assurance
qd	every day
qh	every hour
q (2, 3, 4)h	every 2, 3, or 4 hours
qid	four times a day
qn	every night
qns	quantity not sufficient
qod	every other day
qs	of sufficient quantity
qt	quart
R	registration
	right
RBC	red blood cell
RBC/hpf	red blood cells per high power field
RBCM	red blood cell mass
RBCV	red blood cell volume
RBRVS	Resource-Based Relation Value Scale
REM	rapid eye movement
resp	respiration
Rh	rhesus (factor)
Rh-	rhesus negative
Rh+	rhesus positive
RHD	rheumatic heart disease
RLQ	right lower quadrant
RMA	registered medical assistant
RNA	ribonucleic acid
R/O	rule out
ROA	received on account
ROM	range of motion
	read-only memory
ROS	review of systems
RT	radiation therapy
RUQ	right upper quadrant
Rx	prescription
S	subjective data (POMR)
$\bar{s}$	without
SA	sinoatrial
S&A	sugar and acetone (urine)
SBE	shortness of breath on exertion
	subacute bacterial endocarditis
SC	subcutaneous
SE	standard error

sed rate	sedimentation rate
segs	segmented neutrophils
seq	sequela
SF	scarlet fever
	spinal fluid
SG	specific gravity
SH	social history
SIDS	sudden infant death syndrome
sig	instructions, directions
sigmoid	sigmoidoscopy
SMA 12/60	Sequential Multiple Analyzer (12-test serum profile)
SOAP	subjective data, objective data, assessment, and plan
SOB	shortness of breath
sol	solution
solv	solvent
SOP	standard operating procedure
SOS	if necessary
spec	specimen
sp gr	secific gravity
spont ab	spontaneous abortion
SR	sedimentation rate
SS	signs and symptoms
$\overline{ss}$	one-half
Staph	Staphylococcus
stat	immediately
STD	sexually transmitted disease
Strep	Streptococcus
subcut	subcutaneous
supp	suppository
surg	surgery
sx	signs
	symptoms
sym	symptoms
syr	syrup
T	temperature
T_3	tri-iodothyronine
T_4	thyroxine
T&A	tonsillectomy and adenoidectomy
tab	tablet
TB	tuberculin
tbs	tablespoon
	tuberculosis
TC	throat culture
	tissue culture
	total capacity
	total cholesterol
ther	therapy
therap	therapeutic
TIA	transient ischemic attack
tid	three times a day
tinct	tincture
TLC	tender loving care
TMJ	temporomandibular joint
top	topically
TOPV	trivalent oral poliovirus vaccine

TP	total protein	URI	upper respiratory infection	WBC	white blood cell
TPR	temperature, pulse, and respiration	urol	urology	WC	white cell
		URQ	upper right quadrant	WDWN	well developed, well nourished
tr	tincture	URT	upper respiratory tract		
trig	triglycerides	URTI	upper respiratory tract infection	WHO	World Health Organization
TSH	thyroid stimulating hormone			WN	well nourished
tsp	teaspoon	USP	United States Pharmacopoeia	WNF	well-nourished female
TUR	transurethral resection of the bladder	UT	urinary tract	WNL	within normal limits
		UTI	urinary tract infection	WNM	well-nourished male
tus	cough	UV	ultraviolet	WO	written order
T&X	type and crossmatch			w/o	without
		vac	vaccine	wt	weight
U	unit	vag	vagina		
UA	urinalysis		vaginal	x	multiply by
UB-92	Uniform Bill-92	VD	venereal disease	XR	x-ray
UCG	urinary chorionic gonadotropin	VDRL	Venereal Disease Research Library		
UCHD	usual childhood diseases			YOB	year of birth
ULQ	upper left quadrant	vit	vitamin	yr	year
ung	ointment	vit cap	vital capacity		
URC	usual, reasonable, customary	vol	volume		
urg	urgent	VS	vital signs		

Symbols

*	birth
†	death
♂	male
♀	female
+	positive
−	negative
±	positive or negative, indefinite
÷	divide by
=	equal to
>	greater than
<	less than
×	multiply by
#	number, pound
'	foot, minute
"	inch, second
ℳ	minum
ʒ	dram
℥	ounce
μ	micron
○	pint
@	at

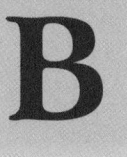

TOP 200 DRUGS BY RETAIL SALES IN 2000

B

Top 200 Brand-Name Drugs by Retail Sales in 2000

Rank	Product	Total retail dollars (000)	Rank	Product	Total retail dollars (000)	Rank	Product	Total retail dollars (000)
1	Prilosec	$4,102,195	36	Synthroid	$649,256	71	Relafen	$351,595
2	Lipitor	3,692,657	37	Flovent	647,980	72	Serzone	349,127
3	Prevacid	2,832,602	38	Accutane	636,246	73	Cardura	344,406
4	Prozac	2,567,107	39	Flonase	618,714	74	Xalatan	340,492
5	Zocor	2,207,042	40	Avandia	617,629	75	Glucotrol XL	321,631
6	Celebrex	2,015,508	41	Ortho Tri-Cyclen	616,997	76	Detrol	319,193
7	Zoloft	1,890,416	42	Ultram	601,465	77	Seroquel	318,844
8	Paxil	1,807,955	43	Plavix	599,512	78	Humulin N	317,017
9	Claritin	1,667,347	44	Biaxin	588,366	79	Lotensin	316,922
10	Glucophage	1,629,157	45	Vasotec	584,418	80	Viracept	315,510
11	Norvasc	1,597,091	46	Pepcid	568,684	81	Avonex	313,114
12	Augmentin	1,584,397	47	Actos	550,674	82	Valtrex	311,102
13	Vioxx	1,517,993	48	Accupril	500,796	83	Allegra-D	310,369
14	Zyprexa	1,418,411	49	Enbrel	500,363	84	Adderall	307,423
15	Pravachol	1,203,474	50	Claritin D 24HR	493,420	85	Procrit	298,764
16	Premarin Tabs	1,146,808	51	Lamisil Oral	487,920	86	Claritin RediTabs	298,253
17	Neurontin	1,131,678	52	Ceftin	455,965	87	Cardizem CD	283,968
18	Oxycontin	1,052,771	53	Combivir	452,844	88	K-Dur 20	276,161
19	Cipro	1,023,657	54	Serevent	448,923	89	Diovan	270,144
20	Zithromax Z-Pak	961,579	55	BuSpar Dividose	434,023	90	Remeron	266,707
21	Risperdal	959,707	56	Prinivil	431,342	91	BuSpar	265,349
22	Wellbutrin SR	850,934	57	Coumadin Tabs	407,565	92	Zerit	264,738
23	Zestril	833,359	58	Claritin D 12HR	403,071	93	Hyzaar	264,128
24	Effexor XR	815,816	59	Evista	398,590	94	Ziac	258,299
25	Allegra	810,001	60	Cozaar	395,292	95	Zithromax Susp	252,501
26	Viagra	809,377	61	Nasonex	391,973	96	Miacalcin Nasal	245,241
27	Ambien	798,858	62	Diflucan	386,846	97	Sporanox	244,434
28	Depakote	758,329	63	Aricept	384,059	98	Lotrisone	243,440
29	Levaquin	753,711	64	Procardia XL	383,822	99	Lescol	238,343
30	Imitrex	747,631	65	Cefzil	382,250	100	Xenical	237,004
31	Zyrtec	739,543	66	Adalat CC	376,992	101	Betaseron	236,503
32	Celexa	737,487	67	Aciphex	372,138	102	Asacol	235,117
33	Prempro	711,798	68	Lotrel	353,784	103	Monopril	233,969
34	Fosamax	704,289	69	Toprol XL	353,725	104	Humulin 70/30	229,600
35	Singulair	676,515	70	Duragesic	352,934	105	Combivent	229,550

Rank	Product	Total retail dollars (000)	Rank	Product	Total retail dollars (000)	Rank	Product	Total retail dollars (000)
106	Flomax	$226,845	138	Plendil	$169,716	170	MS Contin	$125,606
107	Zofran	225,673	139	Proscar	166,868	171	Effexor	125,468
108	Axid	225,365	140	Levoxyl	164,919	172	Pulmicort Turbuhaler	122,785
109	Lamictal	221,847	141	Bactroban	163,939	173	Proventil HFA	121,417
110	Baycol	221,383	142	Daypro	163,783	174	Serostim	121,096
111	Topamax	219,865	143	Lanoxin	163,625	175	Clozaril	119,152
112	Mevacor	216,661	144	Alphagan	159,631	176	Gonal-F	119,096
113	Neoral	214,475	145	Diovan HCT	159,351	177	Arava	118,902
114	Neupogen	212,997	146	Amaryl	158,976	178	Lupron Depot	117,045
115	Famvir	205,223	147	Tricor	158,741	179	Vicoprofen Non-Inj	115,382
116	Epivir	205,172	148	Ortho-Cyclen	157,366	180	Covera-HS	115,239
117	Ortho-Novum 7/7/7	203,989	149	Humalog	157,153	181	Loestrin Fe 1/20	113,408
118	Azmacort	203,389	150	Arthrotec	152,530	182	Elocon	113,324
119	Luvox	199,293	151	Patanol	152,199	183	Skelaxin	113,307
120	Coreg	199,166	152	Vancenase AQ DS	150,883	184	Meridia	113,231
121	Zestoretic	198,956	153	Accolat	150,536	185	Nasacort AQ	112,518
122	Tiazac	198,727	154	Cellcept	150,193	186	Dovonex	110,975
123	Avapro	197,428	155	Copaxone	148,844	187	Catapres-TTS	109,703
124	Benzamycin	196,795	156	Zithromax	146,759	188	Zyrtec Syrup	109,389
125	Triphasil	196,589	157	Hytrin	145,267	189	Propulsid	107,279
126	Zomig	190,231	158	Casodex	143,906	190	Tequin	107,197
127	Rebetron 1200 Pen	189,843	159	Xanax	141,572	191	Rezulin	106,720
128	Imitrex Statdose	184,548	160	Tobradex	137,765	192	Rebetron 1000 Pen	106,624
129	Sustiva	183,008	161	Prograf	137,743	193	Stadol NS	105,637
130	Amoxil	176,847	162	Crixivan	137,645	194	Prevpac	105,011
131	Lovenox	175,402	163	Lo/Ovral 28	137,138	195	Loestrin Fe 1.5/30	103,323
132	Ditropan XL	174,058	164	Differin	136,023	196	Phenergan Supp	102,421
133	Atrovent Inh	174,018	165	DDAVP	133,016	197	Viramune	102,348
134	Zantac	172,662	166	Macrobid	131,419	198	Cosopt	102,212
135	Altace	172,308	167	Betapace	130,263	199	Estratest Tabs	101,697
136	Alesse-28	171,698	168	Ziagen	127,284	200	Prandin	100,310
137	Dilantin Kapseals	171,374	169	Zyban	126,122			

Top 200 Generic Drugs by Retail Sales in 2000

Rank	Product	Total retail dollars (000)	Rank	Product	Total retail dollars (000)	Rank	Product	Total retail dollars (000)
1	Hydrocodone/APAP	$935,093	16	Naproxen	$287,162	31	Methylphenidate	$172,863
2	Ranitidine HCl	690,854	17	Isosorbide Mononitrt	286,576	32	Amitriptyline	168,586
3	Atenolol	532,836	18	Carisoprodol	286,430	33	Trimethoprim/Sulfa	168,446
4	Lorazepam	530,084	19	Terazosin	286,378	34	Nifedipine ER	157,299
5	Albuterol Aerosol	501,115	20	Minocycline	278,055	35	Cimetidine	156,799
6	Alprazolam	489,753	21	Amoxicillin	252,789	36	Ipratropium Bromide	154,735
7	Propoxyphene-N/APAP	457,763	22	Ibuprofen	248,035	37	Hydrochlorothiazide	148,603
8	Cephalexin	399,055	23	Metoprolol Tartrate	230,657	38	Gemfibrozil	148,226
9	Tamoxifen	393,067	24	Furosemide Oral	227,718	39	Prednisone Oral	141,904
10	Clonazepam	351,304	25	Acetaminophen w/Cod	216,379	40	Methotrexate	132,550
11	Glyburide	333,348	26	Trimox	214,918	41	Captopril	129,457
12	Cartia XT	331,837	27	Acyclovir Systemic	209,307	42	Diclofenac Sodium	123,457
13	Albuterol Neb Soln	325,017	28	Cyclobenzaprine	192,847	43	Potassium Chloride	121,779
14	Verapamil SR	301,604	29	Warfarin	178,317	44	Clorazepate Dipot	117,470
15	Triamterene w/HCTZ	292,778	30	Trazodone HCl	173,623	45	Medrxyprgsterone Tab	113,414

Rank	Product	Total retail dollars (000)	Rank	Product	Total retail dollars (000)	Rank	Product	Total retail dollars (000)
46	Spironolactone	$113,240	98	Dicyclomine HCl	$48,747	150	Doxazosin	$28,189
47	Clindamycin Systemic	111,649	99	Indapamide	48,395	151	Diltia XT	27,569
48	Doxycycline	110,567	100	Prednisolone Oral	48,313	152	Ketoconazole Topical	26,558
49	Diltiazem CD	109,812	101	Octicair	47,988	153	Levothyroxine	26,415
50	Estradiol Oral	109,688	102	Hydroxyzine	47,063	154	Dexamethasone Oral	26,304
51	Amiodarone	108,066	103	Bupropion	46,855	155	Chlorhexidine Glucon	26,272
52	Enalapril	107,435	104	Nystatin Systemic	46,135	156	Desoximetasone	26,201
53	Hydroxychloroquine	105,895	105	Triamcinln Acet Top	45,627	157	Bromocriptine	26,133
54	Methylprednis Tabs	101,298	106	Baclofen	45,586	158	Enulose	26,002
55	Diazepam	100,210	107	Ketoprofen	45,484	159	Indomethacin SR	25,979
56	Cefaclor	99,915	108	Sucralfate	45,451	160	Haloperidol	25,865
57	Propranolol LA	98,875	109	Theophylline SR	44,118	161	Valproic Acid	25,856
58	Nitroglycerin	97,650	110	Ticlopidine	43,870	162	Phenobarbital	25,548
59	Clonidine	95,919	111	Phenytoin Sodium Ext	43,299	163	Selegiline	25,384
60	Pentoxifylline	95,402	112	Clozapine	43,091	164	Megestrol Tabs	24,555
61	Glipizide	93,619	113	Atenolol Chlorthal	43,068	165	Quinine Sulfate	24,441
62	Temazepam	93,513	114	Guaif/Phenylprop	43,027	166	Clotrimazole Top	24,320
63	Nortriptyline	91,972	115	Lithium Carbonate	42,933	167	Hydroxyurea	24,282
64	Etodolac	90,898	116	Diphenoxylate w/Atro	42,844	168	Naproxen EC	24,185
65	Allopurinol	89,571	117	Nitrofurantoin Mcroc	42,269	169	Lindane	24,164
66	Diltiazem SR	89,489	118	Penicillin VK	41,679	170	Lonox	24,056
67	Glyburide Micronized	79,195	119	Oxybutynin Chloride	41,307	171	Nitroquick	24,030
68	Cefadroxil	76,442	120	Butalbital Cmpd w/Cd	40,364	172	Sulfasalazine	23,899
69	Clobetasol	76,034	121	Hydrocortsn Valerate	39,458	173	Cholestyramine	23,516
70	Morphine Sul Non Inj	74,084	122	Ery-Tab	39,313	174	Digoxin	23,466
71	Carbidopa/Levodopa	73,230	123	Carbidopa/Levdpa ER	39,286	175	Triazolam	23,453
72	Orphenadrine Citrate	70,339	124	Diclofenac Potassium	38,006	176	Acebutolol	23,093
73	Naproxen Sodium	70,150	125	Prednisolne Acet Oph	37,289	177	Clomipramine HCl	22,853
74	Nadolol	69,757	126	Promethazine/Codeine	37,253	178	Lactulose	22,593
75	Oxycodone w/APAP	69,492	127	Guanfacine HCl	36,569	179	Ibuprofen Liquid	21,880
76	Benzonatate	68,749	128	Clomiphene Citrate	36,467	180	Erythromycin Topical	21,769
77	Phentermine	68,626	129	Timolol Maleate XE	36,124	181	Colchicine	21,372
78	Carbamazepine	67,842	130	Indomethacin	35,849	182	Tobramycin Ophth	21,259
79	Methylphenidate SR	67,025	131	Timolol Maleate Oph	35,258	183	Hydroxyzine Pamoate	20,798
80	Labetalol	66,498	132	Sotalol	35,134	184	Ketorolac Oral	20,523
81	Butalbital/APAP/Caf	65,896	133	Desmopressin Acetate	34,621	185	Isosorbide Dinitrate	20,205
82	Azathioprine	64,242	134	Estropipate	34,373	186	Benztropine	20,203
83	Prochlorperaz Mal	63,598	135	Folic Acid	33,673	187	Diclofenac Sodium SR	19,969
84	Propranolol HCl	62,698	136	Sulindac	33,369	188	Diflorasone	19,534
85	Imipramine HCl	61,106	137	Bumetanide Non-Inj	33,250	189	Gentamicin Ophth	18,966
86	Methocarbamol	59,187	138	Hydrocortison Top Rx	33,080	190	Diltiazem	18,792
87	Metronidazole Tabs	58,338	139	Polymyxin B/Trimeth	33,017	191	Pentazocine/Naloxone	18,783
88	Hyoscyamine	58,107	140	Albuterol Oral Liq	32,386	192	Naproxen Delayed Rel	18,730
89	Neomycin/Polymx/HC	57,961	141	Oxazepam	32,333	193	Dipyridamole	18,696
90	Metoclopramide	55,692	142	Clindamycin Topical	31,721	194	Tetracycline	18,627
91	Doxepin	53,206	143	Guaifenesin/Pseudoep	31,040	195	Probenecid	18,305
92	Cromolyn Sod Neb Sln	51,925	144	Phenazopyridine HCl	30,966	196	Methyldopa	18,283
93	Tretinoin	51,616	145	Ketoconazole Syst	30,812	197	Benzoyl Peroxd Acne	18,182
94	Fluocinonide	51,573	146	Bisoprolol/HCTZ	29,235	198	Nystatin/Triamcinoln	17,761
95	Meclizine HCl	51,400	147	Promethazine Tabs	29,058	199	Erythromycin Ethylsc	17,383
96	Piroxicam	51,077	148	Thioridazine HCl	28,833	200	Methadone HCl Non-In	17,188
97	Adipex-P	49,545	149	Guaifenesin Rx	28,595			

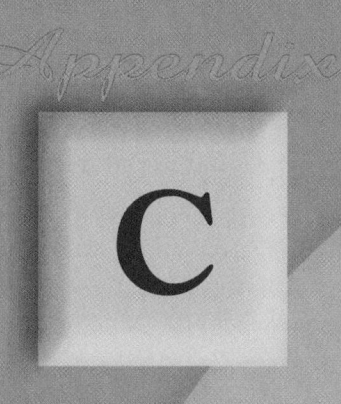

MEDICAL ASSISTANT ROLE DELINEATION CHART

Reprinted with permission of the American Association of Medical Assistants.

*Asterisk denotes advanced skill

ADMINISTRATIVE

Administrative Procedures

- Perform basic clerical functions
- Schedule, coordinate and monitor appointments
- Schedule inpatient/outpatient admissions and procedures
- Understand and apply third-party guidelines
- Obtain reimbursement through accurate claims submission
- Monitor third-party reimbursement
- Perform medical transcription
- Understand and adhere to managed care policies and procedures
- *Negotiate managed care contracts (advanced)*

Practice Finances

- Perform procedural and diagnostic coding
- Apply bookkeeping principles
- Document and maintain accounting and banking records
- Manage accounts receivable
- Manage accounts payable
- Process payroll
- *Develop and maintain fee schedules (advanced)*
- *Manage renewals of business and professional insurance policies (advanced)*
- *Manage personnel benefits and maintain records (advanced)*

CLINICAL

Fundamental Principles

- Apply principles of aseptic technique and infection control
- Comply with quality assurance practices
- Screen and follow up patient test results

Diagnostic Orders

- Collect and process specimens
- Perform diagnostic tests

Patient Care

- Adhere to established triage procedures
- Obtain patient history and vital signs
- Prepare and maintain examination and treatment areas
- Prepare patient for examinations, procedures, and treatments
- Assist with examinations, procedures and treatments
- Prepare and administer medications and immunizations
- Maintain medication and immunization records
- Recognize and respond to emergencies
- Coordinate patient care information with other health care providers

GENERAL (TRANSDISCIPLINARY)

Professionalism

- Project a professional manner and image
- Adhere to ethical principles
- Demonstrate initiative and responsibility
- Work as a team member
- Manage time effectively
- Prioritize and perform multiple tasks
- Adapt to change
- Promote the CMA credential
- Enhance skills through continuing education

Communication Skills

- Treat all patients with compassion and empathy
- Recognize and respect cultural diversity
- Adapt communications to individual's ability to understand
- Use professional telephone technique
- Use effective and correct verbal and written communications
- Recognize and respond to verbal and nonverbal communications
- Use medical terminology appropriately
- Receive, organize, prioritize and transmit information
- Serve as liaison
- Promote the practice through positive public relations

Legal Concepts

- Maintain confidentiality
- Practice within the scope of education, training, and personal capabilities
- Prepare and maintain medical records
- Document accurately

- Use appropriate guidelines when releasing information
- Follow employer's established policies dealing with the health care contract
- Follow federal, state and local legal guidelines
- Maintain awareness of federal and state health care legislation and regulations
- Maintain and dispose of regulated substances in compliance with government guidelines
- Comply with established risk management and safety procedures
- Recognize professional credentialing criteria
- Participate in the development and maintenance of personnel, policy and procedure manuals
- * *Develop and maintain personnel, policy and procedure manuals (advanced)*

Instruction

- Instruct individuals according to their needs
- Explain office policies and procedures
- Teach methods of health promotion and disease prevention
- Locate community resouces and disseminate information
- * *Orient and train personnel (advanced)*
- * *Develop educational materials (advanced)*
- * *Conduct continuing education activities (advanced)*

Operational Functions

- Maintain supply inventory
- Evaluate and recommend equipment and supplies
- Apply computer techniques to support office operations
- * *Supervise personnel (advanced)*
- * *Interview and recommend job applicants (advanced)*
- * *Negotiate leases and prices for equipment and supply contracts (advanced)*

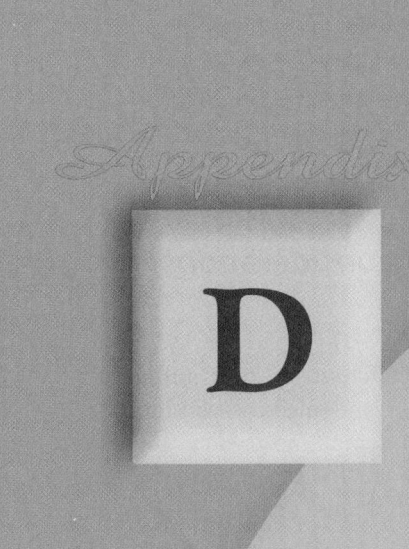

ANSWERS TO CASE STUDY REVIEWS

D

Chapter 5   Coping Skills for the Medical Assistant

Case Study 5-1

1. By being responsible, taking charge of the work environment, and being an inner-directed person, Ellen is more able to achieve her long-term goal of being an office manager. Certainly, she will learn by working closely with and observing Marilyn; there are also specific long-term, skill-building goals Ellen should set to give herself direction. If she gave herself three years to move into the office manager position, Ellen could set one long-term goal for each year. These might include (1) the first year, become proficient in all back-office clinical skills; (2) the second year, add front-office administrative tasks and skills; (3) the third year, begin to focus on office management.

2. Short-term goals break down long-term goals into smaller, more manageable time segments and will help Ellen more easily evaluate her progress. Short-term goals also provide a sense of periodic reward necessary to sustain motivation toward a long-range goal.

   Ellen should review her three long-term goals and determine what short-term goals they include. For example, the first year, Ellen wants to become proficient in all back-office clinical skills; short-term goals may include practicing accuracy when performing clinical duties and understanding which supplies are needed for which procedures. For her second-year goal of developing front-office administrative tasks and skills, Ellen may become proficient on the computer and learn the intricacies of scheduling patients. For the third-year goal that focuses on office management, Ellen can learn team-building skills and develop a procedures manual.

3. Ellen should take an active interest in her profession; she could attend seminars; speak with other medical assistants who are now office managers; read professional journals; and participate in professional organizations. This variety of exposure will enlarge Ellen's perspective and broaden her scope of information.

Case Study 5-2

1. Ellen is demonstrating the classic signs and symptoms of burnout, which include:
   a. she is a perfectionist
   b. she has a decreased sense of humor
   c. she displays frustration and irritability
   d. she is critical of herself and others
   e. she is physically and emotionally exhausted, yet continues to push herself
   f. her work has become a chore
   g. she feels like a failure if everything is not completed at the end of the day to her satisfaction

2. Ellen needs to take time for self-analysis by asking herself some hard questions. These questions must be answered truthfully and completely.

3. Ellen needs to institute some changes.
   a. List negative words or phrases often used, and then substitute neutral replacements.
   b. Create job diversity: Take a different route to work for a change; enter the office through a different door; change work routine where appropriate; investigate the possibility of a different work schedule.
   c. Become creative: Change work area décor by adding a new calendar; change family photo on desk, add a foliage or silk plant to the area.

d. Revisit short- and long-term goals, and make adjustments where necessary; be sure all goals are realistic and attainable.

e. Pay more attention to personal habits: Change eating habits; exercise more; get more rest and sleep; renew old friendships; go to lunch with coworkers.

f. Implement time management techniques.

g. Delegate responsibility to others who are capable.

Chapter 6   The Therapeutic Approach to the Patient with Life-Threatening Illness

Case Study 6-1

1. These questions are intended to help. In this culture, the family is deeply involved.

2. Having such a document would make it easier for everyone involved to know how much information should and can be shared with another.

3. Most all of this concern is related to the culture.

4. Have an honest discussion with everyone involved so it is clear to the staff how the patient would like to have information handled.

Case Study 6-2

1. Bruce should know that the human immunodeficiency virus (HIV) is transmitted between persons through sexual practices (sexual intimacy where body fluids might be exchanged); through direct blood-to-blood contact as in transfusions or needlestick injuries; and through intrauterine transmission. It is not transmitted through touching or other casual contact; AIDS is not an easily contracted disease.

2. AIDS patients and patients with the HIV virus often suffer extreme distress. Certainly, as a health care professional, Bruce needs to be sensitive to their needs and remember they may be both anxious and depressed. He should avoid being fearful and judgmental, but rather should be respectful toward patients with AIDS; while he should practice standard precautions, Bruce should also replace his fear with knowledge based on medical fact. He could be of assistance to HIV-infected or AIDS patients by referring them to support groups, social workers, legal advisors, and by helping the patient build coping skills.

3. Dealing with a large number of AIDS patients can be psychologically exhausting. While Bruce needs to combat his own prejudices, he also needs to be self-nurturing, not by withdrawing from AIDS patients but by giving himself a respite from time to time. If he routinely deals with AIDS patients, Bruce may benefit from a support group of his own that will help him build coping abilities.

Chapter 7   Legal Considerations

Case Study 7-1

1. It is critical that medical charts be kept current at all times. If the physician and medical assistant have maintained an accurate and up-to-date record of patient Boris Bolski's care, Joe can rely on the information in the chart to help him answer any questions. He should study the chart carefully.

Note: At all times, the patient's confidentiality must be respected. Typically, if the patient's attorney has issued the subpoena, the attorney will have the patient sign a release form. If the physician is subpoenaed by someone other than the patient's representative, the physician must be very careful about release of information and should proceed on a case-by-case basis. Certain records, because of their sensitive nature, may require a court order before being released.

2. Information in the chart should contain actual care rendered, dates that it was rendered, and charges made. Joe should note whether any comments were made on the chart that reflect patient input. Joe should also gather and review other material such as consent forms, insurance claim forms, and other documents related to patient care.

3. An expert witness is one who has the knowledge and experience to testify as to a reasonable and expected standard of care. Judges and jurors rely on the testimony of expert witnesses to understand the nature of medical information. Joe should answer questions in a factual way and in terms understood by the lay person.

Chapter 8   Ethical Considerations

Case Study 8-1

1. In most states, physicians and their employees are mandated to report all cases of suspected child abuse. Liz and Dr. Esposito must report the suspected abuse of Henry to the appropriate child protective agency.

2. and 3. Once the suspected abuse is reported, the responsible agency will respond to Henry's needs. However, in the meantime, Liz should take measures to protect and care for Henry, providing a safe environment if possible. While it may be difficult to do so, Liz should also view Juanita Hansen as a victim and seek treatment for her as well as for her son.

Chapter 9 Emergency Procedures and First Aid

Case Study 9-1

1. Wanda must first ascertain whether Annette is having trouble breathing. If she is, Wanda must direct her—and if necessary assist Annette—to receive immediate medical attention at the nearest hospital. If Annette says she is not having any breathing difficulty, Wanda should ask:

   - What are your symptoms?
   - Have you ever experienced an allergic reaction to an insect (specifically yellowjacket) sting before?
   - Do you have hives?
   - Are you experiencing any lightheadedness?
   - Do you have any itching either at the site of the sting or in other body locations?

   From these questions, Wanda needs to determine whether Annette is having a localized reaction, which can result in swelling, itching, and tenderness at the site of the sting, or a generalized reaction, which can be frightening for the patient and dangerous if it involves impairment of breathing functions.

2. If patients are allergic to an insect sting, it is possible that anaphylactic shock may ensue, which can lead to death. The patient must be directed to receive emergency care immediately, which will usually consist of the administration of epinephrine. If Annette must wait for EMS personnel, Wanda should stay with her over the telephone and calm her until EMS personnel arrive. For individuals who present at the ambulatory care setting with an apparent allergic reaction to a sting, the physician will prescribe epinephrine. Attempt to allay patient apprehension and monitor vital signs while waiting for EMS personnel to arrive.

3. Once Annette has received emergency treatment, Wanda can advise her to take certain precautions should she have another, and possibly more severe, reaction to an insect sting. For individuals with a known allergic reaction, the physician will prescribe epinephrine. These individuals should carry the epinephrine with them and self-inject, should they not be able to get immediate emergency care. The patient should then seek immediate emergency treatment. Advise all patients with known allergic reactions to be particularly careful when working or playing outdoors. Insects are not usually aggressive until their nests are approached; however, often these nests are not easy to detect and an individual may approach one without

being aware of its presence. Patients with allergies to insects should always wear shoes out-of-doors, wear light-colored clothing, preferably with long sleeves and pant legs, look before taking a sip from a beverage when outdoors, and inspect lawn areas, shrubbery, and building walls periodically for evidence of nests of stinging insects.

Case Study 9-2

1. Because of the possibility that Mrs. Johnson is experiencing a myocardial infarction, Bruce should get a wheelchair and immediately take Mrs. Johnson into an examination room and notify Dr. Lewis. Bruce should help Mrs. Johnson onto the examination table, place her in semi-Fowler's position, loosen tight clothing, and take her blood pressure, pulse, and respirations. Bruce should activate EMS if Dr. Lewis directed him to. Because Mrs. Johnson is extremely anxious, Bruce must attend to her psychological needs.

2. The equipment, supplies, and medications that Dr. Lewis may want and need to be available for Mrs. Johnson are oxygen tank and mask, electrocardiograph, sphygmomanometer and stethoscope, and nitroglycerine, verapamil, and cardizem from the emergency cart.

3. Once the patient has been stabilized and Dr. Lewis has determined that Mrs. Johnson's symptoms are typical of angina pectoris, Bruce should continue to monitor Mrs. Johnson's vital signs and provide emotional support. He should notify the patient's family and remain with her until family members arrive to take Mrs. Johnson home.

4. Bruce can teach Mrs. Johnson and her family about the importance of using the prescribed form of nitroglycerin (sublingual tablets, transdermal patches) for angina attacks and the need to call Dr. Lewis if the nitroglycerin does not relieve symptoms. He can reinforce the need for regular exercise, a low-fat diet, stress reduction techniques, and no smoking.

Chapter 10 Infection Control, Medical Asepsis, and Sterilization

Case Study 10-1

Include the following in an exposure control plan for blood and/or OPIM:

Exposure determination requires an employer to list all job classifications in which all employees in those jobs are exposed to blood and OPIM in the course of doing their job. Existing job descriptions can be used by the employer to identify the job categories that are at high risk for exposure to blood and/or OPIM. It is important that exposure determination be made without regard to the use of PPE.

The plan must consist of methods of compliance for prevention of exposure, hepatitis B vaccination, past exposure evaluation, communication of hazards to employees, documentation of the bloodborne standard, and a procedure for the determination of the events surrounding the exposure.

The written plan must be employee-accessible, updated at least annually, and modified when necessary and appropriate, especially to reflect a change in employee positions.

Case Study 10-2

By depriving pathogens of their growth requirements, they may be kept from causing an infection. This can be accomplished by providing good lighting since bacteria will die in direct light or sunlight; by providing or withholding oxygen according to the needs of the pathogen (aerobe or anaerobe); by lowering environmental temperature, pathogenic growth is reduced because they favor warm temperatures; and by keeping work surfaces dry, pathogenic growth can be inhibited because they need moisture to grow.

Chapter 11   Taking a Medical History, the Patient's Chart, and Methods of Documentation

Case Study 11-1

1. The medical assistant must be as thorough as possible while respecting the patient's privacy and help Adam understand that the medical history enables the physician to advise patients on how to prevent any future problems.

2. Joe should reassure Adam that patient information is confidential and that his mother has agreed to respect his privacy (since this is the case). Joe can also try to engage Adam in the medical history-taking by inviting Adam's perceptions, such as:

   - What do you expect from this exam?

   - What kind of treatment do you expect?

   Joe should also use his communication skills to get Adam to be responsive; if Joe can develop a relationship with Adam, Adam is more likely to be honest and Joe can be more effective in helping Adam analyze his social behaviors.

3. Joe should not be condemning or judgmental but should help Adam protect himself by following proper

precautions. If Adam has come to respect and trust Joe, he is more likely to accept his opinion. Joe can give Adam some printed material to educate him about HIV infection; reading about the topic may encourage Adam to rethink some of his behaviors.

Some techniques that Joe can use when dealing with sensitive topics include:

- Asking these questions later in the interview;

- Using direct eye contact;

- Posing questions in a matter-of-fact tone;

- "Normalizing" the situation, e.g., saying, "Many students seem to do this. How does it affect you?"

Case Study 11-2

1. *personal data:* Harvey DiAntonio
   45 W. Smith Avenue
   Baltimore, MD 21208
   ph. 667-1870
   Insurance: BC/BS 211678756
   Major Medical—
   Diagnostic #4
   Referred by: Dr. Alan Byers
   DOB 07/08/1954

   chief complaint: Severe "gripping" pain in the anterior mid-chest sometimes radiating to the abdomen, neck, and both arms.

   present illness: Pain occurs with strenuous exercise, walking uphill, shaving, climbing stairs, after a heavy meal, during sexual intercourse. Pain lasts 20 minutes with each episode, does not stop when he ceases activity. Episode last week included dizziness, nausea, and fatigue. Episodes ongoing once or twice per month × 5 months.

   past medical history: Essentially noncontributory. Has not had physical examination for eight years.

   Surgeries: T & A, 1958
   Appendectomy, 1964
   Fractured rib L, 1984
   Usual childhood diseases

   Hospitalization:
   Observation, 1962—Sinai Hospital
   Dx bronchitis

   family history: Both parents deceased, mother age 59—MI, father age 49 ? cause—brother living, hypertension—sister alive and well—two children alive and well (adolescents) *social history:* Firefighter—pump operator—heavy exertion, smokes 1½–2 packs of cigarettes per day, overeats while on duty, hobbies—carpentry, music. Describes self as "fun-loving," "quick tempered," worries about finances. Eligible to retire, but prefers to remain working.

ROS: Well-nourished, well-developed male in no acute distress. Somewhat anxious. Wt. 198 pounds, BP 175/104—T. 98.6—P. 94 (reg.)

HEENT:	normal
Neck	supple
Trachea	midline
Chest	normal in contour—calcium deposit L 6th rib noted on X ray, otherwise neg., probably due to old fracture.
Heart	presystolic gallop
Abdomen	negative
Extremities	negative
Genitalia	negative
Skin	negative
Neurological	negative
Laboratory	Hgb. 11.0 gm
EKG	presystolic atrial sounds, long P–R interval

Impression:

1. angina pectoris

2. anemia

3. hypertension

Plan: nitroglycerin tab sublingually as needed, watch quantity of food intake, low fat 1600 calories, 4 meals/day, avoid extreme cold, sleep 8 hours/night, avoid emotional upsets, no smoking, moderate alcohol intake.

Return in 2 weeks

Chapter 12   Vital Signs and Measurements

Case Study 12-1

1. A normal blood pressure reading for adults would have a systolic reading below 140 and a diastolic reading below 90. Herb's reading of 156/100 is considered hypertension, or a blood pressure that is above normal. Audrey should measure the patient's blood pressure again to confirm that a proper reading was taken. She should also confirm that the cuff size was correct, for a too small cuff can give an artificially high blood pressure reading.

2. Herb is obviously considering but having a difficult time implementing lifestyle changes. Audrey may find that educating Herb about diet and exercise may give him some information that will encourage him to make some changes in his lifestyle. While the high blood pressure may be due to a number of reasons, weight and smoking certainly can contribute to it. Audrey and Herb could pinpoint a long-term goal and then select a few manageable short-term goals to reduce Herb's weight, improve his circulation, and reduce his blood pressure.

3. In reviewing new resources, Audrey discovers that high blood pressure is now considered any reading over 140/90. Previously, she had learned that there were four categories of high blood pressure. In addition to learning new facts, Audrey also discovered the importance of periodically updating her base of information.

Chapter 13   The Physical Examination

Case Study 13-1

1. a. Observation or inspection
   b. Palpation
   c. Percussion
   d. Auscultation
   e. Mensuration
   f. Manipulation

2. Liz should know at least eight common positions that may be required of the patient during the physical examination.

   a. Supine or horizontal recumbent
   b. Dorsal recumbent
   c. Lithotomy
   d. Fowler's
   e. Knee-chest
   f. Prone
   g. Sims'
   h. Trendelenburg

3. Liz should know the basic components of an exam as observed by the physician and how each is an indicator of patient well-being.

   a. Patient appearance, including skin color, grooming, behavior. Patient appearance is also observed by the medical assistant during the patient history.
   b. Gait, including limp, dragging of one leg, balance, or a wide-based walk. Gait can indicate a problem with neurological functioning.

c. Stature, including height and trunk and limb proportion.

d. Posture; a person in pain may have postural abnormalities.

e. Body movements, including both voluntary and involuntary movements.

f. Speech, including loss of voice, difficulty speaking, using wrong speech patterns, and using words in the wrong order.

g. Breath odors, which can indicate specific diseases such as diabetes or liver disease.

h. Nutrition, to discover the cause of overweight or underweight conditions or edema.

i. Skin and appendages, including abnormal skin color or skin conditions.

Case Study 13-2

1. Positioning and draping Mrs. Mason for a complete physical exam won't be different from any other patient who has a complete basic physical exam. Keep in mind Mrs. Mason's age and assist as necessary with positioning and draping. Protect her privacy while helping her to undress in preparation for the exam. Because Mrs. Mason has arthritis, she has limited mobility and needs assistance. Remain with her throughout and assist her onto the examination table and into the various positions for the exam.

   To position Mrs. Mason for the pelvic examination, she will not be able to assume lithotomy position due to her arthritic knees. The pelvic exam can be done with Mrs. Mason in either the dorsal recumbent or Sim's position.

   Be certain she is covered with a drape for warmth and privacy. A diamond shape placement of the drape for either dorsal recumbent or Sims' will facilitate viewing the pelvic area without undue patient exposure.

2. Because of Mrs. Mason's age and frail condition, special consideration should be given to her safety. Assist her on and off the table being certain at the conclusion of the exam that she remain seated on the edge of the exam table while you assess her readiness to get down from the table. Check blood pressure, pulse, and skin color before allowing her to step down. Help her to get dressed, remain with her throughout, and assist her into the physician's office and later out to the reception area to her waiting niece.

3. Since Mrs. Mason is experiencing vaginal spotting, Dr. King will perform a pelvic examination. Prepare the appropriate equipment and supplies necessary to do the pelvic exam.

Chapter 14   Obstetrics and Gynecology

Case Study 14-1

1. The initial prenatal visit is of utmost importance because it is a time for health promotion and patient education. A thorough history will be taken, and a physical exam will include abdominal, pelvic, vaginal, and breast examinations. Pelvic measurements are taken to be certain that Maria's pelvis size is sufficiently adequate to deliver her baby vaginally. Numerous laboratory tests are performed. Time will be spent promoting good health for mother-to-be and her fetus. Liz will stress the importance of healthy habits for Maria to practice. Such topics as proper nutrition, regular exercise, dental care, rest, and sleep will be addressed. Body changes and newborn and infant care are discussed at this visit. The dangers of using alcohol, tobacco, and other drugs, either over-the-counter or prescription, are stressed.

2. Dr. King will watch for signs and symptoms of such diseases and conditions as the following:

Condition/Disease	Signs and Symptoms
Pre-eclampsia	Edema, hypertension, albuminuria, headache, vision changes, rapid weight gain
Hyperemesis gravidarum	Severe, unrelenting nausea and vomiting with possible dehydration
Vaginitis/STD	Vaginal discharge
Threatened abortion	Vaginal bleeding, abdominal pain, or cramping
Possible ectopic pregnancy	A one-sided pelvic or abdominal pain

There are other diseases and conditions pregnant women may experience as well as those listed. Dr. King will be on the alert for signs and symptoms of anything that seems to be out of the ordinary.

3. Some procedures and tests that may be done during the initial prenatal visit include:

- Pelvimetry
- Urinalysis
- Complete blood count (CBC)
- Rh factor
- Blood type
- Rubella titer
- Hepatitis B and C
- Venereal disease research laboratory (VDRL)

- Pap smear
- Gonorrhea and chlamydia cultures

4. Liz may include in her discussion with Maria the importance of good nutrition and what it entails, dental care, rest, relaxation, regular exercise, and sleep. She will caution Maria about drugs (alcohol, over-the-counter, prescription, tobacco, and street drugs) and their ability to cross over the placenta into the fetal circulation. Anticipated body changes, newborn and infant care, and breast-feeding are all part of patient education and health promotion that Maria will be taught.

Case Study 14-2

1. Rest for 24 hours after the procedure.

2. Do not lift heavy objects for approximately two weeks.

3. Leave vaginal pack in place for 24 hours or as directed by physician. Do not insert a tampon unless told to do so by physician.

4. Report any bleeding greater than an average menstrual period.

Case Study 14-3

1. An abdominal and pelvic examination will be done on Annette, therefore, a gynecological examination set-up will be necessary. There is a discharge, so a wet mount procedure will also be done.

2. Most likely the causative microorganism is trichomonas vaginalis. It is a parasite.

3. If the diagnosis is trichomonas, Dr. King is likely to prescribe medication by mouth (Flagyl) and treat both partners.

Chapter 15 Pediatrics

Case Study 15-1

1. Otitis media is an inflammation of the middle ear that frequently follows an upper respiratory tract infection in children. The eustachian tubes of a child are shaped differently than mature tubes. They are shorter and are more prone to having pathogens lodge and grow in the tubes. The infection can travel up the eustachian tube to the middle ear. Antibiotics are used to treat otitis media.

Case Study 15-2

1. When a child has an upper respiratory infection and is showing signs of possible otitis media, vaporizers and decongestants should be used to help prevent otitis media.

Chapter 16 Male Reproductive System

Case Study 16-1

1. First, a digital rectal examination will be done, then a prostate-specific antigen (PSA) blood test, a urinalysis, and a urine culture. Perhaps an intravenous pyelogram will be ordered also. The rectal examination allows Dr. Woo to palpate the prostate gland for enlargement. The PSA blood test measures the amount of a specific protein that is elevated in prostate cancer cases. If the PSA is within normal range, it can help rule out prostate cancer, although a biopsy is necessary to confirm a diagnosis. A urinalysis and culture will show an infection that is not unusual with BPH. An intravenous pyelogram is helpful in determining kidney, ureter, and bladder damage from BPH.

2. The preliminary tests Dr. Woo might order are urinalysis, urine culture, and intravenous pyelogram.

Case Study 16-2

1. Dr. King's workup of Mr. Toomey will include an examination to determine if the testicle is painful, swollen, or inflamed. If there are none of these symptoms, Dr. King most likely will suggest Mr. Toomey have a biopsy of the mass in the right testicle. This will determine whether the lesion is benign or malignant.

Chapter 17 Gerontology

Case Study 17-1

1. Slower movements and decreased flexibility are due to changes in the muscles and joints. The muscles become weaker, and muscle fibers decrease in size and number. Loss of neurons that control muscle function results in slower movements. The wear and tear of everyday living causes worn out joints. Synovial fluid decreases leading to stiffness and immobility.

2. The activities of daily living (ADL) are affected by Mrs. Robinson's problems. It will be difficult or impossible to brush her teeth, comb her hair, use the toilet, feed herself, or bathe herself.

3. Dr. King might suggest some passive and active range of motion exercises to help increase her flexibility and decrease muscle stiffness. (See Chapter 21.)

Case Study 17-2

1. The number of taste buds decrease, and the sense of smell diminishes. Food tastes bland and unappetizing.

2. Dangers to watch for when taste and smell are no longer as acute are:

- Accidentally eating spoiled food, which can cause food poisoning
- Oversalting foods in an attempt to make it taste better
- Weight loss and malnutrition may result
- Gas leaks may go undetected causing loss of consciousness and death
- The inability to hear a smoke alarm resulting in smoke inhalation, severe burns, or death from fire

Chapter 18   Examinations and Procedures of Body Systems

Case Study 18-1

1. The medical assistant's responsibilities include:
   a. Position the patient as requested by the physician.
   b. Clean and dry area to be casted. Note any bruises, swelling, or redness.
   c. Pad bony prominences.
   d. Provide correct width of stockinette for area.
   e. Provide correct width of webril.
   f. Place bandage in container of warm water for 5 seconds. Remove from water and gently squeeze out excess water.
   g. Assist physician with application of cast material.
   h. Comfort and reassure patient as needed.
   i. Give cast care instructions in writing.

2. a. Notify the physician if the following occur:
   - A bad odor coming from the cast
   - Numbness, tingling, severe pain, difficulty moving, severe swelling, cold fingers or toes
   - A burning sensation over a bony area
   - Bleeding or pink to red discoloration on the cast

   b. The following should be verbal and written instructions:
   - Allow casting material to dry by exposing it to air and keeping it uncovered, even at night. Applying pressure prior to drying can result in damage under the pressure area.
   - Elevate right arm to aid in reducing swelling and pain.
   - Observe fingers and toes for color and temperature changes, decreased sensation, and tingling. May indicate cast is too tight.
   - Do not place objects into cast to scratch irritated skin. A break in the skin will provide breeding ground for bacteria. Do not use cream or powder.
   - Do not get cast wet. This could cause malformation of the wrist and arm. Cover with waterproof covering when showering or bathing.
   - Clean cast with a damp cloth.
   - Use water-soluble marking pens if decorating the cast, allowing cast to breathe.
   - Do not cut or trim cast.

Case Study 18-2

1. Anita should be told the following:
   - Seal lips tightly around the mouthpiece.
   - Maintain good posture throughout the test.
   - Inhale deeply and quickly; exhale quickly and forcibly until no more air can be expelled.
   - Do no use bronchodilators for 24 hours before the test.
   - Maximum effort is required for accurate results.

Chapter 19   Assisting with Minor Surgery

Case Study 19-1

1. Wanda should try to gently educate the sisters about the cyst removal procedure in order to allay any apprehension. She will need to ask questions regarding Cele's general state of health and determine whether Cele has any known allergies. Wanda should note the date of Cele's last tetanus booster. Wanda will also need to explain the need for a signed consent form, which is standard protocol before any minor surgery. Costs are sometimes discussed but because the sisters are covered by Medicare and because Inner City accepts Medicare assignment, their only costs may be that of any prescription drugs.

2. The procedure should be fairly routine, especially because the cyst is not inflamed. However, the sisters still need to be instructed about what to expect during the procedure, approximately how long it will take, whether Cele needs to maintain a special diet before the procedure, and whether a special diet is needed after the procedure. If Dottie knows these specifics beforehand, she can shop and prepare for Cele's minor surgery, which will probably make her feel less nervous about being the caregiver.

3. Wanda should give Cele and Dottie specific wound care instructions. She should provide written as well as verbal instructions and tell the sisters to check regularly for symptoms of infection. Wanda should also provide a telephone number that Dottie can call both during and

after hours. Wanda should call the sisters within the first postoperative day to check on Cele's condition. Wanda can also provide for a community agency, such as the Visiting Nurse Association, to check on the sisters and teach Dottie how to check for infection or help with any other problems that can arise.

Case Study 19-2

1. Patient preparation for excision of a nevus:
   a. Wash hands and greet patient.
   b. Offer restroom facilities.
   c. Escort to procedure area.
   d. Check to see if patient followed preoperative instructions.
   e. Review postoperative instructions.
   f. Check for signed consent form.
   g. Have patient remove clothing from waist up. Provide gown, drape, and pillow.
   h. Position patient comfortably.
   i. Prepare patient's skin for surgery.

2. Postoperative care for Letisha consists of:
   a. Check vital signs.
   b. Allow patient to rest if necessary. Remain with patient for her safety.
   c. Assist patient off table and assist her to dress.
   d. Review written instructions with Letisha and caregiver.
   e. Schedule follow-up appointment.
   f. Document postoperative instructions in patient's record.

3. The excised nevus will be carefully placed in a labeled biopsy container with a preservative (formalin). A laboratory requisition or request form will be attached to the specimen container. The specimen will be sent or taken to the laboratory, and documentation will be made in the patient's record.

Chapter 20   Diagnostic Imaging

Case Study 20-1

1. The purpose of the GI series is to study the esophagus, stomach, and small intestine for ulcers, tumors, hiatal hernia, and esophageal varices.

2. Preparation for GI series consists of:

   The day prior to X ray: light evening meal, NPO after midnight.

   The day of test: NPO postprocedure, increase fluid intake, take a laxative as prescribed.

Case Study 20-2

1. Mr. Brunnelle is told that the actual X rays belong to the hospital where they were taken and processed and although he has paid for them, they are not his. He can, however, have a copy of the radiologist's reports of the results of all of the X rays.

2. X rays are best left on-site so that they are accessible for future use to be compared with more recent films of the same body part. Also, this eliminates the possibility of their being lost if they were removed from the site at which they were taken.

Chapter 21   Rehabilitation and Therapeutic Modalities

Case Study 21-1

1. Before beginning any transfer, certain precautions must be observed:

   - The equipment must be stable and firm. Lock the brakes of the wheelchair and be sure the examination table will not move during transfer.

   - Check that there are no obstructions.

   - Take small shuffling steps. Avoid crossing the feet.

   - Adjust the transfer surface to about the same height as the wheelchair.

   - Position the equipment on the patient's stronger side. Take advantage of the patient's assistance in lifting and moving.

   - Always use a gait belt. Never lift the patient by the arms or under the armpits.

   - Never have the patients put their arms around your neck.

   - Both medical assistant and patient should wear nonslip footwear.

   - Be sure the patient understands the process involved in the transfer.

   - Practice good body mechanics.

2. For a one-person transfer, the medical assistant should follow the principles in (1) above and:

   a. Place the wheelchair next to the examination table and lock the brakes.

   b. Place the gait belt around the patient's waist.

   c. Move the wheelchair footrests out of the way or remove if possible; have patient place feet on floor.

d. Position the stool in front of the examination table and as close to the wheelchair as possible.

e. Have patient move to edge of wheelchair; stand in front of patient with feet apart.

f. The medical assistant should bend at hips and knees, grasp the gait belt, and have patient place hand on armrests of wheelchair to push up. The patient can use his strong leg to push as well.

g. Have the patient step onto the stool with the foot closest to the table and pivot. His back is now to the examination table.

h. The patient should grasp the stool handle with one hand and place the other hand on the table.

i. Ease the patient onto the table and position as necessary.

j. Move the wheelchair and stool out of the way.

3. a. Position the wheelchair next to the examination table. Lock the brakes.

b. Position the stool next to the wheelchair.

c. Assist the patient to a sitting position. Place the gait belt snugly around patient's waist.

d. Place your one arm under the patient's arm and around his shoulders, and the other arm under his knees. Pivot the patient so his legs are dangling over the side of the table.

e. Move so you are directly in front of the patient.

f. Grasp the patient by placing your hands under the gait belt. Plant your feet shoulder's width apart and bend your knees.

g. Pull the patient slightly toward you so his feet come down onto the stool. Signal the patient to push off the table, grasping the stool handle for support.

h. Have the patient step onto the floor with his strong leg and pivot so his back is to the chair.

i. Have the patient grasp the armrests of the wheelchair.

j. Lower the patient into the wheelchair and make him comfortable.

k. Lower the footrests and place the patient's feet on them.

Case Study 21-2

Tell Mr. Schwarz to obtain a commercial ice pack or to use an ice bag for the ankle. A commercial pack is pliable and will conform to the shape of the ankle better than an ice bag. Cover the pack with a cloth before applying to the ankle. Leave in place about 30 minutes, and then remove and reapply for another 30 minutes. Report to the physician signs of redness or paleness of skin color, tingling, or increase in pain. Keep the leg elevated as much as possible, and continue ice pack application for about 24 hours.

Chapter 22   Nutrition in Health and Disease

Case Study 22-1

1. Wanda needs to gently educate Anita about the pregnant woman's need to increase various nutrients. Wanda could explain that during pregnancy the growth of the fetus, growth of the placenta, increase in adipose tissue, increased volume of blood, and growth of breast tissue all create the need for additional nutrients. Wanda should try to persuade Anita that pregnancy is an important time for both fetus and mother and that it is normal and healthy for the mother to gain weight.

2. The need during pregnancy is not just for extra calories but for specific nutrients, so Wanda should provide Anita with a range of foods that she can choose from, especially since Anita seems to be a picky eater. The foods should reflect the fact that protein requirements are nearly double during pregnancy; that vitamins are needed in higher quantities than usual; and that calcium, phosphorus, and iron are needed in such high quantities that a vitamin supplement is usually necessary.

3. Anita should be taught that her baby is more likely to be normal and healthy if she has good nutritional habits during her pregnancy. If the problem is one of not having access to healthy foods, the physician may prescribe a nutritional supplement in addition to the vitamin supplement Anita is probably taking. Wanda may want to gather some informational brochures that Anita can read and may even put her in touch with support groups that may encourage and support Anita in her pregnancy. Wanda could also review the list of important nutrients and their food sources and, together with Anita, compose a nutritious but easy-to-make menu.

Case Study 22-2

Mrs. Johnson's activity level, number of calories per day, and dosage of insulin would have to be considered. The diabetic diet consists of a specific number of grams of carbohydrates, protein, and fat. Various foods can be exchanged (derived from a food exchange list) to have a wide selection of foods that come from each of the basic five food groups.

The patient needs to know how to select the correct foods in the correct quantities, how to incorporate a daily exercise routine, and the importance of taking insulin at the appropriate time of the day. The overall goal is geared toward providing sufficient calories to maintain normal body weight, while providing adequate nutrition. Lifestyle is also taken into consideration as well as the patient's ability to comply with the prescribed diabetic diet. The prescribed amount of food should be eaten at prescribed times during the day. Meals should not be skipped.

Encourage the patient to learn more about diabetes by enrolling in a class about the disease at a local hospital.

Chapter 23   Basic Pharmacology

Case Study 23-1

1. Audrey should advise Maria to discard any medication—prescription or nonprescription—that is not used. Most medications lose their potency after a period of time and others become toxic. Maria should discard the leftover suppositories and buy a new supply.

2. Sometimes, an infection or other condition will clear up before a patient finishes all medication and the patient discontinues use. Audrey should tell Maria that in this and other cases, medication should be taken exactly as directed for the prescribed number of days, etc.

3. To discover whether another form of medication might be available for Maria's yeast infection, Audrey consults the PDR. She finds that medications are available that can be taken by mouth, intravenously, or applied topically but that the suppository is the most effective form. The student should consult the PDR to discover what Audrey learned during her research.

Case Study 23-2

Since Dr. King keeps controlled substances on the premises, Joe Guerrero, the certified medical assistant, has the legal responsibility to do the following:

1. Monitor the physician's DEA registration renewal date.

2. Maintain legally designated records.

3. Provide security for all drugs, in particular, controlled substances.

4. Provide security for prescription pads.

5. Destroy expired drugs and document properly.

6. Know and understand federal and state laws that regulate drugs including controlled substances.

Chapter 24   Calculation of Medication Dosage and Medication Administration

Case Study 24-1

1. The size syringe used would be a U-100 insulin syringe.

2. The medication label would indicate 100 units per milliliter. If you use the correct syringe, a U-100 syringe, and draw up 10 units of insulin, the correct dose will be accurately measured.

3. Route of administration for insulin is 90 degree angle with a SC needle. Specifics for insulin administration require that you (a) rotate your site for each injection, (b) give subcutaneously at 90 degree angle, (c) do not massage the injection site following administration, and (d) be certain that insulins are compatible before mixing together in the same syringe.

4. (a) Encourage her to attend diabetes education classes at local hospital or clinic. (b) Stress the importance of monitoring blood and urine for glucose levels. (c) Stress importance of adhering to the diet as prescribed by the physician. (d) Encourage her to engage in regular exercise.

Case Study 24-2

1. BSA of child = 0.74

$$\frac{0.74(m^2)}{1.7(m^2)} \times \text{adult dose} = \text{child's dose}$$

$$\frac{0.74}{1.7} \times \frac{400}{1} = \text{child's dose}$$

$$\frac{0.74}{1.7} \times \frac{400}{1} = \frac{400 \times 0.74}{1.7} =$$

$$\frac{296}{1.7} = 173.55 \text{ or } 174 \text{ mg}$$

2. $\dfrac{\text{Desired}}{\text{On Hand}} \times \text{quantity} = \text{dose}$

$$\frac{174 \text{ mg}}{400 \text{ mg}} \times 1 \text{ ml} = \text{dose}$$

0.44 ml to be administered

3. Give 0.44 ml of erythromycin 400 mg/ml subcutaneously into the vastus lateralis muscle at a 45° angle using a 23–25 gauge ⅝ inch needle.

Chapter 25   Electrocardiography

Case Study 25-1

1. Call emergency medical services—911—for transport to the hospital emergency room. Under Dr. Rice's direction, Wanda would prepare to administer oxygen and other medications as directed, frequently check blood pressure and pulse, place patient in Semi-Fowlers position, assist Dr. Rice as needed, comfort and reassure the patient, and perform CPR if necessary.

2. Wanda can explain (using either hand-drawn pictures or an anatomical model of the heart) the location of the coronary arteries on the myocardium of the heart and their significance as the major supplier of oxygenated blood to the heart itself. She could explain that the lining of the arteries build up with fatty deposits that harden over time and begin to block the flow of blood to the heart. Blood flow to the heart muscle is diminished (especially during periods of increased activity) and the heart's muscle tissue responds by symptoms of pain or pressure beneath the sternum into the neck, jaw, shoulder and/or throat. Rest usually relieves the pain of angina. Pain that does not subside may indicate a complete obstruction of the coronary arteries. No blood flow to nourish the heart muscle results in a heart attack, a much more serious situation that requires immediate medical attention.

Some strategies and healthy habits about which Wanda can remind Mrs. Johnson are (a) avoid tobacco, (b) take medications as prescribed, (c) report unusual symptoms or problems to Dr. Rice, (d) eat a low-fat, low-cholesterol, low-sodium diet, (e) exercise regularly with Dr. Rice's permission, (f) get adequate rest, (g) keep weight under control and at an acceptable level, (h) encourage family members to take a CPR course, and (i) practice stress reduction behaviors.

3. Some resources that can benefit Mrs. Johnson are:

- American Heart Association. Educational materials to learn about arteriosclerotic heart disease, and ways to prevent and manage it.

- American Diabetes Association. Educational materials and classes held in local clinics and hospitals regarding the relationship between diabetes and heart disease. Balance among exercise, diet, and insulin is stressed.

- American Dietetic Association. Educational materials on proper diet for diabetic control and prevention of further fatty deposits on artery linings of the heart.

- American Red Cross. Classes available to learn CPR. Patient and family members benefit from learning CPR in the event a patient suffers a myocardial infarction and goes into cardiac arrest.

- Weight control centers such as Weight Watchers® to learn healthy eating and exercise behaviors for weight reduction and control. Portion control, low-fat, low-sodium food choices are stressed.

- YWCA. Under Dr. Rice's direction, Mrs. Johnson could enroll in a regularly scheduled exercise class to strengthen her heart, lower blood cholesterol levels, and help reduce emotional stress. Yoga and/or meditation classes are also available for stress reduction.

Case Study 25-2

1. The symptoms that Mr. Matthews has been experiencing—palpitations, fast and slow heartbeats, and dizziness—are symptoms of cardiac arrhythmia. Since Mr. Matthews' resting ECG showed no evidence of arrhythmia, Dr. Abbott ordered a Holter monitor in order to record Mr. Matthews' cardiac activity for a 24-hour period. By going about his normal activities while wearing the monitor, should Mr. Matthews again experience similar symptoms, the monitor will pick up the abnormality.

2. Instructions to Mr. Matthews include:
   a. Keep a daily diary of all activities, symptoms, and emotions and note the time they occur.
   b. Do not shower or swim. The recording could be interrupted and the monitor damaged.
   c. Do not handle the electrodes. It could cause artifacts to occur.
   d. Do not remove recorder from its case.
   e. Do not use an electric blanket. It can cause interference, another artifact.
   f. Depress the event marker only briefly and when experiencing a significant symptom. Overuse of the marker can mask the ECG tracing.

3. Activities that should be recorded in the patient's diary include:
   a. Eating meals
   b. Sexual activity
   c. Medications taken
   d. Times of sleep
   e. Smoking
   f. Bowel movements
   g. Physical exercise

Chapter 27   Introduction to the Medical Laboratory

Case Study 27-1

1. No, because the accuracy of the test can be compromised by the patient not fasting.

2. Explain the purpose of the test and the importance of fasting to obtain accurate results. Give the patient written information about the diet. Have the patient repeat the instructions.

3. Perhaps enlist the help of a family member or friend.

Chapter 28   Phlebotomy: Venipuncture and Capillary Puncture

Case Study 28-1

1. Immediately remove the needle and stop the patient from falling. Lower the patient's head and arms. Wipe the patient's forehead and back of the neck with a cold compress if necessary. Pass an ammonia inhalant 4 to 5 inches away from the patient's nose. If the patient still does not respond, notify a physician, move the patient to the floor, and place a pillow under his legs.

2. Liz could have had Wayne lie down and used a pillow to help support his arm to keep it straight for easier venous access.

3. Take the time to ask patient about previous venipuncture experiences, put patient at ease, allay patient's fears, and persuade patient to allow blood to be drawn. Have patient assume the reclining position, which is best for apprehensive patients and patients who may faint.

Chapter 29   Hematology

Case Study 29-1

1. The test results may be affected in the following ways:

   - Falsely increased because of heat from incubator
   - Falsely increased because of vibrations from opening and closing the incubator door
   - Falsely increased due to heat from the sunlight
   - Falsely decreased due to low temperatures by the window during cool periods

2. Normal Westergren ESR values:

   - Males: 0–15 mm/hr.
   - Females: 0–20 mm/hr.

3. Test conditions should be controlled to avoid excessive heat or cold, drafts, and vibrations.

Chapter 30   Urinalysis

Case Study 30-1

1. To aid in the diagnosis of a urinary tract disorder. The presence of abnormal urine sediment cells and microorganisms can be determined when the specimen is examined microscopically.

2. Wanda should look for the presence of white blood cells, bacteria, yeast cells, or parasites.

3. WBC—report as cells per high-power field; e.g., 10/HPF; bacteria—report as few, moderate, many, loaded; yeast cells—report as amount per HPF; parasites—check with physician or someone else more familiar with these organisms before reporting.

Chapter 31   Basic Microbiology

Case Study 31-1

1. Possible reasons for a negative test: a good swab was not obtained, the sides of the mouth and tongue were swabbed by mistake; incorrect swab was used, could be cotton or contain a chemical that would interfere with the test; the test and materials were outdated; directions for the test were not followed; the child does not have strep throat.

2. A throat culture can be set up.

3. A proper throat culture is obtained by swabbing the back of the throat in the red area while trying to avoid the sides of the mouth and tongue. Set up a swab on a blood agar plate in CO_2 atmosphere.

Chapter 32   Specialty Laboratory Tests

Case Study 32-1

1. Anna should review the specific procedure in the office procedures manual to be sure she knows all aspects of the procedure. Anna should also let the office manager or one of the physicians know that she feels uncomfortable performing this procedure. They may be able to (1) review the procedure with Anna to give guidance and answer any specific questions; (2) they may actually accompany Anna while she does the procedure; or (3) they may perform the procedure with Anna attending. It is important to let your supervisor know of any concerns about performing clinical

procedures. Inadequate or inaccurate performance can cause risks to patients and to the practice.

2. If the practice is relying on Anna to perform all clinical duties, Anna may not be as valuable to the practice if she is unwilling to perform procedures expected of her, within the scope of her training. Rather than telling her supervisor that she is not capable or willing to do the procedure, however, Anna should let them know she does not feel confident she knows the procedure well enough to do it correctly and she should let her supervisor know that she is *willing* to try with help.

3. Anna could help make the procedure an effective one by:
   a. making sure all necessary equipment and supplies are on hand and within easy access;
   b. making sure she knows *why* the test is necessary so that she can accurately explain the procedure to the parents, especially if they have questions. If Anna knows answers to their questions she will feel more confident;
   c. requesting the parents' assistance to hold and reassure the baby as much as possible;
   d. using a steady, quick, and accurate motion when actually performing the heelstick; a slow stick of the lancet will cause more distress to the infant and will not produce a better sample;
   e. realize and expect that the infant will cry when the heelstick is performed. Anna should not be upset by this and she should also let the parents know this will happen so they are not upset.

Chapter 33 The Medical Assistant as Office Manager

Case Study 33-1

1. Answers will vary, but the groups should discuss and incorporate the teamwork approach to plan and implement a solution.

2. The team previously should have identified the resources available and met to brainstorm possible problems that could occur and what their solutions might be.

3. The office manager should remain calm and try to keep the argument from escalating. Other patients may be present as well; they should not be disturbed. One of the duties of the office manager is to supervise personnel, so she would want to be supportive of the staff while being understanding of the patients' feelings.

Case Study 33-2

1. Answers will vary, but pros may include that this management style communicates purpose and direction of tasks, solicits participation of others, inspires subordinates, encourages open communication, empowers others, serves as a role model, and is a continuous learner. Cons may include that she may be thought of as one who tattles to higher authorities.

2. Answers will vary.

3. Answers will vary.

Chapter 34 The Medical Assistant as Human Resources Manager

Case Study 34-1

1. Jane should be up-front with Bruce and state that it has been noticed that he frequently takes longer lunches than he is allotted. The two should work on an action plan to correct this situation, and a re-evaluation should be scheduled.

2. Although evaluations may involve more than the office manager or human resource manager and the employee, it probably would not be appropriate to involve the employee's peer or fellow worker. It may affect work relationships and cause hard feelings.

3. Jane should end the formal evaluation on a positive note by stating her confidence in the individual to make any changes necessary, offering assistance where needed, and thanking the employee for participating. End with a positive statement about some portion of the employee's performance.

Chapter 35 Preparing for Medical Assisting Credentials

Case Study 35-1

1. Juan must request the application from the AAMA Certification Department or the Program Coordinator and be sure to complete the correct application. Juan should read all the instructions carefully before completing the application form. The application must be free from errors and each item must be completed in full. The application must be postmarked by March 1 for him to be allowed to take the June examination.

2. Answers will vary, but here is one sample schedule:

March—Form study group. Contact people to see if they are interested. Set up a regular meeting time at least one time per week. Purchase study guides.

April—Increase study group meetings to two times per week. Begin to review course textbooks and tests.

May—Increase study group meetings to three times per week. Study independently two or three times per week also.

3. Juan should be careful to approach people he knows will take the examination seriously. He does not necessarily have to ask only those who are his friends.

Case Study 35-2

1. Nancy must be of good moral character and have graduated from an accredited high school or acceptable equivalent. Nancy must determine the appropriate requirement she satisfies and have been employed in the profession of medical assisting for a minimum of five years, no more than two years of which may have been as an instructor in a postsecondary medical assistant program.

2. Since most examinations may be scheduled within three days of application completion, Nancy should begin her study schedule several months prior to January to allow plenty of time to study each of the categories covered on the test.

3. Nancy should begin early to find a study partner(s). The study partner(s) should take the examination seriously and have a similar date in mind for sitting for the exam. The partner(s) should also agree to and be committed to the study schedule. Meeting once or twice a week helps keep the group focused. Independent study should be done throughout the week. During the independent study time, each group member could write 25 questions relevant to the weeks' study topic. When the group meets, a discussion of the study topic could take place and then copies of the questions distributed for answering. The questions could be corrected and discussion of any questionable or missed answers could take place.

Chapter 36   Employment Strategies

Case Study 36-1

1. The functional resume is probably the best resume style for Eun Mee to follow. The advantages of the functional style are that it allows areas of experience to be sorted into areas of function. This is useful when reentering the job market after an absence, when you have a variety of different, apparently unconnected work experiences, and when you have volunteer work experience.

2. Vital information should include full name, address including street number, city, state, and zip code, and telephone number including area code.

3. Accomplishment statements simply state your accomplishments and what you have done in previous employment settings. They are a way of tooting your own horn to help prospective employers realize your capabilities. Accomplishment statements should begin with power verbs and give a brief description of what you did and the demonstrable results that were produced. An example would be "During my experience as a sales representative, I serviced numerous customers who, as a result of my responsiveness to their needs, asked for me personally when they returned to the store for purchases."

Case Study 36-2

1. The candidate should bring an extra application, cover letter, resume, and reference sheet.

2. Arriving early will give Eun Mee time to collect her thoughts and become composed. It will also demonstrate good work habits to the employer: punctuality.

3. The candidate should wait patiently until the employer calls her in and wait for the employer's cues. The candidate should return a firm handshake and wait to be offered a seat.

GLOSSARY OF TERMS

abduction motion away from the midline of the body (Ch. 21).

ABO blood group genetically determined system of antigens found on the surface of erythrocytes. The population can be divided into four ABO blood groups: A, B, AB, and O (Ch. 32).

abortion expulsion of the products of conception before viability (Ch. 14).

abuse misuse; excessive or improper use, especially of narcotics or psychoactive drugs (Ch. 23).

accomplishment statements statements that begin with a power verb and give a brief description of what you did, and the demonstrable results that were produced (Ch. 36).

accreditation process whereby recognition is granted to an educational program for maintaining standards that qualify its graduates for professional practice; to provide with credentials (Ch. 1).

accredited recognized as being outstanding (Ch. 4).

Accrediting Bureau of Health Education Schools (ABHES) entity accrediting institutions for the American Medical Technologists (Ch. 35).

Acetest® product used to test for the presence of abnormal amounts of acetone (ketones) in urine (Ch. 30).

acetone colorless, inflammable liquid. Found in the blood and urine of diabetics as a result of the breakdown of fatty acids (Ch. 26).

acid/base balance condition that occurs when the net rate at which the body produces acids or bases is equal to the net rate at which acids or bases are excreted (Ch. 30).

acquired immunodeficiency syndrome (AIDS) disorder of the immune system caused by a human immunodeficiency virus (HIV), a retrovirus that destroys the body's ability to fight infection. As the disease progresses, the individual becomes overcome by disorders, including cancers and opportunistic infections. There is no known cure for AIDS (Ch. 6, 10).

active listening received message is paraphrased back to the sender to verify the correct message was decoded (Ch. 4).

activities of daily living (ADL) activities usually performed during a typical day that involve caring for oneself, such as eating and brushing teeth (Ch. 21).

acupuncture treatment to relieve pain and disease by puncturing the skin with thin needles at specific points (Ch. 2, 3).

additive any material placed in a tube that maintains or facilitates the integrity and function of the specimen (Ch. 28).

adduction motion toward the midline of the body (Ch. 21).

administer to give a medication (Ch. 23, 24).

aegis sponsorship or protection (Ch. 26).

aerobic organism that requires oxygen for growth (Ch. 31).

aerosols particles from potentially infectious materials that may be released in the air (Ch. 31).

afebrile without fever (Ch. 12).

agenda printed list of topics to be discussed during a meeting, sometimes giving time allocation (Ch. 33).

agent person representing another (Ch. 7).

agglutination antigen-antibody reaction in which a solid antigen clumps with a solid antibody (Ch. 32).

airborne transmission spread of disease-causing microorganisms over long distances through the air (Ch. 10).

akinesia absence or loss of voluntary muscle movement (Ch. 18).

alimentary canal digestive tract, made up of all the organs through which food passes throughout the body, from mouth to anus (Ch. 18).

aliquot part of the whole specimen that has been taken off for use or storage (Ch. 28).

allergy acquired hypersensitivity to a substance (allergen) that does not normally cause a reaction (Ch. 11, 19).

allied health professionals health care providers with a range of educational backgrounds and skills who support, complement, or assist physicians and who are a critical part of the health care team (Ch. 2).

allopathic   method of treating disease with remedies that produce effects different from those caused by the disease itself. Most traditional physicians today are considered allopathic physicians (Ch. 3).

alveoli   air sacs of the lungs that exchange carbon dioxide and oxygen (Ch. 18).

ambulation   ability to walk (Ch. 21).

ambulatory care setting   health care environment where services are provided on an outpatient basis. Ambulatory is from the Latin and means "capable of walking." Examples include the solo-physician's office, the group practice, the urgent care center, and the health maintenance organization (Ch. 1, 2).

American Association of Medical Assistants (AAMA)   premier organization dedicated to serving the interests of certified medical assistants (Ch. 35).

amino acid   basic structural unit of protein (Ch. 22).

amniocentesis   surgical puncture of the amniotic sac to remove fluid for laboratory analysis (Ch. 10, 14).

amoebic dysentery   infectious intestinal disease caused by amebas and characterized by inflammation of the mucous membrane of the colon (Ch. 10).

amorphous   shapeless; possessing no definite form (Ch. 30).

amplified   made larger or enlarged. The amplifier of the electrocardiograph enlarges the electrical impulse activity and the recording can be read more easily (Ch. 25).

amplitude   amount, extent, size abundance, or fullness (Ch. 25).

anaerobic   organism that needs little or no oxygen for growth (Ch. 31).

anaphylaxis   hypersensitive state of the body to a foreign protein or drug (Ch. 23).

ancillary services   professional occupational companies hired to complete a specific job (Ch. 33).

anesthesia   loss of feeling or sensation; an anesthetic is any mechanism that causes anesthesia (Ch. 19).

angiogram   series of X rays of a blood vessel(s) following injection of a radiopaque substance (Ch. 25).

anisocytosis   marked variation in the size of cells (Ch. 29).

anomaly   abnormality; marked deviation from normal (Ch. 14).

antagonistic   two entities that work against each other (Ch. 15).

antibacterial   capable of destroying bacteria, often applied to a wound in the form of an ointment or cream (Ch. 19).

antibody   specific chemical produced by B cells of the immune system in response to an antigen (Ch. 10, 32).

anticoagulant   chemical in a blood tube that prevents the clotting of the blood by removing the calcium from the blood or by stopping the formation of thrombin (Ch. 28).

antigen   substance such as bacteria or other agents that the body recognizes as foreign; the stimulus for antibody production (Ch. 10, 32).

antioxidant   something that prevents oxidation (Ch. 22).

antiserum   serum containing antibodies (Ch. 32).

aphasia   inability to communicate through speech or other methods. Often caused by brain dysfunction (Ch. 18).

apical   pertaining to the apex of the heart. A site for measuring heart rate with a stethoscope (Ch. 12).

apnea   cessation or absence of normal spontaneous breathing (Ch. 24).

appendicular skeleton   skeleton that consists of the pectoral and pelvic girdles and the upper and lower extremities. The pelvic girdle attaches the upper extremities to the trunk (Ch. 18).

application/cover letter   letter used to introduce yourself and your resume to a prospective employer with the goal of obtaining an interview (Ch. 36).

application form   form devised by a prospective employer to collect information relative to qualifications, education, and experience in employment (Ch. 36).

approximate   to bring together the edges of a wound (Ch. 19).

arrhythmia   deviation from the normal pattern or rhythm of the heartbeat (Ch. 12, 25).

arteriosclerosis   hardening of the arteries caused by buildup of plaque, a deposit of fatty substances on the artery lining (Ch. 17).

artifact   anything artificially produced (Ch. 25).

ascorbic acid   Vitamin C (Ch. 22).

asepsis   protecting against infection caused by pathogenic microorganisms (Ch. 3).

aseptic   freedom from any infectious material; absence of microorganisms (Ch. 18).

aspirate   to remove by suction (Ch. 10).

assay   analysis of a substance to determine constituents and relative proportion of each (Ch. 27).

assistive device   any device used to help patients to walk (Ch. 21).

asymptomatic   without symptoms (Ch. 27).

ataxia   defective muscular coordination, primarily seen when attempting voluntary muscular movements (Ch. 13).

atrophy   decrease in size or ability of a part of the body due to disease, inactivity, or other condition (Ch. 21).

attribute   inherent characteristic (Ch. 1).

augment   to add or increase (Ch. 25).

auricle   The external ear, also called pinna (Ch. 18).

axial skeleton   consists of bones that lie around the center of the body (Ch. 18).

baccalaureate   degree of bachelor conferred by colleges and universities (Ch. 1).

balance   amount owed (N); to verify posting accuracy (V) (Ch. 15).

bandage   nonsterile gauze or other material applied over a sterile dressing to protect and/or immobilize (Ch. 19).

barrier   obstacle that exists to protect an individual from contact with blood or other potentially infected materials. Called personal protective equipment (PPE), barriers include gloves, masks, face shields, laboratory coats, protective eyewear, and gowns (Ch. 10).

Bartholin gland   one of two small mucous glands located near the vaginal opening at base of labia majora (Ch. 14).

basal metabolic rate (BMR)   level of energy required when the body is at rest (Ch. 22).

baseline known or initial measurement against which future measurements are compared (Ch. 12, 27); also, flat, horizontal line that separates the various waves of the ECG cycle (Ch. 25).

basophil granulocytic white blood cell with dark purple cytoplasmic granules. It is the least common of the white blood cells (Ch. 29).

benchmark making a comparison among different organizations relative to how they accomplish tasks, such as office computerization, organizing file systems, and employee remuneration (Ch. 33).

benefit remuneration that is in addition to the salary (Ch. 33).

Betadine® brand of povidone-iodine solution used as a skin antiseptic. Betadine is also available in a scrub (soap) solution (Ch. 19).

bias slant toward a particular belief (Ch. 4).

bilirubin orange-yellow pigment that forms from the breakdown of hemoglobin in broken down red blood cells. Bilirubin usually travels in the bloodstream to the liver, where it is converted to a water-soluble form and is excreted into the bile (Ch. 30, 32).

biochemical tests tests that show biochemical properties and reactions of bacteria to achieve identification of microorganisms; often performed in solid and liquid media (Ch. 31).

bioethics branch of medical ethics concerned with moral issues resulting from high technology and sophisticated medical research. Social issues such as genetic engineering, abortion, and fetal tissue research raise important bioethical questions (Ch. 8).

biohazard material that has been in contact with body fluid and is capable of transmitting disease (Ch. 10).

biopsy removal of a small piece of living tissue from an organ or other part of the body for microscopic examination to confirm or establish a diagnosis (Ch. 27).

bipolar having two poles or processes (Ch. 25).

bloodborne means of transmission of an infectious disease (such as HIV and HBV) via human blood (Ch. 10).

bloodborne pathogen microorganism capable of causing disease found in blood or components of blood (Ch. 10).

blood urea nitrogen (BUN) nitrogen in the blood in the form of urea. The level of nitrogen in the blood is an indicator of kidney function (Ch. 22).

body fluid any secretion or excretion from the human body such as vaginal, cerebral-spinal, synovial, pleural, pericardial, peritoneal, amniotic, sputum, and saliva (Ch. 26).

body language nonverbal communication that includes unconscious body movements, gestures, and facial expressions that accompany verbal messages (Ch. 4).

body mechanics practice of using certain key muscle groups together with correct body alignment to avoid injury when lifting or moving heavy or awkward objects (Ch. 21).

body substance isolation (BSI) type of precaution developed by a hospital that requires special handling of all bodily fluids (Ch. 10).

bond binding agreement with an employee ensuring recovery of financial loss should funds be stolen or embezzled (Ch. 33).

bradycardia (sinus) slow (below 60 beats per minute), but regular heartbeat (Ch. 12, 25).

bradypnea abnormally slowed respiratory rate (Ch. 12).

brainstorming process of developing ideas through a synergistic interaction among participants in an environment free of criticism (Ch. 33).

Braxton-Hicks irregular, intermittent, and painless uterine contractions; also known as false labor (Ch. 14).

bronchi bifurcates from the trachea into each lung that terminate in the bronchial tubes (Ch. 18).

broth tubes tubes filled with a broth substance that will support the growth of certain microorganisms (Ch. 31).

bruits sound of venous or arterial origin heard on auscultation (Ch. 13).

BSA body surface area. A highly accurate method for calculating medication dosages for infants and children up to twelve years of age (Ch. 24).

bubonic plague infectious disease with a high fatality rate transmitted to humans from infected rats and ground squirrels by the bite of the rat flea (Ch. 3).

buccal relating to cheek or mouth (Ch. 23).

buffer words expendable words used while answering the telephone (Ch. 4).

buffy coat layer of white blood cells and platelets that forms at the interface between the plasma and red blood cells in a tube of blood containing an anticoagulant (Ch. 28).

bullet points asterisk or dot followed by a descriptive phrase; helps the reader identify important points easily (Ch. 36).

burnout a state of fatigue or frustration brought about by a devotion to a cause, a way of life, or a relationship that failed to produce the expected reward (Ch. 5).

calculi stones found in the urethra, bladder, ureters, or kidneys; an abnormality (Ch. 18).

calibration determination of the accuracy of an instrument by comparing the information provided with an accepted standard known to be accurate (Ch. 25, 26).

calorie unit of heat. The large Calorie (which is always capitalized) is used in discussion of human nutrition. The large Calorie is also expressed as the kilogram calorie (kcal), equal to 1,000 small calories (Ch. 22).

cannula the blunting member in a Bio-Plexus Punctur-Guard® needle (Ch. 28).

carbuncle necrotizing infection of skin and tissue composed of a cluster of boils (Ch. 18).

carcinoma in situ cancer that does not extend beyond the basement membrane (Ch. 14).

cardiac catheterization passage of a catheter into the heart through an arm or leg vein and blood vessels leading into the heart. The purpose is to obtain cardiac blood samples, detect abnormalities, and determine intracardiac pressure. Contrast medium can be injected and a coronary artery angiogram can be performed (Ch. 25).

cardiac cycle period from the beginning of one heartbeat to the beginning of the next succeeding beat, including systole and diastole. One complete heartbeat (Ch. 25).

cardiopulmonary resuscitation (CPR)   combination of rescue breathing and chest compressions performed by a trained individual on a patient experiencing cardiac arrest (Ch. 9).

cardioversion   conversion of a pathological cardiac rhythm (arrhythmia) such as ventricular fibrillation, to normal sinus rhythm (Ch. 25).

career objective   expresses your career goal and the position for which you are applying (Ch. 36).

career orientation objective   related to one's personal career goals or career growth (Ch. 28).

carotene   Vitamin A (Ch. 22).

carrier   person who harbors a pathogenic organism, and who is capable of transmitting the organism to others (Ch. 10).

casts   tiny structures usually formed by deposits of protein or other substances on the walls of renal tubules; in urine, they can indicate kidney disease (Ch. 30).

catalyst   substance that allows a chemical reaction to proceed at a much quicker rate and without as much energy input (Ch. 22).

catheterization   insertion of a catheter tube into the body for evacuating fluids or injecting fluids into body cavities. In urinary catheterization, the tube is inserted through the urethra into the bladder for withdrawal of urine (Ch. 13).

cautery   destruction of tissue by burning (Ch. 14, 19).

cell-mediated immunity   the regulatory activities of T cells during the specific immune response (Ch. 10).

cellulose   type of indigestible fiber made of carbohydrates found in plants (Ch. 22).

centrifugal hematology analysis   method of testing components of whole blood using centrifugation, fluorescent microscopy, and a micrometer (Ch. 29).

centrifuge   device that spins tubes using centrifugal force to separate the fluid portion of blood from the formed elements (Ch. 28).

certification   guarantees as being true or as represented by or as meeting a standard (Ch. 1, 35).

certification examination   standardized means of evaluating medical assistant competency (Ch. 35).

certified medical assistant (CMA)   a medical assistant who has successfully completed the AAMA's national certification examination and earned the status of being certified (Ch. 1, 35).

cervical punch biopsy   a biopsy of the uterine cervix using an instrument, the end of which is a punch (Ch. 14).

cesarean section   delivery of fetus through surgical incision into the uterus (Ch. 14).

charisma   personality and appearance characteristics that influence people to support the person possessing it; magnetism (Ch. 33).

chart   patient's file of medical history and treatment kept by the physician (Ch. 11).

check cell slides   important part of quality control testing, where preinoculated slides with known organisms are used to test whether or not a stain procedure yields correct results (Ch. 31).

chemotherapeutic agents   agents used in the treatment of diseases; the application of chemical reagents that are toxic to pathogenic microorganisms. Commonly used to describe agents (chemicals) used in the treatment of certain malignancies (Ch. 26).

Cheyne-Stokes   regular pattern of irregular breathing rate often seen in children or may be seen in brain dysfunction (Ch. 12).

chlamydia   a bacteria that causes the most prevalent sexually transmitted disease (Ch. 14).

cholecalciferol   Vitamin D (Ch. 22).

cholesterol   sterol lipid that is widely distributed in animal tissues. Cholesterol is produced in the liver and is a component of bile (Ch. 32).

choriocarcinoma   very rare malignant neoplasm, usually of the uterus or of an ectopic pregnancy. The exact cause is unknown (Ch. 32).

choroid layer   highly vascular membrane covering the posterior of the eye between the sclera and retina (Ch. 18).

chronological resume   resume format used when you have employment experience (Ch. 36).

circadian rhythm   pattern based on a 24-hour cycle emphasizing the repetition of certain physiologic phenomena such as eating and sleeping (Ch. 30).

circumduction   circular motion of a body part (Ch. 21).

civil law   law related to actions between individuals (Ch. 7).

claustrophobia   fear of being confined in any space (Ch. 20).

clinical chemistry   analysis and study of blood, body fluids, excreta, and tissues in the diagnosis and treatment of disease (Ch. 27).

clinical diagnosis   identification of a disease by history, lab studies, and symptoms (Ch. 11, 27).

Clinitest®   reagent tablet test that confirms the presence of reducing sugars in the urine (Ch. 30).

closed fracture   uncomplicated fracture in which the bone does not break the skin (Ch. 18).

closed questions   questions answered with a yes or no (Ch. 4).

clustering   grouping together of nonverbal messages into statements or conclusions (Ch. 4).

cobalamin   Vitamin B$_{12}$ (Ch. 22).

coenzyme   substance that enhances a catalyst (Ch. 22).

cognition   awareness with perception, reasoning, judgment, intuition, and memory (Ch. 17).

colonoscopy   visual examination of the colon with a lighted scope (Ch. 18).

colposcopy   visual examination of vaginal and cervical tissues using a colposcope following abnormal Pap smear. A magnifying lens and powerful lights are used (Ch. 14).

combination placement   externship completed in more than one facility (Ch. 28).

comedone   blackhead; usually the result of blocked sebaceous glands caused by acne (Ch. 18).

communicable   contagious. Capable of being transmitted from one person to another either directly or indirectly (Ch. 10, 26).

communication cycle   involves sending and receiving messages even when unconsciously aware of them (Ch. 4).

compensation   overemphasizing of characteristics to make up for a real or imagined failure or handicap (Ch. 4).

competency   legally qualified or adequate (Ch. 1).

complete blood count (CBC) battery of hematological tests consisting of hemoglobin, hematocrit, total white blood cell and red blood cell counts, differential white blood cell count, and the erythrocyte indices (Ch. 29).

compliance to act in accordance with conditions laid down (Ch. 1).

compounding combining two or more substances in definite proportions (Ch. 24).

concentration method method used in parasitology to identify parasites; consists of flotation and sedimentation methods (Ch. 31).

condenser directs the beam of light from the source to the specimen (Ch. 27).

conditions statements of the circumstances under which the objective will be achieved and with what supplies and equipment (Ch. 28).

condyloma a wart-like lesion of viral origin found on external genitalia or perianal region (Ch. 14).

conflict resolution solving problems between coworkers or any two parties (Ch. 24).

congenital being born with; existing at time of birth (Ch. 14).

congruency the verbal message and the nonverbal message must agree (Ch. 4).

constrict to become smaller in diameter (Ch. 28).

contact tracker form used to keep track of employment contact information such as name of employer, name of contact person, address and telephone number, date of first contact, resume sent, interview date, follow-up information, and dates (Ch. 36).

contact transmission spread of disease-causing microorganisms by directly or indirectly touching the source of the infection or by touching an object or environmental surface (Ch. 10).

contaminate to make something unclean; often used to describe a sterile area being made "unsterile" or exposing a clean area to a pathogenic substance (Ch. 10, 19).

continuing education units (CEU) method for earning points toward recertification (Ch. 35).

contracting acquiring an infection from pathogens (Ch. 10).

contracture fibrosis of connective tissue in skin, fascia, muscle, or joint that prevents normal mobility of the related tissue or joint (Ch. 21).

contraindication any symptom or circumstance that indicates that the use of a particular drug is inappropriate when it would otherwise be advisable. For example, the use of alcoholic beverages is a contraindication when the drug Flagyl® is prescribed (Ch. 23).

control test test of a sample of known results to be used to compare with the results of a patient's sample (Ch. 27).

Council on Accreditation of Allied Health Education Programs (CAAHEP) national, voluntary, specialized, not-for-profit corporation (Ch. 28).

countershock application of an electric current to the heart directly or indirectly in order to alter a disturbance in cardiac rhythm (Ch. 25).

counterstain stain that is used in a staining process after the initial staining has been applied and rinsed off with a decolorizer (Ch. 31).

coupling agent an agent used when ultrasonography is used; enhances penetration of sound waves through tissue (Ch. 14).

creatinine waste product formed in muscle that is excreted by the kidneys; elevated in blood and urine when kidney function is abnormal (Ch. 30).

credentialed testimonials showing that a person is entitled to credit or has a right to exercise official power (Ch. 1).

crepitation grating sound heard on movement of ends of a broken bone (Ch. 9).

criminal law law related to wrongs committed against the welfare and safety of society as a whole (Ch. 7).

criterion level of acceptable performance (Ch. 28).

critical values test results that indicate a potentially life-threatening or greatly debilitating situation that must be reported to the physician immediately (Ch. 30).

cryosurgery the destruction of tissue by application of extreme cold, silver nitrate, and carbon dioxide (Ch. 14).

cryotherapy use of cold to treat a physical condition (Ch. 21).

cryptorchidism undescended testicle (Ch. 26).

crystals found in normal urine sediment having no particular significance; a few should be noted as they may indicate disease states (Ch. 30).

culture social behavior patterns and beliefs (Ch. 6).

cultures microorganisms cultivated in a nutrient medium (Ch. 30, 31).

Cushing's syndrome hypersecretion of the adrenal cortex producing excessive glucocorticoids. The condition may be due to a tumor or hyperfunction of the anterior pituitary (Ch. 32).

cyanmethemoglobin stable hemoglobin compound used to measure concentration of blood hemoglobin (Ch. 29).

cyanosis discoloration of the skin due to abnormal amounts of reduced hemoglobin in the blood caused by decreased oxygen and increased carbon dioxide in the blood (Ch. 13).

cystitis inflammation of the bladder (Ch. 17).

cytology science that deals with the formation, structure, and function of cells (Ch. 27).

cytoscopy visual examination of the urethra and bladder following insertion of a cytoscope, a lighted scope especially designed for the examination of these areas (Ch. 18).

debridement removal of dead or damaged tissue or foreign debris (Ch. 11).

declination form written formal refusal (Ch. 10).

decode to translate into language that is easily understood; to interpret (Ch. 4).

decolorizer substance used to remove the first stain applied in a differential staining process (Ch. 31).

defendant person who defends action brought in litigation (Ch. 7).

defense mechanism behavior that protects the psyche from guilt, anxiety, or shame (Ch. 4).

defibrillation stopping fibrillation of the heart by use of drugs or by physical means (Ch. 25).

defibrillator a machine that delivers an electric current in order to alter a disturbance in cardiac rhythm (Ch. 25).

dementia   impairment of intellectual function that is progressive and interferes with normal activities (Ch. 6, 27).

demyelination   destruction of the nerve fibers; often a factor in multiple sclerosis (Ch. 18).

denial   rejection of or refusal to acknowledge (Ch. 4).

deoxygenated   blood that is high in carbon dioxide, low in oxygen, and pumped through the heart to the lungs where the carbon dioxide is exchanged for oxygen (Ch. 25).

depolarize   process of reducing to a nonpolarized condition. Generation of an electrical current is enhanced. Electrical activity generated when the atria or ventricles contract (Ch. 25).

dermatitis   inflammation of the skin characterized by redness, itching, and skin lesions (Ch. 10).

dermatophytes   category of fungi causing infections of hair, skin, and nails (Ch. 31).

diabetes mellitus   chronic disorder of carbohydrate metabolism characterized by hyperglycemia and resulting from inadequate production or utilization of insulin (Ch. 22).

diagnosis   determination of disease or condition (Ch. 27).

diaphragm   a lens or other object that opens and closes to increase or decrease the amount of light on the object being illuminated (Ch. 27).

diastole   one component of blood pressure measurement representing the lowest amount of pressure exerted during the cardiac cycle; the force exerted on the arterial walls during cardiac relaxation (Ch. 12, 25).

differential diagnosis   diagnosis based on comparison of symptoms of similar diseases (Ch. 27).

digestion   breaking down of food into smaller particles. It can be either physical or chemical (Ch. 22).

dilate   to enlarge in diameter (Ch. 28).

dilation   expansion of an orifice or organ (Ch. 14).

disinfection   use of chemicals or boiling water to free an item from infectious materials but not their spores (Ch. 10).

dislocation   displacement of a bone or joint from its normal position (Ch. 18).

dispense   prepare and give out a medication to be taken at a later time (Ch. 23, 24).

displacement   displacing negative feelings onto something or someone else with no significance to the situation (Ch. 4).

disposition   temperament, character, personality (Ch. 1).

diuretic   substance that causes less water to be reabsorbed by the kidney, and therefore causes water to be excreted from the body (Ch. 22).

DNA   deoxyribonucleic acid; important nucleus material that carries genetic codes (Ch. 31).

doctrine   principle of law established through past decisions (Ch. 7).

documentation   providing factual support through written information (Ch. 10).

dorsiflexion   moving the foot upward at the ankle joint (Ch. 21).

dosimeter   a device for measuring X-ray output (Ch. 20).

dressing   sterile gauze or other material applied directly to a wound to absorb secretions and to protect (Ch. 19).

droplet transmission   method of spreading disease from respiratory secretions through the air. Spread is usually confined to within three feet of the infected patient (Ch. 10).

durable power of attorney for health care   legal form that allows a designated person to act on another's behalf in regard to health care choices (Ch. 6, 7).

dysmenorrhea   painful menses (Ch. 14).

dyspareunia   painful intercourse (Ch. 14).

dysplasia   abnormal development of tissue (Ch. 14).

dyspnea   shortness of breath or labored/difficult breathing (Ch. 12).

dysuria   painful or difficult urination (Ch. 18).

echocardiography   noninvasive diagnostic method that uses ultrasound to visualize internal cardiac structure, including valves (Ch. 20).

eclampsia   complication of pregnancy that includes general edema, hypertension, proteinuria, and convulsions (Ch. 14).

ectopic pregnancy   pregnancy outside the uterus (Ch. 14, 32).

edematous   abnormal accumulation of fluid in the tissues resulting in swelling (Ch. 28).

educational history   listing of places of learning and degrees or certificates earned (Ch. 24).

effacement   thinning and shortening of the cervical canal during labor to permit passage of fetus (Ch. 14).

electrocardiogram   record of the electrical activity of the heart; showing P, QRS, and T waves (Ch. 25).

electrocardiograph   instrument for recording the electrical activity of the heart (Ch. 25).

electrocardiography   process of recording the electrical activity originating in the heart (Ch. 25).

electrode   also known as a sensor. Used to conduct electricity from the body to the electrocardiograph (Ch. 25).

electrolyte   conductor of electricity whose components are important in maintaining fluid and acid-base balance (Ch. 22, 25, 27).

elimination   removal of fecal waste from the body through the anus (Ch. 15).

emaciation   state of being extremely lean (Ch. 18).

emancipated minor   persons under age 18 who are financially responsible for themselves and free of parental care (Ch. 7).

embezzle   to appropriate fraudulently to one's own use (Ch. 33).

Emergency Medical Services (EMS)   Emergency Medical Services (EMS) system is a local network of police, fire, and medical personnel trained to respond to emergency situations. In many communities the system is activated by calling 911 (Ch. 9).

empathy   ability to be objectively aware of and have insight into another's feelings, emotions, and behaviors, and to be aware of the significance and meaning of these to the other person (Ch. 1, 17).

emphysema   chronic pulmonary disease characterized by dilated and damaged alveoli (Ch. 12).

emulate   imitate a characteristic of an individual in order to equal or surpass the original (Ch. 33).

encode (encoding)   creating a message to be sent (Ch. 4).

endometriosis tissue that resembles the endometrium invades various locations in the pelvic cavity and elsewhere (Ch. 14).

endoscopy visual examination of body cavities with a lighted scope (Ch. 10, 18).

engineering controls physical or mechanical devices that isolate or remove health hazards from the workplace (Ch. 10).

enterobacteriaceae family of bacteria that contains genuses that are nonpathogenic and pathogenic to the intestinal and urinary tract (Ch. 31).

eosinophil granulocytic white blood cell with red eosin stained granules in the cytoplasm. It is elevated in cases of allergies (Ch. 29).

epidemiology field of science that studies the history, cause, and patterns of infectious diseases (Ch. 10).

epinephrine hormone also known as adrenaline. Epinephrine is manufactured as a chemical (pharmaceutical preparation) and is often mixed with local anesthetics for use as a vasoconstrictor in minor surgery (Ch. 19).

epistaxis nosebleed (Ch. 10).

Epstein-Barr virus (EBV) virus that is believed to be the cause of infectious mononucleosis and is implicated in such conditions as African Burkitt's lymphoma and nasopharyngeal carcinoma (Ch. 22).

equilibrium state of balance between opposing forces (Ch. 18).

erosion an eating away of tissue (Ch. 18).

erythema redness or inflammation of the skin or mucous membranes that is the result of dilatation and congestion of superficial capillaries (Ch. 18).

erythrocyte red blood cell, one of the formed elements of the blood (Ch. 28, 29).

erythrocyte indices three equations that provide information about the sizes and hemoglobin content of red blood cells. These include the MCV, MCH, and MCHC (Ch. 29).

erythrocyte sedimentation rate measurement of how far the red cells in a sample of blood fall in one hour (Ch. 29).

erythropoietin hormone that causes production of new red blood cells (Ch. 29).

esophageal varices tortuous dilation of the esophageal vein associated with any condition that causes obstruction of drainage from the esophageal veins into the portal vein of the liver. Seen in cirrhosis of the liver and alcoholism (Ch. 20).

ethics defined in terms of what is morally right and wrong; ethics will differ from person to person; often defined by a code or creed as in the Code of Ethics from the American Association of Medical Assistants (AAMA) (Ch. 8).

ethyl alcohol alcohol, used to make a solution (Ch. 26).

eupnea normal breathing (Ch. 12).

evaluation assessment; significance or value of a situation (Ch. 18); also, assessment of an employee's job performance (Ch. 34).

eversion moving a body part outward (Ch. 21).

excoriated abrasion of the epidermis by trauma, chemicals, burns, or other causes (Ch. 10).

excretion waste matter. The elimination of waste products from the body (Ch. 10, 26).

exit interview opportunity for departing employees to provide their positive and negative opinions of the position and facility (Ch. 34).

expectorate to bring up material from the lungs (Ch. 31).

expert witness individual with highly specialized knowledge and skills in a particular area who testifies to a standard of care (Ch. 7).

expressed contract written or verbal contract that specifically describes what each party in the contract will do (Ch. 7).

extension straightening of a body part (Ch. 21).

external respiration ventilation of the lungs when the exchange of oxygen and carbon dioxide takes place (Ch. 18).

externship transition stage between the classroom and actual employment; may also be referred to as internship or practicum (Ch. 1, 33).

extracellular pertaining to the environment outside of a body cell (Ch. 22).

exudate accumulated fluid in a cavity; an oozing of pus (Ch. 15, 19).

facial expressions various aspects of facial anatomy that send nonverbal messages (Ch. 4).

facilitate to make an action or process easier (Ch. 1).

fastidious bacteria bacteria that require a specialized medium to grow and multiply (Ch. 31).

fat-soluble pertaining to substances that are hydrophobic and therefore dissolve better in fat (Ch. 22).

febrile having a fever (Ch. 12).

Federal Register federal government agency from which written CLIA '88 documents may be obtained (Ch. 26).

feedback receiver's way of ensuring that the message that was understood is the same as the message that was sent (Ch. 4).

fenestrated drape a type of drape with an opening, usually round, that can be placed with the opening over a particular body area; used in surgery and for proctological exams (Ch. 13).

first aid immediate (or first) care provided to persons who are suddenly ill or injured; first aid is typically followed by more comprehensive care and treatment (Ch. 9).

flexion bending of a body part (Ch. 21).

fluoroscope a device consisting of a screen; mounts separately or with an X-ray tube that shows the images of objects interposed between the table and the screen (Ch. 20).

folic acid one of the B-complex vitamins (Ch. 22).

fomite substance that absorbs and transmit infectious material, e.g., contaminated items such as equipment (Ch. 10).

forensic pertaining to the law (Ch. 26).

formaldehyde colorless gas combined with methanol and used as a solution, such as a disinfectant, astringent, or a preservative for histologic specimen (Ch. 26).

fractures break in a bone. There are several types of fractures, but all are classified as either open fractures or closed fractures (Ch. 9).

frenulum of the tongue, a fold of mucus membrane located under the tongue attaching the tongue to the floor of the mouth (Ch. 12).

frequency   urinating frequently (Ch. 18).

friable   easily broken (Ch. 19).

fringe benefit   benefit above and beyond salary to which an employee may be entitled. Examples include health and life insurance, paid vacation, sick days, personal days, and tuition reimbursement for courses related to employment (Ch. 2, 33).

fulgaration   destruction by electric current (Ch. 14).

fume hood   type of hood or barrier used in the laboratory to capture chemical vapors and fumes and move them away from health care workers and into a building's exhaust fan system (Ch. 26).

functional resume   resume format used to highlight specialty areas of accomplishment and strengths (Ch. 36).

furuncle   localized, suppurative staphylococcal skin infection originating in a gland or hair follicle (Ch. 18).

gait   manner or style of walking including rhythm and speed (Ch. 21).

gait belt   safety belt worn by the patient around the waist that provides a firm handhold for the caregiver when transferring the patient or when assisting in ambulation (Ch. 21).

galvonometer   mechanism in the electrocardiograph that changes the voltage into a mechanical motion for recording purposes (Ch. 25).

genetic engineering   alteration, manipulation, replacement, or repair of genetic material (Ch. 8).

genitalia   the reproductive organs, internal and external (Ch. 14).

genus   first Greek or Latin name given to a microorganism; always capitalized (Ch. 31).

geriatrics   the branch of medicine concerned with the problems of aging (Ch. 17).

gerontology   the scientific study of the problems associated with aging (Ch. 17).

gestation   period of development from fertilization to birth (Ch. 14).

gestures/mannerisms   movement of various body parts while communicating (Ch. 4).

glucose   simple sugar that is a major source of energy in the human body; monitoring of blood glucose levels in urine and blood is a vital diagnostic test in diabetes and other disorders; also a test on a reagent strip (Ch. 27, 30).

glycogen   carbohydrate form used for storage of sugar in the body (Ch. 22).

goal   result or achievement toward which effort is directed (Ch. 5).

"going bare"   said of a physician who does not carry professional liability insurance (Ch. 33).

goniometer   instrument used to measure the angle of a joint's range of motion (Ch. 18, 21).

goniometry   measurement of joint motion (Ch. 21).

Gram stain   most common stain used in microbiology to observe gross morphological features of bacteria; a differential stain, allowing differentiation between Gram-negative and Gram-positive organisms (Ch. 31).

gravidy   total number of pregnancies a woman has had regardless of duration, including a present one (Ch. 14).

guaiac   used to test for occult blood in feces (Ch. 18).

Guthrie screening test   diagnostic test for the detection of phenylketonuria (PKU) (Ch. 32).

health maintenance organization (HMO)   type of managed care operation that is typically set up as a for-profit corporation with salaried employees. HMOs "with walls" offer a range of medical services under one roof; HMOs "without walls" typically contract with physicians in the community to provide patient services for an agreed-upon fee (Ch. 2).

Heimlich maneuver   abdominal thrusts designed to overcome breathing difficulties in patients who are choking (Ch. 9).

hemacytometer (also spelled hemocytometer)   precisely etched glass slide and coverslip used as a counting chamber for blood cells (Ch. 29).

hematemesis   vomiting blood (Ch. 18).

hematochezia   presence of bright red blood in feces (Ch. 18).

hematocrit   percentage of red blood cells within a specimen of anticoagulated whole blood (Ch. 29).

hematology   study of blood and the blood-forming tissues (Ch. 27, 29).

hematoma   accumulation of blood around the venipuncture site during or after venipuncture caused by the leakage of blood from where the needle punctured the vein (Ch. 18, 21, 28).

hematuria   abnormal presence of blood in urine, symptomatic of many disorders of the genitourinary system and renal diseases (Ch. 18, 30).

hemiplegia   paralysis of one side of the body (Ch. 21).

hemoconcentration   pooling of blood at the location of the venipuncture caused by leaving the tourniquet on the arm longer than one minute, resulting in inaccurate blood samples (Ch. 28).

hemoglobin   molecule with the red blood cell that transports oxygen (Ch. 29).

hemoglobinopathy   inherited disease resulting from the formation of an abnormal hemoglobin molecule (Ch. 29).

hemolysis   rupturing of the red blood cells during the process of blood collection. The serum or plasma becomes contaminated and has a reddish color (Ch. 28).

hemolytic anemia   anemia due to lysis of RBC (Ch. 32).

hemophilia   hereditary blood disease characterized by the blood's failure to clot, causing abnormal bleeding (Ch. 8).

hematopoiesis   formation of blood cells (Ch. 29).

heterophile antibody   antibody that reacts with other than the specific antigens as seen in infectious mononucleosis (Ch. 32).

Hibeclens®   brand of antiseptic soap solution (Ch. 19).

hierarchy   the order of significance or control; ranking of importance (Ch. 33).

hierarchy of needs   needs that are arranged in a specific order or rank; sequential arrangement. Associated with Abraham Maslow (Ch. 4).

high-density lipoprotein (HDL)   lipoprotein in the blood composed primarily of protein; removes cholesterol from peripheral tissues and transports them to the liver for excretion (Ch. 32).

histology   study of biopsied tissue samples for the determination of disease (Ch. 27).

holding media specific media used in the transport of microorganisms to support the life of the organisms until they can be put on nutrient medium in the laboratory (Ch. 31).

holistic in medicine, used to identify a specific approach that treats the "whole" body, mind, and spirit (Ch. 2).

homeostasis state of equilibrium of internal environment (Ch. 22).

hospital-based laboratories hospital-owned labs which perform most tests required by the hospital and local communities (Ch. 27).

human chorionic gonadotrophin (HCG) hormone secreted by the trophoblast after fertilization of the ovum. It may be detected in the blood and urine of pregnant women (Ch. 14, 32).

human immunodeficiency virus (HIV) AIDS virus; it is a retrovirus that ultimately destroys immune system cells (Ch. 6, 10).

human relations objectives relate to improving communication and interpersonal skills (Ch. 28).

humoral immunity immunity mediated by antibodies in body fluids such as plasma and lymph (Ch. 10).

hyaline transparent, clear; hyaline casts are transparent and often hard to see in urine (Ch. 30).

hydatidiform mole development of cysts and rapid growth of the uterus with bleeding (Ch. 32).

hydrogen peroxide antibacterial solution that has a mechanical cleansing action (Ch. 19).

hydronephrosis collection of urine in renal pelvis. This is caused by an obstruction and may result in a cyst. (Ch. 18).

hyperemesis gravidarum severe nausea and vomiting during pregnancy with inability to eat; may lead to severe dehydration (Ch. 14).

hyperextension position of maximum extension, or extending a body part beyond its normal limits (Ch. 21).

hyperglycemia increased levels of blood glucose. Hyperglycemia does not necessarily mean that the patient is diabetic but may be an indication of prediabetes (Ch. 22).

hyperpnea increased respiratory rate and depth as seen in exercise pain, fever, and hysteria (Ch. 12).

hypertension blood pressure that is consistently above 140/90 (Ch. 12).

hyperthermia body temperature above normal range; an unusually high fever (Ch. 17).

hyperventilation ventilation rate that is greater than metabolically necessary, potentially leading to alkalosis (Ch. 12).

hypochromic less color than normal (Ch. 29).

hypoglycemia state of having a lower than normal blood glucose level (Ch. 28, 32).

hypotension abnormally low blood pressure resulting in inadequate tissue profusion and oxygenation (Ch. 12).

hypothermia extremely dangerous cold-related condition that can result in death if the individual does not receive care and if the progression of hypothermia is not reversed. Symptoms include shivering, cold skin, and confusion (Ch. 9, 17).

hypoventilation decrease in respiration rate with shallow depth of respiration (Ch. 12).

hypoxemia lack of oxygen in the blood (Ch. 24).

hysterosalpingogram x-ray of uterus and fallopian tubes using a contrast medium (Ch. 14).

Ictotest® confirmatory test for bilirubin (Ch. 30).

immune system body's strong line of defense against invading microorganisms. The body recognizes foreign substances such as microorganisms and produces substances to fight them off. Antibodies, white blood cells, digestive enzymes, and resistance of the skin are some examples (Ch. 10).

immunity ability of the body to resist specific pathogens and their toxins (Ch. 10).

immunoassay measurement of reaction of antigen with specific antibody (Ch. 32).

immunoglobulins family of proteins capable of acting as antibodies, thereby protecting individuals from pathogenic microorganisms; also, antibodies produced by the cells of the immune system (Ch. 10).

immunohematology study of blood group antigens and antibodies; blood banking (Ch. 27).

immunology the study of the components of the immune system and their function (Ch. 27).

immunosuppressed referring to a patient whose immune system is unhealthy due to disease, medication, genetics, and so on; these patients can be particularly susceptible to attack by microorganisms (Ch. 10, 31).

impedance principle method employed in hematology instrumentation that uses a diluted sample to measure resistance of an electrical current to formed elements in the blood (Ch. 29).

implied consent consent assumed by the health care provider, typically in an emergency that threatens the patient's life. Implied consent also occurs in more subtle ways in the health care environment; e.g., when a patient willingly rolls up the sleeve to receive an injection (Ch. 7).

implied contract contract indicated by actions rather than words (Ch. 7).

improvise to make, invent, or arrange in an offhand manner (Ch. 1).

incinerate to destroy by fire (Ch. 10).

incompetence legally, a person who is insane, inadequate, or not an adult (Ch. 7).

incontinence uncontrollable loss of urine (Ch. 17).

independent physician association (IPA) independent network of physicians in private practice who contract with the association to treat patients for an agreed-upon fee (Ch. 2).

indirect statements means of eliciting a response from a patient by turning a question into a statement of interest (Ch. 4).

infarction area of tissue in an organ or part that becomes necrotic (dead) following cessation of blood supply (Ch. 25).

infection invasion of pathogens into living tissue (Ch. 19).

infection control methods to eliminate or reduce the transmission of infectious microorganisms (Ch. 10).

infectious agent pathogen responsible for a specific infectious disease (Ch. 10).

infectious mononucleosis acute infectious disease primarily affecting the lymphoid tissue caused by the Epstein-Barr virus (Ch. 32).

infectious waste items that have come in contact with patient blood and/or body fluids. Contaminated items (Ch. 10).

inflammatory response body's defense against the threat of infection or trauma. Characterized by redness, pain, heat, and swelling (Ch. 10, 19).

informed consent consent given by the patient who is made aware of any procedure to be performed, its risks, expected outcomes, and alternatives (Ch. 7, 19).

ingestion taking in of food, drugs, etc. into the body by mouth (Ch. 18).

inner-directed people people who decide for themselves what they want to do with their lives (Ch. 5).

inoculate to place colonies of microorganisms onto nutrient media (Ch. 31).

insulin hormone secreted by beta cells of the islets of Langerhans of the pancreas essential for the proper metabolism of glucose (Ch. 32).

integrate to incorporate into a larger unit; to form or blend into a whole (Ch. 1).

integrative medicine bringing together of two or more treatment modalities so they function as a harmonious whole; as seen in alternative forms of health care (Ch. 2).

integrity normal structure without damage (Ch. 28).

internal respiration passage of oxygen from the blood into the cells (Ch. 18).

Internet worldwide computer network available via modem that connects universities, government laboratories, companies, and individuals around the world (Ch. 33).

internship transition stage between classroom and employment (Ch. 1).

interview meeting in which you and the interviewer discuss employment opportunities and strengths you can contribute to the organization (Ch. 36).

interview techniques methods of encouraging the best communication between professionals and the patient (Ch. 4).

intravenous pyelogram X-ray studies of the kidneys, ureters, and bladder using a contrast medium (Ch. 16).

introjection identification with another person or with some object (Ch. 4).

invasive procedure surgical technique or procedure that penetrates healthy tissue. The potential for pathogenic microorganisms to enter the body exists (Ch. 10, 27).

inversion moving a body part inward (Ch. 21).

involuntary dismissal termination of employment based on poor job performance or violation of office policies (Ch. 34).

involution return of the uterus to normal size and shape after childbirth (Ch. 14).

ionizing radiation X-ray beams (Ch. 20).

ischemia local and temporary lack of blood to an organ or part due to obstruction of circulation (Ch. 25).

isoelectric having equal electrical potentials. It is represented on the ECG as the flat horizontal line, the baseline (Ch. 25).

isolation separating a patient with certain infections or communicable diseases from other individuals (Ch. 10).

isolation categories system of seven categories developed by the Centers for Disease Control (CDC) that isolates patients according to known infections. These categories have been condensed into three transmission-based precautions based on air, contact, and droplet routes of transmission (Ch. 10).

isopropyl alcohol 70 percent alcohol solution commonly used as a disinfectant (Ch. 19).

itinerary detailed written plan of a proposed trip (Ch. 33).

jaundice yellow discolorization of the skin and sclera caused by excess bilirubin in the blood (Ch. 10, 13).

job description outline of tasks, duties, and responsibilities for every position in the office (Ch. 34).

ketoacidosis accumulation of ketones in the body, occurring primarily as a complication of diabetes mellitus; if left untreated, it could cause coma (Ch. 30).

ketone chemical compound produced during an increased metabolism of fat; also, test on a reagent strip (Ch. 30).

kinesics study of body language (Ch. 4).

Kirby Bauer manual sensitivity test involving streaking a plate of media with an isolated organism and applying antibiotic disks; the plate is later read to discern which antibiotics will destroy the organism (Ch. 31).

kit commercially packaged materials needed to perform laboratory tests (Ch. 26).

kwashiorkor severe protein deficiency in infants and children (Ch. 22).

labyrinthitis inflammation of inner ear or labyrinth (Ch. 9, 13).

lackluster dull, lacking in sheen (Ch. 9).

Lamaze technique consisting of breathing exercises to facilitate delivery (Ch. 14).

latex beads tiny latex beads coated with antibodies or antigens that react with antigens or antibodies in the test sample in an agglutination reaction. The latex beads may be colored to make the reaction easier to visualize (Ch. 32).

lead a conductor attached to an electrocardiograph. Consists of limb leads and chest leads (Ch. 25).

lesion injury or wound. A circumscribed area of tissue that has been altered pathologically (Ch. 10, 18).

letter of reference letter usually written by an employee's past employer describing the employee's performance, attitude, or qualifications. This letter is presented to a potential employer when applying for a new job (Ch. 34).

letter of resignation letter informing the current employer of the employee's decision to resign from a current position (Ch. 34).

leukocyte white blood cell, one of the formed elements of blood (Ch. 28, 29).

leukocyte esterase test on a reagent strip that indicates the presence of white blood cells in the urinary tract (Ch. 30).

leukorrhea whitish or yellowish mucous discharged from the cervical canal or vagina. Usually normal unless there is an increase in amount or variation in color (Ch. 10).

liability   legal responsibility (Ch. 33).

libel   false and malicious writing about another constituting a defamation of character (Ch. 7).

libido   sexual drive (Ch. 6).

license   permission by competent authority (the state) to engage in a profession; permission to act (Ch. 1).

licensure   granting of licenses to practice a profession (Ch. 1).

ligature   length of suture thread without a needle, used for tying off vessels during surgery (Ch. 19).

lipemia   excessive amount of fat (lipids) in the blood, resulting in a blood sample that has a milky appearance (Ch. 28).

liquid nitrogen   commonly and incorrectly referred to as dry ice, liquid nitrogen is a very volatile freezing agent used to destroy unwanted tissue such as warts (Ch. 19).

litigation   court action (Ch. 7).

litigious   prone to engage in lawsuits (Ch. 1).

living will   document allowing a person to make choices related to treatment in a life-threatening illness (Ch. 6).

lochia   discharge from the uterus of blood, mucus, and tissue during the period following childbirth (Ch. 10, 14).

long-range goals   achievements that may take three to five years to accomplish (Ch. 5).

low-density lipoprotein (LDL)   lipoprotein in the blood composed primarily of cholesterol. The cholesterol carried by LDL may be deposited in peripheral tissues and is associated with an increased risk of heart disease (Ch. 32).

luer   device that screws into an evacuated tube holder. The part inside the holder has a needle to puncture the tube top, the part outside the holder fits into a tubing port (Ch. 28).

lumbar puncture   surgical puncture of the lumbar area of the intervertebral spaces to aspirate cerebrospinal fluid for laboratory analysis (Ch. 10, 31).

lymphocyte   white blood cell with a dense non-segmented nucleus and lacking granules in the cytoplasm (Ch. 29).

macrocytic   term which describes a larger than normal cell (Ch. 29).

macular degeneration   degeneration of the macula area of the retina caused by aging; a leading cause of visual impairment in people over 50, making it difficult to do fine work (Ch. 17).

major mineral   mineral that is required in large amounts by the body (Ch. 22).

malabsorption   inadequate absorption of nutrients from the intestinal tract (Ch. 18).

malaise   discomfort, uneasiness, or indisposition, often indicative of infection (Ch. 18).

malaria   acute infectious disease caused by the presence of protozoan parasites within the red blood cells; usually comes from the bite of a female mosquito (Ch. 10).

malpractice   professional negligence (Ch. 7, 33).

managed care   strategies designed to reduce the cost of health care by managing an insured's health care benefits (Ch. 2).

managed care operation   any health care setting or delivery system that is designed to reduce the cost of care while still providing access to care (Ch. 2).

managed competition   medical care in which physicians and hospitals compete for patients (Ch. 2).

mandate   formal order to obey certain rules and regulations (Ch. 7, 26).

Mantoux test   test for tuberculosis involving the intracutaneous injection of PPD (Ch. 32).

marasmus   protein-calorie malnutrition seen in first year of life (Ch. 22).

marketing   process by which the provider of services makes the consumer aware of the scope and quality of those services. Marketing tools might include public relations, brochures, patient education seminars, and newsletters (Ch. 33).

masking   attempt to conceal or repress true feelings or the message (Ch. 4).

Mayo stand/instrument tray   portable metal tray table used for setting up small sterile fields for minor surgery and procedures (Ch. 19).

medical asepsis   clean and free from infection (Ch. 10, 26).

melena   tarry stools due to blood in feces (Ch. 18).

meniscus   curvature appearing in a liquid's upper surface when a liquid is placed in a container (Ch. 24, 30).

menses   menstruation (Ch. 10).

mentor   person assigned or requested to assist in training, guiding, or coaching another (Ch. 34).

message   content being communicated (Ch. 4).

metabolism   total of all changes, chemical and physical, that take place in the body (Ch. 22).

microbiology   branch of biology dealing with the study of microscopic forms of life (Ch. 27, 31).

microcyctic   term describing a smaller than normal cell (Ch. 29).

microorganism   microscopic living creature capable of transmission and reproduction in specific circumstances (Ch. 10).

microscopy   inspection with a microscope (Ch. 26).

midstream collection   urine sample collected in the middle of a flow of urine (Ch. 30).

minor   person who has not reached the age of majority, usually 18 years (Ch. 7).

minutes   written record of topics discussed and actions taken during meeting sessions (Ch. 33).

modalities   physical agents such as heat, cold, light, water, and electricity used to treat muscular or joint malfunction (Ch. 21).

modes of communication   speaking, listening, gestures, or body language, and writing. Also called channels of communication (Ch. 4).

monocyte   white blood cell without cytoplasmic granules that has a large convoluted non-segmented nucleus (Ch. 29).

morbidity   number of cases of disease in a specific population (Ch. 10).

mordant   substance that causes dye to adhere to an object; iodine is a mordant in Gram stain (Ch. 31).

morphology   form and structure of an organism (Ch. 31).

mortality   the ratio of the number of deaths to a given population (Ch. 10).

mounting   process of applying in sequence a portion of each of the twelve leads of the ECG recording onto a commercially prepared mounting form or plain sheet of paper as part of the patient's permanent record (Ch. 25).

moxibustion   ancient Chinese method of treatment that uses a powdered plant substance on the skin to raise a blister (Ch. 3).

multigravida   a woman who has been pregnant more than once (Ch. 14).

multiparous   pertaining to women who have had two or more pregnancies (Ch. 14).

muscle testing   method of testing the motion, strength, and task potential of a muscle or group of muscles, their tendons, and associated tissues (Ch. 21).

mycobacteria   special types of bacteria, also called acid-fast, that grow only on specialized media; tuberculosis is caused by a mycobacterium (Ch. 31).

mycology   study of fungi (Ch. 27, 31).

myringotomy   incision into the tympanic membrane; part of the treatment for otitis media (Ch. 15).

Nagele's rule   usual method for calculating expected date of birth (Ch. 14).

National Board of Medical Examiners (NBME)   consultants for the certification examination (Ch. 35).

nebulizer   instrument used to produce a fine spray of medication (Ch. 18).

negligence   failure to exercise a certain standard of care (Ch. 7, 33).

nematode   round worm (Ch. 31).

neonatal   pertaining to newborn (Ch. 14).

networking   process in which people of similar interests exchange information in social, business, or professional relationships (Ch. 34).

neutrophil   the most common type of granulocytic white blood cell (Ch. 29).

niacin   one of the B-complex vitamins (Ch. 22).

nitrogenous   waste products in the blood indicating kidney disease (Ch. 18).

nocturia   increased voiding at night (Ch. 18).

nomogram   graph that shows the relationship among numerical values. Body surface area (BSA) of a patient can be estimated by its use (Ch. 24).

noncompliant   failure to follow a required command or instruction (Ch. 7).

noninvasive   procedures that do not require entering the body or puncturing the skin (Ch. 20, 25).

normal flora   microorganisms that are normally present in a specific site (Ch. 10, 31).

normal sinus rhythm   term used to describe the heart's rhythm when it is within the normal range (Ch. 25).

normocytic   term that describes a normal sized cell (Ch. 29).

nosocomial   hospital-acquired (Ch. 31).

not current status   effective January 2003, all CMAs employed or seeking employment must have current certified status to use the CMA credential (Ch. 35).

nullipara   a woman who has not carried a pregnancy to the stage of viability (Ch. 14).

nutrient   ingested substance that helps the body stay in its homeostatic state (Ch. 22).

nutrition   study of the bringing of nutrients into the body and how the body uses these nutrients (Ch. 22).

objective   a patient sign that is visible, palpable, or measurable by an observer (Ch. 11); also, magnifying lens that is closest to the object being viewed with a microscope (Ch. 27).

obturator   tool that obstructs or closes a cavity or opening. The internal portion of an examination instrument that facilitates the entry of the instrument into the body; it is then withdrawn, permitting visualization of the internal area (Ch. 18).

occluder   instrument used to obstruct or close off an eye (Ch. 18).

occlusion   closure of a passage (Ch. 9).

oliguria   decrease in urine output (Ch. 18).

one-site placement   externship completed at only one facility (Ch. 28).

open-ended questions   questions that encourage verbalization and response; questions that seek a response beyond a simple yes or no (Ch. 4).

ophthalmoscope   instrument for examination of the interior of the eye (Ch. 18).

optic nerve   second cranial nerve that carries impulses for the sense of sight (Ch. 18).

orchiectomy   surgical excision of a testicle (Ch. 16).

orthopnea   difficulty breathing in any position other than an upright position (Ch. 12).

oscilloscope   an electronic device used for recording electrical activity of the heart, brain, and muscular tissues (Ch. 20, 25).

ossicle   small bone; often refers to any of the three small bones of the ear (Ch. 18).

otoscope   instrument used to examine the external ear canal and tympanic membrane (Ch. 18).

outer-directed people   people who let events, other people, or environmental factors dictate their behavior (Ch. 5).

ova   eggs of parasites (Ch. 31).

oval window   opening in the middle ear. The base of the stapes, one of the ear ossicles, fits into this opening (Ch. 18).

overtime   money paid at a rate of not less than one and one-half times the regular rate of pay after a forty-hour work week is completed (Ch. 34).

oxidation   process of a substance combining with oxygen (Ch. 22).

oxygenated   containing high levels of oxygen (Ch. 28).

oxytocin   a pituitary hormone that stimulates the muscles of the uterus to contract, thus inducing labor (Ch. 14).

palliative   measures taken to relieve symptoms of disease (Ch. 10, 20).

pallor   lack of color, paleness (Ch. 13).

palpate   to search for a vein using the fingertips with a pressure and release touch (Ch. 28).

paradigm   internalized example or pattern that may influence your perspective (Ch. 33).

parasitology study of organisms (parasites and/or their eggs) that live within or upon another organism and at the expense of that organism (Ch. 27, 31).

parasympathetic nervous system part of the autonomic nervous system that returns the body to its normal state after stress has subsided (Ch. 5).

parenteral injection of a liquid substance into the body via a route other than the alimentary canal (Ch. 10, 24).

parity carrying a pregnancy to the point of viability regardless of the outcome (Ch. 14).

partnership in this text, the collaboration of two or more physicians who share the costs and liabilities of a medical practice (Ch. 2).

parturition the process of giving birth (Ch. 14).

patent open, not blocked (Ch. 14).

pathogen disease-producing microorganism (Ch. 10, 31).

patient service centers satellite lab facilities located in convenient areas for patients where specimens can be collected or dropped off (Ch. 27).

pelvic inflammatory disease infection of uterus, fallopian tubes, and adjacent pelvic structures; most common causes are gonorrhea and chlamydia; spread as sexually transmitted diseases (Ch. 14).

perception conscious awareness of one's own feelings and the feelings of others (Ch. 4).

perforation a hole caused by ulceration (Ch. 18).

performance objectives what is expected to be performed to demonstrate accomplishment (Ch. 28).

peripheral nerve nerves and ganglia away from the spinal cord (Ch. 18).

peritonitis inflammation of the peritoneum (Ch. 18).

pernicious anemia chronic anemia caused by lack of hydrochloric acid in the stomach; weakness, fatigue, tingling of extremities, and even heart failure can result; vitamin B_{12} injections are the treatment for this condition (Ch. 17).

petri dish plastic dish into which agar is placed for the purpose of growing bacteria (Ch. 31).

pH scale that indicates the relative alkalinity or acidity of a solution; measurement of hydrogen ion concentration (Ch. 30).

pharmacology study of drugs; the science concerned with the history, origin, sources, physical and chemical properties, and uses of drugs and their effects on living organisms (Ch. 23).

pharmacopeia book describing drugs and their preparation or a collection or stock of drugs (Ch. 3).

phenylketonuria (PKU) recessive, inherited disease in which the body is unable to oxidize phenylalanine to tyrosine (Ch. 32).

phlebotomy process of collecting blood (Ch. 10, 28).

physician's directive another name for a living will (Ch. 6).

physicians' office laboratories (POL) laboratories within physicians' offices where common office lab tests are performed (Ch. 27).

placenta abruptio sudden and abrupt separation of the placenta from uterine wall (Ch. 14).

placenta previa placenta lies low in uterus and can partially or completely cover the cervical os (Ch. 14).

plaintiff person bringing charges in litigation (Ch. 7).

plantar flexion moving the foot downward at the ankle (Ch. 21).

plasma fluid portion of blood from a tube containing anticoagulant. This fluid contains fibrinogen (Ch. 28).

pluralistic (pluralism) society where there are several distinct ethnic, religious, or cultural groups that coexist with one another (Ch. 3).

poikilocytosis condition where red blood cells show marked variations in shape (Ch. 29).

polychromatic stain stain containing both acid and basic dyes that is used to stain formed elements of the blood (Ch. 29).

polycystic situation of many (poly) or multiple cysts (Ch. 18).

polyp tumor with a stem found in nose, uterus, bladder, colon, or rectum (Ch. 18).

position physical stance of two individuals while communicating (Ch. 4).

posture relates to the position of the body or parts of the body; the pose taken while communicating (Ch. 4).

potentiate to increase potency or action (Ch. 23).

power verbs action words used to describe your attributes and strengths (Ch. 36).

practicum transitional stage providing opportunity to apply theory learned in the classroom to a health care setting through practical, hands-on experience (Ch. 1, 33).

precipitate substance in the form of fine particles that separates from a solution if allowed to stand for a period of time (Ch. 24).

precordial pertaining to the area on the anterior surface of the body overlying the heart (Ch. 25).

pre-eclampsia a complication of pregnancy characterized by generalized edema, hypertension, and proteinuria (Ch. 14).

preferred provider organization (PPO) organization of physicians who network together to offer discounts to purchasers of heath care insurance (Ch. 2).

prejudice opinion or judgment that is formed before all the facts are known (Ch. 4).

prenatal time period between fertilization and birth (Ch. 14).

presbycusis progressive loss of hearing caused by the normal aging process (Ch. 17).

prescribe to order or recommend the use of a drug, diet, or other form of therapy (Ch. 23).

preservative chemical added to food to keep it fresh longer (Ch. 22).

primary container container that directly contains the specimen (Ch. 28).

primigravida a woman pregnant for the first time (Ch. 14).

probation period of time during which the employee and supervisory personnel may determine if both the environment and the position are satisfactory for the employee (Ch. 34).

problem-oriented medical record (POMR) a type of patient chart recordkeeping that uses a sheet at a prominent location in the chart to list vital identification data. Patient medical problems are identified by a number that corresponds to the charting; e.g., bronchitis is #1, a broken wrist is #2, and so forth (Ch. 4, 11).

procedures manual   manual providing detailed information relative to the performance of tasks within the job description (Ch. 33).

processed food   food that is no longer in a whole, natural state; cooked or packaged with parts removed or ingredients added (Ch. 22).

professional liability insurance   insurance policy designed to protect assets in the event a claim for damages resulting from negligence is filed and awarded (Ch. 33).

proficiency testing   sample tests performed in a clinical laboratory to determine with what degree of accuracy tests are being performed. Testing samples are checked in the same manner as patient specimens (Ch. 26).

profile   categories of groups of tests related by body system or body function (Ch. 27).

profit sharing   sharing in the financial profits, gains, and benefits of an organization (Ch. 33).

projection   act of placing one's own feelings upon another (Ch. 4).

pronation   moving the arm so the palm is down (Ch. 21).

proprietary   privately owned and managed facility, a profit-making organization (Ch. 1).

prostaglandin   modulator of biochemical activity in tissues (Ch. 14).

proteinuria   protein in the urine (Ch. 18).

protozoa   one-celled animals divided into four groups: amebae, flagellates, ciliates, and coccidia (Ch. 31).

pruritis   itchiness (Ch. 23).

psychomotor retardation   slowing of physical and mental responses; may be seen in depression (Ch. 6).

puerperium   the period of time from the end of the third stage of labor until involution of uterus is complete, usually 3 to 6 weeks (Ch. 14).

pulmonary edema   accumulation of serous fluid in the air vesicles and interstitial tissues of the lungs (Ch. 26).

purified protein derivative (PPD)   filtrate obtained from Mycobacterium cultures used for intradermal testing for tuberculosis (Ch. 32).

pyorrhea   discharge of pus from the gums, around the teeth (Ch. 13).

pyrexia   fever (Ch. 12).

pyridoxine   Vitamin B_6 (Ch. 22).

pyuria   pus in the urine (Ch. 18).

qualitative test   analysis to identify quality or characteristics of components, such as size, shape, and maturity of cells (Ch. 27).

quality assurance (QA)   process to provide accurate, complete, consistent healthcare documentation in a timely manner while making every reasonable effort to resolve inconsistencies, inaccuracies, risk management issues, and other problems (Ch. 24).

quality control   measures used to monitor the processing of laboratory specimens. Includes proper use, storage, handling, stability,

expiration dates, and indications for measuring precision and accuracy of analytic processes (Ch. 26, 30, 31).

quantitative test   analysis that can identify quantity or actual number counts such as counting the number of blood cells (Ch. 27).

radioactive   emits rays or particles from nucleus (Ch. 20).

radiograph   the film on which an image is produced through exposure to X-rays (Ch. 20).

radiolucent   allowing X rays to pass through. A dark area appears on the radiograph (Ch. 20).

radionuclides   atoms that disintegrate by emitting electromagnetic radiation (Ch. 20).

radiopaque   impenetrable to X rays. A light area appears on the radiograph (Ch. 20).

radiopharmaceuticals   radioactive chemicals used in testing the location, size, outline, or function of tissue, organs, vessels, or body fluids (Ch. 20).

rales   abnormal bubbling or crackling sound heard by auscultation during the inspiratory phase of respiration (Ch. 12).

range of motion (ROM)   amount of movement that is present in a joint (Ch. 21).

ratchets   locking mechanisms on the handles of many surgical instruments (Ch. 19).

rationalization   act of justification, usually illogically, that one uses to keep from facing the truth of the situation (Ch. 4).

reagent   chemical substance that detects or synthesizes other substances in a chemical reaction; used in laboratory analyses because it is known to react in a specific way (Ch. 27, 30, 31).

reagent test strip   narrow strip of plastic on which pads containing reagents are attached; used in the urinalysis chemical examination to detect glucose, bilirubin, ketones, specific gravity, blood, pH, urobilinogen, nitrites, and leukocyte esterase (Ch. 30).

receiver   recipient of the sender's message (Ch. 4).

recertification   documentation admitted to support continued education for maintaining a professional credential (Ch. 35).

reference laboratories   independent, regionally located labs used by hospitals for complex, expensive or specialized tests (Ch. 27).

references   individuals who have known or worked with you long enough to make an honest assessment and recommendation regarding your background history (Ch. 36).

reference values   also referred to as normal value, normal range, or reference range; range of values that includes 95 percent of test results for a normal healthy population (Ch. 37).

refractometer   instrument that measures the refractive index of a substance or solution; used in the urinalysis physical examination to measure the urine specimen's specific gravity (Ch. 30).

registered medical assistant (RMA)   credential awarded for successfully passing the AMT examination (Ch. 1, 35).

regression   moving back to a former stage to escape conflict or fear (Ch. 6).

regulated waste   any waste that contains infectious material that would pose a threat due to possible transmission of pathogenic microorganisms (Ch. 10).

rehabilitation medicine field of medical disciplines that seeks to restore an individual or body part to normal or near normal function following an illness or injury using physical and mechanical agents (Ch. 21).

reimbursement payment (Ch. 26).

repolarization re-establishment of a polarized state in a muscle following contraction (Ch. 25).

repression coping with an overwhelming situation by temporarily forgetting it; temporary amnesia (Ch. 4).

requisition request form sent with a specimen specifying tests to be performed on the specimen; most common tests are separated into logical categories with additional space for writing special requests (Ch. 26, 27).

rescue breathing performed on individuals in respiratory arrest, rescue breathing is a mouth-to-mouth (using appropriate protective equipment) or mouth-to-nose procedure that provides oxygen to the patient until emergency personnel arrive (Ch. 9).

residual amount of urine remaining in bladder immediately after voiding; seen with hyperplasia of prostate (Ch. 16).

resistance ability of the immune system to resist or withstand an infectious disease (Ch. 10).

resume written summary data sheet or brief account of qualifications and progress in your chosen career (Ch. 34, 36).

retention urine held in the bladder; inability to empty the bladder (Ch. 16).

retrolental fibroplasia disease of blood vessels of retina in newborns (Ch. 24).

retrovirus common name for some viruses that contain reverse transcriptase (Ch. 8).

revalidation maintaining current RMA status (Ch. 35).

Rh factor blood factor indicating the presence or absence of the Rh antigen on the surface of human erythrocytes (Ch. 32).

rhonchi sounds during breathing similar to wheezes (Ch. 12).

rhythm strip ECG recording of a single lead, usually lead II, that is used to determine the rhythm of the heart beat. An arrhythmia can more easily be seen in a rhythm strip because it is run longer per physician's request (Ch. 25).

riboflavin Vitamin B_2 (Ch. 22).

ribonucleic acid (RNA) nucleic acid in all living cells; sometimes takes the place of DNA in certain viruses (Ch. 8).

risk management techniques adhered to in the ambulatory care setting that keep the practice, its environment, and its procedures as safe for the patient as possible. Proper risk management also reduces the possibility of negligence that leads to torts and malpractice suits (Ch. 7, 33).

roadblocks (to communication) verbal or nonverbal messages that block the communication cycle (Ch. 4).

rotation turning a body part around its axis (Ch. 21); also, opportunity to spend two or three weeks in a variety of health care settings (Ch. 28).

salary review informing the employee of their revised base pay rate (Ch. 34).

sanitization cleaning or scrubbing contaminated instruments or fomites to remove tissue, debris, or other contaminants (Ch. 10).

saturated fat fat that comes from an animal source and that contains more cholesterol than unsaturated fat, which comes from vegetable sources (Ch. 22).

scabies infectious skin disease caused by the itch mite (Sarcoptes scabiei) which is transmitted by direct contact with infected persons (Ch. 10).

scleroderma slowly progressing disease characterized by deposition of fibrous connective tissue in the skin and in internal organs (Ch. 13).

screening preliminary examination used to detect the most characteristic signs of a disorder that may entail further investigation (Ch. 30).

search engine specialized computer program designed to find specific information on the Internet (Ch. 33).

secretion substance produced by the cells of glandular organs from materials in the blood (Ch. 10, 26).

sediment insoluble material that settles to the bottom of a liquid; material examined in the urinalysis microscopic examination (Ch. 30).

self-actualization being all that you can be; developing your full potential and experiencing fulfillment (Ch. 5, 33).

semen thick, viscid secretion discharged from the urethra of males at orgasm. It is a mixed product containing various fluids and spermatozoa (Ch. 32).

sender the individual beginning the communication cycle (Ch. 4).

senile mental and/or physical weakness sometimes associated with aging (Ch. 17).

sensitivity test in which an organism is placed with antibiotics to determine which antibiotic will effectively kill the organism with the smallest dose (Ch. 31).

septicemia invasion of pathogenic bacteria into the bloodstream (Ch. 3).

serum liquid portion of blood obtained after blood has been allowed to clot (Ch. 9, 28).

shadow follow a supervisor or delegated subordinate in order to learn facility protocol (Ch. 33).

sharps needles or scalpels or other sharp instruments that are capable of causing a penetrating or puncture wound of the skin (Ch. 10).

shock condition in which the circulatory system is not providing enough blood to all parts of the body, causing the body's organs to fail to function properly (Ch. 9).

short-range goals long-range goals are dissected and reassembled into smaller, more manageable time segments (Ch. 5).

sickle cell anemia an inherited disorder that may shorten life span (Ch. 14).

silver nitrate caustic astringent antiseptic. As a weak liquid, it is applied to the eyes of newborns to prevent infections at birth. In the medical office, it is most often seen as a solid substance impregnated onto the end of a wooden applicator. Silver nitrate applicator sticks contain hydrochloric acid and other chemicals and are commonly used to cauterize small blood vessels in the nose or other mucous membranes (Ch. 19).

sitz bath a bath to sit in (Ch. 19).

skills acquisition objective   concerned with the development of new on-the-job skills or learning new tasks or concepts (Ch. 28).

skills application/development objective   improvement and development of skills already learned (Ch. 28).

slander   false and malicious words about another constituting a defamation of character (Ch. 7).

SOAP   acronym for patient progress notes based on subjective impressions (S), objective clinical evidence (O), assessment or diagnosis (A), and plans for further studies (P) (Ch. 11).

sodium hydroxide   chemical used to chemically burn and destroy tissue; usually in a liquid state when used in minor surgery (Ch. 19).

sodium hypochlorite   household bleach (Ch. 10).

sole proprietorship   medical practice that is owned by only one individual (Ch. 2).

sonographer   professionally trained individual capable of performing the ultrasound examination (Ch. 25).

source-oriented medical record (SOMR)   a type of patient chart record keeping that includes separate sections for different sources of patient information, such as laboratory reports, pathology reports, and progress notes (Ch. 11).

species   second Greek or Latin name given to microorganisms; the species name is not capitalized (Ch. 31).

specific gravity   ratio of weight of a given volume of a substance to the weight of the same volume of distilled water at the same temperature; test often performed during the urinalysis physical examination (can also appear on the reagent strip) (Ch. 30).

spill kit   commercially packaged materials containing supplies and equipment needed to clean up a spill of a biohazardous substance (Ch. 10).

spirometry   test to measure the air capacity of the lungs (Ch. 18).

splint   any device used to immobilize a body part. Often used by EMS personnel (Ch. 9).

sprain   injury to a joint, often an ankle, knee, or wrist, that involves a tearing of the ligaments. Most sprains are minor and heal quickly; others are more severe, include swelling, and may not heal properly if the patient continues to put stress on the sprained joint (Ch. 9).

sputum   substance from the respiratory tract expelled by coughing (Ch. 10).

stab culture   culture where the microorganism is stabbed into tubed solid media (Ch. 31).

standard   rules established to measure quality, weight, extent, or value (Ch. 10, 36).

standard precautions   precautions developed in 1996 by the Centers for Disease Control and Prevention (CDC) that augment universal precautions and body substance isolation practices. They provide a wider range of protection and are used any time there is contact with blood, moist body fluid (except perspiration), mucous membranes, or nonintact skin. They are designed to protect all health care providers, patients, and visitors (Ch. 9, 10).

status asthmaticus   severe episode of asthma that does not respond to ordinary treatment (Ch. 24).

statute   law enacted by a legislative body (Ch. 7).

stertorous   snoring sound heard with labored breathing (Ch. 12).

stomatitis   inflammation of the mouth associated with radiation therapy. Can include swelling, redness, halitosis, ulcerations (Ch. 20).

strain   injury to the soft tissue between joints that involves the tearing of muscles or tendons. Strains often occur in the neck, back, or thigh muscles (Ch. 9).

stratum corneum   horny, outermost layer of the skin, epidermis, composed of dead cells converted to keratin that continually flakes away (Ch. 18).

stress   body's response to change; can be manifested in a variety of ways, including changes in blood pressure, heart rate, and onset of headache (Ch. 5).

strictures   narrowing of a tube-like structure such as the esophagus or urethra (Ch. 19).

stridor   crowing sound heard on inspiration, the result of an upper airway obstruction (Ch. 12).

stylus   heated slender wire of the electrocardiograph that melts the wax off of the ECG paper during the recording (Ch. 25).

subjective   symptom that is felt by the patient but not observable by others (Ch. 11).

sublimation   redirecting a socially unacceptable impulse into one that is socially acceptable (Ch. 4).

subordinate   in an organization, a person under the direction of (reporting to) a person of greater authority (Ch. 33).

subpoena   written command designating a person to appear in court under penalty for failure to appear (Ch. 7).

supernatant   urine that appears above the sediment when centrifuged; poured off before sediment is examined in the urinalysis microscopic examination (Ch. 30).

supination   moving the arm so the palm is up (Ch. 21).

suppressed immune system   term used to describe an immune system unable to function normally due to the presence of a disease such as AIDS (Ch. 10, 26).

suppurative   producing or associated with the generation of pus (Ch. 15).

surgery cards   written reference for surgeries and procedures (Ch. 19).

surgical asepsis   procedures that render objects sterile; techniques to maintain sterile conditions during invasive procedures (Ch. 19).

surrogate   substitute; someone who substitutes for another (Ch. 8).

suture   surgical material or thread; may describe the act of sewing with the surgical thread and needle (Ch. 19).

swaged   a surgical needle attached to a length of suture material (Ch. 19).

symmetry   correspondence in shape, size, and position of body parts on opposites of the body (Ch. 13).

sympathetic nervous system   large part of the atuonomic nervous system that prepares the body for fight-or-flight (Ch. 5).

syncope   fainting (Ch. 9, 25).

systole   one component of blood pressure measurement representing the highest amount of pressure exerted during the cardiac cycle; the force exerted on the arterial walls during cardiac contraction (Ch. 12, 25).

T cell type of white blood cell that provides immunity (Ch. 10).

tachycardia pulse rate greater than 100 beats per minute (Ch. 12).

tachycardia, sinus abnormally rapid heartbeat greater than 100 beats/minute. A type of cardiac arrhythmia (Ch. 25).

tachypnea abnormal increased rate of breathing (Ch. 12).

Tamm-Horsfall mucoprotein secreted by the epithelial cells of the renal tubules (Ch. 30).

targeted resume resume format utilized when focusing on a clear, specific job target (Ch. 36).

task force for test construction committee of professionals whose responsibility is to update the CMA examination annually to reflect changes in medical assistants' responsibilities and to include new developments in medical knowledge and technology (Ch. 35).

taut to pull or draw tight a surface, such as skin (Ch. 24).

taxonomy classification of organisms into appropriate categories (Ch. 31).

Tay-Sachs an inherited disease that is usually fatal (Ch. 14).

teamwork persons synergistically working together (Ch. 33).

territoriality represents the distance at which we feel comfortable while communicating with others (Ch. 4).

test cable accessory device that attaches between the Holter monitor and the electrocardiograph to check for correct waveform and lack of artifact (Ch. 25).

tetrads group of four similarly related entities (Ch. 31).

thalassemia a hereditary anemia that may be fatal (Ch. 14).

therapeutic communication use of specific and well-defined professional communication skills to create a feeling of comfort for patients even when difficult or unpleasant information must be exchanged (Ch. 4).

thermolabile easily affected by heat (Ch. 10).

thermotherapy use of heat to treat a physical condition (Ch. 21).

thiamin vitamin B_1 (Ch. 22).

thixotropic separator gel gel material capable of forming an interface between the cells and fluid portion of the blood as a result of centrifugation (Ch. 28).

thoracentesis surgical puncture of the thoracic cavity to aspirate fluid (Ch. 10).

thrombocyte (platelet) cellular fragment of megataryocyte; plays an important role in blood coagulation, hemostasis, and clot formation (Ch. 28, 29).

tine test skin test for tuberculosis (Ch. 32).

tinnitus ringing or buzzing sound in the ear (Ch. 13).

titer measurement of amount of antibody present against a particular antigen (Ch. 14).

tocopherol vitamin E (Ch. 22).

tort wrongful act that results in injury to one person by another (Ch. 7).

touch physically making contact with others (Ch. 4).

tourniquet device used to facilitate vein prominence (Ch. 28).

trace mineral mineral required by the body in small amounts (Ch. 22).

tracing graphic record usually of an event that changes with time as with the electrical activity of the heart (Ch. 25).

transducer device that converts one form of energy to another. During an ultrasound procedure, the transducer picks up echoes and converts them to electrical energy. The energy is transformed into a picture on a television monitor or printed on paper. Photographs of the image can be taken (Ch. 20, 25).

transient ischemic attack temporary interference with blood flow to brain; may last only a few moments or several hours; neurological symptoms occur (Ch. 17).

transilluminator instrument used to inspect a cavity or organ by passing a light through the walls (Ch. 16).

transmission spread of infectious disease by direct contact, indirect contact, inhalation, ingestion, or bloodborne contact (Ch. 10).

transmission-based precautions second tier of Centers for Disease Control and Prevention (CDC) guidelines that applies to specific categories of patients and that include air, contact, and droplet precautions. Transmission-based precautions are always used in addition to standard precautions (Ch. 10).

transurethral resection removal of prostate tissue using a device inserted through the urethra (Ch. 16).

triage process to determine and prioritize patients' needs and the likely benefit from immediate medical attention. From the French *trier*, meaning "to sort" (Ch. 2, 9).

trichomoniasis infestation with a Trichomonas parasite which may be transmitted through sexual intercourse (Ch. 10).

triglycerides form of fat in the bloodstream that functions to store energy (Ch. 32).

trimester three months; one-third of the gestational period of pregnancy (Ch. 14).

tuberculosis infectious disease caused by the bacterium, *Mycobacterium tuberculosis* (Ch. 32).

turbid opaque, lacking clarity (Ch. 30).

tympanostomy placement of a tube through the tympanic membrane to allow ventilation of the middle ear; part of the treatment for otitis media (Ch. 15).

typhus (typhoid) acute infectious disease that causes severe headache, rash, high fever, and progressive neurologic involvement. Prevalent where conditions are unsanitary and congested (Ch. 3).

ultrasonography process of placing a handheld transducer against a body area to be tested. The transducer sends sound waves through the skin and the various internal organs. When echoes are formed and sent back the transducer converts them into electrical energy. This energy is transformed into a picture for a monitor, or printed on paper. Photographs of the images can be taken and become part of the patient's permanent record (Ch. 25).

ultrasound use of high-frequency sound waves for therapeutic reasons to generate heat in deep tissue (Ch. 21).

unipolar having or pertaining to one pole process (Ch. 25).

unit dose premeasured amount of medication, individually packaged on a per-dose basis (Ch. 24).

universal emergency medical identification symbol   identification sometimes carried by individuals to identify health problems they may have (Ch. 9).

universal precautions   guidelines established by the Centers for Disease Control and Prevention (CDC) for the protection of health care workers from infectious diseases (Ch. 10).

urea   principal end product of protein metabolism (Ch. 30).

uremia   toxic condition of the blood caused by the kidneys' inability to filter waste products from the blood (Ch. 18).

urgency   the need to urinate immediately (Ch. 18).

urinalysis   examination of the physical, chemical, and microscopic properties of urine (Ch. 27, 30).

urinometer   device to measure specific gravity; consists of a float with a calibrated stem (Ch. 30).

urobilinogen   colorless compound produced in the intestine after the breakdown by bacteria of bilirubin (Ch. 30).

urochrome   yellow pigment that gives color to urine (Ch. 30).

urticaria   hives (Ch. 23).

vaccine   pharmacologic agent capable of producing artificial active immunity (Ch. 10).

Vacutainer®   brand of vacuum tube used in phlebotomy to obtain a venous blood sample for analysis (Ch. 10).

vasoconstriction   narrowing or constricting of blood vessels (Ch. 21).

vasodilation   widening or dilating of blood vessels (Ch. 21).

vector   a carrier of disease, usually an insect, that is the causative organism of disease from infected to noninfected individuals (Ch. 10).

venipuncture   opening a vein to obtain a blood sample (Ch. 28).

vertigo   the sensation of moving around in space; dizziness, lightheadedness (Ch. 13).

vesicle   blister or elevation on the skin (Ch. 18).

viable   able to live, grow, and develop after birth; usually 24 weeks or greater than one pound (Ch. 14).

virology   study of viruses (Ch. 31).

virulence   an organism's relative power and degree of pathogenicity (Ch. 10).

viscosity   degree of thickness of a liquid (Ch. 28).

vitiligo   skin disorder characterized by smooth white spots on various areas of the body (Ch. 13).

volatile   easily evaporated (Ch. 19).

waived (tests)   used to describe a category of clinical laboratory tests that are simple, unvarying, and require a minimum of judgment and interpretation (Ch. 26).

water-soluble   pertaining to substances that are hydrophilic and therefore dissolve better in water (Ch. 22).

Web site   a remote computer that stores World Wide Web documents consisting of Web pages (Ch. 33).

wheal   slight elevation of skin that can be produced as a result of an intradermal injection (Ch. 24, 32).

wheezes   high-pitched musical sound heard on expiration, often the result of an obstruction or narrowing of respiratory passages (Ch. 12).

Wood's lamp   light source used to fluoresce certain fungal cultures; used to aid in the identification of dermatophytes (Ch. 31).

work history   outline of previous employment positions, employers, positions, duties, and responsibilities. Listed with the most recent position first (Ch. 34).

work practice controls   measures used in the workplace that consist of physical equipment and mechanical devices to control employee exposure to bloodborne pathogens and other potentially infectious materials. Examples are sharps disposal containers, handwashing facilities, PPE, eyewash stations, and so on (Ch. 10).

work statement   concise description of the work you plan to accomplish (Ch. 33).

wound   a break in the continuity of soft parts of body structures caused by violence or trauma to tissues. In an open wound, skin is broken as in a laceration, abrasion, avulsion, or incision. In a closed wound, skin is not broken as in contusion, ecchymosis, or hematoma (Ch. 9).

yellow fever   acute infectious disease where a person develops jaundice, vomits, hemorrhages, and has a fever; caused mostly by mosquitoes (Ch. 3).

INDEX

Note: Page references in **bold type** refer to boxes, procedures, figures, and tables.

A

AAMA *See* American Association of Medical Assistants
Abbreviations
  charting, **199**
Abdomen, physical examination and, **245**, 246
Abdominal thrust, 111–112
ABO blood typing, 765–766
Abortion, 262–263
  ethical issues concerning, 89–90
Abrasions, 100
Abscesses, **136, 353**
  described, **354**
Absorption
  drug, 506
  poison, 108
Abuse
  child, 77
  elderly, 77
  ethical issues concerning, 88
AC (Alternating current), ECG interference and, 578
Accomplishment statements, 847–848
Accreditation, American Association of Medical Assistants and, 8
Accuracy, resumes and, 848
Acetest®, 707
Acid-fast
  organisms, **737**
  stains, 736–737
Acidosis, **110**
Acne, **353**
  described, **354**
Acquired active immunity, 139
Acquired immunodeficiency syndrome. *See* AIDS
Activities of daily living (ADL), 445
Acupuncture, **25**, 30
Acute Hepatitis Panel, **622**
Acute stage, infections, 140
Acute stress response, 771
Acute viral hepatitis diseases, 142

ADA (Americans with Disabilities Act), 77, 78–79
ADL (Activities of daily living), 445
Administer, defined, 504
Administrative forms, patient history and, 185
Adolescents
  ethical issues concerning, **85**
  nutritional needs of, 488
Adrenalin, **511**
Adson forceps, 393, **394**
Adults
  calculating, dosage for, 526–527
  CPR (cardiopulmonary resuscitation) for, **123–124**
  ethical issues concerning, **85**
  Heimlich maneuver
    on conscious, **114**
    on unconscious, **114–116**
  rescue breathing for, **120**
Adverse reaction, 508
Advertising, ethics and, 87
Advisory Council for Elimination of Tuberculosis, 769
Afebrile, defined, 208
AFP (Alpha fetal protein), 262
Agar, described, 739
Age
  cultural calculation of, **191**
  drug dosage and, 518
Agglutination inhibition test
  defined, 761–762
  infectious mononucleosis, 764–765
  pregnancy testing and, 761–762
Aging
  cardiovascular system and, 314–315
  complications of, preventing, 315
  facts about, 313
  gastrointestinal system, 315
  integumentary system and, 314
  musculoskeletal system and, 314
  nervous system and, 314
  physiological changes during, 313–315, 316
  reproductive system and, 315
  urinary tract and, 315
  see also Elderly

AIDS, 77, 140, **141**, 142, 344
  described, **272**
  ethical issues concerning, 90
  patients with, therapeutic response to, 62–63
  transmission of, **729**
Air casts, 346
Airborne Precautions, **148**
Alarm, adaptation to stress and, 52
Aliquot specimen, defined, 646
Allergenic extracts, administration of, 544–545
Allergy testing, skin, 354
Allied health professionals, **21–22**
Alligator-type forceps, 393, **394**
Allopathic medicine, 30
Alm retractor, **398**
Alpha fetal protein (AFP), 262
Alphatocopherol, **481**
Alternating current (AC), ECG interference and, 578
Alternative health care therapies, role of, 24
AMA (American Medical Association)
  ethical guidelines, 87–89
  Principles of Medical Ethics, 84, 85, **86**
Ambulation, defined, 449
Ambulatory health care, settings, 4, 16–18
American Association of Blood Banks, **599**
American Association of Medical Assistants (AAMA)
  accreditation and, 8
  certification and, 8–9
  certification examination, 834
    format/content of, 835–836
    preparing for, 834–835
  Code of Ethics, 84, 85, **86**
    keys to, 86–87
  continuing education verification form, **839**
  creed, **86**
  examination, application process, 836
  founding of, 7–8
  liability insurance and, 805
  Role Delineation Chart, 9, 12, Appendix C
American Diabetes Society, 109
American Medical Association (AMA)
  ethical guidelines, 87
  Principles of Medical Ethics, 84, 85, **86**

American Medical Technologists Institute for Education (AMTIE), 839
American Osteopathic Association, **599**
American Society of Histocompatibility and Immunogenetics, **599**
Americans with Disabilities Act (ADA), 77, 78–79
Amino acids, 478–479
Aminophylline, **511**
Amniocentesis
 defined, 149
 pregnancy and, 262
Amoebic dysentery, 136
Amorphous, defined, 708
Amphetamines, abuse of, 511
Ampule, defined, 534
AMTIE (American Medical Technologists Institute for Education), 839
Anaerobic equipment, microbiology laboratory and, 726
Analgesic drugs, defined, **507**
Anemias, **351**
 described, **352**
Aneroid manometers, **215**, 216
Anesthesia
 office surgery, 403, **403**
Anesthesiologist assistant, 21
Anesthetics drugs, defined, **507**
Angina pectoris, 350
 described, **351**
Angiography, **434**
Animals, as a source of drugs, 499
Anisocytosis cells, 678
Ankle, bandage wrapping technique, **401**
Anorexia nervosa, **328**
Anoscopes, 396
Anterioposterior view, 435
Anterior chamber, eye, defined, 336
Antianemic drugs, defined, **507**
Antianxiety drugs, **507**
Antiarrhythmic drugs, **507**
Antibacterial creams/ointments, surgical, 400
Antibiotic agents, 134
Antibodies, 138
Anticholinergic drugs, **507**
Anticoagulant drugs, **507**
Anticoagulants, 642
Anticonvulsant drugs, **507**
Antidepressant drugs, **507**
Antidiarrheal drugs, **507**
Antiemetic drugs, **507**
Antigens, in ABO/RH blood factors, **766**
Antihistamine drugs, **507**
Antihypertensive drugs, **507**
Anti-inflammatory drugs, **507**
Antimanic drugs, **507**
Antineoplastic drugs, **507**
Antioxidants, 483
Antipsychotic drugs, **507**
Antipyretic drugs, **507**
Antiserum, hCG, 762
Antitussive drugs, **507**
Anvil (incus), 340
APGAR score, 283
Apical pulse, 213
 measuring, **228–229**
API® System, 745
Apnea, defined, 214
Apothecary measures, 523
Appendages, physical examination and, 243
Appendicitis, **328**
Appendicular skeleton, 344

Applicants
 interviewing, 816–818
 questions, **817**
Application employment form
 cover letters, 852
 completing, 852, 854
Aquamatic K-pad®, 459
Arms, physical examination and, **244**
Arrhythmias, cardiac, 579–581
Arteries
 arm, **639**
 versus veins, **637**
Arteriosclerosis, 489–490
 defined, 314–315
Arthritis
 rheumatoid, **345**
 described, **346**
Arthritis Panel, **622**
Artifacts
 alternating current (AC), 578
 charting, 198
 in urine, 709
 interrupted baseline, 579
 somatic tremor, 578
 wandering baseline, 579
Artificial active immunity, 139
Artificial insemination/surrogacy, ethical issues concerning, 90
ASAP, defined, 625
Ascorbic acid, **482**, 483
Asepsis
 medical, 163–165
 appropriate use of, 164
 reducing infection risk using, 32
 sterile, 165–170
Asian cultures
 aversion to talking about death, **190**
 calculating age in, **191**
Aspirate, defined, 149
Aspirating medication
 from ampule, **554–555**
 from a vial, **552–553**
Aspiration joint fluid, **419–420**
Assistive devices, 449–455
 canes, 453–454
 described, **450**
 crutches, described, **450**
 defined, 449
 walkers, 449
 described, **450**
 fitting a, **450**
 wheelchairs, 454–455
Asthma, 343
 described, **344**
 pediatrics and, 294
Astigmatism, **337**, **339**
Atherosclerosis, 489–490
Athletic trainer, 21
Atrial arrhythmias, 580
 fibrillation, 580
Atrophy, muscles, lack of exercise and, 456
Attitude, 5
Attributes, of professionals, 4–7
Audiometry, assisting with, **367–368**
Auditory, measuring ability of, 341–342
Aural temperature, 211
 pediatric, 291
 taking, using tympanic thermometer, **224**
Auricle, 340
Auscultation, described, 238
Autoclave, 166–170
 described, 725

loading the, 167
maintenance/cleaning of, 167–168
materials/supplies, **178–179**
 labeling for, 169–170
 wrapping instruments, **176–177**
 wrapping techniques, 170
 wrapping/packaging for, 168–169
quality control/assurance for, 168
rules for an, **167**
tape, 169
Automated hematology, instrumentation and quality control, 681–682
Automatic ECG machines, 572
Avulsion, 100, **405**
Axial skeleton, 344
Axillary crutches, 450, 450–451
 assisting patients with, **466–467**
 measuring for, 451–452
Axillary temperature, 211
 measuring, **226–227**
 pediatric, 291

B
Bacillary dysentery, **136**
Bacilli, described, 735
Back
 pain, 345
 described, **346**
Bacteria
 acid-fast, **737**
 described, 135–136
 dyes (stains), 735–737
 acid-fast, 736–737
 differential, 735–736
 simple, 735
 growth requirements of, **738**
 identifying characteristics of, **744**
 in urine, 708
 microscopic examination of, 734–737
 infectious bacteria culture, **737–738**
 shapes of, 734–735
Bacterial cell, defined, 724
Bacteriological smear, preparing, **750**
Bandage scissors, 391
Bandages
 changing, 413–414
 emergencies and, 101
 surgical, 400, **403**
 wrapping techniques, **401**
Banting, Frederick G., 33
Barbiturates, abuse of, 511
Barium
 enema, 331, **434**
 swallow, 331, **335**, **434**
Barrier-free accommodations, 78
Bartholin's gland, infection, **271**
Basal metabolic rate (BMR), 479
Baseline values, defined, 617
Basic Metabolic Panel, **622**
Basophil, described, 677
Battery, 73–74
BBL®, 764
Behavior, ethical, 7
Bell's palsy, **348**
 described, **349**
Benadryl, **511**
Benedict's test, 708
Benefits, managing, 804
Benign hypertension, 217
Benign hypertrophy of the prostate, elderly and, 315
Best, Charles, 33

Beta Hemolytic Streptococcus Group A, screening for, 744–745
Betadine®, 400
Biases, 40
"Big E" chart, 293
Bile solubility, bacteria, 742
Bilirubin, 766
    confirmatory testing of, 708
Biochemical tests, 742–744
    identification systems, 744–746
    tube, 743–744
Bioethics
    defined, 85
    dilemmas concerning, 89
Biofeedback, **25**
Biohazard labels, **159**
    symbol on, **728**
Bio-Plexus Puncture-Guard® needle, 640
Biopsy, kidney, 325
Biotin, **482**
Biotransformation, drug, 506
Blackwell, Elizabeth, 31
Bleeding
    control of, **112–113**
    external, 109
    internal, 110
Blind, sighted guide techniques, 317–318
Blood
    arteries versus veins, **637**
    capillary, 652
    cells, 666
    cellular elements of, **638**
    circulation of, 567
    collecting samples of, 638–639
        venipuncture, 641–644
    culture, 734
    disease transmission and, 97
    glucose in
        fasting, 770–771
        glycosylated hemoglobin and, 773
        measuring, **784**
        reference values for, **771**
        testing for, 770–773
    hazard communication for, 159
    infection control and, 146, 149–150
    reagent test strips and, 706
    smear
        counting stained differential, 677
        divisions of leukocytes from, **678**
        examination of, 677–679
        making a differential, 676
        preparation of a differential, **689–690**
        staining, 676
        staining a differential, **690–691**
    specimen collecting, 628
    stroke and, 110
    system, 351–352
        disorders of, **351**
        laboratory tests of, 352
    tubes, **638**
        guide, **643**
    typing, 765–766
    urinary tract test, 323
    see also Phlebotomy
Blood and Other Potentially Infectious Material (OPIM), 151–152
Blood banking department
    described, 621
    laboratory tests, **620**
Blood pressure, 215–217
    high, 489
    measuring, 216–217, **230**
        equipment, 215–216
    pediatric, 292

readings
    abnormal, 217–218
    normal, 217
    recording measurement of, 217
Blood urea nitrogen (BUN). *See* BUN (blood urea nitrogen)
Bloodborne pathogens, 152
    avoiding exposure to, 162–163
Bloodborne Pathogen Standard, 151–159, **160**
BMR (Basal metabolic rate), 479
Body fluids
    disease transmission and, 97
    infection control and, 146, 149–150
Body language, 42–44
Body mechanics
    principles of, 445–448
    posture, 445–446
Body movements, patient, 242–243
Body Substance Isolation (BSI), 146
Body surface area (BSA), dosage calculations and, 528
Body weight, dosage calculations and, 529
Boil, **353**
    described, **354**
Bond, defined, **805**
Bones
    fractures of, 106
    injuries to, 107
Botulism, **136**
Bowel movements, defined, 330
Bozeman forceps, **395**
Brachial pulse, 212
Bradycardia, defined, 213
Bradypnea, defined, 214
Brand name, of drugs, 499
Braxton-Hicks contractions, 264
Breast feeding, encouraged, 260–261
Breasts
    cancer of, **271**
    fibrocystic, **271**
    physical examination and, **245**, 246
    review of systems (ROS), 194–195
    self-examination of, 265, **206**
        instructing patient in, **275**
Breath odors, physical examination and, 243
Breathing
    emergencies, 111–112
    examination of, 266
    sounds, 214
Broken glass, disposal of, 156
Bronchitis, **343**
    described, **344**
Bronchodilator drugs, **507**
Broth tube inoculation, **755**
Bruises, 405
BSA (Body surface method), dosage calculations and, 528–529
BSI (Body Substance Isolation), 146
Budgetary needs analysis, personal, 846
Buffer words, 48
Bulimia, **328**
BUN (Blood urea nitrogen)
    reference values for, **775**
    test for, 325, 775
Burnout
    assessing risk of, **55**
    combating, 55
    described, 54
    preventing, 55
    workplace, 54
Burns, 101–102
    caring for, 103
    degrees of, 102

electrical, 105
first aid for, 104, **104–105**
solar radiation and, 105
Bursitis, **345**
Butterfly collection system, 650

C

Ca (Calcium), 484
CAAHEP (Committee on Accreditation of Allied Health Education Programs), 797–798
Calcium (Ca), 484
Calculi
    renal, **324**
        cystoscopy and, 325
Calibration, defined, 604
Callus, **353**
    described, **354**
Calories
    calculations of percentages of, **480**
    defined, 479
Cambodia, diet of, **492**
Cancer
    breast, **271**
    cervical, **271**
    colon, **328**
    diet and, 490–491
    lung, **343**
        described, **344**
    ovarian, 270
    skin, **353**
        described, **354**
    urinary bladder, **324**
Candida albicans, 749
    in urine, 708
Candidiasis, **271**
    described, **272**
Candle jar, 726
Canes, 453–454
    assisting patients with, **467**
    described, **450**
Capillary
    blood, composition of, 652
    puncture, 652–654
        collecting blood sample, 653–654
        order of draw, 654
        performing, 653
        preparation for, 653
        procedure for, **660–661**
        sites, 652–653
Carbohydrates, 477–478
    energy from, 479
Carbuncle, **353**
    described, **354**
Cardiac
    arrhythmias, 579–581, **582**
    catheterization, 585
    cycle, 568–569
    diagnostic tests, 582–584
    myocardial infarctions, 350, 579
Cardinal signs. *See* Vital signs
Cardiopulmonary resuscitation (CPR), 111, 112
    for adults, **123–124**
    for children, **125**
    for infants, **126**
Cardiovascular system
    disease of, diet for, 489–490
    elderly and, 314–315
    review of systems (ROS), 194–195
Cardiovascular technologist, 21
Cardioversion, 582
Carotene, **481**, 483

Carotid pulse, 212
Carpal tunnel syndrome, **344**
   described, **346**
Carpujet®, 535
Carrying, safely, 446–447
Cartridge needle, defined, 534
Casting, fractures, 346–347
Casts
   care of, 347
   plaster-of-Paris, assisting with, **376**
   removal of, 346–347
   removal procedures, **377**
   types of, 346
Catalase, bacteria, 742–743
Cataracts, **337**
   elderly and, 313
Catheterization
   urinary tract and, 326–327
      equipment, 327
      female patient, **355–356**
      male patient, **357–358**
Cautery, 387
CC (Chief complaint)
   medical history and, 192
CDC (Centers for Disease Control and Prevention), 598
   role of, 142, 145–150
   standard precautions and, 97
Cell-mediated immunity, 138
Cellophane tape swab, preparing/using, **748**
Cells
   blood, 666
   structure of, 724
Centers for Disease Control and Prevention (CDC), 598
   role of, 142, 145–150
   standard precautions and, 97
Centrifuge, microhematocrit, **670**
Cerebral vascular accident (CVA), 110, **348**
   described, **349**
Cerebrospinal fluid (CSF), specimen collecting, 734
Certificate for Provider-Performed Microscopy (PPM) Procedures, CLIA '88 (Clinical Laboratory Improvement Amendments of 1988), 601
Certificate of Accreditation, 602
Certificate of Compliance, 602
Certificate of Registration, 602
Certificate of Waiver, CLIA '88 (Clinical Laboratory Improvement Amendments of 1988), 601
Certification
   American Association of Medical Assistants (AAMA), 8–9
      examination, 834–836
   Certified medical assistant (CMA), examination, 836–839
Certified medical assistant (CMA), 8
   certification examination, 836–839
Cerumen, 340
Cervical
   cancer, **271**
   post biopsy, **273**
   punch biopsy, 273
Cervix, post cryosurgery, **273**
CEUs (Continuing education units), CMA (Certified medical assistant), 838
Chalazion, **337**
Channels, communication, 40–41
Charges, ethical issues concerning, 88
Charging, abbreviations used in, 198, **199**
Charisma, management and, 793

Charting
   correcting errors, 198
   methods of, 195–199
Charts
   organization of, 199
Checks
   payroll, preparing, 803–804
Chemical
   inventory form, **607**
   names of drugs, 499
   sterilization, 165–166, 399
      "cold," 421–422
   tissue destruction, 387
   warning colors, 610, **611**
   warning label determination, **610**
Chemical Hygiene Plan, 606–612
Chemical Hygiene Plan, requirements of, 611–612
Chemicals, avoiding exposure to, 612
Cherokee, attitudes toward illness of, 31
Chest
   circumference, measuring, 290
   measuring circumference of, 219
   physical examination and, **244**, 246
Cheyne-Stokes, defined, 214
Chickenpox, **141**
Chief complaint (CC)
   medical history and, 192
Children, 483
   abuse of, 77, 294
      ethical issues concerning, **85**
   calculating dosages for, 527–529
   CPR (cardiopulmonary resuscitation) for, **125**
   failure to thrive, 285
   Heimlich maneuver
      on conscious, **116**
      on unconscious, **114–115**
   rescue breathing for, **121**
   screening, visual acuity, 292–293
   see also Pediatric
Chinese diet, **491**
Chlamydia, **136**, **271**
   described, **272**
Chloride (Cl), 484
Choking, Heimlich maneuver and, 111–112
Cholangiography, **434**
Cholecalciferol, **481**, 483
Cholecystitis, **328**
Cholecystography, **434**
Cholelithiasis, **328**
Cholera, transmission of, **729**
Cholesterol
   chemistry of, 773–774
   functions of, 774
   reference values for
      HDL, **774**
      total, **773**
   testing for, 773–774, **784**
   transport, lipoproteins and, 774
Chorionic villi sampling (CVS), 262
Choroid layer, defined, 336
Chromium, 484
Chronological
   resume, 849
Circadian rhythm, 702
Circulatory system, 350–351
   anatomy/physiology of, 637–639
   disorders of, **350**
      described, **351**
Citrate, 743–744
   tubes, **744**
Civil law, 69
Civil Rights Act of 1964, 824

Cl (Chloride), 484
Clamps, 392–395
Clean-catch urine collection method, 702
CLIA '88 (Clinical Laboratory Improvement Amendments of 1988), 598–606
   accrediting agencies under, **599**
   aftermath of, 605
   analyses list, **601**
   contents of the law, 601–605
   impact of on medical assistants, 605–606
   intention of, 599–600
   program description, 600
   regulation for Quality Control in Automated Hematology, 605
   testing categories, 600–601
   urine testing and, 700
Clinical chemistry department
   described, 621
   laboratory tests, **620**
Clinical laboratory
   scientist, **21**, 618–619
   technician, **21**, 619
Clinical Laboratory Improvement Amendments of 1988 (CLIA '88), 598–606
   accrediting agencies under, **599**
   aftermath of, 605
   analyses list, **601**
   contents of the law, 601–605
   impact of on medical assistants, 605–606
   intention of, 599–600
   program description, 600
   regulation for Quality Control in Automated Hematology, 605
   testing categories, 600–601
Clinical thermometers, 208
Clinitest®, 708
Closed
   fractures, **347**
   questions, 47
   wounds, 100, 405
Clostridia, gram-positive, gas gangrene and, **136**
Clostridial myonecrosis, **136**
Clostridium
   botulinum, **136**
   tetani, **136**
CLT (Clinical laboratory technician), 619
Clustering
   nonverbal communication and, 44
CMA. See Certified medical assistant
Coagulase, bacteria, 743
Cobalamin, 483
Cocaine, abuse of, 511
Cocci, defined, 734
Cochlea, 341
Code of Ethics
   American Association of Medical Assistants, 84, 85
   Association of Medical Assistants (AAMA), **86**
      keys to, 86–87
Code of Medical Ethics, 87–88
Cognitive functioning, defined, 316
Cold
   common, pediatrics and, 294
   compresses/packs, 460
   therapy with, 457–458
Cold-related illnesses, 107
College of American Pathologists, **599**
Colles fracture, 106, **347**
Colon, cancer, 328
Colonoscopy, 331
Colony count streak, **741**
Color blindness, 337

Color Slide® II Mononucleosis Test, 764
Color vision, 340
    testing, **364–365**
Colposcopy, 270, 272–273
Coma, diabetic, **110**
Comminuted fracture, 106, **347**
Commission on Office Laboratory Accreditation, **599**
Committee on Accreditation of Allied Health Education Programs (CAAHEP), 797–798
Common cold, pediatrics and, 294
Communicable diseases, transmission of, **729**
Communicate, ability to, 7
Communication
    congruency in, 44–45
    cultural influence on, 39–40
    cycle, 40–41
    facial expression and, 43
    five Cs of, 41–42
    importance of, 39
    modes of, 40–41
    nonverbal, 42–44
    position and, 44
    posture and, 43–44
    roadblocks to, 45–46
    skills, as management quality, 791
    technology and, 45
    territoriality and, 43
    verbal, 41–42
Compazine, **511**
Compendium of Drug Therapy, 505
Compensation, as defense mechanism, 46
Complaint
    medical history and, 192
    subjective, 192
Complete abortion, 262
Complete blood count, 668
    described, **352**
Compound fracture, 106
Comprehensive Metabolic Panel, **622**
Compresses
    cold, 460
    hot, 458
Computerized tomography (CT), 437
Computer-modified records, 196–198
Conduction, heat loss by, 207
Condylomata, described, **272**
Confidentiality
    ethical issues concerning, 87–88
    law, 76
Conflict resolution, 827
Congenital passive immunity, 139
Congestive heart failure, **350**
    described, **351**
Congruency, communication and, 44–45
Conjunctivitis, **337, 339**
Connective tissues, disorders of, **345**
Consent
    implied, 75
    informed, 74–75
        form, **75**
Contact Precautions, **148**
Contaminated, defined, 165
Continuing education
    American Association of Medical Assistants and, 9
    units (CEUs), 838
    verification form, **839**
Continuous fever
    chart of, **209**
    defined, 208
Contraception, described, 265
Contraceptive drugs, **508**

Contractions, Braxton-Hicks, 264
Contracts, in law, termination of, 71
Contractures, joints, lack of exercise and, 456
Contraindications, defined, 506
Contrast media, diagnostic imaging and, 433
Control plan
    exposure, 152
        Bloodborne Pathogen Standard, **161–162**
        office work practice, **153**
Control tests, laboratory, 623
Controlled Substance Act of 1970, 500
Controlled substances
    medical assistants role/responsibilities with, 502
    prescription for, 518
    schedules, 500
    storage of, 502
Contusion, 405
Convalescent stage, infections, 140
Convection, heat loss by, 207
Copper, 484
Cornea
    abrasion of, **337**
    defined, 336
Corns, **353**
    described, **354**
Coronary
    artery disease, **350**
    heart disease, described, **351**
Corporations, described, **17**
Cover letters, employment application, 852, **853**
CPR (cardiopulmonary resuscitation), 111, 112
    for adults, **123–124**
    for children, **125**
    for infants, **126**
Creams, surgical, 400, **403**
Crepitation, defined, 106
Crile hemostatic forceps, 393
Crile-Wood needle holder, 393
Criminal law, 69
Crisis, body temperature, defined, 208
Crohn's disease, **328**
Crosswait, C. Bruce, 41
Crutches, 450–453
    assisting patients with, **466–467**
    described, **450**
    walking-gaits, 452–453
Cryosurgery, 273, 388
Crystalline zinc, **525**
Crystals, in urine, 709
CT (Computerized tomography), 437
Cultural
    awareness, displaying, 190–191
    heritage in medicine, 30
Culture
    defined, 60, 701
    diet and, 491–493
    life-threatening illness and, 60–61
    media, 738–739
        classifications of, 739
        inoculating, 740
        streaking, 740–741
    primary, 741
Curative, use of drugs, 499
Current Options of the Council on Ethical and Judicial Affairs of the American Medical Association, 87–88
Cushing's syndrome, 771
CVA (Cerebral vascular accident). *See* Cerebral vascular accident (CVA), 110
CVS (Chorionic villi sampling), 262

Cyanmethemoglobin, 669
Cyanosis, defined, 243
Cystitis, **324**
Cystography, **434**
Cystoscopy, urinary tract and, 325
Cysts, ovarian, 270
Cytochrome oxidase, bacteria, 743
Cytology department
    described, 621
    laboratory tests, **620**
Cytotechnologist, **21**

D

DACUM Competencies, 9
Da Vinci, Leonardo, 31
Death and dying
    cultural aversion to discussing, **190**
    ethical issues concerning, 90
Debridement, defined, 192
Declining stage, infections, 140
Decongestant drugs, **508**
Deep
    tissue, modalities, 460–461
    wounds, defined, 405
Deep slant/slant, **755–756**
Defamation of character, 74
Defendant, in law, 69
Defense mechanisms, 46–47
Defibrillation, 582
Defibrillator, 582
Deltoid muscle, site selection/injection angle, 540–541, **542**
Dementia
    defined, 316
    ethical issues concerning, **85**
Demographic data forms, 185
Denial, as defense mechanism, 46
Deoxyribonucleic acid (DNA), defined, 724
Department of Health and Human Services (HHS), 598
Department of Labor, 598
Dependability, 5
Depressed fracture, 106
Dermatitis, **353**
    described, **354**
Dermatophytosis, **353**
    described, **354**
Dermis, described, 352
Designation of health care surrogate, 78
Desk Reference for Nonprescription Drugs, 505
Dextrose, **511**
Diabetes mellitus, 109
    diet for, 489
    insulin dosage and, 525
Diabetic
    coma, causes/symptoms of, **110**
    retinopathy, **337**
Diagnostic
    use of drugs, 499
Diagnostic imaging
    computerized tomography (CT), 437
    contrast media, 433
    fluoroscopy, 436
    magnetic resonance imaging (MRI), 438
    patient
        positioning, 435
        preparation for, 433–434
    positron emission tomography (PET), 437
    ultrasonography, 436–437
Diagnostic medical sonographer, **22**
Diarrhea
    defined, 330
    shigellosis, **136**

Diary
    patient activity, 584
Diastole
    defined, 569
    pressure, defined, 215
Diet
    culture and, 491–493
    therapeutic, 488–491
Differential
    bacteria stains, 735–736
    blood test, described, 352
    diagnosis, defined, 617
    media, 739
Digestion
    defined, 476
    nutrition and, 476
Digestive system, 328–335, **477**
    conditions/disorders of, 330–331
    diagnostic tests of, 331
        sigmoidoscopy, 331–332
    disorders, **328–329**
    fecal occult blood test, 334
    X-ray studies of, 335
        patient preparation, **336**
Digital
    thermometers, 208
        using, **222–223**
Digoxin, **511**
Dilation, defined, 264
Dilators, 396–398
Diphtheria, transmission of, **729**
Disease transmission, **729–731**
    blood, body fluids and, 97
Diseases, infectious. See Infectious diseases
Disinfection
    chemical, of instruments, **174–175**
    medical asepsis and, 164–165
Dislocation, of joints, described, **346**
Dispense, defined, 504
Displacement, as defense mechanism, 46–47
Disposable
    electrodes, ECG, 573–574
    syringes, 535
    thermometers, 208
Distribution, drug, 506
Diuretic drugs, **508**
Diuril, **511**
Diverticulitis, **328, 331**
DNA (deoxyribonucleic acid), defined, 724
Doctrines, negligence and, 73
Domestic violence, 77
Dorsal recumbent position, 239
    placing patient in, **248–249**
Dorsalis pedis pulse, 212
Dorsogluteal
    site selection/injection angle, 539–540, **541**
Dosage
    calculating
        body surface method, 528–529
        for adults, 526–527
        for children, 527–529
        formulary method, 524–525
        insulin, 525
        kilogram of body weight method, 529
        proportional method, 524
Dosimeter, 433
Drabkin's reagent, 669
Draping, during physical examinations,
    239–241
Dressing forceps, 393
Dressings
    changing, 413–414
    emergencies and, 101
    surgical, 400, **403**

Droplet Precautions, **149**
Drug abuse
    injections and, 108
    urinary drug screening and, 325
Drug dosage, 518–519
    calculating, 520–529
    ratio, 520–521
Drug Enforcement Agency (DEA), registra-
    tion with, **501**
Drug proportion
    understanding, 521
Drug ratio
    expressed as
        a decimal, 521
        a fraction, 520–521
        a quotient, 520
    understanding, 520–521
Drug screening, 76–77
Drugs
    abuse of, 511–512
    actions of, 506–508
    administration of. See Medications
    classifications of, 506
    disposal of, 503–504
    emergency, 510–511
    forms of, 509–510
    genetically engineered, 500
    history/source of, 499–500
    interaction of, 508
    medical use of, 499
    names of, 499
    nonprescription, 503
        guidelines for patients taking, **503**
    office management of, 504
    prescription, 502
        guidelines for patients taking, **502**
    references/standards of, 505–506
    regulations/classifications of, 500–505
    routes of, 508–509
    storage/handling of, 510
    synthetic, 500
    undesirable actions of, 508
Dry
    cold therapies, 460
    heat sterilization, 165
    heat therapies, 459
Duckbill ear forceps, 393, **394**
Duodenal ulcer, **328,** 330
Durable power of attorney, 61, 78
Dyes, bacterial, 735–737
Dying and death, ethical issues concerning,
    90
Dysmenorrhea, defined, 266
Dyspareunia, defined, 266

E

Ear specula, 396
Eardrum, 340
Ears, 340–342
    cross section of, **341**
    disorders of, **341**
    instillation, **370**
    irrigating, performing, **368–369**
    physical examination and, **244,** 246
    review of systems (ROS), 194–195
Eastern Orthodox, diet, **492**
Ecchymosis, 405
ECG. See Electrocardiography, 566–567
Echocardiogram, 436
Echocardiography, 585
Eclampsia, 263
Edematous, defined, 647–648
Education

    medical, 31
    medical assistant, 9–10
    office personnel and, 826–827, **829**
Effacement, defined, 264
Egypt, medical treatment in ancient, 32
EIA (Enzyme immunoassay test)
    pregnancy testing and, 762
    test for hCG, **763**
EKG. See Electrocardiography, 566–567
Elbow, bandage wrapping technique, **402**
Elderly
    abuse, 77
    ethical issues concerning, **85**
    memory-impaired, medical assistant and,
        316–317
    nutritional needs during, 488
    societal bias against, 312
    visually impaired, medical assistant and,
        317–318
    see also Aging
Electrical
    burns, 105
    tissue destruction, 387
Electrocardiography
    described, 566–567
    equipment/supplies for, 572–574
        care of, 574
        electrolyte, 572–573
        paper, 572
    facsimile transmissions using, 572
    heart rate, on ECG graph paper, 569–570
    interference, causes of alternating current
        (AC), 578
    interference/artifacts, 577–579
        somatic, 578
    interpretive, 572
    leads
        augmented, 576
        chest/precordial, 576
        coding, 574
        placement, 574–576
        standard limp/bipolar, 575–576
    sensors/electrodes, 573
    standard resting, 576–577
    standardization of, 576
    telephone transmissions, 572
    tracing, mounting, 577
    types of, 570–572
Electrodes, electrocardiography and, 573
Electrolyte, electrocardiography and,
    572–573
Electrolyte Panel, **622**
Electrolytes, 483
Electromyography, 456
Electroneurodiagnostic technologist, **22**
Electrosurgery, 387
Elimination
    drug, 506, 508
    heat loss by, 207
Emancipated minor, 75
Emergency, 95
    arm splint, applying, **113**
    bleeding, 109–110
        control of, **112–113**
    blood, body fluids, disease transmission
        and, 97
    breathing, 111–112
    burns and, 101–102
    cerebral vascular accident (CVA), 110
    choking, infant back blows/chest thrusts
        for, **117–119**
    common, 99–100
        shock, 99–100
    CPR (cardiopulmonary resuscitation)

for adults, **123–124**
for children, **125**
for infants, **126**
diabetes, 109
dressings/bandages, 101
drugs, 510–511
fainting, 109
Good Samaritan laws and, 97
heart attack, 110–111
heat/cold related illnesses, 107
Heimlich maneuver
    for conscious adult, **114**
    for conscious child, **116**
    for unconscious adult/child, **114–115**
hemorrhage, 109–110
insect stings, 108
musculoskeletal injuries, 105–107
poisoning, 107–108
preparation for, medical crash tray/cart,
    98–99
preparing for, 97–99
recognizing an, 95
rescue breathing
    for adults, **120**
    for children, **121**
    for infants, **122–123**
responding to, 95–96
    primary survey, 96
seizures, 109
sudden illness, 108–109
tourniquets and, 100–101
using
    emergency medical services system, 97
    telephone no. 911, 97
wounds, 100–105
Emergency medical technician, **22**
Emergency visit, by patients, 189
Empathy, 5
Emphysema, **343**
    defined, 214
    described, **344**
Employee
    exposure classification record, **153**
    information/training of, 159
    responsibilities, Bloodborne Pathogen
        Standard, **162**
    supervising, 794–796
Employee Eligibility Verification Form, **825**
Employee Vaccination Form, Hepatitis B,
    158
Employment strategies
    application/cover letters, 852, **853**
    budgetary needs analysis, 846
    contact tracker, 846
    interview process, 855–856
    job analysis/research, 844–846
    look of success, 854
    resume, preparation of, 847–852
    self-assessment, 844
Endometriosis, 269–270, **271**
Endoscopy, digestive system, 331
Enema, barium, 331
Energy
    balance, 479–480
    nutrients, 477–480
Engineering controls
    Bloodborne Pathogen Standard, **160**
    exposure and, 154–155
    exposure prevention and, 152
Enriched media, 739
Enteric
    fever, **136**
    precautions, 145
Enterobius vermicularis, 748

Enterotube®, 745
Enzyme immunoassay (EIA) test
    pregnancy testing and, 762
    test for hCG, **763**
Eosin, 676
Eosinophil, described, 677
Epidemiology, defined, 134
Epidermis, described, 352
Epilepsy, 109, **348**
    described, **349**
Epistaxis, 109, **337**
    defined, 149
Epstein-Barr virus (EBV)
    infectious mononucleosis and, 763
    transmission of, 763
Equal Pay Act of 1963, 824
Equipment
    management, 804–805
Ergonomic Hazards, 613
Ergonomics, 613
Erythrocyte sedimentation rate (SED),
    described, 352
Erythrocytes, **638**, 666
    calculating, 675
    counts, 671–675
        normal, **675**
        Unopette® method, **687–688**
    in urine, 708
    indices, 679
        using to diagnose, 679
    sedimentation rates (ESR), 679–681,
        692–693
        using to diagnose, 681
Erythropoietin, 669
Eskimos, attitudes toward illness by, 31
Esophagogastro-duodenoscopy, 331, **332**
Essential hypertension, 217, **350**
    described, **351**
Estraderm®, 509
Ethics
    abortion, 89–90
    abuse, 88–89
    advertising, 87
    AIDS, 90
    American Medical Association (AMA),
        code of ethics, 87–89
    artificial insemination/surrogacy, 90
    Association of Medical Assistants
        (AAMA), code of ethics, 86–87
    behavior and, 7
    bioethics
        defined, 85
        dilemmas, 89
    confidentiality, 87–88
    defined, 84
    dying and death, 90
    fetal tissue research, 89–90
    genetic engineering/manipulation, 90
    HIV (Human immunodeficiency
        virus), 90
    issues concerning, **85**
    media relations, 87
    medical
        records, 88
        resources allocation, 89
    professional
        fees/charges, 88
        rights/responsibilities, 88
Eukaryote, defined, 724
European diet, **491**
Evacuated tube system, 641–642
    specimen collecting, 649
Evaporation, heat loss by, 207
Examination. *See* Physical examination

Exercise tolerance ECG, 584–585
Exercises, therapeutic, 455–457
Exhaustion, adaptation to stress and, 53
Expectorant drugs, **508**
Expert witness, defined, 72
Exposure
    bloodborne pathogens, avoiding,
        162–163
    Bloodborne Pathogen Standard, compo-
        nents of, **162**
    control plan, 152
        Bloodborne Pathogen Standard, **161**
        office work practice, **153**
    controls, engineering/work practice, 152,
        154–155
    determination, 152
    follow-up after, 157
    preventing, methods of compliance,
        152–159
    standard precautions, 152
Exposure Classification Record, **153**
Exposure control plan, 152
    Bloodborne Pathogen Standard, **161**
    office work practice, **153**
Expressed contract, 69
External
    auditory canal, 340
    bleeding, 109–110
    ear, 340
    otitis, 337
    respiration, 343
Externship, preparation for, 10
Exudate, defined, 294
Eyeballs, cross section of, **338**
Eyes, 335–340
    curing lens, 510
    disorders of, **338**
    instillation, **365**
    irrigating, performing, **366–367**
    patch dressing application, **366**
    physical examination and, **244**, 245
    protection, Bloodborne Pathogen
        Standard, **160**
    review of systems (ROS), 194–195
    visual pathways of, **338**

F

Facial expression, communication and, 43
Facilities management, 804–805
Facsimile (fax) machines
    ECG transmissions using, 572
Failure to thrive, infants/child, 285
Fainting, 109
Fairmindedness, as management quality,
    791
False labor, 264
Family medical history, 193
Fasting blood glucose, 770–771
Fasting/timed specimens, urine, 701–702
Fats, 478
    energy from, 479
Fat-soluble vitamins, **482**
Febrile, defined, 208
Fecal occult blood test, 334
    procedure for, **360–362**
Feces, specimen collecting, 628
Federal Drug Abuse Prevention, Treatment,
    and Rehabilitation Act, 76–77
Feedback, 41
Fees
    ethical issues concerning, 88
Feet
    physical examination and, **245**

Female
  genitalia
    exterior, **326**
    physical examination and, **245**, 246
  reproductive system, diseases/conditions of, **271–272**
Femoral pulse, 212
Fetal heart rate, test for, 262
Fetal tissue research, ethical issues concerning, 89–90
Fever
  defined, 208
  types of, **209**
Fiber, nutrition and, 485
Fibrillation
  atrial, 580
  ventricular, 581
Fibrocystic breasts, **271**
  described, **272**
Fibromyalgia, **345**
Fight-or-flight, adaptation to stress and, 53
Files
  see Medical records
Films
  filing, 439
  flat, 438
Financial management, 801–804
Finer finger bandage scissors, 391
Fingerstick, **660–661**
First aid, purpose of, 95
First-degree burns, 102–103
  response guide for, **104**
Flat plates, 438
Flexibility, 5
Flexion tests, 344
Fluoroscopy, 436
Folacin, **482**
Foley catheter, **327**
Folic acid, 483
Follow-up
  by telephone, 857
  letter, 856–857
Food labels, readings, 485–486
Food poisoning, **141**
  botulism, **136**
  Salmonellosis, **136**
  staphylococcal infection and, **136**
Food Pyramid Guide, **480**
Foot, bandage wrapping technique, **401**
Forceps, 392–395
  sterile transfer, using, 408
Forearm crutches, **450**, 451
Forester forceps, 393, **395**
Forms, patient information, 185–189
Formulary method
  calculating dosages, 524
    for adults, 527
Four-point alternating gait, 452–453, **453**
Fowler's position, 240
  placing patient in, **249**
Fractures, 106, 346–347
  described, **346**
  types of, **347**
Fringe benefits, defined, 804
Frostbite, 107
Fulgurated, defined, 265
Functional resume, 850
Fungi, described, 136
Furuncle, **353**
  described, **354**

G
Gait
  belt, 448
  crutch-walking, 452
  four-point alternating, 452–453
  patient, 242
  three-point, 452
  two-point, 452
Gamete intrafallopian transfer (GIFT), 264
Gas gangrene, **136**
GAS (Hans Selye's General Adaptation Syndrome), 52, **53**
Gas pack jar, 726
Gas sterilization, 165
Gastric ulcer, **328**, 330
Gastritis, **329**, 330
Gastroenteritis, **141**, **328**, 330
Gastrointestinal system
  elderly and, 315
  review of systems (ROS), 194–195
Gastroscopy, 331
Gender, drug dosage and, 519
General Health Panel, **622**
Generic name, of drugs, 499
Genetic engineering/manipulation
  ethical issues concerning, 90
  of pharmaceuticals, 500
Genital warts, **271**
  ethical issues concerning, described, **272**
Genitalia
  physical examination and, 246
  female, **245**, 246
  male, **245**, 246
Geriatric patient, medical assistant and, 316–318
Gerontology, defined, 312
Gestational diabetes, 263
Gestures, communication and, 44
Giemsa's stain, 676
GIFT (Gamete intrafallopian transfer), 264
Glaucoma, **337**
  elderly and, 313
Glomerulonephritis, **324**
Glomerulus, defined, 698
Gloves
  applying sterile, **409–410**
  Bloodborne Pathogen Standard, **160**
  removing contaminated, procedure for, **173–174**
Glucose
  blood
    automated methods of testing, 771–772
    fasting, 770–771
    measuring, **784**
    photometry analysis, 772
    reference values for, **771**
    testing for, 770–773
    testing profiles, 772
  reagent test strips and, 706
  tolerance test, 771
Glycosylated hemoglobin, 773
Goals
  defined, 56
  long-range/short-range, 56–57
  relieving stress through setting, 55–57
"Going bare," defined, 805
Goniometry, defined, 455
Gonococcal disease, transmission of, **729**
Gonorrhea, **136**, **271**
  described, **272**
Good Samaritan law, 77
  emergencies and, 97
Gout, **345**
  described, **346**

Gram stain, 726, **751**
  procedure for, **736**
Gram-negative bacterial, nosocomial (hospital-acquired) infection, **136**
Gravidy, defined, 261
Greeks, attitudes toward illness by, 31
Greenstick fracture, 106, **347**
Group medical practices, 16–17
Guaiac
  hemoccult test, **335**
  slides, 334
Guthrie screening test, 767
  factors affecting, 768
Gynecological
  cervical punch biopsy, 273
  cryosurgery, 273
  diseases/conditions
    endometriosis, 269–270
    infertility, 269
    menopause, 269
    ovarian cancer, 270
    ovarian cysts, 270
    pelvic inflammatory disease, 270
  examination, 265–269
    assisting with, 267–269, **275–276**
    colposcopy and, 270, 272–273
    pap smear equipment, 268
  laparoscopy, **273**, 274
  month-end, 269–274
Gynecology, defined, 258

H
H. influenzae, **136**
H. pylori, ulcers and, **330**
Hammer (malleus), 340
Handling, specimen, 626–627
Hands, physical examination and, **244**
Handwashing
  for surgical asepsis, 385
  medical and surgical, differences between, **387**
  medical asepsis and, 163
Hans Selye's General Adaptation Syndrome (GAS), 52, **53**
Hartman ear forceps, 393
Hartman nasal dressing forceps, 393, **394**
HAV (Hepatitis A virus), **144**
Hazard Communications Standard, 606
HBV (Hepatitis B virus). *See* Hepatitis B, **144**
HCFA (Health Care Financing Administration), 598
  CLIA implementation of, 600
  organ- and disease-oriented panels, **622**
HCFA-116, **602**, **603**
hCG (Human chorionic gonadotropin), 761
  EIA test for, **763**
HCV (Hepatitis C virus), **144**
HDL (High-density lipoprotein), 774
HDV (Hepatitis D virus), **144**
Head
  circumference, measuring, 290
  physical examination and, **244**, 245
Headache, described, **349**
Healing process, wounds, 404–406
Health and safety guidelines, **599**
Health Care Financing Administration (HCFA), 598
  CLIA implementation of, 600
  organ- and disease-oriented panels, **622**
Health care professionals
  allied, **21–22**
  role of, 19
Health care providers, regulation of, 11–12

Health care specialties, **21**
Health care surrogate, 78
    form, **79**
Health care team, 18–25
Health care therapies, role of integrative or
    alternative, 24
Health history. *See* Medical history, 189
Health information administrator, **22**
Health information technician, **22**
Health maintenance organizations (HMOs),
    17–18
Health unit coordinator (HUC), 23
Hearing, elderly and, 313–314
Heart
    anatomy of, 567–568
    attacks, 110–111, **350**
    electrical conduction system of, 568–569
    healthy behaviors for, **579**
    physical examination and, **245**
    pulse rate range, children, **291**
    rate, on ECG graph paper, 569–570
Heat
    cramps, 107
    exhaustion, 107
    modalities, moist/dry, 458–459
    stroke, 107
    therapy with, 457–458
Heat sterilization, dry, 165
Heating pads/packs, 459
Heat-related illnesses, 107
Hegar uterine dilators, 396, **398**
Height
    as vital sign, 218
    measuring, **231**
        devices, 289
        infant/child, 285–289
Heimlich maneuver, 111–112, 325, 582–584
    on conscious
        adult, **114**
        child, **114–116**
Hema-3, **676**
Hemacytometer, 672
    filling, **673**
Hematemesis, 330
Hematocrit
    defined, 668
    determination test, 668–671
    normal, values of, **671**
    packed cell column, **670**
Hematological tests, 667–679
    complete blood count (CBC), 668
    hematocrit determination, 668–671
    hemoglobin determination, 668–671
Hematology
    automated, instrumentation and quality
        control, 681–682
    defined, 666
    instruments
        not requiring sample dilutions, 682
        requiring sample dilutions, 682
    request form, **668**
Hematology department
    described, 621
    laboratory tests, **620**
Hematological tests, infectious mono-
        nucleosis, 763
Hematoma, 405
    defined, 647
Hematopoiesis, defined, 666, 667
Hemiplegia, defined, 448
Hemoconcentration, defined, 647
HemoCue® Blood Glucose System, 771, 772
Hemoglobin
    defined, 668

determination test, 668–671
    using a spectrophotometer, **683**
    using hemoglobin analyzer, **684**
normal
    molecule, **669**
    values of, **669**
Hemoglobinopathies, 669
Hemolytic
    anemia, 766
    streptococci, **136**, 329
Hemorrhoids, **329**
    thrombectomy of, **420–421**
Hemostatic
    drugs, **508**
    forceps, 392
Hemostats, 392–395
Hepatic Function Panel, **622**
Hepatitis, **329**
Hepatitis A, transmission of, **729**
Hepatitis B, 140, **141**, 142, 271
    Employee Vaccination Form, **158**
    facts about, **143**
    symptoms of, 142
    transmission of, 142, **729**
    vaccination, Bloodborne Pathogen Stan-
        dard, **161**
    vaccines, 157
Hepatitis C, transmission of, **729**
Hepatitis diseases, acute viral, 142
Hepatitis viruses, described, **144**
Hernia, hiatal, **329**
Herniated disk, **345**
    described, **346**
Herpes Simplex II, described, **272**
Herpes zoster, **348**
    described, **349**, **354**
Heterophile antibodies, 764
HEV (Hepatitis E virus), **144**
HHS (Department of Health and Human
        Services), 598
Hiatal hernia, **329**
Hibeclens®, 400
Hierarchy of needs, 45
High-density lipoprotein (HDL), 774
Hindu diet, **492**
Hippocrates, 33
Hippocratic Oath, 33, **34**
Hirschman
    anoscope, **397**
    protoscope, **397**
Histidine, 478–479
Histology department
    described, 621
    laboratory tests, **620**
HIV (Human immunodeficiency virus), 62,
        271
    ethical issues concerning, 90
    informed consent and, 77
    transmission of, 142
HMOs (Health care organizations), 17–18
Hodgkin's disease, **351**
    described, **352**
Holding media, defined, 723
Holism, **25**
Holter monitor, 582–584
    application, **590–591**
    electrode placement, **584**
Homeopathy, **25**
Homeostasis, 698
    defined, 476
Hookworm, transmission of, **730**
Hordeolum, **339**
Horedeolum, **337**
Horizontal recumbent position, 239

Hospital-based laboratories, 618
Hot compresses/packs, 458
Hot soaks, 458
Household measures, 523
Housekeeping, Bloodborne Pathogen
        Standard, **160**
HUC (Health unit coordinator), 23
Human chorionic gonadotropin (HCG), 761
Human immunodeficiency virus (HIV), 62, 77
Human resources manager
    conflict resolution and, 827
    discrimination and, 826
    office personnel
        chemically dependent/emotionally ill,
            826
        dismissing, 822–824
        interviewing applicants, 816–818,
            829
        orienting/training new, 819
        performance evaluation of, 819–822
        providing training/education to,
            826–827, **829**
        recruiting, 815
        salary review, 822
        selecting, 818–819
        temporary, 824, 826
    personnel laws, complying with, 824
    personnel records and, 824
    smoking policy, 826
    tasks of, 814–815
    see also Managers
Humoral immunity, 138
Humulin R, **525**
Hydrazoic acid, red blood counts and, 672
Hydrocortisone, **511**
Hydrogen peroxide, 400
Hydronephrosis, IVP (Intravenous pyelo-
        gram) and, 325
Hyperemesis gravidarum, placenta, abruptio
        and, 263
Hyperopia, **337**, **339**
Hyperpnea, defined, 214
Hypertension, 217, 489
Hyperthermia, elderly and, 314
Hyperventilation, defined, 214
Hypnotherapy, **25**
Hypnotic drugs, **508**
Hypochromic cells, 678
Hypodermis, described, 352
Hypoglycemic drugs, **508**
Hypotension, 217–218
Hypothermia, 107
    elderly and, 314
Hypoventilation, defined, 214
Hysterosalpingogram, defined, 264
Hysterosalpingography, **434**

I
Ice packs, 460
Ictotest®, 708
Idea-oriented personality, as management
        style, 792
Illness
    attitudes toward, 31–32
    life-threatening, 60–61
    present, medical history and, 192
    sudden, 108–109
IM (Infectious mononucleosis). *See* Mono-
        nucleosis
Imaging, diagnostic. *See* Diagnostic imaging
Immigration Reform Act, 824
Immune system, 138–139
    purpose of, 138

Immunity, 138–139
    natural barriers to, 139
Immunization, 139
    administration guidelines, **284**
    schedule, **283**
    scheduling books and, 284
Immunoglobulins, 138
Immunohematology department
    described, 621
    laboratory tests, **620**
Immunology department
    described, 621
    laboratory tests, **620**
Impacted fracture, 106, **347**
Impetigo, **353**
    described, **354**
Implantable devices, 510
Implied
    consent, 75
    contract, 69
In and out catheter, **327**
In vitro fertilization (IVF), 264
Incinerator, microbiology laboratory and,
        727
Incisions, 100, **405**
    repairing, **412–413**
Incompetence, 75
Incomplete
    abortion, 263
    fracture, 106
Incubation stage, infections, 140
Incubator, microbiology laboratory and, 726
Incus, 340
Independent physician association (IPA),
        18
India, diet of, **492**
Indirect statements, 47
Individual medical practices, 16
Indole, bacteria, 743
Induced abortion, 263
Indwelling catheter, **327**
Infancy, nutritional needs during, 488
Infants
    conscious/choking, back blows/chest
            thrusts for, **117**
    CPR (cardiopulmonary resuscitation) for,
            126
    ethical issues concerning, **85**
    failure to thrive, 285
    measuring, height/weight, 285–289
    rescue breathing for, **122–123**
    screening
        for hearing impairment, 292
        visual acuity, 292–293
    unconscious, back blows/chest thrusts for,
            118–119
    urine sample, collecting, 292
Infection
    chain of, 134–137
    control, 142
    immune system/immunity and, 138–139
    incision/drainage of localized, **418–419**
    inflammatory response to, 138
    portal of
        entry, 137
        exit, 137
    process of, 134
    reservoir, reservoir, 137
    susceptible host, 137
    transmission of, 137
Infection control
    blood and, 146, 149–150
    body fluids and, 146, 149–150
Infections, Bartholin's gland, **271**

Infectious agents, 134–136
    bacteria, 135–136
    fungi, 136
    parasites, 136
    rickettsia, 136
    viruses, 134–135
Infectious diseases
    impact of, 133–134
    transmission of, 140
Infectious diseases, stages of, 140
Infectious mononucleosis (IM), **351**
    agglutination test for, 764–765
    diagnosis of, 763
    hematological test for, 763
    laboratory tests and, 762–765
    serological test for, 764
    slide test for, 764, **778**
        interpreting, 765
    symptoms of, 763
    treatment of, 763
Infectious waste
    defined, 150
    disposal of, 150
Infertility, 269
Inflammation, defined, 138, 405
Inflammatory response, 138
Influenza, **141, 343**
    described, **344**
    transmission of, **730**
Information, Bloodborne Pathogen Standard,
        161
Informed consent, 74–75, 404
    form, **75**
    HIV (Human immunodeficiency virus)
            and, 77
Ingestion, poison, 107
Inhalation
    medication administration by, 545–547
    poison, 107–108
Initiative, 5
Injectable anesthetics, 403
Injections
    administration guidelines for, 542–544
    allergic extracts, 544–545
    drug abuse, 108
    equipment/supplies for, 534–539
    hazards associated with, 534
    intradermal, 534
        administration of, **550–551**
    intramuscular, 534
    route selection, reasons for, 534
    site selection/injection angle, 539–541
    subcutaneous, 533
        administration of, **550–551, 556**
Inner ear, 340–341
Inner-directed people, stress and, 55
Inoculating equipment
    loop, 726, **727**
    microbiology laboratory and, 726
    needle, 726, **727**
Insect stings, 108
Instruments
    chemical disinfection of, **174–175**
    laboratory validations of, 624
    steam sterilization of, **178–179**
Insulatard NPH, **526**
Insulin
    calculating dosage of, 525
    intermediate/long acting, **526**
    precautions when administering, **526**
    rapid acting, **525**
    shock, **110**
Insurance
    liability, 805

Integrative health care therapies, role of, 24
Integumentary system, 352–354
    aging and, 314
    disorders of, **353**
        described, **354**
Intermittent fever
    chart of, **209**
    defined, 208
Internal
    bleeding, 110
    respiration, 343
Interpretive electrocardiograph, 572
Interrupted baseline artifacts, 579
Interview
    employment, 855–856
        follow-up, 856–857
    techniques, 47
Intradermal injection, 534
    administration of, **550–551, 558–559**
    site selection/injection angle, **540**
Intradermal test, 354
Intramuscular injection, 534
    administration of, **550–551, 557**
    site selection/injection angle, 539–540
    Z-track method of, 544, **562**
Intravenous pyelogram (IVP), 325, **434**
Introjection, as defense mechanism, 46
Invasion of privacy, 74
Inventories, managing, 804
Involutes, defined, 261
Ionizing radiation, 438
IPA (Independent physician association), 18
Ipecac syrup, **511**
Iris
    defined, 336
    scissors, 392
Iron, 484
    deficiency anemia, described, **352**
Ishihara color graph, 340
    testing color vision with, **364–365**
Islamic diet, **492**
Isolation categories, 145
Isopropyl alcohol, 400
Italia diet, **491**
Itinerary, travel, 796–797
IVF (In vitro fertilization), 264
IVP (Intravenous pyelogram), 325, **434**

J

Jaeger chart, 339
Japanese diet, **492**
Jaundice, 142
Jenner, Edward, 32
Jewish diet, **492**
Job
    analysis/research, 844–846
    descriptions, 815–816
Joint Commission on Accreditation of
        Healthcare Organizations, **599**
Joints, injuries to, 107
Joseph skin hooks, **398**
*Journal of Continuing Education Topics &
        Issues*, 839

K

Kelly
    anoscope, **397**
    hemostats, 392–393
Ketoacidosis, urine odor and, 704
Ketones
    confirmatory testing of, 707
    reagent test strips and, 706

Kidneys
  biopsy of, 325
  defined, 698
Killed pathogen vaccines, 139
Kinesics, 42
Kirby Bauer method, 746
Knee, bandage wrapping technique, **401**
Knee-chest position, 240
  placing patient in, **250**
Koch, Robert, 32–33, 133
Korotkoff sounds, 216
Kwashiorkor, 479
Kyphosis, **345**
  described, **346**

L

Labels, Bloodborne Pathogen Standard, **161**
Laboratory, 616–617
  departments, 619–622
  manual page, sample, **626**
  medical assistant's role in, 624
  microscopes, 628–630
  microscopic examination of, bacteria,
    734–737
  personnel, 618–619
  quality control/assurance for, 623–624
  quality control programs, 700
  requisitions/reports, 624–625
  specialty tests
    infectious mononucleosis, 762–765
    pregnancy testing and, 761–762
  specimen collection requirements,
    732–734
  tests
    blood glucose, 770–773
    blood typing/groups/factors, 765–766
    BUN (Blood urea nitrogen), 775
    categories of, **620**
    chemistry profile, **623**
    cholesterol, 773–774
    digestive system, 328–329
    phenylketonuria (PKU) test, 767–768
    prenatal visit, 260
    profiles of, 621
    purposes of, 617
    semen analysis, 766–767
    triglycerides, 774–775
    tuberculosis, 768–770
  types of, 618
Labyrinthitis, 246
Lacerations, 100, **405**
  suturing, **412–413**
Lactation, nutritional needs during, 486–487
Lacto-ova vegetarians, **492**
Lacto-vegetarians, **492**
Laos, diet of, **492**
Laparoscopy, **273**, 274
Larry probe, **397**
Laryngitis, **343**
  described, **344**
Laser surgery, 388
Lateral view, 435
Latex beads, agglutination inhibition test
  and, 761–762
Latex sensitivity, **146**
Latter Day Saints, diet, **492**
Laundry
  Bloodborne Pathogen Standard, **161**
  contaminated, disposal of, 156
  facility, Bloodborne Pathogen Standard,
    161
Law
  abuse and, 77

Americans with Disabilities Act, 77,
    78–79
  battery, 73–74
  confidentiality, 76
  contracts in, 69, 71
  criminal/civil, 69
  defamation of character, 74
  emancipated minor, 75
  Good Samaritan law, 77
  incompetence, 75
  medical records and, 74–76
  minor, 75
  patient rights, 69, **70**
  public duties and, 76–77
  standard of care and, 72
  statute of limitations, 76
  subpoenas, 75
  torts, 72–73
Law lateral view, 435
Lawn streak, **741**
Laxative drugs, **508**
LDL (Low-density lipoprotein), 774
Leaders
  described, **793**
  managers versus, **793**
Learning, desire for, 6
Leg, lower, bandage wrapping technique, **401**
Legionella pneumophila, **136**
Legionnaires' disease, **136**
Legs, physical examination and, **245**
Lens, eye, defined, 336
Lente, **526**
Leonardo da Vinci, 31
Leprosy, transmission of, **730**
Leukemia, 351
  described, **352**
Leukocytes, **638**, 666
  counts, 671–675
    differential, **691–692**
    manual dilution, 671
    normal, **675**, 677
    Unopette® method, **686–687**
    using high-power magnification,
      674–675
    using low-power magnification, 672–673
  differential, 675–677
  divisions of, **678**
  identification guide, **677**
  in urine, 708
  reagent test strips and, 706
Leukorrhea, 149
Libel, 74
License, described, 11
Licensed practical nurse (LPN), 23
Licensure, comparison of requirements, 11
Life-threatening illness, 60–61
  choices in, 61–62
  cultural perspective on, 60–61
  medical assistant and, 63
Lifting
  safely, 446–447
  techniques, 448
Ligation, defined, 265
Ligature, defined, 388–389
Lipid panel, **622**
Lipoproteins, cholesterol transport and, 774
Listening skills, 41
Lister bandage scissors, 391
Lister, Joseph, 32
Lithotomy position, 239–240
Live attenuated pathogens vaccines, 139
Liver function studies, described, 352
Living will, 61, 78
  form, **78**

Lochia, 264
  alba, 264–265
  defined, 149
  rubra, 264
  serosa, 264
Lockjaw, **136**
Long arm cast, 347
Long-range goals, 56–57
Lordosis, **345**
  described, **346**
Low-density lipoprotein (LDL), 774
Lower GI series, 331, **434**
LPN (Licensed practical nurse), 23
LPT (Phlebotomist), 24
LSD (lysergic acid diethylamide), abuse of,
    511
Lucae bayonet-type forceps, 393, **394**
Lumbar puncture, assisting with, **377–378**
Lungs
  cancer of, **343**
    described, **344**
  physical examination and, **244**
Lymph
  importance of, 351
  systems, 351–352
    disorders of, **351**
Lymphedema, **351**
  described, **352**
Lysergic acid diethylamide (LSD), abuse of,
    511
Lysis, defined, 208

M

Macular degeneration, elderly and, 313
Magnesium (Mg), 484
Magnetic resonance imaging (MRI), 438
Malaria, 136
Male, 340
  genitalia, physical examination and, **245**,
    246
Malignant hypertension, 217
Malleus, 340
Malpractice, defined, 72, 805
Mammography, **434**
Managed care, operations, 17–18
Managed care organizations (MCOs)
  impact of operations of, 18
Management
  medical practice, **17**
Managers
  benefits management and, 804
  described, **793**
  facility/equipment management, 804–805
  figuring taxes, 804
  leaders versus, **793**
  liability coverage/bonding, 805
  marketing functions, 799–801
  medical assistant. *See* Medical assistant
  payroll processing and, 803
  procedures manual and, 798–799
  qualities of, 791–792
  records/financial management, 801–804
  risk management and, 805
  student practicums and, 797–798
  styles of, 792–793
  supervising people, 794–796
  time management and, 798
  travel arrangements and, 796–797
  see also Human resources manager
Manipulation, described, 238
Mannerisms, communication and, 44
Mantoux test, 769–770
  procedure for, **782–783**

Marasmus, 479
Marijuana, abuse of, 511
Marketing
    brochures, 800
        office, 800–801
    defined, 799
    managers and, 799–801
    newsletters, 801
    press releases and, 801
    seminars, 799–800
    special events and, 801
    tools, **800**
Mask, oxygen administration by, 547
Masking, defined, **44**
Maslow, Abraham, 45
Maslow's hierarchy of needs, 45
Material Safety Data Sheet (MSDS),
    608–609
Mayo dissecting scissors, 391, **392**, 395
MCOs (Managed care organizations)
    impact of operations of, 18
Measles, transmission of, **730**
Measures. *See* Weights and measures
Media
    culture
        classifications of, 739
        inoculating, 740
        streaking, 740–741
    ethical issues concerning, 87
    microbiology laboratory and, 727
        culture, 738–739
    recommendations for, suspected
        pathogens, **740**
Medical asepsis, 163–165
    appropriate use of, 164
    handwash procedure, **170–171**
Medical assistant, **22**, 814–815
    career opportunities for, 11
    described, 619
    education of, 9–10
    geriatric patient and, 316–318
    life-threatening illness and, 63
    Role Delineation Chart, 9, 11,
        Appendix C
    role of, 18–19
    value of, 25
    see also Human resources manager;
        Managers
Medical assisting
    definition of, 8
    historical perspective of, 7–8
Medical crash tray/cart, 98–99
Medical education, 31
Medical forms, medical history and, 186–189
Medical history
    administrative/demographic data forms,
        185
    chief complaint, 192
    computerized, 189
    cross-cultural model, 185
    family, 193
    forms, completing, 189–192
    function of, 185
    medical forms, 186–189
    past, 192
    patient information forms, 185–189
    present illness, 192
    review of systems (ROS), 194–195
    social history and, 193–194
    see also Patient records
Medical illustrator, **22**
Medical laboratory. *See* Laboratory
Medical laboratory technologist (MLT), 23
Medical practice, management, **17**

Medical records, 74–76
    Bloodborne Pathogen Standard, **161**
    charting methods, 195–199
    computer
        modified, 196–198
        contents of, 195
    ethical issues concerning, 88
    occupational exposure and, 159
    see also Medical history; Patient records
Medical resources, allocation of, 89
Medical specialists, 30–31
Medical treatments, 32–33
Medications
    administration of, 529–533, 545–547
        legal/ethical considerations, 517
        oral, 533
        parenteral, 533–545
    dosage calculations and, *see* Dosage
    errors in, 532
    label on, 519
    measured in units, 524–529
        formulary method, 524–525
        proportional method, 524
    oral, administration of, **548–549**
    order for, 517
    patient assessment and, 532–533
    powder, reconstituting for administration,
        559–561
    "six rights" of, 530–532
    withdrawing from
        ampule, **552–553**
        vial, **552–553**
Medicine
    card, **530**
    cultural heritage in, 30
    new frontiers in, 34
    significant contributions to, 33
Meeting
    agendas, **795**
        preparing, **806**
Meetings, staff, 795–796
Melanoma, **353**
    described, 354
Memory-impaired older adults, medical
        assistant, 316–317
Ménière's disease, **337**
Meningitis
    described, **349**
    meningococcal, transmission of, **730**
Meningococcal meningitis, **136**
Meniscus, defined, 704
Menopause, 269
Menses, defined, 149
Menstruation, defined, 149
Mercury
    manometers, **215**, 216
    thermometers, 208
        taking rectal temperature with, **225**
    using, **220–221**
Message, in communications, 40–41
Metabolism, defined, 479
Metal sensors/electrodes, ECG, 573
Metered dose, instructing patient in,
    374–375
*Methods for Antimicrobial Susceptibility Tests for
    Anaerobic Bacteria*, 746
*Methods for Dilution Antimicrobial Susceptibility
    Tests for Bacteria That Grow Aerobi-
    cally*, 746
Methylene blue, 676
Metric system
    conversion, 523–524
    guidelines, 521–522
    prefixes, 522

Mexican diet, **491**
Mg (Magnesium), 484
Michelangelo, 31
Microbiology
    biochemical tests, 742–744
    classification of, 723–724
    collection procedures, 729, 732–734
    culture. *See* Culture
    defined, 722
    department/laboratory
        described, 621
        equipment/supplies for, 725–727
        medical assistant's role in, 723
        quality control of, 728–729
        tests, **620**
        work area, 728
    mycology, 749
    parasitology, 747–749
    sensitivity testing, 746–747
    specimens
        handling, 728
        safety handling of, 727–728
    spills/waste, disposal of, 728
Microcytic cells, 678
Microhematocrit
    centrifuge, **670**
    procedure for using, **685–686**
    sealing clay, **670**
    tube with blood, **670**
Microscopes, 628–630
    described, 725
    using, **631–632**
Microtainer®, 653
Middle ear, 340
Middle Eastern diet, **491**
Midstream urine collection method, 702
Miltex skin hooks, **397**
Minerals, as a source of drugs, 499–500
Minor, defined, 75
Missed abortion, 262
Mitral valve stenosis, **350**
    described, 351
Mixtard, **525**
MLT (Medical Laboratory Technologist), 23
Moderate complexity tests, provider-
        performed microscopy tests, 600–601
Moles, **353**
    described, **354**
Molybdenum, 484
Mononucleosis
    infectious, 762–765
        agglutination test for, 764–765
        diagnosis of, 763
        hematological test for, 763
        interpreting slide test for, 765
        slide test for, 764, **778**
        symptoms of, 763
        treatment of, 763
Monoslide™ Test, 764
Monospot® Slide Test, 764
Monosticon Dri-Dot®, 764
Morphology, defined, 739
Mormon, diet, **492**
Mosquito hemostatic forceps, 392
Motility, bacteria, 743
Mouth
    physical examination and, **244**, 246
    review of systems (ROS), 194–195
Moxibustion, 30
MRI (Magnetic resonance imaging), 438
Multichannel ECG, 571
Multigravida, defined, 261
Multiple sclerosis, **348**
    described, **349**

Mumps, transmission of, **730**
Muscle relaxant drugs, **508**
Muscles
  disorders of, **345**
    described, **346**
  electrostimulation of, 456
  injuries to, 107
  testing, 455–456
Musculoskeletal injuries, 105–107
Musculoskeletal system, 344–347
  disorders of, **344–345**
    described, **346**
  elderly and, 314
Mycobacteria, resistance in, 769
Mycobacterium tuberculosis, **136**
Mycology, 749
  defined, 724
Myocardial infarction, **350**, 579
  described, **351**
Myopia, **337**, 339
Myringotomy, defined, 294

N

N. meningitidis, **136**
Na (Sodium), 484
Nagel's rule, defined, 262
Narcan, **511**
Nasal
  cannula, oxygen administration by,
    373–374, 546–547
  catheter, oxygen administration by, 547
  examination, assisting with, **370–371**
  irrigating, assisting with, **371**
Nasal polyps, **337**
National Board of Medical Examiners
    (NBME), 836
National Fire Protection Association, chemi-
    cal warning colors, 610, **611**
Native Americans
  attitudes toward illness by, 31
  aversion to talking about death, **190**
  diets of, **491**
Naturopathy, **25**
Navaho, attitudes toward illness by, 31
NBME (National Board of Medical Examin-
    ers), 836
Neck
  physical examination and, **244**, 246
  review of systems (ROS), 194–195
Needle holders, 392–395, **396**
Needles, 538–539
  contaminated, disposal of, 156
  gauges of, **640**
  parts of, 538
  safe disposal of, 538–539
  suture, 389
  venipuncture, 640
Needlestick, 150
Negligence, defined, 72, 805
Neisseria gonorrhoeae, **136**, 271
  described, **272**
Nematode, described, 748
Nephron
  defined, 698
  parts of, **699**
Neurological
  physical examination and, **245**
  review of systems (ROS), 194–195
Neurological system, 347–350
  disorders of, **348**
    described, **349**
  screening, 349–350
    assisting with, **379**

Neutrophil, described, 677
Nevus. See Moles
Newsletters, marketing and, 801
Niacin, **482**, 483
Nicoderm®, 509
Nicotinic acid, **482**
Nitrites, reagent test strips and, 706
Nitro Dur®, 509, **510**
Nitroglycerin, **511**
Nomenclature, microbiology, 724
Nondisposable syringes, 535
Nonprescription drugs, 503
  guidelines for patients taking, **503**
Nonverbal communication, 42–44
Normal flora, 136
Normochromic cells, 678
Nose
  physical examination and, **244**, 246
  review of systems (ROS), 194–195
  swab, 734
Nosebleed, 109, 149
Nosocomial (hospital-acquired) infection,
    136, 724
Novolin, **525**
Novolin L, **526**
Novolin N, **526**
NP (Nurse practitioner), 23
NPH, **526**
Nuclear medicine, 440
Nuclear medicine technologist, **22**
Nullipara, 261
Nurse practitioner (NP), 23
Nurses, 23
Nutrients
  minerals, 483–485
  types of, 476–485
    energy, 477–480
Nutrition
  defined, 476
  digestion and, 476
  physical examination and, 243
  stages of life and, 486–488
Nutrition label, items on, 486

O

OB/GYN physician, 258
Objective sign, defined, 192
Objectivity, as management quality,
    792
Oblique fracture, **347**
Oblique view, 435
Obstetric Panel, **622**
Obstetrics
  defined, 258
  described, 259–265
Obturator, 332
Occlusion, stroke and, 110
*The Occupational Exposure to Hazardous
    Chemicals in the Laboratory Standard,*
    606
Occupational Safety and Health Act,
    824
Occupational Safety and Health
    Administration. See OSHA
Occupational therapist, **22**
Occupational therapy assistant, **22**
Occupational therapy, described, **445**
Office brochures, 800–801
Office personnel
  chemical dependencies/emotional
    problems and, 826
  interviewing applicants, 816–818,
    829

orienting/training new, 819
performance evaluation of, 819–822
personnel records and, 824
providing training/education to, **829**
selecting applicants, 818–819
smoking policy and, 826
temporary, 824, 826
Office policy manual, 815
  preparing, **828**
Office surgery, 406
  anesthetics, 403
  assisting with, **411–412**
  described, 383–384
  patient care/preparation, 404–406
  preparation for, 406–408
  procedures performed, 386–387
  process, 406
  salary review, 822
  setup, 406
  supplies/equipment, 399–400, **403**
Ointments, surgical, 400, **403**
Onset of fever, defined, 208
Open wounds, 100
Open-ended questions, 47
Operating scissors, 391
Ophthalmic medical technician/
    technologist, 22
Ophthalmoscope, 340
OPIM (Blood and Other Potentially
    Infectious Material), 151–152
Oral medications
  administration of, 533, **548–549**
  equipment/supplies for, 533
Oral strip thermometer, using, taking oral
    temperature with, **221–222**
Oral temperature, 210–211
  pediatric, 291
  taking, using mercury thermometer,
    220–221
  using
    digital thermometer, **222–223**
    oral strip thermometer, **221–222**
Organization skills, as management quality,
    792
Orthopnea, defined, 214
Orthotist, **22**
OSHA (Occupational Safety and Health
    Administration, 150–163
  Bloodborne Pathogen Standard,
    151–159
  regulations, 606–612
    students and, 612
  regulations/students, 159, 162–163
Osteoarthritis, **345**
  described, **346**
Osteoporosis, **345**
  described, **346**
Otitis media, **337**
  pediatric, 293–294
  Streptococcal infection and, **136**
Otosclerosis, **337**
Otoscope, 342, 396
Outer-directed people, stress and, 55
Ovarian
  cancer, 270
  cysts, 270
Overtime, defined, 824
Oxygen
  administering, by nasal cannula,
    373–374
  administration of, 545–547
    delivery methods, 546–547
  safety precautions, 547
Oxytocin, labor and, 264

P

P (Phosphorus), 484
Packs
  cold, 460
  hot, 458
  ice, 460
Paget's disease, described, **346**
Pain
  back, **345**
    described, **346**
  cultural perspective on, 61
Pallor, defined, 243
Palpated
  defined, 647
  systolic blood pressure, 292
Palpation, described, 237
Pantothenic acid, **482**
Pap smear, 268–269
  assisting with, **275–276**
  frequency of, 265
  results, 269
PAPNET, 268
Paraffin wax bath, 459
Paramedic, **22**
Parasites
  common, 748–749
  described, 136
  in urine, 708
Parasitology, 747–749
  defined, 724
  department
    described, 621
    laboratory tests, **620**
  examination methods, 747
  specimen collecting, 747
Parenteral medications
  defined, 533
  equipment/supplies for, 534–539
  hazards associated with, 534
  route selection, reasons for, 534
  site selection/injection angle, 539–541
Parity, defined, 261
Parkinson's disease, described, **349**
Parliamentary Procedure, 795
Paroxysmal atrial tachycardia (PAT), 580
Partnerships, described, **17**
Parturition, 264
Passive immunity, 139
Pasteur, Louis, 32, 133
PAT (Paroxysmal atrial tachycardia), 580
Patch test, 354
Patency, defined, 269
Pathogenic toxin vaccines, 139
Pathogens, recommended media for, **740**
Patient
  information forms, medical history,
    185–189
  service centers, 618
Patient Self-Determination Act, 61–62
Patients
  activity diary, 584
  AIDS, therapeutic response to, 62–63
  appearance of, 242
  assisting
    to ambulate, **466–467**
    to stand and walk, **464**
  assisting to ambulate, 449
  discharged by physician, 71
  education brochures, 800
  falling, care of, **465**
  handling difficult, 191
  no longer needs treatment, 72
  physician withdraws from, 71
  transferring, 448–449

from examination table to wheelchair,
    463
  from wheelchair to examination table,
    461–463
Patient's Bill of Rights, 69, **70**
Patients records. *See also* Medical history
Patients records, importance of, 195
Patients rights, 69, **70**
Payroll
  processing, 803–804
PDR (*Physicians' Desk Reference*), **505**
  using, 505–506
Pediatrics
  child abuse and, 294
  described, 282–284
  developmental patterns, 285
  disorders/diseases of
    asthma, 294
    common cold, 294
    otitis media, 293–294
    pediculosis, 294
    tonsillitis, 294
  growth patterns, 285
  measuring
    chest circumference, 290
    child, height/weight, 285–289
    head circumference, 289
  pulse, heart rate range, **291**
  screening
    for hearing impairment, 292
    visual acuity, 292–293
  urine sample, collecting, 292
  vaccines, preparation for administration of,
    284
  vital signs
    blood pressure, 292
    pulse, 291
    respirations, 291
    temperature, 290–291
Pediculosis, pediatrics and, 294
Pelvic examination, assisting with, **275–276**
Pelvic inflammatory disease (PID), 270, **271**
  described, **272**
  impaired fertility and, 264
PEM (Protein-energy malnutrition), 479
People skills, managers, 791
People-oriented personality, as management
    style, 792
Peptic ulcers, 330
Perception, communication and, 45
Percussion, described, 237
Performance review, office personnel,
    819–822
*Performance Standards for Antimicrobial Disc
    Susceptibility Tests*, 746
Pericarditis, 350
  described, **351**
Peritonitis, defined, 330
Pernicious anemia
  defined, 315
  described, **352**
Personal protective equipment (PPE), 152,
    155–156
  Bloodborne Pathogen Standard, **160**
  microbiology laboratory and, 727–728
Personal visit, by patients, 189
Personalities, management style and,
    792–793
Personnel records, maintaining, 824
PET (Positron emission tomography), 437
Peter, Laurence, 55
The Peter Principle, 55
Petri dish, described, 739
pH, reagent test strips and, 706

Pharmacist (RPh), 23–24
Pharmacology, defined, 498
Pharyngitis, **343**, **493**
  described, 344
Phenylketonuria (PKU)
  blood specimen for, 780–781
  described, 767
  filter paper test card, **768**
  test, 767–768
    blood, 768
  urinalysis for, 768
  urine specimen for, **781**
Phlebotomist (LPT), 24
Phlebotomy
  defined, 162, 636
  medical assistant's role in, 637
  see also Blood
Phosphorus (P), 484
Physical attributes, of professionals, 6
Physical disabilities, prevalence of,
    444–445
Physical examination
  assisting with, **252–253**
  auscultation and, 238
  components of, 242–247
    body movements, 242–243
    breath odors, 243
    examination sequence, 243–247
    gait, 242
    nutrition, 243
    patient appearance, 242
    posture, 242
    skin/appendages, 243
    speech, 243
    stature, 242
  equipment/supplies for, 241, **242**
  manipulation and, 238
  observation/inspection and, 236
  palpation and, 237
  percussion and, 237
  positioning/draping during, 239–241
Physical therapist (PT), 24
Physical therapy assistant (PTA), 24
Physical therapy, described, **445**
Physician assistant, **22**
Physician-assisted suicide, ethical issues
    concerning, **85**
Physicians' Desk Reference (PDR), 505
  using, 505–506
Physician's directives, 61, 78
  form, **78**
Physicians' office laboratories (POLS), 618
Physician's splinter forceps, 393
Phytonadione, **481**
"Pick-ups" (forceps), 393
PID (Pelvic inflammatory disease), 270, **271**
  described, **272**
  impaired fertility and, 264
Pinna, 340
Pinworms, **329**, **748**
PKU (Phenylketonuria)
  blood specimen for, obtaining, **780–781**
  described, 767
  filter paper test card, **768**
  test, 767–768
    blood, 768
  urinalysis for, 768
  urine specimen for, **781**
Placenta
  abruptio, 263–264
  previa, 263
Plain films, 438
Plaintiff, in law, 69
Plants, as a source of drugs, 499

Plasma
  defined, 666
  specimen collecting, 628
Plaster-of-Paris casts, 346
  assisting with, **376**
Platelet count, **638**
  described, 352
Platelets, 666
Platform crutches, **450**, 451
Pleurisy, 343
  described, **344**
PMS (Premenstrual syndrome), described, **272**
Pneumonia, 343
  described, **344**
  Legionnaires' disease, **136**
  Streptococcal infection and, **136**
  transmission of, **730**
POCT (Point-of-care testing), 618
Poikilocytosis cells, 678
Point-of-care testing (POCT), 618
Poisoning, 107–108
Policy manual, preparing, **828**
Poliomyelitis, transmission of, **730**
POLS (Physicians' office laboratories), 618
Polychromatic stains, 676
Polycystic kidneys, **324**
  IVP (Intravenous pyelogram) and, 325
POMR (Problem-oriented medical record), 196
Popliteal pulse, 212
Portable ambulatory electrocardiograph, 582–584
  electrode placement, **584**
Portal of exit, infections, 137
Position, communication and, 44
Positioning, during physical examinations, 239–241
Positron emission tomography (PET), 437
Posterior cavity, eye, defined, 336
Posterior chamber, eye, defined, 336
Posterior sclera, defined, 336
Posteroanterior view, 435
Post-exposure follow-up, Bloodborne Pathogen Standard, **161**
Postoperative instructions, 404
Postpartum, pregnancy and, 264–265
Postprandial
  defined, 771
  two-hour blood glucose, 771
Posture, 445–446
  communication and, 43–44
  patient, 242
Potassium hydroxide (KOH), preparation of, 737
Potts fracture, **347**
Powder medications, reconstituting for administration, 559–561
Power verbs, 847–848
PPD (Purified protein derivative), 769
PPE (Personal protective equipment). *See* Personal protective equipment (PPE), Bloodborne Pathogen Standard
PPM (*Certificate for Provider-Performed Microscopy Procedures*), CLIA '88 (Clinical Laboratory Improvement Amendments of 1988), 601
PPO (Preferred provider organization), 18
Practice, scope of, 11–12
Pratt
  rectal probe, 397
  uterine dilators, 398
Preferred provider organization (PPO), 18

Pregnancy
  complications of, 262–264
  defined, 259
  eclampsia and, 263
  gestational diabetes and, 263
  hyperemesis gravidarum, 263
  impaired fertility and, 264
  interruption of, 262–263
  normal uterine, 259
  nutritional needs during, 486–487
  parturition and, 264
  patient education, 260–261
  placenta previa and, 263
  postpartum period and, 264–265
  signs/symptoms of, serious conditions in, **261**
  tests, procedure for, **776–777**
Pregnancy tests, **718–719**
  agglutination inhibition, 761–762
  commercial/home, 761
  enzyme immunoassay (EIA) test, 762
  quality control, 761
  slide test, 761–762
  testing methods, 761
  urine and, 32
Prejudices, 40
Premature ventricular contractures (PVCs), 580–581
Premenstrual syndrome (PMS), described, **272**
Prenatal visit
  assisting with, **274**
  health history and, 261
  initial, 259–261
    laboratory tests at, **260**
  subsequent, 262
    tests/procedures during, 262
Presbyacusia, defined, 314
Presbycusis, defined, 314
Presbyopia, **337, 339**
Prescribe, defined, 504
Prescription drugs, 502
  guidelines for patients taking, 502
Prescriptions
  abbreviations/symbols used with, 518, **519**
  controlled substances and, 518
  described, 517–518
Present illness, medical history and, 192
Press releases, 801
Preventative maintenance, laboratory, 623–624
Preventative use of drugs, 499
Primary container, 645
Primary hypertension, 217
Primigravida, defined, 263
Principles of Medical Ethics, American Medical Association (AMA), 84, 85, **86**
Probes, 396–398
Problem-oriented medical record (POMR), 196
Problems, using teams to solve, 794
Problem-solving skills
  as management quality, 792
Procedures
  administering injections
    intradermal, 550–551, 558–559
    intramuscular, **557**
    intramuscular Z-track, **562**
    subcutaneous, 550–551
  administering oxygen, by nasal cannula, **373–374**
  assisting patient, stand and walk, **464**
  audiometry, assisting with, 368–369

autoclave
  instrument steam sterilization, **178–179**
  wrapping instruments for, **176–177**
bacteriological smear, preparing, **750**
blood
  glucose, measuring, **784**
  smear slide, preparation of a differential, **689–690**
  specimen for, PKU (Phenylketonuria), **780–781**
breast self-examination, instructing patient in, **275**
broth tube inoculation, **755**
capillary puncture, 660–661
chemical "cold" sterilization, 421–422
chemical disinfection, of instruments, **174–175**
cholesterol testing, **784**
color vision test, performing, **364–365**
deep inoculation/slant, **755–756**
differential white blood count, **691–692**
digital thermometer, using, **222–223**
dorsal recumbent position, placing patient in, **248–249**
dressings/bandages, changing, **413–414**
ear, instillation, **370**
ears, irrigating, **368–369**
electrocardiogram
  single-channel, **586–588**
  twelve-lead, **589**
erythrocyte sedimentation rate (ESR), **692–693**
eye
  instillation, performing, **365**
  irrigation, **366–367**
  patch dressing application, **366**
Fowler's position, placing patient in, **249**
gloves, applying sterile, **409–410**
gram stain, **751**
gynecologic/pelvic examination, assisting with, **275–276**
hemorrhoid thrombectomy, **420–421**
Holter monitor, application, **590–591**
incision, repairing, **412–413**
infants/child
  measuring, **297**
  measuring respiration rate, **298**
  taking an apical pulse of, **298**
  taking rectal temperature, **297**
  taking urine sample, **299**
infections, incision/drainage of localized, **418–419**
infectious mononucleosis, slide test for, **778**
interviewing job applicants, **829**
job description, preparing, **828**
joint fluid, aspiration of, **419–420**
knee-chest position, 250
  placing patient in, **250–251**
lumbar puncture, assisting with, **377–378**
Mantoux test, **782–783**
measuring
  height, **231**
  radial pulse, **227–228**
  weight, **231–232**
medical asepsis handwash, **170–171**
meeting agendas, preparing, **806**
mercury thermometer
  taking rectal temperature with, **225**
  using, **220–221**
metered dose, instructing patient in, **374–375**
microhematocrit, using, **685–686**
microscopes, using, **631–632**

Procedures (*continued*)
  nasal
    examination, 370–371
    instillation, 372
    irrigating, 371
  office surgery, assisting with, 411–412
  oral medications administration,
    548–549
  oral strip thermometer, using, 221–222
  patients
    assisting to ambulate, 466–467
    care of falling, 465
  plaster-of-Paris casts, assisting with, 376
  policy manual, developing/maintaining,
    828
  positioning patient in supine position, 247
  powder medications, reconstituting for
    administration, 559–561
  pregnancy tests, 776–777
  prenatal visits, assisting with, 274
  procedures manual, developing/maintain-
    ing, 808–809
  proctosigmoidoscopy, assisting with,
    359–360
  range of motion exercises, 468–472
  rectal temperature
    taking using digital thermometer, 226
    taking using mercury thermometer, 225
  red blood counts, Unopette® method,
    687–688
  removal of casts, 377
  removing contaminated gloves, 173–174
  sanitization of instruments, 172
  sebaceous cyst excision, 417
  semen analysis, 779
  Sims' (lateral) position, placing patient in,
    251
  skin closure strips, applying sterile, 416
  skin surgery, preparation for, 422–423
  specimen inoculation, dilution streaking,
    754
  spirometry testing, 375
  sputum specimen, obtaining, 372–373
  sterile field, setting up/covering, 423–424
  sterile pack, opening, 425–427
  sterile solution, pouring, 427–428
  student practicums, supervising,
    807–808
  sutures, removing, 415
  suturing lacerations, 412–413
  taking
    apical pulse, 228–229
    axillary temperature, 226–227
    blood pressure, 230
    medical history, 200–201
    radial pulse, 227–228
    respiration rate, 229
  throat culture, obtaining, 749–750
  transferring patient
    from examination table to wheelchair,
     463
    from wheelchair to examination table,
     461–463
  travel arrangements, making, 806–807
  Trendelenburg position, placing patient in,
    252
  tympanic thermometers, using, 224
  upper arm veins, finding, 654–655
  urinalysis
    chemical, 714–715
    performing, 718–719
  urinary catheterization
    female patient, 355–356
    male patient, 357–358
  urine
    assessing clarity of, 713
    assessing color of, 712
    assessing volume of, 712
    drug screening, 355
    microscopic examination of sediment,
     717
    testing for sugar, 716
    using refractometer to measure specific
     gravity of, 713–714
  venipuncture
    by butterfly needle, 659–660
    by evacuated tube, 657–658
    by syringe, 655–656
  visual acuity
    measuring near, 363–364
    testing, 362–363
  wet mount, hanging drop slide preparation,
    752–753
  white blood count, Unopette® method,
    686–687
  Ziehl-Neelsen stain, 751–752
Procedures manual, 798–799
  developing/maintaining, 808–809
Proctologic position, 240–241
Proctosigmoidoscopy
  assisting with, 359–360
  setup for, 332
Procuring, specimen, 626–627
Prodromal stage, infections, 140
Professional Development, 41
Professional fees, ethical issues concerning,
  88
Professional liability insurance, 805
The Professional Medical Assistant (PMA),
  839, 845
Professional rights/responsibilities, ethical
  issues concerning, 88
Professionals, attributes of, 4–7
Proficiency testing, laboratory, 623
Projection, as defense mechanism, 46
Prone position, 241, 435
  placing patient in, 250–251
Prophylactic, use of drugs, 499
Proportion, drug, understanding, 521
Proportional method
  calculating dosages, 524–525
  for adults, 527
Prostaglandin, labor and, 264
Prostate, benign hypertrophy of, elderly and,
  315
Prosthetist, 22
Protamine zinc insulin (PZI), 526
Protective clothing, Bloodborne Pathogen
  Standard, 160
Protective equipment
  personal, 152, 155–156, 160
    microbiology laboratory and, 727–728
Protective isolation, 145
Protein-energy malnutrition (PEM), 479
Proteins, 478–479
  confirmatory testing of, 707
  energy from, 479
  reagent test strips and, 706
Protoscopes, 396
Provider-performed microscopy tests,
  600–601
Psoriasis, 353
  described, 354
Psychological
  changes in aging, 316
  review of systems (ROS), 194–195
Psychological suffering, range of, 62
PT (Physical therapist), 24

PTA (Physical therapy assistant), 24
Public duties, 76–77
Puerperium, defined, 259
Puerto Rico, diet of, 491
Pulmonary tuberculosis, 136
Pulse, 212–213
  measuring, 213
  pediatric, 291
  rates, 213
  recording, 213
Punctures, 100, 405
  defined, 405
Punctur-Guard®, 640
Pupil, defined, 336
Purified protein derivative (PPD), 769
PVCs (Premature ventricular contractures),
  580–581
Pyelography
  intravenous, 434
  retrograde, 434
Pyelonephritis, 324
Pyorrhea, 246
Pyrexia, defined, 208
Pyridoxine, 482, 483
PZI (Protamine zinc insulin), 526

Q
Quality control
  microbiology laboratory and, 728–729
  pregnancy tests, 761
  programs, 700
  reagent test strips and, 706

R
Rabies, 348
  described, 349
Radial pulse, 212
  measuring, 227–228
Radiation
  heat loss by, 207
  safety, 432–433
Radiation therapist, 22
Radiation therapy, 439–440
Radioallergosorbent test (RAST), 354
Radiographer, 22
Radiographs, described, 432
Radiolucent, defined, 433
Radiopaque, defined, 433
Rales, defined, 214
Random (spot) specimen
  urine, 701
    collection method, 702
Range of motion (ROM), 455
  exercises, 456–457, 468–472
Rapid strep test, 744–745
RAST (Radioallergosorbent), 354
Ratchets, defined, 389
Ratio, drug, understanding, 520–521
Rationalization, as defense mechanism,
  46–47
r/b System®, 746
RD (Registered dietitian), 23
Reagent test strip
  defined, 705
  quality control of, 706
  sensitivity of, 707
  tests using, 706
Reagents, defined, 700
Receiver, in communications, 41
Recertification
  CMA (Certified medical assistant), 838
Records management, 801–804
Records. *See* Medical records

Rectal examinations, 247
Rectal temperature, 211
  pediatric, 291
  taking
    using digital thermometer, **222–223**
    using mercury thermometer, **225**
Red blood cells, **638**, 666
  calculating, 675
  counts, 671–675
    normal, **675**
    Unopette® method, **687–688**
  in urine, 708
  indices, 679
    using to diagnose, 679
Reducing sugars, confirmatory testing of, 708
Reference laboratories, 618
Reference values, defined, 617
References, for resumes, 848
Reflexes, physical examination and, 247
Refractometer, 704, 705
Refrigerator, microbiology laboratory and, 727
Registered dietitian (RD), 23
Registered medical assistant (RMA), 9
  examination, format/content of, 835–836
Registered nurse (RN), 23
Registration, comparison of requirements, **11**
Regression, as defense mechanism, 46
Regulated waste containers (non-sharp),
    Bloodborne Pathogen Standard, **161**
Rehabilitation medicine
  described, 445
  medical assistant's role in, 445
Rehabilitation therapists, 445
Release of information form, **193**
Remittent fever
  chart of, **209**
  defined, 208
Renal
  calculi, **324**
    cystoscopy and, 325
  epithelial cells, in urine, 708
Renal Function Panel, **622**
Replacement, use of drugs, 499
Reports, filing, 439
Repression, as defense mechanism, 46
Reproductive system
  elderly and, 315
  female, diseases/conditions of, **271–272**
Requisition, laboratory work, 624–625
Res ipsa loquitur, 73
Rescue breathing, 112
  for adults, **120**
  for children, **121**
  for infants, **122–123**
Resistance, 138–139
Respiration, 213–214, **344**
  abnormalities, 214
  breath sounds, 214
  internal/external, 343
  measuring rate of, **229**
  pediatric, 291
  rate, 214
Respiratory isolation, 145
Respiratory system, 343
  disorders of, **343**
  review of systems (ROS), 194–195
Respiratory therapist, **22**
Respiratory therapy technician, **22**
Respondeat superior, 73
Resume
  power verbs, **847–848**
  preparation of, 847–852
  vital information on, 852

Retina
  defined, 336
  detachment of, **337**
Retinol, **481**
Retinopathy, diabetic, **337**
Retractors, 396–398
Retrograde pyelography, **434**
Return-to-normal, adaptation to stress and, 53
Review of systems (ROS), 194–195
Reye's syndrome, 348
  described, **349**
Rh blood typing, 766
Rheumatic fever, **350**
  described, **351**
Rheumatoid arthritis, **345**
  described, **346**
Rhonchi, defined, 214
Riboflavin, **482**, 483
Rickets, **345**
  described, **346**
Rickettsia, described, 136
Right lateral view, 435
Right to know laws, 606
Rigid sigmoidoscopes, 396
Risk management, 73, 805
RMA (Registered medical assistant), 9
RN (Registered nurse), 23
Robert's Rules of Order, 795
Rochester Ochsner hemostatic forceps, 393
Role
  ambiguity, burnout and, 54
  conflict, burnout and, 54
  overload, burnout and, 54
Role Delineation Chart, 9, 11, Appendix C
ROM (Range of motion), 455
  exercises, 456–457, **468–472**
Roman Catholic, diet, **492**
Romans, attitudes toward illness by, 31
ROS (Review of systems), 194–195
Rouleaux, defined, 681
Round window (inner ear), 341
Round worm, 748
RPh (Pharmacist), 23–24
RU 486, 265
Rubella, transmission of, **730**
Rubeola, transmission of, **731**

S

S pneumoniae, **136**
Safety hood, microbiology laboratory and, 725–726
Safety needles, 640
Safety Training Form, **611**
Saliva, defined, 149
Salmonella, **136**
Salmonellosis, **136**
Sanitization
  defined, 163
  medical asepsis and, 163–164
  procedure for, instruments, **172**
Scabies, 136
Scalpels
  handles of, **392**
  surgical, **391**, **392**
Schilling test, described, 352
Sciatica, 348
  described, **349**
Scissors
  iris, **391**, **392**
  Mayo dissecting, **392**
  surgical, **391**, **392**
  suture, **391**, **392**

Sclera, defined, 335
Scleroderma, 245, **353**
  described, **354**
Scoliosis, **345**
  described, **346**
Scope of practice, 11–12
Scopes, 396–398
Scratch test, 354
Sebaceous cyst, excision of, **417**
Second degree burns, 102–103
  response guide for, **104**
Secondary hypertension, 217
SED (Erythrocyte sedimentation rate),
    described, 352
Sediment
  urine, 708–711
    abnormal cells/microorganisms, 708–709
    components of, 708
Sedimentation rates
  erythrocyte (ESR), 679–681
  erythrocyte sedimentation rate (ESR), **692–693**
  using to diagnose, 681
Sediplast®, 681
Seizures, 109
Selective media, 739
Selenium, 484
Self-assessment, 844
  worksheet, **845**
Semen analysis, 766–767
  altering factors in, 767
  composition of, 767
  procedure for, **779**
  reference values for, **766**
Semicircular canals, 340
Semilente, 525
Seminars, marketing, 799–800
Semmeweis, Phillipp, 32
Sender, communication, 40
Senior adults. *See* Elderly, 85
Sensitive topics, dealing with, 191–192
Sensors, electrocardiography and, 573
Sensory system, 335–342
  color vision, 340
  disorders of, **337**
  eye, 335–340
  visual acuity, measuring, 337–340
Separator gel tube, **643**
Serological tests, infectious mononucleosis, 764
Serology department
  described, 621
  laboratory tests, 620
Serum blood, specimen collecting, 627–628
Serum urea nitrogen concentration
  drugs affecting, **775**
  factors affecting, **775**
Seventh Day Adventist, diet, **492**
Sexually transmitted diseases, **271**
  Chlamydia, **136**, **271**
    described, **272**
  Condylomata, **271**
    described, **272**
  Gonorrhea, **136**, **271**
  Neisseria gonorrhoeae, described, **272**
  Syphilis and, **136**
Sharps containers
  Bloodborne Pathogen Standard, **160**
  syringe/needle disposal, 538–539
Shigella, **136**
Shigellosis, **136**

Shock, 99–100
    insulin, **110**
    signs/symptoms of, 99
    treatment of, 100
    types of, 99
Short arm cast, 346
Short-range goals, 56–57
Shoulder, bandage wrapping technique, **402**
Sick-baby, 283, 285
Sick-child, 283, 285
Sickle cell anemia
    CVS (Chorionic villi sampling) and, 262
    described, **352**
Side effect, defined, 508
Sighted guide techniques, **317–318**
Sigmoidoscopes, rigid, 396
Sigmoidoscopy, 331–332
Sign, objective, 192
Simple
    fracture, 106
    stains, bacteria, 735
Simple fracture, **347**
Sims' (lateral) position, 241
    placing patient in, **251**
Sims uterine sound, **397**
Single-channel ECG, 570, **571, 586–588**
Sinus
    bradycardia, 579
    rhythm, 579
    tachycardia, 579
Sinuses, review of systems (ROS), 194–195
Sinusitis, **337**
Sitting, crutches and, 453
Skeleton, 344
    disorders of, described, **346**
Skin
    allergy testing, 354
    cancer, 353
        described, **354**
    closure strips, applying sterile, **416**
    cross section of, **353**
    hooks, 396
    minor surgery on, preparation for,
        422–423
    physical examination and, 243, **244**
    review of systems (ROS), 194–195
Skin test, for TB, 769–770
Slander, 74
Slide test, pregnancy testing and, 761–762
SLR (Supine straight leg rising) test, 344
Smear, blood. *See* Blood, smear
Smell, aging and, 314
Smoking policy, 826
Snellen "E" chart, **293**
    using, **362–363**
SOAP charting method, 198
Social history, medical history and,
        193–194
Sodium azide, red blood counts and, 672
Sodium (Na), 484
Solar radiation, burns from, 105
Sole proprietorships, described, **17**
Solutions
    pouring sterile, 427–428
    surgical, 400, **403**
Somatic tremor artifacts, 578
SOMR (Source-oriented medical record),
        195–196
Sonographer, 585
Source-oriented medical record (SOMR),
        195–196
Southeast Asian diet, **492**
Spasm, muscles, described, **346**
Specific gravity, reagent test strips and, 706

Specimen
    chilling, tests requiring, **652**
    collecting, 626–628
        butterfly system of, 650
        evacuated tube, 649
        feces, 628
        patient reactions, 650
        plasma/whole blood, 628
        quality control/assurance for, **651**
        serum blood, 627–628
        trays, 644
        urine, 628
    identification, 645
    inoculating, dilution streaking, **754**
    laboratory values, factors affecting,
        651–652
    processing/sending to laboratory, 627
    procuring/storage/handling of, 626–627
    rejection criteria, 651
Specula, 396–398
Speech
    patient, 243
    physical examination and, 243
    therapy, described, **445**
Sperm, in urine, 709
Sphygmomanometers, 215–216
Spills, microbiology, disposal of, 728
Spinal curvatures, **345**
    described, **346**
Spiral fracture, 106
Spirilla, described, 735
Spirometry, 343
    testing, **375**
Splinter forceps, 393, **395**
Sponge forceps, **395**
Sponges, surgical, 399–400, **403**
Spontaneous abortion, 262
Sports medicine, described, **445**
Sprains, 105
    muscle/connective tissue, **345**
    described, **346**
Spread streak, **741**
Sputum
    defined, 149
    specimen collecting, 734
    specimen, obtaining, **372–373**
St. Benedict of Nursia, 31
Staff meetings, 795–796
Staff members, supporting, 796
Stains
    bacterial, 735–737
    blood, 676
    use of, **735**
Standard of care, negligence and, 72
Standard Precautions, 145, 146, **147** 152,
        599
*Standards and Guidelines for an Accredited
    Education Program for the Medical
    Assistant,* 8, 10
Standing, crutches and, 453
Stapes, 340
Staphylococcal infection, **136**
Staphylococci, **136**
STAT, defined, 625
Stature, patient, 242
Statute of limitations, 76
Steam sterilization, 166–170
Sterile
    asepsis, 165–170
    field, setting up/covering, 423–424
    pack, opening, 425–427
    principles, 385
    solution, pouring, 427–428
    techniques. *See* Surgical asepsis

    transfer forceps, using, 408
    tray setups, guidelines for, **406**
Sterilization, 165–170
    chemical, 165–166
        "cold," 399, 421–422
    defined, 265
Stertorous respiration, defined, 214
Stirrup (stapes), 340
Stool, specimen collecting, 734
Storage
    specimen, 626–627
Strains, 105–106
    muscle/connective tissue, **345**
Strep throat, **136**
Streptococcal
    infection, **136**
    sore throat, transmission of, **731**
Streptococcus
    screening for, 744–745
        packaged systems, 745
Streptococcus pneumoniae, 742
Stress
    adaptation to, 52–53
    coping with, 53–54
    described, 52
    goal setting to relieve, 55–57
    treadmill test, 584–585
Strict isolation, 145
Stridor, defined, 214
Stroke, 110
Student practicums
    managers and, 797–798
    supervising, **807–808**
Stye, **337, 339**
Subculture, 741–742
Subcutaneous connective tissue, described,
        352
Subcutaneous injections, 533
    administration of, **550–551, 556**
Subjective complaint, defined, 192
Sublimation, as defense mechanism, 46
Subpoena duces tecum, 75
Subpoenas, 75
Substances, controlled. *See* Controlled
        substances, 502
Sudden illness, 108–109
Suicide, physician assisted, ethical issues
        concerning, **85**
Sunburn, 105
Supine position, 239, 435
    placing patient in, **247**
Supine straight leg rising (SLR) test, 344
Suppurative otitis media, 293
Suprapubic catheter, 327
Surgeon's assistant, **22**
Surgery
    alternative methods, 387–388
    instruments, 389–399
        categories/uses of, 389–398
        scissors/scalpels, 391, **392**
        structure of, 389, **390**
    minor office
        anesthetics, 403
        assisting with, **411–412**
        described, 383–384
        patient care/preparation, 404–406
        preparation for, 406–408
        procedures performed, 386–387
        setup, 406
        supplies/equipment, **403**
Surgical
    asepsis, 165, 385
        handwashing for, 385
    blades, 392

dressings/bandages, 400
solutions/creams/ointments, 400
specialties, 19–20
sponges, 399–400
wicks, 399–400
Surgical technologist, **22**
Suture
defined, 388–389
materials/supplies, 388–389
needles, 389
removal of, **415**
scissors, **392**
Suturing, lacerations, **412–413**
Swing-through gait, 453
Swing-to gait, 453
Symmetry, defined, 236
Synthetic casts, 346
Synthetic drugs, 500
Syphilis, **136**
described, **272**
transmission of, **731**
Syringes, 534–537
contaminated, disposal of, 156
hand position, correct, **648**
order of filling, **649**
parts of, **536**, 537
specimen collecting, 648–649
types/uses of, 537
venipuncture, 640
Systole
defined, 569
pressure, defined, 215

T

Tachycardia, defined, 213
Tachypnea, defined, 214
Tamm-Horsfall, 711
Targeted resume, 851
Task Force for Test Construction, 836
Taste, aging and, 314
Taxes, figuring, 804
Taxonomy
defined, 723–724
microbiology, 723–724
Tay-Sachs
CVS (Chorionic villi sampling) and, 262
TB (Tuberculosis), **141, 343**
cause of, 769
described, **344**, 768–769
diagnosis of, 769
Mantoux test, **782–783**
screening for
Mantoux test, 769–770
skin testing, 769
tests for, 768–770
transmission of, **731**
infectious, 769
Teamwork, importance of, 793–794
Technical expertise, as management quality, 792
Technology, communication and, 45
Telephone
ECG transmissions using, 572
reference check, **818**
techniques, 47
Telephone calls
contact, by patients, 189
Temperature (body)
as vital sign, 207–212
measuring, 210–211
pediatric, 290–291
recording, 210
terms used to describe, 208

Temporal pulse, 212
Temporary employees, 824, 826
Tendonitis, **345**
described, **346**
Terminal illness. *See* Life-threatening illness, 32
Territoriality, 43
Tetanus, **136**
transmission of, **731**
Thailand, diet of, **492**
Thalassemia
CVS (Chorionic villi sampling) and, 262
Therapeutic
communication, cultural influence on, 39–40
diets, 488–491
exercises, 455–457
types of, 456
modalities, 457–461
heat and cold, 457–458
moist/dry heat, 458–459
touch, 25
use of drugs, 499
Therapies, health care, role of, 24
Thermometers
cleaning/storing, 211–212
digital, using, **222–223**
oral strip, using, **221–222**
types of, 208, 210
using, mercury, **220–221**
Thiamin, **481**, 483
Things-oriented personality, as management style, 792
Third degree burns, 103
response guide for, **105**
Thixotrophic separator gel, 642
tubes, **643**
Thoracentesis, defined, 149
Threatened abortion, 263
Three-point gait, 452, **453**
Threshold substances, 699
Throat
culture
obtaining, **749–750**
taking a, 732–733, **733**
physical examination and, **244**, 246
review of systems (ROS), 194–195
specimen collecting, requirements, 732
Thrombocyte, **638**, 666
Thrombophlebitis, **350**
described, **351**
Thumb forceps, 393
Thyroid fever, **136**
TIA (Transient ischemic attack), 314
Tic douloureux, **348**
described, **349**
Time management, 798
Tinnitus
defined, 246
Tissue
destruction
chemical, 387
electrical, 387
Title VII of the Civil Rights Act, 824
Tocopherol, 483
Tonsillitis, **343**
described, **344**
pediatrics and, 294
Topical spray anesthetics, 403
TORCH Panel, **622**
Torts, 72–73
Touch, communication and, 44
Tourniquets, 642–644
use of, 100–101

Towel clamps, 393, **395**
Toxicology screening, urine sample and, 325
Trace minerals, 484
Trachoma, transmission of, **731**
Trade name, of drugs, 499
Training
Bloodborne Pathogen Standard, **161**
components, Bloodborne Pathogen Standard, **161**
office personnel and, 826–827, **829**
records, Bloodborne Pathogen Standard, 161
Tranquilizer drugs, **508**
Transderm Scop®, 509
Transducer, 585
Transferring, patients, 448–449
Transient ischemic attack (TIA), 314
Transmission-Based Precautions, 145, 146, **599**
Transverse fracture, **347**
Trauma disorders, cumulative, 613
Travel
making arrangements for, 796–797, **806**
via the Internet, **807**
Treadmill stress test, 584–585
Treatments, medical, 32–33
Trendelenburg position, 241
placing patient in, **252**
Treponema pallidum, **136**
Triage, described, 95
Trichomonas, described, **272**
Trichomonas hominis, 749
Trichomonas vaginalis, 749
in urine, 708
Trichomoniasis, 136, **271**
described, **272**
Triglycerides
factors influencing, **775**
reference values for, **774**
tests for, 774–775
Triple sugar iron agar (TSI), 743
Truthfulness, as management quality, 791
TSI (Triple sugar iron agar), 743
Tuberculosis (TB), **141, 343**
cause of, 769
described, **344**, 768–769
diagnosis of, 769
Mantoux test, **782–783**
screening for
Mantoux test, 769–770
skin testing, 769
tests for, 768–770
transmission of, **731**
infectious, 769
Tubex®, 535
Tubular gauze bandage, 400
Tubule, defined, 698
Tuning fork, testing hearing with, 341, **342**
Turbid, defined, 704
Twelve-lead electrocardiogram, **589**
Twenty-four-hour specimen, urine, 702
Two-point gait, 452
Tympanic
cavity, 340
membrane, 340
thermometers, 208, 210, **224**
Tympanometry, 342
Tympanostomy, defined, 294

U

Ulcer, gastric, 330
Ulcers
duodenal, **328**, 330

Ulcers (*continued*)
  gastric, **328**
  peptic, 330
Ultralente, **526**
Ultrasonic cleaning, 399
Ultrasonography, 585
  pregnancy and, 262
Ultrasound, deep tissue treatment and,
    460–461
United States Adopted Names Council, 499
*United States Pharmacopoeia/National Formu-
    lary*, 505
Universal Blood and Body Fluid Precautions,
    599
Universal Precautions, 145, **599**
Unopette®, 671
Upper GI series, 331, **335**, **434**
Urea nitrogen reference values, **775**
Urgent care centers, 17
Urinalysis, 698
  chemical examination, **714–715**
  for PKU, 768
  performing, **718–719**
Urinalysis department
  described, 621
  laboratory tests, **620**
Urinary catheterization
  female patient, **355–356**
  male patient, **357–358**
Urinary drug screening, 325
Urinary tract, **699**
  bladder, cancer of, **324**
  catheterization, 326–327
  cystoscopy and, 325
  defined, 698
  diagnostic tests of, 323–328
  disorders, **324**
  elderly and, 315
  infections, **324**
    staphylococcal infection and, **136**
  intravenous pyelogram (IVP), 325
  review of systems (ROS), 194–195
  signs/symptoms of, 323
Urine
  ammonium biurate in, **710**
  amorphous phosphates in, **710**
  artifacts in, 709, **710**
  bacteria in, 708, **709**
  blood cells in, 708, **709**
  calcium phosphate in, **710**
  casts in, 711
  composition of, 699–700
  containers, 701–703
  crystals in, 709, **710**
  examination of, 703–705
    chemical, 705–708
    clarity of, **713**
    color, 704, **712**
    confirmatory testing, 707–708
    odor, 704
    sediment, 708–711
    specimen volume, 704, **712**
    testing for sugar, **716**
    transparency, 704
  examination, specific gravity, 704–705
  filtration of, 698–699
  formation of, 698–699
  parasites in, 708–709
  pregnancy testing and, 32
  reabsorption and, 699
  renal epithelial cells in, 708, **709**
  secretion of, 699
  specimens
    collecting, 628, 701–703

collecting, from an infant, 292
collecting, requirements, 732
collection methods, 702
handling precautions, **700**
  sperm in, 709, **710**
  squamous epithelial cells in, **709**
  substances in, **700**
  toxicology screening, 325
  yeast in, **709**
Urinometer, 704–705
Urobilinogen, defined, 706
U.S. Southern diet, **491**

V

Vaccination schedule, **283**, 284
Vaccines
  administration guidelines, **284**
  classifications of, 139
  hepatitis B, 157
  preparation for administration of, 284
Vacutainer®, 641
Vaginal discharge, normal, 149
Vaginitis, 271
  described, **272**
Valium, **511**
Varicella, **141**
Varicose veins, **350**
  described, **351**
Vasectomy, defined, 265
Vasodilator drugs, **508**
Vasopressor drugs, **508**
Vastus lateralis site, site selection/injection
    angle, 541, **543**
Vegans, **493**
Vegetarians, diet of, **492**
Veins
  superficial arm, **639**
  upper arm, finding, **654–655**
  versus arteries, **637**
Velosulin, **525**
Venipuncture, 638–639
  by evacuated tube, procedure, **655–656**
  by syringe, procedure, **655–656**
  equipment, 641–644
  identification, patient/specimen, 645–646
  patient
    approaching, 645
    positioning, 646
  patient reactions, 650
  performing a safe, 647–648
  site selection, 646–647
  steps in, **644**
  technique, 644–652
  unsuccessful, 650–651
Ventricles, 567
Ventricular arrhythmias, 580–581
  fibrillation, 581
  tachycardia, 581
Ventrogluteal site, site selection/injection
    angle, 540, **542**
Verbal communication, 41–42
Vertigo, 246
Verucca. *See* Warts
Vial
  defined, 534
  withdrawing medication from, **552–553**
Vietnam, diet of, **492**
Virapap, 268
Virology, defined, 724
Virtues forceps, 393
Viruses
  described, 134–135
  hepatitis, **144**

Vision
  aging and, 313
  color, 340
Visual acuity
  measuring, 337–340
    near, **363–364**
  pediatric, screening for, 292–293
  testing, **362–363**
Visually impaired
  older adult, medical assistant and,
    317–318
  sighted guide techniques, **317–318**
Vital signs, 206
  accuracy of, importance of, 206
  blood pressure, 215–217
  chest, measuring circumference of,
    219
  height/weight, 218–219
  pulse, 212–213
  respiration, 213–214
  temperature, 207–212
Vitamin A, **481**, 483
Vitamin B1, **481**
Vitamin B2, **482**
Vitamin B3, **482**
Vitamin B5, **482**
Vitamin B6, **482**, 483
Vitamin B12, **482**, 483
Vitamin C, **482**, 483
Vitamin D, **481**, 483
Vitamin E, **481**, 483
Vitamin K, **481**
Vitamins, 480–483
Vitiligo, defined, 243
Volkman retractors, **397**

W

W-2 form, **803**
W-4 form, **802**
Waived tests, 600
Walkers, 449
  assisting patients with, **466**
  fitting a, 450
Walter forceps, 393
Walther urethral sound, **397**
Wandering baseline artifacts, 579
Warts, 353
  described, **354**
  genital, **271**
    described, **272**
Waste
  containers, regulated (non-sharp),
    Bloodborne Pathogen Standard,
    161
  infectious
    defined, 150
    disposal of, 150
  microbiology, disposal of, 728
Water, nutrition and, 485
Water-soluble vitamins, **482**
Web mount, hanging drop slide preparation,
    752–753
Weight
  as vital sign, 219
  control of, 488–489
  drug dosage and, 518–519
  measuring, **231–232**
    devices, 289
    infant/child, 285–289
  significance of, 219
Weights and measures
  apothecary measurements, 523
  household measures, 523

metric system
    conversion, 523–524
    guidelines, 521–522
    prefixes, 522
Welch sensors/electrodes, ECG, 573
Well-baby, 283–285
Well-child, 283–285
Westergren method, erythrocyte sedimentation rate (ESR), 680–681
Wheelchairs, 454–455
    transferring patient
        from examination table to wheelchair, **463**
        from wheelchair to examination table, **461–463**
Wheezes, defined, 214
White blood cells, **638**, 666
    counts, 671–675
        differential, **691–692**
        manual dilution, 671
        normal, **675**, 677
        Unopette® method, **686–687**

using high-power magnification, 674–675
    using low-power magnification, 672–673
    differential, 675–677
    identification guide, **677**
    in urine, 708
Whooping cough, transmission of, **731**
Wicks, surgical, 399–400, **403**
Wilkes, Mary, 41
Williams, Maxine, first AAMA president, 7
Wintrobe macrohematocrit, **670**
Wintrobe method, erythrocyte sedimentation rate (ESR), 680
Work areas, cleanliness of, 156
Work Practice Controls, Bloodborne Pathogen Standard, **160**
Work practice controls, exposure prevention and, 152, 154–155
Wounds, 100–105
    care of, 404–406
    closed, 100, 405

culturing, 734
    open, 100, **405**
Wound/skin precautions, 145
Wright's stain, 676
Wrist, bandage wrapping technique, **402**

X
X-rays
    described, 432
    machines, 432

Y
Yeast, in urine, 708

Z
Zen macrobiotic diets, **493**
Ziehl-Neelsen stain, **751–752**
Zinc, 484
Z-track intramuscular injections, 544, **562**

Delmar's Medical Assisting Clinical Skills CD-ROM

Set-Up Instructions

1. Insert disk into CD-ROM player.
2. From the Start Menu, choose *RUN*.
3. In the *Open* text box, enter **d:setup.exe** then click the *OK* button. (Substitute the letter of your CD-ROM drive for **d:**)
4. Follow the installation prompts from there.

System Requirements

100 Mhz Intel Pentium

Microsoft® Windows® 95 or later

32 MB or more of RAM

Approx. 8 MB free disk space

SVGA monitor with 24-bit (16 million colors) display

4x or faster CD-ROM drive

Sound card and speakers

License Agreement for Delmar Thomson Learning Educational Software/Data

You, the customer, and Delmar Thomson Learning incur certain benefits, rights, and obligations to each other when you open this package and use the software/data it contains. BE SURE YOU READ THE LICENSE AGREEMENT CAREFULLY, SINCE BY USING THE SOFTWARE/DATA YOU INDICATE YOU HAVE READ, UNDERSTOOD, AND ACCEPTED THE TERMS OF THIS AGREEMENT.

Your rights:

1. You enjoy a non-exclusive license to use the software/data on a single microcomputer in consideration for payment of the required license fee (which may be included in the purchase price of an accompanying print component), or receipt of this software/data, and your acceptance of the terms and conditions of this agreement.

2. You acknowledge that you do not own the aforesaid software/data. You also acknowledge that the software/data is furnished "as is" and contains copyrighted and/or proprietary and confidential information of Delmar Thomson Learning or its licensors.

There are limitations on your rights:

1. You may not copy or print the software/data for any reason whatsoever, except to install it on a hard drive on a single microcomputer and to make one archival copy, unless copying or printing is expressly permitted in writing or statements recorded on the disk(s).

2. You may not revise, translate, convert, disassemble or otherwise reverse engineer the software/data except that you may add to or rearrange any data recorded on the media as part of the normal use of the software/data.

3. You may not sell, license, lease, rent, loan, or otherwise distribute or network the software/data except that you may give the software/data to a student or and instructor for use at school or temporarily at home.

Should you fail to abide by the Copyright Law of the United States as it applies to this software/data, your license to use it will become invalid. You agree to erase or otherwise destroy the software/data immediately after receiving note of Delmar Thomson Learning termination of this agreement for violation of its provisions.

Delmar Thomson Learning gives you a LIMITED WARRANTY covering the enclosed software/data. The LIMITED WARRANTY follows this License.

This license is the entire agreement between you and Delmar Thomson Learning interpreted and enforced under New York law.

This warranty does not extend to the software or information recorded on the media. The software and information are provided "AS IS."

Any statements made about the utility of the software or information are not to be considered as express or implied warranties. Delmar Thomson Learning will not be liable for incidental or consequential damages of any kind incurred by you, the consumer, or any other user.

Some states do not allow the exclusion or limitation of incidental or consequential damages, or limitations on the duration of implied warranties, so the above limitation or exclusion may not apply to you. This warranty gives you specific legal rights, and you may also have other rights which vary from state to state. Address all correspondence to Delmar Thomson Learning, Box 15015, Albany, NY 12212 Attention: Technology Department.

LIMITED WARRANTY

Delmar Thomson Learning warrants to the original licensee/purchaser of this copy of microcomputer software/data and the media on which it is recorded that the media will be free from defects in material and workmanship for ninety (90) days from the date of original purchase. All implied warranties are limited in duration to this ninety (90) day period. THEREAFTER, ANY IMPLIED WARRANTIES, INCLUDING IMPLIED WARRANTIES OF MERCHANTABILITY AND FITNESS FOR A PARTICULAR PURPOSE, ARE EXCLUDED. THIS WARRANTY IS IN LIEU OF ALL OTHER WARRANTIES, WHETHER ORAL OR WRITTEN, EXPRESS OR IMPLIED.

If you believe the media is defective, please return it during the ninety-day period to the address shown below. Defective media will be replaced without charge provided that it has not been subjected to misuse or damage.

This warranty does not extend to the software or information recorded on the media. The software and information are provided "AS IS." Any statements made about the utility of the software or information are not to be considered as express or implied warranties.

Limitation of liability: Our liability to you for any losses shall be limited to direct damages and shall not exceed the amount you paid for the software. In no event will we be liable to you for any indirect, special, incidental, or consequential damages (including loss of profits) even if we have been advised of the possibility of such damages.

Some states do not allow the exclusion or limitation of incidental or consequential damages, or limitations on the duration of implied warranties, so the above limitation or exclusion may not apply to you. This warranty gives you specific legal rights, and you may also have other rights which vary from state to state. Address all correspondence to Delmar Thomson Learning, Box 15015, Albany, NY 12212 Attention: Technology Department.

Online Learning Center with PowerWeb

www.mhhe.com/hill

Discover more international business exercises and research tools, plus study aids tailored to the text, by logging onto the Online Learning Center.

- Self-grading quizzes

- Chapter review material

- GlobalEDGE™/CIBER Research Tasks—use web resources to solve international business problems

- Build Your Management Skills—interactive exercises

- PowerWeb—links to current articles related to international business topics

- Business Around the World Atlas—click on an area on the map to access regional data

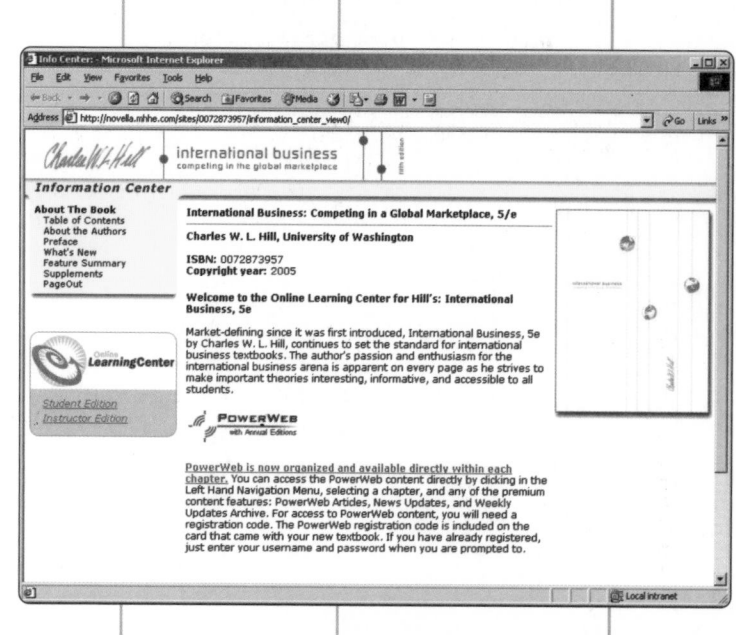

Competing in the Global Marketplace

Fifth Edition

International Business

Charles W. L. Hill

University of Washington

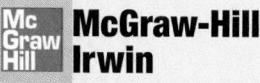

McGraw-Hill
Irwin

Boston   Burr Ridge, IL   Dubuque, IA   Madison, WI   New York   San Francisco   St. Louis
Bangkok   Bogotá   Caracas   Kuala Lumpur   Lisbon   London   Madrid   Mexico City
Milan   Montreal   New Delhi   Santiago   Seoul   Singapore   Sydney   Taipei   Toronto

The McGraw·Hill Companies

McGraw-Hill
Irwin

INTERNATIONAL BUSINESS: COMPETING IN THE GLOBAL MARKETPLACE Published by McGraw-Hill/Irwin, a business unit of The McGraw-Hill Companies, Inc., 1221 Avenue of the Americas, New York, NY, 10020. Copyright © 2005, 2003, 2000, 1997, 1994 by The McGraw-Hill Companies, Inc. All rights reserved. No part of this publication may be reproduced or distributed in any form or by any means, or stored in a database or retrieval system, without the prior written consent of The McGraw-Hill Companies, Inc., including, but not limited to, in any network or other electronic storage or transmission, or broadcast for distance learning.

Some ancillaries, including electronic and print components, may not be available to customers outside the United States.

This book is printed on acid-free paper.

1 2 3 4 5 6 7 8 9 0 WCK/WCK 0 9 8 7 6 5 4

ISBN 0-07-287395-7

Editorial director: *John E. Biernat*
Sponsoring editor: *Ryan Blankenship*
Managing developmental editor: *Laura Hurst Spell*
Marketing manager: *Lisa Nicks*
Producer, Media technology: *Damian Moshak*
Project manager: *Laura Griffin*
Production supervisor: *Debra R. Sylvester*
Designer: *Kami Carter*
Photo research coordinator: *Jeremy Cheshareck*
Senior supplement producer: *Susan Lombardi*
Senior digital content specialist: *Brian Nacik*
Typeface: *10.5/12 Goudy*
Compositor: *Carlisle Communications, Ltd.*
Printer: *Quebecor World Versailles Inc.*

Library of Congress Cataloging-in-Publication Data
Hill, Charles W. L.
    International business: competing in the global marketplace / Charles W. L. Hill.—5th ed.
      p. cm.
    Includes bibliographical references and index.
    ISBN 0-07-287395-7 (alk. paper)
    1. International business enterprises—Management. 2. Competition, International. I.
  Title.
  HD62.4. H55 2005
  658'.049—dc22   2003058739

INTERNATIONAL EDITION ISBN 0-07-111311-8
Copyright © 2005. Exclusive rights by The McGraw-Hill Companies, Inc. for manufacture and export. This book cannot be re-exported from the country to which it is sold by McGraw-Hill. The International Edition is not available in North America.

www.mhhe.com

About the Author

Charles W. L. Hill is the Hughes M. Blake Professor of International Business at the School of Business, University of Washington. Professor Hill received his Ph.D. from the University of Manchester's Institute of Science and Technology (UMIST) in Britain. In addition to the University of Washington, he has served on the faculties of UMIST, Texas A&M University, and Michigan State University.

Professor Hill has published over 40 articles in peer reviewed academic journals, including the *Academy of Management Journal*, *Academy of Management Review*, *Strategic Management Journal*, and *Organization Science*. He has also published two college texts: one on strategic management and the other on international business. Professor Hill has served on the editorial boards of several academic journals, including the *Strategic Management Journal* and *Organization Science*. Between 1993 and 1996 he was consulting editor at the *Academy of Management Review*.

Professor Hill teaches in the MBA, Executive MBA, Management, and Ph.D. programs at the University of Washington. He has received awards for teaching excellence in the MBA, Executive MBA, and Management programs. He has also taught customized executive programs.

Professor Hill works on a consulting basis with a number of organizations. His clients have included ATL, Boeing, BF Goodrich, Hexcel, House of Fraser, Microsoft, Seattle City Light, Tacoma City Light, Thompson Financial Services, and Wizards of the Coast.

Brief Contents

Preface   xxi

Part 1   Introduction and Overview
Chapter 1   Globalization   2

Part 2   Country Factors
Chapter 2   National Differences in Political Economy   40

Chapter 3   Differences in Culture   88

Cases   Nike: The Sweatshop Debate   128

         Qualcomm's Chinese Odyssey   132

         Royal Dutch/Shell: Human Rights in Nigeria   136

Part 3   The Global Trade and Investment Environment
Chapter 4   International Trade Theory   142

Chapter 5   The Political Economy of International Trade   178

Chapter 6   Foreign Direct Investment   212

Chapter 7   The Political Economy of Foreign Direct Investment   238

Chapter 8   Regional Economic Integration   266

Cases   Starbucks   302

         The Politics of Trade in Steel   302

         The Softwood Lumber Dispute   303

         Comparing Ghana and South Korea   306

         Managed Trade: The U.S. and Japanese
Semiconductor Industries, 1970–2002   307

         Dixon Ticonderoga: Victim of Globalization?   311

Part 4   The Global Monetary System
Chapter 9   The Foreign Exchange Market   314

Chapter 10   The International Monetary System   342

Chapter 11   The Global Capital Market   378

Cases   Money Change   402

         Bailing Out Brazil   403

         The International Monetary Fund   405

Part 5   The Strategy and Structure of International Business

Chapter 12   The Strategy of International Business   408

Chapter 13   The Organization of International Business   438

Chapter 14   Entry Strategy and Strategic Alliances   478

Cases   BP: Creating a Global Brand   514

                    Restructuring Exide   514

                    Philips versus Matsushita: A New Century, a New Round   517

Part 6   Business Operations

Chapter 15   Exporting, Importing, and Countertrade   534

Chapter 16   Global Manufacturing and Materials Management   554

Chapter 17   Global Marketing and R&D   582

Chapter 18   Global Human Resource Management   616

Chapter 19   Accounting in the International Business   644

Chapter 20   Financial Management in the International Business   666

Case   Cretors & Co.   694

Glossary   695

Index   708

Contents

Preface xxi

Part 1
Introduction and Overview

Chapter 1
Globalization   2

Opening Case
Wal-Mart's Global Expansion   3

Introduction   4

What Is Globalization?   6
The Globalization of Markets   6
The Globalization of Production   7

The Emergence of Global Institutions   8

Drivers of Globalization   9
Declining Trade and Investment Barriers   9
The Role of Technological Change   12

Management Focus
Homer Simpson—A Global Brand!   15

The Changing Demographics of the
Global Economy   16

The Changing World Output and World Trade Picture   16
The Changing Foreign Direct Investment Picture   18
The Changing Nature of the Multinational Enterprise   19

Management Focus
Wipro Ltd.—The New Face of Global Competition   21

The Changing World Order   22
The Global Economy of the 21st Century   23

The Globalization Debate   24
Antiglobalization Protests   24
Globalization, Jobs, and Incomes   25

Country Focus
Protesting Globalization in France   26

Globalization, Labor Policies, and the Environment   27
Globalization and National Sovereignty   29
Globalization and the World's Poor   29

Managing in the Global Marketplace   31

Chapter Summary   32

Critical Discussion Questions   33

Research Task globalEDGE™ globaledge.msu.edu   35

Closing Case
Ecuadorean Valentine Roses   36

Part 2
Country Factors

Chapter 2
National Differences in Political Economy   40

Opening Case
India's Changing Political Economy   41

Introduction   42

Political Systems   43
Collectivism and Individualism   43
Democracy and Totalitarianism   46

Economic Systems   47
Market Economy   47
Command Economy   48
Mixed Economy   48

Legal Systems   49
Different Legal Systems   49
Differences in Contract Law   50
Property Rights   51
The Protection of Intellectual Property   53

Country Focus
40 Years of Corruption in Nigeria   54

Management Focus
Drug Patents and the AIDS Epidemic in
South Africa   56

Product Safety and Product Liability   57

The Determinants of Economic Development   57
Differences in Economic Development   57
Broader Conceptions of Development: Amartya Sen   62
Political Economy and Economic Progress   62
Geography, Education, and Economic Development   66

States in Transition   66
The Spread of Democracy   67
The New World Order and Global Terrorism   69
The Spread of Market-Based Systems   71
The Nature of Economic Transformation   73

Country Focus
Privatization in Taiwan   74

Implications   76

Focus On Managerial Implications   77

Chapter Summary   82

Critical Discussion Questions   83

Research Task globalEDGE™ globaledge.msu.edu   86

Closing Case
Piracy in the Video Game Market   86

Chapter 3
Differences in Culture   88

Opening Case
Guanxi—**Ties That Bind**   89

Introduction   90

What Is Culture?   91
Values and Norms   91
Culture, Society, and the Nation-State   92
The Determinants of Culture   93

Social Structure   93
Individuals and Groups   94
Social Stratification   96

Religious and Ethical Systems   98
Christianity   98
Islam   100
Hinduism   102

Country Focus
Islamic Banking in Pakistan   103

Buddhism   104
Confucianism   104

Language   106
Spoken Language   106
Unspoken Language   107

Education   107

Culture and the Workplace   108

Cultural Change   113

Management Focus
Matsushita's and Japan's Changing Culture   114

Focus On Managerial Implications   116
Cross-Cultural Literacy   117
Culture and Competitive Advantage   117
Culture and Business Ethics   119

Chapter Summary   121

Critical Discussion Questions   122

Research Task globalEDGE™ globaledge.msu.edu   124

Closing Case
McDonald's and Hindu Culture   125

Cases
Nike: The Sweatshop Debate   128

Qualcomm's Chinese Odyssey   132

Royal Dutch/Shell: Human Rights in Nigeria   136

Part 3
The Global Trade and Investment Environment

Chapter 4
International Trade Theory   142

Opening Case
The Hollowing Out of the U.S. Knowledge-Based Economy   143

Introduction   144

An Overview of Trade Theory   144
The Benefits of Trade   144
The Pattern of International Trade   145

Country Focus
Crawfish Wars   146

Trade Theory and Government Policy   147

Mercantilism   147

Absolute Advantage   148

Comparative Advantage   150
The Gains from Trade   151
Qualifications and Assumptions   153
Simple Extensions of the Ricardian Model   153

Management Focus
Free Trade and REI   155

Heckscher-Ohlin Theory   157
The Leontief Paradox   158

The Product Life-Cycle Theory   159
Evaluating the Product Life-Cycle Theory   160

New Trade Theory   162

The Aerospace Example   163

Implications   164

National Competitive Advantage: Porter's Diamond   165
Factor Endowments   166
Demand Conditions   166
Related and Supporting Industries   167
Firm Strategy, Structure, and Rivalry   167
Evaluating Porter's Theory   168

Management Focus
The Rise of Finland's Nokia   168

Focus On Managerial Implications   169
Location   169
First-Mover Advantagers   170
Government Policy   171

Chapter Summary   172

Critical Discussion Questions   173

Research Task globalEDGE™ globaledge.msu.edu   175

Closing Case
The Rise of the Indian Software Industry   175

Chapter 5
The Political Economy of International Trade   178

Opening Case
Agricultural Subsidies and Development   179

Introduction   180

Instruments of Trade Policy   180
Tariffs   181
Subsidies   181

Country Focus
The Costs of Protectionism in the United States   182

Import Quotas and Voluntary Export Restraints   183
Local Content Requirements   184
Administrative Policies   185

Management Focus
Navigating around Import Quotas   185

Antidumping Policies   186

The Case for Government Intervention   186
Political Arguments for Intervention   187

Country Focus
Trade in Hormone-Treated Beef   189

Economic Arguments for Intervention   191

The Revised Case for Free Trade   193
Retaliation and Trade War   193
Domestic Politics   193

Development of the World Trading System   194
From Smith to the Great Depression   194
1947–1979: GATT, Trade Liberalization, and Economic Growth   195
1980–1993: Disturbing Trends   195
The Uruguay Round and the World Trade Organization   196
WTO: Experience to Date   197

Country Focus
Shrimps, Turtles, and the WTO   200

The Future of the WTO: Unresolved Issues and the Doha Round   202

Focus On Managerial Implications   205
Trade Barriers and Firm Strategy   205
Policy Implications   206

Chapter Summary   207

Critical Discussion Questions   208

Research Task globalEDGE™ globaledge.msu.edu   210

Closing Case
Is a Tax Break an Export Subsidy?   210

Chapter 6
Foreign Direct Investment   212

Opening Case
Starbucks' Foreign Direct Investment   213

Introduction   214

Foreign Direct Investment in the World Economy   215
Trends in FDI   215
The Direction of FDI   217

Country Focus
Foreign Direct Investment in China   218

The Source of FDI   220
The Form of FDI: Acquisitions versus Green-Field Investments   221

Management Focus
Cemex's Foreign Acquisitions   222

Horizontal Foreign Direct Investment   223
Transportation Costs   224
Market Imperfections (Internalization Theory)   224
Strategic Behavior   226
The Product Life Cycle   227
Location-Specific Advantages   228

Vertical Foreign Direct Investment   229
Strategic Behavior   229
Market Imperfections   230

Focus On Managerial Implications   231

Chapter Summary   233

Critical Discussion Questions   234

Research Task globalEDGE™ globaledge.msu.edu   236

Closing Case
Ford and General Motors in Russia   236

Chapter 7
The Political Economy of Foreign Direct Investment 238

Opening Case
Foreign Direct Investment and the Irish Miracle 239

Introduction 240

Political Ideology and Foreign Direct Investment 240
The Radical View 240
The Free Market View 241
Pragmatic Nationalism 242

Management Focus
FDI by Volvo in South Korea 243

Summary 244

The Benefits of FDI to Host Countries 244
Resource-Transfer Effects 244
Employment Effects 246

Country Focus
Foreign Direct Investment in Venezuela's Petroleum Industry 247

Balance-of-Payments Effects 248
Effect on Competition and Economic Growth 250

The Costs of FDI to Host Countries 251
Adverse Effects on Competition 251
Adverse Effects on the Balance of Payments 252
National Sovereignty and Autonomy 252

The Benefits and Costs of FDI to Home Countries 252
Benefits of FDI to the Home Country 253
Costs of FDI to the Home Country 253
International Trade Theory and FDI 253

Government Policy Instruments and FDI 254
Home-Country Policies 254
Host-Country Policies 255
International Institutions and the Liberalization of FDI 256

Focus On Managerial Implications 257
The Nature of Negotiation 257
Bargaining Power 259

Chapter Summary 260

Critical Discussion Questions 261

Research Task globalEDGE™ globaledge.msu.edu 263

Closing Case
Toyota in France 263

Chapter 8
Regional Economic Integration 266

Opening Case
Increasing Competition in the European Automobile Market 267

Introduction 268

Levels of Economic Integration 269

The Case for Regional Integration 271
The Economic Case for Integration 271
The Political Case for Integration 271
Impediments to Integration 272

Country Focus
NAFTA and the U.S. Textile Industry 272

The Case against Regional Integration 273

Regional Economic Integration in Europe 274
Evolution of the European Union 274
Political Structure of the European Union 275

Management Focus
The European Commission and Media Industry Mergers 277

The Single European Act 278
The Establishment of the Euro 279
Enlargement of the European Union 282

Regional Economic Integration in the Americas 284
The North American Free Trade Agreement 285
The Andean Pact 287
MERCOSUR 288
Central American Common Market and CARICOM 289
Free Trade Area of the Americas 289

Regional Economic Integration Elsewhere 290
Association of Southeast Asian Nations 290
Asia Pacific Economic Cooperation 290
Regional Trade Blocs in Africa 291

Focus On Managerial Implications 292
Opportunities 292
Threats 293

Management Focus
Atag Holdings 294

Chapter Summary 295

Critical Discussion Questions 296

Research Task globalEDGE™ globaledge.msu.edu 297

Closing Case
Deutsche Bank's Pan-European Retail Banking Strategy 298

Cases

Starbucks 302

The Politics of Trade in Steel 302

The Softwood Lumber Dispute 303

Comparing Ghana and South Korea 306

Managed Trade: The U.S. and Japanese
Semiconductor Industries, 1970–2002 307

Dixon Ticonderoga: Victim of Globalization? 311

Part 4
The Global Monetary System

Chapter 9
The Foreign Exchange Market 314

Opening Case
Axis Hedges the Euro 315

Introduction 316

The Functions of the Foreign Exchange Market 316
Currency Conversion 317

Management Focus
George Soros—The Man Who Moved Currency
Markets 318

Insuring against Foreign Exchange Risk 318

The Nature of the Foreign Exchange Market 322

Economic Theories of Exchange
Rate Determination 323
Prices and Exchange Rates 323
Interest Rates and Exchange Rates 329
Investor Psychology and Bandwagon Effects 330
Summary 331

Exchange Rate Forecasting 331
The Efficient Market School 331

Country Focus
Why Did the Korean Won Collapse? 332

The Inefficient Market School 332
Approaches to Forecasting 333

Currency Convertibility 334
Convertibility and Government Policy 334
Countertrade 335

Focus On Managerial Implications 336

Chapter Summary 336

Critical Discussion Questions 337

Research Task globalEDGE™ globaledge.msu.edu 339

Closing Case
The Collapse of the Thai Baht in 1997 339

Chapter 10
The International Monetary System 342

Opening Case
Turkey's 18th IMF Program 343

Introduction 344

The Gold Standard 346
Mechanics of the Gold Standard 346
Strength of the Gold Standard 347
The Period between the Wars, 1918–1939 347

The Bretton Woods System 348
The Role of the IMF 348
The Role of the World Bank 349

The Collapse of the Fixed Exchange Rate System 350

The Floating Exchange Rate Regime 351
The Jamaica Agreement 351
Exchange Rates since 1973 351

Fixed versus Floating Exchange Rates 353
The Case for Floating Exchange Rates 353
The Case for Fixed Exchange Rates 354
Who Is Right? 355

Exchange Rate Regimes in Practice 356
Pegged Exchange Rates 356
Currency Boards 357

Country Focus
Argentina's Currency Board 358

Crisis Management by the IMF 359
Financial Crises in the Post–Bretton Woods Era 359
Mexican Currency Crisis of 1995 360
Russian Ruble Crisis 361

Management Focus
The 1995 Mexican Peso Crisis and the Automobile
Industry 362

The Asian Crisis 364
Evaluating the IMF's Policy Prescriptions 368

Focus On Managerial Implications 370
Currency Management 370
Business Strategy 370
Corporate–Government Relations 371

Chapter Summary 372

Critical Discussion Questions 373

Research Task globalEDGE™ globaledge.msu.edu 374

Closing Case
The Tragedy of the Congo (Zaire) 374

Chapter 11
The Global Capital Market 378

Opening Case
China Mobile 379

Introduction 380

Benefits of the Global Capital Market 380
Functions of a Generic Capital Market 380
Attractions of the Global Capital Market 381

Management Focus
Deutsche Telekom Taps the Global Capital Market 383

Growth of the Global Capital Market 386
Information Technology 386
Deregulation 387
Global Capital Market Risks 388

Country Focus
Did the Global Capital Market Fail Mexico? 388

The Eurocurrency Market 390
Genesis and Growth of the Market 390
Attractions of the Eurocurrency Market 391
Drawbacks of the Eurocurrency Market 392

The Global Bond Market 392
Attractions of the Eurobond Market 393

The Global Equity Market 394

Foreign Exchange Risk and the Cost of Capital 394

Focus On Managerial Implications 395

Chapter Summary 396

Critical Discussion Questions 397

Research Task globalEDGE™ globaledge.msu.edu 398

Closing Case
The Surging Samurai Bond Market 398

Cases
Money Change 402

Bailing Out Brazil 403

The International Monetary Fund 405

Part 5
The Strategy and Structure of
International Business

Chapter 12
The Strategy of International Business 408

Opening Case
Global Strategy at MTV Networks 409

Introduction 410

Strategy and the Firm 410
Value Creation 411
The Firm as a Value Chain 413
Strategy in International Business 415

Profiting from Global Expansion 416
Location Economies 417
Experience Effects 418
Leveraging Core Competencies 421
Leveraging Subsidiary Skills 422

Pressures for Cost Reductions and Local
Responsiveness 422
Pressures for Cost Reductions 423
Pressures for Local Responsiveness 424

Management Focus
Tailoring World Cars to the U.S. Market 425

Strategic Choices 427
International Strategy 428
Multidomestic Strategy 429
Global Strategy 429
Transnational Strategy 429

Management Focus
IKEA 430

Summary 433

Chapter Summary 433

Critical Discussion Questions 434

Research Task globalEDGE™ globaledge.msu.edu 436

Closing Case
Global Strategy at General Motors 436

Chapter 13
The Organization of International
Business 438

Opening Case
Organizational Change at Unilever 439

Introduction 440

Organizational Architecture   441

Organizational Structure   444
   *Vertical Differentiation: Centralization
   and Decentralization*   444
   Horizontal Differentiation: The Design of Structure   446

Management Focus
The International Division at Abbott Laboratories   449

Management Focus
The Rise and Fall of Dow Chemical's
Matrix Structure   452

   Integrating Mechanisms   453

Control Systems and Incentives   458
   Types of Control Systems   458
   Incentive Systems   459
   *Control Systems, Incentives, and Strategy in the International
   Business*   460

Management Focus
Organizational Culture and Incentive
at Lincoln Electric   461

Processes   463

Organizational Culture   464
   Creating and Maintaining Organizational Culture   465
   *Organizational Culture and Performance in the International
   Business*   466

Synthesis: Strategy and Architecture   468
   Multidomestic Firms   468
   International Firms   469
   Global Firms   469
   Transnational Firms   469
   Environment, Strategy, Architecture, and Performance   470

Organizational Change   470
   Organizational Inertia   471
   Implementing Organizational Change   472

Chapter Summary   473

Critical Discussion Questions   474

Research Task globalEDGE™ globaledge.msu.edu   474

Closing Case
Organizational Change at Royal Dutch/Shell   476

Chapter 14
Entry Strategy and Strategic Alliances   478

Opening Case
Diebold   479

Introduction   480

Basic Entry Decisions   481

Which Foreign Markets?   481
Timing of Entry   482
Scale of Entry and Strategic Commitments   482
Summary   483

Management Focus
International Expansion at ING Group   484

Management Focus
The Jollibee Phenomenon—A Philippine
Multinational   486

Entry Modes   486
   Exporting   487
   Turnkey Projects   488
   Licensing   488

Management Focus
The Evolution of the Fuji-Xerox Joint Venture   490

   Franchising   492
   Joint Ventures   493
   Wholly Owned Subsidiaries   494

Selecting an Entry Mode   495
   Core Competencies and Entry Mode   496
   Pressures for Cost Reductions and Entry Mode   497

Establishing a Wholly Owned Subsidiary: Green-Field
Venture or Acquisition?   497
   Pros and Cons of Acquisitions   497
   Pros and Cons of Green-Field Ventures   499
   Green-Field Venture or Acquisition?   500

Strategic Alliances   500
   The Advantages of Strategic Alliances   500
   The Disadvantages of Strategic Alliances   501

Making Alliances Work   502
   Partner Selection   502
   Alliance Structure   502
   Managing the Alliance   504

Chapter Summary   505

Critical Discussion Questions   506

Research Task globalEDGE™ globaledge.msu.edu   509

Closing Case
Merrill Lynch in Japan   510

Cases
BP: Creating a Global Brand   514

Restructuring Exide   514

**Philips versus Matsushita: A New Century,
a New Round**   517

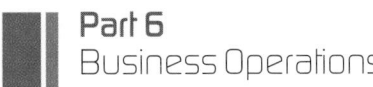

Part 6
Business Operations

Chapter 15
Exporting, Importing, and Countertrade   534

Opening Case
Megahertz Communications   535

Introduction   536

The Promise and Pitfalls of Exporting   536

Improving Export Performance   537
An International Comparison   538
Information Sources   538
Utilizing Export Management Companies   539
Exporting Strategy   539

Management Focus
Exporting Strategy at 3M   540

Management Focus
Red Spot Paint & Varnish   541

Export and Import Financing   541
Lack of Trust   542
Letter of Credit   543
Draft   544
Bill of Lading   545
A Typical International Trade Transaction   545

Export Assistance   546
Export–Import Bank   546
Export Credit Insurance   546

Countertrade   547
The Incidence of Countertrade   547
Types of Countertrade   548
The Pros and Cons of Countertrade   549

Chapter Summary   550

Critical Discussion Questions   551

Research Task globalEDGE™ globaledge.msu.edu   551

Closing Case
Artais Weather Check   552

Chapter 16
Global Manufacturing and Materials Management   554

Opening Case
Competitive Advantage at Dell Computer   555

Introduction   556

Strategy, Manufacturing, and Materials Management   556

Where to Manufacture   558
Country Factors   559
Technological Factors   559

Management Focus
Philips in China   560

Product Factors   564
Locating Manufacturing Facilities   564

The Strategic Role of Foreign Factories   565

Management Focus
Hewlett-Packard in Singapore   567

Make-or-Buy Decisions at the Boeing Company   568
The Advantages of Make   568
The Advantages of Buy   570
Trade-offs   572
Strategic Alliances with Suppliers   572

Managing a Global Supply Chain   573
The Role of Just-in-Time Inventory   573
The Role of Organization   574
The Role of Information Technology and the Internet   575

Chapter Summary   577

Critical Discussion Questions   578

Research Task globalEDGE™ globaledge.msu.edu   578

Closing Case
Li & Fung   580

Chapter 17
Global Marketing and R&D   582

Opening Case
Marketing Coca-Cola in China   583

Introduction   584

The Globalization of Markets and Brands   584

Market Segmentation   585

Management Focus
Marketing to Black Brazil   586

Product Attributes   587
Cultural Differences   587
Economic Development   588
Product and Technical Standards   588

Distribution Strategy   589
Differences between Countries   589
Choosing a Distribution Strategy   591

Communication Strategy   592
Barriers to International Communication   592

Management Focus
Overcoming Cultural Barriers to Selling Tampons   594

Push versus Pull Strategies   595

Management Focus
Unilever—Selling to India's Poor   596

Global Advertising   597

Pricing Strategy   598
Price Discrimination   598
Strategic Pricing   601
Regulatory Influences on Prices   602

Configuring the Marketing Mix   603

Management Focus
Castrol Oil in Vietnam   604

New-Product Development   605
The Location of R&D   605
Integrating R&D, Marketing, and Production   607
Cross-Functional Teams   608

Focus On Managerial Implications   608

Chapter Summary   610

Critical Discussion Questions   610

Research Task globalEDGE™ globaledge.msu.edu   611

Closing Case
Procter & Gamble in Japan   613

Chapter 18
Global Human Resource Management   616

Opening Case
Molex   617

Introduction   618

The Strategic Role of International HRM   619

Staffing Policy   620
Types of Staffing Policy   621
Expatriate Managers   623

Management Focus
Managing Expatriates at Royal Dutch/Shell   626

Training and Management Development   628
Training for Expatriate Managers   629
Repatriation of Expatriates   629
Management Development and Strategy   630

Management Focus
Monsanto's Repatriation Program   631

Performance Appraisal   631

Performance Appraisal Problems   632
Guidelines for Performance Appraisal   632

Compensation   632
National Differences in Compensation   632
Expatriate Pay   634

Management Focus
Executive Pay Policies for Global Managers   635

International Labor Relations   637

The Concerns of Organized Labor   637
The Strategy of Organized Labor   638
Approaches to Labor Relations   638

Chapter Summary   639

Critical Discussion Questions   640

Research Task globalEDGE™ globaledge.msu.edu   640

Closing Case
**Degrussa: Strategy and Human
Resources in China**   643

Chapter 19
Accounting in the International Business   644

Opening Case
**The Adoption of International Accounting
Standards in Germany**   645

Introduction   646

Country Differences in Accounting Standards   647
Relationship between Business and Providers of Capital   647
Political and Economic Ties with Other Countries   649
Inflation Accounting   649
Level of Development   649
Culture   649
Accounting Clusters   650

National and International Standards   650
Lack of Comparability   650
International Standards   652

Management Focus
The Consequences of Different
Accounting Standards   653

Multinational Consolidation and Currency
Translation   654

Consolidated Financial Statements   654

Management Focus
Novartis Joins the International Accounting Club   655

Currency Translation   657
Current U.S. Practice   658

Accounting Aspects of Control Systems 658
  Exchange Rate Changes and Control Systems 659
  Transfer Pricing and Control Systems 660
  Separation of Subsidiary and Manager Performance 661

Chapter Summary 662

Critical Discussion Questions 663

Research Task globalEDGE™ globaledge.msu.edu 663

Closing Case
China's Evolving Accounting System 664

Chapter 20
Financial Management in the
International Business 666

Opening Case
**Global Treasury Management at
Procter & Gamble** 667

Introduction 668

Investment Decisions 669
  Capital Budgeting 669
  Project and Parent Cash Flows 670
  Adjusting for Political and Economic Risk 670

Management Focus
Black Sea Energy Ltd. 671

  Risk and Capital Budgeting 672

Financing Decisions 673
  Source of Financing 673
  Financial Structure 673

Global Money Management: The
Efficiency Objective 674
  Minimizing Cash Balances 674
  Reducing Transaction Costs 675

Global Money Management: The Tax Objective 675

Moving Money across Borders: Attaining
Efficiencies and Reducing Taxes 676
  Dividend Remittances 676
  Royalty Payments and Fees 677
  Transfer Prices 677
  Fronting Loans 679

Techniques for Global Money Management 680
  Centralized Depositories 680
  Multilateral Netting 681

Managing Foreign Exchange Risk 683
  Types of Foreign Exchange Exposure 683
  *Tactics and Strategies for Reducing Foreign
  Exchange Exposure* 685
  *Developing Policies for Managing Foreign
  Exchange Exposure* 686

Chapter Summary 687

Critical Discussion Questions 688

Research Task globalEDGE™ globaledge.msu.edu 689

Closing Case
Motorola's Global Cash Management System 689

Case
Cretors & Co. 694

Glossary 695

Photo Credits 706

Index 708

List of Maps

Map   **2.1**   Gross National Income per Capita, 2001   58

Map   **2.2**   Purchasing Power Parity, 2001   60

Map   **2.3**   Growth in Gross Domestic Product, 1991–2001   61

Map   **2.4**   The Human Development Index, 2001   63

Map   **2.5**   Political Freedom in 2002   68

Map   **2.6**   Global Distribution of Economic Freedom, 2003   72

Map   **3.1**   World Religions   99

Map   **3.2**   Percentage of Gross National Product Spent on Education   109

Map   **3.3**   Adult Illiteracy Rates   110

Map   **8.1**   European Union Countries and Applicants   275

Map   **8.2**   The Shape of the EU after Enlargement   283

Map   **8.3**   Economic Integration in the Americas   284

Map   **8.4**   APEC Members   291

Map   **8.5**   The Trade Blocs in Africa   292

Map   **19.1**   Accounting Clusters   651

Preface

International Business: Competing in the Global Market-place is intended for the first international business course at either the undergraduate or the MBA level. My goal in writing this book has been to set the standard for international business textbooks: I have attempted to write a book that (1) is comprehensive and up-to-date, (2) goes beyond an uncritical presentation and shallow explanation of the body of knowledge, (3) maintains a tight, integrated flow between chapters, (4) focuses on managerial implications, and (5) makes important theories accessible and interesting to students.

Comprehensive and Up-to-Date

To be comprehensive, an international business textbook must:

- Explain how and why the world's countries differ.
- Present a thorough review of the economics and politics of international trade and investment.
- Explain the functions and form of the global monetary system.
- Examine the strategies and structures of international businesses.
- Assess the special roles of an international business's various functions.

This textbook does all these things. Too many other textbooks pay scant attention to the strategies and structures of international businesses and to the implications of international business for firms' various functions. This omission is a serious deficiency because the students in these international business courses will soon be international managers, and they will be expected to understand the implications of international business for their organization's strategy, structure, and functions. This book pays close attention to these issues.

Comprehensiveness and relevance also require coverage of the major theories. Although many international business textbooks do a reasonable job of reviewing long-established theories (e.g., the theory of comparative advantage and Vernon's product life-cycle theory) they often tend to ignore important newer work. It has always been my goal to incorporate the insights gleaned from recent academic work into the text. Consistent with this goal, over the years I have added insights from the following research:

- The new trade theory and strategic trade policy.
- The work of Nobel Prize–winning economist Amartya Sen on economic development.

- Samuel Huntington's influential thesis on the "clash of civilizations."
- The new growth theory of economic development championed by Paul Romer and Gene Grossman.
- Empirical work by Jeffrey Sachs and others on the relationship between international trade and economic growth.
- Michael Porter's theory of the competitive advantage of nations.
- Robert Reich's work on national competitive advantage.
- The work of Nobel Prize winner Douglas North and others on national institutional structures and the protection of property rights.
- The market imperfections approach to foreign direct investment that has grown out of Ronald Coase and Oliver Williamson's work on transaction cost economics.
- Bartlett and Ghoshal's research on the transnational corporation.
- The writings of C. K. Prahalad and Gary Hamel on core competencies, global competition, and global strategic alliances.

I have incorporated all relevant state-of-the-art work at the appropriate points in this book. For example, in Chapter 2, "National Differences in Political Economy," reference is made to the new growth theory, to the work of North and others on national institutional structures and property rights, and to the work of Sen. In Chapter 4, "International Trade Theory," in addition to such standard theories as the theory of comparative advantage and the Heckscher-Ohlin theory, there is detailed discussion of the new trade theory and Porter's theory of national competitive advantage. The empirical work on the relationship between trade and economic growth is also examined in this chapter. In Chapter 5, "The Political Economy of International Trade," the pros and cons of strategic trade policy are discussed. In Chapter 6, "Foreign Direct Investment," the market imperfections approach is reviewed. Chapters 12, 13, and 14, which deal with the strategy and structure of international business, draw extensively on the work of Bartlett, Ghoshal, Hamel, and Prahalad.

In addition to including leading-edge theory, in light of the fast-changing nature of the international business environment, every effort is being made to ensure that the book is as up-to-date as possible when it goes to press.

A significant amount has happened in the world since the first edition of this book was published in 1993. The Uruguay Round of GATT negotiations was successfully concluded, and the World Trade Organization was established. In 2001, the WTO embarked upon another major round of talks aimed to reduce barriers to trade, the Doha round. The European Union moved forward with its post-1992 agenda to achieve a closer economic and monetary union, including the establishment of a common currency in January 1999. The North American Free Trade Agreement passed into law, and Chile indicated its desire to become the next member of the free trade area. The Asia Pacific Economic Cooperation forum (APEC) emerged as the kernel of a possible future Asia Pacific free trade area. The former Communist states of Eastern Europe and Asia continued on the road to economic and political reform. As they did, the euphoric mood that followed the collapse of communism in 1989 was slowly replaced with a growing sense of realism about the hard path ahead for many of these countries. The global money market continued its meteoric growth. By 2002, over $1.5 trillion per day was flowing across national borders. The size of such flows fueled concern about the ability of short-term speculative shifts in global capital markets to destabilize the world economy. These fears were fanned by the well-publicized financial problems of a number of organizations that traded derivatives through the global money market, such as Baring's Bank. The World Wide Web emerged from nowhere to become the backbone of an emerging global network for electronic commerce. The world continued to become more global. Several Asian Pacific economies, including most notably China, continued to grow their economies at a rapid rate. New multinationals continued to emerge from developing nations in addition to the world's established industrial powers. Increasingly, the globalization of the world economy affected a wide range of firms of all sizes, from the very large to the very small. And, unfortunately, in the wake of the September 11, 2001, terrorist attacks on the United States, global terrorism and the attendant geopolitical risks emerged as a threat to global economic integration and activity.

Reflecting this rapid pace of change, in this edition of the book I have tried to ensure that all material and statistics are as up-to-date as possible as of 2003. However, being absolutely up-to-date is impossible since change is always with us. What is current today may be outdated tomorrow. Accordingly, I have established a home page for this book on the World Wide Web at www.mhhe.com/hill. From this home page, the reader can access regular updates of chapter material and reports on topical developments that are relevant to students of international business. I hope readers find this a useful addition to the support material for this book.

What's New in the Fifth Edition

The success of the first four editions of *International Business* was based in part upon the incorporation of leading-edge research into the text, the use of the up-to-date examples and statistics to illustrate global trends and enterprise strategy, and the discussion of current events within the context of the appropriate theory. Building on these strengths, my goals for the fifth revision have been threefold:

1. Incorporate new insights from recent scholarly research wherever appropriate.
2. Make sure the content of the text covers all appropriate issues.
3. Make sure the text is as up-to-date as possible with regard to current events, statistics, and examples.

As part of the revision process, *changes have been made to every chapter in the book.* All statistics have been updated to incorporate the most recently available data. New examples, several cases, and boxes have been added and older examples updated to reflect new developments. New material has been inserted wherever appropriate to reflect recent academic work or important current events. For example, Chapter 2 now contains a section on "The New World Order and Global Terrorism," which discusses the nature of global terrorism and its implication for international business in the wake of the September 11, 2001, attacks on the United States. Chapter 5 has been updated to discuss the new round of talks sponsored by the WTO that are aimed at reducing barriers to trade, particularly in agriculture (the Doha round). Chapter 6 now discusses the slump in foreign direct investment flows that took place in 2001 and 2002. The section on the European Union in Chapter 8 has been revised to reflect the plans to admit 10 more member states into the EU on May 1, 2004. In Chapter 12, there have been additions to the section discussing how multinationals can gain a competitive advantage by leveraging skills between subsidiaries. This addition reflects the substantial academic research addressing this issue that has been published in recent years.

Beyond Uncritical Presentation and Shallow Explanation

Many issues in international business are complex and thus necessitate considerations of pros and cons. To demonstrate this to students, I have adopted a critical approach that presents the arguments for and against economic theories, government policies, business strategies, organizational structures, and so on.

Related to this, I have attempted to explain the complexities of the many theories and phenomena unique to international business so the student might fully comprehend the statements of a theory or the reasons a phenomenon is the way it is. These theories and phenomena are typically explained in more depth in this book than they are in competing textbooks, the rationale being that a shallow explanation is little better than no explanation. In international business, a little knowledge is indeed a dangerous thing.

Integrated Progression of Topics

Many textbooks lack a tight, integrated flow of topics from chapter to chapter. In this book students are told in Chapter 1 how the book's topics are related to each other. Integration has been achieved by organizing the material so that each chapter builds on the material of the previous ones in a logical fashion.

Part One, Chapter 1, provides an overview of the key issues to be addressed and explains the plan of the book.

Part Two, Chapters 2 and 3, focuses on national differences in political economy and culture. Most international business textbooks place this material later, but I believe it is vital to discuss national differences first. After all, many of the central issues in international trade and investment, the global monetary system, international business strategy and structure, and international business operations arise out of national differences in political economy and culture. To fully understand these issues, students must first appreciate the differences in countries and cultures.

Part Three, Chapters 4 through 8, investigates the political economy of international trade and investment. The purpose of this part is to describe and explain the trade and investment environment in which international business occurs.

Part Four, Chapters 9 through 11, describes and explains the global monetary system, laying out in detail the monetary framework in which international business transactions are conducted.

Part Five, Chapters 12 through 14, shifts attention from the environment to the firm. Here the book examines the strategies and structures that firms adopt to compete effectively in the international business environment.

Part Six, Chapters 15 through 20, narrows the focus further to investigate business operations. These chapters explain how firms can perform their key functions—manufacturing, marketing, R&D, human resource management, accounting, and finance—in order to compete and succeed in the international business environment.

Throughout the book, the relationship of new material to topics discussed in earlier chapters is pointed out to the students to reinforce their understanding of how the material comprises an integrated whole.

Focus On Managerial Implications

Many international business textbooks fail to discuss the implications of the various topics for the actual practice of international business. This does not serve the needs of business school students who will soon be practicing managers. Accordingly, the usefulness of this book's material in the practice of international business is discussed explicitly. In particular, at the end of each chapter in Parts Two, Three, and Four—where the focus is on the environment of international business, as opposed to particular firms—there is a section titled Focus On Managerial Implications. In this section, the managerial implications of the material discussed in the chapter are clearly explained. For example, Chapter 4, "International Trade Theory," ends with a detailed discussion of the various trade theories' implications for international business management.

In addition, each chapter begins with a case that illustrates the relevance of chapter material for the practice of international business. Chapter 2, "National Differences in Political Economy," for example, opens with a case that describes how changes in the political and economic institutions of India are making it a more attractive location for international businesses to operate.

I have also added a closing case to each chapter. These cases are also designed to illustrate the relevance of chapter material for the practice of international business. The closing case to Chapter 2, for example, looks at the battle against piracy in the global market for video games. This case helps to illustrate the important role that national differences in the protection of intellectual property rights can play in international business.

Another tool that I have used to focus on managerial implications are Management Focus boxes. There is at least one Management Focus in each chapter. Like the opening case, the purpose of these boxes is to illustrate the relevance of chapter material for the practice of international business. The Management Focus in Chapter 2, for example, looks at how the South African government has adopted laws that allow the sale of cheap generic versions of patented medicines, including powerful new drugs for treating AIDS, without permission from the patent owners, which in this case are large multinational pharmaceutical firms.

New to this edition are GlobalEdge Research Tasks that appear at the end of each chapter. Created by the CIBER Group at Michigan State University headed by Tomas Hult and Tunga Kiyak, these application exercises challenge students to research, collect, and analyze data acting as a manager working for an international firm. From exploring differences in business etiquette to using data sources such as the *World Investment Directory* to identifying tariff restrictions in different countries, these exercises will expose students to the types of sources and tools international managers use to make informed business decisions.

Accessible and Interesting

The international business arena is fascinating and exciting, and I have tried to communicate my enthusiasm for it to the student. Learning is easier and better if the subject matter is communicated in an interesting, informative, and accessible manner. One technique I have used to achieve this is weaving interesting anecdotes into the narrative of the text—stories that illustrate theory. The opening cases and focus boxes are also used to make the theory being discussed in the text both accessible and interesting.

Each chapter has two kinds of focus boxes—a Management Focus box (described above) and a Country Focus box. Country Focus boxes provide background on the political, economic, social, or cultural aspects of countries grappling with an international business issue. In Chapter 2, for example, one Country Focus box discusses the process of privatizing state-owned businesses in Taiwan.

Just how accessible and interesting this book actually is will be revealed by time and student feedback. I am confident, however, that this book is far more accessible to students than its competitors. For those of you who view such a bold claim with skepticism, I urge you to read the sections in Chapter 1 on the globalization of the world economy, the changing nature of international business, and how international business is different.

Acknowledgments

Numerous people deserve to be thanked for their assistance in preparing this book. First, thank you to all the people at McGraw-Hill/Irwin who have worked with me on this project:

John Biernat, Editorial Director

Ryan Blankenship, Sponsoring Editor

Laura Hurst Spell, Managing Development Editor

Lisa Nicks, Marketing Manager

Laura Griffin, Project Manager

Debra R. Sylvester, Production Supervisor

Kami Carter, Designer

Jeremy Cheshareck, Photo Research Coordinator

Second, my thanks go to the reviewers, who provided good feedback that helped shape this book.

Sergio Castello, University of Mobile

Howard Ellis, Millersville University

Diane D. Hathaway, University of Cincinnati

Kanata A. Jackson, Hampton University

H. Lynn Moretz, Central Piedmont Community College

Joseph W. Leonard, Miami University

Behnam Nakhai, Millersville University

Mike W. Peng, The Ohio State University

Kenneth R. Tillery, Middle Tennessee State University

Berry K. Wilson, Pace University

Guided Tour

Cases, focus boxes, and exercises throughout the book make theories accessible and interesting and show how theory relates to the practice of international business.

Opening Case

India's Changing Political Economy

After gaining independence from Britain in 1947, India adopted a democratic system of government. The economic system that developed in India after 1947 was a mixed economy characterized by a large number of state-owned enterprises (of which there were almost 300 in 1991), centralized planning, and subsidies. This system constrained the growth of the private sector. Private companies could expand only with government permission. Under this system, dubbed the "License Raj," private companies often had to wait months for government approval of routine business activities, such as expanding production or hiring a new director. It could take years to get permission to diversify into a new product. Much of heavy industry, such as auto, chemical, and steel production, was reserved for state-owned enterprises. Production quotas and high import tariffs also stunted the development of a healthy private sector, as did restrictive labor laws that made it difficult to fire employees. Access to foreign exchange was limited, investment by foreign firms was severely restricted, land use was strictly controlled, and the government routinely managed prices as opposed to letting them be set by market forces.

By the early 1990s, it was clear that after 40 years of near stagnation, this system was incapable of delivering the kind of economic progress that many Southeastern Asian nations had started to enjoy. In 1994, India's economy was still smaller than Belgium's, despite having a population of 950 million. Its GDP per capita was a paltry $310; less than half the population could read; only 6 million had access to telephones; only 14 percent had access to clean sanitation; the World Bank estimated that some 40 percent of the world's desperately poor lived in India; and only 2.3 percent of the population had a household income in excess of $2,484.

In 1991, the lack of progress led the government to embark on an ambitious economic reform program. Much of the industrial licensing system was dismantled, and several areas once closed to the private sector were opened, including electricity generation, parts of the oil industry, steelmaking, air transport, and some areas of the telecommunications industry. Investment by foreign companies, formerly allowed only grudgingly and subject to arbitrary ceilings, was suddenly welcomed. Approval was made automatic for foreign equity stakes of up to 51 percent in an Indian enterprise, and 100 percent foreign ownership was allowed under certain circumstances. Raw materials and many industrial goods could be freely imported, and the maximum tariff that could be levied on imports was reduced from 400 percent to 65 percent. The top income tax rate was also reduced, and corporate tax

fell from 57.5 percent to 46 percent in 1994, and then to 35 percent in 1997.

The government also announced plans to start privatizing India's state-owned businesses, some 40 percent of which were losing money in the early 1990s. The privatization program has had a bumpy record in India, often slowed by political opposition. In 1999, there were still some 240 state-owned enterprises scattered across many sectors of the economy that accounted for 15 percent of India's gross domestic product. Nevertheless, by the early 2000s the program was progressing at a fairly rapid pace with about 30 state-owned enterprises privatized in 2002 alone.

Judged by some measures, the response to these economic reforms has been impressive. The economy expanded at an annual rate of about 6.1 percent throughout the 1990s. Despite the slowdown in global economic activity after 2000, India still managed to grow 5.5 percent annually during 2000–2002. Foreign investment, a key indicator of the economy's attractiveness, jumped from $150 million in 1991 to an estimated $3.5 billion in 1997, hit a record $5 billion in 2001, and was forecast to exceed this in 2002. Some sectors of the economy have done particularly well, such as the information technology sector in which India has emerged as a vibrant global center for software development. The export revenue of India's software services market reached $6.2 billion in 2002, up from less than $500 million in the mid-1990s.

However, the country still has a long way to go. Attempts to further reduce import tariffs have been stalled by political opposition from employers, employees, and politicians, who fear that if barriers come down, a flood of inexpensive Chinese products will enter India. There has also been strong resistance to reforming many of India's laws that make it difficult for private business to operate efficiently. For example, labor laws make it almost impossible for firms with more than 100 employees to fire workers. Other laws mandate that certain products can be manufactured only by small companies, effectively prohibiting companies in these industries from attaining the scale required to compete internationally.

Also, a decade of reform has done little to solve India's crippling poverty problem. Although the Indian middle class grew richer during the 1990s, by 2002 some 40 percent of India's nearly 1 billion people still lived in abject poverty, earning less than $1 a day, a figure little changed from 1990. By 2002, the gross domestic product per capita of India was still only $450, which ranked India at 164 among the world's nations; 44 percent of the adult population was illiterate; 19 percent of Indians had no

Chapter 2

National Differences in Political Economy

Introduction
Political Systems
  Collectivism and Individualism
  Democracy and Totalitarianism
Economic Systems
  Market Economy
  Command Economy
  Mixed Economy
Legal Systems
  Different Legal Systems
  Differences in Contract Law
  Property Rights
  The Protection of Intellectual Property
  Product Safety and Product Liability
The Determinants of Economic Development
  Differences in Economic Development
  Broader Conceptions of Development:
  Amartya Sen
  Political Economy and Economic Progress
  Geography, Education, and Economic Development
States in Transition
  The Spread of Democracy
  The New World Order and Global Terrorism
  The Spread of Market-Based Systems
  The Nature of Economic Transformation
  Implications
Focus on Managerial Implications
  Attractiveness
  Ethics and Regulations
Chapter Summary
Critical Discussion Questions
Closing Case: Piracy in the Video Game Market

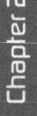
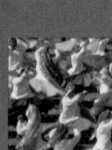
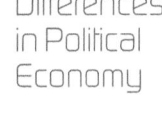
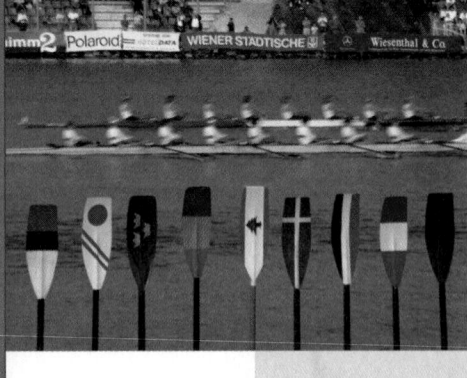
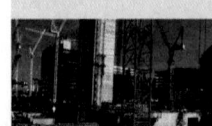

Cases

2. Market Potential Indicators (MPI) is an indexing study conducted by the Michigan State Univer-

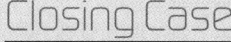

Closing Case

Piracy in the Video Game Market

Over the past decade, the video game industry has grown into a global colossus worth more than $20 billion a year in revenues. For the three biggest players in the industry, Sony with its PlayStation II, Microsoft with X-box, and Nintendo with GameCube, this potentially represents a huge growth engine, but the engine is threatened by a rise in piracy, which cost the industry an estimated $2 billion in 2001.

The piracy problem is particularly serious in East Asia, excluding Japan, where video game consoles are routinely "chipped"—sold with modified chips, called "mod-chips," that override the console's security system, allowing it to play illegally copied games and CDs. Importers or resellers, who charge a small markup for making the modification, illegally install the mod-chips. In some regions, Hong Kong for example, it is almost impossible to find a console that hasn't been modified.

Because they allow users to play illegally copied games, consoles with mod-chips installed offer a gaping gateway for software pirates, and they directly threaten the profitability of console and game makers. The big three in the industry all follow a razor-and-razor-blades business model, where the console (razor) is sold at a loss, and profit is made on the sale of the game (razor blades). In the case of Microsoft's X-box, estimates suggest that the company loses as much as $200 on each X-box it sells. To make profits, Microsoft collects royalties on the sale of games developed under license, in addition to producing and selling some games itself. Each game typically retails for about $50, and Microsoft must sell 6 to 12 games to each X-box user to recoup the $200 loss on the initial sale and start making a profit. If those users are purchasing pirated games and playing them on "chipped" X-box consoles, Microsoft collects nothing in royalties and may never reach breakeven. Sony and Nintendo face similar problems. In East Asia,

Each chapter concludes with a Closing Case demonstrating the relevance of the chapter material to the practice of international business.

▊ Video Case: Starbucks ▞

Synopsis of the Video

This video describes the relationships that Starbucks has built with its coffee suppliers. Starbucks is the world's largest seller of premium-brewed coffee with more than 6,300 stores worldwide in 27 countries. Starbucks has to ensure a consistent supply of premium-grade coffee beans for its roasters. The problem is complicated by the volatility of coffee prices on the world market. The volatile pricing environment can make it difficult for small growers of premium coffee to cover their costs, particularly when excess supply on the world market drives prices down. To help stabilize prices, Starbucks and other companies guarantee a minimum purchase price in advance.

Starbucks signs long-term contracts with growers of high-grade specialty coffee in developed nations. In recent years, it has paid as much as twice the market price for premium coffee. Starbucks is able to do this because the differentiated nature of its product means it can pass on high prices for coffee to its consumers in the form of higher prices. The company also provides farmers with credit to tide them over when they are not generating any income from the sale of coffee.

Beginning in 2000, Starbucks also started selling Fair Trade Coffee in its stores. According to Global Exchange, an international human rights organization, "Few Americans realize that agriculture workers in the

sumers that coffee was purchased under Fair Trade conditions. To become Fair Trade certified, coffee importers must meet certain criteria, which include paying a minimum price per pound of $1.26, providing credit to farmers, and providing technical assistance such as help transitioning to organic farming.[1] However, only a small percentage of Starbucks' total coffee purchase is "fair trade" coffee. According to Starbucks, this is because only 2 percent of the farmers it deals with can adhere to fair trade principles.

In addition to its foray into the Fair Trade market, Starbucks has partnered with Conservation International to promote growing coffee in an environmentally sustainable manner. For example, the coffee trees may be planted in rows shaded by trees. While this means that less land can be devoted to coffee bushes, it also means that the area sustains a more diverse biology, and the farmers have to use less fertilizer. Coffee grows easily among shade trees and other vegetation. The trees keep nitrogen in the soil, and their leaves provide natural mulch for coffee plants, reducing the need for chemical fertilizers and herbicides. The mix of plants prevents erosion and protects the coffee from harsh weather.

Case Discussion Questions

1. Why is it important for Starbucks to ensure a consistent supply of high-grade specialty coffee?

Video Case

NEW! For use with corresponding videos in the video package, these end-of-part cases explore current issues and examine how various companies, such as Starbucks and BP, compete in the international business market.

▊ The Softwood Lumber Dispute

Introduction

"It's the biggest trade dispute on the planet," says Pierre Pettigrew, Canada's trade minister in 2003. Pettigrew was referring to a 20 year dispute between Canada and the United States over exports of Canadian softwood lumber to the United States. The numbers involved suggest that Pettigrew has a point. In 2001, Canada exported softwood lumber products to the United States valued at $6.5 billion. That was before May 2002, when the U.S. Commerce Department imposed countervailing duties averaging 27 percent on Canadian lumber imports. The imposition of duties was a response to pressure from U.S. lumber producers who claim that Canadian producers have been unfairly dumping lumber on the U.S. market at prices below costs, thereby driving U.S. lumber producers out of business.

It's not the first time this claim has been made. Three times over the last two decades U.S. lumber producers have lobbied for protection, three times the U.S. government has responded by imposing tariffs on Canadian lumber imports into the United States, and three times the Canadians have appealed to U.S. and international trade panels, and each time the Canadians have won on appeal. Will it be any different this time? That now depends on a ruling by the World Trade Organization, which in October 2002 decided to investigate a Canadian complaint that the U.S. tariffs violate WTO rules.

mental programs, which are not reflected in the low stumpage fees and which increase production costs in Canada. Additionally, the Canadians have long claimed that low prices of Canadian lumber reflect their more efficient mills, allowing them to sell lumber cheaper and still make profits. Whatever the reason for Canada's price advantage, Canadian lumber has steadily increased its share of the U.S. market and in 2001 accounted for 38 percent of all softwood lumber used in the United States.

The most recent dispute can be traced to a 1996 Softwood Lumber Agreement (SLA) between Canada and the United States. Under the SLA, imports of Canadian lumber up to 14.7 billion board feet annually were allowed into the United States free of tariffs. The next 650 million board feet were subject to a tariff of $50 per thousand board feet, and all greater quantities were subject to a tariff of $100 per thousand board feet. The tariffs were designed to protect U.S. lumber producers from losing market share to the Canadians. The Canadians acquiesced to the SLA, even though they disagreed with it on principle, in an effort to buy trade peace.

The SLA was scheduled to expire March 31, 2001. In advance of the expiration, intense lobbying activity occurred. Among those pushing for the agreement to expire were a broad coalition of lumber-using groups in the United States, including the National Association of Home Builders, the National Lumber and Building Material Dealers Association, Home Depot, and affordable housing groups. The groups asked that the SLA not be re-

Case

Longer, end-of-part cases allow for more in-depth study of international companies.

Focus Boxes and Exercises

Country Focus

Privatization in Taiwan

Taiwan has the fifth largest economy in Asia and a well-earned reputation as an entrepreneurial powerhouse. Despite this, wide swaths of its corporate landscape are dominated by state-owned enterprises, including the banking, telecommunications, oil, and steel industries. According to many analysts, state ownership is responsible for a number of economic ills in Taiwan, including low productivity and government budget deficits. For example, estimates suggest that government-controlled banks currently have 30 percent too many staff members given their level of business. Executives at state-owned companies complain bitterly about strict oversight of budgeting and procurement that they say hampers their ability to compete. Government companies must submit spending plans to the legislature for approval more than a year ahead, leaving them unable to respond to quickly changing markets and giving politicians a unique opportunity to meddle in the running of the business. In an effort to correct this, in 1996 the government set a timetable for the privatization of 47 state-owned companies by 2002. By the end of 2002, however, 17 of these companies, including many of the largest, still remained in government hands.

There has been some progress. About 30 companies have been privatized since 1996, including 11 financial institutions, and some have been shut down. Sales of government-owned enterprises to private investors raised some $11.5 billion between 1996 and 2001. But this track record overstates the success of the privatization program. In many of these companies, the state is still the largest single shareholder and able to exercise control by pointing to enable private and decial decisions.

unemployment will result; and the weak state of Asian stock markets since the 1997 Asian financial crisis, which has made it difficult to attract investors to buy stock in newly privatized entities. These problems were vividly illustrated in 2001 when the state tried to sell two-thirds of its 99.9 percent stake in Chunghwa Telecom, Taiwan's largest telecommunications provider. Vocal opposition from employees and labor unions, along with political infighting in the legislature, delayed the proposed offering of stock to private investors for several years. In the interim, new private telecommunications providers, including wireless companies, have cut into Chunghwa Telecom's former monopoly, making the company less attractive to investors. Also, a rule prohibiting foreign investors from owning more than 20 percent of the company limited the pool of foreign investors interested in the sale. In a humiliating setback, the government was able to sell only 5 percent of the company's stock.

The failure of the Chunghwa Telecom offerings may have revitalized the privatization program. The government is now facing a rising budget deficit and realizes that the sale of state-owned enterprises could help to plug the gap. There has been a leadership shake-up at the ministry responsible for privatization, and ambitious new plans have been drafted, which, if they transpire, may result in the sale of substantial state assets over the next few years. However, the opposition against privatization remains a problem. For example, Chang Shu-jung, the head of the 16,000-employee union at the state-owned Chinese Petroleum, still vocally opposes the privatization of a company that he asserts is a national asset.

Country Focus

Each **Country Focus** example provides background on the political, economic, social or cultural aspects of countries grappling with an international business issue.

Management Focus

Drug Patents and the AIDS Epidemic in South Africa

In December 1997, the government of South Africa passed a law that authorized two controversial practices. One, called parallel importing, allowed importers in South Africa to purchase drugs from the cheapest source available, regardless of whether the patent holders had given their approval or not. The other practice, called compulsory licensing, permitted the South African government to license local companies to produce cheaper versions of drugs whose patents are held by foreign companies. The law seems to violate international agreements to protect property rights, including the World Trade Organization TRIPS agreement. South Africa, however, insisted the law was necessary given its own health crisis and the high cost of patented medicines. South Africa is wrestling with an AIDS crisis of enormous proportions. Some 4.5 million of South Africa's 45 million people are infected with the HIV virus, more than in any other country.

Foreign drug manufacturers saw the law as an unbridled attempt to expropriate their intellectual property rights, and 39 foreign companies quickly filed a lawsuit in the country to try to block implementation of the law. Foreign pharmaceutical companies fear that South Africa is the thin end of the wedge, and if the law is allowed to stand, other countries will follow suit. Many U.S. companies also fear that if poor countries such as South Africa are allowed to buy low-priced drugs in violation of intellectual property laws, American and European consumers will soon demand the same. Drug companies argue that because drug development is a very expensive, time-consuming, and risky process, they need the protection of intellectual patents.

ital. If drug companies could not count on high prices for their few successful products, the drug development process would dry up.

However, the drug companies do recognize that countries such as South Africa face special health challenges and lack the money to pay developed world prices. Accordingly, there is a long history in the industry of pricing drugs low in the developing world or giving them away. For example, AIDS drugs are sold to developing nations at an 80 to 90 percent discount over their prices in the United States. The South African government thought this was not good enough. The government has been supported by various human rights and AIDS organizations, which have cast the case as an attempt by the prosperous multinational drug companies of the West to maintain their intellectual property rights in the face of desperate attempts by an impoverished government to stem a deadly crisis. For their part, the drug companies have stated that the case has little to do with AIDS and is really about the right of South Africa to break international law.

While the drug companies may have international law on their side, the tie-in with the AIDS epidemic has clearly put them on the public relations defensive. After a blizzard of negative publicity, and little support from Western governments that wished to avoid this political "hot potato," in May 2002 the drug companies settled out of court with the South African government. Although the terms of the settlement were kept confidential, it was widely interpreted in the media as a defeat for the drug companies and a reaffirmation of the ability of the South African to enforce compulsory licenses.

Management Focus

Management Focus examples further illustrate the relevance of chapter material for the practice of international business.

multipolar world dominated by a number of civilizations. In such a world, much of the economic promise inherent in the global shift toward market-based economic systems may evaporate in the face of conflicts between civilizations. While the long-term potential for economic gain from investment in the world's new market economies is large, the risks associated with any such investment are also substantial. It would be foolish to ignore these.

Focus On Managerial Implications

 The implications for international business of the material discussed in this chapter fall into two broad categories. First, the political, economic, and legal environment of a country clearly influences the attractiveness of that country as a market and/or investment site. The benefits, costs, and risks associated with doing business in a country are a function of that country's political, economic, and legal systems. Second, the political, economic, and legal systems of a country can raise important ethical issues that have implications for the practice of international business. Here we consider each of these issues.

Attractiveness

The overall attractiveness of a country as a market and/or investment site depends on balancing the likely long-term benefits of doing business in that country against the likely costs and risks. Below we consider the determinants of benefits, costs, and risks.

Benefits In the most general sense, the long-run monetary benefits of doing business in a country are a function of the size of the market, the present wealth (purchasing power) of consumers in that market, and the likely future wealth of consumers. While some markets are very large when measured by number of consumers (e.g., China and India), low living standards may imply limited purchasing power and, therefore, a relatively small market when measured in economic terms. While international businesses need to be aware of this distinction, they also need to keep in mind the likely future prospects of a country. In 1960, for example, South Korea was viewed as just another impoverished Third World nation. By 2000 it was the world's 12th largest economy, measured in terms of GDP. International firms that recognized South

---

64. Jo-Ann Mort, "Sweated Shopping," *The Guardian*, September 8, 1997, p. 11.
65. Details can be found at http://www.oecd.org/EN/home/0,,EN-home-31-nodirectorate-no-no-no-31,00.html.
66. Bardhan Pranab, "Corruption and Development," *Journal of Economic Literature* 36 (September 1997), pp. 1320–46.
cratic Corruption and Endogenous Economic Growth," *Journal of Political Economy* 107 (December 1999), pp. 270–92.
68. P. Mauro, "Corruption and Growth," *Quarterly Journal of Economics*, no. 110 (1995), pp. 681–712.

Research Task  globaledge.msu.edu

Use the globalEDGE site to complete the following exercises:

1. The *Freedom in the World* survey evaluates the state of political rights and civil liberties around the world. Provide a description of this survey and a ranking, in terms of "freedom", of the leaders and laggards of the world. What factors are taken into consideration in this survey when forming the rankings?

2. Market Potential Indicators (MPI) is an indexing study conducted by the Michigan State University Center for International Business Education and Research (MSU-CIBER) to compare emerging markets on a variety of dimensions. Provide a description of the indicators used in the indexing procedure. Which of the indicators would have greater importance for a company that markets laptop computers? Considering the MPI rankings, which developing countries would you advise this company to enter first?

Piracy in the Video Game Market

Over the past decade, the video game industry has grown into a global colossus worth more

Because they allow users to play illegally copied games, consoles with mod-chips installed offer a gaping

---

Supplements
For the Instructor

With this teaching package, you'll have everything you need for engaging, multimedia presentations.

Instructor's Resource CD

An updated **Instructor's Manual and Video Guide** (prepared by Ratee Apana of the University of Cincinnati) includes course outlines, chapter overviews and teaching suggestions, lecture outlines with cues for showing PowerPoint slides, ideas for student exercises and projects, teaching notes for all cases in the book, and video notes.

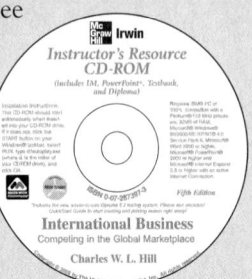

Videos

A new video collection features original business documentaries as well as PBS and NBC News footage that tie in to cases in the text. Featured titles include "Starbucks: Building Relationships with Coffee Growers," "Creating a Global Brand Featuring BP," "The Politics of Trade in Steel," and "Bailing Out Brazil," to name just a few.

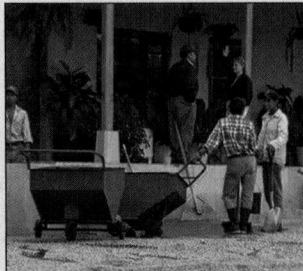

Test Bank

The **Test Bank** (prepared by Amit Shah of Frostburg State University) contains about 100 questions per chapter, each tagged with the level of difficulty, correct answer, and page reference to the text. In addition to traditional true-false and multiple-choice questions, now you can make full use of course technology with a new set of dynamic questions that incorporate graphics, animations, and links (prepared by Howard Cochran of Belmont University).

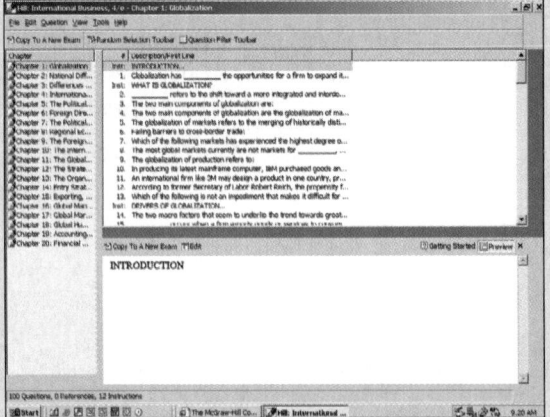

PowerPoint

Over 500 revamped **PowerPoint** slides (also prepared by Ratee Apana) feature original materials not found in the text in addition to reproductions of key text figures, tables, and maps.

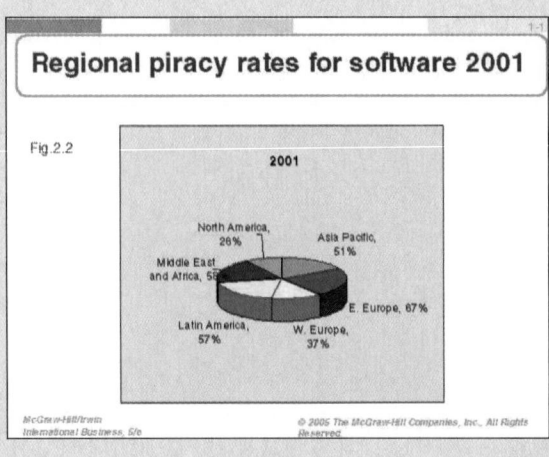

Regional piracy rates for software 2001

For the Student

Student CD

Each new copy of the book is packaged with a free CD that augments the text with video cases, an interactive exercise, and the Global Business Plan Project. Eight up-to-date video cases on such topics as "Starbucks: Building Relationships with Coffee Growers" and "Cretors: Exporting Popcorn Products to Global Markets" allow students to watch videos, read short related cases, and answer discussion questions. In the interactive exercise, students work through a dynamic graphic demonstration of Hofstede's cultural dimensions, then apply the concept to solving a business problem. Finally, the Global Business Plan Project, designed by Les Dlabay of Lake Forest College for use in his own international business class, helps students put the pieces together by guiding them through the creation of a plan to launch a new global business venture.

Online Learning Center with PowerWeb: www.mhhe.com/hill

From the book website, students can access chapter review materials, self-tests, key term flash cards, Internet exercises, Web links, and more. With each new book, students also receive access to the *International Business* PowerWeb site, which offers current articles, weekly updates, informative and timely world news, refereed Web links, research tools, study tools, and interactive exercises.

A password-protected portion of the book website is available to adopters of the book, offering additional online and downloadable teaching resources.

International Business with the *Financial Times*

Keep students on top of today's global economy with the insightful, unbiased reporting of *Financial Times*. Order this packet and your students will receive a 15-week (6 issues per week) subscription at a specially discounted rate. Students enjoy the full benefits of a *Financial Times* subscription, including access to FT.com In-Depth, an online portal featuring breaking news, special reports, portfolio tools and more. Free subscription for adopting instructors. If you'd like your students to receive this package, order **ISBN 0073667439.**

International Business with the *Wall Street Journal*

This package lets you provide a 15-week subscription to the *Wall Street Journal* for students at a specially discounted rate. In addition to their subscription, students will receive a "How to Use the *Wall Street Journal*" handbook. Order **ISBN 0073643254.**

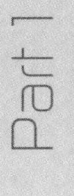

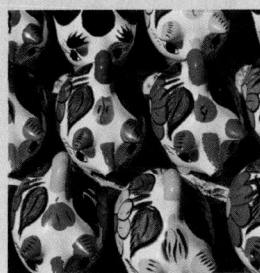

Part 1

Introduction and Overview

Chapter 1
Globalization

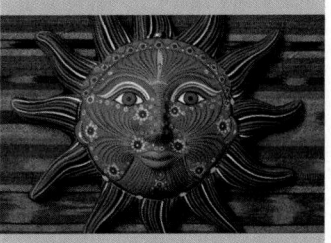

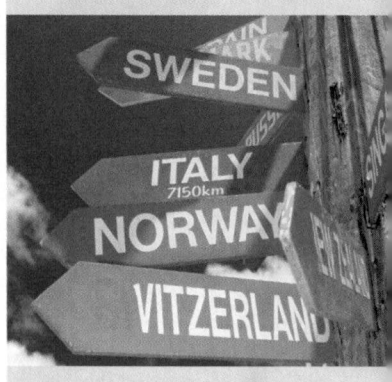

Globalization

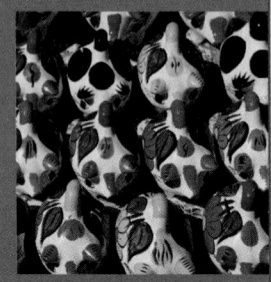

Introduction
What Is Globalization?
  The Globalization of Markets
  The Globalization of Production
The Emergence of Global Institutions
Drivers of Globalization
  Declining Trade and Investment
  Barriers
  The Role of Technological Change
The Changing Demographics of the
Global Economy
  The Changing World Output and World
  Trade Picture
  The Changing Foreign Direct
  Investment Picture
  The Changing Nature of the
  Multinational Enterprise
  The Changing World Order
  The Global Economy of the 21st
  Century
The Globalization Debate
  Antiglobalization Protests
  Globalization, Jobs, and Incomes
  Globalization, Labor Policies, and the
  Environment
  Globalization and National Sovereignty
  Globalization and the World's Poor
Managing in the Global Marketplace
Chapter Summary
Critical Discussion Questions
Closing Case: Ecuadorean Valentine
Roses

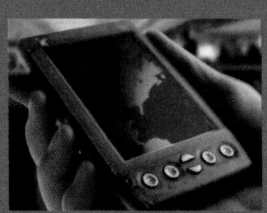

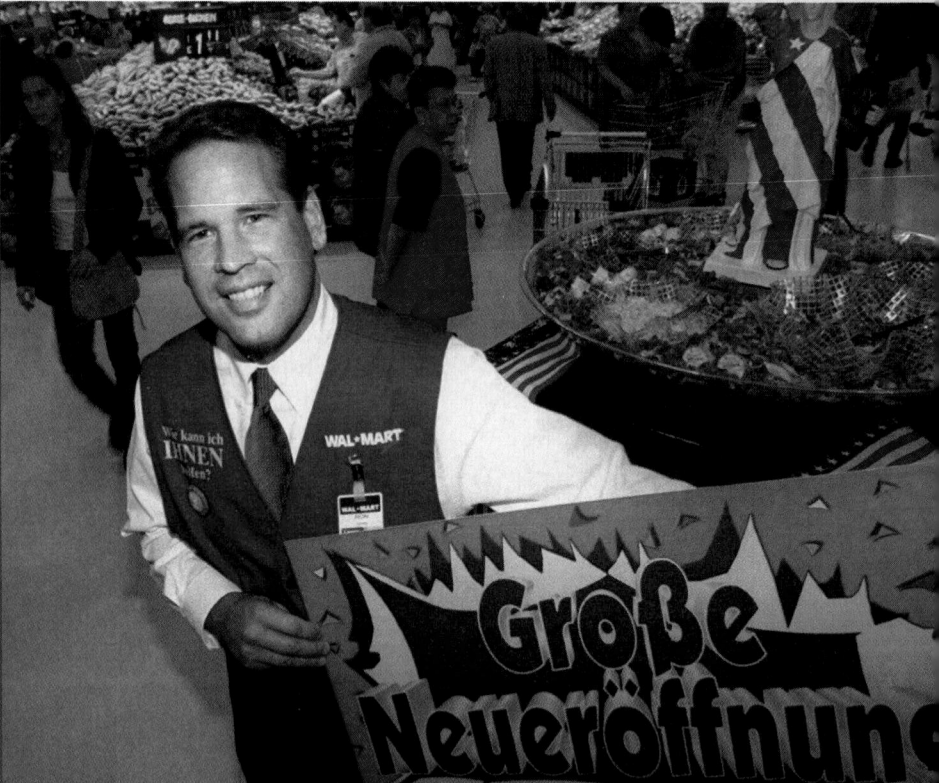

Wal-Mart's Global Expansion

Established in Arkansas in 1962 by Sam Walton, Wal-Mart has grown rapidly to become the largest retailer in the world with 2002 sales of $218 billion, 1.3 million associates (Wal-Mart's term for employees), and some 4,500 stores. Until 1991, Wal-Mart's operations were confined to the United States, where it established a competitive advantage based upon a combination of efficient merchandising and progressive human relations policies. Among other things, Wal-Mart was a leader in the implementation of information systems to track product sales and inventory, it developed one of the most efficient distribution systems in the world, and was one of the first companies to promote widespread stock ownership among employees. These practices led to high productivity that enabled Wal-Mart to drive down its operating costs, which it passed on to consumers in the form of everyday low prices, a strategy that enabled the company to gain market share first in general merchandising, where it now dominates, and later in food retailing, where it is taking market share from established supermarkets.

By 1990, however, Wal-Mart realized that its opportunities for growth in the United States were becoming more limited. By 1995 the company would be active in all 50 states. Management calculated that by the early 2000s, its domestic growth opportunities would be constrained by market saturation. So the company decided to expand globally. Initially, the critics scoffed. Wal-Mart, they said, was too American a company. While its retailing practices were well-suited to America, they would not work in other countries where infrastructure was different, where consumer tastes and preferences varied, and where established retailers already dominated.

Unperturbed, Wal-Mart started to expand internationally in 1991 by opening its first stores in Mexico. The Mexican operation was established as a joint venture with Cifera, the largest local retailer. Initially, Wal-Mart made a number of missteps that seemed to prove the critics right. Wal-Mart had problems replicating its efficient distribution system in Mexico. Poor infrastructure, crowded roads, and a lack of leverage with local suppliers, many of which could not or would not deliver directly to Wal-Mart's stores or distribution centers, resulted in stocking problems and raised costs and prices. Initially, prices at Wal-Mart in Mexico were some 20 percent above prices for comparable products in the company's U.S. stores, which limited Wal-Mart's ability to gain market share. There were also problems with merchandise selection. Initially, many of the stores in Mexico carried items that were popular in the United States. These included ice skates, riding lawn mowers, leaf blowers, and fishing tackle. These items did not sell well in Mexico, so managers would slash prices to move inventory, only to find that the company's automated information systems would immediately order more inventory to replenish the depleted stock.

By the mid-1990s, however, Wal-Mart had learned from its early mistakes and adapted its Mexican operations to match the local environment. A partnership with a Mexican trucking company dramatically improved the distribution system, while more careful stocking practices meant that the Mexican stores sold merchandise that appealed more to local tastes and preferences. As Wal-Mart's presence grew, many of Wal-Mart's suppliers built factories near its Mexican distribution centers so that they could better serve the company, which helped to further drive down inventory and logistics costs. Today, Mexico is a jewel in Wal-Mart's international operations. In 1998, Wal-Mart acquired a controlling interest in Cifera. By 2002, Wal-Mart was more than twice the size of its nearest rival in Mexico with 600 stores and revenues of more than $10 billion.

The Mexican experience proved to Wal-Mart that it could compete outside the United States. It has subsequently expanded into eight other countries. In Canada, Britain, Germany, Japan, and South Korea, Wal-Mart entered by acquiring existing retailers and then transferring its information systems, logistics, and management expertise. In Brazil, Argentina, and China, Wal-Mart established its own stores. As a result of these moves, by 2002 the company had over 1,200 stores outside the United States, 303,000 associates, and generated international revenues of more than $35 billion.

Initially undertaken as a response to market saturation in the United States, Wal-Mart's international expansion has been aided by three developments. First, as barriers to cross-border investment fell during the 1990s, it became possible for Wal-Mart to enter foreign nations on a significant scale. Wal-Mart's 1996 entry into China, for example, where it now has 26 stores, would not have been possible a decade earlier. Second, by expanding internationally Wal-Mart has been able to reap significant economies of scale from its global buying power. Many of Wal-Mart's key suppliers have long been international companies; for example, General Electric (appliances), Unilever (food products), and Procter & Gamble (personal care products) are all major Wal-Mart suppliers that have long had their own global operations. By building international reach, Wal-Mart has used its enhanced size to demand deeper discounts from the local operations of its global suppliers, increasing the company's ability to lower prices to consumers, gain market share, and ultimately earn greater profits. Third, advances in information systems, particularly the spread of Internet-based software, have enabled Wal-Mart to exert considerable control over its global operations, tracking individual store sales, inventory, pricing, and profit data on a daily basis.

Wal-Mart realized that if it didn't expand internationally, other global retailers would beat it to the punch. In fact, Wal-Mart faces significant global competition from Carrefour of France, Ahold of Holland, and Tesco from the United Kingdom. Carrefour, the world's second largest retailer, is perhaps the most global of the lot. The pioneer of the hypermarket concept now operates in 26 countries and generates more than 50 percent of its sales outside France. Compared to this, Wal-Mart is a laggard with just 17 percent of its sales generated from international operations. However, there is still room for significant global expansion. The global retailing market is still very fragmented. The top 25 retailers controlled just 18 percent of worldwide retail sales in 2002, although forecasts suggest the figure could reach 40 percent by 2009, with Latin America, Southeast Asia, and Eastern Europe being the main battlegrounds.

Sources: A. de Rocha and L. A. Dib, "The Entry of Wal-Mart into Brazil," *International Journal of Retail and Distribution Management* 30 (2002), pp. 61–73; "Wal-Mart: Mexico's Biggest Retailer," *Chain Store Age,* June 2001, pp. 52–54; M. N. Hamilton, "Global Food Fight," *Washington Post,* November 19, 2000, p. H1; "Global Strategy—Why Tesco Will Beat Carrefour," *Retail Week,* April 6, 2001, p. 14; "Shopping All over the World," *The Economist,* June 19, 1999, pp. 59–61; M. Flagg, "In Asia, Going to the Grocery Increasingly Means Heading for a European Retail Chain," *Wall Street Journal,* April 24, 2001, p. A21; and Wal-Mart website.

Introduction

A fundamental shift is occurring in the world economy. We are moving away from a world in which national economies were relatively self-contained entities, isolated from each other by barriers to cross-border trade and investment; by distance, time zones, and language; and by national differences in government regulation, culture, and business systems. And we are moving toward a world in which barriers to cross-border trade and investment are tumbling; perceived distance is shrinking due to advances in transportation and telecommunications technology; material culture is starting to look similar the world over; and national economies are merging into an interdependent global economic system. The process by which this is occurring is commonly referred to as globalization.

In this interdependent global economy, an American might drive to work in a car designed in Germany that was assembled in Mexico by DaimlerChrysler from components made in the United States and Japan that were fabricated from Korean steel and Malaysian rubber. She may have filled the car with gasoline at a BP service station owned by a British multinational company. The gasoline could have been made from oil pumped out of a well off the coast of Africa by a French oil company that transported it to the United States in a ship owned by a Greek shipping line. While driving to work, the American might talk to her stockbroker on a Nokia cell phone that was designed in Finland and assembled in Texas using chip sets produced in Taiwan that were designed by Indian engineers working at a firm in San Diego, California, called Qualcomm. She could tell the stockbroker to purchase shares in Deutsche Telekom, a German telecommunications firm transformed from a former state-owned monopoly into a global company by an energetic Israeli CEO. She may turn on the car radio, which was made in Malaysia by a Japanese firm, to hear a popular hip-hop song composed by a Swede and sung by a group of Danes in English who signed a record contract with a French music company to promote their record in America. The driver might pull into a drive-through coffee stall run by a Korean immigrant and order "single-tall-non-fat latte" and chocolate-covered biscotti. The coffee beans come from Brazil and the chocolate from Peru, while the biscotti was made locally using an old Italian recipe. After the song ends, a news announcer might inform the American listener that antiglobalization protests at a meeting of heads of state in Davos, Switzerland, have turned violent. One protester has been killed. The announcer then turns to the next item, a story about how an economic slowdown in America has sent Japan's Nikkei stock market index to 17-year lows.

This is the world we live in. It is a world where the volume of goods, services, and investment crossing national borders expanded faster than world output every year during the last two decades of the 20th century. It is a world where more than $1.2 billion in foreign exchange transactions are made every day. It is a world in which international institutions such as the World Trade Organization and gatherings of leaders from the world's most powerful economies have called for even lower barriers to cross-border trade and investment. It is a world where the symbols of material and popular culture are increasingly global: from Coca-Cola and McDonald's to Sony PlayStations, Nokia cell phones, MTV shows, and Disney films. It is a world in which products are made from inputs that come from all over the world. It is a world in which an economic crisis in Asia can cause a recession in the United States, and a slowdown in the United States really did help drive Japan's Nikkei index in 2002 to lows not seen since 1985. It is also a world in which a vigorous and vocal minority is protesting against globalization, which they blame for a list of ills, from unemployment in developed nations to environmental degradation and the Americanization of popular culture. And yes, these protests really have turned violent.

For businesses, this is in many ways the best of times. Globalization has increased the opportunities for a firm to expand its revenues by selling around the world and reduce its costs by producing in nations where key inputs are cheap. Since the collapse of communism at the end of the 1980s, the pendulum of public policy in nation after nation has swung toward the free market end of the economic spectrum. Regulatory and administrative barriers to doing business in foreign nations have come down, while those nations have often transformed their economies, privatizing state-owned enterprises, deregulating markets, increasing competition, and welcoming investment by foreign businesses. This has allowed businesses both large and small, from both advanced nations and developed nations, to expand internationally.

Wal-Mart, profiled in the opening case, is something of a late mover in this development. In some industries, such as commercial jet aircraft, automobiles, petroleum, household products, semiconductor chips, and computers, companies have been expanding globally for decades. Retailing has been primarily local in orientation, but in a testament to the scope and pace of globalization, led by companies such as Wal-Mart and Carrefour of France, this too is now changing. Falling barriers to cross-border investment have made this possible. Rapid economic growth in developing nations and market saturation at home have made globalization a strategic imperative for established retailers seeking to grow their business. Companies like Wal-Mart believe that they must move aggressively now lest they lose the initiative to early movers such as Carrefour. They see their strategic advantage in terms of building a global brand, realizing economies of scale, and leveraging skills across national borders. In this, they are no different from companies in other industries that have already gone global.

At the same time, going global is not without problems. This too was evident in the opening case. The grand strategic vision of retailers such as Wal-Mart has often run up against the hard reality that for all the superficial similarities in material and popular culture and in business systems, doing business in foreign nations still has unique challenges. Because of different tastes and preferences, what sells in the United States may not sell in China, business processes that give a retailer a competitive advantage in America may be difficult to implement in Mexico, and a brand that means something in Kansas may mean little in Indonesia.

The tension evident in the opening case between the economic opportunities associated with going global and the challenges associated with doing business across borders is important in international business. We shall consider this tension repeatedly in this book. To begin with, however, we need to look more closely at the process of globalization. We need to understand what is driving this process, appreciate how it is changing the face of international businesses, and better comprehend why globalization has become a flash point for debate, demonstration, and conflict over the future direction of our civilization.

▋ What Is Globalization?

As used in this book, **globalization** refers to the shift toward a more integrated and interdependent world economy. Globalization has several different facets including the globalization of markets and the globalization of production.

▎The Globalization of Markets

The globalization of markets refers to the merging of historically distinct and separate national markets into one huge global marketplace. Falling barriers to cross-border trade have made it easier to sell internationally. It has been argued for some time that the tastes and preferences of consumers in different nations are beginning to converge on some global norm, thereby helping to create a global market.[1] Consumer products such as Citicorp credit cards, Coca-Cola soft drinks, Sony PlayStation video games, and McDonald's hamburgers are frequently held up as prototypical examples of this trend. Firms such as Citicorp, Coca-Cola, McDonald's, and Sony are more than just benefactors of this trend; they are also facilitators of it. By offering a standardized product worldwide, they help to create a global market.

A company does not have to be the size of these multinational giants to facilitate, and benefit from, the globalization of markets. In the United States, for example, nearly 89 percent of firms that exported in 2001 were small businesses that employed less than 100 people. Their share of total U.S. exports grew steadily over the last decade to reach 21 percent by 2001.[2] Firms with less than 500 employees accounted for 97 percent of all U.S. exporters and almost 30 percent of all exports by value.[3] Typical of these is Hytech, a New York-based manufacturer of solar panels that generates 40 percent of its $3 million in annual sales from exports to five countries, or B&S Aircraft Alloys, another New York company whose exports account for 40 percent of its $8 million annual revenues.[4] The situation is similar in several other nations. In Germany, for example, companies with less than 500 employees account for about 30 percent of that nation's exports.[5]

Despite the global prevalence of Citicorp credit cards and McDonald's hamburgers, it is important not to push too far the view that national markets are giving way to the global market. As we shall see in later chapters, very significant differences still exist between national markets along many relevant dimensions, including consumer tastes and preferences, distribution channels, culturally embedded value systems, business systems, and legal regulations. These differences frequently require that marketing strategies, product features, and operating practices be customized to best match conditions in a country. For example, automobile companies will promote different car models depending on a range of factors such as local fuel costs, income levels, traffic congestion, and cultural values. Similarly, as we saw in the opening case, global retailers such as Wal-Mart may still need to vary their product mix from country to country depending on local tastes and preferences.

The most global markets currently are not markets for consumer products—where national differences in tastes and preferences are still often important enough to act as a brake on globalization—but markets for industrial goods and materials that serve a universal need the world over. These include the markets for commodities such as aluminum, oil, and wheat; the markets for industrial products such as microprocessors, DRAMs (computer memory chips), and commercial jet aircraft; the markets for computer software; and the markets for financial assets from U.S. Treasury bills to eurobonds and futures on the Nikkei index or the Mexican peso.

In many global markets, the same firms frequently confront each other as competitors in nation after nation. Coca-Cola's rivalry with Pepsi is a global one, as are the rivalries between Ford and Toyota, Boeing and Airbus, Caterpillar and Komatsu, and Nintendo and Sega. If one firm moves into a nation that is not currently served by its rivals, those rivals are sure to follow to prevent their competitor from gaining an advantage.[6] The opening case revealed that retailers such as Wal-Mart, Carrefour, and Tesco are starting to engage in a global rivalry. As firms follow each other around the world, they bring with them many of the assets that served them well in other national markets—including their products, operating strategies, marketing strategies, and brand names—creating some homogeneity across markets. Thus, greater uniformity replaces diversity. Due to such developments, in an increasing number of industries it is no longer meaningful to talk about "the German market," "the American market," "the Brazilian market," or "the Japanese market"; for many firms there is only the global market.

The Globalization of Production

The globalization of production refers to the sourcing of goods and services from locations around the globe to take advantage of national differences in the cost and quality of factors of production (such as labor, energy, land, and capital). By doing this, companies hope to lower their overall cost structure and/or improve the quality or functionality of their product offering, thereby allowing them to compete more effectively. Consider the Boeing Company's commercial jet airliner, the 777. Eight Japanese suppliers make parts for the fuselage, doors, and wings; a supplier in Singapore makes the doors for the nose landing gear; three suppliers in Italy manufacture wing flaps; and so on.[7] Part of Boeing's rationale for outsourcing so much production to foreign suppliers is that these suppliers are the best in the world at their particular activity. A global web of suppliers yields a better final product, which enhances the chances of Boeing winning a greater share of total orders for aircraft than its global rival, Airbus Industrie. Boeing also outsources some production to foreign countries to increase the chance that it will win significant orders from airliners based in that country.

The global dispersal of productive activities is not limited to giants such as Boeing. Many much smaller firms are also getting into the act. Consider Swan Optical, a U.S.-based manufacturer and distributor of eyewear. With annual sales of $20 million to $30 million, Swan is hardly a giant, yet Swan manufactures its eyewear in low-cost factories in Hong Kong and China that it jointly owns with a Hong Kong–based partner. Swan also has a minority stake in eyewear design houses in Japan, France, and Italy. The company has dispersed its manufacturing and design processes to different locations around the world to take advantage of favorable skill bases and cost structures. Foreign investments in Hong Kong and then China have helped Swan lower its cost structure, while investments in Japan, France, and Italy have helped it produce designer eyewear for which it can charge a premium price. By dispersing its manufacturing and design activities, Swan established a competitive advantage for itself in the global marketplace for eyewear, just as Boeing has tried to do by dispersing some of its activities to other countries.[8]

Robert Reich, who served as secretary of labor in the Clinton administration, has argued that as a consequence of the trend exemplified by Boeing and Swan Optical, in many industries it is becoming irrelevant to talk about American products, Japanese products, German products, or Korean products. Increasingly, according to Reich, the outsourcing of productive activities to different suppliers results in the creation of products that are global in nature; that is, "global products."[9] But as with the globalization of markets, one must be careful not to push the globalization of production too far. As we will see in later chapters, substantial impediments still make it difficult for firms to achieve the optimal dispersion of their productive activities to locations around the globe. These impediments include formal and informal barriers to trade between countries, barriers to foreign direct investment, transportation costs, and issues associated with economic and political risk.

Nevertheless, we are traveling down the road toward a future characterized by the increased globalization of markets and production. Modern firms are important actors in this drama, by their very actions fostering increased globalization. These firms, however, are merely responding in an efficient manner to changing conditions in their operating environment—as well they should.

■ The Emergence of Global Institutions

As markets globalize and an increasing proportion of business activity transcends national borders, there is a need for institutions to help manage, regulate, and police the global marketplace, and to promote the establishment of multinational treaties to govern the global business system. Over the past half century, a number of important global institutions have been created to help perform these functions. These institutions include the General Agreement on Tariffs and Trade (the GATT), and its successor, the World Trade Organization (WTO); the International Monetary Fund (IMF) and its sister institution, the World Bank; and the United Nations (UN). All these institutions were created by voluntary agreement between individual nation-states, and their functions are enshrined in international treaties.

The **World Trade Organization** (like the GATT before it) is primarily responsible for policing the world trading system and making sure nation-states adhere to the rules laid down in trade treaties signed by WTO member states. As of April 2003, some 146 nations that collectively accounted for 97 percent of world trade were members of the WTO, thereby giving the organization enormous scope and influence. The WTO is also responsible for facilitating the establishment of additional multinational agreements between WTO member states. Over its entire history, and that of the GATT before it, the WTO has promoted the lowering of barriers to cross-border trade and investment. In doing so, the WTO has been the instrument of its member states, which have sought to create a more open global business system unencumbered by barriers to trade and investment between countries. Without an institution such as the WTO, the globalization of markets and production is unlikely to have proceeded as far as it has. However, as we shall see in this chapter and in Chapter 5 when we take a close look at the WTO, critics charge that the WTO is usurping the national sovereignty of individual nation-states.

The **International Monetary Fund** and the **World Bank** were both created in 1944 by 44 nations that met at Bretton Woods, New Hampshire. The task of the IMF was to maintain order in the international monetary system, and that of the World Bank was to promote economic development. In the 60 years since their creation, both institutions have emerged as significant players in the global economy. The World Bank is the less controversial of the two sister institutions. It has focused on making low interest rate loans to cash-strapped governments in poor nations that wish to undertake significant infrastructure investments (such as building dams or road systems).

The IMF is often seen as the lender of last resort to nation-states whose economies are in turmoil and currencies are losing value against those of other nations. Repeatedly during the last decade, for example, the IMF has stepped in to lend money to the governments of troubled states including Argentina, Indonesia, Mexico, Russia, South Korea, Thailand, and Turkey to name but a few of the more high profile cases. The IMF loans come with strings attached; in return for loans, the IMF requires nation-states to adopt specific economic policies aimed at returning their troubled economies to stability and growth. These "strings" have generated the most debate, for some critics charge that the IMF's policy recommendations are often inappropriate, while others maintain that, like the WTO, by telling national governments what economic policies they must adopt, the IMF is usurping the sovereignty of nation-states. We shall look at the debate over the role of the IMF in Chapter 10.

The **United Nations** was established on October 24, 1945, by 51 countries committed to preserving peace through international cooperation and collective security. Today nearly every nation in the world belongs to the United Nations; membership now totals 191 countries. When states become members of the United Nations, they agree to accept the obligations of the UN Charter, an international treaty that sets out basic principles of international relations. According to the charter, the UN has four purposes: to maintain international peace and security, to develop friendly relations among nations, to cooperate in solving international problems and in promoting respect for human rights, and to be a center for harmonizing the actions of nations. Although the UN is perhaps best known for its peacekeeping role, one of the UN's central mandates is the promotion of higher standards of living, full employment, and conditions of economic and social progress and development—all issues that are central to the creation of a vibrant global economy. As much as 70 percent of the work of the UN system is devoted to accomplishing this mandate. To do so, the UN works closely with other international institutions such as the World Bank. Guiding the work is the belief that eradicating poverty and improving the well-being of people everywhere are necessary steps in creating conditions for lasting world peace.[10]

Drivers of Globalization ■

Two macro factors seem to underlie the trend toward greater globalization.[11] The first is the decline in barriers to the free flow of goods, services, and capital that has occurred since the end of World War II. The second factor is technological change, particularly the dramatic developments in recent years in communication, information processing, and transportation technologies.

∣Declining Trade and Investment Barriers

During the 1920s and 30s, many of the nation-states of the world erected formidable barriers to international trade and foreign direct investment. **International trade** occurs when a firm exports goods or services to consumers in another country. **Foreign direct investment** occurs when a firm invests resources in business activities outside its home country. Many of the barriers to international trade took the form of high tariffs on imports of manufactured goods. The typical aim of such tariffs was to protect domestic industries from foreign competition. One consequence, however, was "beggar thy neighbor" retaliatory trade policies with countries progressively raising trade barriers against each other. Ultimately, this depressed world demand and contributed to the Great Depression of the 1930s.

Having learned from this experience, the advanced industrial nations of the West committed themselves after World War II to removing barriers to the free flow of goods, services, and capital between nations.[12] This goal was enshrined in the General Agreement on Tariffs and Trade (GATT). Under the umbrella of GATT, eight rounds of negotiations among member states (now numbering 146) have worked to lower barriers to the free flow of goods and services. The most recent round of negotiations, known as the Uruguay Round, was completed in December 1993. The Uruguay Round further reduced trade barriers; extended GATT to cover services as well as manufactured goods; provided enhanced protection for patents, trademarks, and copyrights; and established the World Trade Organization (WTO) to police the international trading system.[13] Table 1.1 summarizes the impact of GATT agreements on average tariff rates for manufactured goods. As can be seen, average tariff rates have fallen significantly since 1950 and now stand at 3.9 percent.

In late 2001, the WTO launched a new round of talks aimed at further liberalizing the global trade and investment framework. For this meeting, it picked the remote location of Doha in the Gulf state of Qatar. At Doha, the member states of the WTO

Table 1.1

Average Tariff Rates on
Manufactured Products as
Percent of Value

Source: 1913–1990 data from "Who
Wants to Be a Giant?" *The Economist:
A Survey of the Multinationals,*
June 24, 1995, pp. 3–4. Copyright ©
The Economist Books, Ltd.

	1913	1950	1990	2000
France	21%	18%	5.9%	3.9%
Germany	20	26	5.9	3.9
Italy	18	25	5.9	3.9
Japan	30	—	5.3	3.9
Holland	5	11	5.9	3.9
Sweden	20	9	4.4	3.9
Britain	—	23	5.9	3.9
United States	44	14	4.8	3.9

staked out an agenda. The talks are scheduled to last three years, although if history is any guide, they could last much longer. The agenda includes cutting tariffs on industrial goods, services, and agricultural products; phasing out subsidies to agricultural producers; reducing barriers to cross-border investment (FDI); and limiting the use of antidumping laws. The biggest gain may come from discussion on agricultural products; average agricultural tariff rates are still around 40 percent, and rich nations spend some $300 billion a year in subsidies to support their farm sectors. The world's poorer nations have the most to gain from any reduction in agricultural tariffs and subsidies, since such reforms would give them access to the markets of the developed world.[14]

In addition to reducing trade barriers, many countries have also been progressively removing restrictions to foreign direct investment (FDI). According to the United Nations, some 95 percent of the 1,393 changes made between 1991 and 2001 worldwide in the laws governing foreign direct investment created a more favorable environment for FDI. The desire of governments to facilitate FDI has also been reflected in a dramatic increase in the number of bilateral investment treaties designed to protect and promote investment between two countries. As of 2002, there were 2,099 such treaties in the world involving more than 160 countries, a 10-fold increase from the 181 treaties that existed in 1980.[15]

Such trends facilitate both the globalization of markets and the globalization of production. The lowering of barriers to international trade enables firms to view the world, rather than a single country, as their market. The lowering of trade and investment barriers also allows firms to base production at the optimal location for that activity. Thus, a firm might design a product in one country, produce component parts in two other countries, assemble the product in yet another country, and then export the finished product around the world.

The lowering of trade barriers has facilitated the globalization of production. According to data from the World Trade Organization, the volume of world trade has grown faster than the volume of world output since 1950.[16] From 1950 to 2002, world trade expanded over 20-fold, outstripping world output, which grew by sevenfold. As suggested by Figure 1.1, the growth in world trade seems to have accelerated since 1990.

However, 2001 brought a sudden slowdown in this long-term trend. The volume of world trade fell by 1 percent in 2001, the first decline in two decades, while world output grew by a sluggish 1 percent.[17] Although the volume of world trade grew again by 2.5 percent in 2002, this was well below the average rate of 6.7 percent achieved during the 1990s.[18] The global economic slowdown that occurred in 2001 and 2002 along with the economic aftermath of the September 11, 2001, terrorist attacks on the United States were the major reasons for the slowdown in the growth of world trade. If history is any guide, the slowdown will be modest and short lived,

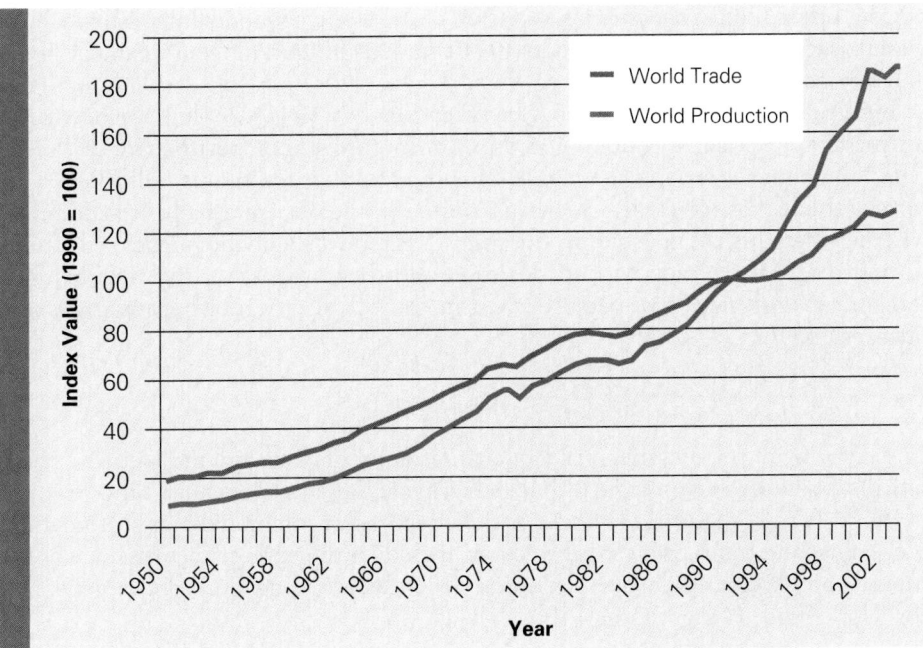

Figure 1.1

Volume of World Trade
and Production,
1950–2002

Source: World Trade Organization,
"International Trade Statistics,
2002," WTO press release, April 22,
2002. Reprinted by permission from
the International Bank for Reconstruction and Development. © by
the World Bank.

although the effects of the Iraq conflict and global severe acute respiratory syndrome (SARS) epidemic were expected to result in sluggish trade and output growth during 2003 as well.

Notwithstanding the recent slowdown in growth, the data summarized in Figure 1.1 imply two things. First, more firms are doing what Boeing does with the 777: dispersing parts of their overall production process to different locations around the globe to drive down production costs and increase product quality. Second, the economies of the world's nation-states are becoming more intertwined. As trade expands, nations are becoming increasingly dependent on each other for important goods and services.

The evidence also suggests that foreign direct investment is playing an increasing role in the global economy as firms ranging in size from Boeing to Swan Optical increase their cross-border investments. The average yearly outflow of FDI increased from about $25 billion in 1975 to a record $1.3 trillion in 2000.[19] However, like world trade, the flow of FDI also fell in 2001, to $735 billion, and to an estimated $534 billion in 2002, for the same underlying reasons.[20] Despite the slowdown in 2001 and 2002, the flow of FDI not only accelerated over the last quarter century, but it also accelerated faster than the growth in world trade. For example, between 1990 and 2000, the total flow of FDI from all countries increased about fivefold, while world trade grew by some 82 percent and world output by 23 percent.[21] As a result of the strong FDI flow, by 2001 the global stock of FDI exceeded $6.6 trillion. In total, 65,000 parent companies had 850,000 affiliates in foreign markets that collectively produced an estimated $19 trillion in global sales, nearly twice as high as the value of global exports.[22]

The globalization of markets and production and the resulting growth of world trade, foreign direct investment, and imports all imply that firms are finding their home markets under attack from foreign competitors. This is true in Japan, where U.S. companies such as Kodak, Procter & Gamble, and Merrill Lynch are expanding their presence. It is true in the United States, where Japanese automobile firms have taken market share away from General Motors and Ford. And it is true in Europe, where the once-dominant Dutch company Philips has seen its market share in the consumer electronics industry taken by Japan's JVC, Matsushita, and Sony. The bottom line is that the growing integration of the world economy into a single, huge marketplace is increasing the intensity of competition in a range of manufacturing and service industries.

But declining trade barriers can't be taken for granted. As we shall see in the following chapters, demands for "protection" from foreign competitors are still often heard in countries around the world, including the United States. Although a return to the restrictive trade policies of the 1920s and 30s is unlikely, it is not clear whether the political majority in the industrialized world favors further reductions in trade barriers. If trade barriers decline no further, at least for the time being, a temporary limit may have been reached in the globalization of both markets and production.

The Role of Technological Change

The lowering of trade barriers made globalization of markets and production a theoretical possibility. Technological change has made it a tangible reality. Since the end of World War II, the world has seen major advances in communication, information processing, and transportation technology, including the explosive emergence of the Internet and World Wide Web. In the words of Renato Ruggiero, director general of the World Trade Organization,

> Telecommunications is creating a global audience. Transport is creating a global village. From Buenos Aires to Boston to Beijing, ordinary people are watching MTV, they're wearing Levi's jeans, and they're listening to Sony Walkmans as they commute to work.[23]

Microprocessors and Telecommunications

Perhaps the single most important innovation has been development of the microprocessor, which enabled the explosive growth of high-power, low-cost computing, vastly increasing the amount of information that can be processed by individuals and firms. The microprocessor also underlies many recent advances in telecommunications technology. Over the past 30 years, global communications have been revolutionized by developments in satellite, optical fiber, and wireless technologies, and now the Internet and the World Wide Web. These technologies rely on the microprocessor to encode, transmit, and decode the vast amount of information that flows along these electronic highways. The cost of microprocessors continues to fall, while their power increases (a phenomenon known as Moore's Law, which predicts that the power of microprocessor technology doubles and its cost of production falls in half every 18 months).[24] As this happens, the costs of global communications are plummeting, which lowers the costs of coordinating and controlling a global organization. Thus, between 1930 and 1990, the cost of a three-minute phone call between New York and London fell from $244.65 to $3.32.[25] By 1998 it had plunged to just 36 cents for consumers, and much lower rates were available for businesses.[26]

The Internet and World Wide Web

The rapid growth of the Internet and the associated World Wide Web (which utilizes the Internet to communicate between World Wide Web sites) is the latest expression of this development. In 1990, fewer than 1 million users were connected to the Internet. By 1995 the figure had risen to 50 million. In 2002 it grew to between 580 and 655 million. By the year 2005, forecasts suggest that the Internet may have over 1.12 billion users, or about 18 percent of the world's population.[27] In July 1993, some 1.8 million host computers were connected to the Internet (host computers host the Web pages of local users). By January 2003 the number of host computers had increased to 172 million, and the number is still growing rapidly.[28] In the United States, where Internet usage is most advanced, 60 percent of the population had Internet access at home by 2002.[29] The rate of growth in Internet adoption is now slowing in the United

States as the market becomes more saturated. The rate of increase in total Internet usage is also slowing. However, most observers believe that this is due to the dominance of slow connections to the Internet (telephone lines), and they believe that once high-speed connections become more widely available (such as cable modems that can transmit data 1,000 times faster than a slow telephone line with a conventional modem), we will see a sharp upswing in the volume of traffic on the Web. In 2002, the number of U.S. households with high speed "broadband" connections surged 59 percent to 33 million.[30]

The Internet and World Wide Web (WWW) promise to develop into the information backbone of the global economy. According to Forrester Research, the value of Web-based transactions hit $657 billion in 2000, from virtually nothing in 1994, and could grow to $6.8 trillion by 2004, with the United States accounting for 47 percent of all Web-based transactions (see Figure 1.2).[31] Many of these transactions are not business-to-consumer transactions (e-commerce), but business-to-business (or

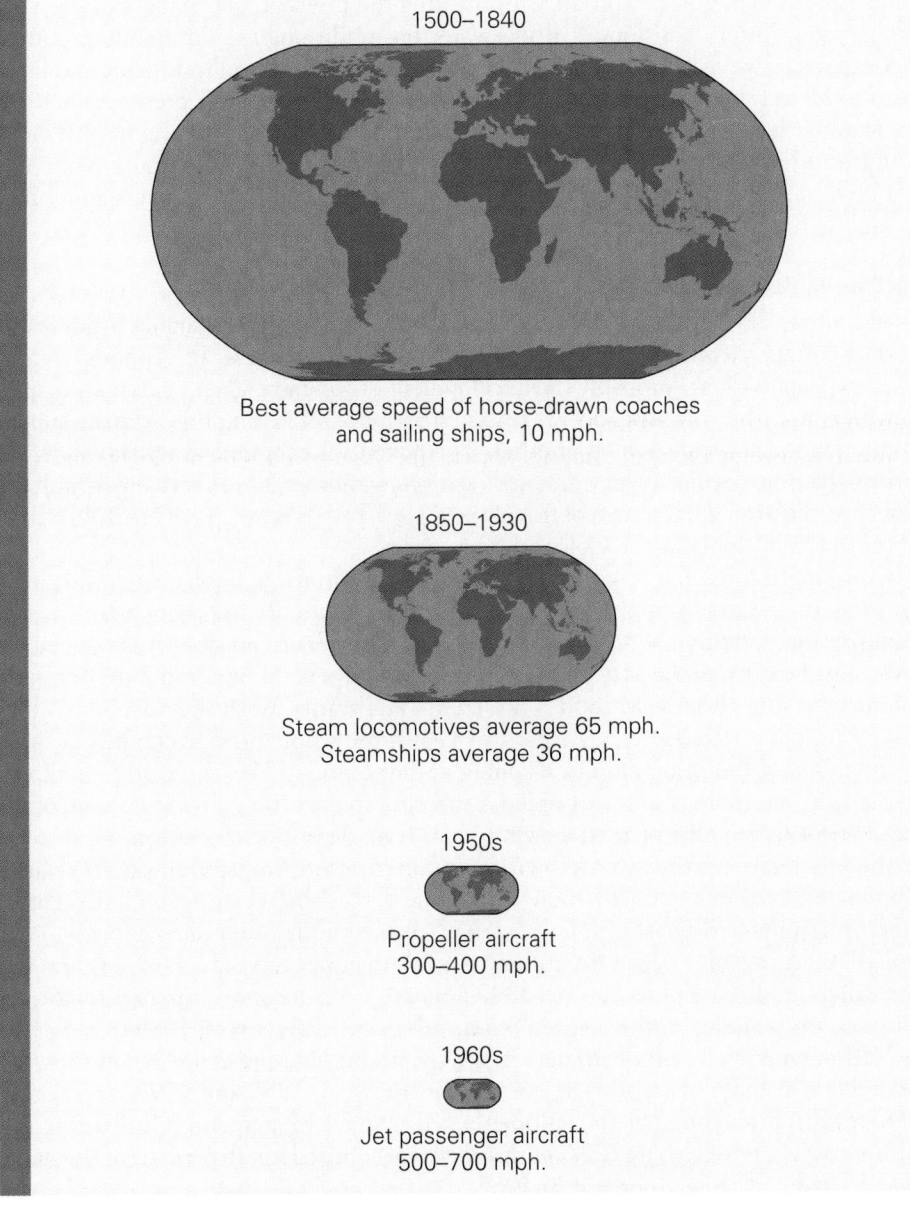

1500–1840

Best average speed of horse-drawn coaches
and sailing ships, 10 mph.

1850–1930

Steam locomotives average 65 mph.
Steamships average 36 mph.

1950s

Propeller aircraft
300–400 mph.

1960s

Jet passenger aircraft
500–700 mph.

Figure 1.2

The Shrinking Globe

Source: P. Dicken, *Global Shift* (New York: Guilford Press, 1992), p. 104.

e-business) transactions. The greatest current potential of the Web seems to be in the business-to-business arena.

Included in the expanding volume of Web-based traffic is a growing percentage of cross-border trade. Viewed globally, the Web is emerging as an equalizer. It rolls back some of the constraints of location, scale, and time zones.[32] The Web allows businesses, both small and large, to expand their global presence at a lower cost than ever before. One example is a small California-based start-up, Cardiac Science, which makes defibrillators and heart monitors. In 1996, Cardiac Science was itching to break into international markets but had little idea of how to establish an international presence. By 1998, the company was selling to customers in 46 countries and foreign sales accounted for $1.02 million of its $1.2 million revenues. By 2002 revenues had surged on the back of new product introductions to $50 million, some $17.5 million of which came from sales to customers in 50 countries. Although some of this business was developed through conventional export channels, a good percentage of it came from "hits" to the company's website, which, according to the company's CEO, "attracts international business people like bees to honey."[33] Similarly, 10 years ago no one would have thought that a small British company based in Stafford would have been able to build a global market for its products by utilizing the Internet, but that is exactly what Bridgewater Pottery has done.[34] Bridgewater has traditionally sold premium pottery through exclusive distribution channels, but the company found it difficult and laborious to identify new retail outlets. Since establishing an Internet presence in 1997, Bridgewater has conducted a significant amount of business with consumers in other countries who could not be reached through existing channels of distribution or could not be reached cost effectively. The Web makes it much easier for buyers and sellers to find each other, wherever they may be located and whatever their size.

Transportation Technology

In addition to developments in communication technology, several major innovations in transportation technology have occurred since World War II. In economic terms, the most important are probably the development of commercial jet aircraft and superfreighters and the introduction of containerization, which simplifies transshipment from one mode of transport to another. The advent of commercial jet travel, by reducing the time needed to get from one location to another, has effectively shrunk the globe (see Figure 1.2). In terms of travel time, New York is now "closer" to Tokyo than it was to Philadelphia in the Colonial days.

Containerization has revolutionized the transportation business, significantly lowering the costs of shipping goods over long distances. Before the advent of containerization, moving goods from one mode of transport to another was very labor-intensive, lengthy, and costly. It could take days and several hundred longshoremen to unload a ship and reload goods onto trucks and trains. With the advent of widespread containerization in the 1970s and 1980s, the whole process can be executed by a handful of longshoremen in a couple of days. Since 1980, the world's containership fleet has more than quadrupled, reflecting in part the growing volume of international trade and in part the switch to this mode of transportation. As a result of the efficiency gains associated with containerization, transportation costs have plummeted, making it much more economical to ship goods around the globe, thereby helping to drive the globalization of markets and production. Between 1920 and 1990, the average ocean freight and port charges per ton of U.S. export and import cargo fell from $95 to $29 (in 1990 dollars).[35] The cost of shipping freight per ton-mile on railroads in the United States fell from 3.04 cents in 1985 to 2.3 cents in 2000, largely as a result of efficiency gains from the widespread use of containers.[36] An increased share of cargo now goes by air. Between 1955 and 1999, average air transportation revenue per ton kilometer fell by over 80 percent.[37] Reflecting the falling cost of air freight, by 2000 air shipments accounted for 28 percent of the value of U.S. trade, up from 7 percent in 1965.

Homer Simpson—A Global Brand!

If a poll were held to identify the world's favorite dysfunctional family, the Simpsons would probably win hands down. The Fox Broadcasting Company production that documents the life and times of Homer and his irreverent clan is the most decorated and longest running animated TV show in history. Some 60 million viewers in more than 70 countries tune in to watch the weekly antics of the Simpsons. The show seems to have universal appeal, with the audience split 50/50 between adults and children, and with audience ratings running high in countries as diverse as Spain and Japan. *Time* magazine named "The Simpsons" the 20th century's best TV show, and the chair of the philosophy department at the University of Manitoba wrote an article claiming "The Simpsons" is the deepest show on television.

Whatever the sources of the show's appeal, there is no question that Homer and his family have become a powerful global brand. Not only do Fox and its parent News Corporation benefit from the huge syndication rights of the show, but they also have made a significant sum from licensing the characters. Since the inception of the show in 1990, "The Simpsons" has generated over $1.2 billion in retail sales from tie-in merchandise, much of it outside the United States. In 2002, about 60 large brand and marketing partners around the world used the Simpsons to sell everything from toilet paper in Germany, Kit Kat bars and potato chips in the United Kingdom, El Cortes Bart Simpson dolls in Spain, and Intel microprocessors in the United States. Clinton Cards, a British greeting card retailer, used Father's Day in 2000 as the perfect opportunity to find the British father whose behavior most resembles that of Homer Simpson. The competition was rolled out across all of the company's 692 stores and supported by TV advertising.

So what's next for the Simpsons? Fox has been careful to manage the licensing deals so that Homer and clan don't suffer from overexposure or aren't used in inappropriate ways. According to Matt Groening, the show's creator, " 'The Simpsons' is a commercial enterprise and we embrace the capitalistic nature of this project. What we try to do with 'The Simpsons' is not do a label slap—that is, we don't just slap their drawings on the side of a product. We try to make each item witty, and sometimes we comment on the absurdity of the item itself." In short, Fox tries to make sure that "The Simpsons" characters are used in a way that is consistent with the irreverent nature of the show itself. "If we didn't do this," notes a Fox spokesman, "we would lose credibility with the fans, and we have to make sure that doesn't happen."

Source: D. Finnigan, "Homer Improvement," *Brandweek*, November 27, 2000, pp. 22–25; "The Simpsons—Picking a Winner," *Marketing*, June 29, 2000, pp. 28–29; and T. Chapman, "Licensing Done Right," *Marketing Magazine*, December 2, 2002, p. 14.

Implications for the Globalization of Production

As transportation costs associated with the globalization of production declined, dispersal of production to geographically separate locations became more economical. As a result of the technological innovations discussed above, the real costs of information processing and communication have fallen dramatically in the past two decades. These developments make it possible for a firm to create and then manage a globally dispersed production system, further facilitating the globalization of production.

A worldwide communications network has become essential for many international businesses. For example, Dell Computer uses the Internet to coordinate and control a globally dispersed production system to such an extent that it holds only three days' worth of inventory at its assembly locations. Dell's Internet-based system records orders for computer equipment as they are submitted by customers via the company's website, then immediately transmits the resulting orders for components to various suppliers around the world, who have a real-time look at Dell's order flow and can adjust their production schedules accordingly. Given the low cost of airfreight, Dell can use air transportation to speed up the delivery of critical components to meet unanticipated demand shifts without delaying the shipment of final product to consumers. Dell has also used modern communications technology to outsource its customer service operations to India. When U.S. customers call Dell with a service inquiry, they are routed to Bangalore in India, where English-speaking service personnel handle the call.

The development of commercial jet aircraft has also helped knit together the worldwide operations of many international businesses. Using jet travel, an American manager need spend a day at most traveling to her firm's European or Asian operations. This enables her to oversee a globally dispersed production system.

Implications for the Globalization of Markets

In addition to the globalization of production, technological innovations have also facilitated the globalization of markets. As noted above, low-cost transportation has made it more economical to ship products around the world, thereby helping to create global markets. Low-cost global communications networks such as the World Wide Web are helping to create electronic global marketplaces. In addition, low-cost jet travel has resulted in the mass movement of people between countries. This has reduced the cultural distance between countries and is bringing about some convergence of consumer tastes and preferences. At the same time, global communication networks and global media are creating a worldwide culture. U.S. television networks such as CNN, MTV, and HBO are now received in many countries, and Hollywood films are shown the world over. In any society, the media are primary conveyors of culture; as global media develop, we must expect the evolution of something akin to a global culture. A logical result of this evolution is the emergence of global markets for consumer products. The first signs of this are already apparent. It is now as easy to find a McDonald's restaurant in Tokyo as it is in New York, to buy a Sony Walkman in Rio as it is in Berlin, and to buy Levi's jeans in Paris as it is in San Francisco. The accompanying Management Focus, "Homer Simpson—A Global Brand," illustrates the power of the media to create global market opportunities.

Despite these trends, we must be careful not to overemphasize their importance. While modern communication and transportation technologies are ushering in the "global village," very significant national differences remain in culture, consumer preferences, and business practices. A firm that ignores differences between countries does so at its peril. We shall stress this point repeatedly throughout this book and elaborate on it in later chapters.

▪ The Changing Demographics of the Global Economy

Hand in hand with the trend toward globalization has been a fairly dramatic change in the demographics of the global economy over the past 30 years. As late as the 1960s, four stylized facts described the demographics of the global economy. The first was U.S. dominance in the world economy and world trade picture. The second was U.S. dominance in world foreign direct investment. Related to this, the third fact was the dominance of large, multinational U.S. firms on the international business scene. The fourth was that roughly half the globe—the centrally planned economies of the Communist world—was off-limits to Western international businesses. As will be explained below, all four of these qualities either have changed or are now changing rapidly.

The Changing World Output and World Trade Picture

In the early 1960s, the United States was still by far the world's dominant industrial power. In 1963, for example, the United States accounted for 40.3 percent of world output. By 2000, the United States accounted for 27 percent of world output, still by far the world's largest industrial power but down significantly in relative size since the 1960s (see Table 1.2). Nor was the United States the only developed nation to see its relative stand-

Country	Share of World Output, 1963‡	Share of World Output, 2001–2002	Share of World Exports, 2002
United States	40.3%	21.5%	11.9%
Japan	5.5	7.55	6.6
Germany*	9.7	4.64	9.3
France	6.3	3.27	5.2
United Kingdom	6.5	3.23	4.4
Italy	3.4	3.0	3.9
Canada	3.0	1.96	4.2
China†	NA	12.77	4.6
South Korea	NA	1.98	1.5

Table 1.2

The Changing Pattern of World Output and Trade

*1963 figure for Germany refers to the former West Germany.

†Figures for China include Hong Kong.

‡Output is measured by gross national product at purchasing power parity.

Sources: Export data from World Trade Organization, *International Trade Trends and Statistics, 2002*; world output data from CIA *World Factbook, 2003*.

ing slip. The same occurred to Germany, France, and the United Kingdom, all nations that were among the first to industrialize. This decline in the U.S. position was not an absolute decline, since the U.S. economy grew at a robust average annual rate of more than 3 percent from 1963 to 2000 (the economies of Germany, France, and the United Kingdom also grew during this time). Rather, it was a relative decline, reflecting the faster economic growth of several other economies, particularly in Asia. For example, as can be seen from Table 1.2, from 1963 to 2002, China's share of world output increased from a trivial amount to 12.77 percent. Other countries that markedly increased their share of world output included Japan, Thailand, Malaysia, Taiwan, and South Korea.

By the end of the 1980s, the U.S. position as the world's leading exporter was threatened. Over the past 30 years, U.S. dominance in export markets has waned as Japan, Germany, and a number of newly industrialized countries such as South Korea and China have taken a larger share of world exports. During the 1960s, the United States routinely accounted for 20 percent of world exports of manufactured goods. But as Table 1.2 shows, the U.S. share of world exports of manufactured goods had slipped to 11.9 percent by 2002. Despite the fall, the United States still remained the world's largest exporter, ahead of Germany and Japan.

In 1997 and 1998, the dynamic economies of the Asian Pacific region were hit by a serious financial crisis that threatened to slow their economic growth rates for several years. Despite this, their powerful growth may continue over the long run, as will that of several other important emerging economies in Latin America (e.g., Brazil) and Eastern Europe (e.g., Poland). Thus, a further relative decline in the share of world output and world exports accounted for by the United States and other long-established developed nations seems likely. By itself, this is not bad. The relative decline of the United States reflects the growing economic development and industrialization of the world economy, as opposed to any absolute decline in the health of the U.S. economy, which entered the new millennium stronger than ever.

If we look 20 years into the future, most forecasts now predict a rapid rise in the share of world output accounted for by developing nations such as China, India, Indonesia, Thailand, South Korea, Mexico, and Brazil, and a commensurate decline in the share enjoyed by rich industrialized countries such as Great Britain, Germany, Japan, and the United States. The World Bank, for example, has estimated that if current trends continue, by 2020 the Chinese economy could be larger than that of the United States, while the economy of India will approach that of Germany. The World Bank also estimates that today's developing nations may account for more than 60 percent of world economic activity by 2020, while today's rich nations, which currently account for over 55 percent of world economic activity, may account for only about

Figure 1.3

Percentage Share of Total
FDI Stock, 1980–2001

Source: United Nations, *World Investment Report, 2002* (New York
and Geneva: United Nations, 2002).

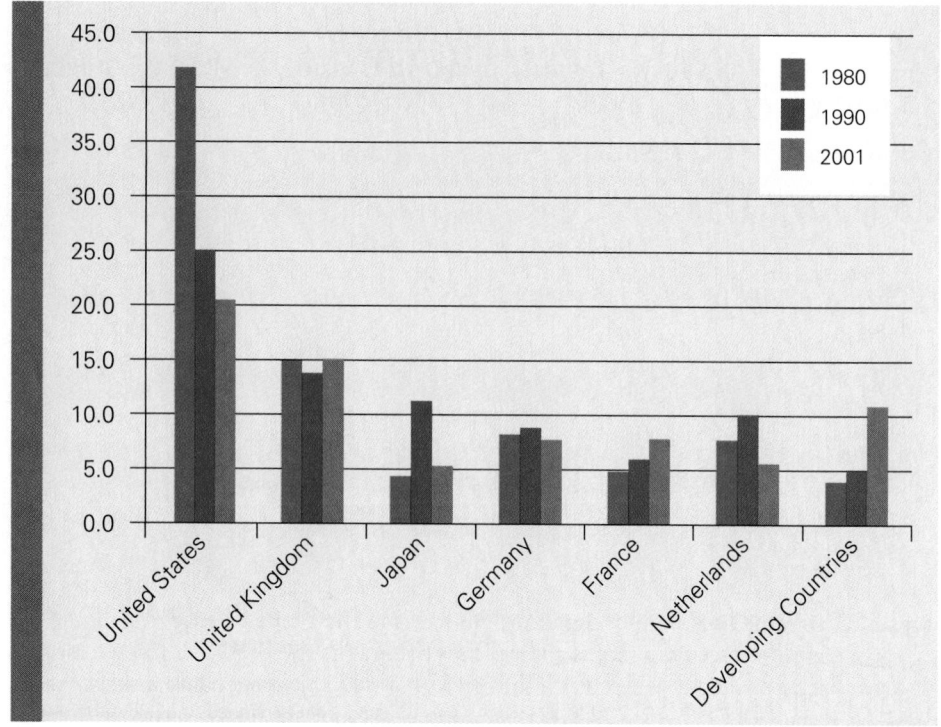

38 percent by 2020.[38] Forecasts are not always correct, but these suggest that a shift in
the economic geography of the world is now under way, although the magnitude of
that shift is still not totally evident. For international businesses, the implications of
this changing economic geography are clear: Many of tomorrow's economic opportunities may be found in the developing nations of the world, and many of tomorrow's
most capable competitors will probably also emerge from these regions.

The Changing Foreign Direct Investment Picture

Reflecting the dominance of the United States in the global economy, U.S. firms accounted for 66.3 percent of worldwide foreign direct investment flows in the 1960s. British
firms were second, accounting for 10.5 percent, while Japanese firms were a distant eighth,
with only 2 percent. The dominance of U.S. firms was so great that books were written
about the economic threat posed to Europe by U.S. corporations.[39] Several European governments, most notably that of France, talked of limiting inward investment by U.S. firms.

However, as the barriers to the free flow of goods, services, and capital fell, and as
other countries increased their shares of world output, non-U.S. firms increasingly began to invest across national borders. The motivation for much of this foreign direct investment by non-U.S. firms was the desire to disperse production activities to optimal
locations and to build a direct presence in major foreign markets. Thus, beginning in the
1970s, European and Japanese firms began to shift labor-intensive manufacturing operations from their home markets to developing nations where labor costs were lower. In
addition, many Japanese firms invested in North America and Europe—often as a hedge
against unfavorable currency movements and the possible imposition of trade barriers.
For example, Toyota, the Japanese automobile company, rapidly increased its investment
in automobile production facilities in the United States and Europe during the late
1980s and early 1990s. Toyota executives believed that an increasingly strong Japanese
yen would price Japanese automobile exports out of foreign markets; therefore, production in the most important foreign markets, as opposed to exports from Japan, made
sense. Toyota also undertook these investments to head off growing political pressures in
the United States and Europe to restrict Japanese automobile exports into those markets.

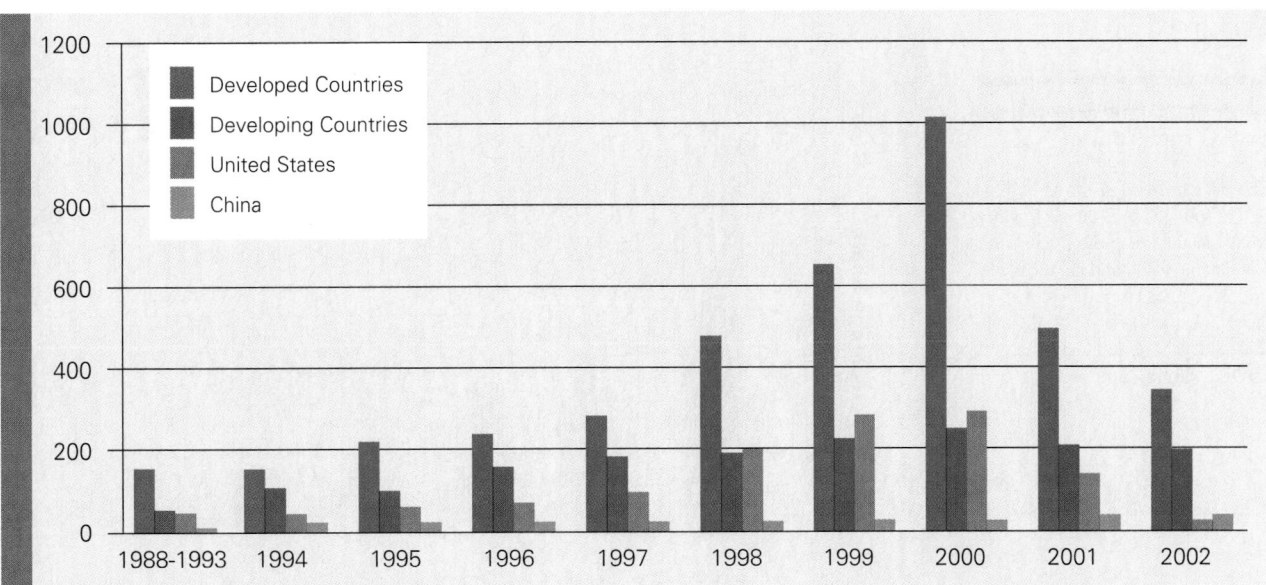

Figure 1.4

FDI Inflows, 1994–2002 (in $ billions)

Source: United Nations, *World Investment Report, 2002* (New York and Geneva: United Nations, 2002), and United Nations, "UNCTAD Predicts 27% Drop in FDI Flows This Year," United Nations press release TAD/INF/PR/63, November 24, 2002. Figures for 2002 are preliminary estimates.

One consequence of these developments is illustrated in Figure 1.3, which shows how the stock of foreign direct investment by the world's six most important national sources— the United States, the United Kingdom, Japan, Germany, France, and the Netherlands— changed between 1980 and 2001. (The stock of foreign direct investment refers to the total cumulative value of foreign investments.) Figure 1.3 also shows the stock accounted for by firms from developing economies. The share of the total stock accounted for by U.S. firms declined substantially from about 42 percent in 1980 to 21 percent in 2001. Meanwhile, the shares accounted for by Japan, France, other developed nations, and the world's developing nations increased markedly. The rise in the share for developing nations reflects a growing trend for firms from these countries, such as South Korea, to invest outside their borders. In 2001, firms based in developing nations accounted for 11.8 percent of the stock of foreign direct investment, up from only 3.1 percent in 1980.

Figure 1.4 illustrates two other important trends—the sustained growth in cross-border flows of foreign direct investment that occurred during the 1990s, and the emerging importance of developing nations as the destination of foreign direct investment. Throughout the 1990s, the amount of investment directed at both developed and developing nations increased dramatically, a trend that reflects the increasing internationalization of business corporations. A surge in foreign direct investment into developed nations from 1998 to 2000 was followed by a slump in 2001–2002 associated with a slowdown in global economic activity. Investment directed at developing nations, however, held up relatively well, averaging around $200 billion annually between 1998 and 2002, with China taking the most important share of this. As we shall see later in this book, the sustained flow of foreign investment into developing nations is a very important stimulus for economic growth in those countries, and bodes well for the future of countries such as China, Mexico, and Brazil, all leading beneficiaries of this trend.

❙ The Changing Nature of the Multinational Enterprise

A **multinational enterprise** is any business that has productive activities in two or more countries. Since the 1960s, there have been two notable trends in the

Figure 1.5

National Origin of Largest
Multinational Corporations,
1973, 1991, 2000

Source: Data for 1973 from N. Hood
and J. Young, *The Economics of the
Multinational Enterprise* (New York:
Longman, 1973), and data for 1991
and 2000 from United Nations,
*World Investment Reports 1992 and
2002* (New York and Geneva:
United Nations, 2002).

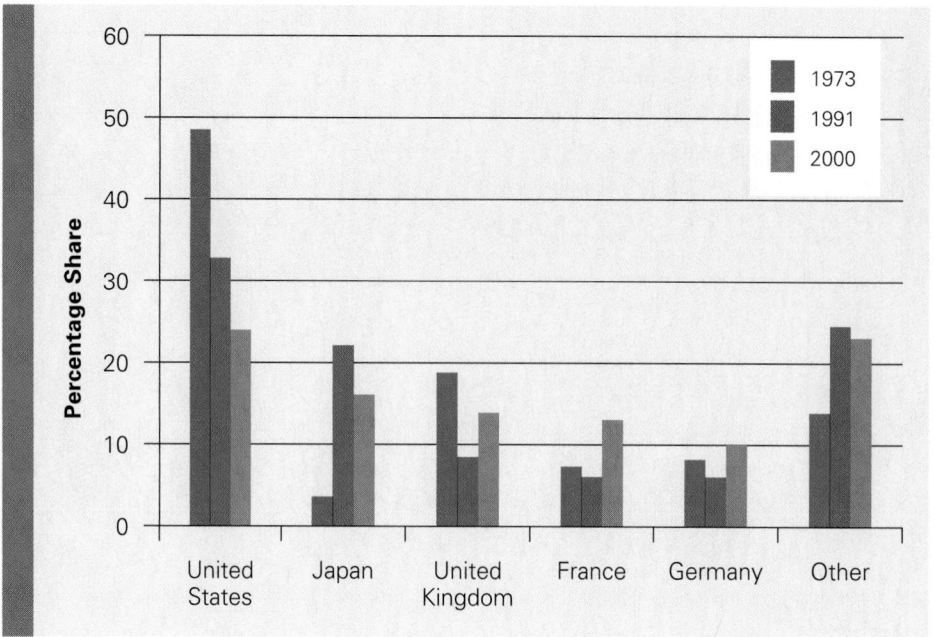

demographics of the multinational enterprise: (1) the rise of non-U.S. multinationals, particularly Japanese multinationals, and (2) the growth of mini-multinationals.

Non-U.S. Multinationals

In the 1960s, global business activity was dominated by large U.S. multinational corporations. With U.S. firms accounting for about two-thirds of foreign direct investment during the 1960s, one would expect most multinationals to be U.S. enterprises. According to the data summarized in Figure 1.5, in 1973, 48.5 percent of the world's 260 largest multinationals were U.S. firms. The second largest source country was the United Kingdom, with 18.8 percent of the largest multinationals. Japan accounted for only 3.5 percent of the world's largest multinationals at the time. The large number of U.S. multinationals reflected U.S. economic dominance in the three decades after World War II, while the large number of British multinationals reflected that country's industrial dominance in the early decades of the 20th century.

By 2000, however, things had shifted significantly. U.S. firms accounted for 24 percent of the world's 100 largest multinationals, followed by Japan with 16 percent. Britain was third with 14 percent.[40] Although the 1973 data summarized in Figure 1.5 are not strictly comparable with the later data, they illustrate the trend. (The 1973 figures are based on the largest 260 firms, whereas the later figures are based on the largest 100 multinationals.) The globalization of the world economy together with Japan's rise to the top rank of economic powers has resulted in a relative decline in the dominance of U.S. (and, to a lesser extent, British) firms in the global marketplace.

According to UN data, the ranks of the world's largest 100 multinationals are still dominated by firms from developed economies.[41] However, for the first time three firms from developing economies entered the UN's list of the 100 largest multinationals. They were Hutchison Whampoa of Hong Kong, China, which ranked 48 in terms of foreign assets; Petroleos de Venezuela of Venezuela, which ranked 84; and Cemex of Mexico, which came in at 100.[42] If we look at smaller firms, it is evident that there has been growth in the number of multinationals from developing economies. At the start of the 2000s, the largest 50 multinationals from developing economies had foreign sales of $103 billion out of total sales of $453 billion and employed 483,129 people outside of their home countries. Some 22 percent of these companies came from Hong Kong, 16.7 percent from Korea, 8.8 percent from China, and 7.6 percent

Management Focus

Wipro Ltd—The New Face of Global Competition

Fifteen years ago, Wipro Ltd. of India was a jumbled conglomerate selling everything from cooking oil and personal care products to knockoffs of Dell microcomputers and light-bulbs. Now it is a fast-growing information technology company at the forefront of India's rapidly expanding tech sector. In 2002, Wipro generated more than $900 million in sales, the majority from export contracts in information technology services. Its sales have grown by 26 percent a year since 1997, and that growth shows no sign of slowing.

Wipro's move into technology began in the early 1990s when the company started to sell its software programming expertise to foreign companies looking to reduce the software development costs. India has a solid base of technology-focused universities and colleges that turn out many engineers every year. While software programmers in the United States often command over $100,000 a year, similarly skilled individuals in India can be had for as little as $2 an hour, and programmers at Wipro on average earn $8,000 a year. That might not sound like a lot, but in India, where the annual per capita income is still under $500, it can translate into a very good living.

Today Wipro's 15,000 technology employees write software, integrate back-office solutions, design semiconductors, debug applications, take orders, and field help calls for some of the biggest companies in the world. Its customers include General Electric, Hewlett-Packard, Home Depot, Nokia, Sony, and Weyerhaeuser. By using the Internet, Wipro can maintain and manage software applications for companies all over the world in real time. Typical is Wipro's relationship with Weyerhaeuser, one of the world's largest timber companies. Wipro's involvement with Weyerhaeuser began in 1999 when two employees conducted a modest on-site analysis at Weyerhaeuser's U.S. headquarters just south of Seattle. By 2003, Wipro was supporting a broad array of Weyerhaeuser's informa-

tion systems including logistics, sales, and human resource applications from Bangalore, India. Overall, Wipro estimates that it can save its clients as much as 40 percent of the cost of maintaining such systems. In a highly competitive global economy, the imperative for companies such as Weyerhaeuser to outsource to outfits like Wipro is compelling.

Wipro, however, is not content to remain in the low-margin end of the software business. Increasingly the company is moving upstream into high value-added applications. For example, in 2002 Wipro signed a deal to design and engineer tape storage devices for Storage Technology. By 2004, Wipro will take over responsibility for all development work on this product line from 200 employees in Minneapolis. Wipro is also moving rapidly into high value-added software services, such as establishing global supply chain or billing systems for large corporations, a business that is currently dominated by Western consulting outfits such as IBM, EDS, and Accenture.

As Wipro expands its business, it is also taking steps to become a more global company. Around the world, Wipro has been hiring local nationals to lead its push into outsourcing deals. By 2005, the company hopes that three-quarters of the employees that customers see will be local nationals. Wipro is also buying local companies to give it instant industry presence. In November 2002, for example, Wipro paid $26 million for American Management Systems, buying not just credibility but also 90 consultants and 50 existing client relationships in the energy business. While these consultants will manage contact with U.S. customers, software development work will be moved back to Bangalore.

Source: K. H. Hammonds, "The New Face of Global Competition," *Fast Company*, February 2003, pp. 90–97; M. Kripalani and P. Engardio, "The Live Wire of Indian High Tech," *Business Week*, January 20, 2003, pp. 70–71; and F. Hayes, "Outsourcing Angst," *Computer World*, March 17, 2003, p. 11.

from Brazil. We can reasonably expect more growth of new multinational enterprises from the world's developing nations. Firms from developing nations can be expected to emerge as important competitors in global markets, thus further shifting the axis of the world economy away from North America and Western Europe and threatening the long dominance of Western companies. One such rising competitor, Wipro of India, is profiled in the accompanying Management Focus.

The Rise of Mini-Multinationals

Another trend in international business has been the growth of medium-size and small multinationals (mini-multinationals).[43] When people think of international businesses, they tend to think of firms such as Exxon, General Motors, Ford, Fuji, Kodak, Matsushita, Procter & Gamble, Sony, and Unilever—large, complex multinational corporations with operations that span the globe. Although most international trade and investment is still conducted by large firms, many medium-size and small businesses are becoming increasingly involved in international trade and investment. We have already discussed several examples in this chapter—Swan Optical, Bridgewater Pottery, and Cardiac Science—and we have noted how the rise of the Internet is lowering the barriers that small firms face in building international sales.

For another example, consider Lubricating Systems, Inc., of Kent, Washington. Lubricating Systems, which manufactures lubricating fluids for machine tools, employs 25 people and generates sales of $6.5 million. It's hardly a large, complex multinational, yet more than $2 million of the company's sales are generated by exports to a score of countries from Japan to Israel and the United Arab Emirates. Lubricating Systems also has set up a joint venture with a German company to serve the European market.[44] Consider also Lixi, Inc., a small U.S. manufacturer of industrial X-ray equipment; 70 percent of Lixi's $4.5 million in revenues comes from exports to Japan.[45] Or take G. W. Barth, a manufacturer of cocoa-bean roasting machinery based in Ludwigsburg, Germany. Employing just 65 people, this small company has captured 70 percent of the global market for cocoa-bean roasting machines.[46] International business is conducted not just by large firms but also by medium-size and small enterprises.

The Changing World Order

Between 1989 and 1991 a series of remarkable democratic revolutions swept the Communist world. For reasons that are explored in more detail in Chapter 2, in country after country throughout Eastern Europe and eventually in the Soviet Union itself, Communist governments collapsed like the shells of rotten eggs. The Soviet Union is now history, having been replaced by 15 independent republics. Czechoslovakia has divided itself into two states, while Yugoslavia dissolved into a bloody civil war among its five successor states.

Many of the former Communist nations of Europe and Asia seem to share a commitment to democratic politics and free market economics. If this continues, the opportunities for international businesses may be enormous. For half a century, these countries were essentially closed to Western international businesses. Now they present a host of export and investment opportunities. Just how this will play out over the next 10 to 20 years is difficult to say. The economies of most of the former Communist states are still in poor condition, and their continued commitment to democracy and free market economics cannot be taken for granted. Disturbing signs of growing unrest and totalitarian tendencies continue to be seen in many Eastern European states. Thus, the risks involved in doing business in such countries are high, but, then, so may be the returns.

In addition to these changes, more quiet revolutions have been occurring in China and Latin America. Their implications for international businesses may be just as profound as the collapse of communism in Eastern Europe. China suppressed its own pro-democracy movement in the bloody Tiananmen Square massacre of 1989. Despite this, China continues to move progressively toward greater free market reforms. If what is occurring in China continues for two more decades, China may move from Third World to industrial superpower status even more rapidly than Japan did. If China's gross domestic product (GDP) per capita grows by an average of 6 percent to 7 percent, which is slower than the 8 percent growth rate achieved during the last decade, then by 2020 this nation of 1.273 billion people could boast an average income per capita of about $13,000, roughly equivalent to that of Spain's today.

The potential consequences for international business are enormous. On the one hand, with nearly 1.3 billion people, China represents a huge and largely untapped market. Reflecting this, between 1983 and 2002, annual foreign direct investment in China increased from less than $2 billion to $50 billion. On the other hand, China's new firms are proving to be very capable competitors, and they could take global market share away from Western and Japanese enterprises. Thus, the changes in China are creating both opportunities and threats for established international businesses.

As for Latin America, both democracy and free market reforms also seem to have taken hold. For decades, most Latin American countries were ruled by dictators, many of whom seemed to view Western international businesses as instruments of imperialist domination. Accordingly, they restricted direct investment by foreign firms. In addition, the poorly managed economies of Latin America were characterized by low growth, high debt, and hyperinflation—all of which discouraged investment by international businesses. Now much of this seems to be changing. Throughout most of Latin America, debt and inflation are down, governments are selling state-owned enterprises to private investors, foreign investment is welcomed, and the region's economies have expanded. These changes have increased the attractiveness of Latin America, both as a market for exports and as a site for foreign direct investment. At the same time, given the long history of economic mismanagement in Latin America, there is no guarantee that these favorable trends will continue. As in the case of Eastern Europe, substantial opportunities are accompanied by substantial risks.

The Global Economy of the 21st Century

The last quarter century has seen rapid changes in the global economy. Barriers to the free flow of goods, services, and capital have been coming down. The volume of cross-border trade and investment has been growing more rapidly than global output, indicating that national economies are becoming more closely integrated into a single, interdependent, global economic system. As their economies advance, more nations are joining the ranks of the developed world. A generation ago, South Korea and Taiwan were viewed as second-tier developing nations. Now they boast large economies, and their firms are major players in many global industries from shipbuilding and steel to electronics and chemicals. The move toward a global economy has been further strengthened by the widespread adoption of liberal economic policies by countries that had firmly opposed them for two generations or more. Thus, in keeping with the normative prescriptions of liberal economic ideology, in country after country we are seeing state-owned businesses privatized, widespread deregulation adopted, markets opened to more competition, and commitment increased to removing barriers to cross-border trade and investment. This suggests that over the next few decades, countries such as the Czech Republic, Poland, Brazil, China, India, and South Africa may build powerful market-oriented economies. In short, current trends indicate that the world is moving rapidly toward an economic system that is more favorable for the practice of international business.

But it is always hazardous to take established trends and use them to predict the future. The world may be moving toward a more global economic system, but globalization is not inevitable. Countries may pull back from the recent commitment to liberal economic ideology if their experiences do not match their expectations. There have been periodic signs, for example, of a retreat from liberal economic ideology in Russia. Russia has experienced considerable economic pain as it tries to shift from a centrally planned economy to a market economy. If Russia's hesitation were to become more permanent and widespread, the liberal vision of a more prosperous global economy based on free market principles might not occur as quickly as many hope. Clearly, this would be a tougher world for international businesses to compete in.

Also, greater globalization brings with it risks of its own. This was starkly demonstrated in 1997 and 1998 when a financial crisis in Thailand spread first to other East

Asian nations and then in 1998 to Russia and Brazil. Ultimately the crisis threatened to plunge the economies of the developed world, including the United States, into a recession. We explore the causes and consequences of this and other similar global financial crises in Chapters 9 and 10. Even from a purely economic perspective, globalization is not all good. The opportunities for doing business in a global economy may be significantly enhanced, but as we saw in 1997–98, the risks associated with global financial contagion are also greater. Still, as explained later in this book, firms can exploit the opportunities associated with globalization, while at the same time reducing the risks through appropriate hedging strategies.

The Globalization Debate

Is the shift toward a more integrated and interdependent global economy a good thing? Many influential economists, politicians, and business leaders seem to think so.[47] They argue that falling barriers to international trade and investment are the twin engines driving the global economy toward greater prosperity. They say increased international trade and cross-border investment will result in lower prices for goods and services. They believe that globalization stimulates economic growth, raises the incomes of consumers, and helps to create jobs in all countries that participate in the global trading system. The arguments of those who support globalization are covered in detail in Chapters 4, 5, 6, and 7. As we shall see, there are good theoretical reasons for believing that declining barriers to international trade and investment do stimulate economic growth, create jobs, and raise income levels. As described in Chapters 5 and 6, empirical evidence lends support to the predictions of this theory. However, despite the existence of a compelling body of theory and evidence, globalization has its critics.[48] Some of these critics have become increasingly vocal and active, taking to the streets to demonstrate their opposition to globalization. Here we look at the rising tide of protests against globalization and briefly review the main themes of the debate concerning the merits of globalization. In later chapters we elaborate on many of the points mentioned below.

Antiglobalization Protests

Street demonstrations against globalization date to December 1999, when more than 40,000 protesters blocked the streets of Seattle in an attempt to shut down a World Trade Organization meeting being held in the city. The demonstrators were protesting against a wide range of issues, including job losses in industries under attack from foreign competitors, downward pressure on the wage rates of unskilled workers, environmental degradation, and the cultural imperialism of global media and multinational enterprises, which was seen as being dominated by what some protesters called the "culturally impoverished" interests and values of the United States. All of these ills, the demonstrators claimed, could be laid at the feet of globalization. The World Trade Organization was meeting to try to launch a new round of talks to cut barriers to cross-border trade and investment. As such, it was seen as a promoter of globalization and a legitimate target for the antiglobalization protesters. The protests turned violent, transforming the normally placid streets of Seattle into a running battle between "anarchists" and Seattle's bemused and poorly prepared police department. Pictures of brick-throwing protesters and armored police wielding their batons were duly recorded by the global media, which then circulated the images around the world. Meanwhile, the World Trade Organization meeting failed to reach agreement, and although the protests outside the meeting halls had little to do with that failure, the impression took hold that the demonstrators had succeeded in derailing the meetings.

Emboldened by the experience in Seattle, antiglobalization protesters have turned up at almost every major meeting of a global institution. In February 2000, they demonstrated at the World Economic Forum meetings in Davos, Switzerland, and vented their frustrations against global capitalism by trashing that hated symbol of U.S. imperialism, a McDonald's restaurant. In April 2000, demonstrators disrupted talks being held at the World Bank and International Monetary Fund, and in September 2000, 12,000 demonstrated at the annual meeting of the World Bank and IMF in Prague. In April 2001, demonstrations and police firing tear gas and water cannons overshadowed the "Summit of the Americas" meeting in Quebec City, Canada. In June 2001, 40,000 protesters marched against globalization at the European Union summit in Göteborg, Sweden. The march was peaceful until a core of masked anarchists wielding cobblestones created bloody mayhem. In July 2001, antiglobalization protests in Genoa, Italy, where the heads of the eight largest economies were meeting (the so-called G8 meetings), turned violent, and in the now familiar ritual of running battles between protesters and police, a protester was killed, giving the antiglobalization movement its first martyr. Smaller scale protests have occurred in several countries, such as France, where antiglobalization protesters destroyed a McDonald's restaurant in August 1999 to protest the impoverishment of French culture by American imperialism (see the accompanying Country Focus for details).

While violent protests may give the antiglobalization effort a bad name, it is clear from the scale of the demonstrations that support for the cause goes beyond a core of anarchists. Large segments of the population in many countries believe that globalization has detrimental effects on living standards and the environment. Both theory and evidence suggest that many of these fears are exaggerated, but this may not have been communicated clearly and both politicians and businesspeople need to do more to counter these fears. Many protests against globalization are tapping into a general sense of loss at the passing of a world in which barriers of time and distance, and vast differences in economic institutions, political institutions, and the level of development of different nations, produced a world rich in the diversity of human cultures. This world is now passing into history. However, while the rich citizens of the developed world may have the luxury of mourning the fact that they can now see McDonald's restaurants and Starbucks coffeehouses on their vacations to exotic locations such as Thailand, fewer complaints are heard from the citizens of those countries, who welcome the higher living standards that progress brings.

Globalization, Jobs, and Income

One concern frequently voiced by opponents of globalization is that falling barriers to international trade destroy manufacturing jobs in wealthy advanced economies such as the United States and the United Kingdom. The critics argue that falling trade barriers allow firms to move their manufacturing activities to countries where wage rates are much lower.[49] D. L. Bartlett and J. B. Steele, two journalists for the *Philadelphia Inquirer* who gained notoriety for their attacks on free trade, cite the case of Harwood Industries, a U.S. clothing manufacturer that closed its U.S. operations, where it paid workers $9 per hour, and shifted manufacturing to Honduras, where textile workers receive 48 cents per hour.[50] Because of moves such as this, argue Bartlett and Steele, the wage rates of poorer Americans have fallen significantly over the past quarter of a century.

Supporters of globalization reply that critics such as Bartlett and Steele miss the essential point about free trade—the benefits outweigh the costs.[51] They argue that free trade will result in countries specializing in the production of those goods and services that they can produce most efficiently, while importing goods that they cannot produce as efficiently. When a country embraces free trade, there is always some dislocation—lost textile jobs at Harwood Industries, for example—but the whole economy is better off as a result. According to this view, it makes little sense for the United States to produce textiles at home when they can be produced at a lower cost in Honduras or China (which, unlike Honduras, is a major source of U.S. textile imports). Importing

Country Focus

Protesting Globalization in France

One night in August 1999, 10 men under the leadership of local sheep farmer and rural activist Jose Bove crept into the town of Millau in central France and vandalized a McDonald's restaurant under construction, causing an estimated $150,000 worth of damage. These were no ordinary vandals, however, at least according to their supporters, for the "symbolic dismantling" of the McDonald's outlet had noble aims, or so it was claimed. The attack was initially presented as a protest against unfair American trade policies. The European Union had banned imports of hormone-treated beef from the United States, primarily because of fears that hormone-treated beef might lead to health problems (although EU scientists had concluded there was no evidence of this). After a careful review, the World Trade Organization stated the EU ban was not allowed under trading rules that the EU and United States were party to, and that the EU would have to lift it or face retaliation. The EU refused to comply, so the U.S. government imposed a 100 percent tariff on imports of certain EU products, including French staples such as foie gras, mustard, and Roquefort cheese. On farms near Millau, Bove and others raised sheep whose milk was used to make Roquefort. They felt incensed by the American tariff and decided to vent their frustrations on McDonald's.

Bove and his compatriots were arrested and charged. They quickly became a focus of the emerging antiglobalization movement in France that was protesting everything from a loss of national sovereignty and "unfair" trade policies that were trying to force hormone-treated beef on French consumers, to the invasion of French culture by alien American values, so aptly symbolized by McDonald's. Lionel Jospin, France's prime minister, called the cause of Jose Bove "just." Allowed to remain free pending his trial, Bove traveled to Seattle in December to protest against the World Trade Organization, where he was feted as a hero of the antiglobalization movement. Back in France, Bove's July 2000 trial drew some 40,000 supporters to the small town of Millau, where they camped outside the courthouse and waited for the verdict. Bove was found guilty and sentenced to three months in jail, far less than the maximum possible sentence of five years. His supporters wore T-shirts claiming, "The world is not merchandise, and neither am I."

About the same time in the Languedoc region of France, California winemaker Robert Mondavi had reached agreement with the mayor and council of the village of Aniane and regional authorities to turn 125 acres of wooded hillside belonging to the village into a vineyard. Mondavi planned to invest $7 million in the project and hoped to produce top-quality wine that would sell in Europe and the United States for $60 a bottle. However, local environmentalists objected to the plan, which they claimed would destroy the area's unique ecological heritage. Jose Bove, basking in sudden fame, offered his support to the opponents, and the protests started. In May 2001, the Socialist mayor who had approved the project was defeated in local elections in which the Mondavi project had become the major issue. He was replaced by a Communist, Manuel Diaz, who denounced the project as a capitalist plot designed to enrich wealthy U.S. shareholders at the cost of his villagers and the environment. Following Diaz's victory, Mondavi announced he would pull out of the project. A spokesman noted, "It's a huge waste, but there are clearly personal and political interests at play here that go way beyond us."

So are the French opposed to foreign investment? The experience of McDonald's and Mondavi seems to suggest so, as does the associated news coverage, but look closer and a different reality seems to emerge. McDonald's has over 800 restaurants in France and continues to do well there. The level of foreign investment in France reached record levels in the late 1990s and 2000. In 2000, France recorded 563 major inward investment deals, a record, and American companies accounted for the largest number, some 178. French enterprises are also investing across borders at record levels. Given all of the talk about American cultural imperialism, it is striking that a French company, Vivendi, acquired two of the propagators of American cultural values: Universal Pictures and publisher Houghton Mifflin. And French politicians seem set on removing domestic barriers that make it difficult for French companies to compete effectively in the global economy.

Sources: "Behind the Bluster," *The Economist,* May 26, 2001; "The French Farmers' Anti-global Hero," *The Economist,* July 8, 2000; C. Trueheart, "France's Golden Arch Enemy?" *Toronto Star,* July 1, 2000; and J. Henley, "Grapes of Wrath Scare Off U.S. Firm," *The Economist,* May 18, 2001, p. 11.

textiles from China leads to lower prices for clothes in the United States, which enables consumers to spend more of their money on other items. At the same time, the increased income generated in China from textile exports increases income levels in that country, which helps the Chinese to purchase more products produced in the United States, such as pharmaceuticals from Amgen, Boeing jets, Intel-based computers, Microsoft software, and Cisco routers. In this manner, supporters of globalization argue that free trade benefits all countries that adhere to a free trade regime.

Supporters of globalization do concede that the wage rate enjoyed by unskilled workers in many advanced economies may have declined in recent years.[52] For example, data for the Organization for Economic Cooperation and Development suggest that since 1980 the lowest 10 percent of American workers have seen a drop in their real wages (adjusted for inflation) of about 20 percent, while the top 10 percent have enjoyed a real pay increase of around 10 percent.[53] In the same vein, a Federal Reserve study found that in the seven years preceding 1996, the earnings of the best-paid 10 percent of U.S. workers rose in real terms by 0.6 percent annually while the earnings of the 10 percent at the bottom of the heap fell by 8 percent. In some areas, the fall was much greater.[54] Similar trends can be seen in many other countries.

However, while globalization critics argue that the decline in unskilled wage rates is due to the migration of low-wage manufacturing jobs offshore and a corresponding reduction in demand for unskilled workers, supporters of globalization see a more complex picture. They maintain that the declining real wage rates of unskilled workers owes far more to a technology-induced shift within advanced economies away from jobs where the only qualification was a willingness to turn up for work every day and toward jobs that require significant education and skills. They point out that many advanced economies report a shortage of highly skilled workers and an excess supply of unskilled workers. Thus, growing income inequality is a result of the wages for skilled workers being bid up by the labor market, and the wages for unskilled workers being discounted. If one agrees with this logic, a solution to the problem of declining incomes is to be found not in limiting free trade and globalization, but in increasing society's investment in education to reduce the supply of unskilled workers.[55]

Some research also suggests that the evidence of growing income inequality may be suspect. Robert Lerman of the Urban Institute believes that the finding of inequality is based on inappropriate calculations of wage rates. Reviewing the data using a different methodology, Lerman has found that far from income inequality increasing, an index of wage rate inequality for all workers actually fell by 5.5 percent between 1987 and 1994.[56] If future research supports this finding—and it may not— the argument that globalization leads to growing income inequality may lose much of its punch. During the last few years of the 1990s, the income of the worst-paid 10 percent of the population actually rose twice as fast as that of the average worker, suggesting that the high employment levels of these years have triggered a rise in the income of the lowest paid.[57]

Globalization, Labor Policies, and the Environment

A second source of concern is that free trade encourages firms from advanced nations to move manufacturing facilities to less developed countries that lack adequate regulations to protect labor and the environment from abuse by the unscrupulous.[58] Globalization critics often argue that adhering to labor and environmental regulations significantly increases the costs of manufacturing enterprises and puts them at a competitive disadvantage in the global marketplace vis-à-vis firms based in developing nations that do not have to comply with such regulations. Firms deal with this cost disadvantage, the theory goes, by moving their production facilities to nations that do not have such burdensome regulations or that fail to enforce the regulations they have.

If this is the case, one might expect free trade to lead to an increase in pollution and result in firms from advanced nations exploiting the labor of less developed nations.[59]

Figure 1.6

Environmental Performance and Income

Source: *Environmental Performance and Income* (Paris: OECD, 2000).

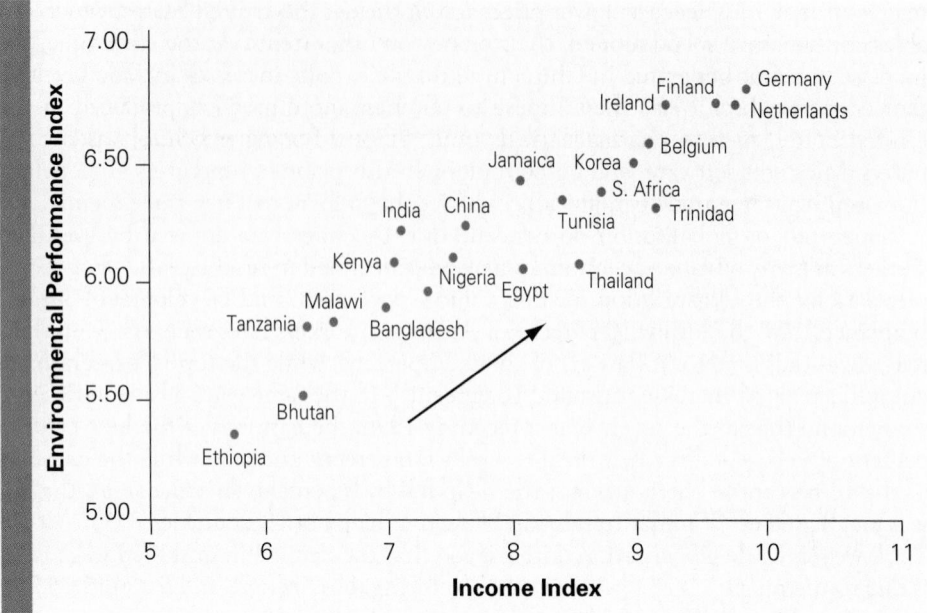

This argument was used repeatedly by those who opposed the 1994 formation of the North American Free Trade Agreement (NAFTA) between Canada, Mexico, and the United States. They painted a picture of U.S. manufacturing firms moving to Mexico in droves so that they would be free to pollute the environment, employ child labor, and ignore workplace safety and health issues, all in the name of higher profits.[60]

Supporters of free trade and greater globalization express doubts about this scenario. They argue that tougher environmental regulations and stricter labor standards go hand in hand with economic progress.[61] In general, as countries get richer, they enact tougher environmental and labor regulations.[62] Because free trade enables developing countries to increase their economic growth rates and become richer, this should lead to tougher environmental and labor laws. In this view, the critics of free trade have got it backward—free trade does not lead to more pollution and labor exploitation, it leads to less. By creating wealth and incentives for enterprises to produce technological innovations, the free market system and free trade could make it easier for the world to cope with problems of pollution and population growth. Indeed, while pollution levels are rising in the world's poorer countries, they have been falling in developed nations. In the United States, for example, the concentration of carbon monoxide and sulphur dioxide pollutants in the atmosphere decreased by 60 percent between 1978 and 1997, while lead concentrations decreased by 98 percent—and these reductions have occurred against a background of sustained economic expansion.[63] Drawn from a study undertaken for the Organization for Economic Cooperation and Development, Figure 1.6 shows there is a positive relationship between the income levels in a country and the environmental performance of that country as measured by various indicators.

Supporters of free trade also point out that it is possible to tie free trade agreements to the implementation of tougher environmental and labor laws in less developed countries. NAFTA, for example, was passed only after side agreements had been negotiated that committed Mexico to tougher enforcement of environmental protection regulations. Thus, supporters of free trade argue that factories based in Mexico are now cleaner than they would have been without the passage of NAFTA.[64]

They also argue that business firms are not the amoral organizations that critics suggest. While there may be some rotten apples, most business enterprises are staffed by managers who are committed to behave in an ethical manner and would be unlikely to move production offshore just so they could pump more pollution into the atmosphere or exploit labor. Furthermore, the relationship between pollution, labor exploitation, and production costs may not be that suggested by critics. In general, a well-treated labor force is productive, and it is productivity rather than base wage rates that often has the greatest influence on costs. The vision of greedy managers who shift production to low-wage countries to exploit their labor force may be misplaced.

Globalization and National Sovereignty

Another concern voiced by critics of globalization is that today's increasingly interdependent global economy shifts economic power away from national governments and toward supranational organizations such as the World Trade Organization, the European Union, and the United Nations. As perceived by critics, unelected bureaucrats now impose policies on the democratically elected governments of nation-states, thereby undermining the sovereignty of those states and limiting the nation-state's ability to control its own destiny.[65]

The World Trade Organization (WTO) is a favorite target of those who attack the headlong rush toward a global economy. As noted earlier, the WTO was founded in 1994 to police the world trading system established by the General Agreement on Tariffs and Trade. The WTO arbitrates trade disputes between the 146 states that are signatories to the GATT. The arbitration panel can issue a ruling instructing a member state to change trade policies that violate GATT regulations. If the violator refuses to comply with the ruling, the WTO allows other states to impose appropriate trade sanctions on the transgressor. As a result, according to one prominent critic, U.S. environmentalist and consumer rights advocate Ralph Nader:

> Under the new system, many decisions that affect billions of people are no longer made by local or national governments but instead, if challenged by any WTO member nation, would be deferred to a group of unelected bureaucrats sitting behind closed doors in Geneva (which is where the headquarters of the WTO are located). The bureaucrats can decide whether or not people in California can prevent the destruction of the last virgin forests or determine if carcinogenic pesticides can be banned from their foods; or whether European countries have the right to ban dangerous biotech hormones in meat . . . At risk is the very basis of democracy and accountable decision making.[66]

In contrast to Nader's rhetoric, many economists and politicians maintain that the power of supranational organizations such as the WTO is limited to what nation-states collectively agree to grant. They argue that bodies such as the United Nations and the WTO exist to serve the collective interests of member states, not to subvert those interests. Supporters of supranational organizations point out that the power of these bodies rests largely on their ability to persuade member states to follow a certain action. If these bodies fail to serve the collective interests of member states, those states will withdraw their support and the supranational organization will quickly collapse. In this view, real power still resides with individual nation-states, not supranational organizations.

Globalization and the World's Poor

Critics of globalization argue that despite the supposed benefits associated with free trade and investment, over the last hundred years or so the gap between the rich and poor nations of the world has gotten wider. In 1870 the average income per capita in the world's 17 richest nations was 2.4 times that of all other countries. In 1990 the same group was 4.5 times as rich as the rest.[67] While recent history has shown that some of the world's poorer nations are capable of rapid periods of economic growth—witness the transformation that has occurred in some Southeast Asian nations such as South Korea, Thailand, and Malaysia—there appear to be strong forces for stagnation among the world's poorest nations. A quarter of the countries with a GDP per capita of less than $1,000 in 1960 had growth rates of less than zero from 1960 to 1995, and a third had growth rates of less than 0.05 percent.[68] Critics argue that if globalization is such a positive development, this divergence between the rich and poor should not have occurred.

Although the reasons for economic stagnation vary, several factors stand out, none of which have anything to do with free trade or globalization.[69] Many of the world's poorest countries have suffered from totalitarian governments, economic policies that destroyed wealth rather than facilitated its creation, scant protection for property rights, and war. Such factors help explain why countries such as Afghanistan, Cambodia, Cuba, Haiti, Iraq, Libya, Nigeria, Sudan, Vietnam, and Zaire have failed to improve the economic lot of their citizens during recent decades. A complicating factor is the rapidly expanding populations in many of these countries. Without a major change in government, population growth may exacerbate their problems. Promoters of free trade argue that the best way for these countries to improve their lot is to lower their barriers to free trade and investment and to implement economic policies based on free market economics.[70]

Many of the world's poorer nations are being held back by large debt burdens. Of particular concern are the 40 or so "highly indebted poorer countries" (HIPCs), which are home to some 700 million people. Among these countries on average, the government debt burden is equivalent to 85 percent of the value of the economy, as measured by gross domestic product, and the annual costs of serving government debt consumes 15 percent of the country's export earnings.[71] Servicing such a heavy debt load leaves the governments of these countries with little left to invest in important public infrastructure projects, such as education, health care, roads, and power. The result is the HIPCs are trapped in a cycle of poverty and debt that inhibits economic development. Free trade alone, some argue, is not sufficient to help these countries bootstrap themselves out of poverty. Instead, large-scale debt relief is needed for the world's poorest nations to give them the opportunity to restructure their economies and start the long climb toward prosperity. Supporters of debt relief also argue that new democratic governments in poor nations should not be forced to honor debts that were incurred and mismanaged long ago by their corrupt and dictatorial predecessors.

In the late 1990s, a debt relief movement began to gain ground among the political establishment in the world's richer nations.[72] Fueled by high-profile endorsements ranging from Irish rock star Bono (who has been a tireless and increasingly effective advocate for debt relief), to Pope John Paul II, the Dalai Lama, and influential Harvard economist Jeffrey Sachs, the debt relief movement was instrumental in persuading the United States to enact legislation in 2000 that provided $435 million in debt relief for HIPCs. More importantly perhaps, the United States also backed an IMF plan to sell some of its gold reserves and use the proceeds to help with debt relief. The IMF and World Bank have now picked up the banner and are actively embarked on a systematic debt relief program.

For such a program to have a lasting effect, however, debt relief must be matched by wise investment in public projects that boost economic growth (such as education), and by the adoption of economic policies that facilitate investment and trade. The rich nations of the world can also help by reducing barriers to the importation of products from the world's poorer nations, particularly tariffs on imports of agricultural products and textiles. Debt relief is not new—it has been tried before.[73] Too often in the past, however, the short-term benefits were squandered by corrupt governments who used their newfound financial freedom to make unproductive investments in military infrastructure or grandiose projects that did little to foster long-run economic development. Developed nations contributed to past failures by refusing to open their markets to the products of poor nations. If such a scenario can be avoided this time, the entire world will benefit.

Managing in the Global Marketplace ■

Much of this book is concerned with the challenges of managing in an international business. An international business is any firm that engages in international trade or investment. A firm does not have to become a multinational enterprise, investing directly in operations in other countries, to engage in international business, although multinational enterprises are international businesses. All a firm has to do is export or import products from other countries. As the world shifts toward a truly integrated global economy, more firms, both large and small, are becoming international businesses. What does this shift toward a global economy mean for managers within an international business?

As their organizations increasingly engage in cross-border trade and investment, it means managers need to recognize that the task of managing an international business differs from that of managing a purely domestic business in many ways. At the most fundamental level, the differences arise from the simple fact that countries are different. Countries differ in their cultures, political systems, economic systems, legal systems, and levels of economic development. Despite all the talk about the emerging global village, and despite the trend toward globalization of markets and production, as we shall see in this book, many of these differences are very profound and enduring.

Differences between countries require that an international business vary its practices country by country. Marketing a product in Brazil may require a different approach than marketing the product in Germany; managing U.S. workers might require different skills than managing Japanese workers; maintaining close relations with a particular level of government may be very important in Mexico and irrelevant in Great Britain; the business strategy pursued in Canada might not work in South Korea; and so on. Managers in an international business must not only be sensitive to these differences, but they must also adopt the appropriate policies and strategies for coping with them. Much of this book is devoted to explaining the sources of these differences and the methods for successfully coping with them.

A further way in which international business differs from domestic business is the greater complexity of managing an international business. In addition to the problems that arise from the differences between countries, a manager in an international business is confronted with a range of other issues that the manager in a domestic business never confronts. An international business must decide where in the world to site its production activities to minimize costs and to maximize value added. Then it must decide how best to coordinate and control its globally dispersed production activities (which, as we shall see later in the book, is not a trivial problem). An international business also must decide which foreign markets to enter and which to avoid. It also must choose the appropriate mode for entering a particular foreign country. Is it best to export its product to the foreign country? Should the firm allow a local company to produce its product under license in that country? Should the firm enter into a joint venture with a local firm to produce its product in that country? Or should the firm set up a wholly owned subsidiary to serve the market in that country? As we shall see, the choice of entry mode is critical because it has major implications for the long-term health of the firm.

Conducting business transactions across national borders requires understanding the rules governing the international trading and investment system. Managers in an international business must also deal with government restrictions on international trade and investment. They must find ways to work within the limits imposed by specific governmental interventions. As this book explains, even though many governments are nominally committed to free trade, they often intervene to regulate cross-border trade and investment. Managers within international businesses must develop strategies and policies for dealing with such interventions.

Cross-border transactions also require that money be converted from the firm's home currency into a foreign currency and vice versa. Since currency exchange rates vary in response to changing economic conditions, an international business must develop policies for dealing with exchange rate movements. A firm that adopts a wrong policy can lose large amounts of money, while a firm that adopts the right policy can increase the profitability of its international transactions.

In sum, managing an international business is different from managing a purely domestic business for at least four reasons: (1) countries are different, (2) the range of problems confronted by a manager in an international business is wider, and the problems themselves more complex than those confronted by a manager in a domestic business, (3) an international business must find ways to work within the limits imposed by government intervention in the international trade and investment system, and (4) international transactions involve converting money into different currencies.

In this book we examine all these issues in depth, paying close attention to the different strategies and policies that managers pursue to deal with the various challenges created when a firm becomes an international business. Chapters 2 and 3 explore how countries differ from each other with regard to their political, economic, legal, and cultural institutions. Chapters 4 to 8 look at the international trade and investment environment within which international businesses must operate. Chapters 9 to 11 review the international monetary system. These chapters focus on the nature of the foreign exchange market and the emerging global monetary system. Chapters 12 to 14 explore the strategy and structure of international businesses. Chapters 15 to 20 look at the management of various functional operations within an international business, including production, marketing, human relations, accounting, and finance. By the time you complete this book, you should have a good grasp of the issues that managers working within international business have to grapple with on a daily basis, and you should be familiar with the range of strategies and operating policies available to compete more effectively in today's rapidly emerging global economy.

ChapterSummary

This chapter sets the scene for the rest of the book. We have seen how the world economy is becoming more global, and we have reviewed the main drivers of globalization and argued that they seem to be thrusting nation-states toward a more tightly integrated global economy. We have looked at how the nature of international business is changing in response to the changing global economy; we have discussed some concerns raised by rapid globalization; and we have reviewed implications of rapid globalization for individual managers. The chapter made these major points.

1. Over the past two decades, we have witnessed the globalization of markets and production.

2. The globalization of markets implies that national markets are merging into one huge marketplace. However, it is important not to push this view too far.

3. The globalization of production implies that firms are basing individual productive activities at the optimal world locations for the particular activities. As a consequence, it is increasingly irrelevant to talk about American products, Japanese products, or German prod-

ucts, since these are being replaced by "global" products.

4. Two factors seem to underlie the trend toward globalization: declining trade barriers and changes in communication, information, and transportation technologies.

5. Since the end of World War II, there has been a significant lowering of barriers to the free flow of goods, services, and capital. More than anything else, this has facilitated the trend toward the globalization of production and has enabled firms to view the world as a single market.

6. As a consequence of the globalization of production and markets, in the last decade world trade has grown faster than world output, foreign direct investment has surged, imports have penetrated more deeply into the world's industrial nations, and competitive pressures have increased in industry after industry.

7. The development of the microprocessor and related developments in communication and information processing technology have helped firms link their worldwide operations into so-

phisticated information networks. Jet air travel, by shrinking travel time, has also helped to link the worldwide operations of international businesses. These changes have enabled firms to achieve tight coordination of their worldwide operations and to view the world as a single market.

8. In the 1960s, the U.S. economy was dominant in the world, U.S. firms accounted for most of the foreign direct investment in the world economy, U.S. firms dominated the list of large multinationals, and roughly half the world—the centrally planned economies of the Communist world—was closed to Western businesses.

9. By the mid-1990s, the U.S. share of world output had been cut in half, with major shares now being accounted for by Western European and Southeast Asian economies. The U.S. share of worldwide foreign direct investment had also fallen, by about two-thirds. U.S. multinationals were now facing competition from a large number of Japanese and European multinationals. In addition, the emergence of mini-multinationals was noted.

10. The most dramatic environmental trend has been the collapse of Communist power in Eastern Europe, which has created enormous long-run opportunities for international businesses. In addition, the move toward free market economies in China and Latin America is creating opportunities (and threats) for Western international businesses.

11. The benefits and costs of the emerging global economy are being hotly debated among businesspeople, economists, and politicians. The debate focuses on the impact of globalization on jobs, wages, the environment, working conditions, and national sovereignty.

12. Managing an international business is different from managing a domestic business for at least four reasons: (*i*) countries are different, (*ii*) the range of problems confronted by a manager in an international business is wider and the problems themselves more complex than those confronted by a manager in a domestic business, (*iii*) managers in an international business must find ways to work within the limits imposed by governments' intervention in the international trade and investment system, and (*iv*) international transactions involve converting money into different currencies.

Critical Discussion Questions

1. Describe the shifts in the world economy over the past 30 years. What are the implications of these shifts for international businesses based in Great Britain? North America? Hong Kong?

2. "The study of international business is fine if you are going to work in a large multinational enterprise, but it has no relevance for individuals who are going to work in small firms." Evaluate this statement.

3. How have changes in technology contributed to the globalization of markets and production? Would the globalization of production and markets have been possible without these technological changes?

4. "Ultimately, the study of international business is no different from the study of domestic business. Thus, there is no point in having a separate course on international business." Evaluate this statement.

5. How might the Internet and the associated World Wide Web affect international business activity and the globalization of the world economy?

6. If current trends continue, China may be the world's largest economy by 2050. Discuss the possible implications of such a development for

   a. The world trading system.

   b. The world monetary system.

   c. The business strategy of today's European and U.S.-based global corporations.

Notes

1. T. Levitt, "The Globalization of Markets," *Harvard Business Review*, May–June 1983, pp. 92–102.

2. U.S. Department of Commerce, "A Profile of U.S. Exporting Companies, 2000–2001," February 2003. Report available at http://www.census.gov/foreign-trade/aip/index.html#profile.

3. Ibid.

4. C. M. Draffen, "Going Global: Export Market Proves Profitable for Region's Small Businesses," *Newsday*, March 19, 2001, p. C18.

5. W. J. Holstein, "Why Johann Can Export, but Johnny Can't," *Business Week*, November 4, 1991, pp. 64–65.

6. See F. T. Knickerbocker, *Oligopolistic Reaction and Multinational Enterprise* (Boston: Harvard Business School Press, 1973), and R. E. Caves, "Japanese Investment in the U.S.: Lessons for the Economic Analysis of Foreign Investment," *The World Economy* 16 (1993), pp. 279–300.

7. I. Metthee, "Playing a Large Part," *Seattle Post-Intelligencer*, April 9, 1994, p. 13.

8. C. S. Tranger, "Enter the Mini-Multinational," *Northeast International Business*, March 1989, pp. 13–14.

9. R. B. Reich, *The Work of Nations* (New York: A. A. Knopf, 1991).

10. United Nations, "The UN in Brief," http://www.un.org/Overview/brief.html.

11. J. A. Frankel, "Globalization of the Economy," National Bureau of Economic Research, Working Paper No. 7858, 2000.

12. J. Bhagwati, *Protectionism* (Cambridge, MA: MIT Press, 1989).

13. F. Williams, "Trade Round Like This May Never Be Seen Again," *Financial Times*, April 15, 1994, p. 8.

14. W. Vieth, "Major Concessions Lead to Success for WTO Talks," *Los Angeles Times*, November 14, 2001, p. A1, and "Seeds Sown for Future Growth," *The Economist*, November 17, 2001, pp. 65–66.

15. United Nations, World Investment Report, 2002 (New York and Geneva: United Nations, 2002).

16. World Trade Organization, *International Trade Trends and Statistics, 2002* (Geneva: WTO, 2002).

17. World Trade Organization, *Annual Report 2002* (Geneva: WTO Secretariat, May 2002).

18. WTO Press Release, "Trade Recovered in 2002, but Uncertainty Continues," April 22, 2003.

19. United Nations, *World Investment Report, 2001* (New York and Geneva: United Nations, 2001), and UN press release, "World FDI Flows Exceed US $1.1 Trillion in 2000," December 7, 2000.

20. United Nations, *World Investment Report, 2002* (New York and Geneva: United Nations, 2002), and United Nations, "UNCTAD Predicts 27% Drop in FDI Flows This Year," United Nations Press Release TAD/INF/PR/63 date 24/10/2002.

21. World Trade Organization, *Annual Report 2000* (Geneva: WTO, 2000), and United Nations, *World Investment Report, 2001* (New York and Geneva: United Nations, 2001).

22. United Nations, *World Investment Report, 2002*.

23. World Trade Organization, "Beyond Borders: Managing a World of Free Trade and Deep In-

terdependence," press release 55, September 10, 1996.

24. Moore's Law is named after Intel founder Gordon Moore.

25. Frankel, "Globalization of the Economy."

26. J. G. Fernald and V. Greenfield, "The Fall and Rise of the Global Economy", *Chicago Fed Letters*, April 2001, pp. 1–4.

27. Data compiled from various sources and listed by CyberAtlas at http://cyberatlas.internet.com/big_picture/.

28. Data on the number of host computers can be found at http://www.nw.com/zone/WWW/report.html.

29. CyberAtlas at http://cyberatlas.internet.com/big_picture/.

30. Ibid.

31. Http://www.forrester.com/ER/Press/ForrFind/0,1768,0,00.html.

32. For a counterpoint, see "Geography and the Net: Putting It in Its Place," *The Economist*, August 11, 2001, pp. 18–20.

33. M. Dickerson, "All Those Inflated Expectations Aside, Many Firms Are Finding the Internet Invaluable in Pursuing International Trade," *Los Angeles Times*, October 14, 1998, p. 10. The company's website is http://www.cardiacscience.com.

34. A. Stewart, "Easier Access to World Markets," *Financial Times*, December 3, 1997, p. 8.

35. Frankel, "Globalization of the Economy."

36. Data from Bureau of Transportation Statistics, 2001.

37. Fernald and Greenfield, "The Fall and Rise of the Global Economy."

38. "War of the Worlds," *The Economist: A Survey of the Global Economy*, October 1, 1994, pp. 3–4.

39. Ibid.

40. United Nations, *World Investment Report, 2002*.

41. Ibid.

42. Ibid.

43. S. Chetty, "Explosive International Growth and Problems of Success among Small and Medium Sized Firms," *International Small Business Journal*, February 2003, pp. 5–28.

44. R. A. Mosbacher, "Opening Up Export Doors for Smaller Firms," *Seattle Times*, July 24, 1991, p. A7.

45. "Small Companies Learn How to Sell to the Japanese," *Seattle Times*, March 19, 1992.

46. Holstein, "Why Johann Can Export but Johnny Can't."

47. J. E. Stiglitz, *Globalization and Its Discontents* (New York: W. W. Norton, 2003).

48. See, for example, Ravi Batra, *The Myth of Free Trade* (New York: Touchstone Books, 1993); William Greider, *One World, Ready or Not: The Manic Logic of Global Capitalism* (New York: Simon and Schuster, 1997); and D. Radrik, *Has Globalization Gone Too Far?* (Washington, DC: Institution for International Economics, 1997).

49. James Goldsmith, "The Winners and the Losers," in *The Case against the Global Economy*, ed. J. Mander and E. Goldsmith (San Francisco: The Sierra Book Club, 1996).

50. D. L. Bartlett and J. B. Steele, "America: Who Stole the Dream," *Philadelphia Inquirer*, September 9, 1996.

51. For example, see Paul Krugman, *Pop Internationalism* (Cambridge, MA: MIT Press, 1996).

52. Peter Gottschalk and Timothy M. Smeeding, "Cross-National Comparisons of Earnings and Income Inequality," *Journal of Economic Literature* 35 (June 1997), pp. 633–87, and Susan M. Collins, *Exports, Imports, and the American Worker* (Washington, DC: Brookings Institution, 1998).

53. Organization for Economic Cooperation and Development, "Income Distribution in OECD Countries," OECD Policy Studies, no. 18 (October 1995).

54. "A Survey of Pay. Winner and Losers," *The Economist*, May 8, 1999, pp. 5–8.

55. See Krugman, *Pop Internationalism*, and D. Belman and T. M. Lee, "International Trade and the Performance of US Labor Markets," in *U.S. Trade Policy and Global Growth*, ed. R. A. Blecker (New York: Economic Policy Institute, 1996).

56. See Robert Lerman, "Is Earnings Inequality Really Increasing? Economic Restructuring and the Job Market," Brief No. 1 (Washington, DC: Urban Institute, March 1997).

57. "A Survey of Pay. Winner and Losers."

58. E. Goldsmith, "Global Trade and the Environment."

59. P. Choate, *Jobs at Risk: Vulnerable U.S. Industries and Jobs under NAFTA* (Washington, DC: Manufacturing Policy Project, 1993).

60. Ibid.

61. B. Lomborg, *The Skeptical Environmentalist* (Cambridge: Cambridge University Press, 2001).

62. H. Nordstrom and S. Vaughan, *Trade and the Environment, World Trade Organization Special Studies No. 4* (Geneva: WTO, 1999).

63. Figures are from "Freedom's Journey: A Survey of the 20th Century. Our Durable Planet," *The Economist*, September 11, 1999, p. 30.

64. Krugman, *Pop Internationalism*.

65. R. Kuttner, "Managed Trade and Economic Sovereignty," in *U.S. Trade Policy and Global Growth*, ed. R. A. Blecker (New York: Economic Policy Institute, 1996).

66. Ralph Nader and Lori Wallach, "GATT, NAFTA, and the Subversion of the Democratic Process," in *US Trade Policy and Global Growth*, ed. R. A. Blecker (New York: Economic Policy Institute, 1996), pp. 93–94.

67. Lant Pritchett, "Divergence, Big Time," *Journal of Economic Perspectives* 11, no. 3 (Summer 1997), pp. 3–18.

68. Ibid.

69. W. Easterly, "How Did Heavily Indebted Poor Countries Become Heavily Indebted?" *World Development*, October 2002, pp. 1677–96.

70. See D. Ben-David, H. Nordstrom, and L. A. Winters, *Trade, Income Disparity and Poverty. World Trade Organization Special Studies No. 5* (Geneva: WTO, 1999).

71. William Easterly, "Debt Relief," *Foreign Policy*, November–December 2001, pp. 20–26.

72. Jeffrey Sachs, "Sachs on Development: Helping the World's Poorest," *The Economist*, August 14, 1999, pp. 17–20.

73. Easterly, "Debt Relief."

Research Task | globalEDGE™   globaledge.msu.edu

Use the globalEDGE™ site to complete the following exercises:

1. Your company has developed a new product that is expected to achieve high penetration rates in all the countries where it is introduced, regardless of the average income status of the local populace. Considering the costs of the product launch, the management team has decided to initially introduce the product only in countries that have a sizeable population base. You are required to prepare a preliminary report with the top ten countries of the world in terms of population size. Since growth opportunities are another major

concern, the average population growth rates should also be listed for management's consideration.

2. You are working for a company that is considering investing in a foreign country. Management has requested a report regarding the attractiveness of alternative countries based on the potential re-

turn of FDI. Accordingly, the ranking of the top 25 countries in terms of FDI attractiveness is a crucial ingredient for your report. A colleague mentioned a potentially useful tool called the "FDI Confidence Index," which is updated periodically. Find this index, and provide additional information regarding how the index is constructed.

Closing Case

Ecuadorean Valentine Roses

It is 6:20 A.M. February 7, 2003, in the Ecuadorean town of Cayambe, and Maria Pacheco has just been dropped off for work by the company bus. She pulls on thick rubber gloves, wraps an apron over her white, traditional embroidered dress, and grabs her clippers, ready for another long day. Any other time of year, Maria would work until 2 P.M., but it's a week before Valentine's Day, and Maria along with her 84 co-workers at the farm are likely to be busy until 5 P.M. By then, Maria will have cut more than 1,000 rose stems.

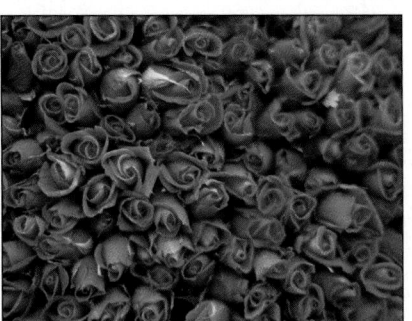

A few days later, after they have been refrigerated and shipped via aircraft, the roses Maria cut will be selling for premium prices in stores from New York to London. Ecuadorean roses are quickly becoming the Rolls-Royce of roses. They have huge heads and unusually vibrant colors, including 10 different reds, from bleeding heart crimson to a rosy lover's blush.

Most of Ecuador's 460 or so rose farms are located in the Cayambe and Cotopaxi regions, 10,000 feet up in the Andes about an hour's drive from the capital, Quito. The rose bushes are planted in huge flat fields at the foot of snow-capped volcanoes that rise to more than 20,000 feet. The bushes are protected by 20-foot-high canopies of plastic sheeting. The combination of intense sunlight, fertile volcanic soil, an equatorial location, and high altitude makes for ideal growing conditions, allowing roses to flower almost year-round.

Ecuador's rose industry started some 20 years ago, and has been expanding rapidly since. Ecuador is now the world's fourth largest producer of roses. Roses are the nation's fifth largest export, with customers all over the world. Rose farms generate $240 million in sales and support tens of thousands in jobs. In Cayambe, the population has increased in 10 years from 10,000 to 70,000, primarily as a result of the rose industry. The revenues and taxes from rose growers have helped to pave roads, build schools, and construct sophisticated irrigation systems. This year construction will begin on an international airport between Quito

and Cayambe from which Ecuadorean roses will begin their journey to flower shops all over the world.

Maria works Monday to Saturday, and earns $210 a month, which she says is an average wage in Ecuador and substantially above the country's $120 a month minimum wage. The farm also provides her with health care and a pension. By employing women such as Maria, the industry has fostered a social revolution in which mothers and wives have more control over their family's spending, especially on schooling for their children.

For all of the benefits that roses have bought to Ecuador, where the gross national income per capita is only $1,080 a year, the industry has come under fire from environmentalists. Large growers have been accused of misusing a toxic mixture of pesticides, fungicides, and fumigants to grow and export unblemished pest-free flowers. Reports claim that workers often fumigate roses in street clothes without protective equipment. Some doctors and scientists claim that many of the industry's 50,000 employees have serious health problems as a result of exposure to toxic chemicals. A 1999 study published by the International Labor Organization claimed that women in the industry had more miscarriages than average and that some 60 percent of all workers suffered from headaches, nausea, blurred vision, and fatigue. Still, the critics acknowledge that their studies have been hindered by a lack of access to the farms, and they do not know what the true situation is. The International Labor Organization has also claimed that some rose growers in Ecuador use child labor, a claim that has been strenuously rejected by both the growers and Ecuadorean government agencies.

In Europe, consumer groups have urged the European Union to press for improvements in environmental safeguards. In response, some Ecuadorean growers have joined a voluntary program aimed at helping customers identify responsible growers. The certification signifies that the grower has distributed protective gear, given training in using chemicals, and hired doctors to visit workers at least weekly. Other environmental groups have pushed for stronger sanctions, including trade sanctions, against

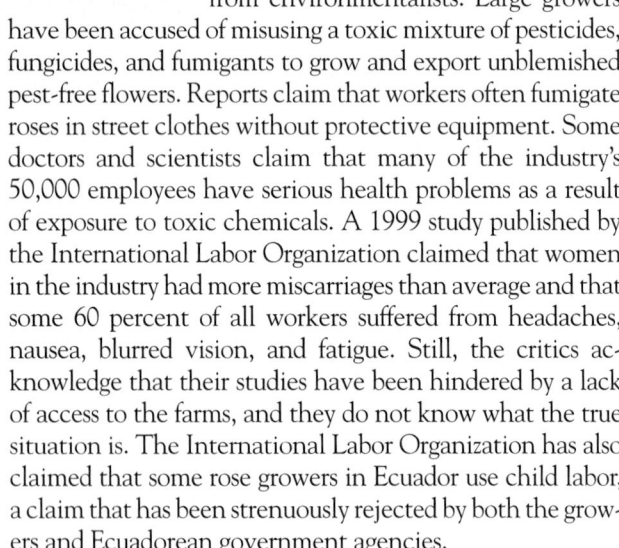

Ecuadorean rose growers that are not environmentally certified by a reputable agency. On February 14, however, most consumers are oblivious to these issues; they simply want to show their appreciation to their wives and girlfriends with a perfect bunch of roses.

Case Discussion Questions

1. How has participation in the international rose trade helped Ecuador's economy and its people? How has the rise of Ecuador as a center for rose growing benefited consumers in developed nations who purchase the roses? What do the answers to these questions tell you about the benefits of international trade?

2. Why do you think that Ecuador's rose industry only began to take off 20 years ago? Why do you think it has grown so rapidly?

3. To what extent can the alleged health problems among workers in Ecuador's rose industry be laid at the feet of consumers in the developed world and their desire for perfect Valentine's Day roses?

4. Do you think governments in the developed world should place trade sanctions on Ecuador roses if reports of health issues among Ecuadorean rose workers are verified? What else might they do to improve the situation in Ecuador?

Sources: G. Thompson, "Behind Roses' Beauty, Poor and Ill Workers," *New York Times*, February 13, 2003, pp. A1, A27; J. Stuart, "You've Come a Long Way Baby," *The Independent*, February 14, 2003, p. 1; V. Marino, "By Any Other Name, It's Usually a Rosa," *New York Times*, May 11, 2003, p. A9; and A. DePalma, "In Trade Issue, the Pressure Is on Flowers," *New York Times*, January 24, 2002, p. 1.

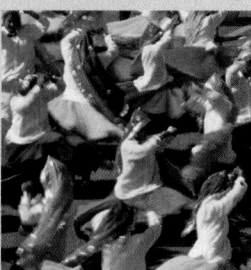

Part 2

Country Factors

Chapter 2
National Differences in Political Economy

Chapter 3
Differences in Culture

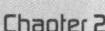

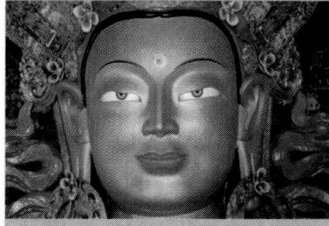

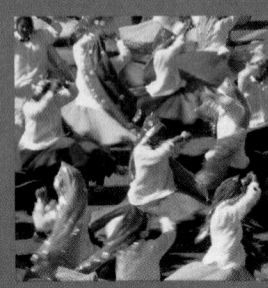

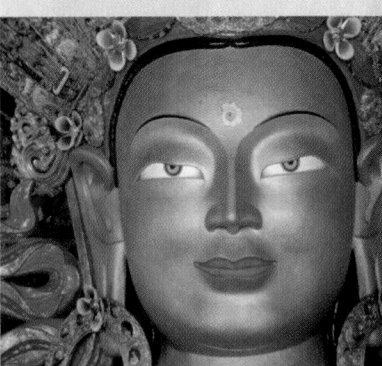

Chapter 2

National Differences in Political Economy

Introduction
Political Systems
  Collectivism and Individualism
  Democracy and Totalitarianism
Economic Systems
  Market Economy
  Command Economy
  Mixed Economy
Legal Systems
  Different Legal Systems
  Differences in Contract Law
  Property Rights
  The Protection of Intellectual Property
  Product Safety and Product Liability
The Determinants of Economic
Development
  Differences in Economic Development
  Broader Conceptions of Development:
  Amartya Sen
  Political Economy and Economic
  Progress
  Geography, Education, and Economic
  Development
States in Transition
  The Spread of Democracy
  The New World Order and Global
  Terrorism
  The Spread of Market-Based Systems
  The Nature of Economic
  Transformation
  Implications
Focus on Managerial Implications
  Attractiveness
  Ethics and Regulations
Chapter Summary
Critical Discussion Questions
Closing Case: Piracy in the Video Game
Market

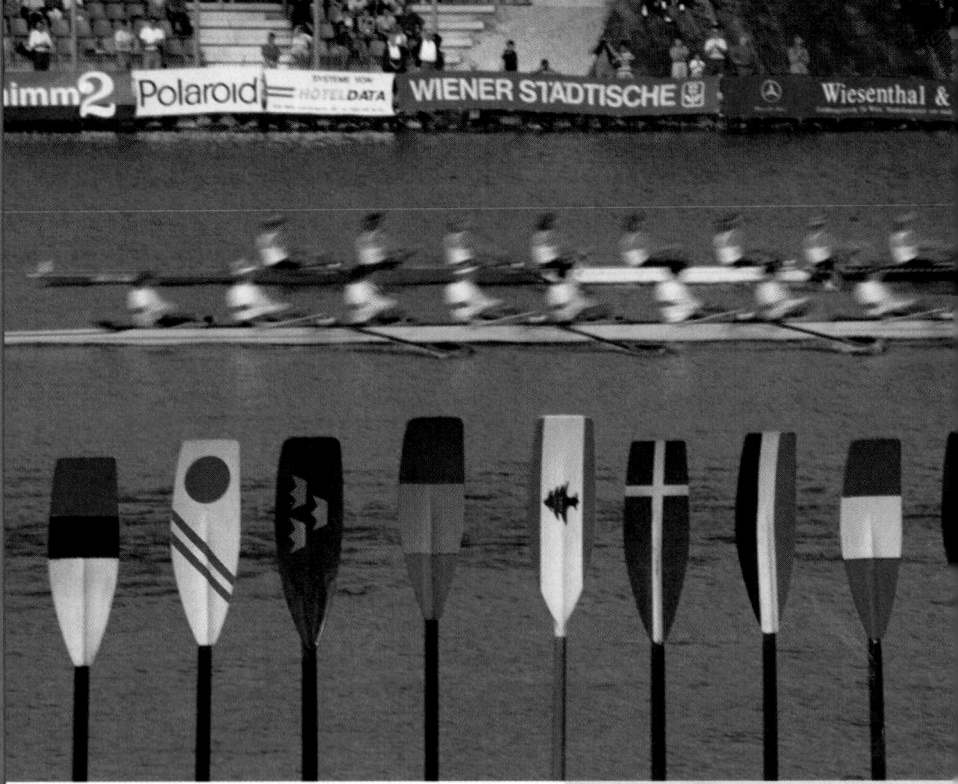

India's Changing Political Economy

After gaining independence from Britain in 1947, India adopted a democratic system of government. The economic system that developed in India after 1947 was a mixed economy characterized by a large number of state-owned enterprises (of which there were almost 300 in 1991), centralized planning, and subsidies. This system constrained the growth of the private sector. Private companies could expand only with government permission. Under this system, dubbed the "License Raj," private companies often had to wait months for government approval of routine business activities, such as expanding production or hiring a new director. It could take years to get permission to diversify into a new product. Much of heavy industry, such as auto, chemical, and steel production, was reserved for state-owned enterprises. Production quotas and high import tariffs also stunted the development of a healthy private sector, as did restrictive labor laws that made it difficult to fire employees. Access to foreign exchange was limited, investment by foreign firms was severely restricted, land use was strictly controlled, and the government routinely managed prices as opposed to letting them be set by market forces.

By the early 1990s, it was clear that after 40 years of near stagnation, this system was incapable of delivering the kind of economic progress that many Southeastern Asian nations had started to enjoy. In 1994, India's economy was still smaller than Belgium's, despite having a population of 950 million. Its GDP per capita was a paltry $310; less than half the population could read; only 6 million had access to telephones; only 14 percent had access to clean sanitation; the World Bank estimated that some 40 percent of the world's desperately poor lived in India; and only 2.3 percent of the population had a household income in excess of $2,484.

In 1991, the lack of progress led the government to embark on an ambitious economic reform program. Much of the industrial licensing system was dismantled, and several areas once closed to the private sector were opened, including electricity generation, parts of the oil industry, steelmaking, air transport, and some areas of the telecommunications industry. Investment by foreign companies, formerly allowed only grudgingly and subject to arbitrary ceilings, was suddenly welcomed. Approval was made automatic for foreign equity stakes of up to 51 percent in an Indian enterprise, and 100 percent foreign ownership was allowed under certain circumstances. Raw materials and many industrial goods could be freely imported, and the maximum tariff that could be levied on imports was reduced from 400 percent to 65 percent. The top income tax rate was also reduced, and corporate tax fell from 57.5 percent to 46 percent in 1994, and then to 35 percent in 1997.

The government also announced plans to start privatizing India's state-owned businesses, some 40 percent of which were losing money in the early 1990s. The privatization program has had a bumpy record in India, often slowed by political opposition. In 1999, there were still some 240 state-owned enterprises scattered across many sectors of the economy that accounted for 15 percent of India's gross domestic product. Nevertheless, by the early 2000s the program was progressing at a fairly rapid pace with about 30 state-owned enterprises privatized in 2002 alone.

Judged by some measures, the response to these economic reforms has been impressive. The economy expanded at an annual rate of about 6.1 percent throughout the 1990s. Despite the slowdown in global economic activity after 2000, India still managed to grow 5.5 percent annually during 2000–2002. Foreign investment, a key indicator of the economy's attractiveness, jumped from $150 million in 1991 to an estimated $3.5 billion in 1997, hit a record $5 billion in 2001, and was forecast to exceed this in 2002. Some sectors of the economy have done particularly well, such as the information technology sector in which India has emerged as a vibrant global center for software development. The export revenue of India's software services market reached $6.2 billion in 2002, up from less than $500 million in the mid-1990s.

However, the country still has a long way to go. Attempts to further reduce import tariffs have been stalled by political opposition from employers, employees, and politicians, who fear that if barriers come down, a flood of inexpensive Chinese products will enter India. There has also been strong resistance to reforming many of India's laws that make it difficult for private business to operate efficiently. For example, labor laws make it almost impossible for firms with more than 100 employees to fire workers. Other laws mandate that certain products can be manufactured only by small companies, effectively prohibiting companies in these industries from attaining the scale required to compete internationally.

Also, a decade of reform has done little to solve India's crippling poverty problem. Although the Indian middle class grew richer during the 1990s, by 2002 some 40 percent of India's nearly 1 billion people still lived in abject poverty, earning less than $1 a day, a figure little changed from 1990. By 2002, the gross domestic product per capita of India was still only $450, which ranked India at 164 among the world's nations; 44 percent of the adult population was illiterate; 19 percent of Indians had no access to safe water supplies; 25 percent had no access to health services; 71 percent had no access to sanitation; and 16 percent of the population was not expected to survive to age 40!

Sources: "A Survey of India: The Tiger Steps Out," *The Economist,* January 21, 1995; P. Moore, "Three Steps Forward," *Euromoney,* September 1997, pp. 190–95; "India's Breakthrough Budget?" *The Economist,* March 3, 2001; Shankar Aiyar, "Reforms: Time to Just Do It," *India Today,* January 24, 2000, p. 47; "America's Pain, India's Gain," *The Economist,* January 11, 2003, p. 57; and Joanna Slater, "In Once Socialist India, Privatizations Are Becoming More Like Routine Matters," *Wall Street Journal,* July 5, 2002, p. A8.

◼ Introduction

As noted in Chapter 1, international business is much more complicated than domestic business because countries differ in many ways. Countries have different political, economic, and legal systems. Cultural practices can vary dramatically from country to country, as can the education and skill level of the population, and countries are at different stages of economic development. All these differences can and do have major implications for the practice of international business. They have a profound impact on the benefits, costs, and risks associated with doing business in different countries; the way in which operations in different countries should be managed; and the strategy international firms should pursue in different countries. A main function of this chapter and the next is to develop an awareness of and appreciation for the significance of country differences in political systems, economic systems, legal systems, and national culture. Another function of this chapter and the next is to describe how the political, economic, legal, and cultural systems of many of the world's nation-states are evolving and to explain the implications of these changes for the practice of international business.

The opening case illustrates the changes occurring in the political and economic systems of one nation, India. As in many other countries, since the early 1990s political and economic ideology in India has shifted away from state planning and toward a free market orientation. One consequence of this shift in ideology has been adoption of an economic reform program that includes as its main elements the privatization of state-owned enterprises, the removal of subsidies, the repeal of laws that hamstring private business practice, and the removal of barriers to foreign investment and trade. This program has made India a more attractive location for international businesses, thus increasing foreign investment in India.

However, as the opening case makes clear, while the Indian program has had some success, it has also run into roadblocks and has yet to alleviate the poverty that afflicts so much of the nation's population. Advocates of economic reform will claim that India's program has so far achieved only partial success because political opposition has significantly slowed the pace of reform. There is probably much truth to this claim. At the same time, the combination of political and cultural legacies and current realities in India is such that rapid reform would be difficult even under the most pro-reform government. This is not unique to India. The pace of reform in many countries is determined by the interplay between the economic goals of the reformers and the political and cultural realities of the country.

The Indian example suggests that the economic, political, legal, and cultural systems of a country are not independent of each other. After all, politicians write the laws that help to shape economic activity in a nation-state, and politicians, like all of us, are influenced by the prevailing culture or cultures of their nation. To understand the economic prospects of a nation such as India and to appreciate its importance to international business, we must also understand the interplay between the political, economic, legal, and cultural systems prevailing in that country.

This chapter focuses on how the political, economic, and legal systems of countries differ. Collectively we refer to these systems as constituting the political economy of a country. We use the term **political economy** to stress that the political, economic, and legal systems of a country are not independent of each other. They interact and influence each other, and in doing so they affect the level of economic well-being in a country. In addition to reviewing these systems, we also explore how differences in political economy influence the benefits, costs, and risks associated with doing business in different countries, and how they affect management practice and strategy. In the next chapter we will look at how differences in culture influence the practice of international business. The political economy and culture of a nation are not independent of each other. As will become apparent in Chapter 3, culture can exert an impact on political economy—on political, economic, and legal systems in a nation—and the converse can also hold true.

Political Systems ■

The economic and legal systems of a country are shaped by its political system.[1] As such, it is important that we understand the nature of different political systems before discussing economic and legal systems. By **political system** we mean the system of government in a nation. Political systems can be assessed according to two related dimensions. The first is the degree to which they emphasize collectivism as opposed to individualism. The second dimension is the degree to which they are democratic or totalitarian. These dimensions are interrelated; systems that emphasize collectivism tend toward totalitarian, while systems that place a high value on individualism tend to be democratic. However, a large gray area exists in the middle. It is possible to have democratic societies that emphasize a mix of collectivism and individualism. Similarly, it is possible to have totalitarian societies that are not collectivist.

Collectivism and Individualism

The term **collectivism** refers to a political system that stresses the primacy of collective goals over individual goals.[2] When collectivism is emphasized, the needs of society as a whole are generally viewed as being more important than individual freedoms. In such circumstances, an individual's right to do something may be restricted on the grounds that it runs counter to "the good of society" or to "the common good." Advocacy of collectivism can be traced to the ancient Greek philosopher Plato (427–347 B.C.), who in *The Republic* argued that individual rights should be sacrificed for the good of the majority and that property should be owned in common. Plato did not equate collectivism with equality; he believed that society should be stratified into classes, with those best suited to rule (which for Plato, naturally, were philosophers and soldiers) administering society for the benefit of all. In modern times, the collectivist mantle has been picked up by socialists.

Socialism

Modern socialists trace their intellectual roots to Karl Marx (1818–1883), although socialist thought clearly predates Marx (elements of it can be traced back to Plato). Marx argued that the few benefit at the expense of the many in a capitalist society where individual freedoms are not restricted. While successful capitalists accumulate considerable wealth, Marx postulated that the wages earned by the majority of workers in a capitalist society would be forced down to subsistence levels. Marx argued that capitalists expropriate for their own use the value created by workers, while paying workers only subsistence wages in return. Put another way, according to Marx, the pay of workers does not reflect the full value of their labor. To correct this perceived wrong, Marx advocated state ownership of the basic means of production, distribution, and exchange (i.e., businesses). His logic was that if the state owned the means of production, the state could ensure that workers were fully compensated for their labor. Thus, the idea is to manage state-owned enterprise to benefit society as a whole, rather than individual capitalists.[3]

In the early 20th century, the socialist ideology split into two broad camps. The **communists** believed that socialism could be achieved only through violent revolution and totalitarian dictatorship, while the **social democrats** committed themselves to achieving socialism by democratic means and turned their backs on violent revolution and dictatorship. Both versions of socialism waxed and waned during the 20th century. The communist version of socialism reached its high point in the late 1970s, when the majority of the world's population lived in communist states. The countries under Communist Party rule at that time included the former Soviet Union; its Eastern European client nations (e.g., Poland, Czechoslovakia, Hungary); China; the Southeast Asian nations of Cambodia, Laos, and Vietnam; various African nations (e.g., Angola, Mozambique); and the Latin American nations of Cuba and Nicaragua. By the mid-1990s, however, communism was in retreat worldwide. The Soviet Union had collapsed and been replaced by a collection of 15 republics, most of which were at least nominally structured as democracies. Communism was swept out of Eastern Europe by the largely bloodless revolutions of 1989. Many believe it is now only a matter of time before communism collapses in China, the last major Communist power left. Although China is still nominally a communist state with substantial limits to individual political freedom, in the economic sphere the country has moved sharply away from strict adherence to communist ideology.[4] Apart from China, communism hangs on only in some small states, such as North Korea and Cuba.

Social democracy also seems to have passed a high-water mark, although the ideology may prove to be more enduring than communism. Social democracy has had perhaps its greatest influence in a number of democratic Western nations including Australia, Great Britain, France, Germany, Norway, Spain, and Sweden, where social democratic parties have from time to time held political power. Other countries where social democracy has had an important influence include India and Brazil. Consistent with their Marxists roots, many social democratic governments nationalized private companies in certain industries, transforming them into state-owned enterprises to be run for the "public good rather than private profit." In Great Britain, for example, by the end of the 1970s, state-owned companies had a monopoly in the telecommunications, electricity, gas, coal, railway, and shipbuilding industries, as well as substantial interests in the oil, airline, auto, and steel industries.

However, experience has demonstrated that state ownership of the means of production can run counter to the public interest. In many countries, state-owned companies have performed poorly. Protected from significant competition by their monopoly position and guaranteed government financial support, many state-owned companies became increasingly inefficient. In the end, individuals found themselves paying for the luxury of state ownership through higher prices and higher taxes. As a consequence, a number of Western democracies voted many social democratic parties out of office in the late 1970s and early 1980s. They were succeeded by political parties, such as Britain's Conservative Party and Germany's Christian Democratic Party, that were more committed to free market economics. These parties devoted considerable effort to selling state-owned enterprises to private investors (a process referred to as **privatization**). Even when social democratic parties have regained the levers of power, as in Great Britain in 1997 when the left-leaning Labor Party won control of the government, they now seem to be committed to greater private ownership.

Individualism

Individualism is the opposite of collectivism. In a political sense, individualism refers to a philosophy that an individual should have freedom in his or her economic and political pursuits. In contrast to collectivism, individualism stresses that the interests of the individual should take precedence over the interests of the state. Like collectivism, individualism can be traced to an ancient Greek philosopher, in this case Plato's disciple Aristotle (384–322 B.C.). In contrast to Plato, Aristotle argued that individual diversity and private ownership are desirable. In a passage that might have been taken from a speech by contemporary politicians who adhere to a free market ideology, he argued that private property is more highly productive than communal property and will thus stimulate progress. According to Aristotle, communal property receives little care, whereas property that is owned by an individual will receive the greatest care and therefore be most productive.

Individualism was reborn as an influential political philosophy in the Protestant trading nations of England and the Netherlands during the 16th century. The philosophy was refined in the work of a number of British philosophers including David Hume (1711–1776), Adam Smith (1723–1790), and John Stuart Mill (1806–1873). The philosophy of individualism exercised a profound influence on those in the American colonies who sought independence from Great Britain. Individualism underlies the ideas expressed in the Declaration of Independence. In more recent years, several Nobel prize-winning economists, including Milton Friedman, Friedrich von Hayek, and James Buchanan, have championed the philosophy.

Individualism is built on two central tenets. The first is an emphasis on the importance of guaranteeing individual freedom and self-expression. As John Stuart Mill put it,

> The sole end for which mankind are warranted, individually or collectively, in interfering with the liberty of action of any of their number is self-protection . . . The only purpose for which power can be rightfully exercised over any member of a civilized community, against his will, is to prevent harm to others. His own good, either physical or moral, is not a sufficient warrant . . . The only part of the conduct of any one, for which he is amenable to society, is that which concerns others. In the part which merely concerns himself, his independence is, of right, absolute. Over himself, over his own body and mind, the individual is sovereign.[5]

The second tenet of individualism is that the welfare of society is best served by letting people pursue their own economic self-interest, as opposed to some collective body (such as government) dictating what is in society's best interest. Or as Adam Smith put it in a famous passage from *The Wealth of Nations*, an individual who intends his own gain is

> led by an invisible hand to promote an end which was no part of his intention. Nor is it always worse for the society that it was no part of it. By pursuing his own interest he frequently promotes that of the society more effectually than when he really intends to promote it. I have never known much good done by those who effect to trade for the public good.[6]

The central message of individualism, therefore, is that individual economic and political freedoms are the ground rules on which a society should be based. This puts individualism in conflict with collectivism. Collectivism asserts the primacy of the collective over the individual, while individualism asserts the opposite. This underlying ideological conflict has shaped much of the recent history of the world. The Cold War, for example, was essentially a war between collectivism, championed by the now-defunct Soviet Union, and individualism, championed by the United States.

In practical terms, individualism translates into an advocacy for democratic political systems and free market economics. Viewed this way, we can see that since the late 1980s the waning of collectivism has been matched by the ascendancy of individualism. Democratic ideals and free market economics have swept away socialism and communism in many states. The changes of the past few years go beyond the revolutions in Eastern Europe and the former Soviet Union to include a move toward greater individualism in Latin America and in some of the social democratic states of the West (e.g., Great Britain and Sweden). This is not to claim that individualism has finally won a long battle with collectivism. It has clearly not. But as a guiding political philosophy, individualism has been on the ascendancy. This represents good news for international business, since in direct contrast to collectivism, the pro-business and pro-free trade values of individualism create a favorable environment within which international business can thrive.

| Democracy and Totalitarianism

Democracy and totalitarianism are at different ends of a political dimension. **Democracy** refers to a political system in which government is by the people, exercised either directly or through elected representatives. **Totalitarianism** is a form of government in which one person or political party exercises absolute control over all spheres of human life and opposing political parties are prohibited. The democratic–totalitarian dimension is not independent of the collectivism–individualism dimension. Democracy and individualism go hand in hand, as do the communist version of collectivism and totalitarianism. However, gray areas exist; it is possible to have a democratic state where collective values predominate, and it is possible to have a totalitarian state that is hostile to collectivism and in which some degree of individualism—particularly in the economic sphere—is encouraged. For example, China also has seen a move toward greater individual freedom in the economic sphere, but the country is still ruled by a totalitarian dictatorship.

Democracy

The pure form of democracy, as originally practiced by several city-states in ancient Greece, is based on a belief that citizens should be directly involved in decision making. In complex, advanced societies with populations in the tens or hundreds of millions this is impractical. Most modern democratic states practice what is commonly referred to as **representative democracy.** In a representative democracy, citizens periodically elect individuals to represent them. These elected representatives then form a government, whose function is to make decisions on behalf of the electorate. A representative democracy rests on the assumption that if elected representatives fail to perform this job adequately, they will be voted down at the next election.

To guarantee that elected representatives can be held accountable for their actions by the electorate, an ideal representative democracy has a number of safeguards that are typically enshrined in constitutional law. These include (1) an individual's right to freedom of expression, opinion, and organization; (2) a free media; (3) regular elections in which all eligible citizens are allowed to vote; (4) universal adult suffrage; (5) limited terms for elected representatives; (6) a fair court system that is independent from the political system; (7) a nonpolitical state bureaucracy; (8) a nonpolitical police force and armed service; and (9) relatively free access to state information.[7]

Totalitarianism

In a totalitarian country, all of the constitutional guarantees on which representative democracies are built—such as an individual's right to freedom of expression and organization, a free media, and regular elections—are denied to the citizens. In most totalitarian states, political repression is widespread and those who question the right of the rulers to rule find themselves imprisoned, or worse.

Four major forms of totalitarianism exist in the world today. Until recently the most widespread was **communist totalitarianism.** As discussed earlier, communism is a version of collectivism that advocates that socialism can be achieved only through totalitarian dictatorship. Communism, however, is in decline worldwide and many of the old Communist dictatorships have collapsed since 1989. The major exceptions to this trend (so far) are China, Vietnam, Laos, North Korea, and Cuba, although all of these states exhibit clear signs that the Communist Party's monopoly on political power is under attack.

A second form of totalitarianism might be labeled **theocratic totalitarianism.** Theocratic totalitarianism is found in states where political power is monopolized by a party, group, or individual that governs according to religious principles. The most common form of theocratic totalitarianism is based on Islam and is exemplified by states such as Iran and Saudi Arabia. These states limit freedom of political and religious expression while the laws of the state are based on Islamic principles.

A third form of totalitarianism might be referred to as **tribal totalitarianism.** Tribal totalitarianism has arisen from time to time in African countries such as Zimbabwe, Tanzania, Uganda, and Kenya. The borders of most African states reflect the administrative boundaries drawn by the old European colonial powers, rather than tribal realities. Consequently, the typical African country contains a number of tribes. Tribal totalitarianism occurs when a political party that represents the interests of a particular tribe (and not always the majority tribe) monopolizes power. Such one-party states still exist in Africa.

A fourth major form of totalitarianism might be described as **right-wing totalitarianism.** Right-wing totalitarianism generally permits some individual economic freedom but restricts individual political freedom on the grounds that it would lead to the rise of communism. One common feature of most right-wing dictatorships is an overt hostility to socialist or communist ideas. Many right-wing totalitarian governments are backed by the military, and in some cases the government may be made up of military officers. The fascist regimes that ruled Germany and Italy in the 1930s and 1940s were right-wing totalitarian states. Until the early 1980s, right-wing dictatorships, many of which were military dictatorships, were common throughout Latin America. They were also found in several Asian countries, particularly South Korea, Taiwan, Singapore, Indonesia, and the Philippines. Since the early 1980s, however, this form of government has been in retreat. Most Latin American countries are now genuine multiparty democracies. Similarly, South Korea, Taiwan, and the Philippines have become functioning democracies.

Economic Systems ■

The previous section shows that there is a connection between political ideology and economic systems. In countries where individual goals are given primacy over collective goals, we are more likely to find free market economic systems. In contrast, in countries where collective goals are given preeminence, the state may have taken control over many enterprises, and markets in such countries are likely to be restricted rather than free. We can identify three broad types of economic systems—a market economy, a command economy, and a mixed economy.

❚ Market Economy

In a pure market economy all productive activities are privately owned, as opposed to being owned by the state. The goods and services that a country produces, and the quantity in which they are produced, are not planned by anyone. Production is determined by the interaction of supply and demand and signaled to producers through the price system. If demand for a product exceeds supply, prices will rise, signaling producers to produce more. If supply exceeds demand, prices will fall, signaling producers to produce less. In this system consumers are sovereign. The purchasing patterns of consumers, as signaled to producers through the mechanism of the price system, determine what is produced and in what quantity.

For a market to work in this manner there must be no restrictions on supply. A restriction on supply occurs when a market is monopolized by a single firm. In such circumstances, rather than increase output in response to increased demand, a monopolist might restrict output and let prices rise. This allows the monopolist to take a greater profit margin on each unit it sells. Although this is good for the monopolist, it is bad for the consumer, who has to pay higher prices. It also is probably bad for the welfare of society. Since a monopolist has no competitors, it has no incentive to search for ways to lower production costs. Rather, it can simply pass on cost increases to consumers in the form of higher prices. The net result is that the monopolist is likely to become increasingly inefficient, producing high-priced, low-quality goods, while society suffers as a consequence.

Given the dangers inherent in monopoly, the role of government in a market economy is to encourage vigorous competition between private producers. Governments do this by outlawing monopolies and restrictive business practices designed to monopolize a market (antitrust laws serve this function in the United States). Private ownership also encourages vigorous competition and economic efficiency. Private ownership ensures that entrepreneurs have a right to the profits generated by their own efforts. This gives entrepreneurs an incentive to search for better ways of serving consumer needs. That may be through introducing new products, by developing more efficient production processes, by better marketing and after-sale service, or simply through managing their businesses more efficiently than their competitors. In turn, the constant improvement in product and process that results from such an incentive has been argued to have a major positive impact on economic growth and development.[8]

Command Economy

In a pure command economy, the goods and services that a country produces, the quantity in which they are produced, and the prices at which they are sold are all planned by the government. Consistent with the collectivist ideology, the objective of a command economy is for government to allocate resources for "the good of society." In addition, in a pure command economy, all businesses are state owned, the rationale being that the government can then direct them to make investments that are in the best interests of the nation as a whole, rather than in the interests of private individuals. Historically, command economies were found in communist countries where collectivist goals were given priority over individual goals. Since the decline of communism in the late 1980s, the number of command economies has fallen dramatically. Some elements of a command economy were also evident in a number of democratic nations led by socialist-inclined governments. France and India both experimented with extensive government planning and state ownership, although government planning has fallen into disfavor in both countries.

While the objective of a command economy is to mobilize economic resources for the public good, the opposite seems to have occurred. In a command economy, state-owned enterprises have little incentive to control costs and be efficient, because they cannot go out of business. Also, the abolition of private ownership means there is no incentive for individuals to look for better ways to serve consumer needs; hence, dynamism and innovation are absent from command economies. Instead of growing and becoming more prosperous, such economies tend to be characterized by stagnation.

Mixed Economy

Between market economies and command economies can be found mixed economies. In a mixed economy, certain sectors of the economy are left to private ownership and free market mechanisms while other sectors have significant state ownership and government planning. India, which was profiled in the opening case, has a mixed economy. Mixed economies were once very common throughout much of the world, although they are becoming much less so. Not too long ago, Great Britain, France, and Sweden were mixed economies, but extensive privatization has reduced state ownership of businesses in all three nations. As we saw in the opening case, a similar trend can be observed in India and in many other countries where there was once a large state sector, such as Brazil and Italy.

In mixed economies, governments also tend to take into state ownership troubled firms whose continued operation is thought to be vital to national interests. The

French automobile company Renault was state owned until recently. The government took over the company when it ran into serious financial problems. The French government reasoned that the social costs of the unemployment that might result if Renault collapsed were unacceptable, so it nationalized the company to save it from bankruptcy. Renault's competitors weren't thrilled by this move, since they had to compete with a company whose costs were subsidized by the state.

Legal Systems

The **legal system** of a country refers to the rules, or laws, that regulate behavior along with the processes by which the laws are enforced and through which redress for grievances is obtained. The legal system of a country is of immense importance to international business. A country's laws regulate business practice, define the manner in which business transactions are to be executed, and set down the rights and obligations of those involved in business transactions. The legal environments of countries differ in significant ways. As we shall see, differences in legal systems can affect the attractiveness of a country as an investment site and/or market.

Like the economic system of a country, the legal system is influenced by the prevailing political system (although it is also strongly influenced by historical tradition). The government of a country defines the legal framework within which firms do business—and often the laws that regulate business reflect the rulers' dominant political ideology. For example, collectivist-inclined totalitarian states tend to enact laws that severely restrict private enterprise, while the laws enacted by governments in democratic states where individualism is the dominant political philosophy tend to favor private enterprise and consumers.

Here we focus on several issues that illustrate how legal systems can vary—and how such variations can affect international business. First, we look at some basic differences in legal systems. Next we look at contract law. Third, we look at the laws governing property rights with particular reference to patents, copyrights, and trademarks. Fourth, we look at laws covering product safety and product liability.

Different Legal Systems

Three main types of legal systems—or legal tradition—are in use around the world: common law, civil law, and theocratic law.

Common Law

The common law system evolved in England over hundreds of years. It is now found in most of Great Britain's former colonies, including the United States. The **common law system** is based on tradition, precedent, and custom. *Tradition* refers to a country's legal history, *precedent* to cases that have come before the courts in the past, and *custom* to the ways in which laws are applied in specific situations. When law courts interpret common law, they do so with regard to these characteristics. This gives a common law system a degree of flexibility that other systems lack. Judges in a common law system have the power to *interpret* the law so that it applies to the unique circumstances of an individual case. In turn, each new interpretation sets a precedent that may be followed in future cases. As new precedents arise, laws may be altered, clarified, or amended to deal with new situations.

Civil Law

A **civil law system** is based on a very detailed set of laws organized into codes. When law courts interpret civil law, they do so with regard to these codes. More than 80 countries, including Germany, France, Japan, and Russia, operate with a civil law system. A civil law system tends to be less adversarial than a common law system because the judges rely upon detailed legal codes rather than tradition, precedent, and custom, which they interpret. A different way of looking at this is that judges under a civil law system have less *flexibility* than those under a common law system. Judges in a common law system have the power to *interpret* the law, while judges in a civil law system have the power only to *apply* the law.

Theocratic Law

A **theocratic law system** is one in which the law is based on religious teachings. Islamic law is the most widely practiced theocratic legal system in the modern world, although usage of both Hindu and Jewish law persisted into the 20th century. Islamic law is primarily a moral rather than a commercial law and is intended to govern all aspects of life.[9] The foundation for Islamic law is the holy book of Islam, the Koran, along with the Sunnah, or decisions and sayings of the Prophet Muhammad, and the writings of Islamic scholars who have derived rules by analogy from the principles established in the Koran and the Sunnah. Since the Koran and Sunnah are holy documents, the basic foundations of Islamic law cannot be changed. However, in practice Islamic jurists and scholars are constantly debating the application of Islamic law to the modern world. In reality, many Muslim countries have legal systems that are a blend of Islamic law and a common or civil law system.

Although Islamic law is primarily concerned with moral behavior, it has been extended to cover certain commercial activities. An example is the payment or receipt of interest, which is considered usury and outlawed by the Koran. To the devout Muslim, acceptance of interest payments is seen as a very grave sin; the giver and the taker are equally damned. This is not just a matter of theology; in several Islamic states it has also become a matter of law. In the 1990s, for example, Pakistan's Federal Shariat Court, the highest Islamic law-making body in the country, pronounced interest to be un-Islamic and therefore illegal and demanded that the government amend all financial laws accordingly. In 1999, Pakistan's Supreme Court ruled that Islamic banking methods should be used in the country after July 1, 2001.[10] By 2002, some 150 Islamic financial institutions in the world collectively managed over $200 billion in assets. In addition to Pakistan, Islamic banks are found in many of the Gulf states, Egypt, and Malaysia.[11]

❘ Differences in Contract Law

The difference between common law and civil law systems can be illustrated by the approach of each to contract law (remember, most theocratic legal systems also have elements of common or civil law). A **contract** is a document that specifies the conditions under which an exchange is to occur and details the rights and obligations of the parties involved. Many business transactions are regulated by some form of contract. **Contract law** is the body of law that governs contract enforcement. The parties to an agreement normally resort to contract law when one party believes the other has violated either the letter or the spirit of an agreement.

Because common law tends to be relatively ill specified, contracts drafted under a common law framework tend to be very detailed with all contingencies spelled out. In civil law systems, however, contracts tend to be much shorter and less specific because many of the issues typically covered in a common law contract are already covered in a civil code. As can be imagined, this implies that it is more expensive to draw up contracts in a common law jurisdiction, and that resolving contract disputes can be very adversarial in common law systems. On the other hand, common law systems have the advantage of greater flexibility and allow for judges to interpret a contract dispute in light of the prevailing situation. International businesses need to be sensitive to these differences since approaching a contract dispute in a state with a civil law system as if it had a common law system may backfire (and vice versa).

When contract disputes arise in international trade, there is always the question of which country's laws apply. To try to resolve this issue, a number of countries, including the United States, have ratified the **United Nations Convention on Contracts for the International Sale of Goods (CISG).** The CISG establishes a uniform set of rules governing certain aspects of the making and performance of commercial contracts between sellers and buyers who have their places of business in different nations. By adopting the CISG, a nation indicates it will treat the convention's rules as part of its law. The CISG applies automatically to all contracts for the sale of goods between different firms based in countries that have ratified the convention, unless the parties to the contract explicitly opt out. One problem with the CISG, however, is that only 61 nations have ratified the convention as of 2002 (the CISG went into effect in 1988).[12] Many of the world's larger trading nations, including Japan and the United Kingdom, have not ratified the CISG.

When firms do not wish to accept the CISG, they often opt for arbitration by a recognized arbitration court to settle contract disputes. The most well known of these is the International Court of Arbitration of the International Chamber of Commerce in Paris. In 2001, this court handled 566 requests for arbitration involving 1,492 parties from 116 countries.[13] The size of the disputes ranged from $50,000 to more than $1 billion.

Property Rights

In a legal sense, the term *property* refers to a resource over which an individual or business holds a legal title; that is, a resource is owned. Resources include land, buildings, equipment, capital, mineral rights, businesses, and intellectual property (such as patents, copyrights, and trademarks). **Property rights** refer to the bundle of legal rights over the use to which a resource is put and over the use made of any income that may be derived from that resource.[14] Countries differ significantly in the extent to which their legal system protects property rights. Although almost all countries have laws on their books that protect property rights, in many countries these laws are not well enforced by the authorities and property rights are violated. Property rights can be violated in two ways—through private action and through public action.

Private Action

Private action refers to theft, piracy, blackmail, and the like by private individuals or groups. While theft occurs in all countries, a weak legal system allows for a much higher level of criminal action in some than in others. For example, in the chaotic period in Russia following the collapse of communism, an outdated legal system, coupled with a weak police force and judicial system, offered both domestic and foreign businesses scant protection from blackmail by the "Russian Mafia." Successful business owners in Russia often had to pay "protection money" to the Mafia or face violent retribution, including bombings and assassinations (about 500 contract killings of businessmen occurred in 1995 and again in 1996).[15] Ivan Kivelidi, a banker and founder of the Russian Business Roundtable, was murdered by poison applied to the rim of his coffee cup. Vladislav Listiev, the head of Channel 1, Russia's largest nationwide TV network, announced in 1996 that he was going to remove unsavory elements (i.e., Mafia) from the network. Soon afterward he was gunned down by professional assassins outside his apartment building.[16]

While the situation in Russia has improved significantly since the mid-1990s, that country is not alone in having Mafia problems. The Mafia has a long history in the United States (Chicago in the 1930s was similar to Moscow in the 1990s). In Japan, the local version of the Mafia, known as the *yakuza*, runs protection rackets, particularly in the food and entertainment industries.[17] However, there was (and perhaps still is) a big difference between the magnitude of such activity in Russia and its limited impact in Japan and the United States. This difference arose because the legal enforcement apparatus, such as the police and court system, was so weak in Russia following the collapse of communism. Many other countries have had problems similar to or even greater than those experienced by Russia.

Figure 2.1

Rankings of Perceived
Corruption by Country
in 2000–2002

Source: Transparency International,
"Global Corruption Report 2003,"
www.transparency.org.

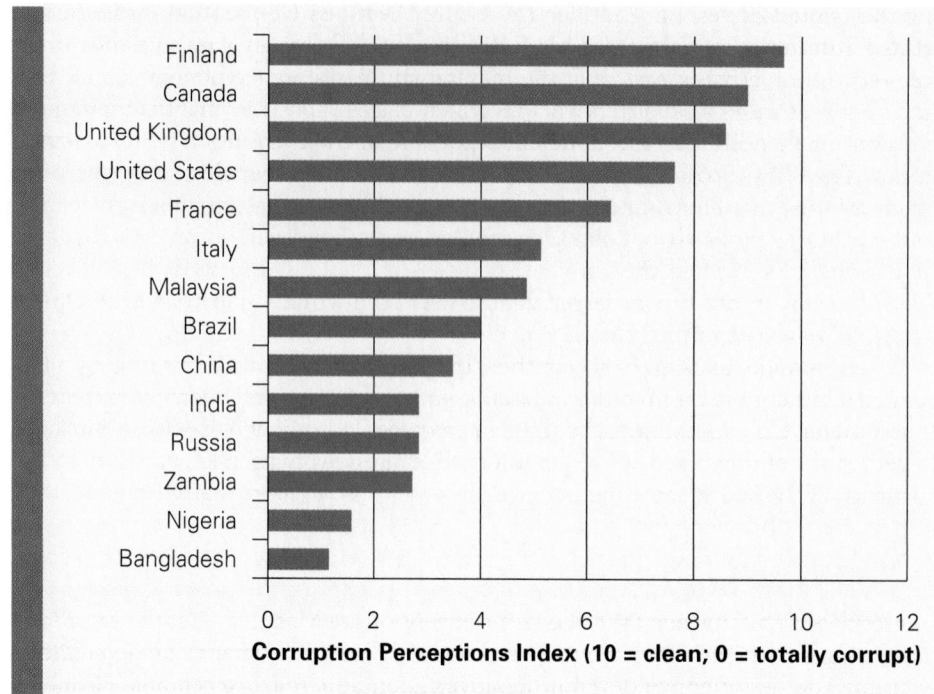

Public Action and Corruption

Public action to violate property rights occurs when public officials, such as politicians and government bureaucrats, extort income or resources from property holders. This can be done through a number of legal mechanisms such as levying excessive taxation, requiring expensive licenses or permits from property holders, or taking assets into state ownership without compensating the owners. It can also be done through illegal means, or corruption, by demanding bribes from businesses in return for the rights to operate in a country, industry, or location.[18] For example, the government of the late Ferdinand Marcos in the Philippines was famous for demanding bribes from foreign businesses wishing to set up operations in that country.[19] The same was true of government officials in Indonesia under the rule of ex-President Suharto.

Corruption has been well documented in every society, from the banks of the Congo River to the palace of the Dutch royal family, from Japanese politicians to Brazilian bankers, and from Indonesian government officials to the New York City Police Department. No society is immune to corruption. However, there are systematic differences in the extent of corruption across countries. In some countries, the rule of law is such that corruption is kept to a minimum. Corruption is seen and treated as illegal and, when discovered, violators are punished by the full force of the law. Unfortunately, in other countries, the rule of law is weak and corruption by bureaucrats and politicians is rife. Corruption is so endemic in some countries that politicians and bureaucrats regard it as a perk of office and openly flout laws against corruption. Transparency International, an independent nonprofit organization dedicated to exposing and fighting corruption, has measured the level of corruption among public officials in different countries.[20] As can be seen in Figure 2.1, the organization rated countries such as Finland and Canada as "very clean," while countries such as Russia, India, and Nigeria are seen as corrupt. Bangladesh ranked last out of all 102 countries in the survey, while Finland ranked first.

Economic evidence suggests that high levels of corruption significantly reduce the foreign direct investment, level of international trade, and economic growth rate in a country.[21] By siphoning off profits, corrupt politicians and bureaucrats reduce the returns to business investment and, hence, reduce the incentive that both domestic and foreign businesses have to invest in that country. The lower level of investment that results has a negative impact on economic growth. Thus, we would expect countries such as Nigeria and Russia to have a much lower economic growth rate than might otherwise have been the case. A detailed example of the negative effect that corruption can have on economic progress is given in the accompanying Country Focus, which looks at the impact of corruption on economic growth in Nigeria.

Foreign Corrupt Practices Act

The **Foreign Corrupt Practices Act** was passed in the United States during the 1970s following revelations that U.S. companies had bribed government officials in foreign countries in an attempt to win lucrative contracts. This law prohibits bribing a foreign government official in order to obtain or maintain business over which that foreign official has authority, and the law requires all publicly traded companies (whether or not they are involved in international trade) to keep records that are detailed enough to allow someone reviewing the records to determine whether a violation of the act has occurred.

The United States is unique in having this kind of law. Other countries have been far less willing to regulate how their firms do business abroad. The U.S. law is circumscribed with language that allows for exceptions.[22] Most notably, the act allows facilitating or expediting payments (also known as "grease payments") to expedite or to secure the performance of a routine governmental action. Acceptable payments might include, for example, payments made to speed up the issuance of permits or licenses, process paperwork, or just get vegetables off the dock and on their way to market. Congress's explanation for this exception to the general antibribery provisions of the act is the fact that while grease payments are, technically, bribes, they are distinguishable from (and, apparently, less offensive than) bribes used to obtain or maintain business, since they merely facilitate performance of duties that the recipients are already obligated to perform.

The Protection of Intellectual Property

Intellectual property refers to property that is the product of intellectual activity, such as computer software, a screenplay, a music score, or the chemical formula for a new drug. Ownership rights over intellectual property are established through patents, copyrights, and trademarks. A **patent** grants the inventor of a new product or process exclusive rights for a defined period to the manufacture, use, or sale of that invention. **Copyrights** are the exclusive legal rights of authors, composers, playwrights, artists, and publishers to publish and disperse their work as they see fit. **Trademarks** are designs and names, often officially registered, by which merchants or manufacturers designate and differentiate their products (e.g., Christian Dior clothes). In the high-technology "knowledge" economy of the 21st century, intellectual property has become an increasingly important source of economic value for businesses. Protecting intellectual property has also become increasingly problematic, particularly if it can be rendered in a digital form and then copied and distributed at very low cost via pirated CDs or over the Internet (e.g., computer software, music and video recordings).[23]

The philosophy behind intellectual property laws is to reward the originator of a new invention, book, musical record, clothes design, restaurant chain, and the like, for his or her idea and effort. Such laws are a very important stimulus to innovation and creative work. They provide an incentive for people to search for novel ways of doing things, and they reward creativity. For example, consider innovation in the pharmaceutical industry. A patent will grant the inventor of a new drug a 20-year monopoly in production of that drug. This gives pharmaceutical firms an incentive to undertake the expensive, difficult, and time-consuming basic research required to generate new drugs (it can cost $500 million in R&D and take 12 years to get a new drug on the market).

Country Focus

40 Years of Corruption in Nigeria

When Nigeria gained independence from Great Britain in 1960, there were hopes that the country might emerge as an economic heavyweight in Africa. Not only was Nigeria Africa's most populous country, but it was also blessed with abundant natural resources, particularly oil, which rose sharply in value in the 1970s following two rounds of oil price increases engineered by the Organization of Petroleum Exporting Countries (OPEC). Between 1970 and 2000, Nigeria earned more than $300 billion from the sale of oil, but at the end of this period it remained one of the poorest countries in the world. In 2000, gross national product per capita was just $300, 40 percent of the adult population was illiterate, life expectancy at birth was only 50 years, and the country was begging for relief on $30 billion in debt. The Human Development Index compiled by the United Nations ranked Nigeria 151 out of 174 countries covered.

What went wrong? Although there is no simple answer, a number of factors seem to have conspired to damage economic activity in Nigeria. The country is composed of several competing ethnic, tribal, and religious groups, and the conflict between them has limited political stability and led to political strife, including a brutal civil war in the 1970s. With the legitimacy of the government always in question, political leaders often purchased support by legitimizing bribes and by raiding the national treasury to reward allies. Civilian rule after independence was followed by a series of military dictatorships, each of which seemed more corrupt and inept than the last (the country returned to civilian rule in 1999).

The most recent military dictator, Sani Abacha, openly and systematically plundered the state treasury for his own personal gain. His most blatant scam was the Petroleum Trust Fund, which he set up in the mid-1990s ostensibly to channel extra revenue from an increase in fuel prices into much-needed infrastructure projects and other investments. The fund was not independently audited and almost none of the money that passed through it was properly accounted for. It was, in fact, a vehicle for Abacha and his supporters to spend a sum that in 1996 was equivalent to some 25 percent of the total federal budget. Abacha, aware of his position as an unpopular and unelected leader, lavished money on personal security and handed out bribes to those whose support he coveted. With examples like this at the very top of the government, it is not surprising that corruption could be found throughout the political and bureaucratic apparatus.

Some of the excesses were simply astounding. In the 1980s, an aluminum smelter was built on the orders of the government, which wanted to industrialize Nigeria. The cost of the smelter was $2.4 billion, some 60 to 100 percent higher than the cost of comparable plants elsewhere in the developed world. This high cost was widely interpreted to reflect the bribes that had to be paid to local politicians by the international contractors that built the plant. The smelter has never operated at more than a fraction of its intended capacity. Another example of corruption in Nigeria was the cement scandal of the early 1980s. At that time, the president announced a grand public housing project. Public officials promptly ordered vast quantities of cement from foreign contractors, taking a percentage of each contract in the form of a kickback. They ordered far more cement than was needed and more than Nigerian ports could cope with. Soon ships loaded with cement formed a line that stretched for several miles outside of Lagos harbor and that took months to unload. Meanwhile, the officials responsible were making a fortune from selling cement import licenses.

Sources: "A Tale of Two Giants," *The Economist, Nigeria: A Survey*, January 15, 2000, p. 5; J. Coolidge and S. Rose Ackerman, "High Level Rent Seeking and Corruption in African Regimes," *World Bank Policy Research Working Paper # 1780*, June 1997; and D. L. Bevan, P. Collier, and J. W. Gunning, *Nigeria and Indonesia: The Political Economy of Poverty, Equity and Growth* (Oxford: Oxford University Press, 1999).

Without the guarantees provided by patents, it is unlikely that companies would commit themselves to extensive basic research.[24]

The protection of intellectual property rights differs greatly from country to country. While many countries have stringent intellectual property regulations on their books, the enforcement of these regulations has often been lax. This has been the case even among some of the 96 countries that have signed the **Paris Convention for the Protection of Industrial Property,** an important international agreement to protect intellectual property. Weak enforcement encourages the piracy of intellectual property.

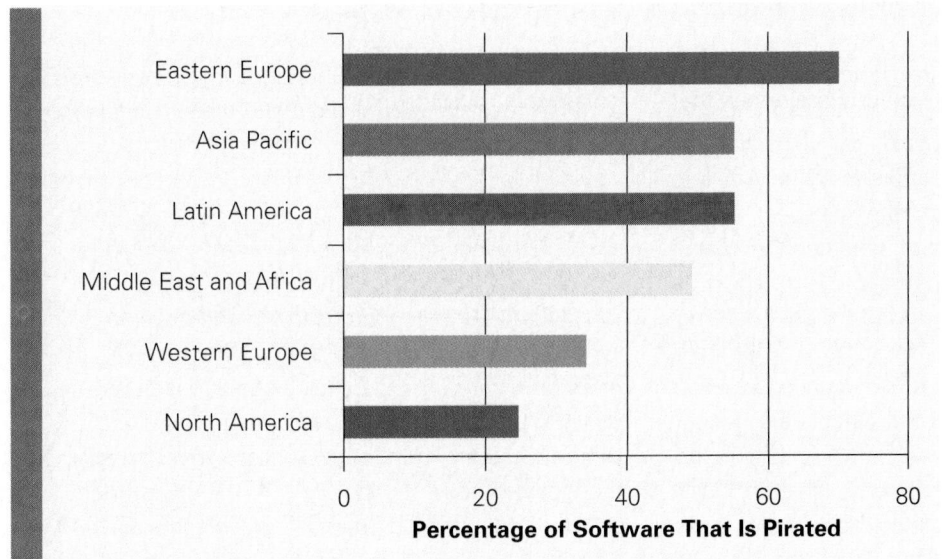

Figure 2.2

Regional Piracy Rates for Software in 2002

Source: Business Software Alliance, Eighth Annual Global Piracy Study, June 2003.

China and Thailand have recently been among the worst offenders in Asia. Pirated computer software is widely available in China. Similarly, the streets of Bangkok, Thailand's capital, are lined with stands selling pirated copies of Rolex watches, Levi's blue jeans, videotapes, and computer software.

Piracy in music recordings is rampant. The International Federation of the Phonographic Industry claims that 40 percent of all CDs and cassettes around the globe were illegally produced and sold in 2001, suggesting that piracy costs the industry more than $4.3 billion annually.[25] The computer software industry also suffers from lax enforcement of intellectual property rights. Estimates suggest that violations of intellectual property rights cost computer software firms revenues equal to $13.08 billion in 2002.[26] According to the Business Software Alliance, a software industry association, in 2002 some 39 percent of all software applications used in the world were pirated. The worst region was Eastern Europe, where the piracy rate was 71 percent (see Figure 2.2). One of the worst countries was China, where the piracy rate in 2002 ran 92 percent and cost the industry over $2.4 billion in lost sales, up from $444 million in 1995. Although the piracy rate was much lower in the United States, the value of sales lost was more significant because of the size of the market, reaching an estimated $2 billion in 2002.[27]

International businesses have a number of possible responses to violations of their intellectual property. Firms can lobby their respective governments to push for international agreements to ensure that intellectual property rights are protected and that the law is enforced. Partly as a result of such actions, international laws are being strengthened. As we shall see in Chapter 5, the most recent world trade agreement, which was signed in 1994, for the first time extends the scope of the General Agreement on Tariffs and Trade (GATT) to cover intellectual property. Under the new agreement, known as the **Trade Related Aspects of Intellectual Property Rights** (or **TRIPS**), as of 1995 a council of the World Trade Organization is overseeing enforcement of much stricter intellectual property regulations. These regulations oblige WTO members to grant and enforce patents lasting at least 20 years and copyrights lasting 50 years. Rich countries had to comply with the rules within a year. Poor countries, in which such protection generally was much weaker, had 5 years' grace, and the very poorest have 10 years.[28] (For further details of the TRIPS agreement, see Chapter 5.)

While many governments are increasing their enforcement of intellectual property rights and abiding by international agreements such as the WTO's TRIPS agreement,

Drug Patents and the AIDS Epidemic in South Africa

In December 1997, the government of South Africa passed a law that authorized two controversial practices. One, called parallel importing, allowed importers in South Africa to purchase drugs from the cheapest source available, regardless of whether the patent holders had given their approval or not. The other practice, called compulsory licensing, permitted the South African government to license local companies to produce cheaper versions of drugs whose patents are held by foreign companies. The law seems to violate international agreements to protect property rights, including the World Trade Organization TRIPS agreement. South Africa, however, insisted the law was necessary given its own health crisis and the high cost of patented medicines. South Africa is wrestling with an AIDS crisis of enormous proportions. Some 4.5 million of South Africa's 45 million people are infected with the HIV virus, more than in any other country.

Foreign drug manufacturers saw the law as an unbridled attempt to expropriate their intellectual property rights, and 39 foreign companies quickly filed a lawsuit in the country to try to block implementation of the law. Foreign pharmaceutical companies fear that South Africa is the thin end of the wedge, and if the law is allowed to stand, other countries will follow suit. Many U.S. companies also fear that if poor countries such as South Africa are allowed to buy low-priced drugs in violation of intellectual property laws, American and European consumers will soon demand the same. Drug companies argue that because drug development is a very expensive, time-consuming, and risky process, they need the protection of intellectual property laws to maintain the incentive to innovate. It can take $500 million and 12 years to develop a drug and bring it to market. Only one in five compounds that enter clinical trials actually become marketed drugs—the rest fail in trials due to poor efficacy or unfavorable side effects—and of those that make it to market, only 3 out of 10 earn profits that exceed their costs of cap-

ital. If drug companies could not count on high prices for their few successful products, the drug development process would dry up.

However, the drug companies do recognize that countries such as South Africa face special health challenges and lack the money to pay developed world prices. Accordingly, there is a long history in the industry of pricing drugs low in the developing world or giving them away. For example, AIDS drugs are sold to developing nations at an 80 to 90 percent discount over their prices in the United States. The South African government thought this was not good enough. The government has been supported by various human rights and AIDS organizations, which have cast the case as an attempt by the prosperous multinational drug companies of the West to maintain their intellectual property rights in the face of desperate attempts by an impoverished government to stem a deadly crisis. For their part, the drug companies have stated that the case has little to do with AIDS and is really about the right of South Africa to break international law.

While the drug companies may have international law on their side, the tie-in with the AIDS epidemic has clearly put them on the public relations defensive. After a blizzard of negative publicity, and little support from Western governments that wished to avoid this political "hot potato," in May 2002 the drug companies settled out of court with the South African government. Although the terms of the settlement were kept confidential, it was widely interpreted in the media as a defeat for the drug companies and a reaffirmation of the ability of the South African to enforce compulsory licensing.

Sources: H. Cooper, R. Zimmerman, and L. McGinley. "Patents Pending—AIDS Epidemic Traps Drug Firms in a Vise," *Wall Street Journal,* March 2, 2001, p. A1; R. Block, "Big Drug Firms Defend Right to Patent on AIDS Drugs in South African Courts," *Wall Street Journal,* March 6, 2001, p. A3; J. Jeter, "Trial Opens in South Africa AIDS Drug Suit," *Washington Post,* March 6, 2001, p. A1; and J. Nurton, "Overcoming the AIDS Hurdle," *Managing Intellectual Property,* June 2002, pp. 39–40.

some have recently taken a counterposition and seem to support the selective violation of intellectual property rights within their borders. In the late 1990s, the government of South Africa passed a law that allowed the country to import cheap generic versions of patented medicines, including powerful new drugs for treating AIDS, without permission from the patent owner. In 2001, this law became the focus of a legal battle between multinational drug companies seeking to protect their intellectual property rights, AIDS activists demanding access to inexpensive treatments for the poor, and the government of South Africa. The details of this case are discussed in the accompanying Management Focus. The case illustrates the difficult issues that international businesses can confront in nations that have different ideas about the value of intellectual property.

In addition to lobbying governments, firms may want to file lawsuits on their own behalf. They may also choose to stay out of countries where intellectual property laws are lax, rather than risk having their ideas stolen by local entrepreneurs (such reasoning partly underlay decisions by Coca-Cola Co. and IBM to pull out of India in the early 1970s). Firms also need to be on the alert to ensure that pirated copies of their products produced in countries where intellectual property laws are lax do not turn up in their home market or in third countries. U.S. computer software giant Microsoft, for example, discovered that pirated Microsoft software, produced illegally in Thailand, was being sold worldwide as the real thing (including in the United States). In addition, Microsoft has encountered significant problems with pirated software in China.

Product Safety and Product Liability

Product safety laws set certain safety standards to which a product must adhere. Product liability involves holding a firm and its officers responsible when a product causes injury, death, or damage. Product liability can be much greater if a product does not conform to required safety standards. There are both civil and criminal product liability laws. Civil laws call for payment and monetary damages. Criminal liability laws result in fines or imprisonment. Both civil and criminal liability laws are probably more extensive in the United States than in any other country, although many other Western nations also have comprehensive liability laws. Liability laws are typically least extensive in less developed nations. A boom in product liability suits and awards in the United States resulted in a dramatic increase in the cost of liability insurance. Many business executives argue that the high costs of liability insurance make American businesses less competitive in the global marketplace.

In addition to the competitiveness issue, country differences in product safety and liability laws raise an important ethical issue for firms doing business abroad. When product safety laws are tougher in a firm's home country than in a foreign country and/or when liability laws are more lax, should a firm doing business in that foreign country follow the more relaxed local standards or should it adhere to the standards of its home country? While the ethical thing to do is undoubtedly to adhere to home-country standards, firms have been known to take advantage of lax safety and liability laws to do business in a manner that would not be allowed back home.

The Determinants of Economic Development ■

The political, economic, and legal systems of a country can have a profound impact on the level of economic development and hence on the attractiveness of a country as a possible market and/or production location for a firm. Here we look first at how countries differ in their level of development. Then we look at how political economy affects economic progress.

Differences in Economic Development

Different countries have dramatically different levels of economic development. One common measure of economic development is a country's gross national income per head of population. GNI is regarded as a yardstick for the economic activity of a country; it measures the total annual income received by residents of a nation (GNI superseded gross national product, or GNP). Map 2.1 summarizes the GNI per capita of the world's nations in 2001. As can be seen, countries such as Japan, Sweden, Switzerland,

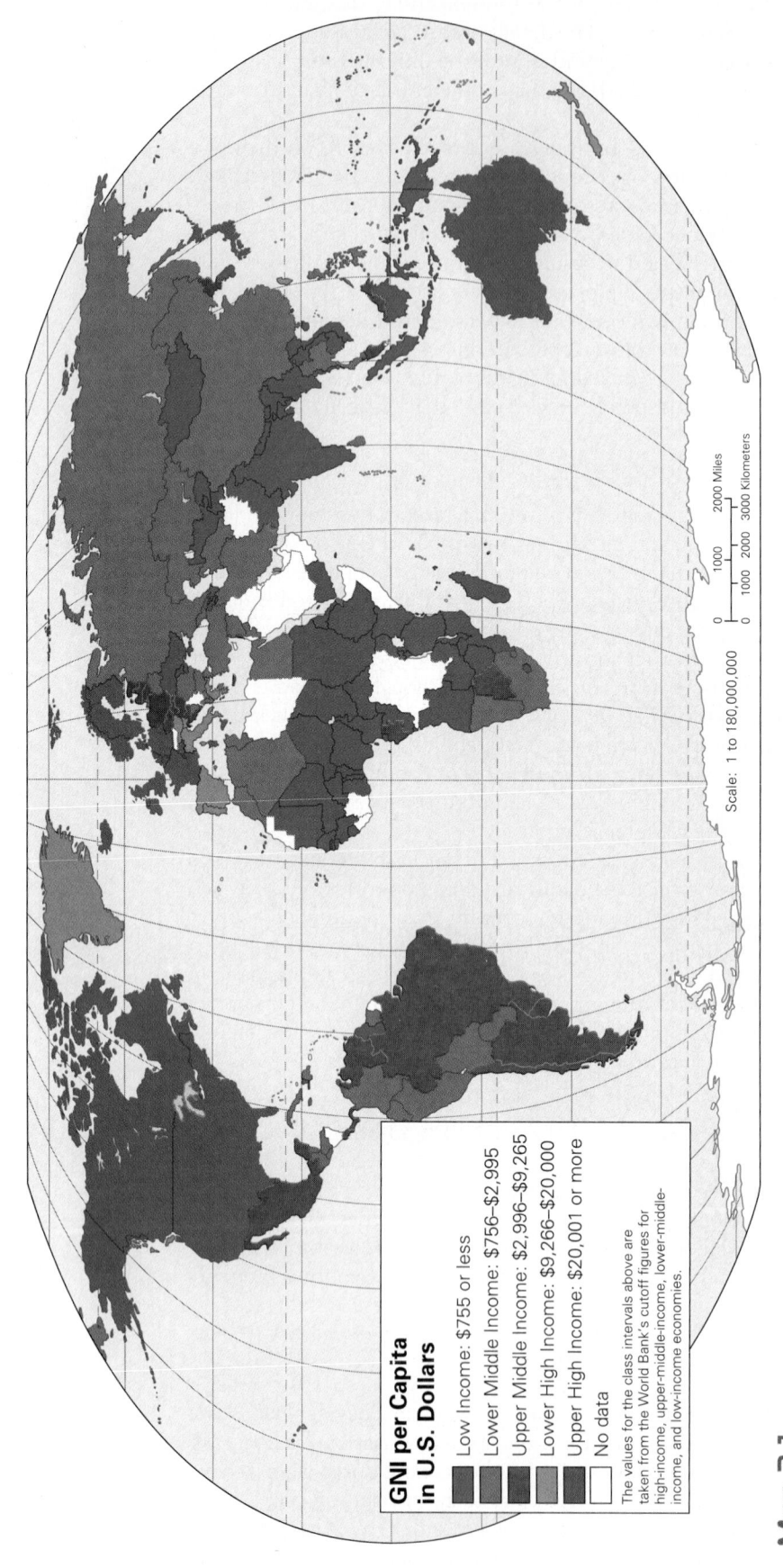

**GNI per Capita
in U.S. Dollars**

Low Income: $755 or less

Lower Middle Income: $756–$2,995

Upper Middle Income: $2,996–$9,265

Lower High Income: $9,266–$20,000

Upper High Income: $20,001 or more

No data

The values for the class intervals above are taken from the World Bank's cutoff figures for high-income, upper-middle-income, lower-middle-income, and low-income economies.

Scale: 1 to 180,000,000

0   1000   2000   2000 Miles

0   1000   2000   3000 Kilometers

Map 2.1

Gross National Income per Captia, 2001

Source: World Bank, World Development Indicators Online, 2003.

Country	GNI per Capita	PPP per Capita	GDP Growth Rate (%) 1991–2001
Brazil	$3,060	$7,450	2.54%
China	$890	$4,260	9.82
Germany	$23,700	$25,530	1.64
India	$460	$2,480	5.5
Japan	$35,990	$27,430	1.2
Nigeria	$290	$830	2.8
Poland	$4,240	$9,280	3.5
Russia	$1,750	$8,660	−3.1
Switzerland	$36,970	$31,320	1.0
United Kingdom	$24,230	$24,460	2.3
United States	$34,870	$34,870	3.0

Table 2.1

PPP Index and GNI and GDP Data for Selected Countries, 2001

Source: World Bank, World Development Indicators Online, 2003.

and the United States are among the richest on this measure, while the large countries of China and India are among the poorest. Japan, for example, had a 2001 GNI per head of $35,990, whereas China achieved only $890 and India, $460. One of the world's poorest countries, Mozambique, had a GNI per capita of only $210, while one of the world's richest, Switzerland, came in at $36,970.32

However, GNI per capita figures can be misleading because they don't consider differences in the cost of living. For example, although the 2001 GNI per capita of Switzerland, at $36,970, exceeded that of the United States, which was $34,870, the higher cost of living in Switzerland meant that American citizens could actually afford more goods and services than Swiss citizens. To account for differences in the cost of living, one can adjust GNI per capita by purchasing power. Referred to as a **purchasing power parity** (PPP) adjustment, it allows for a more direct comparison of living standards in different countries. The base for the adjustment is the cost of living in the United States. The PPP for different countries is then adjusted up (or down) depending upon whether the cost of living is lower (or higher) than in the United States. For example, in 2001 while the GNI per capita for China was $890, the PPP per capita was $4,260, suggesting that the cost of living was lower in China and that $890 in China would buy as much as $4,260 in United States. Table 2.1 gives the GNI per capita measured at PPP in 2001 for a selection of countries, along with their GNI per capita and their growth rate in gross domestic product (GDP) from 1991 to 2001. Map 2.2 summarizes the GNI PPP per capita in 2001 for the nations of the world.

As can be seen, there are striking differences in the standard of living. Table 2.1 suggests that the average Indian citizen can afford to consume only 7 percent of the goods and services consumed by the average U.S. citizen. Given this, one might conclude that, despite having a population of 1 billion, India is unlikely to be a very lucrative market for the consumer products produced by many Western international businesses. However, this is not quite the correct conclusion to draw, because India has a fairly wealthy middle class, despite its large number of very poor people.

Unfortunately, the GNI and PPP data give a static picture of development. They tell us, for example, that China is much poorer than the United States, but they do not tell us if China is closing the gap. To assess this, we have to look at the economic growth rates achieved by countries. Table 2.1 gives the rate of growth in gross domestic product (GDP) achieved by a number of countries between 1991 and 2001. Map 2.3 summarizes the growth rate in GDP from 1990 to 2000. Although countries such as China

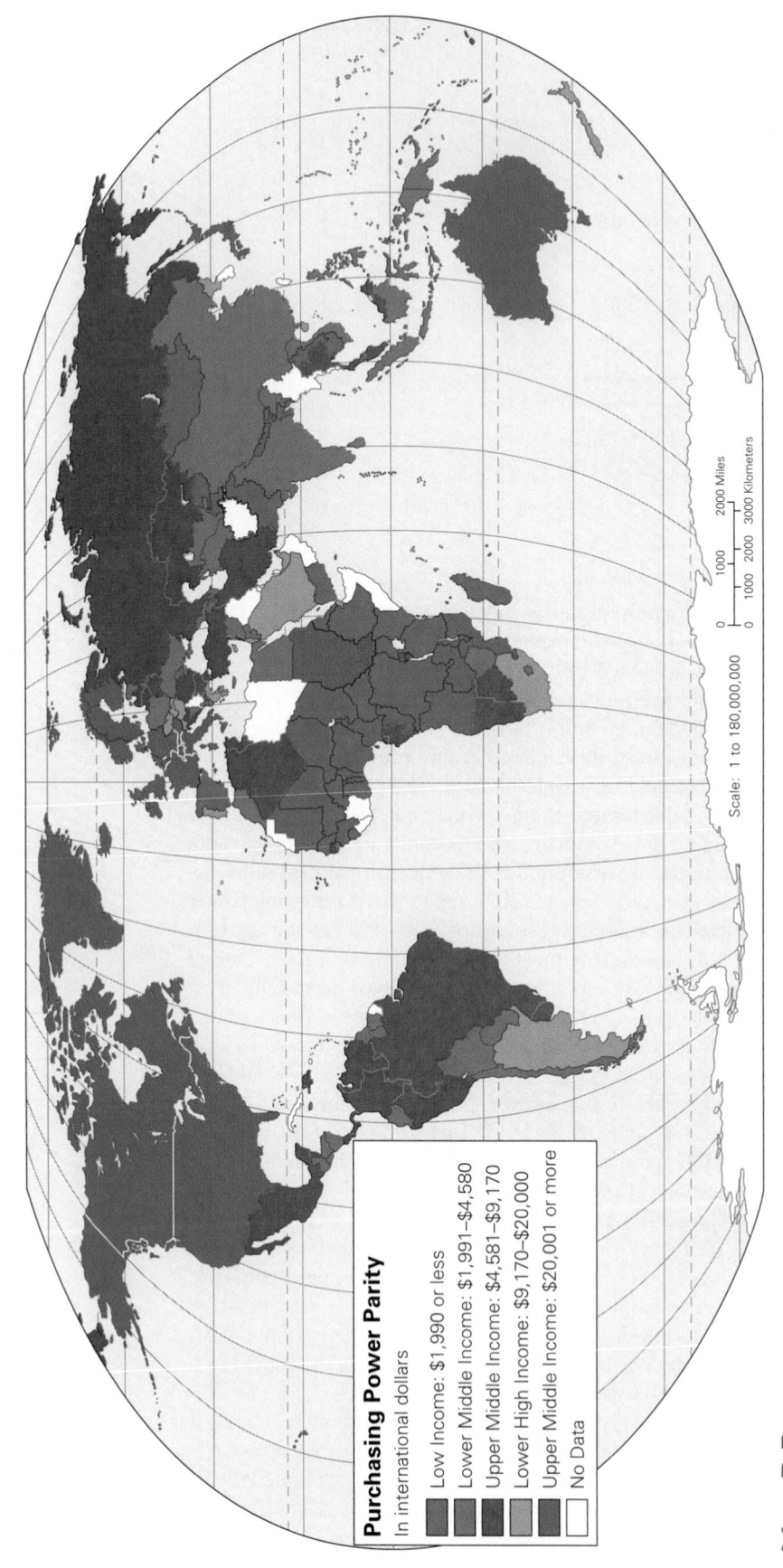

Purchasing Power Parity

In international dollars

Low Income: $1,990 or less

Lower Middle Income: $1,991–$4,580

Upper Middle Income: $4,581–$9,170

Lower High Income: $9,170–$20,000

Upper Middle Income: $20,001 or more

No Data

Scale: 1 to 180,000,000

0   1000   2000 Miles

0   1000   2000   3000 Kilometers

Map 2.2

Purchasing Power Parity, 2001

Source: World Bank, World Development Indicators Online, 2003. Reprinted by permission from the International Bank for Reconstruction and Development. © 2001 by the World Bank.

Map 2.3

Growth in Gross Domestic Product, 1991–2001

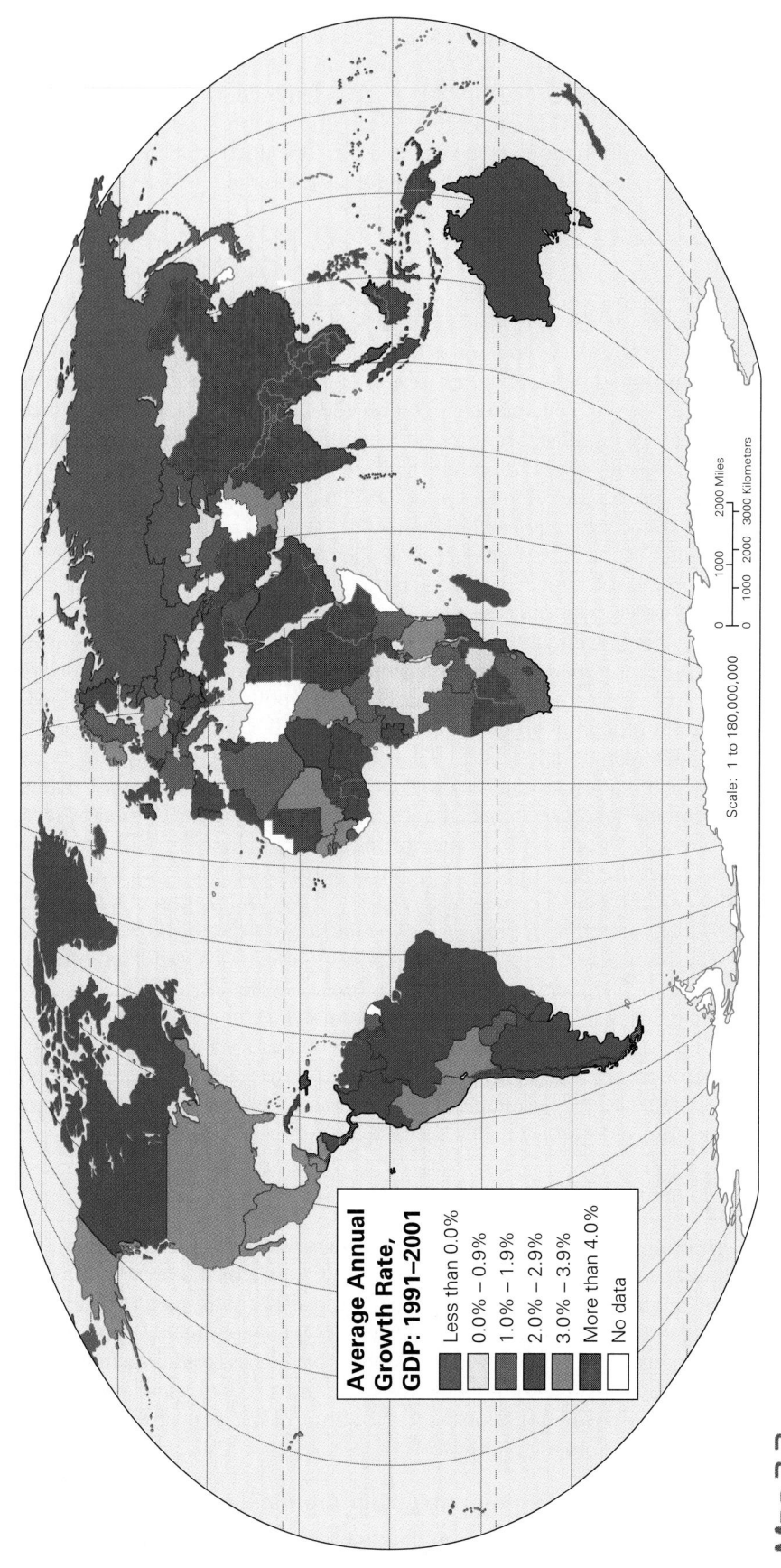

Average Annual Growth Rate, GDP: 1991–2001

- Less than 0.0%
- 0.0% – 0.9%
- 1.0% – 1.9%
- 2.0% – 2.9%
- 3.0% – 3.9%
- More than 4.0%
- No data

Scale: 1 to 180,000,000

0   1000   2000 Miles
0   1000   2000   3000 Kilometers

Source: World Bank, World Development Indicators Online, 2003. Reprinted by permission from the International Bank for Reconstruction and Development. © 2001 by the World Bank.

and India are currently very poor, their economies are growing more rapidly than those of many advanced nations. Thus, in time they may become advanced nations and be huge markets for the products of international businesses. Given their potential, international businesses might want to get a foothold in these markets now. Even though their current contributions to an international firm's revenues might be small, their future contributions could be much larger. One might also note, however, that Table 2.1 indicates that Russia's economy shrank substantially between 1991 and 2001.

Broader Conceptions of Development: Amartya Sen

The Nobel Prize–winning economist Amartya Sen has argued that development should be assessed less by material output measures such as GNI per capita and more by the capabilities and opportunities that people enjoy.[29] According to Sen, development should be seen as a process of expanding the real freedoms that people experience. Hence, development requires the removal of major impediments to freedom: poverty as well as tyranny, poor economic opportunities as well as systematic social deprivation, neglect of public facilities as well as the intolerance of repressive states. In Sen's view, development is not just an economic process, but it is a political one too, and to succeed requires the "democratization" of political communities to give citizens a voice in the important decisions made for the community. This perspective leads Sen to emphasize basic health care, especially for children, and basic education, especially for women. Not only are these factors desirable for their instrumental value in helping to achieve higher income levels, but they are also beneficial in their own right. People cannot develop their capabilities if they are chronically ill or woefully ignorant.

Sen's influential thesis has been picked up by the United Nations, which has developed the **Human Development Index** (HDI) to measure the quality of human life in different nations. The HDI is based on three measures: life expectancy at birth (which is a function of health care), educational attainment (which is measured by a combination of the adult literacy rate and enrollment in primary, secondary, and tertiary education), and whether average incomes, based on PPP estimates, are sufficient to meet the basic needs of life in a country (adequate food, shelter, and health care). As such, the HDI comes much closer to Sen's conception of how development should be measured than narrow economic measures such as GNI per capita—although Sen's thesis suggests that political freedoms should also be included in the index, and they are not. The Human Development Index is scaled from 0 to 1. Countries scoring less than 0.5 are classified as having low human development (the quality of life is poor), those scoring from 0.5 to 0.8 are classified as having medium human development, while those countries that score above 0.8 are classified as having high human development. Map 2.4 summarizes the Human Development Index scores for 2001, the most recent year for which data are available.

Political Economy and Economic Progress

It is often argued that a country's economic development is a function of its economic and political systems. What then is the nature of the relationship between political economy and economic progress? This question has been the subject of vigorous debate among academics and policymakers for some time. Despite the long debate, this remains a question for which it is not possible to give an unambiguous answer. However, it is possible to untangle the main threads of the academic arguments and make a few broad generalizations as to the nature of the relationship between political economy and economic progress.

Innovation and Entrepreneurship Are the Engines of Growth

There is fairly wide agreement that innovation and entrepreneurial activity are the engines of long-run economic growth.[30] Those who make this argument define innova-

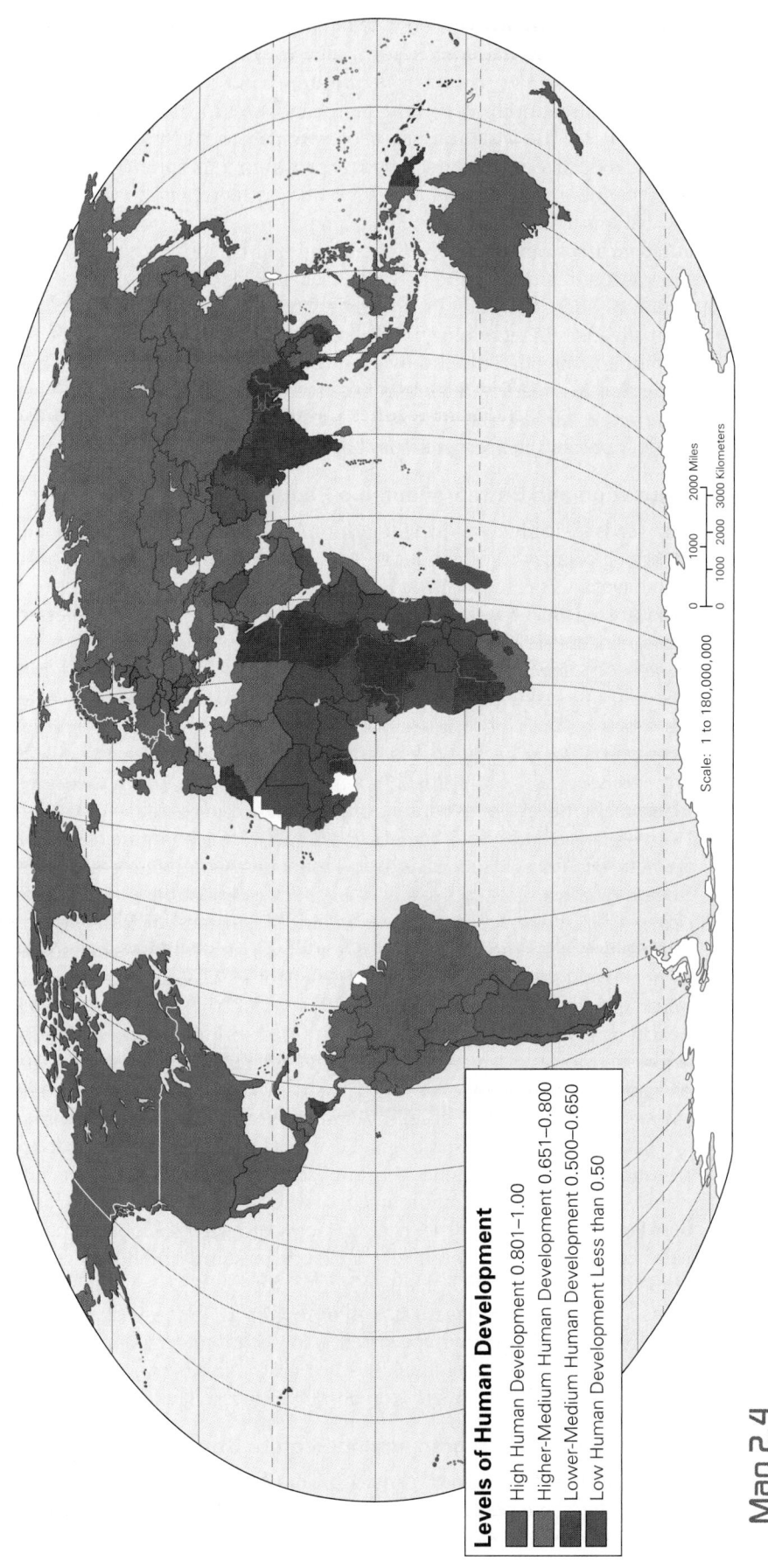

Map 2.4

The Human Development Index, 2001

Levels of Human Development

High Human Development 0.801–1.00

Higher-Medium Human Development 0.651–0.800

Lower-Medium Human Development 0.500–0.650

Low Human Development Less than 0.50

Scale: 1 to 180,000,000

0　　1000　　2000　3000 Kilometers

0　　1000　　2000 Miles

Source: United Nations, Human Development Report, 2003, Human Development Index.

tion broadly to include not just new products, but also new processes, new organizations, new management practices, and new strategies. Thus, Toys "R" Us's strategy of establishing large warehouse-style toy stores and then engaging in heavy advertising and price discounting to sell the merchandise can be classified as an innovation because Toys "R" Us was the first company to pursue this strategy. It also sees innovation as the product of entrepreneurial activity. Often, entrepreneurs first commercialize innovative new products and processes, and entrepreneurial activity provides much of the dynamism in an economy. For example, the economy of the United States has benefited greatly from a high level of entrepreneurial activity, which has resulted in rapid innovation in products and process. Firms such as Cisco Systems, Dell Computer Corporation, Microsoft, and Oracle were all founded by entrepreneurial individuals to exploit advances in technology, and all these firms created significant economic value by helping to commercialize innovations in products and processes. Thus, one can conclude that if a country's economy is to sustain long-run growth, the business environment must be conducive to the consistent production of product and process innovations and to entrepreneurial activity.

Innovation and Entrepreneurship Require a Market Economy

This leads logically to a further question—What is required for the business environment of a country to be conducive to innovation and entrepreneurial activity? Those who have considered this issue highlight the advantages of a market economy.[31] It has been argued that the economic freedom associated with a market economy creates greater incentives for innovation and entrepreneurship than either a planned or a mixed economy. In a market economy, any individual who has an innovative idea is free to try to make money out of that idea by starting a business (by engaging in entrepreneurial activity). Similarly, existing businesses are free to improve their operations through innovation. To the extent that they are successful, both individual entrepreneurs and established businesses can reap rewards in the form of high profits. Thus, market economies contain enormous incentives to develop innovations.

In a planned economy, the state owns all means of production. Consequently, entrepreneurial individuals have little economic incentive to develop valuable new innovations, since it is the state, rather than the individual, that captures most of the gains. The lack of economic freedom and incentives for innovation was probably a main factor in the economic stagnation of so many former Communist states and led ultimately to their collapse at the end of the 1980s. Similar stagnation occurred in many mixed economies in those sectors where the state had a monopoly (such as health care and telecommunications in Great Britain). This stagnation provided the impetus for the widespread privatization of state-owned enterprises that we witnessed in many mixed economies during the mid-1980s and is still going on today (privatization refers to the process of selling state-owned enterprises to private investors).

A study of 102 countries over a 20-year period provided evidence of a strong relationship between economic freedom (as provided by a market economy) and economic growth.[32] The study found that the more economic freedom a country had between 1975 and 1995, the more economic growth it achieved and the richer its citizens became. The six countries that had persistently high ratings of economic freedom from 1975 to 1995 (Hong Kong, Switzerland, Singapore, the United States, Canada, and Germany) were also all in the top 10 in terms of economic growth rates. In contrast, no country with persistently low economic freedom achieved a respectable growth rate. For the 16 countries for which the index of economic freedom declined the most during 1975–95, gross domestic product fell at an annual rate of 0.6 percent.

Innovation and Entrepreneurship Require Strong Property Rights

Strong legal protection of property rights is another requirement for a business environment to be conducive to innovation, entrepreneurial activity, and hence economic growth.[33] Both individuals and businesses must be given the opportunity to profit from innovative ideas. Without strong property rights protection, businesses and individuals run the risk that the profits from their innovative efforts will be expropriated, either by criminal elements or by the state. The state can expropriate the profits from innovation through legal means, such as excessive taxation, or through illegal means, such as demands from state bureaucrats for kickbacks in return for granting an individual or firm a license to do business in a certain area (i.e., corruption). According to the Nobel Prize–winning economist Douglass North, throughout history many governments have displayed a tendency to engage in such behavior. Inadequately enforced property rights reduce the incentives for innovation and entrepreneurial activity—since the profits from such activity are "stolen"—and hence reduce the rate of economic growth.

The Required Political System

There is a great deal of debate as to the kind of political system that best achieves a functioning market economy with strong protection for property rights.[34] People in the West tend to associate a representative democracy with a market economic system, strong property rights protection, and economic progress. Building on this, we tend to argue that democracy is good for growth.[35] However, some totalitarian regimes have fostered a market economy and strong property rights protection and have experienced rapid economic growth. Four of the fastest-growing economies of the past 30 years—South Korea, Taiwan, Singapore, and Hong Kong—had one thing in common at the start of their economic growth: undemocratic governments! At the same time, countries with stable democratic governments, such as India, experienced sluggish economic growth for long periods. In 1992, Lee Kuan Yew, Singapore's leader for many years, told an audience, "I do not believe that democracy necessarily leads to development. I believe that a country needs to develop discipline more than democracy. The exuberance of democracy leads to undisciplined and disorderly conduct which is inimical to development."[36] Others have argued that many of the current problems in Eastern Europe and the states of the former Soviet Union arose because democracy arrived before economic reform, making it more difficult for elected governments to introduce the policies that, while painful in the short run, were needed to promote rapid economic growth. China, which maintains a totalitarian government, has moved rapidly toward a market economy.

However, those who argue for the value of a totalitarian regime miss an important point: If dictators made countries rich, then much of Africa, Asia, and Latin America should have been growing rapidly during 1960–1990, and this was not the case. Only a certain kind of totalitarian regime is capable of promoting economic growth. It must be a dictatorship that is committed to a free market system and strong protection of property rights. Also, there is no guarantee that a dictatorship will continue to pursue such progressive policies. Dictators are rarely so benevolent. Many are tempted to use the apparatus of the state to further their own private ends, violating property rights and stalling economic growth. Given this, it seems likely democratic regimes are far more conducive to long-term economic growth than are dictatorships, even benevolent ones. Only in a well-functioning, mature democracy are property rights truly secure.[37] We should not forget Amartya Sen's arguments that we reviewed earlier. Totalitarian states, by limiting human freedom, also suppress human development and therefore are detrimental to progress.

Economic Progress Begets Democracy

While it is possible to argue that democracy is not a necessary precondition for a free market economy in which property rights are protected, subsequent economic growth often leads to establishment of a democratic regime. Several of the fastest growing Asian economies adopted more democratic governments during the last two decades, including South Korea and Taiwan. Thus, while democracy may not always be the cause of initial economic progress, it seems to be one consequence of that progress.

A strong belief that economic progress leads to adoption of a democratic regime underlies the fairly permissive attitude that many Western governments have adopted toward human rights violations in China. Although China has a totalitarian government in which human rights are abused, many Western countries have been hesitant to criticize the country too much for fear that this might hamper the country's march toward a free market system. The belief is that once China has a free market system, democracy will follow. Whether this optimistic vision comes to pass remains to be seen.

Geography, Education, and Economic Development

While a country's political and economic system is probably the big locomotive driving its rate of economic development, other factors are also important. One that has received attention recently is geography.[38] But the belief that geography can influence economic policy, and hence economic growth rates, goes back to Adam Smith. The influential Harvard University economist Jeffrey Sachs argues

> that throughout history, coastal states, with their long engagements in international trade, have been more supportive of market institutions than landlocked states, which have tended to organize themselves as hierarchical (and often military) societies. Mountainous states, as a result of physical isolation, have often neglected market-based trade. Temperate climes have generally supported higher densities of population and thus a more extensive division of labor than tropical regions.[39]

Sachs's point is that by virtue of favorable geography, certain societies were more likely to engage in trade than others and were thus more likely to be open to and develop market-based economic systems, which in turn would promote faster economic growth. He also argues that, irrespective of the economic and political institutions a country adopts, adverse geographical conditions, such as the high rate of disease, poor soils, and hostile climate that afflict many tropical countries, can have a negative impact on development. Together with colleagues at Harvard's Institute for International Development, Sachs tested for the impact of geography on a country's economic growth rate between 1965 and 1990. He found that landlocked countries grew more slowly than coastal economies and that being entirely landlocked reduced a country's growth rate by roughly 0.7 percent per year. He also found that tropical countries grew 1.3 percent more slowly each year than countries in the temperate zone.

Education emerges as another important determinant of economic development (a point that Amartya Sen emphasizes). The general assertion is that nations that invest more in education will have higher growth rates because an educated population is a more productive population. Some rather striking anecdotal evidence suggests this is true. In 1960, Pakistanis and South Koreans were on equal footing economically. However, just 30 percent of Pakistani children were enrolled in primary schools, while 94 percent of South Koreans were. By the mid-1980s, South Korea's GNP per person was three times that of Pakistan's.[40] A survey of 14 statistical studies that looked at the relationship between a country's investment in education and its subsequent growth rates concluded investment in education did have a positive and statistically significant impact on a country's rate of economic growth.[41] Similarly, the work by Sachs discussed above suggests that investments in education help explain why some countries in Southeast Asia, such as Indonesia, Malaysia, and Singapore, have been able to overcome the disadvantages associated with their tropical geography and grow far more rapidly than tropical nations in Africa and Latin America.

States in Transition

The political economy of many of the world's nation-states has changed radically since the late 1980s. Two trends have been evident. First, during the late 1980s and early 1990s, a wave of democratic revolutions swept the world. Totalitarian governments collapsed and were replaced by democratically elected governments that were typically more committed to free market capitalism than their predecessors had been. The change was most dramatic in Eastern Europe, where the collapse of communism brought an end to the Cold War and led to the breakup of the Soviet Union, but similar changes were occurring throughout the world during the same period. Across much of Asia, Latin America, and Africa there was a marked shift toward greater democracy. Second, there has been a strong move away from centrally planned and mixed economies and toward a more free market economic model. We shall look first at the spread of democracy and then turn our attention to the spread of free market economics.

The Spread of Democracy

One notable development of the past 15 years has been the spread of democracy (and, by extension, the decline of totalitarianism). Map 2.5 reports on the extent of totalitarianism in the world as determined by Freedom House.[42] This map charts political freedom in 2003, on a scale from 1 for the highest degree of political freedom to 7 for the lowest. Among the criteria that Freedom House uses to determine ratings for political freedom are the following:

- Free and fair elections of the head of state and legislative representatives.
- Fair electoral laws, equal campaigning opportunities, and fair polling.
- The right to organize into different political parties.
- A parliament with effective power.
- A significant opposition that has a realistic chance of gaining power.
- Freedom from domination by the military, foreign powers, totalitarian parties, religious hierarchies, or any other powerful group.
- A reasonable amount of self-determination for cultural, ethnic, and religious minorities.

Factors contributing to a low rating (i.e., to totalitarianism) include military or foreign control, the denial of self-determination to major population groups, a lack of decentralized political power, and an absence of democratic elections.

As of December 2002, Freedom House classified some 89 countries as "free," accounting for some 44 percent of the world's population. In these countries, a broad range of political rights is respected. Another 55 countries accounting for 21 percent of the world's population were classified as "partly free," while 48 countries representing some 35 percent of the world's population were classified as "not free." The number of democracies in the world has increased from 69 nations in 1987 to 121, the highest total in history. (Not all democracies are "free," according to Freedom House, because some democracies still restrict certain political and civil liberties.) Almost 55 percent of the world's population now lives under democratic rule. Many of these newer democracies are to be found in Eastern Europe and Latin America, although there have also been some notable gains in Africa during this time, such as in South Africa. Notable entrants into the ranks of the world's democracies include Mexico, which held its first fully free and fair presidential election in 2000 after free and fair parliamentary and state elections in 1997 and 1998; Senegal, where free and fair presidential elections led to a peaceful transfer of power; and Yugoslavia, where a democratic election took place despite attempted fraud by the incumbent.

Three main reasons account for the spread of democracy.[43] First, many totalitarian regimes failed to deliver economic progress to the vast bulk of their populations. The collapse of communism in Eastern Europe, for example, was precipitated by the growing gulf between the vibrant and wealthy economies of the West and the stagnant economies of the Communist East. In looking for alternatives to the socialist model, the populations of these countries could not have failed to notice that most of the world's strongest economies were governed by representative democracies. Today, the economic success of many of the newer democracies, such as Poland and the Czech

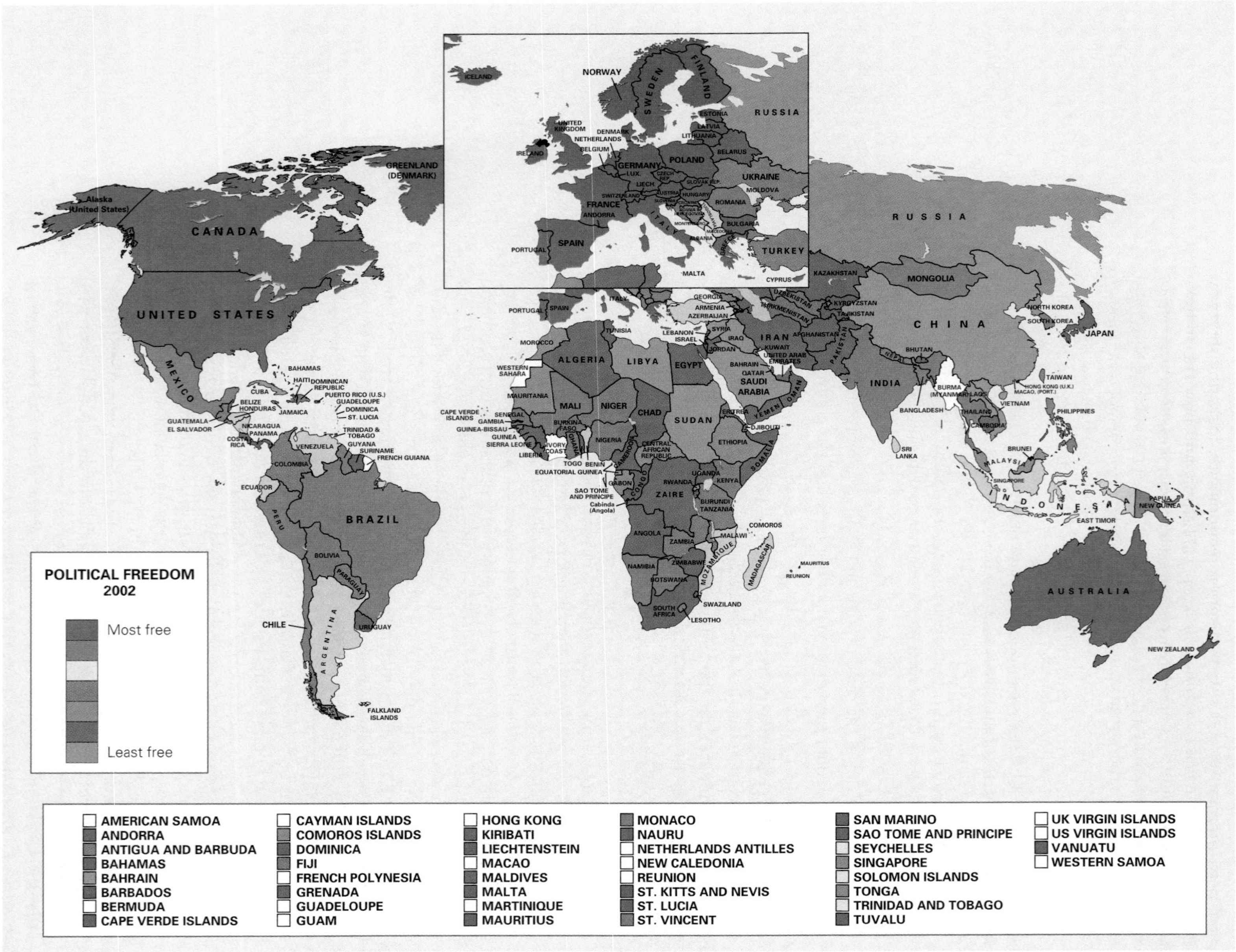

Map 2.5

Political Freedom in 2002

POLITICAL FREEDOM 2002

Most free

Least free

Source: Map data from Freedom House, Freedom in the World 2003: The Annual Survey of Political Rights and Civil Liberties. http://www.freedomhouse.org.

Republic in the former Communist bloc, the Philippines and Taiwan in Asia, and Chile in Latin America, has strengthened the case for democracy as a key component of successful economic advancement.

Second, new information and communication technologies, including shortwave radio, satellite television, fax machines, desktop publishing, and now the Internet, have broken down the ability of the state to control access to uncensored information. These technologies have created new conduits for the spread of democratic ideals and information from free societies. Today the Internet is allowing democratic ideals to penetrate closed societies as never before. In response, some governments have tried to restrict citizens' access to the Internet; for example, China limits access to government employees and those affiliated with universities.[44]

Third, in many countries the economic advances of the last quarter century have led to the emergence of increasingly prosperous middle and working classes who have pushed for democratic reforms. This was certainly a factor in the democratic transformation of South Korea. Entrepreneurs and other business leaders, eager to protect their property rights and ensure the dispassionate enforcement of contracts, are another force pressing for more accountable and open government.

Having said this, it would be naive to conclude that the global spread of democracy will continue unchallenged. There have been several reversals. In the former Soviet republic of Belarus, for example, President Alexander Lukashenko dissolved a democratically elected parliament and harassed the press. In the African nation of Niger, a military coup deposed a democratically elected government. In Asia, China's Marxist–Leninist leaders continue to advocate the virtues of authoritarian paths to "democracy" and to denounce Western democracies as an unacceptable model.

Also, democracy is still rare in large parts of the world. In Sub-Saharan Africa, just 11 nations, 23 of the total, are electoral democracies. Among the 27 post-Communist countries in East and Central Europe, 8 are still not electoral democracies and Freedom House classifies only 12 of these states as "free." And there are no democracies among the 16 Arabic states of the Middle East and North Africa.

The New World Order and Global Terrorism

The end of the Cold War and the "new world order" that followed the collapse of communism in Eastern Europe and the former Soviet Union, taken together with the collapse of many authoritarian regimes in Latin America, have given rise to intense speculation about the future shape of global geopolitics. Author Francis Fukuyama has argued that "we may be witnessing . . . the end of history as such: that is, the end point of mankind's ideological evolution and the universalization of Western liberal democracy as the final form of human government."[45] Fukuyama goes on to say that the war of ideas may be at an end and that liberal democracy has triumphed.

Others have questioned Fukuyama's vision of a more harmonious world dominated by a universal civilization characterized by democratic regimes and free market capitalism. In a controversial book, the influential political scientist Samuel Huntington argues that there is no "universal" civilization based on widespread acceptance of Western liberal democratic ideals.[46] Huntington maintains that while many societies may be modernizing—they are adopting the material paraphernalia of the modern world, from automobiles to Coca-Cola and MTV—they are not becoming more Western. On the contrary, Huntington theorizes that modernization in non-Western societies can result in a retreat toward the traditional, such as the resurgence of Islam in many traditionally Muslim societies:

> The Islamic resurgence is both a product of and an effort to come to grips with
> modernization. Its underlying causes are those generally responsible for
> indigenization trends in non-Western societies: urbanization, social
> mobilization, higher levels of literacy and education, intensified
> communication and media consumption, and expanded interaction with

Western and other cultures. These developments undermine traditional village and clan ties and create alienation and an identity crisis. Islamist symbols, commitments, and beliefs meet these psychological needs, and Islamist welfare organizations, the social, cultural and economic needs of Muslims caught in the process of modernization. Muslims feel a need to return to Islamic ideas, practices, and institutions to provide the compass and the motor of modernization.[47]

Thus, the rise of Islamic fundamentalism is portrayed as a response to the alienation produced by modernization.

In contrast to Fukuyama, Huntington sees a world that is split into different civilizations, each of which has its own value systems and ideology. In addition to Western civilization, Huntington predicts the emergence of strong Islamic and Sinic (Chinese) civilizations, as well as civilizations based on Japan, Africa, Latin America, Eastern Orthodox Christianity (Russian), and Hinduism (Indian). Huntington also sees the civilizations as headed for conflict, particularly along the "fault lines" that separate them, such as Bosnia (where Muslims and Orthodox Christians have clashed), Kashmir (where Muslims and Hindus clash), and the Sudan (where a bloody war between Christians and Muslims has persisted for decades). Huntington predicts conflict between the West and Islam and between the West and China. He bases his predictions on an analysis of the different value systems and ideology of these civilizations, which in his view tend to bring them into conflict with each other. While some commentators originally dismissed Huntington's thesis, in the aftermath of the terrorist attacks on the United States on September 11, 2001, Huntington's views received new attention.

If Huntington's views are even partly correct—and there is little doubt that the events of September 11 added more weight to his thesis—they have important implications for international business. They suggest many countries may be increasingly difficult places in which to do business, either because they are shot through with violent conflicts or because they are part of a civilization that is in conflict with an enterprise's home country. Huntington's views are speculative and controversial. It is not clear that his predictions will come to pass. More likely is the evolution of a global political system that is positioned somewhere between Fukuyama's universal global civilization based on liberal democratic ideals and Huntington's vision of a fractured world. That would still be a world, however, in which geopolitical forces periodically limit the ability of business enterprises to operate in certain foreign countries.

In Huntington's thesis, global terrorism is a product of the tension between civilizations and the clash of value systems and ideology. Others point to terrorism's roots in long-standing conflicts that seem to defy political resolution, the Palestinian, Kashmir, and Northern Ireland conflicts being the most obvious examples. Also, a substantial amount of terrorist activity in some parts of the world, such as Colombia, has been interwoven with the illegal drug trade. The attacks of September 11 created the impression that global terror is on the rise. As U.S. Secretary of State Colin Powell has maintained, terrorism represents one of the major threats to world peace and economic progress in the 21st century. However, the vivid and horrific events of September 11, 2001, and the fact that they took place on U.S. soil, may have unduly shaped our perspective of a phenomenon that has long been with us. According to data from the U.S. Department of State, the number of terrorist attacks worldwide was substantially higher in the late 1980s than in recent years (see Figure 2.3). There were, for example, 666 terrorist incidents worldwide in 1987, 348 in 2001,[48] and 199 in 2002 (the sharp fall in terrorist attacks in 2003 was probably due to U.S.-led anti-terrorism efforts). This is not to deny the psychological and economic shock of the events of September 11, or the tragic loss of human life and the serious threat posed by the combination of determined and sophisticated terrorists, rogue states, and weapons of mass destruction. Terrorism has long been with us, and it has not yet derailed global trends toward greater political and economic freedom; nor should it.

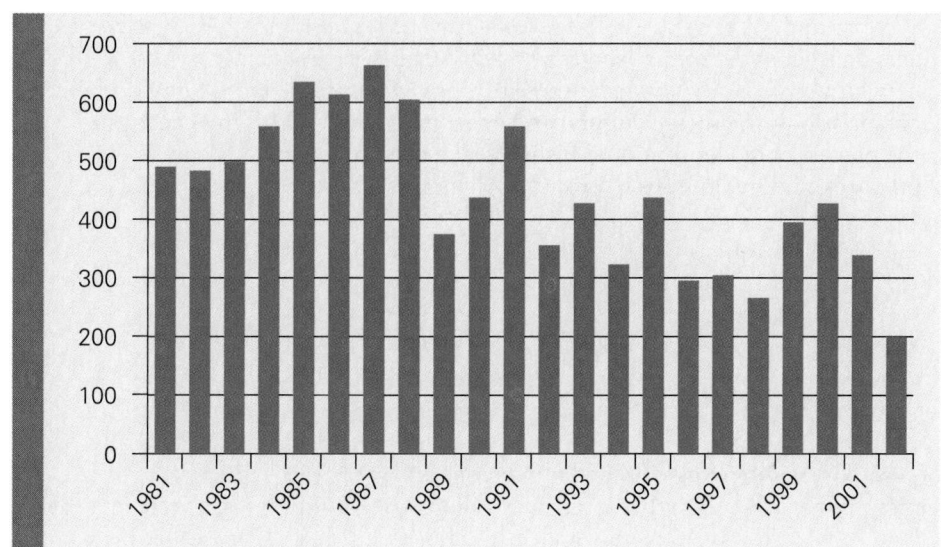

Figure 2.3

Total International Terrorist
Attacks, 1981–2002

Source: U.S. Department of State,
Patterns of Global Terrorism 2002,
April 2003.

The Spread of Market-Based Systems

Paralleling the spread of democracy since the 1980s has been the transformation from centrally planned command economies to market-based economies. More than 30 countries that were in the former Soviet Union or the Eastern European Communist bloc are now changing their economic systems. A complete list of countries would also include Asian states such as China and Vietnam, as well as African countries such as Angola, Ethiopia, and Mozambique.[49] There has been a similar shift away from a mixed economy. Many countries in Asia, Latin America, and Western Europe have sold state-owned businesses to private investors (privatization) and deregulated their economies to promote greater competition.

The underlying rationale for economic transformation has been the same the world over. In general, command and mixed economies failed to deliver the kind of sustained economic performance that was achieved by countries adopting market-based systems, such as the United States, Switzerland, Hong Kong, and Taiwan. As a consequence, even more states have gravitated toward the market-based model. Map 2.6, based on data from the Heritage Foundation, a conservative U.S. research foundation, gives some idea of the degree to which the world has shifted toward market-based economic systems. The Heritage Foundation's index of economic freedom is based on 10 indicators, such as the extent to which the government intervenes in the economy, trade policy, the degree to which property rights are protected, foreign investment regulations, and taxation rules. A country can score between 1 (most free) and 5 (least free) on each of these indicators. The lower a country's average score across all 10 indicators, the more closely its economy represents the pure market model. According to the 2003 index, which is summarized in Map 2.6, the world's freest economies are (in rank order) Hong Kong, Singapore, Luxembourg, New Zealand, Ireland, Denmark, and the United States. The United Kingdom is ranked 9, Japan is ranked at 35; France at 40; Mexico, 56; Brazil, 72; India, 119, China, 127; Russia, 135; while the command economies of Cuba, Laos, Iraq, and North Korea are to be found at the bottom of the rankings.[50]

Economic freedom does not necessarily equate with political freedom, as detailed in Map 2.6. For example, 3 of the top 16 countries in the Heritage Foundation index, Hong Kong, Singapore, and Bahrain, cannot be classified as politically free. Hong Kong was reabsorbed into Communist China in 1997, and the first thing Beijing did was shut down Hong Kong's freely elected legislature. Singapore is ranked as only "partly free" on Freedom House's index of political freedom due to practices such as

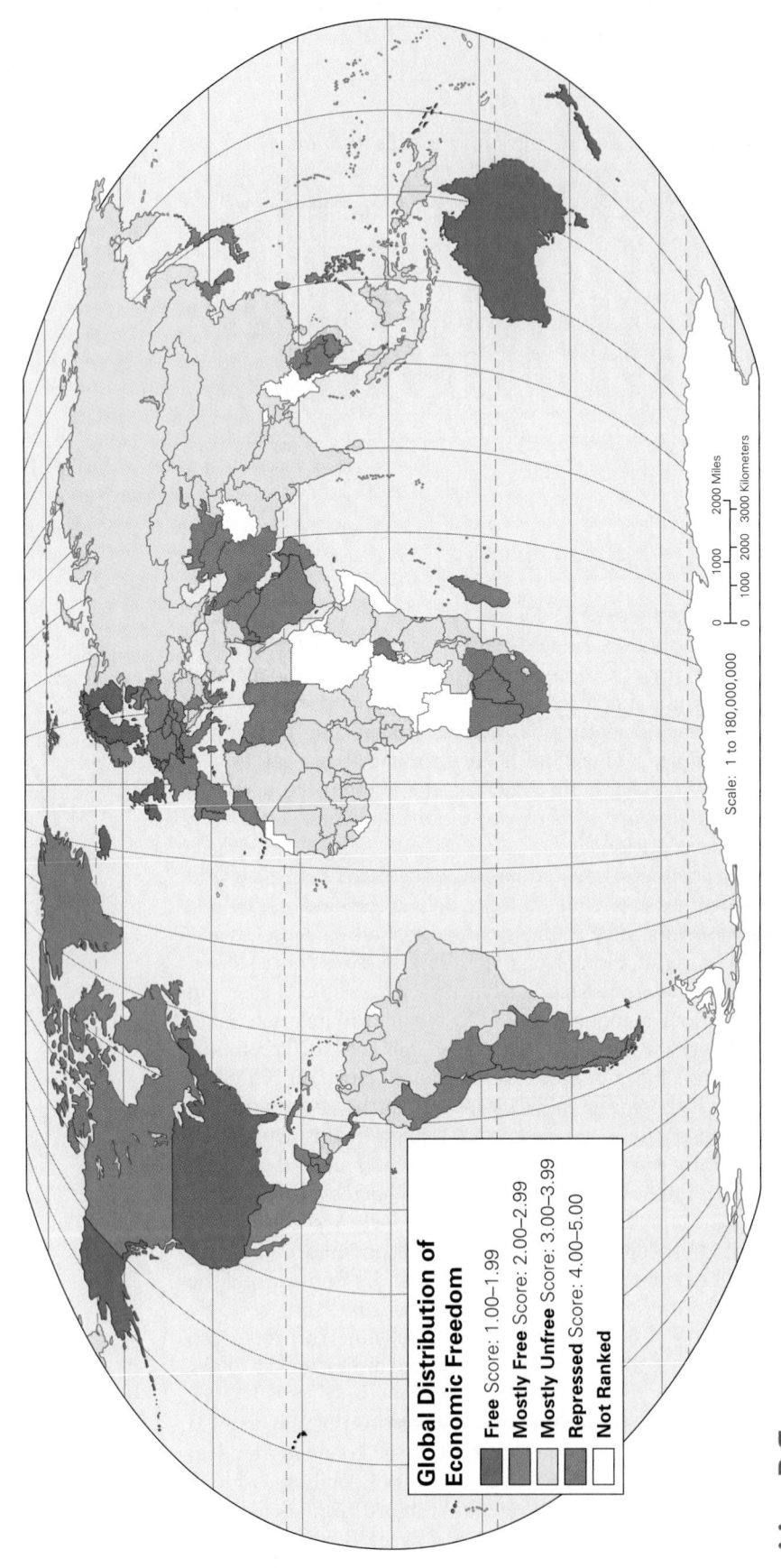

Map 2.6

Global Distribution of Economic Freedom, 2003

Global Distribution of
Economic Freedom

Free Score: 1.00–1.99

Mostly Free Score: 2.00–2.99

Mostly Unfree Score: 3.00–3.99

Repressed Score: 4.00–5.00

Not Ranked

Scale: 1 to 180,000,000

2000 Miles

1000

0

1000   2000   3000 Kilometers

0   1000   2000

Source: Heritage Foundation, 2003 *Index of Economic Freedom.* http://www.heritage.org:so/index/countries/maps&charts/list1.gif.

widespread press censorship, while Bahrain is classified as "least free" due to the monopolization of political power by a hereditary monarchy.

The Nature of Economic Transformation

The shift toward a market-based economic system often entails a number of steps: deregulation, privatization, and creation of a legal system to safeguard property rights.[51] We shall review each before looking at the track record of states engaged in economic transformation.

Deregulation

Deregulation involves removing legal restrictions to the free play of markets, the establishment of private enterprises, and the manner in which private enterprises operate. Before the collapse of communism, the governments in most command economies exercised tight control over prices and output, setting both through detailed state planning. They also prohibited private enterprises from operating in most sectors of the economy, severely restricted direct investment by foreign enterprises, and limited international trade. Deregulation in these cases involved removing price controls, thereby allowing prices to be set by the interplay between demand and supply; abolishing laws regulating the establishment and operation of private enterprises, and relaxing or removing restrictions on direct investment by foreign enterprises and international trade.

In mixed economies, the role of the state was more limited, but here too, in certain sectors the state set prices, owned businesses, limited private enterprise, restricted investment by foreigners, and restricted international trade. For these countries, deregulation has involved the same kind of initiatives that we have seen in former command economies, although the transformation has been easier because there was always a vibrant private sector in these countries. India is a good example of a mixed economy that is currently deregulating large areas of its economy (see the opening case for details). Deregulation has involved reforming the industrial licensing system that made it difficult to establish private enterprises, opening areas that were once closed to the private sector, removing limits on foreign ownership of Indian assets, and lowering barriers to international trade.

Privatization

Hand in hand with deregulation has come a sharp increase in privatization. **Privatization** transfers the ownership of state property into the hands of private individuals, frequently by the sale of state assets through an auction.[52] Privatization is seen as a way to unlock gains in economic efficiency by giving new private owners a powerful incentive—the reward of greater profits—to search for increases in productivity, to enter new markets, and to exit losing ones.[53]

The privatization movement started in Great Britain in the early 1980s when then Prime Minister Margaret Thatcher started to sell state-owned assets such as the British telephone company, British Telecom (BT). In a pattern that has been repeated around the world, this sale was linked with the deregulation of the British telecommunications industry. By allowing other firms to compete head to head with BT, deregulation ensured that privatization did not simply replace a state-owned monopoly with a private monopoly. The accompanying Country Focus looks at privatization in Taiwan, and the opening case discussed privatization in India. As these two examples suggest, privatization has become a worldwide movement. In Africa, for example, Mozambique and Zambia are leading the way with very ambitious privatization plans. Zambia put more than 145 state-owned companies up for sale, while Mozambique has already sold scores of enterprises, ranging from tea plantations to a chocolate factory. The most dramatic privatization programs, however, have occurred in the economies of the former Soviet Union and its Eastern European satellite states.

Country Focus

Privatization in Taiwan

Taiwan has the fifth largest economy in Asia and a well-earned reputation as an entrepreneurial powerhouse. Despite this, wide swaths of its corporate landscape are dominated by state-owned enterprises, including the banking, telecommunications, oil, and steel industries. According to many analysts, state ownership is responsible for a number of economic ills in Taiwan, including low productivity and government budget deficits. For example, estimates suggest that government-controlled banks currently have 30 percent too many staff members given their level of business. Executives at state-owned companies complain bitterly about strict oversight of budgeting and procurement that they say hampers their ability to compete. Government companies must submit spending plans to the legislature for approval more than a year ahead, leaving them unable to respond to quickly changing markets and giving politicians a unique opportunity to meddle in the running of the business. In an effort to correct this, in 1996 the government set a timetable for the privatization of 47 state-owned companies by 2002. By the end of 2002, however, 17 of these companies, including many of the largest, still remained in government hands.

There has been some progress. About 30 companies have been privatized since 1996, including 11 financial institutions, and some have been shut down. Sales of government-owned enterprises to private investors raised some $11.5 billion between 1996 and 2001. But this track record overstates the success of the privatization program. In many of these companies, the state is still the largest single shareholder and able to exercise control by appointing top management and board members. Many of these "privatized" companies are still vulnerable to political influence and, as a result, have not moved quickly to cut excess staff and boost their productivity.

There are several reasons for the slow pace of privatization in Taiwan, including powerful labor unions that have opposed privatization plans at every turn; political opposition from factions in Taiwan's legislature, where many politicians have objected to proposed sales on the grounds that the price is too low or that

unemployment will result; and the weak state of Asian stock markets since the 1997 Asian financial crisis, which has made it difficult to attract investors to buy stock in newly privatized entities. These problems were vividly illustrated in 2001 when the state tried to sell two-thirds of its 99.9 percent stake in Chunghwa Telecom, Taiwan's largest telecommunications provider. Vocal opposition from employees and labor unions, along with political infighting in the legislature, delayed the proposed offering of stock to private investors for several years. In the interim, new private telecommunications providers, including wireless companies, have cut into Chunghwa Telecom's former monopoly, making the company less attractive to investors. Also, a rule prohibiting foreign investors from owning more than 20 percent of the company limited the pool of foreign investors interested in the sale. In a humiliating setback, the government was able to sell only 5 percent of the company's stock.

The failure of the Chunghwa Telecom offerings may have revitalized the privatization program. The government is now facing a rising budget deficit and realizes that the sale of state-owned enterprises could help to plug the gap. There has been a leadership shake-up at the ministry responsible for privatization, and ambitious new plans have been drafted, which, if they transpire, may result in the sale of substantial state assets over the next few years. However, the opposition against privatization remains a problem. For example, Chang Shu-jung, the head of the 16,000-employee union at the state-owned Chinese Petroleum, still vocally opposes the privatization of a company that she states is "an essential national asset," and she claims to have the backing of powerful factions in the Taiwanese legislature. "They have been trying to privatize Chinese Petroleum for years," she says, "and it hasn't happened. And we don't plan to let them do it next year either."

Sources: J. Dean, "Privatizing Taiwan," *Far Eastern Economic Review*, December 19, 2002, pp. 42–45; J. Baum, "Testing the Waters," *Far Eastern Economic Review*, August 31, 2000, pp. 43–44; and M. Montagu-Pollock, "A Landmark Year," *Asiamoney*, January 2001, pp. 31–32.

In the Czech Republic, three-quarters of all state-owned enterprises were privatized between 1989 and 1996, helping to push the share of gross domestic product accounted for by the private sector up from 11 percent in 1989 to 60 percent in 1995. In Russia, where the private sector had been almost completely repressed before 1989, 50 percent of GDP was in private hands by 1995, again much as a result of privatization. And in Poland the private sector accounted for 59 percent of GDP in 1995, up from 20 percent in 1989.[54]

As privatization has proceeded around the world, it has become increasingly clear that simply selling state-owned assets to private investors is not enough to guarantee economic growth. Studies of privatization in central Europe have shown that the process often fails to deliver predicted benefits if the newly privatized firms continue to receive subsidies from the state and if they are protected from foreign competition by barriers to international trade and foreign direct investment.[55] In such cases, the newly privatized firms are sheltered from competition and continue acting like state monopolies. When these circumstances prevail, the newly privatized entities often have little incentive to restructure their operations to become more efficient. For privatization to work, it must also be accompanied by a more general deregulation and opening of the economy. Thus, when Brazil decided to privatize the state-owned telephone monopoly, Telebras Brazil, the government also split the company into four independent units that were to compete with each other and removed barriers to foreign direct investment in telecommunications services. This action ensured that the newly privatized entities would face significant competition and thus would have to improve their operating efficiency to survive.

The ownership structure of newly privatized firms also is important.[56] Many former command economies, for example, lack the legal regulations regarding corporate governance that are found in advanced Western economies. In advanced market economies, boards of directors are appointed by shareholders to make sure managers consider the interests of shareholders when making decisions and try to manage the firm in a manner that is consistent with maximizing the wealth of shareholders. However, some former Communist states lack laws requiring corporations to establish effective boards. In such cases, managers with a small ownership stake can often gain control over the newly privatized entity and run it for their own benefit, while ignoring the interests of other shareholders. Sometimes these managers are the same Communist bureaucrats who ran the enterprise before privatization. Because they have been schooled in the old ways of doing things, they often hesitate to take drastic action to increase the efficiency of the enterprise. Instead, they continue to run the firm as a private fiefdom, seeking to extract whatever economic value they can for their own betterment (in the form of perks that are not reported) while doing little to increase the economic efficiency of the enterprise so that shareholders benefit. Such developments seem less likely to occur, however, if a foreign investor takes a stake in the newly privatized entity. The foreign investor, who usually is a major provider of capital, is often able to use control over a critical resource (money) to push through needed change.

Legal Systems

As noted earlier in this chapter, a well-functioning market economy requires laws protecting private property rights and providing mechanisms for contract enforcement. Without a legal system that protects property rights, and without the machinery to enforce that system, the incentive to engage in economic activity can be reduced substantially by private and public entities, including organized crime, that expropriate the profits generated by the efforts of private-sector entrepreneurs. This has become a problem in many former Communist states. When communism collapsed, many of these countries lacked the legal structure required to protect property rights, all property having been held by the state. Although many states have made big strides toward instituting the required system, it will be years before the legal system is functioning as smoothly as it does in the West. For example, in most Eastern European nations, the title to urban and agricultural property is often uncertain because of incomplete and inaccurate records, multiple pledges on the same property, and unsettled claims resulting from demands for restitution from owners in the pre-Communist era. Also, while most countries have improved their commercial codes, institutional weaknesses still undermine contract enforcement. Court capacity is often inadequate, and procedures for resolving contract disputes out of court are often inadequate or poorly developed.[57]

The Rocky Road

In practice, the road that must be traveled to reach a market-based economic system has often turned out to be rocky.[58] This has been particularly true for the states of Eastern Europe in the post-Communist era. In this region, economic and political chaos has sometimes accompanied the move toward greater political and economic freedom.[59] Most Eastern European states began to liberalize their economies in the heady days of the early 1990s. They dismantled decades of price controls, allowed widespread private ownership of businesses, and permitted much greater competition. Most also planned to sell state-owned enterprises to private investors. However, given the vast number of such enterprises and how inefficient many were, making them unappealing to private investors, most privatization efforts moved forward slowly. In this new environment, many inefficient state-owned enterprises found that they could not survive without a guaranteed market. The newly democratic governments often continued to support these money-losing enterprises to stave off massive unemployment. The resulting subsidies to state-owned enterprises led to ballooning budget deficits that were typically financed by printing money. Printing money, along with the lack of price controls, often led to hyperinflation. In 1993, the inflation rate was 21 percent in Hungary, 38 percent in Poland, 841 percent in Russia, and a staggering 10,000 percent in the Ukraine. Since then, however, many governments have instituted tight monetary policies and brought down their inflation rates.

Another consequence of the shift toward a market economy was collapsing output as inefficient state-owned enterprises failed to find buyers for their goods. Real gross domestic product fell dramatically in many post-Communist states between 1990 and 1994. However, the corner has been turned in several countries. Poland, the Czech Republic, and Hungary now all boast growing economies and relatively low inflation. But some countries, such as Russia and the Ukraine, still find themselves grappling with major economic problems.

A World Bank study suggests that the post-Communist states that have been most successful at transforming their economies followed an economic policy best described as "shock therapy." In these countries—which include the Czech Republic, Hungary, and Poland—prices and trade were liberated quickly, inflation was held in check by tight monetary policy, and the privatization of state-owned industries was implemented rapidly. Among the 26 economies of Eastern Europe and the former Soviet Union, the World Bank found a strong positive correlation between the imposition of such shock therapy and subsequent economic growth. Speedy reformers suffered smaller falls in output and returned to growth more quickly than those such as Russia and the Ukraine that moved more slowly.[60] Rapid transformation may cause considerable dislocation for a number of years, but in the long run it seems to yield the greatest gains.

Implications

The global changes in political and economic systems discussed above have several implications for international business. The ideological conflict between collectivism and individualism that so defined the 20th century is less in evidence today. The West won the Cold War, and Western ideology has never been more widespread than it was at the beginning of the millennium. Although command economies still remain and totalitarian dictatorships can still be found around the world, the tide has been running in favor of free markets and democracy.

The implications for business are enormous. For almost 50 years, half of the world was off-limits to Western businesses. Now all that is changing. Many of the national markets of Eastern Europe, Latin America, Africa, and Asia may still be undeveloped and impoverished, but they are potentially enormous. With a population of more than 1.2 billion, the Chinese market alone is potentially bigger than that of the United States, the European Union, and Japan combined! Similarly India, with its 1 billion people, is a potentially huge future market. Latin America has another 400 million potential consumers. It is unlikely that China, Russia, Poland, or any of the other states now moving toward a free market system will attain the living standards of the West anytime soon. Nevertheless, the upside potential is so large that companies need to consider making inroads now.

However, just as the potential gains are large, so are the risks. There is no guarantee that democracy will thrive in the newly democratic states of Eastern Europe, particularly if these states have to grapple with severe economic setbacks. Totalitarian dictatorships could return, although they are unlikely to be of the communist variety. Although the bipolar world of the Cold War era has vanished, it may be replaced by a multipolar world dominated by a number of civilizations. In such a world, much of the economic promise inherent in the global shift toward market-based economic systems may evaporate in the face of conflicts between civilizations. While the long-term potential for economic gain from investment in the world's new market economies is large, the risks associated with any such investment are also substantial. It would be foolish to ignore these.

Focus On Managerial Implications

The implications for international business of the material discussed in this chapter fall into two broad categories. First, the political, economic, and legal environment of a country clearly influences the attractiveness of that country as a market and/or investment site. The benefits, costs, and risks associated with doing business in a country are a function of that country's political, economic, and legal systems. Second, the political, economic, and legal systems of a country can raise important ethical issues that have implications for the practice of international business. Here we consider each of these issues.

Attractiveness

The overall attractiveness of a country as a market and/or investment site depends on balancing the likely long-term benefits of doing business in that country against the likely costs and risks. Below we consider the determinants of benefits, costs, and risks.

Benefits In the most general sense, the long-run monetary benefits of doing business in a country are a function of the size of the market, the present wealth (purchasing power) of consumers in that market, and the likely future wealth of consumers. While some markets are very large when measured by number of consumers (e.g., China and India), low living standards may imply limited purchasing power and, therefore, a relatively small market when measured in economic terms. While international businesses need to be aware of this distinction, they also need to keep in mind the likely future prospects of a country. In 1960, for example, South Korea was viewed as just another impoverished Third World nation. By 2000 it was the world's 12th largest economy, measured in terms of GDP. International firms that recognized South Korea's potential in 1960 and began to do business in that country may have reaped greater benefits than those that wrote off South Korea.

By identifying and investing early in a potential future economic star, international firms may build brand loyalty and gain experience in that country's business practices. These will pay back substantial dividends if that country achieves sustained high economic growth rates. In contrast, late entrants may find that they lack the brand loyalty and experience necessary to achieve a significant presence in the market. In the language of business strategy, early entrants into potential future economic stars may be able to reap substantial first-mover advantages, while late entrants may fall victim to late-mover disadvantages.[61] (**First-mover advantages** are the advantages that accrue to early entrants into a market. **Late-mover disadvantages** are the handicap that late entrants might suffer from.)

A country's economic system and property rights regime are reasonably good predictors of economic prospects. Countries with free market economies in which property rights are well protected tend to achieve greater economic growth rates than command economies and/or economies where property rights are poorly protected. It follows that a country's economic system and property rights regime, when taken together with market size (in terms of population), probably constitute reasonably good indicators of the potential long-run benefits of doing business in a country.

Costs   A number of political, economic, and legal factors determine the costs of doing business in a country. With regard to political factors, the costs of doing business in a country can be increased by a need to pay off the politically powerful to be allowed by the government to do business. The need to pay what are essentially bribes is greater in closed totalitarian states than in open democratic societies where politicians are held accountable by the electorate (although this is not a hard-and-fast distinction). Whether a company should actually pay bribes in return for market access should be determined on the basis of the legal and ethical implications of such action. We discuss this consideration below.

With regard to economic factors, one of the most important variables is the sophistication of a country's economy. It may be more costly to do business in relatively primitive or undeveloped economies because of the lack of infrastructure and supporting businesses. At the extreme, an international firm may have to provide its own infrastructure and supporting business, which obviously raises costs. When McDonald's decided to open its first restaurant in Moscow, it found that to serve food and drink indistinguishable from that served in McDonald's restaurants elsewhere, it had to vertically integrate backward to supply its own needs. The quality of Russian-grown potatoes and meat was too poor. Thus, to protect the quality of its product, McDonald's set up its own dairy farms, cattle ranches, vegetable plots, and food processing plants within Russia. This raised the cost of doing business in Russia, relative to the cost in more sophisticated economies where high-quality inputs could be purchased on the open market.

As for legal factors, it can be more costly to do business in a country where local laws and regulations set strict standards with regard to product safety, safety in the workplace, environmental pollution, and the like (since adhering to such regulations is costly). It can also be more costly to do business in a country like the United States, where the absence of a cap on damage awards has meant spiraling liability insurance rates. It can be more costly to do business in a country that lacks well-established laws for regulating business practice (as is the case in many of the former Communist nations). In the absence of a well-developed body of business contract law, international firms may find no satisfactory way to resolve contract disputes and, consequently, routinely face large losses from contract violations. Similarly, local laws that fail to adequately protect intellectual property can lead to the "theft" of an international business's intellectual property, and lost income.

Risks   As with costs, the risks of doing business in a country are determined by a number of political, economic, and legal factors. **Political risk** has been defined as the likelihood that political forces will cause drastic changes in a country's business environment that adversely affect the profit and other goals of a particular business enterprise.[62] So defined, political risk tends to be greater in countries experiencing social unrest and disorder or in countries where the underlying nature of a society increases the likelihood of social unrest. Social unrest typically finds expression in strikes, demonstrations, terrorism, and violent conflict. Such unrest is more likely to be found in countries that contain more than one ethnic nationality, in countries where competing ideologies are battling for political control, in countries where economic mismanagement has created high inflation and falling living standards, or in countries that straddle the "fault lines" between civilizations, such as Bosnia.

Social unrest can result in abrupt changes in government and government policy or, in some cases, in protracted civil strife. Such strife tends to have negative economic implications for the profit goals of business enterprises. For example, in the aftermath of the 1979 Islamic revolution in Iran, the Iranian assets of numerous U.S. companies were seized by the new Iranian government without compensation. Similarly, the violent disintegration of the Yugoslavian federation into warring states, including Bosnia, Croatia, and Serbia, precipitated a collapse in the local economies and in the profitability of investments in those countries.

On the economic front, economic risks arise from economic mismanagement by the government of a country. **Economic risks** can be defined as the likelihood that economic mismanagement will cause drastic changes in a country's business environment that adversely affect the profit and other goals of a particular business enterprise. Economic risks are not independent of political risk. Economic mismanagement may give rise to significant social unrest and hence political risk. Nevertheless, economic risks are worth emphasizing as a separate category because there is not always a one-to-one relationship between economic mismanagement and social unrest. One visible indicator of economic mismanagement tends to be a country's inflation rate. Another tends to be the level of business and government debt in the country.

In Asian states such as Indonesia, Thailand, and South Korea, businesses increased their debt rapidly during the 1990s, often at the bequest of the government, which was encouraging them to invest in industries deemed to be of "strategic importance" to the country. The result was overinvestment, with more industrial (factories) and commercial capacity (office space) being built than could be justified by demand conditions. Many of these investments turned out to be uneconomic. The borrowers failed to generate the profits necessary to service their debt payment obligations. In turn, the banks that had lent money to these businesses suddenly found that they had rapid increases in nonperforming loans on their books. Foreign investors, believing that many local companies and banks might go bankrupt, pulled their money out of these countries, selling local stock bonds, and currency. This action precipitated the 1997–98 financial crisis in Southeast Asia. The crisis included a precipitous decline in the value of Asian stock markets, which in some cases exceeded 70 percent; a similar collapse in the value of many Asian currencies against the U.S. dollar; an implosion of local demand; and a severe economic recession that will affect many Asian countries for years to come. In short, economic risks were rising throughout Southeast Asia during the 1990s. Astute foreign businesses and investors, seeing this situation, limited their exposure in this part of the world. More naive businesses and investors lost their shirts!

On the legal front, risks arise when a country's legal system fails to provide adequate safeguards in the case of contract violations or to protect property rights. When legal safeguards are weak, firms are more likely to break contracts and/or steal intellectual property if they perceive it as being in their interests to do so. Thus, **legal risks** might be defined as the likelihood that a trading partner will opportunistically break a contract or expropriate property rights. When legal risks in a country are high, an international business might hesitate entering into a long-term contract or joint-venture agreement with a firm in that country. For example, in the 1970s when the Indian government passed a law requiring all foreign investors to enter into joint ventures with Indian companies, U.S. companies such as IBM and Coca-Cola closed their investments in India. They believed that the Indian legal system did not provide for adequate protection of intellectual property rights, creating the very real danger that their Indian partners might expropriate the intellectual property of the American companies—which for IBM and Coca-Cola amounted to the core of their competitive advantage.

Overall Attractiveness The overall attractiveness of a country as a potential market and/or investment site for an international business depends on balancing the benefits, costs, and risks associated with doing business in that country. Generally, the costs and risks associated with doing business in a foreign country are typically lower in economically advanced and politically stable democratic nations and greater in less developed and politically unstable nations. The calculus is complicated, however, by the fact that the potential long-run benefits are not dependent only upon a nation's current stage of economic development or political stability. Rather, the benefits depend on likely future economic growth rates. Economic growth appears to be a function of a free market system and a country's capacity for growth (which may be greater in less developed nations). This leads one to conclude that, other things being equal, the benefit–cost–risk trade-off is likely to be most favorable in politically stable developed and developing nations that have free market systems and no dramatic upsurge in either inflation rates or private-sector debt. It is likely to be least favorable in politically unstable developing nations that operate with a mixed or command economy or in developing nations where speculative financial bubbles have led to excess borrowing.

Ethics and Regulations

Country differences give rise to some important and contentious ethical issues. Three important issues facing much debate in recent years are (1) the ethics of doing business in nations that violate human rights, (2) the ethics of doing business in countries with very lax labor and environmental regulations, and (3) the ethics of corruption.

Ethics and Human Rights One major ethical dilemma facing firms from democratic nations is whether they should do business in totalitarian countries, such as China, that routinely violate the human rights of their citizens. There are two sides to this issue. Some argue that investing in totalitarian countries provides comfort to dictators and can help prop up repressive regimes that abuse basic human rights. For instance, Human Rights Watch, an organization that promotes the protection of basic human rights around the world, has argued that the progressive trade policies adopted by Western nations toward China have done little to deter human rights abuses.[63] According to Human Rights Watch, the Chinese government stepped up its repression of political dissidents in 1996 after the Clinton administration removed human rights as a factor in determining China's trade status with the United States. Without investment by Western firms and the support of Western governments, many repressive regimes would collapse and be replaced by more democratically inclined governments, critics such as Human Rights Watch argue. Firms that have invested in Chile, China, Iraq, and South Africa have all been the direct targets of such criticisms. The 1994 dismantling of the apartheid system in South Africa has been credited to economic sanctions by Western nations, including a lack of investment by Western firms. This, say those who argue against investment in totalitarian countries, is proof that investment boycotts can work (although decades of U.S.-led investment boycotts against Cuba and Iran, among other countries, have failed to have a similar impact).

In contrast, some argue that Western investment, by raising the level of economic development of a totalitarian country, can help change it from within. They note that economic well-being and political freedoms often go hand in hand. Thus, when arguing against attempts to apply trade sanctions to China in the wake of the violent 1989 government crackdown on pro-democracy demonstrators, the U.S. government claimed that U.S. firms should continue to be allowed to invest in mainland China because greater political freedoms would follow the resulting economic growth. The Clinton administration used similar logic as the basis for its 1996 decision decoupling human rights issues from trade policy considerations.

Since both positions have some merit, it is difficult to arrive at a general statement of what firms should do. Unless mandated by government (as in the case of investment in South Africa) each firm must make its own judgments about the ethical implications of investing in totalitarian states on a case-by-case basis. The more repressive the regime, however, and the less amenable it seems to be to change, the greater the case for not investing.

Ethics and Regulations A second important ethical issue is whether an international firm should adhere to the same standards of product safety, work safety, and environmental protection that are required in its home country. This is of particular concern to many firms based in Western nations, where product safety, worker safety, and environmental protection laws are among the toughest in the world. Should Western firms investing in less developed countries adhere to tough Western standards, even though local regulations don't require them to do so? This issue has taken on added importance in recent years following revelations that Western enterprises have been using child labor or very poorly paid "sweatshop" labor in developing nations. Companies criticized for using sweatshop labor include the Gap, Disney, Wal-Mart, and Nike.[64]

Again there is no easy answer. While on the face of it the argument for adhering to Western standards might seem strong, on closer examination the issue becomes more complicated. What if adhering to Western standards would make the foreign investment unprofitable, thereby denying the foreign country much-needed jobs? What is the ethical thing to do? To adhere to Western standards and not invest, thereby denying people jobs, or to adhere to local standards and invest, thereby providing jobs and income? As with many ethical dilemmas, there is no easy answer. Each case needs to be assessed on its own merits.

Ethics and Corruption A final ethical issue concerns bribes and corruption. Should an international business pay bribes to corrupt government officials to gain market access to a foreign country? To most Westerners, bribery seems to be a corrupt and morally repugnant way of doing business, so the answer might initially be no. Some countries have laws on their books that prohibit their citizens from paying bribes to foreign government officials in return for economic favors. As noted earlier, the Foreign Corrupt Practices Act prohibits U.S. companies from making "corrupt" payments to foreign officials to obtain or retain business, although many other developed nations lack similar laws. In

1997, trade and finance ministers from the member states of the Organization for Economic Cooperation and Development (OECD), an association of the world's 20 or so most powerful economies, adopted the Convention on Combating Bribery of Foreign Public Officials in International Business Transactions.[65] The convention obliges member states to make the bribery of foreign public officials a criminal offense.

In many parts of the world, payoffs to government officials are a part of life. One can argue that not investing ignores the fact that such investment can bring substantial benefits to the local populace in terms of income and jobs. From a pragmatic standpoint, the practice of giving bribes, although a little evil, might be the price that must be paid to do a greater good (assuming the investment creates jobs where none existed before and assuming the practice is not illegal). Several economists advocate this reasoning, suggesting that in the context of pervasive and cumbersome regulations in developing countries, corruption may actually improve efficiency and help growth! These economists theorize that in a country where preexisting political structures distort or limit the workings of the market mechanism, corruption in the form of black-marketeering, smuggling, and side payments to government bureaucrats to "speed up" approval for business investments may actually enhance welfare.[66] Arguments such as this persuaded the U.S. Congress to exempt certain "grease payments" from the Foreign Corrupt Practices Act.

However, other economists have argued that corruption reduces the returns on business investment and leads to low economic growth.[67] In a country where corruption is common, unproductive bureaucrats who demand side payments for granting the enterprise permission to operate may siphon off the profits from a business activity. This reduces the incentive that businesses have to invest and may hurt a country's economic growth rate. One economist's study of the connection between corruption and growth in 70 countries found that corruption had a significant negative impact on a country's economic growth rate.[68] Given the debate and the complexity of this issue, one again might conclude that generalization is difficult. Yes, corruption is bad, and yes, it may harm a country's economic development, but yes, there are also cases where side payments to government officials can remove the bureaucratic barriers to investments that create jobs. This pragmatic stance ignores, however, that corruption tends to "corrupt" both the bribe giver and the bribe taker. Corruption feeds on itself, and once an individual has started to walk down the road of corruption, pulling back may be difficult if not impossible. This strengthens the moral case for never engaging in corruption, no matter how compelling the benefits might seem.

ChapterSummary

This chapter has reviewed how the political, economic, and legal systems of different countries vary. The potential benefits, costs, and risks of doing business in a country are a function of its political, economic, and legal systems. The chapter made these specific points:

1. Political systems can be assessed according to two dimensions: the degree to which they emphasize collectivism as opposed to individualism, and the degree to which they are democratic or totalitarian.

2. Collectivism is an ideology that views the needs of society as being more important than the needs of the individual. Collectivism translates into an advocacy for state intervention in economic activity and, in the case of communism, a totalitarian dictatorship.

3. Individualism is an ideology that is built on an emphasis of the primacy of individual's freedoms in the political, economic, and cultural realms. Individualism translates into an advocacy for democratic ideals and free market economics.

4. Democracy and totalitarianism are at different ends of the political spectrum. In a representa-

tive democracy, citizens periodically elect individuals to represent them and political freedoms are guaranteed by a constitution. In a totalitarian state, political power is monopolized by a party, group, or individual, and basic political freedoms are denied to citizens of the state.

5. There are three broad types of economic systems: a market economy, a command economy, and a mixed economy. In a market economy, prices are free of controls and private ownership is predominant. In a command economy, prices are set by central planners, productive assets are owned by the state, and private ownership is forbidden. A mixed economy has elements of both a market economy and a command economy.

6. Differences in the structure of law between countries can have important implications for the practice of international business. The degree to which property rights are protected can vary dramatically from country to country, as can product safety and product liability legislation and the nature of contract law.

7. The rate of economic progress in a country seems to depend on the extent to which that country has a well-functioning market economy in which property rights are protected.

8. Many countries are now in a state of transition. There is a marked shift away from totalitarian governments and command or mixed economic systems and toward democratic political institutions and free market economic systems.

9. The attractiveness of a country as a market and/or investment site depends on balancing the likely long-run benefits of doing business in that country against the likely costs and risks.

10. The benefits of doing business in a country are a function of the size of the market (population), its present wealth (purchasing power), and its future growth prospects. By investing early in countries that are currently poor but are nevertheless growing rapidly, firms can gain first-mover advantages that will pay back substantial dividends in the future.

11. The costs of doing business in a country tend to be greater where political payoffs are required to gain market access, where supporting infrastructure is lacking or underdeveloped, and where adhering to local laws and regulations is costly.

12. The risks of doing business in a country tend to be greater in countries that are (1) politically unstable, (2) subject to economic mismanagement, and (3) lacking a legal system to provide adequate safeguards in the case of contract or property rights violations.

13. Country differences give rise to several ethical dilemmas, including (a) should a firm do business in a repressive totalitarian state, (b) should a firm conform to its home product, workplace, and environmental standards when they are not required by the host country, and (c) should a firm pay bribes to government officials to gain market access?

Critical Discussion Questions

1. Free market economies stimulate greater economic growth, whereas state-directed economies stifle growth! Discuss.

2. A democratic political system is an essential condition for sustained economic progress. Discuss.

3. What is the relationship between corruption in a country (i.e., bribe taking by government officials) and economic growth? Is corruption always bad?

4. The Nobel Prize–winning economist Amartya Sen argues that the concept of development should be broadened to include more than just economic development. What other factors does Sen think should be included in an assessment of development? How might adoption of Sen's views influence government policy? Do you think Sen is correct that development is about more than just economic development? Explain.

5. During the late 1980s and early 1990s, China was routinely cited by various international organiza-

tions such as Amnesty International and Freedom Watch for major human rights violations, including torture, beatings, imprisonment, and executions of political dissidents. Despite this, in the late 1990s and early 2000s, China received record levels of foreign direct investment, mainly from firms based in democratic societies such as the United States, Japan, and Germany. Evaluate this trend from an ethical perspective. If you were the CEO of a firm that had the option of making a potentially very profitable investment in China, what would you do?

6. You are the CEO of a company that has to choose between making a $100 million investment in Russia or the Czech Republic. Both investments promise the same long-run return, so your choice is driven by risk considerations. Assess the various risks of doing business in each of these nations. Which investment would you favor and why?

Notes

1. Although as we shall see, there is not a strict one-to-one correspondence between political systems and economic systems. A. O. Hirschman, "The On-and-Off-Again Connection between Political and Economic Progress," *American Economic Review* 84, no. 2 (1994), pp. 343–48.

2. For a discussion of the roots of collectivism and individualism, see H. W. Spiegel, *The Growth of Economic Thought* (Durham, NC: Duke University Press, 1991). An easily assessible discussion of collectivism and individualism can be found in M. Friedman and R. Friedman, *Free to Choose* (London: Penguin Books, 1980).

3. For a classic summary of the tenets of Marxism details, see A. Giddens, *Capitalism and Modern Social Theory* (Cambridge: Cambridge University Press, 1971).

4. For details see "A Survey of China," *The Economist*, March 18, 1995.

5. J. S. Mill, *On Liberty* (London: Longman's, 1865), p. 6.

6. A. Smith, *The Wealth of Nations, Vol. 1* (London: Penguin Books), p. 325.

7. R. Wesson, *Modern Government—Democracy and Authoritarianism*, 2nd ed. (Englewood Cliffs, NJ: Prentice Hall, 1990).

8. For a detailed but accessible elaboration of this argument, see Friedman and Friedman, *Free to Choose*. Also see P. M. Romer, "The Origins of Endogenous Growth," *Journal of Economic Perspectives* 8, no. 1 (1994), pp. 2–32.

9. T. W. Lippman, *Understanding Islam* (New York: Meridian Books, 1995).

10. "Islam's Interest," *The Economist*, January 18, 1992, pp. 33–34.

11. Rodney Wilson, "Islamic Banking," *Economic Record*, September 2002, pp. 373–74.

12. This information can be found on the UN's treaty website at http://untreaty.un.org/ENGLISH/bible/englishinternetbible/partI/chapterX/treaty17.asp.

13. International Court of Arbitration, http://www.iccwbo.org/index_court.asp.

14. D. North, *Institutions, Institutional Change, and Economic Performance* (Cambridge: Cambridge University Press, 1991).

15. P. Klebnikov, "Russia's Robber Barons," *Forbes*, November 21, 1994, pp. 74–84; C. Mellow, "Russia: Making Cash from Chaos," *Fortune*, April 17, 1995, pp. 145–51; and "Mr Tatum Checks Out," *The Economist*, November 9, 1996, p. 78.

16. "Godfather of the Kremlin?" *Fortune*, December 30, 1996, pp. 90–96.

17. K. van Wolferen, *The Enigma of Japanese Power* (New York: Vintage Books, 1990), pp. 100–05.

18. P. Bardhan, "Corruption and Development: A Review of the Issues," *Journal of Economic Literature*, September 1997, pp. 1320–46.

19. K. M. Murphy, A. Shleifer, and R. Vishny, "Why Is Rent Seeking So Costly to Growth," *American Economic Review* 83, no. 2 (1993), pp. 409–14.

20. http://www.transparency.de/.

21. J. Coolidge and S. Rose Ackerman, "High Level Rent Seeking and Corruption in African Regimes," *World Bank Policy Research Working Paper #1780*, June 1997; Murphy, Shleifer, and Vishny, "Why Is Rent Seeking So Costly to Growth"; M. Habib and L. Zurawicki, "Corruption and Foreign Direct Investment," *Journal of International Business Studies* 33 (2002), pp. 291–307; and J. E. Anderson and D. Marcouiller, "Insecurity and the Pattern of International Trade," *Review of Economics and Statistics* 84 (2002), pp. 342–52.

22. Dale Stackhouse and Kenneth Ungar, "The Foreign Corrupt Practices Act: Bribery, Corruption, Record Keeping and More," *Indiana Lawyer*, April 21, 1993.

23. For an interesting discussion of strategies for dealing with the low cost of copying and distributing digital information, see the chapter on rights management in C. Shapiro and H. R. Varian, *Information Rules* (Boston: Harvard Business School Press, 1999).

24. Douglass North has argued that the correct specification of intellectual property rights is one factor that lowers the cost of doing business and, thereby, stimulates economic growth and development. See North, *Institutions, Institutional Change, and Economic Performance*.

25. International Federation of the Phonographic Industry, Fighting Piracy, 2001, www.ifpi.org.

26. Business Software Alliance, *Eighth Annual BSA Global Software Piracy Study*, June 2003. Available from http://www.bsa.org.

27. Ibid.

28. "Trade Tripwires," *The Economist*, August 27, 1994, p. 61.

29. A. Sen, *Development as Freedom* (New York: Alfred A. Knopf, 1999).

30. G. M. Grossman and E. Helpman, "Endogenous Innovation in the Theory of Growth," *Journal of*

Economic Perspectives 8, no. 1 (1994), pp. 23–44, and P. M. Romer, "The Origins of Endogenous Growth," *Journal of Economic Perspectives* 8, no. 1 (1994), pp. 3–22.

31. F. A. Hayek, *The Fatal Conceit: Errors of Socialism* (Chicago: University of Chicago Press, 1989).

32. James Gwartney, Robert Lawson, and Walter Block, *Economic Freedom of the World: 1975–1995* (London: Institute of Economic Affairs, 1996).

33. North, *Institutions, Institutional Change and Economic Performance.* See also Murphy, Shleifer, and Vishny, "Why Is Rent Seeking So Costly to Growth?" Also see K. E. Maskus, *Intellectual Property Rights in the Global Economy* (Institute for International Economics, 2000)

34. Hirschman, "The On-and-Off-Again Connection between Political and Economic Progress," and A. Przeworski and F. Limongi, "Political Regimes and Economic Growth," *Journal of Economic Perspectives* 7, no. 3 (1993), pp. 51–59.

35. As an example, see "Why Voting Is Good for You," *The Economist*, August 27, 1994, pp. 15–17.

36. Ibid.

37. For details of this argument, see M. Olson, "Dictatorship, Democracy, and Development," *American Political Science Review*, September 1993.

38. For example, see Jarad Diamond's Pulitzer Prize–winning book, *Guns, Germs, and Steel* (New York: W. W. Norton, 1997). Also see J. Sachs, "Nature, Nurture and Growth," *The Economist*, June 14, 1997, pp. 19–22.

39. Sachs, "Nature, Nurture and Growth."

40. "What Can the Rest of the World Learn from the Classrooms of Asia?" *The Economist*, September 21, 1996, p. 24.

41. J. Fagerberg, "Technology and International Differences in Growth Rates," *Journal of Economic Literature* 32 (September 1994), pp. 1147–75.

42. See The Freedom House Survey Team, "Freedom in the World: 2001–2002" and associated materials. Available at http://www.freedomhouse.org/research/freeworld/2002/essay2002.pdf

43. Freedom House, "Democracies Century: A Survey of Political Change in the Twentieth Century, 1999." Available at http://www.freedomhouse.org.

44. L. Conners, "Freedom to Connect," *Wired*, August 1997, pp. 105–06.

45. F. Fukuyama, "The End of History," *The National Interest* 16 (Summer 1989), p. 18.

46. S. P. Huntington, *The Clash of Civilizations and the Remaking of World Order* (New York: Simon & Schuster, 1996).

47. Ibid., p. 116.

48. United States Department of State, *Patterns of Global Terrorism* 2002 (Washington, DC: U.S. State Department, April 2003).

49. S. Fisher, R. Sahay, and C. A. Vegh, "Stabilization and the Growth in Transition Economies: the Early Experience," *Journal of Economic Perspectives* 10 (Spring 1996), pp. 45–66.

50. G. P. O'Driscoll, K. R. Holmes, and M. Kirkpatrick, *2002 Index of Economic Freedom*. (Washington, DC; Heritage Foundation, 2002).

51. International Monetary Fund, *World Economic Outlook: Focus on Transition Economies* (Geneva: IMF, October 2000).

52. J. C. Brada, "Privatization Is Transition—Is It?" *Journal of Economic Perspectives*, Spring 1996, pp. 67–86.

53. See S. Zahra et al., "Privatization and Entrepreneurial Transformation," *Academy of Management Review* 3, no. 25 (2000), pp. 509–24.

54. Fischer, Sahay, and Vegh, "Stabilization and Growth in Transition Economies."

55. J. Sachs, C. Zinnes, and Y. Eilat, "The Gains from Privatization in Transition Economies: Is Change of Ownership Enough?" *CAER Discussion Paper No. 63* (Cambridge, MA: Harvard Institute for International Development, 2000).

56. J. Nellis, "Time to Rethink Privatization in Transition Economies?" *Finance and Development* 36, no. 2 (1999), pp. 16–19.

57. M. S. Borish and M. Noel, "Private Sector Development in the Visegrad Countries," *World Bank*, March 1997.

58. See S. Fisher and R. Sahay, "The Transition Economies after Ten Years," *IMF Working Paper 00/30* (Washington, DC: International Monetary Fund, 2000).

59. International Monetary Fund, *World Economic Outlook: Focus on Transition Economies* (Washington, DC: International Monetary Fund).

60. "Lessons of Transition," *The Economist*, June 29, 1996, p. 81, and P. K. Mitra and M. Selowsky, "Lessons from a Decade of Transition in Eastern Europe and the Former Soviet Union," *Finance and Development*, June 2002.

61. For a discussion of first-mover advantages, see M. Liberman and D. Montgomery, "First-Mover Advantages," *Strategic Management Journal* 9 (Summer Special Issue, 1988), pp. 41–58.

62. S. H. Robock, "Political Risk: Identification and Assessment," *Columbia Journal of World Business*, July–August 1971, pp. 6–20.

63. Steven L. Myers, "Report Says Business Interests Overshadow Rights," *New York Times*, December 5, 1996, p. A8.

64. Jo-Ann Mort, "Sweated Shopping," *The Guardian*, September 8, 1997, p. 11.

65. Details can be found at http://www.oecd.org/EN/home/0,,EN-home-31-nodirectorate-no-no-no-31,00.html.

66. Bardhan Pranab, "Corruption and Development," *Journal of Economic Literature* 36 (September 1997), pp. 1320–46.

67. A. Shleifer and R. W. Vishny, "Corruption," *Quarterly Journal of Economics*, no. 108 (1993), pp. 599–617, and I. Ehrlich and F. Lui, "Bureaucratic Corruption and Endogenous Economic Growth," *Journal of Political Economy* 107 (December 1999), pp. 270–92.

68. P. Mauro, "Corruption and Growth," *Quarterly Journal of Economics*, no. 110 (1995), pp. 681–712.

Research Task | globalEDGE™   globaledge.msu.edu

Use the globalEDGE™ site to complete the following exercises:

1. The *Freedom in the World* survey evaluates the state of political rights and civil liberties around the world. Provide a description of this survey and a ranking, in terms of "freedom," of the leaders and laggards of the world. What factors are taken into consideration in this survey when forming the rankings?

2. Market Potential Indicators (MPI) is an indexing study conducted by the Michigan State University Center for International Business Education and Research (MSU-CIBER) to compare emerging markets on a variety of dimensions. Provide a description of the indicators used in the indexing procedure. Which of the indicators would have greater importance for a company that markets laptop computers? Considering the MPI rankings, which developing countries would you advise this company to enter first?

Closing Case

Piracy in the Video Game Market

Over the past decade, the video game industry has grown into a global colossus worth more than $20 billion a year in revenues. For the three biggest players in the industry, Sony with its PlayStation II, Microsoft with X-box, and Nintendo with GameCube, this potentially represents a huge growth engine, but the engine is threatened by a rise in piracy, which cost the industry an estimated $2 billion in 2001.

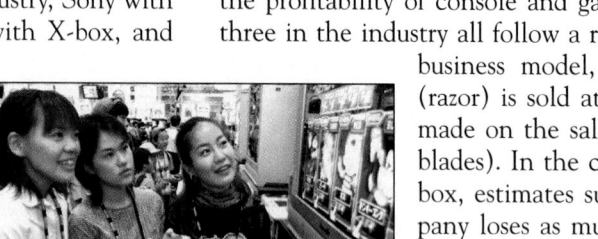

The piracy problem is particularly serious in East Asia, excluding Japan, where video game consoles are routinely "chipped"—sold with modified chips, called "mod-chips," that override the console's security system, allowing it to play illegally copied games and CDs. Importers or resellers, who charge a small markup for making the modification, illegally install the mod-chips. In some regions, Hong Kong for example, it is almost impossible to find a console that hasn't been modified.

Because they allow users to play illegally copied games, consoles with mod-chips installed offer a gaping gateway for software pirates, and they directly threaten the profitability of console and game makers. The big three in the industry all follow a razor-and-razor-blades business model, where the console (razor) is sold at a loss, and profit is made on the sale of the game (razor blades). In the case of Microsoft's X-box, estimates suggest that the company loses as much as $200 on each X-box it sells. To make profits, Microsoft collects royalties on the sale of games developed under license, in addition to producing and selling some games itself. Each game typically retails for about $50, and Microsoft must sell 6 to 12 games to each X-box user to recoup the $200 loss on the initial sale and start making a profit. If those users are purchasing pirated games and playing them on "chipped" X-box consoles, Microsoft collects nothing in royalties and may never reach breakeven. Sony and Nintendo face similar problems. In East Asia, some 70 precent of game software sold in the region may be pirated thanks to the popularity of "chipped" consoles and the low price of pirated games, which may sell for one-third of the price of the legal game.

Historically, the big video game companies tried to deal with the piracy problem in East Asia by ignoring the market. Sony launched its PlayStation II in East Asia two years after its Japanese launch, and Microsoft delayed its East Asian launch for a year after it launched elsewhere in the world. But this tactic is increasingly questionable in a region where there may soon be more gamers than in the United States. Industry estimates suggest that Asian gamers will spend some $7.6 billion on videogame software in 2004, much of it on low-priced pirated games, compared to $7.4 billion in the United States.

Another tactic that both Sony and Microsoft are now using is to regularly alter the hardware specifications of its consoles, rendering the existing mod-chips useless. But the companies have found that this is just a temporary solution, for within a few weeks the new system is cracked, and mod-chips made to override the new specifications are available on the market.

A third tactic is to push the local authorities to legally enforce existing intellectual property rights law that in theory outlaws the mod-chip practice. In late 2002, Microsoft, Sony, and Nintendo joined forces to sue a Hong Kong company called Lik Sang, which sold mod-chips

through its website and is one of the world's largest distributors of the chips. Some observers question the value of this, however, for they argue that if Lik Sang is shut down, many others in Hong Kong may be willing to take its place. They argue that concerted government action is needed to stop the pirates, and so far East Asian governments have not been quick to act.

Case Discussion Questions

1. How important is East Asia to the long-term future of the video game companies, Microsoft, Sony, and Nintendo?

2. How big a threat are software piracy and "mod-chips" to the profitability of the video game businesses of these companies?

3. What strategies or tactics might the companies pursue to stop piracy? How successful do you think these strategies might be?

4. What role might international institutions, such as the World Trade Organization, play in solving this particular problem?

Sources: S. Yoon, "The Mod Squad," *East Asian Economic Review*, November 7, 2002, pp. 34–36; R. Cunningham, "Controversy as Sony Loses Mod-Chip Verdict," *Managing Intellectual Property*, September 2002, pp. 15–18; and A. Pham, "Video Game Losses Nearly $2 Billion," *Los Angeles Times*, February 18, 2002, p. C8.

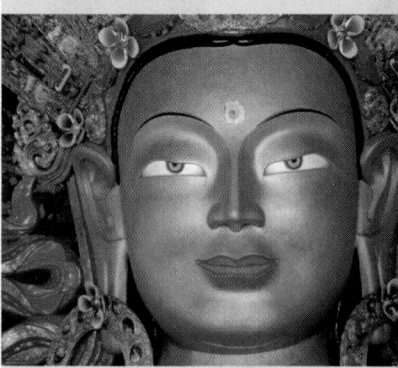

Chapter 3

Differences in Culture

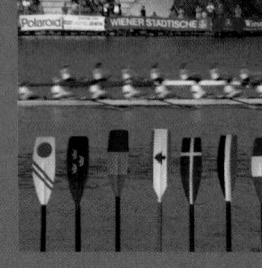

Introduction
What Is Culture?
  Values and Norms
  Culture, Society, and the Nation-State
  The Determinants of Culture
Social Structure
  Individuals and Groups
  Social Stratification
Religious and Ethical Systems
  Christianity
  Islam
  Hinduism
  Buddhism
  Confucianism
Language
  Spoken Language
  Unspoken Language
Education
Culture and the Workplace
Cultural Change
Focus on Managerial Implications
  Cross-Cultural Literacy
  Culture and Competitive Advantage
  Culture and Business Ethics
Chapter Summary
Critical Discussion Questions
Closing Case: McDonald's and Hindu
Culture

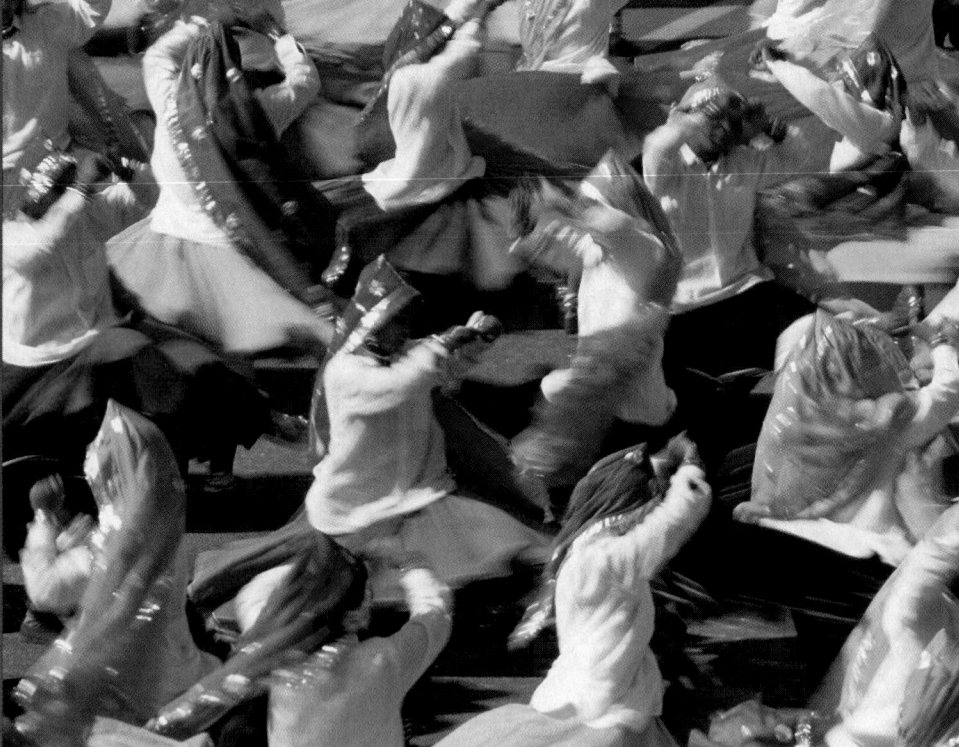

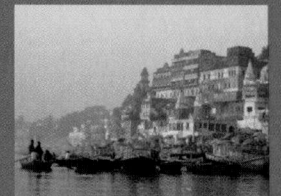

Guanxi—Ties That Bind

In 1992, McDonald's Corporation opened its first restaurant in Beijing, China, after a decade of market research. The restaurant, then the largest McDonald's in the world, was located on the corner of Wangfujing Street and the Avenue of Eternal Peace, just two blocks from Tiananmen Square, the very heart of China's capital. The choice of location seemed auspicious, and within two years, sales at the restaurant were surpassing all expectations. Then the Beijing city government dropped a bombshell; officials abruptly informed McDonald's that it would have to vacate the location to make way for a commercial, residential, and office complex planned by Hong Kong developer Li Ka-shing. At the time, McDonald's still had 18 years to run on its 20-year lease. A stunned McDonald's did what any good Western company would do—it took the Beijing city government to court to try to enforce the lease. The court refused to enforce the lease, and McDonald's had to move. Chinese observers had a simple explanation for the outcome. McDonald's, they said, lacked the *guanxi* of Li Ka-shing. Given this, the company could not expect to prevail. Company executives should have accepted the decision in good grace and moved on, but instead, McDonald's filed a lawsuit—a move that would only reduce what *guanxi* McDonald's might have with the city government!

This example illustrates a basic difference between doing business in the West and doing business in China. In the advanced economies of the West, business transactions are conducted and regulated by the centuries-old framework of contract law, which specifies the rights and obligations of parties to a business contract and provides mechanisms for seeking to redress grievances should one party in the exchange fail to live up to the legal agreement. In the West, McDonald's could have relied on the courts to enforce its legal contract with the city government. In China, this approach didn't work. China does not have the same legal infrastructure. Personal power and relationships or connections, rather than the rule of law, have always been the key to getting things done in China. Decades of Communist rule stripped away the basic legal infrastructure that did exist to regulate business transactions. Power, relationships, and connections are an important, and some say necessary, influence on getting things done and enforcing business agreements in China. The key to understanding this process is the concept of *guanxi*.

Guanxi literally means relationships, although in business settings it can be better understood as "connections." McDonald's lost its lease in central Beijing because it lacked the *guanxi* enjoyed by the powerful Li Ka-shing. The concept of *guanxi* is deeply rooted in Chinese culture, particularly the Confucian philosophy of valuing social hierarchy and reciprocal obligations. Confucian ideology has a 2,000-year-old history in China, and more than half a century of Communist rule has done little to dent its influence on everyday life in China. Confucianism stresses the importance of relationships, both within the family and between master and servant. Confucian ideology teaches that people are not created equal. In Confucian thought, loyalty and obligations to one's superiors (or to family) is regarded as a sacred duty, but at the same time, this loyalty has its price. Social superiors are obligated to reward the loyalty of their social inferiors by bestowing "blessings" upon them; thus, the obligations are reciprocal.

Today, Chinese will often cultivate a *guanxiwang*, or "relationship network," for help. Reciprocal obligations are the glue that holds such networks together. If those obligations are not met—if favors done are not paid back or reciprocated—the reputation of the transgressor is tarnished and he or she will be less able to draw on their *guanxiwang* for help in the future. Thus, the implicit threat of social sanctions is often sufficient to ensure that favors are repaid, that obligations are met, and that relationships are honored. In a society that lacks a rule-based legal tradition, and thus legal ways of redressing wrongs such as violations of business agreements, *guanxi* is an important mechanism for building long-term business relationships and getting business done in China. There is a tacit acknowledgment that if you have the right *guanxi*, legal rules can be broken, or at least bent. Li Ka-shing had the right *guanxi*; McDonald's apparently did not.

As they have come to understand this, many Western businesses have tried to build *guanxi* to grease the wheels required to do business in China. Increasingly, *guanxi* has become a commodity that is for sale to foreigners. Many of the sons and daughters of high-ranking government officials have set up "consulting" firms and offered to mobilize their *guanxiwang* or those of their parents to help Western companies navigate their way through Chinese bureaucracy. Taking advantage of such services, however, requires good ethical judgment. There is a fine line between relationship building, which may require doing favors to meet obligations, and bribery. Consider the case of a lucrative business contract that was under consideration for more than a year between a large Chinese state-owned enterprise and two competing multinational firms. After months of negotiations, the Chinese elected to continue discussions with just one of the competitors—the one that had recently hired the son of the principal Chinese negotiator at a significant salary. This occurred even though the favored firm's equipment was less compatible with Chinese equipment already in place than that offered by the multinational that was rejected. The clear implication is that the son of the negotiator had mobilized his *guanxiwang* to help his new employer gain an advantage in the contract negotiations. While hiring the son of the principal negotiator may be viewed as good business practice by some in the context of Chinese culture, others might argue that this action was ethically suspect and could be viewed as little more than a thinly concealed bribe.

Sources: S. D. Seligman, "Guanxi: Grease for the Wheels of China," *China Business Review,* September–October 1999, pp. 34–38; L. Dana, "Culture Is the Essence of Asia," *Financial Times,* November 27, 2000, p. 12; L. Minder, "McDonald's to Close Original Beijing Store," *USA Today,* December 2, 1996, p. 1A; and M. W. Peng, *Business Strategies in Transition Economies* (Thousand Oaks, CA: Sage Publications, 2000).

■ Introduction

International business is different because countries are different. In Chapter 2 we saw how national differences in political, economic, and legal systems influence the benefits, costs, and risks associated with doing business in different countries. In this chapter, we will explore how differences in culture across and within countries can affect international business. Several themes run through this chapter.

The first theme is that business success in a variety of countries requires cross-cultural literacy. By **cross-cultural literacy,** we mean an understanding of how cultural differences across and within nations can affect the way in which business is practiced. In these days of global communications, rapid transportation, and global markets, when the era of the global village seems just around the corner, it is easy to forget just how different various cultures really are. Underneath the veneer of modernism, deep cultural differences often remain. Westerners in general, and Americans in particular, are quick to conclude that because people from other parts of the world also wear blue jeans, listen to Western popular music, eat at McDonald's, and drink Coca-Cola, they also accept the basic tenets of Western (or American) culture. But this is not true. Increasingly, the Chinese are embracing the material products of modern society. Anyone who has visited Shanghai, for example, cannot fail to be struck by how modern the city seems, with its skyscrapers, department stores, and freeways. But as the opening case demonstrates, beneath the veneer of Western modernism, long-standing cultural traditions rooted in a 2,000-year-old ideology continue to have an important influence on the way business is transacted in China. In China, *guanxi*, or relationships backed by reciprocal obligations, are central to getting business done. As the opening case demonstrates, firms that lack sufficient *guanxi*, as McDonald's apparently did, may find themselves at a disadvantage when doing business in China. In this chapter, we shall argue that it is important for foreign businesses to gain an understanding of the culture, or cultures, that prevail in those countries where they do business.

The opening case also illustrates another important theme that we shall develop further in this chapter: The old adage of "when in Rome do as the Romans do" may have ethical ramifications. Prevailing cultural mores in a country may put a foreign business in a difficult ethical position. For example, while it is important to build *guanxi* in China, there is a thin line between giving gifts to support the establishment of relationships, which is culturally normal behavior, and bribery or corruption, which is viewed dimly in the West and against the law in some nations such as the United States, where the Foreign Corrupt Practices Act makes it illegal for a U.S. company to bribe government officials to gain business in a foreign nation.

Another theme developed in this chapter is that a relationship may exist between culture and the cost of doing business in a country or region. Different cultures are more or less supportive of the capitalist mode of production and may increase or lower the costs of doing business. For example, some observers have argued that cultural factors lowered the costs of doing business in Japan and helped to explain Japan's rapid economic ascent during the 1960s, 70s, and 80s.[1] By the same token, cultural factors can sometimes raise the costs of doing business. Historically, class divisions were an important aspect of British culture, and for a long time, firms operating in Great Britain found it difficult to achieve cooperation between management and labor. Class divisions led to a high level of industrial disputes in that country during the 1960s and 1970s and raised the costs of doing business in Great Britain relative to the costs in countries such as Switzerland, Norway, Germany, or Japan, where class conflict was historically less prevalent.

The British example, however, brings us to the final theme we will explore in this chapter: Culture is not static. It can and does evolve, although the rate at which culture can change is the subject of some dispute. Important aspects of British culture have changed significantly over the past 20 years, and this is reflected in weaker class distinctions and a lower level of industrial disputes. Between 1991 and 2000, the number of days lost per 1,000 workers due to strikes in the United Kingdom was on average 23 each year, significantly less than in the United States (where the figure was 53), France (where 77 days were lost), and Canada (where 189 were lost).[2] Similarly, there is evidence of changes in the culture of Japan, with the traditional Japanese emphasis on group identification giving way to greater emphasis on individualism.

What Is Culture?

Scholars have never been able to agree on a simple definition of culture. In the 1870s, the anthropologist Edward Tylor defined culture as "that complex whole which includes knowledge, belief, art, morals, law, custom, and other capabilities acquired by man as a member of society."[3] Since then hundreds of other definitions have been offered. Geert Hofstede, an expert on cross-cultural differences and management, defined culture as "the collective programming of the mind which distinguishes the members of one human group from another . . . Culture, in this sense, includes systems of values; and values are among the building blocks of culture."[4] Another definition of culture comes from sociologists Zvi Namenwirth and Robert Weber who see culture as a system of ideas and argue that these ideas constitute a design for living.[5]

Here we follow both Hofstede and Namenwirth and Weber by viewing culture as a system of values and norms that are shared among a group of people and that when taken together constitute a design for living. By **values** we mean abstract ideas about what a group believes to be good, right, and desirable. Put differently, values are shared assumptions about how things ought to be.[6] By **norms** we mean the social rules and guidelines that prescribe appropriate behavior in particular situations. We shall use the term **society** to refer to a group of people who share a common set of values and norms. While a society may be equivalent to a country, some countries harbor several "societies" (i.e., they support multiple cultures), and some societies embrace more than one country.

Values and Norms

Values form the bedrock of a culture. They provide the context within which a society's norms are established and justified. They may include a society's attitudes toward such concepts as individual freedom, democracy, truth, justice, honesty, loyalty, social obligations, collective responsibility, the role of women, love, sex, marriage, and so on. Values are not just abstract concepts; they are invested with considerable emotional significance. People argue, fight, and even die over values such as freedom. Values also often are reflected in the political and economic systems of a society. As we saw in Chapter 2, democratic free market capitalism is a reflection of a philosophical value system that emphasizes individual freedom.

Norms are the social rules that govern people's actions toward one another. Norms can be subdivided further into two major categories: folkways and mores. **Folkways** are the routine conventions of everyday life. Generally, folkways are actions of little moral significance. Rather, folkways are social conventions concerning things such as the appropriate dress code in a particular situation, good social manners, eating with the correct utensils, neighborly behavior, and the like. While folkways define the way people are expected to behave, violation of folkways is not normally a serious matter. People who violate folkways may be thought of as eccentric or ill-mannered, but they are not usually considered to be evil or bad. In many countries, foreigners may initially be excused for violating folkways.

A good example of folkways concerns attitudes toward time in different countries. People are very time conscious in the United States. Americans tend to arrive a few minutes early for business appointments. When invited for dinner to someone's home, it is considered polite to arrive on time or just a few minutes late. The concept of time can be very different in other countries. It is not necessarily a breach of etiquette to arrive a little late for a business appointment; it might even be considered more impolite to arrive early. Arriving on time for a dinner engagement can be very bad manners. In Great Britain, for example, when someone says, "Come for dinner at 7:00 P.M.," what he means is "come for dinner at 7:30 to 8:00 P.M." The guest who arrives at 7:00 P.M. is likely to find an unprepared and embarrassed host. Similarly, when an Argentinean says, "Come for dinner anytime after 8:00 P.M." what she means is don't come at 8:00 P.M.—it's far too early!

Mores are norms that are seen as central to the functioning of a society and to its social life. They have much greater significance than folkways. Accordingly, violating mores can bring serious retribution. Mores include such factors as indictments against theft, adultery, incest, and cannibalism. In many societies, certain mores have been enacted into law. Thus, all advanced societies have laws against theft, incest, and cannibalism. However, there are also many differences between cultures as to what is perceived as mores. In America, for example, drinking alcohol is widely accepted, whereas in Saudi Arabia the consumption of alcohol is viewed as violating important social mores and is punishable by imprisonment (as some Western citizens working in Saudi Arabia have found out).

Culture, Society, and the Nation-State

We have defined a society as a group of people that share a common set of values and norms; that is, people who are bound together by a common culture. However, there is not a strict one-to-one correspondence between a society and a nation-state. Nation-states are political creations. They may contain a single culture or several cultures. While the French nation can be thought of as the political embodiment of French culture, the nation of Canada has at least three cultures—an Anglo culture, a French-speaking "Quebecois" culture, and a Native American culture. Similarly, many African nations have important cultural differences between tribal groups, as exhibited in the early 1990s when Rwanda dissolved into a bloody civil war between two tribes, the Tutsis and Hutus. Africa is not alone in this regard. India is composed of many distinct cultural groups. During the Gulf War, the prevailing view presented to Western audiences was that Iraq was a homogenous Arab nation. But the chaos that followed the war revealed several different societies within Iraq, each with its own culture. The Kurds in the north do not view themselves as Arabs and have their own distinct history and traditions. Then there are two Arab societies: the Shiites in the South and the Sunnis who populate the middle of the country and who ruled Iraq (the terms *Shiites* and *Sunnis* refer to different sects within the religion of Islam). Among the southern Sunnis is another distinct society of 500,000 "Marsh Arabs" who live at the confluence of the Tigris and Euphrates rivers, pursuing a way of life that dates back 5,000 years.[7]

At the other end of the scale, we can speak of cultures that embrace several nations. Several scholars, for example, argue that we can speak of an Islamic society or culture that is shared by the citizens of many different nations in the Middle East, Asia, and

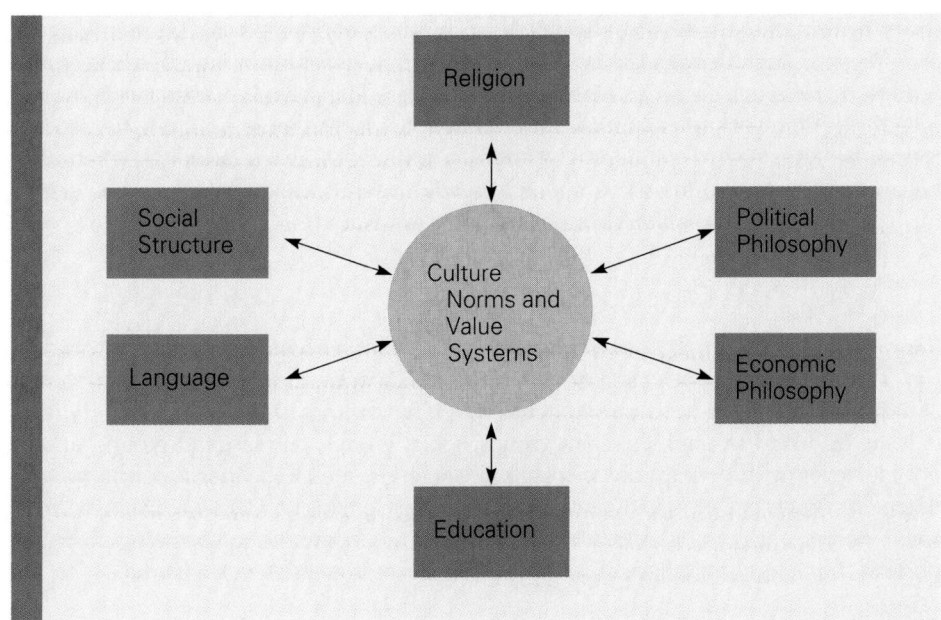

Figure 3.1

The Determinants of
Culture

Africa. As you will recall from the last chapter, this view of expansive cultures that embrace several nations underpins Samuel Huntington's view of a world that is fragmented into different civilizations including Western, Islamic, and Sinic (Chinese) civilizations.[8]

To complicate things further, it is also possible to talk about culture at different levels. It is reasonable to talk about "American society" and "American culture," but there are several societies within America, each with its own culture. One can talk about Afro-American culture, Cajun culture, Chinese-American culture, Hispanic culture, Indian culture, Irish-American culture, and Southern culture. The point is that the relationship between culture and country is often ambiguous. One cannot always characterize a country as having a single homogenous culture, and even when one can, one must also often recognize that the national culture is a mosaic of subcultures.

The Determinants of Culture

The values and norms of a culture do not emerge fully formed. They are the evolutionary product of a number of factors, including the prevailing political and economic philosophy, the social structure of a society, and the dominant religion, language, and education (see Figure 3.1). We discussed political and economic philosophy at length in Chapter 2. Such philosophy clearly influences the value systems of a society. For example, the values found in Communist North Korea toward freedom, justice, and individual achievement are clearly different from the values found in the United States, precisely because each society operates according to a different political and economic philosophy. Below we will discuss the influence of social structure, religion, language, and education. The chain of causation runs both ways. While factors such as social structure and religion clearly influence the values and norms of a society, the values and norms of a society can influence social structure and religion.

Social Structure

A society's "social structure" refers to its basic social organization. Although social structure consists of many different aspects, two dimensions are particularly important when explaining differences between cultures. The first is the degree to which the basic unit of social organization is the individual, as opposed to the group. In general, Western societies tend to emphasize the primacy of the individual, while groups tend to figure much larger in many other societies. The second dimension is the degree to which a society is stratified into classes or castes. Some societies are characterized by a relatively high degree of social stratification and relatively low mobility between strata (e.g., Indian), while other societies are characterized by a low degree of social stratification and high mobility between strata (e.g., American).

▌Individuals and Groups

A **group** is an association of two or more individuals who have a shared sense of identity and who interact with each other in structured ways on the basis of a common set of expectations about each other's behavior.[9] Human social life is group life. Individuals are involved in families, work groups, social groups, recreational groups, and so on. However, while groups are found in all societies, societies differ according to the degree to which the group is viewed as the primary means of social organization.[10] In some societies, individual attributes and achievements are viewed as being more important than group membership, while in other societies the reverse is true.

The Individual

In Chapter 2, we discussed individualism as a political philosophy. However, individualism is more than just an abstract political philosophy. In many Western societies, the individual is the basic building block of social organization. This is reflected not just in the political and economic organization of society, but also in the way people perceive themselves and relate to each other in social and business settings. The value systems of many Western societies, for example, emphasize individual achievement. The social standing of individuals is not so much a function of whom they work for, as of their individual performance in whatever work setting they choose.

The emphasis on individual performance in many Western societies has both beneficial and harmful aspects. In the United States, the emphasis on individual performance finds expression in an admiration of "rugged individualism" and entrepreneurship. One benefit of this is the high level of entrepreneurial activity in the United States and other Western societies. New products and new ways of doing business (e.g., personal computers, photocopiers, computer software, biotechnology, supermarkets, and discount retail stores) have repeatedly been created in the United States by entrepreneurial individuals. One can argue that the dynamism of the U.S. economy owes much to the philosophy of individualism.

Individualism also finds expression in a high degree of managerial mobility between companies, and this is not always a good thing. While moving from company to company may be good for individual managers, who are trying to build impressive résumés, it is not necessarily a good thing for American companies. The lack of loyalty and commitment to an individual company, and the tendency to move on when a better offer comes along, can result in managers who have good general skills but lack the knowledge, experience, and network of interpersonal contacts that come from years of working within the same company. An effective manager draws on company-specific experience, knowledge, and a network of contacts to find solutions to current problems, and American companies may suffer if their managers lack these attributes.

One positive aspect of high managerial mobility is that executives are exposed to different ways of doing business. The ability to compare business practices helps U.S. executives identify how good practices and techniques developed in one firm might be profitably applied to other firms.

The emphasis on individualism may also make it difficult to build teams within an organization to perform collective tasks. If individuals are always competing with each other on the basis of individual performance, it may be difficult for them to cooperate. One study of U.S. competitiveness by the Massachusetts Institute of Technology concluded that U.S. firms are being hurt in the global economy by a failure to achieve co-operation both within a company (e.g., between functions; between management and labor) and between companies (e.g., between a firm and its suppliers). Given the emphasis on individualism in the American value system, this failure is not surprising.[11] So the emphasis on individualism in the United States, while helping to create a dynamic entrepreneurial economy, may raise the costs of doing business due to its adverse impact on managerial stability and cooperation.

The Group

In contrast to the Western emphasis on the individual, the group is the primary unit of social organization in many other societies. For example, in Japan, the social status of an individual is determined as much by the standing of the group to which he or she belongs as by his or her individual performance.[12] In traditional Japanese society, the group was the family or village to which an individual belonged. Today the group has frequently come to be associated with the work team or business organization to which an individual belongs. In a now classic study of Japanese society, Nakane has noted how this expresses itself in everyday life:

> When a Japanese faces the outside (confronts another person) and affixes some position to himself socially he is inclined to give precedence to institution over kind of occupation. Rather than saying, "I am a typesetter" or "I am a filing clerk," he is likely to say, "I am from B Publishing Group" or "I belong to S company."[13]

Nakane goes on to observe that the primacy of the group to which an individual belongs often evolves into a deeply emotional attachment in which identification with the group becomes all important in one's life. One central value of Japanese culture is the importance attached to group membership. This may have beneficial implications for business firms. Strong identification with the group is argued to create pressures for mutual self-help and collective action. If the worth of an individual is closely linked to the achievements of the group (e.g., firm), as Nakane maintains is the case in Japan, this creates a strong incentive for individual members of the group to work together for the common good. Some argue that the success of Japanese enterprises in the global economy during the 1970s and 1980s was based partly on their ability to achieve close cooperation between individuals within a company and between companies. This found expression in the widespread diffusion of self-managing work teams within Japanese organizations, the close cooperation between different functions within Japanese companies (e.g., between manufacturing, marketing, and R&D), and the co-operation between a company and its suppliers on issues such as design, quality control, and inventory reduction.[14] In all of these cases, cooperation is driven by the need to improve the performance of the group (i.e., the business firm).

The primacy of the value of group identification also discourages managers and workers from moving from company to company. Lifetime employment in a particular company was long the norm in certain sectors of the Japanese economy (estimates suggest that between 20 and 40 percent of all Japanese employees have formal or informal lifetime employment guarantees). Over the years, managers and workers build up knowledge, experience, and a network of interpersonal business contacts. All these things can help managers perform their jobs more effectively and achieve cooperation with others.

However, the primacy of the group is not always beneficial. Just as U.S. society is characterized by a great deal of dynamism and entrepreneurship, reflecting the primacy of values associated with individualism, some argue that Japanese society is characterized by a corresponding lack of dynamism and entrepreneurship. Although it is not clear how this will play itself out in the long run, the United States could continue to create more new industries than Japan and continue to be more successful at pioneering radically new products and new ways of doing business.

Social Stratification

All societies are stratified on a hierarchical basis into social categories—that is, into **social strata.** These strata are typically defined on the basis of characteristics such as family background, occupation, and income. Individuals are born into a particular stratum. They become a member of the social category to which their parents belong. Individuals born into a stratum toward the top of the social hierarchy tend to have better life chances than individuals born into a stratum toward the bottom of the hierarchy. They are likely to have a better education, better health, a better standard of living, and better work opportunities. Although all societies are stratified to some degree, they differ in two related ways that are of interest to us here. First, they differ from each other with regard to the degree of mobility between social strata, and second, they differ with regard to the significance attached to social strata in business contexts.

Social Mobility

The term **social mobility** refers to the extent to which individuals can move out of the strata into which they are born. Social mobility varies significantly from society to society. The most rigid system of stratification is a caste system. A caste system is a closed system of stratification in which social position is determined by the family into which a person is born, and change in that position is usually not possible during an individual's lifetime. Often a caste position carries with it a specific occupation. Members of one caste might be shoemakers, members of another might be butchers, and so on. These occupations are embedded in the caste and passed down through the family to succeeding generations. Although the number of societies with caste systems diminished rapidly during the 20th century, one partial example still remains. India has four main castes and several thousand subcastes. Even though the caste system was officially abolished in 1949, two years after India became independent, it is still an important force in rural Indian society where occupation and marital opportunities are still partly related to caste.

A **class system** is a less rigid form of social stratification in which social mobility is possible. A class system is a form of open stratification in which the position a person has by birth can be changed through his or her own achievements and/or luck. Individuals born into a class at the bottom of the hierarchy can work their way up, while individuals born into a class at the top of the hierarchy can slip down.

While many societies have class systems, social mobility within a class system varies from society to society. For example, some sociologists have argued that Britain has a more rigid class structure than certain other Western societies, such as the United States.[15] Historically, British society was divided into three main classes: the upper class, which was made up of individuals whose families for generations had wealth, prestige, and occasionally power; the middle class, whose members were involved in professional, managerial, and clerical occupations; and the working class, whose members earned their living from manual occupations. The middle class was further subdivided into the upper-middle class, whose members were involved in important managerial occupations and the prestigious professions (e.g., lawyers, accountants, doctors), and the lower-middle class, whose members were involved in clerical work (e.g., bank tellers) and the less prestigious professions (e.g., schoolteachers).

Historically, the British class system exhibited significant divergence between the life chances of members of different classes. The upper and upper-middle classes typically sent their children to a select group of private schools, where they wouldn't mix with lower-class children, and where they picked up many of the speech accents and social norms that marked them as being from the higher strata of society. These same private schools also had close ties with the most prestigious universities, such as Oxford and Cambridge. Until recently, Oxford and Cambridge guaranteed to reserve a certain number of places for the graduates of these private schools. Having been to a prestigious university, the offspring of the upper and upper-middle classes then had an excellent chance of being offered a prestigious job in companies, banks, brokerage firms, and law firms run by members of the upper and upper-middle classes.

In contrast, the members of the British working and lower-middle classes typically went to state schools. The majority left at 16, and those who went on to higher education found it more difficult to get accepted at the best universities. When they did, they found that their lower-class accent and lack of social skills marked them as being from a lower social stratum, which made it more difficult for them to get access to the most prestigious jobs.

Because of this, the class system in Britain perpetuated itself from generation to generation, and mobility was limited. Although upward mobility was possible, it could not normally be achieved in one generation. While an individual from a working-class background may have established an income level that was consistent with membership in the upper-middle class, he or she may not have been accepted as such by others of that class due to accent and background. However, by sending his or her offspring to the "right kind of school," the individual could ensure that his or her children were accepted.

According to many commentators, modern British society is now rapidly leaving this class structure behind and moving toward a classless society. However, sociologists continue to dispute this finding and present evidence that this is not the case. For example, a study reported that in the mid-1990s, state schools in the London suburb of Islington, which has a population of 175,000, had only 79 candidates for university, while one prestigious private school alone, Eton, sent more than that number to Oxford and Cambridge.[16] This, according to the study's authors, implies that "money still begets money." They argue that a good school means a good university, a good university means a good job, and "merit" has only a limited chance of elbowing its way into this tight little circle.

The class system in the United States is less extreme than in Britain and mobility is greater. Like Britain, the United States has its own upper, middle, and working classes. However, class membership is determined to a much greater degree by individual economic achievements, as opposed to background and schooling. Thus, an individual can, by his or her own economic achievement, move smoothly from the working class to the upper class in a lifetime. Successful individuals from humble origins are highly respected in American society.

Significance

From a business perspective, the stratification of a society is significant if it affects the operation of business organizations. In American society, the high degree of social mobility and the extreme emphasis on individualism limits the impact of class background on business operations. The same is true in Japan, where most of the population perceives itself to be middle class. In a country such as Great Britain, however, the relative lack of class mobility and the differences between classes have resulted in the emergence of class consciousness. **Class consciousness** refers to a condition where people tend to perceive themselves in terms of their class background, and this shapes their relationships with members of other classes.

This has been played out in British society in the traditional hostility between upper-middle-class managers and their working-class employees. Mutual antagonism and lack of respect historically made it difficult to achieve cooperation between management and labor in many British companies and resulted in a relatively high level of industrial disputes. However, as noted earlier, the last two decades have seen a dramatic reduction in industrial disputes, which bolsters the arguments of those who claim that the country is moving toward a classless society (the level of industrial disputes in the United Kingdom is now lower than in the United States). An antagonistic relationship between management and labor, and the resulting lack of cooperation and high level of industrial disruption, tends to raise the costs of production in countries characterized by significant class divisions. In turn, this can make it more difficult for companies based in such countries to establish a competitive advantage in the global economy.

Religious and Ethical Systems

Religion may be defined as a system of shared beliefs and rituals that are concerned with the realm of the sacred.[17] **Ethical systems** refer to a set of moral principles, or values, that are used to guide and shape behavior. Most of the world's ethical systems are the product of religions. Thus, we can talk about Christian ethics and Islamic ethics. However, there is a major exception to the principle that ethical systems are grounded in religion. Confucianism and Confucian ethics influence behavior and shape culture in parts of Asia, yet it is incorrect to characterize Confucianism as a religion.

The relationship between religion, ethics, and society is subtle and complex. While there are thousands of religions in the world today, in terms of numbers of adherents four dominate—Christianity with 1.7 billion adherents, Islam with 1 billion adherents, Hinduism with 750 million adherents (primarily in India), and Buddhism with 350 million adherents (see Map 3.1). Although many other religions have an important influence in certain parts of the modern world (for example, Judaism, which has 18 million adherents), their numbers pale in comparison with these dominant religions (however, as the precursor of both Christianity and Islam, Judaism has an indirect influence that goes beyond its numbers). We will review these four religions, along with Confucianism, focusing on their business implications. Some scholars have argued that the most important business implications of religion center on the extent to which different religions shape attitudes toward work and entrepreneurship and the degree to which the religious ethics affect the costs of doing business in a country.

It is hazardous to make sweeping generalizations about the nature of the relationship between religion and ethical systems and business practice. As we shall see, while some scholars argue that there is a relationship between religious and ethical systems and business practice in a nation, in a world where nations with Catholic, Protestant, Muslim, Hindu, and Buddhist majorities all show evidence of entrepreneurial activity and sustainable economic growth, it is important to view such proposed relationships with a degree of skepticism. While the proposed relationships may exist, their impact is probably small compared to the impact of economic policy.

Christianity

Christianity is the most widely practiced religion in the world. Approximately 20 percent of the world's people identify themselves as Christians. The vast majority of Christians live in Europe and the Americas, although their numbers are growing rapidly in Africa. Christianity grew out of Judaism. Like Judaism, it is a monotheistic religion (monotheism is the belief in one god). A religious division in the 11th century led to the establishment of two major Christian organizations—the Roman Catholic church and the Orthodox church. Today the Roman Catholic church accounts for more than half of all Christians, most of whom are found in Southern Europe and Latin America. The Orthodox church, while less influential, is still of major importance in several countries (e.g., Greece and Russia). In the 16th century, the Reformation led to a further split with Rome; the result was Protestantism. The nonconformist nature of Protestantism has facilitated the emergence of numerous denominations under the Protestant umbrella (e.g., Baptist, Methodist, Calvinist).

Economic Implications of Christianity: The Protestant Work Ethic

Some sociologists have argued that of the main branches of Christianity—Catholicism, Orthodox, and Protestantism—the latter has the most important economic implications. In 1904, a German sociologist, Max Weber, made a connection between Protestant ethics and "the spirit of capitalism" that has since become fa-

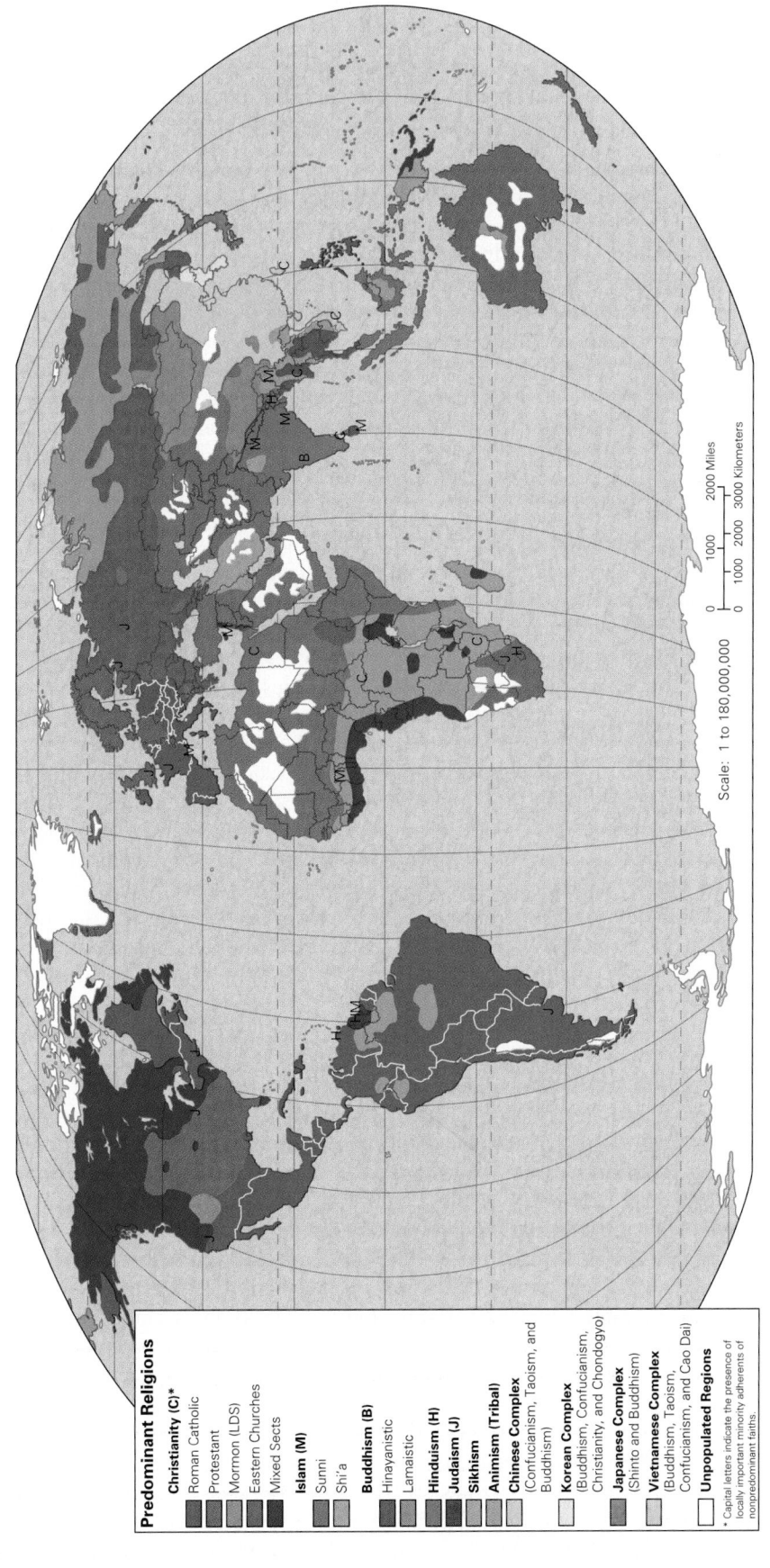

Map 3.1

World Religions

Predominant Religions

Christianity (C)*
Roman Catholic
Protestant
Mormon (LDS)
Eastern Churches
Mixed Sects

Islam (M)
Sunni
Shi'a

Buddhism (B)
Hinayanistic
Lamaistic

Hinduism (H)
Judaism (JJ)
Sikhism
Animism (Tribal)
Chinese Complex
(Confucianism, Taoism, and Buddhism)

Korean Complex
(Buddhism, Confucianism, Christianity, and Chondogyo)

Japanese Complex
(Shinto and Buddhism)

Vietnamese Complex
(Buddhism, Taoism, Confucianism, and Cao Dai)

Unpopulated Regions

* Capital letters indicate the presence of locally important minority adherents of nonpredominant faiths.

Scale: 1 to 180,000,000

0   1000   2000 Miles

0   1000   2000   3000 Kilometers

Source: From *Student Atlas of World Geography*, Second Edition by John L. Allen. Copyright © 2001 by McGraw-Hill Companies. Reprinted by permission of McGraw-Hill/Dushkin, a division of the McGraw-Hill Companies, Guilford, CT 06437.

mous.[18] Weber noted that capitalism emerged in Western Europe. He also noted that in Western Europe:

> Business leaders and owners of capital, as well as the higher grades of skilled labor, and even more the higher technically and commercially trained personnel of modern enterprises, are overwhelmingly Protestant.[19]

According to Weber, there was a relationship between Protestantism and the emergence of modern capitalism. Weber argued that Protestant ethics emphasize the importance of hard work and wealth creation (for the glory of God) and frugality (abstinence from worldly pleasures). According to Weber, this kind of value system was needed to facilitate the development of capitalism. Protestants worked hard and systematically to accumulate wealth. However, their ascetic beliefs suggested that rather than consuming this wealth by indulging in worldly pleasures, they should invest it in the expansion of capitalist enterprises. Thus, the combination of hard work and the accumulation of capital, which could be used to finance investment and expansion, paved the way for the development of capitalism in Western Europe and subsequently in the United States. In contrast, Weber argued that the Catholic promise of salvation in the next world, rather than this world, did not foster the same kind of work ethic.

Protestantism also may have encouraged capitalism's development in another way. By breaking away from the hierarchical domination of religious and social life that characterized the Catholic church for much of its history, Protestantism gave individuals significantly more freedom to develop their own relationship with God. The right to freedom of form of worship was central to the nonconformist nature of early Protestantism. This emphasis on individual religious freedom may have paved the way for the subsequent emphasis on individual economic and political freedoms and the development of individualism as an economic and political philosophy. As we saw in Chapter 2, such a philosophy forms the bedrock on which entrepreneurial free market capitalism is based. Building on this, some scholars claim there is a connection between individualism, as inspired by Protestantism, and the extent of entrepreneurial activity in a nation.[20] Again, one must be careful not to generalize too much from this historical sociological view. While nations with a strong Protestant tradition such as Britain, Germany, and the United States were early leaders in the industrial revolution, in the modern world there is clearly significant and sustained entrepreneurial activity and economic growth in nations with Catholic or Orthodox majorities.

Islam

With nearly 1 billion adherents, Islam is the second largest of the world's major religions. Islam dates back to 610 A.D. when the prophet Mohammed began spreading the word, although the Muslim calendar begins in 622 A.D. when, to escape growing opposition, Mohammed left Mecca for the oasis settlement of Yathrib, later known as Madina. Adherents of Islam are referred to as Muslims. Muslims constitute a majority in more than 35 countries and inhabit a nearly contiguous stretch of land from the northwest coast of Africa, through the Middle East, to China and Malaysia in the Far East.

Islam has roots in both Judaism and Christianity (Islam views Jesus Christ as one of God's prophets). Like Christianity and Judaism, Islam is a monotheistic religion. The central principle of Islam is that there is but the one true omnipotent God. Islam requires unconditional acceptance of the uniqueness, power, and authority of God and the understanding that the objective of life is to fulfill the dictates of his will in the hope of admission to paradise. According to Islam, worldly gain and temporal power are an illusion. Those who pursue riches on earth may gain them, but those who forgo worldly ambitions to seek the favor of Allah may gain the greater treasure—entry into paradise. Other major principles of Islam include: (1) honoring and respecting parents, (2) respecting the rights of others, (3) being generous but not a squanderer, (4) avoiding killing except for justifiable causes, (5) not committing adultery, (6) dealing justly and equitably with others, (7) being of pure heart and mind, (8) safeguarding the possessions of orphans, and (9) being humble and unpretentious.[21] There are obvious parallels here with many of the central principles of both Judaism and Christianity.

Islam is an all-embracing way of life governing the totality of a Muslim's being.[22] As God's surrogate in this world, a Muslim is not a totally free agent but is circumscribed by religious principles—by a code of conduct for interpersonal relations—in social and economic activities. Religion is paramount in all areas of life. The Muslim lives in a social structure that is shaped by Islamic values and norms of moral conduct. The ritual nature of everyday life in a Muslim country is striking to a Western visitor. Among other things, orthodox Muslim ritual requires prayer five times a day (it is not unusual for business meetings to be put on hold while the Muslim participants engage in their daily prayer ritual), requires that women should be dressed in a certain manner, and forbids the consumption of either pork or alcohol.

Islamic Fundamentalism

The past two decades have witnessed the growth of a social movement often referred to as "Islamic fundamentalism."[23] In the West, Islamic fundamentalism is associated in the media with militants, terrorists, and violent upheavals, such as the bloody conflict occurring in Algeria, the killing of foreign tourists in Egypt, or the September 11, 2001, attacks on the World Trade Center and Pentagon in the United States. This characterization is at best misleading. Just as "Christian fundamentalists" in the West are motivated by sincere and deeply held religious values firmly rooted in their faith, so are "Islamic fundamentalists." The violence that the Western media associates with Islamic fundamentalism is perpetrated by a very small minority of radical "fundamentalists" who have hijacked the religion to further their own political and violent ends. (Some Christian "fundamentalists" have done the exactly the same, including Jim Jones and David Koresh). The vast majority of Muslims point out that Islam teaches peace, justice, and tolerance, not violence and intolerance, and that Islam explicitly repudiates the violence that a radical minority practices.

The rise of fundamentalism has no one cause. In part, it is a response to the social pressures created in traditional Islamic societies by the move toward modernization and by the influence of Western ideas, such as liberal democracy, materialism, equal rights for women, and attitudes toward sex, marriage, and alcohol. In many Muslim countries, modernization has been accompanied by a growing gap between a rich urban minority and an impoverished urban and rural majority. For the impoverished majority, modernization has offered little in the way of tangible economic progress, while threatening the traditional value system. Thus, for a Muslim who cherishes his traditions and feels that his identity is jeopardized by the encroachment of alien Western values, Islamic fundamentalism has become a cultural anchor.

Fundamentalists demand a rigid commitment to traditional religious beliefs and rituals. The result has been a marked increase in the use of symbolic gestures that confirm Islamic values. In areas where fundamentalism is strong, women are once again wearing floor-length, long-sleeved dresses and covering their hair; religious studies have increased in universities; the publication of religious tracts has increased; and more religious orations are heard in public.[24] Also, the sentiments of some fundamentalist groups are increasingly anti-Western. Rightly or wrongly, Western influence is blamed for a range of social ills, and many fundamentalists' actions are directed against Western governments, cultural symbols, businesses, and even individuals.

In several Muslim countries, fundamentalists have gained political power and have used this to try to make Islamic law (as set down in the Koran, the bible of Islam) the law of the land. There are good grounds for this in Islam. Islam makes no distinction between church and state. It is not just a religion; Islam is also the source of law, a guide to statecraft, and an arbiter of social behavior. Muslims believe that every human endeavor is within the purview of the faith—and this includes political activity—

because the only purpose of any activity is to do God's will.[25] (Muslims are not unique in this view; it is also shared by some Christian fundamentalists.) The Muslim fundamentalists have been most successful in Iran, where a fundamentalist party has held power since 1979, but they also have had an influence in many other countries, such as Algeria, Afghanistan (where the Taliban established an extreme fundamentalist state until removed by the U.S.-led coalition in 2002), Egypt, Pakistan, the Sudan, and Saudi Arabia.

Economic Implications of Islam

The Koran establishes some explicit economic principles.[26] Many of the economic principles of Islam are pro-free enterprise. The Koran speaks approvingly of free enterprise and of earning legitimate profit through trade and commerce (the prophet Mohammed was once a trader). The protection of the right to private property is also embedded within Islam, although Islam asserts that all property is a favor from Allah (God), who created and so owns everything. Those who hold property are regarded as trustees, rather than owners in the Western sense of the word. As trustees they are entitled to receive profits from the property but are admonished to use it in a righteous, socially beneficial, and prudent manner. This reflects Islam's concern with social justice. Islam is critical of those who earn profit through the exploitation of others. In the Islamic view of the world, humans are part of a collective in which the wealthy and successful have obligations to help the disadvantaged. Put simply, in Muslim countries, it is fine to earn a profit, so long as that profit is justly earned and not based on the exploitation of others for one's own advantage. It also helps if those making profits undertake charitable acts to help the poor. Furthermore, Islam stresses the importance of living up to contractual obligations, of keeping one's word, and of abstaining from deception.

Given the Islamic proclivity to favor market-based systems, Muslim countries are likely to be receptive to international businesses as long as those businesses behave in a manner that is consistent with Islamic ethics. Businesses that are perceived as making an unjust profit through the exploitation of others, by deception, or by breaking contractual obligations are unlikely to be welcomed in an Islamic country. In addition, in Islamic countries where fundamentalism is on the rise, hostility toward Western-owned businesses is likely to increase.

In the previous chapter, we noted that one economic principle of Islam prohibits the payment or receipt of interest, which is considered usury. This is not just a matter of theology; in several Islamic states, it is also becoming a matter of law. In 1992, for example, Pakistan's Federal Shariat Court, the highest Islamic law-making body in the country, pronounced interest to be un-Islamic and therefore illegal and demanded that the government amend all financial laws accordingly. In 1999, Pakistan's Supreme Court ruled that Islamic banking methods should be used in the country after July 1, 2001.[27] The accompanying Country Focus looks at how Pakistan's banks are dealing with this issue.

Hinduism

Hinduism has approximately 750 million adherents, most of whom are on the Indian subcontinent. Hinduism began in the Indus Valley in India over 4,000 years ago, making it the world's oldest major religion. Unlike Christianity and Islam, its founding is not linked to a particular person. Nor does it have an officially sanctioned sacred book such as the Bible or the Koran. Hindus believe that a moral force in society requires the acceptance of certain responsibilities, called *dharma*. Hindus believe in reincarnation, or rebirth into a different body after death. Hindus also believe in *karma*, the spiritual progression of each person's soul. A person's karma is affected by the way he or she lives. The moral state of an individual's karma determines the challenges he or she will face in their next life. By perfecting the soul in each new life, Hindus believe that an individual can eventually achieve *nirvana*, a state of complete spiritual perfection that renders reincarnation no longer necessary. Many Hindus believe that the way to

Country Focus

Islamic Banking in Pakistan

The Koran clearly condemns interest, which is called *riba* in Arabic, as exploitative and unjust. For many years, banks operating in Islamic countries conveniently ignored this condemnation, but starting about 25 years ago with the establishment of an Islamic bank in Egypt, Islamic banks started to open in predominantly Muslim countries. There are now some 170 Islamic financial institutions worldwide managing over $150 billion in assets and making an average return on capital of more than 16 percent. Even conventional banks are entering the market—both Citigroup and HSBC, two of the world's largest financial institutions, now offer Islamic financial services. Until mid-2001, only Iran and the Sudan enforced Islamic banking conventions, but in many other countries, customers could choose between conventional banks and Islamic banks.

In July 2001, Pakistan became the third country to require its banks to adopt Islamic methods. The transition to Islamic banking in Pakistan may determine the fate of Islamic banking elsewhere in the world. Conventional banks make a profit on the spread between the interest rate they have to pay to depositors and the higher interest rate they charge borrowers. Because Islamic banks cannot pay or charge interest, they must find a different way of making money. Pakistan's banks are set to experiment with two different Islamic banking methods—the *mudarabah* and the *murabaha*.

A *mudarabah* contract is similar to a profit-sharing scheme. Under *mudarabah*, when an Islamic bank lends money to a business, rather than charging that business interest on the loan, it takes a share in the profits that are derived from the investment. Similarly, when a business (or individual) deposits money at an Islamic bank in a savings account, the deposit is treated as an equity investment in whatever activity the bank uses the capital for. Thus, the depositor receives a share in the profit from the bank's investment (as opposed to interest payments) according to an agreed-on ratio. Some Muslims claim this is a more ef-ficient system than the Western banking system, since it encourages both long-term savings and long-term investment. However, there is no hard evidence of this, and many believe that a *mudarabah* system is less efficient than a conventional Western banking system.

The second Islamic banking method, the *murabaha* contract, is the most widely used among the world's Islamic banks. It seems set to become the most popular method in Pakistan, primarily because it is the easiest to implement. In a *murabaha contract,* when a firm wishes to purchase something using a loan—let's say a piece of equipment that costs $1,000—the firm tells the bank after having negotiated the price with the equipment manufacturer. The bank then buys the equipment for $1,000, and the borrower buys it back from the bank at some later date for, say, $1,100, a price that includes a $100 markup for the bank. A cynic might point out that such a markup is functionally equivalent to an interest payment, and it is the similarity between this method and conventional banking that makes it so much easier to adopt.

Whichever method is most widely used, observers expect the transition from traditional to Islamic banking to be challenging. One fear is that there could be large-scale withdrawals by depositors, driven by worries that they could suffer in the absence of fixed interest rates. Another concern is that the country needs to have a tight regulatory regime to ensure that unscrupulous borrowers using a *mudarabah* contract do not declare themselves bankrupt, even when their businesses are running a profit. A third concern is that the uncertainty created by the transition will scare off foreign investors, leaving Pakistan starved of capital.

Sources: "Forced Devotion," *The Economist*, February 17, 2001, pp. 76–77; "Islamic Banking Marches On," *The Banker*, February 1, 2000; and F. Bokhari, "Bankers Fear Introduction of Islamic System Will Prompt Big Withdrawals," *Financial Times*, March 6, 2001, p. 4.

achieve nirvana is to lead a severe ascetic lifestyle of material and physical self-denial, devoting life to a spiritual rather than material quest.

Economic Implications of Hinduism

Max Weber, who is famous for expounding on the Protestant work ethic, also argued that the ascetic principles embedded in Hinduism do not encourage the kind of entrepreneurial activity in pursuit of wealth creation that we find in Protestantism.[28] According to Weber, traditional Hindu values emphasize that individuals should not be judged by their material achievements, but by their spiritual achievements. Hindus perceive the pursuit of material well-being as making the attainment of nirvana more difficult. Given the emphasis on an ascetic lifestyle, Weber thought that devout Hindus would be less likely to engage in entrepreneurial activity than devout Protestants.

Mahatma Gandhi, the famous Indian nationalist and spiritual leader, was certainly the embodiment of Hindu asceticism. It has been argued that the values of Hindu asceticism and self-reliance that Gandhi advocated had a negative impact on the economic development of post-independence India.[29] But one must be careful not to read too much into Weber's arguments. Modern India is a very entrepreneurial society and millions of hardworking entrepreneurs form the economic backbone of India's rapidly growing economy.

Historically, Hinduism also supported India's caste system. The concept of mobility between castes within an individual's lifetime makes no sense to traditional Hindus. Hindus see mobility between castes as something that is achieved through spiritual progression and reincarnation. An individual can be reborn into a higher caste in his next life if he achieves spiritual development in this life. In so far as the caste system limits individuals' opportunities to adopt positions of responsibility and influence in society, the economic consequences of this religious belief are somewhat negative. For example, within a business organization, the most able individuals may find their route to the higher levels of the organization blocked simply because they come from a lower caste. By the same token, individuals may get promoted to higher positions within a firm as much because of their caste background as because of their ability. However, the caste system, which has been abolished in India, and its influence are now fading into history.

Buddhism

Buddhism was founded in India in the sixth century B.C. by Siddhartha Gautama, an Indian prince who renounced his wealth to pursue an ascetic lifestyle and spiritual perfection. Siddhartha achieved *nirvana* but decided to remain on earth to teach his followers how they too could achieve this state of spiritual enlightenment. Siddhartha became known as the Buddha (which means "the awakened one"). Today Buddhism has 350 million followers, most of whom are found in Central and Southeast Asia, China, Korea, and Japan. According to Buddhism, there is suffering everywhere that originates in people's desires for pleasure. Cessation of suffering can be achieved by following a path for transformation. Siddhartha offered the Noble Eightfold Path as a route for transformation. This emphasizes right seeing, thinking, speech, action, living, effort, mindfulness, and meditation. Unlike Hinduism, Buddhism does not support the caste system. Nor does Buddhism advocate the kind of extreme ascetic behavior that is encouraged by Hinduism. Nevertheless, like Hindus, Buddhists stress the afterlife and spiritual achievement rather than involvement in this world.

Because of this, the emphasis on wealth creation that is embedded in Protestantism is not found in Buddhism. Thus, in Buddhist societies, we do not see the same kind of historical cultural stress on entrepreneurial behavior that Weber claimed could be found in the Protestant West. But unlike Hinduism, the lack of support for the caste system and extreme ascetic behavior suggests that a Buddhist society may represent a more fertile ground for entrepreneurial activity than a Hindu culture.

Confucianism

Confucianism was founded in the fifth century B.C. by K'ung-Fu-tzu, more generally known as Confucius. For more than 2,000 years until the 1949 Communist revolution, Confucianism was the official ethical system of China. While observance of Confucian ethics has been weakened in China since 1949, more than 200 million people still follow the teachings of Confucius, principally in China, Korea, and Japan. Confucianism teaches the importance of attaining personal salvation through right action. Although not a religion, Confucian ideology has become deeply embedded in the culture of these countries over the centuries, and through that, has an impact on the lives of many millions more. Confucianism is built around a comprehensive ethical code that sets down guidelines for relationships with others. The need for high moral and ethical conduct and loyalty to others are central to Confucianism. Unlike religions, Confucianism is not concerned with the supernatural and has little to say about the concept of a supreme being or an afterlife.

Economic Implications of Confucianism

Some scholars maintain that Confucianism may have economic implications as profound as those Weber argued were to be found in Protestantism, although they are of a different nature.[30] Their basic thesis is that the influence of Confucian ethics on the culture of China, Japan, South Korea, and Taiwan, by lowering the costs of doing business in those countries, may help explain their economic success. In this regard, three values central to the Confucian system of ethics are of particular interest—loyalty, reciprocal obligations, and honesty in dealings with others.

In Confucian thought, loyalty to one's superiors is regarded as a sacred duty—an absolute obligation. In modern organizations based in Confucian cultures, the loyalty that binds employees to the heads of their organization can reduce the conflict between management and labor that we find in more class-conscious societies. Cooperation between management and labor can be achieved at a lower cost in a culture where the virtue of loyalty is emphasized in the value systems.

However, in a Confucian culture, loyalty to one's superiors, such as a worker's loyalty to management, is not blind loyalty. The concept of reciprocal obligations also comes into play. Confucian ethics stress that superiors are obliged to reward the loyalty of their subordinates by bestowing blessings on them. If these "blessings" are not forthcoming, then neither will be the loyalty. As we saw in the opening case, in China this Confucian ethic is central to the concept of *guanxi,* which refers to relationship networks supported by reciprocal obligations. Similarly, in Japan this ethic finds expression in the concept of lifetime employment. The employees of a Japanese company are loyal to the leaders of the organization, and in return the leaders bestow on them the "blessing" of lifetime employment. The lack of mobility between companies implied by the lifetime employment system suggests that, over the years, managers and workers build up knowledge, experience, and a network of interpersonal business contacts. All of these can help managers and workers perform their jobs more effectively and cooperate with others in the organization. One result is the company's improved economic performance.

A third concept found in Confucian ethics is the importance attached to honesty. Confucian thinkers emphasize that, although dishonest behavior may yield short-term benefits for the transgressor, in the long run dishonesty does not pay. The importance attached to honesty has major economic implications. When companies can trust each other not to break contractual obligations, the costs of doing business are lowered. Expensive lawyers are not needed to resolve contract disputes. In a Confucian society, there may be less hesitation to commit substantial resources to cooperative ventures than in a society where honesty is less pervasive. When companies adhere to Confucian ethics, they can trust each other not to violate the terms of cooperative agreements. Thus, the costs of achieving cooperation between companies may be lower in societies such as Japan relative to societies where trust is less pervasive.

For example, it has been argued that the close ties between the automobile companies and their component parts suppliers in Japan are facilitated by a combination of trust and reciprocal obligations. These close ties allow the auto companies and their suppliers to work together on a range of issues, including inventory reduction, quality control, and design. The competitive advantage of Japanese auto companies such as Toyota may in part be explained by such factors.[31] Similarly, the opening case showed how the combination of trust and reciprocal obligations is central to the workings and persistence of *guanxi* networks in China. Someone seeking and receiving help through a *guanxi* network is then obligated to return the favor and faces social sanctions if that obligation is not reciprocated when it is called upon. If they do not return the favor, their reputation will be tarnished and they will be unable to draw on the resources of the network in the future. It is claimed that these relationship-based networks can be more important in helping to enforce agreements between businesses than the Chinese legal system. Some claim that *guanxi* networks are a substitute for the legal system.[32]

Language

One obvious way in which countries differ is language. By language, we mean both the spoken and the unspoken means of communication. Language is one of the defining characteristics of a culture.

Spoken Language

Language does far more than just enable people to communicate with each other. The nature of a language also structures the way we perceive the world. The language of a society can direct the attention of its members to certain features of the world rather than others. The classic illustration of this phenomenon is that whereas the English language has but one word for snow, the language of the Inuit (Eskimos) lacks a general term for it. Instead, because distinguishing different forms of snow is so important in the lives of the Inuit, they have 24 words that describe different types of snow (e.g., powder snow, falling snow, wet snow, drifting snow).[33]

Because language shapes the way people perceive the world, it also helps define culture. In countries with more than one language, one also often finds more than one culture. Canada has an English-speaking culture and a French-speaking culture. Tensions between the two run quite high, with a substantial proportion of the French-speaking minority demanding independence from a Canada "dominated by English speakers." The same phenomenon can be observed in many countries. Belgium is divided into Flemish and French speakers, and tensions between the two groups exist; in Spain, a Basque-speaking minority with its own distinctive culture has been agitating for independence from the Spanish-speaking majority for decades; on the Mediterranean island of Cyprus, the culturally diverse Greek- and Turkish-speaking populations of the island engaged in open conflict in the 1970s, and the island is now partitioned into two parts. While it does not necessarily follow that language differences create differences in culture and, therefore, separatist pressures (e.g., witness the harmony in Switzerland, where four languages are spoken), there certainly seems to be a tendency in this direction.[34]

Chinese is the "mother tongue" of the largest number of people, followed by English and Hindi, which is spoken in India (see Figure 3.2). However, the most widely spoken language in the world is English, followed by French, Spanish, and Chinese (i.e., many people speak English as a second language). English is increasingly becoming the language of international business. When a Japanese and a German businessperson get together to do business, it is almost certain that they will communicate in English. However, while English is widely used, learning the local language yields considerable advantages. Most people prefer to converse in their own language and being able to speak the local language can build rapport, which may be very important for a business deal. International businesses that do not understand the local language can make major blunders through improper translation. For example, the Sunbeam Corporation used the English words for its "Mist-Stick" mist-producing hair curling iron when it entered the German market, only to discover after an expensive adver-

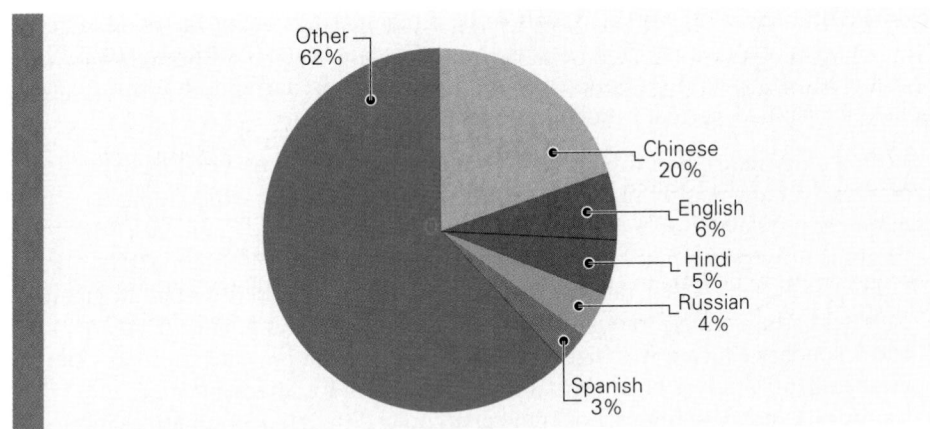

Figure 3.2

Percentage of the World's Population for Whom This Is a First Language

Source: *The Economist Atlas* (London: The Economist Books, 1991), p. 116. Copyright © 1989 and © 1991 The Economist Books, Ltd.

tising campaign that *mist* means excrement in German. General Motors was troubled by the lack of enthusiasm among Puerto Rican dealers for its new Chevrolet Nova. When literally translated into Spanish, *Nova* meant star. However, when spoken it sounded like "no va," which in Spanish means "it doesn't go." General Motors changed the name of the car to Caribe.[35]

Unspoken Language

Unspoken language refers to nonverbal communication. We all communicate with each other by a host of nonverbal cues. The raising of eyebrows, for example, is a sign of recognition in most cultures, while a smile is a sign of joy. Many nonverbal cues, however, are culturally bound. A failure to understand the nonverbal cues of another culture can lead to a communication failure. For example, making a circle with the thumb and the forefinger is a friendly gesture in the United States, but it is a vulgar sexual invitation in Greece and Turkey. Similarly, while most Americans and Europeans use the thumbs-up gesture to indicate that "it's all right," in Greece the gesture is obscene.

Another aspect of nonverbal communication is personal space, which is the comfortable amount of distance between you and someone you are talking to. In the United States, the customary distance apart adopted by parties in a business discussion is five to eight feet. In Latin America, it is three to five feet. Consequently, many North Americans unconsciously feel that Latin Americans are invading their personal space and can be seen backing away from them during a conversation. In turn, the Latin American may interpret such backing away as aloofness. The result can be a regrettable lack of rapport between two businesspeople from different cultures.

Education

Formal education plays a key role in a society. Formal education is the medium through which individuals learn many of the language, conceptual, and mathematical skills that are indispensable in a modern society. Formal education also supplements the family's role in socializing the young into the values and norms of a society. Values and norms are taught both directly and indirectly. Schools generally teach basic facts about the social and political nature of a society. They also focus on the fundamental obligations of citizenship. Cultural norms are also taught indirectly at school. Respect for others, obedience to authority, honesty, neatness, being on time, and so on, are all part of the "hidden curriculum" of schools. The use of a grading system also teaches children the value of personal achievement and competition.[36]

From an international business perspective, one important aspect of education is its role as a determinant of national competitive advantage.[37] The availability of a pool of skilled and educated workers seems to be a major determinant of the likely economic success of a country. In analyzing the competitive success of Japan since 1945, for example, Michael Porter notes that after the war, Japan had almost nothing except for a pool of skilled and educated human resources.

> With a long tradition of respect for education that borders on reverence, Japan possessed a large pool of literate, educated, and increasingly skilled human resources . . . Japan has benefited from a large pool of trained engineers. Japanese universities graduate many more engineers per capita than in the United States . . . A first-rate primary and secondary education system in Japan operates based on high standards and emphasizes math and science. Primary and secondary education is highly competitive . . . Japanese education provides most students all over Japan with a sound education for later education and training. A Japanese high school graduate knows as much about math as most American college graduates.[38]

Porter's point is that Japan's excellent education system is an important factor explaining the country's postwar economic success. Not only is a good education system a determinant of national competitive advantage, but it is also an important factor guiding the location choices of international businesses. It would make little sense to base production facilities that require highly skilled labor in a country where the education system was so poor that a skilled labor pool wasn't available, no matter how attractive the country might seem on other dimensions. It might make sense to base production operations that require only unskilled labor in such a country.

The general education level of a country is also a good index of the kind of products that might sell in a country and of the type of promotional material that should be used. For example, a country such as Pakistan where more than 70 percent of the population is illiterate is unlikely to be a good market for popular books. Promotional material containing written descriptions of mass-marketed products is unlikely to have an effect in a country where almost three-quarters of the population cannot read. It is far better to use pictorial promotions in such circumstances.

Maps 3.2 and 3.3 provide important data on education worldwide. Map 3.2 shows the percentage of a country's GNP that is devoted to education. Map 3.3 shows adult illiteracy rates in 2001. Although there is not a perfect one-to-one correspondence between the percentage of GNP devoted to education and the quality of education, the overall level of spending indicates a country's commitment to education. Note that the United States spends more of its GNP on education than many other advanced industrialized nations, including Germany and Japan. Despite this, the quality of U.S. education is often argued to be inferior to that offered in many other industrialized countries.

◼ Culture and the Workplace

Of considerable importance for an international business with operations in different countries is how a society's culture affects the values found in the workplace. Management process and practices may need to vary according to culturally determined work-related values. For example, if the cultures of the United States and France result in different work-related values, an international business with operations in both countries should vary its management process and practices to take these differences into account.

Probably the most famous study of how culture relates to values in the workplace was undertaken by Geert Hofstede.[39] As part of his job as a psychologist working for IBM, Hofstede collected data on employee attitudes and values for more than 100,000 individuals from 1967 to 1973. These data enabled him to compare dimensions of culture across 40 countries. Hofstede isolated four dimensions that he claimed summarized

Map 3.2

Percentage of Gross National Product Spent on Education

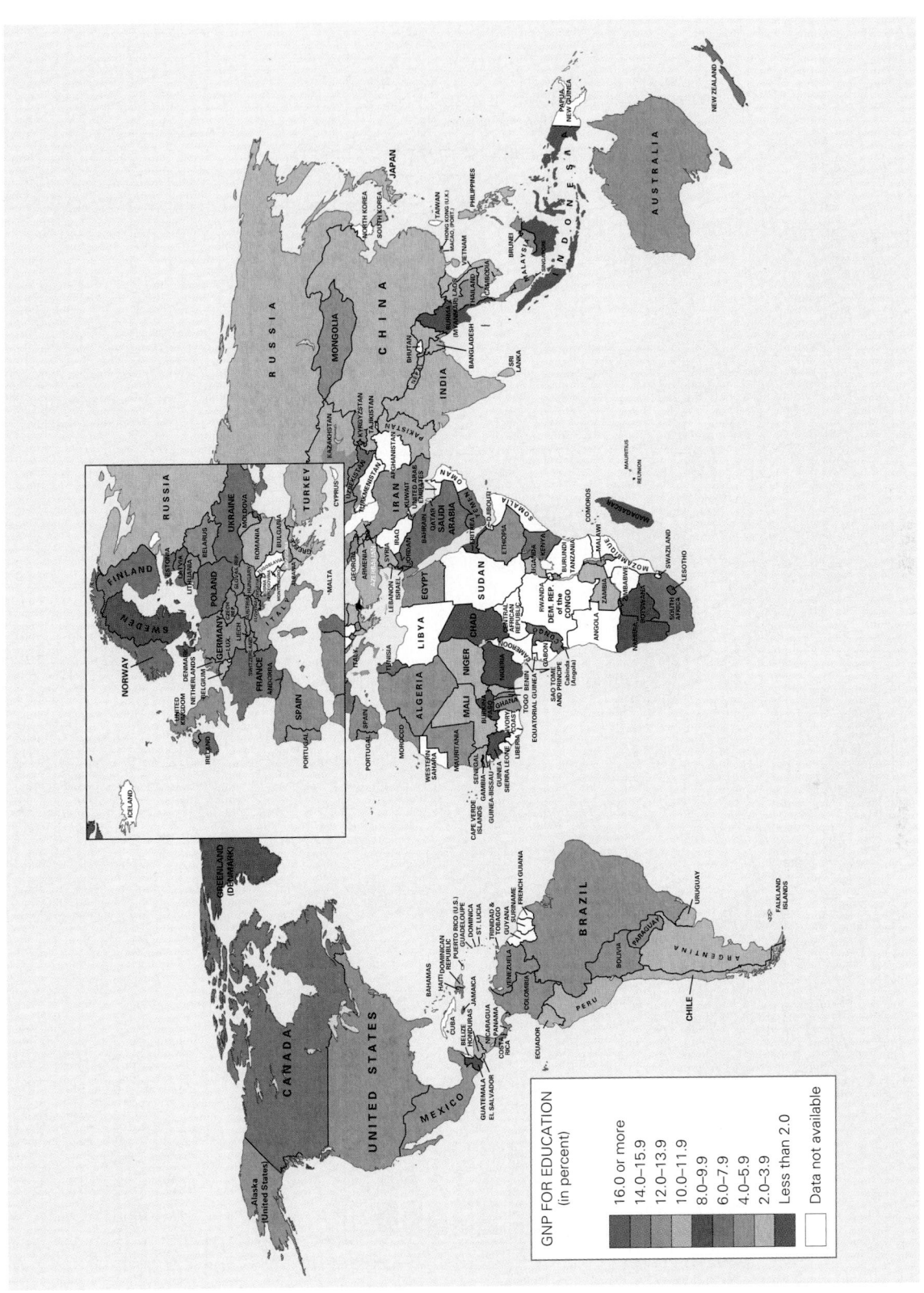

GNP FOR EDUCATION
(in percent)

16.0 or more
14.0–15.9
12.0–13.9
10.0–11.9
8.0–9.9
6.0–7.9
4.0–5.9
2.0–3.9
Less than 2.0
Data not available

Source: Map data are from World Bank, *World Development Report 2000–2001*, pp. 284–85. Reprinted by permission from the International Bank for Reconstruction and Development. © 2001 by the World Bank.

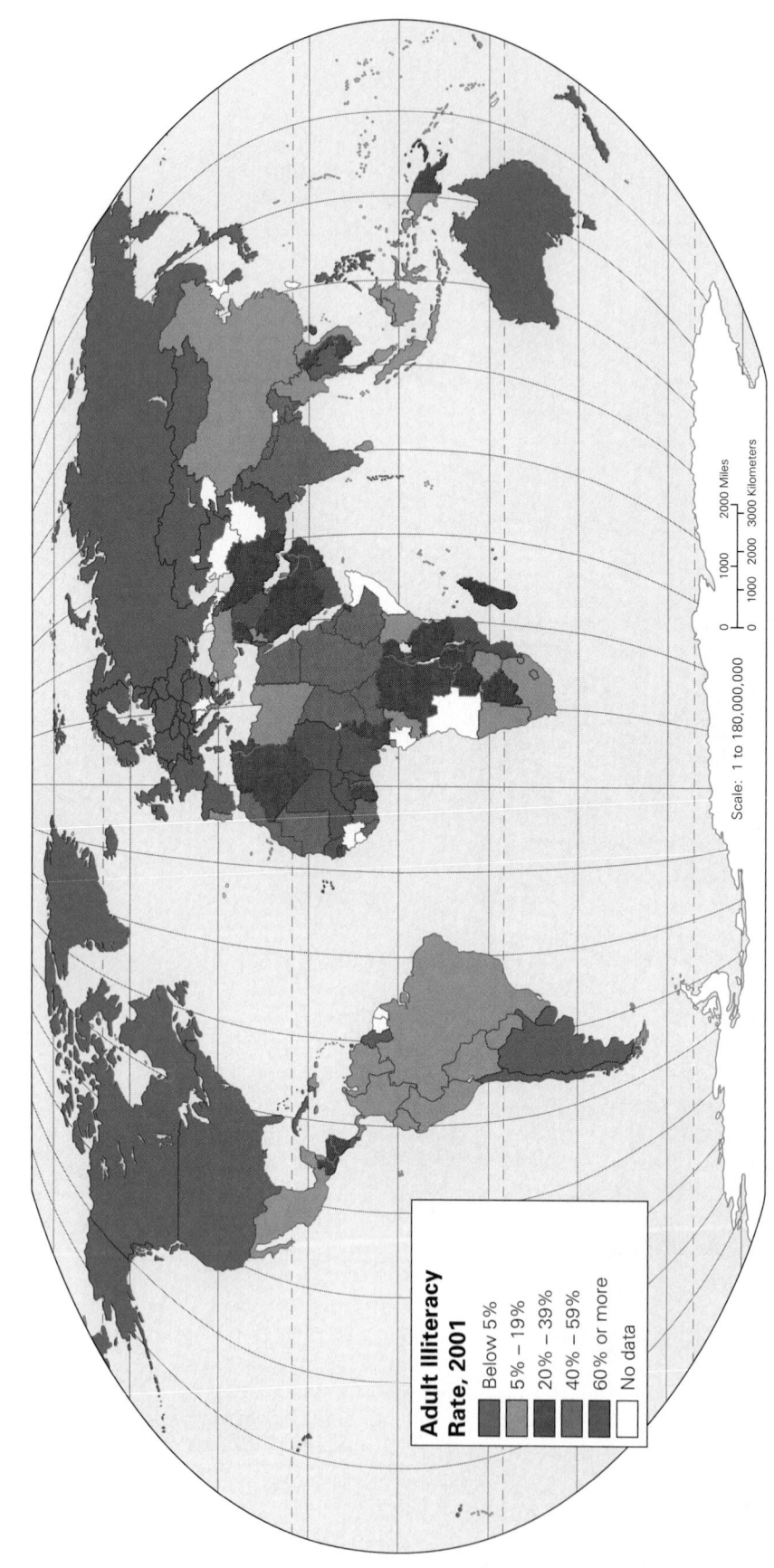

Adult Illiteracy Rate, 2001

Below 5%
5% – 19%
20% – 39%
40% – 59%
60% or more
No data

Scale: 1 to 180,000,000

0   1000   2000 Miles
0   1000   2000   3000 Kilometers

Map 3.3

Adult Illiteracy Rates

Source: From *Student Atlas of World Geography*, Second Edition, by John L. Allen, Copyright © 2001 by The McGraw-Hill Companies, Inc. Reprinted by permission of McGraw Hill/Dushkin, a division of The McGraw-Hill Companies.

different cultures—power distance, uncertainty avoidance, individualism versus collectivism, and masculinity versus femininity.

Hofstede's **power distance** dimension focused on how a society deals with the fact that people are unequal in physical and intellectual capabilities. According to Hofstede, high power distance cultures were found in countries that let inequalities grow over time into inequalities of power and wealth. Low power distance cultures were found in societies that tried to play down such inequalities as much as possible.

The **individualism versus collectivism** dimension focused on the relationship between the individual and his or her fellows. In individualistic societies, the ties between individuals were loose and individual achievement and freedom were highly valued. In societies where collectivism was emphasized, the ties between individuals were tight. In such societies, people were born into collectives, such as extended families, and everyone was supposed to look after the interest of his or her collective.

Hofstede's **uncertainty avoidance** dimension measured the extent to which different cultures socialized their members into accepting ambiguous situations and tolerating uncertainty. Members of high uncertainty avoidance cultures placed a premium on job security, career patterns, retirement benefits, and so on. They also had a strong need for rules and regulations; the manager was expected to issue clear instructions, and subordinates' initiatives were tightly controlled. Lower uncertainty avoidance cultures were characterized by a greater readiness to take risks and less emotional resistance to change.

Hofstede's **masculinity versus femininity** dimension looked at the relationship between gender and work roles. In masculine cultures, sex roles were sharply differentiated and traditional "masculine values," such as achievement and the effective exercise of power, determined cultural ideals. In feminine cultures, sex roles were less sharply distinguished, and little differentiation was made between men and women in the same job.

Hofstede created an index score for each of these four dimensions that ranged from 0 to 100 and scored high for high individualism, high power distance, high uncertainty avoidance, and high masculinity. He averaged the score for all employees from a given country. Table 3.1 summarizes these data for 20 selected countries. Western nations such as the United States, Canada, and Britain score high on the individualism scale and low on the power distance scale. At the other extreme are a group of Latin American and Asian countries that emphasize collectivism over individualism and score high on the power distance scale. Table 3.1 also reveals that Japan's culture has strong uncertainty avoidance and high masculinity. This characterization fits the standard stereotype of Japan as a country that is male dominant and where uncertainty avoidance exhibits itself in the institution of lifetime employment. Sweden and Denmark stand out as countries that have both low uncertainty avoidance and low masculinity (high emphasis on "feminine" values).

Hofstede's results are interesting for what they tell us in a very general way about differences between cultures. Many of Hofstede's findings are consistent with standard Western stereotypes about cultural differences. For example, many people believe Americans are more individualistic and egalitarian than the Japanese (they have a lower power distance), who in turn are more individualistic and egalitarian than Mexicans. Similarly, many might agree that Latin countries such as Mexico place a higher emphasis on masculine value—they are machismo cultures—than the Nordic countries of Denmark and Sweden.

However, one should be careful about reading too much into Hofstede's research. It has been criticized on a number of points.[40] First, Hofstede assumes there is a one-to-one correspondence between culture and the nation-state, but as we saw earlier, many countries have more than one culture. Hofstede's results do not capture this distinction. Second, the research may have been culturally bound. The research team was composed of Europeans and Americans. The questions they asked of IBM employees and their analysis of the answers may have been shaped by their own cultural biases and concerns. So it is not surprising that Hofstede's results confirm Western stereotypes, since it was Westerners who undertook the research!

Table 3.1

Work-Related Values for 20 Selected Countries

Source: G. Hofstede, *Culture's Consequences*. Copyright 1980 by Sage Publications. Reprinted by permission of Sage Publications. Cited in G. Hofstede, "The Cultural Relativity of Organizational Practices and Theories," *Journal of International Business Studies* 14 (Fall 1983), pp. 75–89. Reprinted by permission of Dr. Geert Hofstede.

	Power Distance	Uncertainty Avoidance	Individualism	Masculinity
Argentina	49	86	46	56
Australia	36	51	90	61
Brazil	69	76	38	49
Canada	39	48	80	52
Denmark	18	23	74	16
France	68	86	71	43
Germany (F.R.)	35	65	67	66
Great Britain	35	35	89	66
Indonesia	78	48	14	46
India	77	40	48	56
Israel	13	81	54	47
Japan	54	92	46	95
Mexico	81	82	30	69
Netherlands	38	53	80	14
Panama	95	86	11	44
Spain	57	86	51	42
Sweden	31	29	71	5
Thailand	64	64	20	34
Turkey	66	85	37	45
United States	40	46	91	62

Third, Hofstede's informants worked not only within a single industry, the computer industry, but also within one company, IBM. At the time, IBM was renowned for its own strong corporate culture and employee selection procedures, making it possible that the employees' values were different in important respects from the values of the cultures from which those employees came. Also, certain social classes (such as unskilled manual workers) were excluded from Hofstede's sample. A final caution is that Hofstede's work is now beginning to look dated. Cultures do not stand still; they evolve, albeit slowly. What was a reasonable characterization in the 1960s and 1970s may not be so today.

Still, just as it should not be accepted without question, Hofstede's work should not be dismissed entirely either. It represents a starting point for managers trying to figure out how cultures differ and what that might mean for management practices. Also, several other scholars have found strong evidence that differences in culture affect values and practices in the workplace, and Hofstede's basic results have been replicated using more diverse samples of individuals in different settings.[41] Still, managers should use the results with caution, for they are not necessarily accurate.

Hofstede subsequently expanded his original research to include a fifth dimension that he argued captured additional cultural differences not brought out in his earlier work.[42] He referred to this dimension as "Confucian dynamism" (sometimes called "long-term orientation"). According to Hofstede, **Confucian dynamism** captures attitudes toward time, persistence, ordering by status, protection of face, respect for tradition, and reciprocation of gifts and favors. The label refers to these "values" being derived from Confucian teachings. As might be expected, East Asian countries such as Japan, Hong Kong, and Thailand scored high on Confucian dynamism, while nations such as the United States and Canada scored low. Hofstede and his associates went on to argue that their evidence suggested that nations with higher economic growth rates scored high on Confucian dynamism and low on individualism—the implication being Confucianism is good for growth. However, subsequent studies have shown that this finding does not hold up under more sophisticated statistical analysis.[43] During the past decade, countries with high individualism and low Confucian dynamics such as the United States have attained high growth rates, while some Confucian cultures such as Japan have had stagnant economic growth. In reality, while culture might influence the economic success of a nation, it is just one of many factors, and while its importance should not be ignored, it should not be overstated either. The factors discussed in Chapter 2—economic, political, and legal systems—are probably more important than culture in explaining differential economic growth rates over time.

Cultural Change

Culture is not a constant; it evolves over time.[44] Changes in value systems can be slow and painful for a society. In the 1960s, for example, American values toward the role of women, love, sex, and marriage underwent significant changes. Much of the social turmoil of that time reflected these changes. Change, however, does occur and can often be quite profound. For example, at the beginning of the 1960s, the idea that women might hold senior management positions in major corporations was not widely accepted. Many scoffed at the idea. Today, it is a reality and few in the mainstream of American society question the development or the capability of women in the business world. American culture has changed (although it is still more difficult for women to gain senior management positions than men). Similarly, the value systems of many ex-Communist states, such as Russia, are undergoing significant changes as those countries move away from values that emphasize collectivism and toward those that emphasize individualism. While social turmoil is an inevitable outcome of such a shift, the shift will still probably occur.

Some claim that a major cultural shift is occurring in Japan, with a move toward greater individualism.[45] The model Japanese office worker, or "salaryman," is pictured as being loyal to his boss and the organization to the point of giving up evenings, weekends, and vacations to serve the organization, which is the collective of which he is a member. However, a new generation of office workers does not seem to fit this model. An individual from the new generation is more direct than the traditional Japanese. He acts more like a Westerner, a *gaijian*. He does not live for the company and will move on if he gets the offer of a better job. He is not keen on overtime, especially if he has a date. He has his own plans for his free time, and they may not include drinking or playing golf with the boss.[46]

A more detailed example of the changes occurring in Japan is given in the Management Focus, which looks at the impact of Japan's changing culture on Matsushita, one of Japan's most traditional firms. Several studies have suggested that economic advancement and globalization may be important factors in societal change.[47] For example, there is evidence that economic progress is accompanied by a shift in values away from collectivism and toward individualism.[48] Thus, as Japan has become richer, the cultural emphasis on collectivism has declined and greater individualism is being witnessed. One reason for this shift may be that richer societies exhibit less need for social and material support structures built on collectives, whether the collective is the extended family or the paternalistic company. People are better able to take care of their own needs. As a result, the importance attached to collectivism declines, while greater economic freedoms lead to an increase in opportunities for expressing individualism.

Matsushita's and Japan's Changing Culture

Established in 1920, the consumer electronics giant Matsushita was at the forefront of the rise of Japan to the status of major economic power during the 1970s and 1980s. Like many other long-standing Japanese businesses, Matsushita was regarded as a bastion of traditional Japanese values based on strong group identification, reciprocal obligations, and loyalty to the company. Several commentators attributed Matsushita's success, and that of the Japanese economy, to the existence of Confucian values in the workplace. At Matsushita, employees were taken care of by the company from "cradle to the grave." Matsushita provided them with a wide range of benefits including cheap housing, guaranteed lifetime employment, seniority-based pay systems, and generous retirement bonuses. In return, Matsushita expected, and got, loyalty and hard work from its employees. To Japan's postwar generation, struggling to recover from the humiliation of defeat, it seemed like a fair bargain. The employees worked hard for the greater good of Matsushita, and Matsushita reciprocated by bestowing "blessings" on employees.

However, culture does not stay constant. According to some observers, the generation born after 1964 lacked the same commitment to traditional Japanese values as their parents. They grew up in a world that was richer, where Western ideas were beginning to make themselves felt, and where the possibilities seemed greater. They did not want to be tied to a company for life, to be a "salaryman." These trends came to the fore in the 1990s, when the Japanese economy entered an economic slump from which it has yet to recover. As the decade progressed, one Japanese firm after another was forced to change its traditional ways of doing business. Slowly at first, troubled companies started to lay off older workers, effectively abandoning lifetime employment guarantees. As younger people saw this happening, they concluded that loyalty to a company might not be reciprocated, effectively undermining one of the central bargains made in postwar Japan.

Matsushita was one of the last companies to turn its back on Japanese traditions, but in 1998 after years of poor performance, it too modified traditional practices. First, Matsushita changed the pay scheme for its 11,000 managers. In the past, the traditional twice-a-year bonuses had been based almost entirely on seniority, but now Matsushita said they would be based on performance. In 1999, Matsushita announced that this process would be made transparent; managers would be shown what their performance rankings were and how these fed into pay bonuses. As elementary as this might sound in the West, for Matsushita it represented the beginning of a revolution in human resource practices.

The culture of societies may also change as they become richer because economic progress affects a number of other factors, which in turn impact on culture. For example, increased urbanization and improvements in the quality and availability of education are both a function of economic progress, and both can lead to declining emphasis on the traditional values associated with poor rural societies. A 25-year study of values in 78 countries, known as the World Values Survey, coordinated by the University of Michigan's Institute for Social Research, has documented how values change, and linked these to changes in a country's level of economic development.[49] According to this research, as countries get richer there is a shift away from "traditional values" linked to religion, family, and country, and toward "secular rational" values. Traditionalists say religion is important in their lives. They have a strong sense of national pride, think children should be taught to obey, and that the first duty of a child is to make his or her parents proud. They say abortion, euthanasia, divorce, and suicide are never justified. At the other end of this spectrum are "secular rational" values that emphasize the opposite qualities.

Another category looked at by the World Values Survey is quality of life attributes. At one end of this spectrum are "survival values," the values people hold when the struggle for survival is of paramount importance. These values tend to stress that economic and physical security are more important than self-expression. People who can-

About the same time Matsushita took aim at the lifetime employment system and the associated perks. Under the new system, recruits were given the choice of three employment options. First, they could sign on to the traditional option. Under this, they were eligible to live in subsidized company housing, go free to company-organized social events, and buy subsidized services such as banking from group companies. They would also still receive a retirement bonus equal to two years' salary. Under a second scheme, employees could forgo the guaranteed retirement bonus in exchange for higher starting salaries and keep perks such as cheap company housing. Under a third scheme, they would lose both the retirement bonus and the subsidized services, but they would start on a still higher salary. In its first two years of operation, only 3 percent of recruits chose the third option—suggesting there is still a hankering for the traditional paternalistic relationship—but 41 percent took the second option.

In other ways Matsushita's designs are grander still. As the company has moved into new industries such as software engineering and network communications technology, it has begun to sing the praises of democratization of employees, and it has sought to encourage individuality, initiative taking, and risk seeking among its younger employees. But while such changes may be easy to articulate, they are hard to implement. For all of its talk, Matsushita has still not changed its lifetime employment commitment to those hired under the traditional system; nor does it seem likely to do so anytime soon. This was underlined in early 2001 when, in response to continued poor performance, Matsushita announced it would close 30 factories in Japan, cut 1,000 marketing jobs, and sell a "huge amount of assets" over the next three years. While this seemed to indicate a final break with the lifetime employment system, the company also said that unneeded marketing staff would not be laid off but instead would be transferred to higher growth areas such as health care.

With so many of its managers a product of the old way of doing things, a skeptic might question the ability of the company to turn its intentions into a reality. As growth has slowed, Matsushita has had to cut back on its hiring, but its continued commitment to long-standing employees means that the average age of its workforce is rising. In the 1960s it was around 25; now it is 35, a trend that might counteract Matsushita's attempts to revolutionize the workplace, for surely those who benefited from the old system will not give way easily to the new.

Sources: "Putting the Bounce Back into Matsushita," *The Economist,* May 22, 1999, pp. 67–68; "In Search of the New Japanese Dream," *The Economist,* February 19, 2000, pp. 59–60; and P. Landers, "Matsushita to Restructure in Bid to Boost Thin Profits," *Wall Street Journal,* December 1, 2000, p. A13.

not take food or safety for granted tend to be xenophobic, they are wary of political activity, have authoritarian tendencies, and believe that men make better political leaders than women. "Self-expression" or "well-being" values are the opposite; they stress the importance of diversity, belonging, and participation in political processes.

As countries get richer, there seems to be a shift from "traditional" to "secular rational" values, and from "survival values" to "well-being" values. The shift, however, takes time, primarily because individuals are socialized into a set of values when they are young and find it difficult to change as they grow older. Substantial changes in values are linked to generations, with younger people typically being in the vanguard of a significant change in values. Figure 3.3 illustrates the position of a number of countries on these dimensions, and shows how they have changed over time.

With regard to globalization, some have argued that advances in transportation and communication technologies, the dramatic increase in trade that we have witnessed since World War II, and the rise of global corporations such as Hitachi, Disney, Microsoft, and Levi Strauss, whose products and operations can be found around the globe, are creating the conditions for the merging of cultures.[50] With McDonald's hamburgers in China, Levi's in India, Sony Walkmans in South Africa, and MTV everywhere helping to foster a ubiquitous youth culture, some argue that the conditions for less cultural variation have been created. At the same time, one must

Figure 3.3

Changing Values

Source: http://wvs.isr.umich.edu/
wvs-fig.html.

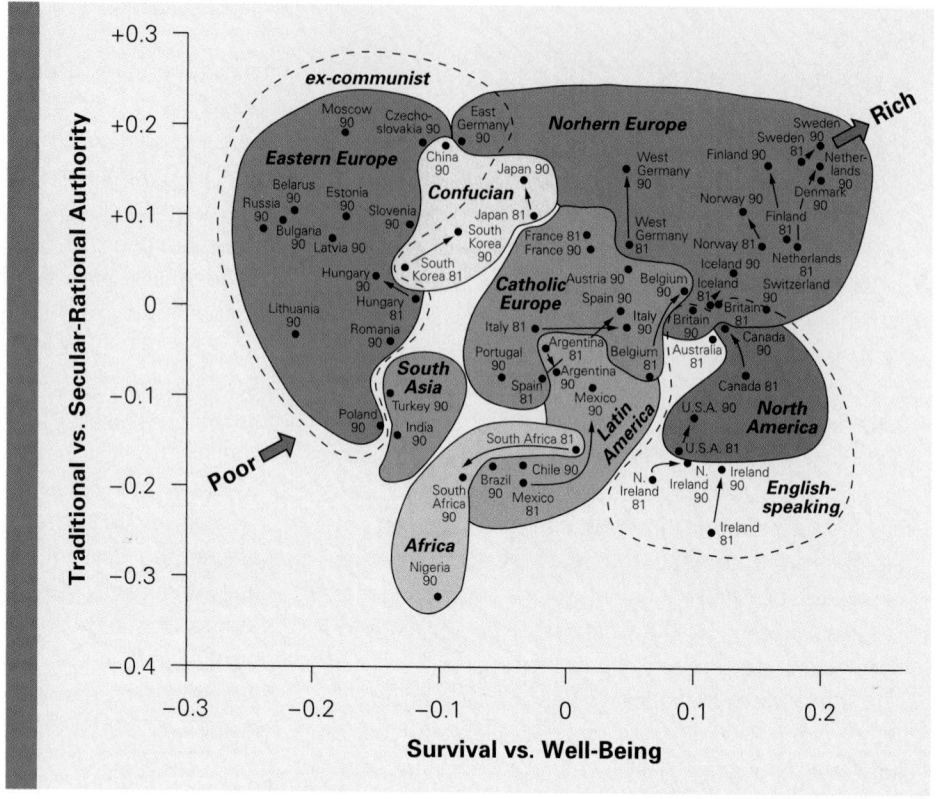

not ignore important countertrends, such as the shift toward Islamic fundamental-ism in several countries; the separatist movement in Quebec, Canada; or the continuing ethnic strains and separatist movements in Russia. Such countertrends in many ways are a reaction to the pressures for cultural convergence. In an increasingly modern and materialistic world, some societies are trying to reemphasize their cultural roots and uniqueness. Cultural change is not unidirectional, with national cultures converging toward some homogenous global entity. Also, while some elements of culture change quite rapidly—particularly the use of material symbols—other elements change only slowly if at all. Thus, just because people the world over wear blue jeans and eat at McDonald's, one should not assume that they have also adopted American values—for more often than not, they have not.

Focus On Managerial Implications

International business is different from national business because countries and societies are different. In this chapter, we have seen just how different societies can be. Societies differ because their cultures vary. Their cultures vary because of profound differences in social structure, religion, language, education, economic philosophy, and political philosophy. Three important implications for international business flow from these differences. The first is the need to develop cross-cultural literacy. There is a need not only to appreciate that cultural differences exist, but also to appreciate what such differences mean for international business. A second implication looks at the connection between culture and ethics in decision making. A third implication for international business centers on the connection between culture and national competitive advantage. In this section, we will explore these issues in greater detail.

Cross-Cultural Literacy

One of the biggest dangers confronting a company that goes abroad for the first time is the danger of being ill-informed. International businesses that are ill-informed about the practices of another culture are likely to fail. Doing business in different cultures requires adaptation to conform with the value systems and norms of that culture. Adaptation can embrace all aspects of an international firm's operations in a foreign country. The way in which deals are negotiated, the appropriate incentive pay systems for salespeople, the structure of the organization, the name of a product, the tenor of relations between management and labor, the manner in which the product is promoted, and so on, are all sensitive to cultural differences. What works in one culture might not work in another.

To combat the danger of being ill-informed, international businesses should consider employing local citizens to help them do business in a particular culture. They must also ensure that home-country executives are cosmopolitan enough to understand how differences in culture affect the practice of international business. Transferring executives overseas at regular intervals to expose them to different cultures will help build a cadre of cosmopolitan executives. An international business must also be constantly on guard against the dangers of ethnocentric behavior. Ethnocentrism is a belief in the superiority of one's own ethnic group or culture. Hand in hand with ethnocentrism goes a disregard or contempt for the culture of other countries. Unfortunately, ethnocentrism is all too prevalent; many Americans are guilty of it, as are many French people, Japanese people, British people, and so on. Ugly as it is, ethnocentrism is a fact of life, one that international businesses must be on continual guard against.

Culture and Competitive Advantage

One theme that continually surfaces in this chapter is the relationship between culture and national competitive advantage. Put simply, the value systems and norms of a country influence the costs of doing business in that country. The costs of doing business in a country influence the ability of firms to establish a competitive advantage in the global marketplace. We have seen how attitudes toward cooperation between management and labor, toward work, and toward the payment of interest are influenced by social structure and religion. It can be argued that the class-based conflict between workers and management in class-conscious societies, when it leads to industrial disruption, raises the costs of doing business in that society. Similarly, we have seen how some sociologists have argued that the ascetic "other-worldly" ethics of Hinduism may not be as supportive of capitalism as the ethics embedded in Protestantism and Confucianism. Also, Islamic laws banning interest payments may raise the costs of doing business by constraining a country's banking system.

Japan presents us with an interesting example of how culture can influence competitive advantage. Some scholars have argued that the culture of modern Japan lowers the costs of doing business relative to the costs in most Western nations. Japan's emphasis on group affiliation, loyalty, reciprocal obligations, honesty, and education all boost the competitiveness of Japanese companies. The emphasis on group affiliation and loyalty encourages individuals to identify strongly with the companies in which they work. This tends to foster an ethic of hard work and cooperation between management and labor "for the good of the company." Similarly, reciprocal obligations and honesty help foster an atmosphere of trust between companies and their suppliers. This encourages them to enter into long-term relationships with each other to work on inventory reduction, quality control, and joint design—all of which have been shown to improve an organization's competitiveness. This level of cooperation has often been lacking in the West, where the relationship between a company and its suppliers tends to be a short-term one structured around competitive bidding, rather than one based on long-term mutual commitments. In addition, the availability of a pool of highly skilled labor, particularly engineers, has helped Japanese enterprises develop cost-reducing process innovations that have boosted their productivity.[51] Thus, cultural factors may help explain the competitive advantage enjoyed by many Japanese businesses in the global marketplace. The rise of Japan as an economic power during the second half of the 20th century may be in part attributed to the economic consequences of its culture.

It has also been argued that the Japanese culture is less supportive of entrepreneurial activity than, say, American society. In many ways, entrepreneurial activity is a product of an individualistic mind-set, not a classic characteristic of the Japanese. This may explain why American enterprises, rather than Japanese corporations, dominate industries where entrepreneurship and innovation are highly valued, such as computer software and biotechnology. Of course, there are obvious and significant exceptions to this generalization. Masayoshi Son recognized the potential of software far faster than any of Japan's corporate giants; set up his company, Softbank, in 1981; and has since built it into Japan's top software distributor. Similarly, dynamic entrepreneurial individuals established major Japanese companies such as Sony and Matsushita. But these examples may be the exceptions that prove the rule, for as yet there has been no surge in entrepreneurial high-technology enterprises in Japan equivalent to what has occurred in the United States.

For the international business, the connection between culture and competitive advantage is important for two reasons. First, the connection suggests which countries are likely to produce the most viable competitors. For example, one might argue that U.S. enterprises are likely to see continued growth in aggressive, cost-efficient competitors from those Pacific Rim nations where a combination of free market economics, Confucian ideology, group-oriented social structures, and advanced education systems can all be found (e.g., South Korea, Taiwan, Japan, and increasingly China).

Second, the connection between culture and competitive advantage has important implications for the choice of countries in which to locate production facilities and do business. Consider a hypothetical case when a company has to choose between two countries, A and B, for locating a production facility. Both countries are characterized by low labor costs and good access to world markets. Both countries are of roughly the same size (in terms of population) and both are at a similar stage of economic development. In country A, the education system is undeveloped, the society is characterized by a marked stratification between the upper and lower classes, and there are six major linguistic groups. In country B, the education system is well developed, there is a lack of social stratification, group identification is valued by the culture, and there is only one linguistic group. Which country makes the best investment site?

Country B probably does. In country A, conflict between management and labor, and between different language groups, can be expected to lead to social and industrial disruption, thereby raising the costs of doing business.[52] The lack of a good education system can also be expected to work against the attainment of business goals.

The same kind of comparison could be made for an international business trying to decide where to push its products, country A or B. Again, country B would be the logical choice because cultural factors suggest that in the long run, country B is the nation most likely to achieve the greatest level of economic growth.

But as important as culture is, it is probably far less important than economic, political, and legal systems in explaining differential economic growth between nations. Cultural differences are significant, but we should not overemphasize their importance in the economic sphere. For example, earlier we noted that Max

Weber argued that the ascetic principles embedded in Hinduism do not encourage entrepreneurial activity. While this is an interesting academic thesis, recent years have seen an increase in entrepreneurial activity in India, particularly in the information technology sector where India is rapidly becoming an important global player. The ascetic principles of Hinduism and caste-based social stratification have apparently not held back entrepreneurial activity in this sector!

Culture and Business Ethics

Many ethical principles are universally held across cultures. For example, basic moral principles such as don't kill or don't steal apply everywhere, despite differences in local culture. Similarly, in all cultures it is regarded as unethical to unilaterally and without reason break a business agreement. As Adam Smith pointed out more than 200 years ago, if people cannot trust each other to honor agreements, business activity will not take place, and economic growth will not occur. A certain level of faith that agreements will be honored—that parties to a transaction will do the ethical thing—is required to encourage economic activity no matter what the culture. In the West, the legal system, and particularly the system of contract law, evolved to help assure people that agreements will be honored, but it is important to recognize that the legal system is designed to deal only with the exceptions to the general principle (which is embedded in our culture) that one should honor agreements. In nations that lack a similar legal tradition, other institutions have emerged to help assure people that business agreements will be honored. As we pointed out in the opening case, *guanxi* networks may fulfill that role in China. Individuals who break agreements will have their reputation tarnished and will be unable to draw on the *guanxi* network in the future. Whether we are talking about China or the West, however, the basic principle remains the same—it is unethical to break business agreements without good reason, and those that do will face sanctions (either legal or cultural).

Although many ethical principles are universal, some are culturally bound.[53] When this is the case, international businesses may be confronted with difficult ethical dilemmas. For example, *guanxi* networks are often supported by the idea of reciprocal gift giving. But if a Western company gives a "gift" to a government official, as an attempt to build a relationship with that individual that may be useful in the future, that company may subsequently be accused of bribery and supporting corruption. What then is the ethical thing to do?

One response to such a dilemma is to argue that because customs vary from country to country, businesses should adopt the customs (and by extension, ethical practices) of the country in which it is currently doing business. This is the *relativist* or "when in Rome" approach to business ethics. It is also a dangerously flawed approach.[54] It would suggest, for example, that if slavery is practiced in a country, it is OK to practice slavery when doing business in that nation! Obviously, this is not the case. Similarly, as several Western businesses have discovered, just because local sweatshops in parts of Asia employ child labor and pay them below subsistence wages, it doesn't follow that one should adopt the same practices. Ethical values are not like a coat that one puts on in certain seasons and certain places and takes off elsewhere. You cannot leave your ethics behind as you venture around the globe. This suggests that one answer to the question "Whose ethics do you use in international business?" is "Your ethics."[55]

But what should "your ethics" be? The answer is somewhat clearer than it used to be. Organizations such as the United Nations have pushed hard to get countries to ratify agreements that have clear ethical implications. An important example is the Universal Declaration of Human Rights, which has been ratified by almost every country and lays down basic principles that should always be adhered to irrespective of the culture in which one is doing business. For example, Article 23 of this declaration states:

1. Everyone has the right to work, to free choice of employment, to just and favorable conditions of work, and to protection against unemployment.

2. Everyone, without any discrimination, has the right to equal pay for equal work.

3. Everyone who works has the right to just and favorable remuneration ensuring for himself and his family an existence worthy of human dignity, and supplemented, if necessary, by other means of social protection.

4. Everyone has the right to form and to join trade unions for the protection of his interests.

Clearly, the rights to "just and favorable work conditions," "equal pay for equal work," and remuneration that ensures an "existence worthy of human dignity" embodied in Article 23 imply that it is unethical to employ child labor in sweatshop settings and pay less than subsistence wages, even if that happens to be common practice in some countries. But does that mean one should not employ children per se, or buy from suppliers who employ children, even if that is common in a certain country? Here the ethical thing to do becomes less clear. If the choice for the child is between living on the streets and begging for food or working in an apparel factory for subsistence wages, what should a firm do? Should it continue to sanction the employment of child labor as a lesser evil? Again probably not, but neither should the firm simply wash its hands of the situation. If a firm already has a relationship with a supplier who is employing child labor and that fact is suddenly uncovered, walking away from that relationship because of moral outrage may do more harm than good to the children whose interests the firm wishes to protect. In such circumstances, the ethical thing to do may be to find a way of improving the children's lives.

For example, when Levi Strauss found that one of its suppliers employed child labor, it did not terminate the relationship. Instead, it discovered that many of the women who worked in the factory brought their children to work with them because there was no local school, and because the pittance that the children earned kept the family's income above subsistence level. So Levi Strauss built a school for the children under 14, and it paid the parents the additional money that their children would otherwise have earned. This was a small price for Levi Strauss to pay, but it made a big difference in the lives of the affected children.

Gray areas will always exist that require managers to use their own moral judgment to solve ethical dilemmas, but those judgments should be made with regard to a high ethical code. Consider again the example of "gift giving" to support relationships. What is the ethical thing to do? Should one respond to the cultural expectation that a gift should be given, and do so to try to build a relationship that might pay dividends in the future? In nations such as China, where reciprocal gift giving is common and helps to cement *guanxi* relationships, this is not an unreasonable approach, although it may conflict with Western notions of fair play.[56] For example, consider a situation where two Western companies are competing with each other to win a supply contract from a Chinese firm. Imagine that the firm that wins the contract is not the lowest bidder but is the firm that employed the son of the CEO of the Chinese firm as a consultant to advise it on the negotiations. The losing company might believe that principles of fair play have been violated here, but this is not necessarily so. Rather, the winning firm has simply recognized that relationships matter in China and employed an individual with connections to help it win the contract. By employing the son of the CEO, the firm that won the bid helped someone in the CEO's *guanxiwang*, which increased the probability that this "gift" or gesture would be reciprocated.

The practice becomes obviously problematic, however, when government officials are the recipients of the gifts, either directly or indirectly, for then the gifts can be construed as bribery. As was noted in the last chapter, bribery is dangerous, even if it is culturally sanctioned, because the practice can corrupt both the bribe taker and the bribe giver. There is a dividing line between corruption and legitimate gift giving to support business transactions. It is a line that a manager with a strong moral compass should be able to recognize.

Reflecting on such dilemmas, the ethicist Thomas Donaldson has argued that when thinking through ethical problems in international business, firms should be guided by three principles.[57]

1. Respect for core human values (human rights), which determine the absolute moral threshold for all business activities.
2. Respect for local tradition.
3. The belief that context matters when deciding what is right and what is wrong.

Donaldson's point is that respect of core human values must be the starting point for all ethical decisions. Once those are assured, businesses must also respect local cultural differences, which he defines as traditions and context. Thus, Donaldson argues that "gift giving" is not unethical, even though some Western businesses might feel that it is wrong. Gift giving does not violate core human values and is important in the context of some cultures such as China and Japan. By the same token, Donaldson would condemn as unethical decisions that clearly violate core human values. Employing child labor at less than subsistence wages would fall into that category.

ChapterSummary

We have looked at the nature of social culture and studied some implications for business practice. The chapter made these major points:

1. Culture is a complex whole that includes knowledge, beliefs, art, morals, law, customs, and other capabilities acquired by people as members of society.

2. Values and norms are the central components of a culture. Values are abstract ideals about what a society believes to be good, right, and desirable. Norms are social rules and guidelines that prescribe appropriate behavior in particular situations.

3. Values and norms are influenced by political and economic philosophy, social structure, religion, language, and education.

4. The social structure of a society refers to its basic social organization. Two main dimensions along which social structures differ are the individual–group dimension and the stratification dimension.

5. In some societies, the individual is the basic building block of social organization. These societies emphasize individual achievements above all else. In other societies, the group is the basic building block of social organization. These societies emphasize group membership and group achievements above all else.

6. All societies are stratified into different classes. Class-conscious societies are characterized by low social mobility and a high degree of stratification. Less class-conscious societies are characterized by high social mobility and a low degree of stratification.

7. Religion may be defined as a system of shared beliefs and rituals that is concerned with the realm of the sacred. Ethical systems refer to a set of moral principles, or values, that are used to guide and shape behavior. The world's major religions are Christianity, Islam, Hinduism, and Buddhism. Although not a religion, Confucianism has an impact on behavior that is as profound as that of many religions. The value systems of different religious and ethical systems have different implications for business practice.

8. Language is one defining characteristic of a culture. It has both spoken and unspoken dimensions. In countries with more than one spoken language, we tend to find more than one culture.

9. Formal education is the medium through which individuals learn skills and are socialized into the values and norms of a society. Education plays an important role in the determination of national competitive advantage.

10. Geert Hofstede studied how culture relates to values in the workplace. Hofstede isolated four dimensions that he claimed summarized different cultures: power distance, uncertainty avoidance, individualism versus collectivism, and masculinity versus femininity.

11. Culture is not a constant; it evolves. Economic progress and globalization seem to be two important engines of cultural change.

12. One danger confronting a company that goes abroad for the first time is being ill-informed. To develop cross-cultural literacy, international busi-

nesses need to employ host-country nationals, build a cadre of cosmopolitan executives, and guard against the dangers of ethnocentric behavior.

13. The value systems and norms of a country can affect the costs of doing business in that country.

14. Although many ethical principles are universal, some are culturally bounded. What is not ethical in one country might be common in another. Despite this, the "when in Rome" approach to business ethics is dangerous. International businesses need to adhere to a consistent set of ethics derived from a high moral code.

Critical Discussion Questions

1. Outline why the culture of a country might influence the costs of doing business in that country. Illustrate your answer with examples.

2. Do you think that business practices in an Islamic country are likely to differ from business practices in the United States, and if so, how?

3. What are the implications for international business of differences in the dominant religion and/or ethical system of a country?

4. Choose two countries that appear to be culturally diverse. Compare the cultures of those countries and then indicate how cultural differences influence (a) the costs of doing business in each country, (b) the likely future economic development of that country, (c) business practices, and (d) business ethics.

5. It is unreasonable to expect Western businesses active in developing nations to adhere

to the same ethical standards they use at home. Discuss!

6. A Western firm is trying to get a license from the government of a developing nation to set up a factory in that country. The firm knows that the factory will bring many benefits to the country. It will provide jobs in an area where unemployment is high, and it will produce exports for the country, allowing that nation to earn valuable foreign exchange. So far, the government official with whom the firm is negotiating has been noncommittal, neither rejecting nor approving the request, but simply asking for more and more information. The firm has been told that relationships are important in this country, and that if it hired the daughter of the government official as a consultant, she could use her influence to get the license application approved, to everyone's betterment. What should the firm do?

Notes

1. See R. Dore, *Taking Japan Seriously* (Stanford, CA: Stanford University Press, 1987).

2. Data come from the Cologne Institute of the German Economy. Reported in C. Rhoades and S. Miller, "Daimler, Porsche to Be Targeted in German Strike," *Wall Street Journal*, May 6, 2002, p. A15.

3. E. B. Tylor, *Primitive Culture* (London: Murray, 1871).

4. Geert Hofstede, *Culture's Consequences: International Differences in Work Related Values* (Beverly Hills, CA: Sage Publications, 1984), p. 21.

5. J. Z. Namenwirth and R. B. Weber, *Dynamics of Culture* (Boston: Allen & Unwin, 1987), p. 8.

6. R. Mead, *International Management: Cross Cultural Dimensions* (Oxford: Blackwell Business, 1994), p. 7.

7. "Iraq: Down But Not Out," *The Economist*, April 8, 1995, pp. 21–23.

8. S. P. Huntington, *The Clash of Civilizations* (New York, Simon & Schuster, 1996).

9. M. Thompson, R. Ellis, and A. Wildavsky, *Cultural Theory* (Boulder, CO: Westview Press, 1990).

10. M. Douglas, "Cultural Bias," in *Active Voice* (London: Routledge, 1982), pp. 183–254.

11. M. L. Dertouzos, R. K. Lester, and R. M. Solow, *Made in America* (Cambridge, MA: MIT Press, 1989).

12. C. Nakane, *Japanese Society* (Berkeley, CA: University of California Press, 1970).

13. Ibid.

14. For details, see M. Aoki, *Information, Incentives, and Bargaining in the Japanese Economy* (Cambridge: Cambridge University Press, 1988); and Dertouzos, Lester, and Solow, *Made in America*.

15. For an excellent historical treatment of the evolution of the English class system, see E. P. Thompson, *The Making of the English Working Class* (London: Vintage Books, 1966). See also R. Miliband, *The State in Capitalist Society* (New York: Basic Books, 1969), especially Chapter 2. For more recent studies of class in British societies, see Stephen Brook, *Class: Knowing Your Place in Modern Britain* (London: Victor Gollancz, 1997); A. Adonis and S. Pollard, *A Class Act: The Myth of Britain's Classless Society* (London: Hamish Hamilton, 1997); and J. Gerteis and M. Savage, "The Salience of Class in Britain and America: A Comparative Analysis," *British Journal of Sociology*, June 1998.

16. Adonis and Pollard, *A Class Act: The Myth of Britain's Classless Society*.

17. N. Goodman, *An Introduction to Sociology* (New York: HarperCollins, 1991).

18. M. Weber, *The Protestant Ethic and the Spirit of Capitalism* (New York: Charles Scribner's Sons, 1958, original 1904–1905). For an excellent review of Weber's work, see A. Giddens, *Capitalism and Modern Social Theory* (Cambridge: Cambridge University Press, 1971).

19. Weber, *The Protestant Ethic and the Spirit of Capitalism*, p. 35.

20. A. S. Thomas and S. L. Mueller, "The Case for Comparative Entrepreneurship," *Journal of International Business Studies* 31, no. 2 (2000), pp. 287–302, and S. A. Shane, "Why Do Some Societies Invent More Than Others?" *Journal of Business Venturing* 7 (1992), pp. 29–46.

21. See S. M. Abbasi, K. W. Hollman, and J. H. Murrey, "Islamic Economics; Foundations and Practices," *International Journal of Social Economics* 16, no. 5 (1990), pp. 5–17; and R. H. Dekmejian, *Islam in Revolution: Fundamentalism in the Arab World* (Syracuse: Syracuse University Press, 1995).

22. T. W. Lippman, *Understanding Islam* (New York: Meridian Books, 1995).

23. Dekmejian, *Islam in Revolution*.

24. M. K. Nydell, *Understanding Arabs* (Yarmouth, ME: Intercultural Press, 1987).

25. Lippman, *Understanding Islam*.

26. The material in this section is based largely on Abbasi, Hollman, and Murrey, "Islamic Economics; Foundations and Practices."

27. "Islam's Interest," *The Economist*, January 18, 1992, pp. 33–34.

28. For details of Weber's work and views, see Giddens, *Capitalism and Modern Social Theory*.

29. See, for example, the views expressed in "A Survey of India: The Tiger Steps Out," *The Economist*, January 21, 1995.

30. See R. Dore, *Taking Japan Seriously* (Stanford, CA: Stanford University Press, 1987), and C. W. L. Hill, "Transaction Cost Economizing as a Source of Comparative Advantage: The Case of Japan," *Organization Science* 6 (1995).

31. See Aoki, *Information, Incentives, and Bargaining in the Japanese Economy*, and J. P. Womack, D. T. Jones, and D. Roos, *The Machine That Changed the World* (New York: Rawson Associates, 1990).

32. For examples of this line of thinking, see the work by Mike Peng and his associates, M. W. Peng and P. S. Heath, "The Growth of the Firm in Planned Economies in Transition," *Academy of Management Review* 21 (1996), pp. 492–528; M. W. Peng, *Business Strategies in Transition Economies* (Thousand Oaks, CA: Sage, 2000); and M. W. Peng and Y. Luo, "Managerial Ties and Firm Performance in a Transition Economy," *Academy of Management Journal*, June 2000, pp. 486–501.

33. This hypothesis dates back to two anthropologists, Edward Sapir and Benjamin Lee Whorf. See E. Sapir, "The Status of Linguistics as a Science," *Language* 5 (1929), pp. 207–14, and B. L. Whorf, *Language, Thought, and Reality* (Cambridge, MA: MIT Press, 1956).

34. In fact, the tendency has been documented empirically. See A. Annett, "Social Fractionalization, Political Instability, and the Size of Government," *IMF Staff Papers* 48 (2001), pp. 561–92.

35. D. A. Ricks, *Big Business Blunders: Mistakes in Multinational Marketing* (Homewood, IL: Dow Jones-Irwin, 1983).

36. N. Goodman, *An Introduction to Sociology*.

37. M. E. Porter, *The Competitive Advantage of Nations* (New York: Free Press, 1990).

38. Ibid., pp. 395–97.

39. G. Hofstede, "The Cultural Relativity of Organizational Practices and Theories," *Journal of International Business Studies*, Fall 1983, pp. 75–89.

40. For a more detailed critique, see R. Mead, *International Management: Cross-Cultural Dimensions* (Oxford: Blackwell, 1994), pp. 73–75.

41. For example, see W. J. Bigoness and G. L. Blakely, "A Cross-National Study of Managerial Values," *Journal of International Business Studies*, December 1996, p. 739; D. H. Ralston, D. H. Holt, R. H. Terpstra, and Y. Kai-Cheng, "The Impact of National Culture and Economic Ideology on Managerial Work Values," *Journal of International Business Studies* 28, no. 1 (1997), pp. 177–208; and P. B. Smith, M. F. Peterson, and Z. Ming Wang, "The Manager as a Mediator of Alternative Meanings," *Journal of International Business Studies* 27, no. 1 (1996), pp. 115–37.

42. G. Hofstede and M. H. Bond, "The Confucius Connection," *Organizational Dynamics* 16, no. 4 (1988), pp. 5–12, and G. Hofstede, *Culture's Consequences: Comparing Values, Behaviors, Institutions and Organizations across Nations* (Thousand Oaks, CA: Sage, 2001).

43. R. S. Yeh and J. J. Lawerence, "Individualism and Confucian Dynamism," *Journal of International Business Studies* 26, no. 3 (1995), pp. 655–66.

44. For evidence of this, see R. Inglehart. "Globalization and Postmodern Values," *The Washington Quarterly*, Winter 2000, pp. 215–28.

45. Mead, *International Management: Cross-Cultural Dimensions*, chap. 17.

46. "Free, Young, and Japanese," *The Economist*, December 21, 1991.

47. Namenwirth and Weber, *Dynamics of Culture*, and Inglehart, "Globalization and Postmodern Values."

48. G. Hofstede, "National Cultures in Four Dimensions," *International Studies of Management and Organization* 13, no. 1, pp. 46–74.

49. See Inglehart, "Globalization and Postmodern Values." For updates, go to http://wvs.isr.umich.edu/index.html.

50. Hofstede, "National Cultures in Four Dimensions."

51. See Aoki, *Information, Incentives, and Bargaining in the Japanese Economy*; Dertouzos, Lester, and Solow, *Made in America*; and Porter, *The Competitive Advantage of Nations*, pp. 395–97.

52. For empirical work supporting such a view, see Annett, "Social Fractionalization, Political Instability, and the Size of Government."

53. J. Goodwin and D. Goodwin, "Ethical Judgements across Cultures," *Journal of Business Ethics* 18, no. 3 (February 1999), pp. 267–81.

54. T. Donaldson, "Values in Tension: Ethics Away from Home," *Harvard Business Review*, September–October 1996.

55. R. T. DeGeorge, "Ethics in International Business—A Contradiction in Terms?" *Business Credit*, September 2000, pp. 50–52.

56. S. Lovett, L. C. Simmons, and R. Kali, "Guanxi versus the Market: Ethics and Efficiency," *Journal of International Business Studies* 30, no. 2 (1999), pp. 231–48.

57. Donaldson, "Values in Tension: Ethics Away from Home."

Research Task | globalEDGE™   globaledge.msu.edu

Use the globalEDGE™ site to complete the following exercises:

1. You are preparing for a business trip to Venezuela where you will need to interact extensively with local professionals. Therefore, you may consider collecting information regarding local culture and business habits prior to your departure. Prepare a short description of the most striking cultural characteristics that may affect business interactions in this country.

2. Asian cultures exhibit significant differences in business etiquette when compared to Western cultures. For example, in Thailand it is considered offensive to show the sole of the shoe or foot to another. Using the globalEDGE site, find five additional tips regarding the business etiquette of a specific Asian country of your choice.

McDonald's and Hindu Culture

In many ways, McDonald's Corporation has written the book on global expansion. Every day, on average, somewhere around the world 4.2 new McDonald's restaurants are opened. By 2003, the company had 30,000 restaurants in 121 countries that collectively served 46 million customers each day.

One of the latest additions to McDonald's list of countries entered by the famous golden arches had been India, where McDonald's started to establish restaurants in the late 1990s. Although India is a poor nation, the large and relatively prosperous middle class, estimated to number between 150 and 200 million, attracted McDonald's. India, however, offered McDonald's unique challenges. For thousands of years, India's Hindu culture has revered the cow. Hindu scriptures state that the cow is a gift of the gods to the human race. The cow represents the Divine Mother that sustains all human beings. Cows give birth to bulls that are harnessed to pull plows, cow milk is highly valued and used to produce yogurt and ghee (a form of butter), cow urine has a unique place in traditional Hindu medicine, and cow dung is used as fuel. Some 300 million of these animals roam India, untethered, revered as sacred providers. They are everywhere, ambling down roads, grazing in rubbish dumps, and resting in temples—everywhere, that is, except on your plate, for Hindus do not eat the meat of the scared cow.

McDonald's is the world's largest user of beef. Since its founding in 1955, countless animals have died to produce Big Macs. How can a company whose fortunes are built upon beef enter a country where the consumption of beef is a grave sin? Use pork instead? But there are some 140 million Muslims in India, and Muslims don't eat pork. This leaves chicken and mutton. McDonald's responded to this cultural food dilemma by creating an Indian version of its Big Mac—the "Maharaja Mac"—which is made from mutton. Other additions to the menu conform to local sensibilities such as the "McAloo Tikki Burger," which is made from chicken. All foods are strictly segregated into vegetarian and nonvegetarian lines to conform with preferences in a country where many Hindus are vegetarian. According to the head of McDonald's Indian operations, "We had to reinvent ourselves for the Indian palate."

For a while, this seemed to work. Then in 2001 McDonald's was blindsided by a class action lawsuit brought against it in the United States by three Indian businessmen living in Seattle. The businessmen, all vegetarians and two of whom were Hindus, sued McDonald's for "fraudulently concealing" the existence of beef in McDonald's French fries! McDonald's had said it used only 100 percent vegetable oil to make French fries, but the company soon admitted that it used a "minuscule" amount of beef extract in the oil. McDonald's settled the suit for $10 million and issued an apology, which read, "McDonald's sincerely apologizes to Hindus, vegetarians, and others for failing to provide the kind of information they needed to make informed dietary decisions at our U.S. restaurants." Going forward, the company pledged to do a better job of labeling the ingredients of its food and to find a substitute for the beef extract used in its oil.

However, news travels fast in the global society of the 21st century, and the revelation that McDonald's used beef extract in its oil was enough to bring Hindu nationalists onto the streets in Delhi, where they vandalized one McDonald's restaurant, causing $45,000 of damage; shouted slogans outside of another; picketed the company's headquarters; and called on India's prime minister to close McDonald's 27 stores in the country. McDonald's Indian franchise holders quickly issued denials that they used oil that contained beef extract, and Hindu extremists responded by stating they would submit McDonald's oil to laboratory tests to see if they could detect beef extract.

The negative publicity seemed to have little impact on McDonald's long-term plans in India, however. The company continued to open restaurants, and by 2003 had 38 in the country and announced plans to open another 80 by 2005. When asked why they frequented McDonald's restaurants, Indian customers noted that their children enjoyed the "American" experience, the food was of a consistent quality, and the toilets were always clean!

Case Discussion Questions

1. What lessons does the experience of McDonald's in India hold for other foreign fast-food chains and retail stores?

2. Is there anything that McDonald's could have done to have foreseen or better prepared itself for the negative publicity associated with the revelation that it used beef extract in its frying oil?

3. How far should a firm such as McDonald's go in localizing its product to account for cultural differences? At some point, might it not lose an advantage by doing so?

Sources: Luke Harding, "Give Me a Big Mac—But Hold the Beef," *The Guardian*, December 28, 2000, p. 24; Luke Harding, "Indian McAnger," *The Guardian*, May 7, 2001, p. 1; and A. Dhillon, "India Has No Beef with Fast Food Chains," *Financial Times*, March 23, 2002, p. 3.

Cases

Nike: The Sweatshop Debate   128

Qualcomm's Chinese Odyssey   132

Royal Dutch/Shell: Human Rights
in Nigeria   136

Nike: The Sweatshop Debate 🎥

Introduction

Nike is in many ways the quintessential global corporation. Established in 1972 by former University of Oregon track star Phil Knight, Nike is now one of the leading marketers of athletic shoes and apparel on the planet. The company has $10 billion in annual revenues and sells its products in some 140 countries. Nike does not do any manufacturing. Rather, it designs and markets its products, while contracting for their manufacture from a global network of 600 factories scattered around the globe that employ some 550,000 people.[1] This huge corporation has made Knight into one of the richest people in America. The Nike marketing phrase "Just Do It!" has become as recognizable in popular culture as its "swoosh" logo or the faces of its celebrity sponsors, such as Michael Jordan and Tiger Woods.

For all of its successes, the company has been dogged for more than a decade by repeated and persistent accusations that its products are made in sweatshops where workers, many of them children, slave away in hazardous conditions for less than subsistence wages. Nike's wealth, its detractors claim, has been built upon the backs of the world's poor. To many, Nike has become a symbol of the evils of globalization—a rich Western corporation exploiting the world's poor to provide expensive shoes and apparel to the pampered consumers of the developed world. Nike's "Niketown" stores have become standard targets for antiglobalization protesters. Several nongovernmental organizations, such as San Franciso–based Global Exchange, a human rights organization dedicated to promoting environmental, political, and social justice around the world, have targeted Nike for repeated criticism and protests.[2] News organizations such as CBS's "48 Hours" hosted by Dan Rather have run exposés on working conditions in foreign factories that supply Nike. Students on the campuses of several major U.S. universities with which Nike has lucrative sponsorship deals have protested against the ties, citing Nike's use of sweatshop labor.

For its part, Nike has taken steps to counter the protests. Yes, it admits, there have been problems in some overseas factories. But the company has signaled a commitment to improving working conditions. It requires that foreign subcontractors meet minimum thresholds for working conditions and pay. It has arranged for factories to be examined by independent auditors. It has terminated contracts with factories that do not comply with its standards. But for all this effort, the company continues to be a target of protests and a symbol of dissent.

The Case against Nike

Typical of the exposés against Nike was a "48 Hours" report that aired October 17, 1996.[3] Reporter Roberta Baskin visited a Nike factory in Vietnam. With a shot of the factory, her commentary began:

> The signs are everywhere of an American invasion in search of cheap labor. Millions of people who are literate, disciplined, and desperate for jobs. This is Nike Town near what use to be called Saigon, one of four factories Nike doesn't own but subcontracts to make a million shoes a month. It takes 25,000 workers, mostly young women, to "Just Do It."
>
> But the workers here don't share in Nike's huge profits. They work six days a week for only $40 a month, just 20 cents an hour.

Baskin interviewed one factory worker, a young woman named Lap. Baskin told viewers:

> Her basic wage, even as sewing team leader, still doesn't amount to the minimum wage . . . She's down to 85 pounds. Like most of the young women who make shoes, she has little choice but to accept the low wages and long hours. Nike says that it requires all subcontractors to obey local laws; but Lap has already put in much more overtime than the annual legal limit: 200 hours.

Baskin then asked Lap what would happen if she was sick or had something she needed to take care of, such as a sick relative, and needed to leave the factory? Through a translator, Lap replied:

> It is not possible if you haven't made enough shoes. You have to meet the quota before you can go home.

The clear implication of the story was that Nike was at fault here for allowing such working conditions to persist in the Vietnam factory, which was owned by a Korean company.

Another attack on Nike's subcontracting practices came in June 1996 from Made in the USA, a foundation largely financed by labor unions and domestic apparel manufacturers that oppose free trade with low-wage countries. According to Joel Joseph, chairman of the foundation, a popular line of high-priced Nike sneakers, the "Air Jordans," were put together by 11-year-olds in Indonesia making 14 cents per hour. A Nike spokeswoman, Donna Gibbs, countered that this was false. According to Gibbs, the average worker made 240,000 rupiah ($103) a month working a maximum 54-hour week, or about 45 cents per hour. Gibbs also noted that Nike had staff members in each factory monitoring conditions to make sure the factory obeyed local minimum wage and child labor laws.[4]

Another example of the criticism against Nike is the following extract from a newsletter published by Global Exchange:[5]

> During the 1970s, most Nike shoes were made in South Korea and Taiwan. When workers there gained new freedom to organize and wages began to rise, Nike looked for "greener pastures." It found them in Indonesia and China, where Nike started producing in the 1980s, and most recently in Vietnam.
>
> The majority of Nike shoes are made in Indonesia and China, countries with governments that prohibit independent unions and set the minimum wage at rock bottom. The Indonesian government admits that the minimum wage there does not provide enough to supply the basic needs of one person, let alone a family. In early 1997 the entry-level wage was a miserable $2.46 a day. Labor groups estimate that a livable wage in Indonesia is about $4.00 a day.
>
> In Vietnam the pay is even less—20 cents an hour, or a mere $1.60 a day. But in urban Vietnam, three simple meals cost about $2.10 a day, and then of course there is rent, transportation, clothing, health care, and much more. According to Thuyen Nguyen of Vietnam Labor Watch, a living wage in Vietnam is at least $3 a day.

In another attack on Nike's practices, in September 1997 Global Exchange published a report on working conditions in four Nike and Reebok subcontractors in southern China.[6] Global Exchange, in conjunction with two Hong Kong human rights groups, had interviewed workers at the factories in 1995 and again in 1997. According to Global Exchange, in one factory, a Korean-owned subcontractor for Nike, workers as young as 13 earning as little as 10 cents an hour toiled up to 17 hours daily in enforced silence. Talking during work was not allowed, with violators fined $1.20 to $3.60, according to the report. The practices were in violation of Chinese labor law, which states that no child under 16 may work in a factory, and the Chinese minimum wage requirement of $1.90 for an eight-hour day. Nike condemned the study as erroneous, stating that the report incorrectly stated the wages of workers and made irresponsible accusations.

Global Exchange, however, continued to be a major thorn in Nike's side. In November 1997, the organization obtained and then leaked a confidential report by Ernst & Young of an audit that Nike had commissioned of a factory in Vietnam owned by a Nike subcontractor.[7] The factory had 9,200 workers and made 400,000 pairs of shoes a month. The Ernst & Young report painted a dismal picture of thousands of young women, most under age 25, laboring 10 1/2 hours a day, six days a week, in excessive heat and noise and in foul air, for slightly more than $10 a week. The report also found that workers with skin or breathing problems had not been transferred to departments free of chemicals and that more than half the workers who dealt with dangerous chemicals did not wear protective masks or gloves. It claimed workers were exposed to carcinogens that exceeded local legal standards by 177 times in parts of the plant and that 77 percent of the employees suffered from respiratory problems.

Put on the defensive yet again, Nike called a news conference and pointed out that it had commissioned the report and had acted on it.[8] The company stated it had formulated an action plan to deal with the problems cited in the report, and had slashed overtime, improved safety and ventilation, and reduced the use of toxic chemicals. The company also asserted that the report showed that its internal monitoring system had performed exactly as it should have. According to one spokesman:

> This shows our system of monitoring works . . . We have uncovered these issues clearly before anyone else, and we have moved fairly expeditiously to correct them.

Nike's Responses

Unaccustomed to playing defense, Nike formulated a number of strategies and tactics to deal with the problems of working conditions and pay at subcontractors. In 1996, Nike hired Andrew Young, onetime U.S. ambassador to the United Nations and former Atlanta mayor, to assess working conditions in subcontractors' plants around the world. Young released a mildly critical report of Nike in mid-1997. After completing a two-week tour that covered 15 factories in three countries, Young informed Nike it was doing a good job in treating workers, though it should do better. According to Young, he did not see

> sweatshops, or hostile conditions . . . I saw crowded dorms . . . but the workers were eating at least two meals a day on the job and making what I was told were subsistence wages in those cultures.[9]

Young was widely criticized by human rights and labor groups for not taking his own translators and for doing slipshod inspections, an assertion he repeatedly denied.

In 1996, Nike joined a presidential task force designed to find a way of banishing sweatshops in the shoe and clothing industries. The task force included industry leaders such as Nike, representatives from human rights groups, and labor leaders. In April 1997, the task force announced an agreement for workers rights that U.S. companies could agree to when manufacturing abroad. The accord limited the work week to 60 hours and called for paying at least the local minimum wage in foreign factories. The task force also agreed to establish an independent monitoring association—later named the Fair Labor Association (FLA)—to assess whether companies are abiding by the code.[10]

The FLA now includes among its members the Lawyers Committee for Human Rights, the National Council of Churches, the International Labor Rights Fund, some 135 universities (universities have extensive licensing agreements with sports apparel companies such as Nike), and companies such as Nike, Reebok, and Levi Strauss.

In early 1997, Nike also began to commission independent organizations such as Ernst & Young to audit the factories of its subcontractors. In September 1997, Nike tried to show its critics that it was involved in more than just a public relations exercise when it terminated its relationship with four Indonesian subcontractors, stating that they had refused to comply with the company's standard for wage levels and working conditions. Nike identified one of the subcontractors, Seyon, which manufactured specialty sports gloves for Nike. Nike said that Seyon refused to meet a 10.7 percent increase in the monthly wage, to $70.30, declared by the Indonesian government in April 1997.[11]

On May 12, 1998, in a speech given at the National Press Club, Phil Knight spelled out in detail a series of initiatives designed to improve working conditions for the 500,000 people that make products for Nike.[12] Among the initiatives Knight highlighted were the following:

> We have effectively changed our minimum age limits from the ILO (International Labor Organization) standards of 15 in most countries and 14 in developing countries to 18 in all footwear manufacturing and 16 in all other types of manufacturing (apparel, accessories, and equipment.). Existing workers legally employed under the former limits were grandfathered into the new requirements.
>
> During the past 13 months we have moved to a 100 percent factory audit scheme, where every Nike contract factory will receive an annual check by PricewaterhouseCoopers teams who are specially trained on our Code of Conduct Owner's Manual and audit/monitoring procedures. To date they have performed about 300 such monitoring visits. In a few instances in apparel factories they have found workers under our age standards. Those factories have been required to raise their standards to 17 years of age, to require three documents certifying age, and to redouble their efforts to ensure workers meet those standards through interviews and records checks.
>
> Our goal was to ensure workers around the globe are protected by requiring factories to have no workers exposed to levels above those mandated by the permissible exposure limits (PELs) for chemicals prescribed in the OSHA indoor air quality standards.[13]

These moves were applauded in the business press, but they were greeted with a skeptical response from Nike's long-term adversaries in the debate over the use of foreign labor. While conceding that Nike's policies were an improvement, one critic writing in the *New York Times* noted:

> Mr. Knight's child labor initiative is . . . a smoke screen. Child labor has not been a big problem with Nike, and Philip Knight knows that better than anyone. But public relations is public relations. So he announces

that he's not going to let the factories hire kids, and suddenly that's the headline.

> Mr. Knight is like a three-card monte player. You have to keep a close eye on him at all times.
>
> The biggest problem with Nike is that its overseas workers make wretched, below-subsistence wages. It's not the minimum age that needs raising, it's the minimum wage. Most of the workers in Nike factories in China and Vietnam make less than $2 a day, well below the subsistence levels in those countries. In Indonesia the pay is less than $1 a day.
>
> The company's current strategy is to reshape its public image while doing as little as possible for the workers. Does anyone think it was an accident that Nike set up shop in human rights sinkholes, where labor organizing was viewed as a criminal activity and deeply impoverished workers were willing, even eager, to take their places on assembly lines and work for next to nothing?[14]

Other critics question the value of Nike's auditors, PricewaterhouseCoopers (PwC). Dara O'Rourke, an assistant professor at MIT, followed the PwC auditors around several factories in China, Korea, and Vietnam. He concluded that although the auditors found minor violations of labor laws and codes of conduct, they missed major labor practice issues including hazardous working conditions, violations of overtime laws, and violation of wage laws. The problem, according to O'Rourke, was that the auditors had limited training and relied on factory managers for data and to set up worker interviews, all of which were performed in the factories. The auditors, in other words, were getting an incomplete and somewhat sanitized view of conditions in the factory.[15]

The Controversy Continues

Fueled perhaps by the unforgiving criticisms of Nike that continued after Phil Knight's May 1998 speech, beginning in 1998 and continuing into 2001, a wave of protests against Nike occurred on many university campuses. The moving force behind the protests was the United Students Against Sweatshops (USAS). The USAS argued that the Fair Labor Association (FLA), which grew out of the presidential task force on sweatshops, was an industry tool, and not a truly independent auditor of foreign factories. The USAS set up an alternative independent auditing organization, the Workers Rights Consortium (WRC), which they charged with auditing factories that produce products under collegiate licensing programs (Nike is a high profile supplier of products under these programs). The WRC is backed, and partly funded, by labor unions and refuses to cooperate with companies, arguing that doing so would jeopardize its independence.

By mid-2000, the WRC had persuaded some 48 universities to join the organization, including all nine campuses of the University of California system, the University of Michigan, and the University of Oregon, Phil Knight's alma mater. When Knight heard that the University of Oregon would join the WRC, as opposed to the FLA, he withdrew a planned $30 million donation to the university.[16] Despite this, in November 2000, the University of Washington announced it too would join the WRC, although it would also retain its membership in the FLA.[17]

Nike continued to push forward with its own initiatives, updating progress on its website. In April 2000, in response to pressure that it was still hiding poor working conditions, Nike announced it would release the complete reports of all independent audits of its subcontractors' plants. Global Exchange continued to criticize the company, arguing in mid-2001 that the company was not living up to Knight's 1998 promises, and that it was intimidating workers from speaking out about abuses.[18]

Case Discussion Questions

1. Should Nike be held responsible for working conditions in foreign factories that it does not own, but where subcontractors make products for Nike?

2. What labor standards regarding safety, working conditions, overtime, and the like should Nike hold foreign factories to: those prevailing in that country, or those prevailing in the United States?

3. An income of $2.28 a day, the base pay of Nike factory workers in Indonesia, is double the daily income of about half the working population. Half of all adults in Indonesia are farmers, who receive less than $1 a day.[19] Given this, is it correct to criticize Nike for the low pay rates of its subcontractors in Indonesia?

4. Could Nike have handled the negative publicity over sweatshops better? What might it have done differently, not just from a public relations perspective, but also from a policy perspective?

5. Do you think Nike needs to make any changes to its current policy? If so what? Should Nike make changes even if they hinder the ability of the company to compete?

6. Is the WRC right to argue that the FLA is a tool of industry?

7. If sweatshops are a global problem, what might be a global solution to this problem?

Notes

1. From Nike's corporate website at http://www.nikebiz.com.

2. From http://www.globalexchange.org.

3. "Boycott Nike," CBS News "48 Hours," October 17, 1996.

4. D. Jones, "Critics Tie Sweatshop Sneakers to 'Air Jordan,'" *USA Today*, June 6, 1996, p. 1B.

5. Global Exchange Special Report, Nike Just Don't Do It, http://www.globalexchange.org/education/publications/newsltr6.97p2.html#nike.

6. V. Dobnik, "Chinese Workers Abused Making Nikes, Reeboks," *Seattle Times*, September 21, 1997, p. A4.

7. S. Greenhouse, "Nike Shoeplant in Vietnam Is Called Unsafe for Workers," *New York Times*, November 8, 1997.

8. S. Greenhouse, "Nike Shoeplant in Vietnam Is Called Unsafe for Workers."

9. V. Dobnik, "Chinese Workers Abused Making Nikes, Reeboks."

10. W. Bounds and H. Stout, "Sweatshop Pact: Good Fit or Threadbare?" *Wall Street Journal*, April 10, 1997, p. A2.

11. Associated Press, "Nike Gives Four Factories the Boot," *Los Angeles Times*, September 23, 1997, p. 20.

12. Archived at http://www.nikebiz.com/labor/speech_trans.shtml.

13. OSHA is the United States Occupational Safety and Health Administration.

14. B. Herbert, "Nike Blinks," *New York Times*, May 21, 1998.

15. Dara O'Rourke, "Monitoring the Monitors: A Critique of the PricewaterhouseCoopers (PwC) Labor Monitoring," Department of Urban Studies and Planning, MIT.

16. L. Lee and A. Bernstein, "Who Says Student Protests Don't Matter?" *Business Week*, June 12, 2000, pp. 94–96.

17. R. Deen, "UW to Join Anti-sweatshop Group," *Seattle Post-Intelligencer*, November 20, 2000, p. B2.

18. "Rights Group Says Nike Isn't Fulfilling Promises," *Wall Street Journal*, May 16, 2001.

19. Figures from P. Kenel, "The Sweatshop Dilemma," *Christian Science Monitor*, August 21, 1996, p. 20.

Qualcomm's Chinese Odyssey

Company and Industry Background

Qualcomm was founded in 1985 by Dr. Irwin Jacobs, a former engineering professor. Under his leadership, the company developed a digital communications technology for wireless phones known as code division multiple access (CDMA). Introduced in 1989, CDMA was to become one of the three main technologies used in digital wireless phones. CDMA and the two other main digital wireless communications technologies, TDMA (which stands for time division multiple access) and GSM (which is a form of TDMA and stands for global system for mobile communications) are the digital technologies used to transmit a wireless phone user's voice or data over radio waves using the wireless phone operator's network. CDMA works by converting speech into digital information, which is then transmitted in the form of a radio signal over the phone network. These digital wireless phone networks are complete phone systems comprised primarily of base stations, or cells, which are geographically placed throughout a service or coverage area. Once communication between a wireless phone user and a base station is established, the system detects the movement of the wireless phone user and the communication is handed off to another base station, or cell, as the user moves throughout the service area.

Qualcomm has more than 800 patents on CDMA and essentially owns this standard for digital wireless phones. Qualcomm licenses its technology to equipment manufacturers in return for royalties on the sale of any equipment, such as base stations and handsets. The equipment manufacturers sell the equipment to service providers. Thus, for example, Qualcomm might license its technol-

ogy to Motorola, which then makes base stations and handsets that are based on CDMA technology. In turn, Motorola might sell the CDMA equipment to a service provider, such as Verizon, which offers wireless phone service to consumers in the United States. Every time Motorola makes a sale, Qualcomm collects a royalty based on a percentage of the price of that equipment (Qualcomm has not reported that figure, but it is believed to be 4 percent of the value of the equipment). Qualcomm also makes and sells "chipsets" based on CDMA technology to equipment manufacturers that then place those chipsets into base stations and handsets. Some 90 percent of CDMA phones contain chipsets manufactured by Qualcomm. In 2002, Qualcomm generated record revenues of $3.79 billion and net profits of $1.21 billion.

The great advantage claimed for CDMA over competing standards is that it uses radio spectrum more efficiently than GSM or TDMA. Qualcomm states that CDMA equipment has three times the capacity of comparable GSM or TDMA equipment, thereby enabling service operators to offer the same capacity with a lower investment in network equipment such as base stations. Because the wireless service industry is very price competitive, any technology that promises to lower costs for service operators should gain an advantage in the marketplace. However, CDMA was a latecomer to the digital communications market, and by 2002 was still in third place behind TDMA and GSM with 13 percent of the world market. In the early 1990s, the European Union backed GSM as the standard for digital communications technology. At the time, Europe led the world in the adoption of wireless phone technology. Also, since Euro-

Figure 1

Number of Wireless Subscribers Worldwide (in Millions)

Source: EMC press releases (http://www.emc-database.com) and Qualcomm 10K reports.

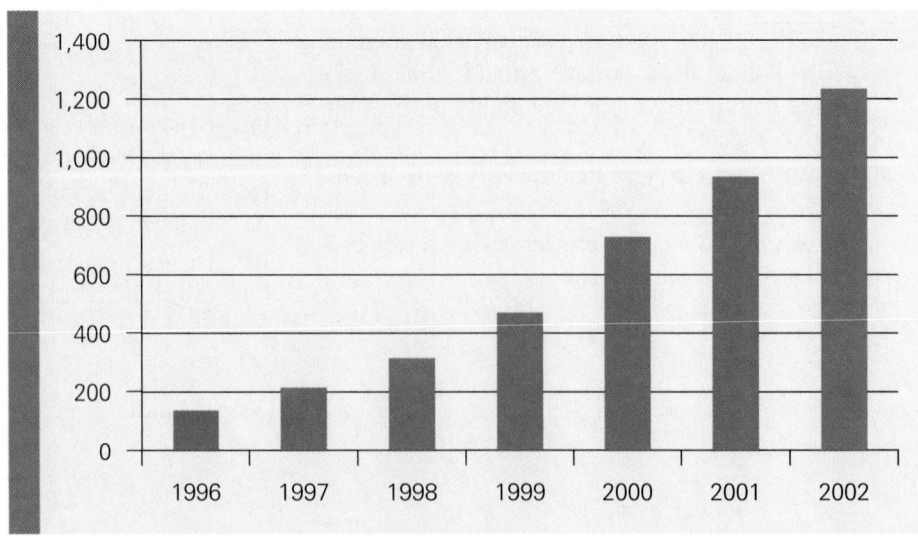

pean firms such as Ericsson and Nokia were major suppliers of GSM equipment, this decision benefited them.

Although CDMA equipment can in theory handle more data traffic than comparable TDMA or GSM equipment, the larger installed base of TDMA and GSM subscribers means that companies making this equipment benefit from substantial economies of scale, which to some extent nullifies the cost advantage associated with CDMA technology and helps explain the continued dominance of these standards. Because far more GSM handsets are sold than CDMA handsets, economies of scale mean that GSM handsets are less expensive than CDMA handsets.

By the end of 2002, there were more than 1.2 billion wireless subscribers worldwide, and some 140 million used CDMA technology. Forecasts called for the total number of wireless subscribers to grow to 2 billion by 2006. Among the different wireless technologies, CDMA was registering the fastest growth rate. In the year ending June 2002, the number of CDMA subscribers grew by 32 percent worldwide. CDMA is now the most widely used technology in the United States, where 43 percent of the nation's 141 million wireless phone subscribers in 2002 used CDMA equipment. CDMA also has a large and growing presence in Latin America, where 24 million subscribers in 15 countries used CDMA phones in 2002. In Asia Pacific, there were some 45 million CDMA subscribers by mid-2002. The laggard in CDMA penetration is Europe, where GSM dominates and CDMA technology had less than 10 million subscribers in 2002.

The future success of Qualcomm will be driven by two related factors. First, there is a shift to a new generation of technology, known in the industry as 3G, or third-generation wireless technology. This new generation of digital wireless technology is designed to handle much greater amounts of data at rapid download speeds, enabling subscribers to download multimedia applications, such as streaming video or audio, onto their wireless phones, effectively turning the handsets into small computers that are connected to the Internet and able to access it from anyplace at anytime. Two versions of CDMA technology have been developed for 3G, CDMA2000 and WCDMA. While Qualcomm developed CDMA2000, WCDMA was developed by rival telecommunications firms Nokia and Ericsson. However, Qualcomm's patents cover both versions of the technology, and the firm will earn royalties no matter which version is used by a particular service carrier, although Qualcomm favors CDMA2000 and reportedly makes greater royalties from this variant of the technology. Both CDMA 3G technologies will have to compete with a 3G version of the popular GSM technology, know as GPRS, which was introduced in 2002.

The second factor driving Qualcomm's success is the penetration of CDMA technology into developing markets where there is still large potential for new subscriber adoptions, particularly in the Asia Pacific region. Industry forecasts suggest the number of wireless phone subscribers in this region will grow from 232 million in 2000 to 761 million in 2005. Top among these expanding developing markets are China, with its 1.2 billion people, and India. In both nations, wireless penetration is currently low but growing rapidly. Given the large population base in these markets, the standard that dominates here may be the standard that dominates worldwide. China and India have thus become the main battlegrounds for the future of digital wireless technology, and Qualcomm's future depends upon the outcome of this battle.

The Early Days: Great Wall

Qualcomm's Irwin Jacobs was quick to recognize the importance of China in Qualcomm's future. He began making business trips to China in 1992 to try to persuade China's fledgling telecommunications providers to adopt CDMA technology. In 1994 it began to look as if he might make some headway. At the time, the People's Liberation Army, China's army, was keen to develop a secure communications network. CDMA is a civilian application of a technology developed for secure military transmissions and is well-suited to this application. Also, the Chinese army happened to own the spectrum that CDMA uses, the 800 MHz band. By building a commercial CDMA network with its spare spectrum, the army figured it could dominate the nascent mobile phone market in China, and use the profits and expertise gained from that business to modernize its own communications network.

When the army announced in 1994 that it would deploy a CDMA network, China's top telephone official, Wu Jichuan, the minister of Posts and Telecommunications, was caught off guard. Wu Jichuan saw telecommunications as a national priority and favored state-owned China Telecommunications Corp. He had allowed the company to charge high long-distance rates, and then had forced it to use the profits to bring telecommunications services to remote villages. He had little use for competition from the army that might sap China Telecom's profits and derail his plans.

To deal with the threat, the canny Wu invited the army into his camp, proposing that it form a 50/50 joint venture with China Telecomm to build a CDMA network. Called "Great Wall," the venture won a license to run an experimental CDMA network in four cities—creating a potential boom in demand for CDMA equipment and a royalty stream for Qualcomm. However, Wu also ordered China Telecom to roll out as fast as possible a separate, nationwide digital network based on GSM. Coincidentally, the ministry of Posts and Telecommunications happened to own the 900 MHz radio spectrum used by the GSM technology. Wu then refused to issue permits to the army to allow it to expand its network beyond four cities. By 1998 it was clear that Great Wall's expansion plans had been stymied by Wu, with a corresponding loss of opportunity for Qualcomm.

China Unicom

However, the story was far from over. In the late 1990s, China separated out two wireless phone operators from China Telecomm—China Mobile and China Unicom. Although both were initially state owned, the idea was to sell some equity to private investors and set the two entities up as competitors in China's wireless phone market. While China Mobile inherited the bulk of existing networks and subscribers, China Unicom was left to choose its own technology, opening the door for Qualcomm to get back into China.

Irwin Jacobs had also been working the political angle in the interim. China's leadership decided in the late 1990s that it needed to become a member of the World Trade Organization (WTO) if it was to participate in the global economy of the 21st century. If China was to enter the WTO, it would have to win the support of major trading nations that were already members, including the United States. Behind the scenes, Jacobs lobbied the U.S. government, urging it to pressure China to adopt CDMA technology as one of the conditions for U.S. support of China's entry into the WTO. For a while the efforts were fruitless, but in March 1999 Chinese Premier Zhu Rongi decided to offer the United States what it had long wanted—a commitment to use CDMA technology in return for U.S. support of China's entry into the WTO. The premier proposed that China Unicom work with Qualcomm and others to roll out a CDMA network in China.

However, before this deal could be finalized, Qualcomm had to negotiate a licensing framework with Wu's ministry, which had been renamed the Ministry of Information. But the negotiations dragged on, with Qualcomm demanding a higher royalty rate on sales of CDMA equipment than Wu was allowed to sanction. In the end, Wu ordered Unicom to negotiate directly with Qualcomm. For Unicom, this represented a problem. The company was trying to become profitable so that it could start selling equity to private investors and gain a listing on the Hong Kong and New York stock exchanges. It had already started to roll out a wireless network based on GSM and was not too happy about being ordered to make duplicate investments in a CDMA network. Reports suggest that like Wu, Unicom insisted that Qualcomm lower its royalty rate or nothing would happen. In the end, Qualcomm relented (the royalty agreement has not been made public), and in February 2000 Unicom announced that a deal had been reached and it would soon start construction on a CDMA network for 10 million subscribers.

The issue was far from resolved, however. At the signing ceremony, it was clear that something was wrong—Wu and other cabinet officials declined to attend. In a private meeting between Wu and Jacobs it became clear why—Wu was exerting his influence again, and this time he was insisting that Qualcomm must transfer the design for the chips that run the CDMA system to a Chinese firm. This was something that Qualcomm had never done and was unlikely to now. Jacobs said the request could not be met. A few days later, China Unicom withdrew its request for bids on a CDMA network, but denied that the project was on hold. But in June 2000, after the U.S. House of Representatives had approved a bill enabling China to enter the WTO, Unicom confirmed that it would continue to use a GSM network, but the company held out the possibility that it would use 3G equipment based on CDMA.

According to news reports, while politics played a part in the Unicom decision, so did pressure from local equipment manufacturers, many of whom were joint ventures between Chinese companies and foreigners, such as Ericsson, Nokia, and Motorola. Many of these joint ventures had already made investments to produce GSM equipment and were not ready to produce CDMA equipment. Some of these manufacturers reportedly pressured Unicom to stick with GSM, or at the very least, slow down the rollout of CDMA networks.

After so many years trying to break into China, Irwin Jacobs was not about to give up. In October 2000, Jacobs visited with Premier Zhu Rongi in Beijing. The meeting was private, but it is speculated that Qualcomm lowered the royalty rate that Chinese equipment manufacturers would have to pay the company to 2.65 percent of handset sales, substantially lower than the 4 percent rate reportedly paid to Qualcomm elsewhere in the world. Soon after the meeting, China Unicom reversed course, announcing it would build a CDMA network to support 10 million subscribers, although it would now be mid-2002 before that network started to generate significant handset sales, and thus royalties for Qualcomm, not 2001 as originally hoped. Analysts speculated that the small size of the network would make it hard for Qualcomm to get its favored 3G technology, CDMA2000, widely adopted in China.

By April 2001, it looked as if Qualcomm had finally cracked the Chinese market. Then, one day before China Unicom was due to sign contracts with equipment suppliers to supply its planned CDMA network, the deal was delayed again. No reason was given. Some speculated that a rise in political tension between the United States and China was to blame. A U.S. surveillance plane had been forced down by the Chinese air force, who accused the United States of spying on China. Thrown into the mix were heightened tensions between the United States and China over the future of Taiwan.

Whatever the reason, a month later Chinese President Jiang Zemin appeared to give the green light to the deal when he told a gathering of foreign business leaders that CDMA could increase competition in China. Shortly after, Unicom signed contracts to build a CDMA network with a capacity of 15.15 million subscribers.

The Rollout of CDMA in China

After years of back and forth, China Unicom turned on its CDMA network in January 2002 following a $2.5 billion investment in equipment. Its year-end target for 2002 was 7 million subscribers, but by June 2002 the number stood at a meager 700,000, while China now had 160 million wireless subscribers, the majority using GSM equipment. Critics were quick to claim that the slow rollout demonstrated Unicom's lack of commitment to CDMA, which some view as being forced on them by Chinese politicians. Unicom executives disagreed, and claimed the decision was sound business because CDMA network equipment is cheaper than GSM equipment. Unicom and Qualcomm executives did concede that they had priced CDMA phones too high in an attempt to recoup the higher cost of CDMA handsets, which cost $350 each, some $100 more than GSM phones.

By the second half of 2002, however, the rollout of CDMA service accelerated. In October 2002, China Unicom reported that it had more than 4 million CDMA subscribers, and that it was encountering rapid growth and should hit 7 million by year-end. In March 2003, China Unicom announced that it planned to add over 11 million subscribers to its CDMA network by the end of 2003. In May 2003, Qualcomm announced that China Unicom had over 10 million CDMA subscribers in China. At the same time, however, subscriptions to its GSM networks were also growing. At the end of 2002, China Unicom had 52 million subscribers in China, while China Mobile had 123 million. Both companies were growing rapidly, but China Unicom was catching up to its larger rival, a fact that some now started to attribute to the rollout of its CDMA network.

Meanwhile, Qualcomm continued to show its commitment to China. In 2002, the company opened a 43,000-square-foot research center in China to focus on the development of 3G CDMA technology and applications for the Chinese market, and in June 2003 the company announced it would invest $100 million in Chinese equipment companies to help them develop CDMA equipment. Jacobs also predicted that, looking forward to 3G rollout in China, China Unicom would move its networks to CDMA2000, while China Mobile would adopt WCDMA technology. Either way, Qualcomm would benefit.

Case Discussion Questions

1. If CDMA is the better technology, as Qualcomm claims, why does GSM have a larger share of wireless subscribers worldwide? To what extent do political decisions explain the global leadership of GSM? To what extent do economic factors? Are the economic and political factors independent of each other?

2. What does Qualcomm's experience in China tell you about the difficulties of doing business in this nation? Do you think China is unique in this regard, or can one expect similar problems in other nations?

3. How important is China to Qualcomm's future? Given this, do you think it was right for Qualcomm to accept a lower royalty rate in China than elsewhere?

4. Do you think Qualcomm could have done anything different to accelerate the adoption of CDMA technology in China? How politically savvy has the company been? What lessons can be derived from Qualcomm's experience about the importance of business–government relations in foreign nations?

5. What should Qualcomm do strategically and politically to make sure that CDMA technology, and CDMA2000 in particular, diffuses rapidly in China?

Sources

1. Biers, D., and K. Wilhem. "A Cautious Courtship." *Far Eastern Economic Review*, December 7, 2000, pp. 50–51.

2. Einhorn, B. "Will China Ever Be Qualcomm's Dream Come True?" *Business Week*, June 24, 2002, p. 138.

3. EMC Market data at http://www.emc-database.com/.

4. "Face Value: Qualcomm's Dr Strangelove," *The Economist*, June 17, 2000, p. 67.

5. Forney, M. "Walled Out—For Qualcomm, China Has Beckoned Twice and Then Hung Up." *Wall Street Journal*, July 13, 2000, p. A1.

6. Kripalani, M., and B. Einhorn. "Go East Young Chipmaker." *Business Week*, December 30, 2002, p. 46.

7. Pottinger, M. "China Signs Contracts for CDMA Equipment." *Wall Street Journal*, May 16, 2001, p. A14.

8. Qualcomm 10K statements for 2002.

9. Qualcomm press releases at http://www.qualcomm.com/press/.

Royal Dutch/Shell: Human Rights in Nigeria

Introduction

In 1995, a Nigerian military tribunal, in what most observers decried as a sham trial, ordered the execution of noted author and playwright Ken Saro-Wiwa and eight other members of the Movement for the Survival of the Ogoni People. The Ogoni are a 500,000-member ethnic group of farmers and fishermen that live in Nigeria's coastal plain. For several years, the Ogoni had been waging a vigorous political campaign against Nigeria's military rulers and the giant oil company Royal Dutch/Shell. They had been seeking greater self-determination, rights to the revenue stemming from oil exploration on traditional Ogoni lands, and compensation for the environmental degradation to their land caused by frequent oil spills from fractured pipelines. Shell had been pumping oil from Ogoni lands since the late 1950s. In 1994, four Ogoni chiefs who advocated cooperation rather than confrontation with Nigeria's military government were lynched by a mob of Ogoni youth. Though he was not present, Saro-Wiwa, a leader of the protest movement, was arrested and subsequently sentenced to death along with eight other Ogoni activists.

Despite intensive international pressure that included appeals to Shell to use its influence in the country to gain clemency for the convicted, the executions went ahead as scheduled on November 10, 1995. After the executions, Shell was criticized in the Western media for its apparent unwillingness to pressure Nigeria's totalitarian regime. The incident started some soul-searching at Shell about the social and environmental responsibility of a multinational corporation in societies such as Nigeria that fall short of Western standards for the protection of human rights and the environment.

Background

In 1961, the African nation of Nigeria won independence from Britain. At that time, many believed that Nigeria had the potential to become one of the engines of economic growth in Africa. The country was blessed with abundant natural resources, particularly oil and gas; was a net exporter of foodstuffs; and had a large population that by African standards was well educated (today Nigeria has the largest population in Africa, with over 110 million people). By the mid-1990s, much of that potential was still to be realized. Thirty-five years after winning independence, Nigeria was still heavily dependent on the oil sector. Oil production accounted for 30 percent of GDP, 95 percent of foreign exchange earnings, and about 80 percent of the government's budget revenues. The largely subsistence agricultural sector had failed to keep up with rapid population growth, and Nigeria, once a large net exporter of food, now had to import food. GDP per capita was a paltry $230, one-quarter of what it was in 1981, and the country was creaking under $40 billion of external debt. Nigeria had been unable to garner financial assistance from institutions such as the International Monetary Fund because of the government's unwillingness to account for how it used the revenues from oil taxes.

Political problems partly explained Nigeria's economic malaise. The country has suffered from internal strife among some of the more than 250 ethnic groups that constitute the nation. In the 1960s, the country was racked by a particularly nasty civil war. In December 1983, the civilian government of the country was replaced in a coup by a military regime that proceeded to rule by decree. In 1993, democratic elections were held in Nigeria, but the military government nullified the results, declaring there had been widespread ballot fraud.

Royal Dutch/Shell is the main foreign oil producer operating in Nigeria. The company was formed at the start of the 20th century when Holland's Royal Dutch Company, which had substantial oil operations in Indonesia, merged with Britain's Shell Transport and Trading to create one of the world's first multinational oil companies. Shell is now the world's largest oil company with annual revenues that exceed $130 billion. The company has been operating in Nigeria since 1937, and by the mid-1990s was pumping about half of Nigeria's oil. Nigerian oil accounts for about 11 to 12 percent of the company's global output and generates net income for Shell of around $200 million per year.

Problems in the Ogoni Region

In 1958, Royal Dutch/Shell struck oil on Ogoni lands. By some estimates, the company has extracted some $30 billion worth of oil from the region since then. Despite this, the Ogoni remain desperately poor. Most live in palm-roofed mud huts and practice subsistence agriculture. Of Shell's 5,000 employees in Nigeria, in 1995 only 85 were Ogoni. Because they are a powerless minority among Nigeria's 110 million people, the Ogoni are often overlooked when it comes to the allocation of jobs either in government or the private sector.

Starting in 1982, the Nigerian government supposedly directed 1.5 percent of the oil revenue it received back to the communities where the oil was produced. In 1992, the percentage was increased to 3 percent. The Ogoni, however, claim they have seen virtually none of this money. Most appears to have been spent in the tribal lands of the ruling majority or has vanished in corrupt deals. Although there were 96 oil wells, two refineries, a petrochemical complex, and a fertilizer plant in the Ogoni region in 1994, the lone hospital was an unfinished concrete shell and the government schools, unable to pay teachers, were rarely open.

In addition to the lack of returns from oil production in their region, the Ogoni claim that their lands have suffered from environmental degradation, much of which could be laid at the feet of Shell. Ogoni activists claim that Shell's poor environmental safeguards have resulted in numerous oil spills and widespread contamination of the soil and groundwater. A Shell spokesman, interviewed in 1994, seemed to acknowledge there might be some basis to these complaints. He stated, "Some of the facilities installed during the last 30 years, whilst acceptable at the time, aren't as we would build them today. Given the age of some of these lines (oil pipelines), regrettably oil spills have occurred from time to time."[1] However, the same spokesman also blamed many of the more recent leaks in the Ogoni region on deliberate sabotage. The sabotage, he stated, had one of two motives—to back up claims for compensation and to support claims of environmental degradation.

On hearing of these claims, Ken Saro-Wiwa called them preposterous. Saro-Wiwa argued that although uneducated youths, frustrated and angry, may have damaged some Shell installations in one or two incidents, "the people would never deliberately spill oil on their land because they know the so-called compensation is paltry and the land is never restored."[2] To support his position, Saro-Wiwa pointed to a spill from the 1960s near a settlement called Ebubu that still had not been cleaned up. In response, Shell stated that the spill occurred during the civil war in the 1960s, and cleanup work was completed in 1990. Subsequently, sunken oil reappeared at the surface, but Shell claims it was unable to do anything about this because of threats made against its employees in the region. In January 1993, out of concern for their safety, Shell barred its employees from entering the region.

In April 1993, the Ogoni organized their first protests against Shell and the government. Ogoni farmers stood in front of earthmoving equipment that was laying a pipeline for Shell through croplands. Although Shell stated that the land had been acquired by legal means and that full compensation had been paid to the farmers and the local community, some of the locals remained unhappy about what they viewed as continuing exploitation of their land. Seeing a threat to the continuity of its oil operations, Shell informed the Nigerian government about the protest. Units from the Nigerian military soon arrived, and shots were fired into the crowd of protesters, killing one Ogoni man and wounding several others.

Subsequently, in a series of murky incidents, Nigerian soldiers stormed Ogoni villages, saying they were quelling unrest between neighboring Ogoni tribes. The Ogoni claimed the raids were punishment for obstructing Shell. They stated that the military had orders to use minor land disputes, which had long been settled with little violence, as an excuse to lay entire villages to waste. A feared unit of the mobile police with the nickname "Kill and Go" conducted some of the raids. Although details are sketchy, it has been reported that hundreds of people lost their lives in the violence. The cycle of violence ultimately culminated in the killing of the Ogoni chiefs who argued for compromise with the Nigerian government. This provided the government with the justification to arrest Ken Saro-Wiwa and eight associates in the Movement for the Survival of the Ogoni People.

Nigeria and Shell under Pressure

Saro-Wiwa's arrest achieved the goal that the protests and bloodshed had not; it focused international attention on the plight of the Ogoni people, the heavy-handed policies of the Nigerian government, and Shell's activities in Nigeria. Several human rights organizations immediately pressured Shell to use its influence to gain the release of Saro-Wiwa. They also urged Shell to put on hold plans to start work on a $3.5 billion liquefied natural gas project in Nigeria. The project was structured as a joint venture with the Nigerian government. Shell's central role in the project gave it considerable influence over the government, or so human rights activists believed.

Shell stated that it deplored the heavy-handed approach taken by the Nigerian government toward the Ogoni people and regretted the pain and loss suffered by Ogoni communities. The company also indicated it was using "discreet diplomacy" to try to influence the Nigerian government. Nigeria's military leadership, however, was in no mood to listen to discreet diplomacy from Shell or anyone else. After a trial by a military tribunal that was derided as nothing more than a kangaroo court, Saro-Wiwa and his associates were sentenced to death by hanging. The sentence was carried out shortly after sunrise November 10, 1995.

Aftermath

In the wake of Saro-Wiwa's hanging, a storm of protest erupted around the world. The heads of state of the 52-nation British Commonwealth, meeting in New Zealand at the time of Saro-Wiwa's execution, suspended Nigeria and stated they would expel the country if it did not return to democratic rule within two years. U.S. President

Bill Clinton recalled the U.S. ambassador to Nigeria and banned the sale of military equipment, on top of aid cuts made in protest at Saro-Wiwa's arrest. British Prime Minister John Major banned arms sales to Nigeria and called for the widest possible embargo. Ambassadors from the 15-nation European Union were recalled, and the EU suspended all aid to Nigeria.

But no country halted purchases of Nigerian oil or sales of oil service equipment to Nigeria. The United States, which imports 40 percent of Nigeria's daily output of 2 million barrels, was silent on the question of an oil embargo. Similarly, no Western country—many of which had national companies working in the Nigerian oil industry—indicated they would impose an embargo on sales to, or purchase from, the Nigerian oil industry. Alone among major public figures, South African President Nelson Mandela called for a ban on Shell. The call was echoed by several environmental groups, including Greenpeace and Friends of the Earth, both of which urged their supporters to boycott Shell products. However, South Africa never enacted a formal ban, and the boycott calls met with only limited success.

For its part, Shell indicated it would go ahead with its plans for a liquefied natural gas operation in Nigeria in partnership with the Nigerian government. In a public notice published in British newspapers, Shell stated, "It has been suggested that Shell should pull out of Nigeria's liquefied natural gas project. But if we do so now, the project will collapse, maybe forever. So let's be clear who gets hurt if the project gets cancelled. A cancellation would certainly hurt the thousands of Nigerians who will be working on the project, and the tens of thousands benefiting in the local economy."[3]

In November 1996, the Center for Constitutional Rights filed a federal lawsuit in the U.S. District Court in Manhattan on behalf of relatives of Saro-Wiwa who were now residing in the United States. The lawsuit accused Royal Dutch/Shell of being part of a conspiracy that led to Saro-Wiwa's hanging. Shell denied the allegations and stated they would be refuted in court.

In May 1997, at the annual general meeting of Shell Transport and Trading in London, a group of 18 institutional investors tabled a resolution that would have required Shell to establish an independent external body to monitor its environmental and human rights policies. John Jennings, the outgoing chairman of the company, told reporters after the meeting that proxy votes from shareholders were running 10 to 1 against the resolution.

One reason for the defeat of the shareholder resolution was that the company had already indicated it was taking steps to reform its culture and improve its own monitoring of environmental and human rights policies. Before the shareholder meeting, the company issued its own report on its policies in Nigeria, in which the company admitted that it needed to improve its monitoring of environmental and human rights policies. Under the leadership of its new head, Mark Moody-Stuart, Shell subsequently stated that it expected its companies to express support for fundamental human rights in line with the legitimate role of business and to give proper regard to health, safety, and the environment consistent with their commitment to sustainable development. The company also embraced the UN Universal Declaration of Human Rights, pledged to set up socially responsible management systems, and promised to develop training procedures to help management deal with human rights dilemmas.

Commenting on these steps, a spokesman for Human Rights Watch stated, "I'm prepared to give them some credit that they realized they had to look at what their own operations were and how to respond. They acknowledged that big companies have social responsibility, and that's a pretty big step for the multinational corporations."[4]

Due to ongoing threats, Shell continued to keep its employees out of the Ogoni region and as of 2002 this was still the case. There are oil reserves of approximately 300 million barrels in the region, but Shell is unable to tap them for fear that it will again awaken hostility to the company. The pipelines that Shell left behind have been attacked by thieves, who cut the lines with hacksaws or blowtorches. A 25-foot section of lines goes for 10,000 Nigerian naira, or about $87, more than the monthly wage of many public-sector workers. As the lines are cut, leftover oil pours onto the ground contributing to environmental degradation. Shell has stated repeatedly that it would like to send its workers back into the region to clean up the environmental mess, but it cannot do so for fears about their safety.

Leaders of the Ogoni people continue to regard Shell with hostility. In 2001, Ledum Mittee, Ken Saro-Wiwa's successor as leader of the Movement for the Survival of the Ogoni People, stated: "I am overwhelmed by the suggestion that Shell has changed and wants to be loved. There is absolutely nothing in the company's actions in Nigeria to justify this. People in Ogoni and most other places here in the delta think of Shell as a company that is insensitive to people and their environment. They see it as an ally to oppression. The change in rhetoric from Shell over the years has not been matched by a change in actions in Nigeria. Shell is excellent at public relations but it is terrible at turning words into reality." Privately, some Shell executives suggest that it serves the interests of the Movement for the Survival of the Ogoni People to keep the spotlight on Shell and note that the environmental degradation in the Ogoni region is a "convenient showpiece for the world's press to keep the suffering of the Ogoni people alive in the media."[5]

Case Discussion Questions

1. Does Shell bear some responsibility for the problems in the Ogoni region of Nigeria?

2. What steps might Shell have taken to nip some of the protests against it in the bud, or even preempt them?

3. Could the company have done more to gain clemency for Ken Saro-Wiwa? What? Should it have done more?

4. Was the response of Western governments to the execution of Ken Saro-Wiwa about right, too excessive, or too mild? What should have been the appropriate response?

5. In the wake of Saro-Wiwa's execution, was Shell correct to push ahead with the liquefied natural gas project in Nigeria?

6. Do you think it is possible for a company such as Shell to reform itself from within, or would it have been better for Shell to establish an external body to monitor its human rights and environmental policies?

7. A decade after Shell pulled its people out of the Ogoni region, they have yet to return despite the region's rich oil reserves. Some have suggested that it serves the political interests of the Movement for the Survival of the Ogoni People to have Shell cast in the villain's role. Do you think this is true? Is there anything Shell can do about this? Who suffers most from Shell's continued absence in the Ogoni region?

Notes

1. G. Brooks, "Slick Alliance," *Wall Street Journal*, May 6, 1994, p. A1.

2. Ibid.

3. P. Beckett, "Shell Boldly Defends Its Role in Nigeria," *Wall Street Journal*, November 27, 1995, p. A9.

4. J. Vidal, "What Happens When Disaster Strikes?" *The Guardian*, July 9, 2001, pp. 2, 10.

5. S. Moore, "For Shell, Nigerian Debacle Isn't End of the Line," *Wall Street Journal*, January 10, 2002, p. A10.

Sources

1. Beckett, P. "Shell Boldly Defends Its Role in Nigeria." *Wall Street Journal*, November 27, 1995, p. A9.

2. Brooks, G. "Slick Alliance." *Wall Street Journal*, May 6, 1994, p. A1.

3. Corzine, R. "Shell Discovers Time and Tide Wait for No Man." *Financial Times*, March 10, 1998, p. 17.

4. Corzine, R., and Boulton. "Shell Defends Its Ethics on Eve of General Meeting." *Financial Times*, May 14, 1997, p. 29.

5. Hamilton, H. "Shell's New Worldview." *Washington Post*, August 2, 1998, p. H1.

6. Hoagland, J. "Shell's Game in Nigeria." *Washington Post*, November 5, 1995, p. C7.

7. Hudson, R., and M. Rose. "Shell Is Pressured to Scrap Its Plans for a New Plant in Nigeria amid Protests." *Wall Street Journal*, November 14, 1995, p. A11.

8. Kamm, T. "Executions Raise Sanction Threat." *Wall Street Journal*, November 13, 1995, p. A10.

9. "Multinationals and Their Morals." *The Economist*, December 2, 1995, p. 18.

10. Moore, S. "For Shell, Nigerian Debacle Isn't End of the Line." *Wall Street Journal*, January 10, 2002, p. A10.

11. Vidal, J. "What Happens When Disaster Strikes?" *The Guardian*, July 9, 2001, pp. 2, 10.

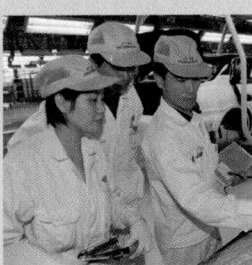

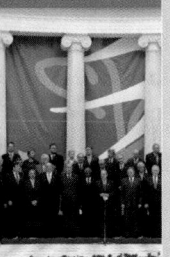

Part 3

The Global Trade and Investment Environment

Chapter 4
International Trade Theory

Chapter 5
The Political Economy of International Trade

Chapter 6
Foreign Direct Investment

Chapter 7
The Political Economy of Foreign Direct Investment

Chapter 8
Regional Economic Integration

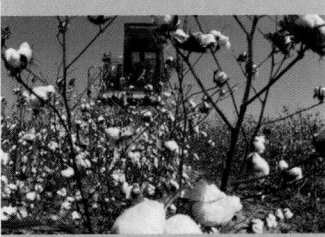

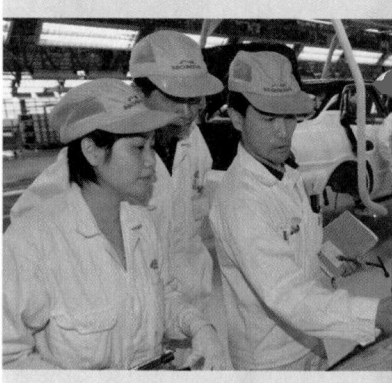

Chapter 4

International Trade Theory

Introduction
An Overview of Trade Theory
  The Benefits of Trade
  The Pattern of International Trade
  Trade Theory and Government Policy
Mercantilism
Absolute Advantage
Comparative Advantage
  The Gains from Trade
  Qualifications and Assumptions
  Simple Extensions of the Ricardian Model
Heckscher-Ohlin Theory
  The Leontief Paradox
The Product Life-Cycle Theory
  Evaluating the Product Life-Cycle Theory
New Trade Theory
  The Aerospace Example
  Implications
National Competitive Advantage:
Porter's Diamond
  Factor Endowments
  Demand Conditions
  Related and Supporting Industries
  Firm Strategy, Structure, and Rivalry
  Evaluating Porter's Theory
Focus on Managerial Implications
  Location
  First-Mover Advantages
  Government Policy
Chapter Summary
Critical Discussion Questions
Closing Case: The Rise of the Indian Software Industry

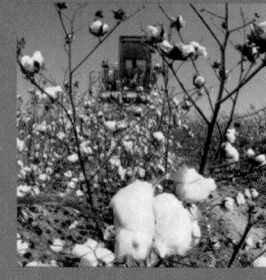

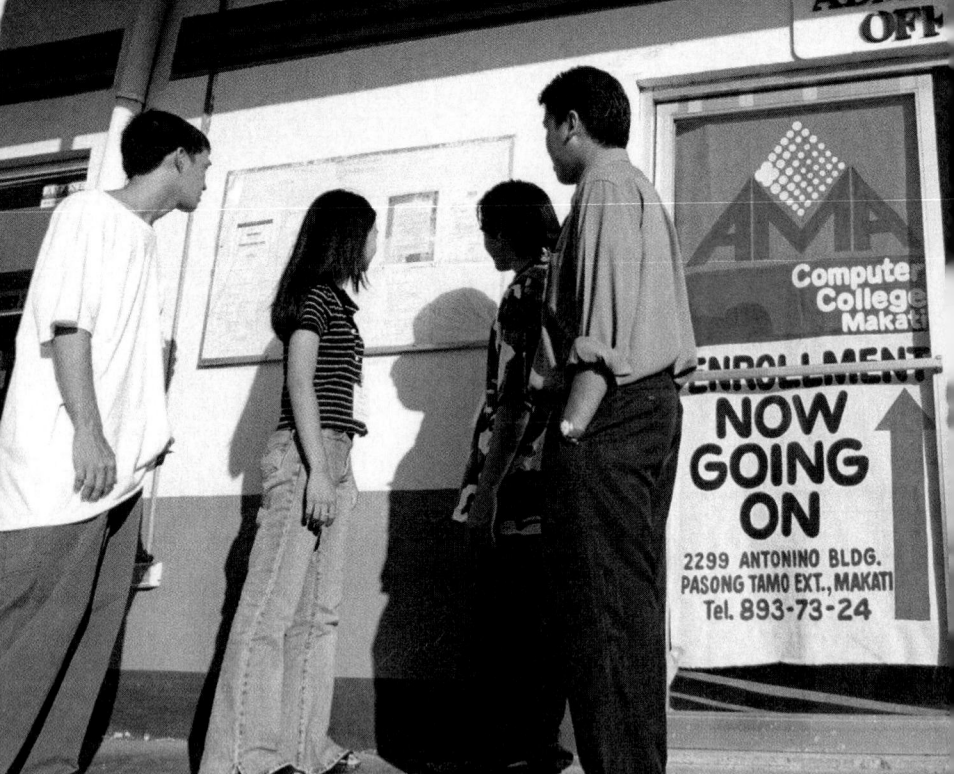

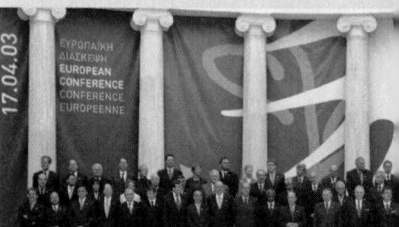

The Hollowing Out of the U.S. Knowledge-Based Economy

Economists have long argued that free trade produces gains for all countries that participate in a free trading system, but as the next wave of globalization sweeps through the U.S. economy, many people are wondering if this is true, particularly those who stand to lose their jobs as a result of this wave of globalization. In the popular imagination for much of the past quarter century, free trade was associated with the movement of low-skill, blue-collar manufacturing jobs out of rich countries such as the United States and toward low-wage countries— textiles to Costa Rica, athletic shoes to the Philippines, steel to Brazil, electronic products to Malaysia, and so on. While many observers bemoaned the "hollowing out" of U.S. manufacturing, economists stated that high-skilled and high-wage, white-collar jobs associated with the knowledge-based economy would stay in the United States. Computers might be assembled in Malaysia, so the argument went, but they would continue to be designed in Silicon Valley by high-skilled U.S. engineers.

Recent developments have some people questioning this assumption. As the global economy slowed after 2000 and corporate profits slumped, many American companies responded by moving knowledge-based jobs to developing nations where they could be performed for a fraction of the cost. During the long economic boom of the 1990s, Bank of America had to compete with other organizations for the scarce talents of information technology specialists, driving annual salaries to more than $100,000. But with business under pressure, between 2002 and early 2003 the bank cut nearly 5,000 jobs from its 25,000-strong, U.S.-based information technology workforce. Some of these jobs are being transferred to India, where work that costs $100 an hour in the United States can be done for $20 an hour.

One beneficiary of Bank of America's downsizing is Infosys Technologies Ltd., a Bangalore, India, information technology firm where 250 engineers now develop information technology applications for the bank. Other Infosys employees are busy processing home loan applications for Greenpoint Mortgage of Novato, California. Nearby in the offices of another Indian firm, Wipro Ltd., five radiologists interpret 30 CT scans a day for Massachusetts General Hospital that are sent over the Internet. At yet another Bangalore business, engineers earn $10,000 a year designing leading-edge semiconductor chips for Texas Instruments. Nor is India the only beneficiary of these changes. Accenture, a large U.S. management consulting and information technology firm, recently moved 5,000 jobs in software development and accounting to the Philippines. Also in the Philippines, Procter & Gamble employs 650 professionals who prepare the company's global tax returns. The work used to

be done in the United States, but now it is done in Manila, with just final submission to local tax authorities in the United States and other countries handled locally.

Some architectural work also is being outsourced to lower-cost locations. Flour Corp., a California-based construction company, employs some 1,200 engineers and draftsmen in the Philippines, Poland, and India to turn layouts of industrial facilities into detailed specifications. For a Saudi Arabian chemical plant Flour is designing, 200 young engineers based in the Philippines earning less than $3,000 a year collaborate in real time over the Internet with elite U.S. and British engineers who make up to $90,000 a year. Why does Flour do this? According to the company, the answer is simple. Doing so reduces the prices of a project by 15 percent, giving the company a cost-based competitive advantage in the global market for construction design.

The companies that outsource such skilled jobs clearly benefit from lower costs. Developing nations such as India and the Philippines with a good supply of well-educated, skilled, and (by global standards) low-cost labor also benefit. However, some observers wonder whether the United States will suffer from the loss of highly skilled and high paying jobs?

Economists schooled in international trade theory think not. They believe that although some individuals suffer from the transfer of jobs overseas—unemployed former Bank of America workers, for example—the nation as a whole benefits. They support this contention with three arguments. First, they point out that while some of the more routine skilled jobs are going overseas (lower-level architectural design work, for example), most managerial, marketing, and cutting-edge research and development jobs are staying in the country, precisely because America has a comparative advantage in these areas. Second, economists argue that the lower price of services that results from such outsourcing means that the average American consumer can afford to consume more of these services, or can use any savings to consume more of other goods and services, thereby boosting their economic well-being. Third, economists believe that any economic growth occurring in India, the Philippines, and the like as a result of this trend will ultimately benefit the United States, since consumers in those countries will be able to purchase more American goods and services. If the economists' theories are correct, concerns over the recent trend to outsource knowledge-based work may be exaggerated. If the theories are wrong, the living standards of Americans could decline significantly over the next few decades.

Source: (1) P. Engardio, A. Bernstein, and M. Kripalani, "Is Your Job Next?" Business Week, February 3, 2003, pp. 50–60. (2) Anonymous, "America's Pain, India's Gain," The Economist, January 11, 2003, p. 57.

Introduction

The opening case goes to the heart of a debate that has been played out many times over the past half century. Some argue that free trade leads to a migration of jobs overseas and will ultimately create higher unemployment and lower living standards. To these people, the recent trend for companies to outsource high paying, "knowledge-based" jobs to low-wage locations, such as India, is a very disturbing development. But those schooled in economic theory, and particularly in international trade theory, argue that free trade ultimately benefits *all* countries that participate in a free trade system. Those who take this position concede that some individuals lose as a result of a shift to free trade, but in the aggregate they argue that the gains outweigh the losses.

This argument is not just an abstract academic one. It has shaped the economic policy of many nations for the past 50 years and is the driver behind the formation of the World Trade Organization and regional trade blocs such as the European Union and the North American Free Trade Agreement (NAFTA). The 1990s, in particular, saw a global move toward greater free trade. It is crucially important to understand, therefore, what these theories are and why they have been so successful in shaping the economic policy of so many nations and the competitive environment that international businesses must compete in.

This chapter has two goals that go to the heart of this debate. The first is to review a number of theories that explain why it is beneficial for a country to engage in international trade. The second goal is to explain the pattern of international trade that we observe in the world economy. With regard to the pattern of trade, we will be primarily concerned with explaining the pattern of exports and imports of goods and services between countries. We will not be concerned with the pattern of foreign direct investment between countries; that is discussed in Chapter 7.

An Overview of Trade Theory

We open this chapter with a discussion of mercantilism. Propagated in the 16th and 17th centuries, mercantilism advocated that countries should simultaneously encourage exports and discourage imports. Although mercantilism is an old and largely discredited doctrine, its echoes remain in modern political debate and in the trade policies of many countries. Next we will look at Adam Smith's theory of absolute advantage. Proposed in 1776, Smith's theory was the first to explain why unrestricted free trade is beneficial to a country. **Free trade** refers to a situation where a government does not attempt to influence through quotas or duties what its citizens can buy from another country, or what they can produce and sell to another country. Smith argued that the invisible hand of the market mechanism, rather than government policy, should determine what a country imports and what it exports. His arguments imply that such a laissez-faire stance toward trade was in the best interests of a country. Building on Smith's work are two additional theories that we shall review. One is the theory of comparative advantage, advanced by the 19th-century English economist David Ricardo. This theory is the intellectual basis of the modern argument for unrestricted free trade. In the 20th century, Ricardo's work was refined by two Swedish economists, Eli Heckscher and Bertil Ohlin, whose theory is known as the Heckscher-Ohlin theory.

The Benefits of Trade

The great strength of the theories of Smith, Ricardo, and Heckscher-Ohlin is that they identify with precision the specific benefits of international trade. Common sense suggests that some international trade is beneficial. For example, nobody would suggest that Iceland should grow its own oranges. Iceland can benefit from trade by exchanging some of the products that it can produce at a low cost (fish) for some products that it cannot produce at all (oranges). Thus, by engaging in international trade, Icelanders are able to add oranges to their diet of fish.

The theories of Smith, Ricardo, and Heckscher-Ohlin go beyond this common-sense notion, however, to show why it is beneficial for a country to engage in international trade *even for products it is able to produce for itself*. This is a difficult concept for people to grasp. For example, many people in the United States believe that American consumers should buy products produced in the United States by American companies whenever possible to help save American jobs from foreign competition. Such thinking apparently underlay a 2002 decision by President Bush to protect American steel producers from competition from lower-cost foreign producers.

The same kind of nationalistic sentiments can be observed in many other countries. However, the theories of Smith, Ricardo, and Heckscher-Ohlin tell us that a country's economy may gain if its citizens buy certain products from other nations that could be produced at home. The gains arise because international trade allows a country to specialize in the manufacture and export of products that can be produced most efficiently in that country, while importing products that can be produced more efficiently in other countries. So it may make sense for the United States to specialize in the production and export of commercial jet aircraft, since the efficient production of commercial jet aircraft requires resources that are abundant in the United States, such as a highly skilled labor force and cutting-edge technological know-how. On the other hand, it may make sense for the United States to import textiles from Mexico since the efficient production of textiles requires a relatively cheap labor force—and cheap labor is not abundant in the United States.

Of course, this economic argument is often difficult for segments of a country's population to accept. With their future threatened by imports, U.S. textile companies and their employees have tried hard to persuade the government to limit the importation of textiles by demanding quotas and tariffs. Similarly, as the Country Focus illustrates, with their future threatened by Chinese imports, producers of crawfish in Louisiana lobbied the U.S. government for protection in the form of tariffs that raised the price of imported Chinese crawfish. Although such import controls may benefit particular groups, such as textile businesses and their employees or unprofitable steel mills and their employees, the theories of Smith, Ricardo, and Heckscher-Ohlin suggest that the economy as a whole is hurt by such action. Limits on imports are often in the interests of domestic producers, but not domestic consumers (as the feature on the crawfish industry makes clear).

The Pattern of International Trade

The theories of Smith, Ricardo, and Heckscher-Ohlin also help to explain the pattern of international trade that we observe in the world economy. Some aspects of the pattern are easy to understand. Climate and natural-resource endowments explain why Ghana exports cocoa, Brazil exports coffee, Saudi Arabia exports oil, and China exports crawfish. But much of the observed pattern of international trade is more difficult to explain. For example, why does Japan export automobiles, consumer electronics, and machine tools? Why does Switzerland export chemicals, watches, and jewelry? David Ricardo's theory of comparative advantage offers an explanation in terms of international differences in labor productivity. The more sophisticated Heckscher-Ohlin theory emphasizes the interplay between the proportions in which the factors of production (such as land, labor, and capital) are available in different countries and the proportions in which they are needed for producing particular goods. This explanation rests on the assumption that countries have varying endowments of the various factors of production. Tests of this theory, however, suggest that it is a less powerful explanation of real-world trade patterns than once thought.

One early response to the failure of the Heckscher-Ohlin theory to explain the observed pattern of international trade was the *product life-cycle theory*. Proposed by

Crawfish Wars

Once upon a time, Louisiana was owned by the French. Napoleon sold the territory to the United States when Thomas Jefferson was president, but many of the French stayed on. Over time, their descendants developed the distinctive Cajun culture that today is celebrated in the United States for its unique cuisine and music. At the heart of that cuisine can be found the venerable crawfish, as Louisianians call the crayfish. The crawfish is a fresh-water crustacean native to the bayous of Louisiana. A central ingredient of crawfish pie, bisque, etouffee, and gumbo, the crawfish is to Cajun Louisiana what wine is to France: a culinary symbol of its culture. It is also a major industry that generates $300 million per year in revenues for Louisiana crawfish farmers—or at least it did until the Chinese appeared.

In the early 1990s, development of the Chinese industry was encouraged by Louisiana importers to meet the growing demand for crawfish. In China, the crawfish industry proved to be attractive for entrepreneurial farmers. Chinese crawfish first started to appear on the Louisiana scene in 1991. Although old-time Cajuns were quick to claim that the Chinese crawfish had a markedly inferior taste, consumers didn't seem to notice the difference. More importantly perhaps, they liked the price, which ran between $2 and $3 per pound depending on the season, compared to $5 to $8 per pound for native Louisiana crawfish. With the significant price advantage, sales of Chinese imports skyrocketed from 353,000 pounds in 1992 to 5.5 million pounds in 1996. By 1996, Louisiana state officials estimated that 3,000 jobs had been lost in the local industry, mostly minimum-wage crawfish peelers, due to market share gains made by the Chinese.

This was too much for the Louisiana industry to stomach. In 1996, Louisiana's Crawfish Promotion and Research Board filed a petition with the International Trade Commission, an arm of the U.S. government, requesting an antidumping action. The petition claimed that Chinese crawfish producers were dumping their product, selling at below cost to drive Louisiana producers out of business. The industry requested that a 200 percent to 300 percent import tax be placed on Chinese crawfish. The State of Louisiana appropriated $350,000 from state funds to support the action.

Lawyers representing the Chinese crawfish industry claimed that lower production costs in China were the reason for the low prices—not dumping. One Louisiana-based importer of Chinese crawfish pointed out that 27 processing plants in China supplied his company. Workers at these plants were given housing and other amenities and paid 15 cents per hour, or $9 for a 60-hour week. The lawyers also said Chinese crawfish have been good for American consumers, who have saved money and benefited from a steadier supply, and good for Louisiana cuisine, because it is has become less expensive to cook. The lawyers pointed out that the action was not in the interests of American consumers, since it was nothing more than an attempt by Louisiana producers to reestablish their lucrative monopoly on the production of crawfish, a monopoly that would enable them to extract higher prices from consumers.

However, the International Trade Commission was deaf to such arguments. The commission deemed that China was a "nonmarket economy" since it was not yet a member of the World Trade Organization (something that changed in 2001). The commission then used prices in a "market economy," Spain, to establish a benchmark for a "fair market value" for crawfish. Since Spanish crawfish sell for approximately twice the price of Chinese crawfish and about the same price as Louisiana crawfish, the commission concluded that the Chinese were dumping (selling below costs of production). In August 1997, the commission levied a 110 to 123 percent duty on imports of Chinese crawfish, effectively negating the price advantage enjoyed by Chinese producers. In the interests of protecting American jobs, the commission sided with Louisiana producers and against American consumers, who would now have to pay higher prices for crawfish. Under commission regulations, the ruling would stay in place for five years, after which the legitimacy of the import duty must be reevaluated.

Sources: Donna St. George, "Crawfish Wars: Cajun Country Vs China," *New York Times,* May 7, 1997, pp. B1, B10; P. Passell, "Protecting America's Shores from Those Chinese Crawfish," *New York Times,* August 28, 1997, p. D2; N. Dunne, "Shellfish Imports Stick in the Cajun Craw," *Financial Times,* August 21, 1997, p. 16; and B. Thevenot, "Getting Pinched," *The Times Picayune,* March 11, 2000, p. C1.

Country Focus

Raymond Vernon, this theory suggests that early in their life cycle, most new products are produced in and exported from the country in which they were developed. As a new product becomes widely accepted internationally, however, production starts in other countries. As a result, the theory suggests, the product may ultimately be exported back to the country of its original innovation.

In a similar vein, during the 1980s economists such as Paul Krugman of the Massachusetts Institute of Technology developed what has come to be known as the *new trade theory*. New trade theory stresses that in some cases countries specialize in the production and export of particular products not because of underlying differences in factor endowments, but because in certain industries the world market can support only a limited number of firms. (This is argued to be the case for the commercial aircraft industry.) In such industries, firms that enter the market first are able to build a competitive advantage that is subsequently difficult to challenge. Thus, the observed pattern of trade between nations may be due in part to the ability of firms within a given nation to capture first-mover advantages. The United States dominates in the export of commercial jet aircraft because American firms such as Boeing were first movers in the world market. Boeing built a competitive advantage that has subsequently been difficult for firms from countries with equally favorable factor endowments to challenge.

In a work related to the new trade theory, Michael Porter of the Harvard Business School developed a theory, referred to as the theory of national competitive advantage, that attempts to explain why particular nations achieve international success in particular industries. In addition to factor endowments, Porter points out the importance of country factors such as domestic demand and domestic rivalry in explaining a nation's dominance in the production and export of particular products.

Trade Theory and Government Policy

Although all these theories agree that international trade is beneficial to a country, they lack agreement in their recommendations for government policy. Mercantilism makes a crude case for government involvement in promoting exports and limiting imports. The theories of Smith, Ricardo, and Heckscher-Ohlin form part of the case for unrestricted free trade. The argument for unrestricted free trade is that both import controls and export incentives (such as subsidies) are self-defeating and result in wasted resources. Both the new trade theory and Porter's theory of national competitive advantage can be interpreted as justifying some limited government intervention to support the development of certain export-oriented industries. We will discuss the pros and cons of this argument, known as strategic trade policy, as well as the pros and cons of the argument for unrestricted free trade, in Chapter 5.

Mercantilism ◼

The first theory of international trade emerged in England in the mid-16th century. Referred to as *mercantilism*, its principle assertion was that gold and silver were the mainstays of national wealth and essential to vigorous commerce. At that time, gold and silver were the currency of trade between countries; a country could earn gold and silver by exporting goods. By the same token, importing goods from other countries would result in an outflow of gold and silver to those countries. The main tenet of **mercantilism** was that it was in a country's best interests to maintain a trade surplus, to export more than it imported. By doing so, a country would accumulate gold and silver and, consequently, increase its national wealth and prestige. As the English mercantilist writer Thomas Mun put it in 1630:

> The ordinary means therefore to increase our wealth and treasure is by foreign trade, wherein we must ever observe this rule: to sell more to strangers yearly than we consume of theirs in value.[1]

Consistent with this belief, the mercantilist doctrine advocated government intervention to achieve a surplus in the balance of trade. The mercantilists saw no virtue in a large volume of trade. Rather, they recommended policies to maximize exports and minimize imports. To achieve this, imports were limited by tariffs and quotas, while exports were subsidized.

The classical economist David Hume pointed out an inherent inconsistency in the mercantilist doctrine in 1752. According to Hume, if England had a balance-of-trade surplus with France (it exported more than it imported) the resulting inflow of gold and silver would swell the domestic money supply and generate inflation in England. In France, however, the outflow of gold and silver would have the opposite effect. France's money supply would contract, and its prices would fall. This change in relative prices between France and England would encourage the French to buy fewer English goods (because they were becoming more expensive) and the English to buy more French goods (because they were becoming cheaper). The result would be a deterioration in the English balance of trade and an improvement in France's trade balance, until the English surplus was eliminated. Hence, according to Hume, in the long run no country could sustain a surplus on the balance of trade and so accumulate gold and silver as the mercantilists had envisaged.

The flaw with mercantilism was that it viewed trade as a zero-sum game. (A **zero-sum game** is one in which a gain by one country results in a loss by another.) It was left to Adam Smith and David Ricardo to show the shortsightedness of this approach and to demonstrate that trade is a **positive-sum game,** or a situation in which all countries can benefit. The mercantilist doctrine is by no means dead.[2] For example, Jarl Hagelstam, a director at the Finnish Ministry of Finance, has observed that in most trade negotiations:

> The approach of individual negotiating countries, both industrialized and developing, has been to press for trade liberalization in areas where their own comparative competitive advantages are the strongest, and to resist liberalization in areas where they are less competitive and fear that imports would replace domestic production.[3]

Hagelstam attributes this strategy by negotiating countries to a neo-mercantilist belief held by the politicians of many nations. This belief equates political power with economic power and economic power with a balance-of-trade surplus. Thus, the trade strategy of many nations is designed to simultaneously boost exports and limit imports.

▮ Absolute Advantage

In his 1776 landmark book *The Wealth of Nations*, Adam Smith attacked the mercantilist assumption that trade is a zero-sum game. Smith argued that countries differ in their ability to produce goods efficiently. In his time, the English, by virtue of their superior manufacturing processes, were the world's most efficient textile manufacturers. Due to the combination of favorable climate, good soils, and accumulated expertise, the French had the world's most efficient wine industry. The English had an *absolute advantage* in the production of textiles, while the French had an *absolute advantage* in the production of wine. Thus, a country has an **absolute advantage** in the production of a product when it is more efficient than any other country in producing it.

According to Smith, countries should specialize in the production of goods for which they have an absolute advantage and then trade these for goods produced by other countries. In Smith's time, this suggested that the English should specialize in the production of textiles while the French should specialize in the production of wine. England could get all the wine it needed by selling its textiles to France and buying wine in exchange. Similarly, France could get all the textiles it needed by selling wine to England and buying textiles in exchange. Smith's basic argument, therefore, is that a coun-

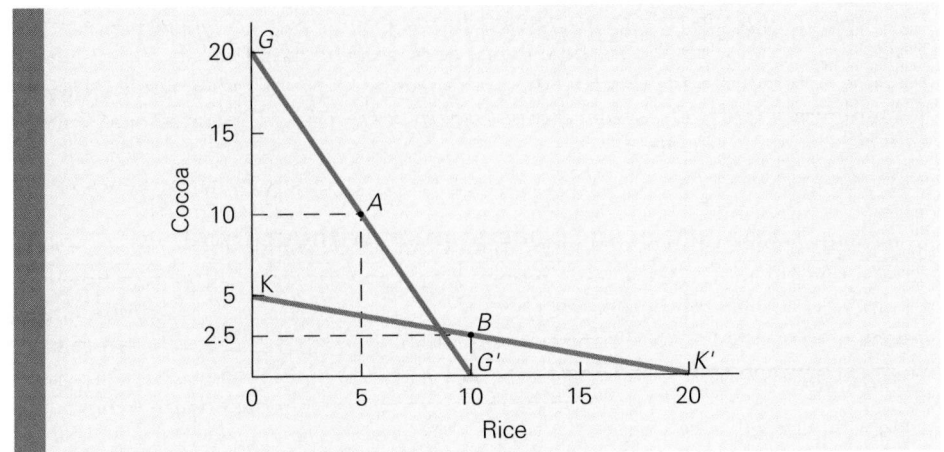

Figure 4.1

The Theory of Absolute Advantage

try should never produce goods at home that it can buy at a lower cost from other countries. Smith demonstrates that, by specializing in the production of goods in which each has an absolute advantage, both countries benefit by engaging in trade.

Consider the effects of trade between two countries, Ghana and South Korea. The production of any good (output) requires resources (inputs) such as land, labor, and capital. Assume that Ghana and South Korea both have the same amount of resources and that these resources can be used to produce either rice or cocoa. Assume further that 200 units of resources are available in each country. Imagine that in Ghana it takes 10 resources to produce one ton of cocoa and 20 resources to produce one ton of rice. Thus, Ghana could produce 20 tons of cocoa and no rice, 10 tons of rice and no cocoa, or some combination of rice and cocoa between these two extremes. The different combinations that Ghana could produce are represented by the line GG' in Figure 4.1. This is referred to as Ghana's production possibility frontier (PPF). Similarly, imagine that in South Korea it takes 40 resources to produce one ton of cocoa and 10 resources to produce one ton of rice. Thus, South Korea could produce 5 tons of cocoa and no rice, 20 tons of rice and no cocoa, or some combination between these two extremes. The different combinations available to South Korea are represented by the line KK' in Figure 4.1, which is South Korea's PPF. Clearly, Ghana has an absolute advantage in the production of cocoa. (More resources are needed to produce a ton of cocoa in South Korea than in Ghana.) By the same token, South Korea has an absolute advantage in the production of rice.

Now consider a situation in which neither country trades with any other. Each country devotes half of its resources to the production of rice and half to the production of cocoa. Each country must also consume what it produces. Ghana would be able to produce 10 tons of cocoa and 5 tons of rice (point A in Figure 4.1), while South Korea would be able to produce 10 tons of rice and 2.5 tons of cocoa. Without trade, the combined production of both countries would be 12.5 tons of cocoa (10 tons in Ghana plus 2.5 tons in South Korea) and 15 tons of rice (5 tons in Ghana and 10 tons in South Korea). If each country were to specialize in producing the good for which it had an absolute advantage and then trade with the other for the good it lacks, Ghana could produce 20 tons of cocoa, and South Korea could produce 20 tons of rice. Thus, by specializing, the production of both goods could be increased. Production of cocoa would increase from 12.5 tons to 20 tons, while production of rice would increase from 15 tons to 20 tons. The increase in production that would result from specialization is therefore 7.5 tons of cocoa and 5 tons of rice. Table 4.1 summarizes these figures.

By engaging in trade and swapping one ton of cocoa for one ton of rice, producers in both countries could consume more of both cocoa and rice. Imagine that Ghana and South Korea swap cocoa and rice on a one-to-one basis; that is, the price of one

Table 4.1

Absolute Advantage
and the Gains from Trade

Resources Required to Produce 1 Ton of Cocoa and Rice		
	Cocoa	**Rice**
Ghana	10	20
South Korea	40	10
Production and Consumption without Trade		
	Cocoa	**Rice**
Ghana	10.0	5.0
South Korea	2.5	10.0
Total production	12.5	15.0
Production with Specialization		
	Cocoa	**Rice**
Ghana	20.0	0.0
South Korea	0.0	20.0
Total production	20.0	20.0
Consumption After Ghana Trades 6 Tons of Cocoa for 6 Tons of South Korean Rice		
	Cocoa	**Rice**
Ghana	14.0	6.0
South Korea	6.0	14.0
Increase in Consumption as a Result of Specialization and Trade		
	Cocoa	**Rice**
Ghana	4.0	1.0
South Korea	3.5	4.0

ton of cocoa is equal to the price of one ton of rice. If Ghana decided to export 6 tons of cocoa to South Korea and import 6 tons of rice in return, its final consumption after trade would be 14 tons of cocoa and 6 tons of rice. This is 4 tons more cocoa than it could have consumed before specialization and trade and 1 ton more rice. Similarly, South Korea's final consumption after trade would be 6 tons of cocoa and 14 tons of rice. This is 3.5 tons more cocoa than it could have consumed before specialization and trade and 4 tons more rice. Thus, as a result of specialization and trade, output of both cocoa and rice would be increased, and consumers in both nations would be able to consume more. Thus, we can see that trade is a positive-sum game; it produces net gains for all involved.

Comparative Advantage

David Ricardo took Adam Smith's theory one step further by exploring what might happen when one country has an absolute advantage in the production of all goods.[4] Smith's theory of absolute advantage suggests that such a country might derive no ben-

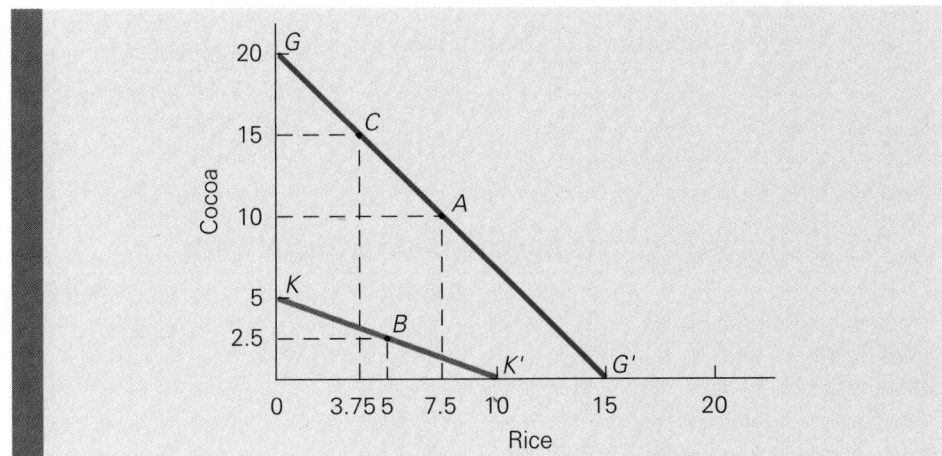

Figure 4.2

The Theory of
Comparative Advantage

efits from international trade. In his 1817 book *Principles of Political Economy*, Ricardo
showed that this was not the case. According to Ricardo's theory of **comparative advantage,** it makes sense for a country to specialize in the production of those goods that
it produces most efficiently and to buy the goods that it produces less efficiently from
other countries, even if this means buying goods from other countries that it could produce more efficiently itself.[5] While this may seem counterintuitive, the logic can be
explained with a simple example.

Assume that Ghana is more efficient in the production of both cocoa and rice; that
is, Ghana has an absolute advantage in the production of both products. In Ghana it
takes 10 resources to produce one ton of cocoa and 13 1/3 resources to produce one ton
of rice. Thus, given its 200 units of resources, Ghana can produce 20 tons of cocoa and
no rice, 15 tons of rice and no cocoa, or any combination in between on its PPF (the
line GG' in Figure 4.2). In South Korea it takes 40 resources to produce one ton of cocoa and 20 resources to produce one ton of rice. Thus, South Korea can produce 5 tons
of cocoa and no rice, 10 tons of rice and no cocoa, or any combination on its PPF (the
line KK' in Figure 4.2). Again assume that without trade, each country uses half of its
resources to produce rice and half to produce cocoa. Thus, without trade, Ghana will
produce 10 tons of cocoa and 7.5 tons of rice (point A in Figure 4.2), while South Korea will produce 2.5 tons of cocoa and 5 tons of rice (point B in Figure 4.2).

In light of Ghana's absolute advantage in the production of both goods, why should
it trade with South Korea? Although Ghana has an absolute advantage in the production of both cocoa and rice, it has a comparative advantage only in the production
of cocoa: Ghana can produce 4 times as much cocoa as South Korea, but only 1.5 times
as much rice. Ghana is *comparatively* more efficient at producing cocoa than it is at producing rice.

Without trade the combined production of cocoa will be 12.5 tons (10 tons in
Ghana and 2.5 in South Korea), and the combined production of rice will also be
12.5 tons (7.5 tons in Ghana and 5 tons in South Korea). Without trade each country must consume what it produces. By engaging in trade, the two countries can increase their combined production of rice and cocoa, and consumers in both nations
can consume more of both goods.

The Gains from Trade

Imagine that Ghana exploits its comparative advantage in the production of cocoa to
increase its output from 10 tons to 15 tons. This uses up 150 units of resources, leaving
the remaining 50 units of resources to use in producing 3.75 tons of rice (point C in Figure 4.2). Meanwhile, South Korea specializes in the production of rice, producing

Table 4.2

Comparative Advantage and the Gains from Trade

Resources Required to Produce 1 Ton of Cocoa and Rice		
	Cocoa	**Rice**
Ghana	10	13.33
South Korea	40	20

Production and Consumption without Trade		
	Cocoa	**Rice**
Ghana	10.0	7.5
South Korea	2.5	5.0
Total production	12.5	12.5

Production with Specialization		
	Cocoa	**Rice**
Ghana	15.0	3.75
South Korea	0.0	10.0
Total production	15.0	13.75

Consumption After Ghana Trades 4 Tons of Cocoa for 4 Tons of South Korean Rice		
	Cocoa	**Rice**
Ghana	11.0	7.75
South Korea	4.0	6.0

Increase in Consumption as a Result of Specialization and Trade		
	Cocoa	**Rice**
Ghana	1.0	0.25
South Korea	1.5	1.0

10 tons. The combined output of both cocoa and rice has now increased. Before specialization, the combined output was 12.5 tons of cocoa and 12.5 tons of rice. Now it is 15 tons of cocoa and 13.75 tons of rice (3.75 tons in Ghana and 10 tons in South Korea). The source of the increase in production is summarized in Table 4.2.

Not only is output higher, but both countries also can now benefit from trade. If Ghana and South Korea swap cocoa and rice on a one-to-one basis, with both countries choosing to exchange 4 tons of their export for 4 tons of the import, both countries are able to consume more cocoa and rice than they could before specialization and trade (see Table 4.2). Thus, if Ghana exchanges 4 tons of cocoa with South Korea for 4 tons of rice, it is still left with 11 tons of cocoa, which is 1 ton more than it had before trade. The 4 tons of rice it gets from South Korea in exchange for its 4 tons of cocoa, when added to the 3.75 tons it now produces domestically, leaves it with a total of 7.75 tons of rice, which is .25 of a ton more than it had before specialization. Similarly, after swapping 4 tons of rice with Ghana, South Korea still ends up with 6 tons of rice, which is more than it had before specialization. In addition, the 4 tons of cocoa it receives in exchange is 1.5 tons more than it produced before trade. Thus, consumption of cocoa and rice can increase in both countries as a result of specialization and trade.

The basic message of the theory of comparative advantage is that *potential world production is greater with unrestricted free trade than it is with restricted trade.* Ricardo's theory suggests that consumers in all nations can consume more if there are no restrictions on trade. This occurs even in countries that lack an absolute advantage in the production of any good. In other words, to an even greater degree than the theory of absolute advantage, *the theory of comparative advantage suggests that trade is a positive-sum game in which all countries that participate realize economic gains.* As such, this theory provides a strong rationale for encouraging free trade. So powerful is Ricardo's theory that it remains a major intellectual weapon for those who argue for free trade.

Qualifications and Assumptions

The conclusion that free trade is universally beneficial is a rather bold one to draw from such a simple model. Our simple model includes many unrealistic assumptions:

1. We have assumed a simple world in which there are only two countries and two goods. In the real world, there are many countries and many goods.

2. We have assumed away transportation costs between countries.

3. We have assumed away differences in the prices of resources in different countries. We have said nothing about exchange rates, simply assuming that cocoa and rice could be swapped on a one-to-one basis.

4. We have assumed that resources can move freely from the production of one good to another within a country. In reality, this is not always the case.

5. We have assumed constant returns to scale; that is, that specialization by Ghana or South Korea has no effect on the amount of resources required to produce one ton of cocoa or rice. In reality, both diminishing and increasing returns to specialization exist. The amount of resources required to produce a good might decrease or increase as a nation specializes in production of that good.

6. We have assumed that each country has a fixed stock of resources and that free trade does not change the efficiency with which a country uses its resources. This static assumption makes no allowances for the dynamic changes in a country's stock of resources and in the efficiency with which the country uses its resources that might result from free trade.

7. We have assumed away the effects of trade on income distribution within a country.

Given these assumptions, can the conclusion that free trade is mutually beneficial be extended to the real world of many countries, many goods, positive transportation costs, volatile exchange rates, immobile domestic resources, nonconstant returns to specialization, and dynamic changes? Although a detailed extension of the theory of comparative advantage is beyond the scope of this book, economists have shown that the basic result derived from our simple model can be generalized to a world composed of many countries producing many different goods.[6] Despite the shortcomings of the Ricardian model, research suggests that the basic proposition that countries will export the goods that they are most efficient at producing is borne out by the data.[7] However, once all the assumptions are dropped, the case for unrestricted free trade, while still positive, has been argued by some economists associated with the "new trade theory" to lose some of its strength.[8] We return to this issue later in this chapter and in the next.

Simple Extensions of the Ricardian Model

Let us explore the effect of relaxing three of the assumptions identified above in the simple comparative advantage model. Below we relax the assumption that resources move freely from the production of one good to another within a country, the assumption of constant returns to specialization, and the assumption that trade does not change a country's stock of resources or the efficiency with which those resources are utilized.

Immobile Resources

In our simple comparative model of Ghana and South Korea, we assumed that producers (farmers) could easily convert land from the production of cocoa to rice, and vice versa. While this assumption may hold for some agricultural products, resources do not always shift quite so easily from producing one good to another. A certain amount of friction is involved. For example, embracing a free trade regime for an advanced economy such as the United States often implies that the country will produce less of some labor-intensive goods, such as textiles, and more of some knowledge-intensive goods, such as computer software or biotechnology products. Although the country as a whole will gain from such a shift, textile producers will lose. A textile worker in South Carolina is probably not qualified to write software for Microsoft. Thus, the shift to free trade may mean that she becomes unemployed or has to accept another less attractive job, such as working at a fast-food restaurant. For an example of how the shift toward free trade can impact an individual enterprise and its employees, look at the Management Focus profiling how the outdoor equipment cooperative REI is adjusting its own production activities to deal with a move toward greater free trade in textiles in the U.S. economy.

Resources do not always move easily from one economic activity to another. The process creates friction and human suffering too. While the theory predicts that the benefits of free trade outweigh the costs by a significant margin, this is of cold comfort to those who bear the costs. Accordingly, political opposition to the adoption of a free trade regime typically comes from those whose jobs are most at risk. In the United States, for example, textile workers and their unions have long opposed the move toward free trade precisely because this group has much to lose from free trade. Governments often ease the transition toward free trade by helping to retrain those who lose their jobs as a result. The pain caused by the movement toward a free trade regime is a short-term phenomenon, while the gains from trade once the transition has been made are both significant and enduring.

Diminishing Returns

The simple comparative advantage model developed above assumes constant returns to specialization. By constant returns to specialization we mean the units of resources required to produce a good (cocoa or rice) are assumed to remain constant no matter where one is on a country's production possibility frontier (PPF). Thus, we assumed that it always took Ghana 10 units of resources to produce one ton of cocoa. However, it is more realistic to assume diminishing returns to specialization. Diminishing returns to specialization occurs when more units of resources are required to produce each additional unit. While 10 units of resources may be sufficient to increase Ghana's output of cocoa from 12 tons to 13 tons, 11 units of resources may be needed to increase output from 13 to 14 tons, 12 units of resources to increase output from 14 tons to 15 tons, and so on. Diminishing returns implies a convex PPF for Ghana (see Figure 4.3), rather than the straight line depicted in Figure 4.2.

It is more realistic to assume diminishing returns for two reasons. First, not all resources are of the same quality. As a country tries to increase its output of a certain good, it is increasingly likely to draw on more marginal resources whose productivity is not as great as those initially employed. The result is that it requires ever more resources to produce an equal increase in output. For example, some land is more productive than other land. As Ghana tries to expand its output of cocoa, it might have to utilize increasingly marginal land that is less fertile than the land it originally used. As yields per acre decline, Ghana must use more land to produce one ton of cocoa.

A second reason for diminishing returns is that different goods use resources in different proportions. For example, imagine that growing cocoa uses more land and less

Management Focus

Free Trade and REI

Recreational Equipment Inc. (REI) is a buyers' cooperative that has grown into one of the major suppliers of outdoor equipment in the United States and has a rapidly growing international business. Started in Seattle in 1938 by Lloyd Anderson, the company provided high-quality climbing gear at a low price to members of the cooperative. For its first 37 years, REI operated a single store in Seattle, but in 1975 the cooperative started opening stores in other cities. Today REI has become a $740 million-a-year business with 60 stores worldwide, 6,600 employees, revenue growth of 6 to 8 percent annually, and a goal of opening three to five retail outlets per year. REI also has one of the most profitable Internet sites in the retail industry, which registered revenues of $116 million in 2001, up 26 percent from a year earlier. Despite the growth, REI is still organized as a cooperative with 1.7 million active members. All members receive a dividend check at the end of each year that amounts to about 10 percent of the value of their purchases during the year (one does not have to be a member to shop at REI).

To supply some of its own product needs, REI long had two subsidiaries. One of these, Thaw, supplied REI with a range of gear, including tents, backpacks, sleeping bags, and clothing, for 33 years. In the 1990s, Thaw concentrated on producing clothing items made out of fleece for REI's stores. Unfortunately for Thaw's 200 employees, the economics of manufacturing garments in the United States have been changing for several years. Following passage of the North American Free Trade Agreement (NAFTA) in 1993, all tariffs on trade in textile garments between the United States and Mexico were dropped. In the following years, an increasing number of textile operations shut down in the United States and moved to Mexico, attracted by lower labor costs. Wage rates for textile workers in Mexico run about $5 to $10 a day, compared to $8 to $10 an hour at Thaw's operation. For a labor-intensive operation such as garment production, these wage differentials are significant.

Given these economics, in mid-2000, REI announced it would be closing its Thaw subsidiary and sourcing its fleece products from Mexico. By shifting its production to Mexico, REI expected to reduce the cost of its fleece items by 20 percent. That means lower prices for REI's members and other customers and bigger profits for REI, which translates into larger dividend checks for REI's members. It also means that its Thaw employees will be out of a job. To assist its former employees at Thaw, REI added funds to federal money to assist with job retraining, unemployment benefits, and health insurance.

The events at Thaw are being repeated across the country. Since 1993, about 450,000 jobs have been lost in the U.S. garment industry as production has moved to low-wage countries such as Mexico. Former textile workers, most of whom are low skilled, have found it difficult to find alternative full-time employment. The Department of Labor estimates that between 1995 and 1997, 58 percent of unemployed textile workers failed to find full-time jobs, while for the 42 percent that did, their average wage dropped by some 20 percent. As painful as this has been for textile workers, the U.S. consumer has gained from lower prices, and U.S. companies in many other industries have seen their sales to Mexico boom as trade barriers have come down. Thus, while a strong case can be made that NAFTA has benefited the majority of U.S. citizens and Mexicans alike, it has inflicted pain on some groups, such as U.S. textile workers, and forces some companies, such as REI, to make difficult managerial decisions.

Sources: R. T. Nelson, "REI's Globalization," *Seattle Times,* May 14, 2000, pp. D1, D2; E. Chabrow, "REI Gets Head Start in Clicks and Mortar Race," *Information Week,* May 1, 2000; and J. Ozretich, "Largest 100 Private Companies: REI Climbs Back into Prominence after Down Years," *Puget Sound Business Journal,* June 14, 2002, p. 59.

labor than growing rice, and that Ghana tries to transfer resources from rice production to cocoa production. The rice industry will release proportionately too much labor and too little land for efficient cocoa production. To absorb the additional resources of labor and land, the cocoa industry will have to shift toward more labor-intensive methods of production. The effect is that the efficiency with which the cocoa industry uses labor will decline, and returns will diminish.

Figure 4.3

Ghana's PPF under
Diminishing Returns

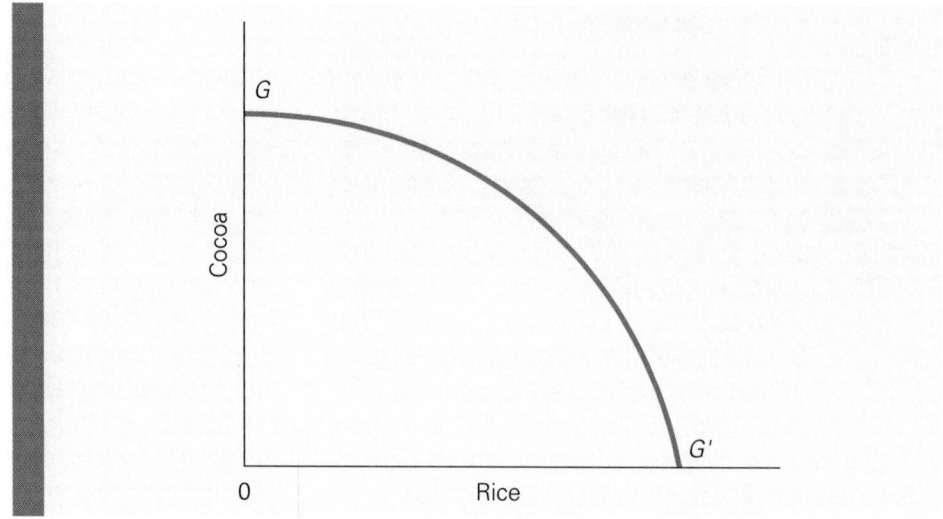

Diminishing returns show that it is not feasible for a country to specialize to the degree suggested by the simple Ricardian model outlined earlier. Diminishing returns to specialization suggest that the gains from specialization are likely to be exhausted before specialization is complete. In reality, most countries do not specialize but instead produce a range of goods. However, the theory predicts that it is worthwhile to specialize until that point where the resulting gains from trade are outweighed by diminishing returns. Thus, the basic conclusion that unrestricted free trade is beneficial still holds, although because of diminishing returns, the gains may not be as great as suggested in the constant returns case.

Dynamic Effects and Economic Growth

Our simple comparative advantage model assumed that trade does not change a country's stock of resources or the efficiency with which it utilizes those resources. This static assumption makes no allowances for the dynamic changes that might result from trade. If we relax this assumption, it becomes apparent that opening an economy to trade is likely to generate dynamic gains of two sorts.[9] First, free trade might increase a country's stock of resources as increased supplies of labor and capital from abroad become available for use within the country. This is occurring now in Eastern Europe, where many Western businesses are investing significant capital in the former Communist countries.

Second, free trade might also increase the efficiency with which a country uses its resources. Gains in the efficiency of resource utilization could arise from a number of factors. For example, economies of large-scale production might become available as trade expands the size of the total market available to domestic firms. Trade might make better technology from abroad available to domestic firms; better technology can increase labor productivity or the productivity of land. (The so-called green revolution had this effect on agricultural outputs in developing countries.) Also, opening an economy to foreign competition might stimulate domestic producers to look for ways to increase their efficiency. Again, this phenomenon is arguably occurring in the once-protected markets of Eastern Europe, where many former state monopolies are increasing the efficiency of their operations to survive in the competitive world market.

Dynamic gains in both the stock of a country's resources and the efficiency with which resources are utilized will cause a country's PPF to shift outward. This is illustrated in Figure 4.4, where the shift from PPF$_1$ to PPF$_2$ results from the dynamic gains that arise from free trade. As a consequence of this outward shift, the country in Figure 4.4 can produce more of both goods than it did before introduction of free trade. The theory suggests that opening an economy to free trade not only results in static

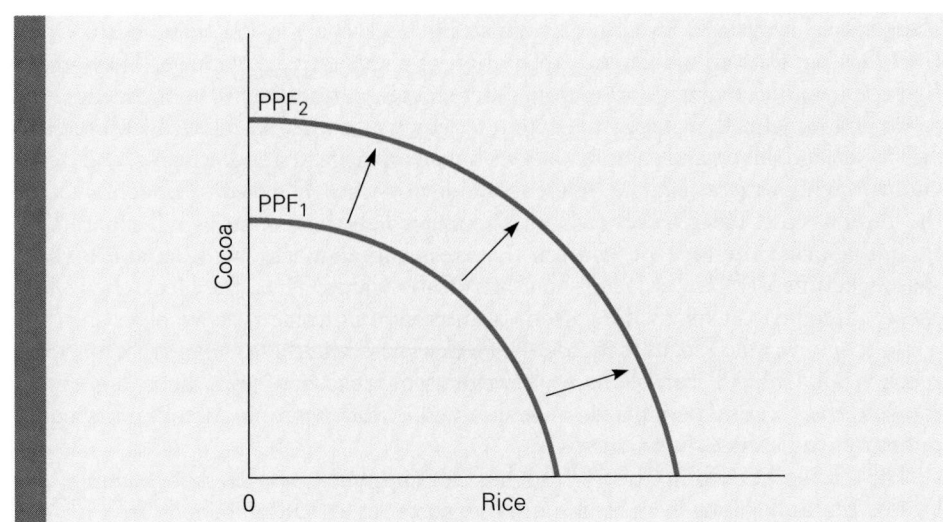

Figure 4.4

The Influence of Free
Trade on the PPF

gains of the type discussed earlier, but also results in dynamic gains that stimulate economic growth. If this is so, the case for free trade becomes stronger.

Evidence for the Link between Trade and Growth

Many economic studies have looked at the relationship between trade and economic growth.[10] In general, these studies suggest that, as predicted by the theory, countries that adopt a more open stance toward international trade enjoy higher growth rates than those that close their economies to trade. Jeffrey Sachs and Andrew Warner created a measure of how "open" to international trade an economy was and then looked at the relationship between "openness" and economic growth for a sample of more than 100 countries from 1970 to 1990.[11] Among other findings, they reported:

> We find a strong association between openness and growth, both within the group of developing and the group of developed countries. Within the group of developing countries, the open economies grew at 4.49 percent per year, and the closed economies grew at 0.69 percent per year. Within the group of developed economies, the open economies grew at 2.29 percent per year, and the closed economies grew at 0.74 percent per year.[12]

The message of this study seems clear: Adopt an open economy and embrace free trade, and over time your nation will be rewarded with higher economic growth rates. Higher growth will raise income levels and living standards. This last point has been confirmed by a study that looked at the relationship between trade and growth in incomes. The study, undertaken by Jeffrey Frankel and David Romer, found that on average, a one percentage point increase in the ratio of a country's trade to its gross domestic product increases income per person by at least one-half percent.[13] For every 10 percent increase in the importance of international trade in an economy, average income levels will rise by at least 5 percent. Despite the short-term adjustment costs associated with adopting a free trade regime, trade would seem to produce greater economic growth and higher living standards in the long run, just as the theory of Ricardo would lead us to expect.[14]

Heckscher–Ohlin Theory ■

Ricardo's theory stresses that comparative advantage arises from differences in productivity. Thus, whether Ghana is more efficient than South Korea in the production of cocoa depends on how productively it uses its resources. Ricardo stressed labor productivity and argued that differences in labor productivity between nations underlie the notion of comparative advantage. Swedish economists Eli Heckscher (in 1919) and Bertil Ohlin (in 1933) put forward a different explanation of comparative advantage. They argued that comparative advantage arises from differences in national factor endowments.[15] By factor endowments they meant the extent to which a country is endowed with such resources as land, labor, and capital. Nations have varying factor endowments, and different factor endowments explain differences in factor costs. The more abundant a factor, the lower its cost. The Heckscher-Ohlin theory predicts that countries will export those goods that make intensive use of factors that are locally abundant, while importing goods that make intensive use of factors that are locally scarce. Thus, the Heckscher-Ohlin theory attempts to explain the pattern of international trade that we observe in the world economy. Like Ricardo's theory, the Heckscher-Ohlin theory argues that free trade is beneficial. Unlike Ricardo's theory, however, the Heckscher-Ohlin theory argues that the pattern of international trade is determined by differences in factor endowments, rather than differences in productivity.

The Heckscher-Ohlin theory also has commonsense appeal. For example, the United States has long been a substantial exporter of agricultural goods, reflecting in part its unusual abundance of arable land. In contrast, China excels in the export of goods produced in labor-intensive manufacturing industries, such as textiles and footwear. This reflects China's relative abundance of low-cost labor. The United States, which lacks abundant low-cost labor, has been a primary importer of these goods. Note that it is relative, not absolute, endowments that are important; a country may have larger absolute amounts of land and labor than another country, but be relatively abundant in one of them.

The Leontief Paradox

The Heckscher-Ohlin theory has been one of the most influential theoretical ideas in international economics. Most economists prefer the Heckscher-Ohlin theory to Ricardo's theory because it makes fewer simplifying assumptions. Because of its influence, the theory has been subjected to many empirical tests. Beginning with a famous study published in 1953 by Wassily Leontief (winner of the Nobel Prize in economics in 1973), many of these tests have raised questions about the validity of the Heckscher-Ohlin theory.[16] Using the Heckscher-Ohlin theory, Leontief postulated that since the United States was relatively abundant in capital compared to other nations, the United States would be an exporter of capital-intensive goods and an importer of labor-intensive goods. To his surprise, however, he found that U.S. exports were less capital intensive than U.S. imports. Since this result was at variance with the predictions of the theory, it has become known as the Leontief paradox.

No one is quite sure why we observe the Leontief paradox. One possible explanation is that the United States has a special advantage in producing new products or goods made with innovative technologies. Such products may be less capital intensive than products whose technology has had time to mature and become suitable for mass production. Thus, the United States may be exporting goods that heavily use skilled labor and innovative entrepreneurship, such as computer software, while importing heavy manufacturing products that use large amounts of capital. Some more recent empirical studies tend to confirm this.[17] Tests of the Heckscher-Ohlin theory using data for a large number of countries tend to confirm the existence of the Leontief paradox.[18]

This leaves economists with a difficult dilemma. They prefer the Heckscher-Ohlin theory on theoretical grounds, but it is a relatively poor predictor of real-world international trade patterns. On the other hand, the theory they regard as being too limited, Ricardo's theory of comparative advantage, actually predicts trade patterns with greater accuracy. The best solution to this dilemma may be to return to the Ricardian idea that trade patterns are largely driven by international differences in productivity. Thus, one might argue that the United States exports commercial aircraft and imports automobiles not because its factor endowments are especially suited to aircraft manufacture and not suited to automobile manufacture, but because the United States is more efficient at producing aircraft than automobiles. A key assumption in the Heckscher-Ohlin theory is that technologies are the same across countries. This may not be the case. Differences in technology may lead to differences in productivity, which in turn, drives international trade patterns.[19] Thus, Japan's success in exporting automobiles in the 1970s and 1980s was based not just on the relative abundance of capital, but also on its development of innovative manufacturing technology that enabled it to achieve higher productivity levels in automobile production than other countries that also had abundant capital. The most recent empirical work strongly suggests that this theoretical explanation may be correct.[20] The new research shows that once differences in technology across countries are controlled for, countries do indeed export those goods that make intensive use of factors that are locally abundant, while importing goods that make intensive use of factors that are locally scarce. In other words, once the impact of differences of technology on productivity is controlled for, the Heckscher-Ohlin seems to gain predictive power.

The Product Life-Cycle Theory ▪

Raymond Vernon initially proposed the product life-cycle theory in the mid-1960s.[21] Vernon's theory was based on the observation that for most of the 20th century a very large proportion of the world's new products had been developed by U.S. firms and sold first in the U.S. market (e.g., mass-produced automobiles, televisions, instant cameras, photocopiers, personal computers, and semiconductor chips). To explain this, Vernon argued that the wealth and size of the U.S. market gave U.S. firms a strong incentive to develop new consumer products. In addition, the high cost of U.S. labor gave U.S. firms an incentive to develop cost-saving process innovations.

Just because a new product is developed by a U.S. firm and first sold in the U.S. market, it does not follow that the product must be produced in the United States. It could be produced abroad at some low-cost location and then exported back into the United States. However, Vernon argued that most new products were initially produced in America. Apparently, the pioneering firms believed it was better to keep production facilities close to the market and to the firm's center of decision making, given the uncertainty and risks inherent in introducing new products. Also, the demand for most new products tends to be based on nonprice factors. Consequently, firms can charge relatively high prices for new products, which obviates the need to look for low-cost production sites in other countries.

Vernon went on to argue that early in the life cycle of a typical new product, while demand is starting to grow rapidly in the United States, demand in other advanced countries is limited to high-income groups. The limited initial demand in other advanced countries does not make it worthwhile for firms in those countries to start producing the new product, but it does necessitate some exports from the United States to those countries.

Over time, demand for the new product starts to grow in other advanced countries (e.g., Great Britain, France, Germany, and Japan). As it does, it becomes worthwhile for foreign producers to begin producing for their home markets. In addition, U.S. firms might set up production facilities in those advanced countries where demand is growing. Consequently, production within other advanced countries begins to limit the potential for exports from the United States.

As the market in the United States and other advanced nations matures, the product becomes more standardized, and price becomes the main competitive weapon. As this occurs, cost considerations start to play a greater role in the competitive process. Producers based in advanced countries where labor costs are lower than in the United States (e.g., Italy, Spain) might now be able to export to the United States. If cost pressures become intense, the process might not stop there. The cycle by which the

United States lost its advantage to other advanced countries might be repeated once more, as developing countries (e.g., Thailand) begin to acquire a production advantage over advanced countries. Thus, the locus of global production initially switches from the United States to other advanced nations and then from those nations to developing countries.

The consequence of these trends for the pattern of world trade is that over time the United States switches from being an exporter of the product to an importer of the product as production becomes concentrated in lower-cost foreign locations. Figure 4.5 shows the growth of production and consumption over time in the United States, other advanced countries, and developing countries.

Evaluating the Product Life-Cycle Theory

Historically, the product life-cycle theory is an accurate explanation of international trade patterns. Consider photocopiers; the product was first developed in the early 1960s by Xerox in the United States and sold initially to U.S. users. Originally Xerox exported photocopiers from the United States, primarily to Japan and the advanced countries of Western Europe. As demand began to grow in those countries, Xerox entered into joint ventures to set up production in Japan (Fuji-Xerox) and Great Britain (Rank-Xerox). In addition, once Xerox's patents on the photocopier process expired, other foreign competitors began to enter the market (e.g., Canon in Japan, Olivetti in Italy). As a consequence, exports from the United States declined, and U.S. users began to buy some of their photocopiers from lower-cost foreign sources, particularly Japan. More recently, Japanese companies have found that manufacturing costs are too high in their own country, so they have begun to switch production to developing countries such as Singapore and Thailand. As a result, initially the United States and now several other advanced countries (e.g., Japan and Great Britain) have switched from being exporters of photocopiers to being importers. This evolution in the pattern of international trade in photocopiers is consistent with the predictions of the product life-cycle theory that mature industries tend to go out of the United States and into low-cost assembly locations.

However, the product life-cycle theory is not without weaknesses. Viewed from an Asian or European perspective, Vernon's argument that most new products are developed and introduced in the United States seems ethnocentric. Although it may be true that during U.S. global dominance (from 1945 to 1975), most new products were introduced in the United States, there have always been important exceptions. These exceptions appear to have become more common in recent years. Many new products are now introduced in Japan (e.g., videogame consoles). With the increased globalization and integration of the world economy discussed in Chapter 1, a growing number of new products (e.g., laptop computers, compact disks, and digital cameras) are now introduced simultaneously in the United States, Japan, and the advanced European nations. This may be accompanied by globally dispersed production, with particular components of a new product being produced in those locations around the globe where the mix of factor costs and skills is most favorable (as predicted by the theory of comparative advantage).

Consider laptop computers, which were introduced simultaneously in a number of major national markets by Toshiba. Although various components for Toshiba laptop computers are manufactured in Japan (e.g., display screens, memory chips), other components are manufactured in Singapore and Taiwan and still others (e.g., hard drives and microprocessors) are manufactured in the United States. All the components are shipped to Singapore for final assembly, and the completed product is then shipped to the major world markets (the United States, Western Europe, and Japan). The pattern of trade associated with this new product is both different from and more complex than the pattern predicted by Vernon's model. Trying to explain this pattern using the product life-cycle theory would be very difficult. The

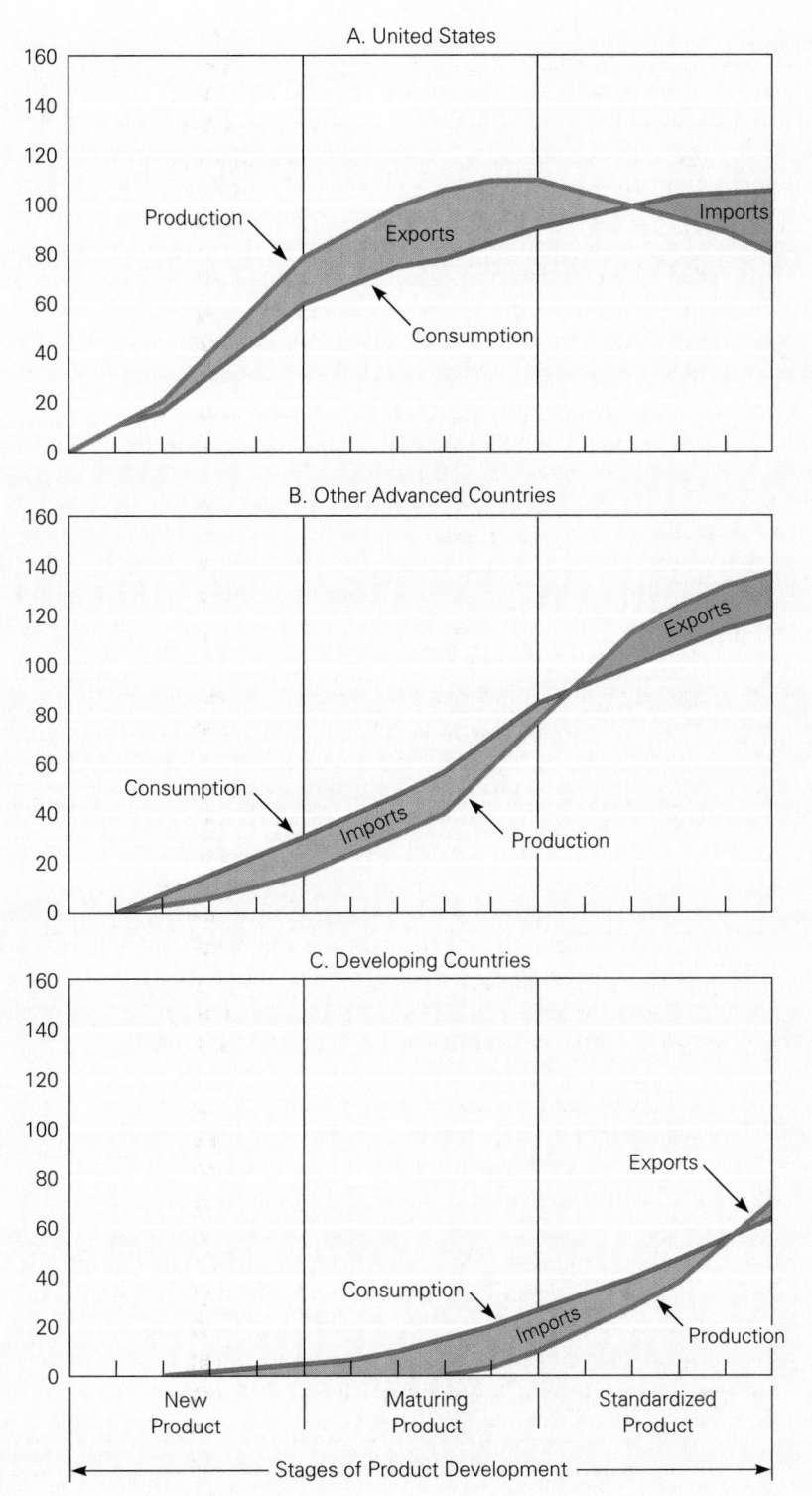

Figure 4.5

The Product Life-Cycle Theory

Source: Adapted from R. Vernon and L. T. Wells, *The Economic Environment of International Business.* 4th ed., © 1986. Reprinted by permission of Pearson Education, Inc. Upper Saddle River, N.J.

theory of comparative advantage might better explain why certain components are produced in certain locations and why the final product is assembled in Singapore. Although Vernon's theory may be useful for explaining the pattern of international trade during the brief period of American global dominance, its relevance in the modern world is limited.

New Trade Theory

The new trade theory began to emerge in the 1970s when a number of economists were questioning the assumption of diminishing returns to specialization used in international trade theory (see Figure 4.3).[22] They argued that increasing returns to specialization might exist in some industries. Economies of scale represent one particularly important source of increasing returns. **Economies of scale** are unit cost reductions associated with a large scale of output. If international trade results in a country specializing in the production of a certain good, and if there are economies of scale in producing that good, as output of that good expands, unit costs will fall. In such a case, there will be increasing returns to specialization, not diminishing returns! Put differently, as a country produces more of the good, due to the realization of economies of scale, productivity will increase and unit costs will fall.

New trade theory argues that in industries where there are economies of scale, both the variety of goods that a country can produce and the scale of production are limited by the size of the market. The domestic market may not be big enough to allow producers to realize economies of scale for certain products, and accordingly, those products may not be produced, thus limiting the variety of products available to consumers. Alternatively, they may be produced, but in such low volumes that unit costs and prices are higher. When nations trade with each other and form a single world market that is bigger than individual national markets, individual firms in a nation may be able to better attain scale economies. The implication, according to new trade theory, is that each nation may be able to specialize in producing a narrower range of products than it would in the absence of trade, yet by buying goods that it does not make from other countries, each nation can simultaneously increase the *variety* of goods available to its consumers and *lower the costs* of those goods—thus trade offers an opportunity for mutual gain even when countries do not differ in their resource endowments or technology.

Suppose there are two countries, each with an annual market for 1 million automobiles. By trading with each other, these countries can create a combined market for 2 million cars. In this combined market, due to the ability to better realize economies of scale, more varieties (models) of cars can be produced, and cars can be produced at a lower average cost, than in either market alone. For example, demand for a sports car may be limited to 55,000 units in each national market, while a total output of at least 100,000 per year may be required to realize significant scale economies. Similarly, demand for a minivan may be 80,000 units in each national market, and again a total output of at least 100,000 per year may be required to realize significant scale economies. Faced with limited domestic market demand, firms in each nation may decide not to produce a sports car, since the costs of doing so at such low volume are too great. Although they may produce minivans, the cost of doing so will be higher, as will prices, than if significant economies of scale had been attained. Once the two countries decide to trade however, a firm in one nation may specialize in producing sports cars, while a firm in the other nation may produce minivans. The combined demand for 110,000 sports cars and 160,00 minivans allows each firm to realize scale economies. Consumers in this case benefit from having access to a product (sports cars) that was not available before international trade, and from the lower price for a product (minivans) that could not be produced at the most efficient scale before international trade. Trade is thus mutually beneficial because it allows for the specialization of production, the realization of scale economies, the production of a greater variety of products, and lower prices.

New trade theory also argues that if the output required to realize significant scale economies represents a substantial proportion of total world demand for that product, the world market may be able to support only a limited number of firms based in a limited number of countries producing that product. Those firms that enter the world market first may gain an advantage that may be difficult for other firms to match. Thus, a country may dominate in the export of a particular product where scale economies are important, and where the volume of output required to gain scale economies represents a significant proportion of world output, because it is home to a firm that was an early mover in this industry.

The Aerospace Example

The commercial aerospace industry, which is currently dominated by just two firms, Boeing and Airbus (although there are several niche players), is a good example of this theory. Economies of scale in this industry come from the ability to spread fixed costs over a large output. The fixed costs of developing a new commercial jet airliner are astronomical. Boeing spent an estimated $5 billion to develop its Boeing 777 jetliner. A major source of scale economies is the ability to spread these fixed costs over a large output. If Boeing makes only 100 of the Boeing 777, its fixed costs will amount to $50 million per unit (i.e., $5 billion divided by 100). If the variable costs such as labor, equipment, and parts equal $80 million per aircraft, the total cost of each aircraft would be $130 million (i.e., $80 million in per unit variable costs plus $50 million in per unit fixed costs). If Boeing makes 500 of these aircraft, the fixed costs fall to $10 million per unit (i.e., $5 billion divided by 500), bringing the total cost of each aircraft to just $90 million (i.e., $80 million plus $10 million). The economies of scale here are significant, with average unit costs falling by $40 million as output expands from 100 units to 500 units.

In addition to economies of scale, learning effects also exist in this industry. These too may result in increasing returns to specialization. **Learning effects** are cost savings that come from learning by doing. Labor, for example, learns by repetition how best to carry out a task. Labor productivity increases over time and variable unit costs fall as individuals learn the most efficient way to perform a particular task. Learning effects tend to be more significant when a technologically complex task is repeated because there is more to learn. Thus, learning effects will be more significant in an assembly process involving 1,000 complex steps than in an assembly process involving 100 simple steps—and assembling a commercial jetliner involves more complex steps than perhaps any other product. Learning effects were first documented in the aerospace industry where it was found that each time accumulated output of airframes was doubled, unit costs declined to 80 percent of their previous level.[23] Thus, the fourth airframe typically cost only 80 percent of the second airframe to produce, the eighth airframe only 80 percent of the fourth, the 16th only 80 percent of the eighth, and so on. This observation implies that the $80 million in per unit variable costs required to build a 777 will decline over time as output expands, primarily because of gains in labor productivity. Thus, while variable costs per unit might be $80 million by the time 100 aircraft have been manufactured, by the time 500 aircraft have been manufactured, they may have fallen to $60 million per unit.

Combine learning effects with our earlier calculation of the decline in unit fixed costs, and our analysis suggests that as output of 777s expands from 100 to 500 units, unit costs will fall from $130 million ($80 million variable costs and $50 million fixed costs per unit), to $70 million ($60 million variable costs plus $10 million fixed costs per unit). Obviously, increasing returns to specialization are very important in this industry. Just how important they are can be appreciated by the fact that the list price for a new Boeing 777 is about $120 million. Thus, if Boeing sells only 100 aircraft it will not make any money on this product. If it sells 500 aircraft, due to scale economies and learning effects it will make acceptable profits.

World demand is large enough to support only a limited number of aircraft producers at high output levels. Forecasts suggest that the global market for long-range aircraft with a seating capacity of about 300, such as the 777, will be about 1,500 aircraft between 1997 and 2008. If we assume that Boeing has to sell about 500 aircraft to make a decent return on its investment, this suggests that the world market is large enough to support only three producers profitably!

Implications

New trade theory has important implications. The theory suggests that nations may benefit from trade even when they do not differ in resource endowments or technology. Trade allows a nation to specialize in the production of certain products, attaining scale economies and lowering the costs of producing those products, while buying products that it does not produce from other nations that are similarly specialized. By this mechanism, the variety of products available to consumers in each nation is increased, while the average costs of those products should fall, as should their price, freeing resources to produce other goods and services.

The theory also suggests that a country may predominate in the export of a good simply because it was lucky enough to have one or more firms among the first to produce that good. Underpinning this argument is the notion of **first-mover advantages,** which are the economic and strategic advantages that accrue to early entrants into an industry.[24] Because they are able to gain economies of scale and learning effects, the early entrants in an industry may get a lock on the world market that discourages subsequent entry. First movers' ability to benefit from increasing returns creates a barrier to entry. In the commercial aircraft industry, for example, the fact that Boeing and Airbus are already in the industry and have the benefits of economies of scale and learning effects discourages new entry and reenforces the dominance of America and Europe in the trade of commercial jet aircraft. This dominance is further reenforced because global demand may not be sufficient to profitably support another producer in the industry. So although Japanese firms might be able to compete in the market, they have decided not to enter the industry but to ally themselves as major subcontractors with primary producers (e.g., Mitsubishi Heavy Industries is a major subcontractor for Boeing on the 767 and 777 programs).

New trade theory is at variance with the Heckscher-Ohlin theory, which suggests that a country will predominate in the export of a product when it is particularly well endowed with those factors used intensively in its manufacture. New trade theorists argue that the United States leads in exports of commercial jet aircraft not because it is better endowed with the factors of production required to manufacture aircraft, but because one of the first movers in the industry, Boeing, was a U.S. firm. The new trade theory is not at variance with the theory of comparative advantage. Economies of scale and learning effects both increase the efficiency of resource utilization, and hence increase productivity. Thus, the new trade theory identifies an important source of comparative advantage.

It is perhaps too early to say how useful this theory is in explaining trade patterns, although empirical studies seem to support the predictions of the theory that trade increases the specialization of production within an industry, increases the variety of products available to consumers, and results in lower average prices.[25] With regard to first-mover advantages and international trade, a study by Harvard business historian Alfred Chandler suggests the existence of first-mover advantages is an important factor in explaining the dominance of firms from certain nations in specific industries.[26] The number of firms is very limited in many global industries, including the chemical industry, the heavy construction-equipment industry, the heavy truck industry, the tire industry, the consumer electronics industry, the jet engine industry, and the computer software industry.

Perhaps the most contentious implication of the new trade theory is the argument that it generates for government intervention and strategic trade policy.[27] New trade theorists stress the role of luck, entrepreneurship, and innovation in giving a firm first-mover advantages. According to this argument, the reason Boeing was the first mover in commercial jet aircraft manufacture—rather than firms like Great Britain's De-Havilland and Hawker Siddely, or Holland's Fokker, all of which could have been—was that Boeing was both lucky and innovative. One way Boeing was lucky is that DeHavilland shot itself in the foot when its Comet jet airliner, introduced two years

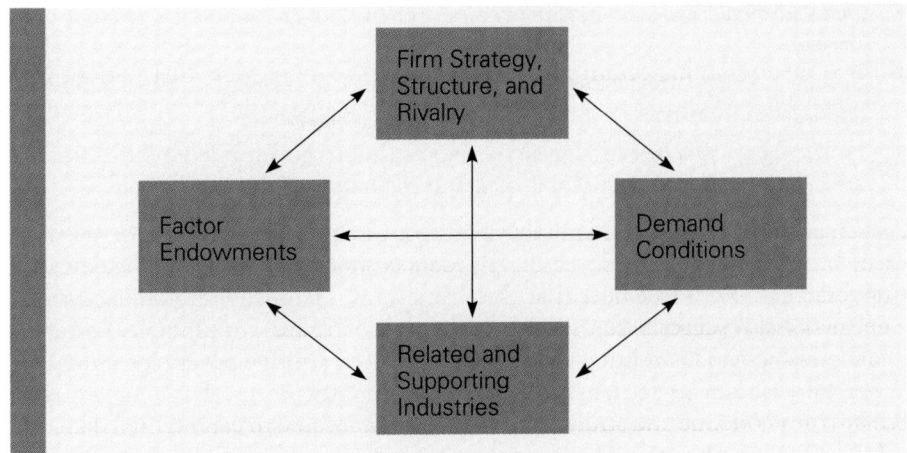

Figure 4.6

Determinants of National
Competitive Advantage:
Porter's Diamond

Reprinted by permission of the *Harvard Business Review*. "The Competitive Advantage of Nations" by Michael E. Porter, March–April 1990, p. 77. Copyright © 1990 by The President and Fellows of Harvard College; all rights reserved.

earlier than Boeing's first jet airliner, the 707, was found to be full of serious technological flaws. Had DeHavilland not made some serious technological mistakes, Great Britain might now be the world's leading exporter of commercial jet aircraft! Boeing's innovativeness was demonstrated by its independent development of the technological know-how required to build a commercial jet airliner. Several new trade theorists have pointed out, however, that Boeing's R&D was largely paid for by the U.S. government; the 707 was a spinoff from a government-funded military program. Herein lies a rationale for government intervention. By the sophisticated and judicious use of subsidies, could a government increase the chances of its domestic firms becoming first movers in newly emerging industries, as the U.S. government apparently did with Boeing? If this is possible, and the new trade theory suggests it might be, then we have an economic rationale for a proactive trade policy that is at variance with the free trade prescriptions of the trade theories we have reviewed so far. We will consider the policy implications of this issue in Chapter 5.

National Competitive Advantage: Porter's Diamond

In 1990, Michael Porter of the Harvard Business School published the results of an intensive research effort that attempted to determine why some nations succeed and others fail in international competition.[28] Porter and his team looked at 100 industries in 10 nations. Like the work of the new trade theorists, Porter's work was driven by a belief that existing theories of international trade told only part of the story. For Porter, the essential task was to explain why a nation achieves international success in a particular industry. Why does Japan do so well in the automobile industry? Why does Switzerland excel in the production and export of precision instruments and pharmaceuticals? Why do Germany and the United States do so well in the chemical industry? These questions cannot be answered easily by the Heckscher-Ohlin theory, and the theory of comparative advantage offers only a partial explanation. The theory of comparative advantage would say that Switzerland excels in the production and export of precision instruments because it uses its resources very productively in these industries. Although this may be correct, this does not explain why Switzerland is more productive in this industry than Great Britain, Germany, or Spain. Porter tries to solve this puzzle.

Porter theorizes that four broad attributes of a nation shape the environment in which local firms compete, and these attributes promote or impede the creation of competitive advantage (see Figure 4.6). These attributes are

- *Factor endowments*—a nation's position in factors of production such as skilled labor or the infrastructure necessary to compete in a given industry.

- *Demand conditions*—the nature of home demand for the industry's product or service.
- *Relating and supporting industries*—the presence or absence of supplier industries and related industries that are internationally competitive.
- *Firm strategy, structure, and rivalry*—the conditions governing how companies are created, organized, and managed and the nature of domestic rivalry.

Porter speaks of these four attributes as constituting the *diamond*. He argues that firms are most likely to succeed in industries or industry segments where the diamond is most favorable. He also argues that the diamond is a mutually reinforcing system. The effect of one attribute is contingent on the state of others. For example, Porter argues favorable demand conditions will not result in competitive advantage unless the state of rivalry is sufficient to cause firms to respond to them.

Porter maintains that two additional variables can influence the national diamond in important ways: chance and government. Chance events, such as major innovations, can reshape industry structure and provide the opportunity for one nation's firms to supplant another's. Government, by its choice of policies, can detract from or improve national advantage. For example, regulation can alter home demand conditions, antitrust policies can influence the intensity of rivalry within an industry, and government investments in education can change factor endowments.

Factor Endowments

Factor endowments lie at the center of the Heckscher-Ohlin theory. While Porter does not propose anything radically new, he does analyze the characteristics of factors of production. He recognizes hierarchies among factors, distinguishing between basic factors (e.g., natural resources, climate, location, and demographics) and advanced factors (e.g., communication infrastructure, sophisticated and skilled labor, research facilities, and technological know-how). He argues that advanced factors are the most significant for competitive advantage. Unlike the naturally endowed basic factors, advanced factors are a product of investment by individuals, companies, and governments. Thus, government investments in basic and higher education, by improving the general skill and knowledge level of the population and by stimulating advanced research at higher education institutions, can upgrade a nation's advanced factors.

The relationship between advanced and basic factors is complex. Basic factors can provide an initial advantage that is subsequently reinforced and extended by investment in advanced factors. Conversely, disadvantages in basic factors can create pressures to invest in advanced factors. An obvious example of this phenomenon is Japan, a country that lacks arable land and mineral deposits and yet through investment has built a substantial endowment of advanced factors. Porter notes that Japan's large pool of engineers (reflecting a much higher number of engineering graduates per capita than almost any other nation) has been vital to Japan's success in many manufacturing industries.

Demand Conditions

Porter emphasizes the role home demand plays in upgrading competitive advantage. Firms are typically most sensitive to the needs of their closest customers. Thus, the characteristics of home demand are particularly important in shaping the attributes of domestically made products and in creating pressures for innovation and quality. Porter argues that a nation's firms gain competitive advantage if their domestic consumers are sophisticated and demanding. Such consumers pressure local firms to meet high standards of product quality and to produce innovative products. Porter notes that Japan's sophisticated and knowledgeable buyers of cameras helped stimulate the Japanese camera industry to improve product quality and to introduce innovative models. A similar example can be found in the wireless telephone equipment industry, where sophisticated and demanding local customers in Scandinavia helped push

Nokia of Finland and Ericsson of Sweden to invest in cellular phone technology long before demand for cellular phones took off in other developed nations. The case of Nokia is reviewed in more depth in the accompanying Management Focus.

Related and Supporting Industries

The third broad attribute of national advantage in an industry is the presence of suppliers or related industries that are internationally competitive. The benefits of investments in advanced factors of production by related and supporting industries can spill over into an industry, thereby helping it achieve a strong competitive position internationally. Swedish strength in fabricated steel products (e.g., ball bearings and cutting tools) has drawn on strengths in Sweden's specialty steel industry. Technological leadership in the U.S. semiconductor industry until the mid-1980s provided the basis for U.S. success in personal computers and several other technically advanced electronic products. Similarly, Switzerland's success in pharmaceuticals is closely related to its previous international success in the technologically related dye industry.

One consequence of this process is that successful industries within a country tend to be grouped into clusters of related industries. This was one of the most pervasive findings of Porter's study. One such cluster is the German textile and apparel sector, which includes high-quality cotton, wool, synthetic fibers, sewing machine needles, and a wide range of textile machinery. Such clusters are important, because valuable knowledge can flow between the firms within a geographic cluster, benefiting all within that cluster. Knowledge flows occur when employees move between firms within a region and when national industry associations bring employees from different companies together for regular conferences or workshops.[29]

Firm Strategy, Structure, and Rivalry

The fourth broad attribute of national competitive advantage in Porter's model is the strategy, structure, and rivalry of firms within a nation. Porter makes two important points here. First, different nations are characterized by different management ideologies, which either help them or do not help them to build national competitive advantage. For example, Porter notes the predominance of engineers in top management at German and Japanese firms. He attributes this to these firms' emphasis on improving manufacturing processes and product design. In contrast, Porter notes a predominance of people with finance backgrounds leading many U.S. firms. He links this to U.S. firms' lack of attention to improving manufacturing processes and product design, particularly during the 1970s and 80s. He also argues that the dominance of finance has led to a corresponding overemphasis on maximizing short-term financial returns. According to Porter, one consequence of these different management ideologies has been a relative loss of U.S. competitiveness in those engineering-based industries where manufacturing processes and product design issues are all-important (e.g., the automobile industry).

Porter's second point is that there is a strong association between vigorous domestic rivalry and the creation and persistence of competitive advantage in an industry. Vigorous domestic rivalry induces firms to look for ways to improve efficiency, which makes them better international competitors. Domestic rivalry creates pressures to innovate, to improve quality, to reduce costs, and to invest in upgrading advanced factors. All this helps to create world-class competitors. Porter cites the case of Japan:

> Nowhere is the role of domestic rivalry more evident than in Japan, where it is all-out warfare in which many companies fail to achieve profitability. With goals that stress market share, Japanese companies engage in a continuing struggle to outdo each other. Shares fluctuate markedly. The process is prominently covered in the business press. Elaborate rankings measure which companies are most popular with university graduates. The rate of new product and process development is breathtaking.[30]

The Rise of Finland's Nokia

The mobile telephone equipment industry is one of the great growth stories of recent years. The number of wireless subscribers has been expanding rapidly. By the end of 2002, there were over 1 billion wireless subscribers worldwide, up from less than 10 million in 1990. Forecasts suggest that by 2004, the number could reach 1.5 billion.

Nokia is a dominant player in the market for mobile telephone sales. Nokia's roots are in Finland, not normally a country that comes to mind when one talks about leading-edge technology companies. In the 1980s, Nokia was a rambling Finnish conglomerate with activities that embraced tire manufacturing, paper production, consumer electronics, and telecommunication equipment. By 2002 it had transformed itself into a focused telecommunications equipment manufacturer with a global reach, sales of over $30 billion, and earnings of more than $5 billion. How has this former conglomerate emerged to take a global leadership position in wireless telecommunication equipment? Much of the answer lies in the history, geography, and political economy of Finland and its Nordic neighbors.

The story starts in 1981 when the Nordic nations got together to create the world's first international mobile telephone network. They had good reason to become pioneers; in the sparsely populated and inhospitably cold areas, it cost far too much to lay a traditional wireline telephone service. Yet the same geographic features make telecommunications all the more valuable; people driving through the Arctic winter and owners of remote northern houses need a telephone to summon help if things go wrong. As a result, Sweden, Norway, and Finland became the first nations to take wireless telecommunications seriously. They found, for example, that while it cost up to $800 per subscriber to bring a traditional wireline service to remote locations in the far north, the same locations could be linked by wireless telephones for only $500 per person. As a consequence, by 1994, 12 percent of Scandinavians owned wireless phones, compared with less than 6 percent in the United States, the world's second most developed market. This leadership has continued. By the end of 2002, 85 percent of the population in Finland owned a wireless phone, compared with 55 percent in the United States.

Nokia, as a longtime telecommunication equipment supplier, was well positioned to take advantage of this development. Other forces were also at work in Finland that helped Nokia develop its competitive edge. Unlike virtually every other developed nation, Finland has

---

A similar point about the stimulating effects of strong domestic competition can be made with regard to the rise of Nokia of Finland to global preeminence in the market for cellular telephone equipment. For details, see the Management Focus.

Evaluating Porter's Theory

Porter contends that the degree to which a nation is likely to achieve international success in a certain industry is a function of the combined impact of factor endowments, domestic demand conditions, related and supporting industries, and domestic rivalry. He argues that the presence of all four components is usually required for this diamond to boost competitive performance (although there are exceptions). Porter also contends that government can influence each of the four components of the diamond—either positively or negatively. Factor endowments can be affected by subsidies, policies toward capital markets, policies toward education, and so on. Government can shape domestic demand through local product standards or with regulations that mandate or influence buyer needs. Government policy can influence supporting and related industries through regulation and influence firm rivalry through such devices as capital market regulation, tax policy, and antitrust laws.

If Porter is correct, we would expect his model to predict the pattern of international trade that we observe in the real world. Countries should be exporting products from those industries where all four components of the diamond are favorable, while importing in those areas where the components are not favorable. Is he correct? We never had a national telephone monopoly. Instead, the country's telephone services have long been provided by about 50 autonomous local telephone companies, whose elected boards set prices by referendum (which naturally means low prices). This army of independent and cost-conscious telephone service providers prevented Nokia from taking anything for granted in its home country. With typical Finnish pragmatism, they were willing to buy from the lowest-cost supplier, whether that was Nokia, Ericsson, Motorola, or someone else. This situation contrasted sharply with that prevailing in most developed nations until the late 1980s and early 1990s; domestic telephone monopolies typically purchased equipment from a dominant local supplier or made it themselves. Nokia responded to this competitive pressure by doing everything possible to drive down its manufacturing costs while still staying at the leading edge of wireless technology.

The consequences of these forces are clear. Nokia is now the leader in digital wireless technology, which is the wave of the future. Many now regard Finland as the lead market for wireless telephone services. If you want to see the future of wireless, you don't go to New York or San Francisco, you go to Helsinki, where Finns use their wireless handsets not just to talk to each other, but also to browse the Web, execute e-commerce transac-tions, control household heating and lighting systems, or purchase Coke from a wireless-enabled vending machine. Nokia has gained this lead because Scandinavia started switching to digital technology five years before the rest of the world. Spurred on by its cost-conscious Finnish customers, Nokia now has the lowest cost structure of any cellular phone equipment manufacturer in the world, making it a more profitable enterprise than Motorola, its leading global rival. It cost Nokia an average of $114 to make and sell each phone in the third quarter of 2002, compared with about $131 a year earlier. Its closest rival, Motorola Inc., of Schaumburg, Ill., spent an average of $139 to make and sell each phone in the third quarter.

Sources: "Lessons from the Frozen North," *The Economist*, October 8, 1994, pp. 76–77; G. Edmondson, "Grabbing Markets from the Giants," *Business Week, Special Issue: 21st Century Capitalism,* 1995, p. 156; company news releases; "A Finnish Fable," *The Economist,* October 14, 2000; "To the Finland Base Station," *The Economist,* October 9, 1999, pp. 23–27; "A Survey of Telecommunications," *The Economist,* October 9, 1999; M. Newman, "The U.S. Starts to Catch Up," *Wall Street Journal,* September 23, 2002, p. R6; and D. Pringle, "How Nokia Thrives by Breaking the Rules," *Wall Street Journal,* January 3, 2003, p. A7.

simply do not know. Porter's theory has not yet been subjected to independent empirical testing. Much about the theory rings true, but the same can be said for the new trade theory, the theory of comparative advantage, and the Heckscher-Ohlin theory. It may be that each of these theories, which complement each other, explains something about the pattern of international trade.

Focus On Managerial Implications

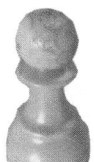

Why does all this matter for business? There are at least three main implications for international businesses of the material discussed in this chapter: location implications, first-mover implications, and policy implications.

Location

Underlying most of the theories we have discussed is the notion that different countries have particular advantages in different productive activities. Thus, from a profit perspective, it makes sense for a firm to disperse its productive activities to those countries where, according to the theory of international trade, they can be performed most efficiently. If design can be performed most efficiently in France, that is where design facilities should be located; if the manufacture of basic components can be performed most efficiently in Singapore, that is where they should be manufactured; and if final assembly can be performed most efficiently in China, that is where final assembly should be performed. The result is a global web of productive activities, with different activities being performed in different locations around the globe depending on considerations of comparative advantage, factor endowments, and the like. If the firm does not do this, it may find itself at a competitive disadvantage relative to firms that do.

Consider the production of a laptop computer, a process with four major stages: (1) basic research and development of the product design, (2) manufacture of standard electronic components (e.g., memory chips), (3) manufacture of advanced components (e.g., flat-top color display screens and microprocessors), and (4) final assembly. Basic R&D requires a pool of highly skilled and educated workers with good backgrounds in microelectronics. The two countries with a comparative advantage in basic microelectronics R&D and design are Japan and the United States, so most producers of laptop computers locate their R&D facilities in one, or both, of these countries. (Apple, IBM, Motorola, Texas Instruments, Toshiba, and Sony all have major R&D facilities in both Japan and the United States.)

The manufacture of standard electronic components is a capital-intensive process requiring semiskilled labor, and cost pressures are intense. The best locations for such activities today are places such as Singapore, Taiwan, Malaysia, and South Korea. These countries have pools of relatively skilled, moderate-cost labor. Thus, many producers of laptop computers have standard components, such as memory chips, produced at these locations.

The manufacture of advanced components such as microprocessors and display screens is a capital-intensive process requiring skilled labor. Because cost pressures are not so intense at this stage, these components can be—and are—manufactured in countries with high labor costs that also have pools of highly skilled labor (primarily Japan and the United States).

Finally, assembly is a relatively labor-intensive process requiring only low-skilled labor, and cost pressures are intense. As a result, final assembly may be carried out in a country such as Mexico, which has an abundance of low-cost, low-skilled labor. A laptop computer produced by a U.S. manufacturer may be designed in California, have its standard components produced in Taiwan and Singapore, its advanced components produced in Japan and the United States, its final assembly in Mexico, and be sold in the United States or elsewhere in the world. By dispersing production activities to different locations around the globe, the U.S. manufacturer is taking advantage of the differences between countries identified by the various theories of international trade.

First-Mover Advantages

According to the new trade theory, firms that establish a first-mover advantage with regard to the production of a particular new product may subsequently dominate global trade in that product. This is particularly true in industries where the global market can profitably support only a limited number of firms, such as the aerospace market, but early commitments also seem to be important in less concentrated industries such as the market for cellular telephone equipment (see the Management Focus on Nokia). For the individual firm, the clear message is that it pays to invest substantial financial resources in trying to build a first-mover, or early-mover, advantage, even if that means several years of substantial losses before a new venture becomes profitable—the idea being to preempt the available demand, gain cost advantages related to volume, build an enduring brand ahead of later competitors, and, consequently, establish a long-term sustainable competitive advantage. Although the details of how to achieve this are beyond the scope of this book, many publications offer strategies for exploiting first-mover advantages, and for avoiding the traps associated with pioneering a market (first-mover disadvantages).[31]

Government Policy

The theories of international trade also matter to international businesses because firms are major players on the international trade scene. Business firms produce exports, and business firms import the products of other countries. Because of their pivotal role in international trade, businesses can exert a strong influence on government trade policy, lobbying to promote free trade or trade restrictions. The theories of international trade claim that promoting free trade is generally in the best interests of a country, although it may not always be in the best interest of an individual firm. Many firms recognize this and lobby for open markets.

For example, when the U.S. government announced in 1991 its intention to place a tariff on Japanese imports of liquid crystal display (LCD) screens, IBM and Apple Computer protested strongly. Both IBM and Apple pointed out that (1) Japan was the lowest-cost source of LCD screens, (2) they used these screens in their own laptop computers, and (3) the proposed tariff, by increasing the cost of LCD screens, would increase the cost of laptop computers produced by IBM and Apple, thus making them less competitive in the world market. In other words, the tariff, designed to protect U.S. firms, would be self-defeating. In response to these pressures, the U.S. government reversed its posture.

Unlike IBM and Apple, however, businesses do not always lobby for free trade. In the United States, for example, restrictions on imports of steel are the result of direct pressure by U.S. firms on the government. In some cases, the government has responded to pressure by getting foreign companies to agree to "voluntary" restrictions on their imports, using the implicit threat of more comprehensive formal trade barriers to get them to adhere to these agreements (historically, this has occurred in the automobile industry). In other cases, the government used what are called "antidumping" actions to justify tariffs on imports from other nations (these mechanisms will be discussed in detail in the next chapter).

As predicted by international trade theory, many of these agreements have been self-defeating, such as the voluntary restriction on machine tool imports agreed to in 1985. Due to limited import competition from more efficient foreign suppliers, the prices of machine tools in the United States rose to higher levels than would have prevailed under free trade. Because machine tools are used throughout the manufacturing industry, the result was to increase the costs of U.S. manufacturing in general, creating a corresponding loss in world market competitiveness. Shielded from international competition by import barriers, the U.S. machine tool industry had no incentive to increase its efficiency. Consequently, it lost many of its export markets to more efficient foreign competitors. As a consequence of this misguided action, the U.S. machine tool industry shrank during the period when the agreement was in force. For anyone schooled in international trade theory, this was not surprising.[32] A similar scenario may be unfolding now in the U.S. steel industry, where tariff barriers erected by the government have raised the cost of steel to important U.S. users, such as automobile companies and appliance makers, making their products more uncompetitive.

Finally, Porter's theory of national competitive advantage also contains policy implications. Porter's theory suggests that it is in the best interest of business for a firm to invest in upgrading advanced factors of production; for example, to invest in better training for its employees and to increase its commitment to research and development. It is also in the best interests of business to lobby the government to adopt policies that have a favorable impact on each component of the national diamond. Thus, according to Porter, businesses should urge government to increase investment in education, infrastructure, and basic research (since all these enhance advanced factors) and to adopt policies that promote strong competition within domestic markets (since this makes firms stronger international competitors, according to Porter's findings).

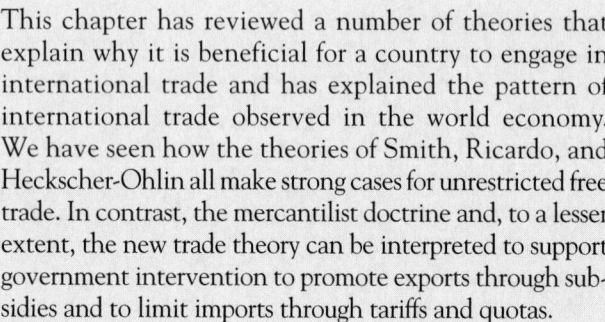

Chapter Summary

This chapter has reviewed a number of theories that explain why it is beneficial for a country to engage in international trade and has explained the pattern of international trade observed in the world economy. We have seen how the theories of Smith, Ricardo, and Heckscher-Ohlin all make strong cases for unrestricted free trade. In contrast, the mercantilist doctrine and, to a lesser extent, the new trade theory can be interpreted to support government intervention to promote exports through subsidies and to limit imports through tariffs and quotas.

In explaining the pattern of international trade, the second objective of this chapter, we have seen that with the exception of mercantilism, which is silent on this issue, the different theories offer largely complementary explanations. Although no one theory may explain the apparent pattern of international trade, taken together, the theory of comparative advantage, the Heckscher-Ohlin theory, the product life-cycle theory, the new trade theory, and Porter's theory of national competitive advantage do suggest which factors are important. Comparative advantage tells us that productivity differences are important; Heckscher-Ohlin tells us that factor endowments matter; the product life-cycle theory tells us that where a new product is introduced is important; the new trade theory tells us that increasing returns to specialization and first-mover advantages matter; and Porter tells us that all these factors may be important insofar as they impact the four components of the national diamond.

The chapter made these major points

1. Mercantilists argued that it was in a country's best interests to run a balance-of-trade surplus. They viewed trade as a zero-sum game, in which one country's gains cause losses for other countries.

2. The theory of absolute advantage suggests that countries differ in their ability to produce goods efficiently. The theory suggests that a country should specialize in producing goods in areas where it has an absolute advantage and import goods in areas where other countries have absolute advantages.

3. The theory of comparative advantage suggests that it makes sense for a country to specialize in producing those goods that it can produce most efficiently, while buying goods that it can produce relatively less efficiently from other countries—even if that means buying goods from other countries that it could produce more efficiently itself.

4. The theory of comparative advantage suggests that unrestricted free trade brings about increased world production; that is, that trade is a positive-sum game.

5. The theory of comparative advantage also suggests that opening a country to free trade stimulates economic growth, which creates dynamic gains from trade. The empirical evidence seems to be consistent with this claim.

6. The Heckscher-Ohlin theory argues that the pattern of international trade is determined by differences in factor endowments. It predicts that countries will export those goods that make intensive use of locally abundant factors and will import goods that make intensive use of factors that are locally scarce.

7. The product life-cycle theory suggests that trade patterns are influenced by where a new product is introduced. In an increasingly integrated global economy, the product life-cycle theory seems to be less predictive than it was between 1945 and 1975.

8. New trade theory states that trade allows a nation to specialize in the production of certain goods, attaining scale economies and lowering the costs of producing those goods, while buying goods that it does not produce from other nations that are similarly specialized. By this mechanism, the variety of goods available to consumers in each nation is increased, while the average costs of those goods should fall.

9. New trade theory also states that in those industries where substantial economies of scale imply that the world market will profitably support only a few firms, countries may predominate in the export of certain products simply because they had a firm that was a first mover in that industry.

10. Some new trade theorists have promoted the idea of strategic trade policy. The argument is that government, by the sophisticated and judicious use of subsidies, might be able to increase the chances of domestic firms becoming first movers in newly emerging industries.

11. Porter's theory of national competitive advantage suggests that the pattern of trade is influenced by four attributes of a nation: (*a*) factor endowments, (*b*) domestic demand conditions, (*c*) relat-

ing and supporting industries, and (*d*) firm strategy, structure, and rivalry.

12. Theories of international trade are important to an individual business firm primarily because they can help the firm decide where to locate its various production activities.

13. Firms involved in international trade can and do exert a strong influence on government policy toward trade. By lobbying government, business firms can promote free trade or trade restrictions.

Critical Discussion Questions

1. Mercantilism is a bankrupt theory that has no place in the modern world. Discuss.

2. Japan is a neo-mercantilist nation. It protects industries where it has no competitive advantage in the world economy, while demanding that other countries open up those markets where Japanese producers have a competitive advantage. Discuss this statement.

3. Unions in developed nations often oppose imports from low-wage countries and advocate trade barriers to protect jobs from what they often characterize as "unfair" import competition. Is such competition "unfair"? Do you think that this argument is in the best interests of (*a*) the unions, (*b*) the people they represent, and/or (*c*) the country as a whole?

4. Drawing on the theory of comparative advantage to support your arguments, outline the case for free trade.

5. What are the potential costs of adopting a free trade regime? Do you think govern-

ments should do anything to reduce these costs? What?

6. Using the new trade theory and Porter's theory of national competitive advantage, outline the case for government policies that would build national competitive advantage in a particular industry. What kinds of policies would you recommend that the government adopt? Are these policies at variance with the basic free trade philosophy?

7. The world's poorest countries are at a competitive disadvantage in every sector of their economies. They have little to export. They have no capital; their land is of poor quality; they often have too many people given available work opportunities; and they are poorly educated. Free trade cannot possibly be in the interests of such nations! Discuss.

8. In general, policies designed to limit competition from low-cost foreign competitors do not help a country to achieve greater economic growth. Discuss this statement.

Notes

1. H. W. Spiegel, *The Growth of Economic Thought* (Durham, NC: Duke University Press, 1991).

2. G. de Jonquieres, "Mercantilists Are Treading on Thin Ice," *Financial Times*, July 3, 1994, p. 16.

3. Jarl Hagelstam, "Mercantilism Still Influences Practical Trade Policy at the End of the Twentieth Century," *Journal of World Trade*, 1991, pp. 95–105.

4. S. Hollander, *The Economics of David Ricardo* (Buffalo: The University of Toronto Press, 1979).

5. D. Ricardo, *The Principles of Political Economy and Taxation* (Homewood, IL: Irwin, 1967, first published in 1817).

6. For example, R. Dornbusch, S. Fischer, and P. Samuelson, "Comparative Advantage: Trade

and Payments in a Ricardian Model with a Continuum of Goods," *American Economic Review* 67 (December 1977), pp. 823–39.

7. B. Balassa, "An Empirical Demonstration of Classic Comparative Cost Theory," *Review of Economics and Statistics*, 1963, pp. 231–38.

8. See P. R. Krugman, "Is Free Trade Passé?" *Journal of Economic Perspectives* 1 (Fall 1987), pp. 131–44.

9. P. Samuelson, "The Gains from International Trade Once Again," *Economic Journal* 72 (1962), pp. 820–29.

10. For example, J. D. Sachs and A. Warner, "Economic Reform and the Process of Global Integration," *Brookings Papers on Economic Activity*,

1995, pp. 1–96; J. A. Frankel and D. Romer, "Does Trade Cause Growth?" *American Economic Review* 89, no. 3 (June 1999), pp. 379–99; and D. Dollar and A. Kraay, "Trade, Growth and Poverty," Working Paper, Development Research Group, World Bank, June 2001. Also, for an accessible discussion of the relationship between free trade and economic growth, see T. Taylor, "The Truth about Globalization," *Public Interest*, Spring 2002, pp. 24–44.

11. Sachs and Warner, "Economic Reform and the Process of Global Integration."

12. Ibid., pp. 35–36.

13. Frankel and Romer, "Does Trade Cause Growth?"

14. A recent skeptical review of the empirical work on the relationship between trade and growth questions these results. See Francisco Rodriguez and Dani Rodrik, "Trade Policy and Economic Growth: A Skeptics Guide to the Cross-National Evidence," *National Bureau of Economic Research*, Working Paper Series Number 7081, April 1999. Even these authors, however, cannot find any evidence that trade hurts economic growth or income levels.

15. B. Ohlin, *Interregional and International Trade* (Cambridge: Harvard University Press, 1933). For a summary, see R. W. Jones and J. P. Neary, "The Positive Theory of International Trade," in *Handbook of International Economics*, R. W. Jones and P. B. Kenen, eds. (Amsterdam: North Holland, 1984).

16. W. Leontief, "Domestic Production and Foreign Trade: The American Capital Position Re-Examined," *Proceedings of the American Philosophical Society* 97 (1953), pp. 331–49.

17. R. M. Stern and K. Maskus, "Determinants of the Structure of U.S. Foreign Trade," *Journal of International Economics* 11 (1981), pp. 207–44.

18. See H. P. Bowen, E. E. Leamer, and L. Sveikayskas, "Multicountry, Multifactor Tests of the Factor Abundance Theory," *American Economic Review* 77 (1987), pp. 791–809.

19. D. Trefler, "The Case of the Missing Trade and Other Mysteries," *American Economic Review* 85 (December 1995), pp. 1029–46.

20. D. R. Davis and D. E. Weinstein, "An Account of Global Factor Trade," *American Economic Review*, December 2001, pp. 1423–52.

21. R. Vernon, "International Investments and International Trade in the Product Life Cycle," *Quarterly Journal of Economics*, May 1966, pp. 190–207, and R. Vernon and L. T. Wells, *The Economic Environment of International Business*, 4th ed. (Englewood Cliffs, NJ: Prentice Hall, 1986).

22. For a good summary of this literature, see E. Helpman and P. Krugman, *Market Structure and Foreign Trade: Increasing Returns, Imperfect Competition, and the International Economy* (Boston: MIT Press, 1985). Also see P. Krugman, "Does the New Trade Theory Require a New Trade Policy?" *World Economy* 15, no. 4, (1992), pp. 423–41; and P. R. Krugman, "Increasing Returns, Imperfect Competition and the Positive Theory of International Trade," in *Handbook of International Economics*, vol. 3, G. M. Grossman and K. Rogoff, eds. (Amsterdam: North-Holland, 1997), pp. 1243–77.

23. A. A. Alchian, "Reliability of Progress Curves in Airframe Production," *Econometrica* 31 (1963), pp. 679–93.

24. M. B. Lieberman and D. B. Montgomery, "First-Mover Advantages," *Strategic Management Journal* 9 (Summer 1988), pp. 41–58, and W. T. Robinson and Sungwook Min, "Is the First to Market the First to Fail?" *Journal of Marketing Research* 29 (2002), pp. 120–28.

25. J. R. Tybout, "Plant and Firm Level Evidence on New Trade Theories," *National Bureau of Economic Research*, Working Paper Series Number 8418, August 2001. Paper available at http://www.nber.org.

26. A. D. Chandler, *Scale and Scope* (New York: Free Press, 1990).

27. Krugman, "Does the New Trade Theory Require a New Trade Policy?"

28. M. E. Porter, *The Competitive Advantage of Nations* (New York: Free Press, 1990). For a good review of this book, see R. M. Grant, "Porter's Competitive Advantage of Nations: An Assessment," *Strategic Management Journal* 12 (1991), pp. 535–48.

29. B. Kogut, ed., *Country Competitiveness: Technology and the Organizing of Work* (New York: Oxford University Press, 1993).

30. Porter, *The Competitive Advantage of Nations*, p. 121.

31. Lieberman and Montgomery, "First-Mover Advantages." See also Robinson and Min, "Is the First to Market the First to Fail?"; W. Boulding and M. Christen, "First Mover Disadvantage," *Harvard Business Review*, October 2001, pp. 20–21; and R. Agarwal and M. Gort, "First Mover Advantage and the Speed of Competitive Entry," *Journal of Law and Economics* 44 (2001), pp. 131–59.

32. C. A. Hamilton, "Building Better Machine Tools," *Journal of Commerce*, October 30, 1991, p. 8, and "Manufacturing Trouble," *The Economist*, October 12, 1991, p. 71.

Research Task | globalEDGE™ globaledge.msu.edu

Use the globalEDGE™ site to complete the following exercises:

1. *WTO's International Trade Statistics* is an annual report that provides comprehensive, comparable, and up-to-date statistics on trade in merchandise and commercial services. This report allows for an assessment of world trade flows by country, region, and main product groups or service categories. Using the most recent statistics available, identify the top five countries that lead in the export and import of merchandise, respectively.

2. Your company is interested in importing Australian wine to the United States. As part of the initial analysis, you want to identify the strengths of the Australian wine industry. Provide a short description of the current status of Australian wine exports by variety, and a list of the top importing countries of Australian wines.

Closing Case

The Rise of the Indian Software Industry

As a relatively poor country, India is not normally thought off as a nation capable of building a major presence in a high-technology industry, such as computer software. In little over a decade, however, the Indian software industry has astounded its skeptics and emerged from obscurity to become an important force in the global software industry. Between 1991–92 and 2001–02, sales of Indian software companies grew at a compound rate in excess of 50 percent annually. In 1991–92, the industry had sales totaling $388 million. By 2002 they were around $8 billion. By the early 2000s, more than 900 software companies in India employed 200,000 software engineers, the third largest concentration of such talent in the world.

Much of this growth was powered by exports. In 1985, Indian software exports were worth less than $10 million. They surged to $1.8 billion in 1997 and hit a record $6.2 billion in 2002, with some two-thirds of those exports going to the United States. The future looks very bright. Powered by continued export-led growth, India's National Association of Software and Service Companies projects that total software revenues generated by Indian companies will hit $21 billion by 2008. As a testament to this growth, many foreign software companies are now investing heavily in Indian software development operations including Microsoft, IBM, Oracle, and Computer Associates, the four largest U.S.-based software houses. Equally significantly, two out of every five global companies now source their software services from India.

Most of the current growth of the Indian software industry has been based on contract or project-based work for foreign clients. Many Indian companies, for example, maintain applications for their clients, convert code, or migrate software from one platform to another. Increasingly, Indian companies are also involved in important development projects for foreign clients. For example, TCS, India's largest software company, has an alliance with Ernst & Young under which TCS will develop and maintain customized software for Ernst & Young's global clients. TCS also has a development alliance with Microsoft under which the company developed a paperless national share depository system for the Indian stock market based on Microsoft's Windows operating system and SQL Server database technology. Indian companies are also moving aggressively into e-commerce projects. From almost zero in 1997, e-commerce or e-business projects now account for about 10 percent of all software development and service work in India and are projected to reach 20 percent within two years.

The Indian software industry has emerged despite a poor information technology infrastructure. In 2000, India had just five personal computers per 1,000 people, compared to 588 per 1,000 in the United States, 32 telephone lines per 1,000 people compared to 700 per 1,000 in the United States, and Internet users numbered around 5 million, compared to almost 100 million in the United States. But sales of personal computers are starting to take off, and the rapid growth of mobile telephones in India's main cities is to some extent compensating for the lack of fixed telephone lines.

In explaining the success of their industry, India's software entrepreneurs point to a number of factors. Although the general level of education in India is low, India's important middle class is highly educated and its top educational institutions are world class. Also, India has always emphasized engineering. Another great plus from an international perceptive is that English is the working language throughout much of middle-class India—a remnant from the days of the British raja. Then there is the wage rate. American software engineers are increasingly scarce, and the basic salary has been driven up to one of the highest for any occupational group in the country, with programmers earning $90,000 per year. Programmers in India, in contrast, earn about $5,800 per year, which is very low by international standards but high by Indian standards. Salaries for programmers are rising rapidly in India, but so is productivity. In 1992, productivity was around $21,000 per software engineer. By 2000, the figure had risen to $65,000. As a consequence of these factors, in 2002 work done in India for U.S. software companies amounted to $25 to $35 an hour, compared to $75 to $100 per hour for software development done in the United States.

Another factor helping India is that satellite communications have removed distance as an obstacle to doing business for foreign clients. Because software is nothing more than a stream of zeros and ones, it can be transported at the speed of light and negligible cost to any point in the world. In a world of instant communication, India's geographical position between Europe and the United States has given it a time zone advantage. Indian companies have been able to exploit the rapidly expanding international market for outsourced software services, including the expanding market for remote maintenance. Indian engineers can fix software bugs, upgrade systems, or process data overnight while their users in Western companies are asleep.

To maintain their competitive position, Indian software companies are now investing heavily in training and leading-edge programming skills. They have also been enthusiastic adopters of international quality standards, particularly ISO 9000 certification. Indian companies are also starting to make forays into the application and shrink-wrapped software business, primarily with applications aimed at the domestic market. It may only be a matter of time, however, before Indian companies start to compete head to head with companies such as Microsoft, Oracle, PeopleSoft, and SAP in the applications business.

Case Discussion Questions

1. To what extent does the theory of comparative advantage explain the rise of the Indian software industry?

2. To what extent does the Heckscher-Ohlin theory explain the rise of the Indian software industry?

3. Use Michael Porter's diamond to analyze the rise of the Indian software industry. Does this analysis help explain the rise of this industry?

4. Which of the above theories—comparative advantage, Heckscher-Ohlin, or Porter's—gives the best explanation of the rise of the Indian software industry? Why?

Sources: P. Taylor, "Poised for Global Growth," *Financial Times: India's Software Industry*, December 3, 1997, pp. 1, 8; P. Taylor, "An Industry on the Up and Up," *Financial Times: India's Software Industry*, December 3, 1997, p. 3; Krishna Guha, "Strategic Alliances with Global Partners," *Financial Times: India's Software Industry*, December 3, 1997, p. 6; "Indian SW Industry to Touch $13 Billion in 2001–02," *Computers Today*, December 15, 2000, pp. 14–17; World Bank, *World Development Indicators, 2002*; "America's Pain, India's Gain," *The Economist*, January 11, 2003, p. 57; and S. Rai, "India Is Regaining Contracts with the United States," *New York Times*, December 25, 2002, p. W1.

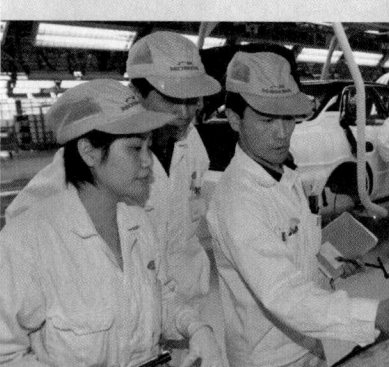

Chapter 5

The Political Economy of International Trade

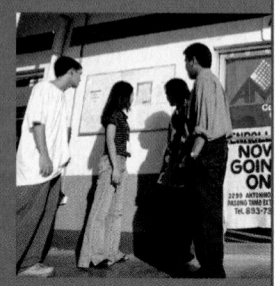

Introduction
Instruments of Trade Policy
   Tariffs
   Subsidies
   Import Quotas and Voluntary Export
   Restraints
   Local Content Requirements
   Administrative Policies
   Antidumping Policies
The Case for Government Intervention
   Political Arguments for Intervention
   Economic Arguments for Intervention
The Revised Case for Free Trade
   Retaliation and Trade War
   Domestic Politics
Development of the World Trading
System
   From Smith to the Great Depression
   1947–1979: GATT, Trade Liberalization,
   and Economic Growth
   1980–1993: Disturbing Trends
   The Uruguay Round and the World
   Trade Organization
   WTO: Experience to Date
   The Future of the WTO: Unresolved
   Issues and the Doha Round
Focus on Managerial Implications
   Trade Barriers and Firm Strategy
   Policy Implications
Chapter Summary
Critical Discussion Questions
Closing Case: Is a Tax Break an Export
Subsidy?

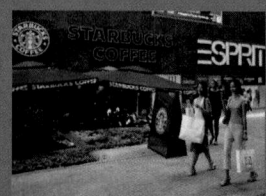

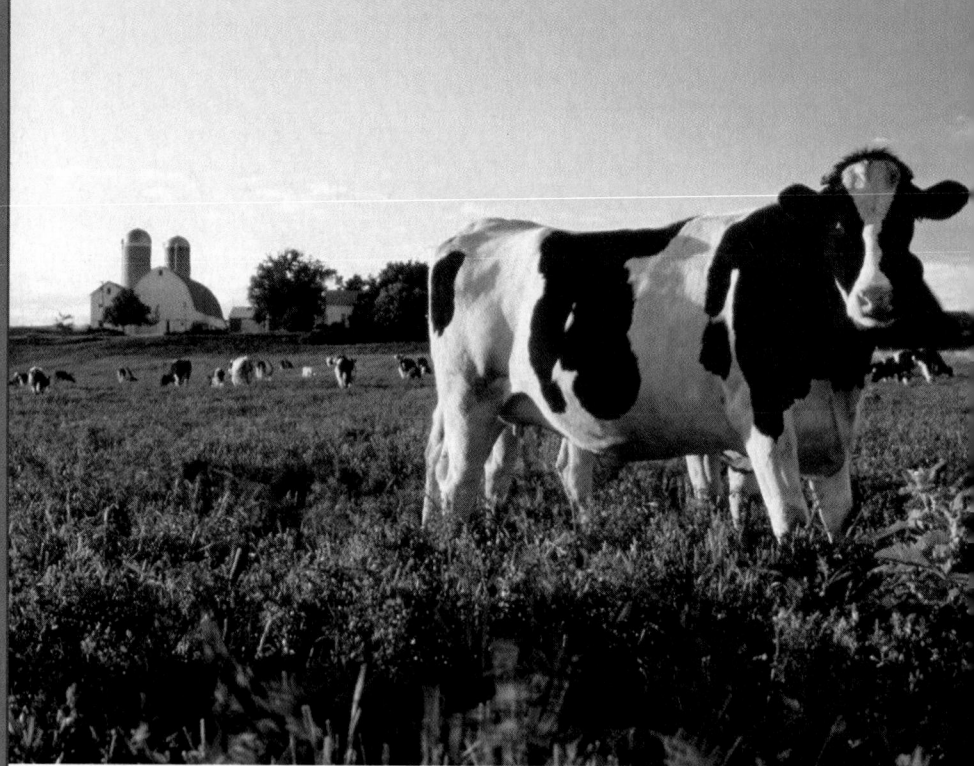

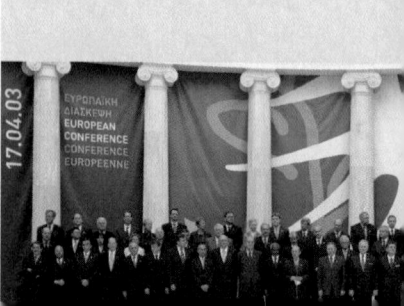

Agricultural Subsidies and Development

For decades the rich countries of the developed world have lavished subsidies on their farmers, typically guaranteeing them a minimum price for the products they produce. The aim has been to protect farmers in the developed world from the potentially devastating effects of low commodity prices. Although they are small in numbers, farmers tend to be politically active, and winning their support is important for many politicians. The politicians often claim that their motive is to preserve a historic rural lifestyle, and see subsidies as a way of doing this.

This logic has resulted in financial support estimated to exceed $300 billion a year for farmers in rich nations. The European Union, for example, has set a minimum price for butter of euros 3,282 per ton. If the world price for butter falls below that amount, the EU will make up the difference to farmers in the form of a direct payment or subsidy. In total, EU dairy farmers receive roughly $15 billion a year in subsidies to produce milk and butter, or about $2 a day for every cow in the EU—a figure that is more than the daily income of half the world's population.

The EU is not alone in this practice. In the United States, subsidies are given to a wide range of crop and dairy farmers. Typical is the guarantee that U.S. cotton farmers will receive at least $0.70 for every pound of cotton they harvest. If world cotton prices fall below this level, the government makes up the difference, writing a check to the farmers. In 2001, U.S. cotton farmers received some $3.4 billion in subsidy checks.

One consequence of such subsidies is to create surplus production. That surplus is then sold on world markets, where the extra supply depresses prices, making it much harder for producers in the developing world to sell their output at a profit. For example, EU subsidies to sugar beet producers amount to more than $4,000 an acre. With a minimum price guarantee that exceeds their costs of production, EU farmers plant more sugar beet than the EU market can absorb. The surplus, some 6 million tons per year, is dumped on the world market, where it depresses world prices. Estimates suggest that if the EU stopped dumping its surplus production on world markets, sugar prices would increase by 20 percent. That would make a big difference for developing nations such as South Africa, which exports roughly half of its 2.6 million tons of annual sugar production. With a 20 percent rise in world prices, the South African economy would reap about $40 million more from sugar exports.

American subsidies to cotton farmers have a similar effect. Brazilian officials contend that by creating surplus production in the United States that is then dumped on the world market, U.S. cotton subsidies have depressed world prices for cotton by more than 50 percent since the mid-1990s. Low cotton prices cost Brazil some $640 million in lost export earnings in 2001. India, another big cotton producer, has estimated that U.S. cotton subsidies reduced its export revenue from cotton by some $1 billion in 2001. According to the charitable organization Oxfam, the U.S. government spends about three times as much on cotton subsidies as it does on foreign aid for all of Africa. In 2001, the African nation of Mali lost about $43 million in export revenues due to plunging cotton prices, significantly more than the $37 million in foreign aid it received from the United States that year.

Overall, the United Nations has estimated that while developed nations give about $50 billion a year in foreign aid to the developing world, agricultural subsidies cost producers in the developing world some $50 billion in lost export revenues, effectively canceling out the effect of the aid. As one UN official has noted, "It's no good building up roads, clinics, and infrastructure in poor areas if you don't give them access to markets and engines for growth." Similarly, Oxfam has taken the unusual position for a charity of coming out strongly in support of the elimination of agricultural subsidies and price supports to developing world producers. By increasing world prices and shifting production from high-cost, protected producers in Europe and America to lower-cost producers in the developing world, Oxfam claims that consumers in rich nations would benefit from lower domestic prices and the elimination of taxes required to pay for the subsidies, while producers in the developing world would gain from fairer competition, expanded markets, and higher world prices. In the long run, the greater economic growth that would occur in agriculturally dependent developing nations would be to everyone's benefit.

Sources: E. L. Andrews. "Rich Nations Are Criticized for Enforcing Trade Barriers," *New York Times,* September 30, 2002, p. A1; R. Thurrow and G. Winestock, "Bittersweet: How an Addiction to Sugar Subsidies Hurts Development," *Wall Street Journal,* September 16, 2002, p. A1; and Oxfam, "Milking the CAP," Oxfam Briefing Paper Number 34, 2002, http://www.maketradefair.com/assets/english/DairyPaper.pdf.

Introduction

Our review of the classical trade theories of Smith, Ricardo, and Heckscher-Ohlin in Chapter 4 showed us that in a world without trade barriers, trade patterns are determined by the relative productivity of different factors of production in different countries. Countries will specialize in products that they can make most efficiently, while importing products that they can produce less efficiently. Chapter 4 also laid out the intellectual case for free trade. Remember, **free trade** refers to a situation where a government does not attempt to restrict what its citizens can buy from another country or what they can sell to another country. As we saw in Chapter 4, the theories of Smith, Ricardo, and Heckscher-Ohlin predict that the consequences of free trade include both static economic gains (because free trade supports a higher level of domestic consumption and more efficient utilization of resources) and dynamic economic gains (because free trade stimulates economic growth and the creation of wealth).

In this chapter we look at the political reality of international trade. While many nations are nominally committed to free trade, they tend to intervene in international trade to protect the interests of politically important groups. The opening case illustrates the nature of such political realities. The case describes how politicians in both the European Union and the United States have lavished subsidies on farmers, partly in an attempt to win votes. This effectively raises the price of farm products to domestic consumers and stimulates excess production of farm products in the EU and United States. The excess production is then dumped on world markets, depressing world prices and the export earnings of farmers in developing nations. Subsidies to the farm sector in the developed world have distorted international trade flows and helped to retard the economic growth of agriculturally dependent developing nations.

In this chapter, we explore the political and economic reasons that governments have for intervening in international trade. When governments intervene, they often do so by restricting imports of goods and services into their nation, while adopting policies that promote exports. Normally their motives are to protect domestic producers and jobs from foreign competition while increasing the foreign market for products of domestic producers. However, in recent years, "social" issues have intruded into the decision-making calculus. In the United States, for example, there is a movement to try to ban imports of goods from countries that do not abide by the same labor, health, and environmental regulations as the United States.

We start this chapter by describing the range of policy instruments that governments use to intervene in international trade. This is followed by a detailed review of the various political and economic motives that governments have for intervention. In the third section of this chapter we consider how the case for free trade stands up in view of the various justifications given for government intervention in international trade. Then we look at the emergence of the modern international trading system, which is based on the General Agreement on Tariffs and Trade (GATT) and its successor, the World Trade Organization (WTO). The GATT and WTO are the creations of a series of multinational treaties. The most recent was completed in 1995, involved more than 120 countries, and resulted in the creation of the WTO. The purpose of these treaties has been to lower barriers to the free flow of goods and services between nations. Like the GATT before it, the WTO promotes free trade by limiting the ability of national governments to adopt policies that restrict imports into their nations. In the final section of this chapter, we discuss the implications of this material for business practice.

Instruments of Trade Policy

Trade policy uses seven main instruments: tariffs, subsidies, import quotas, voluntary export restraints, local content requirements, administrative policies, and antidumping duties. Tariffs are the oldest and simplest instrument of trade policy. As we shall see later in this chapter, they are also the instrument that GATT and WTO have been most successful in limiting. A fall in tariff barriers in recent decades has been accompanied by a rise in nontariff barriers, such as subsidies, quotas, voluntary export restraints, and antidumping duties.

Tariffs

A **tariff** is a tax levied on imports. Tariffs fall into two categories. **Specific tariffs** are levied as a fixed charge for each unit of a good imported (for example, $3 per barrel of oil). **Ad valorem tariffs** are levied as a proportion of the value of the imported good. The European Union has imposed such a tariff on imports of bananas from Latin America; the tariff amounts to 15 to 20 percent by value on the first 2.5 million tons of imports of bananas from Latin America.

A tariff raises the cost of imported products. In most cases, tariffs are put in place to protect domestic producers from foreign competition. In March 2002, when the U.S. steel industry was losing market share to foreign steelmakers, the U.S. government placed a tariff ranging from 8 to 30 percent by value on a range of steel imports. While the principal objective of most tariffs is to protect domestic producers and employees against foreign competition, they also raise revenue for the government. Until the income tax was introduced, for example, the U.S. government raised most of its revenues from tariffs.

The important thing to understand about a tariff is who suffers and who gains. The government gains, because the tariff increases government revenues. Domestic producers gain, because the tariff affords them some protection against foreign competitors by increasing the cost of imported foreign goods. Consumers lose because they must pay more for certain imports. Thus, following the imposition of the steel tariff in March 2002, a number of U.S. steel consumers, ranging from appliance makers to automobile companies, objected that the steel tariffs would raise their costs of production and make it more difficult for them to compete in the global marketplace. Whether the gains to the government and domestic producers exceed the loss to consumers depends on various factors such as the amount of the tariff, the importance of the imported good to domestic consumers, the number of jobs saved in the protected industry, and so on.

Although detailed consideration of these issues is beyond the scope of this book, two conclusions can be derived from a more advanced analysis.[1] First, tariffs are unambiguously pro-producer and anti-consumer. While they protect producers from foreign competitors, this restriction of supply also raises domestic prices. For example, a study by Japanese economists calculated that tariffs on imports of foodstuffs, cosmetics, and chemicals into Japan in 1989 cost the average Japanese consumer about $890 per year in the form of higher prices.[2] Almost all studies that have looked at this issue find that import tariffs impose significant costs on domestic consumers in the form of higher prices.[3] For another example, see the accompanying Country Focus, which looks at the cost to U.S. consumers of tariffs on imports into the United States.

Second, tariffs reduce the overall efficiency of the world economy. They reduce efficiency because a protective tariff encourages domestic firms to produce products at home that, in theory, could be produced more efficiently abroad. The consequence is an inefficient utilization of resources. For example, tariffs on the importation of rice into South Korea have caused the land of South Korean rice farmers to be used in an unproductive manner. It would make more sense for the South Koreans to purchase their rice from lower-cost foreign producers and to utilize the land now employed in rice production in some other way, such as growing foodstuffs that cannot be produced more efficiently elsewhere or for residential and industrial purposes.

Subsidies

A **subsidy** is a government payment to a domestic producer. Subsidies take many forms including cash grants, low-interest loans, tax breaks, and government equity participation in domestic firms. By lowering production costs, subsidies help domestic producers

Country Focus

The Costs of Protectionism in the United States

The United States likes to think of itself as a nation committed to unrestricted free trade. In their negotiations with trading partners such as China, the European Union, and Japan, U.S. trade representatives can often be heard claiming that the U.S. economy is an open one with few import tariffs. However, while it is true that tariffs on the importation of goods into the United States are low when compared to those found in many other nations, they still exist. One study concluded that these tariffs cost U.S. consumers about $32 billion per year during the 1980s. A more recent study suggested that in 1996, import protection cost U.S. consumers $223.4 billion in higher prices.

Gary Hufbauer and Kim Elliott of the Institute for International Economics undertook the earlier study. They looked at the effect of import tariffs on economic activity in 21 industries with annual sales of $1 billion or more that the U.S. protected most heavily from foreign competition. The industries included apparel, ceramic tiles, luggage, and sugar. In most of these industries, import tariffs had originally been imposed to protect U.S. firms and employees from the effects of low-cost foreign competitors. The typical reasoning behind the tariffs was that without such protection, U.S. firms in these industries would go out of business and substantial unemployment would result. So the tariffs were presented as having positive effects for the U.S. economy, not to mention the U.S. Treasury, which benefited from the associated revenues.

The study found, however, that while these import tariffs saved about 200,000 jobs in the protected industries that would otherwise have been lost to foreign competition, they also cost U.S. consumers about $32 billion per year in the form of higher prices. Even when the proceeds from the tariff that accrued to the U.S. Treasury were added into the equation, the total cost to the nation of this protectionism still amounted to $10.2 billion per year, or over $50,000 per job saved.

The two economists argued that these figures understated the tariffs' true cost to the nation. They maintained that by making imports less competitive with American-made products, tariffs allowed domestic producers to charge more than they might otherwise because they did not have to compete with low-priced imports. By dampening competition, these tariffs removed an incentive for firms in the protected industries to become more efficient, thereby retarding economic progress. Further, the study's authors noted that if the tariffs had not been imposed, some of the $32 billion freed up every year would have been spent on other goods and services, and growth in these areas would have created additional jobs, thereby offsetting the loss of 200,000 jobs in the protected industries.

In a 1999 study, Howard Wall used a different methodology to provide updated estimates on the impact of protectionism on trade volume and prices. Wall found that while the United States imported more than $723 billion in merchandise from countries outside of NAFTA in 1996, it would have imported over $111 billion more if it had a policy of pure free trade. (NAFTA is the North American Free Trade Agreement signed by Canada, Mexico, and the United States.) Wall concluded that the higher prices resulting from import protection cost U.S. consumers some $223.4 billion in 1996, or 3.4 percent of GDP. However, Wall's estimates also suggest that the United States suffered from trade barriers in other countries. While the United States exported $499 billion of goods in 1996, according to Wall, it would have exported an additional $130 billion of goods to non-NAFTA countries had those countries not had trade barriers.

Sources: G. Hufbauer and K. A. Elliott, *Measuring the Costs of Protectionism in the United States* (Washington, DC: Institute for International Economics, 1993), and H. J. Wall, "Using the Gravity Model to Estimate the Costs of Protectionism," *Federal Reserve Bank of St. Louis Review,* January–February 1999, pp. 33–40.

in two ways: They help producers compete against foreign imports, and subsidies help them gain export markets.

As discussed in the opening case, agriculture tends to be one of the largest beneficiaries of subsidies in most countries. At the beginning of the 21st century, in Japan, agricultural subsidies amounted to a staggering 62 percent of the value of gross farm receipts, or $21,000 per farmer. In the European Union, where the Common Agricultural Policy (CAP) has long provided subsidies to help farmers stay in business, subsidies amount to 43 percent of the value of gross farm receipts, or $19,000 per farmer. In the United States, subsidies were 22 percent of gross farm receipts, which again amounts to $19,000 per farmer. In Canada, subsidies were 18 percent of gross farm receipts, or $8,000 per farmer.[4] In 2002, the European Union was paying $43 billion annually in farm subsidies. Not to be outdone, in May 2002 President George W. Bush signed into law a bill that contained subsidies of over $180 billion for U.S. farmers spread out over a number of years.

Outside of agriculture, subsidies are much lower, but they are still significant. One study found that government subsidies to manufacturing industries in most industrialized countries amounted to between 2 percent and 3.5 percent of the value of industrial output. The average rate of subsidy in the United States was 0.5 percent, in Japan it was 1 percent, and in Europe it ranged from just below 2 percent in Great Britain and West Germany to as much as 6 to 7 percent in Sweden and Ireland.[5] These figures, however, almost certainly underestimate the true value of subsidies, because the numbers are based only on cash grants and ignore other kinds of subsidies (e.g., equity participation or low-interest loans).

The main gains from subsidies accrue to domestic producers, whose international competitiveness is increased as a result of them. Advocates of strategic trade policy (which, as you will recall from Chapter 4, is an outgrowth of the new trade theory) favor subsidies to help domestic firms achieve a dominant position in those industries where economies of scale are important and the world market is not large enough to profitably support more than a few firms (e.g., aerospace, semiconductors). According to this argument, subsidies can help a firm achieve a first-mover advantage in an emerging industry (just as U.S. government subsidies, in the form of substantial R&D grants, allegedly helped Boeing). If this is achieved, further gains to the domestic economy arise from the employment and tax revenues that a major global company can generate.

Subsidies must be paid for. Governments typically pay for subsidies by taxing individuals. Therefore, whether subsidies generate national benefits that exceed their national costs is debatable. In practice, many subsidies are not that successful at increasing the international competitiveness of domestic producers. Rather, they tend to protect the inefficient and promote excess production. Agricultural subsidies (1) allow inefficient farmers to stay in business, (2) encourage countries to overproduce heavily subsidized agricultural products, (3) encourage countries to produce products that could be grown more cheaply elsewhere and imported, and, therefore, (4) reduce international trade in agricultural products. One recent study estimated that if advanced countries abandoned subsidies to farmers, global trade in agricultural products would be 50 percent higher and the world as a whole would be better off to the tune of $160 billion.[6] This increase in wealth arises from the more efficient use of agricultural land.

Import Quotas and Voluntary Export Restraints

An **import quota** is a direct restriction on the quantity of some good that may be imported into a country. The restriction is usually enforced by issuing import licenses to a group of individuals or firms. For example, the United States has a quota on cheese imports. The only firms allowed to import cheese are certain trading companies, each of which is allocated the right to import a maximum number of pounds of cheese each year. In some cases, the right to sell is given directly to the governments of exporting countries. This is the case for sugar and textile imports in the United States.

A variant on the import quota is the voluntary export restraint (VER). A **voluntary export restraint** is a quota on trade imposed by the exporting country, typically at the request of the importing country's government. One of the most famous examples is the limitation on auto exports to the United States enforced by Japanese automobile producers in 1981. A response to direct pressure from the U.S. government, this VER limited Japanese imports to no more than 1.68 million vehicles per year. The agreement was revised in 1984 to allow 1.85 million Japanese vehicles per year. The agreement was allowed to lapse in 1985, but the Japanese government indicated its intentions at that time to continue to restrict exports to the United States to 1.85 million vehicles per year.[7]

Foreign producers agree to VERs because they fear far more damaging punitive tariffs or import quotas might follow if they do not. Agreeing to a VER is seen as a way of making the best of a bad situation by appeasing protectionist pressures in a country.

As with tariffs and subsidies, both import quotas and VERs benefit domestic producers by limiting import competition. As with all restrictions on trade, quotas do not benefit consumers. An import quota or VER always raises the domestic price of an imported good. When imports are limited to a low percentage of the market by a quota or VER, the price is bid up for that limited foreign supply. In the case of the automobile industry, for example, the VER increased the price of the limited supply of Japanese imports. According to a study by the U.S. Federal Trade Commission, the automobile industry VER cost U.S. consumers about $1 billion per year between 1981 and 1985. That $1 billion per year went to Japanese producers in the form of higher prices.[8] The extra profit that producers make when supply is artificially limited by an import quota is referred to as a **quota rent.**

If a domestic industry lacks the capacity to meet demand, an import quota can raise prices for *both* the domestically produced and the imported good. This happened in the U.S. sugar industry, where an import quota has long limited the amount foreign producers can sell in the U.S. market. According to one study, as a result of import quotas the price of sugar in the United States has been as much as 40 percent greater than the world price.[9] These higher prices have translated into greater profits for U.S. sugar producers, who have lobbied politicians to keep the lucrative agreement. They argue U.S. jobs in the sugar industry will be lost to foreign producers if the quota system is scrapped.

Another industry that has long operated with import quotas is the textile industry, which has a complex set of multinational agreements that govern the amount one country can export to others. In this industry, quotas on imports into the United States have restricted the supply of certain apparel products and increased their price by as much as 70 percent.[10] Quotas also encourage firms to engage in strategic actions designed to circumvent quotas. The accompanying Management Focus looks at how one company, Hong Kong-based Esquel, has altered the geographic distribution of its production system to circumvent quotas on the importation of certain textile products into the United States. The United States is not alone in imposing quotas on textile imports. Most other developed nations have similar quotas. Under a World Trade Organization agreement struck in 1995, many of the quotas on textile products are scheduled to be phased out by 2005.

Local Content Requirements

A **local content requirement** is a requirement that some specific fraction of a good be produced domestically. The requirement can be expressed either in physical terms (e.g., 75 percent of component parts for this product must be produced locally) or in value terms (e.g., 75 percent of the value of this product must be produced locally). Local content regulations have been widely used by developing countries to shift their manufacturing base from the simple assembly of products whose parts are manufactured elsewhere into the local manufacture of component parts. They have also been used in developed countries to try to protect local jobs and industry from foreign competition. For example, a little-known law in the United States, the Buy America Act, specifies that government agencies must give preference to American products when putting contracts for equipment out to bid unless the foreign products have a significant price advantage. The law specifies a product as "American" if 51 percent of the materials by value are produced domestically. This amounts to a local content requirement. If a foreign company, or an American one for that matter, wishes to win a contract from a U.S. government agency to provide some equipment, it must ensure that at least 51 percent of the product by value is manufactured in the United States.

Navigating around Import Quotas

The Hong Kong–based Esquel Group, founded in 1976, is the world's largest manufacturer of men's cotton shirts, with annual sales of about $500 million. Esquel produces about 48 million shirts and 5 million pairs of pants a year. Its customers include the premier brands in the United States—Polo Ralph Lauren, Tommy Hilfiger, Brooks Brothers, Hugo Boss, Nordstrom, Eddie Bauer, Abercrombie and Fitch, and Lands' End. Soon after it began production, Esquel found its growth opportunities limited by Hong Kong's quota rights. A quota right is a right to export a prespecified amount of a certain product into a country. Hong Kong's total quota right for shirts in 2000 was 36 million, meaning that it could export 36 million shirts to other countries. With growth limited by restrictive quota rights, Esquel switched production to mainland China, which at the time did not have any quota restrictions. In no time, Esquel was shipping 12 million shirts per year from China to Europe and the United States. However, as Chinese textile products began to grab an ever-larger share of the European and U.S. markets, domestic U.S. and European producers lobbied for and got quotas imposed on imports from China. This meant it was time for Esquel to shift production location yet again, this time to Malaysia, which had quota rights that exceeded domestic production. Esquel quickly built up a large export position in men's and women's shirts, but, as Malaysian textiles began to make inroads into the U.S. market, the United States placed tight quota restrictions on Malaysia too. So Esquel made another shift in production location, this time to Mauritius, an island in the Indian Ocean that had unused quota rights.

Mauritius is so far from anywhere that under normal circumstances, no one would think of locating major production facilities there, but its unused quota rights made it a valuable location. Currently, Esquel grows extra-long staple cotton in western China and spins the yarn there and in Guangdong in southern China. It then loads the fiber and accessories on boats to Mauritius, where the materials are assembled into products for the United States and Europe. One drawback with Mauritius, apart from its geographic isolation, is that although it is rich in quota rights, it is short in labor to exploit those rights. So Esquel imported 2,000 factory workers from China to Mauritius to make its textile products.

This is not the last word in Esquel's efforts to exploit quota rights. Under the 1994 North American Free Trade Agreement, Mexico has quota-free and duty-free access to the U.S. market. Under another law, Caribbean countries have unlimited access to the U.S. apparel market for fabric made and woven in the United States. Esquel has yet to take advantage of the Mexican opening, although it is weighing its options, but it has already taken advantage of the Caribbean opening. The company built a plant in Jamaica, and, finding the local labor inadequate, imported 700 workers from China to staff the plant. Next stop is Maldives, another island nation in the Indian Ocean with unused quota rights. Esquel plans to produce 200,000 knit shirts and cotton pants in Maldives for export to the United States and Europe, again using imported Chinese labor.

Source: A. Tanzer, "The Great Quota Hustle," *Forbes*, March 6, 2000, pp. 119–25.

From the point of view of a domestic producer of parts, local content regulations provide protection in the same way an import quota does: by limiting foreign competition. The aggregate economic effects are also the same; domestic producers benefit, but the restrictions on imports raise the prices of imported components. In turn, higher prices for imported components are passed on to consumers of the final product in the form of higher final prices. So as with all trade policies, local content regulations tend to benefit producers and not consumers.

Administrative Policies

In addition to the formal instruments of trade policy, governments of all types sometimes use informal or administrative policies to restrict imports and boost exports. **Administrative trade policies** are bureaucratic rules that are designed to make it difficult for imports to enter a country. Some would argue that the Japanese are the masters of this kind of trade barrier. In recent years Japan's formal tariff and nontariff barriers have been among the lowest in the world. However, critics charge that the country's informal administrative barriers to imports more than compensate for this. For example, the Netherlands exports tulip bulbs to almost every country in the world except Japan. In Japan, customs inspectors insist on checking every tulip bulb by cutting it vertically down the middle, and even Japanese ingenuity cannot put them back together again! Federal Express has had a tough time expanding its global express shipping services into Japan because Japanese customs inspectors insist on opening a large proportion of express packages to check for pornography, a process that can delay an "express" package for days. Japan is not the only country that engages in such policies. France required that all imported videotape recorders arrive through a small customs entry point that was both remote and poorly staffed. The resulting delays kept Japanese VCRs out of the French market until a VER agreement was negotiated.[11] As with all instruments of trade policy, administrative instruments benefit producers and hurt consumers, who are denied access to possibly superior foreign products.

Antidumping Policies

In the context of international trade, **dumping** is variously defined as selling goods in a foreign market at below their costs of production, or as selling goods in a foreign market at below their "fair" market value. There is a difference between these two definitions; the "fair" market value of a good is normally judged to be greater than the costs of producing that good because the former includes a "fair" profit margin. Dumping is viewed as a method by which firms unload excess production in foreign markets. Some dumping may be the result of predatory behavior, with producers using substantial profits from their home markets to subsidize prices in a foreign market with a view to driving indigenous competitors out of that market. Once this has been achieved, so the argument goes, the predatory firm can raise prices and earn substantial profits.

An alleged example of dumping occurred in 1997, when two South Korean manufacturers of semiconductors, LG Semicon and Hyundai Electronics, were accused of selling dynamic random access memory chips (DRAMs) in the U.S. market at below their costs of production. This action occurred in the middle of a worldwide glut of chip-making capacity. It was alleged that the firms were trying to unload their excess production in the United States.

Antidumping policies are designed to punish foreign firms that engage in dumping. The ultimate objective is to protect domestic producers from "unfair" foreign competition. Although antidumping policies vary somewhat from country to country, the majority are similar to the policies used in the United States. If a domestic producer believes that a foreign firm is dumping production in the U.S. market, it can file a petition with two government agencies, the Commerce Department and the International Trade Commission. In the Korean DRAM case, Micron Technology, a U.S. manufacturer of DRAMs, filed the petition. The government agencies then investigate the complaint. If they find a complaint has merit, the Commerce Department may impose an antidumping duty on the offending foreign imports (antidumping duties are often called **countervailing duties**). These duties, which represent a special tariff, can be fairly substantial and stay in place for up to five years. For example, after reviewing Micron's complaint, the Commerce Department imposed 9 percent and 4 percent countervailing duties on LG Semicon and Hyundai DRAM chips, respectively.

The Case for Government Intervention

Now that we have reviewed the various instruments of trade policy that governments can use, it is time to look at the case for government intervention in international trade. Arguments for government intervention take two paths—political and economic. Political arguments for intervention are concerned with protecting the interests of certain groups within a nation (normally producers), often at the expense of other groups (normally consumers). Economic arguments for intervention are typically concerned with boosting the overall wealth of a nation (to the benefit of all, both producers and consumers).

Political Arguments for Intervention

Political arguments for government intervention cover a range of issues including protecting jobs, protecting industries deemed important for national security, retaliating to unfair foreign competition, protecting consumers from "dangerous" products, furthering the goals of foreign policy, and protecting the human rights of individuals in exporting countries.

Protecting Jobs and Industries

Perhaps the most common political argument for government intervention is that it is necessary for protecting jobs and industries from foreign competition. Voluntary export restraints that offered some protection to the U.S. automobile, machine tool, and steel industries during the 1980s were motivated by such considerations. Similarly, Japan's quotas on imports of rice are aimed at protecting jobs in that country's agricultural sector. The same motive underlay establishment of the Common Agricultural Policy (CAP) by the European Union. The CAP was designed to protect the jobs of Europe's politically powerful farmers by restricting imports and guaranteeing prices. However, the higher prices that resulted from the CAP have cost Europe's consumers dearly. This is true of most attempts to protect jobs and industries through government intervention. As we saw earlier in the chapter, the VER in the automobile industry raised the price of Japanese imports, at a cost of $1 billion per year to U.S. consumers.

In addition to hurting consumers, trade controls may sometimes hurt the very producers they are intended to protect. The VER agreement in the U.S. machine tool industry turned out to be self-defeating. By limiting Japanese and Taiwanese machine tool imports, the VER raised the prices of machine tools purchased by U.S. manufacturers to levels above those prevailing in the world market. In turn, this raised the capital costs of the U.S. manufacturing industry in general, thereby decreasing its international competitiveness.

National Security

Countries sometimes argue that it is necessary to protect certain industries because they are important for national security. Defense-related industries often get this kind of attention (e.g., aerospace, advanced electronics, semiconductors, etc.). Although not as common as it used to be, this argument is still made. Those in favor of protecting the U.S. semiconductor industry from foreign competition, for example, argue that semiconductors are now such important components of defense products that it would be dangerous to rely primarily on foreign producers for them. In 1986, this argument helped persuade the federal government to support Sematech, a consortium of 14 U.S. semiconductor companies that accounted for 90 percent of the U.S. industry's revenues. Sematech's mission was to conduct joint research into manufacturing techniques that can be parceled out to members. The government saw the venture as so critical that Sematech was specially protected from antitrust laws. Initially, the U.S. government provided Sematech with $100 million per year in subsidies. By the mid-1990s, however, the U.S. semiconductor industry had regained its leading market position, largely through the personal computer boom and demand for microprocessor chips made by Intel. In 1994, the consortium's board voted to seek an end to federal funding, and since 1996 the consortium has been funded entirely by private money.[12]

Retaliation

Some argue that governments should use the threat to intervene in trade policy as a bargaining tool to help open foreign markets and force trading partners to "play by the rules of the game." The U.S. government has used the threat of punitive trade sanctions to try to get the Chinese government to enforce its intellectual property laws. Lax enforcement of these laws had given rise to massive copyright infringements in China that had been costing U.S. companies such as Microsoft hundreds of millions of dollars per years in lost sales revenues. After the United States threatened to impose 100 percent tariffs on a range of Chinese imports, and after harsh words between officials from the two countries, the Chinese agreed to tighter enforcement of intellectual property regulations.[13]

If it works, such a politically motivated rationale for government intervention may liberalize trade and bring with it resulting economic gains. It is a risky strategy, however. A country that is being pressured may not back down and instead may respond to the imposition of punitive tariffs by raising trade barriers of its own. This is exactly what the Chinese government threatened to do when pressured by the United States, although it ultimately did back down. If a government does not back down, however, the results could be higher trade barriers all around and an economic loss to all involved.

Protecting Consumers

Many governments have long had regulations in place to protect consumers from "unsafe" products. The indirect effect of such regulations often is to limit or ban the importation of such products. In 1998, the U.S. government decided to permanently ban imports of 58 types of military-style assault weapons. (The United States already prohibited the sale of such weapons in the United States by U.S.-based firms.) The ban was motivated by a desire to increase public safety. It followed on the heels of a rash of random and deadly shootings by deranged individuals using such weapons, including one in President Clinton's home state of Arkansas that left four children and a schoolteacher dead.[14]

The accompanying Country Focus describes how the European Union banned the sale and importation of hormone-treated beef. The ban was motivated by a desire to protect European consumers from the possible health consequences of meat from animals treated with growth hormones.

The conflict over the importation of hormone-treated beef into the European Union may prove to be a taste of things to come. In addition to the use of hormones to promote animal growth and meat production, the science of biotechnology has made it possible to genetically alter many crops so that they are resistant to common herbicides, produce proteins that are natural insecticides, have dramatically improved yields, or can withstand inclement weather conditions. A new breed of genetically modified tomatoes has an antifreeze gene inserted into its genome and can thus be grown in colder climates than hitherto possible. Another example is a genetically engineered cotton seed produced by Monsanto. The seed has been engineered to express a protein that provides protection against three common insect pests: the cotton bollworm, tobacco budworm, and pink bollworm. Use of this seed reduces or eliminates the need for traditional pesticide applications for these pests. As enticing as such innovations sound, they have met with intense resistance from consumer groups, particularly in Europe. The fear is that the widespread use of genetically altered seed corn could have unanticipated and harmful effects on human health and may result in "genetic pollution." (An example of genetic pollution would be when the widespread use of crops that produce "natural pesticides" stimulates the evolution of "super-bugs" that are resistant to those pesticides.) Such concerns have led Austria and Luxembourg to outlaw the importation, sale, or use of genetically altered organisms. Sentiment against genetically altered organisms also runs strongly in several other European countries, most notably Germany and Switzerland. It seems likely, therefore, that the

Trade in Hormone-Treated Beef

In the 1970s, scientists discovered how to synthesize certain hormones and use them to promote the growth rate of livestock animals, reduce the fat content of meat, and increase milk production. Bovine somatotropin (BST), a growth hormone produced by beef cattle, was first synthesized by the biotechnology firm Genentech. Injections of BST could be used to supplement an animal's own hormone production and increase its growth rate. These hormones soon became popular among farmers, who found that they could cut costs and help satisfy consumer demands for leaner meat. Although several of these hormones occurred naturally in animals, consumer groups in several countries soon raised concerns about the practice. They argued that the use of hormone supplements was unnatural and that the health consequences of consuming hormone-treated meat were unknown but might include hormonal irregularities and cancer.

The European Union (EU) responded to these concerns in 1989 by banning the use of growth-promoting hormones in the production of livestock and the importation of hormone-treated meat. The ban was controversial because a reasonable consensus existed among scientists that the hormones posed no health risk. Before the ban, a number of these hormones had passed licensing procedures in several EU countries. As part of this process, research had been assembled that appeared to show that consuming hormone-treated meat had no effect on human health. Although the EU banned hormone-treated meat, many other countries did not, including big meat-producing countries such as Australia, Canada, New Zealand, and the United States. The use of hormones soon became widespread in these countries. According to trade officials outside the EU, the European ban constituted an unfair restraint on trade. As a result of this ban, exports of meat to the EU fell. For example, U.S. red meat exports to the EU declined from $231 million in 1988 to $98 million in 1994. The complaints of meat exporters were bolstered in 1995 when Codex Alimentarius, the international food standards body of the UN's Food and Agriculture Organization and the World Health Organization, approved the use of growth hormones. In making this decision, Codex reviewed the scientific literature and found no evidence of a link between the consumption of hormone-treated meat and human health problems, such as cancer.

Fortified by such decisions, in 1995 the United States pressed the EU to drop the ban on the import of hormone-treated beef. The EU refused, citing "consumer concerns about food safety." In response, both Canada and the United States independently filed formal complaints with the World Trade Organization. The United States was joined in its complaint by a number of other countries, including Australia and New Zealand. The WTO created a trade panel of three independent experts. After reviewing evidence and hearing from a range of experts and representatives of both parties, the panel in May 1997 ruled that the EU ban on hormone-treated beef was illegal because it had no scientific justification. The panel also noted that the EU was inconsistent in its application of the ban. The EU takes a very strict view on the use of growth-promoting hormones in the beef sector, where it has a substantial surplus and is not internationally competitive, while it still allows the use of some growth hormones for pork production, where the EU has no substantial surplus and does not compete in international markets. The EU immediately indicated it would appeal the finding to the WTO court of appeals. The WTO court heard the appeal in November 1997 and in February 1998 agreed with the findings of the trade panel that the EU had not presented any scientific evidence to justify the hormone ban.

This ruling left the EU in a difficult position. Legally, the EU had to lift the ban or face punitive sanctions, but the ban had wide public support in Europe. The EU feared that lifting the ban could produce a consumer backlash. Instead the EU did nothing, so in February 1999 the United States asked the WTO for permission to impose punitive sanctions on the EU. The WTO responded by allowing the United States to impose punitive tariffs valued at $120 million on EU exports to the United States. The EU decided to accept these tariffs, rather than lift the ban on hormone-treated beef, and as of 2003, the ban and punitive tariffs were still in place.

Sources: C. Southey, "Hormones Fuel a Meaty EU Row," *Financial Times,* September 7, 1995, p. 2; E. L. Andrews, "In Victory for U.S., European Ban on Treated Beef Is Ruled Illegal," *New York Times,* May 9, 1997, p. A1; F. Williams and G. de Jonquieres, "WTO's Beef Rulings Give Europe Food for Thought," *Financial Times,* February 13, 1998, p. 5; World Trade Organization, *EC Measures concerning Meat and Meat Products,* August 18, 1997; R. Baily, "Food and Trade: EU Fear Mongers' Lethal Harvest," *Los Angeles Times,* August 18, 2002, p. M3; and "The US-EU Dispute over Hormone Treated Beef," *The Kiplinger Agricultural Letter,* January 10, 2003.

World Trade Organization will be drawn into the conflict between those that want to expand the global market for genetically altered organisms, such as Monsanto, and those that want to limit it, such as Austria and Luxembourg.[15]

Furthering Foreign Policy Objectives

Governments sometimes use trade policy to support their foreign policy objectives.[16] A government may grant preferential trade terms to a country it wants to build strong relations with. Trade policy has also been used several times to pressure or punish "rogue states" that do not abide by international law or norms. Iraq labored under extensive trade sanctions since the UN coalition defeated the country in the 1991 Gulf War until the 2003 invasion of Iraq by United States-led forces. The theory is that such pressure might persuade the "rogue state" to mend its ways or it might hasten a change of government. In the case of Iraq, the sanctions were seen as a way of forcing that country to comply with several UN resolutions. The United States has maintained long-running trade sanctions against Cuba. Their principal function is to impoverish Cuba in the hope that the resulting economic hardship will lead to the downfall of Cuba's Communist government and its replacement with a more democratically inclined (and pro-U.S.) regime. The United States also has trade sanctions in place against Libya and Iran, both of which it accuses of supporting terrorist action against U.S. interests.

Other countries can undermine any unilateral trade sanctions. The U.S. sanctions against Cuba, for example, have not stopped other Western countries from trading with Cuba. The U.S. sanctions have done little more than help create a vacuum into which other trading nations, such as Canada and Germany, can and have stepped. In an attempt to put a halt to this and further tighten the screws on Cuba, in 1996 the U.S. Congress passed the **Helms-Burton Act.** This act allows Americans to sue foreign firms that use property in Cuba confiscated from them after the 1959 revolution. A similar act, the **D'Amato Act,** aimed at Libya and Iran was also passed that year.

The passage of Helms-Burton elicited protests from America's trading partners, including the European Union, Canada, and Mexico, all of which claim the law violates their sovereignty and is illegal under World Trade Organization rules. For example, Canadian companies that have been doing business in Cuba for years see no reason they should suddenly be sued in U.S. courts when Canada does not restrict trade with Cuba. They are not violating Canadian law and they are not U.S. companies, so why should they be subject to U.S. law? Despite such protests, the law is still on the books in the United States, although the U.S. government has been less than enthusiastic about enforcing it—probably because it is unenforceable.

Protecting Human Rights

Protecting and promoting human rights in other countries is an important element of foreign policy for many democracies. Governments sometimes use trade policy to try to improve the human rights policies of trading partners. For years the most obvious example of this was the annual debate in the United States over whether to grant most favored nation (MFN) status to China. MFN status allows countries to export goods to the United Status under favorable terms. Under MFN rules, the average tariff on Chinese goods imported into the United States is 8 percent. If China's MFN status were rescinded, tariffs would probably rise to about 40 percent. Trading partners who are signatories of the World Trade Organization, as most are, automatically receive MFN status. However, China did not join the WTO until 2001, so historically the decision of whether to grant MFN status to China was a real one. The decision was made more difficult by the perception that China had a poor human rights record. As indications of the country's disregard for human rights, critics of China often point to the 1989 Tiananmen Square massacre, China's continuing subjugation of Tibet (which China occupied in the 1950s), and the squashing of political dissent in China (there are an estimated 1,700 political prisoners in China).[17] These critics argued that it was wrong for the United States to grant MFN status to China, and that instead, the United States should withhold MFN status until China showed measurable improvement in its human rights record. To put it differently, the critics argued that trade policy should be used as a political weapon to force China to change its internal policies toward human rights.

But others contend that limiting trade with such countries would make matters worse, not better. They argue that the best way to change the internal human rights stance of a country is to engage it through international trade. At its core, the argument is simple: Growing bilateral trade raises the income levels of both countries, and as a state becomes richer, its people begin to demand—and generally receive—better treatment with regard to their human rights. This is a variant of the argument in Chapter 2 that economic progress begets political progress (if political progress is measured by the adoption of a democratic government that respects human rights). This argument ultimately won the day in 1999 when the Clinton administration blessed China's application to join the WTO and announced that trade and human rights issues should be decoupled.

Economic Arguments for Intervention

With the development of the new trade theory and strategic trade policy (see Chapter 4), the economic arguments for government intervention have undergone a renaissance in recent years. Until the early 1980s, most economists saw little benefit in government intervention and strongly advocated a free trade policy. This position has changed at the margins with the development of strategic trade policy, although as we will see in the next section, there are still strong economic arguments for sticking to a free trade stance.

The Infant Industry Argument

The infant industry argument is by far the oldest economic argument for government intervention. Alexander Hamilton first proposed it in 1792. According to this argument, many developing countries have a potential comparative advantage in manufacturing, but new manufacturing industries cannot initially compete with well-established industries in developed countries. To allow manufacturing to get a toehold, the argument is that governments should temporarily support new industries (with tariffs, import quotas, and subsidies) until they have grown strong enough to meet international competition.

This argument has had substantial appeal for the governments of developing nations during the past 50 years, and the GATT has recognized the infant industry argument as a legitimate reason for protectionism. Nevertheless, many economists remain very critical of this argument. They make two main points. First, protection of manufacturing from foreign competition does no good unless the protection helps make the industry efficient. In case after case, however, protection seems to have done little more than foster the development of inefficient industries that have little hope of ever competing in the world market. Brazil, for example, built up the world's 10th largest auto industry behind tariff barriers and quotas. Once those barriers were removed in the late 1980s, however, foreign imports soared, and the industry was forced to face up to the fact that after 30 years of protection, the Brazilian industry was one of the world's most inefficient.[18]

Second, the infant industry argument relies on an assumption that firms are unable to make efficient long-term investments by borrowing money from the domestic or international capital market. Consequently, governments have been required to subsidize long-term investments. Given the development of global capital markets over the past 20 years, this assumption no longer looks as valid as it once did. Today, if a developing country really does have a potential comparative advantage in a manufacturing industry, firms in that country should be able to borrow money from the capital markets to finance the required investments. Given financial support, firms based in countries with a potential comparative advantage have an incentive to go through the necessary initial losses in order to make long-run gains without requiring government protection. Many Taiwanese and South Korean firms did this in industries such as textiles, semiconductors, machine tools, steel, and shipping. Thus, given efficient global capital markets, the only industries that would require government protection would be those that are not worthwhile.

Strategic Trade Policy

Some new trade theorists have proposed the strategic trade policy argument.[19] We reviewed the basic argument in Chapter 4 when we considered the new trade theory. The new trade theory argues that in industries where the existence of substantial scale economies implies that the world market will profitably support only a few firms, countries may predominate in the export of certain products simply because they had firms that were able to capture first-mover advantages. The dominance of Boeing in the commercial aircraft industry is attributed to such factors.

The strategic trade policy argument has two components. First, it is argued that by appropriate actions, a government can help raise national income if it can somehow ensure that the firm or firms to gain first-mover advantages in such an industry are domestic rather than foreign enterprises. Thus, according to the strategic trade policy argument, a government should use subsidies to support promising firms that are active in newly emerging industries. Advocates of this argument point out that the substantial R&D grants that the U.S. government gave Boeing in the 1950s and 60s probably helped tilt the field of competition in the newly emerging market for passenger jets in Boeing's favor. (Boeing's 707 jet airliner was derived from a military plane.) Similar arguments are now made with regard to Japan's dominance in the production of liquid crystal display screens (used in laptop computers). Although these screens were invented in the United States, the Japanese government, in cooperation with major electronics companies, targeted this industry for research support in the late 1970s and early 80s. The result was that Japanese firms, not U.S. firms, subsequently captured the first-mover advantages in this market.

The second component of the strategic trade policy argument is that it might pay government to intervene in an industry if it helps domestic firms overcome the barriers to entry created by foreign firms that have already reaped first-mover advantages. This argument underlies government support of Airbus Industrie, Boeing's major competitor. Formed in 1966 as a consortium of four companies from Great Britain, France, Germany, and Spain, Airbus had less than 5 percent of the world commercial aircraft market when it began production in the mid-1970s. By 2002 it had increased its share to over 50 percent, threatening Boeing's long-term dominance of the market. How did Airbus achieve this? According to the U.S. government, the answer is a $13.5 billion subsidy from the governments of Great Britain, France, Germany, and Spain.[20] Without this subsidy, Airbus would have never been able to break into the world market. In another example, the rise to dominance of the Japanese semiconductor industry, despite the first-mover advantages enjoyed by U.S. firms, is attributed to intervention by the Japanese government. In this case the government did not subsidize the costs of domestic manufacturers. Rather, it protected the Japanese home market while pursuing policies that ensured Japanese companies got access to the necessary manufacturing and product know-how.

If these arguments are correct, they support a rationale for government intervention in international trade. Governments should target technologies that may be important in the future and use subsidies to support development work aimed at commercializing those technologies. Furthermore, government should provide export subsidies until the domestic firms have established first-mover advantages in the world market. Government support may also be justified if it can help domestic firms overcome the first-mover advantages enjoyed by foreign competitors and emerge as viable competitors in the world market (as in the Airbus and semiconductor examples). In this case, a combination of home-market protection and export-promoting subsidies may be called for.

The Revised Case for Free Trade ■

The strategic trade policy arguments of the new trade theorists suggest an economic justification for government intervention in international trade. This justification challenges the rationale for unrestricted free trade found in the work of classic trade theorists such as Adam Smith and David Ricardo. In response to this challenge to economic orthodoxy, a number of economists—including some of those responsible for the development of the new trade theory, such as Paul Krugman of MIT—point out that although strategic trade policy looks nice in theory, in practice it may be unworkable. This response to the strategic trade policy argument constitutes the revised case for free trade.[21]

Retaliation and Trade War

Krugman argues that a strategic trade policy aimed at establishing domestic firms in a dominant position in a global industry is a beggar-thy-neighbor policy that boosts national income at the expense of other countries. A country that attempts to use such policies will probably provoke retaliation. In many cases, the resulting trade war between two or more interventionist governments will leave all countries involved worse off than if a hands-off approach had been adopted in the first place. If the U.S. government were to respond to the Airbus subsidy by increasing its own subsidies to Boeing, for example, the result might be that the subsidies would cancel each other out. In the process, both European and U.S. taxpayers would end up supporting an expensive and pointless trade war, and both Europe and the United States would be worse off.

Krugman may be right about the danger of a strategic trade policy leading to a trade war. The problem, however, is how to respond when one's competitors are already being supported by government subsidies; that is, how should Boeing and the United States respond to the subsidization of Airbus? According to Krugman, the answer is probably not to engage in retaliatory action, but to help establish rules of the game that minimize the use of trade-distorting subsidies. This is what the World Trade Organization seeks to do.

Domestic Politics

Governments do not always act in the national interest when they intervene in the economy; politically important interest groups often influence them. The European Union's support for the Common Agricultural Policy (CAP), which arose because of the political power of French and German farmers, is an example. The CAP benefited inefficient farmers and the politicians who relied on the farm vote, but not consumers in the EU, who end up paying more for their foodstuffs. Thus, a further reason for not embracing strategic trade policy, according to Krugman, is that such a policy is almost certain to be captured by special interest groups within the economy, who will distort it to their own ends. Krugman concludes that in the United States:

> To ask the Commerce Department to ignore special-interest politics while formulating detailed policy for many industries is not realistic: to establish a blanket policy of free trade, with exceptions granted only under extreme pressure, may not be the optimal policy according to the theory but may be the best policy that the country is likely to get.[22]

Development of the World Trading System

There are strong economic arguments for supporting unrestricted free trade. While many governments have recognized the value of these arguments, they have been unwilling to unilaterally lower their trade barriers for fear that other nations might not follow suit. Consider the problem that two neighboring countries, say, Brazil and Argentina, face when considering whether to lower barriers to trade between them. In principle, the government of Brazil might be in favor of lowering trade barriers, but it might be unwilling to do so for fear that Argentina will not do the same. Instead, the government might fear that the Argentineans will take advantage of Brazil's low barriers to enter the Brazilian market, while at the same time continuing to shut Brazilian products out of their market through high trade barriers. The Argentinean government might feel that it faces exactly the same dilemma. The essence of the problem is a lack of trust. Both governments recognize that their respective nations will benefit from lower trade barriers between them, but neither government is willing to lower barriers for fear that the other might not follow.[23]

Such a deadlock can be resolved if both countries negotiate a set of rules to govern cross-border trade and lower trade barriers. But who is to monitor the governments to make sure they are playing by the trade rules? And who is to impose sanctions on a government that cheats? Both governments could set up an independent body whose function is to act as a referee. This referee could monitor trade between the countries, make sure that no side cheats, and impose sanctions on a country if it does cheat in the trade game.

While it might sound unlikely that any government would compromise its national sovereignty by submitting to such an arrangement, since World War II an international trading framework has evolved that has exactly these features. For its first 50 years, this framework was known as the General Agreement on Tariffs and Trade (GATT). Since 1995, it has been known as the World Trade Organization (WTO). Here we look at the evolution and workings of the GATT and WTO. We set the scene with a brief discussion of the pre-GATT history of world trade.

From Smith to the Great Depression

As we saw in Chapter 4, the theoretical case for free trade dates to the late 18th century and the work of Adam Smith and David Ricardo. Free trade as a government policy was first officially embraced by Great Britain in 1846, when the British Parliament repealed the Corn Laws. The Corn Laws placed a high tariff on imports of foreign corn. The objectives of the Corn Laws tariff were to raise government revenues and to protect British corn producers. There had been annual motions in Parliament in favor of free trade since the 1820s when David Ricardo was a member. However, agricultural protection was withdrawn only as a result of a protracted debate when the effects of a harvest failure in Great Britain were compounded by the imminent threat of famine in Ireland. Faced with considerable hardship and suffering among the populace, Parliament narrowly reversed its long-held position.

During the next 80 years or so, Great Britain, as one of the world's dominant trading powers, pushed the case for trade liberalization; but the British government was a voice in the wilderness. Its major trading partners did not reciprocate the British policy of unilateral free trade. The only reason Britain kept this policy for so long was that as the world's largest exporting nation, it had far more to lose from a trade war than did any other country.

By the 1930s, however, the British attempt to stimulate free trade was buried under the economic rubble of the Great Depression. The Great Depression had roots in the failure of the world economy to mount a sustained economic recovery after the end of World War I in 1918. Things got worse in 1929 with the U.S. stock market collapse and the subsequent run on the U.S. banking system. Economic problems were compounded in 1930 when the U.S. Congress passed the Smoot-Hawley tariff. Aimed at avoiding rising unemployment by protecting domestic industries and diverting consumer demand away from foreign products, the **Smoot-Hawley tariff** erected an enormous wall of tariff barriers. Almost every industry was rewarded with its "made-to-order" tariff. A particularly odd aspect of the Smoot-Hawley tariff-raising binge was that the United States was running a balance-of-payment surplus at the time and it was the world's largest creditor nation. The Smoot-Hawley tariff had a damaging effect on employment abroad. Other countries reacted to the U.S. action by raising their own tariff barriers. U.S. exports tumbled in response, and the world slid further into the Great Depression.[24]

1947–1979: GATT, Trade Liberalization, and Economic Growth

The economic damage caused by the beggar-thy-neighbor trade policies that the Smoot-Hawley tariff ushered in exerted a profound influence on the economic institutions and ideology of the post–World War II world. The United States emerged from the war both victorious and economically dominant. After the debacle of the Great Depression, opinion in the U.S. Congress had swung strongly in favor of free trade. Under U.S. leadership, GATT was established in 1947.

The GATT was a multilateral agreement whose objective was to liberalize trade by eliminating tariffs, subsidies, import quotas, and the like. From its foundation in 1947 until it was superseded by the WTO, the GATT's membership grew from 19 to more than 120 nations. The GATT did not attempt to liberalize trade restrictions in one fell swoop; that would have been impossible. Rather, tariff reduction was spread over eight rounds. The most recent, the Uruguay Round, was launched in 1986 and completed in December 1993. In these rounds, mutual tariff reductions were negotiated among all members, who then committed themselves not to raise import tariffs above negotiated rates. GATT regulations were enforced by a mutual monitoring mechanism. If a country felt that one of its trading partners was violating a GATT regulation, it could ask the Geneva-based bureaucracy that administered the GATT to investigate. If GATT investigators found the complaints to be valid, member countries could be asked to pressure the offending party to change its policies. In general, such pressure was sufficient to get an offending country to change its policies. If it were not, the offending country could have been expelled from the GATT.

In its early years, the GATT was by most measures very successful. For example, the average tariff declined by nearly 92 percent in the United States between the Geneva Round of 1947 and the Tokyo Round of 1973–79. Consistent with the theoretical arguments first advanced by Ricardo and reviewed in Chapter 4, the move toward free trade under the GATT appeared to stimulate economic growth. From 1953 to 1963, world trade grew at an annual rate of 6.1 percent, and world income grew at an annual rate of 4.3 percent. Performance from 1963 to 1973 was even better; world trade grew at 8.9 percent annually, and world income grew at 5.1 percent annually.[25]

1980–1993: Disturbing Trends

During the 1980s and early 1990s, the world trading system erected by the GATT came under strain as pressures for greater protectionism increased around the world. Three reasons caused the rise in such pressures during the 1980s. First, the economic success of Japan strained the world trading system. Japan was in ruins when the GATT was created. By the early 1980s, however, it had become the world's second largest economy and its largest exporter. Japan's success in such industries as automobiles and semiconductors by itself might have been enough to strain the world trading system. Things were made worse, however, by the widespread perception in the West that despite low tariff rates and subsidies, Japanese markets were closed to imports and foreign investment by administrative trade barriers.

Second, the world trading system was strained by the persistent trade deficit in the world's largest economy, the United States. Although the deficit peaked in 1987 at more than $170 billion, by the end of 1992 the annual rate was still running about $80 billion. From a political perspective, the matter was worsened in 1992 by the United States' $45 billion trade deficit with Japan, a country perceived as not playing by the rules. The consequences of the U.S. deficit included painful adjustments in industries such as automobiles, machine tools, semiconductors, steel, and textiles, where domestic producers steadily lost market share to foreign competitors. The resulting unemployment gave rise to renewed demands in the U.S. Congress for protection against imports.

A third reason for the trend toward greater protectionism was that many countries found ways to get around GATT regulations. Bilateral voluntary export restraints (VERs) circumvent GATT agreements, because neither the importing country nor the exporting country complain to the GATT bureaucracy in Geneva—and without a complaint, the GATT bureaucracy can do nothing. Exporting countries agreed to VERs to avoid more damaging punitive tariffs. One of the best-known examples is the VER between Japan and the United States, under which Japanese producers promised to limit their auto imports into the United States as a way of defusing growing trade tensions. According to a World Bank study, 13 percent of the imports of industrialized countries in 1981 were subjected to nontariff trade barriers such as VERs. By 1986, this figure had increased to 16 percent. The most rapid rise was in the United States, where the value of imports affected by nontariff barriers (primarily VERs) increased by 23 percent between 1981 and 1986.[26]

The Uruguay Round and the World Trade Organization

Against the background of rising pressures for protectionism, in 1986 the GATT members embarked on their eighth round of negotiations to reduce tariffs, the Uruguay Round (so named because it occurred in Uruguay). This was the most difficult round of negotiations yet, primarily because it was also the most ambitious. Until then, GATT rules had applied only to trade in manufactured goods and commodities. In the Uruguay Round, member countries sought to extend GATT rules to cover trade in services. They also sought to write rules governing the protection of intellectual property, to reduce agricultural subsidies, and to strengthen the GATT's monitoring and enforcement mechanisms.

The Uruguay Round dragged on for seven years before an agreement was reached December 15, 1993. The agreement was formally signed by member states at a meeting in Marrakech, Morocco, on April 15, 1994. It went into effect July 1, 1995. The Uruguay Round contained the following provisions:

1. tariffs on industrial goods were to be reduced by more than one-third, and tariffs were to be scrapped on over 40 percent of manufactured goods;
2. average tariff rates imposed by developed nations on manufactured goods were to be reduced to less than 4 percent of value, the lowest level in modern history;
3. agricultural subsidies were to be substantially reduced;
4. for the first time GATT fair trade and market access rules were to be extended to cover a wide range of services;
5. GATT rules were also to be extended to provide enhanced protection for patents, copyrights, and trademarks (intellectual property);
6. barriers on trade in textiles were to be significantly reduced over 10 years; and
7. a World Trade Organization (WTO) was to be created to implement the GATT agreement.

Services and Intellectual Property

In the long run, the extension of GATT rules to cover services and intellectual property may be particularly significant. Until 1995, GATT rules applied only to industrial goods (i.e., manufactured goods and commodities). In 2001, world trade in services amounted to $1,460 billion (compared to world trade in goods of $5,984 billion).[27] Extension of GATT rules to this important trading arena could significantly increase both the total share of world trade accounted for by services and the overall volume of world trade. The extension of GATT rules to cover intellectual property will make it much easier for high-technology companies to do business in developing nations where intellectual property rules have historically been poorly enforced (see Chapter 2 for details). High-technology companies now have a mechanism to force countries to prohibit the piracy of intellectual property.

The World Trade Organization

The clarification and strengthening of GATT rules and the creation of the World Trade Organization also hold out the promise of more effective policing and enforcement of GATT rules. The WTO acts as an umbrella organization that encompasses the GATT along with two new sister bodies, one on services and the other on intellectual property. The WTO's General Agreement of Trade in Services (GATS) has taken the lead to extending free trade agreements to services. The WTO's Agreement on Trade Related Aspects of Intellectual Property Rights (TRIPS) is an attempt to narrow the gaps in the way intellectual property rights are protected around the world, and to bring them under common international rules. WTO has taken over responsibility for arbitrating trade disputes and monitoring the trade policies of member countries. While the WTO operates on the basis of consensus as the GATT did, in the area of dispute settlement, member countries will no longer be able to block adoption of arbitration reports. Arbitration panel reports on trade disputes between member countries will be automatically adopted by the WTO unless there is a consensus to reject them. Countries that have been found by the arbitration panel to violate GATT rules may appeal to a permanent appellate body, but its verdict is binding. If offenders fail to comply with the recommendations of the arbitration panel, trading partners have the right to compensation or, in the last resort, to impose (commensurate) trade sanctions. Every stage of the procedure is subject to strict time limits. Thus, the WTO has something that the GATT never had—teeth.[28]

WTO: Experience to Date

By 2003, the WTO had 145 members, including China, which joined at the end of 2001. Another 25 countries, including the Russian Federation and Saudi Arabia, were negotiating for membership into the organization. Since its formation, the WTO has remained at the forefront of efforts to promote global free trade. Its creators expressed the hope that the enforcement mechanisms granted to the WTO would make it a more effective policeman of global trade rules than the GATT had been. The great hope was that the WTO might emerge as an effective advocate and facilitator of future trade deals, particularly in areas such as services. The experience so far has been encouraging, although the collapse of WTO talks in Seattle in late 1999 raised a number of questions about the future direction of the WTO.

WTO as a Global Policeman

The first few years in the life of the WTO suggest that its policing and enforcement mechanisms are having a positive effect. Between 1995 and early 2003, more than 280 trade disputes between member countries were brought to the WTO.[29] This record compares with a total of 196 cases handled by the GATT over almost half a century. Of the cases brought to the WTO, three-fourths had been resolved by late 2002 following informal consultations between the disputing countries. Resolving the remainder has involved more formal procedures, but these have been largely successful. In general, the countries involved have adopted the WTO's recommendations. The fact that countries are using the WTO represents an important vote of confidence in the organization's dispute resolution procedures.

Expanding Trade Agreements

As explained above, the Uruguay Round of GATT negotiations extended global trading rules to cover trade in services. The WTO was given the role of brokering future agreements to open up global trade in services. The WTO was also encouraged to extend its reach to encompass regulations governing foreign direct investment, something the GATT had never done. Two of the first industries targeted for reform were the global telecommunication and financial services industries.

The WTO tackled telecommunications first. The goal of the WTO was to get countries to agree to open their telecommunication markets to competition, allowing foreign operators to purchase ownership stakes in domestic telecommunication providers and establishing a set of common rules for fair competition. The benefits claimed for such agreements were threefold.

First, advocates argued that inward investment and increased competition would stimulate the modernization of telephone networks around the world and lead to higher quality service. Second, supporters maintained that the increased competition would benefit customers through lower prices. Estimates suggested that a deal would soon reduce the average cost of international telephone calls by 80 percent and save users $1,000 billion over three years.[30] Third, the WTO argued that trade in other goods and services invariably depends on flows of information matching buyers to sellers. As telecommunication services improve in quality and decline in price, international trade increases in volume and becomes less costly for traders. Telecommunication reform, therefore, should promote cross-border trade in other goods and services.

A deal was reached February 15, 1997. Under the pact, 68 countries accounting for more than 90 percent of world telecommunication revenues pledged to start opening their markets to foreign competition and to abide by common rules for fair competition in telecommunications. Most of the world's biggest markets, including the United States, European Union, and Japan, were fully liberalized by January 1, 1998, when the pact went into effect. All forms of basic telecommunication service are covered, including voice telephony, data and fax transmissions, and satellite and radio communications. Many telecommunication companies responded positively to the deal, pointing out that it would give them a much greater ability to offer their business customers "one-stop shopping"—a global, seamless service for all their corporate needs and a single bill.[31]

Fresh from success in brokering a telecommunication agreement, in 1997 the WTO embarked on a series of negotiations to liberalize the global financial services industry. The financial services industry includes banking, securities businesses, insurance, asset management services, and the like. The global financial services industry is enormous. The sector executes $1.2 trillion a day in foreign exchange transactions. International financing extended by banks around the world reporting to the Bank for International Settlements is estimated at $6.4 trillion, including $4.6 trillion net international lending. Total world banking assets are put at more than $20 trillion, insurance premiums at $2 trillion, stock market capitalization at over $10 trillion, and market value of listed bonds at about $10 trillion. In addition, practically every international trade in goods or services requires credit, capital, foreign exchange, and insurance.[32]

Participants in the negotiations wanted to see more competition in the sector, both to allow firms greater opportunities abroad and to encourage greater efficiency. Developing countries need the capital and financial infrastructure for their development. But governments also have to ensure that the system is sound and stable because of the economic shocks that can be caused if exchange rates, interest rates, or other market conditions fluctuate excessively. They also have to avoid economic crises caused by bank failures. Therefore, government intervention in prudential safeguards is an important condition underpinning financial market liberalization.

An agreement was reached December 14, 1997.[33] The deal covers more than 95 percent of the world's financial services market. Under the agreement, which took effect at the beginning of March 1999, 102 countries pledged to open to varying degrees their banking, securities, and insurance sectors to foreign competition. In common with the telecommunication deal, the accord covers not just cross-border trade but also foreign direct investment. Seventy countries agreed to dramatically lower or eradicate barriers to foreign direct investment in their financial services sector. The United States and the European Union, with minor exceptions, are fully open to inward investment by foreign banks, insurance, and securities companies. As part of the deal, many Asian countries made important concessions that allow significant foreign participation in their financial services sectors for the first time.

The WTO in Seattle: A Watershed?

At the end of November 1999, representatives from the WTO's member states met in Seattle, Washington. The goal of the meeting was to launch a new round of talks—dubbed "the millennium round"—aimed at further reducing barriers to cross-border trade and investment. Prominent on the agenda was an attempt to get the assembled countries to agree to work toward the reduction of barriers to cross-border trade in agricultural products and cross-border trade and investment in services.

These expectations were dashed on the rocks of a hard and unexpected reality. The talks ended December 3, 1999, without any agreement being reached. Inside the meeting rooms, the problem was an inability to reach consensus on the primary goals for the next round of talks. A major stumbling block was friction between the United States and the European Union over whether to endorse the aim of ultimately eliminating subsidies to agricultural exporters. The United States wanted the elimination of such subsidies to be a priority. The EU, with its politically powerful farm lobby and long history of farm subsidies, was unwilling to take this step. Another stumbling block was related to efforts by the United States to write "basic labor rights" into the law of the world trading system. The United States wanted the WTO to allow governments to impose tariffs on goods imported from countries that did not abide by what the United States saw as fair labor practices. Representatives from developing nations reacted angrily to this proposal, suggesting that it was simply an attempt by the United States to find a legal way of restricting imports from poorer nations.

While the disputes inside the meeting rooms were acrimonious, it was events outside that captured the attention of the world press. The WTO talks proved to be a lightning rod for a diverse collection of organizations from environmentalists and human rights groups to labor unions. For various reasons, these groups are opposed to free trade. All these organizations argued that the WTO is an undemocratic institution that was usurping the national sovereignty of member states and making decisions of great importance behind closed doors. They took advantage of the Seattle meetings to voice their opposition, which the world press recorded. Environmentalists expressed concern about the impact that free trade in agricultural products might have on the rate of global deforestation. They argued that lower tariffs on imports of lumber from developing nations will stimulate demand and accelerate the rate at which virgin forests are logged, particularly in nations such as Malaysia and Indonesia. They also pointed to the adverse impact that some WTO rulings have had on environmental policies. For example, the WTO had recently blocked a U.S. rule that ordered shrimp nets be equipped with a device that allows endangered sea turtles to escape. The WTO found the rule discriminated against foreign importers who lacked such nets.[34] Environmentalists argued that the rule was necessary to protect the turtles from extinction (see the accompanying Country Focus for details).

Shrimps, Turtles, and the WTO

There are seven species of sea turtles in the world; six of them are on the list of endangered species in the United States. A major cause of the decline of sea turtles has been poor fishing practices, particularly by shrimp boats. An estimated 150,000 sea turtles are trapped and drown in the nets of shrimp boats each year. In an effort to limit this carnage, in 1989 the U.S. Congress passed a law that required shrimp boats to be equipped with a turtle-excluder device. This is a simple grate that fits over the mouth of shrimp trawling nets and prevents sea turtles from becoming trapped. The law also banned the importation of shrimp from countries that fail to mandate the use of turtle-excluder devices.

As with many such laws, the U.S. government dragged its heels on enforcing the import ban. It wasn't until 1996 that the United States placed an embargo on the importation of shrimp from countries that failed to mandate the use of excluder devices. Even then, it did so only because environmental groups in the United States had brought a lawsuit against the government to compel it to enforce its own law. Three countries were targeted by the 1996 ban—India, Pakistan, and Malaysia. The three responded to the ban by filing a complaint with the World Trade Organization. They were joined by Thailand, which decided as a matter of principle to pursue the WTO case (Thailand had already satisfied the United States that its turtle protection methods were adequate).

As is normal in such cases, the WTO formed an independent arbitration panel composed of three experts from countries not involved in the dispute. The panel was charged with reviewing the U.S. position to see whether it conflicted with WTO rules. In its defense, the United States claimed there are provisions in the WTO rules for taking restrictive measures if they are related "to the conservation of exhaustible natural resources and if such measures are made effective in conjunction with restrictions on domestic production or consumption." The United States was supported in its case by a number of environmental organizations, including the World Wildlife Fund (WWF). In a brief submitted to the panel, the WWF argued that marine turtles are migratory animals, a global resource that should be subject to stewardship by international society. Even though no multilateral body or resolution had authorized the United States to enact its ban, the WWF claimed that the United States acted in a manner consistent with its obligations and took reasonable measures that reflected the will of the international community.

For their part, the four countries that brought the complaint argued that the U.S. ban represented an unfair restraint on trade that was illegal under WTO rules. According to these countries, the United States was violating WTO rules by applying domestic legislation outside of its boundaries and by applying it in a discriminatory manner. Influential voices in all these countries accused the United States of hypocrisy. An

Human rights activists see WTO rules as outlawing the ability of nations to stop imports from countries where child labor is used or working conditions are hazardous. Similarly, labor unions oppose trade laws that allow imports from low-wage countries and result in a loss of jobs in high-wage countries. They buttress their position by arguing that American workers are losing their jobs to imports from developing nations that do not have adequate labor standards.

Supporters of the WTO and free trade dismiss these concerns. They have repeatedly pointed out that the WTO exists to serve the interests of its member states, not subvert them. The WTO lacks the ability to force any member nation to take an action that it is opposed to. The WTO can allow member nations to impose retaliatory tariffs on countries that do not abide by WTO rules, but that is the limit of its power. Furthermore, supporters argue, it is rich countries that pass strict environmental laws and laws governing labor standards, not poor ones. In their view, free trade, by raising living standards in developing nations, will be followed by the passage of such laws in these nations. Using trade regulations to try to impose such practices on developing nations, they believe, will produce a self-defeating backlash.

Many representatives from developing nations, who make up about 107 of the WTO's 145 members, also reject the position taken by environmentalists and advocates of huarticle in *The Hindu,* an Indian newspaper, stated, "Compared to what the U.S. as a nation is doing to another global shared resource, the world's climate and atmosphere, what complainant nations like India are doing to the marine turtle is a contemptuously small problem . . . The U.S. leadership has, unfortunately, always put its national interests before global concerns in its global environmental policies. Its behavior on the climate change issue is one example. Its refusal to sign the bio-diversity treaty is another. Its refusal to pay dues to the United Nations is yet another."

The World Trade Organization panel on April 6, 1998, ruled that the ban was in violation of WTO rules and would need to be amended. According to the WTO, by enacting a targeted ban against just three countries, the United States had acted in a discriminatory manner, which was in violation of WTO accords. Further, the WTO stated that if the United States wished to impose such a ban, it should be a blanket ban against imports from all countries that fail to use a turtle-excluder device, not just a targeted list of countries.

The environmental movement reacted to the WTO ruling with dismay. A Sierra Club spokesman noted, "This is the clearest slap at environmental protection to come out of the WTO to date." Similarly, a spokeswoman for the Washington, D.C.–based Center for Marine Conservation stated, "It is unthinkable that we should not be allowed to mitigate the impacts of our own shrimp markets on endangered sea turtles. This

entire life form is threatened with extinction." However, this reaction, which was widely reported in the press, seems to have been based on a failure to read and/or understand the WTO's ruling. The ruling actually stated that under certain circumstance it was all right for the United States to restrict imports for environmental reasons, but only if such restrictions were applied in a nondiscriminatory manner. The problem with the U.S. ban as it stood was that it had targeted a select group of countries—it was discriminatory.

In response, the United States revised the law so that it restricted shrimp imports from any country that failed to use a turtle-excluder device on its shrimp boats. The import ban, however, stayed in place. Malaysia responded by filing a complaint in October 2000 with the WTO, arguing that the United States was still in violation of WTO rules. In October 2001, the WTO rejected Malaysia's complaint, effectively confirming that the amended U.S. ban was consistent with WTO rules.

Sources: A. Aggarwal and S. Narain, "Politics of Conservation," *The Hindu,* October 26, 1997, p. 26; J. H. Cushman, "Trade Group Strikes a Blow at U.S. Environmental Law," *New York Times,* April 7, 1998, p. D1; "WTO Ruling in Turtle Protection Dispute," *Bangkok Post,* March 18, 1998; J. Maggs, "WTO Shrimp Ruling Heightens Environment vs. Trade Debate," *Journal of Commerce,* April 7, 1998, p. 3A; and "Malaysia Swims against the Tide over U.S. Shrimps Import Ban," *New Straits Times Press* (Malaysia), October 25, 2001, p. 2.

man and labor rights. Poor countries, which depend on exports to boost their economic growth rates and work their way out of poverty, fear that rich countries will use environmental concerns, human rights, and labor-related issues to erect barriers to the products of the developing world. They believe that attempts to incorporate language about the environment or labor standards in future trade agreements will amount to little more than trade barriers by another name.[35] If this were to occur, they argue that the effect would be to trap the developing nations of the world in a grinding cycle of poverty and debt.

These pro-trade arguments fell on deaf ears. As the WTO representatives gathered in Seattle, environmentalists, human rights activists, and labor unions marched in the streets. Some of the more radical elements in these organizations, together with groups of anarchists who were philosophically opposed to "global capitalism" and "the rape of the world by multinationals," succeeded not only in shutting down the opening ceremonies of the WTO, but also in sparking violence in the normally peaceful streets of Seattle. A number of demonstrators engaged in property damage and looting and the police responded with tear gas, rubber bullets, pepper spray, and baton charges. When it was all over, 600 demonstrators had been arrested, millions of dollars in property had been damaged in downtown Seattle, and the global news media had their headline: "WTO Talks Collapse amid Violent Demonstrations."

What happened in Seattle is notable because it may have been a watershed of sorts In the past, previous trade talks were pursued in relative obscurity with only interested economists, politicians, and businesspeople paying much attention. Seattle demonstrated that the issues surrounding the global trend toward free trade have moved to center stage in the popular consciousness. The debate on the merits of free trade and globalization has become mainstream. Whether further liberalization occurs, therefore, may depend on the importance that popular opinion in countries such as the United States attaches to issues such as human rights and labor standards, job security, environmental policies, and national sovereignty. It will also depend on the ability of advocates of free trade to articulate in a clear and compelling manner the argument that, in the long run, free trade is the best way of promoting adequate labor standards, of providing more jobs, and of protecting the environment. Exactly how this debate will play out remains to be seen, but given recent trends it would not be surprising if labor rights and environmental considerations played a much larger role in the next round of global trade talks, which was finally launched in 2001.

The Future of the WTO: Unresolved Issues and the Doha Round

There is still a lot to be done on the international trade front. Three issues at the forefront of the current agenda of the WTO are the increase in antidumping policies, the high level of protectionism in agriculture, and the lack of strong protection for intellectual property rights in many nations. We shall look at each in turn before discussing the latest attempt to launch a round of talks between WTO members aimed at reducing trade barriers, the Doha Round.

Antidumping Actions

Antidumping actions have proliferated in recent years. WTO rules allow countries to impose antidumping duties on foreign goods that are being sold cheaper than at home, or below their cost of production, when domestic producers can show that they are being harmed. Unfortunately, the rather vague definition of what constitutes "dumping" has proved to be a loophole that many countries are exploiting to pursue protectionism. In the United States, for example, 26 antidumping cases were launched in 1998, up from 16 cases in the prior year. In 1999, the United States launched 47 cases, as it did in 2000. In 2001, the United States launched another 76 antidumping actions. There has also been a rise in cases filed by the European Union and India.[36]

Between January 1995 and December 2002, WTO members had reported implementation of some 2,160 antidumping actions to the WTO. India initiated the largest number of antidumping actions, some 331; the EU initiated 267 over the same period, and the United States 292(see Figure 5.1). Together these three countries accounted for almost half of all cases between 2000 and 2002. Antidumping actions seem to be concentrated on certain sectors of the economy. Basic metal industries (e.g., aluminum and steel) accounted for 687 of the 2,160 antidumping cases between 1995 and 2002, followed by chemicals (393), plastics (258), and machinery and electrical equipment (194).[37] In sum, four sectors account for some 70 percent of all antidumping actions reported to the WTO. Not surprisingly perhaps, since 1995 these four sectors have been characterized by periods of intense competition and excess productive capacity, which in turn has led to low prices and profits (or losses) for firms in those industries. It is not unreasonable, therefore, to hypothesize that the high level of antidumping actions in these industries represents an attempt by beleaguered manufacturers to use the political process in their nations to seek protection from foreign competitors, who they claim are engaging in unfair competition. While there may well be merit to some of these claims, the process can become very politicized as representatives of businesses and their employees lobby government officials to "protect domestic jobs from unfair foreign competition," and government officials, mindful of the

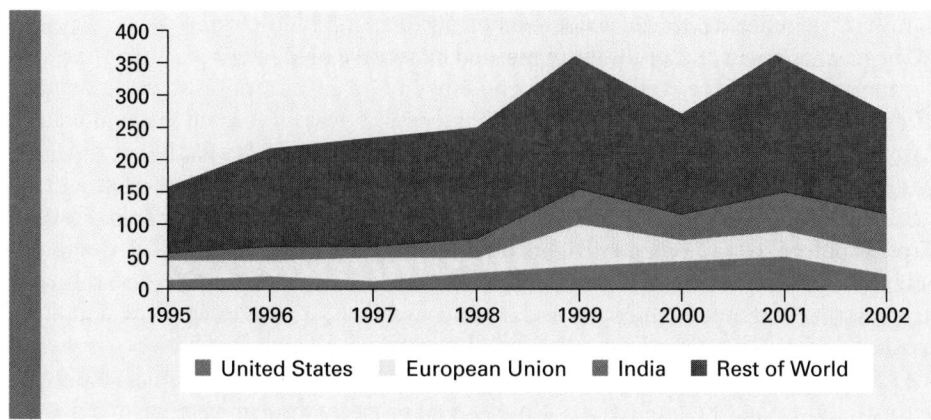

Figure 5.1

Antidumping Cases by
WTO Members,
1995–2002

Source: WTO data at http://www.
wto.org/english/tratop_e/adp_e/adp_
stattab2_e.htm.

need to get votes in future elections, oblige by pushing for antidumping actions. The WTO is clearly worried by this trend, suggesting that it reflects persistent protectionist tendencies and pushing members to strengthen the regulations governing the imposition of antidumping duties.

Protectionism in Agriculture

Another recent focus of the WTO has been the high level of tariffs and subsidies in the agricultural sector of many economies. Tariff rates on agricultural products are generally much higher than tariff rates on manufactured products or services. In 2000, for example, the average tariff rates on nonagricultural products were 4.4 percent for Canada, 4.5 percent for the European Union, 4.0 percent for Japan, and 4.7 percent for the United States. On agricultural products, however, the average tariff rates were 22.9 percent for Canada, 17.3 percent for the European Union, 18.2 percent for Japan, and 11 percent for the United States.[38] The implication is that consumers in these countries are paying significantly higher prices than necessary for agricultural products imported from abroad, which leaves them with less money to spend on other goods and services.

The historically high tariff rates on agricultural products reflect a desire to protect domestic agriculture and traditional farming communities from foreign competition. In addition to high tariffs, agricultural producers also benefit from substantial subsidies (see the opening case). According to estimates from the OECD, on average government subsidies account for some 20 percent of the cost of agricultural production in Canada, 24 percent in the United States, 49 percent in the European Union, and 64 percent in Japan.[39] In total, OECD countries spend more than $300 billion a year in subsidies to agricultural producers.

Not surprisingly, the combination of high tariff barriers and significant subsidies introduces significant distortions into the production of agricultural products, and international trade of those products. The net effect is to raise prices to consumers, reduce the volume of agricultural trade, and encourage the overproduction of products that are heavily subsidized (with the government typically buying the surplus). Since global trade in agriculture currently amounts to 10.5 percent of total merchandized trade, or about $700 billion per year, the WTO argues that removing tariff barriers and subsidies could significantly boost the overall level of trade, lower prices to consumers, and raise global economic growth by freeing consumption and investment resources for more productive uses. The biggest defenders of the existing system have been the advanced nations of the world, who want to protect their agricultural sectors from competition by low-cost producers in developing nations. In contrast, developing nations have been pushing hard for reforms that would allow their producers greater access to the protected markets of the developed nations. Estimates suggest that removing all subsidies on agricultural production alone in OECD countries could return to the developing nations of the world three times more than all foreign aid that they currently receive from the OECD nations.[40] In other words, free trade in agriculture could help to jump-start economic growth among the world's poorer nations and alleviate global poverty.

Protecting Intellectual Property

Another issue that has become increasingly important to the WTO has been protecting intellectual property. As noted earlier, the 1995 Uruguay agreement that established the WTO also contained an agreement to protect intellectual property (the Trade Related Aspects of Intellectual Property Rights (or TRIPS agreement). The TRIPS regulations oblige WTO members to grant and enforce patents lasting at least 20 years and copyrights lasting 50 years. Rich countries had to comply with the rules within a year. Poor countries, in which such protection generally was much weaker, had 5 years' grace, and the very poorest had 10 years. The basis for this agreement was a strong belief among signatory nations that the protection of intellectual property through patents, trademarks, and copyrights must be an essential element of the international trading system. Inadequate protections for intellectual property reduce the incentive for innovation. Because innovation is a central engine of economic growth and rising living standards, the argument has been that a multilateral agreement is needed to protect intellectual property.

Without such an agreement, there has been a fear that producers in a country, let's say India, might market imitations of patented innovations pioneered in a different country, let's say the United States. This can affect international trade in two ways. First, it reduces the export opportunities in India for the original innovator in the United States. Second, to the extent that the Indian producer is able to export its pirated imitation to third countries, it also reduces the export opportunities for the U.S. inventor in those countries. Also, one can argue that because the size of the total world market for the innovator is reduced, its incentive to pursue risky and expensive innovations is also reduced. The net effect would be less innovation in the world economy and less economic growth.

Something very similar to this has been occurring in the pharmaceutical industry, with Indian drug companies making copies of patented drugs discovered elsewhere. In 1970, the Indian government stopped recognizing product patents on drugs, but elected to continue respecting process patents. This permitted Indian companies to reverse-engineer Western pharmaceuticals without paying licensing fees. As a result, foreigners' share of the Indian drug market fell from 75 percent in 1970 to 30 percent in 2000. For example, an Indian company sells a version of Bayer's patented antibiotic Cipro for $0.12 a pill, versus the $5.50 it costs in the United States. Under the WTO TRIPS agreement, India has agreed to adopt and enforce the international drug patent regime by 2005.[41]

As noted in Chapter 2, intellectual property rights violation is also an endemic problem in several other industries, most notably computer software and music. The WTO believes that reducing piracy rates in areas such as drugs, software, and music recordings would have a significant impact on the volume of world trade and increase the incentive for producers to invest in the creation of intellectual property. In a world without piracy, there would be more new drugs, computer software, and music recordings produced every year. In turn, this would boost economic and social welfare, and global economic growth rates. It is thus in the interests of the member states of the WTO to make sure that intellectual property rights are respected and enforced among its member states. While the 1995 Uruguay agreement that created the WTO did make some headway with the TRIPS agreement, some believe these requirements do no go far enough and further commitments are necessary.

Launching a New Round of Talks: Doha

Antidumping actions, trade in agricultural products, and better enforcement of intellectual property laws were three of the issues the WTO wanted to tackle at the 1999 meetings in Seattle, but as noted earlier, those meetings were derailed. In late 2001, the WTO tried again to launch a new round of talks between member states aimed at further liberalizing the global trade and investment framework. For this meeting, it picked the remote location of Doha in the Gulf state of Qatar, no doubt with an eye on the difficulties that antiglobalization protesters would have in getting there. Unlike the Seattle meetings, at Doha, the member states of the WTO agreed to launch a new round of talks and staked out an agenda. The talks are scheduled to last three years, although if history is any guide, they could last much longer.

The agenda agreed upon at Doha should be seen as a game plan for negotiations over the next few years. The agenda includes cutting tariffs on industrial goods and services, phasing out subsidies to agricultural producers, reducing barriers to cross-border investment (FDI), and limiting the use of antidumping laws. Some difficult compromises were made to reach agreement on this agenda. The EU and Japan had to give significant ground on the issue of agricultural subsidies, which are used extensively by both entities to support politically powerful farmers. The United States bowed to pressure from virtually every other nation to negotiate revisions of antidumping rules, which the United States has used extensively to protect its steel producers from foreign competition. Europe had to scale back its efforts to include environmental policy in the trade talks, primarily because of pressure from developing nations that see environmental protection policies as trade barriers by another name. Excluded from the agenda was any language pertaining to attempts to tie trade to labor standards in a country.

Countries with big pharmaceutical sectors acquiesced to demands from African, Asian, and Latin American nations on the issue of drug patents. Specifically, the language in the agreement declares that WTO regulation on intellectual property "does not and should not prevent members from taking measures to protect public health." This language was meant to assure the world's poorer nations that they can make or buy generic equivalents to fight such killers as AIDS and malaria.

Clearly, it is one thing to agree to an agenda, and quite another to reach a consensus on a new treaty. Nevertheless, there are some potential winners in this agreement. These include low-cost agricultural producers in the developing world and developed nations such as Australia and the United States. If the talks are successful, agricultural producers in these nations will ultimately see the global markets for their goods expand. Developing nations also gain from the lack of language on labor standards, which many saw as an attempt by rich nations to erect trade barriers. The sick and poor of the world also benefit from guaranteed access to cheaper medicines. There are also clear losers in this agreement, including EU and Japanese farmers, U.S. steelmakers, environmental activists, and pharmaceutical firms in the developed world. These losers can be expected to lobby their government hard during the ensuing years to make sure that the final agreement is more in their favor.[42]

Focus On Managerial Implications

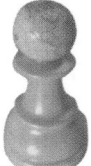

What are the implications of all of this for business practice? Why should the international manager care about the political economy of free trade or about the relative merits of arguments for free trade and protectionism? There are two answers to this question. The first concerns the impact of trade barriers on a firm's strategy. The second concerns the role that business firms can play in promoting free trade and/or trade barriers.

Trade Barriers and Firm Strategy

To understand how trade barriers affect a firm's strategy, consider first the material in Chapter 4. Drawing on the theories of international trade, we discussed how it makes sense for the firm to disperse its various production activities to those countries around the globe where they can be performed most efficiently. Thus, it may make sense for a firm to design and engineer its product in one country, to manufacture components in another, to perform final assembly operations in yet another country, and then export the finished product to the rest of the world.

Clearly, trade barriers are a constraint on a firm's ability to disperse its productive activities in such a manner. First, and most obviously, tariff barriers raise the costs of exporting products to a country (or of exporting partly finished products between countries). This may put the firm at a competitive disadvantage viv-à-vis indigenous competitors in that country. In response, the firm may then find it economical to locate production facilities in that country so that it can compete on an even footing with indigenous competitors. Second, quotas and voluntary export restraints may limit a firm's ability to serve a country from locations outside of that country. Again, the response by the firm might be to set up production facilities in that country—even though it may result in higher production costs. Such reasoning was one of the factors behind the rapid expansion of Japanese automaking capacity in the United States during the 1980s and 1990s. This followed the establishment of a VER agreement between the United States and Japan that limited U.S. imports of Japanese automobiles.

Third, to conform to local content regulations, a firm may have to locate more production activities in a given market than it would otherwise. Again, from the firm's perspective, the consequence might be to raise costs above the level that could be achieved if each production activity was dispersed to the optimal location for that activity. And finally, even when trade barriers do not exist, the firm may still want to locate some production activities in a given country to reduce the threat of trade barriers being imposed in the future.

All the above effects are likely to raise the firm's costs above the level that could be achieved in a world without trade barriers. The higher costs that result need not translate into a significant competitive disadvantage relative to other foreign firms, however, if the countries imposing trade barriers do so to the imported products of all foreign firms, irrespective of their national origin. But when trade barriers are targeted at exports from a particular nation, firms based in that nation are at a competitive disadvantage to firms of other nations. The firm may deal with such targeted trade barriers by moving production into the country imposing barriers. Another strategy may be to move production to countries whose exports are not targeted by the specific trade barrier, which is what the Esquel Group did to circumvent quota limits (see the Management Focus).

Finally, the threat of antidumping action limits the ability of a firm to use aggressive pricing to gain market share in a country. Firms in a country can also make strategic use of antidumping measures to limit aggressive competition from low-cost foreign producers. For example, the U.S. steel industry has been very aggressive in bringing antidumping actions against foreign steelmakers, particularly in times of weak global demand for steel and excess capacity. For example, in 1998 and 1999, the United States faced a surge in low-cost steel imports as a severe recession in Asia left producers there with excess capacity. The U.S. producers filed several complaints with the International Trade Commission. One argued that Japanese producers of hot rolled steel were selling it at below cost in the United States. The ITC agreed and levied tariffs ranging from 18 percent to 67 percent on imports of certain steel products from Japan.[43]

Policy Implications

As noted in Chapter 4, business firms are major players on the international trade scene. Because of their pivotal role in international trade, firms can and do exert a strong influence on government policy toward trade. This influence can encourage protectionism or it can encourage the government to support the WTO and push for open markets and freer trade among all nations. Government policies with regard to international trade can have a direct impact on business.

Consistent with strategic trade policy, examples can be found of government intervention in the form of tariffs, quotas, antidumping actions, and subsidies helping firms and industries establish a competitive advantage in the world economy. In general, however, the arguments contained in this chapter and in Chapter 4 suggest that government intervention has three drawbacks. Intervention can be self-defeating, since in practice it tends to protect the inefficient rather than help firms become efficient global competitors. Intervention is dangerous; it may invite retaliation and trigger a trade war. Finally, intervention is unlikely to be well-executed, given the opportunity for such a policy to be captured by special-interest groups. Does this mean that business should simply encourage government to adopt a laissez-faire free trade policy?

Most economists would probably argue that the best interests of international business are served by a free trade stance, but not a laissez-faire stance. It is probably in the best long-run interests of the business community to encourage the government to aggressively promote greater free trade by, for example, strengthening the WTO. Business probably has much more to gain from government efforts to open protected markets to imports and foreign direct investment than from government efforts to support certain domestic industries in a manner consistent with the recommendations of strategic trade policy.

This conclusion is reinforced by a phenomenon we touched on in Chapter 1—the increasing integration of the world economy and internationalization of production that has occurred over the past two decades. We live in a world where many firms of all national origins increasingly depend for their competitive advantage on globally dispersed production systems. Such systems are the result of freer trade. Freer trade has brought great advantages to firms that have exploited it and to consumers who benefit from the resulting lower prices. Given the danger of retaliatory action, business firms that lobby their governments to engage in protectionism must realize that by doing so they may be denying themselves the opportunity to build a competitive advantage by constructing a globally dispersed production system. By encouraging their governments to engage in protectionism, their own activities and sales overseas may be jeopardized if other governments retaliate. This does not mean that a firm should never seek protection in the form of antidumping actions and the like, but it should review its options carefully and think through the larger consequences.

ChapterSummary

The objective of this chapter was to describe how the reality of international trade deviates from the theoretical ideal of unrestricted free trade reviewed in Chapter 4. Consistent with this objective, in this chapter we have reported the various instruments of trade policy, reviewed the political and economic arguments for government intervention in international trade, reexamined the economic case for free trade in light of the strategic trade policy argument, and looked at the evolution of the world trading framework. While a policy of free trade may not always be the theoretically optimal policy (given the arguments of the new trade theorists), in practice it is probably the best policy for a government to pursue. In particular, the long-run interests of business and consumers may be best served by strengthening international institutions such as the WTO. Given the danger that isolated protectionism might escalate into a trade war, business probably has far more to gain from government efforts to open protected markets to imports and foreign direct investment (through the WTO) than from government efforts to protect domestic industries from foreign competition.

The chapter made these major points:

1. The effect of a tariff is to raise the cost of imported products. Gains accrue to the government (from revenues) and to producers (who are protected from foreign competitors). Consumers lose because they must pay more for imports.

2. By lowering costs, subsidies help domestic producers to compete against low-cost foreign imports and to gain export markets. However, subsidies must be paid for by taxpayers. They also tend to be captured by special interests that use them to protect the inefficient.

3. An import quota is a direct restriction imposed by an importing country on the quantity of some

good that may be imported. A voluntary export restraint (VER) is a quota on trade imposed from the exporting country's side. Both import quotas and VERs benefit domestic producers by limiting import competition, but they result in higher prices, which hurts consumers.

4. A local content requirement calls for some specific fraction of a good to be produced domestically. Local content requirements benefit the producers of component parts, but they raise prices of imported components, which hurts consumers.

5. An administrative policy is an informal instrument or bureaucratic rule that can be used to restrict imports and boost exports. Such policies benefit producers but hurt consumers, who are denied access to possibly superior foreign products.

6. There are two types of arguments for government intervention in international trade: political and economic. Political arguments for intervention are concerned with protecting the interests of certain groups, often at the expense of other groups, or with promoting goals with regard to foreign policy, human rights, consumer protection, and the like. Economic arguments for intervention are about boosting the overall wealth of a nation.

7. The most common political argument for intervention is that it is necessary to protect jobs. However, political intervention often hurts consumers and it can be self-defeating.

8. Countries sometimes argue that it is important to protect certain industries for reasons of national security.

9. Some argue that government should use the threat to intervene in trade policy as a bargaining tool to open up foreign markets. This can be a risky policy; if it fails, the result can be higher trade barriers.

10. The infant industry argument for government intervention contends that to let manufacturing get a toehold, governments should temporarily support new industries. In practice, however, governments often end up protecting the inefficient.

11. Strategic trade policy suggests that with subsidies, government can help domestic firms gain first-mover advantages in global industries where economies of scale are important. Government subsidies may also help domestic firms overcome barriers to entry into such industries.

12. The problems with strategic trade policy are twofold: (a) such a policy may invite retaliation, in which case all will lose, and (b) strategic trade policy may be captured by special-interest groups, which will distort it to their own ends.

13. The Smoot-Hawley tariff, introduced in 1930, erected an enormous wall of tariff barriers to imports. Other countries responded by adopting similar tariffs, and the world slid further into the Great Depression

14. The GATT was a product of the postwar free trade movement. The GATT was successful in lowering trade barriers on manufactured goods and commodities. The move toward greater free trade under the GATT appeared to stimulate economic growth.

15. The completion of the Uruguay Round of GATT talks and the establishment of the World Trade Organization have strengthened the world trading system by extending GATT rules to services, increasing protection for intellectual property, reducing agricultural subsidies, and enhancing monitoring and enforcement mechanisms.

16. Trade barriers act as a constraint on a firm's ability to disperse its various production activities to optimal locations around the globe. One response to trade barriers is to establish more production activities in the protected country.

17. Business may have more to gain from government efforts to open protected markets to imports and foreign direct investment than from government efforts to protect domestic industries from foreign competition.

Critical Discussion Questions

1. Do you think governments should take human rights considerations into account when granting preferential trading rights to countries? What are the arguments for and against taking such a position?

2. Whose interests should be the paramount concern of government trade policy—the interests of producers (businesses and their employees) or those of consumers?

3. Given the arguments relating to the new trade theory and strategic trade policy, what kind of trade policy should business be pressuring government to adopt?

4. You are an employee of a U.S. firm that produces personal computers in Thailand and then exports them to the United States and other countries for sale. The personal computers were originally pro-

duced in Thailand to take advantage of relatively low labor costs and a skilled workforce. Other possible locations considered at the time were Malaysia and Hong Kong. The U.S. government decides to impose punitive 100 percent ad valorem tariffs on imports of computers from Thailand to punish the country for administrative trade barriers that restrict U.S. exports to Thailand. How do you think your firm should re-spond? What does this tell you about the use of targeted trade barriers?

5. Some economists argue that reducing barriers to trade in agricultural products will do more to stimulate the economic development of the world's less developed countries than foreign aid could ever do. Is this view correct? Who will benefit from free trade in agricultural products? Who will lose?

Notes

1. For a detailed welfare analysis of the effect of a tariff, see P. R. Krugman and M. Obstfeld, *International Economics: Theory and Policy* (New York: HarperCollins, 2000), chap. 8.

2. Y. Sazanami, S. Urata, and H. Kawai, *Measuring the Costs of Protection in Japan* (Washington, DC: Institute for International Economics, 1994).

3. J. Bhagwati, *Protectionism* (Cambridge, MA: MIT Press, 1988), and "Costs of Protection," *Journal of Commerce*, September 25, 1991, p. 8A.

4. "A Not So Perfect Market," *The Economist: Survey of Agriculture and Technology*, March 25, 2000, pp. 8–10.

5. "From the Sublime to the Subsidy," *The Economist*, February 24, 1990, p. 71.

6. The study was undertaken by Kym Anderson of the University of Adelaide. See "A Not So Perfect Market."

7. R. W. Crandall, *Regulating the Automobile* (Washington, DC: Brookings Institution, 1986).

8. Quoted in Krugman and Obstfeld, *International Economics*.

9. G. Hufbauer and Z. A. Elliott, *Measuring the Costs of Protectionism in the United States* (Washington, DC: Institute for International Economics, 1993).

10. A. Tanzer, "The Great Quota Hustle," *Forbes*, March 6, 2000, pp. 119–25.

11. Bhagwati, *Protectionism*, and "Japan to Curb VCR Exports," *New York Times*, November 21, 1983, p. D5.

12. Alan Goldstein, "Sematech Members Facing Dues Increase; 30% Jump to Make Up for Loss of Federal Funding," *Dallas Morning News*, July 27, 1996, p. 2F.

13. N. Dunne and R. Waters, "U.S. Waves a Big Stick at Chinese Pirates," *Financial Times*, January 6, 1995, p. 4.

14. John Broder, "Clinton to Impose Ban on 58 Types of Imported Guns," *New York Times*, April 6, 1998, p. A1.

15. Bill Lambrecht, "Monsanto Softens Its Stance on Labeling in Europe," *St. Louis Post-Dispatch*, March 15, 1998, p. E1.

16. Peter S. Jordan, "Country Sanctions and the International Business Community," *American Society of International Law Proceedings of the Annual Meeting* 20, no. 9 (1997), pp. 333–42.

17. "Waiting for China; Human Rights and International Trade," *Commonwealth*, March 11, 1994, and "China: The Cost of Putting Business First," *Human Rights Watch*, July 1996.

18. "Brazil's Auto Industry Struggles to Boost Global Competitiveness," *Journal of Commerce*, October 10, 1991, p. 6A.

19. For reviews, see J. A. Brander, "Rationales for Strategic Trade and Industrial Policy," in *Strategic Trade Policy and the New International Economics*, ed. P. R. Krugman (Cambridge, MA: MIT Press, 1986); P. R. Krugman, "Is Free Trade Passé?" *Journal of Economic Perspectives* 1 (1987), pp. 131–44; and P. R. Krugman, "Does the New Trade Theory Require a New Trade Policy?" *World Economy* 15, no. 4 (1992), pp. 423–41.

20. "Airbus and Boeing: The Jumbo War," *The Economist*, June 15, 1991, pp. 65–66.

21. For details see Krugman, *Is Free Trade Passé?* and Brander, "Rationales for Strategic Trade and Industrial Policy."

22. Krugman, *Is Free Trade Passé?*

23. This dilemma is a variant of the famous prisoner's dilemma, which has become a classic metaphor for the difficulty of achieving cooperation between self-interested and mutually suspicious entities. For a good general introduction, see A. Dixit and B. Nalebuff, *Thinking Strategically: The Competitive Edge in Business, Politics, and Everyday Life* (New York: W. W. Norton & Co., 1991).

24. Note that the Smoot-Hawley tariff did not cause the Great Depression. However, the beggar-thy-neighbor trade policies that it ushered in

certainly made things worse. See Bhagwati, *Protectionism*.

25. Ibid.

26. World Bank, *World Development Report* (New York: Oxford University Press, 1987).

27. World Trade Organization, *International Trade Statistics 2002* (Geneva: WTO, 2002).

28. Frances Williams, "WTO—New Name Heralds New Powers," *Financial Times*, December 16, 1993, p. 5, and Frances Williams, "Gatt's Successor to Be Given Real Clout," *Financial Times*, April 4, 1994, p. 6.

29. Information provided on WTO website at http://www.wto.org/english/tratop_e/dispu_e/dispu_status_e.htm.

30. Alan Cane, "Getting Through: Why Telecommunications Talks Matter," *Financial Times*, February 14, 1997.

31. Frances Williams, "Telecoms: World Pact Set to Slash Costs of Calls," *Financial Times*, February 17, 1997.

32. WTO press brief, "Financial Services," September 1996.

33. G. De Jonquieres, "Happy End to a Cliff Hanger," *Financial Times*, December 15, 1997, p. 15.

34. Jim Carlton, "Greens Target WTO Plan for Lumber," *Wall Street Journal*, November 24, 1999, p. A2.

35. Kari Huus, "WTO Summit Leaves Only Discontent," MSNBC, December 3, 1999 (www.msnbc.com).

36. WTO statistics on the WTO antidumping web site at http://www.wto.org/english/tratop_e/adp_e/adp_e.htm.

37. Ibid.

38. *Annual Report by the Director General* (Geneva: World Trade Organization, 2001).

39. Ibid.

40. World Trade Organization, *Annual Report 2002* (Geneva: WTO, 2002).

41. A. Tanzer, "Pill Factory to the World," *Forbes*, December 10, 2001, pp. 70–72.

42. W. Vieth, "Major Concessions Lead to Success for WTO Talks," *Los Angeles Times*, November 14, 2001, p. A1, and "Seeds Sown for Future Growth," *The Economist*, November 17, 2001, pp. 65–66.

43. "Punitive Tariffs Are Approved on Imports of Japanese Steel," *New York Times*, June 12, 1999, p. A3.

Research Task | globalEDGE™   globaledge.msu.edu

Use the globalEDGE™ site to complete the following exercises:

1. Your company is considering exporting its products to Egypt. Yet, management's current knowledge of this country's trade policies and barriers is limited. Conduct a web research to identify Egypt's current import policies with respect to fundamental issues such as tariffs and restrictions; prepare an executive summary of your findings.

2. The number of member nations of the World Trade Organization is increasing constantly. Additionally, some of the non-member countries have observer status, which requires accession negotiations to begin within five years of attaining the preliminary position. Identify the current total number of WTO members. Also, prepare a list of the observer countries.

Closing Case

Is a Tax Break an Export Subsidy?

The U.S. economy was facing a surging trade deficit in 1971. Alarmed by this, then-President Nixon concocted a special income tax break for U.S. exporters. The corporate deduction, known as the Foreign Sales Corporation (FSC), produced large tax savings for U.S. exporters, although it is questionable as to whether those had an impact on the trade deficit. In 1999 and 2000, however, the FSC moved to center stage in a trade dispute between the United States and the European Union that ended up at the World Trade Organization.

The FSC tax break allows exporters to avoid paying corporate income tax on exports of manufactured goods, the sales of which are channeled through shell companies, known as foreign sales corporations, which are registered in offshore tax havens such as Bermuda. While this sounds fairly arcane, the benefits are not. Estimates suggest that some 6,000 U.S. companies saved about $3.5 billion in income taxes in 1998 as a result of the FSC. Two of the major beneficiaries include Boeing and General Electric. Boeing saved $130 million in taxes in 1998 as a result of the FSC, 12 percent of its total earnings that year, while General Electric saved $150 million.

In 1998, the European Union filed a complaint with the WTO claiming that the FSC constituted an illegal export subsidy that was in clear violation of WTO rules. The United States was a bit taken aback by this action, arguing that it had an unwritten "gentleman's agreement" with the EU that neither entity would attack each other's tax systems in trade courts. Furthermore, the United States stated that tax codes had always been seen as "internal matters" that fell outside the jurisdiction of trade policy. The EU replied that this was a hypocritical stance. The United States had already challenged the EU at the WTO on other policies that are normally considered "internal matters," such as food safety and environmental regulations. (The United States had complained to the WTO about the EU policy to ban hormone-treated beef, which the EU implemented for safety and environmental reasons.) Given this, why should tax codes be any different? After hearing the evidence, a WTO arbitration panel in February 2000 agreed with the EU, arguing that the tax break was illegal because it applied just to exports and was thus technically an export subsidy and in violation of WTO rules. The United States was given until October 1, 2000, to revise the code or face the possibility of punitive sanctions. The prospect of trade sanctions sent Treasury officials, tax lawyers, members of Congress, and business lobbyists into a frenzy to fashion a fix for the FSC. After working in secret for several months, the Ways and Means Committee of the House of Representatives formulated a bill to amend the FSC. While the bill did scrap many of the FSC provisions, it not only retained the tax break given to export sales, but also expanded the break, adding $1.5 billion to the projected $25 billion cost of the tax write-off to the U.S. Treasury. In reaching this decision, the politicians argued that the reason for retaining the tax break was to compensate for the EU practice of granting European exporters a rebate on the value-added taxes they normally have to pay.

The Europeans were quick to point out that trade rules allow rebates on consumption taxes such as the European value-added tax and on U.S. excise taxes and state sales taxes, but specifically not on income tax. Moreover, the Europeans do not exempt their corporations from paying income tax on export revenue. The EU signaled that if the revised FSC code were passed, it would challenge it in the WTO and seek permission to impose punitive tariffs worth $4.04 billion on U.S. exports to the EU. That threat got the attention of Congress, which scrambled to amend the legislation. In mid-November 2000, the U.S. Congress passed an amended bill that repealed the FSC, but replaced it with a new system that offered up to $6 billion a year in tax breaks to large exporters such as Boeing and Microsoft. The United States claimed the new scheme would bring it into compliance with WTO rules. The EU countered that the new code was no better than the FSC, since it still maintained a tax break for export income. Two days later it filed a brief with the WTO seeking permission to impose punitive tariffs of $4.04 billion on U.S. exports.

In late December 2000, the WTO agreed to set up a panel to review the new U.S. tax code. At the same time, the WTO gave the EU permission to impose sanctions against the United States if the revised code is found to be in violation of WTO rules. Suddenly, an arcane debate over tax codes had moved to center stage in the trade debate and risked sparking a trade war between the world's two largest trading entities. After several delays, the WTO finally issued its ruling in August 2002. The EU ruled that the tax break to U.S. corporations was indeed an export subsidy, and granted the EU the right to impose $4 billion in penalties in the form of retaliatory tariffs on U.S. exports to the EU. The EU, however, made it clear that it would not impose the sanctions immediately, and would instead give the United States time to change its tax laws. The U.S. government reluctantly indicated it would change the offending law.

Sources: A. Entous, "Congress Oks Bill to Avert Trade War with EU," *Reuters,* November 14, 2000; G. Winestock, "EU Aims for Huge Sanctions on the U.S.," *Wall Street Journal,* November 20, 2000, p. A2; and P. Magnusson, "The Tax Break Could Trigger a Trade War," *Business Week,* September 4, 2000, pp. 103–04; and E. L. Andrews, "Trade Panel Says Europe Can Impose Penalties on the U.S," *New York Times,* August 31, 2002, p. A1.

Case Discussion Questions

1. How does the FSC item in the U.S. tax code constitute an export subsidy?

2. Do you think that "internal matters" such as tax codes and food safety laws should be excluded from consideration by the World Trade Organization?

3. Why do you think the U.S. Congress was apparently so reluctant to scrap the FSC?

4. What do you think might occur if the U.S. government fails to amend its tax laws? Would the EU impose sanctions? What would the U.S. response be?

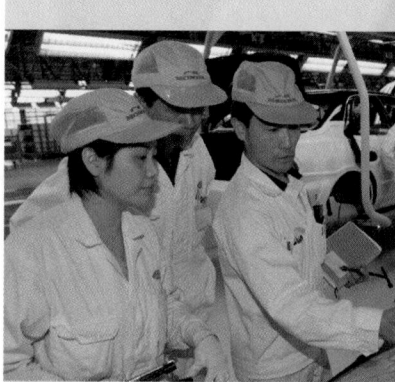

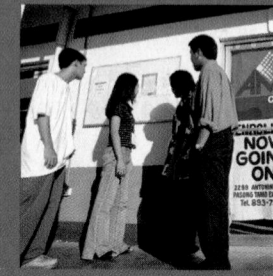

Chapter 6

Foreign Direct Investment

Introduction
Foreign Direct Investment in the World
Economy
  Trends in FDI
  The Direction of FDI
  The Source of FDI
  The Form of FDI: Acquisitions versus
  Green-Field Investments
Horizontal Foreign Direct Investment
  Transportation Costs
  Market Imperfections (Internalization
  Theory)
  Strategic Behavior
  The Product Life Cycle
  Location-Specific Advantages
Vertical Foreign Direct Investment
  Strategic Behavior
  Market Imperfections
Focus on Managerial Implications
Chapter Summary
Critical Discussion Questions
Closing Case: Ford and General Motors
in Russia

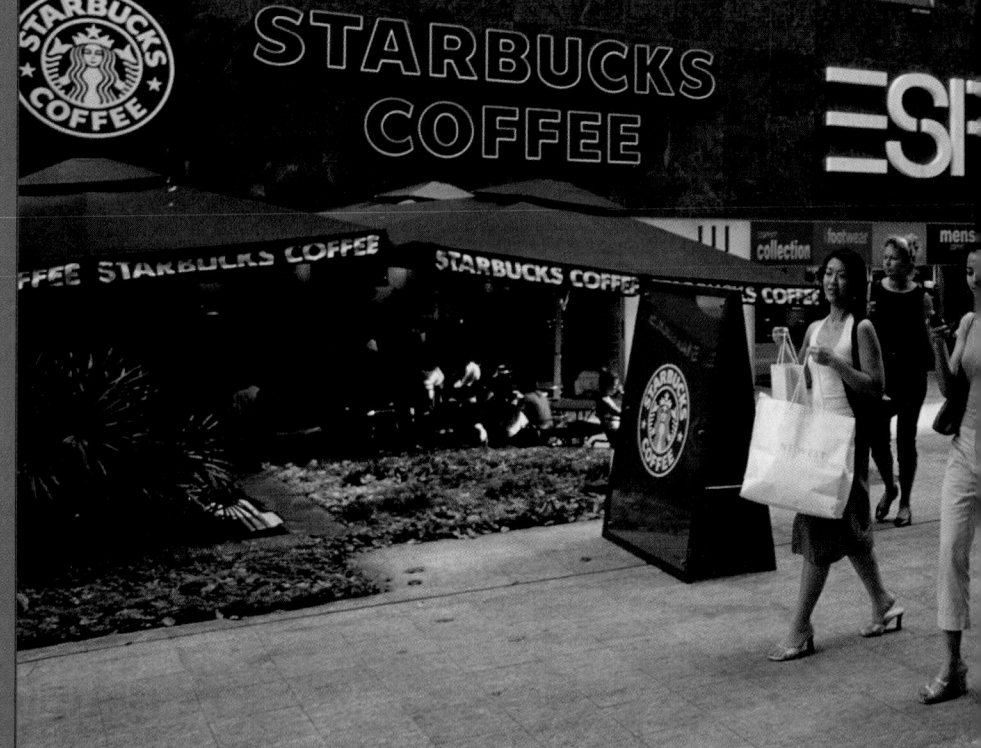

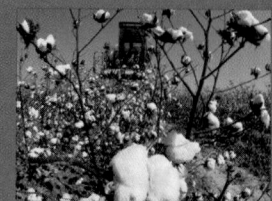

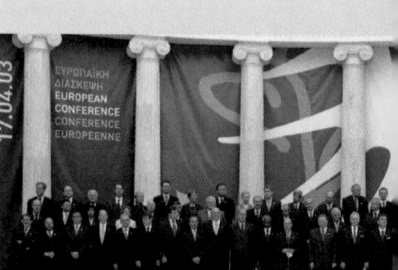

Starbucks' Foreign Direct Investment

Thirty years ago Starbucks was a single store in Seattle's Pike Place Market selling premium roasted coffee. Today it is a global roaster and retailer of coffee with more than 6,000 stores, an increasing proportion of which are to be found outside the United States. Starbucks Corporation set out on its current course in the 1980s when the company's director of marketing, Howard Schultz, came back from a trip to Italy enchanted with the Italian coffeehouse experience. Schultz, who later became CEO, persuaded the company's owners to experiment with the coffeehouse format—and the Starbucks experience was born. The basic strategy was to sell the company's own premium roasted coffee, along with freshly brewed espresso-style coffee beverages, a variety of pastries, coffee accessories, teas, and other products, in a tastefully designed coffeehouse setting. The company also stressed providing superior customer service. Reasoning that motivated employees provide the best customer service, Starbucks executives devoted much attention to employee hiring and training programs and progressive compensation policies that gave even part-time employees stock option grants and medical benefits. The formula met with spectacular success in the United States, where Starbucks went from obscurity to one of the best known brands in the country in a decade.

In 1995, with almost 700 stores across the United States, Starbucks began exploring foreign opportunities. Its first target market was Japan. Although Starbucks had resisted a franchising strategy in North America, where its stores are company owned, Starbucks initially decided to license its format in Japan. However, the company also realized that a pure licensing agreement would not give Starbucks the control needed to ensure that the Japanese licensees closely followed Starbucks' successful formula. So the company established a joint venture with a local retailer, Sazaby Inc. Each company held a 50 percent stake in the venture, Starbucks Coffee of Japan. Starbucks initially invested $10 million in this venture, its first foreign direct investment. The Starbucks format was then licensed to the venture, which was charged with taking over responsibility for growing Starbucks' presence in Japan.

To make sure the Japanese operations replicated the North American "Starbucks experience," Starbucks transferred some employees to the Japanese operation. The licensing agreement required all Japanese store managers and employees to attend training classes similar to those given to U.S. employees. The agreement also required that stores adhere to the design parameters established in the United States. In 2001, the company introduced a stock option plan for all Japanese employees, making it the first company in Japan to do so. Skeptics doubted that Starbucks would be able to replicate its North American success overseas, but by early 2003, Starbucks had more than 310 stores in Japan and plans to continue opening them at a brisk pace.

After getting its feet wet in Japan, the company embarked on an aggressive foreign investment program. In 1998, it purchased Seattle Coffee, a British coffee chain with 60 retail stores, for $84 million. An American couple, originally from Seattle, had started Seattle Coffee with the intention of establishing a Starbucks-like chain in Britain. In the late 1990s, Starbucks opened stores in Taiwan, China, Singapore, Thailand, New Zealand, South Korea, and Malaysia.

In Asia, Starbucks' most common strategy was to license its format to a local operator in return for initial licensing fees and royalties on store revenues. Starbucks also sold coffee and related products to the local licensees, who then resold them to customers. As in Japan, Starbucks insisted on an intensive employee training program and strict specifications regarding the format and layout of the store. However, Starbucks became disenchanted with some of the straight licensing arrangements and converted several into joint-venture arrangements or wholly owned subsidiaries. In Thailand, for example, Starbucks initially entered into a licensing agreement with Coffee Partners, a local Thai company. Under the terms of the licensing agreement, Coffee Partners was required to open at least 20 Starbucks coffee stores in Thailand within five years. However, Coffee Partners found it difficult to raise funds from Thai banks to finance this expansion. In July 2000, Starbucks acquired Coffee Partners for about $12 million. Its goal was to gain tighter control over the expansion strategy in Thailand. A similar development occurred in South Korea, where Starbucks initially licensed its format to ESCO Korea Ltd. in 1999. Although ESCO soon had 10 very successful stores open, Starbucks felt that ESCO would not be able to achieve the company's aggressive growth targets, so in December 2000 it converted its licensing arrangement into a joint venture with Shinsegae, the parent company of ESCO. The joint venture enabled Starbucks to exercise greater control over the growth strategy in South Korea and to help fund that operation, while gaining the benefits of a local operating partner.

By October 2000, Starbucks had invested some $52 million in foreign joint ventures. By the end of 2002, Starbucks had more than 1,200 stores in 27 countries outside of North America and was initiating aggressive expansion plans into Europe. The company's plans called for opening some 650 stores in six European countries, including the coffee cultures of France and Italy, by 2005. As its first entry point on the European Continent (Starbucks had 150 stores in Great Britain), Starbucks chose Switzerland. Drawing on its experience in Asia, the company entered into a joint venture with a Swiss company, Bon Appetit Group, Switzerland's largest food service company. Bon Appetit was to hold a majority stake in the venture, and Starbucks would license its format to the Swiss company using an agreement similar to those it had used successfully in Asia.

Sources: Starbucks 10K, various years; C. McLean, "Starbucks Set to Invade Coffee-Loving Continent," *Seattle Times,* October 4, 2000, p. E1; J. Ordonez, "Starbucks to Start Major Expansion in Overseas Market," *Wall Street Journal,* October 27, 2000, p. B10; and S. Homes and D. Bennett, "Planet Starbucks," *Business Week,* September 9, 2002, pp 99–110.

▇ Introduction

This chapter is concerned with foreign direct investment (FDI). **Foreign direct investment** occurs when a firm invests directly in facilities to produce and/or market a product in a foreign country. When Starbucks invested $10 million in Starbucks Coffee of Japan in 1996, it was engaging in its first foreign direct investment. According to the U.S. Department of Commerce, FDI occurs whenever a U.S. citizen, organization, or affiliated group takes an interest of 10 percent or more in a foreign business entity (all of Starbucks' foreign investments were for more than 10 percent of the equity of a business). Once a firm undertakes FDI, it becomes a **multinational enterprise** (the meaning of multinational being "more than one country").

FDI takes on two main forms. The first is a **green-field investment,** which involves the establishment of a wholly new operation in a foreign country. The second involves acquiring or merging with an existing firm in the foreign country. Acquisitions can be a minority (where the foreign firm takes a 10 percent to 49 percent interest in the firm's voting stock), majority (foreign interest of 50 percent to 99 percent), or full outright stake (foreign interest of 100 percent).[1] There is an important distinction between FDI and **foreign portfolio investment** (FPI). Foreign portfolio investment is investment by individuals, firms, or public bodies (e.g., national and local governments) in foreign financial instruments (e.g., government bonds, foreign stocks). FPI does not involve taking a significant equity stake in a foreign business entity (i.e., the equity stake is less than 10 percent). FPI is determined by different factors than FDI and raises different issues. Accordingly, we discuss FPI in Chapter 11 in our review of the international capital market.

In Chapter 4, we considered several theories that sought to explain the pattern of trade between countries. These theories focus on why countries export some products and import others. None of these theories addresses why a firm might decide to invest directly in production facilities in a foreign country, rather than exporting its domestic production to that country or licensing a foreign entity to produce its product in return for licensing fees. The theories we reviewed in Chapter 4 do not explain the pattern of foreign direct investment between countries. They do not explain, for example, why Starbucks chose to acquire Seattle Coffee in Great Britain, rather than simply license the Starbucks formula to a British firm. The theories we explore in this chapter seek to do just this.

Our central objective will be to identify the economic rationale that underlies foreign direct investment. Firms often view exports and FDI as substitutes for each other. For example, when deciding to serve the North American market, Toyota had to choose between exporting and foreign direct investment in North American production facilities. Although Toyota initially served the North American market through exports, increasingly it has turned to FDI. Toyota now has the capability to produce 600,000 cars a year in North America. This chapter attempts to understand the conditions under which firms such as Toyota prefer FDI to exporting. We will review various theories regarding these conditions.

These theories also need to explain why it is preferable for a firm to engage in FDI rather than licensing. **Licensing** occurs when a domestic firm, the licensor, licenses to a foreign firm, the licensee, the right to produce its product, to use its production processes, or to use its brand name or trademark. In return for giving the licensee these rights, the licensor collects royalty fees on every unit the licensee sells or on total licensee revenues. The advantage claimed for licensing over FDI is that the licensor does not have to pay for opening a foreign market; the licensee does that. Nor does the licensor have to bear the risks associated with opening a foreign market. However, despite these attractions, many firms are reluctant to engage in straight licensing arrangements, preferring to make some kind of foreign direct investment. Thus, in the opening case we saw that Starbucks originally considered a straight licensing strategy for entering the Japanese market but ultimately entered through a joint venture, which required some direct investment. Similarly, while the company did initially license its format in several Asian countries, such as Thailand and South Korea, there too it has switched to a direct investment strategy, acquiring its Thai licensee and entering into a joint venture with its South Korean licensee. What is the theoretical rationale for such a decision? The opening case hints that the need for control was a consideration. We shall develop the theoretical explanation in this chapter, and as we shall see, the need for control is an important factor in explaining the decision.

In the remainder of the chapter, we first look at the growing importance of FDI in the world economy. Next we look at the theories that have been used to explain horizontal foreign direct investment. **Horizontal foreign direct investment** is FDI in the same industry in which a firm operates at home. Starbucks' acquisition of Seattle Coffee in Britain is an example of horizontal FDI. After reviewing horizontal FDI, we consider the theories that help to explain vertical foreign direct investment. **Vertical foreign direct investment** is investment in an industry that provides inputs for a firm's domestic operations, or it may be FDI in an industry abroad that sells the outputs of a firm's domestic operations. Finally, we review the implications of these theories for business practice.

Foreign Direct Investment in the World Economy ■

When discussing foreign direct investment, it is important to distinguish between the flow of FDI and the stock of FDI. The **flow of FDI** refers to the amount of FDI undertaken over a given time period (normally a year). The **stock of FDI** refers to the total accumulated value of foreign-owned assets at a given time. We also talk of **outflows of FDI,** meaning the flow of FDI out of a country, and **inflows of FDI,** meaning the flow of FDI into a country.

Trends in FDI

The past 20 years have seen a marked increase in both the flow and stock of FDI in the world economy. The average yearly flow of FDI increased from about $25 billion in 1975 to a record $1.3 trillion in 2000, before slumping dramatically in 2001 to $735 billion and to an estimated $534 billion in 2002 (see Figure 6.1).[2] Between 1975 and 2001 the flow of FDI not only accelerated but also accelerated faster than the growth in world trade. For example, between 1990 and 2001, the total flow of FDI from all countries increased about 365 percent, while world trade grew by some 75 percent and world output by 26 percent (see Figure 6.2).[3] As a result of the strong FDI flow, by 2001 the global stock of FDI exceeded $6.6 trillion. In total, 65,000 parent companies had 850,000 affiliates in foreign markets that collectively produced an estimated $19 trillion in global sales, nearly twice as high as the value of global exports.[4]

FDI has grown more rapidly than world trade and world output for several reasons. Despite the general decline in trade barriers that we have witnessed over the past 30 years, business firms still fear protectionist pressures. Executives see FDI as

Figure 6.1

FDI Outflows, 1982–2002

Source: *United Nations, World Investment Report, 2002* (New York and Geneva: United Nations, 2002), and United Nations, "UNCTAD Predicts 27% Drop in FDI Flows This Year," United Nations Press Release TAD/INF/PR/63, October 24, 2002.

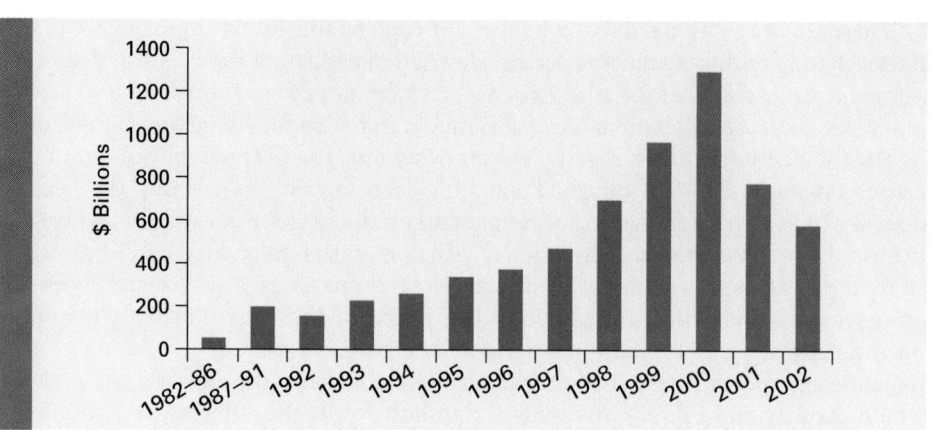

Figure 6.2

Growth in World Exports, World GDP, and FDI, 1990–2001 (index = 100 in 1990)

Source: United Nations, *World Investment Report, 2002* (New York and Geneva: United Nations, 2001), and World Trade Organization, *International Trade Statistics 2002* (Geneva: WTO, 2002).

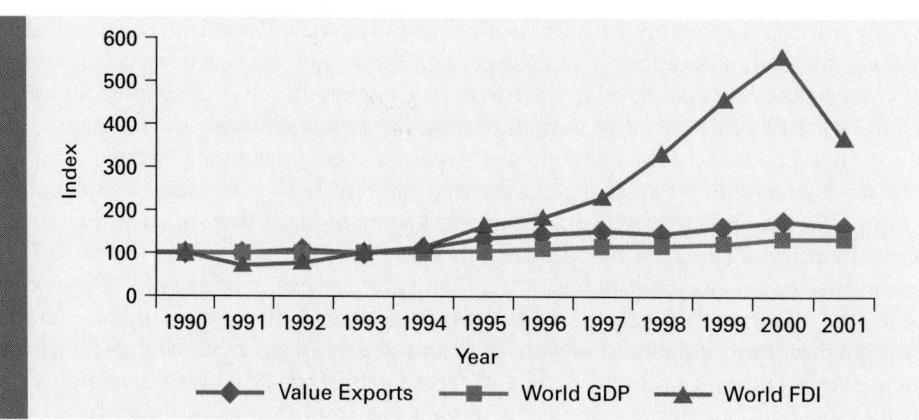

a way of circumventing future trade barriers. Much of the Japanese automobile companies' investment in the United States during the 1980s and early 1990s was driven by a desire to reduce exports from Japan, thereby alleviating trade tensions between the two nations. Also, much of the recent increase in FDI is being driven by the dramatic political and economic changes that have been occurring in many of the world's developing nations. The general shift toward democratic political institutions and free market economies that we discussed in Chapter 2 has encouraged FDI. Across much of Asia, Eastern Europe, and Latin America, economic growth, economic deregulation, privatization programs that are open to foreign investors, and the removal of many restrictions on FDI have made these countries more attractive to foreign investors. According to the United Nations, some 95 percent of the 1,393 changes made between 1991 and 2001 worldwide in the laws governing foreign direct investment created a more favorable environment for FDI. The desire of governments to facilitate FDI has also been reflected in a dramatic increase in the number of bilateral investment treaties designed to protect and promote investment between two countries. As of 2002, there were 2,099 such treaties in the world involving more than 160 countries, a 10-fold increase from the 181 treaties that existed in 1980.[5]

The globalization of the world economy, a phenomenon that we first discussed in Chapter 1, is also having a positive impact on the volume of FDI. Firms such as Starbucks now see the whole world as their market, and they are undertaking FDI in an attempt to make sure they have a significant presence in many regions of the world. For reasons that we shall explore later in this book, many firms now believe it is important to have production facilities based close to their major customers. This, too, is creating pressures for greater FDI.

Slumping FDI: 2001 and 2002

In contrast to the long-term trend, between 2000 and 2002 the value of FDI slumped almost 60 percent from $1.3 trillion to about $543 billion (see Figure 6.1). The most notable decline was in the levels of cross-border mergers and acquisitions. In 2000, there were some 7,900 cross-border deals totaling $1.1 trillion. In 2001, the number of cross-border mergers and acquisitions fell to less than 6,000 deals that were valued at $594 billion, and initial figures suggest another 45 percent decline in 2002. The overall decline in FDI was also most pronounced in developed nations, where FDI flows fell in half to $503 billion in 2001, and then to an estimated $340 billion in 2002. In comparison, FDI into developing nations declined from $240 billion in 2000 to $205 billion in 2001 and an estimated $185 billion in 2002.[6]

The slowdown in FDI flows observed in 2001 and 2002 will probably be temporary. It appears to reflect three related developments: (1) the general slowdown in the growth rate of the world economy; (2) heightened geopolitical uncertainty following the September 11, 2001, attack on the United States; and (3) the bursting of the stock market bubble in the United States, which limited the ability of many companies to raise additional capital to finance aggressive FDI activity, particularly mergers and acquisitions. The surge in FDI during 1999 and 2000 was a product of the late 1990s stock market bubble, and in retrospect represented an unsustainable short-term peak in FDI activity. As noted, much of the FDI activity during this period took the form of mergers and acquisitions, and many of these were financed by issuing new shares on world stock markets. With global stock markets in a depressed state, this seems unlikely to be repeated soon.

Nevertheless, surveys undertaken by the United Nations and other institutions in late 2001 suggest that most corporations plan to continue with their foreign investment plans over the next five years. Among the nations that are likely to benefit from increased FDI inflows between 2001 and 2005, China seems likely to see the largest percentage increase. In 2001, China was the largest recipient of FDI among developing nations, with inflows of $46.8 billon, and in 2002 the country received an estimated $50 billion in additional FDI. Many firms planned to accelerate their investment in China following the country's December 2001 entry into the WTO. For example, in late 2001 one-quarter of large Japanese firms stated they would increase their investment in China following WTO entry or had already done so in anticipation of WTO entry.[7]

The Direction of FDI

Historically, most FDI has been directed at the developed nations of the world as firms based in advanced countries invested in the others' markets (see Figure 6.3). The United States has often been the favorite target for FDI inflows. This trend continued in the late 1990s, when the United States remained the largest recipient of foreign direct investment.[8] In 2000, the United States was again the largest national recipient of FDI, accounting for $281 billion of the $1.3 trillion in global FDI, while Western Europe was the largest single regional recipient of FDI, with $633 billion in inflows.[9] In 2001, the totals for the United States and Western Europe dropped to $124 billion and $323 billion, respectively, reflecting the drop in economic activity.[10] Historically, the United States has been an attractive target for FDI because of its large and wealthy domestic markets, its dynamic and stable economy, a favorable political environment, and the openness of the country to FDI. Investors included firms based in Britain, Japan, Germany, Holland, and France.

Although developed nations in general, and the United States in particular, still account for the largest share of FDI inflows, there has been some increase of FDI into the world's developing nations (see Figure 6.3). From 1985 to 1990, the annual inflow of FDI into developing nations averaged $27.4 billion, or 17.4 percent of the total global flow. By 1997, the inflow into developing nations had risen to $149 billion, or 37 percent of

Foreign Direct Investment in China

Beginning in late 1978, China's leadership decided to move the economy away from a centrally planned system to one that was more market driven, while still maintaining the rigid political framework of Communist Party control. The strategy had a number of key elements, including a switch to household responsibility in agriculture instead of the old collectivization, increases in the authority of local officials and plant managers in industry, establishment of small- to medium-scale private enterprises in services and light manufacturing, and increased foreign trade and investment. The result has been two decades of sustained high economic growth rates of between 10 and 11 percent annually compounded.

Starting from a tiny base, foreign investment surged to an annual average rate of $2.7 billion between 1985 and 1990 and then surged to reach $40 billion annually in the late 1990s, making China the second biggest recipient of FDI inflows in the world after the United States. Although world FDI flows slumped in 2001 and 2002, China still attracted close to $50 billion in each year. Over the past 20 years, this inflow has resulted in establishment of 170,000 foreign-funded enterprises in China. The total stock of FDI in China had grown to $395 billion in 2001 ($854 billion in Hong Kong is added to this figure), amounting to 28 percent of China's total GDP and 10 to 14 percent of annualized gross fixed capital formation between 1994 and 2001. FDI inflows have been a major source of investment and economic growth in China since liberalization began, accounting for perhaps as much as 30 percent of the country's growth.

The reasons for the investment are fairly obvious. With a population of 1.3 billion people, China represents the largest potential market in the world. Import tariffs have made it difficult to serve this market via exports, so FDI was required if a company wanted to tap into the country's huge potential. Although China joined the World Trade Organization in 2001, which will ultimately mean a reduction in import tariffs, this will occur only slowly, so this motive for investing in China will persist. Also, many foreign firms believe that doing business in China requires a substantial presence in the country to build *guanxi,* the crucial relationship networks (see Chapter 3 for details). Furthermore, a combination of cheap labor and tax incentives, particularly for enterprises that establish themselves in special economic zones, makes China an attractive base from which to serve Asian or world markets with exports. By 2001, foreign affiliates were accounting for some 50 percent of all exports from China, with rapid growth in exports of high-technology products from China made by the Chinese subsidiaries of companies such as Samsung, Nokia, and Motorola.

Less obvious, at least to begin with, was how difficult it would be for foreign firms to do business in China. Blinded by the size and potential of China's market, many firms have paid scant attention to the complexities of operating a business in this country until after the investment has been made. China may have a huge population, but despite two decades of rapid growth, it is still a poor country where the average income is little more than $750 per year. This lack of purchasing power translates into a weak market for many Western consumer goods from automobiles to

the total. In 2001, the flow into developing nations accounted for 27 percent of the total, and it rose to $185 billion and 35 percent of the total in 2002. Most recent inflows into developing nations have been targeted at the emerging economies of South, East, and Southeast Asia. Driving much of the increase has been the growing importance of China as a recipient of FDI.[11] The reasons for the strong flow of investment into China are discussed in the accompanying Country Focus.

Latin America emerged as the next most important region in the developing world for FDI inflows. In 2000, total inward investments into this region reached about $86 billion, and it remained at that level during 2001 before dropping to $62 billion in 2002. Much of this investment was concentrated on Mexico and Brazil and was a response to reforms in the region, including privatization, the liberalization of regulations governing FDI, and the growing importance of regional free trade areas such as MERCOSUR and NAFTA (which will be discussed in Chapter 8). At the other end of the scale, Africa received the smallest amount of inward investment, about $6 bil-

household appliances. Another problem is the lack of a well-developed transportation infrastructure or distribution system. PepsiCo discovered this problem at its subsidiary in Chongqing. Perched above the Yangtze River in southwest Sichuan province, Chongqing lies at the heart of China's massive hinterland. The Chongqing municipality, which includes the city and its surrounding regions, contains over 30 million people, but according to Steve Chen, the manager of the Pepsi subsidiary, the lack of well-developed road and distribution systems means he can reach only about half of this population with his product.

Other problems include a highly regulated environment that can make it problematic to conduct business transactions and shifting tax and regulatory regimes. For example, in 1997, the Chinese government suddenly scrapped a tax credit scheme that had made it attractive to import capital equipment into China. This immediately made it more expensive to set up operations in the country. There are also difficulties finding qualified personnel to staff operations. The cultural revolution produced a generation of people who lack the basic educational background that is taken for granted in the West. Because of the country's past, few local people understand the complexities of managing a modern industrial enterprise. Then there are problems with local joint-venture partners who are inexperienced, opportunistic, or simply operate according to different goals. One U.S. manager explained that when he laid off 200 people to reduce costs, his Chinese partner hired them all back the next day. When he inquired why they had been hired back, the Chinese partner, which was government owned, explained that as an agency of the government, it had an "obligation" to reduce unemployment.

To continue to attract foreign investment, the Chinese government has committed itself to invest more than $800 billion in infrastructure projects over the next 10 years. This should improve the nation's poor highway system. By giving preferential tax breaks to companies that invest in special regions, such as that around Chongqing, the Chinese have created incentives for foreign companies to invest in China's vast interior where markets are underserved. They have been pursuing a macroeconomic policy that includes an emphasis on maintaining steady economic growth, low inflation, and a stable currency, all of which are attractive to foreign investors. And to deal with the lack of qualified personnel, in the late 1990s, the government instructed universities to establish 30 business schools to train Chinese in basic skills such as accounting, finance, and human resource management. Given these developments, it seems likely that the country will continue to be an important magnet for foreign investors well into the future.

Sources: Interviews by the author while in China, March 1998; L. Sly, "China Losing Its Golden Glow," *Chicago Tribune*, September 15, 1997, p. 1; M. Miller, "Search for Fresh Capital Widens," *South China Morning Post*, April 9, 1998, p. 1; S. Mufson, "China Says Asian Crisis Will Have an Impact," *Washington Post*, March 8, 1998, p. A27; United Nations, *World Investment Report, 2002* (New York and Geneva: United Nations, 2002); and Linda Ng and C. Tuan, "Building a Favorable Investment Environment: Evidence for the Facilitation of FDI in China," *The World Economy*, 2002, pp. 1095–114.

lion in 2002. The inability of Africa to attract greater investment is in part a reflection of the political unrest, armed conflict, and frequent changes in economic policy in the region.[12]

Another way of looking at the importance of FDI inflows is to express them as a percentage of gross fixed capital formation. **Gross fixed capital formation** summarizes the total amount of capital invested in factories, stores, office buildings, and the like. Other things being equal, the greater the capital investment in an economy, the more favorable its future growth prospects are likely to be. Viewed this way, FDI can be seen as an important source of capital investment and a determinant of the future growth rate of an economy. Figure 6.4 summarizes inward flows of FDI as a percentage of gross fixed capital formation by region for 2000 (the latest year for which data are available). During 1996–2000, FDI accounted for about 11 percent of worldwide gross fixed capital formation, up from 4 percent worldwide in the early 1990s. These figures suggest that FDI is becoming an increasingly important source of investment in the world's economies.

Figure 6.3

FDI Flows by Region

Source: United Nations, *World Investment Report, 2002* (New York and Geneva: United Nations, 2002), and United Nations, "UNCTAD Predicts 27% Drop in FDI Flows This Year," United Nations Press Release TAD/INF/PR/63, October 24, 2002.

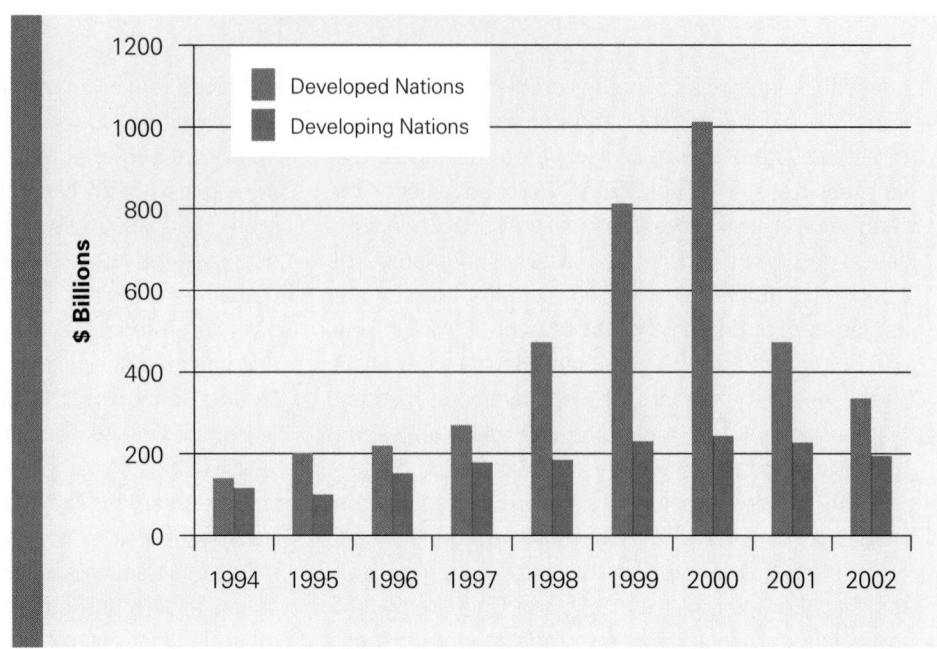

Figure 6.4

Inward FDI Flows as a Percentage of Gross Fixed Capital Formation, 2000

Source: United Nations, *World Investment Report, 2002* (New York and Geneva: United Nations, 2002).

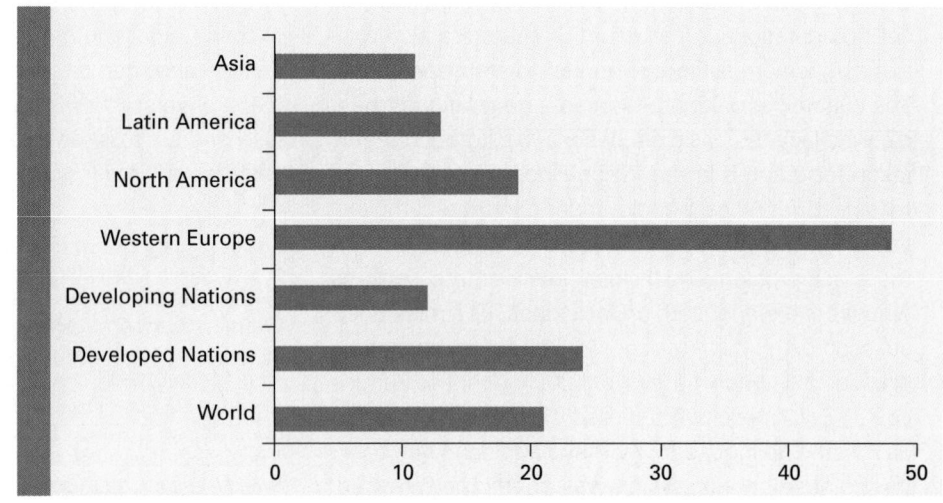

These gross figures hide important individual country differences. For example, in 2000, inward FDI accounted for some 46 percent of gross fixed capital formation in the United Kingdom, 28 percent in Brazil, and 23 percent in Chile, but only 2.3 percent in India, 6.3 percent in Italy, and 0.7 percent in Japan—suggesting that FDI is an important source of investment capital, and thus economic growth, in the first three countries, but not the latter three. These differences can be explained by several factors, including the perceived ease and attractiveness of investing in a nation. To the extent that burdensome regulations limit the opportunities for foreign investment in countries such as Japan and India, these nations may be hurting themselves by limiting their access to needed capital investments. We shall return to and discuss this issue in more detail in Chapter 7.

❙The Source of FDI

Since World War II, the United States has been by far the largest source country for FDI. During the late 1970s, the United States still accounted for about 47 percent of

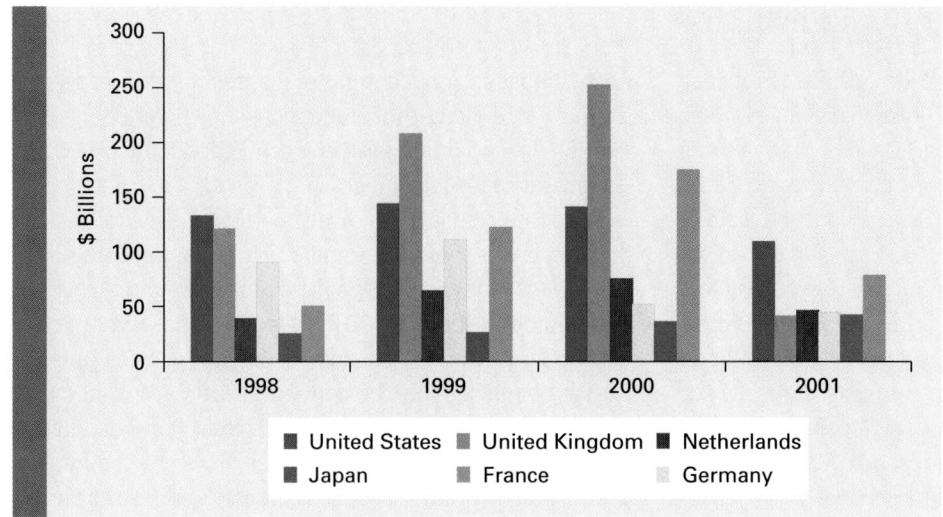

Figure 6.5

FDI Outflows by Select
Country, 1998–2001

Source: United Nations, *World Investment Report, 2002* (New York and Geneva: United Nations, 2002).

all FDI outflows from industrialized countries, while the second-place United Kingdom accounted for about 18 percent. U.S. firms so dominated the growth of FDI in the 1960s and 70s, that the words *American* and *multinational* became almost synonymous. By 1980, 178 of the world's largest 382 multinationals were U.S. firms, and 40 of them were British.[13] During 1985–90, the United States slipped to third place behind Japan and the United Kingdom. Since then the United States regained its dominant position in every year but 1999 and 2000, when the United Kingdom was the largest source country (see Figure 6.5). However, as a percentage of total outward FDI flows, the U.S. share declined to less than 20 percent by 1998–2001. The source of FDI by country remains highly concentrated, with five countries generally accounting for more than two-thirds of all foreign direct investment outflows. The countries illustrated in Figure 6.5 have dominated foreign direct investment outflows for much of the last two decades. As might be expected, these countries also predominate in rankings of the world's largest multinationals. As of 2001, 26 percent of the world's 100 largest multinationals were U.S. enterprises; 17 percent were Japanese; 12 percent were French; 12 percent, German; and 10 percent, British.[14]

The high level of FDI outflows from the United States during 1990–2000 was driven by a combination of factors including a strong U.S. economy; strong corporate profits and cash flow, which have given firms the capital to invest abroad; a booming stock market, which made it easy to raise capital to finance FDI; and a relatively strong currency. Similar factors explain the continued growth of FDI outflows from the United Kingdom during the 1990s.

The Form of FDI: Acquisitions versus Green-Field Investments

FDI can take the form of a green-field investment in a new facility or an acquisition of or a merger with an existing local firm. The data suggest the majority of cross-border investment is in the form of mergers and acquisitions rather than green-field investments. UN estimates indicate that some 70 to 80 percent of all FDI inflows are in the form of mergers and acquisitions. In 2001, for example, mergers and acquisitions accounted for some 78 percent of all FDI inflows.[15] However, there is a marked difference between FDI flows into developed and developing nations. In the case of *developing* nations, only about one-third of FDI is in the form of cross-border mergers and acquisitions. The lower percentage of FDI inflows that is in the form of mergers and acquisitions may simply reflect the fact that there are fewer target firms to acquire in developing nations.

Cemex's Foreign Acquisitions

In little more than a decade, Mexico's largest cement manufacturer, Cemex, has transformed itself from a primarily Mexican operation into the third largest cement company in the world behind Holderbank of Switzerland and Lafarge Group of France with 2001 sales of $6.7 billion and $2.2 billion in cash flow. Cemex has long been a powerhouse in Mexico and currently controls more than 60 percent of the market for cement in that country. Cemex's domestic success has been based in large part on an obsession with efficient manufacturing and a focus on customer service that is second to none in the industry.

Cemex is a leader in using information technology to match production with consumer demand. The company sells ready-mixed cement that can survive for only about 90 minutes before solidifying, so precise delivery is important. But Cemex can never predict with total certainty what demand will be on any given day, week, or month. To better manage unpredictable demand patterns, Cemex developed a system of seamless information technology, including truck-mounted global positioning systems, radio transmit-ters, satellites, and computer hardware, that allows Cemex to control the production and distribution of cement like no other company can, responding quickly to unanticipated changes in demand and reducing waste. The results are lower costs and superior customer service, both differentiating factors for Cemex.

The company also pays lavish attention to its distributors—some 5,000 in Mexico alone—who can earn points toward rewards for hitting sales targets. Those points can then be converted into Cemex stock. High-volume distributors can purchase trucks and other supplies through Cemex at significant discounts. Cemex also is known for its marketing drives that focus on end users, the builders themselves. For example, Cemex trucks drive around Mexican building sites, and if Cemex cement is being used, the construction crews win soccer balls, caps, and T-shirts.

Cemex's international expansion strategy was driven by a number of factors. First, the company wished to reduce its reliance on the Mexican construction market, which was characterized by very volatile demand. Second, the company realized there was tremendous demand for cement in many developing

---

When contemplating FDI, why do firms apparently prefer to acquire existing assets rather than undertake green-field investments? We shall return to this and consider it in greater depth in Chapter 14, so for now we will make only a few basic observations. First, mergers and acquisitions are quicker to execute than green-field investments. This is an important consideration in the modern business world where markets evolve very rapidly. Many firms apparently believe that if they do not acquire a desirable target firm, then their global rivals will. The case of Cemex in the accompanying Management Focus illustrates this. Cemex is the world's third largest cement company and Mexico's largest multinational company. Cemex's rise to global status took less than a decade and has been driven primarily by acquisitions. If Cemex had relied on green-field investments, it could not have become so large so fast.

Second, foreign firms are acquired because those firms have valuable strategic assets, such as brand loyalty, customer relationships, trademarks or patents, distribution systems, production systems, and the like. It is easier and perhaps less risky for a firm to acquire those assets than to build them from the ground up through a green-field investment. Cemex's acquisition of Houston-based cement maker Southland for $2.5 billion is a good example. Cemex wanted quick entry to the growing U.S. construction market, and Southland's production and distribution assets enabled Cemex to achieve this.

Third, firms make acquisitions because they believe they can increase the efficiency of the acquired unit by transferring capital, technology, or management skills. For example, Cemex has developed the best information systems in the global cement industry, which has enabled it to better meet customer needs (see the Management Focus for details). Cemex can increase the efficiency of its acquired units, such as countries, where significant construction was being undertaken or needed. Third, the company believed that it understood the needs of construction businesses in developing nations better than the established multinational cement companies, all of which were from developed nations. Fourth, Cemex believed that it could create significant value by acquiring cement companies in other markets and transferring its skills in customer service, marketing, information technology, and production management to those units.

The company embarked in earnest on its international expansion strategy in the early 1990s. Initially Cemex targeted other developing nations, acquiring established cement makers in Venezuela, Colombia, Indonesia, the Philippines, Egypt, and several other countries. It also purchased two stagnant companies in Spain and turned them around. Then in 2000, it undertook its largest purchase, the $2.5 billion acquisition of Houston-based Southland, one of the largest cement companies in the United States. Cemex entered 2002 with 56 cement plants in 30 countries, most of which were gained through acquisitions. In all cases, Cemex has devoted great attention to transferring its techno-

logical, management, and marketing know-how to acquired units, thereby improving their performance.

The benefits of this strategy have flowed through to the bottom line. From 1991 to 2001, the company's earnings before interest, tax, and depreciation when measured in U.S. dollars grew by more than 20 percent annually. Cash earnings per share also grew by 20 percent a year, while sales grew by 17 percent. Since profits have grown faster than sales, the company must be realizing significant efficiency gains in its acquired units. By 2001, Cemex was number one among the world's four largest cement manufacturers on most measures of financial performance, suggesting that its strategy of entering foreign markets through acquisitions was paying dividends, and it was more profitable than its major competitors.

Sources: C. Piggott, "Cemex's Stratospheric Rise," *Latin Finance,* March 2001, p. 76; J. F. Smith, "Making Cement a Household Word," *Los Angeles Times,* January 16, 2000, p. C1; D. Helft, "Cemex Attempts to Cement Its Future," *The Industry Standard,* November 6, 2000; and Diane Lindquist, "From Cement to Services," *Chief Executive,* November 2002, pp. 48–50.

Southland, by transferring its technological know-how to those units after the acquisition. Thus, there are some fairly compelling arguments for favoring mergers and acquisitions over green-field investments. But many mergers and acquisitions fail to realize their anticipated gains.[16] Chapter 11 further studies this issue.

Horizontal Foreign Direct Investment ■

Horizontal FDI is investment in the same industry abroad as a firm operates in at home. We need to understand why firms go to the trouble of acquiring or establishing operations abroad, when the alternatives of exporting and licensing are available. Other things being equal, FDI is expensive and risky compared to exporting or licensing. FDI is expensive because a firm must bear the costs of establishing production facilities in a foreign country or of acquiring a foreign enterprise. FDI is risky because of the problems associated with doing business in another culture where the "rules of the game" may be very different. Relative to firms native to a culture, there is a greater probability that a firm in a foreign culture will make costly mistakes due to ignorance. When a firm exports, it need not bear the costs of FDI, and the risks associated with selling abroad can be reduced by using a native sales agent. Similarly, when a firm licenses its know-how, it need not bear the costs or risks of FDI. So why do so many firms apparently prefer FDI over either exporting or licensing?

The quick answer is that other things are not equal! A number of factors can alter the relative attractiveness of exporting, licensing, and FDI. We will consider these factors: (1) transportation costs, (2) market imperfections, (3) strategic behavior, (4) the product life cycle, and (5) location advantages.

Transportation Costs

When transportation costs are added to production costs, it becomes unprofitable to ship some products a long distance. This is particularly true of products that have a low value-to-weight ratio and can be produced in almost any location (e.g., cement, soft drinks, etc.). For such products, relative to either FDI or licensing, the attractiveness of exporting decreases. Thus, transportation costs alone help explain why Cemex has undertaken FDI rather than exporting (see the Management Focus). For products with a high value-to-weight ratio, however, transport costs are normally a very minor component of total landed cost (e.g., electronic components, personal computers, medical equipment, computer software, etc.). In such cases, transportation costs have little impact on the relative attractiveness of exporting, licensing, and FDI.

Market Imperfections (Internalization Theory)

Market imperfections provide a major explanation of why firms may prefer FDI to either exporting or licensing. Market imperfections are factors that inhibit markets from working perfectly. The market imperfections explanation of FDI is the one favored by most economists.[17] In the international business literature, the marketing imperfections approach to FDI is typically referred to as internalization theory.

With regard to horizontal FDI, market imperfections arise in two circumstances: when there are impediments to the free flow of products between nations, and when there are impediments to the sale of know-how. (Licensing is a mechanism for selling know-how.) Impediments to the free flow of products between nations decrease the profitability of exporting, relative to FDI and licensing. Impediments to the sale of know-how increase the profitability of FDI relative to licensing. Thus, the market imperfections explanation predicts that FDI will be preferred whenever there are impediments that make both exporting and the sale of know-how difficult and/or expensive.

Impediments to Exporting

Governments are the main source of impediments to the free flow of products between nations. By placing tariffs on imported goods, governments increase the cost of exporting relative to FDI and licensing. Similarly, by limiting imports through the imposition of quotas, governments increase the attractiveness of FDI and licensing. For example, the wave of FDI by Japanese auto companies in the United States during the 1980s was partly driven by protectionist threats from Congress and by quotas on the importation of Japanese cars. For Japanese auto companies, these factors have decreased the profitability of exporting and increased the profitability of FDI.

Impediments to the Sale of Know-How

The competitive advantage that many firms enjoy comes from their technological, marketing, or management know-how. Technological know-how can enable a company to build a better product; for example, Nokia's technological know-how has given it a strong competitive position in the global market for wireless telephone equipment. Alternatively, technological know-how can improve a company's production process vis-à-vis competitors. For example, many claim that Toyota's competitive advantage comes from its superior production system. Marketing know-how can enable a company to better position its products in the marketplace; the competitive advantage of such companies as Kellogg, H. J. Heinz, and Procter & Gamble seems to come from superior marketing know-how. Management know-how with regard to factors such as organizational structure, human relations, control systems, planning systems, inventory management, and so on can enable a company to manage its assets more efficiently than competitors. The competitive advantage of Starbucks, which was profiled in the opening case, seems to come from valuable management knowledge related to the branding and operations of retail coffee stores. Similarly, Cemex has used its technological know-how to better manage customer demand and improve operating efficiencies and its marketing knowledge to build a well-earned reputation for being very customer focused (see Management Focus).

If we view know-how (expertise) as a competitive asset, it follows that the larger the market in which that asset is applied, the greater the profits that can be earned from the asset. Nokia can earn greater returns on its know-how by selling its wireless telephone equipment worldwide than by selling it only in its native Finland. However, this alone does not explain why Nokia undertakes FDI (the company has production locations around the world). For Nokia to favor FDI, two conditions must hold. First, transportation costs and/or impediments to exporting must rule out exporting as an option. Second, there must be some reason Nokia cannot sell its wireless know-how to foreign producers. Since licensing is the main mechanism by which firms sell their know-how, there must be some reason Nokia is not willing to license a foreign firm to manufacture and market its cellular telephone equipment. Other things being equal, licensing might look attractive to such a firm, since it would not have to bear the costs and risks associated with FDI yet it could still earn a good return from its know-how in the form of royalty fees.

According to economic theory, there are three reasons the market does not always work well as a mechanism for selling know-how, or why licensing is not as attractive as it initially appears. First, licensing may result in a firm's giving away its know-how to a potential foreign competitor. For example, in the 1960s, RCA licensed its leading-edge color television technology to a number of Japanese companies, including Matsushita and Sony. At the time, RCA saw licensing as a way to earn a good return from its technological know-how in the Japanese market without the costs and risks associated with FDI. However, Matsushita and Sony quickly assimilated RCA's technology and used it to enter the U.S. market to compete directly against RCA. As a result, RCA is now a minor player in its home market, while Matsushita and Sony have a much bigger market share.

Second, licensing does not give a firm the tight control over manufacturing, marketing, and strategy in a foreign country that may be required to profitably exploit its advantage in know-how. With licensing, control over production, marketing, and strategy is granted to a licensee in return for a royalty fee. However, for both strategic and operational reasons, a firm may want to retain control over these functions. For example, a firm might want its foreign subsidiary to price and market very aggressively, but the licensee may be unable to do this. The opening case showed how this became an issue with Starbucks, which originally pursued a licensing strategy in Thailand, but then acquired the Thai operation because it thought the licensee was not aggressive enough in growing the market and was capital-constrained. In another case, the firm might want the licensee to price and market very aggressively to keep a global competitor in check, but the licensee, which has to make a profit, may be unwilling to do this for the greater good of the licensor. For example, Kodak has used its Japanese subsidiary to launch aggressive attacks against its global competitor, Fuji Film. The idea has been to keep Fuji busy defending its home market, which limits Fuji's ability to launch aggressive attacks in the United States. While Kodak's Japanese subsidiary, which is wholly owned, has to accept such strategic direction from the center, a licensee would be unlikely to accept such an imposition, since such a strategy would allow the licensee to make only a low profit or even take a loss.

Or a firm may want control over the operations of a foreign entity to take advantage of differences in factor costs among countries, producing only part of its final product in a given country, while importing other parts from where they can be produced at lower cost. Again, a licensee would be unlikely to accept such an arrangement because it would limit the licensee's autonomy. When tight control over a foreign entity is desirable, horizontal FDI is preferable to licensing.

Third, a firm's know-how may not be amenable to licensing. This is particularly true of management and marketing know-how. It is one thing to license a foreign firm to manufacture a particular product, but quite another to license the way a firm does business—how it manages its process and markets its products. Consider Toyota, a company whose competitive advantage in the global auto industry is acknowledged to come from its superior ability to manage the overall process of designing, engineering, manufacturing, and selling automobiles; that is, from its management and organizational know-how. Toyota is credited with pioneering the development of a new production process, known as lean production, that enables it to produce higher-quality automobiles at a lower cost than its global rivals.[18] Although Toyota has certain products that can be licensed, its real competitive advantage comes from its management and process know-how. These kinds of skills are difficult to articulate or codify; they cannot be written down in a simple licensing contract. They are organizationwide and have been developed over years. They are not embodied in any one individual, but instead are widely dispersed throughout the company. Toyota's skills are embedded in its organizational culture, and culture is something that cannot be licensed. Thus, as Toyota moves away from its traditional exporting strategy, it has increasingly pursued a strategy of FDI, rather than licensing foreign enterprises to produce its cars.

The same is true of Cemex, which was profiled in the Management Focus. Because it is embedded in organizational processes and managerial skills, Cemex's know-how with regard to management, marketing, and technology might all be difficult to transfer via a licensing contract. Thus, FDI became the logical way for Cemex to expand internationally. Starbucks may also have found it difficult to transfer its management and marketing know-how via a licensing strategy, hence its recent preference for FDI in the form of acquisitions or joint ventures over straight licensing deals (see the opening case).

All of this suggests that when one or more of the following conditions holds, markets fail as a mechanism for selling know-how and FDI is more profitable than licensing: (1) when the firm has valuable know-how that cannot be adequately protected by a licensing contract, (2) when the firm needs tight control over a foreign entity to maximize its market share and earnings in that country, and (3) when a firm's skills and know-how are not amenable to licensing.

Strategic Behavior

Another theory used to explain FDI is based on the idea that FDI flows are a reflection of strategic rivalry between firms in the global marketplace. An early variant of this argument was expounded by F. T. Knickerbocker, who looked at the relationship between FDI and rivalry in oligopolistic industries.[19] An **oligopoly** is an industry composed of a limited number of large firms (e.g., an industry in which four firms control 80 percent of a domestic market would be defined as an oligopoly). A critical competitive feature of such industries is *interdependence* of the major players: What one firm does can have an immediate impact on the major competitors, forcing a response in kind. If one firm in an oligopoly cuts prices, this can take market share away from its competitors, forcing them to respond with similar price cuts to retain their market share. Thus, the interdependence between firms in an oligopoly leads to imitative behavior; rivals often quickly imitate what a firm does in an oligopoly.

Imitative behavior can take many forms in an oligopoly. One firm raises prices, the others follow; someone expands capacity, and the rivals imitate lest they be left at a disadvantage in the future. Knickerbocker argued that the same kind of imitative behavior characterizes FDI. Consider an oligopoly in the United States in which three firms—A, B, and C—dominate the market. Firm A establishes a subsidiary in France. Firms B and C decide that if this investment is successful, it may knock out their export business to France and give firm A a first-mover advantage. Furthermore, firm A might discover some competitive asset in France that it could repatriate to the United States to torment firms B and C on their native soil. Given these possibilities, firms B and C decide to follow firm A and establish operations in France.

Studies that looked at FDI by U.S. firms during the 1950s and 60s show that firms based in oligopolistic industries tended to imitate each other's FDI.[20] The same phenomenon has been observed with regard to FDI undertaken by Japanese firms during the 1980s.[21] For example, Toyota and Nissan responded to investments by Honda in the United States and Europe by undertaking their own FDI in the United States and Europe. More recently, research has shown that models of strategic behavior in a global oligopoly can explain the pattern of FDI in the global tier industry.[22]

Knickerbocker's theory can be extended to embrace the concept of multipoint competition. **Multipoint competition** arises when two or more enterprises encounter each other in different regional markets, national markets, or industries.[23] Economic theory suggests that rather like chess players jockeying for advantage, firms will try to match each other's moves in different markets to try to hold each other in check. The idea is to ensure that a rival does not gain a commanding position in one market and then use the profits generated there to subsidize competitive attacks in other markets. Kodak and Fuji Photo Film Co., for example, compete against each other around the world. If Kodak enters a particular foreign market, Fuji will not be far behind. Fuji feels compelled to follow Kodak to ensure that Kodak does not gain a dominant position in the foreign market that it could then leverage to gain a competitive advantage elsewhere. The converse also holds, with Kodak following Fuji when the Japanese firm is the first to enter a foreign market.

Although Knickerbocker's theory and its extensions can help to explain imitative FDI behavior by firms in oligopolistic industries, it does not explain why the first firm in an oligopoly decides to undertake FDI, rather than to export or license. In contrast, the market imperfections explanation addresses this phenomenon. The imitative theory also does not address the issue of whether FDI is more efficient than exporting or licensing for expanding abroad. Again, the market imperfections approach addresses the efficiency issue. For these reasons, many economists favor the market imperfections explanation for FDI, although most would agree that the imitative explanation tells an important part of the story.

The Product Life Cycle

Raymond Vernon's product life-cycle theory, described in Chapter 4, also is used to explain FDI. Vernon argued that often the same firms that pioneer a product in their home markets undertake FDI to produce a product for consumption in foreign markets. Thus, Xerox introduced the photocopier in the United States, and it was Xerox that set up production facilities in Japan (Fuji-Xerox) and Great Britain (Rank-Xerox) to serve those markets. Vernon's view is that firms undertake FDI at particular stages in the life cycle of a product they have pioneered. They invest in other advanced countries when local demand in those countries grows large enough to support local production (as Xerox did). They subsequently shift production to developing countries when product standardization and market saturation give rise to price competition and cost pressures. Investment in developing countries, where labor costs are lower, is seen as the best way to reduce costs.

Vernon's theory has merit. Firms do invest in a foreign country when demand in that country will support local production, and they do invest in low-cost locations (e.g., developing countries) when cost pressures become intense.[24] However, Vernon's theory fails to explain why it is profitable for a firm to undertake FDI at such times, rather than continuing to export from its home base and rather than licensing a foreign firm to produce its product. Just because demand in a foreign country is large enough to support local production, it does not necessarily follow that local production is the most profitable option. It may still be more profitable to produce at home and export to that country (to realize the scale economies that arise from serving the global market from one location). Alternatively, it may be more profitable for the firm to license a foreign company to produce its product for sale in that country. The product life-cycle theory ignores these options and, instead, simply argues that once a foreign market is large enough to support local production, FDI will occur. This limits its explanatory power and its usefulness to business in that it fails to identify when it is profitable to invest abroad.

Location-Specific Advantages

The British economist John Dunning has argued that in addition to the various factors discussed above, location-specific advantages can help explain the nature and direction of FDI.[25] By **location-specific advantages,** Dunning means the advantages that arise from using resource endowments or assets that are tied to a particular foreign location and that a firm finds valuable to combine with its own unique assets (such as the firm's technological, marketing, or management know-how). Dunning accepts the internalization argument that market failures make it difficult for a firm to license its own unique assets (know-how). Therefore, he argues that combining location-specific assets or resource endowments and the firm's own unique assets often requires FDI. It requires the firm to establish production facilities where those foreign assets or resource endowments are located. (Dunning refers to this argument as the **eclectic paradigm.**)

An obvious example of Dunning's arguments is natural resources, such as oil and other minerals, which are specific to certain locations. Dunning suggests that a firm must undertake FDI to exploit such foreign resources. This explains the FDI undertaken by many of the world's oil companies, which have to invest where oil is located to combine their technological and managerial knowledge with this valuable location-specific resource. Another example is valuable human resources, such as low-cost, highly skilled labor. The cost and skill of labor varies from country to country. Because labor is not internationally mobile, according to Dunning it makes sense for a firm to locate production facilities where the cost and skills of local labor are most suited to its particular production processes.

However, the implications of Dunning's theory go beyond basic resources such as minerals and labor. Consider Silicon Valley, which is the world center for the computer and semiconductor industry. Many of the world's major computer and semiconductor companies, such as Apple Computer, Silicon Graphics, and Intel, are located close to each other in the Silicon Valley region of California. As a result, much of the cutting-edge research and product development in computers and semiconductors occur here. According to Dunning's arguments, knowledge being generated in Silicon Valley with regard to the design and manufacture of computers and semiconductors is available nowhere else in the world. As it is commercialized, that knowledge diffuses throughout the world, but the leading edge of knowledge generation in the computer and semiconductor industries is to be found in Silicon Valley. In Dunning's language, this means Silicon Valley has a location-specific advantage in the generation of knowledge related to the computer and semiconductor industries. In part, this advantage comes from the sheer concentration of intellectual talent in this area, and in part it arises from a network of informal contacts that allows firms to benefit from each other's knowledge generation. Economists refer to such knowledge "spillovers" as **externalities,** and one well-established theory suggests that firms can benefit from such externalities by locating close to their source.[26]

In so far as this is the case, it makes sense for foreign computer and semiconductor firms to invest in research and (perhaps) production facilities so they too can learn about and utilize valuable new knowledge before those based elsewhere, thereby giving them a competitive advantage in the global marketplace.[27] Evidence suggests that European, Japanese, South Korean, and Taiwanese computer and semiconductor firms are investing in the Silicon Valley region, precisely because they wish to benefit from the externalities that arise there.[28] Others have argued that direct investment by foreign firms in the U.S. biotechnology industry has been motivated by desires to gain access to the unique location-specific technological knowledge of U.S. biotechnology firms.[29] Dunning's theory, therefore, seems to be a useful addition to those outlined above, for it helps explain how location factors affect the direction of FDI.[30]

Vertical Foreign Direct Investment ■

Vertical FDI takes two forms. There is **backward vertical FDI** into an industry abroad that provides inputs for a firm's domestic production processes. Historically, most backward vertical FDI has been in extractive industries (e.g., oil extraction, bauxite mining, tin mining, copper mining). The objective has been to provide inputs into a firm's downstream operations (e.g., oil refining, aluminum smelting and fabrication, tin smelting and fabrication). Firms such as Royal Dutch/Shell, British Petroleum (BP), RTZ, Consolidated Gold Field, and Alcoa are among the classic examples of such vertically integrated multinationals.

A second form of vertical FDI is **forward vertical FDI** in which an industry abroad sells the outputs of a firm's domestic production processes. Forward vertical FDI is less common than backward vertical FDI. For example, when Volkswagen entered the U.S. market, it acquired a large number of dealers rather than distribute its cars through independent U.S. dealers.

With both horizontal and vertical FDI, the question that must be answered is why would a firm go to all the trouble and expense of setting up operations in a foreign country? Why, for example, did petroleum companies such as BP and Royal Dutch/ Shell vertically integrate backward into oil production abroad? The location-specific advantages argument helps explain the direction of such FDI; vertically integrated multinationals in extractive industries invest where the raw materials are. However, this argument does not clarify why they did not simply import raw materials extracted by local producers. And why do companies such as Volkswagen feel it is necessary to acquire their own dealers in foreign markets, when in theory it might seem less costly to rely on foreign dealers? There are two basic answers to these kinds of questions. The first is a strategic behavior argument, and the second draws on the market imperfections approach.

❙Strategic Behavior

According to economic theory, by vertically integrating backward to gain control over the source of raw material, a firm can raise entry barriers and shut new competitors out of an industry.[31] Such strategic behavior involves vertical FDI if the raw material is found abroad. A famous example occurred in the 1930s when North American firms such as Alcoa pioneered commercial smelting of aluminum. Aluminum is derived by smelting bauxite. Although bauxite is a common mineral, the percentage of aluminum in bauxite is typically so low that it is not economical to mine and smelt. During the 1930s, only one large-scale deposit of bauxite with an economical percentage of aluminum had been discovered, and it was on the Caribbean island of Trinidad. Alcoa and Alcan vertically integrated backward and acquired ownership of the deposit. This action created a barrier to entry into the aluminum industry. Potential competitors were deterred because they could not get access to high-grade bauxite—it was all owned by Alcoa and Alcan. Those that did enter the industry had to use lower-grade bauxite than Alcan and Alcoa and found themselves at a cost disadvantage. This situation persisted until the 1950s and 1960s, when new high-grade deposits were discovered in Australia and Indonesia.

However, despite the bauxite example, the opportunities for barring entry through vertical FDI seem far too limited to explain the incidence of vertical FDI among the world's multinationals. In most extractive industries, mineral deposits are not as concentrated as in the case of bauxite in the 1930s; new deposits are constantly being discovered. Consequently, any attempt to monopolize all viable raw material deposits is bound to prove very expensive if not impossible.

Another strand of the strategic behavior explanation of vertical FDI sees such investment not as an attempt to build entry barriers, but as an attempt to circumvent the barriers established by firms already doing business in a country. This may explain Volkswagen's decision to establish its own dealer network when it entered the North American auto market. GM, Ford, and Chrysler then dominated the market. Each firm had its own network of dealers. Volkswagen believed that the only way to get quick access to the United States was to promote its cars through company-owned dealerships.

Market Imperfections

As in the case of horizontal FDI, a more general explanation of vertical FDI can be found in the market imperfections approach.[32] The market imperfections approach offers two explanations for vertical FDI. As with horizontal FDI, the first explanation revolves around the idea that there are impediments to the sale of know-how through the market mechanism. The second explanation is based on the idea that investments in specialized assets expose the investing firm to hazards that can be reduced only through vertical FDI.

Impediments to the Sale of Know-How

Consider the case of oil refining companies such as British Petroleum and Royal Dutch/Shell. Historically, these firms pursued backward vertical FDI to supply their British and Dutch oil refining facilities with crude oil. When this occurred in the early decades of the 20th century, neither Great Britain nor the Netherlands had domestic oil supplies. However, why did these firms not just import oil from firms in oil-rich countries such as Saudi Arabia and Kuwait?

Originally, there were no Saudi Arabian or Kuwaiti firms with the technological expertise for finding and extracting oil. BP and Royal Dutch/Shell had to develop this know-how to get access to oil. This alone does not explain FDI, however, for once BP and Shell had developed the necessary know-how, they could have licensed it to Saudi Arabian or Kuwaiti firms. However, as we saw in the case of horizontal FDI, licensing can be self-defeating as a mechanism for the sale of know-how. If the oil refining firms had licensed their prospecting and extraction know-how to Saudi Arabian or Kuwaiti firms, they would have risked giving away their technological know-how to those firms, creating future competitors in the process. Once they had the know-how, the Saudi and Kuwaiti firms might have gone prospecting for oil in other parts of the world, competing directly against BP and Royal Dutch/Shell. Thus, it made more sense for these firms to undertake backward vertical FDI and extract the oil themselves instead of licensing their hard-earned technological expertise to local firms.

Generalizing from this example, the prediction is that backward vertical FDI will occur when a firm has the knowledge and the ability to extract raw materials in another country and there is no efficient producer in that country that can supply raw materials to the firm.

Investment in Specialized Assets

Another strand of the market imperfections argument predicts that vertical FDI will occur when a firm must invest in specialized assets whose value depends on inputs provided by a foreign supplier. In this context, a specialized asset is an asset designed to perform a specific task and whose value is significantly reduced in its next-best use. Consider the case of an aluminum refinery, which is designed to refine bauxite ore and produce aluminum. Bauxite ores vary in content and chemical composition from deposit to deposit. Each type of ore requires a different type of refinery. Running one type of bauxite through a refinery designed for another type increases production costs by 20 to 100 percent.[33] Thus, the value of an investment in an aluminum refinery depends on the availability of the desired kind of bauxite ore.

Imagine that a U.S. aluminum company must decide whether to invest in an aluminum refinery designed to refine a certain type of ore. Assume further that this ore is available only through an Australian mining firm at a single bauxite mine. Using a different type of ore in the refinery would raise production costs by at least 20 percent. Therefore, the value of the U.S. company's investment depends on the price it must pay the Australian firm for this bauxite. Recognizing this, once the U.S. company has invested in a new refinery, what is to stop the Australian firm from raising bauxite prices? Absolutely nothing; and once it has made the investment, the U.S. firm is locked into its relationship with the Australian supplier. The Australian firm can increase bauxite prices, secure in the knowledge that as long as the increase in the total production costs is less than 20 percent, the U.S. firm will continue to buy from it. (It would become economical for the U.S. firm to buy from another supplier only if total production costs increased by more than 20 percent.)

The U.S. firm can reduce the risk of the Australian firm opportunistically raising prices in this manner by buying out the Australian firm. If the U.S. firm can buy the Australian firm, or its bauxite mine, it need no longer fear that bauxite prices will be increased after it has invested in the refinery. In other words, it would make economic sense for the U.S. firm to engage in vertical FDI. In practice, these kinds of considerations have driven aluminum firms to pursue vertical FDI to such a degree that a large percentage of the total volume of bauxite is transferred within vertically integrated firms.[34]

Focus On Managerial Implications

The implications of the theories of horizontal and vertical FDI for business practice are relatively straightforward. First, the location-specific advantages argument associated with John Dunning helps explain the direction of FDI, both with regard to horizontal and vertical FDI. However, the argument does not explain why firms prefer FDI to licensing or to exporting. In this regard, from both an explanatory and a business perspective, perhaps the most useful theory is the market imperfections approach. With regard to horizontal FDI, this approach identifies with some precision how the relative rates of return associated with horizontal FDI, exporting, and licensing vary with circumstances. The theory suggests that exporting is preferable to licensing and horizontal FDI as long as transport costs are minor and tariff barriers are trivial. As transport costs and/or tariff barriers increase, exporting becomes unprofitable, and the choice is between horizontal FDI and licensing. Since horizontal FDI is more costly and more risky than licensing, other things being equal, the theory argues that licensing is preferable to horizontal FDI. Other things are seldom equal, however. Although licensing may work, it is not an attractive option when one or more of the following conditions exist: (a) the firm has valuable know-how that cannot be adequately protected by a licensing contract, (b) the firm needs tight control over a foreign entity to maximize its market share and earnings in that country, and (c) a firm's skills and know-how are not amenable to licensing. Figure 6.6 presents these considerations as a decision tree.

Firms for which licensing is not a good option tend to be clustered in three types of industries:

1. High-technology industries where protecting firm-specific expertise is of paramount importance and licensing is hazardous.

2. Global oligopolies, where competitive interdependence requires that multinational firms maintain tight control over foreign operations so that they have the ability to launch coordinated attacks against their global competitors (as Kodak has done with Fuji).

Figure 6.6

A Decision Framework

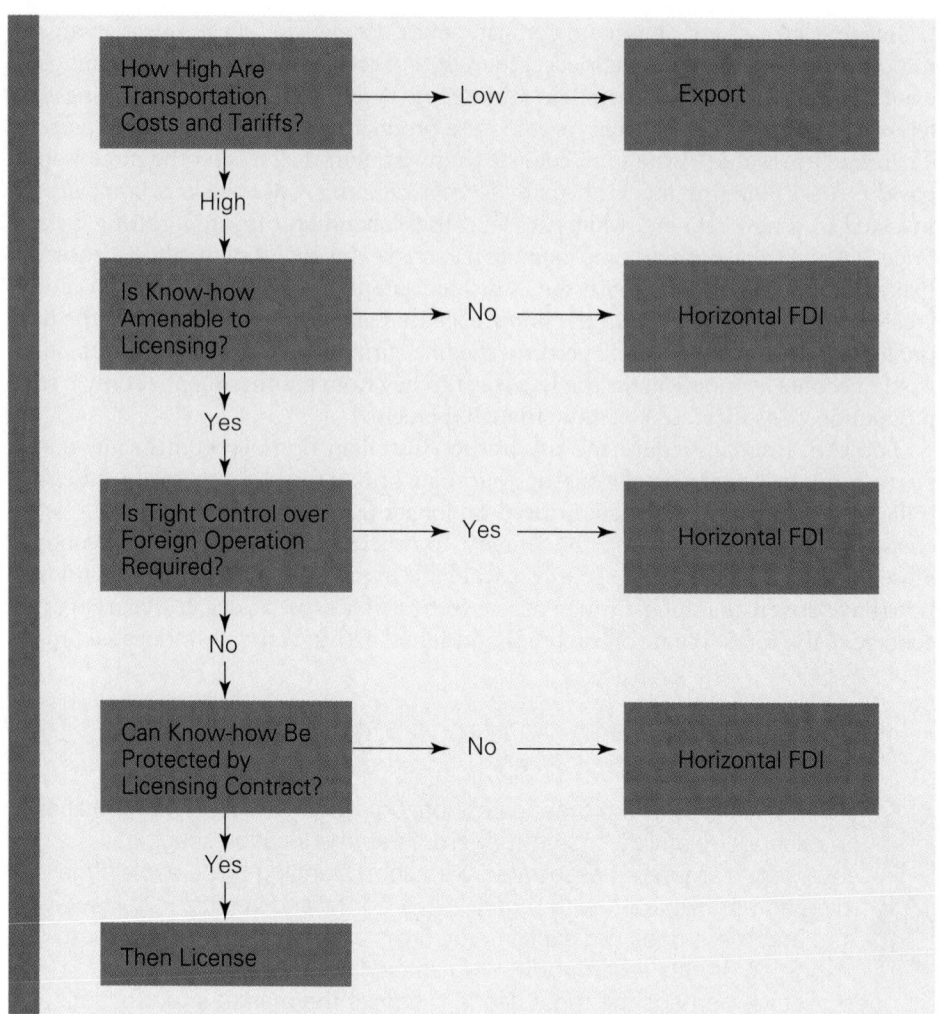

3.   Industries where intense cost pressures require that multinational firms maintain tight control over foreign operations (so they can disperse manufacturing to locations around the globe where factor costs are most favorable to minimize costs).

The majority of the evidence seems to support these conjectures.[35] In addition, licensing is not a good option if the competitive advantage of a firm is based upon managerial or marketing knowledge that is embedded in the routines of the firm, and/or the skills of its managers, and is difficult to codify in a "book of blueprints." This would seem to be the case for firms based in a fairly wide range of industries, and as we have seen from examples in this chapter, includes the likes of Starbucks and Cemex.

Firms for which licensing is a good option tend to be in industries whose conditions are opposite to those specified above. Licensing tends to be more common (and more profitable) in fragmented, low-technology industries in which globally dispersed manufacturing is not an option. Licensing is also easier if the knowledge to be transferred is relatively easy to codify. A good example of an industry where these conditions seem to exist is the fast-food industry. McDonald's has expanded globally by using a franchising strategy. Franchising is essentially the service-industry version of licensing—although it normally involves much longer-term commitments than licensing. With franchising, the firm licenses its brand name to a foreign firm in return for a percentage of the franchisee's profits. The franchising contract specifies the conditions that the franchisee must fulfill if it is to use the franchisor's brand name. Thus, McDonald's allows foreign firms to use its brand name as long as they agree to run their restaurants on exactly the same lines as McDonald's restaurants elsewhere in the world. This strategy makes sense for McDonald's because (a) like many services, fast food cannot be exported, (b) franchising economizes the costs and risks associated with opening foreign markets, (c) unlike technological know-how, brand names are relatively easy to protect using a contract, (d) there is no compelling reason for McDonald's to have tight control over franchisees, and (e) McDonald's know-how, in terms of how to run a fast-food restaurant, is amenable to being specified in a written contract (e.g., the contract specifies the details of how to run a McDonald's restaurant). This said, it is worth noting that McDonald's does undertake some FDI to establish "master franchisors" in each country in which it does business. These master franchisors are normally joint ventures with local companies, and their task is to manage McDonald's franchisees within a particular country.

In contrast to the market imperfections approach, the product life-cycle theory and Knickerbocker's theory of horizontal FDI are perhaps less useful from a business perspective. These two theories are descriptive rather than analytical. They do a good job of describing the historical pattern of FDI, but they do a relatively poor job of identifying the factors that influence the relative profitability of FDI, licensing, and exporting. The issue of licensing as an alternative to FDI is ignored by both these theories.

Finally, with regard to vertical FDI, both the market imperfections approach and the strategic behavior approach have some useful implications for business practice. The strategic behavior approach points out that vertical FDI may be a way of building barriers to entry into an industry. The strength of the market imperfections approach is that it points out the conditions under which vertical FDI might be preferable to the alternatives. Most importantly, the market imperfections approach points to the importance of investments in specialized assets and imperfections in the market for know-how as factors that increase the relative attractiveness of vertical FDI.

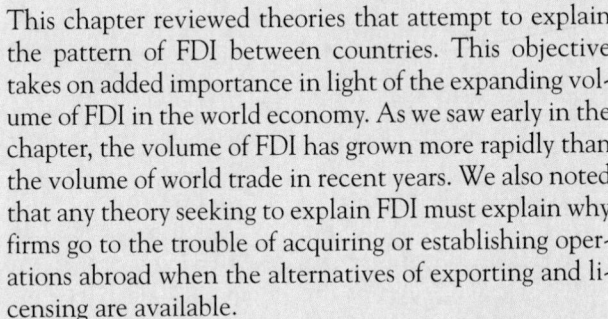

Chapter Summary

This chapter reviewed theories that attempt to explain the pattern of FDI between countries. This objective takes on added importance in light of the expanding volume of FDI in the world economy. As we saw early in the chapter, the volume of FDI has grown more rapidly than the volume of world trade in recent years. We also noted that any theory seeking to explain FDI must explain why firms go to the trouble of acquiring or establishing operations abroad when the alternatives of exporting and licensing are available.

We reviewed a number of theories that attempt to explain horizontal and vertical FDI. With regard to horizontal FDI, it was argued that the market imperfections and location-specific advantages approaches might have the greatest explanatory power and therefore be most useful for business practice. This is not to belittle the explanations for horizontal FDI put forward by Vernon and Knickerbocker, since these theories also have value in

explaining the pattern of FDI in the world economy. Still, both theories are weakened by their failure to explicitly consider the factors that drive the choice among exporting, licensing, and FDI. Finally, with regard to vertical FDI, it was argued that the strategic behavior and market imperfections approaches both have a certain amount of explanatory power.

The chapter made these major points:

1. Foreign direct investment occurs when a firm invests directly in facilities to produce a product in a foreign country. It also occurs when a firm buys an existing enterprise in a foreign country.

2. Horizontal FDI is FDI in the same industry abroad as a firm operates at home. Vertical FDI is FDI in an industry abroad that provides inputs into or sells outputs from a firm's domestic operations.

3. Any theory seeking to explain FDI must explain why firms go to the trouble of acquiring or establishing operations abroad when the alternatives of exporting and licensing are available.

4. Several factors characterized FDI trends over the past 20 years: (a) There has been a rapid increase in the total volume of FDI undertaken; (b) there has been some decline in the relative importance of the United States as a source for FDI, while several other countries have increased their share of total FDI outflows; (c) an increasing share of FDI seems to be directed at the developing nations of Asia and Eastern Europe, while the United States has become a major recipient of FDI; and (d) there has been an increase in the amount of FDI undertaken by firms based in developing nations.

5. High transportation costs and/or tariffs imposed on imports help explain why many firms prefer horizontal FDI or licensing over exporting.

6. Impediments to the sale of know-how explain why firms prefer horizontal FDI to licensing. These impediments arise when: (a) a firm has valuable know-how that cannot be adequately protected by a licensing contract, (b) a firm needs tight control over a foreign entity to maximize its market share and earnings in that country, and (c) a firm's skills and know-how are not amenable to licensing.

7. Knickerbocker's theory suggests that much FDI is explained by imitative strategic behavior by rival firms in an oligopolistic industry. However, this theory does not address the issue of whether FDI is more efficient than exporting or licensing for expanding abroad.

8. Vernon's product life-cycle theory suggests that firms undertake FDI at particular stages in the life cycle of products they have pioneered. However, Vernon's theory does not address the issue of whether FDI is more efficient than exporting or licensing for expanding abroad.

9. Dunning has argued that location-specific advantages are of considerable importance in explaining the nature and direction of FDI. According to Dunning, firms undertake FDI to exploit resource endowments or assets that are location-specific.

10. Backward vertical FDI may be explained as an attempt to create barriers to entry by gaining control over the source of material inputs into the downstream stage of a production process. Forward vertical FDI may be seen as an attempt to circumvent entry barriers and gain access to a national market.

11. The market imperfections approach suggests that vertical FDI is a way of reducing a firm's exposure to the risks that arise from investments in specialized assets.

12. From a business perspective, the most useful theory is probably the market imperfections approach because it identifies how the relative profit rates associated with horizontal FDI, exporting, and licensing vary with circumstances.

Critical Discussion Questions

1. In 2000, inward FDI accounted for some 45 percent of gross fixed capital formation in Ireland, but only 0.3 percent in Japan. What do you think explains this difference in FDI inflows into the two countries?

2. Compare and contrast these explanations of horizontal FDI: the market imperfections approach, Vernon's product life-cycle theory, and Knickerbocker's theory of FDI. Which theory do you think offers the best explanation of the historical pattern of horizontal FDI? Why?

3. Read the opening case on Starbucks. Using the market imperfections approach to FDI, explain Starbucks' approach to expanding its presence in Thailand, Great Britain, and Japan.

4. Compare and contrast these explanations of vertical FDI: the strategic behavior approach and the market imperfections approach. Which theory do you think offers the better explanation of the historical pattern of vertical FDI? Why?

5. You are the international manager of a U.S. business that has just developed a revolutionary new personal computer that can perform the same functions as existing PCs but costs only half as much to manufacture. Several patents protect the unique design of this computer. Your CEO has asked you to formulate a recommendation for how to expand into Western Europe. Your options are (a) to export from the United States, (b) to license a European firm to manufacture and market the computer in Europe, and (c) to set up a wholly owned subsidiary in Europe. Evaluate the pros and cons of each alternative and suggest a course of action to your CEO.

Notes

1. United Nations, *World Investment Report, 2000* (New York and Geneva: United Nations, 2001).

2. United Nations, *World Investment Report, 2002* (New York and Geneva: United Nations, 2002), and United Nations, "UNCTAD Predicts 27% Drop in FDI Flows This Year," United Nations Press Release TAD/INF/PR/63, October 24, 2002.

3. World Trade Organization, *International Trade Statistics, 2002* (Geneva: WTO, 2002), and United Nations, *World Investment Report, 2002.*

4. United Nations, *World Investment Report, 2002.*

5. Ibid.

6. United Nations, *World Investment Report, 2002,* and United Nations, "UNCTAD Predicts 27% Drop in FDI Flows This Year."

7. United Nations, "FDI Downturn in 2001 Touches Almost All Regions," TAD/INF/PR36, United Nations Press Release, January 21, 2002.

8. Ibid.

9. United Nations, *World Investment Report, 2002.*

10. Ibid.

11. United Nations, *World Investment Report, 2002,* and United Nations, "UNCTAD Predicts 27% Drop in FDI Flows This Year."

12. United Nations, "UNCTAD Predicts 27% Drop in FDI Flows This Year."

13. M. Kidron and R. Segal, *The New State of the World Atlas* (New York: Simon & Schuster, 1987).

14. United Nations, *World Investment Report, 2002.*

15. Ibid.

16. See D. J. Ravenscraft and F. M. Scherer, *Mergers, Selloffs and Economic Efficiency* (Washington, DC: The Brookings Institution, 1987). Also A. Seth, K. P. Song, and R. R. Pettit, "Value Creation and Destruction in Cross Border Acquisitions," *Strategic Management Journal* 23 (2002), pp. 921–40.

17. For example, see S. H. Hymer, *The International Operations of National Firms: A Study of Direct Foreign Investment* (Cambridge, MA: MIT Press, 1976); A. M. Rugman, *Inside the Multinationals: The Economics of Internal Markets* (New York: Columbia University Press, 1981); D. J. Teece, "Multinational Enterprise, Internal Governance, and Industrial Organization," *American Economic Review* 75 (May 1983), pp. 233–38; and C. W. L. Hill and W. C. Kim, "Searching for a Dynamic Theory of the Multinational Enterprise: A Transaction Cost

Model," *Strategic Management Journal* (special issue) 9 (1988), pp. 93–104.

18. J. P. Womack, D. T. Jones, and D. Roos, *The Machine That Changed the World* (New York: Rawson Associates, 1990).

19. The argument is most often associated with F. T. Knickerbocker, *Oligopolistic Reaction and Multinational Enterprise* (Boston: Harvard Business School Press, 1973).

20. The studies are summarized in R. E. Caves, *Multinational Enterprise and Economic Analysis,* 2nd ed. (Cambridge, UK: Cambridge University Press, 1996).

21. See R. E. Caves, "Japanese Investment in the US: Lessons for the Economic Analysis of Foreign Investment," *The World Economy* 16 (1993), pp. 279–300; B. Kogut and S. J. Chang, "Technological Capabilities and Japanese Direct Investment in the United States," *Review of Economics and Statistics* 73 (1991), pp. 401–43; and J. Anand and B. Kogut, "Technological Capabilities of Countries, Firm Rivalry, and Foreign Direct Investment," *Journal of International Business Studies,* Third Quarter 1997, pp. 445–65.

22. K. Ito and E. L. Rose, "Foreign Direct Investment Location Strategies in the Tier Industry," *Journal of International Business Studies* 33 (2002), pp. 593–602.

23. H. Haveman and L. Nonnemaker, "Competition in Multiple Geographical Markets," *Administrative Science Quarterly,* 45 (2000), pp. 232–67.

24. For the use of Vernon's theory to explain Japanese direct investment in the United States and Europe, see S. Thomsen, "Japanese Direct Investment in the European Community," *The World Economy* 16 (1993), pp. 301–15.

25. J. H. Dunning, *Explaining International Production* (London: Unwin Hyman, 1988).

26. Paul Krugman, "Increasing Returns and Economic Geography," *Journal of Political Economy* 99, no. 3 (1991), pp. 483–99.

27. J. M. Shaver and F. Flyer, "Agglomeration Economies, Firm Heterogeneity, and Foreign Direct Investment in the United States," *Strategic Management Journal* 21 (2000), pp. 1175–93.

28. J. H. Dunning and R. Narula, "Transpacific Foreign Direct Investment and the Investment Development Path," *South Carolina Essays in International Business,* May 1995.

29. W. Shan and J. Song, "Foreign Direct Investment and the Sourcing of Technological Advantage:

Evidence from the Biotechnology Industry," *Journal of International Business Studies*, Second Quarter 1997, pp. 267–84.

30. For some additional evidence see L. E. Brouthers, K. D. Brouthers, and S. Warner, "Is Dunning's Eclectic Framework Descriptive or Normative?" *Journal of International Business Studies* 30 (1999), pp. 831–844.

31. Caves, *Multinational Enterprise and Economic Analysis.*

32. J. F. Hennart, "Upstream Vertical Integration in the Aluminum and Tin Industries," *Journal*

of *Economic Behavior and Organization* 9 (1988), pp. 281–99; and O. E. Williamson, *The Economic Institutions of Capitalism* (New York: Free Press, 1985). See also G. M. Grossman and E. Helpman, "Outsourcing versus FDI in Industry Equilibrium," NBER Working Paper 9300, October 2002.

33. Hennart, "Upstream Vertical Integration."

34. Ibid.

35. See Caves, *Multinational Enterprise and Economic Analysis.*

Research Task | globalEDGE™   globaledge.msu.edu

Use the globalEDGE™ site to complete the following exercises:

1. The World Investment Directory provides quick electronic access to comprehensive statistics on foreign direct investment (FDI) and the operations of transnational corporations (TNCs). Gather a list of the top transnational corporations in terms of their foreign direct investment; also, identify their home country (i.e., headquarters country). Provide a commentary about the characteristics of countries that have the greatest number of transnational firms.

2. Your company is considering opening a new factory in Latin America, and management is in the process of evaluating the specific country locations for this direct investment. The pool of candidate countries has been narrowed down to Argentina, Mexico, and Brazil. Prepare a short report comparing the foreign direct investment environment and regulations of these three countries.

Closing Case

Ford and General Motors in Russia

In July 2002, Ford Motor Company officially opened its first Russian car factory near St. Petersburg. The factory, which cost some $150 million to build, is 100 percent owned by Ford and represents the first wholly owned investment by a foreign carmaker in Russia. The factory is tiny by international standards; it will employ 800 people and initially will produce 10,000 Ford Focus cars a year. By comparison, a typical auto plant in the developed world produces 200,000 cars a year. If things go well, Ford plans to increase production to 25,000 cars a year by 2007, and if things go really well, the plant may ultimately produce 100,000 vehicles a year. If these plans come to fruition, it could be a boon for the region. Assembly-line workers at the Ford factory will make approximately $220 a month, significantly more than the $134 average wage in Russia, and skilled engineers at the factory may make as much as $600 a month.

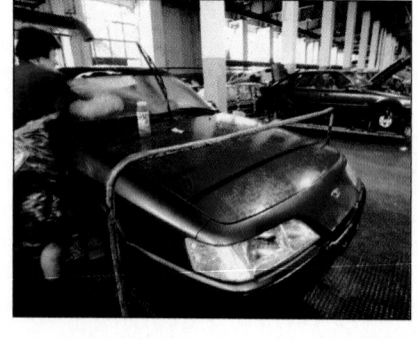

Ford was motivated in part by a desire to gain a foothold in the Russian car market. Although car ownership levels in Russia are very low by international standards—120 cars per 1,000 people compared to 580 per 1,000 in Western Europe—car sales have been rising by 7 to 8 percent a year. In 2002, about 1.5 million new and used cars were bought in Russia, about 1 million of which were Russian cars. New Russian models sell for $5,000 to $8,000. Ford intends to sell its locally produced Ford Focus for about $10,900, a price premium that Ford believes is justified given the poor reputation of Russian cars. An imported Ford Focus currently sells for $14,000 due to transportation costs, import duties, and higher wages at Ford's Western European factories. With the Russian government increasing import duties on finished cars to about 35 percent, and the political climate stabilizing, Ford thought it was time to establish local production.

Although most imported automobile components face a 25 percent duty, in exchange for duty-free status Ford has agreed to make sure that 50 percent of all components for the Ford Focus come from Russia within five years. Initially, however, only 20 percent of components will be sourced locally. To help increase this, Ford plans to invest some $45 million in local suppliers over the next few years to upgrade their capabilities.

Three months after Ford's announcement, General Motors became the second Western company to invest in Russian car factories. Rather than go it alone, however, GM opted to enter a joint venture with AvtoVAZ, Russia's largest auto company, to produce a new version of its popular SUV, the Niva. AvtoVAZ was reportedly looking for a venture partner to both invest capital and provide much-needed technical expertise to help the company upgrade product quality and lower production costs. In recent years, AvtoVAZ has been losing market share to imported used cars. In late 2002, it halted production in its factories for three weeks, despite strong car sales in Russia, while it attempted to move unsold inventory of 60,000 cars.

GM will reportedly invest some $141 million in the AvtoVAZ venture for a 41.5 percent ownership stake. The joint venture plans to produce 75,000 Nivas a year by 2005, each selling for about $8,000. In addition to their being sold locally, there are plans to export the Nivas to the Middle East, Asia, and Latin America. In total, the venture is forecasted to create some 3,500 new jobs.

AvtoVaz has reportedly also been looking for a Western joint-venture partner to launch a new mass-market version of its Lada, but the company is apparently asking for a $500 million investment, and most foreign companies are still hesitant about committing that kind of money. However, other foreign auto companies may soon enter Russia. The Japanese company Isuzu announced in late 2002 that it would team up with Severstal Steel, which has a stake in the UAZ automotive plant, to produce Elf light trucks in Russia. Volkswagen is also reportedly considering setting up a facility in Russia.

Sources: B. Aris, "Ford Drives under the Barrier," *Euromoney*, August 2002, pp. 20–22; J. Daniszewski, "GM Rolls Out Joint Venture with Russia," *Los Angeles Times*, September 24, 2002, p. A3; and G. Chazan, "Russians Want Foreign Wheels," *Wall Street Journal*, December 24, 2002, p. A8.

Case Discussion Questions

1. Why are Ford and GM entering the Russian car market now? Why did they not invest earlier, and why do they not postpone investment until the market is bigger?

2. Why do you think Ford chose to establish a wholly owned subsidiary in Russia, rather than license its production and product technology to a Russian carmaker like AvtoVAZ?

3. Why do you think GM chose to establish a joint venture with AvtoVAZ, rather than a wholly owned subsidiary? What are the risks associated with GM's joint-venture strategy?

4. Which theory of foreign direct investment best explains the sudden increase in interest by foreign auto companies in Russian investment?

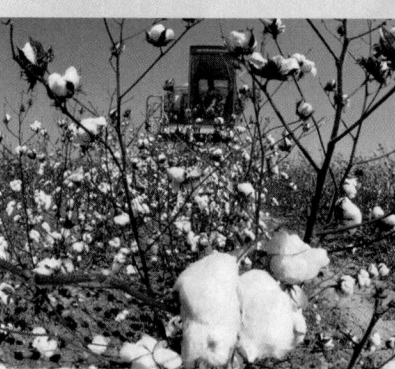

Chapter 7

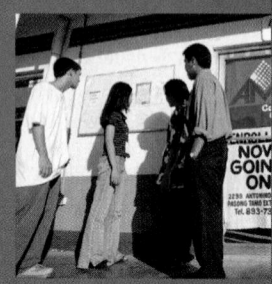

The Political Economy of Foreign Direct Investment

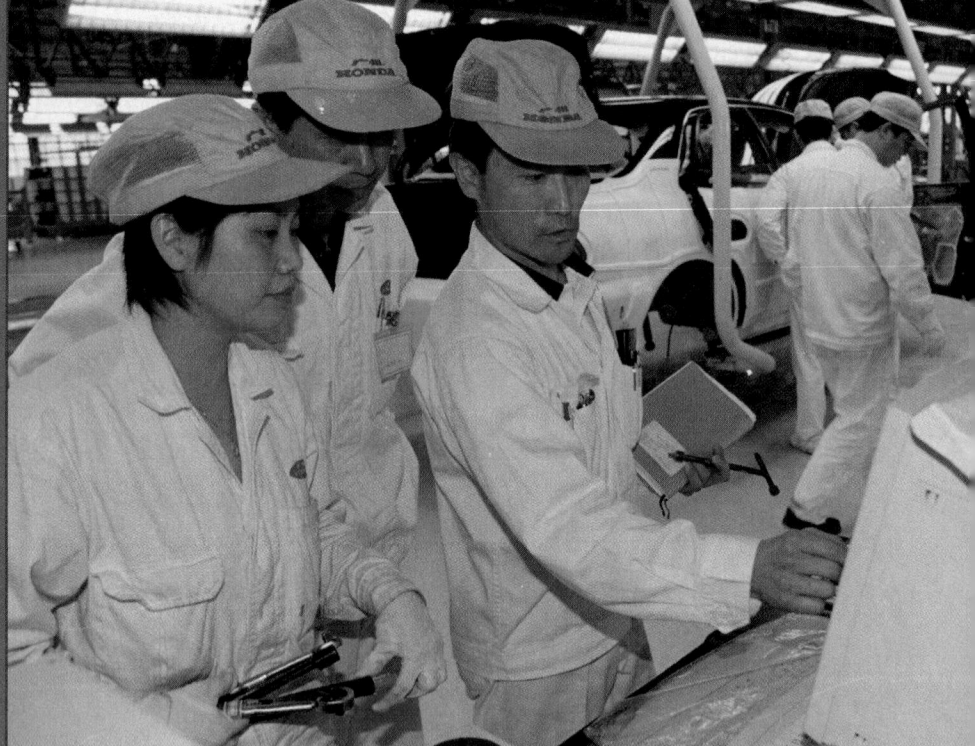

Introduction
Political Ideology and Foreign Direct
Investment
 The Radical View
 The Free Market View
 Pragmatic Nationalism
 Summary
The Benefits of FDI to Host Countries
 Resource-Transfer Effects
 Employment Effects
 Balance-of-Payments Effects
 *Effect on Competition and Economic
 Growth*
The Costs of FDI to Host Countries
 Adverse Effects on Competition
 *Adverse Effects on the Balance
 of Payments*
 National Sovereignty and Autonomy
The Benefits and Costs of FDI to Home
Countries
 Benefits of FDI to the Home Country
 Costs of FDI to the Home Country
 International Trade Theory and FDI
Government Policy Instruments and FDI
 Home-Country Policies
 Host-Country Policies
 *International Institutions and the
 Liberalization of FDI*
Focus on Managerial Implications
 The Nature of Negotiation
 Bargaining Power
Chapter Summary
Critical Discussion Questions
Closing Case: Toyota in France

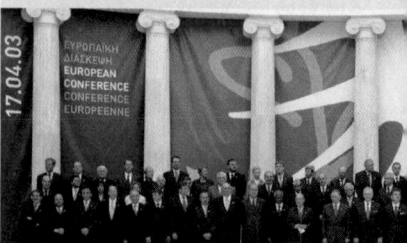

Foreign Direct Investment and the Irish Miracle

During the 1990s and early 2000s, Ireland registered one of the fastest economic growth rates in the developed world. Long an economic backwater in Western Europe famed only for its export of people and its relative poverty, Ireland's GDP grew at an average rate of 7.24 percent per year between 1990 and 2001. At the start of this period, the GDP per capita in Ireland on a purchasing power parity basis was $12,687. By the end of the period, it had reached $32,133, putting it ahead of countries such as Britain ($24,421), Germany ($25,715), and France ($25,074). Driving much of this growth was a rapid expansion in exports from Ireland. In 1985, Ireland exported $10 billion of goods and services. By 2001, the figure had risen to $82.8 billion. Also, the mix of exports from Ireland had changed dramatically during that period, with exports of primary products (agricultural goods) falling from 20.5 percent of the total to 6 percent of the total, while exports of high-technology manufactured products rose from 23 percent to 36 percent.

Driving this export-led boom was an inflow of foreign direct investment. Inward FDI grew from $164 million in 1985 to a record $24 billion in 2000, before dropping off to $9.78 billion in 2001 (the 2001 decline reflected a general slump in global FDI activity). Much of this FDI was undertaken by large multinationals that saw Ireland as a desirable base for exporting to the rest of Europe. Among the major investors were a raft of large American high-technology multinationals, including Intel, Dell Computer, Microsoft, Gateway, Apple, IBM, and EMC, and several major pharmaceutical firms including Johnson & Johnson, Bristol-Myers Squibb, and Eli Lilly. By the early 2000s, the Irish subsidiaries of foreign multinationals were accounting for more than 80 percent of Ireland's exports, with Intel and Dell both exporting more than $4 billion each from Irish factories, Microsoft almost $2.5 billion, and Eli Lilly and Johnson & Johnson more than $1 billion apiece. Two-thirds of Ireland's top exporters are the Irish subsidiaries of foreign multinationals.

How did Ireland become so successful at attracting FDI? First, Ireland benefited from a number of favorable location factors. With Ireland a member of the European Union, subsidiaries based there have preferential access to EU markets. In addition, Ireland was blessed with a highly educated work force including many engineers, relatively low wage rates, low corporate tax rates, good basic infrastructure (e.g., roads, water, electricity, telecommunications), English as the main language (important for American multinationals), and a government that was friendly toward foreign businesses.

The last item became the linchpin in Ireland's success. Since the 1980s, Ireland has implemented an industrialization strategy that relies on FDI to promote dynamic export-led growth. The centerpiece of this strategy has been the country's Investment and Development Agency (IDA), which has been endowed with a large budget to attract FDI (in 2000 this included $160 million in grant money that could be used to attract foreign multinationals). The IDA has helped to coordinate a combination of tax breaks and outright grants that, when linked with other location-specific factors, has helped to attract many multinationals to Ireland. Also, the IDA has been very proactive in seeking out investors from the high-technology sector. The IDA was also early to realize that Ireland was a good location for centralized call centers, and companies such as Dell Computer now have important customer service call centers in Ireland.

More importantly perhaps, the IDA was instrumental in persuading Intel to open its first plant in Ireland in 1990. Subsequently, Intel's investment helped to encourage many other high-technology firms to locate facilities in Ireland. High-technology investments have also been stimulated by an Irish government policy that all royalty income from products developed in Ireland is tax-free. This has created an incentive for foreign multinationals to establish R&D centers in Ireland. By the mid-1990s, the process had become self-sustaining, with the concentration of high-technology enterprises in Ireland attracting other high-technology companies to the country where they could benefit from being close to suppliers, providers of complementary products, and even rivals.

Sources: United Nations, *World Investment Report, 2002* (Geneva: United Nations, 2002); L. Bowman, "Irish Revival," *Strategic Direct Investor,* April 2002, pp. 30–32; World Bank Online database; and E.R.E. O'Higgins, "Government and the Creation of the Celtic Tiger," *Academy of Management Executive 16* (2002), pp. 104–20.

◼ Introduction

Chapter 6 looked at the phenomenon of foreign direct investment (FDI) and reviewed several theories that attempt to explain the economic rationale for FDI, but it did not discuss the role of governments in FDI. Through their choice of policies and their statements and actions, governments can both encourage and restrict FDI. Host governments can encourage FDI by providing incentives for foreign firms to invest in their economies, and they can restrict or discourage FDI through a variety of laws, policies, and statements. In the opening case, we saw how Ireland was able to attract significant FDI during the 1990s, and how this FDI helped to spark an export-led boom in the Irish economy that has raised living standards there.

The government of a source country for FDI also can encourage or restrict FDI by domestic firms. In recent years, the Japanese government has pressured many Japanese firms to undertake FDI. The Japanese government sees FDI as a substitute for exporting and thus as a way of reducing Japan's politically embarrassing balance of payments surplus. In contrast, the U.S. government has, for political reasons, from time to time restricted FDI by domestic firms. For example, in response to a belief that the Iranian government actively supports terrorist organizations, the U.S. government has prohibited U.S. firms from investing in or exporting to Iran.

Historically, one important determinant of a government's policy toward FDI has been its political ideology. Accordingly, this chapter opens with a discussion of how political ideology influences government policy. To a greater or lesser degree, the officials of many governments tend to be pragmatic nationalists who weigh the benefits and costs of FDI and vary their stated policy on a case-by-case basis. After discussing political ideology, we will consider the benefits and costs of FDI. Then we will look at the various policies home and host governments adopt to encourage and/or restrict FDI. The chapter closes with a detailed discussion of the implications of government policy for the business firm. In this closing section, we examine the factors that determine the relative bargaining strengths of a host government and a firm contemplating FDI. We will look at how the negotiations between firm and government are often played out and at how firms can use this knowledge to their advantage.

◼ Political Ideology and Foreign Direct Investment

Historically, ideology toward FDI has ranged from a dogmatic radical stance that is hostile to all FDI at one extreme to an adherence to the noninterventionist principle of free market economics at the other. Between these two extremes is an approach that might be called pragmatic nationalism.

❙ The Radical View

The radical view traces its roots to Marxist political and economic theory. Radical writers argue that the multinational enterprise (MNE) is an instrument of imperialist domination. They see the MNE as a tool for exploiting host countries to the exclusive benefit of their capitalist-imperialist home countries. They argue that MNEs extract profits from the host country and take them to their home country, giving nothing of value to the host country in exchange. They note, for example, that key technology is tightly controlled by the MNE, and that important jobs in the foreign subsidiaries of MNEs go to home-country nationals rather than to citizens of the host country. Because of this, according to the radical view, FDI by the MNEs of advanced capitalist nations keeps the less developed countries of the world relatively backward and dependent on advanced capitalist nations for investment, jobs, and technology. Thus, according to the extreme version of this view, no country should ever permit foreign corporations to undertake FDI, since they can never be instruments of economic development, only of economic domination. Where MNEs already exist in a country, they should be immediately nationalized.[1]

From 1945 until the 1980s, the radical view was very influential in the world economy. Until the collapse of communism between 1989 and 1991, the countries of Eastern Europe were opposed to FDI. Similarly, Communist countries elsewhere, such as China, Cambodia, and Cuba, were all opposed in principle to FDI (although in practice the Chinese started to allow FDI in mainland China in the 1970s). Many socialist countries, particularly in Africa where one of the first actions of many newly independent states was to nationalize foreign-owned enterprises, also embraced the radical position. Countries whose political ideology was more nationalistic than socialistic further embraced the radical position. This was true in Iran and India, for example, both of which adopted tough policies restricting FDI and nationalized many foreign-owned enterprises. Iran is a particularly interesting case because its Islamic government, while rejecting Marxist theory, has essentially embraced the radical view that FDI by MNEs is an instrument of imperialism.

By the end of the 1980s, however, the radical position was in retreat almost everywhere. There seem to be three reasons for this: (1) the collapse of communism in Eastern Europe; (2) the generally abysmal economic performance of those countries that embraced the radical position, and a growing belief by many of these countries that FDI can be an important source of technology and jobs and can stimulate economic growth; and (3) the strong economic performance of those developing countries that embraced capitalism rather than radical ideology (e.g., Singapore, Hong Kong, and Taiwan).

The Free Market View

The free market view traces its roots to classical economics and the international trade theories of Adam Smith and David Ricardo (see Chapter 4). The intellectual case for this view has been strengthened by the market imperfections explanation of horizontal and vertical FDI that we reviewed in Chapter 6. The free market view argues that international production should be distributed among countries according to the theory of comparative advantage. Countries should specialize in the production of those goods and services that they can produce most efficiently. Within this framework, the MNE is an instrument for dispersing the production of goods and services to the most efficient locations around the globe. Viewed this way, FDI by the MNE increases the overall efficiency of the world economy.

Consider a well-publicized decision by IBM in the mid-1980s to move assembly operations for many of its personal computers from the United States to Guadalajara, Mexico. IBM invested about $90 million in an assembly facility with the capacity to produce 100,000 PCs per year, 75 percent of which were exported back to the United States.[2] According to the free market view, moves such as this can be seen as increasing the overall efficiency of resource utilization in the world economy. Mexico, due to its low labor costs, has a comparative advantage in the assembly of PCs. According to the free market view, by moving the production of PCs from the United States to Mexico, IBM frees U.S. resources for use in activities in which the United States has a comparative advantage (e.g., the design of computer software, the manufacture of high-value-added components such as microprocessors, or basic R&D). Also, consumers benefit because the PCs cost less than they would if they were produced domestically. In addition, Mexico gains from the technology, skills, and capital that IBM transfers with its FDI. Contrary to the radical view, the free market view stresses that such resource transfers benefit the host country and stimulate its economic growth. Thus, the free market view argues that FDI is a benefit to both the source country and the host country.

For reasons explored earlier in this book (see Chapter 2), in recent years, the free market view has been ascendant worldwide, spurring a global move toward the removal of restrictions on inward and outward foreign direct investment. An example is South Korea, which started dismantling its restrictive regulations governing inward FDI in the mid-1990s. As described in the accompanying Management Focus, foreign firms are starting to affect competition in certain sectors of the South Korean economy.

As noted earlier in this book, according to the United Nations, between 1991 and 2001, 95 percent of the 1,393 changes made in the laws governing foreign direct investment created a more favorable environment for FDI. However, in practice no country has adopted the free market view in its pure form (just as no country has adopted the radical view in its pure form). Countries such as Britain and the United States are among the most open to FDI, but the governments of these countries both have a tendency to intervene. Britain does so by reserving the right to block foreign takeovers of domestic firms if the takeovers are seen as "contrary to national security interests" or if they have the potential for "reducing competition." (In practice this right is rarely exercised.) U.S. controls on FDI are more limited and largely informal. As noted earlier, for political reasons, the United States will occasionally restrict U.S. firms from undertaking FDI in certain countries (e.g., Cuba and Iran). In addition, there are some limited restrictions on inward FDI. For example, foreigners are prohibited from purchasing more than 25 percent of any U.S. airline or from acquiring a controlling interest in a U.S. broadcast television network. Since 1989, the government has had the right to review foreign investment on the grounds of "national security."

Pragmatic Nationalism

In practice, many countries have adopted neither a radical policy nor a free market policy toward FDI, but instead a policy that can best be described as pragmatic nationalism.[3] The pragmatic nationalist view is that FDI has both benefits and costs. FDI can benefit a host country by bringing capital, skills, technology, and jobs, but those benefits often come at a cost. When a foreign company rather than a domestic company produces products, the profits from that investment go abroad. Many countries are also concerned that a foreign-owned manufacturing plant may import many components from its home country, which has negative implications for the host country's balance-of-payments position.

Recognizing this, countries adopting a pragmatic stance pursue policies designed to maximize the national benefits and minimize the national costs. According to this view, FDI should be allowed only if the benefits outweigh the costs. Japan offers an example of pragmatic nationalism. Until the 1980s, Japan's policy was probably one of the most restrictive among countries adopting a pragmatic nationalist stance. This was due to Japan's perception that direct entry of foreign (especially U.S.) firms with ample managerial resources into the Japanese markets could hamper the development and growth of its own industry and technology.[4] This belief led Japan to block the majority of applications to invest in Japan. However, there were always exceptions to this policy. Firms that had important technology were often permitted to undertake FDI if they insisted that they would neither license their technology to a Japanese firm nor enter into a joint venture with a Japanese enterprise. IBM and Texas Instruments were able to set up wholly owned subsidiaries in Japan by adopting this negotiating position. From the perspective of the Japanese government, the benefits of FDI in such cases— the stimulus that these firms might impart to the Japanese economy—outweighed the perceived costs.

Another aspect of pragmatic nationalism is the tendency to aggressively court FDI believed to be in the national interest by, for example, offering subsidies to foreign MNEs in the form of tax breaks or grants. The countries of the European Union often seem to be competing with each other to attract U.S. and Japanese FDI by offering large tax breaks and subsidies. Britain has been the most successful at attracting Japanese investment in the automobile industry. Nissan, Toyota, and Honda now have major assembly plants in Britain and use the country as their base for serving the rest of Europe—with obvious employment and balance-of-payments benefits for Britain.

FDI by Volvo in South Korea

Historically, South Korea has been largely closed to foreign direct investment. During its 30-year dash from one of the world's poorest nations to one of its richest, South Korea closely adhered to the Japanese model of development, severely restricting foreign ownership of industrial and commercial activities. The walls of fortress Korea began to crumble in the mid-1990s when the government lifted almost all restrictions on foreign entry into the country's retail sector. The move was prompted by a belief that foreign entry would provide much-needed competition and lower prices in the retail sector. Over the next few years, a wave of foreign retailers entered the country, opening 22 large discount stores by the end of 1999. These discounters included Carrefour and Promodes from France, Wal-Mart and Costco from the United States, and Tesco from the United Kingdom. Together they provide a new source of competition for Korea's indigenous discounters, which included E-Mart and Magnet. The entry of foreign competitors with access to significant capital resources stimulated E-Mart and Magnet to increase their operating efficiency and lower prices to keep the foreigners at bay. The main beneficiaries of this development have been South Korean consumers who now enjoy more choice and lower prices than hitherto.

Liberalization of the retail sector, however, was just the first wave of opening up South Korea to foreign direct investment. In 1997, Korea's long period of economic expansion came to an abrupt end when a financial crisis swept across Asia. This produced a sharp drop in economic activity in South Korea. The Korean currency slumped against the dollar, requiring the government to seek $58 billion in aid from the International Monetary Fund. As demand for their products plummeted, dozens of highly leveraged Korean companies found themselves unable to service the debt that they had taken on during the boom years to finance their expansion. Many teetered on the edge of bankruptcy. The South Korean government responded by making the historic decision to remove many of the restrictions to foreign direct investment, including regulations that prohibited foreign firms from making hostile takeovers of Korean enterprises.

The impact was dramatic. FDI in the Korean economy surged from $3 billion in 1997 to $9.3 billion in 2000. The total stock of foreign investment in South Korea soared from $5.2 billion in 1990 to $62.7 billion by the end of the decade. While many Koreans initially viewed the new wave of foreign investment with deep suspicion, and the radical press demonized foreign companies as unwelcome guests feeding off the local market like leeches, it quickly became apparent that the reality was something else. An example was the acquisition of Samsung's money-losing construction equipment division by Sweden's Volvo in February 1998 for $572 million. This was Korea's first major sale of a distressed company to a foreign investor, and both the public and Samsung employees greeted the sale with deep apprehension. Two years later, however, most of those fears had been put to rest.

Volvo immediately launched an ambitious investment program, committing another $200 million to the plant in an attempt to turn the ex-Samsung facility into its main global base for excavators and other construction equipment. The company transferred leading-edge manufacturing technology to the ex-Samsung plant, moved in some of its best managers to oversee the operations, and made the facility its global center for R&D in excavators. Volvo even closed its excavator plant in Sweden, signaling the company's commitment to the South Korean facility. Although some 13 percent of the 1,655 employees at the plant left after the Volvo acquisition, these job reductions were achieved through attrition and not layoffs. Volvo refocused the production of the plant, emphasizing higher quality and higher priced machines that promise better profit margins. The old Korean emphasis on sales volume and market share has been replaced by a focus on product quality, operating efficiency, and profitability. The management hierarchy was significantly reduced, much of the bureaucracy was removed, and decision-making responsibilities were pushed down the line to self-managing work teams. By 2000, the plant was once more making a profit, and capacity utilization had increased from 50 percent to about 70 percent. The ultimate goal is to export 60 percent to 70 percent of the output from the plant, up from 35 percent of production when Samsung owned the plant. The early signs are encouraging; in 2001, exports from the plant had risen by over 40 percent since 1998.

Sources: Charles S. Lee, "Foreign Affair," *Far Eastern Economic Review*, April 29, 1999, pp. 58–60; S. W. Park, "Foreign Retail Chains Take Root in Korea," *Business Korea*, December 1999, pp. 42–43; M. Schuman, "South Korea Enjoys Foreign Investment Boom," *Wall Street Journal*, November 26, 1999, p. A8; and H. Ilbo, "Volvo Helps Korea Secure Global Strength," *Korea Times*, November 24, 2001.

Table 7.1

Political Ideology
toward FDI

Ideology	Characteristics	Host-Government Policy Implications
Radical	Marxist roots Views the MNE as an instrument of imperialist domination	Prohibit FDI Nationalize subsidiaries of foreign-owned MNEs
Free market	Classical economic roots (Smith) Views the MNE as an instrument for allocating production to most efficient locations	No restrictions on FDI
Pragmatic nationalism	Views FDI as having both benefits and costs	Restrict FDI where costs outweigh benefits Bargain for greater benefits and fewer costs Aggressively court beneficial FDI by offering incentives

Summary

The three main ideological positions regarding FDI are summarized in Table 7.1. Recent years have seen a marked decline in the number of countries that adhere to a radical ideology. Although no countries have adopted a pure free market policy stance, an increasing number of countries are gravitating toward the free market end of the spectrum and have liberalized their foreign investment regime. This includes many countries that less than two decades ago were firmly in the radical camp (e.g., the former Communist countries of Eastern Europe and many of the socialist countries of Africa) and several countries that until recently could best be described as pragmatic nationalists with regard to FDI (e.g., Japan, South Korea, Italy, Spain, and most Latin American countries). One result has been the surge in the volume of FDI worldwide, which, as we noted in Chapter 6, has been growing twice as fast as the growth in world trade. Another result has been a dramatic increase in the volume of FDI directed at countries that have recently liberalized their FDI regimes, such as China, India, and Vietnam.

The Benefits of FDI to Host Countries

In this section, we explore the four main benefits of FDI for a host country: the resource-transfer effects, the employment effects, the balance-of-payments effects, and the effects on competition and economic growth. In the next section, we will explore the costs of FDI to host countries. Economists who favor the free market view argue that the benefits of FDI to a host country so outweigh the costs that pragmatic nationalism is a misguided policy. According to the free market view, in a perfect world the best policy would be for all countries to forgo intervening in the investment decisions of MNEs.[5]

Resource-Transfer Effects

Foreign direct investment can make a positive contribution to a host economy by supplying capital, technology, and management resources that would otherwise not be available and thus boost that country's economic growth rate.[6] The accompanying

Country Focus describes how the Venezuelan government has been encouraging FDI in its petroleum industry in an attempt to benefit from resource-transfer effects. The transfer of capital, technology, and management resources was also an important feature of Volvo's acquisition of Samsung's excavation business (see the Management Focus), and is one reason the Irish government has been so keen to encourage FDI (see the opening case).

Capital

Many MNEs, by virtue of their large size and financial strength, have access to financial resources not available to host-country firms. These funds may be available from internal company sources, or, because of their reputation, large MNEs may find it easier to borrow money from capital markets than host-country firms would. This consideration was a factor in the Venezuelan government's decision to invite foreign oil companies to enter into joint ventures with PDVSA, the state-owned Venezuelan oil company, to develop Venezuela's oil industry. Similarly, the desire of the Irish government to encourage FDI by foreign firms is partly based on the belief that they have access to capital resources that Ireland needs (see the opening case).

Technology

As we saw in Chapter 2, the crucial role played by technological progress in economic growth is now widely accepted.[7] Technology can stimulate economic development and industrialization. It can take two forms, both of which are valuable. Technology can be incorporated in a production process (e.g., the technology for discovering, extracting, and refining oil) or it can be incorporated in a product (e.g., personal computers). However, many countries lack the research and development resources and skills required to develop their own indigenous product and process technology. This is particularly true of the world's less developed nations. Such countries must rely on advanced industrialized nations for much of the technology required to stimulate economic growth, and FDI can provide it. As we see in the Country Focus on Venezuela, a lack of relevant technological know-how with regard to the discovery, extraction, and refining of oil was one factor behind the Venezuelan government's decision to invite foreign oil companies into Venezuela.

FDI is not the only way to access advanced technology. Another option is to license that technology from foreign MNEs. The Japanese government, in particular, long favored this strategy. The Japanese government believed that, in the case of FDI, the technology is still ultimately controlled by the foreign MNE. Consequently, it is difficult for indigenous Japanese firms to develop their own, possibly better, technology because they are denied access to the basic technology. With this in mind, the Japanese government has insisted in the past that technology be transferred to Japan through licensing agreements, rather than through FDI. The advantage of licensing is that, in return for royalty payments, host-country firms are given direct access to valuable technology.

The licensing option is generally less attractive to the MNE, however. By licensing its technology to foreign companies, an MNE risks creating a future competitor—as many U.S. firms have learned at great cost in Japan. Given this tension, the mode for transferring technology—licensing or FDI—can be a major negotiating point between an MNE and a host government. Whether the MNE gets its way depends on the relative bargaining powers of the MNE and the host government. In addition to this issue, it can be difficult to transfer technology using a licensing agreement, particularly when the technology is complex and making the technology operational requires substantial experience. In such cases, direct investment is usually preferred to licensing (this issue is discussed in more detail in Chapter 6).

Research supports the view that multinational firms often transfer significant technology when they invest in a foreign country.[8] For example, a study of FDI in Sweden found that foreign firms increased both the labor and total factor productivity of

Swedish firms that they acquired, suggesting that significant technology transfers had occurred (technology typically boosts productivity).[9] Also, a study of FDI by the Organization for Economic Cooperation and Development (OECD) found that foreign investors invested significant amounts of capital in R&D in the countries in which they had invested, suggesting that not only were they transferring technology to those countries, but they may also have been upgrading existing technology or creating new technology in those countries.[10]

Management

Foreign management skills acquired through FDI may also produce important benefits for the host country. Foreign managers trained in the latest management techniques can often help to improve the efficiency of operations in the host country, whether those operations are acquired or green-field developments. This was a factor in Volvo's acquisition of Samsung excavation business, when Volvo's managers took actions to improve the operations and efficiency of the acquired unit (see the Management Focus). Beneficial spin-off effects may also arise when local personnel who are trained to occupy managerial, financial, and technical posts in the subsidiary of a foreign MNE leave the firm and help to establish indigenous firms. Similar benefits may arise if the superior management skills of a foreign MNE stimulate local suppliers, distributors, and competitors to improve their own management skills.

The benefits may be considerably reduced if most management and highly skilled jobs in the subsidiaries are reserved for home-country nationals. The percentage of management and skilled jobs that go to citizens of the host country can be a major negotiating point between an MNE wishing to undertake FDI and a potential host government. In recent years, most MNEs have responded to host-government pressures on this issue by agreeing to reserve a large proportion of management and highly skilled jobs for citizens of the host country.

Employment Effects

Another beneficial employment effect claimed for FDI is that it brings jobs to a host country that would otherwise not be created there. The effects of FDI on employment are both direct and indirect. Direct effects arise when a foreign MNE employs a number of host-country citizens. Indirect effects arise when jobs are created in local suppliers as a result of the investment and when jobs are created because of increased local spending by employees of the MNE. The indirect employment effects are often as large as, if not larger than, the direct effects. For example, when Toyota decided to open a new auto plant in France in 1997, estimates suggested that the plant would create 2,000 direct jobs and perhaps another 2,000 jobs in support industries.[11]

Cynics argue that not all the "new jobs" created by FDI represent net additions in employment. In the case of FDI by Japanese auto companies in the United States, some argue that the jobs created by this investment have been more than offset by the jobs lost in U.S.-owned auto companies, which have lost market share to their Japanese competitors. As a consequence of such substitution effects, the net number of new jobs created by FDI may not be as great as initially claimed by an MNE. The issue of the likely net gain in employment may be a major negotiating point between an MNE wishing to undertake FDI and the host government.

When FDI takes the form of an acquisition of an established enterprise in the host economy as opposed to a green-field investment (as in the case of Volvo's acquisition of Samsung's excavation division), the immediate effect may be to reduce employment as the multinational tries to restructure the operations of the acquired unit to improve its operating efficiency (again, this was the case in Volvo's acquisition of the Samsung division; see the Management Focus). However, even in such cases, research suggests that once the initial period of restructuring is over, enterprises acquired by foreign firms tend to grow their employment base at a faster rate than domestic rivals. For ex-

Country Focus

Foreign Direct Investment in Venezuela's Petroleum Industry

In 1976, Venezuela nationalized its oil industry, effectively closing the sector to foreign investors. The stated goal at the time was to control this important natural resource for the benefit of Venezuela, as opposed to foreign oil companies. The results, however, fell short of expectations. The country's state-owned oil monopoly, Petroleos de Venezuela SA (PDVSA), failed to develop new oil fields to replace the depletion of existing reserves, and the country's oil output was falling by the mid-1980s.

Faced with the prospect of declining export revenues from oil, Venezuela reversed its policy in 1991 and began to open its oil industry to foreign investors. The Venezuelan government turned to foreign investors for three reasons. First, it recognized that PDVSA did not have the capital required to undertake the investment alone. Second, it realized that PDVSA lacked the technological resources and skills of many of the world's major oil companies, particularly in the areas of oil exploration, oil field development, and sophisticated refining. The government understood that if PDVSA was to develop many of Venezuela's oil fields in a timely fashion, it had no alternative but to turn to foreign companies for help. Third, the government believed that PDVSA would be able to use joint ventures with foreign oil companies as a vehicle for learning about modern management techniques in the industry. PDVSA could then use this knowledge to improve the efficiency of its own operations.

The original plan called for the investment of $73 billion in the oil industry. The plan, as outlined by Gustavo Roosen, president of PDVSA, was to develop a crude oil production potential of 4 million barrels per day by 2002 and 7 million barrels per day by 2007 (the country produced about 2.6 million barrels per day in 1991). Of the $73 billion in projected capital spending, PDVSA planned to invest around $45 billion, while foreign oil companies were expected to supply the remaining $28 billion. The first FDI agreement was signed in 1992 with British Petroleum (BP). BP agreed to invest $60 million by 1995 to develop a marginal oil field that it would then be given the rights to for 20 years. Using a BP study, PDVSA identified sectors in eastern Venezuela with strong prospects for large discoveries of crude oil and entered into several ventures with other foreign partners to develop these zones. If commercial quantities of oil are discovered, PDVSA will share future production with its partners. Under the terms of most agreements, PDVSA will receive 35 percent of the earnings from any successful exploration venture. Also, with foreign investors such as Conoco and Total, PDVSA is investing in state-of-the-art refining facilities that can be used to convert heavy crude oil into a lighter, high-value crude oil for export. Finally, PDVSA, Shell, Exxon, and Mitsubishi have entered into a $5.6 billion joint venture to produce liquefied natural gas for export.

By 1997, more than 40 development projects were under way in Venezuela involving cooperation between PDVSA and foreign oil companies. Almost all of the world's major oil companies now had some activities in the country, compared to none before 1991. The country's oil output was also expanding, reaching 3.5 million barrels per day in 1997, up from a low of 1.7 million barrels per day in 1985. By 1999, the once marginally profitable enterprise earned profits of $24 billion, boosted in part by higher oil prices and in part by a 20 percent reduction in operating costs due to productivity gains. In 2000, PDVSA launched another 10-year plan. The plan called for the investment of another $53 billion between 2000 and 2010, with some $31 billion coming from the private sector, and the majority of that from foreign investors.

Sources: J. Mann, "A Little Help from Their Friends," *Financial Times*, November 10, 1993, p. 28; "Venezuela: A Survey," *The Economist*, October 14, 1994; E. Luce, "Oil: Foreign Investment: Finding a Balanced Approach," *Financial Times*, October 21, 1997, p. 6; and "PDVSA Projects $53 Billion in Outlays for 10 Year Plan," *Oil & Gas Journal*, April 17, 2000, pp. 26–27.

ample, an OECD study found that between 1989 and 1996 foreign firms created new jobs at a faster rate than their domestic counterparts.[12] In America, the workforce of foreign firms grew by 1.4 percent per year, compared to 0.8 percent per year for domestic firms. In Britain and France, the workforce of foreign firms grew at 1.7 percent per year, while employment at domestic firms fell by 2.7 percent. The same study found that foreign firms tended to pay higher wage rates than domestic firms, suggesting that the quality of employment was better. Another study looking at FDI in Eastern European transition economies found that although employment fell following the acquisition of an enterprise by a foreign firm, often those enterprises were in competitive difficulties and would not have survived if they had not been acquired. Also, after an initial period of adjustment and retrenchment, employment downsizing was often followed by new investments, and employment either remained stable or increased.[13]

Balance-of-Payments Effects

FDI's effect on a country's balance-of-payments accounts is an important policy issue for most host governments. To understand this concern, we must first familiarize ourselves with balance-of-payments accounting. Then we will examine the link between FDI and the balance-of-payments accounts.

Balance-of-Payments Accounts

A country's **balance-of-payments accounts** track both its payments to and its receipts from other countries. A summary copy of the U.S. balance-of-payments accounts for 2001 is given in Table 7.2. Any transaction resulting in a payment to other countries is entered in the balance-of-payments accounts as a debit and given a negative ($-$) sign. Any transaction resulting in a receipt from other countries is entered as a credit and given a positive ($+$) sign.

Balance-of-payments accounts are divided into two main sections: the current account and the capital account. The **current account** records transactions that pertain to three categories, all of which can be seen in Table 7.2. The first category, *merchandise trade*, refers to the export or import of physical goods (e.g., autos, computers, chemicals). The second category is the export or import of *services* (e.g., intangible products such as banking and insurance services). The third category, *investment income*, refers to income from foreign investments and payments that have to be made to foreigners investing in a country. For example, if a U.S. citizen owns a share of a Finnish company and receives a dividend payment of $5, that payment shows up on the U.S. current account as the receipt of $5 of investment income.

A **current account deficit** occurs when a country imports more goods, services, and income than it exports. A **current account surplus** occurs when a country exports more goods, services, and income than it imports. In recent years, the United States has run a persistent trade deficit. Table 7.2 shows that in 2001 the current account deficit was $393,371 million.

The **capital account** records transactions that involve the purchase or sale of assets. Thus, when a German firm purchases stock in a U.S. company, the transaction enters the U.S. balance of payments as a credit on the capital account. This is because capital is flowing into the country. When capital flows out of the United States, it enters the capital account as a debit.

A basic principle of balance-of-payments accounting is double-entry bookkeeping. Every international transaction automatically enters the balance of payments twice—once as a credit and once as a debit. Imagine that you purchase a car produced in Japan by Toyota for $20,000. Since your purchase represents a payment to another country for goods, it will enter the balance of payments as a debit on the current account. Toyota now has the $20,000 and must do something with it. If Toyota deposits the money at a U.S. bank, Toyota has purchased a U.S. asset—a bank deposit worth $20,000—and the transaction will show up as a $20,000 credit on the capital account. Or Toyota might deposit the cash in a Japanese bank in return for Japanese yen. Now the Japanese bank must decide what to do with the $20,000. Any action that it takes will ultimately result in a credit for the U.S. balance of payments. For example, if the bank lends the $20,000 to a Japanese firm that uses it to import personal computers from the United States, then the $20,000 must be credited to the U.S. balance-of-payments current account. Or the Japanese bank might use the $20,000 to purchase U.S. gov-

Current Account	Credits	Debits
Exports of goods, services, and income	$1,281,793	
Merchandised Goods	718,762	
Services	279,260	
Income receipts on investments	283,771	
Imports of goods, services, and income		−$1,625,701
Merchandised Goods		−1,145,927
Services		−210,385
Income payments on investments		−269,389
Unilateral transfers		−49,463
Balance of current account		−393,371
Capital Account		
U.S. assets abroad		−370,962
Foreign assets in United States	752,806	
Balance on capital account	826	
Statistical discrepancy	10,701	

Table 7.2

U.S. Balance of Payments Accounts for 2001 (figures in $ millions)

Source: U.S Department of Commerce.

ernment bonds, in which case it will show up as a credit on the U.S. balance-of-payments capital account.

Thus, any international transaction automatically gives rise to two offsetting entries in the balance of payments. Because of this, the current account balance and the capital account balance should always add up to zero. (In practice, this does not always occur due to the existence of statistical discrepancies that need not concern us here.)

Governments normally are concerned when their country is running a deficit on the current account of their balance of payments.[14] When a country runs a current account deficit, the money that flows to other countries is then used by those countries to purchase assets in the deficit country. Thus, when the United States runs a trade deficit with Japan, the Japanese use the money that they receive from U.S. consumers to purchase U.S. assets such as stocks, bonds, and the like. Put another way, a deficit on the current account is financed by selling assets to other countries; that is, by a surplus on the capital account. Thus, the U.S. current account deficit during the 1980s and 90s was financed by a steady sale of U.S. assets (stocks, bonds, real estate, and whole corporations) to other countries. Countries that run current account deficits become net debtors.

For example, as a result of financing its current account deficit through asset sales, the United States must deliver a stream of interest payments to foreign bondholders, rents to foreign landowners, and dividends to foreign stockholders. Such payments to foreigners drain resources from a country and limit the funds available for investment within the country. Since investment within a country is necessary to stimulate economic growth, a persistent current account deficit can choke off a country's future economic growth.

FDI and the Balance of Payments

Given the concern about current account deficits, the balance-of-payments effects of FDI can be an important consideration for a host government. There are three potential balance-of-payments consequences of FDI. First, when an MNE establishes a foreign subsidiary, the capital account of the host country benefits from the initial capital inflow. (A debit will be recorded in the capital account of the MNE's home country, since capital is flowing out of the home country.) However, this is a one-time-only effect. Set against this must be the outflow of earnings to the foreign parent company, which will be recorded as a debit on the current account of the host country.

Second, if the FDI is a substitute for imports of goods or services, it can improve the current account of the host country's balance of payments. Much of the FDI by Japanese automobile companies in the United States and United Kingdom, for example, can be seen as substituting for imports from Japan. Thus, the current account of the U.S. balance of payments has improved somewhat because many Japanese companies are now supplying the U.S. market from production facilities in the United States, as opposed to facilities in Japan. Insofar as this has reduced the need to finance a current account deficit by asset sales to foreigners, the United States has clearly benefited from this.

A third potential benefit to the host country's balance-of-payments position arises when the MNE uses a foreign subsidiary to export goods and services to other countries. There are some striking examples of this phenomenon. In the Czech Republic, Skoda, the national automobile company, was a well-established producer and exporter. After its sale to Volkswagen in 1992, however, exports boomed as the new owners redirected the company's sales efforts toward the European Union. The share of exports in Skoda's sales increased from 34 percent in 1990 to 52 percent in 1995 and 80 percent in 1999. The Management Focus provides us with another example of this phenomenon. After acquiring Samsung's excavation division, Volvo made it the global center for its excavation business and redirected its attention toward exports. In addition, as we saw in the opening case, much of the FDI into Ireland has subsequently increased exports from Ireland, as foreign multinationals have used the country as a base for exporting to the rest of the European Union.

According to a recent UN report, inward FDI by foreign multinationals has been a major driver of export-led economic growth in a number of developing and developed nations over the last decade.[15] For example, in China exports have increased from $26 billion in 1985 to over $250 billion by 2001. According to UN data, much of this export growth was due to the presence of foreign multinationals that invested heavily in China during the 1990s. The subsidiaries of foreign multinationals accounted for 50 percent of all exports from that country in 2001, up from 17 percent in 1991. In mobile phones, for example, the Chinese subsidiaries of foreign multinationals—primarily Nokia, Motorola, Ericsson, and Siemens—accounted for 95 percent of China's exports.

Effect on Competition and Economic Growth

Economic theory tells us that the efficient functioning of markets depends on an adequate level of competition between producers. When FDI takes the form of a green-field investment, the result is to establish a new enterprise, increasing the number of players in a market and thus consumer choice. In turn, this can increase the level of competition in a national market, thereby driving down prices and increasing the economic welfare of consumers. Increased competition tends to stimulate capital investments by firms in plant, equipment, and R&D as they struggle to gain an edge over their rivals. The long-term results may include increased productivity growth, product and process innovations, and greater economic growth.[16] Such beneficial effects seem to have occurred in the South Korean retail sector following the liberalization of FDI regulations in 1996. FDI by large Western discount stores, including Wal-Mart, Costco, Carrefour, and Tesco, seems to have encouraged indigenous discounters such as E-Mart to improve the efficiency of their own operations (see the Management Focus). The results have included more competition and lower prices, which benefit South Korean consumers.

FDI's impact on competition in domestic markets may be particularly important in the case of services, such as telecommunications, retailing, and many financial services, where exporting is often not an option because the service has to be produced where it is delivered.[17] For example, under a 1997 agreement sponsored by the World Trade Organization, 68 countries accounting for more than 90 percent of world telecommunications revenues pledged to start opening their markets to foreign investment and competition and to abide by common rules for fair competition in telecommunications. Before this agreement, most of the world's telecommunications markets were closed to foreign competitors and in most countries the market was monopolized by a single carrier, which was often a state-owned enterprise. The agreement has dramatically increased the level of competition in many national telecommunications markets. Three benefits from this agreement have started to occur. First, inward investment has increased competition and stimulated investment in the modernization of telephone networks around the world, leading to better service. Second, the increased competition has resulted in lower prices. Third, trade in other goods and services depends upon flows of information matching buyers to sellers. As telecommunications service improves in quality and declines in price, international trade increases in volume and becomes less costly for traders. Telecommunications reform, therefore, should promote cross-border trade in other goods and services.

The Costs of FDI to Host Countries ■

Three costs of FDI concern host countries. They arise from possible adverse effects on competition within the host nation, adverse effects on the balance of payments, and the perceived loss of national sovereignty and autonomy.

▌Adverse Effects on Competition

Although we have just outlined in the previous section how foreign direct investment can boost competition, host governments sometimes worry that the subsidiaries of foreign MNEs may have greater economic power than indigenous competitors. If it is part of a larger international organization, the foreign MNE may be able to draw on funds generated elsewhere to subsidize its costs in the host market, which could drive indigenous companies out of business and allow the firm to monopolize the market. (Once the market was monopolized, the foreign MNE could raise prices above those that would prevail in competitive markets, with harmful effects on the economic welfare of the host nation.) This concern tends to be greater in countries that have few large firms of their own (generally less developed countries). It tends to be a relatively minor concern in most advanced industrialized nations.

In general, while FDI in the form of green-field investments should increase competition, it is less clear that this is the case when the FDI takes the form of acquisition of an established enterprise in the host nation, as was the case when Volvo acquired Samsung's excavation division (see the Management Focus). Because an acquisition does not result in a net increase in the number of players in a market, the effect on competition may be neutral. When a foreign investor acquires two or more firms in a host country, and subsequently merges them, the effect may be to reduce the level of competition in that market, create monopoly power for the foreign firm, reduce consumer choice, and raise prices. For example, in India, Hindustan Lever Ltd., the Indian subsidiary of Unilever, acquired its main local rival, Tata Oil Mills, to assume a dominant position in the bath soap (75 percent) and detergents (30 percent) markets. Hindustan Lever also acquired several local companies in other markets, such as the ice cream makers Dollops, Kwality, and Milkfood. By combining these companies, Hindustan Lever's share of the Indian ice cream market went from zero in 1992 to 74 percent in 1997.[18] However, while such cases are of obvious concern, there is little evidence that such developments are widespread. In many nations, domestic competition authorities have the right to review and block any mergers or acquisitions that they view as having a detrimental impact on competition. If such institutions are operating effectively, this should be sufficient to make sure that foreign entities do not monopolize a country's markets.

Adverse Effects on the Balance of Payments

The possible adverse effects of FDI on a host country's balance-of-payments position have been hinted at earlier. There are two main areas of concern with regard to the balance of payments. First, as mentioned earlier, set against the initial capital inflow that comes with FDI must be the subsequent outflow of earnings from the foreign subsidiary to its parent company. Such outflows show up as a debit on the capital account. Some governments have responded to such outflows by restricting the amount of earnings that can be repatriated to a foreign subsidiary's home country.

A second concern arises when a foreign subsidiary imports a substantial number of its inputs from abroad, which results in a debit on the current account of the host country's balance of payments. One criticism leveled against Japanese-owned auto assembly operations in the United States, for example, is that they tend to import many component parts from Japan. Because of this, the favorable impact of this FDI on the current account of the U.S. balance-of-payments position may not be as great as initially supposed. The Japanese auto companies have responded to these criticisms by pledging to purchase 75 percent of their component parts from U.S.-based manufacturers (but not necessarily U.S.-owned manufacturers). When the Japanese auto company Nissan invested in the United Kingdom, Nissan responded to concerns about local content by pledging to increase the proportion of local content to 60 percent, and by subsequently raising it to more than 80 percent.

National Sovereignty and Autonomy

Some host governments worry that FDI is accompanied by some loss of economic independence. The concern is that key decisions that can affect the host country's economy will be made by a foreign parent that has no real commitment to the host country, and over which the host country's government has no real control. A quarter of a century ago this concern was expressed by several European countries, who feared that FDI by U.S. MNEs was threatening their national sovereignty. The same concerns surfaced in the United States with regard to European and Japanese FDI during the 1980s and early 1990s. The main fear seems to be that if foreigners own assets in the United States, they can somehow "hold the country to economic ransom." Twenty-five years ago when officials in the French government were making similar complaints about U.S. investments in France, many U.S. politicians dismissed the charge as silly, but when the shoe was on the other foot, some U.S. politicians did not think the notion was silly. However, most economists dismiss such concerns as groundless and irrational. Political scientist Robert Reich has noted that such concerns are the product of outmoded thinking because they fail to account for the growing interdependence of the world economy.[19] In a world where firms from all advanced nations are increasingly investing in each other's markets, it is not possible for one country to hold another to "economic ransom" without hurting itself.

◼ The Benefits and Costs of FDI to Home Countries

FDI also produces costs and benefits to the home (or source) country. Does the U.S. economy benefit or lose from investments by its firms in foreign markets? Does the Swedish economy lose or gain from Volvo's investment in South Korea? Some argue that FDI is not always in the home country's national interest and should be restricted. Others argue that the benefits far outweigh the costs and any restrictions would be contrary to national interests. To understand why people take these positions, let us look at the benefits and costs of FDI to the home (source) country.[20]

Benefits of FDI to the Home Country

The benefits of FDI to the home country arise from three sources. First, and perhaps most important, the capital account of the home country's balance of payments benefits from the inward flow of foreign earnings. Thus, one benefit to Sweden from Volvo's investment in South Korea is the earnings that are subsequently repatriated to Sweden from Korea. FDI can also benefit the current account of the home country's balance of payments if the foreign subsidiary creates demands for home-country exports of capital equipment, intermediate goods, complementary products, and the like.

Second, benefits to the home country from outward FDI arise from employment effects. As with the balance of payments, positive employment effects arise when the foreign subsidiary creates demand for home-country exports of capital equipment, intermediate goods, complementary products, and the like. Thus, Toyota's investment in auto assembly operations in Europe has benefited both the Japanese balance-of-payments position and employment in Japan, because Toyota imports some component parts for its European-based auto assembly operations directly from Japan.

Third, benefits arise when the home-country MNE learns valuable skills from its exposure to foreign markets that can subsequently be transferred back to the home country. This amounts to a reverse resource-transfer effect. Through its exposure to a foreign market, an MNE can learn about superior management techniques and superior product and process technologies. These resources can then be transferred back to the home country, contributing to the home country's economic growth rate.[21] For example, one reason General Motors and Ford invested in Japanese automobile companies (GM owns part of Isuzu, and Ford owns part of Mazda) was to learn about their production processes. If GM and Ford are successful in transferring this know-how back to their U.S. operations, the result may be a net gain for the U.S. economy.

Costs of FDI to the Home Country

Against these benefits must be set the apparent costs of FDI for the source country. The most important concerns center around the balance-of-payments and employment effects of outward FDI. The home country's balance of payments may suffer in three ways. First, the capital account of the balance of payments suffers from the initial capital outflow required to finance the FDI. This effect, however, is usually more than offset by the subsequent inflow of foreign earnings. Second, the current account of the balance of payments suffers if the purpose of the foreign investment is to serve the home market from a low-cost production location. Third, the current account of the balance of payments suffers if the FDI is a substitute for direct exports. Thus, insofar as Toyota's assembly operations in the United States are intended to substitute for direct exports from Japan, the current account position of Japan will deteriorate.

With regard to employment effects, the most serious concerns arise when FDI is seen as a substitute for domestic production. This was the case with Volvo's investment in South Korea and Toyota's investments in Europe. One obvious result of such FDI is reduced home-country employment. If the labor market in the home country is already very tight, with little unemployment, this concern may not be that great. However, if the home country is suffering from unemployment, concern about the export of jobs may arise. For example, one objection frequently raised by U.S. labor leaders to the free trade pact between the United States, Mexico, and Canada (see the next chapter) is that the United States will lose hundreds of thousands of jobs as U.S. firms invest in Mexico to take advantage of cheaper labor and then export back to the United States.[22]

International Trade Theory and FDI

When assessing the costs and benefits of FDI to the home country, keep in mind the lessons of international trade theory (see Chapter 4). International trade theory tells us that home-country concerns about the negative economic effects of offshore production may be misplaced. The term **offshore production** refers to FDI undertaken to serve the home market. Far from reducing home-country employment, such FDI may actually stimulate economic growth (and hence employment) in the home country by freeing home-country resources to concentrate on activities where the home country has a comparative advantage. In addition, home-country consumers benefit if the price of the particular product falls as a result of the FDI. Also, if a company were prohibited from making such investments on the grounds of negative employment effects while its international competitors reaped the benefits of low-cost production locations, it would undoubtedly lose market share to its international competitors. Under such a scenario, the adverse long-run economic effects for a country would probably outweigh the relatively minor balance-of-payments and employment effects associated with offshore production.

Government Policy Instruments and FDI

Before tackling the important issue of bargaining between the MNE and the host government, we need to discuss the policy instruments that governments use to regulate FDI activity by MNEs. Both home (source) countries and host countries have a range of policy instruments that they can use. We will look at each in turn.

Home-Country Policies

Through their choice of policies, home countries can both encourage and restrict FDI by local firms. We look at policies designed to encourage outward FDI first. These include foreign risk insurance, capital assistance, tax incentives, and political pressure. Then we will look at policies designed to restrict outward FDI.

Encouraging Outward FDI

Many investor nations now have government-backed insurance programs to cover major types of foreign investment risk. The types of risks insurable through these programs include the risks of expropriation (nationalization), war losses, and the inability to transfer profits back home. Such programs are particularly useful in encouraging firms to undertake investments in politically unstable countries.[23] In addition, several advanced countries also have special funds or banks that make government loans to firms wishing to invest in developing countries. As a further incentive to encourage domestic firms to undertake FDI, many countries have eliminated double taxation of foreign income (i.e., taxation of income in both the host country and the home country). Last, and perhaps most significant, a number of investor countries (including the United States) have used their political influence to persuade host countries to relax their restrictions on inbound FDI. For example, in response to direct U.S. pressure, Japan relaxed many of its formal restrictions on inward FDI in the 1980s. Now, in response to further U.S. pressure, Japan moved toward relaxing its informal barriers to inward FDI. One beneficiary of this trend has been Toys "R" Us, which, after five years of intensive lobbying by company and U.S. government officials, opened its first retail stores in Japan in December 1991. By 2000, Toys "R" Us had more than 150 stores in Japan and its Japanese operation, in which Toys "R" Us retained a controlling stake, had a listing on the Japanese stock market.

Restricting Outward FDI

Virtually all investor countries, including the United States, have exercised some control over outward FDI from time to time. One common policy has been to limit capital outflows out of concern for the country's balance of payments. From the early 1960s until 1979, for example, Britain had exchange-control regulations that limited the amount of capital a firm could take out of the country. Although the main intent of such policies was to improve the British balance of payments, an important secondary intent was to make it more difficult for British firms to undertake FDI.

In addition, countries have occasionally manipulated tax rules to try to encourage their firms to invest at home. The objective behind such policies is to create jobs at home rather than in other nations. At one time these policies were also adopted by Britain. The British advanced corporation tax system taxed British companies' foreign earnings at a higher rate than their domestic earnings. This tax code created an incentive for British companies to invest at home.

Finally, countries sometimes prohibit national firms from investing in certain countries for political reasons. Such restrictions can be formal or informal. For example, formal U.S. rules prohibited U.S. firms from investing in countries such as Cuba, Libya, and Iran, whose political ideology and actions are judged to be contrary to U.S. interests. Similarly, during the 1980s, informal pressure was applied to dissuade U.S. firms from investing in South Africa. In this case, the objective was to pressure South Africa to change its apartheid laws, which happened during the early 1990s.

Host-Country Policies

Host countries adopt policies designed both to restrict and to encourage inward FDI. As noted earlier in this chapter, political ideology has determined the type and scope of these policies in the past. In the last decade of the 20th century, many countries moved quickly away from a situation where many countries adhered to some version of the radical stance and prohibited much FDI, and toward a situation where a combination of free market objectives and pragmatic nationalism took hold.

Encouraging Inward FDI

It is increasingly common for governments to offer incentives to foreign firms to invest in their countries. Such incentives take many forms, but the most common are tax concessions, low-interest loans, and grants or subsidies. Incentives are motivated by a desire to gain from the resource-transfer and employment effects of FDI. They are also motivated by a desire to capture FDI away from other potential host countries. For example, in the mid-1990s, the governments of Britain and France competed with each other on the incentives they offered Toyota to invest in their respective countries. In the United States, state governments often compete with each other to attract FDI. For example, Kentucky offered Toyota an incentive package worth $112 million to persuade it to build its U.S. automobile assembly plants there. The package included tax breaks, new state spending on infrastructure, and low-interest loans.[24]

Restricting Inward FDI

Host governments use a wide range of controls to restrict FDI in one way or another. The two most common are ownership restraints and performance requirements. Ownership restraints can take several forms. In some countries, foreign companies are excluded from specific fields. For example, they are excluded from tobacco and mining in Sweden and from the development of certain natural resources in Brazil, Finland, and Morocco. In other industries, foreign ownership may be permitted although a significant proportion of the equity of the subsidiary must be owned by local investors. For example, foreign ownership is restricted to 25 percent or less of an airline in the United States. In India, foreign firms were prohibited from owning media businesses until 2001, when the rules were relaxed, allowing foreign firms to purchase up to 26 percent of a foreign newspaper.[25]

The rationale underlying ownership restraints seems to be twofold. First, foreign firms are often excluded from certain sectors on the grounds of national security or competition. Particularly in less developed countries, the feeling seems to be that local firms might not be able to develop unless foreign competition is restricted by a combination of import tariffs and controls on FDI. This is a variant of the infant industry argument discussed in Chapter 5.

Second, ownership restraints seem to be based on a belief that local owners can help to maximize the resource-transfer and employment benefits of FDI for the host country. Until the early 1980s, the Japanese government prohibited most FDI but allowed joint ventures between Japanese firms and foreign MNEs if the MNE had a valuable technology. The Japanese government clearly believed such an arrangement would speed up the subsequent diffusion of the MNE's valuable technology throughout the Japanese economy.

Performance requirements can also take several forms. Performance requirements are controls over the behavior of the MNE's local subsidiary. The most common performance requirements are related to local content, exports, technology transfer, and local participation in top management. As with certain ownership restrictions, the logic underlying performance requirements is that such rules help to maximize the benefits and minimize the costs of FDI for the host country. Virtually all countries employ some form of performance requirements when it suits their objectives. However, performance requirements tend to be more common in less developed countries than in advanced industrialized nations.[26] For example, one study found that some 30 percent of the affiliates of U.S. MNEs in less developed countries were subject to performance requirements, while only 6 percent of the affiliates in advanced countries were faced with such requirements.[27]

International Institutions and the Liberalization of FDI

Until the 1990s, there was no consistent involvement by multinational institutions in the governing of FDI. This changed with the formation of the World Trade Organization in 1995. As noted in Chapter 5, the role of the WTO embraces the promotion of international trade in services. Since many services have to be produced where they are sold, exporting is not an option (for example, one cannot export McDonald's hamburgers or consumer banking services). Given this, the WTO has become involved in regulations governing FDI. As might be expected for an institution created to promote free trade, the thrust of the WTO's efforts has been to push for the liberalization of regulations governing FDI, particularly in services. Under the auspices of the WTO, two extensive multinational agreements were reached in 1997 to liberalize trade in telecommunications and financial services. Both these agreements contained detailed clauses that require signatories to liberalize their regulations governing inward FDI, essentially opening their markets to foreign telecommunications and financial services companies.

However, the WTO has had less success trying to initiate talks aimed at establishing a universal set of rules designed to promote the liberalization of FDI. Led by Malaysia and India, developing nations have so far rejected any attempts by the WTO to start such discussions. In an attempt to make some progress on this issue, the Organization for Economic Cooperation and Development (OECD) in 1995 initiated talks between its members. (The OECD is a Paris-based intergovernmental organization of "wealthy" nations whose purpose is to provide its 29 member states with a forum in which governments can compare their experiences, discuss the problems they share, and seek solutions that can then be applied within their own national contexts. The members include most European Union countries, the United States, Canada, Japan, and South Korea). The aim of the talks was to draft a multilateral agreement on investment (MAI) that would make it illegal for signatory states to discriminate against foreign investors. This would liberalize rules governing FDI between OECD states.

Unfortunately for those promoting the agreement, the talks broke down in early 1998, primarily because the United States refused to sign the agreement. According to the United States, the proposed agreement contained too many exceptions that would weaken its powers. For example, the proposed agreement would not have barred discriminatory taxation of foreign-owned companies, and it would have allowed countries to restrict foreign television programs and music in the name of preserving culture. Also campaigning against the MAI were environmental and labor groups, who criticized the proposed agreement on the grounds that it contained no binding environmental or labor agreements.

Despite these problems, negotiations on a revised MAI treaty might restart in the future. Also, as noted earlier, individual nations have continued to unilaterally remove restrictions to inward FDI as a wide range of countries from South Korea to South Africa try to encourage foreign firms to invest in their economies.[28]

Focus On Managerial Implications

There are a number of fairly obvious implications for business in the material discussed in this chapter. For a start, a host government's attitude toward FDI should be an important variable in deciding where to locate foreign production facilities and where to make a foreign direct investment. Other things being equal, investing in countries that have permissive policies toward FDI is clearly preferable to investing in countries that restrict FDI.

Generally, however, the issue is not this straightforward. Despite the move toward a free market stance in recent years, many countries still have a rather pragmatic stance toward FDI.[29] In such cases, a firm considering FDI may have to negotiate the specific terms of the investment with the host country's government. Such negotiations often center on two broad issues. If the host government is trying to attract FDI, the central issue is likely to be the kind of incentives the host government is prepared to offer to the MNE and what the firm will commit in exchange. If the host government is uncertain about the benefits of FDI and might restrict access, the central issue is likely to be the concessions that the firm must make to go forward with a proposed investment.

In the remainder of this section, we will focus on negotiating with a host government. Increasingly, negotiations between MNEs and host governments are occurring within the framework of broad multilateral agreements to which the host and home countries are signatories.[30] For example, when a U.S. firm is considering investing in the Brazilian telecommunications sector, the 1997 WTO telecommunications agreements sets the parameters under which negotiations can proceed. Because the agreement has removed most impediments to cross-border investments in telecommunications, the scope for bargaining between the MNE and the host government is significantly reduced. The same is true of much cross-border investment in financial services, again due to the establishment of a WTO agreement. In additional, extensive regional agreements such as the European Union (EU) and the North American Free Trade Agreement (NAFTA) now govern FDI flows between countries that are members of the same regional bloc (we discuss these agreements in depth in the next chapter). NAFTA, for example, sets the parameters that govern the conditions under which firms from Canada, Mexico, and the United States can invest in each other's markets. These parameters, which are generally very liberal and remove most restrictions on FDI flows between member states, significantly limit the scope for bargaining. Still, given the failure of both the WTO and the OECD to establish extensive multilateral agreements governing FDI, negotiation between MNEs and host governments remains an important issue in many instances.

The Nature of Negotiation

The objective of any negotiation is to reach an agreement that benefits both parties. Negotiation is both an art and a science. The science of it requires analyzing the relative bargaining strengths of each party and the different strategic options available to each party and assessing how the other party might respond to various bargaining ploys.[31] The art of negotiation incorporates

Figure 7.1

The Context of
Negotiation—the Four Cs

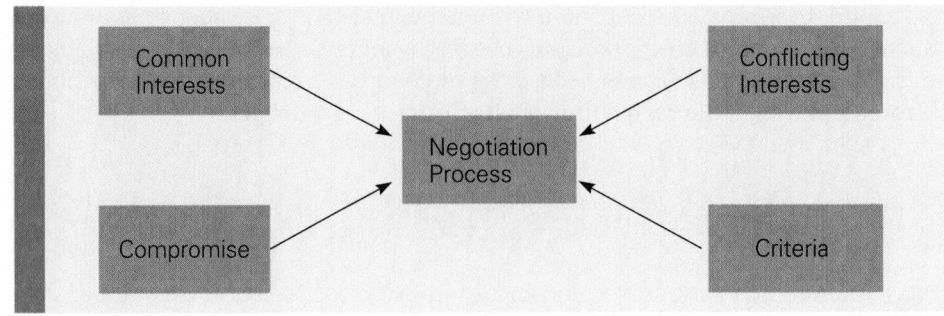

"interpersonal skills, the ability to convince and be convinced, the ability to employ a basketful of bargaining ploys, and the wisdom to know when and how to use them."[32] In the context of international business, the art of negotiation also includes understanding the influence of national norms, value systems, and culture on the approach and likely negotiating tactics of the other party as well as sensitivity to such factors in shaping a firm's approach to negotiations with a foreign government. For example, negotiating with the Japanese government for access is likely to be very different from negotiating with the British government. Consequently, it requires different interpersonal skills and bargaining ploys. We discussed the importance of national differences in society and culture in Chapter 3. It would be well to keep these differences in mind at this juncture.

The negotiation process has been characterized as occurring within the context of "the four Cs": common interests, conflicting interests, compromise, and criteria (see Figure 7.1).[33] To explore this concept, consider the negotiation between IBM and Mexico that occurred in 1984 and 1985 when IBM tried to get permission to establish a facility to manufacture personal computers in Guadalajara, Mexico. At that time, Mexican law required foreign investors to agree to a minimum of 51 percent local ownership of any production facilities established in Mexico (the law was repealed as part of the 1994 North American Free Trade Agreement). The rationale for this law was Mexico's desire to reduce its economic dependence on foreign-owned enterprises, thereby preserving its national sovereignty. As with many such laws, in practice it was used as a bargaining chip by the Mexican government to extract concessions from foreign firms wishing to establish production facilities in Mexico. The government was often willing to waive the 51 percent ownership requirement if a foreign firm would make concessions that increased the beneficial impact of its investment on the Mexican economy.

IBM proposed to invest about $40 million in a state-of-the-art production facility with the capacity to produce 100,000 PCs per year, 75 percent of which would be exported (primarily to the United States). IBM's objective was to take advantage of Mexico's low labor costs to reduce the cost of manufacturing PCs. Given the proprietary nature of the product and process technology involved in the design and manufacture of PCs, IBM wanted to maintain 100 percent ownership of the Guadalajara facility. IBM believed that if it entered into a joint venture with a Mexican firm to produce PCs, as required under Mexican law, it would risk giving away valuable technology to a potential future competitor.

When presenting its case to the Mexican government, IBM stressed the benefits of the proposed investment for the Mexican economy. These included the creation of 80 direct jobs and 800 indirect ones, the transfer of high-technology job skills to Mexico, new direct investment of $7 million (the remaining $33 million required to finance the investment would be raised from the Mexican capital market), and exports of 75,000 personal computers per year. The Mexican government rejected the proposal on the grounds that IBM did not propose to use sufficient local content in the plant and would thus be importing too many parts and materials. IBM twice resubmitted its proposal. Maintaining its insistence on 100 percent ownership, IBM with each proposal increased its commitment to purchase local parts, increased the level of its direct investment, and raised its planned level of exports. The Mexican government agreed to the third proposal, which had extracted significant concessions from IBM.

The final agreement required IBM to invest $91 million (up from $40 million). This money was distributed among expansion of the Guadalajara plant ($7 million), investment in local R&D ($35 million), development of local suppliers ($20 million), expansion of its purchasing and distribution network ($13 million), contributions to a Mexican government-sponsored semiconductor technology center ($12 million), and various other minor investments. In addition, IBM agreed to achieve 82 percent local content by the fourth year of operation and to export 92 percent of the PCs produced. In exchange, the Mexican government waived its 51 percent local ownership requirement and allowed IBM to maintain 100 percent control.[34]

In this example, the common interest of both IBM and Mexico is establishing a new enterprise in Mexico. Conflicting interests arise from such issues as the proportion of component parts that will be procured locally rather than imported, the total amount of investment, the total number of jobs created, and the proportion of output that will be exported. Compromise involves reaching a decision that brings benefits to both parties, even though neither will get all of what it wants. IBM's criteria or objectives are to achieve satisfactory profits and to maintain 100 percent ownership. Mexico's criteria are to achieve satisfactory net benefits from the resource-transfer, employment, and balance-of-payments effects of the investment.

Bargaining Power

The outcome of any negotiated agreement depends on the relative bargaining power of both parties. Each side's bargaining power depends on three factors (see Table 7.3):

- The value each side places on what the other has to offer.
- The number of comparable alternatives available to each side.
- Each party's time horizon.

From the perspective of a firm negotiating the terms of an investment with a host government, the firm's bargaining power is high when the host government places a high value on what the firm has to offer, the number of comparable alternatives open to the firm is great, and the firm has a long time in which to complete the negotiations. The converse also holds. The firm's bargaining power is low when the host government places a low value on what the firm has to offer, few comparable alternatives are open to the firm, and the firm has a short time in which to complete the negotiations.

	Bargaining Power of Firm	
	High	**Low**
Firm's time horizon	Long	Short
Comparable alternatives open to firm	Many	Few
Value placed by host government on investment	High	Low

Table 7.3

Determinants of Bargaining Power

To see how this plays out in practice, consider again the case of IBM and Mexico. IBM was in a fairly strong bargaining position, primarily because Mexico was suffering from a flight of capital out of the country at the time (1985), which made the government eager to attract new foreign investment. But IBM's bargaining power was moderated somewhat by three things. First, despite its symbolic importance, the size of the proposed investment was unlikely to have more than a marginal impact on the Mexican economy, so the economic value placed by Mexico on the investment was not that great. Second, IBM was looking for a low-labor-cost, politically stable location close to the United States. Mexico was obviously the most desirable location given these criteria. Greater distance and higher transportation costs made alternative low-labor-cost locations, such as Taiwan or Singapore, relatively less attractive, while other potential locations in Central America were ruled out because of political instability. Third, given the profusion of low-cost competitors moving into the U.S. personal computer market during the mid-1980s, IBM probably believed it needed to move quickly to establish its own low-cost production facilities. But there was no compelling reason for Mexico to close a deal quickly. Due to all these factors, the Mexican government also held some bargaining power in the negotiations and was able to extract some concessions from IBM. On the other hand, IBM's strong position allowed it to insist that it maintain 100 percent ownership of its Mexican subsidiary. This represented a significant concession from the Mexican government; IBM was the first major company for which Mexico waived its prohibition of majority ownership.

In a similar case during the 1960s, IBM was one of the few firms to get the Japanese government to waive the restriction on FDI that would allow it to establish a wholly owned subsidiary in Japan. IBM was able to do this because it was the only major source of mainframe computer technology at the time, and numerous Japanese companies needed that technology for data processing. The lack of comparable alternatives available to the Japanese enabled IBM to pry open the Japanese market. Similarly, during the 1980s, Toyota extracted significant concessions from the state of Kentucky in the form of tax breaks, low-interest loans, and grants, and Honda received similar concessions from the state of Ohio. At that time, both states were suffering from high unemployment, and the proposed auto assembly plants promised to have a substantial impact on employment. Also, both companies had a number of states from which to choose. Thus, the high value placed by state governments on the proposed investment and the number of comparable alternatives open to each company considerably strengthened the bargaining power of both companies relative to that of the state governments.

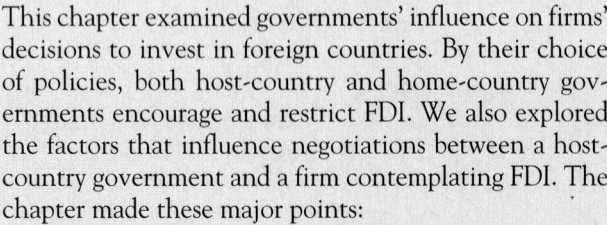

ChapterSummary

This chapter examined governments' influence on firms' decisions to invest in foreign countries. By their choice of policies, both host-country and home-country governments encourage and restrict FDI. We also explored the factors that influence negotiations between a host-country government and a firm contemplating FDI. The chapter made these major points:

1. An important determinant of government policy toward FDI is political ideology. Political ideology ranges from a radical stance that is hostile to FDI to a noninterventionist, free market

stance. Between the two extremes is an approach best described as pragmatic nationalism.

2. The radical view sees the MNE as an imperialist tool for exploiting host countries. According to this view, no country should allow FDI. Due to the collapse of communism, the radical view was in retreat everywhere by the end of the 1990s.

3. The free market view sees the MNE as an instrument for increasing the overall efficiency of resource utilization in the world economy. FDI can be viewed as a way of dispersing the production of

goods and services to those locations around the globe where they can be produced most efficiently.

4. Pragmatic nationalism views FDI as having both benefits and costs. Countries adopting a pragmatic stance pursue policies designed to maximize the benefits and minimize the costs of FDI.

5. The benefits of FDI to a host country arise from resource-transfer effects, employment effects, balance-of-payments effects, and its ability to promote competition.

6. FDI can make a positive contribution to a host economy by supplying capital, technology, and management resources that would otherwise not be available. Such resource transfers can stimulate the economic growth of the host economy.

7. Employment effects arise from the direct and indirect creation of jobs by FDI.

8. Balance-of-payments effects arise from the initial capital inflow to finance FDI, from import substitution effects, and from subsequent exports by the new enterprise.

9. By increasing consumer choice, foreign direct investment can help to increase the level of competition in national markets, thereby driving down prices and increasing the economic welfare of consumers.

10. The costs of FDI to a host country include adverse effects on competition and balance of payments and a perceived loss of national sovereignty.

11. Host governments are concerned that foreign MNEs may have greater economic power than indigenous companies and that they may be able to monopolize the market.

12. Adverse effects on the balance of payments arise from the outflow of a foreign subsidiary's earnings and from the import of inputs from abroad.

13. National sovereignty concerns are raised by FDI because key decisions that affect the host country will be made by a foreign parent that may have no real commitment to the host country and the host government will have no control over them.

14. The benefits of FDI to the home (source) country include improvement in the balance of payments as a result of the inward flow of foreign earnings, positive employment effects when the foreign subsidiary creates demand for home-country exports, and benefits from a reverse resource-transfer effect. A reverse resource-transfer effect arises when the foreign subsidiary learns valuable skills abroad that can be transferred back to the home country.

15. The costs of FDI to the home country include adverse balance-of-payments effects that arise from the initial capital outflow and from the export substitution effects of FDI. Costs also arise when FDI exports jobs abroad.

16. Home countries can adopt policies designed to both encourage and restrict FDI. Host countries try to attract FDI by offering incentives and try to restrict FDI by dictating ownership restraints and requiring that foreign MNEs meet specific performance requirements.

17. A firm considering FDI usually must negotiate the terms of the investment with the host government. The object of any negotiation is to reach an agreement that benefits both parties. Negotiation inevitably involves compromise.

18. The outcome of negotiation is typically determined by the relative bargaining powers of the foreign MNE and the host government. Bargaining power depends on the value each side places on what the other has to offer, the number of comparable alternatives available to each side, and each party's time horizon.

Critical Discussion Questions

1. Read the opening case on FDI in Ireland. How important was FDI to the health of the Irish economy?

2. Explain how the political ideology of a host government might influence the negotiations between the host government and a foreign MNE.

3. Under what circumstances is an MNE in a powerful negotiating position vis-à-vis a host government? What kind of concessions is a firm likely to win in such situations?

4. Under what circumstances is an MNE in a weak negotiating position vis-à-vis a host government?

What kind of concessions is a host government likely to win in such situations?

5. Inward FDI is bad for (i) a developing economy and (ii) a developed economy and should be subjected to strict controls. Discuss.

6. Firms should not be investing abroad when there is a need for investment to create jobs at home. Discuss.

7. Do you think the successful conclusion of a multilateral agreement to liberalize regulations governing FDI will benefit the world economy? Why?

Notes

1. For elaboration see S. Hood and S. Young, *The Economics of the Multinational Enterprise* (London: Longman, 1979), and P. M. Sweezy and H. Magdoff, "The Dynamics of U.S. Capitalism," *New York. Monthly Review Press,* 1972.

2. S. Weiss, "The Long Path to the IBM-Mexico Agreement: An Analysis of Micro-Computer Investment Decisions," Working Paper 3, NYU School of Business, 1989.

3. For an example of this policy as practiced in China, see L. G. Branstetter and R. C. Freenstra, "Trade and Foreign Direct Investment in China: A Political Economy Approach," *Journal of International Economics* 58 (December 2002), pp. 335–58.

4. M. Itoh and K. Kiyono, "Foreign Trade and Direct Investment," in *Industrial Policy of Japan,* ed. R. Komiya, M. Okuno, and K. Suzumura (Tokyo: Academic Press, 1988).

5. See S. Hood and S. Young, *The Economics of the Multinational Enterprise.* Also, Chapter 6 in United Nations, *World Investment Report, 2000* (New York and Geneva; United Nations, 2000).

6. R. E. Lipsey, "Home and Host Country Effects of FDI," National Bureau of Economic Research, Working Paper # 9293, October 2002.

7. P. M. Romer, "The Origins of Endogenous Growth," *Journal of Economic Perspectives* 8, no. 1 (1994), pp. 3–22.

8. X. J. Zhan and T. Ozawa, *Business Restructuring in Asia: Cross Border M&As in Crisis Affected Countries* (Copenhagen: Copenhagen Business School, 2000), I. Costa, S. Robles, and R. de Queiroz, "Foreign Direct Investment and Technological Capabilities," *Research Policy* 31 (2002), pp. 1431–443; B. Potterie and F. Lichtenberg, "Does Foreign Direct Investment Transfer Technology across Borders?" *Review of Economics and Statistics* 83 (2001), pp. 490–97; and K. Saggi, "Trade, Foreign Direct Investment and International Technology Transfer," *World Bank Research Observer* 17 (2002), pp. 191–235.

9. K. M. Moden, "Foreign Acquisitions of Swedish Companies: Effects on R&D and Productivity" (Stockholm: Research Institute of International Economics, 1998, mimeo).

10. "Foreign Friends," *The Economist,* January 8, 2000, pp. 71–72.

11. A. Jack, "French Go into Overdrive to Win Investors," *Financial Times,* December 10, 1997, p. 6.

12. "Foreign Friends."

13. G. Hunya and K. Kalotay, *Privatization and Foreign Direct Investment in Eastern and Central Europe* (Geneva: UNCTAD, 2001).

14. P. Krugman, *The Age of Diminished Expectations* (Cambridge, MA: MIT Press, 1990).

15. United Nations, *World Investment Report, 2002.* (New York and Geneva: United Nations, 2002).

16. R. Ram and K. H. Zang "Foreign Direct Investment and Economic Growth," *Economic Development and Cultural Change* 51 (2002), pp. 205–25.

17. United Nations, *World Investment Report, 1998* (New York and Geneva: United Nations, 1997).

18. United Nations, *World Investment Report, 2000.*

19. R. B. Reich, *The Work of Nations: Preparing Ourselves for the 21st Century* (New York: Alfred A. Knopf, 1991).

20. For a review, see J. H. Dunning, "Re-Evaluating the Benefits of Foreign Direct Investment," *Transnational Corporations* 3, no. 1 (February 1994), pp. 23–51.

21. This idea has recently been articulated, although not quite in this form, by C. A. Bartlett and S. Ghoshal, *Managing across Borders: The Transnational Solution* (Boston: Harvard Business School Press, 1989).

22. P. Magnusson, "The Mexico Pact: Worth the Price?" *Business Week,* May 27, 1991, pp. 32–35.

23. C. Johnston, "Political Risk Insurance," in *Assessing Corporate Political Risk,* ed. D. M. Raddock (Totowa, NJ: Rowan & Littlefield, 1986).

24. M. Tolchin and S. Tolchin, *Buying into America: How Foreign Money Is Changing the Face of Our Nation* (New York: Times Books, 1988).

25. S. Rai, "India to Ease Limits on Foreign Ownership of Media and Tea," *New York Times,* June 26, 2002, p. W1.

26. L. D. Qiu and Z. Tao, "Export, Foreign Direct Investment and Local Content Requirements," *Journal of Development Economics* 66 (October 2001), pp. 101–25.

27. J. Behrman and R. E. Grosse, *International Business and Government: Issues and Institutions* (Columbia, SC: University of South Carolina Press, 1990).

28. G. De Jonquiers and S. Kuper, "Push to Keep Alive Effort to Draft Global Investment Rules," *Financial Times,* April 29, 1988, p. 5.

29. J. H. Dunning, "An Overview of Relations with National Governments," *New Political Economy* 3, no. 2 (1998), pp. 280–84.

30. R. Ramamurti, "The Obsolescing Bargaining Model? MNC-Host Developing Country Relations Revisited," *Journal of International Business Studies* 32, no. 1, (2001), pp. 23–39.

31. For a good introduction, see M. H. Bazerman, *Negotiating Rationally* (New York: Free Press, 1997), and A. Dixit and B. Nalebuff, *Thinking Strategically: The Competitive Edge in Business, Politics, and Everyday Life* (New York: W. W. Norton, 1991).

32. H. Raiffa, *The Art and Science of Negotiation* (Cambridge, MA: Harvard University Press, 1982).

33. J. Fayerweather and A. Kapoor, *Strategy and Negotiation for the International Corporation* (Cambridge, MA: Ballinger, 1976).

34. Behrman and Grosse, *International Business and Government: Issues and Institutions*, and S. Weiss, "The Long Path to the IBM-Mexico Agreement: An Analysis of Microcomputer Investment Negotiations, 1983–1986," Working Paper 3, NYU School of Business, 1989.

Research Task | globalEDGE™   globaledge.msu.edu

Use the globalEDGE™ site to complete the following exercises:

1. The top management of your company is looking for somebody to analyze the current position of the United States in world trade. Remembering that you have learned about the dynamics of the balance of payments in your studies, you decide to prepare the analysis of the latest state of U.S. trade.

2. The Bureau of Economic Analysis is an agency of the U.S. Department of Commerce. It lists data about the U.S. International Accounts, including current investment positions and the amount of direct investment. Prepare a brief report regarding the investment status of other countries in the United States. Which are the leading countries in foreign direct investment?

Closing Case

Toyota in France

The French have always been somewhat ambivalent toward foreign direct investment. In the 1960s and 70s, successive French governments used a mixture of socialist and nationalist rhetoric to spurn foreign investment proposals by companies such as General Motors. These governments took the view that direct investment by foreign multinational enterprises would damage the French economy. Government officials believed strongly in the need for France to build its own indigenous enterprises. They argued that the economic power enjoyed by foreign multinationals gave them the ability to dominate any markets they entered, at the expense of locally grown enterprises. Successive socialist governments in France expressed a desire to control economic activity through extensive planning and the nationalization of private businesses. Letting foreign multinationals into the country was thought to be inconsistent with this goal.

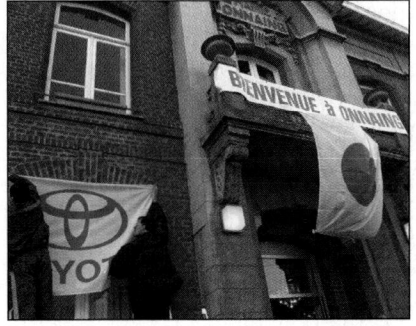

France's policy toward inward foreign direct investment began to change in the early 1980s. Although France's socialist president, François Mitterrand, remained suspicious of direct investment by foreign firms, his successive administrations reduced the bureaucratic obstacles to foreign investment and created a more coherent mechanism for luring inward investment. The change in policy reflected the growing realization that inward investment could have substantial benefits for the French economy, including the creation of jobs, the transfer of valuable technology, and the increase of exports that would bolster France's balance-of-payments position. The shift toward a more liberal attitude accelerated under Mitterrand's successor, Gaullist Jacques Chirac. Chirac, who espoused a free market philosophy with a unique French twist, made encouraging inward investment a priority. The results have been striking. According to UN data, FDI inflows into France surged from an annual average of $13.9 billion between 1988 and 1993 to a record $52.9 billion in 2001. France was one of the few countries that saw FDI inflows increase in 2001. The cumulative stock of FDI in France grew from $86 billion in 1990 to $310 billion by 2001. Among the foreign companies that made major investments in France over this time period were Toyota, IBM, Motorola, and Federal Express Corp.

One noteworthy inward investment was Toyota's December 1997 decision to invest $656.8 million in a car plant in France to produce 150,000 vehicles per year. The investment represents the Japanese company's second major commitment to Europe. Toyota already has extensive operations in the United Kingdom. The decision to locate in France was taken despite intense lobbying from British government officials, who wanted Toyota to expand its UK operations. The investment represents a continuation of Toyota's strategy to replace exports from Japan with direct production in important regional markets. This strategy was originally undertaken to reduce European demands for trade barriers to limit the "flood" of Japanese automobile imports.

Plans called for the car to be produced at Toyota's French plant to have 60 percent European content, thus qualifying it to be classified as "European" under European Union regulations and allowing Toyota to circumvent import duties. By 2001, some 2,000 people were employed at the new plant, and an additional 2,000 jobs were estimated to have been created among suppliers. Toyota has been exporting output from the plant to other countries within the European Union, helping France's balance-of-trade position.

A number of factors motivated Toyota's choice of France as a location for the plant. First, the company hoped that its new plant would help it to increase its market share in France from 1.1 percent in 1997 to around 5 percent. Second, Toyota picked France because the country has long had an indigenous automobile industry, which yields an adequate supply of trained labor and technical expertise, along with a network of experienced subcontractors. Third, the French government reportedly offered considerable subsidies to induce Toyota to invest in the country. These included tax breaks, the waiving of some social security contributions, and financial aid for training the work force. In addition, the city of Valenciennes, where the plant is located, waived or significantly reduced the annual property tax on the site. Estimates suggest that these subsidies reached 10 percent of the value of the investment. Fourth, one of the most important attractions of France was the priority of establishing a presence not only within Europe's single market, but also within the euro single currency zone. Great Britain's continued ambivalence to monetary (and currency) union with other European Union countries was a big hindrance to Toyota investing further in the United Kingdom. As of January 1999, the exchange rate for the French franc was locked against that of several other currencies—including that of Germany—in advance of full monetary and currency union which occurred in 2002.

Early evidence suggested the French investment is paying dividends for Toyota. Sales from the French operation helped Toyota to raise its European market share from 2.5 percent in 1992 to 3.8 percent in 2001. By 2002 the company was selling 660,000 cars in Europe and was planning to sell 800,000 by 2005, the majority of which would be assembled either in the United Kingdom or in France. Leading Toyota's expansion in Europe was the Toyota Yaris, a "super-mini" model produced in France exclusively for the European marketplace.

Case Discussion Questions

1. How would you characterize the shift in French attitudes and policies toward FDI? What do you think has driven this change in attitudes and policies?

2. What are the benefits to the French economy of Toyota's investment in France?

3. How do you think European Union regulations affected Toyota's decision to invest in France?

4. Why do you think Toyota chose France over the United Kingdom as a location for its new plant?

5. Can you see any downside for France of Toyota's investment?

Sources: A. Jack, "French Consider Takeover Defences," *Financial Times*, November 15, 1997, p. 2; R. Graham and H. Simonian, "Toyota Picks France for New Plant," *Financial Times*, December 10, 1997, p. 6; A. Jack, "French Go into Overdrive to Win Investors," *Financial Times*, December 10, 1997, p. 6; "Toyota Thinking Big," *Automotive News Europe*, September 9, 2002, p. 26; "Toyota Focuses on Key Models in Europe," *Automotive News Europe*, July 1, 2002, p. 9; and United Nations, *World Investment Report, 2002* (New York and Geneva: United Nations, 2002).

Chapter 8

Regional
Economic
Integration

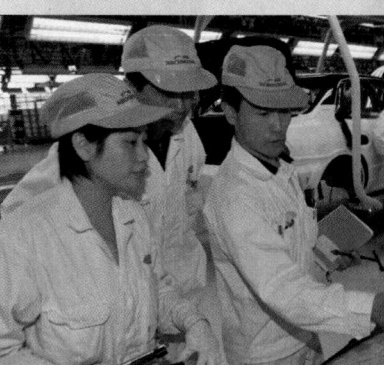

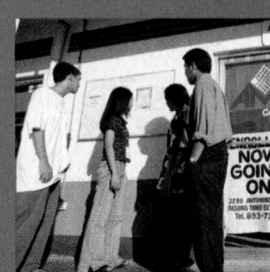

Introduction
Levels of Economic Integration
The Case for Regional Integration
  The Economic Case for Integration
  The Political Case for Integration
  Impediments to Integration
The Case against Regional Integration
Regional Economic Integration in Europe
  Evolution of the European Union
  *Political Structure of the
  European Union*
  The Single European Act
  The Establishment of the Euro
  EU Enlargement
Regional Economic Integration in the
Americas
  *The North American Free
  Trade Agreement*
  The Andean Pact
  MERCOSUR
  *Central American Common Market
  and CARICOM*
  Free Trade Area of the Americas
Regional Economic Integration
Elsewhere
  Association of Southeast Asian Nations
  Asia Pacific Economic Cooperation
  Regional Trade Blocs in Africa
Focus on Managerial Implications
  Opportunities
  Threats
Chapter Summary
Critical Discussion Questions
Closing Case: Deutsche Bank's Pan-
European Retail Banking Strategy

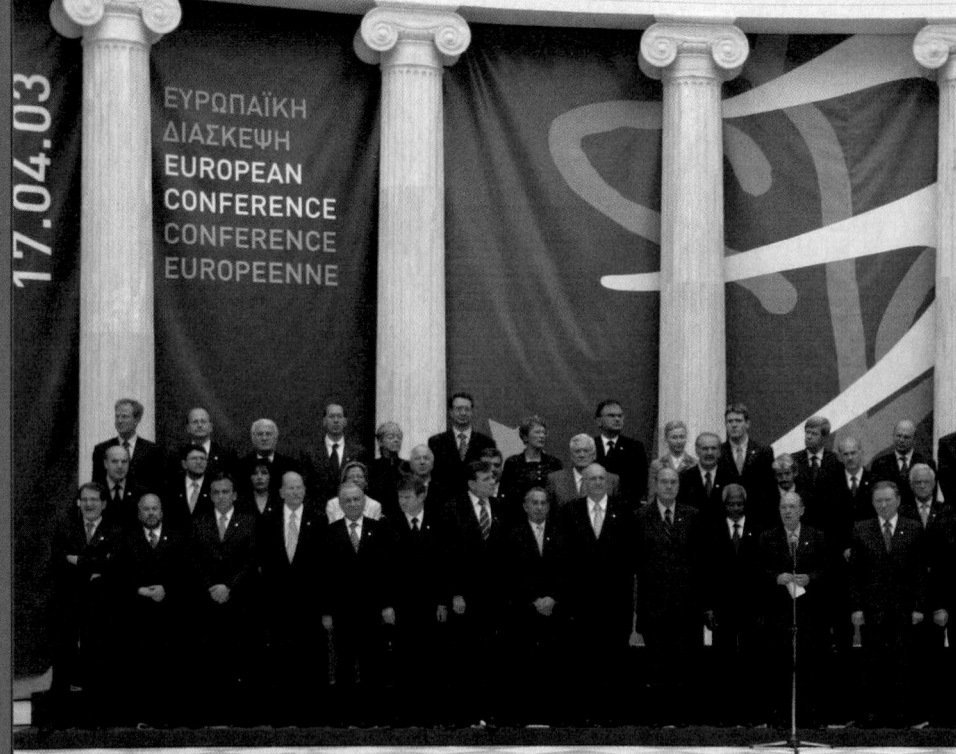

17.04.03

ΕΥΡΩΠΑΪΚΗ
ΔΙΑΣΚΕΨΗ
**EUROPEAN
CONFERENCE**
CONFERENCE
EUROPEENNE

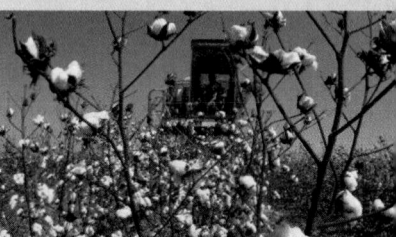

Increasing Competition in the European Automobile Market

The Single European Act became law among the member states of the European Union on January 1, 1993. The goal of the act was to remove barriers to cross-border trade and investment within the confines of the EU, thereby creating a single market instead of a collection of distinct national markets. Among the benefits claimed for this act were an increase in competition and a corresponding reduction in prices. The move toward a single market received another boost January 1, 1999, when the majority of the EU's member states formally adopted the euro as a common currency. As of 2002, 12 of the 15 member states of the EU used the euro as their currency (these 12 countries are referred to as members of the euro zone). It was claimed that the euro would benefit European consumers by making it easier to compare prices across nations, and should in theory lead to the harmonization of prices within the euro zone. For example, due to the adoption of a common currency within a single market, a car sold in Germany should in theory be priced the same as a car sold in France.

In the automobile market the reality has been somewhat different. By the end of 2002, significant variations remained between the prices of the same automobiles in different countries. According to the European Commission, in November 2002 there was a 32.2 percent differential between the price of a Volkswagen Golf in the cheapest and the most expensive national market in the euro zone. There was also a 26.6 percent differential in the price of a Ford Focus, a 26.8 percent differential in the price of a Peugeot 106, and a 22.7 percent differential in the price of an Opel Vectra. In general, the average price differential of cars across countries in the euro zone was 10.1 percent. This, however, represents a marked improvement from November 1999, when the average price differential was 17.5 percent.

Within the euro zone, Germany was the most expensive car market. In Germany, 37 car models are sold to consumers at the highest prices in the euro zone, and 31 of these are between 42 percent and 20 percent more expensive than the cheapest national market within the euro zone. Within the euro zone countries, cars are cheapest in Finland. The United Kingdom is the most expensive car market within the EU (the United Kingdom has not yet adopted the euro), with the average new car costing British consumers $800 more than comparable models sold in cheaper EU markets. The widest price differential found by the European Commission was for the Fiat Seicento, which was priced 59.5 percent higher in the United Kingdom than in Spain.

One reason for the persistence of price differentials within the EU is that since 1985, regulations have allowed automobile manufacturers to restrict competition between car dealers. The "block exemption" clause in EU competition policy allowed automakers to dictate where a dealership could be located, to limit the number of brands that a dealer could sell, and to prohibit a dealer from selling vehicles outside of its home country. For example, Volkswagen might tell a dealer in Belgium that if it wanted to become (or remain) a Volkswagen dealer, it (a) could not sell models made by other car companies, and (b) could not sell Volkswagen cars on its lot to consumers in Germany. This practice effectively allowed automobile companies to restrict competition, segment the European market, and price cars differently in various countries to reflect underlying demand conditions.

In response to persistent complaints from consumers, the European Commission in late 2002 scrapped the block exemption clause and issued a new set of regulations designed to encourage competition within the EU car market. Under the new rules, dealers will be allowed to sell anywhere they want to, open new locations where they choose, and sell more than one brand of car. Thus, a Belgium car dealer will now be able to sell Volkswagen cars to German consumers. In a concession to automobile companies, which lobbied against the proposed revisions, the new rules will be phased in over three years and take full effect in September 2005. Once established, the new rules are expected by analysts to weaken the control that automobile companies have over pricing in different EU countries, increase competition between dealers, and result in lower overall prices and less variation in pricing across countries.

Sources: K. Kelly, "Global Politics Shift Auto Industry Focus," *Ward's Auto World,* November 2002, pp. 39–40; S. Miller, "Benefits of EU Car Sales Rules Are Questionable," *Wall Street Journal,* July 17, 2002, p. A14; and European Commission, "Lastest Commission Report on Car Price Differentials in the European union," European Commission Press Release DN: IP/03/290, February 27, 2003.

Introduction

One notable trend in the global economy in recent years has been the accelerated movement toward regional economic integration. **Regional economic integration** refers to agreements among countries in a geographic region to reduce, and ultimately remove, tariff and nontariff barriers to the free flow of goods, services, and factors of production between each other. The last few years have witnessed an unprecedented proliferation of regional trade arrangements. World Trade Organization members are required to notify the WTO of any regional trade agreements in which they participate. By early 2003, nearly all of the WTO's 145 members had notified the organization of participation in one or more regional trade agreements. From 1948 to 1994, there were 124 notifications to the GATT of regional trade agreements. Since the creation of the WTO in 1995, more than 130 additional arrangements covering trade in goods or services have been created. Not all regional trade agreements notified in the past 50 years are still in force. Most of the discontinued agreements, however, have been superseded by redesigned agreements among the same signatories. Out of the more than 250 agreements or enlargements so far notified to the GATT and the WTO, some 170 are deemed to be currently in force.[1]

Consistent with the predictions of international trade theory, particularly the theory of comparative advantage (see Chapter 4), the belief has been that agreements designed to promote freer trade within regions will produce gains from trade for all member countries. As we saw in Chapter 5, the General Agreement on Tariffs and Trade and its successor, the World Trade Organization, also seek to reduce trade barriers. With more than 140 member states, the WTO has a worldwide perspective. By entering into regional agreements, groups of countries aim to reduce trade barriers more rapidly than can be achieved under the auspices of the WTO.

Nowhere has the movement toward regional economic integration been more successful than in Europe. As noted in the opening case, on January 1, 1993, the European Union effectively became a single market with 340 million consumers. But the EU is not stopping there. The member states of the EU have launched a single currency, they are moving toward a closer political union, and they are now committed to enlarging the EU from the current 15 countries to include another 10 Eastern European states.

Similar moves toward regional integration are being pursued elsewhere in the world. Canada, Mexico, and the United States have implemented the North American Free Trade Agreement (NAFTA). This promises to ultimately remove all barriers to the free flow of goods and services between the three countries. Argentina, Brazil, Paraguay, and Uruguay have implemented a 1991 agreement known as MERCOSUR to start reducing barriers to trade between each other. Moves are also under way to establish a hemispherewide Free Trade Agreement of the Americas (FTAA). Negotiations between 34 countries in the Americas began in 2001 and are scheduled to conclude in 2005. Along similar lines, 21 Pacific Rim countries, including the NAFTA member states, Japan, and China, have been discussing a possible pan-Pacific free trade area under the auspices of the Asia Pacific Economic Cooperation forum (APEC). There are also active attempts at regional economic integration in Central America, the Andean Region of South America, Southeast Asia, and parts of Africa.

A move toward greater regional economic integration can potentially deliver important benefits to consumers and present firms with new challenges. As noted in the opening case for example, the creation of a single EU car market was designed to increase competition, lower prices, and reduce variations in the price of the same car model across nations. As the case documents, however, although a single market was in theory established in January 1993, 10 years later the reality still falls short of the ideal. Nevertheless, the EU is making progress in removing the barriers that have impeded the development of a true single market, and ultimately, a single market for automobiles will probably emerge in the EU. The resulting fall in car prices will benefit consumers, who will have more money to spend on other goods and services. As for automobile companies, the increase in competition and the price pressure that will occur will force them to look for greater efficiencies and should lead to productivity gains.

While the movement toward regional economic integration is generally seen as a good thing, some observers worry that it will lead to a world in which regional trade blocs compete against each other. In this scenario of the future, free trade will exist within each bloc, but each bloc will protect its market from outside competition with high tariffs. The specter of the EU and NAFTA turning into "economic fortresses" that shut out foreign producers with high tariff barriers is worrisome to those who believe in unrestricted free trade. If such a scenario were to materialize, the resulting decline in trade between blocs could more than offset the gains from free trade within blocs.

With these issues in mind, the main objectives of this chapter are as follows: (1) to explore the economic and political debate surrounding regional economic integration, paying particular attention to the economic and political benefits and costs of integration; (2) to review progress toward regional economic integration around the world; and (3) to map the important implications of regional economic integration for the practice of international business. Before tackling these objectives, however, we first need to examine the levels of integration that are theoretically possible.

Levels of Economic Integration

Several levels of economic integration are possible in theory (see Figure 8.1). From least integrated to most integrated, they are a free trade area, a customs union, a common market, an economic union, and, finally, a full political union.

In a **free trade area,** all barriers to the trade of goods and services among member countries are removed. In the theoretically ideal free trade area, no discriminatory tariffs, quotas, subsidies, or administrative impediments are allowed to distort trade between members. Each country, however, is allowed to determine its own trade policies with regard to nonmembers. Thus, for example, the tariffs placed on the products of

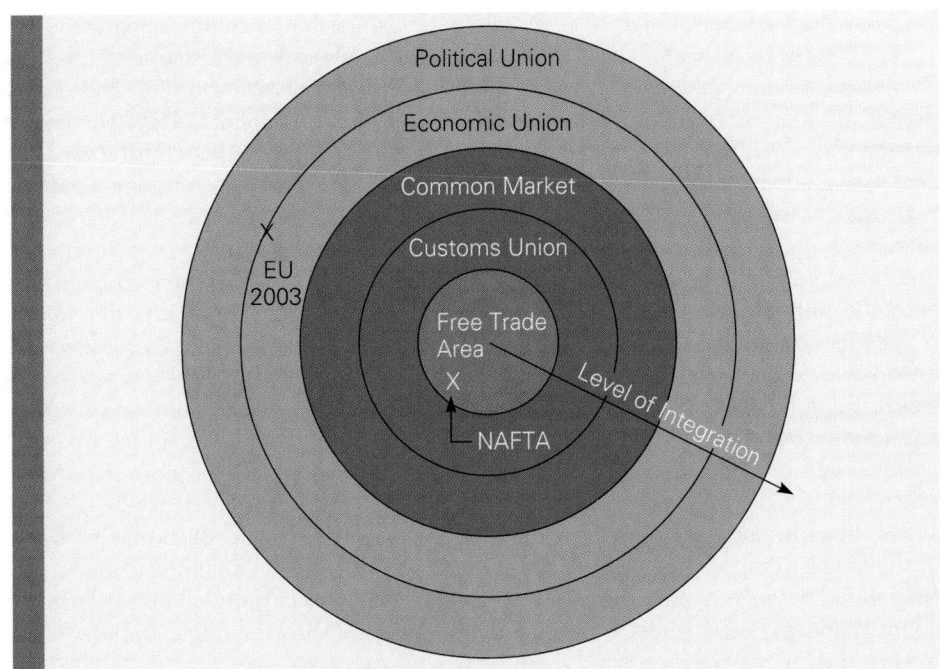

Figure 8.1

Levels of Economic Integration.

nonmember countries may vary from member to member. Free trade agreements are the most popular form of regional economic integration, accounting for almost 90 percent of regional agreements.[2]

The most enduring free trade area in the world is the European Free Trade Association (EFTA). Established in January 1960, EFTA currently joins four countries—Norway, Iceland, Liechtenstein, and Switzerland—down from seven in 1995 (three EFTA members, Austria, Finland, and Sweden, joined the EU on January 1, 1996). EFTA was founded by those Western European countries that initially decided not to be part of the European Community (the forerunner of the EU). Its original members included Austria, Great Britain, Denmark, Finland, and Sweden, all of which are now members of the EU. The emphasis of EFTA has been on free trade in industrial goods. Agriculture was left out of the arrangement, each member being allowed to determine its own level of support. Members are also free to determine the level of protection applied to goods coming from outside EFTA. Other free trade areas include the North American Free Trade Agreement, which we shall discuss in depth later in the chapter.

The customs union is one step further along the road to full economic and political integration. A **customs union** eliminates trade barriers between member countries and adopts a common external trade policy. Establishment of a common external trade policy necessitates significant administrative machinery to oversee trade relations with nonmembers. Most countries that enter into a customs union desire even greater economic integration down the road. The EU began as a customs union and has moved beyond this stage. Other customs unions around the world include the current version of the Andean Pact (between Bolivia, Colombia, Ecuador, and Peru). The Andean Pact established free trade between member countries and imposes a common tariff, of 5 to 20 percent, on products imported from outside.[3]

The next level of economic integration, a **common market** has no barriers to trade between member countries, includes a common external trade policy, and allows factors of production to move freely between members. Labor and capital are free to move because there are no restrictions on immigration, emigration, or cross-border flows of capital between member countries. Establishing a common market demands a significant degree of harmony and cooperation on fiscal, monetary, and employment policies. Achieving this degree of cooperation has proven very difficult. For years the European Union functioned as a common market, although it has now moved beyond this stage. MERCOSUR, the South American grouping of Argentina, Brazil, Paraguay, and Uruguay, hopes to eventually establish itself as a common market.

An economic union entails even closer economic integration and cooperation than a common market. Like the common market, an **economic union** involves the free flow of products and factors of production between member countries and the adoption of a common external trade policy, but it also requires a common currency, harmonization of members' tax rates, and a common monetary and fiscal policy. Such a high degree of integration demands a coordinating bureaucracy and the sacrifice of significant amounts of national sovereignty to that bureaucracy. The EU is an economic union, although an imperfect one since not all members of the EU have adopted the euro, the currency of the EU, and differences in tax rates across countries still remain.

The move toward economic union raises the issue of how to make a coordinating bureaucracy accountable to the citizens of member nations. The answer is through **political union** in which a central political apparatus coordinates the economic, social, and foreign policy of the member states. The EU is on the road toward at least partial political union. The European Parliament, which is playing an ever more important role in the EU, has been directly elected by citizens of the EU countries since the late 1970s. In addition, the Council of Ministers (the controlling, decision-making body of the EU) is composed of government ministers from each EU member. Canada and the United States provide examples of even closer degrees of political union; in each country, independent states were effectively combined into a single nation. Ultimately, the EU may move toward a similar federal structure.

The Case for Regional Integration

The case for regional integration is both economic and political. The case for integration is typically not accepted by many groups within a country, which explains why most attempts to achieve regional economic integration have been contentious and halting. In this section, we examine the economic and political cases for integration and two impediments to integration. In the next section, we look at the case against integration.

The Economic Case for Integration

The economic case for regional integration is straightforward. We saw in Chapter 4 how economic theories of international trade predict that unrestricted free trade will allow countries to specialize in the production of goods and services that they can produce most efficiently. The result is greater world production than would be possible with trade restrictions. We also saw in that chapter how opening a country to free trade stimulates economic growth, which creates dynamic gains from trade. Further, we saw in Chapter 6 how foreign direct investment (FDI) can transfer technological, marketing, and managerial know-how to host nations. Given the central role of knowledge in stimulating economic growth, opening a country to FDI also is likely to stimulate economic growth. In sum, economic theories suggest that free trade and investment is a positive-sum game, in which all participating countries stand to gain.

Given this, the theoretical ideal is a total absence of barriers to the free flow of goods, services, and factors of production among nations. However, as we saw in Chapters 5 and 7, a case can be made for government intervention in international trade and FDI. Because many governments have accepted part or all of the case for intervention, unrestricted free trade and FDI have proved to be only an ideal. Although international institutions such as GATT and the WTO have been moving the world toward a free trade regime, success has been less than total. In a world of many nations and many political ideologies, it is very difficult to get all countries to agree to a common set of rules.

Against this background, regional economic integration can be seen as an attempt to achieve additional gains from the free flow of trade and investment between countries beyond those attainable under international agreements such as the WTO. It is easier to establish a free trade and investment regime among a limited number of adjacent countries than among the world community. Problems of coordination and policy harmonization are largely a function of the number of countries that seek agreement. The greater the number of countries involved, the greater the number of perspectives that must be reconciled, and the harder it will be to reach agreement. Thus, attempts at regional economic integration are motivated by a desire to exploit the gains from free trade and investment.

The Political Case for Integration

The political case for regional economic integration has also loomed large in most attempts to establish free trade areas, customs unions, and the like. Linking neighboring economies and making them increasingly dependent on each other creates incentives for political cooperation between the neighboring states and reduces the potential for violent conflict. In addition, by grouping their economies, the countries can enhance their political weight in the world.

These considerations underlay the 1957 establishment of the European Community (EC), the forerunner of the EU. Europe had suffered two devastating wars in the first half of the 20th century, both arising out of the unbridled ambitions of nation-states. Those who have sought a united Europe have always had a desire to make another outbreak of war in Europe unthinkable. Many Europeans also believed that after World War II the European nation-states were no longer large enough to hold their own in world markets and world politics. The need for a united Europe to deal with

NAFTA and the U.S. Textile Industry

When the North American Free Trade Agreement went into effect in 1994, many expressed fears that one consequence would be large job losses in the U.S. textile industry as companies moved production from the United States to Mexico. NAFTA opponents argued passionately, but unsuccessfully, that the treaty should not be adopted because of the negative impact it would have on employment in the United States.

A quick glance at the data available eight years after the passage of NAFTA suggests the critics had a point. Between 1993 and 2002, employment in the U.S. textile industry fell from about 1 million to 432,000, a 57 percent reduction. Between 1993 and 2001, exports of garments from Mexico to the United States surged from $1.6 billion to $8.95 billion. Such data seem to indicate that the job losses have been due to apparel production migrating from the United States to Mexico. Examples are plentiful. In 1995, Fruit of the Loom Inc., the largest manufacturer of underwear in the United States, said it would close six of its domestic plants and cut back operations at two others, laying off about 3,200 workers, or 12 percent of its U.S. workforce. The company announced the closures were part of its drive to move its operations to cheaper plants abroad, particularly in Mexico. Before

the closures, less than 30 percent of its sewing was done outside the United States, but Fruit of the Loom planned to move the majority of that work to Mexico. Similarly, fabric makers have been moving production to Mexico. Cone Mills of South Carolina, one of the country's largest producers of denim fabric, has reduced its U.S. employment by one-third since 1994, while investing $200 million in two new factories in Mexico. Burlington Industries in 1999 eliminated 2,900 jobs in its North Carolina fabric plants, or 17 percent of its total workforce, while investing heavily in Mexican manufacturing capability.

For textile manufactures, the advantages of locating in Mexico include cheap labor and cheap inputs. Labor rates in Mexico average between $10 and $20 a day, compared to $10 to $12 an hour for U.S. textile workers. Another advantage for denim makers such as Cone Mills is cheap water (water is essential for dyeing cotton yarn with indigo). In Mexico, Cone Mills pays about 30 cents per cubic meter for water, about one-fifth of the rate in South Carolina. In addition, Cone Mills and other fabric makers have been locating in Mexico because many of their customers—garment makers—have already located there and being in the same region reduces transportation costs.

However, job losses in the U.S. textile industry do not mean that the overall effects of NAFTA have been

the United States and the politically alien Soviet Union certainly loomed large in the minds of many of the EC's founders.[4] A long-standing joke in Europe is that the European Commission should erect a statue to Joseph Stalin, for without the aggressive policies of the former dictator of the old Soviet Union, the countries of Western Europe may have lacked the incentive to cooperate and form the EC.

Impediments to Integration

Despite the strong economic and political arguments for integration, it has never been easy to achieve or sustain for two main reasons. First, although economic integration benefits the majority, it has its costs. While a nation as a whole may benefit significantly from a regional free trade agreement, certain groups may lose. Moving to a free trade regime involves painful adjustments. For example, as a result of the 1994 establishment of NAFTA, some Canadian and U.S. workers in such industries as textiles, which employ low-cost, low-skilled labor, lost their jobs as Canadian and U.S. firms moved production to Mexico. The promise of significant net benefits to the Canadian and U.S. economies as a whole is little comfort to those who lose as a result of NAFTA. It is understandable then, that such groups have been at the forefront of opposition to NAFTA and will continue to oppose any widening of the agreement (see the accompanying Country Focus).

A second impediment to integration arises from concerns over national sovereignty. For example, Mexico's concerns about maintaining control of its oil interests negative. Clothing prices in the United States have also fallen since 1994 as textile production shifted from high-cost U.S. producers to lower-cost Mexican producers. This benefits consumers, who now have more money to spend on other items. Denim fabric, which used to sell for $3.20 per yard, now sells for $2.40 per yard. The cost of a typical pair of designer jeans, for example, fell from $55 in 1994 to about $48 today. In 1994, blank T-shirts wholesaled for $24 a dozen. Now they sell for $14 a dozen.

In addition to lower prices, the shift in textile production to Mexico has also benefited the U.S. economy in other ways. First, despite the shift of fabric and apparel production to Mexico, there has been a surge in exports from U.S. fabric and yarn makers, many of which are in the chemical industry. Before the passage of NAFTA, U.S. yarn producers, such as E.I. du Pont, supplied only small amounts of fabric and yarn to Asian producers. However, as apparel production has moved from Asia to Mexico, exports of fabric and yarn to that country have surged. U.S. producers supply 70 percent of the raw material going to Mexican sewing shops. Between 1994 and 2001, U.S. fabric and yarn exports to Mexico, mostly in the form of cut pieces ready for sewing, grew from $760 million to almost $3 billion. In addition, U.S. manufacturers of textile equipment have also seen an increase in their sales as apparel factories in Mexico order textile equipment. Exports of textile equipment to Mexico nearly doubled in 2000 over the 1994 level, to $35.5 million.

Although there have been job losses in the U.S. textile industry, advocates of NAFTA argue that there have been benefits to the U.S. economy in the form of lower clothing prices and an increase in exports from fabric and yarn producers and from producers of textile machinery, to say nothing of the gains in other sectors of the U.S. economy. Trade has been created as a result of NAFTA. The gains from trade are being captured by U.S. consumers and by producers in certain sectors. As always, the establishment of a free trade area creates winners and losers—and the losers have been employees in the textile industry—but advocates argue that the gains outweigh the losses.

Sources: C. Burritt, "Seven Years into NAFTA, Textile Makers Seek a Payoff in Mexico," *Atlanta Journal-Constitution*, December 17, 2000, p. Q1; I. McAllister, "Trade Agreements: How They Affect U.S. Textile," *Textile World*, March 2000, pp. 50–54; J. Millman, "Mexico Weaves More Ties," *Wall Street Journal*, August 21, 2000, p. A12; J. R. Giermanski, "A Fresh Look at NAFTA: What Really Happened?" *Logistics*, September 2002, pp. 43–46; and American Textile Manufactures Institute at http://www.atmi.org/index.asp.

resulted in an agreement with Canada and the United States to exempt the Mexican oil industry from any liberalization of foreign investment regulations achieved under NAFTA. Concerns about national sovereignty arise because close economic integration demands that countries give up some degree of their control over such key policy issues as monetary policy, fiscal policy (e.g., tax policy), and trade policy. This has been a major stumbling block in the EU. To achieve full economic union, the EU introduced a common currency to be controlled by a central EU bank. Although most member states have signed on to such a deal, Great Britain remains an important holdout. A politically important segment of public opinion in that country opposes a common currency on the grounds that it would require relinquishing control of the country's monetary policy to the EU, which many British perceive as a bureaucracy run by foreigners. In 1992, the British won the right to opt out of any single currency agreement, and as of 2003, the British government had yet to reverse its decision.

The Case against Regional Integration ∎

Although the tide has been running strongly in favor of regional free trade agreements in recent years, some economists have expressed concern that the benefits of regional integration have been oversold, while the costs have often been ignored.[5] They point out that the benefits of regional integration are determined by the extent of trade creation, as opposed to trade diversion. **Trade creation** occurs when high-cost domestic producers are replaced by low-cost producers within the free trade area. It may also occur when higher-cost external producers are replaced by lower-cost external producers within the free trade area (see the accompanying Country Focus for an example). **Trade diversion** occurs when lower-cost external suppliers are replaced by higher-cost suppliers within the free trade area. A regional free trade agreement will benefit the world only if the amount of trade it creates exceeds the amount it diverts.

Suppose the United States and Mexico imposed tariffs on imports from all countries, and then they set up a free trade area, scrapping all trade barriers between themselves but maintaining tariffs on imports from the rest of the world. If the United States began to import textiles from Mexico, would this change be for the better? If the United States previously produced all its own textiles at a higher cost than Mexico, then the free trade agreement has shifted production to the cheaper source. According to the theory of comparative advantage, trade has been created within the regional grouping, and there would be no decrease in trade with the rest of the world. Clearly, the change would be for the better. If, however, the United States previously imported textiles from Costa Rica, which produced them more cheaply than either Mexico or the United States, then trade has been diverted from a low-cost source—a change for the worse.

In theory, WTO rules should ensure that a free trade agreement does not result in trade diversion. These rules allow free trade areas to be formed only if the members set tariffs that are not higher or more restrictive to outsiders than the ones previously in effect. However, as we saw in Chapter 5, GATT and the WTO do not cover some nontariff barriers. As a result, regional trade blocs could emerge whose markets are protected from outside competition by high nontariff barriers. In such cases, the trade diversion effects might outweigh the trade creation effects. The only way to guard against this possibility, according to those concerned about this potential, is to increase the scope of the WTO so it covers nontariff barriers to trade. There is no sign that this is going to occur anytime soon, however; so the risk remains that regional economic integration will result in trade diversion.

Regional Economic Integration in Europe

Europe has two trade blocs—the European Union and the European Free Trade Association. Of the two, the EU is by far the more significant, not just in terms of membership (the EU currently has 15 members and is expanding to 25; the EFTA has 4), but also in terms of economic and political influence in the world economy. Many now see the EU as an emerging economic and political superpower of the same order as the United States and Japan. Accordingly, we will concentrate our attention on the EU.[6]

Evolution of the European Union

The EU is the product of two political factors: (1) the devastation on Western Europe of two world wars and the desire for a lasting peace, and (2) the European nations' desire to hold their own on the world's political and economic stage. In addition, many Europeans were aware of the potential economic benefits of closer economic integration of the countries.

The original forerunner of the EU, the European Coal and Steel Community, was formed in 1951 by Belgium, France, West Germany, Italy, Luxembourg, and the Netherlands. Its objective was to remove barriers to intragroup shipments of coal, iron, steel, and scrap metal. With the signing of the Treaty of Rome in 1957, the European Community was established. The name changed again in 1994 when the European Community became the European Union following the ratification of the Maastricht Treaty (discussed later).

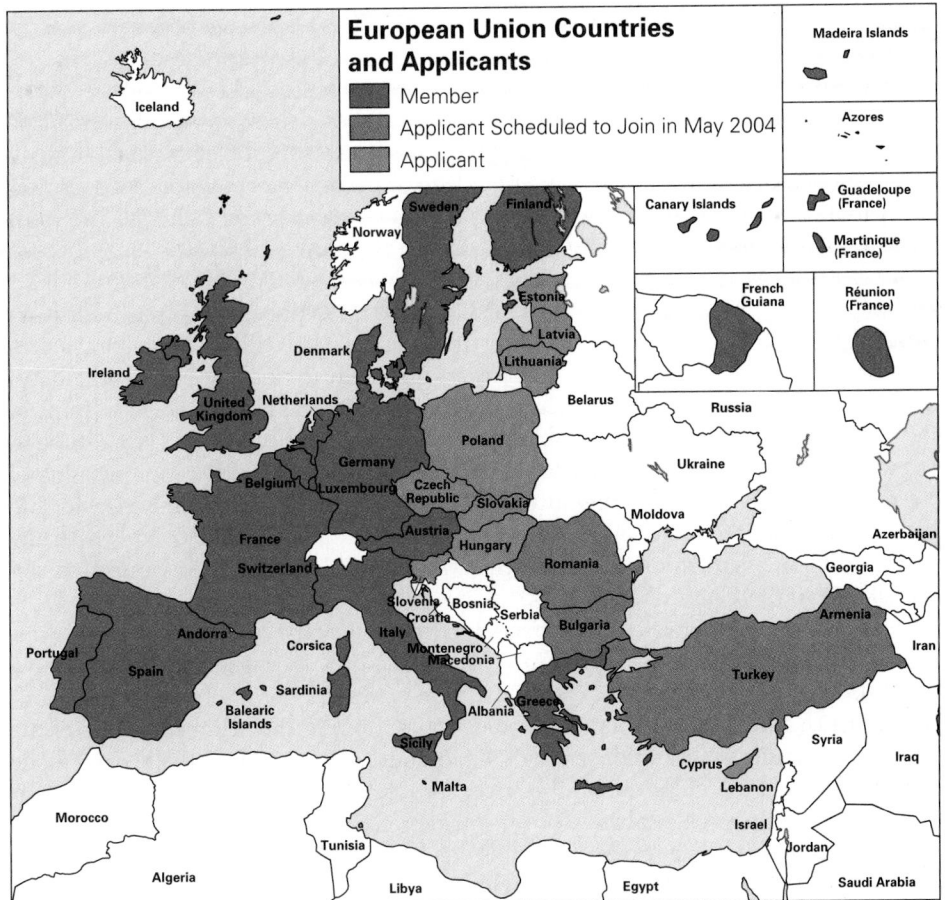

Map 8.1

European Union Countries and Applicants

Source: http://www.europa.eu.int/abc/maps/index_en.htm#. Copyright of the maps is owned by the European Commission but reproduction is authorized.

The Treaty of Rome provided for the creation of a common market. Article 3 of the treaty laid down the key objectives of the new community, calling for the elimination of internal trade barriers and the creation of a common external tariff and requiring member states to abolish obstacles to the free movement of factors of production among the members. To facilitate the free movement of goods, services, and factors of production, the treaty provided for any necessary harmonization of the member states' laws. Furthermore, the treaty committed the EC to establish common policies in agriculture and transportation.

The community grew in 1973, when Great Britain, Ireland, and Denmark joined. These three were followed in 1981 by Greece, in 1986 by Spain and Portugal, and in 1996 by Austria, Finland, and Sweden (see Map 8.1) bringing the total membership to 15 (East Germany became part of the EC after the reunification of Germany in 1990). With a population of 350 million and a GDP greater than that of the United States, the EU through these enlargements became a potential global superpower. Another 10 countries are scheduled to join the EU on May 1, 2004, if the electorates in those countries approve.

Political Structure of the European Union

The economic policies of the EU are formulated and implemented by a complex and still-evolving political structure. The five main institutions in this structure are the European Council, the Council of Ministers, the European Commission, the European Parliament, and the Court of Justice.[7]

The **European Council** is composed of the heads of state of the EU's member nations and the president of the European Commission. Each head of state is normally accompanied by a foreign minister to these meetings. The European Council meets at least twice a year and often resolves major policy issues and sets policy directions.

The **European Commission** is responsible for proposing EU legislation, implementing it, and monitoring compliance with EU laws by member states. Headquartered in Brussels, Belgium, the commission has more than 10,000 employees. It is run by a group of 20 commissioners appointed by each member country for four-year renewable terms. Most countries appoint only one commissioner, although the most populated states—Great Britain, France, Germany, Italy, and Spain—appoint two each. A president and six vice presidents are chosen from among these commissioners for two-year renewable terms. The commission has a monopoly in proposing European Union legislation. The commission starts the legislative ball rolling by making a proposal, which goes to the Council of Ministers and then to the European Parliament. The Council of Ministers cannot legislate without a commission proposal in front of it. The commission is also responsible for implementing aspects of EU law, although in practice much of this must be delegated to member states. Another responsibility of the commission is to monitor member states to make sure they are complying with EU laws. In this policing role, the commission will normally ask a state to comply with any EU laws that are being broken. If this persuasion is not sufficient, the commission can refer a case to the Court of Justice.

The European Commission's role in competition policy has become increasingly important to business in recent years. Since 1990 when the office was formally assigned a role in competition policy, the EU's competition commissioner has been steadily gaining influence as the chief regulator of competition policy in the member nations of the EU. As with antitrust authorities in the United States, which include the Federal Trade Commission and the Department of Justice, the role of the competition commissioner is to ensure that no one enterprise uses its market power to drive out competitors and monopolize markets. The commissioner also reviews proposed mergers and acquisitions to make sure they do not create a dominant enterprise with substantial market power.[8] Between 1990 and 2001, the commission reviewed some 1,857 merger cases. Of these, 18 were rejected, and another 20 were withdrawn after the commission raised substantial objections.[9] For example, in 2000 a proposed merger between Time Warner of the United States and EMI of the United Kingdom, both music recording companies, was withdrawn after the commission expressed concerns that the merger would reduce the number of major record companies from five to four and create a dominant player in the $40 billion global music industry. Similarly, the commission blocked a proposed merger between two U.S. telecommunication companies, WorldCom and Sprint, because their combined holdings of Internet infrastructure in Europe would give the merged companies so much market power that the commission argued the combined company would dominate that market. Another example of the commission's influence over business combinations is given in the accompanying Management Focus, which looks at the commission's role in shaping mergers and joint ventures in the media industry.

The **Council of Ministers** represents the interests of member states. It is clearly the ultimate controlling authority within the EU since draft legislation from the commission can become EU law only if the council agrees. The council is composed of one representative from the government of each member state. The membership, however, varies depending on the topic being discussed. When agricultural issues are being discussed, the agriculture ministers from each state attend council meetings; when transportation is being discussed, transportation ministers attend, and so on. Before 1993, all council issues had to be decided by unanimous agreement between member states. This often led to marathon council sessions and a failure to make progress or reach agreement on commission proposals. In an attempt to clear the resulting logjams, the Single European Act formalized the use of majority voting rules on issues "which have as their object the establishment and functioning of a single market." Most other issues, however, such as tax regulations and immigration policy, still require unanimity among council members if they are to become law.

The European Commission and Media Industry Mergers

In late 1999, U.S. Internet giant AOL announced it would merge with the music and publishing conglomerate Time Warner. Both the U.S. companies had substantial operations in Europe. The European Commissioner for Competition Mario Monti announced that the commission would investigate the impact of the merger on competition in Europe.

The investigation took on a new twist when Time Warner subsequently announced it would form a joint venture with British-based EMI. Time Warner and EMI are two of the top five music publishing companies in the world. The proposed joint venture would have been three times as large as its nearest global competitor. The European Commission now had two concerns. The first was that the joint venture between EMI and Time Warner would reduce the level of competition in the music publishing industry. The second was that a combined AOL–Time Warner would dominate the emerging market for downloading music over the Internet, particularly given the fact that AOL would be able to gain preferential access to the music libraries of both Warner and EMI. This would potentially put other online service providers at a disadvantage. The commission was also concerned that AOL Europe was a joint venture between AOL and Bertelsmann, a German media company that also had considerable music publishing interests. Accordingly, the commission announced it would undertake a separate investigation of the proposed deal between Time Warner and EMI.

Yet another twist occurred in mid-2000 while the AOL, Time Warner, EMI combinations were still under investigation. Vivendi, a French media conglomerate with significant music publishing, television, and Internet activities, announced it was in talks to acquire Seagram, a Canadian company that owned Universal Studios and Polygram Records, along with an alcoholic beverage business. Vivendi's plan was to sell the beverage business and hold on to Universal. Vivendi announced that its proposed acquisition would be a competitive answer to the AOL–Time Warner combination. The European Commission, however, was concerned that Vivendi, which owned Europe's largest pay television service, Canal Plus, and had a 20 percent ownership stake in British Sky Broadcasting, a satellite TV venture, would use its power to dominate the pay television market and dictate the use of Universal films and music, thereby putting competitors in the film and

music business at a disadvantage. Thus, Monti announced that the European Commission would also investigate this deal.

These investigations continued into late 2000 and were resolved by a series of concessions extracted by the European Commission from the various players. First, under pressure from the commission, Time Warner and EMI agreed to drop their proposed joint venture, thereby maintaining the level of competition in the music publishing business. Second, AOL and Time Warner agreed to allow rival Internet service providers access to online music on the same terms as AOL would receive from Warner Music Group for the next five years. Third, AOL agreed to sever all ties with Bertelsmann, and the German company agreed to withdraw from AOL Europe. These developments alleviated the commission's concern that the AOL–Time Warner combination would dominate the emerging market for the digital download of music. With these concessions in hand, the commission approved the AOL–Time Warner merger in early October 2000.

The commission then turned its attention to the proposed deal between Vivendi and Seagram. The commission appeared to buy the argument that the Vivendi–Universal combination was a competitive response to the AOL–Time Warner action, but still it extracted several concessions from Vivendi to ensure that the enlarged company did not abuse its market power. Most importantly, the commission agreed that the proposed acquisition could proceed as long as Vivendi agreed to sell its 20 percent ownership stake in British Sky Broadcasting, a condition to which Vivendi readily agreed.

By late 2000, all these transactions had been completed. The shape of the media business, both in Europe and worldwide, now looked very different, and the European Commission had played a pivotal role in determining the outcome. Its demand for concessions had altered the strategy of several of the players, led to somewhat different combinations than those originally planned, and, the commission believed, preserved competition in the global media business.

Sources: W. Drozdiak, "EU Allows Vivendi Media Deal," *Washington Post,* October 14, 2000, p. E2; D. Hargreaves, "Business as Usual in the New Economy," *Financial Times,* October 6, 2000, p. 1; and D. Hargreaves, "Brussels Clears AOL-Time Warner Deal," *Financial Times,* October 12, 2000, p. 12.

The **European Parliament,** which now has about 630 members, is directly elected by the populations of the member states. The parliament, which meets in Strasbourg, France, is primarily a consultative rather than legislative body. It debates legislation proposed by the commission and forwarded to it by the council. It can propose amendments to that legislation, which the commission and ultimately the council are not obliged to take up but often will. The power of the parliament recently has been increasing, although not by as much as parliamentarians would like. The European Parliament now has the right to vote on the appointment of commissioners as well as veto some laws (such as the EU budget and single-market legislation). One major debate now being waged in Europe is whether the council or the parliament should ultimately be the most powerful body in the EU. There is concern in Europe over the democratic accountability of the EU bureaucracy. Some think the answer to this apparent democratic deficit lies in increasing the power of the parliament, while others think that true democratic legitimacy lies with elected governments, acting through the Council of Ministers.[10]

The **Court of Justice,** which is comprised of one judge from each country, is the supreme appeals court for EU law. Like commissioners, the judges are required to act as independent officials, rather than as representatives of national interests. The commission or a member country can bring other members to the court for failing to meet treaty obligations. Similarly, member countries, companies, or institutions can bring the commission or council to the court for failure to act according to an EU treaty.

The Single European Act

Two revolutions occurred in Europe in the late 1980s. The first was the collapse of communism in Eastern Europe. The second revolution was much quieter, but its impact on Europe and the world may have been just as profound as the first. It was the adoption of the Single European Act by the member nations of the EC in 1987. This act committed the EC countries to work toward establishment of a single market by December 31, 1992.

The Single European Act was born of a frustration among EC members that the community was not living up to its promise. By the early 1980s, it was clear that the EC had fallen short of its objectives to remove barriers to the free flow of trade and investment between member countries and to harmonize the wide range of technical and legal standards for doing business. Against this background, many of the EC's prominent businesspeople mounted an energetic campaign in the early 1980s to end the EC's economic divisions. The EC responded by creating the Delors Commission. Under the chairmanship of Jacques Delors, the former French finance minister and president of the EC Commission, the Delors Commission produced a discussion paper in 1985. This proposed that all impediments to the formation of a single market be eliminated by December 31, 1992. The result was the Single European Act, which was independently ratified by the parliaments of each member country and became EC law in 1987.

The Objectives of the Act

The purpose of the Single European Act was to have one market in place by December 31, 1992. The act proposed the following changes:[11]

- Remove all frontier controls between EC countries, thereby abolishing delays and reducing the resources required for complying with trade bureaucracy.

- Apply the principle of "mutual recognition" to product standards. A standard developed in one EC country should be accepted in another, provided it meets basic requirements in such matters as health and safety.

- Open public procurement to nonnational suppliers, reducing costs directly by allowing lower-cost suppliers into national economies and indirectly by forcing national suppliers to compete.

- Lift barriers to competition in the retail banking and insurance businesses, which should drive down the costs of financial services, including borrowing, throughout the EC.
- Remove all restrictions on foreign exchange transactions between member countries by the end of 1992.
- Abolish restrictions on cabotage—the right of foreign truckers to pick up and deliver goods within another member state's borders—by the end of 1992. Estimates suggested this would reduce the cost of haulage within the EC by 10 to 15 percent.

All those changes were predicted to lower the costs of doing business in the EC, but the single-market program was also expected to have more complicated supply-side effects. For example, the expanded market was predicted to give EC firms greater opportunities to exploit economies of scale. In addition, it was thought that the increase in competitive intensity brought about by removing internal barriers to trade and investment would force EC firms to become more efficient. To signify the importance of the Single European Act, the European Community also decided to change its name to the European Union once the act took effect.

Impact

It is clear that the Single European Act has had a significant impact on the EU economy.[12] The act provided the impetus for the restructuring of substantial sections of European industry. Many firms have shifted from national to pan-European production and distribution systems in an attempt to realize scale economies and better compete in a single market. The results have included faster economic growth than would otherwise have been the case.

However, 10 years after the formation of a single market it is clear that the reality still falls someway short of the ideal. As documented in the opening case, as of 2002 there was still not a fully functioning single market for automobiles in the EU (although that may ultimately change given the new rules introduced in November 2002). The same is true in a number of other industries. The financial services industry, for example, still remains segmented on a national basis due to the presence of different rules in different member nations. Currently, regulations prohibit banks in Britain from selling mortgages to consumers living in Germany, investment specialists in Finland from selling mutual funds in Spain, and French financial institutions from making loans to Italian firms. According to economists, if the barriers between EU nations were removed and a single integrated EU market for financial services created, the EU's economic output would be 0.5 percent to 0.7 percent higher.[13] Thus, although the EU is undoubtedly moving toward a single marketplace, established legal, cultural, and language differences between nations mean that implementation has been uneven. As in the case of the automobile industry, however, progress is being made toward the adoption of a single market

The Establishment of the Euro

In December 1991, leaders of the EC member states met in Maastricht, the Netherlands, to discuss the next steps for the EC. The results of the Maastricht meeting surprised both Europe and the rest of the world. The EC countries had been fighting for months over the issue of a common currency. Although many economists believed a common currency was required to cement a closer economic union, deadlock had been predicted. The British, in particular, had opposed any attempt to establish a common currency. But instead of deadlock, the 12 members signed a treaty that committed them to adopting a common currency by January 1, 1999, and paved the way for closer political cooperation.

The treaty laid down the main elements, if only in embryo, of a future European government: a single currency, the euro; a common foreign and defense policy; a common citizenship; and an EU parliament with teeth. It is now just a matter of waiting, some believe, for a "United States of Europe" to emerge. Of more immediate interest are the implications for business of the establishment of a single currency.[14]

The euro is a currency unit now used by 12 of the 15 member states of the European Union; these 12 states are now members of what is often referred to as the euro zone. The establishment of the euro has rightly been described as an amazing political feat with few historical precedents. Establishing the euro required the participating national governments not only to give up their own currencies, but also to give up control over monetary policy. Governments do not routinely sacrifice national sovereignty for the greater good, indicating the importance that the Europeans attach to the euro. By adopting the euro, the EU has created the second largest currency zone in the world after that of the U.S. dollar. Some believe that ultimately the euro could come to rival the dollar as the most important currency in the world.

Three EU countries, Britain, Denmark, and Sweden, are still sitting on the sidelines. The 12 countries agreeing to the euro locked their exchange rates against each other January 1, 1999. Euro notes and coins were not actually issued until January 1, 2002. In the interim, national currencies circulated in each of the 12 countries. However, in each participating state, the national currency stood for a defined amount of euros. After January 1, 2002, euro notes and coins were issued and the national currencies were taken out of circulation. By mid-2002, all prices and routine economic transactions within the euro zone were in euros.

Benefits of the Euro

Europeans decided to establish a single currency in the EU for a number of reasons. First, they believe that businesses and individuals will realize significant savings from having to handle one currency, rather than many. These savings come from lower foreign exchange and hedging costs. For example, people going from Germany to France will no longer have to pay a commission to a bank to change deutsche marks into francs. Instead, they will be able to use euros. According to the European Commission, such savings could amount to 0.5 percent of the European Union's GDP, or about $40 billion a year.

Second, and perhaps more importantly, the adoption of a common currency will make it easier to compare prices across Europe. This should increase competition because it will be much easier for consumers to shop around. For example, if a German finds that cars sell for less in France than Germany, he may be tempted to purchase from a French car dealer rather than his local car dealer. Alternatively, traders may engage in arbitrage to exploit such price differentials, buying cars in France and reselling them in Germany. The only way that German car dealers will be able to hold onto business in the face of such competitive pressures will be to reduce the prices they charge for cars. As a consequence of such pressures, the introduction of a common currency should lead to lower prices. This should translate into substantial gains for European consumers

Third, faced with lower prices European producers will be forced to look for ways to reduce their production costs to maintain their profit margins. The introduction of a common currency, by increasing competition, should ultimately produce long-run gains in the economic efficiency of European companies.

Fourth, the introduction of a common currency should give a strong boost to the development of a highly liquid pan-European capital market. The development of such a capital market should lower the cost of capital and lead to an increase in both the level of investment and the efficiency with which investment funds are allocated. This could be especially helpful to smaller companies that have historically had difficulty borrowing money from domestic banks. For example, the capital market of Portugal is very small and illiquid, which makes it extremely difficult for bright Portuguese entrepreneurs with a good idea to borrow money at a reasonable price. However, in theory, such companies should soon be able tap a much more liquid pan-European capital market. Currently Europe has no continentwide capital market, such as the NAS-DAQ market in the United States that funnels investment capital to dynamic young growth companies. The euro's introduction could facilitate establishment of such a market. The long-run benefits of such a development should not be underestimated.

Finally, the development of a pan-European euro-denominated capital market will increase the range of investment options open to both individuals and institutions. For example, it will now be much easier for individuals and institutions based in, let's say, Holland to invest in Italian or French companies. This will enable European investors to better diversify their risk, which again lowers the cost of capital, and should also increase the efficiency with which capital resources are allocated.[15]

Costs of the Euro

The drawback, for some, of a single currency is that national authorities have lost control over monetary policy. Thus, it is crucial to ensure that the EU's monetary policy is well managed. The Maastricht Treaty called for establishment of an independent European Central Bank (ECB), similar in some respects to the U.S. Federal Reserve, with a clear mandate to manage monetary policy so as to ensure price stability. The ECB, based in Frankfurt, is meant to be independent from political pressure—although critics question this. Among other things, the ECB sets interest rates and determines monetary policy across the euro zone.

The implied loss of national sovereignty to the ECB underlies the decision by Great Britain, Denmark, and Sweden to stay out of the euro zone for now. Many in these countries are suspicious of the ECB's ability to remain free from political pressure and to keep inflation under tight control.

In theory, the design of the ECB should ensure that it remains free of political pressure. The ECB is modeled on the German Bundesbank, which historically has been the most independent and successful central bank in Europe. The Maastricht Treaty prohibits the ECB from taking orders from politicians. The executive board of the bank, which consists of a president, vice president, and four other members, carries out policy by issuing instructions to national central banks. The policy itself is determined by the governing council, which consists of the executive board plus the central bank governors from the 12 euro zone countries. The governing council votes on interest rate changes. Members of the executive board are appointed for eight-year nonrenewable terms, insulating them from political pressures to get reappointed. Nevertheless, the jury is still out on the issue of the ECB's independence, and it will take some time for the bank to establish its inflation-fighting credentials.

According to critics, another drawback of the euro is that the EU is not what economists would call an optimal currency area. In an optimal currency area, similarities in the underlying structure of economic activity make it feasible to adopt a single currency and use a single exchange rate as an instrument of macroeconomic policy. Many of the European economies in the euro zone, however, are very dissimilar. For example, Finland and Portugal are very dissimilar economies. The structure of economic activity within each country is very different. They have different wage rates, tax regimes, and business cycles, and they may react very differently to external economic shocks. A change in the euro exchange rate that helps Finland may hurt Portugal. Obviously, such differences complicate macroeconomic policy. For example, when euro economies are not growing in unison, a common monetary policy may mean that interest rates are too high for depressed regions and too low for booming regions. It will be interesting to see how the EU copes with the strains caused by such divergent economic performance.

One way of dealing with such divergent effects within the euro zone might be for the EU to engage in fiscal transfers, taking money from prosperous regions and pumping it into depressed regions. Such a move, however, would open a political can of worms. Would the citizens of Germany forgo their "fair share" of EU funds to create jobs for underemployed Portuguese workers?

Several critics believe that the euro puts the economic cart before the political horse. In their view, a single currency should follow, not precede, political union. They argue that the euro will unleash enormous pressures for tax harmonization and fiscal transfers from the center, both policies that cannot be pursued without the appropriate political structure. The most apocalyptic vision that flows from these negative views is that far from stimulating economic growth, as its advocates claim, the euro will lead to lower economic growth and higher inflation within Europe. To quote one critic:

> Imposing a single exchange rate and an inflexible exchange rate on countries that are characterized by different economic shocks, inflexible wages, low labor mobility, and separate national fiscal systems without significant cross-border fiscal transfers will raise the overall level of cyclical unemployment among EMU members. The shift from national monetary policies dominated by the (German) Bundesbank within the European Monetary System to a European Central Bank governed by majority voting with a politically determined exchange rate policy will almost certainly raise the average future rate of inflation.[16]

The Early Experience

Since its establishment January 1, 1999, the euro has had a volatile trading history against the U.S. dollar. After starting life in 1999 at $1.17, the euro steadily fell until it reached a low of 83 cents to the dollar in October 2000, leading critics to claim that the euro was a failure. A major reason for the fall in the value of the euro was that international investors were investing money in booming U.S. stocks and bonds and taking money out of Europe to finance this investment. In other words, they were selling euros to buy dollars so that they could invest money in dollar-denominated assets. This increased the demand for dollars, and decreased the demand for the euro, driving the value of the euro down against the dollar.

The fortunes of the euro began improving in late 2001 when the dollar weakened, and the currency stood at a robust three-year high of $1.10 in early March 2003. One reason for the rise in the value of the euro was that the flow of capital into the United States had stalled as the U.S. financial markets fell.[17] Many investors were now taking money out of the United States, selling dollar-denominated assets such as U.S. stocks and bonds and using the proceeds to purchase euro-denominated assets. Falling demand for U.S. dollars and rising demand for euros translated into a fall in the value of the dollar against the euro. Furthermore, in a vote of confidence in both the euro and the ability of the ECB to manage monetary policy within the euro zone, many foreign central banks added more euros to their supply of foreign currencies during 2002 and 2003. In the first three years of its life, the euro never reached the 13 percent of global reserves made up by the deutsche mark and other former euro zone currencies. The euro didn't jump that hurdle until early 2002, but by 2003 it made up 15 percent of global reserves. Currency specialists expected the growing U.S. current account deficit, at 5 percent, in 2003 to drive the dollar down further, and the euro still higher, over the next two to four years. However, this is a mixed blessing for the EU. A strengthening euro, while a source of pride, will make it harder for euro zone exporters to sell their goods abroad.

Enlargement of the European Union

One major issue facing the EU over the past few years has been that of enlargement. Enlargement of the EU into Eastern Europe has been a possibility ever since the collapse of communism at the end of the 1980s, and by the end of the 1990s, 13 countries had applied to become EU members. To qualify for EU membership the applicants had to privatize state assets, deregulate markets, restructure industries, and tame inflation. They also had to enshrine complex EU laws into their own systems, establish stable democratic governments, and respect human rights.[18] In December 2002, the EU formally agreed to accept the applications of 10 countries (see Map 8.2). Only the Mediterranean island nations of Malta and Cyprus are not in Eastern Europe. They include the Baltic states, the Czech Republic, and the larger nations of Hungary and Poland. Their inclusion in the EU will expand the union to 25 states, stretching from the Atlantic to the borders of Russia; add 23 percent to the landmass of the EU; bring 75 million new citizens into the EU, creating an EU with a population of 450 million people; and create a single continental economy with a GDP of $9.3 trillion that rivals the United States in size.

Before this occurs, however, a number of things have to happen. First, voters in each applicant nation will have their say on joining, and passage is by no means certain. If the referendums are approved, the nations will formally join the EU May 1, 2004. The new members will not be able to adopt the euro until 2007, and free movement of labor between the new and existing members will not be allowed until 2007. Consistent with theories of free trade, the enlargement should create added benefits for all members. However, given the small size of the Eastern European economies (together they only amount to 5 percent of the GDP of current EU members) the initial impact will probably be small. The biggest notable change might be in the EU

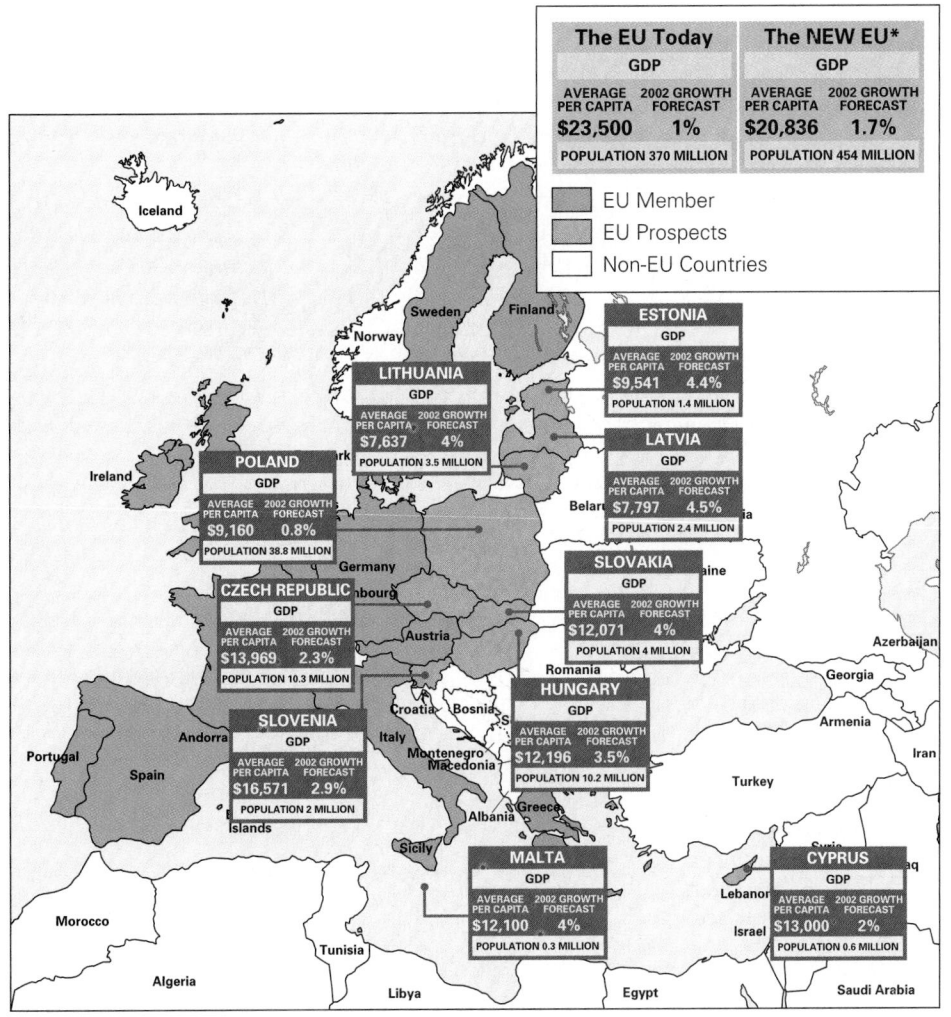

Map 8.2

The Shape of the EU after Enlargement

Source: *Business Week*, November 18, 2002, http://businessweek.com/magazine/content/02_46/b3808711.htm.

bureaucracy and decision-making processes, where budget negotiations among 25 nations are bound to prove more problematic than negotiations among 15 nations.

Left standing at the door for now were Turkey, Romania, and Bulgaria. Turkey, which has long lobbied to join the union, presents the EU with some difficult issues. The country has had a customs union with the EU since 1995, and about half of its international trade is already with the EU. However, full membership has so far been denied because of concerns over human rights issues (particularly Turkish policies toward its Kurdish minority). In addition, there is some suspicion on the Turk side that the EU is not eager to let a primarily Muslim nation of 66 million people that has one foot in Asia join the EU. The EU formally indicated in December 2002 that it would allow the Turkish application to proceed with no further delay in December 2004 if the country improved its human rights record to the satisfaction of the EU.

Regional Economic Integration in the Americas

No other attempt at regional economic integration comes close to the EU in its boldness or its potential implications for the world economy, but regional economic integration is on the rise in the Americas. The most significant attempt is the North American Free Trade Agreement. In addition to NAFTA, several other trade blocs are in the offing in the Americas (see Map 8.3), the most significant of which appear to be the Andean Group and MERCOSUR. There are also plans to establish a hemispherewide Free Trade Area of the Americas (FTAA) by late 2005.

Map 8.3

Economic Integration in the Americas

Source: *The Economist*, April 21, 2001, p. 20.

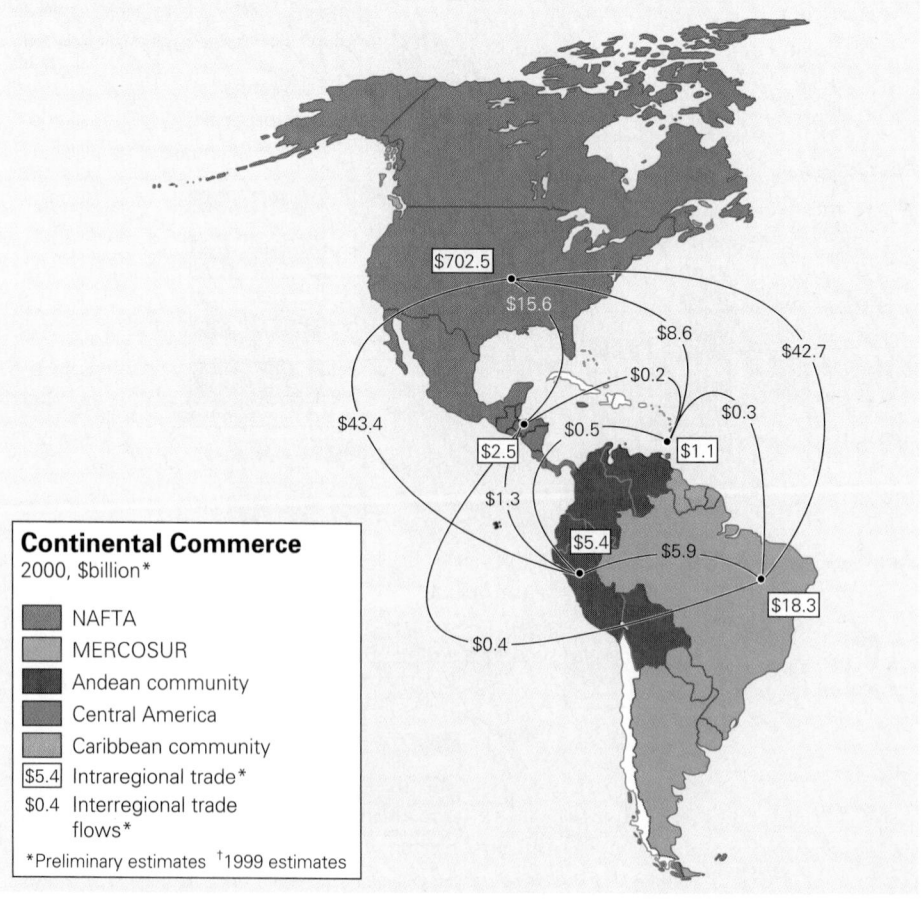

Continental Commerce
2000, $billion*

- NAFTA
- MERCOSUR
- Andean community
- Central America
- Caribbean community
- $5.4 Intraregional trade*
- $0.4 Interregional trade flows*

*Preliminary estimates †1999 estimates

The North American Free Trade Agreement

The governments of the United States and Canada in 1988 agreed to enter into a free trade agreement, which took effect January 1, 1989. The goal of the agreement was to eliminate all tariffs on bilateral trade between Canada and the United States by 1998. This was followed in 1991 by talks among the United States, Canada, and Mexico aimed at establishing a North American Free Trade Agreement for the three countries. The talks concluded in August 1992 with an agreement in principle, and the following year the agreement was ratified by the governments of all three countries.

NAFTA's Contents

The agreement became law January 1, 1994.[19] The contents of NAFTA include the following:

- Abolition within 10 years of tariffs on 99 percent of the goods traded between Mexico, Canada, and the United States.
- Removal of most barriers on the cross-border flow of services, allowing financial institutions, for example, unrestricted access to the Mexican market by 2000.
- Protection of intellectual property rights.
- Removal of most restrictions on foreign direct investment between the three member countries, although special treatment (protection) will be given to Mexican energy and railway industries, American airline and radio communications industries, and Canadian culture.
- Application of national environmental standards, provided such standards have a scientific basis. Lowering of standards to lure investment is described as being inappropriate.
- Establishment of two commissions with the power to impose fines and remove trade privileges when environmental standards or legislation involving health and safety, minimum wages, or child labor are ignored.

The Case for NAFTA

At the time NAFTA was being debated, proponents argued that NAFTA should be viewed as an opportunity to create an enlarged and more efficient productive base for the entire region. Advocates of the agreement acknowledged that one effect of NAFTA would be that some U.S. and Canadian firms would move production to Mexico to take advantage of lower labor costs. (In 2001, the average hourly labor cost in Mexico was still one-tenth of that in the United States and Canada.) Movement of production to Mexico, they argued, was most likely to occur in low-skilled, labor-intensive manufacturing industries where Mexico might have a comparative advantage (e.g., textiles; see the Country Focus). Advocates of NAFTA argued that many would benefit from such a trend. Mexico would benefit from much-needed inward investment and employment. The United States and Canada would benefit because the increased incomes of the Mexicans would allow them to import more U.S. and Canadian goods, thereby increasing demand and making up for the jobs lost in industries that moved production to Mexico. U.S. and Canadian consumers would benefit from the lower prices of products produced in Mexico. In addition, the international competitiveness of U.S. and Canadian firms that move production to Mexico to take advantage of lower labor costs would be enhanced, enabling them to better compete with Asian and European rivals.

The Case against NAFTA

Those who opposed NAFTA claimed that ratification would be followed by a mass exodus of jobs from the United States and Canada into Mexico as employers sought to profit from Mexico's lower wages and less strict environmental and labor laws.

According to one extreme opponent, Ross Perot, up to 5.9 million U.S. jobs would be lost to Mexico after NAFTA. Most economists, however, dismissed these numbers as being absurd and alarmist. They argued that Mexico would have to run a bilateral trade surplus with the United States of close to $300 billion for job loss on such a scale to occur—and $300 billion was the size of Mexico's GDP. In other words, such a scenario seemed implausible.

More sober estimates of the impact of NAFTA ranged from a net creation of 170,000 jobs in the United States (due to increased Mexican demand for U.S. goods and services) and an increase of $15 billion per year to the joint U.S. and Mexican GDP, to a net loss of 490,000 U.S. jobs. To put these numbers in perspective, employment in the U.S. economy was predicted to grow by 18 million from 1993 to 2003. As most economists repeatedly stressed, NAFTA would have a small impact on both Canada and the United States. It could hardly be any other way, since the Mexican economy was only 5 percent of the size of the U.S. economy. Signing NAFTA required the largest leap of economic faith from Mexico rather than Canada or the United States. Falling trade barriers would expose Mexican firms to highly efficient U.S. and Canadian competitors that, when compared to the average Mexican firm, had far greater capital resources, access to highly educated and skilled workforces, and much greater technological sophistication. The short-run outcome was likely to be painful economic restructuring and unemployment in Mexico. But if economic theory is any guide, advocates of NAFTA claimed there would be dynamic gains in the long run in the efficiency of Mexican firms as they adjusted to the rigors of a more competitive marketplace. To the extent that this occurred, they argued, Mexico's long-run rate of economic growth would accelerate, and Mexico might become a major market for Canadian and U.S. firms.[20]

Environmentalists also voiced concerns about NAFTA. They pointed to the sludge in the Rio Grande River and the smog in the air over Mexico City and warned that Mexico could degrade clean air and toxic waste standards across the continent. They pointed out that the lower Rio Grande was the most polluted river in the United States, and that following NAFTA there would be an increase in chemical waste and sewage along its course from El Paso, Texas, to the Gulf of Mexico.

There was also opposition in Mexico to NAFTA from those who feared a loss of national sovereignty. Mexican critics argued that their country would be dominated by U.S. firms that would not really contribute to Mexico's economic growth, but instead would use Mexico as a low-cost assembly site, while keeping their high-paying, high-skilled jobs north of the border.

NAFTA: The First Decade

Studies of NAFTA's early impact suggest that its initial effects were at best muted, and both advocates and detractors may have been guilty of exaggeration.[21] The most comprehensive early study was undertaken by researchers at the University of California, Los Angeles, and funded by various departments of the U.S. government.[22] This study focused on the effects of NAFTA in its first three and a half years. The authors conclude that the growth in trade between Mexico and the United States began to change nearly a decade before the implementation of NAFTA when Mexico unilaterally started to liberalize its own trade regime to conform with GATT standards. The initial period since NAFTA took effect had little impact on trends already in place. The study found that trade growth in those sectors that underwent tariff liberalization in the first two and a half years of NAFTA was only marginally higher than trade growth in sectors not yet liberalized. For example, between 1993 and 1996, U.S. exports to Mexico in sectors liberalized under NAFTA grew by 5.83 percent annually, while exports in sectors not liberalized under NAFTA grew by 5.35 percent. In short, the authors argue that NAFTA had only a marginal impact on the level of trade between the United States and Mexico.

As for NAFTA's much-debated impact on jobs in the United States, the study concluded the impact was positive but very small. The study found that while NAFTA created 31,158 new jobs in the United States, 28,168 jobs were lost due to imports from Mexico, for a net job gain of about 3,000 in the first two years of the NAFTA regime. However, as the report's authors point out, trade flows and employment in 1995 and 1996 were significantly affected by an economic crisis that gripped Mexico in early 1995. Given this, it may have been too early to draw conclusions about the true impact of NAFTA on trade flows and employment.

More recent surveys indicate that NAFTA's overall impact has been small but positive.[23] From 1993 to 2001, trade between NAFTA's partners grew from $297 billion to $622 billion, an increase of 109 percent. Canada and Mexico are now the number one and two trade partners of the United States, suggesting that the economies of the three NAFTA nations have become more closely integrated. There has also been strong productivity growth in all three countries over this period. In Mexico, labor productivity has increased by 50 percent since 1993, and the passage of NAFTA may have contributed to this. However, estimates suggest that employment effects of NAFTA have been small. Perhaps the most significant impact of NAFTA has not been economic, but political. Many observers credit NAFTA with helping to create the background for increased political stability in Mexico. Mexico is now viewed as a stable democratic nation with a steadily growing economy, something that is beneficial to the United States, which shares a 2,000-mile border with the country.[24]

Enlargement

One issue confronting NAFTA is that of enlargement. A number of other Latin American countries have indicated their desire to eventually join NAFTA. The governments of both Canada and the United States are adopting a wait-and-see attitude with regard to most countries. Getting NAFTA approved was a bruising political experience, and neither government is eager to repeat the process soon. Nevertheless, the Canadian, Mexican, and U.S. governments began talks in 1995 regarding Chile's possible entry into NAFTA. As of 2002, however, these talks had yielded little progress, partly because of political opposition in the U.S. Congress to expanding NAFTA. In December 2002, however, the United States and Chile did sign a bilateral free trade pact.

The Andean Pact

The Andean Pact was formed in 1969 when Bolivia, Chile, Ecuador, Colombia, and Peru signed the Cartagena Agreement. The Andean Pact was largely based on the EU model, but it has been far less successful at achieving its stated goals. The integration steps begun in 1969 included an internal tariff reduction program, a common external tariff, a transportation policy, a common industrial policy, and special concessions for the smallest members, Bolivia and Ecuador.

By the mid-1980s, the Andean Pact had all but collapsed and had failed to achieve any of its stated objectives. There was no tariff-free trade between member countries, no common external tariff, and no harmonization of economic policies. Political and economic problems seem to have hindered cooperation between member countries. The countries of the Andean Pact have had to deal with low economic growth, hyperinflation, high unemployment, political unrest, and crushing debt burdens. In addition, the dominant political ideology in many of the Andean countries during this period tended toward the radical/socialist end of the political spectrum. Since such an ideology is hostile to the free market economic principles on which the Andean Pact was based, progress toward closer integration could not be expected.

The tide began to turn in the late 1980s when, after years of economic decline, the governments of Latin America began to adopt free market economic policies. In 1990, the heads of the five current members of the Andean Pact—Bolivia, Ecuador, Peru, Colombia, and Venezuela—met in the Galápagos Islands. The resulting Galápagos Declaration effectively relaunched the Andean Pact. The declaration's objectives included the establishment of a free trade area by 1992, a customs union by 1994, and a common market by 1995.

This last milestone has not been reached. However, there are some grounds for cautious optimism. For the first time, the controlling political ideology of the Andean countries is at least consistent with the free market principles underlying a common market. In addition, since the Galápagos Declaration, internal tariff levels have been reduced by all five members, and a customs union with a common external tariff was established in mid-1994, six months behind schedule.

Significant differences between member countries still exist that may make harmonization of policies and close integration difficult. For example, Venezuela's GNP per person is four times that of Bolivia's, and Ecuador's tiny production-line industries cannot compete with Colombia's and Venezuela's more advanced industries. Such differences are a recipe for disagreement and suggest that many of the adjustments required to achieve a true common market will be painful, even though the net benefits will probably outweigh the costs.[25] To complicate matters even further, in recent years Peru and Ecuador have fought a border war, Venezuela has remained aloof during a banking crisis, and Colombia has suffered from domestic political turmoil and problems related to its drug trade. This has led some to argue that the pact is more "formal than real."[26] The outlook for the Andean Pact started to change in 1998 when the group entered into negotiations with MERCOSUR to establish a South American free trade area. However, these negotiations broke down in 1999, and there has been no progress since.

Mercosur

MERCOSUR originated in 1988 as a free trade pact between Brazil and Argentina. The modest reductions in tariffs and quotas accompanying this pact reportedly helped bring about an 80 percent increase in trade between the two countries in the late 1980s.[27] This success encouraged the expansion of the pact in March 1990 to include Paraguay and Uruguay. The initial aim was to establish a full free trade area by the end of 1994 and a common market sometime thereafter. The four countries of MERCOSUR have a combined population of 200 million. With a market of this size, MERCOSUR could have a significant impact on the economic growth rate of the four economies. In December 1995, MERCOSUR's members agreed to a five-year program under which they hoped to perfect their free trade area and move toward a full customs union.[28]

For its first eight years or so, MERCOSUR seemed to be making a positive contribution to the economic growth rates of its member states. Trade between MERCOSUR's four core members quadrupled between 1990 and 1998. The combined GDP of the four member states grew at an annual average rate of 3.5 percent between 1990 and 1996, a performance that is significantly better than the four attained during the 1980s.[29]

However, MERCOSUR has its critics, including Alexander Yeats, a senior economist at the World Bank, who wrote a stinging critique of MERCOSUR that was "leaked" to the press in October 1996.[30] According to Yeats, the trade diversion effects of MERCOSUR outweigh its trade creation effects. Yeats points out that the fastest growing items in intra-MERCOSUR trade are cars, buses, agricultural equipment, and other capital-intensive goods that are produced relatively inefficiently in the four member countries. In other words, MERCOSUR countries, insulated from outside competition by tariffs that run as high as 70 percent of value on motor vehicles, are investing in factories that build products that are too expensive to sell to anyone but themselves. The result, according to Yeats, is that MERCOSUR countries might not be able to compete globally once the group's external trade barriers come down. In the meantime, capital is being drawn away from more efficient enterprises. In the near term, countries with more efficient manufacturing enterprises lose because MERCOSUR's external trade barriers keep them out of the market.

The leak of the Yeats report caused a storm at the World Bank, which typically does not release reports that are critical of member states (the MERCOSUR countries are members of the World Bank). It also drew strong protests from Brazil, one of the primary targets of the critique. Still, in tacit admission that at least some of the arguments have merit, a senior MERCOSUR diplomat let it be known that external trade barriers will gradually be reduced, forcing member countries to compete globally. Many external MERCOSUR tariffs, which average 14 percent, are lower than they were before the group's creation, and there are plans for a hemispheric Free Trade Area of the Americas to be established by 2005 (which will combine MERCOSUR, NAFTA, and other American nations). If that occurs, MERCOSUR will have no choice but to reduce its external tariffs further.

MERCOSUR hit a significant roadblock in 1998, when its member states slipped into recession and intrabloc trade slumped. Trade fell further in 1999 following a financial crisis in Brazil that led to the devaluation of the Brazilian real, which immediately made the goods of other MERCOSUR members 40 percent more expensive in Brazil, their largest export market. At this point, progress toward establishing a full customs union all but came to a halt. Things deteriorated further in 2001 when Argentina, beset by economic stresses, suggested that the customs union be temporarily suspended. Argentina wanted to suspend MERCOSUR's tariff so that it could abolish duties on imports of capital equipment, while raising those on consumer goods to 35 percent (MERCOSUR had established a 14 percent import tariff on both sets of goods). Brazil agreed to this request, effectively halting MERCOSUR's quest to become a fully functioning customs union.[31] Hope for a revival in the importance of MERCOSUR rose in 2003 when new Brazilian President Lula da Silva announced his support for a revitalized and expanded MERCOSUR modeled after the EU with a larger membership, a common currency, and a democratically elected MERCOSUR parliament.[32]

Central American Common Market and CARICOM

Two other trade pacts in the Americas have not made much progress yet. In the early 1960s, Costa Rica, El Salvador, Guatemala, Honduras, and Nicaragua attempted to set up a Central American common market. It collapsed in 1969 when war broke out between Honduras and El Salvador after a riot at a soccer match between teams from the two countries. Since then the five countries have made some progress toward reviving their agreement, and the proposed common market was given a boost in 2003 when the United States signaled its intention to enter into bilateral free trade negotiations with the group.

A customs union was to have been created in 1991 between the English-speaking Caribbean countries under the auspices of the Caribbean Community. Referred to as CARICOM, it was established in 1973. However, it has repeatedly failed to progress toward economic integration. A formal commitment to economic and monetary union was adopted by CARICOM's member states in 1984, but since then little progress has been made. In October 1991, the CARICOM governments failed, for the third consecutive time, to meet a deadline for establishing a common external tariff.

Free Trade Area of the Americas

At a hemispherewide "Summit of the Americas" in December 1994, a Free Trade Area of the Americas (FTAA) was proposed. It took more than three years for the talks to start, but in April 1998, 34 heads of state traveled to Santiago, Chile, for the second Summit of the Americas where they formally inaugurated talks to establish an FTAA by 2005. The continuing talks have addressed a wide range of economic, political, and environmental issues related to cross-border trade and investment. Although the United States was an early advocate of the FTAA, support from the United States seems to be mixed at this point. Because the United States has by far the largest economy in the region, strong U.S. support is a precondition for establishment of the free trade area. Canada is chairing the crucial first stage of negotiations and hosted the second Summit of the Americas in early 2001. If the FTAA is established, it will have major implications for cross-border trade and investment flows within the hemisphere. The FTAA would open a free trade umbrella over nearly 800 million people who accounted for more than $11 trillion in GDP in 2000. At this point, however, any definitive agreement is still several years away.

Regional Economic Integration Elsewhere

Numerous attempts at regional economic integration have been tried throughout Asia and Africa. However, few exist in anything other than name. Perhaps the most significant is the Association of Southeast Asian Nations (ASEAN). In addition, the Asia Pacific Economic Cooperation (APEC) forum has recently emerged as the seed of a potential free trade region.

Association of Southeast Asian Nations

Formed in 1967, ASEAN includes Brunei, Indonesia, Laos, Malaysia, Myanmar, Philippines, Singapore, Thailand, and Vietnam. Laos, Myanmar, and Vietnam have all joined recently, and their inclusion complicates matters because their economies are so far behind those of the original members. The basic objectives of ASEAN are to foster freer trade between member countries and to achieve cooperation in their industrial policies. Progress has been very limited, however. For example, only 5 percent of intra-ASEAN trade currently consists of goods whose tariffs have been reduced through an ASEAN preferential trade arrangement. Future progress seems limited because the financial crisis that swept through Southeast Asia in 1997 hit several ASEAN countries particularly hard, most notably Indonesia, Malaysia, and Thailand. Until these countries can get back on their economic feet, it is unlikely that much progress will be made.[33]

Asia Pacific Economic Cooperation

Asia Pacific Economic Cooperation (APEC) was founded in 1990 at the suggestion of Australia. APEC currently has 21 member states including such economic powerhouses as the United States, Japan, and China (see Map 8.4). Collectively the 18 member states account for half of the world's GNP, 40 percent of world trade, and most of the growth in the world economy. The stated aim of APEC is to increase multilateral cooperation in view of the economic rise of the Pacific nations and the growing interdependence within the region. U.S. support for APEC was also based on the belief that it might prove a viable strategy for heading off any moves to create Asian groupings from which it would be excluded.

Interest in APEC was heightened considerably in November 1993 when the heads of APEC member states met for the first time at a two-day conference in Seattle. Debate before the meeting speculated on the likely future role of APEC. One view was that APEC should commit itself to the ultimate formation of a free trade area. Such a move would transform the Pacific Rim from a geographical expression into the world's largest free trade area. Another view was that APEC would produce no more than hot air and lots of photo opportunities for the leaders involved. As it turned out, the APEC meeting produced little more than some vague commitments from member states to work together for greater economic integration and a general lowering of trade barriers. However, significantly, member states did not rule out the possibility of closer economic cooperation in the future.[34]

The heads of state met again in November 1994 in Jakarta, Indonesia. This time they agreed to take more concrete steps, and the joint statement at the end of the

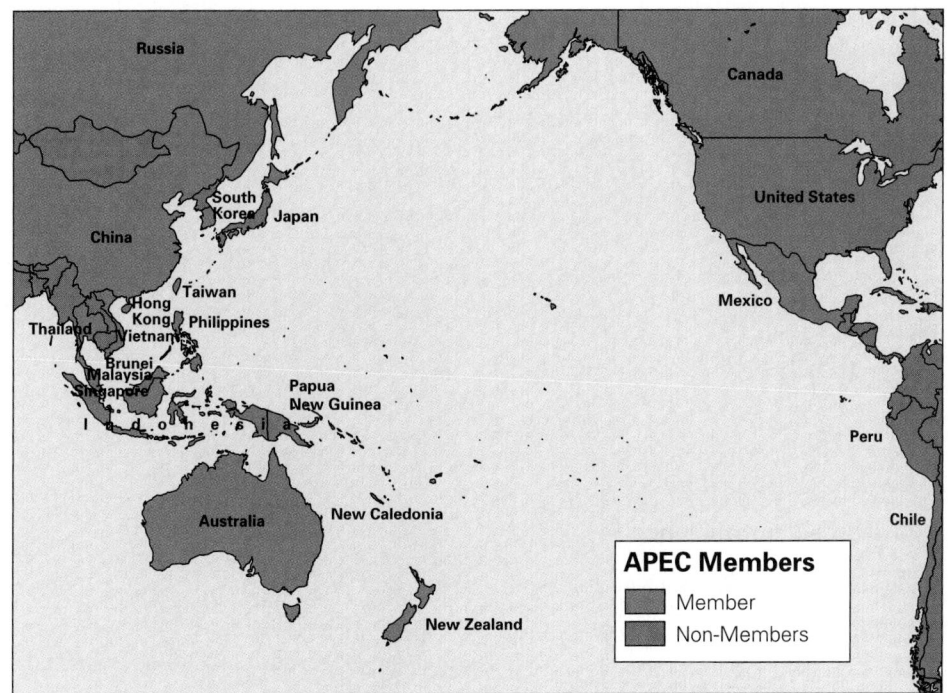

Map 8.4

APEC Members

Source: APEC website.

meeting formally committed APEC's industrialized members to remove their trade and investment barriers by 2010 and for developing economies to do so by 2020. They also called for a detailed blueprint charting how this might be achieved. This blueprint was presented and discussed at the next APEC summit, held in Osaka, Japan, in November 1995.[35] This was followed by further annual meetings. At the 1997 meeting, member states formally endorsed proposals designed to remove trade barriers in 15 sectors, ranging from fish to toys. However, the plan is vague and commits APEC to doing no more than holding further talks. Commenting on the vagueness of APEC pronouncements, the influential Brookings Institution, a U.S.-based economic policy institution, noted that APEC "is in grave danger of shrinking into irrelevance as a serious forum." Despite the slow progress, APEC is worth watching. If it eventually does transform itself into a free trade area, it will probably be the world's largest.[36]

Regional Trade Blocs in Africa

African countries have been experimenting with regional trade blocs for half a century. There are now nine trade blocs on the African continent (see Map 8.5). Many countries are members of more than one group. Although the number of trade groups is impressive, progress toward the establishment of meaningful trade blocs has been slow.

Many of these groups have been dormant for years. Significant political turmoil in several African nations has persistently impeded any meaningful progress. Also, deep suspicion of free trade exists in several African countries. The argument most frequently heard is that because these countries have less developed and less diversified economies, they need to be "protected" by tariff barriers from unfair foreign competition. Given the prevalence of this argument, it has been hard to establish free trade areas or customs unions.

The most recent attempt to reenergize the free trade movement in Africa occurred in early 2001, when Kenya, Uganda, and Tanzania, member states of the East African Community (EAC), committed themselves to relaunching their bloc, 24 years after it collapsed. The three countries, with 80 million inhabitants, intend to establish a customs union, regional court, legislative assembly, and, eventually, a political federation.

Map 8.5

Trade Blocs in Africa

Source: *The Economist*, February 10, 2001, p. 77 ©2001 The Economist Newspapers Ltd. All rights reserved. Reprinted with permission. Further reproduction prohibited. www.economist.com

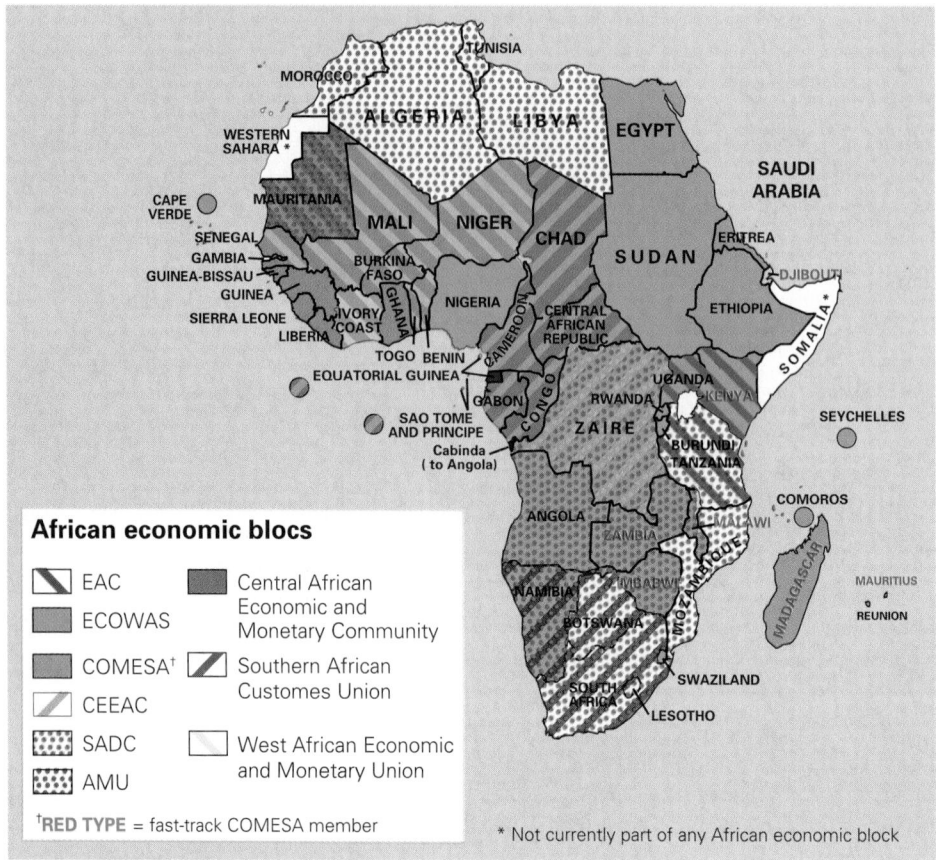

Their program includes cooperation on immigration, road and telecommunication networks, investment, and capital markets. However, while local business leaders welcomed the relaunch as a positive step, they were critical of the EAC's failure in practice to make progress on free trade. At the EAC treaty's signing in November 1999, members gave themselves four years to negotiate a customs union, with a draft slated for the end of 2001. But that fell far short of earlier plans for an immediate free trade zone, shelved after Tanzania and Uganda, fearful of Kenyan competition, expressed concerns that the zone could create imbalances similar to those that contributed to the breakup of the first community.[37] It remains to be seen if these countries can have success this time, but if history is any guide, it will be an uphill road.

Focus On Managerial Implications

Currently the most significant developments in regional economic integration are occurring in the EU and NAFTA. Although some of the Latin American trade blocs, APEC, and the proposed FTAA may have economic significance in the future, at present the EU and NAFTA have more profound and immediate implications for business practice. Accordingly, in this section we will concentrate on the business implications of those two groups. Similar conclusions, however, could be drawn with regard to the creation of a single market anywhere in the world.

Opportunities

The creation of a single market offers significant opportunities because markets that were formerly protected from foreign competition are opened. For example, in Europe before 1992 the large French and Italian markets were among the most protected. These markets are now much more open to foreign competition in the form of both exports and direct investment. Nonetheless, to fully exploit such opportunities, it may pay non-EU firms to set up EU subsidiaries. Many major U.S. firms have long had subsidiaries in Europe. Those that do not would be advised to consider establishing them now, lest they run the risk of being shut out of the EU by nontariff barriers. Non-EU firms have rapidly increased their direct investment in the EU in anticipation of the creation of a single market. Between 1985 and 1989, for example, approximately 37 percent of the FDI inflows into industrialized countries was directed at the EC. By 1991, this figure had risen to 66 percent, and FDI inflows into the EU has been substantial ever since (see Chapter 6).[38]

Additional opportunities arise from the inherent lower costs of doing business in a single market—as opposed to 15 national markets in the case of the EU or 3 national markets in the case of NAFTA. Free movement of goods across borders, harmonized product standards, and simplified tax regimes make it possible for firms based in the EU and the NAFTA countries to realize potentially significant cost economies by centralizing production in those EU and NAFTA locations where the mix of factor costs and skills is optimal. Rather than producing a product in each of the 15 EU countries or the 3 NAFTA countries, a firm may be able to serve the whole EU or North American market from a single location. This location must be chosen carefully, of course, with an eye on local factor costs and skills.

For example, in response to the changes created by EU after 1992, the St. Paul–based 3M Company has been consolidating its European manufacturing and distribution facilities to take advantage of economies of scale. Thus, a plant in Great Britain now produces 3M's printing products and a German factory its reflective traffic control materials for all of the EU. In each case, 3M chose a location for centralized production after carefully considering the likely production costs in alternative locations within the EU. The ultimate goal of 3M is to dispense with all national distinctions, directing R&D, manufacturing, distribution, and marketing for each product group from an EU headquarters.[39] Similarly, Unilever, one of Europe's largest companies, began rationalizing its production in advance of 1992 to attain scale economies. Unilever concentrated its production of dishwashing powder for the EU in one plant, bath soap in another, and so on.[40]

Even after the removal of barriers to trade and investment, enduring differences in culture and competitive practices often limit the ability of companies to realize cost economies by centralizing production in key locations and producing a standardized product for a single multicountry market. Consider the case of Atag Holdings NV, a Dutch maker of kitchen appliances that is profiled in the accompanying Management Focus. Due to enduring differences between nations within the EU's single market, Atag still has to produce various "national brands," which clearly limits the company's ability to attain scale economies.

Threats

Just as the emergence of single markets in the EU and America creates opportunities for business, it also presents a number of threats. For one thing, the business environment within each grouping will become more competitive. The lowering of barriers to trade and investment between countries is likely to lead to increased price competition throughout the EU and NAFTA. For example, before 1992 a Volkswagen Golf cost 55 percent more in Great Britain than in Denmark and 29 percent more in Ireland than in Greece.[41] Over time, such price differentials will vanish in a single market. This is a direct threat to any firm doing business in EU or NAFTA countries. To survive in the tougher single-market

Management Focus

Atag Holdings

Atag Holdings NV is a Dutch company whose main business is kitchen appliances. Atag thought it was well placed to benefit from the single market, but so far it has found it tough going. Atag's plant is just one mile from the German border and near the center of the EU's population. The company thought it could cater to both the "potato" and "spaghetti" belts—marketers' terms for consumers in Northern and Southern Europe—by producing two main product lines and selling these standardized "-euro-products" to "euro-consumers." The main benefit of doing so is the economy of scale derived from mass production of a standardized range of products.

Unfortunately, Atag quickly discovered that the "euro-consumer" is a myth. Consumer preferences vary much more across nations than Atag had thought. Consider ceramic stove tops; Atag planned to market just 2 varieties throughout the EU but has found it needs 11. Belgians, who cook in huge pots, require extra-large burners. Germans like oval pots and burners to fit. The French need small burners and very low temperatures for simmering sauces and broths. Ger-

mans like oven knobs on the top; the French want them on the front. Most Germans and French prefer black and white cookers; the British demand a range of colors including peach, pigeon blue, and mint green.

Despite these problems, foreign sales of Atag's kitchenware increased from 4 percent of total revenues in 1985 to 25 percent a few years after the formation of Europe's single market. But the company now has a much more realistic assessment of the benefits of a single market among a group of countries whose cultures and traditions still differ in deep and often profound ways. Atag now believes its range of designs and product quality, rather than the magic bullet of a "euro-product" designed for a "euro-consumer," will keep the company competitive. At the same time, Atag has to cope with higher costs than would have been the case were it possible to pursue greater product standardization.

Sources: T. Horwitz, "Europe's Borders Fade," *Wall Street Journal*, May 18, 1993, pp. A1, A12; "A Singular Market," *The Economist*, October 22, 1994, pp. 10–16; and "Something Dodgy in Europe's Single Market," *The Economist*, May 21, 1994, pp. 69–70.

environment, firms must take advantage of the opportunities offered by the creation of a single market to rationalize their production and reduce their costs. Otherwise, they will be severely disadvantaged.

A further threat to firms outside these trading blocs arises from the likely long-term improvement in the competitive position of many firms within the areas. This is particularly relevant in the EU, where many firms are currently limited by a high cost structure in their ability to compete globally with North American and Asian firms. The creation of a single market and the resulting increased competition in the EU is beginning to produce serious attempts by many EU firms to reduce their cost structure by rationalizing production. This could transform many EU companies into efficient global competitors. The message for non-EU businesses is that they need to prepare for the emergence of more capable European competitors by reducing their own cost structures.

Another threat to firms outside of trading areas is the threat of being shut out of the single market by the creation of a "trade fortress." The charge that regional economic integration might lead to a fortress mentality is most often leveled at the EU. Although the free trade philosophy underpinning the EU theoretically argues against the creation of any fortress in Europe, there are occasional signs that the EU may raise barriers to imports and investment in certain "politically sensitive" areas, such as autos. Non-EU firms might be well advised, therefore, to set up their own EU operations as quickly as possible. This could also occur in the NAFTA countries, but it seems less likely.

Finally, the emerging role of the European Commission in competition policy suggests the EU is increasingly willing and able to intervene and impose conditions on companies proposing mergers and acquisitions. This is a threat insofar as it limits the ability of firms to pursue the corporate strategy of their choice. As we saw in the Management Focus on the media industry mergers, the commission may require significant concessions from businesses as a precondition for allowing proposed mergers and acquisitions to proceed. While this constrains the strategic options for firms, it should be remembered that in taking such action, the commission is trying to maintain the level of competition in Europe's single market, which should benefit consumers.

ChapterSummary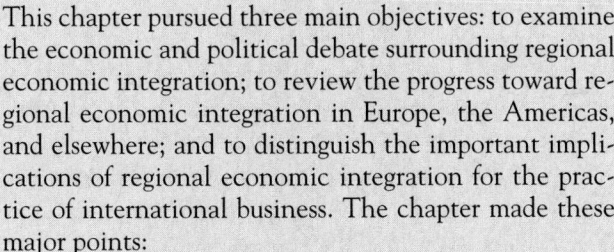

This chapter pursued three main objectives: to examine the economic and political debate surrounding regional economic integration; to review the progress toward regional economic integration in Europe, the Americas, and elsewhere; and to distinguish the important implications of regional economic integration for the practice of international business. The chapter made these major points:

1. A number of levels of economic integration are possible in theory. In order of increasing integration, they include a free trade area, a customs union, a common market, an economic union, and full political union.

2. In a free trade area, barriers to trade between member countries are removed, but each country determines its own external trade policy. In a customs union, internal barriers to trade are removed and a common external trade policy is adopted. A common market is similar to a customs union, except that a common market also allows factors of production to move freely between countries. An economic union involves even closer integration, including the establishment of a common currency and the harmonization of tax rates. A political union is the logical culmination of attempts to achieve ever-closer economic integration.

3. Regional economic integration is an attempt to achieve economic gains from the free flow of trade and investment between neighboring countries.

4. Integration is not easily achieved or sustained. Although integration brings benefits to the majority, it is never without costs for the minority. Concerns over national sovereignty often slow or stop integration attempts.

5. Regional integration will not increase economic welfare if the trade creation effects in the free trade area are outweighed by the trade diversion effects.

6. The Single European Act sought to create a true single market by abolishing administrative barriers to the free flow of trade and investment between EU countries.

7. The Maastricht Treaty aims to take the EU even further along the road to economic union by establishing a common currency. The economic gains from a common currency come from reduced exchange costs, reduced risk associated with currency fluctuations, and increased price competition within the EU.

8. Increasingly, the European Commission is taking an activist stance with regard to competition policy, intervening to restrict mergers and acquisitions that it believes will reduce competition in the EU.

9. Although no other attempt at regional economic integration comes close to the EU in terms of potential economic and political significance, various other attempts are being made in the world. The most notable include NAFTA in North America, the Andean Pact and MERCOSUR in Latin America, ASEAN in Southeast Asia, and perhaps APEC.

10. The creation of single markets in the EU and North America means that many markets that were formerly protected from foreign competition are now more open. This creates major investment and export opportunities for firms within and outside these regions.

11. The free movement of goods across borders, the harmonization of product standards, and the simplification of tax regimes make it possible for firms based in a free trade area to realize potentially enormous cost economies by centralizing production in those locations within the area where the mix of factor costs and skills is optimal.

12. The lowering of barriers to trade and investment between countries within a trade group will probably be followed by increased price competition.

Critical Discussion Questions

1. NAFTA is likely to produce net benefits for the Canadian, Mexican, and U.S. economies. Discuss.

2. What are the economic and political arguments for regional economic integration? Given these arguments, why don't we see more integration in the world economy?

3. What effect is creation of a single market and a single currency within the EU likely to have on competition within the EU? Why?

4. Do you think it is correct for the European Commission to restrict mergers between American companies that do business in Europe? (For example, the European Commission vetoed the proposed merger between WorldCom and Sprint, both U.S. companies, and it carefully reviewed the merger between AOL and Time Warner, again both U.S. companies.)

5. How should a U.S. firm that currently exports only to Western Europe respond to the creation of a single market?

6. How should a firm with self-sufficient production facilities in several EU countries respond to the creation of a single market? What are the constraints on its ability to respond in a manner that minimizes production costs?

7. After a promising start, in the last few years MERCOSUR, the major Latin American trade agreement, has faltered and by 2001 seemed to be in trouble. What problems are hurting MERCOSUR? What can be done to solve these problems?

8. Would establishment of a Free Trade Area of the Americas (FTAA) in 2005 be good for the two most advanced economies in the hemisphere, the United States and Canada? How might the establishment of the FTAA impact the strategy of North American firms?

Notes

1. Information taken from World Trade Organization website and current as of March 2003, www.wto.org.

2. World Trade Organization, *Annual Report, 2002* (Geneva: WTO; 2002).

3. The Andean Pact has been through a number of changes since its inception. The latest version was established in 1991. See "Free-Trade Free for All," *The Economist*, January 4, 1991, p. 63.

4. D. Swann, *The Economics of the Common Market*, 6th ed. (London: Penguin Books, 1990).

5. See J. Bhagwati, "Regionalism and Multilateralism: An Overview," Columbia University Discussion Paper 603, Department of Economics, Columbia University, New York; A. de la Torre and M. Kelly, "Regional Trade Arrangements," Occasional Paper 93, Washington, DC: International Monetary Fund, March 1992; J. Bhagwati, "Fast Track to Nowhere," *The Economist*, October 18, 1997, pp. 21–24; and Jagdish Bhagwati, *Free Trade Today* (Princeton and Oxford: Princeton University Press, 2002).

6. N. Colchester and D. Buchan, *Europower: The Essential Guide to Europe's Economic Transformation in 1992* (London: The Economist Books, 1990); and Swann, *Economics of the Common Market*.

7. Swann, *Economics of the Common Market*; Colchester and Buchan, *Europower: The Essential Guide to Europe's Economic Transformation in 1992*; "The European Union: A Survey," *The Economist*, October 22, 1994; and "The European Community: A Survey," *The Economist*, July 3, 1993.

8. E. J. Morgan, "A Decade of EC Merger Control," *International Journal of Economics and Business*, November 2001, pp. 451–73.

9. European Commission, *XXXI Report on Competition Policy, 2001* (Brussels: European Commission, 2002).

10. "The European Community: A Survey."

11. "One Europe, One Economy," *The Economist*, November 30, 1991, pp. 53–54, and "Market Failure: A Survey of Business in Europe," *The Economist*, June 8, 1991, pp. 6–10.

12. Alan Riley, "The Single Market Ten Years On," *European Policy Analyst*, December 2002, pp. 65–72.

13. P. Hofheinz, "A Capital Idea: The European Union Has a Grand Plan to Make Its Financial Markets More Efficient," *Wall Street Journal*, October 14, 2002, p. R4.

14. See C. Wyploze, "EMU: Why and How It Might Happen," *Journal of Economic Perspectives* 11

(1997), pp. 3–22, and M. Feldstein, "The Political Economy of the European Economic and Monetary Union," *Journal of Economic Perspectives* 11 (1997), pp. 23–42.

15. "One Europe, One Economy," and Feldstein, "The Political Economy of the European Economic and Monetary Union."

16. Feldstein, "The Political Economy of the European Economic and Monetary Union."

17. "Time for Europhoria?" *The Economist*, January 4, 2003, p. 58.

18. Details regarding conditions of membership and the progression of enlargement negotiations can be found at http://europa.eu.int/comm/enlargement/index.htm.

19. "What Is NAFTA?" *Financial Times*, November 17, 1993, p. 6, and S. Garland, "Sweet Victory," *Business Week*, November 29, 1993, pp. 30–31.

20. "NAFTA: The Showdown," *The Economist*, November 13, 1993, pp. 23–36.

21. N. C. Lustog, "NAFTA: Setting the Record Straight," *The World Economy*, 1997, pp. 605–14.

22. R. H. Ojeda, C. Dowds, R. McCleery, S. Robinson, D. Runsten, C. Wolff, and G. Wolff, "NAFTA—How Has It Done? North American Integration Three Years after NAFTA," North American Integration and Development Center at UCLA, December 1996.

23. W. Thorbecke and C. Eigen-Zucchi. "Did NAFTA Cause a Giant Sucking Sound?" *Journal of Labor Research*, Fall 2002, pp. 647–658, and G. Gagne, "North American Free Trade, Canada, and U.S. Trade Remedies: An Assessment after Ten Years," *The World Economy*, 2000, pp. 77–91.

24. J. Cavanagh et al., "Happy Ever NAFTA?" *Foreign Policy*, September–October 2002, pp. 58–65.

25. "NAFTA Is Not Alone," *The Economist*, June 18, 1994, pp. 47–48; B. Sweeney, "First Latin American Customs Union Looms over Venezuela," *Journal of Commerce*, September 26, 1991, p. 5A; and "The Business of the American Hemisphere," *The Economist*, August 24, 1991, pp. 37–38.

26. The comment was made by the Colombian ambassador. See K. G. Hall, "Andean Pact Nations to Work Together at Talks," *Journal of Commerce*, April 8, 1998, p. 2A.

27. "Business of the American Hemisphere."

28. "NAFTA Is Not Alone."

29. "Murky MERCOSUR," *The Economist*, July 26, 1997, pp. 66–67.

30. See M. Philips, "South American Trade Pact Under Fire," *Wall Street Journal*, October 23, 1996, p. A2; A. J. Yeats, *Does MERCOSUR's Trade Performance Justify Concerns about the Global Welfare-Reducing Effects of Free Trade Arrangements? Yes!* (Washington, DC: World Bank, 1996); and D. M. Leipziger et al., "MERCOSUR: Integration and Industrial Policy," *The World Economy*, 1997, pp. 585–604.

31. "Another Blow to MERCOSUR," *The Economist*, March 31, 2001, pp. 33–34.

32. "Lula Lays Out MERCOSUR Rescue Mission," *Latin America Newsletters*, February 4, 2003, p. 7.

33. Anonymous. "Every Man for Himself: Trade in Asia," *The Economist*, November 2, 2002, pp. 43–44.

34. "Aimless in Seattle," *The Economist*, November 13, 1993, pp. 35–36.

35. G. de Jonquieres, "Different Aims, Common Cause," *Financial Times*, November 18, 1995, p. 14.

36. G. de Jonquieres, "APEC Grapples with Market Turmoil," *Financial Times*, November 21, 1997, p. 6; and G. Baker, "Clinton Team Wins Most of the APEC Tricks," *Financial Times*, November 27, 1997, p. 5.

37. M. Turner, "Trio Revives East African Union," *Financial Times*, January 16, 2001, p. 4.

38. United Nations *World Investment Report* (New York and Geneva), various issues.

39. P. Davis, "A European Campaign: Local Companies Rush for a Share of EC Market While Barriers Are Down," *Minneapolis-St. Paul City Business*, January 8, 1990, p. 1.

40. "The Business of Europe," *The Economist*, December 7, 1991, pp. 63–64.

41. E. G. Friberg, "1992: Moves Europeans Are Making," *Harvard Business Review*, May–June 1989, pp. 85–89.

Research Task | globalEDGE™   globaledge.msu.edu

Use the globalEDGE™ site to complete the following exercises:

1. Your company is considering expanding its market by opening new representatives in the European Union. Nevertheless, the size of the investment is significant and the top management wishes to have a clearer picture of the current and probable future economic status of the union. Prepare an executive summary describing

the features you consider as crucial in taking such a decision.

2. The establishment of the Free Trade Area of Americas can be a threat, as well as an opportunity for your company. Using the globalEDGE™ website, identify the countries participating in the negotiations for the FTAA. What are the main themes of the negotiation process?

Deutsche Bank's Pan-European Retail Banking Strategy

In March 2000, Deutsche Bank, Germany's largest bank, announced it would merge with Dresdner Bank, Germany's third largest bank. The stated strategic goal of the merger was to create a European investment and asset management institution that would have the economies of scale required to compete with the top global investment banks, including Citicorp and Merrill Lynch. An important component of the proposed merger was a plan by Deutsche Bank and Dresdner to combine their retail bank operations into Deutsche Bank's retail banking division, Bank 24, and then spin off Bank 24 as an independent entity in which the merged company would have no more than a 10 percent ownership stake. At the time, Bank 24 had some 11 million customers, the majority in Germany but 1.5 million in Italy and another 600,000 in Spain. In addition to its 2,000 retail branches, Bank 24 had also been a pioneer in using the Internet to sell banking services, and by 2000 some 20 percent of all transactions were online. The plan to spin off Bank 24 indicated the two banks had decided to withdraw from retail banking, instead concentrating on the wholesale side of the business (investment banking and money management). Most analysts applauded the proposed deal, noting that retail banking in Germany was a low-margin business that held few attractions, while investment banking was a high-margin business.

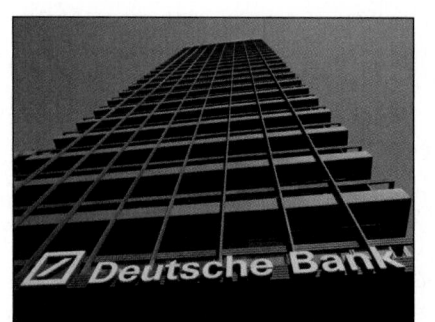

By April 2000, however, the proposed deal had collapsed following significant disagreements between management teams at the two companies. Initially, few thought that this would lead to a change in strategy at Deutsche Bank, but six months later the bank announced it had rethought its retail strategy. Suddenly, Bank 24 was at the heart of a new strategy by Deutsche Bank to build a pan-European retail channel. The change of strategy stemmed from a growing realization that Deutsche Bank's branch and online banking platform provided a powerful sales channel to a rapidly growing "money class"—Europe's highly educated and prosperous 30- and 40-year-olds. Deutsche Bank esti-

mated there are more than 60 million people in this demographic with the European Union. Increasingly, this group is switching their savings from deposit accounts into equities and investment funds as they begin to plan for their retirement. Deutsche Bank realized it could use its retail branch network to sell the investment products churned out by its investment banking and asset management operations. Deutsche Bank also realized that with the advent of the euro, the impediments to the cross-border sale of money management products had been significantly reduced, at least within the euro zone.

To implement the strategy, Deutsche Bank plans to weld Bank 24's operations, which are scattered across seven European countries, into a coherent whole. The model in each country will be the same. The basic idea will be to offer a full range of financial services via branch offices, telephones, and increasingly the Internet. But in an effort to curb costs, the emphasis is likely to be the Internet. Thus, the company wants to grow its retail customer base to 14 million by 2004, while keeping the number of branches constant at 2,000 and reducing total employment by about 10 percent. The geographical distribution of branches will change, however, with some branches in Germany being consolidated or closed, while retail branches are opened in other European countries. The initial plans call for further expansion in Italy, Spain, France, and Belgium, where Bank 24 already has a presence. The company, however, also states that if the concept works, it will move into the Netherlands and the United Kingdom, as well as some non-EU countries, such as Poland and the Czech Republic (both of which have applied to enter the EU). Deutsche Bank also indicated that Bank 24 might make selected acquisitions to establish a larger retail presence in other EU nations.

Another element of the strategy calls for Deutsche Bank to expand the reach of its online brokerage unit, Maxblue, into a pan-European discount broker. Bank 24 will be used to market Maxblue. In late 2000, Maxblue had some 300,000 client accounts, the majority in Germany. The plan calls for this number to grow to 1.5 million by 2004, many of whom would be outside of Germany. If attained, this would give Deutsche Bank a 30 percent share of the online market that is expected to exist by 2004.

Implementing this strategy will require heavy investments, particularly in information technology. Before the change in strategy, Deutsche Bank had budgeted some $110 million for building up Bank 24, including redesigning branches abroad, unifying information technology, and marketing the new look. Now estimates suggest it will take some $250 million of marketing expenditure just to achieve brand recognition across Europe, and significant additional investments will be required in information technology. Despite this investment, Deutsche Bank claims the shift in strategy will boost Bank 24's profits from euro 400 million in 2000 to euro 1 billion by 2004.

Sources: "German Banking," *The Economist*, April 8, 2000; M. Walker, "Deutsche Bank Plans to Make Its Retail Unit a Stock Outlet," *Wall Street Journal*, October 23, 2000, p. A25; and T. Major, "DB24 Reprised to Target Europe's Forty Somethings," *Financial Times*, November 17, 2000, p. 33.

Case Discussion Questions

1. What are the main elements of Deutsche Bank's strategy for Bank 24? Does this strategy hold appeal given (*a*) the creation of a single market in the European Union and (*b*) the introduction of the euro?

2. What potential impediments do you think might get in the way of Deutsche Bank's aspirations to establish a pan-European retail presence and a pan-European discount brokerage?

3. How easy do you think it might be for other European banks to adopt a similar strategy and for U.S. banks to enter Europe and go after the same "money class"? Given this, how competitive do you think this market is likely to be?

4. Deutsche Bank estimated it could more than double the profits of Bank 24 by 2004, while holding the number of branches roughly constant and increasing its customer base from 11 million to 14 million. How realistic do you think this profit goal is given your answers to questions 2 and 3 and the investments apparently required to implement the strategy?

Cases

Video Case: Starbucks   302

The Politics of Trade in Steel   302

The Softwood Lumber Dispute   303

Comparing Ghana and South Korea   306

Managed Trade: The U.S.
and Japanese Semiconductor
Industries, 1970–2002   307

Dixon Ticonderoga—Victim of
Globalization?   311

■ Video Case: Starbucks 🎥

Synopsis of the Video

This video describes the relationships that Starbucks has built with its coffee suppliers. Starbucks is the world's largest seller of premium-brewed coffee with more than 6,300 stores worldwide in 27 countries. Starbucks has to ensure a consistent supply of premium-grade coffee beans for its roasters. The problem is complicated by the volatility of coffee prices on the world market. The volatile pricing environment can make it difficult for small growers of premium coffee to cover their costs, particularly when excess supply on the world market drives prices down. To help stabilize prices, Starbucks and other companies guarantee a minimum purchase price in advance.

Starbucks signs long-term contracts with growers of high-grade specialty coffee in developed nations. In recent years, it has paid as much as twice the market price for premium coffee. Starbucks is able to do this because the differentiated nature of its product means it can pass on high prices for coffee to its consumers in the form of higher prices. The company also provides farmers with credit to tide them over when they are not generating any income from the sale of coffee.

Beginning in 2000, Starbucks also started selling Fair Trade Coffee in its stores. According to Global Exchange, an international human rights organization, "Few Americans realize that agriculture workers in the coffee industry often toil in what can be described as 'sweatshops in the fields.' " . . . Many small coffee farmers receive prices for their coffee that are less than the costs of production, forcing them into a cycle of poverty and debt." To counter this cycle of poverty, the Fair Trade certification mark was developed to assure con-

sumers that coffee was purchased under Fair Trade conditions. To become Fair Trade certified, coffee importers must meet certain criteria, which include paying a minimum price per pound of $1.26, providing credit to farmers, and providing technical assistance such as help transitioning to organic farming.[1] However, only a small percentage of Starbucks' total coffee purchase is "fair trade" coffee. According to Starbucks, this is because only 2 percent of the farmers it deals with can adhere to fair trade principles.

In addition to its foray into the Fair Trade market, Starbucks has partnered with Conservation International to promote growing coffee in an environmentally sustainable manner. For example, the coffee trees may be planted in rows shaded by trees. While this means that less land can be devoted to coffee bushes, it also means that the area sustains a more diverse biology, and the farmers have to use less fertilizer. Coffee grows easily among shade trees and other vegetation. The trees keep nitrogen in the soil, and their leaves provide natural mulch for coffee plants, reducing the need for chemical fertilizers and herbicides. The mix of plants prevents erosion and protects the coffee from harsh weather.

Case Discussion Questions

1. Why is it important for Starbucks to ensure a consistent supply of high-grade specialty coffee?

2. How do long-term contracts help Starbucks to ensure this consistent supply? What is the main drawback associated with signing long-term contracts? Why is this drawback not particularly important for Starbucks?

3. Starbucks has started to sell Fair Trade coffee. What is the difference between "free trade" coffee and "fair trade" coffee? Does it follow that "free trade coffee" is not fair? What do theories of international trade tell us about how "fair" free trade is?

[1]http://www.globalexchange.org/campaigns/fairtrade/coffee/; website accessed June 20, 2003.

■ The Politics of Trade in Steel

In March 2002 President George W. Bush imposed sweeping tariffs ranging from 8 percent to 30 percent on a range of steel imports from foreign producers. The tariffs were scheduled to remain in place until March 2005. The move was an attempt to rescue an industry that has been shrinking for years, but still provides 160,000 jobs in the United States. When the tariffs were announced, 16 American steelmakers were operating under the pro-

tection of the bankruptcy court. Leo Gerard, the president of the United Steelworkers of America, the main labor union in the industry, said the tariffs would protect American jobs by offering the industry a chance for survival. Echoing this, the managers of steel companies said they needed trade protection to give them time to upgrade their mills so that they could better compete with foreign producers.

This wasn't the first time the U.S. steel industry sought, and got, government protection from foreign producers. In fact, the steel industry has received periodic protection of one sort or another for the past 30 years. Despite this, many producers have continued to suffer as more efficient foreign producers and, perhaps just as importantly, efficient nonunionized U.S. mini-mills such as Nucor Steel, have taken market share from old-line unionized steel companies. Mini-mills, which utilize electric arc furnaces to smelt scrap steel, now hold 40 percent of the U.S. steel market, up from nothing in the 1960s, and unlike many older steelmakers, most of the mini-mills are profitable.

The main losers of the Bush tariffs appear to be foreign producers and U.S. consumers. Producers in the European Union were particularly incensed by the tariffs, since more than one-third of their $4 billion worth of steel exports were to be hit by a 30 percent tariff, and they feared that the EU market would now be flooded with steel that other foreign producers diverted from the United States. The EU immediately stated it would seek compensation from the United States, as allowed for by World Trade Organization (WTO) rules. If granted, this would raise the costs to the United States of the Bush tariffs.

In the aftermath of the Bush tariffs, consumers of U.S. steel saw the price of steel jump, which raised their costs and made them more uncompetitive in the global marketplace. In the months following the imposition of tariffs, the price of steel products in the United States rose between 30 percent and 50 percent. Cold rolled steel, which is used by automobile manufacturers among others, was averaging $525 a ton in the United States versus $280 in Japan and $304 in Germany. According to Gary Hufbauer, an economist at the Institute for International Economics, this round of price increases is just the latest in a long line of costs that steel tariffs have imposed on U.S. consumers over the last three decades. Hufbauer has estimated that efforts since the 1970s to protect U.S. steel have cost U.S. steel users some $120 billion in the form of higher prices.

In August 2002, the World Trade Organization told the European Union it could impose some $2 billion in retaliatory tariffs on imports from the United States. With the threat of a trade war looming, and U.S. steel users complaining vociferously to the White House about higher steel prices, the Bush administration announced it would roll back many of the tariffs on EU steel. In response, the EU stated it would not impose retaliatory tariffs. While this action bought some relief to U.S. steel consumers, the higher prices persisted throughout the fall of 2002, and with many tariffs still scheduled to stay in place until 2005, no short-term relief seemed imminent.

Case Discussion Questions

1. Do you believe the Bush administration was correct in imposing tariffs in March 2002 on a wide range of steel imports?

2. Who are the main beneficiaries of protective tariffs such as those imposed on steel imports? Who are the losers?

3. Does the World Trade Organization in this case represent a loss of U.S. national sovereignty? Why do you think the WTO sided with the European Union?

4. If all tariffs on international trade in steel were removed, and subsidies to steel exporters around the world were banned, who would this benefit? Who would lose from such action?

Sources

1. King, N., and R. Guy Matthews. "Errant Shot? So Far Steel Tariffs Do Little of What President Envisioned," *Wall Street Journal*, September 13, 2002, p. A1.

2. "Rust Never Sleeps: Steel." *The Economist*, March 9, 2002, pp. 61–62.

3. "Steel, Rolled." *The Economist*, August 31, 2002, pp. 54–55.

4. "Steel's Tariff Addiction." *The Economist*, August 20, 2002, p. A18.

The Softwood Lumber Dispute

Introduction

"It's the biggest trade dispute on the planet," says Pierre Pettigrew, Canada's trade minister in 2003. Pettigrew was referring to a 20-year dispute between Canada and the United States over exports of Canadian softwood lumber to the United States. The numbers involved suggest that Pettigrew has a point. In 2001, Canada exported softwood lumber products to the United States valued at $6.5 bil-

lion. That was before May 2002, when the U.S. Commerce Department imposed countervailing duties averaging 27 percent on Canadian lumber imports. The imposition of duties was a response to pressure from U.S. lumber producers who claim that Canadian producers have been unfairly dumping lumber on the U.S. market at prices below costs, thereby driving U.S. lumber producers out of business.

It's not the first time this claim has been made. Three times over the last two decades U.S. lumber producers have lobbied for protection, three times the U.S. government has responded by imposing tariffs on Canadian lumber imports into the United States, and three times the Canadians have appealed to U.S. and international trade panels, and each time the Canadians have won on appeal. Will it be any different this time? That now depends on a ruling by the World Trade Organization, which in October 2002 decided to investigate a Canadian complaint that the U.S. tariffs violate WTO rules.

Background

At the heart of the long-standing dispute are differences in forestry practices in the United States and Canada. In the United States, almost all timber is privately owned and sold at auction. In Canada, various provincial governments own about 95 percent of timber producing lands, and these governments set harvest levels, restrict the export of raw logs, and set stumpage rates (or cutting fees) according to market conditions. Lobbyists for the U.S. lumber industry claim that these stumpage rates fall significantly below the prices that would prevail if the lumber was auctioned off as in the United States. The U.S. lumber industry claims that the low stumpage rates in Canada constitute a subsidy. The U.S. industry charges the Canadians set stumpage rates low in an effort to preserve jobs in Canada's timber industry, at the cost of U.S. jobs.

For their part, the Canadians say comparisons between the two countries' timber systems are misleading. Canadian officials argue that their policies require companies to spend additional money on roads and environmental programs, which are not reflected in the low stumpage fees and which increase production costs in Canada. Additionally, the Canadians have long claimed that low prices of Canadian lumber reflect their more efficient mills, allowing them to sell lumber cheaper and still make profits. Whatever the reason for Canada's price advantage, Canadian lumber has steadily increased its share of the U.S. market and in 2001 accounted for 38 percent of all softwood lumber used in the United States.

The most recent dispute can be traced to a 1996 Softwood Lumber Agreement (SLA) between Canada and the United States. Under the SLA, imports of Canadian lumber up to 14.7 billion board feet annually were allowed into the United States free of tariffs. The next 650 million board feet were subject to a tariff of $50 per thousand board feet, and all greater quantities were subject to a tariff of $100 per thousand board feet. The tariffs were designed to protect U.S. lumber producers from losing market share to the Canadians. The Canadians acquiesced to the SLA, even though they disagreed with it on principle, in an effort to buy trade peace.

The SLA was scheduled to expire March 31, 2001. In advance of the expiration, intense lobbying activity oc-

curred. Among those pushing for the agreement to expire were a broad coalition of lumber-using groups in the United States, including the National Association of Home Builders, the National Lumber and Building Material Dealers Association, Home Depot, and affordable housing groups. This group asked that the SLA not be renewed, and that no new restrictions be erected. Their pitch was that free trade in lumber would result in lower prices that would benefit not only lumber-using businesses, but also millions of American home buyers.

The Cato Institute, a Washington, D.C.–based research body, came up with data that backed the position of lumber users. The Cato study concluded that trade restrictions under the SLA had raised the price of lumber in the United States between 20 percent and 35 percent, or $50 to $80 per thousand board feet. As a result, the cost of a new home was some $800 to $1,300 higher than it would have been under a free trade regime. Also, according to an analysis by the U.S. Board of Census, every $1,000 increase in home prices means that an additional 300,000 families in the United States are unable to buy a home. The Cato study thus argued that tariffs on lumber imports act as a regressive tax that keeps the dream of home ownership out of reach of many low-income Americans.

On the other side stood the Coalition for Fair Lumber Imports (CFLI), an association of U.S. timber producers. The CFLI argued that Canadian stumpage rates were one-third to one-fourth of the true market value of lumber cutting fees and constituted a subsidy to Canadian timber producers of C$4.4 billion a year. In the view of the CFLI, the SLA should be strengthened, not allowed to expire. According to the CFLI, between August 2000 and March 2001, while the SLA was still in force, more than 150 lumber mills in the United States were closed, 27 permanently, compared to only 2 permanent closures in Canada. Moreover, in the fourth quarter of 2000, while U.S. production slumped by 15 percent, Canadian producers continued to gain market share in the United States, indicating, claimed the CFLI, that the Canadians were dumping subsidized timber on the U.S. market. The CFLI also dismissed claims that timber tariffs substantially raise home prices. They argued that the cost of lumber in a new home is less than 3 percent of its value, so any tariffs have a trivial impact.

On its website, the CFLI concluded,

> Canada's lumber subsidies are destroying the U.S. lumber industry, threatening its workers with mounting unemployment, and denying many tree farmers a market for their timber crops. The impact of these subsidies is apparent everywhere. Despite a strong home building market, U.S. lumber prices are touching new lows, bankruptcies and mill shutdowns are high and climbing higher, while Canada's share of the U.S. market approaches 35 percent, a near record high.

In response to the CFLI's claims of job losses, the Cato Institute pointed out that in 1999 there were 217,000 jobs in logging and sawmills in the United States, but some 6 million jobs in lumber-using industries such as furniture and home construction. Thus, employment in lumber-using industries exceeded employment in lumber-producing industries by 25 to 1. If Congress really wanted to boost employment in the United States, the Cato Institute study argued, it should allow the SLA to expire because the cheaper lumber would create jobs in lumber-consuming industries. The Cato report also noted that U.S. producers themselves received various government subsidizes that collectively amounted to some $600 million annually. Moreover, the study authors noted that various academic studies have concluded that Canadian stumpage values were within normal price ranges and therefore did not distort the price or quantity of logs or softwood lumber.

Renewed Trade Tensions, 2001–2003

Initially it seemed as if lumber consumers won the day. On March 31, 2001, the U.S. Congress allowed the SLA to expire, effectively allowing for free trade in lumber between Canada and the United States. In April, the CFLI filed with the U.S. Commerce Department a request for a 40 percent countervailing duty on Canadian lumber imports and antidumping duties of up to an additional 40 percent. In its filing, the CFLI claimed that Canadian producers were exporting lumber to the United States at prices ranging from 22.5 percent to 72.9 percent below costs.

In May 2001, the CFLI was joined by a coalition of U.S. environmental groups and Canadian native tribes, who asked the Commerce Department to add an additional 3.5 percent in tariffs, or $160 million a year, on imports from British Columbia to punish that province for its lax protection of fish habitat.

In August 2001, the Commerce Department responded by imposing a 19.3 percent interim countervailing duty on Canadian timber imports. In September 2001, the department added an additional 12.6 percent preliminary antidumping duty, bringing the total duties in Canadian timber imports up to 31.9 percent. In reaching its decisions, the Commerce Department repeated the often-stated opinion that stumpage rates in Canada constituted an unfair subsidy to Canadian producers. In May 2002, the department revised the preliminary tariffs and imposed an average tariff of 27 percent on imports of Canadian lumber. In response, Canada filed a complaint with the World Trade Organization, claiming that the U.S. tariffs were in violation of WTO rules.

In theory, the imposition of tariffs should have hurt Canadian producers, and in a sense they did. But the effects were more complex than expected. In Canada, mills were closed, thousands of workers were laid off, and lumber producers' profits crashed. But the Canadian industry seemed to emerge fitter than ever. With production now concentrated in the more efficient mills that can survive despite the high tariffs, the average costs of production in Canada have fallen by $65 per thousand board feet of lumber, *even after adding on the cost of duties!*

Meanwhile, the duties do not seem to have protected U.S. lumber producers from pain. European timber producers quickly stepped into the gap created by the initial fall in timber exports from Canada, increasing their exports to the United States by more than 90 percent between late 2000 and late 2002. More efficient Canadian producers also started to regain lost market share in 2002. To complicate matters, weak demand for timber in other countries such as Japan helped to depress prices by 10 percent in 2002. By late 2002, it was estimated that due to weak global demand, capacity utilization rates at lumber mills were around 85 percent compared with 91 percent in peak years. Between May 2002 and February 2003, twice as many U.S. mills (114) as Canadian ones (51) shut down or cut their output.

The Next Round

With the lumber industry in trouble on both sides of the border, in early 2003 the Canadians and U.S. officials decided to revisit the issue. At the invitation of the U.S. Department of Commerce, all parties to the dispute met to see if they could resolve the issue. Initial signs were encouraging. The Canadians seemed to indicate they might be willing to change their long-standing stumpage practices and move toward a system that more closely matched the U.S. market-based system. At the same time, the CFLI renewed its calls for protection, now arguing that instead of duties, quotas should be placed to limit imports of Canadian timber. In the meantime, the WTO continues to review the case and will issue a preliminary ruling in 2003.

Case Discussion Question

1. Who benefits from tariffs on Canadian lumber imports? Who loses?

2. Why do you think that lumber producers in the United States have historically been successful at lobbying for tariffs on imports of Canadian lumber?

3. What is the root cause of the 20-year-long timber trade dispute between Canada and the United States? How might this dispute be permanently resolved?

4. If the U.S. government wishes to promote job growth, what should its strategy be toward Canadian lumber imports? Why?

5. What does the recent experience in the U.S. lumber market tell you about the intended and unintended

consequences of imposing tariffs on imports from a specific country?

Sources

1. "A Simple Lesson in Economics: The Softwood Lumber Institute." *The Economist*, February 2003, p. 34.

2. Caffrey, A. "U.S. Tariff on Canadian Lumber Backfires." *Wall Street Journal*, October 21, 2002, p. A2.

3. Chipello, C. J. "Green Groups, Native Tribes Want U.S. to Levy Duties on Canadian Lumber." *Wall Street Journal*, May 10, 2001, p. C16.

4. Chipello, C. J. "U.S. Adds to Import Duties on Canadian Lumber." *Wall Street Journal*, November 1, 2001, p. A15.

5. Coalition for Fair Lumber Imports. Information at http://www.fairlumbercoalition.org/issuebkgrnd_intro.htm.

6. Farnsworth, C. B. "Lumber Agreement Lapses." *Builder*, June 2001, pp. 97–98.

7. Lindsey, B., M. A. Groombridge, and P. Loungani. "Nailing the Homeowner." *Cato Institute*, July 6, 2000.

8. "Stump War." *The Economist*, September 1, 2001, p. 45.

Comparing Ghana and South Korea

Living standards in Ghana and South Korea were roughly comparable in 1970. Ghana's 1970 gross national product (GNP) per head was $250, and South Korea's was $260. By 1998 the situation had changed dramatically. South Korea had a GNP per head of $8,600 and boasted the world's 12th largest economy. Ghana's GNP per capita in 1998 was only $390, while its economy ranked 96 in the world. These differences in economic circumstances were due to vastly different economic growth rates since 1970. Between 1968 and 1998, the average annual growth rate in Ghana's GNP was less than 1.5 percent. In contrast, South Korea achieved a rate of more than 8 percent annually between 1968 and 1998.

In 1957, Ghana became the first of Great Britain's West African colonies to gain independence. Its first president, Kwame Nkrumah, influenced the rest of the continent with his theories of pan-African socialism. For Ghana this meant the imposition of high tariffs on many imports, an import substitution policy aimed at fostering Ghana self-sufficiency in certain manufactured goods, and the adoption of policies that discouraged Ghana's enterprises from engaging in exports. The results were an unmitigated disaster that transformed one of Africa's most prosperous nations into one of the world's poorest. While no simple explanation addresses the difference in growth rates between Ghana and South Korea, part of the answer may be found in the countries' attitudes toward international trade. A now classic study by the World Bank suggests that whereas the South Korean government implemented policies that encouraged companies to engage in international trade, the actions of the Ghanaian government discouraged domestic producers from becoming involved in international trade. As a consequence, in 1980 trade accounted for 18 percent of Ghana's GNP by value compared to 74 percent of South Korea's GNP.

As an illustration of how Ghana's antitrade policies destroyed the Ghanaian economy, consider the government's involvement in the cocoa trade. A combination of favorable climate, good soil, and ready access to world shipping routes has given Ghana an absolute advantage in cocoa production. Quite simply, it is one of the best places in the world to grow cocoa. As a consequence, Ghana was the world's largest producer and exporter of cocoa in 1957. Then the government of the newly independent nation created a state-controlled cocoa marketing board. The board was given the authority to fix prices for cocoa and was designated the sole buyer of all cocoa grown in Ghana. The board held down the prices that it paid farmers for cocoa, while selling the cocoa that it bought from them on the world market at world prices. Thus, it might buy cocoa from farmers at 25 cents a pound and sell it on the world market for 50 cents a pound. In effect, the board was taxing exports by paying farmers considerably less for their cocoa than it was worth on the world market and putting the difference into government coffers. This money was used to fund the government policy of nationalization and industrialization.

One result of the cocoa policy was that between 1963 and 1979, the price paid by the cocoa marketing board to Ghana's farmers increased by a factor of 6, while the price of consumer goods in Ghana increased by a factor of 22, and while the price of cocoa in neighboring countries increased by a factor of 36! In real terms, the Ghanaian farmers were paid less every year for their cocoa by the cocoa marketing board, while the world price increased significantly. Ghana's farmers responded by switching to the production of subsistence foodstuffs that could be sold within Ghana, and the country's production and exports of cocoa plummeted by more than one-third in seven years. At the same time, the Ghanaian government's attempt to build an industrial base through state-run enterprises failed. The resulting drop in Ghana's export earnings plunged the country into recession, led to a decline in its foreign currency reserves, and severely limited its ability to pay for necessary imports.

In contrast, consider the trade policy adopted by the South Korean government. The World Bank has characterized the trade policy of South Korea as "strongly outward-oriented." Unlike in Ghana, the policies of the South Korean government emphasized low import barriers on manufactured goods (but not on agricultural goods) and incentives to encourage South Korean firms to export. Beginning in the late 1950s, the South Korean government progressively reduced import tariffs from an average of 60 percent of the price of an imported good to less than 20 percent in the mid-1980s. On most nonagricultural goods, import tariffs were reduced to zero. In addition, the number of imported goods subjected to quotas was reduced from more than 90 percent in the late 1950s to zero by the early 1980s. Over the same period, South Korea progressively reduced the subsidies given to South Korean exporters from an average of 80 percent of their sales price in the late 1950s to an average of less than 20 percent of their sales price in 1965 and down to zero in 1984. Put another way, with the exception of the agricultural sector (where a strong farm lobby maintained import controls), South Korea moved progressively toward a free trade stance.

South Korea's outward-looking orientation has been rewarded by a dramatic transformation of its economy. Initially, South Korea's resources shifted from agriculture to the manufacture of labor-intensive goods, especially textiles, clothing, and footwear. An abundant supply of cheap but well-educated labor helped form the basis of South Korea's comparative advantage in labor-intensive manufacturing. More recently, as labor costs have risen, the growth areas in the economy have been in the more capital-intensive manufacturing sectors, especially motor vehicles, semiconductors, consumer electronics, and advanced materials. As a result of these developments, South Korea has gone through some dramatic changes. In the late 1950s, 77 percent of the country's employment was in the agricultural sector; today the figure is less than 20 percent. Over the same period the percentage of its GNP accounted for by manufacturing increased from less than 10 percent to more than 30 percent, while the overall GNP grew at an annual rate of more than 9 percent.

Case Discussion Questions

1. Use the theory of comparative advantage to explain how the trade policies adopted by the governments of Ghana and South Korea had an effect on the economic growth rates of both nations?

2. What trade and trade-related policies could the government of Ghana have adopted that would have led to greater economic growth? Why?

3. What trade policies could South Korea have adopted that might have boosted that country's economic growth rates?

Sources

1. "Poor Man's Burden: A Survey of the Third World." *The Economist*, September 23, 1989.

2. Wha-Lee, J. "International Trade, Distortions, and Long-Run Economic Growth." *International Monetary Fund Staff Papers* 40, no. 2 (June 1993), p. 299.

3. World Bank. *World Development Report, 2000*. Oxford: Oxford University Press, 2000, Table 1.

Managed Trade: The U.S. and Japanese Semiconductor Industries, 1970–2002

Introduction

The semiconductor industry was born with the invention of the transistor at Bell Telephone Laboratories in 1947. The transistor was first commercialized in the 1950s by U.S. firms, and it soon became a major component of electronic products. In the 1960s, the transistor was replaced by the integrated circuit. Like the transistor, the integrated circuit was first developed and commercialized by U.S. firms. Today, semiconductors are the main components of numerous electronic products including computers, photocopiers, and telecommunica-

tions equipment. In addition, they are increasingly finding their way into a host of other products from automobiles to machine tools.

Semiconductors can be divided into several broad product groups, the most important of which are memory devices, such as DRAMs (dynamic random access memory chips), and logic chips, such as the microprocessors and microcontrollers. The total world market for semiconductors stood at $35 billion in 1988, reached $91.5 billion in 1994, increased to a record $204 billion in 2000, before slumping to $140.7 billion in 2002 as a result of a global slump in spending on information technology.

U.S. enterprises dominated the world market from the 1950s until the early 1980s. At the height of U.S. success in the mid-1970s, U.S. firms held close to 70 percent of the world market. During the 1980s, however, the market share of U.S. firms plummeted, falling to 29 percent by 1990, while the share held by Japanese producers rose from 24 percent at the end of the 1970s to 49 percent by 1990. By the end of the 1980s, the United States was a net importer of semiconductors, while 5 of the 10 largest semiconductor producers were Japanese. More significantly still, Japanese firms by 1988 had captured more than 80 percent of the world market for the most widely used integrated circuit in digital equipment, the DRAM. Invented by Intel and once produced exclusively by U.S. firms, as of 1988 only two U.S. firms were in the DRAM market, Micron Technologies and Texas Instruments, and Texas Instruments was manufacturing most of its DRAMs in Japan.

However, the late 1980s may have been something of a high-water mark in the global success of Japanese semiconductor firms. By the mid-1990s, the U.S. industry was again gaining global market share. By 1994, U.S. manufacturers had increased their share of the world semiconductor market to 42 percent, while the share taken by Japanese firms stood at 41 percent, down almost 10 percentage points from their high. Also, foreign firms held 22.4 percent of the Japanese semiconductor market in 1994, up from about 14 percent in 1990. As the 1990s progressed, Japan's share of the global market continued to decline. In this case we explore some reasons for the rise of Japan's semiconductor industry and for the subsequent decline in its growth in global market share.

Japan's Industrial Policy

Why were the Japanese so successful in the global semiconductor industry between the 1970s and late 1980s? One argument is that the industrial policy of the Japanese government was the driving force behind Japan's success in semiconductors. During the 1960s and 1970s, the Japanese government, principally through the Ministry of International Trade and Industry (MITI), sought to build a competitive semiconductor industry by limiting foreign competition in the domestic market and acquiring foreign technology and know-how. The foreign investment laws created after World War II (ironically by the U.S. occupation government) required the Japanese government to review for approval all applications for foreign direct investment in Japan. MITI consistently rejected all applications by U.S. semiconductor firms to set up wholly owned subsidiaries in Japan, to set up joint ventures in which the U.S. partner would have a majority stake, or to acquire equity in Japanese semiconductor firms. At the same time, the government limited foreign import penetration of the Japanese market through a

combination of high tariffs and restrictive quotas. Import penetration of the Japanese market was also limited by requirements that Japanese companies get permission from MITI before buying advanced integrated circuits from foreign companies. For example, until 1974, integrated circuits that contained more than 200 circuit elements could not be imported without special permission.

Because U.S. producers were denied direct access to the Japanese semiconductor market, they typically sought indirect access by licensing their product and process know-how to Japanese enterprises. This too was regulated by MITI. MITI's policy was to insist that if a foreign firm was going to license technology in Japan, that technology had to be licensed to all Japanese firms that requested access. In other words, U.S. firms were not able to discriminate between licensees. MITI also conditioned approval of certain deals on the willingness of the involved Japanese firms to diffuse their technological developments, through sublicensing agreements, to other Japanese firms. The net result of these policies was to encourage the rapid diffusion of advanced semiconductor product and process technology throughout the Japanese semiconductor industry.

U.S. firms went along with this policy because it was their only way to get access to the Japanese market. Initially, licensing was a very lucrative arrangement for U.S. firms. By the end of the 1960s, Japanese semiconductor firms were reportedly paying at least 10 percent of their sales revenues as royalties to U.S. firms: 2 percent to General Electric, 4.5 percent to Fairchild, and 3.5 percent to Texas Instruments. The most notable long-run consequence, however, was a transfer of U.S. technological know-how to a number of emerging Japanese competitors. Shielded from foreign competition by import barriers and restrictions on foreign direct investment and armed with state-of-the-art technological know-how, the Japanese firms had only each other to compete with for a share of the rapidly growing Japanese semiconductor market. Stimulated by MITI's insistence that technology be shared among all Japanese semiconductor firms, this competition was intense and based primarily on cost (since everyone had the same technology). The firms that rose to the top in this tough environment, such as NEC, were more than capable of going head-to-head with U.S. semiconductor firms by the mid-1970s.

Trade Agreements

By the mid-1980s, the changing fortunes of the Japanese and U.S. semiconductor industries had given birth to a bitter trade dispute between the two countries. After incurring heavy losses, U.S. firms claimed they were facing unfair competition from Japan. They accused the Japanese of selling semiconductors, and especially DRAMs, in the United States for less than their fair market value while simultaneously shutting U.S. firms out of the important and lucrative Japanese semiconductor market. The dispute was settled by a 1986 trade agreement between the United States and Japan. The agreement specified a fair market value for semiconductors. Japanese companies were not supposed to sell their semiconductors for less than this price outside of Japan. The agreement also sought to increase foreign access to Japan's domestic semiconductor market. In a nonbinding side letter, the Japanese government agreed to help ensure that foreign manufacturers gained more than 20 percent of the Japanese market by the end of 1991, a significant increase from the 8.6 percent share held in 1986.

Although the agreement led to an increase in prices for semiconductors in the United States, foreign producers were still not able to capture a major share of Japan's semiconductor market. By early 1991 when the 1986 agreement was close to expiration, the American Semiconductor Industry Association claimed that foreigners held only a 12 percent share of the Japanese market; the Japanese claimed the foreign share was closer to 17 percent.

In June 1991, the United States and Japan signed a new five-year pact to replace the 1986 agreement. Unlike the previous agreement, this pact formally committed the Japanese to ensuring that foreign producers gained a 20 percent share of their semiconductor market by the end of 1992. In return, the United States agreed to abolish the fair market value system created under the 1986 pact.

This new agreement received a mixed reception on both sides. While most U.S. semiconductor manufacturers approved of the agreement, some analysts and politicians argued that the government should not have abolished the fair market value system. House Democratic Leader Richard Gephardt, for example, criticized the agreement for its lack of specific commitments by Japan to widen its chip market to foreign sellers. Similarly, Clyde Prestowitz, a former U.S. trade official who helped to craft the 1986 agreement, called the pact "a step backwards," primarily because it abolished the fair market value system. The Japanese, in contrast, expressed pleasure that the fair market value system had been removed, but many criticized the formal commitment to a 20 percent market share for foreign companies. For example, a senior official at Toshiba, one of Japan's largest semiconductor manufacturers, noted, "We believe that the agreement infringes the principles of free trade, which shouldn't be limited by an agreement of any kind." Similarly, a senior official from the NEC Corporation said, "As you know, the semiconductor was invented in the U.S. and the U.S. was number one in the world for a long time in semiconductors. The U.S. might be a little complacent about what it has achieved. There has been a lack of effort."

Despite such misgivings, the pact seemed to deliver what it promised. The foreign share of the Japanese semiconductor market reached 20 percent in the fourth quarter of 1992. Although it fell back somewhat in the first half of 1993, foreign producers again gained share in the fourth quarter, pushing their total share for the year to 19.4 percent, up from an average of 16.7 percent for all of 1992. The performance of foreigners was even better in 1994, when they captured more than 22 percent of the Japanese market. In the fourth quarter of 1994, foreign producers gained a record 23.7 percent market share. However, some analysts wondered whether the pact had much to do with the foreign success. They pointed out that the value of the Japanese yen had strengthened by about 40 percent against the U.S. dollar since 1991. With the yen this high, the terms of trade in the Japanese semiconductor market had swung sharply toward foreign producers, which now had a distinct cost advantage over their Japanese rivals.

Also, critics note that in the important DRAM market there has been only a limited U.S. resurgence (in contrast to the market for logic chips, where Intel, Motorola, and others continue to dominate). While both Micron Technology and Texas Instruments—the lone two U.S. DRAM manufacturers—did extremely well during 1994 and 1995, much of the DRAM market share gain in Japan has been made by South Korean firms, particularly Samsung. Samsung, which didn't even produce DRAMs in 1988, accounted for 12.7 percent of the world DRAM market in 1994, ahead of Japan's Hitachi Corp. and NEC, which accounted for 9.7 percent and 9.2 percent, respectively. The Japanese share of the world DRAM market was cut in half between 1988 and 1994 as customers switched to low-cost producers such as market leader Samsung and Micron Technology (which enjoyed a 4.5 percent market share in 1994). As of 1995, these trends showed no sign of slowing down. One 1995 estimate suggested that South Korean firms were reinvesting 30 percent to 55 percent of their semiconductor revenues in new plants and equipment, the Americans were reinvesting 22 percent, while the Japanese were reinvesting only 15 percent. Also, a number of Taiwanese firms had announced aggressive plans to expand their presence in the DRAM business. In the face of this rapid investment in capacity by non-Japanese firms and the apparent reluctance of Japanese firms to invest, many thought it would be difficult for the Japanese producers to keep their 37 percent share of the global DRAM market.

In the summer of 1996, representatives from Japan and the United States met again to renegotiate the 1991 semiconductor agreement, which was due to expire July 31, 1996. This time, the Japanese were determined to oppose any attempt by the United States to continue to impose numerical targets or otherwise interfere in the market mechanism. In making their case, the Japanese pointed out that during the first six months of 1996, the foreign share of the Japanese semiconductor market had risen to more than 30 percent and that two-thirds of that share had been taken by U.S. firms. In the wider global market, Japanese producers were seeing their share being taken by aggressive competitors from South Korea and now Taiwan. Particularly in the DRAM sector, the rise in the value of the Japanese yen had made it increasingly difficult for Japanese firms to compete against the Koreans and Taiwanese.

Publicly, the Americans declared that they would push for another agreement, and they voiced concerns that without some kind of deal, the Japanese market would once more be closed to foreign competition. Privately, however, government officials admitted that Japan's semiconductor industry seemed to be on the wane, and that it would be difficult to renew the agreement, particularly given the rise of new competitors and the profit boom being enjoyed by some of America's own semiconductor companies.

After the customary hard bargaining, which went down to the wire as so many trade deals seem to, an agreement was reached that enabled the U.S. side to save face while basically giving the Japanese what they wanted. Under the deal, U.S. and Japanese industry associations agreed to create an entity to collect data about the sector and deliver it to their governments, which would meet annually to discuss the industry. In the words of one observer, the deal represented "the tiniest of fig leaves . . . The idea that there will be government meetings yearly to review semiconductor trade but with no power to do anything about it means that everyone has decided to smile and go home."[1]

Aftermath

The years after the 1996 agreement were not kind to the semiconductor industry. In 1997, a glut of new capacity in South Korea and Taiwan produced excess memory chips. Prices for DRAMs fell by as much as 70 percent, and most of the world's major producers of memory chips posted significant losses. Among those worst hit were the big five Japanese semiconductor companies NEC, Toshiba, Hitachi, Fujitsu, and Mitsubishi Electric. Throughout 1997–98, the yen continued to gain strength against the currencies of South Korea and Taiwan (the former collapsed in value in late 1997), effectively pricing Japanese firms out of the DRAM market. By late 1998, Japan's share of the global market for DRAMs had shrunk to 30 percent, down from a peak of 80 percent 10 years earlier, and Japan's share was forecasted to fall to 20 percent by 2000. News reports suggested that Hitachi, Fujitsu, and Mitsubishi Electric were contemplating leaving the DRAM market and focusing on niches within the market for logic chips. The big gainers in the DRAM market were Taiwanese firms. Japan's share of the total semi-

conductor market (memory plus logic chips) fell from 36 percent in 1996 to 26.4 percent in 1998, while U.S. firms saw their share of the total increase from 46.2 percent to 53.4 percent over the same period due to strong sales of logic chips (see Figure 1).

The global semiconductor industry quickly recovered from the 1997–98 slowdown, and in 1999 and 2000 global sales surged, hitting a record $204 billion in 2000. However, this boom was short lived. A global economic slowdown in 2001 precipitated a collapse in prices for semiconductors, and global sales contracted by more than 25 percent to $138 billion. Japanese firms were again particularly hard hit. NEC announced 4,000 job cuts and stated it would exit the DRAM business in 2003. Fujitsu reported losses of $1.6 billion in its semiconductor business. Meanwhile, foreigners continued to hold onto their about 30 percent of Japan's semiconductor market in the 1996–2001 period. In the North American market, the share of Japanese firms stood at 11.1 percent in 2001, down from 19 percent in 1996. U.S. firms accounted for 72.5 percent of the market, up from 67.6 percent in 1996.

Case Discussion Questions

1. What factors account for the rise of Japan's semiconductor manufacturers during the 1970s and 1980s?

2. Does the rise of Japanese semiconductor companies during the 1970s and 1980s indicate that government industrial policy can play an important role in facilitating national competitiveness in industries targeted by that policy?

3. What explains the relative decline of Japanese semiconductor firms since 1988? Can it be attributed to the 1991 semiconductor pact or to other economic factors?

4. What are the implications of your answer to question 3 for national trade policy?

Notes

1. M. Nakamoto, "Tough Poker Game for Barshefsky," *Financial Times*, August 5, 1996, p. 3.

Sources

1. "And Then There Were Two." *The Economist*, January 23, 1999, pp. 58–59.

2. Borrus, M., L. A. Tyson, and J. Zysman. "Creating Advantage: How Government Policies Created Trade in the Semiconductor Industry." In *Strategic Trade Policy and the New International Economics*, ed. P. Krugman. Cambridge, MA: MIT Press, 1986.

Figure 1

World Market Share, 1982–2001

Source: Semiconductor Industry Association statistics, www.semichips.org.

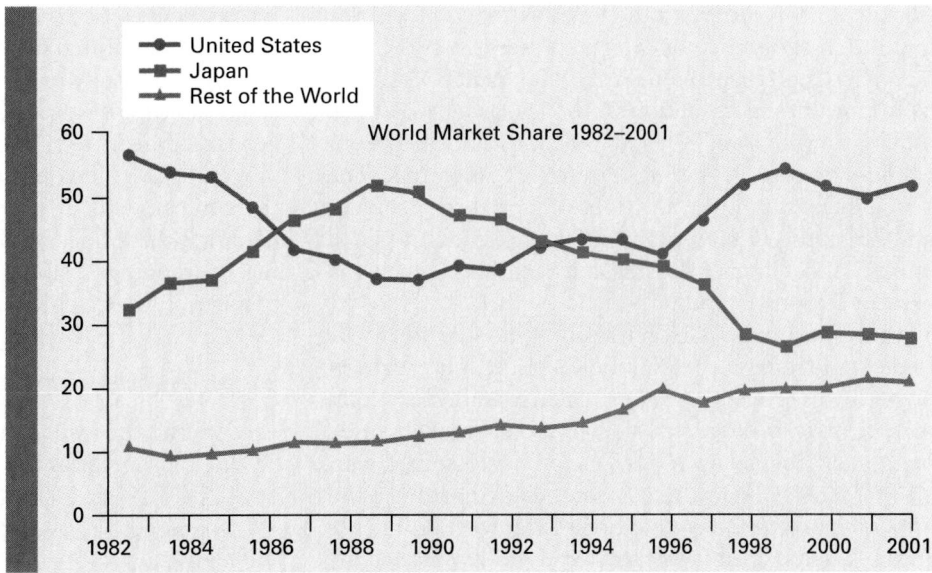

3. Chao, J., and D. Hamilton. "Bad Times Are Just a Memory for DRAM Chip Makers." *Wall Street Journal*, August 28, 1995, p. B4.

4. Darlin, D. "South Korean Chip Firms Play Catch-Up." *Wall Street Journal*, July 29, 1991, p. A5.

5. Davis, B. "Chip Report Eases U.S.-Japan Conflict." *Wall Street Journal*, March 21, 1994, p. A2.

6. Dertouzos, M. L., R. K. Lester, and R. M. Solow. *Made in America.* Cambridge, MA: MIT Press, 1989.

7. Dunne, N. "US and Japan in Agreement on Chips." *Financial Times*, August 3, 1996, p. 3.

8. "Global Sales Heading for 9% Growth Next Year." *Financial Times*, November 13, 1998, p. 6.

9. Nakamoto, M. "Tough Poker Game for Barshefsky." *Financial Times*, August 5, 1996, p. 3.

10. Schlesinger, J. "As U.S. Firms Hail Semiconductor Pact, Some Japan Concerns Have Reservations." *Wall Street Journal*, June 6, 1991, p. A14.

11. Semiconductor Industry Association statistics and forecasts, http://www.semichips.org.

12. "Semiconductor Trade: A Wafer Thin Case." *The Economist*, July 27, 1996, p. 53.

13. "Standard & Poors Industry Surveys." *Electronics*, August 3, 1995.

14. Yamamura, K. "Caveat Emptor: The Industrial Policy of Japan." In *Strategic Trade Policy and the New International Economics*, ed. P. Krugman. Cambridge, MA: MIT Press, 1986.

Dixon Ticonderoga—Victim of Globalization?

Dixon Ticonderoga is one of the oldest public companies in the United States. The company's flagship product is the ubiquitous No.2 yellow pencil, introduced in 1913, which is known to almost anyone who went to school or took standardized tests in the United States. With annual revenues of a little more than $100 million, Dixon is the second largest pencil manufacturer in the country. For most of its history, Dixon has been a prosperous company, but the 1990s proved to be a very difficult decade. It's not that people are no longer buying pencils—in fact, demand for pencils in the United States has soared. Americans bought an estimated 4.2 billion pencils in

1999, a 53 percent jump from 1991. But an increasing proportion of these pencils have been from China.

The problem began in the early 1990s when Chinese manufacturers entered the market with low-priced pencils. The pencil industry fought back, arguing that the Chinese were dumping pencils on the U.S. market at below cost and lobbying Washington for protection. In 1994, when foreign pencil imports accounted for 16 percent of the market, the United States enacted heavy antidumping duties on Chinese pencils, effectively raising their price. Imports fell dramatically, but the Chinese kept making better, cheaper pencils, and after a couple of years imports returned to the levels attained before the imposition of duties. Nor did it stop there. In 1999, U.S. manufacturers shipped some 2.2 billion pencils domestically, down from 2.4 billion in 1991. During that time, imports jumped from 16 percent to more than 50 percent of the market, with China leading the importers. The pencil industry continued to lobby for protection, and in mid-2000, the United States renewed duties on pencil imports from China, imposing import tariffs as high as 53 percent on some brands.

In the meantime, Dixon was not standing still. To try to meet the foreign competition on price, Dixon experimented with cheaper ways to make pencils. The company tried to make pencils out of recycled paper cases, but quickly backed away after the product jammed pencil sharpeners. Then the company looked at the wood used to make pencils—traditionally California incense cedar—and decided it was too expensive for all but the company's premium brand. Now the company uses lower priced Indonesian jelutong wood. As an additional cost-reduction measure instituted in the late 1990s, Dixon started to buy the erasers for its pencils from a Korean supplier, rather than its traditional U.S. supplier.

Despite these steps, the company continued to lose share to imports, and by 1999 it was beginning to lose money, too. Realizing that it could bring in finished pencils cheaper than it could manufacture them in the United States, Dixon established a manufacturing operation in Mexico. The original idea behind the Mexican operation was to supplement its U.S. manufacturing, but in late 2000 the company realized it needed to be more aggressive and switched many of its processes from the United States to Mexico, cutting some 40 jobs at its U.S. facility. In another strategic move, in 2000 Dixon created a wholly owned subsidiary in China. This subsidiary manufactures wooden slats for pencil manufacturing. The slats are then sent to Mexico, where they are turned

into pencils. The lead for the pencils (carbon) is still made in the United States by Dixon, while the erasers are shipped from Korea. The Chinese subsidiary is also responsible for the production and distribution of certain products that are sold internationally. As a result of these moves, by 2002 Dixon's performance was improving, but the company still needed to cut its cost structure. Accordingly, it decided to shut down its U.S. manufacturing operation at Sandusky, Ohio, in 2003 and move production to either Mexico or China.

Case Discussion Questions

1. Why do you think that the Chinese apparently have a cost advantage in the production of pencils?

2. Do you think that lobbying the U.S. government to impose antidumping duties on imports of pencils from China is a good way to protect U.S. jobs? Who benefits most from such duties? Who loses? What alternative policy stance might the government take?

3. Why has Dixon become a multinational company? What are the economic benefits to Dixon of becoming an international business?

4. Now that Dixon has a production operation in China, why does it not simply import finished pencils from China to the United States, instead of making those pencils in Mexico?

Sources

1. Carns, A. "Point Taken: Hard Hit by Imports, American Pencil Icon Tries to Get a Grip." *Wall Street Journal,* November 24, 2000, p. B10.

2. "Dixon Decides to Dissect Options." *Mergers and Acquisitions,* November 2000, p. 34.

3. Dixon Ticonderoga, *Form 10K,* 2002.

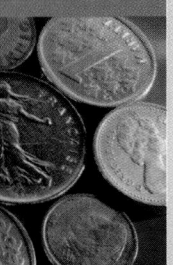

Part 4

The Global
Monetary System

MONEDA	COTIZACIONE
	COMPRA
DOLAR Ee	4600
DOLAR Ch.	4560
PESO ARGENTINO	3000
REAL	1770
PESO URUGUAYO	333
MARCO	1956
FRANCO SUIZO	2612
FRANCO FRANCE	583
LIBRA	6061

Chapter 9
The Foreign Exchange Market

Chapter 10
The International Monetary System

Chapter 11
The Global Capital Market

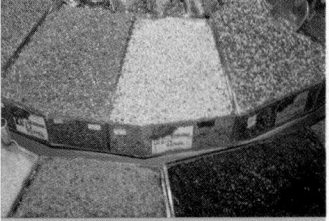

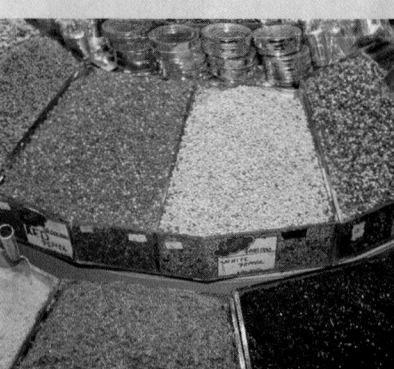

Chapter 9

The Foreign Exchange Market

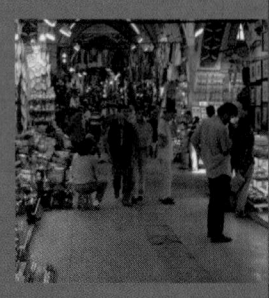

Introduction
The Functions of the Foreign Exchange Market
 Currency Conversion
 Insuring against Foreign Exchange Risk
The Nature of the Foreign Exchange Market
Economic Theories of Exchange Rate Determination
 Prices and Exchange Rates
 Interest Rates and Exchange Rates
 Investor Psychology and Bandwagon Effects
 Summary
Exchange Rate Forecasting
 The Efficient Market School
 The Inefficient Market School
 Approaches to Forecasting
Currency Convertibility
 Convertibility and Government Policy
 Countertrade
Focus on Managerial Implications
Chapter Summary
Critical Discussion Questions
Closing Case: The Collapse of the Thai Baht in 1997

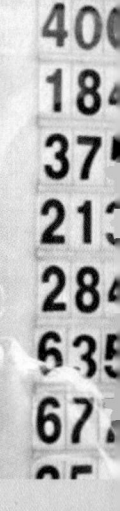

MONEDA	COTIZACIONES	
	COMPRA	V
DOLAR Ef.	4600	46
DOLAR Ch.	4560	46
PESO ARGENTINO	3000	46
REAL	1770	400
PESO URUGUAYO	333	184
MARCO	1956	37
FRANCO SUIZO	2612	213
FRANCO FRANCE	583	284
LIBRA	6061	635
		67

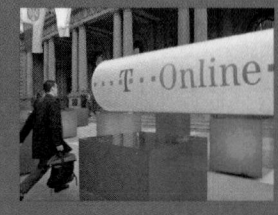

Axis Hedges the Euro

In 1999 when the European Union introduced the euro, Michael Jones, owner and CEO of Axis Ltd., a small manufacturer of wiring components for the aerospace industry, thought it would be a good idea to start pricing sales to European customers in euros (€). During late 1998, Axis entered into multiyear deals with two European aerospace companies to supply wiring. The prices were calculated using an exchange rate of $1=€1.18, which was just a little stronger than the exchange rate for the euro at the time of its introduction in January 1999.

As Jones later noted: "Stupid us! At the time the euro was introduced, no one thought its value would immediately plunge against the dollar. We thought the currency would trade in a narrow range against the dollar, and that pricing in euros was in the best interests of our European customers." However, the euro promptly fell against the dollar, bottoming out at nearly $1=€0.82 in October 2000. For Axis, the plunge was devastating. One of the contracts called for Axis to supply €5 million of wiring to a European customer in 2000. Axis had hoped to generate $5.9 million in revenue at an exchange rate of $1=€1.18 (€5 million × 1.18 = $5.9 million). The company knew that as long as the euro stayed over $1=€1.05 it would be able to make a decent profit on the deal. However, when payment was due, the exchange rate stood at $1=€0.88, and the €5 million deal netted Axis only $4.4 million in revenues. Axis lost money that year due to the adverse movement in foreign exchange rates. The company's 10 top managers all took 20 percent pay cuts, there were no profit-sharing bonuses, and no other employees got a raise.

To make sure that didn't happen again, Jones began to actively hedge against adverse currency movements in 2000. To do this, Axis entered the foreign exchange market, buying currency forward (that is, entering a contract today to buy currency at some point in the future at a predetermined exchange rate). For example, in late 2000,

Axis entered a contract to supply wire to a European customer in the first half of 2001, with payment due in June 2001. The total value of the contract was €2.5 million. At the time, the prevailing dollar/euro exchange rate was $1=€0.90, so the contract would generate $2.25 million in revenues for Axis (€2.5 million × 0.9= $2.25 million). To protect this projected revenue stream from adverse movement in the exchange rate, Axis entered into a forward contract with the foreign exchange desk of its bank to change euros into dollars on July 1, 2001. The bank quoted Axis a rate of $1=€0.94 for making the exchange on that date, which would guarantee Axis $2.35 million. The higher forward rate offered by the bank reflected the view of the foreign exchange market that the euro would appreciate a little against the dollar over the next year.

To Jones, this seemed like a good deal and he entered the contract. But on July 1, the exchange rate stood at $1=€0.85. The foreign exchange market was wrong, and the euro had depreciated against the dollar. Had Axis not entered into the forward exchange contract, its €2.5 million in revenues would have been worth only $2.125 million, not the $2.35 million Axis actually received by executing the forward contract. "It doesn't always work in our favor though," notes Jones. "In 2002, we entered another forward contract to supply wiring through till early 2003. We hedged the exchange rate risk by buying dollars forward on the market at $1=€0.95, which was the forward rate at the time. But guess what! In March 2003, when the customer had to pay, the exchange rate stood at $1=€1.07. Had we not hedged, we would have made a tidy sum on the appreciation in the value of the euro against the dollar, but I cannot stomach the risk associated with that type of speculation anymore. I would rather know what I am getting."[1]

Source: Case from personal interviews by Charles Hill. Name of company and CEO have been changed at the request of the company.

Introduction

This chapter has three main objectives. The first is to explain how the foreign exchange market works. The second is to examine the forces that determine exchange rates, and to discuss the degree to which it is possible to predict future exchange rate movements. The third objective is to map the implications for international business of exchange rate movements and the foreign exchange market. This chapter is the first of three that deal with the international monetary system and its relationship to international business. In the next chapter, we will explore the institutional structure of the international monetary system. The institutional structure is the context within which the foreign exchange market functions. As we shall see, changes in the institutional structure of the international monetary system can exert a profound influence on the development of foreign exchange markets. In the third chapter, we shall look at the growth of the global capital market.

The **foreign exchange market** is a market for converting the currency of one country into that of another country. An **exchange rate** is simply the rate at which one currency is converted into another. We saw in the opening case how Axis used the foreign exchange market to convert euros into U.S. dollars. Without the foreign exchange market, international trade and international investment on the scale that we see today would be impossible; companies would have to resort to barter. The foreign exchange market is the lubricant that enables companies based in countries that use different currencies to trade with each other. On March 7, 2003, the exchange rate between the U.S. dollar and the European euro was $1=€1.10, meaning that $1 bought €0.91.

We know from earlier chapters that international trade and investment have their risks. As the opening case illustrates, some of these risks exist because future exchange rates cannot be perfectly predicted. The rate at which one currency is converted into another can change over time. In January 1999, for example, the U.S. dollar/European euro exchange rate stood at $1=€1.17, by October 2000 it stood at $1=€0.82, and by March 2003 it was up to $1=€1.10. One function of the foreign exchange market is to provide some insurance against the risks that arise from changes in exchange rates, commonly referred to as foreign exchange risk. Although the foreign exchange market offers some insurance against foreign exchange risk, it cannot provide complete insurance. It is not unusual for international businesses to suffer losses because of unpredicted changes in exchange rates. Currency fluctuations can make seemingly profitable trade and investment deals unprofitable, and vice versa. The opening case contains an example of this.

While the existence of foreign exchange markets is a necessary precondition for large-scale international trade and investment, the movement of exchange rates introduces many risks into international trade and investment. Some of these risks can be insured against by using instruments offered by the foreign exchange market, such as the forward exchange contracts discussed in the opening case; others cannot be.

We begin this chapter by looking at the functions and the form of the foreign exchange market. This includes distinguishing among spot exchanges, forward exchanges, and currency swaps. Then we will consider the factors that determine exchange rates. We will also look at how foreign trade is conducted when a country's currency cannot be exchanged for other currencies; that is, when its currency is not convertible. The chapter closes with a discussion of these things in terms of their implications for business.

The Functions of the Foreign Exchange Market

The foreign exchange market serves two main functions. The first is to convert the currency of one country into the currency of another. The second is to provide some insurance against **foreign exchange risk,** by which we mean the adverse consequences of unpredictable changes in exchange rates.[1]

Currency Conversion

Each country has a currency in which the prices of goods and services are quoted. In the United States, it is the dollar ($); in Great Britain, the pound (£); in France, Germany, and other members of the euro zone it is the euro (€); in Japan, the yen (¥); and so on. In general, within the borders of a particular country, one must use the national currency. A U.S. tourist cannot walk into a store in Edinburgh, Scotland, and use U.S. dollars to buy a bottle of Scotch whisky. Dollars are not recognized as legal tender in Scotland; the tourist must use British pounds. Fortunately, the tourist can go to a bank and exchange her dollars for pounds. Then she can buy the whisky.

When a tourist changes one currency into another, she is participating in the foreign exchange market. The exchange rate is the rate at which the market converts one currency into another. For example, an exchange rate of $1 = ¥120 specifies that one U.S. dollar has the equivalent value of 120 Japanese yen. The exchange rate allows us to compare the relative prices of goods and services in different countries. Our U.S. tourist wishing to buy a bottle of Scotch whisky in Edinburgh, may find that she must pay £30 for the bottle, knowing that the same bottle costs $40 in the United States. Is this a good deal? Imagine the current pound/dollar exchange rate is £1.00 = $1.50. Our intrepid tourist takes out her calculator and converts £30 into dollars. (The calculation is 30 × 1.5). She finds that the bottle of Scotch costs the equivalent of $45. She is surprised that a bottle of Scotch whisky could cost less in the United States than in Scotland. (This is true; alcohol is taxed heavily in Great Britain.)

Tourists are minor participants in the foreign exchange market; companies engaged in international trade and investment are major ones. International businesses have four main uses of foreign exchange markets. First, the payments a company receives for its exports, the income it receives from foreign investments, or the income it receives from licensing agreements with foreign firms may be in foreign currencies. To use those funds in its home country, the company must convert them to its home country's currency. Consider the Scotch distillery that exports its whisky to the United States. The distillery is paid in dollars, but since those dollars cannot be spent in Great Britain, they must be converted into British pounds.

Second, international businesses use foreign exchange markets when they must pay a foreign company for its products or services in its country's currency. For example, Dell Computer buys many of the components for its computers from Malaysian firms. The Malaysian companies must be paid in Malaysia's currency, the ringgit, so Dell must convert money from dollars into ringgit to pay them.

Third, international businesses use foreign exchange markets when they have spare cash that they wish to invest for short terms in money markets. For example, consider a U.S. company that has $10 million it wants to invest for three months. The best interest rate it can earn on these funds in the United States may be 2 percent. Investing in a South Korean money market account, however, may earn 12 percent. Thus, the company may change its $10 million into Korean won and invest it in South Korea. Note, however, that the rate of return it earns on this investment depends not only on the Korean interest rate, but also on the changes in the value of the Korean won against the dollar in the intervening period.

Finally, **currency speculation** is another use of foreign exchange markets. Currency speculation typically involves the short-term movement of funds from one currency to another in the hopes of profiting from shifts in exchange rates. Consider again the U.S. company with $10 million to invest for three months. Suppose the company suspects that the U.S. dollar is overvalued against the Japanese yen. That is, the company expects the value of the dollar to *depreciate* (fall) against that of the yen. Imagine the current dollar/yen exchange rate is $1 = ¥120. The company exchanges its $10 million into yen, receiving ¥1.2 billion ($10 million × 120 = ¥1.2 billion). Over the next three months, the value of the dollar depreciates against the yen until $1 = ¥100. Now the company exchanges its ¥1.2 billion back into dollars and finds that it has $12 million.

George Soros—The Man Who Moved Currency Markets

George Soros, a Hungarian-born financier, is the principal partner of the Quantum Group, which controls a series of hedge funds, the largest of which had assets of about $7 billion in late 2002. A **hedge fund** is an investment fund that not only buys financial assets (such as stocks, bonds, and currencies) but also sells them short. **Short selling** occurs when an investor places a speculative bet that the value of a financial asset will decline and then profits from that decline. A common variant of short selling occurs when an investor borrows stock from his broker and sells that stock. The short seller has to ultimately pay back that stock to his broker. However, he hopes that the value of the stock will decline in the intervening period so that the cost of repurchasing the stock to pay back the broker is significantly less than the income he received from the initial sale of the stock. For example, imagine that a short seller borrows 100 units of IBM stock and sells it in the market at $150 per share, yielding a total income of $15,000. In one year, the short seller has to give the 100 units of IBM stock back to his broker. In the intervening period, the value of the IBM stock falls to $50. Consequently, it now costs the short seller only $5,000 to repurchase the 100 units of IBM stock for his broker. The difference between the initial sales price ($150) and the repurchase price ($50) represents the short seller's profit, which in this case is $100

per unit of stock for a total profit of $10,000. Short selling was originally developed as a means of reducing risk (of hedging), but it is often used for speculation.

Along with other hedge funds, the Quantum Fund often takes a short position in currencies that Soros expects to decline in value. For example, if Soros expects the British pound to decline against the U.S. dollar, he may borrow 1 billion pounds from a currency trader and immediately sell those for U.S. dollars. Soros will then hope that the value of the pound will decline against the dollar, so that when he has to repay the 1 billion pounds it will cost him considerably less (in U.S. dollars) than he received from the initial sale.

Since the 1970s, Soros has consistently earned huge returns by making such speculative bets. His most spectacular triumph came in September 1992. He believed the British pound was likely to decline in value against major currencies, particularly the German deutsche mark (this was before the DM was replaced by the euro). The prevailing exchange rate was £1=DM2.80. The British government was obliged by a European Union agreement on monetary policy to try to keep the pound above DM2.77. Soros doubted that the British could do this, so he shorted the pound, borrowing billions of pounds (using the assets of the Quantum Fund as collateral) and immediately began selling them for German deutsche marks. His simultaneous sale of pounds and purchase of marks were so

The company has made a $2 million profit on currency speculation in three months on an initial investment of $10 million!

One of the most famous currency "speculators" is George Soros, whose Quantum Group of "hedge funds" controls about $15 billion in assets. The activities of Soros, who has been spectacularly successful, are profiled in the accompanying Management Focus. In general, however, companies should beware that speculation is a very risky business. The company cannot know for sure what will happen to exchange rates. While a speculator may profit handsomely if his speculation about future currency movements turns out to be correct, he can also lose vast amounts of money if it turns out to be wrong.

Insuring against Foreign Exchange Risk

A second function of the foreign exchange market is to provide insurance to protect against the possible adverse consequences of unpredictable changes in exchange rates (foreign exchange risk). To explain how the market performs this function, we must first distinguish among spot exchange rates, forward exchange rates, and currency swaps.

Spot Exchange Rates

When two parties agree to exchange currency and execute the deal immediately, the transaction is referred to as a spot exchange. Exchange rates governing such "on the large that it helped drive down the value of the pound against the mark. Other currency traders, seeing Soros's market moves and knowing his reputation for making successful currency bets, jumped on the bandwagon and started to sell pounds short and buy deutsche marks. The resulting *bandwagon effect* put enormous pressure on the pound. The British Central Bank, at the request of the British government, spent about £20 billion on September 16, 1992, to try to prop up the value of the pound against the deutsche mark (by selling marks and buying pounds), but to no avail. The pound continued to fall and on September 17, the British government gave up and let the pound decline (it actually fell to £1=DM2.00). Soros made a $1 billion profit in four weeks!

Like all currency speculators, however, George Soros has had his losses. In February 1994, he bet that the Japanese yen would decline in value against the U.S. dollar and promptly shorted the yen. However, the yen defied his expectations and continued to rise, costing his Quantum Fund $600 million. Similarly, a series of incorrect bets in 1987 resulted in losses of more than $800 million for Quantum.

Soros gained a reputation for being able to move currency markets by his actions. This is the consequence not so much of the money that Soros puts into play, but of the bandwagon effect that results when other speculators follow his lead. This reputation resulted in Soros being depicted as the archvillain of the 1997 Asian currency crisis. In 1997, the currencies of Thailand, Malaysia, South Korea, and Indonesia all lost between 50 percent and 70 percent of their value against the U.S. dollar. While the reasons for the crisis are complex, a common feature was excessive borrowing by firms based in these countries. Several Asian leaders, however, most notably Mahathir bin Mohamad, the prime minister of Malaysia, instead blamed the crisis on "criminal speculation" by Soros, who he said had been intent on impoverishing Asian nations. Soros denied that his fund had been involved in shorting Asian currencies.

In 2002, at the age of 72, Soros remained actively involved in running the Quantum Hedge fund. He predicts that over the next few years, the U.S. dollar could lose about a third of its value against other major currencies due to prolonged economic weakness in the United States.

Sources: P. Harverson, "Billion Dollar Man the Money Markets Fear," *Financial Times,* September 30, 1994, p. 10; "A Quantum Dive," *The Economist,* March 15, 1994, pp. 83–84; B. J. Javetski, "Europe's Money Mess," *Business Week,* September 28, 1992, pp. 30–31; "Meltdown," *The Economist,* September 19, 1992, p. 69; T. L. Friedman, "Mahathir's Wrath," *New York Times,* December 18, 1997, p. 27; and J. R. Hagerty, "George Soros Says Dollar May Post Large Decline," *Wall Street Journal,* June 28, 2002, p. C13.

spot" trades are referred to as spot exchange rates. The **spot exchange rate** is the rate at which a foreign exchange dealer converts one currency into another currency on a particular day. Thus, when our U.S. tourist in Edinburgh goes to a bank to convert her dollars into pounds, the exchange rate is the spot rate for that day.

Spot exchange rates are reported daily in the financial pages of newspapers. Table 9.1 shows the dollar exchange rates for currencies traded in the New York foreign exchange market as of 4 P.M. March 7, 2003. Spot exchange rates can also be found on the Web (for example, at http://finance.yahoo.com). An exchange rate can be quoted in two ways: as the price of the foreign currency in terms of dollars (for example, $0.00854 per yen; $1.1006 per euro) or as the price of dollars in terms of the foreign currency (for example, ¥117.10 per dollar; €0.9086 per dollar). The first of these exchange rate quotations (dollar per foreign currency) is said to be in *direct* (or American) terms, the second (foreign currency units per dollar) in *indirect* terms.

Spot rates change continually, often on a day-by-day basis (although the magnitude of the changes over such short time periods will be small). The value of a currency is determined by the interaction between the demand and supply of that currency relative to the demand and supply of other currencies. For example, if lots of people want U.S. dollars and dollars are in short supply, and few people want British pounds and pounds are in plentiful supply, the spot exchange rate for converting dollars into pounds will change. The dollar is likely to appreciate against the pound (or, conversely,

Table 9.1

Foreign Exchange Quotations, June 18, 2003

Source: *Wall Street Journal*, June 19, 2003, p. C12 Copyright© 2003 by DOW JONES & CO. INC. Reproduced with permission of DOW JONES & CO. INC. in textbook and CD-ROM format via the Copyright Clearance Center.

Key Currency Cross Rates

Late New York Trading Wednesday, June 18, 2003

	Dollar	Euro	Pound	SFranc	Peso	Yen	CdnDlr
Canada	1.3367	1.5624	2.2441	1.0102	.12589	.01135	...
Japan	117.81	137.70	197.79	89.032	11.096	...	88.136
Mexico	10.6180	12.4103	17.825	8.0240	...	.09013	7.9433
Switzerland	1.3233	1.5466	2.2215	...	.12463	.01123	.9899
U.K.	.59570	.6962	...	.4501	.05610	.00506	.44562
Euro	.85560	...	1.4363	.64656	.08058	.00726	.64006
U.S.	...	1.1688	1.6788	.75570	.09418	.00849	.74810

Source: Reuters

Exchange Rates

The foreign exchange mid-range rates below apply to trading among banks in amounts of $1 million and more, as quoted at 4 p.m. Eastern time by Reuters and other sources. Retail transactions provide fewer units of foreign currency per dollar.

Country	U.S. $ EQUIVALENT Wed	Tue	CURRENCY PER U.S. $ Wed	Tue
Argentina (Peso)-y	.3568	.3568	2.8027	2.8027
Australia (Dollar)	.6729	.6701	1.4861	1.4923
Bahrain (Dinar)	2.6522	2.6523	.3770	.3770
Brazil (Real)	.3463	.3492	2.8877	2.8637
Canada (Dollar)	.7481	.7469	1.3367	1.3389
1-month forward	.7467	.7455	1.3392	1.3414
3-months forward	.7440	.7427	1.3441	1.3464
6-months forward	.7403	.7389	1.3508	1.3534
Chile (Peso)	.001414	.001421	707.21	703.73
China (Renminbi)	.1208	.1208	8.2781	8.2781
Colombia (Peso)	.0003540	.0003539	2824.86	2825.66
Czech. Rep. (Koruna)				
Commercial rate	.03711	.03761	26.947	26.589
Denmark (Krone)	.1574	.1588	6.3532	6.2972
Ecuador (US Dollar)	1.0000	1.0000	1.0000	1.0000
Egypt (Pound)-y	.1670	.1670	5.9898	5.9898
Hong Kong (Dollar)	.1282	.1282	7.8003	7.8003
Hungary (Forint)	.004365	.004466	229.10	223.91
India (Rupee)	.02150	.02149	46.512	46.533
Indonesia (Rupiah)	.0001215	.0001218	8230	8210
Israel (Shekel)	.2279	.2292	4.3879	4.3630
Japan (Yen)	.008488	.008466	117.81	118.12
1-month forward	.008496	.008474	117.70	118.01
3-months forward	.008511	.008488	117.50	117.81
6-months forward	.008532	.008509	117.21	117.52
Jordan (Dinar)	1.4104	1.4104	.7090	.7090
Kuwait (Dinar)	3.3448	3.3503	.2990	.2985
Lebanon (Pound)	.0006634	.0006634	1507.39	1507.39
Malaysia (Ringgit)-b	.2632	.2632	3.7994	3.7994
Malta (Lira)	2.7315	2.7517	.3661	.3634

Country	U.S. $ EQUIVALENT Wed	Tue	CURRENCY PER U.S. $ Wed	Tue
Mexico (Peso)				
Floating rate	.0942	.0952	10.6180	10.5009
New Zealand (Dollar)	.5842	.5852	1.7117	1.7088
Norway (Krone)	.1432	.1438	6.9832	6.9541
Pakistan (Rupee)	.01734	.01732	57.670	57.737
Peru (new Sol)	.2881	.2878	3.4710	3.4746
Philippines (Peso)	.01872	.01872	53.419	53.419
Poland (Zloty)	.2634	.2684	3.7965	3.7258
Russia (Ruble)-a	.03291	.03292	30.386	30.377
Saudi Arabia (Riyal)	.2666	.2667	3.7509	3.7495
Singapore (Dollar)	.5777	.5787	1.7310	1.7280
Slovak Rep. (Koruna)	.02806	.02837	35.638	35.249
South Africa (Rand)	.1262	.1279	7.9239	7.8186
South Korea (Won)	.0008432	.0008446	1185.96	1183.99
Sweden (Krona)	.1291	.1304	7.7459	7.6687
Switzerland (Franc)	.7557	.7645	1.3233	1.3080
1-month forward	.7563	.7650	1.3222	1.3072
3-months forward	.7572	.7659	1.3207	1.3057
6-months forward	.7585	.7672	1.3184	1.3034
Taiwan (Dollar)	.02899	.02902	34.495	34.459
Thailand (Baht)	.02403	.02407	41.615	41.546
Turkey (Lira)	.00000071	.00000071	1408451	1408451
U.K. (Pound)	1.6788	1.6849	.5957	.5935
1-month forward	1.6752	1.6811	.5969	.5948
3-months forward	1.6678	1.6740	.5996	.5974
6-months forward	1.6577	1.6638	.6032	.6010
United Arab (Dirham)	.2722	.2723	3.6738	3.6724
Uruguay (Peso)				
Financial	.03810	.03800	26.247	26.316
Venezuela (Bolivar)	.000626	.000626	1597.44	1597.44
SDR	1.4234	1.4270	.7025	.7008
Euro	1.1688	1.1797	.8556	.8477

Special Drawing Rights (SDR) are based on exchange rates for the U.S., British, and Japanese currencies. Source: International Monetary Fund.
a-Russian Central Bank rate. b-Government rate. y-Floating rate.

the pound will depreciate against the dollar). Imagine the spot exchange rate is £1 = $1.50 when the market opens. As the day progresses, dealers demand more dollars and fewer pounds. By the end of the day, the spot exchange rate might be £1 = $1.48. The dollar has appreciated, and the pound has depreciated.

Forward Exchange Rates

These changes in spot exchange rates can be problematic for an international business. A U.S. company that imports laptop computers from Japan knows that in 30 days it must pay yen to a Japanese supplier when a shipment arrives. The company will pay the Japanese supplier ¥200,000 for each laptop computer, and the current dollar/yen spot exchange rate is $1 = ¥120. At this rate, each computer costs the importer $1,667 (i.e., 1,667 = 200,000/120). The importer knows she can sell the computers the day they arrive for $2,000 each, which yields a gross profit of $333 on each computer ($2,000 − $1,667). However, the importer will not have the funds to pay the Japanese supplier until the computers have been sold. If over the next 30 days the dollar unexpectedly depreciates against the yen, say, to $1 = ¥95, the importer will still have to pay the Japanese company ¥200,000 per computer, but in dollar terms that would be equivalent to $2,105 per computer, which is more than she can sell the computers for. A depreciation in the value of the dollar against the yen from $1 = ¥120 to $1 = ¥95 would transform a profitable deal into an unprofitable one.

To avoid this risk, the U.S. importer might want to engage in a forward exchange. A **forward exchange** occurs when two parties agree to exchange currency and execute the deal at some specific date in the future. Exchange rates governing such future transactions are referred to as **forward exchange rates.** For most major currencies, forward exchange rates are quoted for 30 days, 90 days, and 180 days into the future. (Forward exchange rate quotations appear in Table 9.1.) In some cases, it is possible to get forward exchange rates for several years into the future. Returning to our computer importer example, let us assume the 30-day forward exchange rate for converting dollars into yen is $1 = ¥110. The importer enters into a 30-day forward exchange transaction with a foreign exchange dealer at this rate and is guaranteed that she will have to pay no more than $1,818 for each computer (1,818 = 200,000/110). This guarantees her a profit of $182 per computer ($2,000 − $1,818). She also insures herself against the possibility that an unanticipated change in the dollar/yen exchange rate will turn a profitable deal into an unprofitable one.

In this example, the spot exchange rate ($1 = ¥120) and the 30-day forward rate ($1 = ¥110) differ. Such differences are normal; they reflect the expectations of the foreign exchange market about future currency movements. In our example, the fact that $1 bought more yen with a spot exchange than with a 30-day forward exchange indicates foreign exchange dealers expected the dollar to depreciate against the yen in the next 30 days. When this occurs, we say the dollar is selling at a *discount* on the 30-day forward market (i.e., it is worth less than on the spot market). Of course, the opposite can also occur. If the 30-day forward exchange rate were $1 = ¥130, for example, $1 would buy more yen with a forward exchange than with a spot exchange. In such a case, we say the dollar is selling at a *premium* on the 30-day forward market. This reflects the foreign exchange dealers' expectations that the dollar will appreciate against the yen over the next 30 days.

Currency Swaps

The above discussion of spot and forward exchange rates might lead you to conclude that the option to buy forward is very important to companies engaged in international trade—and you would be right. By 2001, the last year for which international data are available, forward instruments accounted for some 67 percent of all foreign exchange transactions, while spot exchanges accounted for 33 percent (data are collected every three years; the next set of statistics will be published in 2005).[2] However, the vast majority of these forward exchanges were not forward exchanges of the type we have been discussing, but rather a more sophisticated instrument known as currency swaps.

A **currency swap** is the simultaneous purchase and sale of a given amount of foreign exchange for two different value dates. Swaps are transacted between international businesses and their banks, between banks, and between governments when it is desirable to move out of one currency into another for a limited period without incurring foreign exchange risk. A common kind of swap is spot against forward. Consider a company such as Apple Computer. Apple assembles laptop computers in the United States, but the screens are made in Japan. Apple also sells some of the finished laptops in Japan. So, like many companies, Apple both buys from and sells to Japan. Imagine Apple needs to change $1 million into yen to pay its supplier of laptop screens today. Apple knows that in 90 days it will be paid ¥120 million by the Japanese importer that buys its finished laptops. It will want to convert these yen into dollars for use in the United States. Let us say today's spot exchange rate is $1 = ¥120 and the 90-day forward exchange rate is $1 = ¥110. Apple sells $1 million to its bank in return for ¥120 million. Now Apple can pay its Japanese supplier. At the same time, Apple enters into a 90-day forward exchange deal with its bank for converting ¥120 million into dollars. Thus, in 90 days Apple will receive $1.09 million (¥120 million/110 = $1.09 million). Since the yen is trading at a premium on the 90-day forward market, Apple ends up with more dollars than it started with (although the opposite could also occur). The swap deal is just like a conventional forward deal in one important respect: It enables Apple to insure itself against foreign exchange risk. By engaging in a swap, Apple knows today that the ¥120 million payment it will receive in 90 days will yield $1.09 million.

The Nature of the Foreign Exchange Market

So far we have dealt with the foreign exchange market only as an abstract concept. It is now time to look more closely at the nature of this market. The foreign exchange market is not located in any one place. It is a global network of banks, brokers, and foreign exchange dealers connected by electronic communications systems. When companies wish to convert currencies, they typically go through their own banks rather than entering the market directly. The foreign exchange market has been growing at a rapid pace, reflecting a general growth in the volume of cross-border trade and investment (see Chapter 1). In March 1986, the average total value of global foreign exchange trading was about $200 billion per day. By April 1995, it was more than $1,200 billion per day, and by April 1998, it reached $1,490 billion per day. However, it fell back to $1,200 billion per day in April 2001, largely due to the introduction of the euro, which reduced the number of major trading currencies in the world.[3] The most important trading centers are London (33 percent of activity), New York (14 percent of activity), Tokyo (10 percent of activity), and Singapore (6 percent of activity).[4] Major secondary trading centers include Zurich, Frankfurt, Paris, Hong Kong, San Francisco, and Sydney.

London's dominance in the foreign exchange market is due to both history and geography. As the capital of the world's first major industrial trading nation, London had become the world's largest center for international banking by the end of the 19th century, a position it has retained. Today London's central position between Tokyo and Singapore to the east and New York to the west has made it the critical link between the East Asian and New York markets. Due to the particular differences in time zones, London opens soon after Tokyo closes for the night and is still open for the first few hours of trading in New York.

Two features of the foreign exchange market are of particular note. The first is that the market never sleeps. Tokyo, London, and New York are all shut for only 3 hours out of every 24. During these three hours, trading continues in a number of minor centers, particularly San Francisco and Sydney, Australia. The second feature of the market is the integration of the various trading centers. High-speed computer linkages between trading centers around the globe have effectively created a single market. The integration of financial centers implies there can be no significant difference in exchange rates quoted in the trading centers. For example, if the yen/dollar exchange rate quoted in London at 3 P.M. is ¥120 = $1, the yen/dollar exchange rate quoted in New York at the same time (10 A.M. New York time) will be identical. If the New York yen/dollar exchange rate were ¥125 = $1, a dealer could make a profit through **arbitrage,** buying a currency low and selling it high. For example, if the prices differed in London and New York as given, a dealer in New York could take $1 million and use that to purchase ¥125 million. She could then immediately sell the ¥125 million for dollars in London, where the transaction would yield $1.046666 million, allowing the trader to book a profit of $46,666 on the transaction. If all dealers tried to cash in on the opportunity, however, the demand for yen in New York would rise, resulting in an appreciation of the yen against the dollar such that the price differential between New York and London would quickly disappear. Because foreign exchange dealers are always watching their computer screens for arbitrage opportunities, the few that arise tend to be small, and they disappear in minutes.

Another feature of the foreign exchange market is the important role played by the U.S. dollar. Although a foreign exchange transaction can in theory involve any two currencies, most transactions involve dollars on one side. This is true even when a dealer wants to sell a nondollar currency and buy another. A dealer wishing to sell Korean won for Brazilian real, for example, will usually sell the won for dollars and then use the dollars to buy real. Although this may seem a roundabout way of doing things, it is actually cheaper than trying to find a holder of real who wants to buy won. Because the volume of international transactions involving dollars is so great, it is not hard to find dealers who wish to trade dollars for won or real.

Due to its central role in so many foreign exchange deals, the dollar is a vehicle currency. In April 2001, 90 percent of all foreign exchange transactions involved dollars on one side of the transaction. After the dollar, the most important vehicle currencies were the euro and the British pound—reflecting the importance of these trading entities in the world economy. The euro has replaced the Germany mark as the world's second most important vehicle currency. The British pound used to be second in importance to the dollar as a vehicle currency, but its importance has diminished in recent years. Despite this, London has retained its leading position in the global foreign exchange market.

Economic Theories of Exchange Rate Determination ■

At the most basic level, exchange rates are determined by the demand and supply of one currency relative to the demand and supply of another. For example, if the demand for dollars outstrips the supply of them and if the supply of Japanese yen is greater than the demand for them, the dollar/yen exchange rate will change. The dollar will appreciate against the yen (or the yen will depreciate against the dollar). However, while differences in relative demand and supply explain the determination of exchange rates, they do so only in a superficial sense. This simple explanation does not tell us what factors underlie the demand for and supply of a currency. Nor does it tell us when the demand for dollars will exceed the supply (and vice versa) or when the supply of Japanese yen will exceed demand for them (and vice versa). Neither does it tell us under what conditions a currency is in demand or under what conditions it is not demanded. In this section, we will review economic theory's answers to these questions. This will give us a deeper understanding of how exchange rates are determined.

If we understand how exchange rates are determined, we may be able to forecast exchange rate movements. Because future exchange rate movements influence export opportunities, the profitability of international trade and investment deals, and the price competitiveness of foreign imports, this is valuable information for an international business. Unfortunately, there is no simple explanation. The forces that determine exchange rates are complex, and no theoretical consensus exists, even among academic economists who study the phenomenon every day. Nonetheless, most economic theories of exchange rate movements seem to agree that three factors have an important impact on future exchange rate movements in a country's currency: the country's price inflation, its interest rate, and market psychology.[5]

|Prices and Exchange Rates

To understand how prices are related to exchange rate movements, we first need to discuss an economic proposition known as the law of one price. Then we will discuss the theory of purchasing power parity (PPP), which links changes in the exchange rate between two countries' currencies to changes in the countries' price levels.

The Law of One Price

The **law of one price** states that in competitive markets free of transportation costs and barriers to trade (such as tariffs), identical products sold in different countries must sell for the same price when their price is expressed in terms of the same currency.[6] For example, if the exchange rate between the British pound and the dollar is £1=$1.50, a jacket that retails for $75 in New York should sell for £50 in London (since $75/1.50 = £50). Consider what would happen if the jacket cost £40 in London ($60 in U.S. currency). At this price, it would pay a trader to buy jackets in London and sell them in New York (an example of arbitrage). The company initially could make a profit of

$15 on each jacket by purchasing it for £40 ($60) in London and selling it for $75 in New York (we are assuming away transportation costs and trade barriers). However, the increased demand for jackets in London would raise their price in London, and the increased supply of jackets in New York would lower their price there. This would continue until prices were equalized. Thus, prices might equalize when the jacket cost £44 ($66) in London and $66 in New York (assuming no change in the exchange rate of £1 = $1.50).

Purchasing Power Parity

If the law of one price were true for all goods and services, the purchasing power parity (PPP) exchange rate could be found from any individual set of prices. By comparing the prices of identical products in different currencies, it would be possible to determine the "real" or PPP exchange rate that would exist if markets were efficient. (An **efficient market** has no impediments to the free flow of goods and services, such as trade barriers.)

A less extreme version of the PPP theory states that given relatively efficient markets— that is, markets in which few impediments to international trade exist—the price of a "basket of goods" should be roughly equivalent in each country. To express the PPP theory in symbols, let $P_\$$ be the U.S. dollar price of a basket of particular goods and $P_¥$ be the price of the same basket of goods in Japanese yen. The PPP theory predicts that the dollar/yen exchange rate, $E_{\$/¥}$, should be equivalent to:

$$E_{\$/¥} = P_\$/P_¥$$

Thus, if a basket of goods costs $200 in the United States and ¥20,000 in Japan, PPP theory predicts that the dollar/yen exchange rate should be $200/¥20,000 or $0.01 per Japanese yen (i.e. $1=¥100).

Every year, the newsmagazine *The Economist* publishes its own version of the PPP theorem, which it refers to as the "Big Mac Index." *The Economist* has selected McDonald's "Big Mac" as a proxy for a "basket of goods" because it is produced according to more or less the same recipe in about 120 countries. The Big Mac PPP is the exchange rate that would have hamburgers costing the same in each country. According to *The Economist*, comparing a country's actual exchange rate with the one predicted by the PPP theorem based on relative prices of Big Macs is a test on whether a currency is undervalued or not. This is not a totally serious exercise, as *The Economist* admits, but it does provide us with a useful illustration of the PPP theorem.

The Big Mac index for April 2002 is reproduced in Table 9.2. The first column of the table shows local currency prices of a Big Mac; the second converts them into dollars. The average price of a Big Mac in the United States is $2.49; in Japan it is ¥262, or $2.01 at April 2002 exchange rates. The third column shows the PPP exchange rate implied by these different prices. Thus, the PPP exchange rate for the dollar and yen implied by comparing the prices for Big Macs in Japan and the United States is $1=¥105. Column four gives the actual exchange rate on April 23, 2002 ($1=¥130). Column five compares this to the exchange rate predicted by PPP. This tells us that the Japanese yen is 19 percent undervalued against the dollar and should appreciate against the dollar by that amount according to the PPP theorem. If the Big Mac index were an accurate indicator of PPPs, which it is not, a glance down column five suggests that the U.S. dollar was significantly overvalued against the majority of currencies in early 2002 and would be expected to depreciate in value over the next few months. Interestingly enough, the dollar did decline in value against a wide range of currencies over the next 12 months.

The next step in the PPP theory is to argue that the exchange rate will change if relative prices change. For example, imagine there is no price inflation in the United States, while prices in Japan are increasing by 10 percent a year. At the beginning of

	Big Mac prices		Implied PPP* of the Dollar	Actual Dollar Exchange Rate, April 24, 2002	Under(−)/ Over(+) Valuation against the Dollar, %
	In Local Currency	In Dollars			
United States[†]	$2.49	2.49			
Argentina	Peso 2.50	0.78	1.00	3.13	−68
Australia	A$3.00	1.62	1.20	1.86	−35
Brazil	*Real* 3.60	1.55	1.45	2.34	−38
Britain	£1.99	2.88	1.25[‡]	1.45[‡]	+16
Canada	C$3.33	2.12	1.34	1.57	−15
Chile	Peso 1,400	2.16	562	655	−14
China	Yuan 10.50	1.27	4.22	8.28	−49
Czech Republic	Koruna 56.28	1.66	22.6	34.0	−33
Denmark	DKr24.75	2.96	9.94	8.38	+19
Euro area	€2.67	2.37	0.93[§]	0.89[§]	−5
Hong Kong	HK$11.20	1.40	4.50	7.80	−42
Hungary	Forint 459	1.69	184	272	−32
Indonesia	Rupiah 16,000	1.71	6,426	9,430	−32
Israel	Shekel 12.00	2.51	4.82	4.79	+1
Japan	¥262	2.01	105	130	−19
Malaysia	M$5.04	1.33	2.02	3.8	−47
Mexico	Peso 21.90	2.37	8.80	9.28	−5
New Zealand	NZ$3.95	1.77	1.59	2.24	−29
Peru	New Sol 8.50	2.48	3.41	3.43	−1
Philippines	Peso 65.00	1.28	26.1	51.0	−49
Poland	Zloty 5.90	1.46	2.37	4.04	−41
Russia	Rouble 39.00	1.25	15.7	31.2	−50
Singapore	S$3.30	1.81	1.33	1.82	−27
South Africa	Rand 9.70	0.87	3.90	10.9	−64
South Korea	Won 3,100	2.36	1.245	1.304	−5
Sweden	SKr26.00	2.52	10.4	10.3	+1
Switzerland	SFr6.30	3.81	2.53	1.66	+53
Taiwan	NT$70.00	2.01	28.1	34.8	−19
Thailand	Baht 55.00	1.27	22.1	43.3	−49
Turkey	Lira 4,000,000	3.06	1,606,426	1,324,500	+21
Venezuela	Bolivar 2,500	2.92	1,004	857	+17

Table 9.2

Big Mac Index for April 2002

*Purchasing-power parity: Local price divided by price in United States

[†]Average of New York, Chicago, San Francisco, and Atlanta

[‡]Dollars per pound

[§]Dollars per euro

the year, a basket of goods costs $200 in the United States and ¥20,000 in Japan, so the dollar/yen exchange rate, according to PPP theory, should be $1 = ¥100. At the end of the year, the basket of goods still costs $200 in the United States, but it costs ¥22,000 in Japan. PPP theory predicts that the exchange rate should change as a result. More precisely, by the end of the year:

$$E_{\$/¥} = \$200/¥22,000$$

Thus, ¥1 = $0.0091 (or $1=¥110). Because of 10 percent price inflation, the Japanese yen has *depreciated* by 10 percent against the dollar. One dollar will buy 10 percent more yen at the end of the year than at the beginning.

Money Supply and Price Inflation

In essence, PPP theory predicts that changes in relative prices will result in a change in exchange rates. Theoretically, a country in which price inflation is running wild should expect to see its currency depreciate against that of countries in which inflation rates are lower. If we can predict what a country's future inflation rate is likely to be, we can also predict how the value of its currency relative to other currencies—its exchange rate—is likely to change. The growth rate of a country's money supply determines its likely future inflation rate.[7] Thus, in theory at least, we can use information about the growth in money supply to forecast exchange rate movements.

Inflation is a monetary phenomenon. It occurs when the quantity of money in circulation rises faster than the stock of goods and services; that is, when the money supply increases faster than output increases. Imagine what would happen if everyone in the country was suddenly given $10,000 by the government. Many people would rush out to spend their extra money on those things they had always wanted—new cars, new furniture, better clothes, and so on. There would be a surge in demand for goods and services. Car dealers, department stores, and other providers of goods and services would respond to this upsurge in demand by raising prices. The result would be price inflation.

A government increasing the money supply is analogous to giving people more money. An increase in the money supply makes it easier for banks to borrow from the government and for individuals and companies to borrow from banks. The resulting increase in credit causes increases in demand for goods and services. Unless the output of goods and services is growing at a rate similar to that of the money supply, the result will be inflation. This relationship has been observed time after time in country after country.

So now we have a connection between the growth in a country's money supply, price inflation, and exchange rate movements. Put simply, when the growth in a country's money supply is faster than the growth in its output, price inflation is fueled. The PPP theory tells us that a country with a high inflation rate will see a depreciation in its currency exchange rate. In one of the clearest historical examples, in the mid-1980s, Bolivia experienced hyperinflation—an explosive and seemingly uncontrollable price inflation in which money loses value very rapidly. Table 9.3 presents data on Bolivia's money supply, inflation rate, and its peso's exchange rate with the U.S. dollar during the period of hyperinflation. The exchange rate is actually the "black market" exchange rate, as the Bolivian government prohibited converting the peso to other currencies during the period. The data show that the growth in money supply, the rate of price inflation, and the depreciation of the peso against the dollar all moved in step with each other. This is just what PPP theory and monetary economics predict. Between April 1984 and July 1985, Bolivia's money supply increased by 17,433 percent, prices increased by 22,908 percent, and the value of the peso against the dollar fell by 24,662 percent! In October 1985, the Bolivian government instituted a dramatic stabilization plan—which included the introduction of a new currency and tight control of the money supply—and by 1987 the country's annual inflation rate was down to 16 percent.[8]

Month	Money Supply (billions of pesos)	Price Level Relative to 1982 (average = 1)	Exchange Rate (pesos per dollar)
1984			
April	270	21.1	3,576
May	330	31.1	3.512
June	440	32.3	3,342
July	599	34.0	3,570
August	718	39.1	7,038
September	889	53.7	13,685
October	1,194	85.5	15,205
November	1,495	112.4	18,469
December	3,296	180.9	24,515
1985			
January	4,630	305.3	73,016
February	6,455	863.3	141,101
March	9,089	1,078.6	128,137
April	12,885	1,205.7	167,428
May	21,309	1,635.7	272,375
June	27,778	2,919.1	481,756
July	47,341	4,854.6	885,476
August	74,306	8,081.0	1,182,300
September	103,272	12,647.6	1,087,440
October	132,550	12,411.8	1,120,210

Table 9.3

Macroeconomic Data for Bolivia, April 1984–October 1985

Source: Juan-Antino Morales, "Inflation Stabilization in Bolivia," in *Inflation Stabilization: The Experience of Israel, Argentina, Brazil, Bolivia, and Mexico*, ed. Michael Bruno et al. (Cambridge, MA: MIT Press, 1988).

Another way of looking at the same phenomenon is that an increase in a country's money supply, which increases the amount of currency available, changes the relative demand and supply conditions in the foreign exchange market. If the U.S. money supply is growing more rapidly than U.S. output, dollars will be relatively more plentiful than the currencies of countries where monetary growth is closer to output growth. As a result of this relative increase in the supply of dollars, the dollar will depreciate on the foreign exchange market against the currencies of countries with slower monetary growth.

Government policy determines whether the rate of growth in a country's money supply is greater than the rate of growth in output. A government can increase the money supply simply by telling the country's central bank to issue more money. Governments tend to do this to finance public expenditure (building roads, paying government workers, paying for defense, etc.). A government could finance public expenditure by raising taxes, but since nobody likes paying more taxes and since politicians do not like to be unpopular, they have a natural preference for expanding the money supply. Unfortunately, there is no magic money tree. The inevitable result of excessive growth in money supply is price inflation. However, this has not stopped governments around the world from expanding the money supply, with predictable results. If an international business is attempting to predict future movements in the value of a country's currency on the foreign exchange market, it should examine that country's policy toward monetary growth. If the government seems committed to controlling the rate of growth in money supply, the country's future inflation rate may be low (even if the current rate is high) and its currency should not depreciate too much on the foreign exchange market. If the government seems to lack the political will to control the rate of growth in money supply, the future inflation rate may be high, which is likely to cause its currency to depreciate. Historically, many Latin American governments have fallen into this latter category, including Argentina, Bolivia, and Brazil. More recently, many of the newly democratic states of Eastern Europe made the same mistake.

Empirical Tests of PPP Theory

PPP theory predicts that exchange rates are determined by relative prices, and that changes in relative prices will result in a change in exchange rates. A country in which price inflation is running wild should expect to see its currency depreciate against that of countries with lower inflation rates. This is intuitively appealing, but is it true in practice? There are several good examples of the connection between a country's price inflation and exchange rate position (such as Bolivia). However, extensive empirical testing of PPP theory has yielded mixed results.[9] While PPP theory seems to yield relatively accurate predictions in the long run, it does not appear to be a strong predictor of short-run movements in exchange rates covering time spans of five years or less.[10] In addition, the theory seems to best predict exchange rate changes for countries with high rates of inflation and underdeveloped capital markets. The theory is less useful for predicting short-term exchange rate movements between the currencies of advanced industrialized nations that have relatively small differentials in inflation rates.

The failure to find a strong link between relative inflation rates and exchange rate movements has been referred to as the purchasing power parity puzzle. Several factors may explain the failure of PPP theory to predict exchange rates more accurately.[11] PPP theory assumes away transportation costs and barriers to trade. In practice, these factors are significant and they tend to create significant price differentials between countries. Transportation costs are certainly not trivial for many goods. Moreover, as we saw in Chapter 5, governments routinely intervene in international trade, creating tariff and nontariff barriers to cross-border trade. Barriers to trade limit the ability of traders to use arbitrage to equalize prices for the same product in different countries, which is required for the law of one price to hold. Government intervention in cross-border trade, by violating the assumption of efficient markets, weakens the link between relative price changes and changes in exchange rates predicted by PPP theory.

In addition, the PPP theory may not hold if many national markets are dominated by a handful of multinational enterprises that have sufficient market power to be able to exercise some influence over prices, control distribution channels, and differentiate their product offerings between nations.[12] In fact, this situation seems to prevail in a number of industries. In the detergent industry, two companies, Unilever and Procter & Gamble, dominate the market in nation after nation. In heavy earthmoving equipment, Caterpillar Inc. and Komatsu are global market leaders. In the market for semiconductor equipment, Applied Materials has a commanding market share lead in almost every important national market. Microsoft dominates the market for personal computer operating systems and applications systems around the world, and so on. In such cases, dominant enterprises may be able to exercise a degree of pricing power, setting different prices in different markets to reflect varying demand conditions. This is referred to as price discrimination (we consider the topic from a strategic perspective in Chapter 17). For price discrimination to work, arbitrage must be limited. According to this argument, enterprises with some market power may be able to control distribution channels and therefore limit the unauthorized resale (arbitrage) of products purchased in another national market. They may also be able to limit resale (arbitrage) by differentiating otherwise identical products among nations along some line, such as design or packaging.

For example, even though the version of Microsoft Office sold in China may be less expensive than the version sold in the United States, the use of arbitrage to equalize prices may be limited because few Americans would want a version that was based on Chinese characters. The design differentiation between Microsoft Office for China and for the United States means that the law of one price would not work for Microsoft Office, even if transportation costs were trivial and tariff barriers between the United States and China did not exist. If the inability to practice arbitrage were widespread enough, it would break the connection between changes in relative prices and exchange rates predicted by the PPP theorem and help explain the limited empirical support for this theory.

Another factor of some importance is that governments also intervene in the foreign exchange market in attempting to influence the value of their currencies. We will look at why and how they do this in Chapter 10. For now, the important thing to note is that governments regularly intervene in the foreign exchange market, and this further weakens the link between price changes and changes in exchange rates. One more factor explaining the failure of PPP theory to predict short-term movements in foreign exchange rates is the impact of investor psychology and other factors on currency purchasing decisions and exchange rate movements. We will discuss this issue in more detail later in this chapter.

Interest Rates and Exchange Rates

Economic theory tells us that interest rates reflect expectations about likely future inflation rates. In countries where inflation is expected to be high, interest rates also will be high, because investors want compensation for the decline in the value of their money. This relationship was first formalized by economist Irvin Fisher and is referred to as the Fisher Effect. The **Fisher Effect** states that a country's "nominal" interest rate (i) is the sum of the required "real" rate of interest (r) and the expected rate of inflation over the period for which the funds are to be lent (I). More formally,

$$i = r + I$$

For example, if the real rate of interest in a country is 5 percent and annual inflation is expected to be 10 percent, the nominal interest rate will be 15 percent. As predicted by the Fisher Effect, a strong relationship seems to exist between inflation rates and interest rates.[13]

We can take this one step further and consider how it applies in a world of many countries and unrestricted capital flows. When investors are free to transfer capital between countries, real interest rates will be the same in every country. If differences in real interest rates did emerge between countries, arbitrage would soon equalize them. For example, if the real interest rate in Japan was 10 percent and only 6 percent in the United States, it would pay investors to borrow money in the United States and invest it in Japan. The resulting increase in the demand for money in the United States would raise the real interest rate there, while the increase in the supply of foreign money in Japan would lower the real interest rate there. This would continue until the two sets of real interest rates were equalized. (In practice, differences in real interest rates may persist due to government controls on capital flows; investors are not always free to transfer capital between countries.)

It follows from the Fisher Effect that if the real interest rate is the same worldwide, any difference in interest rates between countries reflects differing expectations about inflation rates. Thus, if the expected rate of inflation in the United States is greater than that in Japan, U.S. nominal interest rates will be greater than Japanese nominal interest rates.

Since we know from PPP theory that there is a link (in theory at least) between inflation and exchange rates, and since interest rates reflect expectations about inflation, it follows that there must also be a link between interest rates and exchange rates. This link is known as the International Fisher Effect (IFE). The International Fisher Effect states that for any two countries, the spot exchange rate should change in an equal amount but in the opposite direction to the difference in nominal interest rates between the two countries. Stated more formally, the change in the spot exchange rate between the United States and Japan, for example, can be modeled as follows:

$$(S_1 - S_2)/S_2 \times 100 = i_\$ - i_\yen$$

where $i_\$$ and $i_\yen$ are the respective nominal interest rates in the United States and Japan, S_1 is the spot exchange rate at the beginning of the period, and S_2 is the spot exchange rate at the end of the period. If the U.S. nominal interest rate is higher than Japan's, reflecting greater expected inflation rates, the value of the dollar against the yen should fall by that interest rate differential in the future. So if the interest rate in the United States is 10 percent and in Japan it is 6 percent, we would expect the value of the dollar to depreciate by 4 percent against the Japanese yen.

Do interest rate differentials help predict future currency movements? The evidence is mixed; as in the case of PPP theory, in the long run, there seems to be a relationship between interest rate differentials and subsequent changes in spot exchange rates. However, considerable short-run deviations occur. Like PPP, the International Fisher Effect is not a good predictor of short-run changes in spot exchange rates.[14]

Investor Psychology and Bandwagon Effects

Empirical evidence suggests that neither PPP theory nor the International Fisher Effect are particularly good at explaining short-term movements in exchange rates. One reason may be the impact of investor psychology on short-run exchange rate movements. Increasing evidence reveals that various psychological factors play an important role in determining the expectations of market traders as to likely future exchange rates.[15] In turn, expectations have a tendency to become self-fulfilling prophecies. We discussed a good example of this mechanism in the Management Focus about George Soros. When Soros shorted the British pound in September 1992, many foreign exchange traders jumped on the bandwagon and did likewise, selling British pounds and purchasing German marks. As the bandwagon effect gained momentum, with more traders selling British pounds and purchasing deutsche marks in expectation of a decline in the pound, their expectations became a self-fulfilling prophecy with massive selling forcing down the value of the pound against the deutsche mark. In other words, the pound declined in value not because of any major shift in macroeconomic fundamentals, but because investors moved in a herd in response to a bet placed by a major speculator, George Soros.

According to a number of studies, investor psychology and bandwagon effects play a major role in determining short-run exchange rate movements.[16] However, these effects can be hard to predict. Investor psychology can be influenced by political factors and by microeconomic events, such as the investment decisions of individual firms, many of which are only loosely linked to macroeconomic fundamentals, such as relative inflation rates. Also, bandwagon effects can be both triggered and exacerbated by the idiosyncratic behavior of politicians. Something like this seems to have occurred in Southeast Asia during 1997 when, one after another, the currencies of Thailand, Malaysia, South Korea, and Indonesia lost between 50 percent and 70 percent of their value against the U.S. dollar in a few months. For a detailed look at what occurred in South Korea, see the accompanying Country Focus. The collapse in the value of the Korean currency did not occur because South Korea had a higher inflation rate than the United States. It occurred because of an excessive buildup of dollar-denominated debt among South Korean firms. By mid-1997 it was clear that these companies were having trouble servicing this debt. Foreign investors, fearing a wave of corporate bankruptcies, took their money out of the country, exchanging won for U.S. dollars. As this began to depress the exchange rate, currency traders jumped on the bandwagon and speculated against the won (selling it short).

Summary

Relative monetary growth, relative inflation rates, and nominal interest rate differentials are all moderately good predictors of long-run changes in exchange rates. They are poor predictors of short-run changes in exchange rates, however, perhaps because of the impact of psychological factors, investor expectations, and bandwagon effects on short-term currency movements. This information is useful for an international business. Insofar as the long-term profitability of foreign investments, export opportunities, and the price competitiveness of foreign imports are all influenced by long-term movements in exchange rates, international businesses would be advised to pay attention to countries' differing monetary growth, inflation, and interest rates. International businesses that engage in foreign exchange transactions on a day-to-day basis could benefit by knowing some predictors of short-term foreign exchange rate movements. Unfortunately, short-term exchange rate movements are difficult to predict.

Exchange Rate Forecasting ■

A company's need to predict future exchange rate variations raises the issue of whether it is worthwhile for the company to invest in exchange rate forecasting services to aid decision making. Two schools of thought address this issue. The efficient market school argues that forward exchange rates do the best possible job of forecasting future spot exchange rates, and, therefore, investing in forecasting services would be a waste of money. The other school of thought, the inefficient market school, argues that companies can improve the foreign exchange market's estimate of future exchange rates (as contained in the forward rate) by investing in forecasting services. In other words, this school of thought does not believe the forward exchange rates are the best possible predictors of future spot exchange rates.

The Efficient Market School

Forward exchange rates represent market participants' collective predictions of likely spot exchange rates at specified future dates. If forward exchange rates are the best possible predictor of future spot rates, it would make no sense for companies to spend additional money trying to forecast short-run exchange rate movements. Many economists believe the foreign exchange market is efficient at setting forward rates.[17] An **efficient market** is one in which prices reflect all available public information. (If forward rates reflect all available information about likely future changes in exchange rates, there is no way a company can beat the market by investing in forecasting services.)

If the foreign exchange market is efficient, forward exchange rates should be unbiased predictors of future spot rates. This does not mean the predictions will be accurate in any specific situation. It means inaccuracies will not be consistently above or below future spot rates; they will be random. Many empirical tests have addressed the efficient market hypothesis. Although most of the early work seems to confirm the hypothesis (suggesting that companies should not waste their money on forecasting services), more recent studies have challenged it.[18] There is some evidence that forward rates are not unbiased predictors of future spot rates, and that more accurate predictions of future spot rates can be calculated from publicly available information.[19]

Why Did the Korean Won Collapse?

In early 1997, South Korea could look back with pride on a 30-year "economic miracle" that had raised the country from the ranks of the poor and given it the world's 11th largest economy. By the end of 1997, the Korean currency, the won, had lost a staggering 67 percent of its value against the U.S. dollar, the South Korean economy lay in tatters, and the International Monetary Fund was overseeing a $55 billion rescue package. This sudden turn of events had its roots in investments made by South Korea's large industrial conglomerates, or *chaebol*, during the 1990s, often at the bequest of politicians. In 1993, Kim Young-Sam, a populist politician, became president of South Korea. Mr. Kim took office during a mild recession and promised to boost economic growth by encouraging investment in export-oriented industries. He urged the *chaebol* to invest in new factories. South Korea enjoyed an investment-led economic boom in 1994–95, but at a cost. The *chaebol,* always reliant on heavy borrowing, built up massive debts that were equivalent, on average, to four times their equity.

As the volume of investments ballooned during the 1990s, the quality of many of these investments declined significantly. The investments often were made on the basis of unrealistic projections about future demand conditions. This resulted in significant excess capacity and falling prices. An example is investments made by South Korean *chaebol* in semiconductor factories. Investments in such facilities surged in 1994 and 1995 when a temporary global shortage of dynamic random access memory chips (DRAMs) led to sharp price increases for this product. However, supply shortages had disappeared by 1996 and excess capacity was beginning to make itself felt, just as the South Koreans started to bring new DRAM factories on stream. The results were predictable; prices for DRAMs plunged and the earnings of South Korean DRAM manufacturers fell by 90 percent, which meant it was difficult for them to make scheduled payments on the debt they had acquired to build the extra capacity. The risk of corporate bankruptcy increased significantly, and not just in the semiconductor industry. South Korean companies were also investing heavily in a wide range of other industries, including automobiles and steel.

Matters were complicated further because much of the borrowing had been in U.S. dollars, as opposed to Korean won. This had seemed like a smart move at the time. The dollar/won exchange rate had been stable at around $1=won850. Interest rates on dollar borrowings were two to three percentage points lower than rates on borrowings in Korean won. Much of this borrowing was in the form of short-term dollar-denominated debt that had to be paid back to the lending institution within one year. While the borrowing strategy seemed to make sense, it involved risk. If the won were to depreciate against the dollar, the size of the debt burden that South Korean companies would have to service would increase when measured in the local currency. Currency depreciation would raise borrowing costs, depress corporate earnings, and increase the risk of bankruptcy. This is exactly what happened.

By mid-1997, foreign investors had become alarmed at the rising debt levels of South Korean companies, particularly given the emergence of excess ca-

The Inefficient Market School

Citing evidence against the efficient market hypothesis, some economists believe the foreign exchange market is inefficient. An **inefficient market** is one in which prices do not reflect all available information. In an inefficient market, forward exchange rates will not be the best possible predictors of future spot exchange rates.

If this is true, it may be worthwhile for international businesses to invest in forecasting services (as many do). The belief is that professional exchange rate forecasts might provide better predictions of future spot rates than forward exchange rates do. However, the track record of professional forecasting services is not that good. An analysis of the forecasts of 12 major forecasting services between 1978 and 1982 concluded the forecasters in general did not provide better forecasts than the forward exchange rates.[20] Also, forecasting services did not predict the 1997 currency crisis that swept through Southeast Asia.

pacity and plunging prices in several areas where the companies had made huge investments, including semiconductors, automobiles, and steel. Given increasing speculation that many South Korean companies would not be able to service their debt payments, foreign investors began to withdraw their money from the Korean stock and bond markets. In the process, they sold Korean won and purchased U.S. dollars. The selling of won accelerated in mid-1997 when two of the smaller *chaebol* filed for bankruptcy, citing their inability to meet scheduled debt payments. The increased supply of won and the increased demand for U.S. dollars pushed down the price of won in dollar terms from around won 840=$1 to won 900=$1.

At this point, the South Korean central bank stepped into the foreign exchange market to try to keep the exchange rate above won 1,000=$1. It used dollars that it held in reserve to purchase won. The idea was to try to push up the price of the won in dollar terms and restore investor confidence in the stability of the exchange rate. This action, however, did not address the underlying debt problem faced by South Korean companies. Against a backdrop of more corporate bankruptcies in South Korea, and the government's stated intentions to take some troubled companies into state ownership, Standard & Poor's, the U.S. credit rating agency, downgraded South Korea's sovereign debt. This caused the Korean stock market to plunge 5.5 percent, and the Korean won to fall to won 930 = $1. According to S&P, "The downgrade of . . . ratings reflects the escalating cost to the government of supporting the country's ailing corporate and financial sectors."

The S&P downgrade triggered a sharp sale of the Korean won. In an attempt to protect the won against what was fast becoming a classic bandwagon effect, the South Korean central bank raised short-term interest rates to over 12 percent, more than double the inflation rate. The bank also stepped up its intervention in the currency exchange markets, selling dollars and purchasing won in an attempt to keep the exchange rate above won 1,000 = $1. The main effect of this action, however, was to rapidly deplete South Korea's foreign exchange reserves. These stood at $30 billion on November 1, but fell to only $15 billion two weeks later. With its foreign exchange reserves almost exhausted, the South Korean central bank gave up its defense of the won November 17. Immediately, the price of won in dollars plunged to around won 1,500=$1, effectively increasing by 60 to 70 percent the amount of won heavily indebted Korean companies had to pay to meet scheduled payments on their dollar-denominated debt. These losses, due to adverse changes in foreign exchange rates, depressed the profits of many firms. South Korean firms suffered foreign exchange losses of more than $15 billion in 1997.

Sources: J. Burton and G. Baker, "The Country That Invested Its Way into Trouble," *Financial Times,* January 15, 1998, p. 8; J. Burton, "South Korea's Credit Rating is Lowered," *Financial Times,* October 25, 1997, p. 3; J. Burton, "Currency Losses Hit Samsung Electronics," *Financial Times,* March 20, 1998, p. 24; and "Korean Firms' Foreign Exchange Losses Exceed US $15 Billion," *Business Korea,* February 1998, p. 55.

Approaches to Forecasting

Assuming the inefficient market school is correct that the foreign exchange market's estimate of future spot rates can be improved, on what basis should forecasts be prepared? Here again, there are two schools of thought. One adheres to fundamental analysis, while the other uses technical analysis.

Fundamental Analysis

Fundamental analysis draws on economic theory to construct sophisticated econometric models for predicting exchange rate movements. The variables contained in these models typically include those we have discussed, such as relative money supply growth rates, inflation rates, and interest rates. In addition, they may include variables related to balance-of-payments positions.

Running a deficit on a balance-of-payments current account (a country is importing more goods and services than it is exporting), creates pressures that result in the depreciation of the country's currency on the foreign exchange market.[21] (For background on the balance of payments, see Chapter 6.) Consider what might happen if the United States was running a persistent current account balance-of-payments deficit. Since the United States would be importing more than it was exporting, people in other countries would be increasing their holdings of U.S. dollars. If these people were willing to hold their dollars, the dollar's exchange rate would not be influenced. However, if these people converted their dollars into other currencies, the supply of dollars in the foreign exchange market would increase (as would demand for the other currencies). This shift in demand and supply would create pressures that could lead to the depreciation of the dollar against other currencies.

This argument hinges on whether people in other countries are willing to hold dollars. This depends on such factors as U.S. interest rates, the return on holding other dollar-denominated assets such as stocks in U.S. companies, and inflation rates. So, in a sense, the balance-of-payments position is not a fundamental predictor of future exchange rate movements. For example, between 1998 and 2001, the U.S. dollar appreciated against most major currencies despite a growing balance-of-payments deficit. Relatively high real interest rates in the United States, coupled with a booming U.S. stock market that attracted inward investment from foreign capital, made the dollar very attractive to foreigners, so they did not convert their dollars into other currencies. On the contrary, they converted other currencies into dollars to invest in U.S. financial assets, such as bonds and stocks, because they believed they could earn a high return by doing so. Capital flows into the United States fueled by foreigners who wanted to buy U.S. stocks and bonds kept the dollar strong. But what makes financial assets such as stocks and bonds attractive? The answer is prevailing interest rates and inflation rates, both of which affect underlying economic growth and the real return to holding U.S. financial assets. Given this, we are back to the argument that the fundamental determinants of exchange rates are monetary growth, inflation rates, and interest rates.

Technical Analysis

Technical analysis uses price and volume data to determine past trends, which are expected to continue into the future. This approach does not rely on a consideration of economic fundamentals. Technical analysis is based on the premise that there are analyzable market trends and waves and that previous trends and waves can be used to predict future trends and waves. Since there is no theoretical rationale for this assumption of predictability, many economists compare technical analysis to fortune-telling. Despite this skepticism, technical analysis has gained favor in recent years.[22]

Currency Convertibility

Until this point we have assumed that the currencies of various countries are freely convertible into other currencies. This assumption is invalid. Many countries restrict the ability of residents and nonresidents to convert the local currency into a foreign currency, making international trade and investment more difficult. Many international businesses have used "countertrade" practices to circumvent problems that arise when a currency is not freely convertible.

Convertibility and Government Policy

Due to government restrictions, a significant number of currencies are not freely convertible into other currencies. A country's currency is said to be **freely convertible** when the country's government allows both residents and nonresidents to purchase unlimited amounts of a foreign currency with it. A currency is said to be **externally**

convertible when only nonresidents may convert it into a foreign currency without any limitations. A currency is **nonconvertible** when neither residents nor nonresidents are allowed to convert it into a foreign currency.

Free convertibility is far from universal. Many countries place some restrictions on their residents' ability to convert the domestic currency into a foreign currency (a policy of external convertibility). Restrictions range from the relatively minor (such as restricting the amount of foreign currency they may take with them out of the country on trips) to the major (such as restricting domestic businesses' ability to take foreign currency out of the country). External convertibility restrictions can limit domestic companies' ability to invest abroad, but they present few problems for foreign companies wishing to do business in that country. For example, even if the Japanese government tightly controlled the ability of its residents to convert the yen into U.S. dollars, all U.S. businesses with deposits in Japanese banks may at any time convert all their yen into dollars and take them out of the country. Thus, a U.S. company with a subsidiary in Japan is assured that it will be able to convert the profits from its Japanese operation into dollars and take them out of the country.

Serious problems arise, however, under a policy of nonconvertibility. This was the practice of the former Soviet Union, and it continued to be the practice in Russia until recently. When strictly applied, nonconvertibility means that although a U.S. company doing business in a country such as Russia may be able to generate significant ruble profits, it may not convert those rubles into dollars and take them out of the country. Obviously this is not desirable for international business.

Governments limit convertibility to preserve their foreign exchange reserves. A country needs an adequate supply of these reserves to service its international debt commitments and to purchase imports. Governments typically impose convertibility restrictions on their currency when they fear that free convertibility will lead to a run on their foreign exchange reserves. This occurs when residents and nonresidents rush to convert their holdings of domestic currency into a foreign currency—a phenomenon generally referred to as **capital flight**. Capital flight is most likely to occur when the value of the domestic currency is depreciating rapidly because of hyperinflation, or when a country's economic prospects are shaky in other respects. Under such circumstances, both residents and nonresidents tend to believe that their money is more likely to hold its value if it is converted into a foreign currency and invested abroad. Not only will a run on foreign exchange reserves limit the country's ability to service its international debt and pay for imports, but it will also lead to a precipitous depreciation in the exchange rate as residents and nonresidents unload their holdings of domestic currency on the foreign exchange markets (thereby increasing the market supply of the country's currency). Governments fear that the rise in import prices resulting from currency depreciation will lead to further increases in inflation. This fear provides another rationale for limiting convertibility.

Countertrade

Companies can deal with the nonconvertibility problem by engaging in countertrade. Countertrade is discussed in detail in Chapter 15, so we will merely introduce the concept here. Countertrade refers to a range of barterlike agreements by which goods and services can be traded for other goods and services. Countertrade can make sense when a country's currency is nonconvertible. For example, consider the deal that General Electric struck with the Romanian government in 1984, when that country's currency was nonconvertible. When General Electric won a contract for a $150 million generator project in Romania, it agreed to take payment in the form of Romanian goods that could be sold for $150 million on international markets. In a similar case, the Venezuelan government negotiated a contract with Caterpillar in 1986 under which Venezuela would trade 350,000 tons of iron ore for Caterpillar heavy construction equipment. Caterpillar subsequently traded the iron ore to Romania in exchange for Romanian farm products, which it then sold on international markets for dollars.[23]

How important is countertrade? One estimate is that 20 to 30 percent of world trade in 1985 involved some form of countertrade agreements. Since then, however, more currencies have become freely convertible, and the percentage of world trade that involves countertrade has fallen to between 10 percent and 20 percent.[24]

Focus On Managerial Implications

This chapter contains a number of clear implications for business. First, it is critical that international businesses understand the influence of exchange rates on the profitability of trade and investment deals. Adverse changes in exchange rates can make apparently profitable deals unprofitable. The risk introduced into international business transactions by changes in exchange rates is referred to as foreign exchange risk.

Means of hedging against foreign exchange risk are available. Forward exchange rates and currency swaps allow companies to insure against this risk.

International businesses must also understand the forces that determine exchange rates. This is particularly true in light of the increasing evidence that forward exchange rates are not unbiased predictors. If a company wants to know how the value of a particular currency is likely to change over the long term on the foreign exchange market, it should look closely at those economic fundamentals that appear to predict long-run exchange rate movements (i.e., the growth in a country's money supply, its inflation rate, and its nominal interest rates). For example, an international business should be very cautious about trading with or investing in a country with a recent history of rapid growth in its domestic money supply. The upsurge in inflation that is likely to follow such rapid monetary growth could lead to a sharp drop in the value of the country's currency on the foreign exchange market, which could transform a profitable deal into an unprofitable one. This is not to say that an international business should not trade with or invest in such a country. Rather, it means an international business should take some precautions before doing so, such as buying currency forward on the foreign exchange market or structuring the deal around a countertrade arrangement.

Complicating this picture is the issue of currency convertibility. The proclivity that many governments seem to have to restrict currency convertibility suggests that the foreign exchange market does not always provide the lubricant necessary to make international trade and investment possible. Given this, international businesses need to explore alternative mechanisms for facilitating international trade and investment that do not involve currency conversion. Countertrade seems the obvious mechanism. We return to the topic of countertrade and discuss it in depth in Chapter 15.

Chapter Summary

This chapter explained how the foreign exchange market works, examined the forces that determine exchange rates, and then discussed the implications of these factors for international business. Given that changes in exchange rates can dramatically alter the profitability of foreign trade and investment deals, this is an area of major interest to international business. The chapter made these major points:

1. One function of the foreign exchange market is to convert the currency of one country into the currency of another.

2. International businesses participate in the foreign exchange market to facilitate international trade and investment, to invest spare cash in short-term money market accounts abroad, and to engage in currency speculation.

3. A second function of the foreign exchange market is to provide insurance against foreign exchange risk.

4. The spot exchange rate is the exchange rate at which a dealer converts one currency into another currency on a particular day.

5. Foreign exchange risk can be reduced by using forward exchange rates. A forward exchange rate is an exchange rate governing future transactions.

6. Foreign exchange risk can also be reduced by engaging in currency swaps. A swap is the simultaneous purchase and sale of a given amount of foreign exchange for two different value dates.

7. The law of one price holds that in competitive markets that are free of transportation costs and barriers to trade, identical products sold in different countries must sell for the same price when their price is expressed in the same currency.

8. Purchasing power parity (PPP) theory states the price of a basket of particular goods should be roughly equivalent in each country. PPP theory predicts that the exchange rate will change if relative prices change.

9. The rate of change in countries' relative prices depends on their relative inflation rates. A country's inflation rate seems to be a function of the growth in its money supply.

10. The PPP theory of exchange rate changes yields relatively accurate predictions of long-term trends in exchange rates, but not of short-term movements. The failure of PPP theory to predict exchange rate changes more accurately may be due to the existence of transportation costs, barriers to trade and investment, and the impact of psychological factors such as bandwagon effects on market movements and short-run exchange rates.

11. Interest rates reflect expectations about inflation. In countries where inflation is expected to be high, interest rates also will be high.

12. The International Fisher Effect states that for any two countries, the spot exchange rate should change in an equal amount but in the opposite direction to the difference in nominal interest rates.

13. The most common approach to exchange rate forecasting is fundamental analysis. This relies on variables such as money supply growth, inflation rates, nominal interest rates, and balance-of-payments positions to predict future changes in exchange rates.

14. In many countries, the ability of residents and nonresidents to convert local currency into a foreign currency is restricted by government policy. A government restricts the convertibility of its currency to protect the country's foreign exchange reserves and to halt any capital flight.

15. Particularly bothersome for international business is a policy of nonconvertibility, which prohibits residents and nonresidents from exchanging local currency for foreign currency. A policy of nonconvertibility makes it very difficult to engage in international trade and investment in the country.

16. One way of coping with the nonconvertibility problem is to engage in countertrade—to trade goods and services for other goods and services.

Critical Discussion Questions

1. The interest rate on South Korean government securities with one-year maturity is 4 percent, and the expected inflation rate for the coming year is 2 percent. The interest rate on U.S. government securities with one-year maturity is 7 percent, and the expected rate of inflation is 5 percent. The current spot exchange rate for Korean won is $1 = W1,200. Forecast the spot exchange rate one year from today. Explain the logic of your answer.

2. Two countries, Great Britain and the United States, produce just one good: beef. Suppose the price of beef in the United States is $2.80 per pound and in Britain it is £3.70 per pound.

   a. According to PPP theory, what should the $/£ spot exchange rate be?

   b. Suppose the price of beef is expected to rise to $3.10 in the United States and to £4.65 in Britain. What should the one-year forward $/£ exchange rate be?

   c. Given your answers to parts a and b, and given that the current interest rate in the United States is 10 percent, what would you expect the current interest rate to be in Britain?

3. You manufacture wine goblets. In mid-June you receive an order for 10,000 goblets from Japan. Payment of ¥400,000 is due in mid-December.

You expect the yen to rise from its present rate of $1 = ¥130 to $1 = ¥100 by December. You can borrow yen at 6 percent a year. What should you do?

Notes

1. For a good general introduction to the foreign exchange market, see R. Weisweiller, *How the Foreign Exchange Market Works* (New York: New York Institute of Finance, 1990). A detailed description of the economics of foreign exchange markets can be found in P. R. Krugman and M. Obstfeld, *International Economics: Theory and Policy* (New York: HarperCollins, 1994).

2. Bank for International Settlements, *Central Bank Survey of Foreign Exchange and Derivatives Market Activity, April 2001* (Basle: Switzerland: BIS, 2002).

3. Ibid.

4. Ibid.

5. For a comprehensive review see M. Taylor, "The Economics of Exchange Rates," *Journal of Economic Literature* 33 (1995), pp. 13–47.

6. Krugman and Obstfeld, *International Economics: Theory and Policy*

7. M. Friedman, *Studies in the Quantity Theory of Money* (Chicago: University of Chicago Press, 1956). For an accessible explanation, see M. Friedman and R. Friedman, *Free to Choose* (London: Penguin Books, 1979), chap. 9.

8. Juan-Antino Morales, "Inflation Stabilization in Bolivia," in *Inflation Stabilization: The Experience of Israel, Argentina, Brazil, Bolivia, and Mexico*, ed. Michael Bruno et al. (Cambridge, MA: MIT Press, 1988); and The Economist, *World Book of Vital Statistics* (New York: Random House, 1990).

9. For reviews and recent articles, see L. H. Officer, "The Purchasing Power Parity Theory of Exchange Rates: A Review Article," International Monetary Fund Staff Papers, March 1976, pp. 1–60; Taylor, "The Economics of Exchange Rates"; H. J. Edison, J. E. Gagnon, and W. R. Melick, "Understanding the Empirical Literature on Purchasing Power Parity," *Journal of International Money and Finance* 16 (February 1997), pp. 1–18; J. R. Edison, "Multi-Country Evidence on the Behavior of Purchasing Power Parity under the Current Float," *Journal of International Money and Finance* 16 (February 1997), pp. 19–36; K. Rogoff, "The Purchasing Power Parity Puzzle," *Journal of Economic Literature* 34 (1996), pp. 647–68; and D. R. Rapach and M. E. Wohar, "Testing the Monetary Model of Exchange Rate Determination: New Evidence from a Century of Data," *Journal of International Economics*, December 2002, pp. 359–85.

10. M. Obstfeld and K. Rogoff, "The Six Major Puzzles in International Economics," National Bureau of Economic Research Working Paper 7777, July 2000.

11. Ibid.

12. See M. Devereux and C. Engel, "Monetary Policy in the Open Economy Revisited: Price Setting and Exchange Rate Flexibility," National Bureau of Economic Research Working Paper 7665, April 2000. Also P. Krugman, "Pricing to Market When the Exchange Rate Changes," in *Real Financial Economics*, ed. S. Arndt and J. Richardson, (Cambridge, MA: MIT Press, 1987).

13. For a summary of the evidence, see the survey by Taylor, "The Economics of Exchange Rates."

14. R. E. Cumby and M. Obstfeld, "A Note on Exchange Rate Expectations and Nominal Interest Differentials: A Test of the Fisher Hypothesis," *Journal of Finance*, June 1981, pp. 697–703.

15. Taylor, "The Economics of Exchange Rates." See also R. K. Lyons, *The Microstructure Approach to Exchange Rates* (Cambridge, MA: MIT Press, 2002).

16. See H. L. Allen and M. P. Taylor, "Charts, Noise, and Fundamentals in the Foreign Exchange Market," *Economic Journal* 100 (1990), pp. 49–59, and T. Ito, "Foreign Exchange Rate Expectations: Micro Survey Data," *American Economic Review* 80 (1990), pp. 434–49.

17. For example, see E. Fama, "Forward Rates as Predictors of Future Spot Rates," *Journal of Financial Economics*, October 1976, pp. 361–77.

18. R. M. Levich, "The Efficiency of Markets for Foreign Exchange," in *International Finance*, ed. G. D. Gay and R. W. Kold (Richmond, VA: Robert F. Dane, Inc., 1983).

19. J. Williamson, *The Exchange Rate System* (Washington, DC: Institute for International Economics, 1983).

20. R. M. Levich, "Currency Forecasters Lose Their Way," *Euromoney*, August 1983, p. 140.

21. Rogoff, "The Purchasing Power Parity Puzzle."

22. C. Engel and J. D. Hamilton, "Long Swings in the Dollar: Are They in the Data and Do Markets Know It?" *American Economic Review*, September 1990, pp. 689–713.

23. J. R. Carter and J. Gagne, "The Do's and Don'ts of International Countertrade," *Sloan Management Review*, Spring 1988, pp. 31–37.

24. D. S. Levine, "Got a Spare Destroyer Lying Around?" *World Trade* 10 (June 1997), pp. 34–35, and Dan West, "Countertrade," *Business Credit*, April 2001, pp. 64–67.

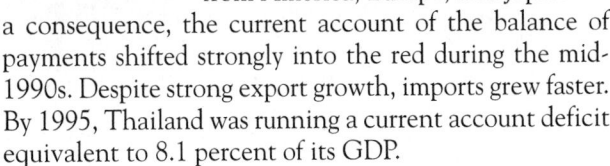

Research Task | globalEDGE™ globaledge.msu.edu

Use the globalEDGE™ site to complete the following exercises:

1. You are assigned the duty of ensuring the availability of 100,000 yen for the payment that is scheduled for next month. Considering that your company possesses only U.S. dollars, identify the spot and forward exchange rates. What are the factors that affect your decision of utilizing spot versus forward exchange rates? Which one would you choose? How many dollars do you have to spend to acquire the amount of yen required?

2. The Big Mac Index compares the purchasing-power parity of 120 countries based on the price of an identical item. Locate the latest edition of this index. Identify the five countries (and the currencies) with the lowest purchasing power parity according to this classification. Which currencies, if any, are overvalued?

Closing Case

The Collapse of the Thai Baht in 1997

During the 1980s and 1990s, Thailand emerged as one of Asia's most dynamic tiger economies. From 1985 to 1995, Thailand achieved an annual average economic growth rate of 8.4 percent, while keeping its annual inflation rate at only 5 percent (comparable figures for the United States over this period were 1.3 percent for economic growth and 3.2 percent for inflation). Much of Thailand's economic growth was powered by exports. From 1990 to 1996, for example, the value of exports from Thailand grew by 16 percent per year compounded. The wealth created by export-led growth fueled an investment boom in commercial and residential property, industrial assets, and infrastructure. As demand for property increased, the value of commercial and residential real estate in Bangkok soared. This fed a building boom the likes of which had never been seen in Thailand. Office and apartment buildings were going up all over the city. Heavy borrowing from banks financed much of this construction, but as long as property values continued to rise, the banks were happy to lend to property companies.

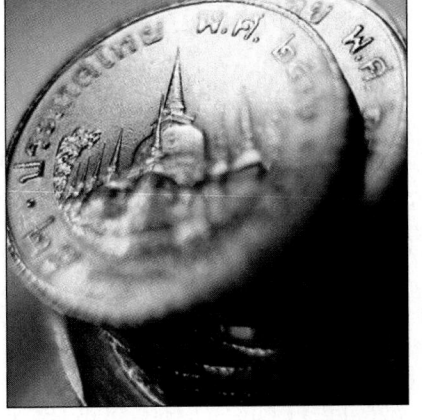

By early 1997, however, it was clear that the boom had produced excess capacity in residential and commercial property. An estimated 365,000 apartment units were unoccupied in Bangkok in late 1996. With another 100,000 units scheduled to be completed in 1997, years of excess demand in the Thai property market had been replaced by excess supply. By one estimate, Bangkok's building boom by 1997 had produced enough excess space to meet its residential and commercial needs for at least five years. At the same time, Thailand's investments in infrastructure, industrial capacity, and commercial real estate were sucking in foreign goods at unprecedented rates. To build infrastructure, factories, and office buildings, Thailand was purchasing capital equipment and materials from America, Europe, and Japan. As a consequence, the current account of the balance of payments shifted strongly into the red during the mid-1990s. Despite strong export growth, imports grew faster. By 1995, Thailand was running a current account deficit equivalent to 8.1 percent of its GDP.

Things started to fall apart February 5, 1997, when Somprasong Land, a Thai property developer, announced it had failed to make a scheduled $3.1 million interest payment on an $80 billion eurobond loan, effectively entering into default. Somprasong Land was the first victim of speculative overbuilding in the Bangkok property market. The Thai stock market had already declined by 45 percent since its high in early 1996, primarily on concerns that several property companies might be forced into bankruptcy. Now one had been. The stock market fell another 2.7 percent on the news, but it was only the beginning. In the aftermath of Somprasong's default, it became clear that, along with several other property developers, many of the country's financial institutions, including Finance One, were also on the brink of default. Finance One, the country's largest financial institution, had pioneered a practice that had become widespread among Thai institutions—issuing bonds denominated in U.S. dollars and using the proceeds to finance lending to the country's booming property developers. In theory, this practice made sense because Finance One was able to exploit the interest rate differential between dollar-denominated debt and Thai debt (i.e., Finance One borrowed in U.S. dollars at a low interest rate and lent in Thai baht at high interest rates). The only problem with this financing strategy was that when the Thai property market began to unravel in 1996 and 1997, the property developers could no longer pay back the cash they had borrowed from Finance One. This made it difficult for Finance One to pay back its creditors. As the effects of overbuilding became evident in 1996, Finance One's nonperforming loans doubled, then doubled again in the first quarter of 1997.

In February 1997, trading in the shares of Finance One was suspended while the government tried to arrange for the troubled company to be acquired by a small Thai bank in a deal sponsored by the Thai central bank. It didn't work, and when trading resumed in Finance One shares in May, they fell 70 percent in a single day. By this time bad loans in the Thai property market were swelling daily and had risen to more than $30 billion. Finance One was bankrupt, and it was feared that others would follow.

It was at this point that currency traders began a concerted attack on the Thai currency. For the previous 13 years, the Thai baht had been pegged to the U.S. dollar at an exchange rate of about $1=Bt25. This peg, however, had become increasingly difficult to defend. Currency traders, looking at Thailand's growing current account deficit and dollar-denominated debt burden, reasoned that demand for dollars in Thailand would rise while demand for baht would fall. (Businesses and financial institutions would be exchanging baht for dollars to service their debt payments and purchase imports.) There were several attempts to force a devaluation of the baht in late 1996 and early 1997. These speculative attacks typically involved traders selling baht short to profit from a future decline in the

value of the baht against the dollar. In this context, short selling involves a currency trader borrowing baht from a financial institution and immediately reselling those baht in the foreign exchange market for dollars. The theory is that if the value of the baht subsequently falls against the dollar, then when the trader has to buy the baht back to repay the financial institution, it will cost her fewer dollars than she received from the initial sale of baht. For example, a trader might borrow Bt100 from a bank for six months. The trader then exchanges the Bt100 for $4 (at an exchange rate of $1=Bt25). If the exchange rate subsequently declines to $1=Bt50, it will cost the trader only $2 to repurchase the Bt100 in six months and pay back the bank, leaving the trader with a 100 percent profit!

In May 1997, short sellers were swarming over the Thai baht. In an attempt to defend the peg, the Thai government used its foreign exchange reserves (which were denominated in U.S. dollars) to purchase baht. It cost the Thai government $5 billion to defend the baht, which reduced its "officially reported" foreign exchange reserves to a two-year low of $33 billion. In addition, the Thai government raised key interest rates from 10 percent to 12.5 percent to make holding baht more attractive, but because this also raised corporate borrowing costs it exacerbated the debt crisis. What the world financial community did not know at this point, was that with the blessing of his superiors, a foreign exchange trader at the Thai central bank had locked up most of Thailand's foreign exchange reserves in forward contracts. The reality was that Thailand had only $1.14 billion in available foreign exchange reserves left to defend the dollar peg. Defending the peg was now impossible.

On July 2, 1997, the Thai government bowed to the inevitable and announced it would allow the baht to float freely against the dollar. The baht immediately lost 18 percent of its value and started a slide that would bring the exchange rate down to $1=Bt55 by January 1998. As the baht declined, the Thai debt bomb exploded. A 50 percent decline in the value of the baht against the dollar doubled the amount of baht required to serve the dollar-denominated debt commitments taken on by Thai financial institutions and businesses. This made more bankruptcies and further pushed down the battered Thai stock market. The Thailand Set stock market index ultimately declined from 787 in January 1997 to a low of 337 in December of that year, and this on top of a 45 percent decline in 1996!

Sources: "Bitter Pill for the Thais," *Straits Times*, July 5, 1997, p. 46; World Bank, *1997 World Development Report* (New York: World Bank, 1997), Table 2; T. Bardacke, "Somprasong Defaults on $80 Million Eurobond," *Financial Times*, February 6, 1997, p. 25; and T. Bardacke, "The Day the Miracle Came to an End," *Financial Times*, January 12, 1998, pp. 6–7.

Case Discussion Questions

1. Identify the main factors that led to the collapse of the Thai baht in 1997.

2. Do you think the sudden collapse of the Thai baht can be explained by the purchasing power parity theorem?

3. What role did speculators play in the fall of the Thai baht? Did they cause its fall?

4. What steps might the Thai government have taken to preempt the financial crisis that swept the nation in 1997?

5. How will the collapse of the Thai baht affect businesses in Thailand, particularly those that purchase inputs from abroad or export finished products?

6. Do you notice any similarities between the collapse of the Thai baht in 1997 and the collapse of the Korean won around the same time (see the Country Focus in this chapter)? What are these similarities? Do you think these two events were related? How?

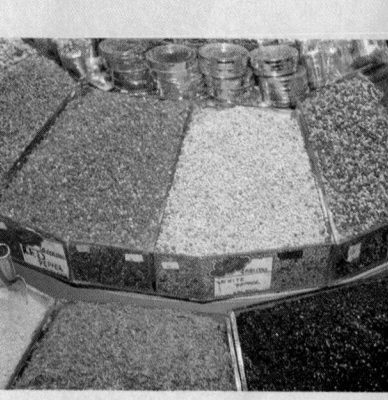

MONEDA	COTIZACIONE
DOLAR Ef	COMPRA
DOLAR Ch.	4600
PESO ARGENTINO	4560
REAL	3000
PESO URUGUAYO	1770
MARCO	333
FRANCO SUIZO	1956
FRANCO FRANCE	2612
LIBRA	583
	6061

The International Monetary System

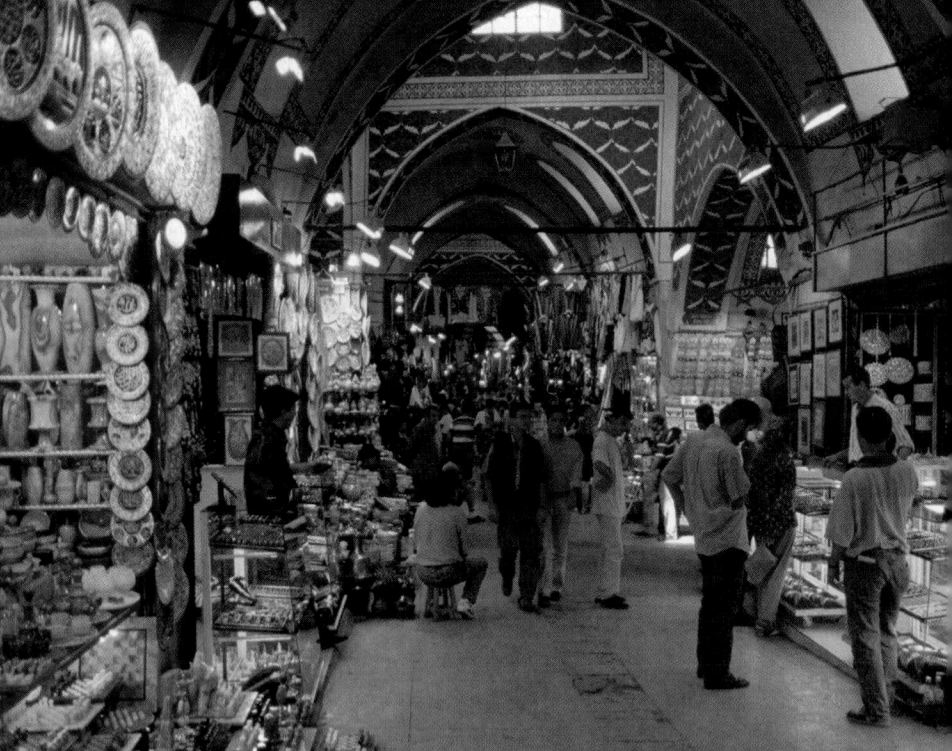

Introduction
The Gold Standard
  Mechanics of the Gold Standard
  Strength of the Gold Standard
  The Period between the Wars,
  1918–1939
The Bretton Woods System
  The Role of the IMF
  The Role of the World Bank
The Collapse of the Fixed Exchange Rate
System
The Floating Exchange Rate Regime
  The Jamaica Agreement
  Exchange Rates since 1973
Fixed versus Floating Exchange Rates
  The Case for Floating Exchange Rates
  The Case for Fixed Exchange Rates
  Who Is Right?
Exchange Rate Regimes in Practice
  Pegged Exchange Rates
  Currency Boards
  Target Zones: The European Monetary
  System in Retrospect
Crisis Management by the IMF
  Financial Crises in the Post–Bretton
  Woods Era
  Mexican Currency Crisis of 1995
  Russian Ruble Crisis
  The Asian Crisis
  Evaluating the IMF's Policy
  Prescriptions
Focus on Managerial Implications
  Currency Management
  Business Strategy
  Corporate–Government Relations
Chapter Summary
Critical Discussion Questions
Closing Case: The Tragedy of the Congo
(Zaire)

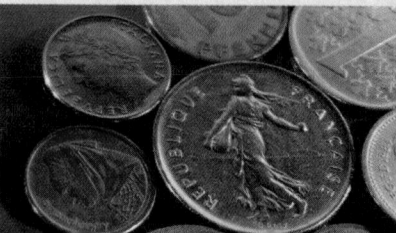

Turkey's 18th IMF Program

In May 2001, the International Monetary Fund (IMF) agreed to lend $8 billion to Turkey to help the country stabilize its economy and halt a sharp slide in the value of its currency. This was the third time in two years that the international lending institution had put together a loan program for Turkey, and it was the 18th program since Turkey became a member of the IMF in 1958.

Many of Turkey's problems stemmed from a large and inefficient state sector and heavy subsidies to various private sectors of the economy such as agriculture. Although the Turkish government started to privatize state-owned companies in the late 1980s, the programs proceeded at a glacial pace, hamstrung by political opposition within Turkey. Instead of selling state-owned assets to private investors, successive governments increased support to unprofitable state-owned industries and raised the wage rates of state employees. Nor did the government cut subsidies to politically powerful private sectors of the economy, such as agriculture. To support state industries and finance subsidies, Turkey issued significant amounts of government debt. To limit the amount of debt, the government simply expanded the money supply to finance spending. The result, predictably, was rampant inflation and high interest rates. During the 1990s, inflation averaged over 80 percent a year while real interest rates rose to more than 50 percent on a number of occasions. Despite this, the Turkish economy continued to grow at a healthy pace of 6 percent annually in real terms, a remarkable achievement given the high inflation rates and interest rates.

By the late 1990s, however, the "Turkish miracle" of sustained growth in the face of high inflation and interest rates was running out of steam. Government debt had risen to 60 percent of gross domestic product, government borrowing was leaving little capital for private enterprises, and the cost of financing government debt was spiraling out of control. Rampant inflation was putting pressure on the Turkish currency, the lira, which at the time was pegged in value to a basket of other currencies. Realizing that it needed to drastically reform its economy, the Turkish government sat down with the IMF in late 1999 to work out a recovery program, adopted in January 2000.

As with most IMF programs, the focus was on bringing down the inflation rate, stabilizing the value of the Turkish currency, and restructuring the economy to reduce government debt. The Turkish government committed itself to reducing government debt by taking a number of steps. These included an accelerated privatization program, using the proceeds to pay down debt; the reduction of agricultural subsidies; reform to make it more difficult

for people to qualify for public pension programs; and tax increases. The government also agreed to rein in the growth in the money supply to better control inflation. To limit the possibility of speculative attacks on the Turkish currency in the foreign exchange markets, the Turkish government and IMF announced that Turkey would peg the value of the lira against a basket of currencies and devalue the lira by a predetermined amount each month throughout 2000, bringing the total devaluation for the year to 25 percent. To ease the pain, the IMF agreed to provide the Turkish government with $5 billion in loans that could be used to support the value of the lira.

Initially the program seemed to be working. Inflation fell to 35 percent in 2000, while the economy grew by 6 percent. By the end of 2000, however, the program was in trouble. Burdened with nonperforming loans, a number of Turkish banks faced default and had been taken into public ownership by the government. When a criminal fraud investigation uncovered evidence that several of these banks had been pressured by politicians into providing loans at below-market interest rates, foreign investors, worried that more banks might be involved, started to pull their money out of Turkey. This sent the Turkish stock market into a tailspin and put enormous pressure on the Turkish lira as foreign investors took their money out of the country. The government raised Turkish overnight interbank lending rates to as high as 1,950 percent to try to stem the outflow of capital, but it was clear that Turkey alone could not halt the flow.

The IMF stepped once more into the breach, December 6, 2000, announcing a quickly arranged $7.5 billion loan program for the country. In return for the loan, the IMF required the Turkish government to close 10 insolvent banks, speed up its privatization plans (which had once more stalled), and cap any pay increases for government workers. The IMF also reportedly urged the Turkish government to let its currency float freely in the foreign exchange markets, but the government refused, arguing that the result would be a rapid devaluation in the lira, which would raise import prices and fuel price inflation. The government insisted that reducing inflation should be its first priority.

This plan started to come apart in February 2001. A surge in inflation and a rapid slowdown in economic growth once more spooked foreign investors. Into this explosive mix waded Turkey's prime minister and president, who engaged in a highly public argument about economic policy and political corruption. This triggered a rapid outflow of capital. The government raised the overnight interbank lending rate to 7,500 percent to try to persuade foreigners to leave their money in the country, but to no avail. Realizing that it would be unable to keep the lira within its planned monthly devaluation range without raising interest rates to absurd levels or seriously depleting the country's foreign exchange reserves, on February 23, 2001, the Turkish government decided to let the lira float freely. The lira immediately dropped 50 percent in value against the U.S. dollar, but ended the day down some 28 percent.

Over the next two months, the Turkish economy continued to weaken as a global economic slowdown affected the nation. Inflation stayed high, and progress at reforming the country's economy remained bogged down by political considerations. By early April, the lira had fallen 40 percent against the dollar since February 23, and the country was teetering on the brink of an economic meltdown. For the third time in 18 months, the IMF stepped in, arranging for another $8 billion in loans. Once more, the IMF insisted that the Turkish government accelerate privatization, close insolvent banks, deregulate its market, and cut government spending. Critics of the IMF, however, claimed this "austerity program" would only slow the Turkish economy and make matters worse, not better. These critics advocated a mix of sound monetary policy and tax cuts to boost Turkey's economic growth.

By 2003, some progress had been made, but it was halting at best. Inflation had fallen from a peak of 68.5 percent in December 2000 to about 30 percent in December 2002, but that was still too high to maintain the value of the lira on foreign exchange markets. The Turkish government had failed to fully comply with IMF mandates on economic policy, causing the institution to hold back a scheduled $1.6 billion in IMF loans until the government passed an "austerity budget," which it did reluctantly in March 2003 after months of public hand-wringing. The slow progress in reforming the economy was causing many to wonder how long it would be before Turkey applied for its 19th IMF loan program.

Sources: P. Blustein, "Turkish Crisis Weakens the Case for Intervention," *Washington Post,* March 2, 2001, p. E1; H. Pope, "Can Turkey Finally Mend Its Economy?" *Wall Street Journal,* May 22, 2001, p. A18; "Turkish Bath," *Wall Street Journal,* February 23, 2001, p. A14; E. McBride, "Turkey—Fingers Crossed," *The Economist,* June 10, 2000, p. SS16–SS17; "Turkey and the IMF," *The Economist,* December 9, 2000, pp. 81–82; G. Chazan, "Turkey's Decision on Aid Is Sinking In," *Wall Street Journal,* March 6, 2003, p. A11.

Introduction

The **international monetary system** refers to the institutional arrangements that countries adopt to govern exchange rates. In Chapter 9 we assumed the foreign exchange market was the primary institution for determining exchange rates and the impersonal market forces of demand and supply determined the relative value of any two currencies (i.e., their exchange rate). Furthermore, we explained that the demand and supply of currencies is influenced by their respective countries' relative inflation rates and interest rates. When the foreign exchange market determines the relative value of a currency, we say that the country is adhering to a **floating exchange rate** regime. The world's four major trading currencies—the U.S. dollar, the European Union's euro, the Japanese yen, and the British pound—are all free to float against each other. Thus, their exchange rates are determined by market forces and fluctuate against each other on a day-to-day, if not minute-to-minute, basis. However, the exchange rates of many currencies are not determined by the free play of market forces; other institutional arrangements are adopted.

The opening case, for example, explained that, until recently, the value of the Turkish lira was pegged to a basket of currencies. Many of the world's smaller nations peg their currencies, primarily to the dollar or the euro. A **pegged exchange rate** means the value of the currency is fixed relative to a reference currency, such as the U.S. dollar, and then the exchange rate between that currency and other currencies is determined by the reference currency exchange rate. Thus, Belize pegs its currency to the dollar, and the exchange rate between the Belizean currency and the euro is determined by the U.S. dollar/euro exchange rate.

Other countries, while not adopting a formal pegged rate, try to hold the value of their currency within some range against an important reference currency such as the U.S. dollar. This is often referred to as a **dirty float.** It is a float because in theory, the value of the currency is determined by market forces, but it is a dirty float (as opposed to a clean float) because the central bank of a country will intervene in the foreign exchange market to try to maintain the value of its currency if it depreciates too rapidly against an important reference currency.

Still other countries have operated with a **fixed exchange rate,** in which the values of a set of currencies are fixed against each other at some mutually agreed on exchange rate. Before the introduction of the euro in 2000, several member states of the European Union operated with fixed exchange rates within the context of the European Monetary System (EMS). For a quarter of a century after World War II, the world's major industrial nations participated in a fixed exchange rate system. Although this system collapsed in 1973, some still argue that the world should attempt to reimpose it.

Pegged exchange rates, dirty floats, and fixed exchange rates all require some degree of government intervention in the foreign exchange market to maintain the value of a currency. A currency may come under pressure when there are significant economic problems in the nation. In the case of Turkey, for example, these included high inflation, excessive government debt, and a crisis in the banking system, all of which led foreign investors to take capital out of the country. As they did, the value of the Turkish currency plunged on foreign exchange markets. A government can try to maintain the value of its currency by using foreign currency held in reserve (foreign exchange reserves) to buy its currency in the market, thereby increasing demand for the currency and raising its price. Thus, as the Turkish lira began to depreciate rapidly in late 2000, the Turkish central bank entered the foreign exchange market, using foreign currency it held in reserve, such as U.S. dollars, Japanese yen, and euros, to purchase lira in an attempt to halt the depreciation in the exchange rate. However, because governments may not have sufficient foreign exchange reserves to defend the value of their currency, they sometimes call on a powerful multinational institution, the International Monetary Fund (IMF), for loans to help them do this. The IMF is another important player in the international monetary system. As we saw in the opening case, the IMF does not simply lend money to a country in trouble. In exchange for the loan, it requires that the government adopt policies designed to correct whatever economic problems caused the depreciation in the nation's currency. Thus, the IMF insisted that Turkey take steps to reduce its inflation rate and government debt and to resolve problems in the country's banking system.

In this chapter, we will explain how the international monetary system works and point out its implications for international business. To understand how the system works, we must review its evolution. We will begin with a discussion of the gold standard and its breakup during the 1930s. Then we will discuss the 1944 Bretton Woods conference. This established the basic framework for the post–World War II international monetary system. The Bretton Woods system called for fixed exchange rates against the U.S. dollar. Under this fixed exchange rate system, the value of most currencies in terms of U.S. dollars was fixed for long periods and allowed to change only under a specific set of circumstances. The Bretton Woods conference also created two major international institutions that play a role in the international monetary system—the International Monetary Fund (IMF) and the World Bank. The IMF was given the task of maintaining order in the international monetary system; the World Bank's role was to promote development.

Today, both these institutions continue to play major roles in the world economy. In 1997 and 1998, for example, the IMF helped several Asian countries deal with the dramatic decline in the value of their currencies that occurred during the Asian financial crisis that started in 1997. By 2002, the IMF had programs in 88 countries, the majority in the developing world, and had committed some $88 billion in loans to these nations.[1] However, debate is growing about the role of the IMF and to a lesser extent the World Bank and the appropriateness of their policies for many developing nations. In the case of Turkey, several prominent critics claim that IMF policy might make things worse, not better, and they point out that despite successive IMF-sponsored austerity programs over the years, the country still has serious economic problems. The debate over the role of the IMF took on new urgency given the institution's extensive involvement in the economies of Asia and Eastern Europe during the latter part of the 1990s. Accordingly, we shall discuss the issue in depth.

The Bretton Woods system of fixed exchange rates collapsed in 1973. Since then, the world has operated with a mixed system in which some currencies are allowed to float freely, but many are either managed by government intervention or pegged to another currency. We will explain the reasons for the failure of the Bretton Woods system as well as the nature of the present system. We will also discuss how pegged exchange rate systems work. Two decades after the breakdown of the Bretton Woods system, the debate continues over what kind of exchange rate regime is best for the world. Some economists advocate a system in which major currencies are allowed to float against each other. Others argue for a return to a fixed exchange rate regime similar to the one established at Bretton Woods. This debate is intense and important, and we will examine the arguments of both sides.

Finally, we will discuss the implications of all this material for international business. We will see how the exchange rate policy adopted by a government can have an important impact on the outlook for business operations in a given country. If government exchange rate policies result in a currency devaluation, for example, exporters based in that country may benefit as their products become more price competitive in foreign markets. Alternatively, importers will suffer from an increase in the price of their products. We will also look at how the policies adopted by the IMF can have an impact on the economic outlook for a country and, accordingly, on the costs and benefits of doing business in that country.

The Gold Standard

The gold standard had its origin in the use of gold coins as a medium of exchange, unit of account, and store of value—a practice that dates to ancient times. When international trade was limited in volume, payment for goods purchased from another country was typically made in gold or silver. However, as the volume of international trade expanded in the wake of the Industrial Revolution, a more convenient means of financing international trade was needed. Shipping large quantities of gold and silver around the world to finance international trade seemed impractical. The solution adopted was to arrange for payment in paper currency and for governments to agree to convert the paper currency into gold on demand at a fixed rate.

Mechanics of the Gold Standard

Pegging currencies to gold and guaranteeing convertibility is known as the **gold standard.** By 1880, most of the world's major trading nations, including Great Britain, Germany, Japan, and the United States, had adopted the gold standard. Given a common gold standard, the value of any currency in units of any other currency (the exchange rate) was easy to determine.

For example, under the gold standard, one U.S. dollar was defined as equivalent to 23.22 grains of "fine" (pure) gold. Thus, one could, in theory, demand that the U.S. government convert that one dollar into 23.22 grains of gold. Since there are 480 grains in an ounce, one ounce of gold cost $20.67 (480/23.22). The amount of a currency needed to purchase one ounce of gold was referred to as the **gold par value.** The British pound was defined as containing 113 grains of fine gold. In other words, one ounce of gold cost £4.25 (480/113). From the gold par values of pounds and dollars, we can calculate what the exchange rate was for converting pounds into dollars; it was £1 = $4.87 (i.e., $20.67/£4.25).

Strength of the Gold Standard

The great strength claimed for the gold standard was that it contained a powerful mechanism for achieving balance-of-trade equilibrium by all countries.[2] A country is said to be in **balance-of-trade equilibrium** when the income its residents earn from exports is equal to the money its residents pay to other countries for imports (the current account of its balance of payments is in balance). Suppose there are only two countries in the world, Japan and the United States. Imagine Japan's trade balance is in surplus because it exports more to the United States than it imports from the United States. Japanese exporters are paid in U.S. dollars, which they exchange for Japanese yen at a Japanese bank. The Japanese bank submits the dollars to the U.S. government and demands payment of gold in return. (This is a simplification of what would occur, but it will make our point.)

Under the gold standard, when Japan has a trade surplus, there will be a net flow of gold from the United States to Japan. These gold flows automatically reduce the U.S. money supply and swell Japan's money supply. As we saw in Chapter 9, there is a close connection between money supply growth and price inflation. An increase in money supply will raise prices in Japan, while a decrease in the U.S. money supply will push U.S. prices downward. The rise in the price of Japanese goods will decrease demand for these goods, while the fall in the price of U.S. goods will increase demand for these goods. Thus, Japan will start to buy more from the United States, and the United States will buy less from Japan, until a balance-of-trade equilibrium is achieved.

This adjustment mechanism seems so simple and attractive that even today, more than 60 years after the final collapse of the gold standard, some people believe the world should return to a gold standard.

The Period between the Wars: 1918–1939

The gold standard worked reasonably well from the 1870s until the start of World War I in 1914, when it was abandoned. During the war, several governments financed part of their massive military expenditures by printing money. This resulted in inflation, and by the war's end in 1918, price levels were higher everywhere. The United States returned to the gold standard in 1919, Great Britain in 1925, and France in 1928.

Great Britain returned to the gold standard by pegging the pound to gold at the prewar gold parity level of £4.25 per ounce, despite substantial inflation between 1914 and 1925. This priced British goods out of foreign markets, which pushed the country into a deep depression. When foreign holders of pounds lost confidence in Great Britain's commitment to maintaining its currency's value, they began converting their holdings of pounds into gold. The British government saw that it could not satisfy the demand for gold without seriously depleting its gold reserves, so it suspended convertibility in 1931.

The United States followed suit and left the gold standard in 1933 but returned to it in 1934, raising the dollar price of gold from $20.67 per ounce to $35 per ounce. Since more dollars were needed to buy an ounce of gold than before, the implication was that the dollar was worth less. This effectively amounted to a devaluation of the dollar relative to other currencies. Thus, before the devaluation, the pound/dollar exchange rate was £1=$4.87, but after the devaluation it was £1 = $8.24. By reducing the price of U.S. exports and increasing the price of imports, the government was trying to create employment in the United States by boosting output. However, a number of other countries adopted a similar tactic, and in the cycle of competitive devaluations that soon emerged, no country could win.

The net result was the shattering of any remaining confidence in the system. With countries devaluing their currencies at will, one could no longer be certain how much gold a currency could buy. Instead of holding onto another country's currency, people often tried to change it into gold immediately, lest the country devalue its currency in the intervening period. This put pressure on the gold reserves of various countries, forcing them to suspend gold convertibility. By the start of World War II in 1939, the gold standard was dead.

The Bretton Woods System

In 1944, at the height of World War II, representatives from 44 countries met at Bretton Woods, New Hampshire, to design a new international monetary system. With the collapse of the gold standard and the Great Depression of the 1930s fresh in their minds, these statesmen were determined to build an enduring economic order that would facilitate postwar economic growth. There was general consensus that fixed exchange rates were desirable. In addition, the conference participants wanted to avoid the senseless competitive devaluations of the 1930s, and they recognized that the gold standard would not assure this. The major problem with the gold standard as previously constituted was that no multinational institution could stop countries from engaging in competitive devaluations.

The agreement reached at Bretton Woods established two multinational institutions—the International Monetary Fund (IMF) and the World Bank. The task of the IMF would be to maintain order in the international monetary system and that of the World Bank would be to promote general economic development. The Bretton Woods agreement also called for a system of fixed exchange rates that would be policed by the IMF. Under the agreement, all countries were to fix the value of their currency in terms of gold but were not required to exchange their currencies for gold. Only the dollar remained convertible into gold—at a price of $35 per ounce. Each country decided what it wanted its exchange rate to be vis-à-vis the dollar and then calculated the gold par value of the currency based on that selected dollar exchange rate. All participating countries agreed to try to maintain the value of their currencies within 1 percent of the par value by buying or selling currencies (or gold) as needed. For example, if foreign exchange dealers were selling more of a country's currency than demanded, that country's government would intervene in the foreign exchange markets, buying its currency in an attempt to increase demand and maintain its gold par value.

Another aspect of the Bretton Woods agreement was a commitment not to use devaluation as a weapon of competitive trade policy. However, if a currency became too weak to defend, a devaluation of up to 10 percent would be allowed without any formal approval by the IMF. Larger devaluations required IMF approval.

The Role of the IMF

The IMF Articles of Agreement were heavily influenced by the worldwide financial collapse, competitive devaluations, trade wars, high unemployment, hyperinflation in Germany and elsewhere, and general economic disintegration that occurred between the two world wars. The aim of the Bretton Woods agreement, of which the IMF was the main custodian, was to try to avoid a repetition of that chaos through a combination of discipline and flexibility.

Discipline

A fixed exchange rate regime imposes discipline in two ways. First, the need to maintain a fixed exchange rate puts a brake on competitive devaluations and brings stability to the world trade environment. Second, a fixed exchange rate regime imposes monetary discipline on countries, thereby curtailing price inflation. For example, consider what would happen under a fixed exchange rate regime if Great Britain rapidly increased its money supply by printing pounds. As explained in Chapter 9, the increase in money supply would lead to price inflation. Given fixed exchange rates, inflation would make British goods uncompetitive in world markets, while the prices of imports would become more attractive in Great Britain. The result would be a widening trade deficit in Great Britain, with the country importing more than it exports. To correct this trade imbalance under a fixed exchange rate regime, Great Britain would be required to restrict the rate of growth in its money supply to bring price inflation back under control. Thus, fixed exchange rates are seen as a mechanism for controlling inflation and imposing economic discipline on countries.

Flexibility

Although monetary discipline was a central objective of the Bretton Woods agreement, it was recognized that a rigid policy of fixed exchange rates would be too inflexible. It would probably break down just as the gold standard had. In some cases, a country's attempts to reduce its money supply growth and correct a persistent balance-of-payments deficit could force the country into recession and create high unemployment. The architects of the Bretton Woods agreement wanted to avoid high unemployment, so they built limited flexibility into the system. Two major features of the IMF Articles of Agreement fostered this flexibility: IMF lending facilities and adjustable parities.

The IMF stood ready to lend foreign currencies to members to tide them over during short periods of balance-of-payments deficits, when a rapid tightening of monetary or fiscal policy would hurt domestic employment. A pool of gold and currencies contributed by IMF members provided the resources for these lending operations. A persistent balance-of-payments deficit can lead to a depletion of a country's reserves of foreign currency, forcing it to devalue its currency. By providing deficit-laden countries with short-term foreign currency loans, IMF funds would buy time for countries to bring down their inflation rates and reduce their balance-of-payments deficits. The belief was that such loans would reduce pressures for devaluation and allow for a more orderly and less painful adjustment.

Countries were to be allowed to borrow a limited amount from the IMF without adhering to any specific agreements. However, extensive drawings from IMF funds would require a country to agree to increasingly stringent IMF supervision of its macroeconomics policies. Heavy borrowers from the IMF must agree to monetary and fiscal conditions set down by the IMF, which typically included IMF-mandated targets on domestic money supply growth, exchange rate policy, tax policy, government spending, and so on.

The system of adjustable parities allowed for the devaluation of a country's currency by more than 10 percent if the IMF agreed that a country's balance of payments was in "fundamental disequilibrium." The term *fundamental disequilibrium* was not defined in the IMF's Articles of Agreement, but it was intended to apply to countries that had suffered permanent adverse shifts in the demand for their products. Without devaluation, such a country would experience high unemployment and a persistent trade deficit until the domestic price level had fallen far enough to restore a balance-of-payments equilibrium. The belief was that devaluation could help sidestep a painful adjustment process in such circumstances.

The Role of the World Bank

The official name for the World Bank is the International Bank for Reconstruction and Development (IBRD). When the Bretton Woods participants established the World Bank, the need to reconstruct the war-torn economies of Europe was foremost in their minds. The bank's initial mission was to help finance the building of Europe's economy by providing low-interest loans. As it turned out, the World Bank was overshadowed in this role by the Marshall Plan, under which the United States lent money directly to European nations to help them rebuild. So the bank turned its attention to "development" and began lending money to Third World nations. In the 1950s, the bank concentrated on public-sector projects. Power stations, road building, and other transportation investments were much in favor. During the 1960s, the bank also began to lend heavily in support of agriculture, education, population control, and urban development.

The bank lends money under two schemes. Under the IBRD scheme, money is raised through bond sales in the international capital market. Borrowers pay what the bank calls a market rate of interest—the bank's cost of funds plus a margin for expenses. This "market" rate is lower than commercial banks' market rate. Under the IBRD scheme, the bank offers low-interest loans to risky customers whose credit rating is often poor.

A second scheme is overseen by the International Development Agency (IDA), an arm of the bank created in 1960. Resources to fund IDA loans are raised through subscriptions from wealthy members such as the United States, Japan, and Germany. IDA loans go only to the poorest countries. Borrowers have 50 years to repay at an interest rate of 1 percent a year.

The Collapse of the Fixed Exchange Rate System

The system of fixed exchange rates established at Bretton Woods worked well until the late 1960s, when it began to show signs of strain. The system finally collapsed in 1973, and since then we have had a managed-float system. To understand why the system collapsed, one must appreciate the special role of the U.S. dollar in the system. As the only currency that could be converted into gold, and as the currency that served as the reference point for all others, the dollar occupied a central place in the system. Any pressure on the dollar to devalue could wreak havoc with the system, and that is what occurred.

Most economists trace the breakup of the fixed exchange rate system to the U.S. macroeconomic policy package of 1965–68.[3] To finance both the Vietnam conflict and his welfare programs, President Lyndon Johnson backed an increase in U.S. government spending that was not financed by an increase in taxes. Instead, it was financed by an increase in the money supply, which led to a rise in price inflation from less than 4 percent in 1966 to close to 9 percent by 1968. At the same time, the rise in government spending had stimulated the economy. With more money in their pockets, people spent more—particularly on imports—and the U.S. trade balance began to deteriorate.

The increase in inflation and the worsening of the U.S. foreign trade position gave rise to speculation in the foreign exchange market that the dollar would be devalued. Things came to a head in the spring of 1971 when U.S. trade figures showed that for the first time since 1945, the United States was importing more than it was exporting. This set off massive purchases of German deutsche marks in the foreign exchange market by speculators who guessed that the mark would be revalued against the dollar. On a single day, May 4, 1971, the Bundesbank (Germany's central bank) had to buy $1 billion to hold the dollar/deutsche mark exchange rate at its fixed exchange rate given the great demand for deutsche marks. On the morning of May 5, the Bundesbank purchased another $1 billion during the first hour of foreign exchange trading! At that point, the Bundesbank faced the inevitable and allowed its currency to float.

In the weeks following the decision to float the deutsche mark, the foreign exchange market became increasingly convinced that the dollar would have to be devalued. However, devaluation of the dollar was no easy matter. Under the Bretton Woods provisions, any other country could change its exchange rates against all currencies simply by fixing its dollar rate at a new level. But as the key currency in the system, the dollar could be devalued only if all countries agreed to simultaneously revalue against the dollar. And many countries did not want this, because it would make their products more expensive relative to U.S. products.

To force the issue, President Nixon announced in August 1971 that the dollar was no longer convertible into gold. He also announced that a new 10 percent tax on imports would remain in effect until U.S. trading partners agreed to revalue their currencies against the dollar. This brought the trading partners to the bargaining table, and in December 1971 an agreement was reached to devalue the dollar by about 8 percent against foreign currencies. The import tax was then removed.

The problem was not solved, however. The U.S. balance-of-payments position continued to deteriorate throughout 1972, while the nation's money supply continued to expand at an inflationary rate. Speculation continued to grow that the dollar was still over-valued and that a second devaluation would be necessary. In anticipation, foreign exchange dealers began converting dollars to deutsche marks and other currencies. After a massive wave of speculation in February 1972, which culminated with European central banks spending $3.6 billion on March 1 to try to prevent their currencies from appreciating against the dollar, the foreign exchange market was closed. When the foreign exchange market reopened March 19, the currencies of Japan and most European countries were floating against the dollar, although many developing countries continued to peg their currency to the dollar, and many do to this day. At that time, the switch to a floating system was viewed as a temporary response to unmanageable speculation in the foreign exchange market. But it is now more than 30 years since the Bretton Woods system of fixed exchange rates collapsed, and the temporary solution looks permanent.

The Bretton Woods system had an Achilles' heel: The system could not work if its key currency, the U.S. dollar, was under speculative attack. The Bretton Woods system could work only as long as the U.S. inflation rate remained low and the United States did not run a balance-of-payments deficit. Once these things occurred, the system soon became strained to the breaking point.

The Floating Exchange Rate Regime ■

The floating exchange rate regime that followed the collapse of the fixed exchange rate system was formalized in January 1976 when IMF members met in Jamaica and agreed to the rules for the international monetary system that are in place today.

The Jamaica Agreement

The Jamaica meeting revised the IMF's Articles of Agreement to reflect the new reality of floating exchange rates. The main elements of the Jamaica agreement include the following:

1. Floating rates were declared acceptable. IMF members were permitted to enter the foreign exchange market to even out "unwarranted" speculative fluctuations.
2. Gold was abandoned as a reserve asset. The IMF returned its gold reserves to members at the current market price, placing the proceeds in a trust fund to help poor nations. IMF members were permitted to sell their own gold reserves at the market price.
3. Total annual IMF quotas—the amount member countries contribute to the IMF—were increased to $41 billion. (Since then they have been increased to $280 billion while the membership of the IMF has been expanded to include 184 countries.) Non-oil-exporting, less developed countries were given greater access to IMF funds.

After Jamaica, the IMF continued its role of helping countries cope with macroeconomic and exchange rate problems, albeit within the context of a radically different exchange rate regime.

Exchange Rates since 1973

Since March 1973, exchange rates have become much more volatile and less predictable than they were between 1945 and 1973.[4] This volatility has been partly due to a number of unexpected shocks to the world monetary system, including:

1. The oil crisis in 1971, when the Organization of Petroleum Exporting Countries (OPEC) quadrupled the price of oil. The harmful effect of this on the U.S. inflation rate and trade position resulted in a further decline in the value of the dollar.

Figure 10.1

Long-Term Exchange Rate Trends, 1970–2001

Source: Data from J. P. Morgan Effective Exchange Rate Index, 1970–2001 (1990 = 100).

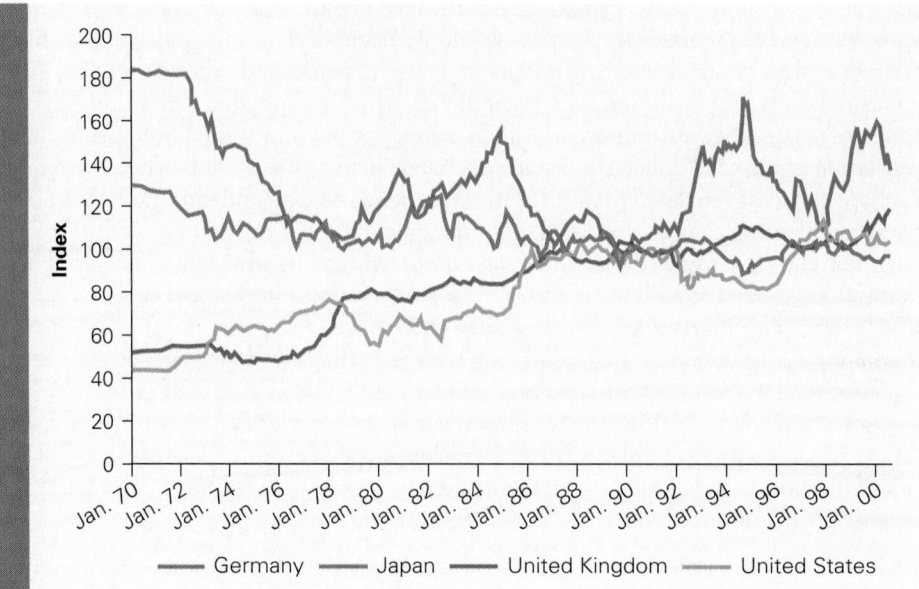

2. The loss of confidence in the dollar that followed the rise of U.S. inflation in 1977 and 1978.

3. The oil crisis of 1979, when OPEC once again increased the price of oil dramatically—this time it was doubled.

4. The unexpected rise in the dollar between 1980 and 1985, despite a deteriorating balance-of-payments picture.

5. The rapid fall of the U.S. dollar against the Japanese yen and German deutsche mark between 1985 and 1987, and against the yen between 1993 and 1995.

6. The partial collapse of the European Monetary System in 1992.

7. The 1997 Asian currency crisis, when the Asian currencies of several countries, including South Korea, Indonesia, Malaysia, and Thailand, lost between 50 percent and 80 percent of their value against the U.S. dollar in a few months.

Figure 10.1 summarizes the volatility of four major currencies—the German mark, Japanese yen, British pound, and U.S. dollar—from 1970 to 2001. The Morgan Guaranty Index, the basis for Figure 10.1, represents the exchange rate of each of these currencies against a weighted basket of the currencies of 19 industrial countries (the index was set equal to 100 in 1990). All four currencies have been quite volatile over the period. The index value of the Japanese yen, for example, has ranged from a low of 44 in 1970 to a high of 170 in June 1995. Similarly, the U.S. dollar index has been as low as 89.3 in 1995 and as high as 158 in 1985.

Perhaps the most interesting phenomena in Figure 10.1 are the rapid rise in the value of the dollar between 1980 and 1985 and its subsequent fall between 1985 and 1988, and the similar rise and fall in the value of the Japanese yen between 1990 and 1998. We will briefly discuss the rise and fall of the dollar, since this tells us something about how the international monetary system has operated in recent years.[5]

The rise in the value of the dollar between 1980 and 1985 is particularly interesting because it occurred when the United States was running a large and growing trade deficit, importing substantially more than it exported. Conventional wisdom would suggest that the increased supply of dollars in the foreign exchange market as a result of the deficit should lead to a reduction in the value of the dollar, but it increased in value. Why? A number of favorable factors temporarily overcame the unfavorable effect of a trade deficit. Strong economic growth in the United States attracted heavy inflows of capital from foreign investors seeking high returns on capital assets. High real interest rates attracted foreign investors seeking high returns on financial assets. At the same time, political turmoil in other parts of the world, along with relatively slow economic growth in the developed countries of Europe, helped create the view that the United States was a good place to invest. These inflows of capital increased the demand for dollars in the foreign exchange market, which pushed the value of the dollar upward against other currencies.

The fall in the value of the dollar between 1985 and 1988 was caused by a combination of government intervention and market forces. The rise in the dollar, which priced U.S. goods out of foreign markets and made imports relatively cheap, had contributed to a dismal trade picture. In 1985, the United States posted a record-high trade deficit of more than $160 billion. This led to growth in demands for protectionism in the United States. In September 1985, the finance ministers and central bank governors of the so-called Group of Five major industrial countries (Great Britain, France, Japan, Germany, and the United States) met at the Plaza Hotel in New York and reached what was later referred to as the Plaza Accord. They announced that it would be desirable for most major currencies to appreciate vis-à-vis the U.S. dollar and pledged to intervene in the foreign exchange markets, selling dollars, to encourage this objective. The dollar had already begun to weaken in the summer of 1985, and this announcement further accelerated the decline.

The dollar continued to decline until early 1987. The governments of the Group of Five even began to worry that the dollar might decline too far, so the finance ministers of the Group of Five met in Paris in February 1987 and reached a new agreement known as the Louvre Accord. They agreed that exchange rates had been realigned sufficiently and pledged to support the stability of exchange rates around their current levels by intervening in the foreign exchange markets when necessary to buy and sell currency. Although the dollar continued to decline for a few months after the Louvre Accord, the rate of decline slowed, and by early 1988 the decline had ended. Except for a brief speculative flurry around the time of the Persian Gulf War in 1991, the dollar was relatively stable for most of the 1990s against most major currencies with the notable exception of the Japanese yen. However, in 2000 and 2001, the dollar began to appreciate against most major currencies, including the euro, even though the United States was once more running a record balance-of-payments deficit.

Thus, we see that in recent history the value of the dollar has been determined by both market forces and government intervention. Under a floating exchange rate regime, market forces have produced a volatile dollar exchange rate. Governments have responded by intervening in the market—buying and selling dollars—in an attempt to limit the market's volatility and to correct what they see as overvaluation (in 1985) or potential undervaluation (in 1987) of the dollar. The frequency of government intervention in the foreign exchange markets explains why the current system is often referred to as a managed-float system or a dirty-float system.

Fixed versus Floating Exchange Rates

The breakdown of the Bretton Woods system has not stopped the debate about the relative merits of fixed versus floating exchange rate regimes. Disappointment with the system of floating rates in recent years has led to renewed debate about the merits of fixed exchange rates. In this section, we review the arguments for fixed and floating exchange rate regimes.[6] We will discuss the case for floating rates before discussing why many commentators are disappointed with the experience under floating exchange rates and yearn for a system of fixed rates.

The Case for Floating Exchange Rates

The case for floating exchange rates has two main elements: monetary policy autonomy and automatic trade balance adjustments.

Monetary Policy Autonomy

It is argued that under a fixed system, a country's ability to expand or contract its money supply as it sees fit is limited by the need to maintain exchange rate parity. Monetary expansion can lead to inflation, which puts downward pressure on a fixed exchange rate (as predicted by the PPP theory; see Chapter 9). Similarly, monetary contraction requires high interest rates (to reduce the demand for money). Higher interest rates lead to an inflow of money from abroad, which puts upward pressure on a fixed exchange rate. Thus, to maintain exchange rate parity under a fixed system, countries were limited in their ability to use monetary policy to expand or contract their economies.

Advocates of a floating exchange rate regime argue that removal of the obligation to maintain exchange rate parity would restore monetary control to a government. If a government faced with unemployment wanted to increase its money supply to stimulate domestic demand and reduce unemployment, it could do so unencumbered by the need to maintain its exchange rate. While monetary expansion might lead to inflation, this would lead to a depreciation in the country's currency. If PPP theory is correct, the resulting currency depreciation on the foreign exchange markets should offset the effects of inflation. Although under a floating exchange rate regime, domestic inflation would have an impact on the exchange rate, it should have no impact on businesses' international cost competitiveness due to exchange rate depreciation. The rise in domestic costs should be exactly offset by the fall in the value of the country's currency on the foreign exchange markets. Similarly, a government could use monetary policy to contract the economy without worrying about the need to maintain parity.

Trade Balance Adjustments

Under the Bretton Woods system, if a country developed a permanent deficit in its balance of trade (importing more than it exported) that could not be corrected by domestic policy, this would require the IMF to agree to a currency devaluation. Critics of this system argue that the adjustment mechanism works much more smoothly under a floating exchange rate regime. They argue that if a country is running a trade deficit, the imbalance between the supply and demand of that country's currency in the foreign exchange markets (supply exceeding demand) will lead to depreciation in its exchange rate. In turn, by making its exports cheaper and its imports more expensive, an exchange rate depreciation should correct the trade deficit.

The Case for Fixed Exchange Rates

The case for fixed exchange rates rests on arguments about monetary discipline, speculation, uncertainty, and the lack of connection between the trade balance and exchange rates.

Monetary Discipline

We have already discussed the nature of monetary discipline inherent in a fixed exchange rate system when we discussed the Bretton Woods system. The need to maintain a fixed exchange rate parity ensures that governments do not expand their money supplies at inflationary rates. While advocates of floating rates argue that each country should be allowed to choose its own inflation rate (the monetary autonomy argument), advocates of fixed rates argue that governments all too often give in to political pressures and expand the monetary supply far too rapidly, causing unacceptably high price inflation. A fixed exchange rate regime would ensure that this does not occur.

Speculation

Critics of a floating exchange rate regime also argue that speculation can cause fluctuations in exchange rates. They point to the dollar's rapid rise and fall during the 1980s, which they claim had nothing to do with comparative inflation rates and the

U.S. trade deficit, but everything to do with speculation. They argue that when foreign exchange dealers see a currency depreciating, they tend to sell the currency in the expectation of future depreciation regardless of the currency's longer-term prospects. As more traders jump on the bandwagon, the expectations of depreciation are realized. Such destabilizing speculation tends to accentuate the fluctuations around the exchange rate's long-run value. It can damage a country's economy by distorting export and import prices. Thus, advocates of a fixed exchange rate regime argue that such a system will limit the destabilizing effects of speculation.

Uncertainty

Speculation also adds to the uncertainty surrounding future currency movements that characterizes floating exchange rate regimes. The unpredictability of exchange rate movements in the post–Bretton Woods era has made business planning difficult, and it makes exporting, importing, and foreign investment risky activities. Given a volatile exchange rate, international businesses do not know how to react to the changes—and often they do not react. Why change plans for exporting, importing, or foreign investment after a 6 percent fall in the dollar this month, when the dollar may rise 6 percent next month? This uncertainty, according to the critics, dampens the growth of international trade and investment. They argue that a fixed exchange rate, by eliminating such uncertainty, promotes the growth of international trade and investment. Advocates of a floating system reply that the forward exchange market insures against the risks associated with exchange rate fluctuations (see Chapter 9), so the adverse impact of uncertainty on the growth of international trade and investment has been overstated.

Trade Balance Adjustments

Those in favor of floating exchange rates argue that floating rates help adjust trade imbalances. Critics question the closeness of the link between the exchange rate and the trade balance. They claim trade deficits are determined by the balance between savings and investment in a country, not by the external value of its currency.[7] They argue that depreciation in a currency will lead to inflation (due to the resulting increase in import prices). This inflation will wipe out any apparent gains in cost competitiveness that come from currency depreciation. In other words, a depreciating exchange rate will not boost exports and reduce imports, as advocates of floating rates claim; it will simply boost price inflation. In support of this argument, those who favor floating rates point out that the 40 percent drop in the value of the dollar between 1985 and 1988 did not correct the U.S. trade deficit. In reply, advocates of a floating exchange rate regime argue that between 1985 and 1992, the U.S. trade deficit fell from more than $160 billion to about $70 billion, and they attribute this in part to the decline in the value of the dollar.

Who Is Right?

Which side is right in the vigorous debate between those who favor a fixed exchange rate and those who favor a floating exchange rate? Economists cannot agree on this issue. From a business perspective, this is unfortunate because business, as a major player on the international trade and investment scene, has a large stake in the resolution of the debate. Would international business be better off under a fixed regime, or are flexible rates better? The evidence is not clear.

We do, however, know that a fixed exchange rate regime modeled along the lines of the Bretton Woods system will not work. Speculation ultimately broke the system, a phenomenon that advocates of fixed rate regimes claim is associated with floating exchange rates! Nevertheless, a different kind of fixed exchange rate system might be more enduring and might foster the stability that would facilitate more rapid growth in international trade and investment. In the next section, we look at potential models for such a system and the problems with such systems.

Figure 10.2

IMF Members' Exchange Rate Policies, 2002

Source: *IMF Annual Report, 2002* (Washington, DC: IMF, 2002).

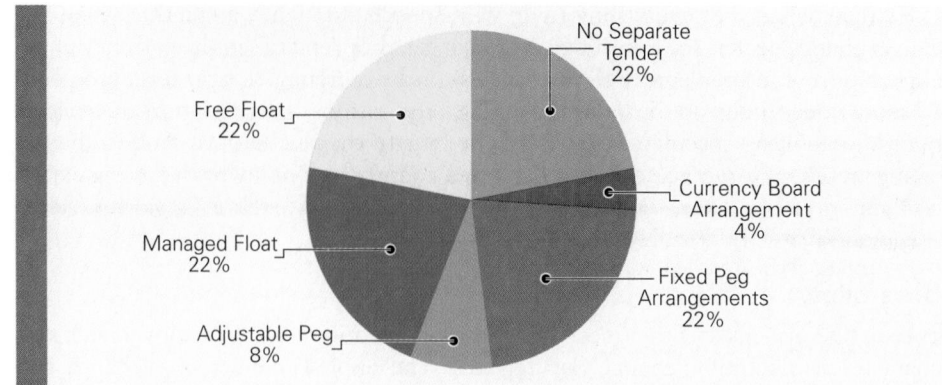

Exchange Rate Regimes in Practice

A number of different exchange rate policies are pursued by governments around the world. These range from a pure "free float" where the exchange rate is determined by market forces to a pegged system that has some aspects of the pre-1973 Bretton Woods system of fixed exchange rates. Figure 10.2 summarizes the exchange rate policies adopted by member states of the IMF in 2002. Some 22 percent of the IMF's 184 members allow their currency to float freely. Another 22 percent intervene in only a limited way (the so-called managed float). A further 22 percent of IMF members now have no separate legal tender of their own. These include the 12 European Union countries that have adopted the euro, and effectively given up their own currencies, along with 28 smaller states mostly in Africa or the Caribbean that have no domestic currency and have adopted a foreign currency as legal tender within their borders, typically the U.S. dollar or the euro. The remaining countries use more inflexible systems, including a fixed peg arrangement (22 percent) under which they peg their currencies to other currencies, such as the U.S. dollar or the euro, or to a basket of currencies. Other countries have adopted a somewhat more flexible system under which their exchange rate is allowed to fluctuate against other currencies within a target zone (an adjustable peg system). In this section, we will look more closely at the mechanics and implications of exchange rate regimes that rely on a currency peg or target zone.

Pegged Exchange Rates

Under a pegged exchange rate regime, a country will peg the value of its currency to that of a major currency so that, for example, as the U.S. dollar rises in value, its own currency rises too. Pegged exchange rates are popular among many of the world's smaller nations. As with a full fixed exchange rate regime, the great virtue claimed for a pegged exchange rate is that it imposes monetary discipline on a country and leads to low inflation. For example, if Belize pegs the value of the Belizean dollar to that of the U.S. dollar so that US$1 = B$1.99 (the peg as of 2002), then the Belizean government must make sure the inflation rate in Belize is similar to that in the United States. If the Belizean inflation rate is greater than the U.S. inflation rate, this will lead to pressure to devalue the Belizean dollar (i.e., to alter the peg). To maintain the peg, the Belizean government would be required to rein in inflation. Of course, for a pegged exchange rate to impose monetary discipline on a country, the country whose currency is chosen for the peg must also pursue sound monetary policy.

Evidence shows that adopting a pegged exchange rate regime moderates inflationary pressures in a country. An IMF study concluded that countries with pegged exchange rates had an average annual inflation rate of 8 percent, compared with 14 percent for intermediate regimes and 16 percent for floating regimes.[8] However, many countries operate with only a nominal peg and in practice are willing to devalue their currency rather than pursue a tight monetary policy. It can be very difficult for a smaller country to maintain a peg against another currency if capital is flowing out of the country and foreign exchange traders are speculating against the currency. Something like this occurred in 1997 when a combination of adverse capital flows and currency speculation forced several Asian countries, including Thailand and Malaysia, to abandon pegs against the U.S. dollar and let their currencies float freely. Malaysia and Thailand would not have been in this position had they dealt with a number of problems that began to arise in their economies during the 1990s, including excessive private-sector debt and expanding current account trade deficits.

Currency Boards

Hong Kong's experience during the 1997 Asian currency crisis added a new dimension to the debate over how to manage a pegged exchange rate. During late 1997 when other Asian currencies were collapsing, Hong Kong maintained the value of its currency against the U.S. dollar at about $15HK = $7.8 despite several concerted speculative attacks. Hong Kong's currency board has been given credit for this success. A country that introduces a **currency board** commits itself to converting its domestic currency on demand into another currency at a fixed exchange rate. To make this commitment credible, the currency board holds reserves of foreign currency equal at the fixed exchange rate to at least 100 percent of the domestic currency issued. The system used in Hong Kong means its currency must be fully backed by the U.S. dollar at the specified exchange rate. This is still not a true fixed exchange rate regime, because the U.S. dollar, and by extension the Hong Kong dollar, floats against other currencies, but it has some features of a fixed exchange rate regime.

Under this arrangement, the currency board can issue additional domestic notes and coins only when there are foreign exchange reserves to back it. This limits the ability of the government to print money and, thereby, create inflationary pressures. Under a strict currency board system, interest rates adjust automatically. If investors want to switch out of domestic currency into, for example, U.S. dollars, the supply of domestic currency will shrink. This will cause interest rates to rise until it eventually becomes attractive for investors to hold the local currency again. In the case of Hong Kong, the interest rate on three-month deposits climbed as high as 20 percent in late 1997, as investors switched out of Hong Kong dollars and into U.S. dollars. The dollar peg, however, held, and interest rates declined again.

Since its establishment in 1983, the Hong Kong currency board has weathered several storms, including the latest. This success persuaded several other countries in the developing world to consider a similar system. Argentina introduced a currency board in 1991, and Bulgaria, Estonia, and Lithuania have all gone down this road in recent years (eight IMF members had currency boards in 2002). Despite growing interest in the arrangement, however, critics are quick to point out that currency boards have their drawbacks.[9] If local inflation rates remain higher than the inflation rate in the country to which the currency is pegged, the currencies of countries with currency boards can become uncompetitive and overvalued. Also, under a currency board system, government lacks the ability to set interest rates. Interest rates in Hong Kong, for example, are effectively set by the U.S. Federal Reserve. In addition, economic collapse in Argentina in 2001 and the subsequent decision to abandon its currency board dampened much of the enthusiasm for this mechanism of managing exchange rates (see the accompanying Country Focus).

Argentina's Currency Board

During the 1990s, Argentina was often held up as an example of a country that was on the fast track to economic prosperity. Between 1991 and 1998, inflation, long the scourge of Argentina, was vanquished, foreign capital poured into the country, and the economy grew at an annual average rate of 5.7 percent, the highest growth rate in the region. Much of the credit for this performance was laid at the feet of President Carlos Menem and his finance minister, Domingo Cavallo. Under their leadership, Argentina in 1991 adopted a currency board that pegged the Argentinean peso at parity to the dollar ($1=1 peso). They also opened the economy to foreign investment and international trade, and they privatized numerous state-owned enterprises.

By 2002, the glory days of the 1990s were a distant memory. In early 2002, after a brutal four-year recession that had pushed unemployment up to 25 percent, Argentina defaulted on its $155 billion public-sector debt, the largest such default by any country in history. The currency board arrangement was abandoned, and the peso fell from parity to 3.5 pesos to the dollar by mid-2002.

Why did the Argentinean economy go so badly astray? According to some critics, the currency board was partly to blame. By adopting a currency board, Argentina renounced both exchange rate and monetary policy (interest rates were in effect set by the U.S. Federal Reserve). This limited the ability of the government to respond to external shocks, and Argentina was hit by several of them. First, prices for commodities stopped rising, depriving the Argentinean economy of a major source of export earnings. Then, the dollar appreciated against other major currencies, and since it was pegged to the dollar, so did the Argentinean peso, pricing many Argentinean goods out of world export markets while making imports cheaper. Finally, Brazil, Argentina's largest trading partner, devalued its currency, making Argentinean exports prohibitively expensive in Brazil. These factors conspired to dramatically slow Argentina's export-led growth and contributed to rapidly rising unemployment.

To make matters worse, from 1996 onward the Argentinean government expanded public-sector spending without increasing taxes. At the same time, the pace of economic reform started to slow. The inevitable result was rising public-sector debt. Investors began to fear that the government would not be able to finance its growing debt, particularly in light of the slowdown in Argentinean exports. Capital started to leave the country, and foreign investors limited their lending to the Argentinean government. In late 2000, Argentina applied to the IMF for help and was granted a $14 billion loan in January 2001 to support the peso and maintain the dollar peg. In return for the IMF loan, the government agreed to reduce public spending. But with Argentinean exports still priced out of world markets, conditions failed to improve. Ordinary Argentines began to lose confidence in the government and the ability of the banking system to finance spiraling public-sector debts. Between July and November 2001, Argentines withdrew some $15 billion from local banks. With their asset base shrinking, the banks could no longer finance government debt, and with foreign financial institutions unwilling to lend more money to the government, the stage was set for Argentina's decision to default on payment of its public-sector debt. The government simply did not have enough money left to finance the debt that it had taken on in the late 1990s, and could not borrow any more.

Shortly afterward, the government abandoned the currency board arrangement, and the peso plunged, reaching a low of 3.5 to the dollar in mid-2002 before rising to about 3 to the dollar in early 2003. In 2002, exports started to pick up, imports declined, the economy expanded for the first time since 1998, albeit by a small amount, unemployment started to fall (it was down to 18 percent by late 2002), and consumer confidence rose. While prices increased by 40 percent in 2002, reflecting the impact of currency devaluation on inflation rates, the rise was less than the depreciation in the currency, and held in check by weak internal demand. By abandoning the currency board, Argentina may have started on the road to economic recovery.

Sources: "Down and Almost Out in Buenos Aires," *The Economist,* November 3, 2001, pp. 43–44; "A Decline without Parallel," *The Economist,* March 2, 2002, pp. 26–28; and "Storm Abated, Outlook Still Unsettled," *The Economist,* January 11, 2003, pp. 26–27.

Crisis Management by the IMF ■

Many observers initially believed that the collapse of the Bretton Woods system in 1973 would diminish the role of the IMF within the international monetary system. The IMF's original function was to provide a pool of money from which members could borrow, short term, to adjust their balance-of-payments position and maintain their exchange rate. Some believed the demand for short-term loans would be considerably diminished under a floating exchange rate regime. A trade deficit would presumably lead to a decline in a country's exchange rate, which would help reduce imports and boost exports. No temporary IMF adjustment loan would be needed. Consistent with this, after 1973, most industrialized countries tended to let the foreign exchange market determine exchange rates in response to demand and supply. No major industrial country has borrowed funds from the IMF since the mid-1970s, when Great Britain and Italy did. Since the early 1970s, the rapid development of global capital markets has allowed developed countries such as Great Britain and the United States to finance their deficits by borrowing private money, as opposed to drawing on IMF funds.

Despite these developments, the activities of the IMF have expanded over the past 30 years. By 2002, the IMF had 184 members, 88 of which had some kind of IMF program in place in June 2002. In 1997, the institution implemented its largest rescue packages, committing more than $110 billion in short-term loans to three troubled Asian countries—South Korea, Indonesia, and Thailand. The IMF's activities have expanded because periodic financial crises have continued to hit many economies in the post–Bretton Woods era, particularly among the world's developing nations. The IMF has repeatedly lent money to nations experiencing financial crises, requesting in return that the governments enact certain macroeconomic policies. Critics of the IMF claim these policies have not always been as beneficial as the IMF might have hoped and in some cases may have made things worse. Following the IMF loans to several Asian economies, these criticisms reached new levels and a vigorous debate is under way as to the appropriate role of the IMF. In this section, we shall discuss some of the main challenges the IMF has had to deal with over the past quarter of a century and review the ongoing debate over the role of the IMF.

| Financial Crises in the Post–Bretton Woods Era

A number of broad types of financial crises have occurred over the past 25 years, many of which have required IMF involvement. A **currency crisis** occurs when a speculative attack on the exchange value of a currency results in a sharp depreciation in the value of the currency or forces authorities to expend large volumes of international currency reserves and sharply increase interest rates to defend the prevailing exchange rate. A **banking crisis** refers to a loss of confidence in the banking system that leads to a run on banks, as individuals and companies withdraw their deposits. A **foreign debt crisis** is a situation in which a country cannot service its foreign debt obligations, whether private-sector or government debt. These crises tend to have common underlying macroeconomic causes: high relative price inflation rates, a widening current account deficit, excessive expansion of domestic borrowing, and asset price inflation (such as sharp increases in stock and property prices).[10] At times, elements of currency, banking, and debt crises may be present simultaneously, as in the 1997 Asian crisis, the 1999–2001 Turkish crisis (see the opening case), and the 2000–2002 Argentinean crisis (see the Country Focus).

To assess the frequency of financial crises, the IMF looked at the macroeconomic performance of a group of 53 countries from 1975 to 1997 (22 of these countries were developed nations, and 31 were developing countries).[11] The IMF found there had been 158 currency crises, including 55 episodes in which a country's currency declined by more than 25 percent. There were also 54 banking crises. The IMF's data, which

Figure 10.3

Incidence of Currency and
Banking Crises,
1975–1997

Source: International Monetary
Fund, *World Economic Outlook,
1998* (Washington, DC: IMF, May
1998), p. 77.

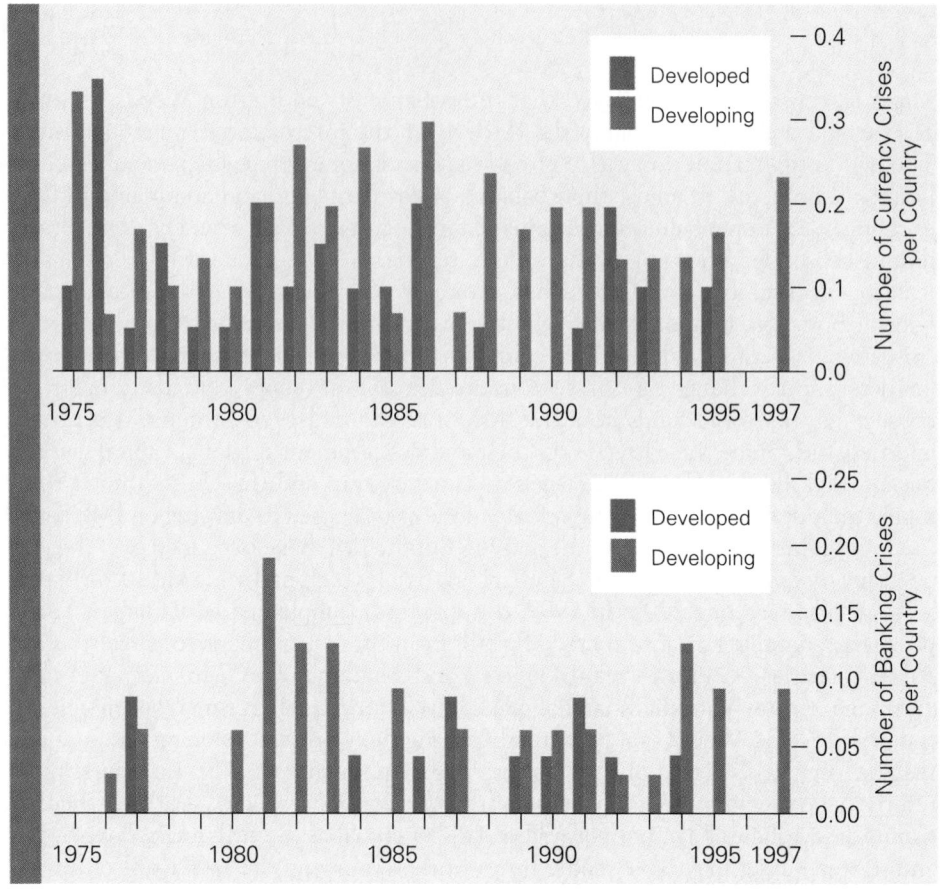

are summarized in Figure 10.3, suggest that developing nations were more than twice
as likely to experience currency and banking crises than developed nations. It is not
surprising, therefore, that most of the IMF's loan activities since the mid-1970s have
been targeted toward developing nations.

Three crises have been of particular significance in terms of IMF involvement since
the early 1990s—the 1995 Mexican currency crisis, the Russian ruble crisis, and the
1997 Asian financial crisis. All these crises were the result of excessive foreign borrowings, a weak or poorly regulated banking system, and high inflation rates. These
factors came together to trigger simultaneous debt and currency crises. Checking the
resulting crises required IMF involvement.

Mexican Currency Crisis of 1995

The Mexican peso had been pegged to the dollar since the early 1980s when the International Monetary Fund had made it a condition for lending money to the Mexican government to help bail the country out of a 1982 financial crisis. Under the
IMF-brokered arrangement, the peso had been allowed to trade within a tolerance
band of plus or minus 3 percent against the dollar. The band was also permitted to
"crawl" down daily, allowing for an annual peso depreciation of about 4 percent against
the dollar. The IMF believed that the need to maintain the exchange rate within a
fairly narrow trading band would force the Mexican government to adopt stringent financial policies to limit the growth in the money supply and contain inflation.

Until the early 1990s, it looked as if the IMF policy had worked. However, the strains
were beginning to show by 1994. Since the mid-1980s, Mexican producer prices had
risen 45 percent more than prices in the United States, and yet there had not been a

corresponding adjustment in the exchange rate. By late 1994, Mexico was running a $17 billion trade deficit, which amounted to some 6 percent of the country's gross domestic product and there had been an uncomfortably rapid expansion in public- and private-sector debt. Despite these strains, Mexican government officials had been stating publicly that they would support the peso's dollar peg at around $1 = 3.5 pesos by adopting appropriate monetary policies and by intervening in the currency markets if necessary. Encouraged by such public statements, $64 billion of foreign investment money poured into Mexico between 1990 and 1994 as corporations and mutual fund money managers sought to take advantage of the booming economy.

However, many currency traders concluded the peso would have to be devalued, and they began to dump pesos on the foreign exchange market. The government tried to hold the line by buying pesos and selling dollars, but it lacked the foreign currency reserves required to halt the speculative tide (Mexico's foreign exchange reserves fell from $6 billion at the beginning of 1994 to less than $3.5 billion at the end of the year). In mid-December 1994, the Mexican government abruptly announced a devaluation. Immediately, much of the short-term investment money that had flowed into Mexican stocks and bonds over the previous year reversed its course, as foreign investors bailed out of peso-denominated financial assets. This exacerbated the sale of the peso and contributed to the rapid 40 percent drop in its value.

The IMF stepped in again, this time arm in arm with the U.S. government and the Bank for International Settlements. Together the three institutions pledged close to $50 billion to help Mexico stabilize the peso and to redeem $47 billion of public- and private-sector debt that was set to mature in 1995. Of this amount, $20 billion came from the U.S. government and another $18 billion came from the IMF (which made Mexico the largest recipient of IMF aid up until that point). Without the aid package, Mexico would probably have defaulted on its debt obligations, and the peso would have gone into free fall. As is normal in such cases, the IMF insisted on tight monetary policies and further cuts in public spending, both of which helped push the country into a deep recession. However, the recession was relatively short-lived, and by 1997 the country was once more on a growth path, had pared down its debt, and had paid back the $20 billion borrowed from the U.S. government ahead of schedule.[12] (The accompanying Management Focus details how this crisis affected the U.S. automobile industry, which was experiencing booming sales in Mexico before the crisis.)

Russian Ruble Crisis

The IMF's involvement in Russia came about as the result of a persistent decline in the value of the Russian ruble, which was the product of high inflation rates and growing public-sector debt. Between January 1992 and April 1995, the value of the ruble against the U.S. dollar fell from $1 = R125 to $1 = R5,130. This fall occurred while Russia was implementing an economic reform program designed to transform the country's crumbling centrally planned economy into a dynamic market economy. The reform program involved a number of steps, including the January 1, 1992, removal of price controls. Prices surged immediately and inflation was soon running at a monthly rate of about 30 percent. For the whole of 1992, the inflation rate in Russia was 3,000 percent. The annual rate for 1993 was approximately 900 percent.

Several factors contributed to Russia's high inflation. Prices had been held at artificially low levels by state planners during the Communist era. At the same time, there was a shortage of many basic goods, so with nothing to spend their money on, many Russians simply hoarded rubles. After the liberalization of price controls, the country was suddenly awash in rubles chasing a still limited supply of goods. The result was to rapidly bid up prices. The inflationary fires that followed price liberalization were stoked by the Russian government itself. Unwilling to face the social consequences of the massive unemployment that would follow if many state-owned enterprises quickly were privatized, the government continued to subsidize the operations of many

Management Focus

The Mexican Peso Crisis and the Automobile Industry

In the euphoria that followed the January 1, 1994, implementation of the North American Free Trade Agreement (NAFTA), no industry looked set to gain more than the auto industry. Because of falling trade barriers and booming demand in Mexico, between January and October 1994, U.S. car exports to Mexico increased 500 percent. For all of 1994, Ford shipped 30,000 vehicles to Mexico, up from 6,000 in 1993. The company planned to ship 50,000 in 1995. General Motors and Chrysler also saw their shipments to Mexico surge in 1994 and were planning for even greater increases in 1995. Forecasts suggested that the number of vehicles sold in Mexico would rise to 1.2 million by 1999, up from 600,000 in 1994. With this growth in mind, not only had auto companies been exporting more to Mexico, but they also had been investing in Mexican-based production capacity both for serving the Mexican market and for exporting elsewhere. Among the biggest foreign investors were Chrysler, Ford, General Motors, Nissan, Mercedes-Benz, and Volkswagen.

In a few short days in December 1994, the euphoric bubble of the post-NAFTA boom was rudely burst by an unexpected decision on the part of the Mexican government to abandon a system of pegging the value of the peso at 3.5 to the dollar. Instead, the government decided to allow the peso to float freely against the dollar. In the weeks that followed this decision, the peso plummeted 40 percent, and by mid-January 1995 it was trading at 5.6 to the dollar.

As with many other industries, the impact on the auto industry was dramatic and immediate. By February 1995, the price of imported autos had risen by 40 percent. There had also been a substantial rise in the price of most autos assembled in Mexico, such as those coming off Ford's Cuautitlan plant, because many of these operations depended on parts imported from the United States and Canada. Demand for autos was further depressed by the Mexican government's economic austerity plan, introduced in March 1995 at the IMF's insistence. The plan tightened credit and raised interest rates.

Demand for autos slumped. Demand for the whole of 1995 was expected to come in between 30 and 50 percent below 1994 levels. Volkswagen, Nissan, Mercedes-Benz, and Ford temporarily closed their Mexican factories in January in expectation of the drop in demand. In other developments, Fiat of Italy pulled out of plans to build a new auto factory in Mexico, while Nissan announced plans to cut its 1995 production in Mexico from 210,000 to 180,000 vehicles. However, while the short-term outlook was grim, many auto companies expected to benefit from the fall in value of the peso in the longer run. Although Volkswagen closed its Mexican plant for two weeks in January 1995, it planned to ship 175,000 Mexican-made vehicles to the United States in 1995, 25,000 more than in 1994. Similarly, the big three U.S. automakers planned to keep their Mexican plants operating at full capacity in the second half of 1995 by boosting exports to the United States.

Sources: J. Darling and D. Nauss, "Stall in the Fast Lane," *Los Angeles Times,* February 19, 1995, p. 1; "Mexico Drops Efforts to Prop Up Peso," *Wall Street Journal,* December 23, 1994, p. A3; and R. Dornbusch, "We Have Salinas to Thank for the Peso Debacle," *Business Week,* January 16, 1995, p. 20.

money-losing establishments. The result was a surge in the government's budget deficit. In the first quarter of 1992, the budget deficit amounted to 1.5 percent of the country's GDP. By the end of 1992, it had risen to 17 percent. Unable or unwilling to finance this deficit by raising taxes, the government found another solution—it printed money, which added fuel to the inflation fire.

With inflation rising, the ruble tumbled. By the end of 1992, the exchange rate was $1 = R480. By the end of 1993, it was $1 = R1,500. As 1994 progressed, it became increasingly evident that due to vigorous political opposition, the government would not be able to bring down its budget deficit as quickly as had been thought. By September the monthly inflation rate was accelerating. October started badly, with the ruble sliding more than 10 percent in value against the U.S. dollar in the first 10 days of the month. On October 11, the ruble plunged 21.5 percent against the dollar, reaching a value of $15=R3,926 by the time the foreign exchange market closed!

Despite the announcement of a tough budget plan that placed tight controls on the money supply, the ruble continued to slide, and by April 1995 the exchange rate stood at $1 = R5,120. However, inflation was again on the way down by mid-1995. In June 1995, the monthly inflation rate was at a yearly low of 6.7 percent. Also, the ruble had recovered to stand at $1 = R4,559 by July 6. On that day the Russian government announced it would intervene in the currency market to keep the ruble in a trading range of R4,300 to R4,900 against the dollar. The Russian government believed it was essential to maintain a relatively stable currency. Government officials announced that the central bank would be able to draw on $10 billion in foreign exchange reserves to defend the ruble against any speculative selling in Russia's relatively small foreign exchange market.

In the world of international finance, $10 billion is small change and it wasn't long before Russia found that its foreign exchange reserves were being depleted. It was at this point that the Russian government requested IMF loans. In February 1996, the IMF obliged with its second largest rescue effort after Mexico, a loan of $10 billion. In return for the loan, Russia agreed to limit the growth in its money supply, reduce public-sector debt, increase government tax revenues, and peg the ruble to the dollar.

The package seemed to have the desired effect initially. Inflation declined from nearly 50 percent in 1996 to about 15 percent in 1997; the exchange rate stayed within its predetermined band; and the balance-of-payments situation remained broadly favorable. In 1997, the Russian economy grew for the first time since the breakup of the former Soviet Union, if only by a modest half of 1 percent of GDP. However, the public-sector debt situation did not improve. The Russian government continued to spend more than it agreed to under IMF targets, while government tax revenues were much lower than projected. Low tax revenues were partly due to falling oil prices (the government collected tax on oil sales), partly due to the difficulties of collecting tax in an economy where so much economic activity was in the "underground economy," and partly due to a complex tax system that was peppered with loopholes. Currently available estimates indicate that in 1997, Russian federal government spending amounted to 18.3 percent of GDP, while revenues were only 10.8 percent of GDP, implying a deficit of 7.5 percent of GDP, which was financed by an expansion in public debt.

The IMF responded by suspending its scheduled payment to Russia in early 1998, pending reform of Russia's complex tax system and a sustained attempt by the Russian government to cut public spending. This put further pressure on the Russian ruble, forcing the Russian central bank to raise interest rates on overnight loans to 150 percent. In June 1998, the U.S. government indicated it would support a new IMF bailout. The IMF was more circumspect, insisting instead that the Russian government push through a package of corporate tax increases and public spending cuts to balance the budget. The Russian government indicated it would do so, and the IMF released a tranche of $640 million that had been suspended. The IMF followed this with an additional $11.2 billion loan designed to preserve the ruble's stability.

Almost as soon as the funding was announced, however, it began to unravel. The IMF loan required the Russian government to take concrete steps to raise personal tax rates, improve tax collections, and cut government spending. A bill containing the required legislative changes was sent to the Russian parliament, where it was emasculated by antigovernment forces. The IMF responded by withholding $800 million of its first $5.6 billion tranche, undermining the credibility of its own program. The Russian stock market plummeted on the news, closing down 6.5 percent. Sales of rubles accelerated. The central bank began hemorrhaging foreign exchange reserves as it tried to maintain the value of the ruble. Foreign exchange reserves fell by $1.4 billion in the first week of August, to $17 billion, while interest rates surged again.

Against this background, on the weekend of August 15–16, top Russian officials huddled to develop a response to the most recent crisis. Their options were limited. The patience of the IMF had been exhausted. Foreign currency reserves were being rapidly depleted. Social tensions in the country were running high. The government faced upcoming redemptions on $18 billion of domestic bonds, with no idea of where the money would come from.

On Monday, August 17, Prime Minister Sergei Kiriyenko announced the results of the weekend's conclave. He said Russia would restructure the domestic debt market, unilaterally transforming short-term debt into long-term debt. In other words, the government had decided to default on its debt commitments. The government also announced a 90-day moratorium on the repayment of private foreign debt and stated it would allow the ruble to decline by 34 percent against the U.S. dollar. In short, Russia had turned its back on the IMF plan. The effect was immediate. Overnight, shops marked up the price of goods by 20 percent. As the ruble plummeted, currency exchange points were prepared to sell dollars only at a rate of 9 rubles per dollar, rather than the new official exchange rate of 6.43 rubles to the dollar. As for Russian government debt, it lost 85 percent of its value in a matter of hours, leaving foreign and Russian holders of debt alike suddenly gaping at a huge black hole in their financial assets.[13]

The Asian Crisis

The financial crisis that erupted across Southeast Asia during the fall of 1997 emerged as the biggest challenge to date for the IMF. Holding the crisis in check required IMF loans to help the shattered economies of Indonesia, Thailand, and South Korea stabilize their currencies. In addition, although they did not request IMF loans, the economies of Japan, Malaysia, Singapore, and the Philippines were also hurt by the crisis.

The seeds of this crisis were sown during the previous decade when these countries were experiencing unprecedented economic growth. Although there were and remain important differences between the individual countries, a number of elements were common to most. Exports had long been the engine of economic growth in these countries. From 1990 to 1996, the value of exports from Malaysia had grown by 18 percent annually, Thai exports had grown by 16 percent per year, Singapore's by 15 percent, Hong Kong's by 14 percent, and those of South Korea and Indonesia by 12 percent annually.[14] The nature of these exports had also shifted in recent years from basic materials and products such as textiles to complex and increasingly high-technology products, such as automobiles, semiconductors, and consumer electronics.

The Investment Boom

The wealth created by export-led growth helped fuel an investment boom in commercial and residential property, industrial assets, and infrastructure. The value of commercial and residential real estate in cities such as Hong Kong and Bangkok started to soar. This fed a building boom the likes of which had never been seen in Asia. Heavy borrowing from banks financed much of this construction. As for industrial assets, the success of Asian exporters encouraged them to make bolder investments in industrial capacity. This was exemplified most clearly by South Korea's giant diversified conglomerates, or *chaebol,* many of which had ambitions to build a major position in the global automobile and semiconductor industries.

An added factor behind the investment boom in most Southeast Asian economies was the government. In many cases, the governments had embarked on huge infrastructure projects. In Malaysia, for example, a new government administrative center was being constructed in Putrajaya for M$20 billion (U.S.$8 billion at the pre-July 1997 exchange rate), and the government was funding the development of a massive high-technology communications corridor and the huge Bakun dam, which at a cost of M$13.6 billion was to be the most expensive power generation plant in the country.[15] Throughout the region, governments also encouraged private businesses to invest in certain sectors of the economy in accordance with "national goals" and "industrialization strategy." In South Korea, long a country where the government played a proactive role in private-sector investments, President Kim Young-Sam urged the *chaebol* to invest in new factories as a way of boosting economic growth. South Korea enjoyed an investment-led economic boom in 1994–95, but at a cost. The *chaebol*, always reliant on heavy borrowings, built up massive debts that were equivalent, on average, to four times their equity.[16]

In Indonesia, President Suharto had long supported investments in a network of an estimated 300 businesses owned by his family and friends in a system known as "crony capitalism." Many of these businesses were granted lucrative monopolies by the president. For example, Suharto announced in 1995 that he had decided to build a national car and the car would be built by a company owned by one of his sons, Hutomo Mandala Putra, in association with Kia Motors of South Korea. To support the venture, a consortium of Indonesian banks was "ordered" by the government to offer almost $700 million in start-up loans to the company.[17]

By the mid-1990s, Southeast Asia was in the grips of an unprecedented investment boom, much of it financed with borrowed money. Between 1990 and 1995, gross domestic investment grew by 16.3 percent annually in Indonesia, 16 percent in Malaysia, 15.3 percent in Thailand, and 7.2 percent in South Korea. By comparison, investment grew by 4.1 percent annually over the same period in the United States and 0.8 percent in all high-income economies.[18] And the rate of investment accelerated in 1996. In Malaysia, for example, spending on investment accounted for a remarkable 43 percent of GDP in 1996.[19]

Excess Capacity

As the volume of investments ballooned during the 1990s, often at the bequest of national governments, the quality of many of these investments declined significantly. The investments often were made on the basis of unrealistic projections about future demand conditions. The result was significant excess capacity. For example, South Korean *chaebol* investments in semiconductor factories surged in 1994 and 1995 when a temporary global shortage of dynamic random access memory chips (DRAMs) led to sharp price increases for this product. However, supply shortages had disappeared by 1996 and excess capacity was beginning to make itself felt, just as the South Koreans started to bring new DRAM factories on stream. The results were predictable; prices for DRAMs plunged, and the earnings of South Korean DRAM manufacturers fell by 90 percent, which meant it was difficult for them to make scheduled payments on the debt they had taken on to build the extra capacity.[20]

In another example, a building boom in Thailand resulted in excess capacity in residential and commercial property. By early 1997, an estimated 365,000 apartment units were unoccupied in Bangkok. With another 100,000 units scheduled to be completed in 1997, years of excess demand in the Thai property market had been replaced by excess supply. By one estimate, Bangkok's building boom had produced enough excess space by 1997 to meet its residential and commercial needs for five years.[21]

The Debt Bomb

By early 1997 what was happening in the South Korean semiconductor industry and the Bangkok property market was being played out elsewhere in the region. Massive investments in industrial assets and property had created excess capacity and plunging prices, while leaving the companies that had made the investments groaning under huge debt burdens that they were now finding it difficult to service.

To make matters worse, much of the borrowing had been in U.S. dollars, as opposed to local currencies. This had originally seemed like a smart move. Throughout the region, local currencies were pegged to the dollar, and interest rates on dollar borrowings were generally lower than rates on borrowings in domestic currency. Thus, it often made economic sense to borrow in dollars if the option was available. However, if the governments could not maintain the dollar peg and their currencies started to depreciate against the dollar, this would increase the size of the debt burden when measured in the local currency. Currency depreciation would raise borrowing costs and could result in companies defaulting on their debt obligations.

Expanding Imports

A final complicating factor was that by the mid-1990s, although exports were still expanding across the region, imports were too. The investments in infrastructure, industrial capacity, and commercial real estate were sucking in foreign goods at unprecedented rates. To build infrastructure, factories, and office buildings, Southeast Asian countries were purchasing capital equipment and materials from America, Europe, and Japan. Many Southeast Asian states saw the current accounts of their balance of payments shift strongly into the red during the mid-1990s. By 1995, Indonesia was running a current account deficit that was equivalent to 3.5 percent of its GDP, Malaysia's was 5.9 percent, and Thailand's was 8.1 percent.[22] With deficits like these, it was increasingly difficult for the governments of these countries to maintain their currencies against the U.S. dollar. If that peg could not be held, the local currency value of dollar-denominated debt would increase, raising the specter of large-scale default on debt service payments. The scene was now set for a potentially rapid economic meltdown.

The Crisis

The Asian meltdown began in mid-1997 in Thailand when it became clear that several key Thai financial institutions were on the verge of default (see the closing case to Chapter 9 for more details). These institutions had been borrowing dollars from international banks at low interest rates and lending Thai baht at higher interest rates to local property developers. However, due to speculative overbuilding, these developers could not sell their commercial and residential property, forcing them to default on their debt obligations. In turn, the Thai financial institutions seemed increasingly likely to default on their dollar-denominated debt obligations to international banks. Sensing the beginning of the crisis, foreign investors fled the Thai stock market, selling their positions and converting them into U.S. dollars. The increased demand for dollars and increased supply of Thai baht, pushed down the dollar/Thai baht exchange rate, while the stock market plunged.

Seeing these developments, foreign exchange dealers and hedge funds started speculating against the baht, selling it short. For the previous 13 years, the Thai baht had been pegged to the U.S. dollar at an exchange rate of about $1 = Bt25. The Thai government tried to defend the peg, but only succeeded in depleting its foreign exchange reserves. On July 2, 1997, the Thai government abandoned its defense and announced it would allow the baht to float freely against the dollar. The baht started a slide that would bring the exchange rate down to $1 = Bt55 by January 1998. As the baht declined, the Thai debt bomb exploded. The 55 percent decline in the value of the baht against the dollar doubled the amount of baht required to serve the dollar-denominated debt commitments taken on by Thai financial institutions and businesses. This increased the probability of corporate bankruptcies and further pushed down the battered Thai stock market. The Thailand Set stock market index ultimately declined from 787 in January 1997 to a low of 337 in December of that year, on top of a 45 percent decline in 1996.

On July 28, the Thai government called in the International Monetary Fund. With its foreign exchange reserves depleted, Thailand lacked the foreign currency needed to finance its international trade and service debt commitments and desperately needed the capital the IMF could provide. It also needed to restore international confidence in its currency and needed the credibility associated with gaining access to IMF funds. Without IMF loans, the baht likely would increase its free fall against the U.S. dollar and the whole country might go into default. The IMF agreed to provide the Thai government with $17.2 billion in loans, but the conditions were restrictive.[23] The IMF required the Thai government to increase taxes, cut public spending, privatize several state-owned businesses, and raise interest rates—all steps designed to cool Thailand's overheated economy. The IMF also required Thailand to close illiquid financial institutions. In December 1997, the government shut 56 financial institutions, laying off 16,000 people and further deepening the recession that now gripped the country.

Following the devaluation of the Thai baht, wave after wave of speculation hit other Asian currencies. One after another in a period of weeks, the Malaysian ringgit, Indonesian rupiah, and the Singaporean dollar were all marked sharply lower. With its foreign exchange reserves down to $28 billion, Malaysia let the ringgit float on July 14, 1997. Before the devaluation, the ringgit was trading at $1 = 2.525 ringgit. Six months later it had declined to $1 = 4.15 ringgit. Singapore followed on July 17, and the Singaporean dollar quickly dropped in value from $1 = S$1.495 before the devaluation to $1 = S$2.68 a few days later. Next up was Indonesia, whose rupiah was allowed to float August 14. For Indonesia, this was the beginning of a precipitous decline in the value of its currency, which was to fall from $1 = 2,400 rupiah in August 1997 to $1 = 10,000 rupiah on January 6, 1998, a loss of 76 percent.

With the exception of Singapore, whose economy is probably the most stable in the region, these devaluations were driven by factors similar to those behind the earlier devaluation of the Thai baht—a combination of excess investment; high borrowings, much of it in dollar-denominated debt; and a deteriorating balance-of-payments position. Although both Malaysia and Singapore were able to halt the slide in their currencies and stock markets without the help of the IMF, Indonesia was not. Indonesia was struggling with a private-sector, dollar-denominated debt of close to $80 billion. With the rupiah sliding precipitously almost every day, the cost of servicing this debt was exploding, pushing more Indonesian companies into technical default.

On October 31, 1997, the IMF announced it had put together a $37 billion rescue deal for Indonesia in conjunction with the World Bank and the Asian Development Bank. In return, the Indonesian government agreed to close a number of troubled banks, reduce public spending, remove government subsidies on basic foodstuffs and energy, balance the budget, and unravel the crony capitalism that was so widespread in Indonesia. But the government of President Suharto appeared to backtrack several times on commitments made to the IMF. This precipitated further declines in the Indonesian currency and stock markets. Ultimately, Suharto caved in and removed costly government subsidies, only to see the country dissolve into chaos as the populace took to the streets to protest the resulting price increases. This unleashed a chain of events that led to Suharto's removal from power in May 1998.

The final domino to fall was South Korea (for further details, see the Country Focus in Chapter 9). During the 1990s, South Korean companies had built up huge debt loads as they invested heavily in new industrial capacity. Now they found they had too much industrial capacity and could not generate the income required to service their debt. South Korean banks and companies had also made the mistake of borrowing in dollars, much of it in the form of short-term loans that would come due within a year. Thus, when the Korean won started to decline in the fall of 1997 in sympathy with the problems elsewhere in Asia, South Korean companies saw their debt obligations balloon. Several large companies were forced to file for bankruptcy. This triggered a decline in the South Korean currency and stock market that was difficult to halt. The South Korean central bank tried to keep the dollar/won exchange rate above $1=W1,000 but found that this only depleted its foreign exchange reserves. On November 17, the South Korean central bank gave up the defense of the won, which quickly fell to $1=W1,500.

With its economy on the verge of collapse, the South Korean government on November 21 requested $20 billion in standby loans from the IMF. As the negotiations progressed, it became apparent that South Korea was going to need far more than $20 billion. Among other problems, the country's short-term foreign debt was found to be twice as large as previously thought at close to $100 billion, while the country's foreign exchange reserves were down to less than $6 billion. On December 3, 1997, the IMF and South Korean government reached a deal to lend $55 billion to the country. The agreement with the IMF called for the South Koreans to open their economy and banking system to foreign investors. South Korea also pledged to restrain the *chaebol* by reducing their share of bank financing and requiring them to publish consolidated financial statements and undergo annual independent external audits. On trade liberalization, the IMF said South Korea would comply with its commitments to the World Trade Organization to eliminate trade-related subsidies and restrictive import licensing and would streamline its import certification procedures, all of which should open the South Korean economy to greater foreign competition.[24]

Evaluating the IMF's Policy Prescriptions

By 2002, the IMF was committing over $88 billion in loans to more than 80 countries struggling with economic and currency crises. All these loan packages came with conditions attached. In general, the IMF insists on a combination of tight macroeconomic policies, including cuts in public spending, higher interest rates, and tight monetary policy. It also often pushes for the deregulation of sectors formerly protected from domestic and foreign competition, privatization of state-owned assets, and better financial reporting from the banking sector. These policies are designed to cool overheated economies by reining in inflation and reducing government spending and debt. Recently, this set of policy prescriptions has come in for tough criticisms from many observers.[25]

Inappropriate Policies

One criticism is that the IMF's "one-size-fits-all" approach to macroeconomic policy is inappropriate for many countries. In the case of the Asian crisis, critics argue that the tight macroeconomic policies imposed by the IMF are not well suited to countries that are suffering not from excessive government spending and inflation, but from a private-sector debt crisis with deflationary undertones.[26] In South Korea, for example, the government had been running a budget surplus for years (it was 4 percent of South Korea's GDP in 1994–1996) and inflation was low at about 5 percent. South Korea had the second strongest financial position of any country in the Organization for Economic Cooperation and Development. Despite this, critics say, the IMF insisted on applying the same policies that it applies to countries suffering from high inflation. The IMF required South Korea to maintain an inflation rate of 5 percent. However, given the collapse in the value of its currency and the subsequent rise in price for imports such as oil, critics claimed inflationary pressures would inevitably increase in South Korea. So to hit a 5 percent inflation rate, the South Koreans would be forced to apply an unnecessarily tight monetary policy. Short-term interest rates in South Korea did jump from 12.5 percent to 21 percent immediately after the country signed its initial deal with the IMF. Increasing interest rates made it even more difficult for companies to service their already excessive short-term debt obligations, and critics used this as evidence to argue that the cure prescribed by the IMF may actually increase the probability of widespread corporate defaults, not reduce them.

The IMF rejected this criticism. According to the IMF, the central task was to rebuild confidence in the won. Once this was achieved, the won would recover from its oversold levels, reducing the size of South Korea's dollar-denominated debt burden when expressed in won, making it easier for companies to service their dollar-denominated debt. The IMF also argued that by requiring South Korea to remove restrictions on foreign direct investment, foreign capital would flow into the country to take advantage of cheap assets. This, too, would increase demand for the Korean currency and help to improve the dollar/won exchange rate.

Korea did recover fairly quickly from the crisis, supporting the position of the IMF. While the economy contracted by 7 percent in 1998, by 2000 it had rebounded and grew at a 9 percent rate (measured by growth in GDP). Inflation, which peaked at 8 percent in 1998, fell to 2 percent by 2000, and unemployment fell from 7 percent to 4 percent over the same period. The won hit a low of $1 = W1,812 in early 1998, but by 2000 was back to an exchange rate of around $1 = W1,200, at which it seems to have stabilized.

Moral Hazard

A second criticism of the IMF is that its rescue efforts are exacerbating a problem known to economists as moral hazard. **Moral hazard** arises when people behave recklessly because they know they will be saved if things go wrong. Critics point out that many Japanese and Western banks were far too willing to lend large amounts of capital to overleveraged Asian companies during the boom years of the 1990s. These critics argue that the banks should now be forced to pay the price for their rash lending policies, even if that means some banks must close.[27] Only by taking such drastic action, the argument goes, will banks learn the error of their ways and not engage in rash lending in the future. By providing support to these countries, the IMF is reducing the probability of debt default and in effect bailing out the banks whose loans gave rise to this situation.

This argument ignores two critical points. First, if some Japanese or Western banks with heavy exposure to the troubled Asian economies were forced to write off their loans due to widespread debt default, the impact would be difficult to contain. The failure of large Japanese banks, for example, could trigger a meltdown in the Japanese financial markets. This would almost inevitably lead to a serious decline in stock markets around the world. That is the very risk the IMF was trying to avoid by stepping in with financial support. Second, it is incorrect to imply that some banks have not had to pay the price for rash lending policies. The IMF has insisted on the closure of banks in South Korea, Thailand, and Indonesia. Foreign banks with short-term loans outstanding to South Korean enterprises have been forced by circumstances to reschedule those loans at interest rates that do not compensate for the extension of the loan maturity.

Lack of Accountability

The final criticism of the IMF is that it has become too powerful for an institution that lacks any real mechanism for accountability.[28] By 2002, the IMF was engaged in loan programs in 88 developing countries that collectively contain 1.4 billion people. The IMF was determining macroeconomic policies in those countries, yet according to critics such as noted Harvard economist Jeffrey Sachs, the IMF, with a staff of less than 1,000, lacks the expertise required to do a good job. Evidence of this, according to Sachs, can be found in the fact that the IMF was singing the praises of the Thai and South Korean governments only months before both countries lurched into crisis. Then the IMF put together a draconian program for South Korea without having deep knowledge of the country. Sachs's solution to this problem is to reform the IMF so it makes greater use of outside experts and its operations are open to greater outside scrutiny.

Observations

As with many debates about international economics, it is not clear which side has the winning hand about the appropriateness of IMF policies. There are cases where one can argue that IMF policies have been counterproductive. In addition, one might question the success of the IMF's involvement in Turkey, given that the country has had to implement 18 IMF programs since 1958! But the IMF can also point to some notable accomplishments, including its success in containing the Asian crisis, which could have rocked the global international monetary system to its core. Similarly, many observers give the IMF credit for its deft handling of politically difficult situations, such as the Russian ruble crisis and Mexican peso crisis, and for successfully promoting a free market philosophy.

Several years after the IMF's intervention, the economies of Asia, Russia, and Mexico had all recovered to some extent. Certainly they had all averted the kind of catastrophic implosion that might have occurred had the IMF not stepped in, and although some countries still faced considerable problems, it is not clear that the IMF should take much blame for this. At the end of the day, the IMF cannot force countries to adopt the policies required to correct economic mismanagement. As the opening case on Turkey illustrates, while a government may commit to taking corrective action in return for an IMF loan, internal political problems may make it difficult for a government to act on that commitment. In such cases, the IMF is caught between a rock and a hard place, for if it decided to withhold money, it might trigger financial collapse and the kind of contagion that it seeks to avoid.

Focus On Managerial Implications

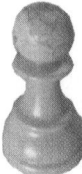

In chapters focusing on the external business environment, the Implications for Business section shows how the concepts apply to the practice of international business. The implications for international businesses of the material discussed in this chapter fall into three main areas: currency management, business strategy, and corporate–government relations.

Currency Management

An obvious implication with regard to currency management is that companies must recognize that the foreign exchange market does not work quite as depicted in Chapter 9. The current system is a mixed system in which a combination of government intervention and speculative activity can drive the foreign exchange market. Companies engaged in significant foreign exchange activities need to be aware of this and to adjust their foreign exchange transactions accordingly. For example, the currency management unit of Caterpillar claims it made millions of dollars in the hours following the announcement of the Plaza Accord by selling dollars and buying currencies that it expected to appreciate on the foreign exchange market following government intervention.

We have seen how under the present system, speculative buying and selling of currencies can create very volatile movements in exchange rates (as exhibited by the rise and fall of the dollar during the 1980s). Contrary to the predictions of the purchasing power parity theory (see Chapter 9), we have seen that exchange rate movements during the 1980s, at least with regard to the dollar, did not seem to be strongly influenced by relative inflation rates. Insofar as volatile exchange rates increase foreign exchange risk, this is not good news for business. On the other hand, as we saw in Chapter 9, the foreign exchange market has developed a number of instruments, such as the forward market and swaps, that can help to insure against foreign exchange risk. Not surprisingly, use of these instruments has increased markedly since the breakdown of the Bretton Woods system in 1973.

Business Strategy

The volatility of the present global exchange rate regime presents a conundrum for international businesses. Exchange rate movements are difficult to predict, and yet their movement can have a major impact on a business's competitive position. Faced with uncertainty about the future value of currencies, firms can utilize the forward exchange market. However, the forward exchange market is far from perfect as a predictor of future exchange rates (see Chapter 9). It is also difficult if not impossible to get adequate insurance coverage for exchange rate changes that might occur several years in the future. The forward market tends to offer coverage for exchange rate changes a few months—not years—ahead. Given this, it makes sense to pursue strategies that will increase the company's strategic flexibility in the face of unpredictable exchange rate movements.

Maintaining strategic flexibility can take the form of dispersing production to different locations around the globe as a real hedge against currency fluctuations. Consider the case of Daimler-Benz (now DaimlerChrysler), Germany's export-oriented automobile and aerospace company. In June 1995, the company stunned the German business community when it announced it expected to post a severe loss in 1995 of about $720 million. The cause was Germany's strong currency, which had appreciated by 4 percent against a basket of major currencies since the beginning of 1995 and had risen by over 30 percent against the U.S. dollar since late 1994. By mid-1995, the exchange rate against the dollar stood at $1 = DM1.38. Daimler's management believed it could not make money with an exchange rate under $1 = DM1.60. Daimler's senior managers concluded that the appreciation of the mark against the dollar was probably permanent, so they decided to move substantial production outside of Germany and increase purchasing of foreign components. The idea was to reduce the vulnerability of the company to future exchange rate movements. The Mercedes-Benz division has begun to implement this move. Even before its acquisition of Chrysler Corporation in 1998, Mercedes planned to produce 10 percent of its cars outside of Germany by 2000, mostly in the United States.[29] Similarly, the move by Japanese automobile companies to expand their productive capacity in the United States and Europe can be seen in the context of the increase in the value of the yen between 1985 and 1995, which raised the price of Japanese exports. For the Japanese companies, building production capacity overseas is a hedge against continued appreciation of the yen (as well as against trade barriers).

Another way of building strategic flexibility involves contracting out manufacturing. This allows a company to shift suppliers from country to country in response to changes in relative costs brought about by exchange rate movements. However, this kind of strategy may work only for low-value-added manufacturing (e.g., textiles), in which the individual manufacturers have few if any firm-specific skills that contribute to the value of the product. It may be less appropriate for high-value-added manufacturing, in which firm-specific technology and skills add significant value to the product (e.g., the heavy equipment industry) and in which switching costs are correspondingly high. For high-value-added manufacturing, switching suppliers will lead to a reduction in the value that is added, which may offset any cost gains arising from exchange rate fluctuations.

The roles of the IMF and the World Bank in the present international monetary system also have implications for business strategy. Increasingly, the IMF has been acting as the macroeconomic policeman of the world economy, insisting that countries seeking significant borrowings adopt IMF-mandated macroeconomic policies. These policies typically include anti-inflationary monetary policies and reductions in government spending. In the short run, such policies usually result in a sharp contraction of demand. International businesses selling or producing in such countries need to be aware of this and plan accordingly. In the long run, the kind of policies imposed by the IMF can promote economic growth and an expansion of demand, which create opportunities for international business.

Corporate–Government Relations

As major players in the international trade and investment environment, businesses can influence government policy toward the international monetary system. For example, intense government lobbying by U.S. exporters helped convince the U.S. government that intervention in the foreign exchange market was necessary. With this in mind, business can and should use its influence to promote an international monetary system that facilitates the growth of international trade and investment. Whether a fixed or floating regime is optimal is a subject for debate. However, exchange rate volatility such as the world experienced during the 1980s and 1990s creates an environment less conducive to international trade and investment than one with more stable exchange rates. Therefore, it would seem to be in the interests of international business to promote an international monetary system that minimizes volatile exchange rate movements, particularly when those movements are unrelated to long-run economic fundamentals.

ChapterSummary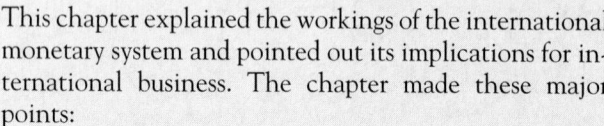

This chapter explained the workings of the international monetary system and pointed out its implications for international business. The chapter made these major points:

1. The gold standard is a monetary standard that pegs currencies to gold and guarantees convertibility to gold.

2. It was thought that the gold standard contained an automatic mechanism that contributed to the simultaneous achievement of a balance-of-payments equilibrium by all countries.

3. The gold standard broke down during the 1930s as countries engaged in competitive devaluations.

4. The Bretton Woods system of fixed exchange rates was established in 1944. The U.S. dollar was the central currency of this system; the value of every other currency was pegged to its value. Significant exchange rate devaluations were allowed only with the permission of the IMF.

5. The role of the IMF was to maintain order in the international monetary system (i) to avoid a repetition of the competitive devaluations of the 1930s and (ii) to control price inflation by imposing monetary discipline on countries.

6. To build flexibility into the system, the IMF stood ready to lend countries funds to help protect their currency on the foreign exchange market in the face of speculative pressure and to assist countries in correcting a fundamental disequilibrium in their balance-of-payments position.

7. The fixed exchange rate system collapsed in 1973, primarily due to speculative pressure on the dollar following a rise in U.S. inflation and a growing U.S. balance-of-trade deficit.

8. Since 1973 the world has operated with a floating exchange rate regime, and exchange rates have become more volatile and far less predictable. Volatile exchange rate movements have helped reopen the debate over the merits of fixed and floating systems.

9. The case for a floating exchange rate regime claims (i) such a system gives countries autonomy regarding their monetary policy and (ii) floating exchange rates facilitate smooth adjustment of trade imbalances.

10. The case for a fixed exchange rate regime claims (i) the need to maintain a fixed exchange rate imposes monetary discipline on a country, (ii) floating exchange rate regimes are vulnerable to speculative pressure, (iii) the uncertainty that accompanies floating exchange rates dampens the growth of international trade and investment, and (iv) far from correcting trade imbalances, depreciating a currency on the foreign exchange market tends to cause price inflation.

11. In today's international monetary system, some countries have adopted floating exchange rates, some have pegged their currency to another currency, such as the U.S. dollar, and some have pegged their currency to a basket of other currencies, allowing their currency to fluctuate within a zone around the basket.

12. In the post-Bretton Woods era, the IMF has continued to play an important role in helping countries navigate their way through financial crises by lending significant capital to embattled governments and by requiring them to adopt certain macroeconomic policies.

13. An important debate is occurring over the appropriateness of IMF-mandated macroeconomic policies. Critics charge that the IMF often imposes inappropriate conditions on developing nations that are the recipients of its loans.

14. The present managed-float system of exchange rate determination has increased the importance of currency management in international businesses.

15. The volatility of exchange rates under the present managed-float system creates both opportunities and threats. One way of responding to this volatility is for companies to build strategic flexibility by dispersing production to different locations around the globe by contracting out manufacturing (in the case of low-value-added manufacturing) and other means.

Critical Discussion Questions

1. Why did the gold standard collapse? Is there a case for returning to some type of gold standard? What is it?

2. What opportunities might current IMF lending policies to developing nations create for international businesses? What threats might they create?

3. Do you think the standard IMF policy prescriptions of tight monetary policy and reduced government spending are always appropriate for developing nations experiencing a currency crisis? How might the IMF change its approach? What would the implications be for international businesses?

4. Debate the relative merits of fixed and floating exchange rate regimes. From the perspective of an international business, what are the most important criteria in a choice between the systems? Which system is the more desirable for an international business?

5. Imagine that Canada, the United States, and Mexico decide to adopt a fixed exchange rate system. What would be the likely consequences of such a system for (a) international businesses and (b) the flow of trade and investment among the three countries?

Notes

1. Updates can be found at the IMF website: http://www.imf.org/external/np/exr/facts/glance.htm

2. The argument goes back to 18th-century philosopher David Hume. See D. Hume, "On the Balance of Trade," reprinted in *The Gold Standard in Theory and in History*, ed. B. Eichengreen (London: Methuen, 1985).

3. R. Solomon, *The International Monetary System, 1945–1981* (New York: Harper & Row, 1982).

4. International Monetary Fund, *World Economic Outlook, 1998* (Washington, DC: IMF, May 1998).

5. For an extended discussion of the dollar exchange rate in the 1980s, see B. D. Pauls, "US Exchange Rate Policy: Bretton Woods to the Present," *Federal Reserve Bulletin*, November 1990, pp. 891–908.

6. For a feel for the issues contained in this debate, see P. Krugman, *Has the Adjustment Process Worked?* (Washington, DC: Institute for International Economics, 1991); "Time to Tether Currencies," *The Economist*, January 6, 1990, pp. 15–16; P. R. Krugman and M. Obstfeld, *International Economics: Theory and Policy* (New York: HarperCollins, 1994); J. Shelton, *Money Meltdown* (New York: Free Press, 1994); and S. Edwards, "Exchange Rates and the Political Economy of Macroeconomic Discipline," *American Economic Review* 86, no. 2 (May 1996), pp. 159–63.

7. The argument is made by several prominent economists, particularly Stanford's Robert McKinnon. See R. McKinnon, "An International Standard for Monetary Stabilization," *Policy Analyses in International Economics* 8 (1984). The details of this argument are beyond the scope of this book. For a relatively accessible exposition, see P. Krugman, *The Age of Diminished Expectations* (Cambridge, MA: MIT Press, 1990).

8. A. R. Ghosh and A. M. Gulde, "Does the Exchange Rate Regime Matter for Inflation and Growth?" *Economic Issues*, no. 2 (1997).

9. "The ABC of Currency Boards," *The Economist*, November 1, 1997, p. 80.

10. International Monetary Fund, *World Economic Outlook, 1998*.

11. Ibid.

12. See P. Carroll and C. Torres, "Mexico Unveils Program of Harsh Fiscal Medicine," *Wall Street Journal*, March 10, 1995, pp. A1, A6, and "Putting Mexico Together Again," *The Economist*, February 4, 1995, p. 65.

13. S. Erlanger, "Russia Will Test a Trading Band for the Ruble," *New York Times*, July 7, 1995, p. 1; C. Freeland, "Russia to Introduce a Trading Band for Ruble against Dollar," *Financial Times*, July 7, 1995, p. 1; J. Thornhill, "Russians Bemused by 'Black Tuesday,'" *Financial Times*, October 12, 1994, p. 4; R. Sikorski, "Mirage of Numbers," *Wall Street Journal*, May 18, 1994, p. 14; "Can Russia Fight Back?" *The Economist*, June 6, 1998,

pp. 47–48; and J. Thornhill, "Russia's Shrinking Options," *Financial Times*, August 19, 1998, p. 19.

14. World Trade Organization, *Annual Report, 1997*, vol. II, table III, p. 69.

15. J. Ridding and J. Kynge, "Complacency Gives Way to Contagion," *Financial Times*, January 13, 1998, p. 8.

16. J. Burton and G. Baker, "The Country That Invested Its Way into Trouble," *Financial Times*, January 15, 1998, p. 8.

17. P. Shenon, "The Suharto Billions," *New York Times*, January 16, 1998, p. 1.

18. World Bank, *1997 World Development Report* (Oxford: Oxford University Press), Table 11.

19. Ridding and Kynge, "Complacency Gives Way to Contagion."

20. Burton and Baker, "The Country That Invested Its Way into Trouble."

21. "Bitter Pill for the Thais," *Straits Times*, July 5, 1997, p. 46.

22. World Bank, *1997 World Development Report*, Table 2.

23. International Monetary Fund, Press Release No. 97/37, August 20, 1997.

24. T. S. Shorrock, "Korea Starts Overhaul; IMF Aid Hits $60 Billion," *Journal of Commerce*, December 8, 1997, p. 3A.

25. See J. Sachs, "Economic Transition and Exchange Rate Regime," *American Economic Review* 86, no. 92 (May 1996), pp. 147–52, and J. Sachs, "Power unto Itself," *Financial Times*, December 11, 1997, p. 11.

26. Sachs, "Power unto Itself."

27. Martin Wolf, "Same Old IMF Medicine," *Financial Times*, December 9, 1997, p. 12.

28. Sachs, "Power unto Itself."

29. P. Gumbel and B. Coleman, "Daimler Warns of Severe 95 Loss Due to Strong Mark," *New York Times*, June 29, 1995, pp. 1, 10, and M. Wolf, "Daimler-Benz Announces Major Losses," *Financial Times*, June 29, 1995, p. 1.

Research Task | globalEDGE™   globaledge.msu.edu

Use the globalEDGE™ site to complete the following exercises:

1. U.S. Department of State provides annual country reports on economic policy and trade practices. Locate these reports and prepare a description of the exchange rate and debt management policies of an emerging market of your choice.

2. The Biz/ed website presents a "Trade Balance and Exchange Rate Simulation" which helps understand how a change in exchange rate influences the trade balance. Locate the online simulator (check under the Academy section of globalEDGE) and identify what the trade balance is assumed to be a function of. Run the simulation to identify how exchange rate changes affect the exports, imports and trade balance.

The Tragedy of the Congo (Zaire)

Closing Case

The Democratic Republic of the Congo, formerly known as Zaire, gained its independence from Belgium in 1960. The central African nation, rich in natural resources such as copper, seemed to have a promising future. If the country had simply sustained its preindependence economic growth rate, its gross national product (GNP) would have been $1,400 per capita by 1997, making it one of the richest countries in Africa. Instead, by 1997, the country was a wreck. Battered by a brutal civil war that led to the ousting of the country's longtime dictator, Mobutu Sese Seko, the economy had shrunk to its 1958 level with a GNP per capita below $100. The annual inflation rate was in excess of 750 percent, an improvement from the 9,800 percent inflation rate recorded in 1994. Consequently, the local currency was almost worthless. Most transactions were made by barter or, for the lucky few, with U.S. dollars. Infant mortality stood at a dismal 106 per 1,000 live births, and life expectancy stood at 47 years, roughly comparable to that of Europe in the Middle Ages.

What were the underlying causes of the economic, political, and social collapse of Zaire? While the story is a complex one, according to several influential critics, some of the blame must be placed at the feet of two multinational lending institutions, the International Monetary Fund (IMF) and the World Bank. Both institutions were established in 1944 at the famous Bretton Woods conference, which paved the way for the post–World War II international monetary system. The IMF was given the task of maintaining order in the international monetary system, while the role of the World Bank was to promote general economic development, particularly among the world's poorer nations. The IMF typically provides loans to countries whose currencies are losing value due to economic mismanagement. In return for these loans, the IMF imposes on debtor countries strict financial policies that are designed to rein in inflation and stabilize their economies. The World Bank has historically provided low interest rate loans to help countries build basic infrastructure. Both institutions are funded by subscriptions from member states, including significant contributions from all of the world's developed nations.

The IMF and the World Bank were major donors to postindependence Zaire. The IMF's involvement with Zaire dates to 1967, when the IMF approved Zaire's first economic stabilization plan, backed by a $27 million line of credit. About the same time, the World Bank began to make low-interest infrastructure loans to the government of Mobutu Sese Seko. This was followed by a series of further plans and loans between 1976 and 1981. At the urging of the IMF, Zaire's currency was devalued five times during this period to help boost exports and reduce imports, while taxes were raised in an effort to balance Zaire's budget. IMF and other Western officials were also placed in key positions at the Zairian central bank, finance ministry, and office of debt management.

Despite all this help, Zaire's economy continued to deteriorate. By 1982, after 15 years of IMF assistance, Zaire had a lower GNP than in 1967 and faced default on its debt. Some critics, including Jeffrey Sachs, the noted development economist from Harvard University, claim that this poor performance could in part be attributed to the policies imposed by the IMF, which included tax hikes, cuts in government subsidies, and periodic competitive currency devaluations. These policies, claim critics, were ill suited to such a poor country and created a vicious cycle of economic decline. The tax hikes simply drove work into the "underground economy" or created a disincentive to work. As a consequence, government tax revenues dwindled and the budget deficit expanded, making it difficult for the government to service its debt obligations. By raising import prices,

the devaluations helped fuel the phenomenon the IMF was trying to control: inflation. In turn, high inflation of both prices and wages soon brought ordinary Zairians into high tax brackets, which drove even more work into the underground economy and further shrank government tax revenues.

When explaining Zaire's malaise, others point to corruption. In 1982, a senior IMF official in Zaire reported that President Mobutu Sese Seko and his cronies were systematically stealing IMF and World Bank loans. Later news reports suggest that Mobutu accumulated a personal fortune of $4 billion by the mid-1980s, making him one of the richest men in the world at that time.

In 1982, Zaire was initially suspended from further use of its IMF credit line. However, the position was reversed in 1983 when a new agreement was negotiated that included an additional $356 million in IMF loans. The loans were linked to a further devaluation of the Zairian currency, more tax hikes, and cuts in government subsidies. The IMF's decision to turn a blind eye to the corruption problem and extend new loans was influenced by pressure from Western politicians who saw Mobutu's pro-Western regime as a bulwark against the spread of Marxism in Africa. By ignoring the corruption, the IMF could claim it was abiding by IMF rules, which stated the institution should offer only economic advice and stay out of internal political issues. The IMF's decision lent credence to Mobutu Sese Seko's government and enabled Zaire to attract more foreign loans. As a consequence, the country's overall foreign debt increased to $5 billion by the mid-1980s, up from $3 billion in 1978.

Unfortunately, the new loans and IMF policies did little to improve Zaire's economic performance, which continued to deteriorate. In 1987, Zaire was forced to abandon its agreement with the IMF due to food riots. The IMF negotiated another agreement for 1989–91, which included further currency devaluation. This also failed to produce any tangible progress. The Zairian economy continued to implode while the country's civil war flared. In 1993, Zaire suspended its debt repayments, effectively going into default. In 1994, the World Bank announced it would shut down its operations in the country. About the same time, the IMF suspended Zaire's membership in the institution, making Zaire ineligible for further loans.

In 1997, after a long civil war, Mobutu Sese Seko was deposed. The new government inherited $14.6 billion of external debt, including debt arrears exceeding $1 billion. At a formal meeting chaired by the World Bank to discuss rescheduling of the country's debt, delegates from the new government claimed that the World Bank, IMF, and other institutions acted irresponsibly by lending money to Mobutu's regime despite evidence of both substantial corruption and Zaire's inability to service such a high level of debt. In an implicit acknowledgment that this may have been the case, the IMF and World Bank began telling debtor countries to stamp out corruption or lose access to IMF and World Bank loans.

Sources: G. Fossedal, "The IMF's Role in Zaire's Decline," *Wall Street Journal*, May 15, 1997, p. 22; J. Burns and M. Holman, "Mobutu Built a Fortune of $4 Billion from Looted Aid," *Financial Times*, May 12, 1997, p. 1; J. D. Sachs and R. I. Rotberg, "Help Congo Now," *New York Times*, May 29, 1997, p. 21; H. Dunphy, "IMF, World Bank Now Make Political Judgements," *Journal of Commerce*, August 21, 1997, p. 3A; and *CIA World Factbook* (Washington, DC: CIA, 1998).

Case Discussion Questions

1. What was the goal of the policies that (*a*) the IMF and (*b*) World Bank adopted toward Zaire? Do you think these policies were appropriate for an impoverished nation? In what ways may IMF policies have contributed to economic problems in Zaire?

2. Do you think the IMF and World Bank should lend money to countries such as Zaire where there is systematic evidence of widespread government corruption?

3. What alternative policies could the IMF and World Bank have adopted in Zaire? How might these policies have helped the country avert the economic and political chaos of the 1990s, which include a prolonged civil war and economic disintegration?

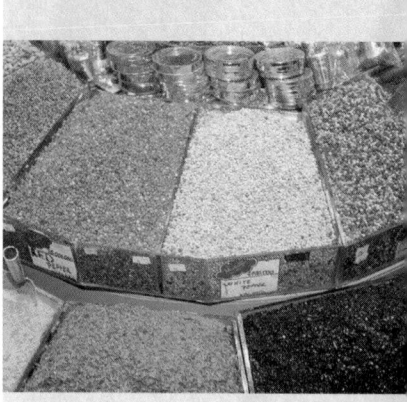

Chapter 11

The Global Capital Market

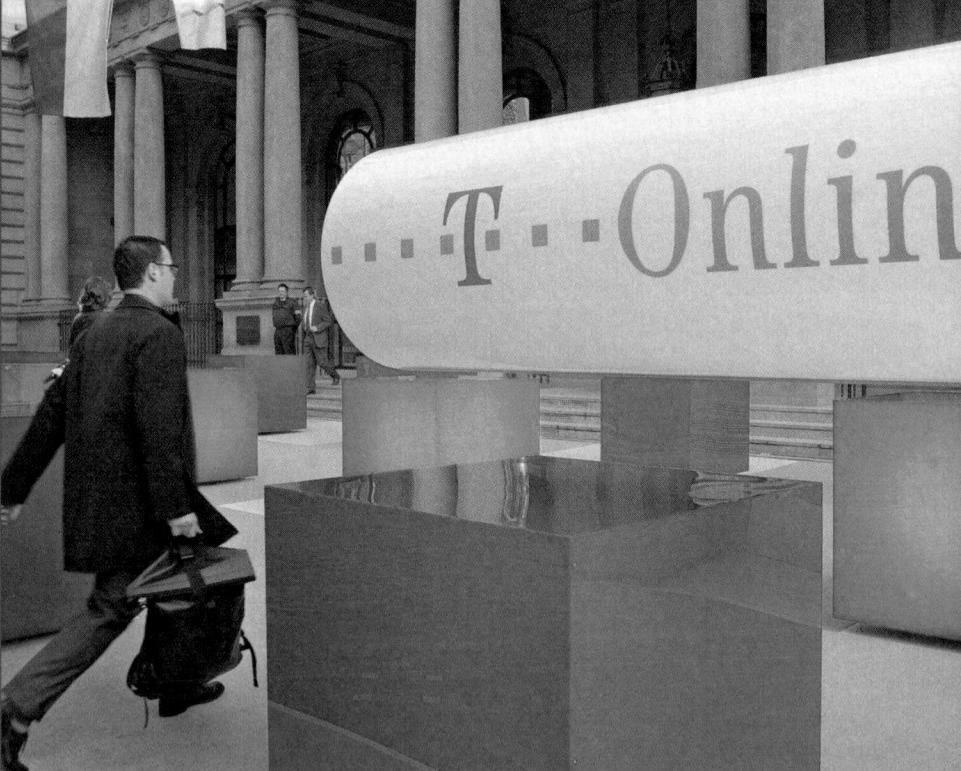

Introduction
Benefits of the Global Capital Market
    Functions of a Generic Capital Market
    Attractions of the Global Capital Market
Growth of the Global Capital Market
    Information Technology
    Deregulation
    Global Capital Market Risks
The Eurocurrency Market
    Genesis and Growth of the Market
    Attractions of the Eurocurrency Market
    Drawbacks of the Eurocurrency Market
The Global Bond Market
    Attractions of the Eurobond Market
The Global Equity Market
Foreign Exchange Risk and the Cost of Capital
Focus on Managerial Implications
Chapter Summary
Critical Discussion Questions
Closing Case: The Surging Samurai Bond Market

MONEDA	COMPRA
DOLAR EE	4600
DOLAR Ch.	4560
PESO ARGENTINO	3000
REAL	1770
PESO URUGUAYO	333
MARCO	1956
FRANCO SUIZO	2612
FRANCO FRANCE	583
LIBRA	6061

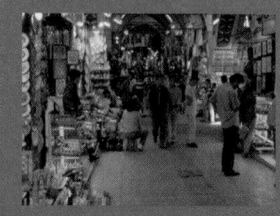

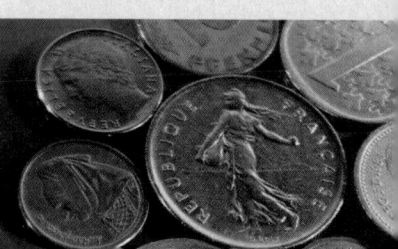

China Mobile

China Mobile (Hong Kong) Ltd. is a Hong Kong–based provider of wireless telephone service and one of the largest providers of mobile telephone service in the world. The company was spun off in 1996 from China Mobile Communications Corporation, a state-owned provider of mobile telephone service in mainland China, which retained a 75 percent ownership stake in China Mobile (Hong Kong) Ltd. The spin-off was part of a strategy by the Chinese government for privatizing its telecommunications network. China Mobile was given the right to expand into mainland China. By September 2000, the company was the largest provider of mobile communications in China with 23.9 million subscribers and a market leadership position in six provinces.

In late 2000, China was finishing up negotiations to enter the World Trade Organization. Under the terms of the WTO agreement, China would progressively have to open its telecommunications market to foreign telecommunications service providers. Galvanized by the impending threat of new competition in its fast-growing market, China Mobile realized it needed to accelerate its expansion into mainland China to preempt foreign competitors. Accordingly, in October 2000, China Mobile reached an agreement to purchase mobile networks in an additional seven provinces from its state-owned parent company. The purchase of these networks would give China Mobile an additional 15.4 million subscribers. It would also give the Hong Kong company a geographically contiguous market covering all the coastal regions of mainland China, a 56 percent share of all cellular subscribers in mainland China, and service coverage of approximately 48 percent of the total population.

The price tag for this deal was $32.8 billion. For China Mobile, a critical question was how to finance the deal. It could issue additional equity or debt in Hong Kong, but Hong Kong's relatively small capital market might not be big enough to absorb a multibillion-dollar offering without driving up the price of the capital to an unacceptably high level. For example, China Mobile might be required to pay a relatively high interest rate in order to sell sufficient bonds in Hong Kong to finance part of its acquisition of the provincial networks, thereby raising its cost of capital. After consulting its underwriters, which included the U.S. companies Goldman Sachs and Merrill Lynch, China Mobile opted for an international offering of equity and debt. The shares of China Mobile were already listed on the New York Stock Exchange as American Depository Receipts (ADRs). Each ADR represented and controlled five shares in the Hong Kong company. China Mobile opted to sell ADRs worth about $6.6 billion and to raise a further $600 million from the sale of five-year convertible bonds. (Convertible bonds can be converted into equity at some future date, in this case after five years. They are considered to be a hybrid between conventional stocks and bonds.) In addition, China Mobile agreed to sell a 2 percent stake in the company to Vodafone PLC, Europe's largest wireless service provider, for $2.5 billion. The remainder of the $32.8 billion purchase price for the mainland wireless networks was to be financed by issuing new shares to state-owned China Mobile Communications Corporation, which would retain for now its 75 percent stake in the company despite the issuing of new equity.

A significant portion of the ADRs would be offered for sale in New York. However, the underwriters also planned to offer ADRs in Asia and Europe. Similarly, the convertible bond issue would be priced in U.S. dollars and offered to global investors. The equity and bond offerings were closed in November 2000. Both offerings were substantially oversubscribed. The equity portion of the offering was 2.6 times oversubscribed. This was a remarkable achievement for what was the largest ever Asian equity issue outside of Japan. In total, China Mobile raised some $8.24 billion, over $1 billion more than planned. Some $690 million came from the sale of convertible bonds, and the remainder from the sale of equity. The convertible bonds carried a 2.25 percent interest rate, significantly less than the 2.75 percent rate initially targeted (as bond prices are bid up, the interest rate offered by the bond goes down). This lowered China Mobile's cost of capital. The oversubscription of the equity portion of the offering had a similar effect. The offering was truly global in nature. While 55 percent of the placement was in the United States, another 25 percent went to Asian investors and 20 percent to European investors.

Sources: China Mobile Hong Kong Ltd., SEC Form F-3, filed October 30, 2000; M. Johnson, "Deal of the Month," *Corporate Finance*, December 2000, p. 10; and "Jumbo Equity Raid Elevates China Mobile to Big League," *Euroweek*, November 3, 2000, pp. 1, 13.

Introduction

The opening case describes how China Mobile overcame the financing constraints imposed by a relatively small and illiquid Hong Kong capital market and raised $8.24 billion by simultaneously selling equity and bonds through several different exchanges, including Hong Kong and New York, to a broad range of international investors. As we saw, China Mobile also lists its shares on the New York Stock Exchange in addition to the Hong Kong Stock Exchange. By successfully tapping into the large and liquid global capital market, the Hong Kong–based company was able to raise more funds than initially planned and lower its cost of capital. (The cost of capital refers to the price of money, such as the interest rate that must be paid to bondholders or the dividends and capital appreciation that stockholders expect to receive.) For example, as noted in the opening case, the convertible bonds carried an interest rate a full half point lower than originally expected, implying a lower cost of capital for China Mobile.

Although China Mobile's international equity and debt offering was among the largest to date, the tactic of selling equity and debt internationally is becoming increasingly common. This represents a sharp break from common practice during much of the 20th century. In the past, substantial regulatory barriers separated national capital markets from each other. These made it difficult for a company based in one country to list its stock on a foreign exchange. These regulatory barriers tumbled during the 1980s and 1990s. By the middle of the last decade, a truly global capital market was emerging. This capital market enabled firms to list their stock on multiple exchanges and to raise funds by issuing equity or debt around the world. For example, in 1994, Daimler-Benz, Germany's largest industrial company, raised $300 million by issuing new shares not in Germany, but in Singapore.[1] In 1996, the German telecommunications provider Deutsche Telekom raised some $13.3 billion by simultaneously listing its shares for sale on stock exchanges in Frankfurt, London, New York, and Tokyo. And in late 2002, China Telecom, China's largest fixed-line phone company, raised $1.4 billion by selling a 10 percent stake in the company to investors in New York and Hong Kong.[2] Like China Mobile, these three companies elected to raise equity through foreign markets because they reasoned that their domestic capital market was too small to supply the requisite funds at a reasonable cost. To lower their cost of capital, they tapped into the large and highly liquid global capital market.

We begin this chapter by looking at the benefits associated with the globalization of capital markets. This is followed by a more detailed look at the growth of the international capital market and the macroeconomic risks associated with such growth. Next, there is a detailed review of three important segments of the global capital market: the eurocurrency market, the international bond market, and the international equity market. As usual, we close the chapter by pointing out some of the implications for the practice of international business.

Benefits of the Global Capital Market

Although this section is about the global capital market, we open it by discussing the functions of a generic capital market. Then we will look at the limitations of domestic capital markets and discuss the benefits of using global capital markets.

Functions of a Generic Capital Market

A capital market brings together those who want to invest money and those who want to borrow money (see Figure 11.1). Those who want to invest money include corporations with surplus cash, individuals, and nonbank financial institutions (e.g., pension funds, insurance companies). Those who want to borrow money include

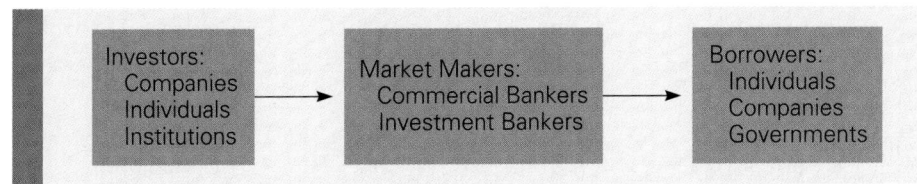

Figure 11.1

The Main Players in a Generic Capital Market

individuals, companies, and governments. Between these two groups are the market makers. **Market makers** are the financial service companies that connect investors and borrowers, either directly or indirectly. They include commercial banks (e.g., Citicorp, U.S. Bancorp) and investment banks (e.g., Merrill Lynch, Goldman Sachs).

Commercial banks perform an indirect connection function. They take cash deposits from corporations and individuals and pay them interest in return. They then lend that money to borrowers at a higher rate of interest, making a profit from the difference in interest rates (commonly referred to as the interest rate spread). Investment banks perform a direct connection function. They bring investors and borrowers together and charge commissions for doing so. For example, Merrill Lynch may act as a stockbroker for an individual who wants to invest some money. Its personnel will advise her as to the most attractive purchases and buy stock on her behalf, charging a fee for the service.

Capital market loans to corporations are either equity loans or debt loans. An **equity loan** is made when a corporation sells stock to investors. The money the corporation receives in return for its stock can be used to purchase plants and equipment, fund R&D projects, pay wages, and so on. A share of stock gives its holder a claim to a firm's profit stream. The corporation honors this claim by paying dividends to the stockholders. The amount of the dividends is not fixed in advance. Rather, it is determined by management based on how much profit the corporation is making. Investors purchase stock both for their dividend yield and in anticipation of gains in the price of the stock, which in theory reflects future dividend yields. Thus, investors may (and often do) purchase equity in companies that do not currently issue dividends to stockholders because they anticipate that the company will do so in the future.Stock prices increase when a corporation is projected to have greater earnings in the future, which increases the probability that it will raise (or initiate) future dividend payments.

A **debt loan** requires the corporation to repay a predetermined portion of the loan amount (the sum of the principal plus the specified interest) at regular intervals regardless of how much profit the company is making. Management has no discretion as to the amount it will pay investors. Debt loans include cash loans from banks and funds raised from the sale of corporate bonds to investors. When an investor purchases a corporate bond, he purchases the right to receive a specified fixed stream of income from the corporation for a specified number of years (i.e., until the bond maturity date).

Attractions of the Global Capital Market

A global capital market benefits both borrowers and investors. It benefits borrowers by increasing the supply of funds available for borrowing and by lowering the cost of capital. It benefits investors by providing a wider range of investment opportunities, thereby allowing them to build portfolios of international investments that diversify their risks.

The Borrower's Perspective: A Lower Cost of Capital

In a purely domestic capital market, the pool of investors is limited to residents of the country. This places an upper limit on the supply of funds available to borrowers. In other words, the liquidity of the market is limited. (China Mobile faced this problem in the opening case.) A global capital market, with its much larger pool of investors, provides a larger supply of funds for borrowers to draw on.

Figure 11.2

Market Liquidity and the
Cost of Capital

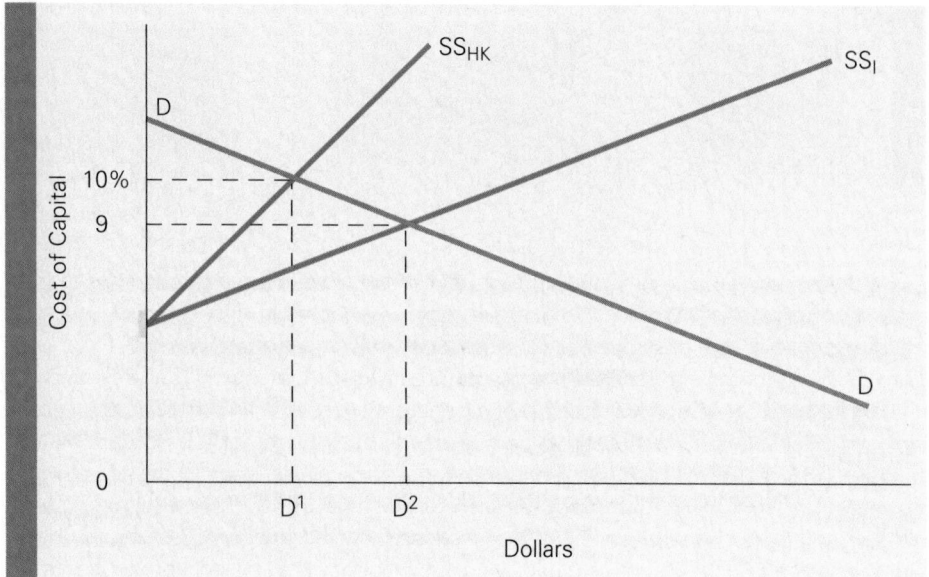

Perhaps the most important drawback of the limited liquidity of a purely domestic capital market is that the cost of capital tends to be higher than it is in an international market. The **cost of capital** is the price of borrowing money, which is the rate of return that borrowers must pay investors. This is the interest rate on debt loans and the dividend yield and expected capital gains on equity loans. In a purely domestic market, the limited pool of investors implies that borrowers must pay more to persuade investors to lend them their money. The larger pool of investors in an international market implies that borrowers will be able to pay less.

The argument is illustrated in Figure 11.2, using the China Mobile example. The vertical axis in the figure is the cost of capital (the price of borrowing money), and the horizontal axis is the amount of money available at varying interest rates. DD is the China Mobile demand curve for borrowings. Note that the China Mobile demand for funds varies with the cost of capital; the lower the cost of capital, the more money China Mobile will borrow. (Money is just like anything else; the lower its price, the more of it people can afford.) SS_{HK} is the supply curve of funds available in the Hong Kong capital market, and SS_I represents the funds available in the global capital market. Note that China Mobile can borrow more funds more cheaply on the global capital market. As Figure 11.2 illustrates, the greater pool of resources in the global capital market—the greater liquidity—both lowers the cost of capital and increases the amount China Mobile can borrow. Thus, the advantage of a global capital market to borrowers is that it lowers the cost of capital.

Problems of limited liquidity are not restricted to less developed nations, which naturally tend to have smaller domestic capital markets. As discussed in the introduction, even very large enterprises based in some of the world's most advanced industrialized nations in recent years have tapped the international capital markets in their search for greater liquidity and a lower cost of capital, such as Germany's Deutsche Telekom.[3] The Deutsche Telekom case is discussed in more detail in the Management Focus.

The Investor's Perspective: Portfolio Diversification

By using the global capital market, investors have a much wider range of investment opportunities than in a purely domestic capital market. The most significant consequence of this choice is that investors can diversify their portfolios internationally, thereby reducing their risk to below what could be achieved in a purely domestic capital market. We will consider how this works in the case of stock holdings, although the same argument could be made for bond holdings.

Management Focus

Deutsche Telekom Taps the Global Capital Market

Based in the world's third largest industrial economy, Deutsche Telekom is one of the world's largest telephone companies. Until late 1996, the company was wholly owned by the German government. However, in the mid-1990s, the German government privatized the utility, selling shares to the public. The privatization effort was driven by two factors: (1) a realization that state-owned enterprises tend to be inherently inefficient, and (2) the impending deregulation of the European Union telecommunication industry in 1998, which promised to expose Deutsche Telekom to foreign competition for the first time. Deutsche Telekom realized that, to become more competitive, it needed massive investments in new telecommunication infrastructure, including fiber optics and wireless, lest it start losing share in its home market to more efficient global competitors. Financing such investments from state sources would have been difficult even under the best of circumstances and almost impossible in the late 1990s, when the German government was trying to limit its budget deficit to meet the criteria for membership in the European monetary union. With the encouragement of the government, Deutsche Telekom hoped to finance its investments in capital equipment through the sale of shares to the public.

From a financial perspective, the privatization looked anything but easy. In 1996, Deutsche Telekom was valued at about $60 billion. If it maintained this valuation as a private company, it would dwarf all others listed on the German stock market. However, many analysts doubted there was anything close to $60 billion available in Germany for investment in Deutsche Telekom stock. One problem was that there was no tradition of retail stock investing in Germany. In 1996, only 1 in 20 German citizens owned shares, compared with 1 in every 4 or 5 in the United States and Great Britain. This lack of retail interest in stock ownership makes for a relatively illiquid stock market. Nor did banks, the traditional investors in company stocks in Germany, seem enthused about underwriting such a massive privatization effort. A further problem was that a wave of privatizations was already sweeping through Germany and the rest of Europe, so Deutsche Telekom would have to compete with many other state-owned enterprises for investors' attention. Given these factors, probably the only way that Deutsche Telekom could raise $60 billion through the German capital market would have been by promising investors a dividend yield that would raise the company's cost of capital above levels that could be serviced profitably.

Deutsche Telekom managers concluded they had to privatize the company in stages and sell a substantial portion of Deutsche Telekom stock to foreign investors. The company's plans called for an initial public offering (IPO) of 713 million shares of Deutsche Telekom stock, representing 25 percent of the company's total value, for about $18.50 per share. With a total projected value in excess of $13 billion, even this "limited" sale of Deutsche Telekom represented the largest IPO in European history and the second largest in the world after the 1987 sale of shares in Japan's telephone monopoly, NTT, for $15.6 billion. Concluding there was no way the German capital market could absorb even this partial sale of Deutsche Telekom equity, the managers of the company decided to simultaneously list shares and offer them for sale in Frankfurt (where the German stock exchange is located), London, New York, and Tokyo, attracting investors from all over the world. The IPO was successfully executed in November 1996 and raised $13.3 billion for the company.

Sources: J. O. Jackson, "The Selling of the Big Pink," *Time,* December 2, 1996, p. 46; S. Ascarelli, "Privatization Is Worrying Deutsche Telekom," *Wall Street Journal,* February 3, 1995, p. A1; "Plunging into Foreign Markets," *The Economist,* September 17, 1994, pp. 86–87; and A. Raghavan and M. R. Sesit, "Financing Boom: Foreign Firms Raise More and More Money in the U.S. Market," *Wall Street Journal,* October 5, 1993, p. A1.

Consider an investor who buys stock in a biotech firm that has not yet produced a new product. Imagine the price of the stock is very volatile—investors are buying and selling the stock in large numbers in response to information about the firm's prospects. Such stocks are risky investments; investors may win big if the firm produces a marketable product, but investors may also lose all their money if the firm fails to come up with a product that sells. Investors can guard against the risk associated with

Figure 11.3

Risk Reduction through
Portfolio Diversification

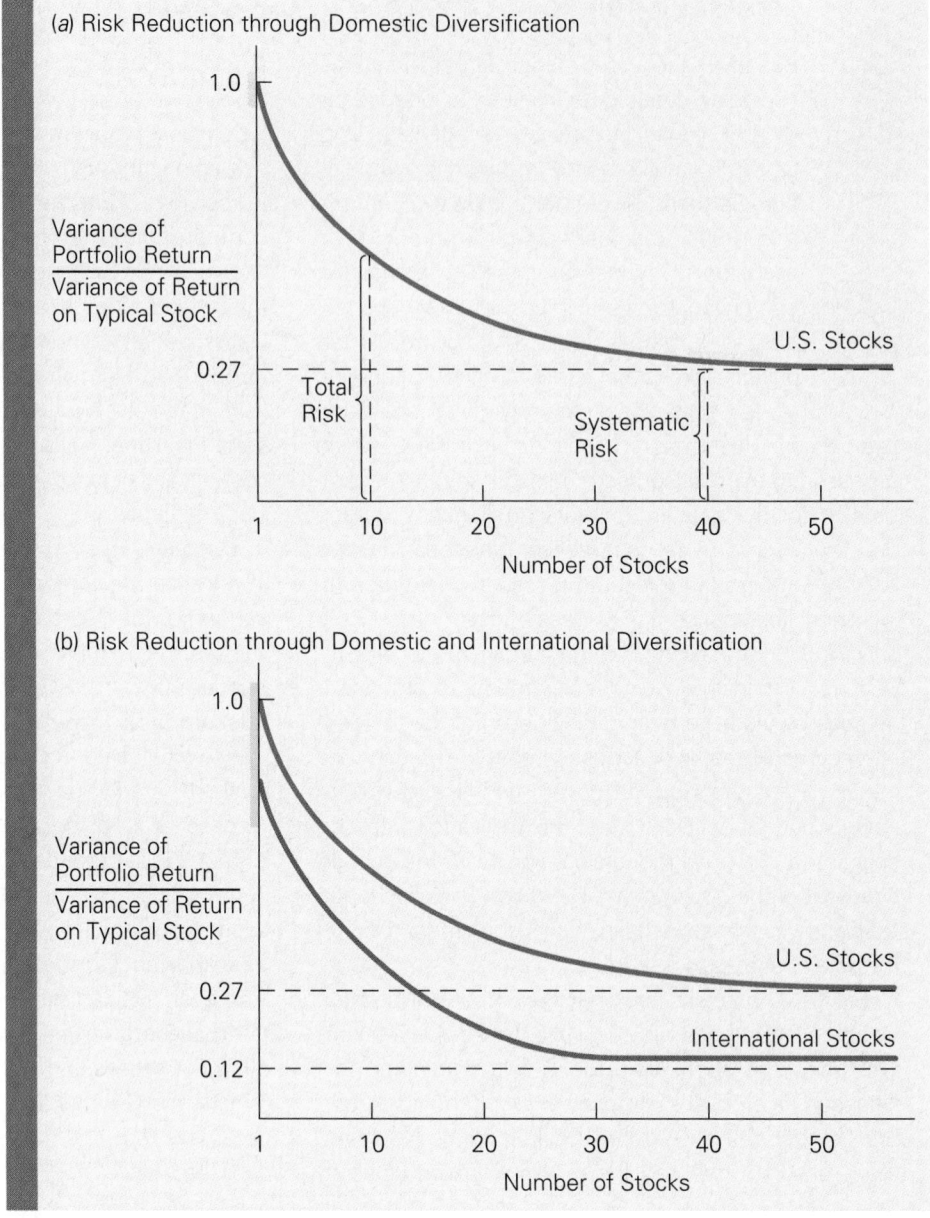

holding this stock by buying other firms' stocks, particularly those weakly or negatively correlated with the biotech stock. By the holding of a variety of stocks in a diversified portfolio, the losses incurred when some stocks fail to live up to their promises are offset by the gains enjoyed when other stocks exceed their promise.

As an investor increases the number of stocks in his portfolio, the portfolio's risk declines. At first this decline is rapid. Soon, however, the rate of decline falls off and asymptotically approaches the systematic risk of the market. **Systematic risk** refers to movements in a stock portfolio's value that are attributable to macroeconomic forces affecting all firms in an economy, rather than factors specific to an individual firm. The systematic risk is the level of nondiversifiable risk in an economy. Figure 11.3 illustrates this relationship for the United States. It suggests that a fully diversified U.S. portfolio is only about 27 percent as risky as a typical individual stock.

By diversifying a portfolio internationally, an investor can reduce the level of risk even further because the movements of stock market prices across countries are not perfectly correlated. For example, one study looked at the correlation between three stock market indexes. The Standard & Poor's 500 (S&P 500) summarized the movement of large U.S. stocks. The Morgan Stanley Capital International Europe, Australia, and Far East Index (EAFE) summarized stock market movements in other developed nations. The third index, the International Finance Corporation Global Emerging Markets Index (IFC), summarized stock market movements in less developed "emerging economies." From 1981 to 1994, the correlation between the S&P 500 and EAFE indexes was 0.45, suggesting they moved together only about 20 percent of the time (i.e., $0.45 \times 0.45 = 0.2025$). The correlation between the S&P 500 and IFC indexes was even lower at 0.32, suggesting they moved together only a little over 10 percent of the time.[4] Another study reported that for 1970–96, the correlation between the U.S. stock market and the U.K. market was 0.51, between the U.S. and French markets it was 0.44, and between the U.S. and Japanese markets it was 0.26.[5]

The relatively low correlation between the movements of stock markets in different countries reflects two basic factors. First, countries pursue different macroeconomic policies and face different economic conditions, so their stock markets respond to different forces and can move in different ways. For example, in 1997, the stock markets of several Asian countries, including South Korea, Malaysia, Indonesia, and Thailand, lost more than 50 percent of their value in response to the Asian financial crisis, while at the same time the S&P 500 increased in value by over 20 percent. Second, different stock markets are still somewhat segmented from each other by capital controls—that is, by restrictions on cross-border capital flows (although such restrictions are declining rapidly). The most common restrictions include limits on the amount of a firm's stock that a foreigner can own and limits on the ability of a country's citizens to invest their money outside that country. For example, until recently it was difficult for foreigners to own more than 30 percent of the equity of South Korean enterprises. Tight restrictions on capital flows make it very hard for Chinese citizens to take money out of their country and invest it in foreign assets. Such barriers to cross-border capital flows limit the ability of capital to roam the world freely in search of the highest risk-adjusted return. Consequently, at any one time, there may be too much capital invested in some markets and too little in others. This will tend to produce differences in rates of return across stock markets.[6] The implication is that by diversifying a portfolio to include foreign stocks, an investor can reduce the level of risk below that incurred by holding just domestic stocks.

Figure 11.3 also illustrates the relationship between international diversification and risk found by a now classic study by Bruno Solnik.[7] According to the figure, a fully diversified portfolio that contains stocks from many countries is less than half as risky as a fully diversified portfolio that contains only U.S. stocks. A fully diversified portfolio of international stocks is only about 12 percent as risky as a typical individual stock, whereas a fully diversified portfolio of U.S. stocks is about 27 percent as risky as a typical individual stock.

An increasingly common perception among investment professionals is that in the past 10 years the growing integration of the global economy and the emergence of the global capital market have increased the correlation between different stock markets, reducing the benefits of international diversification.[8] Today, it is argued, if the U.S. economy enters a recession, and the U.S. stock market declines rapidly, other markets follow suit. A recent study by Solnik suggests there may be some truth to this assertion, but the rate of integration is not occurring as rapidly as the popular perception would lead one to believe. Solnik and his associates looked at the correlation between 15 major stock markets in developed countries between 1971 and 1998. They found that on average, the correlation of monthly stock market returns increased from 66 percent in 1971 to 75 percent in 1998, indicating some convergence over time, but that "the regression results were weak," which suggests this "average" relationship was not strong, and there was considerable variation among countries.[9] The implication here is that international portfolio diversification can still reduce risk. As noted earlier, the correlation between stock market movements in developed and emerging markets seems to be much lower.

The risk-reducing effects of international portfolio diversification would be greater were it not for the volatile exchange rates associated with the current floating exchange rate regime. Floating exchange rates introduce an additional element of risk into investing in foreign assets. As we have said repeatedly, adverse exchange rate movements can transform otherwise profitable investments into unprofitable ones. The uncertainty engendered by volatile exchange rates may be acting as a brake on the otherwise rapid growth of the international capital market.

The Home Bias Puzzle

Generally, investors do not hold as many foreign financial assets in their portfolios as the theory on international portfolio diversification suggests they should. Investors tend to heavily bias their portfolios toward firms located in their country of residence. For example, one study reported that U.S. investors held 94 percent of their investments in domestic equities, Japanese investors held 98 percent, and UK investors 82 percent.[10] This phenomenon is referred to as the *home bias puzzle*.

Several explanations have been offered to explain the home bias puzzle.[11] One is that within a country, more information is available on domestic firms than foreign firms, and so the home bias reflects information asymmetries. Another explanation is that the transaction costs associated with purchasing foreign equities (e.g., commissions that must be paid to stock brokers) are such that the costs of international equity diversification outweigh the benefits. To date, however, this puzzle has not been resolved to the satisfaction of most economists. This tendency of investors to display a preference for domestic equities may be another force that keeps domestic capital markets segmented.

Growth of the Global Capital Market

According to data from the Bank for International Settlements, the global capital market is growing at a rapid pace.[12] By late 2002, the stock of cross-border bank loans stood at $9,446 billion, up from $3,600 billion in 1990. There were $8,780 billion in outstanding international bonds, up from $3,515 billion in 1997 and $620 billion in 1994. International equity offerings peaked in 2000, when they exceeded $314 billion. This compared to $90 billion in 1997 and some $18 billion in 1990. By 2002, international equity offerings had fallen to $102 billion, but this drop must be viewed in light of the general weak performance of global stock markets during the early 2000s, and suggests that the underlying long-term trend is still up.

What factors allowed the international capital market to bloom in the 1980s and 1990s? There seem to be two answers—advances in information technology and deregulation by governments.

Information Technology

Financial services is an information-intensive industry. It draws on large volumes of information about markets, risks, exchange rates, interest rates, creditworthiness, and so on. It uses this information to make decisions about what to invest where, how much to charge borrowers, how much interest to pay to depositors, and the value and riskiness of a range of financial assets including corporate bonds, stocks, government securities, and currencies.

Because of this information intensity, the financial services industry has been revolutionized more than any other industry by advances in information technology since the 1970s. The growth of international communication technology has facilitated instantaneous communication between any two points on the globe. At the same time, rapid advances in data processing have allowed market makers to absorb and process large volumes of information from around the world. According to one study, because of these technological developments, the real cost of recording, transmitting, and processing information fell by 95 percent between 1964 and 1990.[13] With the rapid rise of the Internet and the massive increase in computing power that we have seen since 1990, it seems likely that the cost of recording, transmitting, and processing information has fallen by a similar amount since 1990 and is now a trivial amount.

Such developments have facilitated the emergence of an integrated international capital market. It is now technologically possible for financial services companies to engage in 24-hour-a-day trading, whether it is in stocks, bonds, foreign exchange, or any other financial asset. Due to advances in communications and data processing technology, the international capital market never sleeps. San Francisco closes one hour before Tokyo opens, but during this period trading continues in New Zealand.

But the integration facilitated by technology has a dark side.[14] Shocks that occur in one financial center now spread around the globe very quickly. The collapse of U.S. stock prices on the notorious Black Monday of October 19, 1987, immediately triggered similar collapses in all the world's major stock markets, wiping billions of dollars off the value of corporate stocks worldwide. Similarly, the Asian financial crisis of 1997 sent shock waves around the world and precipitated a sell-off in world stock markets, although the effects of the shock were short lived. Most market participants would argue that the benefits of an integrated global capital market far outweigh any potential costs.

Deregulation

In country after country, financial services have been the most tightly regulated of all industries. Governments around the world have traditionally kept other countries' financial service firms from entering their capital markets. In some cases, they have also restricted the overseas expansion of their domestic financial services firms. In many countries, the law has also segmented the domestic financial services industry. For example, until recently U.S. commercial banks were prohibited from performing the functions of investment banks, and vice versa. Historically, many countries have limited the ability of foreign investors to purchase significant equity positions in domestic companies. They have also limited the amount of foreign investment that their citizens could undertake. In the 1970s, for example, capital controls made it very difficult for a British investor to purchase U.S. stocks and bonds.

Many of these restrictions have been crumbling since the early 1980s. In part, this has been a response to the development of the eurocurrency market, which from the beginning was outside of national control. (This is explained later in the chapter.) It has also been a response to pressure from financial services companies, which have long wanted to operate in a less regulated environment. Increasing acceptance of the free market ideology associated with an individualistic political philosophy also has a lot to do with the global trend toward the deregulation of financial markets (see Chapter 2). Whatever the reason, deregulation in a number of key countries has undoubtedly facilitated the growth of the international capital market.

The trend began in the United States in the late 1970s and early 80s with a series of changes that allowed foreign banks to enter the U.S. capital market and domestic banks to expand their operations overseas. In Great Britain, the so-called Big Bang of October 1986 removed barriers that had existed between banks and stockbrokers and allowed foreign financial service companies to enter the British stock market. Restrictions on the entry of foreign securities houses have been relaxed in Japan, and Japanese banks are now allowed to open international banking facilities. In France, the "Little Bang" of 1987 opened the French stock market to outsiders and to foreign and domestic banks. In Germany, foreign banks are now allowed to lend and manage foreign euro issues, subject to reciprocity agreements.[15] All of this has enabled financial services companies to transform themselves from primarily domestic companies into global operations with major offices around the world—a prerequisite for the development of a truly international capital market. In late 1997, the World Trade Organization brokered a deal that removed many of the restrictions on cross-border trade

Did the Global Capital Market Fail Mexico?

In early 1994, soon after passage of the North American Free Trade Agreement (NAFTA), Mexico was widely admired among the international community as a shining example of a developing country with a bright economic future. Since the late 1980s, the Mexican government had pursued sound monetary, budget, tax, and trade policies. By historical standards, inflation was low, the country was experiencing solid economic growth, and exports were booming. This robust picture attracted capital from foreign investors; between 1991 and 1993, foreigners invested more than $75 billion in the Mexican economy, more than in any other developing nation.

If there was a blot on Mexico's economic report card, it was the country's growing current account (trade) deficit. Mexican exports were booming, but so were its imports. In the 1989–1990 period, the current account deficit was equivalent to about 3 percent of Mexico's gross domestic product. In 1991, it increased to 5 percent, and by 1994 it was running at an annual rate of more than 6 percent. Bad as this might seem, it is not unsustainable and should not bring an economy crashing down. The United States has been running a current account deficit for decades with apparently little in the way of ill effects. A current account deficit will not be a problem for a country as long as foreign investors take the money they earn from trade with that country and reinvest it within the country. This has been the case in the United States for years, and during the early 1990s, it was occurring in Mexico too. Companies such as Ford took the pesos they earned from exports to Mexico and reinvested those funds in productive capacity in Mexico, building auto plants to serve the future needs of the Mexican market and to export elsewhere.

Unfortunately for Mexico, much of the $25 billion annual inflow of capital it received during the early 1990s was not the kind of patient long-term money that Ford was putting into Mexico. Rather, according to economist Martin Feldstein, much of the inflow was short-term capital that could flee if economic conditions changed for the worst. This is what seems to have occurred. In February 1994, the U.S. Federal Reserve began to increase interest rates. This led to a rapid fall in U.S. bond prices. At the same time, the

in financial services. This deal facilitated further growth in the size of the global capital market.

In addition to the deregulation of the financial services industry, many countries beginning in the 1970s started to dismantle capital controls, loosening both restrictions on inward investment by foreigners and outward investment by their own citizens and corporations. By the 1980s, this trend spread from developed nations to the emerging economies of the world as countries across Latin America, Asia, and Eastern Europe started to dismantle decades-old restrictions on capital flows. Between 1985 and 1997 an index of capital controls in emerging markets computed by the IMF has declined from a high of 0.66 to around 0.56 (the index would be 1.0 if all emerging economies had tight capital controls, and 0.0 if they had no controls).

As of 2003, the trends toward deregulation of financial services and removal of capital controls were still firmly in place. Given the benefits associated with the globalization of capital, the growth of the global capital market can be expected to continue for the foreseeable future. While most commentators see this as a positive development, some believe there are serious risks inherent in the globalization of capital.

Global Capital Market Risks

Some observers are concerned that due to deregulation and reduced controls on cross-border capital flows, individual nations are becoming more vulnerable to speculative capital flows. They see this as having a destabilizing effect on national economies.[16] Harvard economist Martin Feldstein, for example, has argued that most of the capital that moves internationally is pursuing temporary gains, and it shifts in and out of countries as quickly as conditions change.[17] He distinguishes between this short-term yen began to appreciate sharply against the dollar. These events resulted in large losses for many managers of short-term capital, such as hedge fund managers and banks, which had been betting on exactly the opposite happening. Many hedge funds had been expecting interest rates to fall, bond prices to rise, and the dollar to appreciate against the yen.

Faced with large losses, money managers tried to reduce the riskiness of their portfolios by pulling out of risky situations. About the same time, events took a turn for the worse in Mexico. An armed uprising in the southern state of Chiapas, the assassination of the leading candidate in the presidential election campaign, and an accelerating inflation rate all helped produce a feeling that Mexican investments were riskier than had been assumed. Money managers began to pull many of their short-term investments out of the country.

As hot money flowed out, the Mexican government realized it could not continue to count on capital inflows to finance its current account deficit. The government had assumed the inflow was mainly composed of patient, long-term money. In reality, much of it appeared to be short-term money. As money flowed out of Mexico, the Mexican government had to commit more foreign reserves to defending the value of the peso against the U.S. dollar, which was pegged at 3.5 to the dollar. Currency speculators entered the picture and began to bet against the Mexican government by selling pesos short. Events came to a head in December 1994 when the Mexican government was essentially forced by capital flows to abandon its support for the peso. Over the next month, the peso lost 40 percent of its value against the dollar, the government was forced to introduce an economic austerity program, and the Mexican economic boom came to an abrupt end.

Sources: Martin Feldstein, "Global Capital Flows: Too Little, Not Too Much," *The Economist,* June 24, 1995, pp. 72–73; R. Dornbusch, "We Have Salinas to Thank for the Peso Debacle," *Business Week,* January 16, 1995, p. 20; and P. Carroll and C. Torres, "Mexico Unveils Program of Harsh Fiscal Medicine," *Wall Street Journal,* March 10, 1995, pp. A1, A6. See also Martin Feldstein and Charles Horioka, "Domestic Savings and International Capital Flows," *Economic Journal* 90 (1980), pp. 314–29.

capital, or "hot money," and "patient money" that would support long-term cross-border capital flows. To Feldstein, patient money is still relatively rare, primarily because although capital is free to move internationally, its owners and managers still prefer to keep most of it at home. Feldstein supports his arguments with statistics that demonstrate that although $1.5 trillion flow through the foreign exchange markets every day, "when the dust settles, most of the savings done in each country stays in that country."[18] Feldstein argues that the lack of patient money is due to the relative paucity of information that investors have about foreign investments. In his view, if investors had better information about foreign assets, the global capital market would work more efficiently and be less subject to short-term speculative capital flows. Feldstein claims that Mexico's economic problems in the mid-1990s were the result of too much hot money flowing in and out of the country and too little patient money. This example is reviewed in detail in the accompanying Country Focus.

A lack of information about the fundamental quality of foreign investments may encourage speculative flows in the global capital market. Faced with a lack of quality information, investors may react to dramatic news events in foreign nations and pull their money out too quickly. Despite advances in information technology, it is still difficult for investors to get access to the same quantity and quality of information about foreign investment opportunities that they can get about domestic investment opportunities. This information gap is exacerbated by varying accounting conventions in different countries, which makes the direct comparison of cross-border investment opportunities difficult for all but the most sophisticated investor (see Chapter 19 for details).

Given the problems created by differences in the quantity and quality of information, many investors have yet to venture into the world of cross-border investing, and those that do are prone to reverse their decision on the basis of limited (and perhaps inaccurate) information. However, if the international capital market continues to grow, financial intermediaries likely will increasingly provide quality information about foreign investment opportunities. Better information should increase the sophistication of investment decisions and reduce the frequency and size of speculative capital flows. Although concerns about the volume of "hot money" sloshing around in the global capital market increased as a result of the Asian financial crisis, IMF research suggests there has not been an increase in the volatility of financial markets over the past 25 years.[19]

According to Martin Feldstein, the Mexican economy was brought down not by currency speculation on the foreign exchange market, but by a lack of long-term patient money. He argued that Mexico offered, and still offers, many attractive long-term investment opportunities, but because of the lack of information on long-term investment opportunities in Mexico, most of the capital flowing into the country from 1991 to 1993 was short-term, speculative money, the flow of which could quickly be reversed. If foreign investors had better information, Feldstein argued, Mexico should have been able to finance its current account deficit from inward capital flows because patient capital would naturally gravitate toward attractive Mexican investment opportunities.

The Eurocurrency Market

A **eurocurrency** is any currency banked outside of its country of origin. Eurodollars, which account for about two-thirds of all eurocurrencies, are dollars banked outside the United States. Other important eurocurrencies include the euro-yen and the euro-pound. The term *eurocurrency* is actually a misnomer because a eurocurrency can be created anywhere in the world; the persistent euro- prefix reflects the European origin of the market. The eurocurrency market has been an important and relatively low-cost source of funds for international businesses.

Genesis and Growth of the Market

The eurocurrency market was born in the mid-1950s when Eastern European holders of dollars, including the former Soviet Union, were afraid to deposit their holdings in the United States lest they be seized by the U.S. government to settle U.S. residents' claims against business losses resulting from the Communist takeover of Eastern Europe. These countries deposited many of their dollar holdings in Europe, particularly in London. Additional dollar deposits came from various Western European central banks and from companies that earned dollars by exporting to the United States. These two groups deposited their dollars in London banks, rather than U.S. banks, because they were able to earn a higher rate of interest (which will be explained).

The eurocurrency market received a major push in 1957 when the British government prohibited British banks from lending British pounds to finance non-British trade, a business that had been very profitable for British banks. British banks began financing the same trade by attracting dollar deposits and lending dollars to companies engaged in international trade and investment. Because of this historical event, London became, and has remained, the leading center of eurocurrency trading.

The eurocurrency market received another push in the 1960s when the U.S. government enacted regulations that discouraged U.S. banks from lending to non-U.S. residents. Would-be dollar borrowers outside the United States found it increasingly difficult to borrow dollars in the United States to finance international trade, so they turned to the eurodollar market to obtain the necessary dollar funds.

The U.S. government changed its policies after the 1973 collapse of the Bretton Woods system (see Chapter 10), removing an important impetus to the growth of the eurocurrency market. However, another political event, the oil price increases engineered by OPEC in 1973–74 and 1979–80, gave the market another big shove. As a

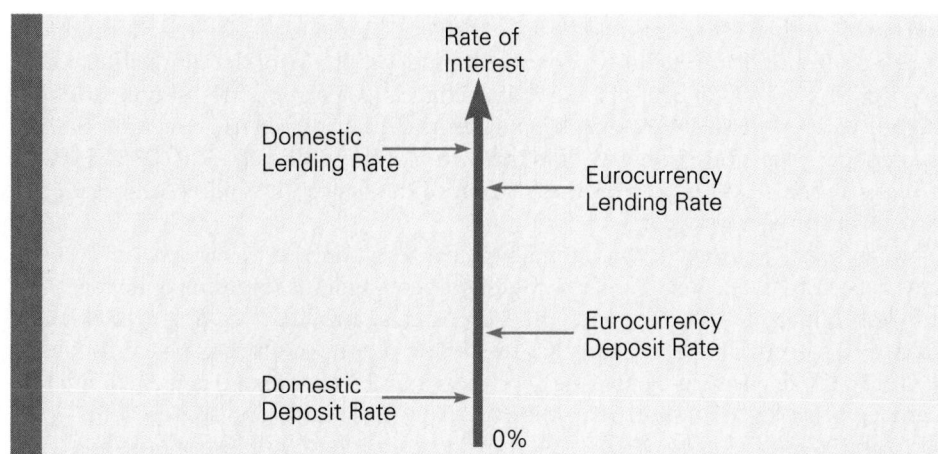

Figure 11.4

Interest Rate Spreads in Domestic and Eurocurrency Markets

result of the oil price increases, the Arab members of OPEC accumulated huge amounts of dollars. They were afraid to place their money in U.S. banks or their European branches, lest the U.S. government attempt to confiscate them. (Iranian assets in U.S. banks and their European branches were frozen by President Carter in 1979 after Americans were taken hostage at the U.S. embassy in Tehran; their fear was not unfounded.) Instead, these countries deposited their dollars with banks in London, further increasing the supply of eurodollars.

Although these various political events contributed to the growth of the eurocurrency market, they alone were not responsible for it. The market grew because it offered real financial advantages—initially to those who wanted to deposit dollars or borrow dollars and later to those who wanted to deposit and borrow other currencies.

Attractions of the Eurocurrency Market

Its lack of government regulation makes the eurocurrency market attractive to both depositors and borrowers. Banks can offer higher interest rates on eurocurrency deposits than on deposits made in the home currency, making eurocurrency deposits attractive to those who have cash to invest. The lack of regulation also allows banks to charge borrowers a lower interest rate for eurocurrency borrowings than for borrowings in the home currency, making eurocurrency loans attractive for those who want to borrow money. In other words, the spread between the eurocurrency deposit rate and the eurocurrency lending rate is less than the spread between the domestic deposit and lending rates (see Figure 11.4). To understand why this is so, we must examine how government regulations raise the costs of domestic banking.

Domestic currency deposits are regulated in all industrialized countries. Such regulations ensure that banks have enough liquid funds to satisfy demand if large numbers of domestic depositors should suddenly decide to withdraw their money. All countries operate with certain reserve requirements. For example, each time a U.S. bank accepts a deposit in dollars, it must place some fraction of that deposit in a non-interest-bearing account at a Federal Reserve Bank as part of its required reserves. Similarly, each time a British bank accepts a deposit in pounds sterling, it must place a certain fraction of that deposit with the Bank of England.

Banks are given much more freedom in their dealings in foreign currencies, however. For example, the British government does not impose reserve requirement restrictions on deposits of foreign currencies within its borders. Nor are the London branches of U.S. banks subject to U.S. reserve requirement regulations, provided those deposits are payable only outside the United States. This gives eurobanks a competitive advantage.

For example, suppose a bank based in New York faces a 10 percent reserve requirement. According to this requirement, if the bank receives a $100 deposit, it can lend out no more than $90 of that and it must place the remaining $10 in a non-interest-bearing account at a Federal Reserve bank. Suppose the bank has annual operating costs of $1 per $100 of deposits and that it charges 10 percent interest on loans. The highest interest the New York bank can offer its depositors and still cover its costs is 8 percent per year. Thus, the bank pays the owner of the $100 deposit (0.08 × $100=) $8, earns (0.10 × $90=) $9 on the fraction of the deposit it is allowed to lend, and just covers its operating costs.

In contrast, a eurobank can offer a higher interest rate on dollar deposits and still cover its costs. The eurobank, with no reserve requirements regarding dollar deposits, can lend out all of a $100 deposit. Therefore, it can earn 0.10 × $100 = $10 at a loan rate of 10 percent. If the eurobank has the same operating costs as the New York bank ($1 per $100 deposit), it can pay its depositors an interest rate of 9 percent, a full percentage point higher than that paid by the New York bank, and still cover its costs. That is, it can pay 0.09 × $100 = $9 to its depositor, receive $10 from the borrower, and be left with $1 to cover operating costs. Alternatively, the eurobank might pay the depositor 8.5 percent (which is still above the rate paid by the New York bank), charge borrowers 9.5 percent (still less than the New York bank charges), and cover its operating costs even better. Thus, the eurobank has a competitive advantage vis-à-vis the New York bank in both its deposit rate and its loan rate.

Clearly, there are strong financial motivations for companies to use the eurocurrency market. By doing so, they receive a higher interest rate on deposits and pay less for loans. Given this, the surprising thing is not that the euromarket has grown rapidly but that it hasn't grown even faster. Why do any depositors hold deposits in their home currency when they could get better yields in the eurocurrency market?

Drawbacks of the Eurocurrency Market

The eurocurrency market has two drawbacks. First, when depositors use a regulated banking system, they know that the probability of a bank failure that would cause them to lose their deposits is very low. Regulation maintains the liquidity of the banking system. In an unregulated system such as the eurocurrency market, the probability of a bank failure that would cause depositors to lose their money is greater (although in absolute terms, still low). Thus, the lower interest rate received on home-country deposits reflects the costs of insuring against bank failure. Some depositors are more comfortable with the security of such a system and are willing to pay the price.

Second, borrowing funds internationally can expose a company to foreign exchange risk. For example, consider a U.S. company that uses the eurocurrency market to borrow euro-pounds—perhaps because it can pay a lower interest rate on euro-pound loans than on dollar loans. Imagine, however, that the British pound subsequently appreciates against the dollar. This would increase the dollar cost of repaying the euro-pound loan and thus the company's cost of capital. This possibility can be insured against by using the forward exchange market (as we saw in Chapter 9), but the forward exchange market does not offer perfect insurance. Consequently, many companies borrow funds in their domestic currency to avoid foreign exchange risk, even though the eurocurrency markets may offer more attractive interest rates.

The Global Bond Market

The global bond market grew rapidly during the past two decades. Bonds are an important means of financing for many companies. The most common kind of bond is a fixed-rate bond. The investor who purchases a fixed-rate bond receives a fixed set of cash payoffs. Each year until the bond matures, the investor gets an interest payment and then at maturity she gets back the face value of the bond.

International bonds are of two types: foreign bonds and eurobonds. Foreign bonds are sold outside the borrower's country and are denominated in the currency of the country in which they are issued. Thus, when Dow Chemical issues bonds in Japanese yen and sells them in Japan, it is issuing foreign bonds. Many foreign bonds have nicknames; foreign bonds sold in the United States are called Yankee bonds, foreign bonds sold in Japan are Samurai bonds, and foreign bonds sold in Great Britain are bulldogs. Companies will issue international bonds if they believe it will lower their cost of capital. For example, in recent years many companies have been issuing Samurai bonds in Japan to take advantage of very low interest rates. In early 2001, 10-year Japanese government bonds yielded 1.24 percent, compared with 5 percent for comparable U.S. government bonds. Against this background, companies found that they could raise debt at a cheaper rate in Japan than in the United States.

Eurobonds are normally underwritten by an international syndicate of banks and placed in countries other than the one in whose currency the bond is denominated. For example, a bond may be issued by a German corporation, denominated in U.S. dollars, and sold to investors outside the United States by an international syndicate of banks. Eurobonds are routinely issued by multinational corporations, large domestic corporations, sovereign governments, and international institutions. They are usually offered simultaneously in several national capital markets, but not in the capital market of the country, nor to residents of the country, in whose currency they are denominated. Historically, eurobonds accounted for the lion's share of international bond issues, but increasingly they are being eclipsed by foreign bonds.

Attractions of the Eurobond Market

Three features of the eurobond market make it an appealing alternative to most major domestic bond markets:

- An absence of regulatory interference.
- Less stringent disclosure requirements than in most domestic bond markets.
- A favorable tax status.

Regulatory Interference

National governments often impose tight controls on domestic and foreign issuers of bonds denominated in the local currency and sold within their national boundaries. These controls tend to raise the cost of issuing bonds. However, government limitations are generally less stringent for securities denominated in foreign currencies and sold to holders of those foreign currencies. Eurobonds fall outside the regulatory domain of any single nation. As such, they can often be issued at a lower cost to the issuer.

Disclosure Requirements

Eurobond market disclosure requirements tend to be less stringent than those of several national governments. For example, if a firm wishes to issue dollar-denominated bonds within the United States, it must first comply with Securities and Exchange Commission (SEC) disclosure requirements. The firm must disclose detailed information about its activities, the salaries and other compensation of its senior executives, stock trades by its senior executives, and the like. In addition, the issuing firm must submit financial accounts that conform to U.S. accounting standards. For non-U.S. firms, redoing their accounts to make them consistent with U.S. standards can be very time consuming and expensive. Therefore, many firms have found it cheaper to issue eurobonds, including those denominated in dollars, than to issue dollar-denominated bonds within the United States.

Favorable Tax Status

Before 1984, U.S. corporations issuing eurobonds were required to withhold for U.S. income tax up to 30 percent of each interest payment to foreigners. This did not encourage foreigners to hold bonds issued by U.S. corporations. Similar tax laws were operational in many countries at that time, and they limited market demand for eurobonds. U.S. laws were revised in 1984 to exempt from any withholding tax foreign holders of bonds issued by U.S. corporations. As a result, U.S. corporations found it feasible for the first time to sell eurobonds directly to foreigners. Repeal of the laws caused other governments—including those of France, Germany, and Japan—to liberalize their tax laws likewise to avoid outflows of capital from their markets. The consequence was an upsurge in demand for eurobonds from investors who wanted to take advantage of their tax benefits.

The Global Equity Market

Although we have talked about the growth of the global equity market, strictly speaking there is no international equity market in the sense that there are international currency and bond markets. Rather, many countries have their own domestic equity markets in which corporate stock is traded. The largest of these domestic equity markets are to be found in the United States, Great Britain, Japan, and Germany. Although each domestic equity market is still dominated by investors who are citizens of that country and companies incorporated in that country, developments are internationalizing the world equity market. Investors are investing heavily in foreign equity markets to diversify their portfolios. Facilitated by deregulation and advances in information technology, this trend seems to be here to stay.

An interesting consequence of the trend toward international equity investment is the internationalization of corporate ownership. Today it is still generally possible to talk about U.S. corporations, British corporations, and Japanese corporations, primarily because the majority of stockholders (owners) of these corporations are of the respective nationality. However, this is changing. Increasingly, U.S. citizens are buying stock in companies incorporated abroad, and foreigners are buying stock in companies incorporated in the United States. Looking into the future, Robert Reich has mused about "the coming irrelevance of corporate nationality."[20]

A second development internationalizing the world equity market is that companies with historic roots in one nation are broadening their stock ownership by listing their stock in the equity markets of other nations. The reasons are primarily financial. Listing stock on a foreign market is often a prelude to issuing stock in that market to raise capital. The idea is to tap into the liquidity of foreign markets, thereby increasing the funds available for investment and lowering the firm's cost of capital. (The relationship between liquidity and the cost of capital was discussed earlier in the chapter.) Firms also often list their stock on foreign equity markets to facilitate future acquisitions of foreign companies. Other reasons for listing a company's stock on a foreign equity market are that the company's stock and stock options can be used to compensate local management and employees, it satisfies the desire for local ownership, and it increases the company's visibility with local employees, customers, suppliers, and bankers. Although firms based in developed nations were the first to start listing their stock on foreign exchanges, increasingly firms from developing countries who find their own growth limited by an illiquid domestic capital market are exploiting this opportunity.

Foreign Exchange Risk and the Cost of Capital

While a firm can borrow funds at a lower cost on the global capital market than on the domestic capital market, foreign exchange risk complicates this picture. Adverse movements in foreign exchange rates can substantially increase the cost of foreign currency loans, which is what happened to many Asian companies during the 1997–98 Asian financial crisis.

Consider a South Korean firm that wants to borrow 1 billion Korean won for one year to fund a capital investment project. The company can borrow this money from a Korean bank at an interest rate of 10 percent, and at the end of the year pay back the loan plus interest, for a total of W1.10 billion. Or the firm could borrow dollars from an international bank at a 6 percent interest rate. At the prevailing exchange rate of $1 = W1,000, the firm would borrow $1 million and the total loan cost would be $1.06 million, or W1.06 billion. By borrowing dollars, the firm could reduce its cost of capital by 4 percent, or W40 million. However, this saving is predicated on the assumption that during the year of the loan, the dollar/won exchange rate stays constant. Instead, imagine that the won depreciates sharply against the U.S. dollar and ends the year at $1 = W1,500. (This occurred in late 1997 when the won declined in value from $1 = W1,000 to $1 = W1,500 in two months.) The firm still has to pay the international bank $1.06 million at the end of the year, but now this costs the company W1.59 billion (i.e., $1.06 × W1,500). As a result of the depreciation in the value of the won, the cost of borrowing in U.S. dollars has soared from 6 percent to 59 percent, a huge rise in the firm's cost of capital. Although this may seem like an extreme example, it happened to many South Korean firms in 1997 at the height of the Asian financial crisis. Not surprisingly, many of them were pushed into technical default on their loans.

Unpredictable movements in exchange rates can inject risk into foreign currency borrowing, making something that initially seems less expensive ultimately much more expensive. The borrower can hedge against such a possibility by entering into a forward contract to purchase the required amount of the currency being borrowed at a predetermined exchange rate when the loan comes due (see Chapter 9 for details). Although this will raise the borrower's cost of capital, the added insurance limits the risk involved in such a transaction. Unfortunately, many Asian borrowers did not hedge their dollar-denominated short-term debt, so when their currencies collapsed against the dollar in 1997, many saw a sharp increase in their cost of capital.

When a firm borrows funds from the global capital market, it must weigh the benefits of a lower interest rate against the risks of an increase in the real cost of capital due to adverse exchange rate movements. Although using forward exchange markets may lower foreign exchange risk with short-term borrowings, it cannot remove the risk. Most importantly, the forward exchange market does not provide adequate coverage for long-term borrowings.

Focus On Managerial Implications

In chapters focusing on the external business environment, the Implications for Business section shows how the concepts apply to the practice of international business.

The implications of the material discussed in this chapter are quite straightforward but no less important for being obvious. The growth of the global capital market has created opportunities for international businesses that wish to borrow and/or invest money. By using the global capital market, firms can often borrow funds at a lower cost than is possible in a purely domestic capital market. This conclusion holds no matter what form of borrowing a firm uses—equity, bonds, or cash loans. The lower cost of capital on the global market reflects greater liquidity and the general absence of government regulation. Government regulation tends to raise the cost of capital in most domestic capital markets. The global market, being transnational, escapes regulation. Balanced against this, however, is the foreign exchange risk associated with borrowing in a foreign currency.

On the investment side, the growth of the global capital market is providing opportunities for firms, institutions, and individuals to diversify their investments to limit risk. By holding a diverse portfolio of stocks and bonds in different nations, an investor can reduce total risk to a lower level than can be achieved in a purely domestic setting. Once again, however, foreign exchange risk is a complicating factor.

The trends noted in this chapter seem likely to continue, with the global capital market continuing to increase in both importance and degree of integration over the next decade. Perhaps the most significant development will be the emergence of a unified capital market within the EU by the end of the decade as those countries continue toward economic and monetary union. Since Europe's capital markets are currently fragmented and relatively introspective (with the major exception of Great Britain's capital market), such a development could pave the way for even more rapid internationalization of the capital market in the early years of the next century. If this occurs, the implications for business are likely to be positive.

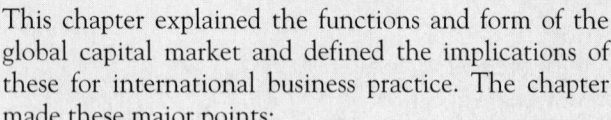

Chapter Summary

This chapter explained the functions and form of the global capital market and defined the implications of these for international business practice. The chapter made these major points:

1. The function of a capital market is to bring those who want to invest money together with those who want to borrow money.

2. Relative to a domestic capital market, the global capital market has a greater supply of funds available for borrowing, and this makes for a lower cost of capital for borrowers.

3. Relative to a domestic capital market, the global capital market allows investors to diversify portfolios of holdings internationally, thereby reducing risk.

4. The growth of the global capital market during recent decades can be attributed to advances in information technology, the widespread deregulation of financial services, and the relaxation of regulations governing cross-border capital flows.

5. A eurocurrency is any currency banked outside its country of origin. The lack of government regulations makes the eurocurrency market attractive to both depositors and borrowers. Because of the absence of regulation, the spread between the eurocurrency deposit and lending rates is less than the spread between the domestic deposit and lending rates. This gives eurobanks a competitive advantage.

6. The global bond market has two classifications: the foreign bond market and the eurobond market. Foreign bonds are sold outside the borrower's country and are denominated in the currency of the country in which they are is-

sued. A eurobond issue is normally underwritten by an international syndicate of banks and placed in countries other than the one in whose currency the bond is denominated. Eurobonds account for the lion's share of international bond issues.

7. The eurobond market is an attractive way for companies to raise funds due to the absence of regulatory interference, less stringent disclosure requirements, and eurobonds' favorable tax status.

8. Foreign investors are investing in other countries' equity markets to reduce risk by diversifying their holdings among nations.

9. Many companies are now listing their stock in the equity markets of other nations, primarily as a prelude to issuing stock in those markets to raise additional capital. Other reasons for listing stock in another country's exchange are to facilitate future stock swaps; to enable the company to use its stock and stock options for compensating local management and employees; to satisfy local ownership desires; and to increase the company's visibility among its local employees, customers, suppliers, and bankers.

10. When borrowing funds from the global capital market, companies must weigh the benefits of a lower interest rate against the risks of greater real costs of capital due to adverse exchange rate movements.

11. One major implication of the global capital market for international business is that companies can often borrow funds at a lower cost of capital in the international capital market than they can in the domestic capital market.

12. The global capital market provides greater opportunities for businesses and individuals to build a truly diversified portfolio of international investments in financial assets, which lowers risk.

Critical Discussion Questions

1. Why has the global capital market grown so rapidly in recent decades? Do you think this growth will continue throughout the next decade? Why?

2. A firm based in Mexico has found that its growth is restricted by the limited liquidity of the Mexican capital market. List the firm's options for raising money on the global capital market. Discuss the pros and cons of each option, and make a recommendation. How might your recommended options be affected if the Mexican peso depreciates significantly on the foreign exchange markets over the next two years?

3. Happy Company wants to raise $2 million with debt financing. The funds are needed to finance working capital, and the firm will repay them with interest in one year. Happy Company's treasurer is considering three options:

   a. Borrowing U.S. dollars from Security Pacific Bank at 8 percent.
   b. Borrowing British pounds from Midland Bank at 14 percent.
   c. Borrowing Japanese yen from Sanwa Bank at 5 percent.

   If Happy borrows foreign currency, it will not cover it; that is, it will simply change foreign currency for dollars at today's spot rate and buy the same foreign currency a year later at the spot rate then in effect. Happy Company estimates the pound will depreciate by 5 percent relative to the dollar and the yen will appreciate 3 percent relative to the dollar in the next year. From which bank should Happy Company borrow?

Notes

1. D. Waller, "Daimler in $250m Singapore Placing," *Financial Times*, May 10, 1994, p. 17.

2. G. Platt, "China Telecom Issue Poorly Received in U.S.," *Global Finance*, January 2003, p. 19.

3. Waller, "Daimler in $250m Singapore Placing."

4. C. G. Luck and R. Choudhury, "International Equity Diversification for Pension Funds," *Journal of Investing* 5, no. 2 (1996), pp. 43–53

5. K. K. Lewis, "Trying to Explain Home Bias in Equities and Consumption," *Journal of Economic Literature*, 37 (1999), pp. 571–608.

6. Ian Domowitz, Jack Glen, and Ananth Madhavan, "Market Segmentation and Stock Prices: Evidence from an Emerging Market," *Journal of Finance* 3, no. 3 (1997), pp. 1059–68.

7. B. Solnik, "Why Not Diversify Internationally Rather Than Domestically?" *Financial Analysts Journal*, July 1974, p. 17.

8. A. Lavine, "With Overseas Markets Now Moving in Sync with U.S. Markets, It's Getting Harder to Find True Diversification Abroad," *Financial Planning*, December 1, 2000, pp. 37–40.

9. B. Solnik and J. Roulet, "Dispersion as Cross Sectional Correlation," *Financial Analysts Journal* 56, no. 1 (2000), pp. 54–61.

10. A. Serrat, "A Dynamic Equilibrium Model of International Portfolio Holdings," *Econometrica*, 69 (2001), pp. 1467–89.

11. For a review, see K. K. Lewis, "Trying to Explain Home Bias in Equities and Consumption," *Journal of Economic Literature*, 37 (1999), pp. 571–608.

12. Bank for International Settlements, *BIS Quarterly Review*, March 2003.

13. T. F. Huertas, "U.S. Multinational Banking: History and Prospects," in *Banks as Multinationals*, ed. G. Jones (London: Routledge, 1990).

14. G. J. Millman, *The Vandals' Crown* (New York: Free Press, 1995).

15. P. Dicken, *Global Shift: The Internationalization of Economic Activity* (London: The Guilford Press, 1992).

16. Ibid.

17. Martin Feldstein, "Global Capital Flows: Too Little, Not Too Much," *The Economist*, June 24, 1995, pp. 72–73.

18. Ibid., p. 73.

19. International Monetary Fund, *World Economic Outlook* (Washington, DC: IMF, 1998).

20. R. Reich, *The Work of Nations* (New York: Alfred A. Knopf, 1991).

Research Task | globalEDGE™   globaledge.msu.edu

Use the globalEDGE™ site to complete the following exercises:

1. The "Global Financial Stability Report" is a semi-annual report published by the IMF. It reports on the developments and trends taking place in the world's capital markets global and tries to identify potential systemic weaknesses that could lead to crises. Locate the latest report and prepare an executive summary of the latest developments in mature markets (major financial centers).

2. IMF's Global Financial Stability Report also contains detailed information regarding the financial markets of emerging countries. Utilize the relevant section of this report to prepare an executive summary of the latest developments in the emerging equity markets.

Closing Case

The Surging Samurai Bond Market

Since Japan's stock market and real estate bubbles imploded in the early 1990s, the country has had to contend with a decade of poor economic performance. The economy has seemingly constantly teetered on the brink of a serious recession, and sustained growth has remained elusive. In an effort to keep the bleak economic clouds at bay, the Bank of Japan has repeatedly lowered interest rates to try to encourage corporate and consumer spending. As a result, by early 2001 Japan had the lowest interest rates in the world. In March 2001, 10-year Japanese government bonds yielded 1.24 percent, compared with 5 percent for comparable U.S. government debt. Despite these low interest rates, many Japanese corporations continue to focus on restructuring and downsizing, rather than investing in new capacity, as they struggle with the sustained hangover from the boom years of the 1980s and early 1990s. Consequently, Japanese corporations have not rushed to take advantage of the low interest rates to issue additional debt. Nor have consumers responded to the lower interest rates by increasing their consumption. Instead, the personal savings rate in Japan remains stubbornly high, even though many Japanese hold the majority of their savings in post office accounts that pay very low interest rates.

However, there is a silver lining to this bleak economic outlook—for foreign corporations and governments. They have increasingly been taking advantage of

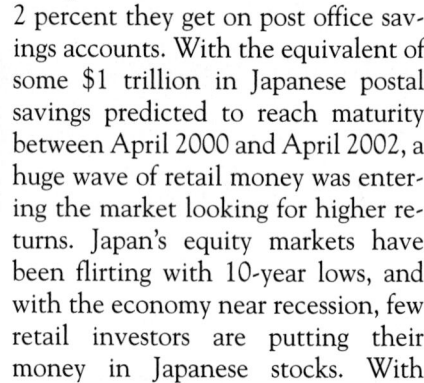

Japan's low interest rate to issue yen-denominated debt. With the yen/dollar exchange rate relatively stable, this seems like a shrewd economic bet. Foreign debt offerings in Japan have been snapped up by yield-hungry retail investors, who are looking for better returns than the 1 to 2 percent they get on post office savings accounts. With the equivalent of some $1 trillion in Japanese postal savings predicted to reach maturity between April 2000 and April 2002, a huge wave of retail money was entering the market looking for higher returns. Japan's equity markets have been flirting with 10-year lows, and with the economy near recession, few retail investors are putting their money in Japanese stocks. With Japanese corporations issuing only a few bonds, there are few investment opportunities there. This leaves foreign bonds as one of the few attractive investment opportunities for retail investors looking for higher yields.

A large number of foreigners took advantage of this opportunity. In 2001, foreigners issuing yen-denominated debt raised some $24 billion in the Japanese bond market, up from $9 billion in 1998. Countries including Croatia, Uruguay, and Brazil have raised money for their treasuries by issuing Samurai bonds. For example, in February 2002, the government of Uruguay issued ¥30 billion of five-year bonds. The interest rate it had to pay on those bonds was just 2.2 percent. In contrast, Uruguay had to pay 7.6 percent for five-year dollar borrowings. Similarly, an increasing number of corporations have been issuing Samurai bonds. In late 2000, Citigroup completed an offering of ¥155 billion ($1.43 billion) in Samurai bonds. Several U.S. investment banks, including Morgan Stanley, Merrill Lynch, and Lehman Brothers also issued Samurai bonds in 2000. In early 2001, the trend continued with a major Samurai bond issue placed by Deutsche Telekom, which offered ¥500 billion ($4.5 billion) in bonds. In addition, Posco, South Korea's largest steel company, came to the market with a ¥30 billion five-year offering. In both cases, these companies chose to raise debt in Japan as opposed to other markets because even factoring in the costs of hedging against fluctuations in the value of the Japanese yen, they could significantly reduce their cost of capital by doing so.

Sources: "Posco to Return to Samurai Market as Yen Offers Cheap Alternative to Dollar Funding," *Euroweek*, January 19, 2001, p. 13; J. Singer, "Japan's Woes Benefit World's Borrowers," *Wall Street Journal*, March 8, 2001, p. A17; and "Samurai Market to Scale New Heights," *Asiamoney*, October 2000, pp. 42–43.

Case Discussion Questions

1. What are the macroeconomic underpinnings of the increase in Samurai bond issues?

2. How might an increase in Japan's rate of economic growth affect the vitality of the Samurai bond market?

3. For a company such as Deutsche Telekom, which issued yen-denominated debt to raise funds for investments outside of Japan, the lower interest rate must be offset against higher costs. What are these higher costs, and what determines their magnitude?

4. What would happen to activity in the Samurai bond market if the yen started to appreciate significantly against the dollar but interest rate differentials between the United States and Japan stayed constant? What would happen if the yen depreciated against the dollar? What does this tell you about the risks of issuing foreign bonds?

Cases

Money Change   402

Bailing Out Brazil   403

The International Monetary Fund   405

Money Change 🎥

On January 1, 2002, the euro completed a three-year transition process and became the only legal tender in 12 of the 15 nations of the European Union (during the previous two years, euros had circulated side by side with historic currencies). For now, Britain, Sweden, and Denmark have stayed out of what is known as the euro zone. Across all 12 countries, prices are now listed in a common currency, the euro, and centuries-old currencies have been retired from circulation. Gone are the French franc, the German deutsche mark, and the Italian lira. Although the change has been emotionally difficult for many people, the European Union did it for solid economic reasons.

First, the EU believed that business and individuals would realize significant savings from having to handle one currency, rather than many. These savings come from lower foreign exchange and hedging costs. According to the European Commission, such savings could amount to 0.5 percent of the European Union's GDP, or about $40 billion a year. Second, the adoption of a common currency will make it easier to compare prices across Europe. This should increase competition because it will be much easier for consumers to shop around, which should translate into substantial gains for European consumers.

Third, faced with lower prices, European producers will be forced to look for ways to reduce their production costs to maintain their profit margins. The introduction of a common currency, by increasing competition, should ultimately produce long-run gains in the economic efficiency of European companies. Fourth, the introduction of a common currency should give a strong boost to the development of a highly liquid pan-European capital market. The development of such a capital market should lower the cost of capital and lead to an increase in both the level of investment and the efficiency with which investment funds are allocated.

Finally, the development of a pan-European, euro-denominated capital market will increase the range of investment options open to both individuals and institutions. For example, it will now be much easier for individuals and institutions based in, let's say, Holland to invest in Italian or French companies. This will enable European investors to better diversify their risk, which again lowers the cost of capital, and should also increase the efficiency with which capital resources are allocated.

What then are the potential costs of switching to the euro? The drawback, for some, of a single currency is that national authorities have lost control over monetary policy. Thus, it is crucial to ensure that the EU's monetary policy is well managed. The EU established an independent European Central Bank (ECB), similar in some respects to the U.S. Federal Reserve, with a clear mandate to set monetary policy so as to ensure price stability. The ECB, based in Frankfurt, is meant to be independent from political pressure—although critics question this. Among other things, the ECB sets interest rates and determines monetary policy across the euro zone.

The implied loss of national sovereignty to the ECB underlies the decision by Great Britain, Denmark, and Sweden to stay out of the euro zone for now. In these countries, many are suspicious of the ECB's ability to remain free from political pressure and to keep inflation under tight control. In theory, the design of the ECB should ensure that it remains free of politics. The ECB is modeled on the German Bundesbank, which historically has been the most independent and successful central bank in Europe. The Maastricht Treaty prohibits the ECB from taking orders from politicians. The executive board of the bank, which consists of a president, vice president, and four other members, carries out policy by issuing instructions to national central banks. The policy itself is determined by the governing council, which consists of the executive board plus the central bank governors from the 12 euro zone countries. The governing council votes on interest rate changes. Members of the executive board are appointed for eight-year nonrenewable terms, insulating them from political pressures to get reappointed. Nevertheless, the jury is still out on the issue of the ECB's independence, and it will take some time for the bank to establish its inflation-fighting credentials.

Another potential drawback of the euro is that the EU is not what economists would call an optimal currency area. In an optimal currency area, similarities in the underlying structure of economic activity make it feasible to adopt a single currency and use a single exchange rate as an instrument of macroeconomic policy. Many of the European economies in the euro zone, however, are very dissimilar. For example, Finland and Portugal are very dissimilar economies. The structure of economic activity within each country is very different. They have different wage rates and tax regimes, different business cycles, and may react very differently to external economic shocks. A change in the euro exchange rate that helps Finland may hurt Portugal. Obviously, such differences complicate macroeconomic policy. For example, when euro economies are not growing in unison, a common monetary policy may mean that interest rates are too high for depressed regions and too low for booming regions.

It will be interesting to see how the EU copes with the strains caused by such divergent economic performance. One way of dealing with such divergent effects within the euro zone might be for the EU to engage in fiscal transfers, taking money from prosperous regions and pumping it into depressed regions. Such a move, however, would open a political can of worms. Would the citizens of Germany forgo their "fair share" of EU funds to create jobs for underemployed Portuguese workers?

Since its establishment on January 1, 1999, the euro has had a volatile trading history against the U.S. dollar. After starting life in 1999 at $1.17, the euro steadily fell until it reached a low of 83 cents to the dollar in October 2000. Its fortunes began improving in late 2001, when the dollar weakened, and the currency stood near a robust three-year high of $1.176 on May 30, 2003. Many foreign central banks are now adding euros to their supply of foreign currencies. In the first three years of its life, the euro never reached the 13 percent of global reserves made up by the deutsche mark and other former euro zone currencies. The euro didn't jump that hurdle until early 2002, but by 2003 it made up 15 percent of global reserves. Currency specialists say the growing U.S. current account deficit, now at 5 percent, is bound to drive the dollar down further, and the euro still higher, over the next two to four years.

Also contributing to the volatility of the euro against the U.S. dollar have been short-term capital flows. In 2000, capital from foreign investors surged into the United States as they tried to cash in on a stock market boom, which pushed up the value of the dollar against other currencies, including the euro. In 2001, that flow began to weaken and it reversed in 2002 as foreign investors took their money out of a weak U.S. stock market, choosing to invest their fund elsewhere. The flow of capital out of dollar-denominated assets (U.S. equities) and into other assets helped to boost the euro against the dollar.

The decline in the value of the dollar against the euro is a mixed blessing for the EU. A strengthening euro, while a source of pride, will make it harder for euro zone exporters to sell their goods abroad.

Case Discussion Questions

1. What are the implications of the establishment of the euro for (a) European consumers, (b) businesses based in the EU, and (c) businesses based elsewhere in the world?

2. In your view, do the advantages of the euro outweigh its perceived disadvantages? Be sure to justify your answer.

3. What are the benefits to Britain, Sweden, and Denmark of staying out of the euro zone? What are the potential costs? Do you think these countries will eventually join the euro zone? Under what circumstances will they join?

4. Look at the relative performance of the euro against the dollar since 2000. What does this tell you, if anything, about the viability if the euro? (The historic exchange rate between the U.S. dollar and euro can be accessed on the Web at http://www.x-rates.com/cgi-bin/hlookup.cgi).

5. What are the implications of the euro gaining ground at the expense of the U.S. dollar as a major reserve currency for the world's central banks?

Sources

1. "Euros Take the Lead." *Euro Week*, January 31 2003, pp. 60–61.

2. Fairlamb, D.

3. Feldstein, M. "The Political Economy of the European Economic and Monetary Union." *Journal of Economic Perspectives* 11 (1997), pp. 23–42.

4. "Market Failure: A Survey of Business in Europe." *The Economist*, June 8, 1991, pp. 6–10.

5. "One Europe, One Economy." *The Economist*, November 30, 1991, pp. 53–54.

6. "Super Euro." *Business Week*, February 2003, p. 54.

7. Wyploze, C. "EMU: Why and How It Might Happen." *Journal of Economic Perspectives* 11 (1997), pp. 3–22.

Bailing Out Brazil 🎥

The International Monetary Fund agreed August 7, 2002, to provide Brazil with $30 billion in funds to help the country come to grips with a financial crisis that had driven its currency, the *real*, down to all-time lows against the U.S. dollar. This was not the first time the IMF had stepped in to help Brazil. The IMF had been actively assisting Brazil since 1998, when it provided $41.5 billion in financial commitments to the country to help it ride out a financial crisis that was driving down the value of the *real* on foreign exchange markets. Four years later, the country was back at the IMF asking for more money.

There were several reasons for the current crisis. First, a global economic slowdown had hurt the economies of South America, slowing exports, reducing foreign direct investment inflows, and leading to an economic recession. Second, earlier in the year, Brazil's neighbor and largest trading partner, Argentina, had defaulted on its government debt. In the first half of 2002, Argentina's economy shrank by almost 20 percent and unemployment surged to 22 percent. With financial chaos in Argentina, Brazilian exports to its neighbor slumped, helping to drive Brazil into a recession. Third, Brazil was scheduled to hold new presidential elections in October 2002, and foreign investors were getting increasingly nervous that a populist left-wing candidate, Luiz Inacio Lula da Silva (know as Lula) would win, replacing President Fernando Henrique Cardoso. As finance minister in the early 1990s, Cardoso had been the mastermind of Brazil's "*real* plan," which succeeded in conquering hyperinflation, a long-term problem in Brazil, and putting the country on a stable growth track. As president, Cardoso had won high marks from the international financial community for adhering rigorously to conditions imposed by the IMF in 1998 in return for its loans. An important part of that plan called for Brazil's government to run a budget surplus and use that to pay down government debt.

If Cardoso was replaced by Lula, as seemed likely, many foreign investors feared that the Brazilian government's commitment to maintain IMF targets on debt levels would be shattered. Publicly, Lula had stated he favored increasing government spending in times of economic crisis. To many, this seems like a recipe for more government debt—debt that in all probability would be financed by printing money, and lead to a resurgence of hyperinflation. Foreign investors feared that this would be unsustainable, and that Brazil would ultimately follow the example of Argentina and default on its government debt. History provided little comfort for the foreign investment community because Brazil had defaulted on its government debt in the 1980s.

Rather than wait for the outcome of the October 2002 election, foreign investors began to pull money out of Brazil in early 2002, while inflows of foreign capital started to dry up. This led to a fall in the value of the *real* against the dollar on foreign exchange markets. Sensing a currency crisis, traders began to sell the Brazilian currency short (effectively betting that it would go down). This put more pressure on the *real*, and its decline against the dollar accelerated, falling by 25 percent by early August from its January levels.

To protect the *real* from further depreciation, the Brazilian central bank started to use its foreign exchange reserves (mainly in the form of U.S. dollars) to buy *real* on the foreign exchange markets. The central bank also raised interest rates, but this had the effect of increasing the costs of serving government debt and implied that to meet IMF-mandated debt targets, the Brazilian government would have to further reduce government spending, taking money out of an economy that was already on the ropes.

It soon became clear that Brazil was in a very difficult position. Its foreign exchange reserves were limited, and high interest rates could be self-defeating. Without further assistance from the IMF, the currency could collapse, plunging Brazil into a financial crisis. If this happened, it could destabilize the entire region, and perhaps throw the global financial system into chaos. With the 10th largest economy, Brazil was not a bit player on the world economic scene.

It was against this background that the IMF decided to extend further loans to Brazil. The $30 billion loan package would be spread out over 15 months. In return for the loans, the Brazilian government agreed to maintain a budget surplus of at least 3.75 percent of GDP, using the surplus to continue retiring debt. However, the IMF did not seek agreement from election candidates, such as Lula, to abide by the terms of the agreement. This led to some skepticism on the part of investors, and the *real* had declined by another 15 percent against the dollar by late September. At this point, Lula stated that if he won the presidential election in October, he would abide by the IMF-mandated debt targets in 2003. This statement helped the currency to stabilize.

Lula did win the presidential election, and his administration was quick to state it would continue to pursue the free market policies of the prior administration and grant operational autonomy to the Brazilian central bank, effectively removing politics from decisions about monetary policy. The new government also indicated that it would adhere to the terms of the IMF rescue package.

Case Discussion Questions

1. Given that Brazil had already received IMF funding in 1998, do you think it should have received funding again in 2002?

2. What would have happened to the Brazilian economy, and the world economy, if the IMF had not stepped in to help Brazil?

3. The terms of the IMF loan call for Brazil to continue to run a budget surplus and use the proceeds to pay down government debt. What are the benefits of this policy prescription? What are the potential drawbacks?

4. What are the implications for international business of a potential financial crisis in Brazil involving a meltdown in the value of the *real*, and the Brazilian government defaulting on its debt?

5. What do you think will happen if Lula breaks the commitment to the IMF and decides to increase government spending?

Sources

1. Hall, K. G. "New Leftist Brazilian President Moves to Calm Investors." Knight Ridder/Tribune News Service, January 3, 2003.

2. "A Matter of Faith: Brazil and the IMF." *The Economist*, August 17, 2002, pp. 56–57.

3. "Race against Time: Brazil." *The Economist*, September 28, 2002, p. 69.

4. " Stopping the Rot in Brazil." *The Economist*, August 3, 2002, pp. 11–12.

The International Monetary Fund 🎥

Since its foundation in 1944, the International Monetary Fund (IMF) has grown to become a major player in the global economic system and on par with other international institutions such as the World Trade Organization and the World Bank. As of 2003, the IMF had some 184 member states, including all of the world's major industrial nations.

The IMF was originally founded to promote stability in the international monetary system, and in particular to help manage the system of fixed exchange rates that was established after World War II. Since the breakdown of the fixed exchange rate system in 1973, however, the role of the IMF has evolved, and now it can be viewed as a lender of last resort to the governments of countries experiencing financial crises. The IMF typically steps in when a country is experiencing a sharp fall in the value of its currency on foreign exchange markets. In exchange for loans that can be used to support the value of its currency, the IMF requires the recipient nations to implement certain macroeconomic policies. The specific policies required by the IMF vary depending upon the nature of the crisis, but they have often included cuts in government spending to reduce the level of public-sector debt and tight controls on the growth of the domestic money supply to help rein in inflation. Historically, excessive government spending coupled with loose control over the domestic money supply, and hence rapid price inflation, have been major causes of financial crises and a fall in the value of a country's currency on the foreign exchange market. These policies usually result in a sharp contraction in the domestic economy of the recipient country, leading to a recession. The IMF's view, however, is that once macroeconomic stability is restored, an economy can embark upon a *sustainable* growth path. In addition to its inflation-fighting policies, the IMF has also been a persistent advocate of policies to deregulate an economy, privatize state-owned businesses, open the economy to foreign investment and international trade, and strengthen the banking system (the belief being that such policies will help a country achieve sustainable economic growth).

The track record of the IMF has been somewhat spotty. While some recipient countries have used IMF loans to great effect, and quickly put their economic house in order, others have failed to do so and returned to the IMF for more loans. An example of a persistently troubled nation would be Turkey, which has had to implement 18 IMF programs since 1958! The spotty record has led critics to question the effectiveness of IMF-mandated policies. Major critics of the IMF, such as Columbia University economist Jeffrey Sachs, have made two main arguments.

First, critics have asserted that the IMF's policy prescriptions are not always appropriate. For example, in the case of South Korea, which borrowed $21 billion from the IMF in the late 1990s, the IMF imposed tight macroeconomic policies, including cuts in government spending and curbs on the growth in the money supply. However, South Korea was not suffering from excessive government spending and inflation, but from excessive private-sector debt with deflationary undertones. Korean companies had borrowed too much money, much of which was denominated in dollars, not Korean won. When the value of the won fell on foreign exchange market, this increased the won that Korean companies had to earn to service their dollar-denominated debt, forcing many into bankruptcy. The government had been running a budget surplus for years (it was 4 percent of South Korea's GDP in 1994–96) and inflation was low at about 5 percent. Despite this, critics say, the IMF insisted on applying the same policies that it applies to countries suffering from high inflation.

The IMF rejected this criticism. According to the IMF, the central task was to rebuild confidence in the Korean won. Once this has had been achieved, the won would recover from its oversold levels, reducing the size of South Korea's dollar-denominated debt burden when expressed in won, making it easier for companies to service their dollar-denominated debt. The IMF also notes that it does tailor policy prescriptions to specific cases. For example, the IMF required South Korea to remove restrictions on foreign direct investment, which would allow foreign capital to flow into the country to take advantage of cheap assets. The idea was to increase demand for the Korean currency and help to improve the dollar/won exchange rate.

South Korea did recover fairly quickly from the crisis. While the economy contracted by 7 percent in 1998, by 2000 it had rebounded and grew at a 9 percent rate (measured by growth in GDP). Inflation, which peaked at 8 percent in 1998, fell to 2 percent by 2000, and unemployment fell from 7 percent to 4 percent over the same period. The won hit a low of $1 = W1,812 in early 1998, but by 2000 was back to an exchange rate of about $1 = W1,200, at which it seems to have stabilized.

The second major criticism of the IMF is that its rescue efforts lead to a problem known as moral hazard. Moral hazard arises when people behave recklessly because they know they will be saved if things go wrong. Critics point out that many Japanese and Western banks were far too willing to lend large amounts of capital to overleveraged Asian companies during the boom years of the 1990s. These critics argue that the banks should have been forced to pay the price for their rash lending policies, even if that meant some banks would fail. Only by taking such drastic action, the argument goes, will banks learn the error of their ways and not engage in rash lending in the future. By providing support to these countries, the IMF is reducing the probability of debt default and in effect bailing out the banks whose loans gave rise to this situation.

For its part, the IMF dismisses this criticism, arguing that the costs of reckless financial policies are such that countries are unlikely to embark upon them just because they believe that the IMF will step in with a rescue package if things go wrong. As an IMF representative states in the video, doing so would be rather like taking out fire insurance and then leaving candles burning in a house. Just because you take out fire insurance, it doesn't mean that you are more reckless about leaving candles burning in a house, and just because the IMF is there to step into the breach in the case of a financial crisis, it doesn't follow that a government will therefore pursue more reckless policies. The IMF also states that historically this has not been a problem, although a critic might wonder how this squares with the experience of countries such as Turkey that have requested multiple loans from the IMF over the years.

Case Discussion Questions

1. What do you think might have happened to the world financial system if the IMF had never been created?

2. Do you think that the criticisms of the IMF are fair? To what extent is there evidence that the IMF (*a*) adopts a one-size-fits-all policy, and (*b*) encourages governments to engage in reckless behavior (moral hazard)?

3. What, if anything, could the IMF do differently to help ensure that countries such as Turkey do not keep returning to the IMF for additional rescue packages?

4. The video case highlights the role of the IMF in promoting stability in Afghanistan and Uganda, both chronically poor nations. In some respects, this suggests that in addition to its role in solving financial crisis, the IMF is starting to play a role in promoting the development of poor nations. Do you think this is appropriate?

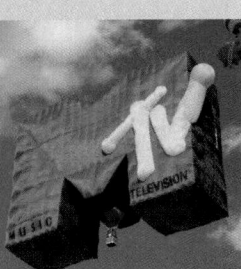

Part 5

The Strategy and Structure
of International Business

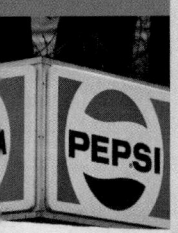

Chapter 12
The Strategy of International Business

Chapter 13
The Organization of International Business

Chapter 14
Entry Strategy and Strategic Alliances

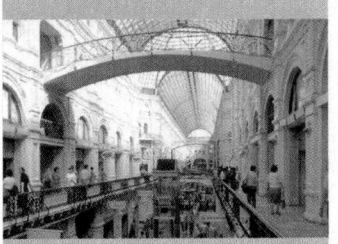

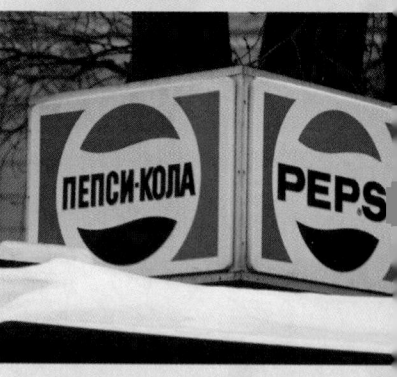

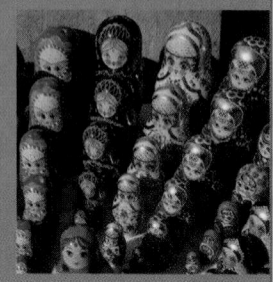

Chapter 12

The Strategy of International Business

Introduction
Strategy and the Firm
  Value Creation
  The Firm as a Value Chain
  Strategy in International Business
Profiting from Global Expansion
  Location Economies
  Experience Effects
  Leveraging Core Competencies
  Leveraging Subsidiary Skills
Pressures for Cost Reductions and Local Responsiveness
  Pressures for Cost Reductions
  Pressures for Local Responsiveness
Strategic Choices
  International Strategy
  Multidomestic Strategy
  Global Strategy
  Transnational Strategy
  Summary
Chapter Summary
Critical Discussion Questions
Closing Case: Global Strategy at General Motors

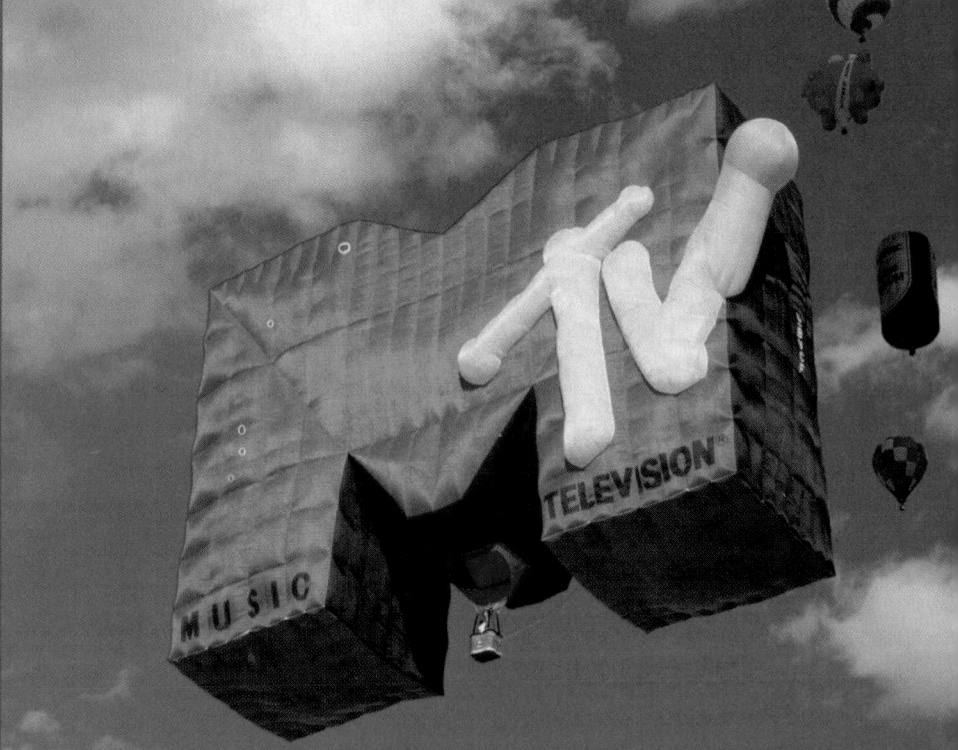

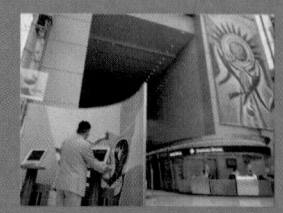

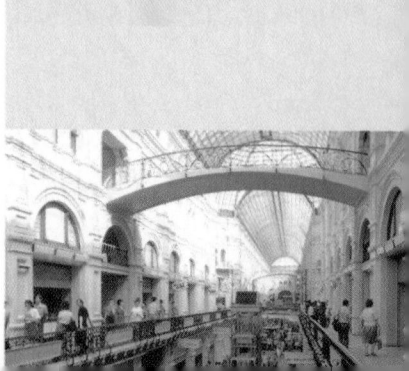

Global Strategy at MTV Networks

MTV Networks has become a symbol of globalization. Established in 1981, the U.S.-based music TV network has been expanding outside of its North American base since it opened MTV Europe in 1987. Now owned by media conglomerate Viacom, MTV Networks, which includes siblings Nickelodeon and VH1, the music station for the aging baby boomers, generated more than $1.4 billion in operating profit in 2002 on annual revenues that exceeded $3 billion. Since 1987, MTV has become the most ubiquitous cable programmer in the world. By March 2003 the network had 30 channels, or distinct feeds, that reached a combined 413 million households in 166 countries. While the United States still leads in number of households, with 85 million, the most rapid growth is elsewhere, particularly in Asia, where nearly two-thirds of the region's 3 billion people are under 35, the middle class is expanding quickly, and TV ownership is spreading rapidly. MTV Networks figures that every second of every day almost 2 million people are watching MTV around the world, the majority outside the United States.

Despite its international success, MTV's global expansion got off to a weak start. In 1987, it piped a single feed across Europe almost entirely composed of American programming with English-speaking veejays. Naively, the network's U.S. managers thought Europeans would flock to the American programming. But while viewers in Europe shared a common interest in a handful of global superstars, who at the time included Madonna and Michael Jackson, their tastes turned out to be surprisingly local. What was popular in Germany might not be popular in Great Britain. Many staples of the American music scene left Europeans cold. MTV suffered as a result. Soon local copycat stations were springing up in Europe that focused on the music scene in individual countries. They took viewers and advertisers away from MTV. As explained by Tom Freston, chairman of MTV Networks, "We were going for the most shallow layer of what united viewers and brought them together. It didn't go over too well."

In 1995, MTV changed its strategy and broke Western Europe into regional feeds, of which there are now eight: one for the United Kingdom and Ireland; another for Germany, Austria, and Switzerland; one for Scandinavia; one for Italy; one for France; one for Spain; one for Holland; and a feed for other European nations including Belgium and Greece. The network adopted the same localization strategy elsewhere in the world. For example, in Asia it has an English-Hindi channel for India, separate Mandrine feeds for China and Taiwan, a Korean feed for South Korea, a Bahasa-language feed for Indonesia, a Japanese feed for Japan, and so on. Digital and satellite technology have made the localization of programming cheaper and easier. MTV Networks can now beam half a dozen feeds off one satellite transponder.

While MTV Networks exercises creative control over these different feeds, and while all the channels have the same familiar frenetic look and feel of MTV in the United States, an increasing share of the programming and content is now local. When MTV opens a local station now, it begins with expatriates from elsewhere in the world to do a "gene transfer" of company culture and operating principles. But once these are established, the network switches to local employees and the expatriates move on. The idea is to "get inside the heads" of the local population and produce programming that matches their tastes. Although as much as 60 percent of the programming still originates in the United States, with staples such as "The Real World" having equivalents in different countries, an increasing share of programming is local in conception. In Italy, "MTV Kitchen" combines cooking with a music countdown. "Erotica" airs in Brazil and features a panel of youngsters discussing sex. The Indian channel produces 21 homegrown shows hosted by local veejays who speak "Hinglish," a city-bred breed of Hindi and English. Hit shows include "MTV Cricket in Control," appropriate for a land where cricket is a national obsession, "MTV Housefull," which hones in on Hindi film stars (India has the biggest film industry outside of Hollywood), and "MTV Bakra," which is modeled after "Candid Camera."

The same local variation is evident in the music videos aired by the different feeds. While some music stars still have global appeal, 70 percent of the video content is now local in most markets. In a direct countertrend to the notion that popular culture is becoming more global and homogenous, William Roedy, the president of MTV's international networks, observes, "People root for the home team, both culturally and musically. Local repertoire is a worldwide trend. There are fewer global megastars." When music tastes do transcend borders, MTV has found that it is often in ways that would have been difficult to predict. Currently, Japanese pop music is all the rage in Taiwan, while soul and hip-hop are big in South Korea.

This localization push has reaped big benefits for MTV, capturing viewers back from local imitators. In India, ratings increased by more than 700 percent between 1996, when the localization push began, and 2000. In turn, localization helps MTV to capture more of those all-important advertising revenues, even from other multinationals such as Coca-Cola, whose own advertising budgets are often locally determined. In Europe, MTV's advertising revenues increased by 60 percent between 1995 and 2002. While the total market for pan-European advertising is valued at just $200 million, the total market for local advertising across Europe is a much bigger pie, valued at $12 billion. MTV now gets 70 percent of its European advertising revenue from local spots, up from 15 percent in 1995. Similar trends are evident elsewhere in the world.

Sources: B. Pulley and A. Tanzer, "Sumner's Gemstone," *Forbes,* February 21, 2000, pp. 107–11; K. Hoffman, "Youth TV's Old Hand Prepares for the Digital Challenge," *Financial Times,* February 18, 2000, p. 8; presentation by Sumner M. Redstone, chairman and CEO, Viacom Inc., delivered to Salomon Smith Barney 11th Annual Global Entertainment Media, Telecommunications Conference, Scottsdale, Arizona, January 8, 2001. Archived at www.viacom.com. Viacom, SEC Form 10-k, filed March 27, 2003.

Introduction

Our primary concern thus far in this book has been with aspects of the larger environment in which international businesses compete. As we have described it in the preceding chapters, this environment has included the different political, economic, and cultural institutions found in nations, the international trade and investment framework, and the international monetary system. Now our focus shifts from the environment to the firm itself and, in particular, to the actions managers can take to compete more effectively as an international business. In this chapter, we look at how firms can increase their profitability by expanding their operations in foreign markets. We discuss the different strategies that firms pursue when competing internationally. We consider the pros and cons of these strategies. We discuss the various factors that affect a firm's choice of strategy. We also look at why firms often enter into strategic alliances with their global competitors, and we discuss the benefits, costs, and risks of strategic alliances. In subsequent chapters, we shall build on the framework established here to discuss a variety of topics including the design of organization structures and control systems for international businesses, strategies for entering foreign markets, the use and misuse of strategic alliances, strategies for exporting, and the various manufacturing, marketing, R&D, human resource, accounting, and financial strategies that are pursued by international businesses.

MTV Networks, profiled in the opening case, gives us a preview of some issues that we will explore in this chapter. When MTV began its global expansion in 1987, its strategy was to transfer its programming and content wholesale from the successful U.S. network. This strategy, which treated the world as a homogenous cultural entity with little variation in local tastes and preferences, was a failure. MTV soon found itself outmaneuvered by local imitators, who captured viewers and advertising revenues from the network by tailoring programming and content to local tastes and preferences. Realizing that it had made a serious strategic error, MTV changed its strategy in 1995 and emphasized localization. At MTV, localization means local programming and local video content hosted by local veejays and aimed at local markets. At the same time, MTV has been careful to ensure that its local channels still have the look and feel of MTV, and that its local operations share a common "genetic code" or set of operating principles. This strategy has enabled MTV to capture more viewers and to grow its advertising revenues at a double-digit rate. Thus, at MTV, the strategy has shifted from one that emphasized global standardization to one that emphasized local responsiveness. As we shall see, finding the correct balance between global standardization and local responsiveness is a major strategic challenge for many multinational enterprises. It is one that MTV appears to have solved, at least for now.

Strategy and the Firm

Before we discuss the strategies that multinational enterprises can pursue, we need to review basic principles of strategy. A firm's **strategy** can be defined as the actions that managers take to attain the goals of the firm. For most firms, the preeminent goal is to maximize long-term profitability. A firm makes a profit if the price it can charge for its output is greater than its costs of producing that output. **Profit (Π)** is thus defined as the difference between total revenues (TR) and total costs (TC), or:

$$\Pi = TR - TC$$

Total revenues (TR) are equal to price (P) times the number of units sold by the firm (Q) or $TR = P \times Q$. Total costs (TC) are equal to cost per unit (C) times the number of units sold or $TC = C \times Q$. Total profit (Π) is equal to profit per unit (π) times the number of units sold, or $\Pi = \pi \times Q$.

Profitability is a ratio or rate of return concept. A simple example would be the rate of return on sales (ROS), which is defined as profit (Π) over total revenues, or:

$$ROS = \Pi/TR$$

Thus, a firm might operate with the goal of maximizing its profitability, as defined by its return on sales (ROS), and its strategy would be the actions that its managers take to attain that goal. A more common goal is to maximize the firm's return on invested capital, or ROI, which is defined as $ROI = \Pi/I$ where I represents the total capital, including both equity and debt, that has been invested in the firm.[1]

Value Creation

Two basic conditions determine a firm's profits (Π): the amount of value customers place on the firm's goods or services (sometimes referred to as perceived value) and the firm's costs of production. In general, the more value customers place on a firm's products, the higher the price the firm can charge for those products. Note, however, that the price a firm charges for a good or service is typically less than the value placed on that good or service by the customer. This is so because the customer captures some of that value in the form of what economists call a consumer surplus.[2] The customer is able to do this because the firm is competing with other firms for the customer's business, so the firm must charge a lower price than it could were it a monopoly supplier. Also, it is normally impossible to segment the market to such a degree that the firm can charge each customer a price that reflects that individual's assessment of the value of a product, which economists refer to as a customer's reservation price. For these reasons, the price that gets charged tends to be less than the value placed on the product by many customers.

Figure 12.1 illustrates these concepts. The value of a product to a consumer is V; the price that the firm can charge for that product given competitive pressures and its ability

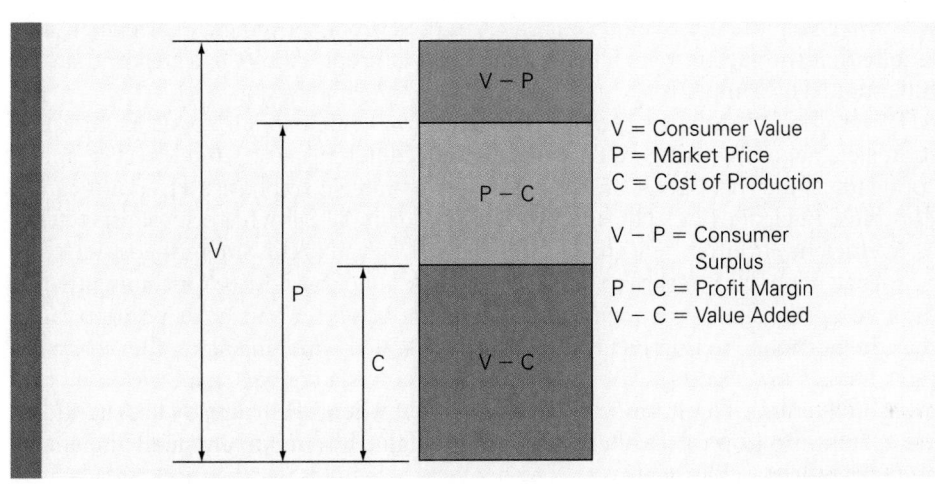

Figure 12.1

Value Creation

Figure 12.2

Strategic Positioning

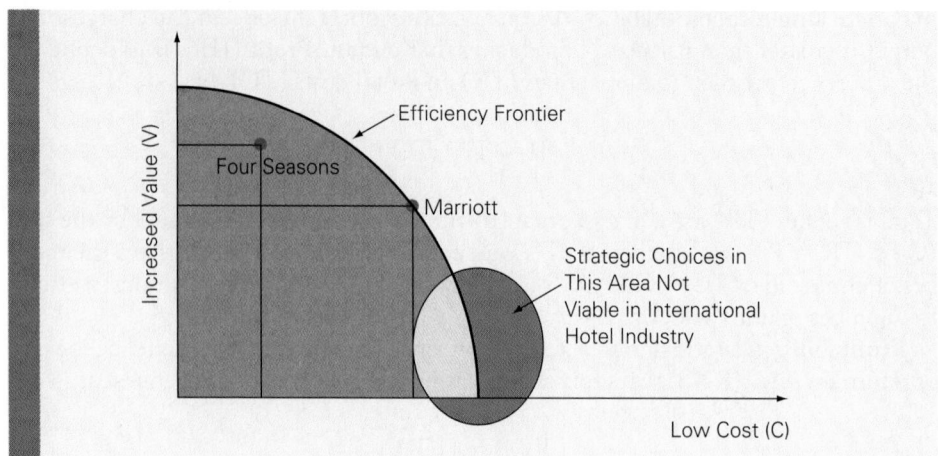

to segment the market is P; and the cost of producing that product is C. The firm's profit per unit sold (π) is equal to P−C, while the consumer surplus is equal to V−P. The firm makes a profit so long as P is greater than C, and its profit will be greater the lower C is *relative* to P. The difference between V and P is in part determined by the intensity of competitive pressure in the marketplace. The lower the intensity of competitive pressure, the higher the price that can be charged relative to V.[3]

The **value creation** by a firm is measured by the difference between V and C (V−C); a company creates value by converting inputs that cost C into a product on which consumers place a value of V. A company can create more value (V − C) either by lowering production costs, C, or by making the product more attractive through superior design, functionality, features, quality, and the like, so that consumers place a greater value on it (V increases) and, consequently, are willing to pay a high price (P increases). This discussion suggests that a firm has high profits when it creates more value for its customers and does so at a lower cost. We refer to a strategy that focuses primarily on lowering production costs as a *low cost strategy*. We refer to a strategy that focuses primarily on increasing the attractiveness of a product as a *differentiation strategy*.[4] Michael Porter has argued that *low cost* and *differentiation* are two basic strategies for creating value and attaining a competitive advantage in an industry.[5] According to Porter, superior profitability goes to those firms that can create superior value, and the way to create superior value is to drive down the cost structure of the business and/or differentiate the product in some way so that consumers value it more and are prepared to pay a premium price. Superior value creation relative to rivals does not necessarily require a firm to have the lowest cost structure in an industry, or to create the most valuable product in the eyes of consumers. However, it does require that the gap between value (V) and cost of production (C) is greater than the gap attained by competitors.

Porter also notes that it is important for a firm to be explicit about its choice of strategic emphasis with regard to value creation (differentiation) and low cost, and to configure its internal operations to support that strategic emphasis.[6] His point can be illustrated in Figure 12.2. The convex curve in Figure 12.2 is what economists refer to as an efficiency frontier. The efficiency frontier shows all of the different positions that a firm can adopt with regard to value creation (V) and low cost (C) assuming that its internal operations are configured efficiently to support a particular position (note that the horizontal axis in Figure 12.2 is reverse scaled—moving along the axis to the right implies lower costs). The efficiency frontier has a convex shape because of diminishing returns. Diminishing returns imply that when a firm already has significant value built into its product offering, increasing value by a relatively small amount requires significant additional costs. The converse also holds, when a firm already has a

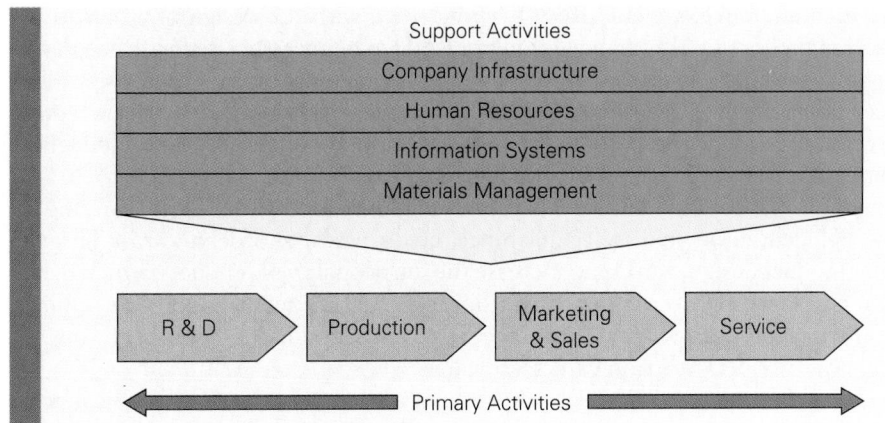

Figure 12.3

The Firm as a Value Chain

low cost structure, it has to give up a lot of value in its product offering to get additional cost reductions.

Two hotel firms with a global presence are plotted on Figure 12.2, Four Seasons and the Marriott International. Four Seasons positions itself as a luxury chain, and emphasizes the value of its product offering, which drives up its costs of operations. Marriott is positioned more in the middle of the market, and emphasizes sufficient value to attract international business travelers, but it is not a luxury chain like Four Seasons. In Figure 12.2, Marriott is shown to be on the efficiency frontier, indicating that its internal operations are well configured to its strategy and run efficiently. Four Seasons is inside the frontier, indicating that its operations are not running as efficiently as they might. This implies that Marriott International should be more profitable than Four Seasons. During the early 2000s, this was the case. In 2002, for example, Marriott earned a ROIC (return on inverted capital) of more than 12 percent, compared to 2.65 percent for Four Seasons.[7]

In sum, Porter emphasizes that it is very important for management to decide where the company wants to be positioned with regard to value (V) and cost (C), to configure operations accordingly, and to manage them efficiently to make sure the firm is operating on the efficiency frontier. However, not all positions on the efficiency frontier are viable. As shown on Figure 12.2, in the international hotel industry, there might not be enough demand to support a chain that emphasizes very low cost and strips all the value out of its product offering. International travelers are relatively affluent and expect a degree of comfort (value) when they travel away from home. Thus, a firm must also choose a strategic position that is viable.

The Firm as a Value Chain

The operations of a firm can be thought of as a value chain composed of a series of distinct value creation activities including production, marketing and sales, materials management, R&D, human resources, information systems, and the firm infrastructure. We can categorize these value creation activities, or operations, as primary activities and support activities (see Figure 12.3).[8] If a firm is to implement its strategy efficiently, and get onto the frontier shown in Figure 12.2, it must manage these activities effectively and in a manner that is consistent with its strategy.

Primary Activities

Primary activities have to do with the design, creation, and delivery of the product; its marketing; and its support and after-sale service. In the value chain illustrated in Figure 12.3, the primary activities are broken into four functions: research and development, production, marketing and sales, and service.

Research and development (R&D) is concerned with the design of products and production processes. Although we think of R&D as being associated with the design of physical products and production processes in manufacturing enterprises, many service companies also undertake R&D. For example, banks compete with each other by developing new financial products and new ways of delivering those products to customers. Online banking and smart debit cards are two examples of new product development in the banking industry. Earlier examples of innovation in the banking industry included automated teller machines, credit cards, and debit cards. Through superior product design, R&D can increase the functionality of products, which makes them more attractive to consumers (raising V). Alternatively, R&D may result in more efficient production processes, thereby cutting production costs (lowering C). Either way, the R&D function can create value.

Production is concerned with the creation of a good or service. For physical products, when we talk about production we generally mean manufacturing. For services such as banking or retail operations, "production" typically occurs when the service is delivered to the customer (for example, when a bank originates a loan for a customer it is engaged in production of the loan). For a media company such as MTV, production involves the creation and delivery of content (programming). The production activity of a firm creates value by performing its activities efficiently so lower costs result (lower C) or by performing them in such a way that a more reliable and higher quality product is produced (which results in higher V).

The marketing and sales functions of a firm can help to create value in several ways. Through brand positioning and advertising, the marketing function can increase the value (V) that consumers perceive to be contained in a firm's product. If these create a favorable impression of the firm's product in the minds of consumers, they increase the price that can be charged for the firm's product. For example, Ford has produced a high value version of its Ford Expedition SUV. Sold as the Lincoln Navigator and priced around $10,000 higher, the Navigator has the same body, engine, chassis, and design as the Expedition, but through skilled advertising and marketing, supported by some fairly minor features changes (e.g., more accessories and the addition of a Lincoln-style engine grille and nameplate), Ford has fostered the perception that the Navigator is a "luxury SUV." This marketing strategy has increased the perceived value (V) of the Navigator relative to the Expedition, and thus enables Ford to charge a higher price for the car (P).

Marketing and sales can also create value by discovering consumer needs and communicating them back to the R&D function of the company, which can then design products that better match those needs. For example, the allocation of research budgets at Pfizer, the world's largest pharmaceutical company, is determined by the marketing function's assessment of the potential market size associated with solving unmet medical needs. Thus, Pfizer is currently directing significant monies to R&D efforts aimed at finding treatments for Alzheimer's disease, principally because marketing has identified the treatment of Alzheimer's as a major unmet medical need.

The role of the enterprise's service activity is to provide after-sale service and support. This function can create a perception of superior value (V) in the minds of consumers by solving customer problems and supporting customers after they have purchased the product. For example, Caterpillar, the U.S.-based manufacturer of heavy earthmoving equipment, can get spare parts to any point in the world within 24 hours, thereby minimizing the amount of downtime its customers have to suffer if their Caterpillar equipment malfunctions. This is an extremely valuable capability in an industry where downtime is very expensive. It has helped to increase the value that customers associate with Caterpillar products and thus the price that Caterpillar can charge for its products.

Support Activities

The support activities of the value chain provide inputs that allow the primary activities to occur (see Figure 12.3). The materials management (or logistics) function controls the transmission of physical materials through the value chain, from procurement through production and into distribution. The efficiency with which this is carried out can significantly reduce cost (lower C), thereby creating more value.

Similarly, the human resource function can help create more value in a number of ways. It ensures that the company has the right mix of skilled people to perform its value creation activities effectively. Recall from the opening case how MTV staffs its foreign operations with local nationals—the idea being that local nationals will have a better feel for the tastes and preferences of local viewers than expatriate managers from the United States. MTV believes that better programming results from this staffing choice. In so far as this improves the fit between MTV's programming and local tastes, and drives viewer ratings, it raises the value (V) to advertisers of a slot on MTV. In turn, this increases the price that MTV can charge for those advertising slots. The human resource function also ensures that people are adequately trained, motivated, and compensated to perform their value creation tasks.

Information systems refer to the electronic systems for managing inventory, tracking sales, pricing products, selling products, dealing with customer service inquiries, and so on. Information systems, when coupled with the communications features of the Internet, can alter the efficiency and effectiveness with which a firm manages its other value creation activities. As we shall see, good information systems are very important in the global arena.

The final support activity is the company infrastructure. By infrastructure we mean the context within which all the other value creation activities occur. The infrastructure includes the organizational structure, control systems, and culture of the firm. Because top management can exert considerable influence in shaping these aspects of a firm, top management should also be viewed as part of the firm's infrastructure. Through strong leadership, top management can consciously shape the infrastructure of a firm and through that the performance of all its value creation activities.

Strategy in International Business

Many international markets are now extremely competitive due to the liberalization of the world trade and investment environment. In industry after industry, capable competitors confront each other around the globe. To be profitable in such an environment, a firm must make a clear and viable strategic choice with regard to its position on the efficiency frontier, and take actions at the operational and strategic level that support this position. Thus, strategy is often concerned with identifying and taking actions that will *lower the costs* of value creation and/or will *differentiate* the firm's product offering through superior design, quality, service, functionality, and so on.

For an example of how this works in an international business, consider Clear Vision, a manufacturer and distributor of eyewear. Started in the 1970s by David Glassman, the firm now generates annual gross revenues of more than $100 million. Not exactly small, but no corporate giant either, Clear Vision is a multinational firm with production facilities on three continents and customers around the world. Clear Vision began its move toward becoming a multinational in the early 1980s. The strong dollar at that time made U.S.-based manufacturing very expensive. Low-priced imports were taking an ever-larger share of the U.S. eyewear market, and Clear Vision realized it could not survive unless it also began to import. Initially the firm bought from independent overseas manufacturers, primarily in Hong Kong. However, the firm became dissatisfied with these suppliers' product quality and delivery. As Clear Vision's volume of imports increased, Glassman decided the best way to guarantee quality and delivery was to set up Clear Vision's own manufacturing operation overseas. Accordingly, Clear Vision found a Chinese partner, and together they opened a manufacturing facility in Hong Kong, with Clear Vision being the majority shareholder.

The choice of the Hong Kong location was influenced by its combination of low labor costs, a skilled workforce, and tax breaks given by the Hong Kong government.

The firm's objective at this point was to lower production costs by locating value creation activities at an appropriate location. After a few years, however, the increasing industrialization of Hong Kong and a growing labor shortage had pushed up wage rates to the extent that it was no longer a low-cost location. In response, Glassman and his Chinese partner moved part of their manufacturing to a plant in mainland China to take advantage of the lower wage rates there. Again, the goal was to lower production costs. The parts for eyewear frames manufactured at this plant are shipped to the Hong Kong factory for final assembly and then distributed to markets in North and South America. The Hong Kong factory now employs 80 people and the China plant between 300 and 400.

At the same time, Clear Vision was looking for opportunities to invest in foreign eyewear firms with reputations for fashionable design and high quality. Its objective was not to reduce production costs but to launch a line of high-quality differentiated, "designer" eyewear. Clear Vision did not have the design capability in-house to support such a line, but Glassman knew that certain foreign manufacturers did. As a result, Clear Vision invested in factories in Japan, France, and Italy, holding a minority shareholding in each case. These factories now supply eyewear for Clear Vision's Status Eye division, which markets high-priced designer eyewear.[9]

Thus, to deal with a threat from foreign competition, Clear Vision adopted a strategy intended to lower its cost structure (lower C): shifting its production from a high-cost location, the United States, to a low-cost location, first Hong Kong and later China. Then Clear Vision adopted a strategy intended to increase the perceived value of its product (increase V) so it could charge a premium price. Reasoning that premium pricing in eyewear depended on superior design, its strategy involved investing capital in French, Italian, and Japanese factories that had reputations for superior design. In sum, Clear Vision's strategies included some actions intended to reduce its costs of creating value and other actions intended to add perceived value to its product through differentiation. The overall goal was to increase the value created by Clear Vision and thus the profit and profitability of the enterprise. To the extent that these strategies were successful, the firm should have attained a higher profit margin and greater profitability than if it had remained a U.S.-based manufacturer of eyewear.

Profiting from Global Expansion

As suggested by the Clear Vision example, expanding globally allows firms to increase their profitability in ways not available to purely domestic enterprises.[10] Firms that operate internationally are able to:

1. Realize location economies by dispersing individual value creation activities to those locations around the globe where they can be performed most efficiently and effectively.

2. Realize greater cost economies from experience effects by serving an expanded global market from a central location, thereby reducing the costs of value creation.

3. Earn a greater return from the firm's distinctive skills or core competencies by leveraging those skills and applying them to new geographic markets.

4. Earn a greater return by leveraging any valuable skills developed in foreign operations and transferring them to other entities within the firm's global network of operations.

As we will see, however, a firm's ability to increase its profitability by pursuing these strategies is to some extent constrained by the need to customize its product offering, marketing strategy, and business strategy to differing national conditions; that is, by the imperative of localization.

Location Economies

We know from earlier chapters that countries differ along a range of dimensions, including the economic, political, legal, and cultural, and that these differences can either raise or lower the costs of doing business in a country. The theory of international trade also teaches us that due to differences in factor costs, certain countries have a comparative advantage in the production of certain products. Japan might excel in the production of automobiles and consumer electronics; the United States in the production of computer software, pharmaceuticals, biotechnology products, and financial services; Switzerland in the production of precision instruments and pharmaceuticals; and South Korea in the production of steel.[11]

What does all this mean for a firm that is trying to survive in a competitive global market? It means that, *trade barriers and transportation costs* permitting, the firm will benefit by basing each value creation activity it performs at that location where economic, political, and cultural conditions, including relative factor costs, are most conducive to the performance of that activity. Thus, if the best designers for a product live in France, a firm should base its design operations in France. If the most productive labor force for assembly operations is in Mexico, assembly operations should be based in Mexico. If the best marketers are in the United States, the marketing strategy should be formulated in the United States. And so on.

Firms that pursue such a strategy can realize what we refer to as **location economies,** the economies that arise from performing a value creation activity in the optimal location for that activity, wherever in the world that might be (transportation costs and trade barriers permitting). Locating a value creation activity in the optimal location for that activity can have one of two effects. *It can lower the costs of value creation and help the firm to achieve a low cost position, and/or it can enable a firm to differentiate its product offering from those of competitors.* In terms of Figure 12.1, it can lower C or increase V, which in general supports higher pricing (P). These considerations were at work in the case of Clear Vision, discussed earlier. Clear Vision moved its manufacturing operations out of the United States, first to Hong Kong and then to mainland China, to take advantage of low labor costs, thereby lowering the costs of value creation (C). At the same time, Clear Vision shifted some design operations from the United States to France and Italy. Clear Vision reasoned that skilled Italian and French designers could probably help the firm better differentiate its product, increasing perceived value (V). In other words, Clear Vision thinks that the optimal location for performing manufacturing operations is China, whereas the optimal locations for performing design operations are France and Italy. The firm has configured its value chain accordingly. By doing so, Clear Vision hopes to be able to simultaneously lower its cost structure and differentiate its product offering. In turn, differentiation should allow Clear Vision to charge a premium price for its product offering.

Creating a Global Web

Generalizing from the Clear Vision example, one result of this kind of thinking is the creation of a **global web** of value creation activities, with different stages of the value chain being dispersed to those locations around the globe where perceived value is maximized or where the costs of value creation are minimized. Consider the case of General Motors' Pontiac Le Mans cited in Robert Reich's *The Work of Nations*.[12] Marketed primarily in the United States, the car was designed in Germany; key components were manufactured in Japan, Taiwan, and Singapore; assembly was performed in South Korea; and the advertising strategy was formulated in Great Britain. The car was designed in Germany because GM believed the designers in its German subsidiary had the skills most suited to the job. (They were the most capable of producing a design that added value.) Components were manufactured in Japan, Taiwan, and Singapore, because favorable factor conditions there—relatively low-cost, skilled labor—suggested that those locations had a comparative advantage in the production of components (which helped reduce the costs of value creation). The car was assembled in South Korea because GM believed that due to its low labor costs, the costs of assembly could be minimized there (also helping to minimize the costs of value creation). Finally, the advertising strategy was formulated in Great Britain because GM believed a particular advertising agency there was the most able to produce an advertising campaign that would help sell the car. (This decision was consistent with GM's desire to maximize the value added.)

In theory, a firm that realizes location economies by dispersing each of its value creation activities to its optimal location should have a competitive advantage vis-à-vis a firm that bases all of its value creation activities at a single location. It should be able to better differentiate its product offering (thereby raising perceived value, V) and lower its cost structure (C) than its single-location competitor. In a world where competitive pressures are increasing, such a strategy may become an imperative for survival (as it seems to have been for Clear Vision).

Some Caveats

Introducing transportation costs and trade barriers complicates this picture. Due to favorable factor endowments, New Zealand may have a comparative advantage for automobile assembly operations, but high transportation costs would make it an uneconomical location from which to serve global markets. A consideration of transportation costs and trade barriers helps explain why many U.S. firms are now shifting their production from Asia to Mexico. Mexico has three distinct advantages over many Asian countries as a location for value creation activities. First, low labor costs relative to the United States make it a good location for labor-intensive production processes. In recent years, wage rates have increased significantly in Japan, Taiwan, and Hong Kong, but they have remained relatively low in Mexico. Second, Mexico's proximity to the large U.S. market reduces transportation costs. This is particularly important in the case of products with high weight-to-value ratios (e.g., automobiles). And third, the North American Free Trade Agreement (see Chapter 8) has removed many trade barriers between Mexico, the United States, and Canada, increasing Mexico's attractiveness as a production site for the North American market. Although value added and the costs of value creation are important, transportation costs and trade barriers also must be considered in location decisions.

Another caveat concerns the importance of assessing political and economic risks when making location decisions. Even if a country looks very attractive as a production location when measured against all the standard criteria, if its government is unstable or totalitarian, the firm might be advised not to base production there. (Political risk is discussed in Chapter 2.) Similarly, if the government appears to be pursuing inappropriate economic policies, that might be another reason for not basing production in that location, even if other factors look favorable.

Experience Effects

The **experience curve** refers to systematic reductions in production costs that have been observed to occur over the life of a product.[13] A number of studies have observed that a product's production costs decline by some quantity about each time accumulated output doubles. The relationship was first observed in the aircraft industry, where each time accumulated output of airframes was doubled, unit costs typically declined to 80 percent of their previous level.[14] Thus, production cost for the fourth airframe would be 80 percent of production cost for the second airframe, the eighth airframe's production costs 80 percent of the fourth's, the sixteenth's 80 percent of the eighth's, and so on. Figure 12.4 illustrates this experience curve relationship between production costs and output. Two things explain this: learning effects and economies of scale.

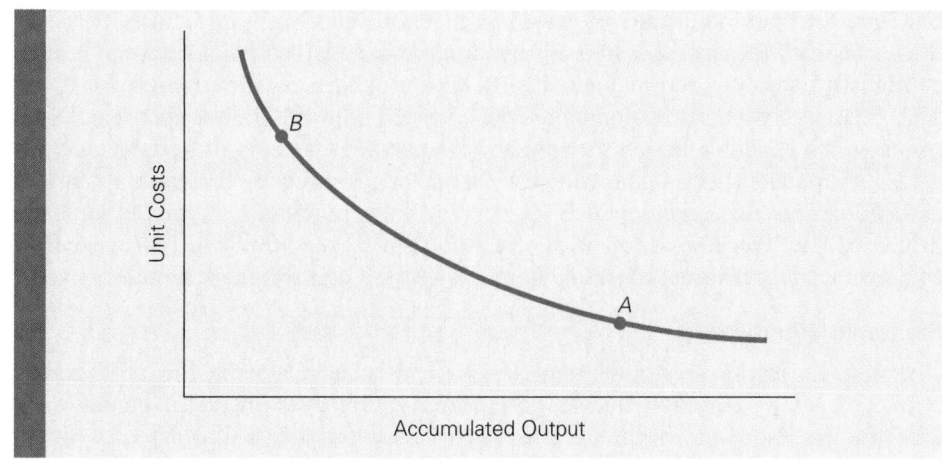

Figure 12.4

The Experience Curve

Learning Effects

Learning effects refer to cost savings that come from learning by doing. Labor, for example, learns by repetition how to carry out a task, such as assembling airframes, most efficiently. Labor productivity increases over time as individuals learn the most efficient ways to perform particular tasks. Equally important, in new production facilities, management typically learns how to manage the new operation more efficiently over time. Hence, production costs eventually decline due to increasing labor productivity and management efficiency.

Learning effects tend to be more significant when a technologically complex task is repeated, because there is more that can be learned about the task. Thus, learning effects will be more significant in an assembly process involving 1,000 complex steps than in one of only 100 simple steps. No matter how complex the task, however, learning effects typically disappear after a while. It has been suggested that they are important only during the start-up period of a new process and that they cease after two or three years.[15] Any decline in the experience curve after such a point is due to economies of scale.

Economies of Scale

Economies of scale refer to the reductions in unit cost achieved by producing a large volume of a product. Economies of scale have a number of sources. One of the most important seems to be the ability to spread fixed costs over a large volume.[16] Fixed costs are the costs required to set up a production facility, develop a new product, and the like, and they can be substantial. For example, the fixed cost of establishing a new production line to manufacture semiconductor chips now exceeds $1 billion. Similarly, according to one estimate, developing a new drug costs about $500 million and takes about 10 years.[17] The only way to recoup such high fixed costs is to sell the product worldwide, which reduces unit costs by spreading them over a larger volume. The more rapidly that cumulative sales volume is built up, the more rapidly fixed costs can be amortized, and the more rapidly unit costs fall.

Another source of scale economies arises from the ability of large firms to employ increasingly specialized equipment or personnel. This theory goes back more than 200 years to Adam Smith, who argued that the division of labor is limited by the extent of the market. As a firm's output expands, it is better able to fully utilize specialized equipment and can justify hiring specialized personnel. For example, consider a metal stamping machine that is used in the production of body parts for automobiles. The machine can be purchased in a customized form, which is optimized for the production of a particular type of body part—say door panels—or a general-purpose form that will produce any kind of body part. The general-purpose form is less efficient and costs more to purchase than the customized form, but it is more flexible. Because these machines are very expensive, costing millions of dollars each, they have to be used continually to recoup a return on their costs. Fully utilized, a machine can turn out about 200,000 units a year. If an automobile company sells only 100,000 cars per year, it will not be worthwhile purchasing the specialized equipment, and it will have to purchase general-purpose machines. This will give it a higher cost structure than a firm that sells 200,000 cars per year, and for which it is economical to purchase a specialized stamping machine. Thus, because a firm with a large output can more fully utilize specialized equipment (and personnel) it should have a lower unit cost than a generalized firm.

Strategic Significance

The strategic significance of the experience curve is clear. Moving down the experience curve allows a firm to reduce its cost of creating value (to lower C in Figure 12.1). The firm that moves down the experience curve most rapidly will have a cost advantage vis-à-vis its competitors. Thus, firm A in Figure 12.4, because it is farther down the experience curve, has a clear cost advantage over firm B.

Many of the underlying sources of experience-based cost economies are plant based. This is true for most learning effects as well as for the economies of scale derived by spreading the fixed costs of building productive capacity over a large output. Thus, one key to progressing downward on the experience curve as rapidly as possible is to increase the volume produced by a single plant as rapidly as possible. Because global markets are larger than domestic markets, a firm that serves a global market from a single location is likely to build accumulated volume more quickly than a firm that serves only its home market or that serves multiple markets from multiple production locations. Thus, serving a global market from a single location is consistent with moving down the experience curve and establishing a low cost position. In addition, to get down the experience curve rapidly, a firm may need to price and market aggressively so demand will expand rapidly. It will also need to build sufficient production capacity for serving a global market. Also, the cost advantages of serving the world market from a single location will be even more significant if that location is the optimal one for performing the particular value creation activity.

Once a firm has established a low cost position, it can act as a barrier to new competition. Specifically, an established firm that is well down the experience curve, such as firm A in Figure 12.4, can price so that it is still making a profit while new entrants, which are farther up the curve, are suffering losses.

The classic example of the successful pursuit of such a strategy concerns the Japanese consumer electronics company Matsushita. Along with Sony and Philips, Matsushita was in the race to develop a commercially viable videocassette recorder in the 1970s. Although Matsushita initially lagged behind Philips and Sony, it was able to get its VHS format accepted as the world standard and to reap enormous experience-curve-based cost economies in the process. This cost advantage subsequently constituted a formidable barrier to new competition. Matsushita's strategy was to build global volume as rapidly as possible. To ensure it could accommodate worldwide demand, the firm increased its production capacity 33-fold from 205,000 units in 1977 to 6.8 million units by 1984. By serving the world market from a single location in Japan, Matsushita was able to realize significant learning effects and economies of scale. These allowed Matsushita to drop its prices 50 percent within five years of selling its first VHS-formatted VCR. As a result, Matsushita was the world's major VCR producer by 1983, accounting for about 45 percent of world production and enjoying a significant cost advantage over its competitors. The next largest firm, Hitachi, accounted for only 11.1 percent of world production in 1983.[18] Today, firms such as Intel are the masters of this kind of strategy. The costs of building a state-of-the-art facility to manufacture microprocessors are so large (easily in excess of $1 billion) that to make this investment pay Intel *must* pursue experience curve effects, serving world markets from a limited number of plants to maximize the cost economies that derive from scale and learning effects.

Leveraging Core Competencies

The term **core competence** refers to skills within the firm that competitors cannot easily match or imitate.[19] These skills may exist in any of the firm's value creation activities—production, marketing, R&D, human resources, general management, and so on. Such skills are typically expressed in product offerings that other firms find difficult to match or imitate, and thus the core competencies are the bedrock of a firm's competitive advantage. They enable a firm to reduce the costs of value creation and/or to create perceived value in such a way that premium pricing is possible. For example, Toyota has a core competence in the production of cars. It is able to produce high-quality, well-designed cars at a lower delivered cost than any other firm in the world. The skills that enable Toyota to do this seem to reside primarily in the firm's production and materials management functions.[20] McDonald's has a core competence in managing fast-food operations (it seems to be one of the most skilled firms in the world in this industry); Toys "R" Us has a core competence in managing high-volume, discount toy stores (it is perhaps the most skilled firm in the world in this business); Procter & Gamble has a core competence in developing and marketing name brand consumer products (it is one of the most skilled firms in the world in this business); Wal-Mart has a core competence in the information systems and logistics required to efficiently manage a large-scale retail operation; MTV has a core competence in managing the programming and delivery of cable TV music and related offerings.

For such firms, global expansion is a way of further exploiting the value creation potential of their skills and product offerings by applying those skills and products in a larger market. The potential for creating value from such a strategy is greatest when the skills and products of the firm are most unique, when the value placed on them by consumers is great, and when there are very few capable competitors with similar skills and/or products in foreign markets. Firms with unique and valuable skills can often realize enormous returns by applying those skills, and the products they produce, to foreign markets where indigenous competitors lack similar skills and products. MTV has built a vibrant global business by leveraging its skills in the programming and delivery of music and related content and applying those skills to local markets where indigenous competitors lacked equivalent skills. The network's success has raised the value that viewers ascribe to MTV and, by extension, the value that advertisers ascribe to an advertising slot on an MTV channel. In turn, this has enabled MTV to command a higher price for advertising slots than competitors.

Historically, U.S. firms such as Kellogg, Coca-Cola, H. J. Heinz, and Procter & Gamble expanded overseas to exploit their skills in developing and marketing name brand consumer products. These skills and the resulting products, which were developed in the U.S. market during the 1950s and 60s, yielded enormous returns when applied to European markets, where most indigenous competitors lacked similar marketing skills and products. Their near-monopoly on consumer marketing skills allowed these U.S. firms to dominate many European consumer product markets during the 1960s and 70s. Similarly, in the 1970s and 80s, many Japanese firms expanded globally to exploit their skills in production, materials management, and new product development—skills that many of their indigenous North American and European competitors seemed to lack at the time. Today, retail companies such as Wal-Mart and financial companies such as Citicorp, Merrill Lynch, and American Express are transferring the valuable skills they developed in their core home market to other developed and emerging markets where indigenous competitors lack those skills. The same can be said of MTV, profiled in the opening case.

Leveraging Subsidiary Skills

Implicit in the discussion of leveraging core competencies is the idea that skills are developed first at home and than transferred to foreign operations. Thus, MTV developed its programming skills in the United States before transferring them to foreign locations. However, for more mature multinationals that have already established a network of subsidiary operations in foreign markets, the development of valuable skills can just as well occur in foreign subsidiaries.[21] Skills can be created anywhere within a multinational's global network of operations, wherever people have the opportunity and incentive to try new ways of doing things. The creation of skills that help to lower the costs of production, or to enhance perceived value and support higher product pricing, is not the monopoly of the corporate center.

Leveraging the skills created within subsidiaries and applying them to other operations within the firm's global network may create value. For example, McDonald's increasingly is finding that its foreign franchisees are a source of valuable new ideas. Faced with slow growth in France, its local franchisees have begun to experiment not only with the menu, but also with the layout and theme of restaurants. Gone are the ubiquitous Golden Arches, gone too are many of the utilitarian chairs and tables and other plastic features of the fast-food giant. Many McDonald's restaurants in France now have hardwood floors, exposed brick walls, and even armchairs. Half of the 930 or so outlets in France have been upgraded to a level that would make them unrecognizable to an American. The menu, too, has been changed to include premier sandwiches, such as a chicken on focaccia bread, priced some 30 percent higher than the average hamburger. In France at least, the strategy seems to be working. Following the change, increases in same store sales rose from 1 percent annually to 3.4 percent. Impressed with the impact, McDonald's executives are now considering adopting similar changes at other McDonald's restaurants in markets where same store sales growth is sluggish, including the United States.[22]

In another example, Hewlett-Packard has decentralized the authority for the design and production of many of its leading-edge ink-jet printers to its operation in Singapore. Hewlett-Packard made this decision after employees in Singapore distinguished themselves by finding ways to reduce production costs through better product design. Hewlett-Packard now views its Singapore subsidiary as an important source for valuable new knowledge about production and product design that can be applied to other activities within the firm's global network of operations.[23]

For the managers of the multinational enterprise, this phenomenon creates important new challenges. First, they must have the humility to recognize that valuable skills can arise anywhere within the firm's global network, not just at the corporate center. Second, they must establish an incentive system that encourages local employees to acquire new skills. This is not as easy as it sounds. Creating new skills involves a degree of risk. Not all new skills add value. For every valuable idea created by a McDonald's subsidiary in a foreign country, there may be several failures. The management of the multinational must install incentives that encourage employees to take the necessary risks. The company must reward people for successes and not sanction them unnecessarily for taking risks that did not pan out. Third, managers must have a process for identifying when valuable new skills have been created in a subsidiary, and finally, they need to act as facilitators, helping to transfer valuable skills within the firm. We shall discuss these issues in more depth in the next chapter.

Pressures for Cost Reductions and Local Responsiveness

Firms that compete in the global marketplace typically face two types of competitive pressure. They face *pressures for cost reductions* and *pressures to be locally responsive* (see Figure 12.5). These competitive pressures place conflicting demands on a firm. Responding to pressures for cost reductions requires that a firm try to minimize its unit costs. Attaining such a goal may necessitate that a firm base its productive activities at the most favorable low-cost location, wherever in the world that might be. It may also necessitate that a firm offer a standardized product to the global marketplace. This

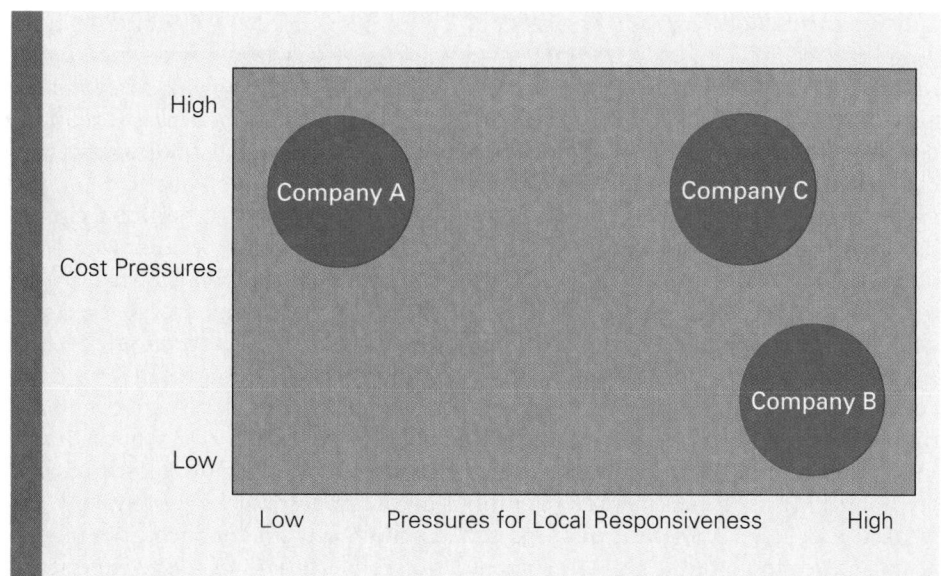

Figure 12.5

Pressures for Cost Reduction and Local Responsiveness

helps the firm spread the fixed costs of developing a product offering over as large a volume as possible, thereby lowering its average unit costs. Offering a standardized product also enables the firm to attain other scale economies and ride down the experience curve as quickly as possible. In contrast, responding to pressures to be locally responsive requires that a firm differentiate its product offering and marketing strategy from country to country in an attempt to accommodate the diverse demands that arise from national differences in consumer tastes and preferences, business practices, distribution channels, competitive conditions, and government policies. Because customizing product offerings to different national requirements can involve significant duplication and a lack of product standardization, the result may be to raise costs.

Some firms, such as company A in Figure 12.5, face high pressures for cost reductions and low pressures for local responsiveness. Others, such as company B, face low pressures for cost reductions and high pressures for local responsiveness. Many others are in the position of company C. They face high pressures for cost reductions and high pressures for local responsiveness. Dealing with these conflicting and contradictory pressures is a difficult strategic challenge for a firm, primarily because being locally responsive can raise costs. In the remainder of this section, we shall look at the source of pressures for cost reductions and local responsiveness. In the next section, we look at the strategies that firms adopt to deal with these pressures.

Pressures for Cost Reductions

In competitive global markets, international businesses often face pressures for cost reductions. Responding to pressures for cost reduction requires a firm to try to lower the costs of value creation by mass producing a standardized product at the optimal location in the world, wherever that might be, to realize location and experience curve economies. Cost reduction pressures can be particularly intense in industries producing commodity-type products where meaningful differentiation on nonprice factors is difficult and price is the main competitive weapon. This tends to be the case for products that serve universal needs. Universal needs exist when the tastes and preferences of consumers in different nations are similar if not identical. This is the case for conventional commodity products such as bulk chemicals, petroleum, steel, sugar, and the like. It also tends to be the case for many industrial and consumer products; for example, handheld calculators, semiconductor chips, personal computers, and liquid crystal display screens. Pressures for cost reductions are also intense in industries where major competitors are based in low-cost locations, where there is persistent excess capacity, and where consumers are powerful and face low switching costs. Many commentators have also argued that the liberalization of the world trade and investment environment in recent decades, by facilitating greater international competition, has generally increased cost pressures.[24]

For example, pressures for cost reductions have been intense in the global tire industry over the past decade. Tires are a commodity–type product where meaningful differentiation is difficult and price is the main competitive weapon. The major buyers of tires, automobile firms, are powerful and face low switching costs, so they have been playing tire firms off against each other in an attempt to get lower prices. And the decline in global demand for automobiles in the early 1990s created serious excess capacity in the tire industry, with as much as 25 percent of world capacity standing idle. The result was a worldwide price war with almost all tire firms suffering heavy losses in the 1990s. In response to the resulting cost pressures, most tire firms are now trying to rationalize their operations in a manner that is consistent with the attainment of a low cost position. This includes moving production facilities to low-cost facilities and offering globally standardized products to try to realize experience curve economies.[25]

Pressures for Local Responsiveness

Pressures for local responsiveness arise from a number of sources including (*i*) differences in consumer tastes and preferences, (*ii*) differences in infrastructure and traditional practices, (*iii*) differences in distribution channels, and (*iv*) host-government demands.

Differences in Consumer Tastes and Preferences

Strong pressures for local responsiveness emerge when consumer tastes and preferences differ significantly between countries, as they may for historic or cultural reasons. In such cases, product and/or marketing messages have to be customized to appeal to the tastes and preferences of local consumers. This typically creates pressure to delegate production and marketing functions to national subsidiaries.

The opening case provided a good example of this. Other things being equal, MTV would probably have preferred to centralize as much programming and content in the United States as possible. Offering standardized programming and content around the world would have allowed MTV to realize scale economies by leveraging its fixed costs of programming and content development over a global viewer base. However, this strategy essentially failed. Instead, to gain viewers in different countries, MTV found that it needs to respond to local tastes and preferences, customizing its programming and content accordingly. Thus, while "MTV Cricket in Control" would be unlikely to wet the appetite of U.S. viewers, it is an important program in India.

The automobile industry in the 1980s and early 1990s moved toward the creation of "world cars." The idea was that global companies such as General Motors, Ford, and Toyota would be able to sell the same basic vehicle the world over, sourcing it from centralized production locations. If successful, the strategy would have enabled automobile companies to reap significant gains from global scale economies. However, this strategy has frequently run aground upon the hard rocks of consumer reality. Consumers in different automobile markets seem to have different tastes and preferences, and these require different types of vehicles. For example, North American consumers show a strong demand for pickup trucks. This is particularly true in the South and West where many families have a pickup truck as a second or third car. But in European countries, pickup trucks are seen purely as utility vehicles and are purchased primarily by firms rather than individuals. As a consequence, the marketing message needs to be tailored to take into account the different nature of demand in North

Management Focus

Tailoring World Cars to the U.S. Market

American consumers love their light pickup trucks. When the last serious recession hit the U.S. automobile market in the early 1990s, sales of light trucks continued to grow through the slowdown at an astonishing 12 percent a year. The lesson was not lost on Toyota, whose Toyota Land Cruiser and Four Runner models did well. But there was a big hole in Toyota's product offerings; the company did not sell a full-size pickup truck to compete with the rugged offerings from General Motors and Ford so beloved by American consumers.

Toyota's first attempt to fix this problem was the T100, a heavy-duty truck launched in the United States in November 1992. But while the T100 had the look of a rugged pickup, it lacked the power. Americans have a thirst for pickups with powerful V8 engines that can haul large loads with ease, but the T100 had only a V6 engine. Plus, in trials it underperformed other smaller pickups with V6 engines—not a good omen. Soon after launch, it was clear that the T100 would do little to help Toyota capture share in the U.S. pickup truck market. By February 1, 1993, Toyota had sold only 2,500 T100s, well short of the 50,000 annual rate it aimed for. Toyota replaced the T100 with a more Americanized product, the Toyota Tundra, in mid-2000. The Toyota Tundra doesn't just look like a heavy-duty pickup truck; it also comes powered to perform like one with a V8 engine. Reflecting the enhanced responsiveness to the U.S. market, Toyota hopes to sell about 100,000 Tundras a year in the United States, but it also recognizes that there will be few opportunities for selling the Tundra outside the United States—it's just too American.

Toyota is not alone in learning this lesson. Another Japanese company, Nissan, decided in 2001 to do what would have been unthinkable a year earlier—let U.S. engineers and planners be completely responsible for the development of most vehicles sold in North America. Among other things, Nissan conducted focus group sessions with American children, asking them for ideas about cup holders, storage, and new features for a range of minivans Nissan planned to launch in 2003. According to a Nissan spokesperson, the company is taking this approach because "we tried for a long time to design cars in Japan and shove them down American consumers throats. It didn't work very well."

Honda took a similar tack with its next-generation sport utility vehicle, the Pilot, which was introduced in 2002. Although Honda has long delegated design work to U.S. engineers, in an attempt to keep costs down, Honda's Japanese management initially wanted its U.S. product designers to base the Pilot on a recycled platform developed in Japan. After some hard lobbying on this issue, the Japanese gave way to the desires of U.S. engineers, who wanted an all-American car. But then the Japanese wanted the Pilot to have just two rows of seats, while the U.S. designers were pushing for a larger vehicle with three rows of seats. The Japanese reasoned that if consumers wanted three rows of seats, they would buy a minivan. To overcome Japanese objections, the American designers flew several of Honda's Japanese executives to the United States and for several days took them to the homes of American families that drove large Ford Expeditions. The Japanese observed how mothers utilized the three rows of seats hauling their children and neighborhood kids to soccer games and how many families used the third row for their dogs. According to the Pilot's designers, had the market research been done in Japan, designers would have missed such characteristic behavior of the American middle class. As a result, they may have designed an SUV that appealed less to the tastes and preferences of the American consumer.

Sources: N. Shirouzu, "Tailoring World Cars to U.S. Tastes," *Wall Street Journal*, January 15, 2001, p. B1, and P. Dean, "Autos: California Style," *Los Angeles Times*, April 1, 1999, p. A9.

America and Europe. The accompanying Management Focus gives some examples of this in the U.S. automobile market.

As a counterpoint, in a now classic article, Harvard Business School Professor Theodore Levitt argued that consumer demands for local customization are on the decline worldwide.[26] According to Levitt, modern communication and transportation technologies have created the conditions for a convergence of the tastes and preferences of consumers from different nations. The result is the emergence of enormous global markets for standardized consumer products. Levitt cites worldwide acceptance of McDonald's hamburgers, Coca-Cola, Levi Strauss jeans, and Sony television sets, all of which are sold as standardized products, as evidence of the increasing homogeneity of the global marketplace.

Levitt's argument, however, has been characterized as extreme by many commentators. For example, Christopher Bartlett and Sumantra Ghoshal have observed that in the consumer electronics industry, consumers reacted to an overdose of standardized global products by showing a renewed preference for products that are differentiated to local conditions.[27] They note that Amstrad, the British computer and electronics firm, got its start by recognizing and responding to local consumer needs. Amstrad captured a major share of the British audio player market by moving away from the standardized inexpensive music centers marketed by global firms such as Sony and Matsushita. Amstrad's product was encased in teak rather than metal cabinets and had a control panel tailor-made to appeal to British consumers' preferences. In response, Matsushita reversed its earlier bias toward standardized global design and placed more emphasis on local customization. Similarly, as we saw in the opening case, to fight off competitive threats from local competitors, MTV customized its programming and content to tastes and preferences in local markets. In direct counterpoint to Levitt's thesis, the music industry seems to have moved away from global megastars and toward more local tastes.

Differences in Infrastructure and Traditional Practices

Pressures for local responsiveness emerge when there are differences in infrastructure and/or traditional practices between countries. In such circumstances, the product may need to be customized to the distinctive infrastructure and practices of different nations. This may necessitate the delegation of manufacturing and production functions to foreign subsidiaries. For example, in North America, consumer electrical systems are based on 110 volts, while in some European countries 240-volt systems are standard. Thus, domestic electrical appliances have to be customized for this difference in infrastructure. Traditional practices also often vary across nations. For example, in Great Britain, people drive on the left side of the road, thus creating a demand for right-hand drive cars, whereas in neighboring France, people drive on the right side of the road, thus creating a demand for left-hand drive cars. Obviously automobiles have to be customized for this difference in traditional practices.

While many of the country differences in infrastructure are rooted in history, some are quite recent. For example, in the wireless telecommunication industry, technical standards vary around the world. A technical standard known as GSM is common in Europe, while an alternative standard, referred to as CDMA, is more common in the United States and parts of Asia. Equipment designed for GSM will not work on a CDMA network, and vice versa. Thus, companies such as Nokia, Motorola, and Ericsson, which manufacture wireless handsets and infrastructure such as switches, need to customize their product offering according to the technical standard prevailing in a given country.

Differences in Distribution Channels

A firm's marketing strategies may have to be responsive to differences in distribution channels between countries. This may necessitate the delegation of marketing functions to national subsidiaries. In Germany, for example, a handful of food retailers dominate the market, but the market is very fragmented in neighboring Italy. Thus, retail chains have considerable buying power in Germany but relatively little in Italy. Dealing with these differences requires different marketing approaches on the part of detergent firms. Similarly, in the pharmaceutical industry, the British and Japanese distribution systems are radically different from the U.S. system. British and Japanese doctors will not accept or respond favorably to an American-style high-pressure sales force. Thus, pharmaceutical firms have to adopt different marketing practices in Great Britain and Japan compared to the United States (soft sell versus hard sell).

Host-Government Demands

Economic and political demands imposed by host-country governments may necessitate a degree of local responsiveness. For example, the politics of health care around the world requires that pharmaceutical firms manufacture in multiple locations. Pharmaceutical firms are subject to local clinical testing, registration procedures, and pricing restrictions, all of which require that the manufacturing and marketing of a drug should meet local requirements. Because governments and government agencies control a significant proportion of the health care budget in most countries, they can demand a high level of local responsiveness.

Threats of protectionism, economic nationalism, and local content rules (which require that a certain percentage of a product be manufactured locally) all dictate that international businesses manufacture locally. Consider Bombardier, the Canadian-based manufacturer of railcars, aircraft, jet boats, and snowmobiles. Bombardier has 12 railcar factories across Europe. Critics of the firm argue that the resulting duplication of manufacturing facilities leads to high costs and explains why Bombardier makes lower profit margins on its railcar operations than on its other business lines. Managers at Bombardier argue that in Europe, informal rules with regard to local content favor people who use local workers. To sell railcars in Germany, they claim, you must manufacture in Germany. The same goes for Belgium, Austria, and France. To address its cost structure in Europe, Bombardier has centralized its engineering and purchasing functions, but it has no plans to centralize manufacturing.[28]

Implications

Pressures for local responsiveness imply that it may not be possible for a firm to realize the full benefits from experience curve and location economies. For example, it may not be possible to serve the global marketplace from a single low-cost location, producing a globally standardized product and marketing it worldwide to achieve experience curve cost economies. The need to customize the product offering to local conditions may work against implementation of such a strategy. As noted earlier, automakers have found that Japanese, American, and European consumers demand different kinds of cars, and that this necessitates producing products that are customized for local markets. In response, Honda, Ford, and Toyota are establishing top-to-bottom design and production facilities in each of these regions to better serve local demands. While such customization brings benefits, it also limits a firm's ability to realize significant experience curve cost economies and location economies.

In addition, pressures for local responsiveness imply that it may not be possible to leverage the skills and products associated with a firm's core competencies wholesale from one nation to another. Concessions often have to be made to local conditions. Despite being depicted as the poster boy for the proliferation of standardized global products, even McDonald's has found it has to customize its product offering (i.e., its menu) to account for national differences in tastes and preferences.

Strategic Choices ▮

Firms use four basic strategies to enter and compete in the international environment: an international strategy, a multidomestic strategy, a global strategy, and a transnational strategy.[29] Each of these strategies has its advantages and disadvantages. The appropriateness of each strategy varies with the extent of pressures for cost reductions and local responsiveness. Figure 12.6 illustrates when each of these strategies is most appropriate. In this section we describe each strategy, identify when it is appropriate, and discuss the pros and cons of each.

Figure 12.6

Four Basic Strategies

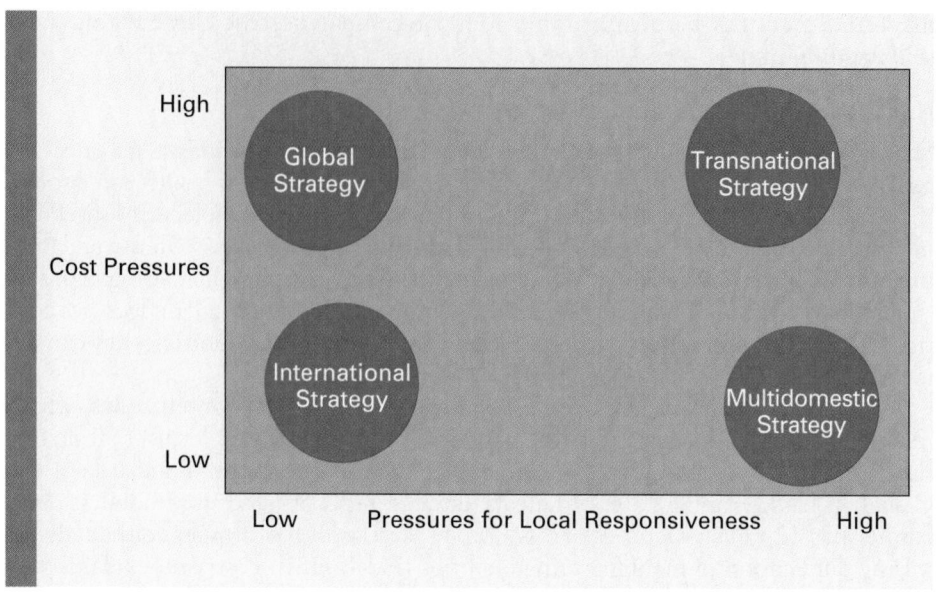

International Strategy

Firms that pursue an international strategy try to create value by transferring valuable skills and products to foreign markets where indigenous competitors lack those skills and products. Most international firms have created value by transferring differentiated product offerings developed at home to new markets overseas. Accordingly, they tend to centralize product development functions at home (e.g., R&D). However, they also tend to establish manufacturing and marketing functions in each major country in which they do business. But while they may undertake some local customization of product offering and marketing strategy, this tends to be limited. In most international firms, the head office retains tight control over marketing and product strategy.

International firms include the likes of Toys "R" Us, McDonald's, IBM, Kellogg, Procter & Gamble, Wal-Mart, and Microsoft. Microsoft, for example, develops the core architecture underlying its products at its Redmond campus in Washington state and also writes the bulk of the computer code there. However, the company does allow national subsidiaries to develop their own marketing and distribution strategy and to customize aspects of the product to account for such basic local differences as language and alphabet. The accompanying Management Focus profiles IKEA, a Swedish retailer that has traditionally pursued an international strategy, transferring its retailing formula developed in Sweden wholesale into other markets. As the feature makes clear, however, this strategy did not work for IKEA once it opened stores in the United States.

An international strategy makes sense if a firm has a valuable core competence that indigenous competitors in foreign markets lack and if the firm faces relatively weak pressures for local responsiveness and cost reductions (as is the case for Microsoft). In such circumstances, an international strategy can be very profitable. However, when pressures for local responsiveness are high, firms pursuing this strategy lose to firms that emphasize customizing the product offering and market strategy to local conditions. IKEA experienced this problem in the United States and subsequently shifted its strategy to accommodate local differences in tastes and preferences (see the Management Focus). Similarly, when MTV expanded into Europe, it pursued an international strategy, but as we saw from the opening case, this strategy failed. In addition, due to the duplication of manufacturing facilities, firms that pursue an international strategy tend to suffer from high operating costs. This makes the strategy inappropriate in manufacturing industries where cost pressures are high.

Multidomestic Strategy

Firms pursuing a multidomestic strategy orient themselves toward achieving maximum local responsiveness. The key distinguishing feature of multidomestic firms is that they extensively customize both their product offering and their marketing strategy to match different national conditions. Consistent with this, they also tend to establish a complete set of value creation activities, including production, marketing, and R&D, in each major national market in which they do business. As a consequence, they are generally unable to realize value from experience curve effects and location economies. Accordingly, many multidomestic firms have a high cost structure. They also tend to do a poor job of leveraging core competencies within the firm.

A multidomestic strategy makes most sense when there are high pressures for local responsiveness and low pressures for cost reductions. The high cost structure associated with the duplication of production facilities makes this strategy inappropriate in industries where cost pressures are intense. Another weakness associated with this strategy is that many multidomestic firms have developed into decentralized federations in which each national subsidiary functions in a largely autonomous manner. This was exemplified by the failure of Philips NV to establish its V2000 VCR format as the standard in the industry during the late 1970s. Its U.S. subsidiary refused to adopt the V2000 format; instead, it bought VHS-format VCRs produced by Matsushita and put its own label on them!

Global Strategy

Firms that pursue a global strategy focus on increasing profitability by reaping the cost reductions that come from experience curve effects and location economies. That is, they are pursuing a low cost strategy. The production, marketing, and R&D activities of firms pursuing a global strategy are concentrated in a few favorable locations. Global firms tend not to customize their product offering and marketing strategy to local conditions because customization raises costs (it involves shorter production runs and the duplication of functions). Instead, global firms prefer to market a standardized product worldwide so they can reap the maximum benefits from the economies of scale that underlie the experience curve. They may also use their cost advantage to support aggressive pricing in world markets.

This strategy makes most sense where there are strong pressures for cost reductions and where demands for local responsiveness are minimal. Increasingly, these conditions prevail in many industrial goods industries. In the semiconductor industry, for example, global standards have created enormous demands for standardized global products. Accordingly, firms such as Intel, Texas Instruments, and Motorola all pursue a global strategy. However, as we noted earlier, these conditions are not found in many consumer goods markets, where demands for local responsiveness remain high (e.g., processed food products). The strategy is inappropriate when demands for local responsiveness are high.

Transnational Strategy

Christopher Bartlett and Sumantra Ghoshal have argued that in today's environment, competitive conditions are so intense that to survive in the global marketplace, firms *must exploit experience-based cost economies and location economies, they must transfer core competencies within the firm, and they must do all of this while paying attention to pressures for local responsiveness.*[30] They note that in the modern multinational enterprise, core competencies do not just reside in the home country. Valuable skills can develop in

IKEA

Established in the 1940s in Sweden by Ingvar Kamprad, IKEA has grown rapidly in recent years to become one of the world's largest retailers of home furnishings. In its initial push to expand globally, IKEA largely ignored the retailing rule that international success involves tailoring product lines closely to national tastes and preferences. Instead, IKEA stuck with the vision, articulated by founder Kamprad, that the company should sell a basic product range that is "typically Swedish" wherever it ventures in the world. The company also remained primarily production oriented; that is, the Swedish management and design group decided what it was going to sell and then presented it to the worldwide public—often with little research as to what the public actually wanted. The company also emphasized its Swedish roots in its international advertising, even insisting on a blue-and-gold color scheme for its stores.

Despite breaking some key rules of international retailing, the formula of selling Swedish-designed products in the same manner everywhere seemed to work. Between 1974 and 2002, IKEA expanded from a company with 10 stores, only one of which was outside Scandinavia, and annual revenues of $210 million to a group with 175 stores in 31 countries and sales of $9.6 billion. In 2002, only 7 percent of sales were generated in Sweden. Of the balance, 21 percent came from Germany, 50 percent from the rest of Europe, and 17 per-

cent from North America. IKEA is beginning to expand in Asia, which generated 3 percent of total sales.

The foundation of IKEA's success has been to offer consumers good value for money. IKEA's approach starts with a global network of suppliers, which now numbers 1,800 firms in 55 countries. An IKEA supplier gains long-term contracts, technical advice, and leased equipment from the company. In return, IKEA demands an exclusive contract and low prices. IKEA's designers work closely with suppliers to build savings into the products from the outset by designing products that can be produced at a low cost. IKEA displays its enormous range of more than 10,000 products in cheap out-of-town stores. It sells most of its furniture as kits for customers to take home and assemble themselves. The firm reaps huge economies of scale from the size of each store and the big production runs made possible by selling the same products all over the world. This strategy allows IKEA to match its rivals on quality, while undercutting them by up to 30 percent on price and still maintaining a healthy after-tax return on sales of about 7 percent.

This strategy worked well until IKEA entered the North American market. Between 1985 and 1996, IKEA opened six stores in North America, but unlike the company's experience across Europe, the stores did not quickly become profitable. As early as 1990, it was clear that IKEA's North American operations were in trouble. Part of the problem was adverse movement in exchange rates. In 1985, the exchange rate was $1=

any of the firm's worldwide operations. Thus, Bartlett and Ghoshal maintain that the flow of skills and product offerings should not be all one way, from home firm to foreign subsidiary, as in the case of firms pursuing an international strategy. Rather, the flow should also be from foreign subsidiary to home country, and from foreign subsidiary to foreign subsidiary—a process they refer to as **global learning**.[31] Bartlett and Ghoshal refer to the strategy pursued by firms that are trying to simultaneously create value in these different ways as a **transnational strategy.**

A transnational strategy makes sense when a firm faces high pressures for cost reductions, high pressures for local responsiveness, and where there are significant opportunities for leveraging valuable skills within a multinational's global network of operations. In some ways, firms that pursue a transnational strategy are trying to simultaneously achieve cost and differentiation advantages. In terms of the framework summarized in Figure 12.1, they are trying to simultaneously lower C and increase V. As attractive as this may sound, the strategy is not easy to pursue. Pressures for local responsiveness and cost reductions place conflicting demands on a firm; being locally responsive raises costs. How can a firm effectively pursue a transnational strategy? Some clues can be derived from the case of Caterpillar. In the 1980s, the need to compete with low-cost competitors such as Komatsu and Hitachi of Japan

8.6 Swedish kronor; by 1990 it was $1=SKr5.8. At this exchange rate, many products imported from Sweden did not look inexpensive to American consumers.

But there was more to IKEA's problems than adverse movements in exchange rates. IKEA's unapologetically Swedish products, which had sold so well across Europe, jarred with American tastes and sometimes physiques. Swedish beds were narrow and measured in centimeters. IKEA did not sell the matching bedroom suites that Americans liked. Its kitchen cupboards were too narrow for the large dinner plates. Its glasses were too small for a nation that added ice to everything. The drawers in IKEA's bedroom chests were too shallow for American consumers, who tend to store sweaters in them. And the company made the mistake of selling European-sized curtains that did not fit American windows. As one senior IKEA manager joked later, "Americans just wouldn't lower their ceilings to fit our curtains."

By 1991, the company's top management realized that if it was going to succeed in North America, it would have to customize its product offering to North American tastes. The company set about redesigning its product range. The drawers on bedroom chests were designed to be two inches deeper, and sales immediately increased by 30 to 40 percent. IKEA now sells American-style king- and queen-size beds, measured in inches, and it sells them as part of complete bedroom suites. It redesigned its kitchen furniture and kitchenware to better appeal to American tastes. IKEA also shifted the emphasis on its textile products to coordinated color schemes, thereby appealing to the sensibilities of North American consumers. The company also boosted the amount of products sourced locally from 15 percent in 1990 to 45 percent in 1997, which makes the company far less vulnerable to adverse exchange rate movements. By 2002, about one-third of IKEA's total product offerings were designed exclusively for the U.S. market.

This break with IKEA's traditional strategy seems to be paying off. Between 1990 and 1994, IKEA's North American sales tripled to $480 million, and they nearly doubled again to about $900 million in 1997 and reached $1.63 billion in 2002. The company claims it has been making a profit in North America since early 1993, although the privately held company does not release precise figures and does admit that its profit rate is lower in America than in Europe. Still, the company is pushing ahead with plans for further expansions in North America, including a goal of opening 50 new stores between 2003 and 2013, which will bring its total to 75.

Sources: "Furnishing the World," *The Economist,* November 19, 1994, pp. 79–80; H. Carnegy, "Struggle to Save the Soul of IKEA," *Financial Times,* March 27, 1995, p. 12; J. Flynn and L. Bongiorno, "IKEA's New Game Plan," *Business Week,* October 6, 1997, pp. 99–102; M. Duff, "IKEA Eyes Aggressive Growth," *DSN Retailing Today,* January 27, 2003, pp. 2–3; and IKEA's website at www.ikea.com.

forced Caterpillar to look for greater cost economies. At the same time, variations in construction practices and government regulations across countries meant that Caterpillar had to remain responsive to local demands. Therefore, as illustrated in Figure 12.7, Caterpillar was confronted with significant pressures for cost reductions and for local responsiveness.

To deal with cost pressures, Caterpillar redesigned its products to use many identical components and invested in a few large-scale component-manufacturing facilities, sited at favorable locations, to fill global demand and realize scale economics. The firm also augmented the centralized manufacturing of components with assembly plants in each of its major global markets. At these plants, Caterpillar added local product features, tailoring the finished product to local needs. By pursuing this strategy, Caterpillar realized many of the benefits of global manufacturing while also responding to pressures for local responsiveness by differentiating its product among national markets.[32] Caterpillar started to pursue this strategy in the early 1980s and by 1997 had doubled output per employee, significantly reducing its overall cost structure. Meanwhile, Komatsu and Hitachi, which are still wedded to a Japan-centric global strategy, have seen their cost advantages evaporate and have been steadily losing market share to Caterpillar.

Figure 12.7

Cost Pressures and Pressures for Local Responsiveness Facing Caterpillar

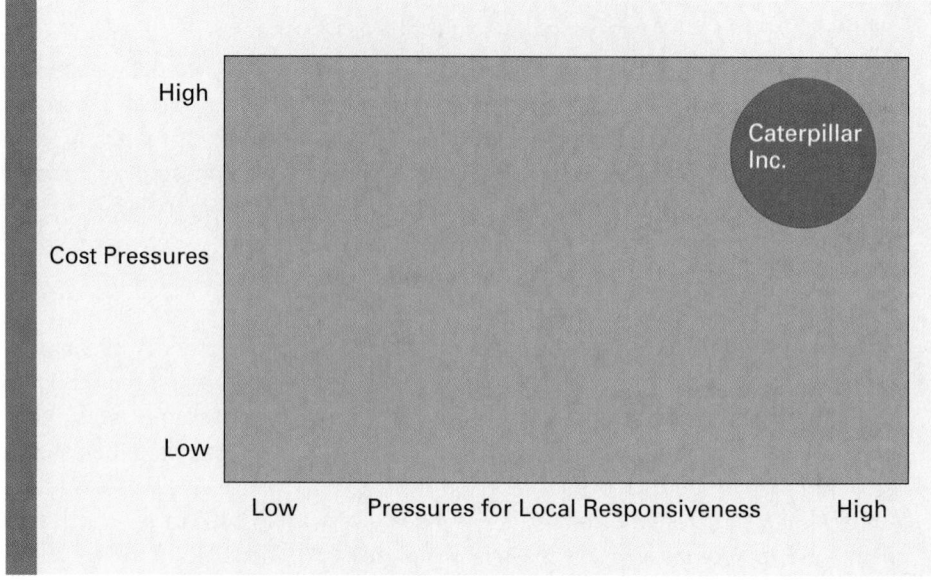

Unilever, once a classic multidomestic firm, has had to shift toward more of a transnational strategy. A rise in low-cost competition, which increased cost pressures, forced Unilever to look for ways of rationalizing its detergent business. During the 1980s, Unilever had 17 largely self-contained detergent operations in Europe alone. The duplication of assets and marketing was enormous. Because Unilever was so fragmented, it could take as long as four years for the firm to introduce a new product across Europe. Now Unilever has integrated its European operation into a single entity, with detergents being manufactured in a handful of cost-efficient plants, and standard packaging and advertising being used across Europe. According to the firm, the result was an annual cost saving of more than $200 million. At the same time, however, due to national differences in distribution channels and brand awareness, Unilever recognizes that it must still remain locally responsive, even while it tries to realize economies from consolidating production and marketing at the optimal locations.[33] One might also argue that the MTV Networks shifted from an international to a transnational strategy in the 1990s (see the opening case). Rather than creating everything in the United States, MTV now tries to strike a balance between the need to maintain uniformity in operating principles and the "frenetic look" of MTV programming across its global operations and the need to customize programming and content to local tastes and preferences.

Bartlett and Ghoshal admit that building an organization that is capable of supporting a transnational strategic posture is a complex and difficult task. Simultaneously trying to achieve cost efficiencies, global learning (the leveraging of skills), and local responsiveness places contradictory demands on an organization. It is important to note that the organizational problems associated with pursuing what are essentially conflicting objectives constitute a major impediment to the pursuit of a transnational strategy. Firms that attempt to pursue a transnational strategy can become bogged down in an organizational morass that only leads to inefficiencies.

Also, Bartlett and Ghoshal may be overstating the case for the transnational strategy. They present the transnational strategy as the only viable strategy. While no one doubts that in some industries the firm that can adopt a transnational strategy will have a competitive advantage, in other industries, global, multidomestic, and international strategies remain viable. In the semiconductor industry, for example, pressures for local customization are minimal and competition is purely a cost game, in which case a global strategy, not a transnational strategy, is optimal. This is the case in

Strategy	Advantages	Disadvantages
Global	Exploit experience curve effects Exploit location economies	Lack of local responsiveness
International	Transfer core competencies to foreign markets	Lack of local responsiveness Inability to realize location economies Failure to exploit experience curve effects
Multidomestic	Customize product offerings and marketing in accordance with local responsiveness	Inability to realize location economies Failure to exploit experience curve effects Failure to transfer core competencies to foreign markets
Transnational	Exploit experience curve effects Exploit location economies Customize product offerings and marketing in accordance with local responsiveness Reap benefits of global learning	Difficult to implement due to organizational problems

Table 12.1

The Advantages and Disadvantages of the Four Strategies

many industrial goods markets where the product serves universal needs. On the other hand, the argument can be made that to compete in certain consumer goods markets, such as the automobile and consumer electronics industry, a firm has to try to adopt a transnational strategy.

Summary

The advantages and disadvantages of each of the four strategies discussed above are summarized in Table 12.1. While a transnational strategy appears to offer the most advantages, implementing a transnational strategy raises difficult organizational issues. As shown in Figure 12.6, the appropriateness of each strategy depends on the relative strength of pressures for cost reductions and for local responsiveness.

Chapter Summary

In this chapter we reviewed basic principles of strategy and the various ways in which firms can profit from global expansion, and we looked at the strategies that firms that compete globally can adopt. The chapter made these major points:

1. A firm's strategy can be defined as the actions that managers take to attain the goals of the firm. For most firms, the preeminent goal is to maximize long-term profitability. Maximizing profitability requires firms to focus on value creation.

2. Due to national differences, it may pay a firm to base each value creation activity it performs at that location where factor conditions are most conducive to the performance of that activity. We refer to this strategy as focusing on the attainment of location economies.

3. By rapidly building sales volume for a standardized product, international expansion can assist a firm in moving down the experience curve.

4. International expansion may enable a firm to earn greater returns by transferring the skills and

product offerings derived from its core competencies to markets where indigenous competitors lack those skills and product offerings.

5. A multinational firm can create additional value by identifying valuable skills created within its foreign subsidiaries and leveraging those skills within its global network of operations.

6. The best strategy for a firm to pursue often depends on a consideration of the pressures for cost reductions and for local responsiveness.

7. Pressures for cost reductions are greatest in industries producing commodity-type products where price is the main competitive weapon.

8. Pressures for local responsiveness arise from differences in consumer tastes and preferences, national infrastructure and traditional practices, distribution channels, and from host-government demands.

9. Firms pursuing an international strategy transfer the skills and products derived from distinctive competencies to foreign markets, while undertaking some limited local customization.

10. Firms pursuing a multidomestic strategy customize their product offering, marketing strategy, and business strategy to national conditions.

11. Firms pursuing a global strategy focus on reaping the cost reductions that come from experience curve effects and location economies.

12. Many industries are now so competitive that firms must adopt a transnational strategy. This involves a simultaneous focus on reducing costs, transferring skills and products, and boosting local responsiveness. Implementing such a strategy may not be easy.

Critical Discussion Questions

1. In a world of zero transportation costs, no trade barriers, and nontrivial differences between nations with regard to factor conditions, firms must expand internationally if they are to survive. Discuss.

2. Plot the position of the following firms on Figure 12.5: Procter & Gamble, IBM, Nokia, Coca-Cola, Dow Chemicals, US Steel, McDonald's. In each case justify your answer.

3. Are the following global industries or multidomestic industries: bulk chemicals, pharmaceuticals, branded food products, moviemaking, television manufacture, personal computers, airline travel?

4. What do you see as the main organizational problems that are likely to be associated with implementation of a transnational strategy?

Notes

1. T. Copeland, T. Koller, and J. Murrin, *Valuation: Measuring and Managing the Value of Companies* (New York: John Wiley & Sons, 1996).

2. The concept of consumer surplus is an important one in economics. For a more detailed exposition, see D. Besanko, D. Dranove, and M. Shanley, *Economics of Strategy* (New York: John Wiley & Sons, 1996).

3. However, P=V only in the special case where the company has a perfect monopoly, and where it can charge each customer a unique price that reflects the value of the product to that customer (i.e., where perfect price discrimination is possible). More generally, except in the limiting case of perfect price discrimination, even a monopolist will see most consumers capture some of the value of a product in the form of a consumer surplus.

4. This point is central to the work of Michael Porter, *Competitive Advantage* (New York: Free Press, 1985). See also chap. 4 in P. Ghemawat, *Commitment: The Dynamic of Strategy* (New York: Free Press, 1991).

5. M. E. Porter, *Competitive Strategy* (New York: Free Press, 1980).

6. M. E. Porter, "What is Strategy?" *Harvard Business Review*, On-point Enhanced Edition Article, February 1, 2000.

7. Figures taken from Value Line Investment Survey.

8. Porter, *Competitive Advantage*.

9. Example is based on C. S. Trager, "Enter the Mini-Multinational," *Northeast International Business*, March 1989, pp. 13–14.

10. Empirical evidence does seem to indicate that, on average, international expansion is linked to greater firm profitability. For some recent examples, see M. A. Hitt, R. E. Hoskisson, and H. Kim, "International Diversification, Effects on Inno-

vation and Firm Performance," *Academy of Management Journal* 40, no. 4 (1997), pp. 767–98, and S. Tallman and J. Li, "Effects of International Diversity and Product Diversity on the Performance of Multinational Firms," *Academy of Management Journal* 39, no. 1 (1996), pp. 179–96.

11. M. E. Porter, *The Competitive Advantage of Nations* (New York: Free Press, 1990).

12. R. B. Reich, *The Work of Nations* (New York: Alfred A. Knopf, 1991).

13. G. Hall and S. Howell, "The Experience Curve from an Economist's Perspective," *Strategic Management Journal* 6 (1985), pp. 197–212.

14. A. A. Alchain, "Reliability of Progress Curves in Airframe Production," *Econometrica* 31 (1963), pp. 697–93.

15. Hall and Howell, "The Experience Curve from an Economist's Perspective."

16. For a full discussion of the source of scale economies, see D. Besanko, D. Dranove, and M. Shanley, *Economics of Strategy* (New York: John Wiley & Sons, 1996).

17. This estimate was provided by the Pharmaceutical Manufacturers Association.

18. "Matsushita Electrical Industrial in 1987," in *Transnational Management*, eds. C. A. Bartlett and S. Ghoshal (Homewood, IL: Richard D. Irwin, 1992).

19. This concept has been popularized by G. Hamel and C. K. Prahalad, *Competing for the Future* (Boston: Harvard Business School Press, 1994). The concept is grounded in the resource-based view of the firm; for a summary, see J. B. Barney, "Firm Resources and Sustained Competitive Advantage," *Journal of Management* 17 (1991), pp. 99–120, and K. R. Conner, "A Historical Comparison of Resource-Based Theory and Five Schools of Thought within Industrial Organization Economics: Do We Have a New Theory of the Firm?" *Journal of Management* 17 (1991), pp. 121–54.

20. J. P. Womack, D. T. Jones, and D. Roos, *The Machine That Changed the World* (New York: Rawson Associates, 1990).

21. See J. Birkinshaw and N. Hood, "Multinational Subsidiary Evolution: Capability and Charter Change in Foreign-Owned Subsidiary Companies," *Academy of Management Review* 23 (October 1998), pp. 773–95; A. K. Gupta and V. J. Govindarajan, "Knowledge Flows within Multinational Corporations," *Strategic Management Journal* 21 (2000), pp. 473–96; V. J. Govindarajan and A. K. Gupta, *The Quest for Global Dominance* (San Francisco: Jossey Bass, 2001); T. S. Frost, J. M. Birkinshaw, and P. C. Ensign, "Centers of Excellence in Multinational Corporations," *Strategic Management Journal* 23 (2002), pp. 997–1018; and U. Andersson, M. Forsgren, and U. Holm, "The Strategic Impact of External Networks," *Strategic Management Journal* 23 (2002), pp. 979–96.

22. S. Leung, "Armchairs, TVs and Espresso: Is It McDonald's?" *Wall Street Journal*, August 30, 2002, p. A1, A6.

23. K. Ferdows, "Making the Most of Foreign Factories," *Harvard Business Review*, March–April 1997, pp. 73–88.

24. C. K. Prahalad and Yves L. Doz, *The Multinational Mission: Balancing Local Demands and Global Vision* (New York: Free Press, 1987). Prahalad and Doz actually talk about local responsiveness rather than local customization.

25. "The Tire Industry's Costly Obsession with Size," *The Economist*, June 8, 1993, pp. 65–66.

26. T. Levitt, "The Globalization of Markets," *Harvard Business Review*, May–June 1983, pp. 92–102.

27. C. A. Bartlett and S. Ghoshal, *Managing across Borders* (Boston: Harvard Business School Press, 1989).

28. C. J. Chipello, "Local Presence Is Key to European Deals," *Wall Street Journal*, June 30, 1998, p. A15.

29. This section is based on Bartlett and Ghoshal, *Managing across Borders*.

30. Bartlett and Ghoshal, *Managing across Borders*.

31. A recent empirical study seems to confirm this hypothesis. See J. Birkinshaw, N. Hood, and S. Jonsson, "Building Firm-Specific Advantages in Multinational Corporations: The Role of Subsidiary Initiative," *Strategic Management Journal* 19 (1998), pp. 221–41.

32. See P. Marsh and S. Wagstyle, "The Hungry Caterpillar," *Financial Times*, December 2, 1997, p. 22, and T. Hout, M. E. Porter, and E. Rudden, "How Global Firms Win Out," *Harvard Business Review*, September–October 1982, pp. 98–108.

33. Guy de Jonquieres, "Unilever Adopts a Clean Sheet Approach," *Financial Times*, October 21, 1991, p. 13.

Research Task | globalEDGE™ globaledge.msu.edu

Use the globalEDGE™ site to complete the following exercises:

1. Several classifications and rankings of multi-national corporations are prepared by a variety of sources. Find one such ranking system and identify the criteria that are used in ranking the top global companies. Extract the list of the highest ranked 25 companies, paying particular attention to the home countries of the companies.

2. The top management of your company, a manufacturer and marketer of laptop computers, has decided to pursue international expansion opportunities in Eastern Europe. In order to achieve some economies of scale, your management is aiming towards a strategy of minimum local adaptation. Focusing on an Eastern European country of your choice, prepare an executive summary that features those aspects of the product where standardization will simply not work, and adaptation to local conditions will be essential.

Closing Case

Global Strategy at General Motors

General Motors is one of the oldest multinational corporations in the world. Founded in 1908, GM established its first international operations in the 1920s. General Motors is now the world's largest industrial corporation and full-line automobile manufacturer with annual revenues in 2002 of $186 billion. The company sells 8.5 million vehicles per year, 3.2 million of which are produced and marketed outside of its North American base. In 2002, GM had a 15 percent share of the world automobile market.

Historically, most of GM's foreign operations have been concentrated in Western Europe. Local brand names

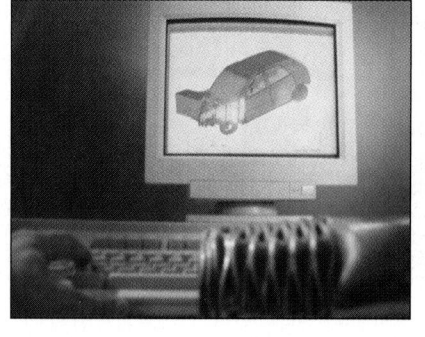

such as Opel, Vauxhall, Saab, and Holden helped the company to capture a 12 percent market share in 2002, second only to that of Ford. Although GM has long had a presence in Latin America and Asia, until recently sales there accounted for only a relatively small fraction of the company's total international business. However, GM's plans call for this to change rapidly over the next few years. Sensing that Asia, Latin America, and Eastern Europe may be the automobile industry's growth markets, in 1997 GM embarked on ambitious plans to invest $2.2 billion in four new manufacturing facilities in Argentina, Poland, China, and Thailand. This expansion goes hand in hand with a sea change in GM's philosophy toward the management of its international operations.

Traditionally, GM saw the developing world as a dumping ground for obsolete technology and outdated models. Just a few years ago, for example, GM's Brazilian factories were churning out U.S.-designed Chevy Chevettes that hadn't been produced in North America

for years. GM's Detroit-based executives saw this as a way of squeezing the maximum cash flow from the company's investments in aging technology. GM managers in the developing world, however, took it as an indication that the center did not view developing world operations as being significant. This feeling was exacerbated by the fact that most operations in the developing world were instructed to carry out manufacturing and marketing plans formulated in the company's Detroit headquarters, rather than being trusted to develop their own.

In contrast, GM's European operations were traditionally managed on an arm's-length basis, with the company's national operations often being allowed to design their own cars and manufacturing facilities and formulate their own marketing strategies. This regional and national autonomy allowed GM's European operations to produce vehicles that were closely tailored to the needs of local customers. However, it also led to costly duplication in design and manufacturing operations and to a failure to share valuable technology, skills, and practices among subsidiaries. Thus, while General Motors exerted tight control over its operations in the developing world, its control over operations in Europe was perhaps too lax. The result was a company whose international operations lacked overall strategic coherence.

GM has been trying to change this since 1997 by switching from its Detroit-centric view of the world to a philosophy that centers of excellence may reside anywhere in the company's global operations. The company is trying to tap these centers of excellence to provide its global operations with the latest technology.

The four new manufacturing plants in the developing world are an embodiment of this new approach. Each is identical, each incorporates state-of-the-art technology, and each has been designed not by Americans, but by a team of Brazilian and German engineers. By building identical plants, GM should be able to mimic Toyota, whose plants are so much alike that a change in a car in Japan can be quickly replicated around the world. The plants are modeled after GM's Eisenach facility in Germany, which is managed by the company's Opel subsidiary. It was at the Eisenach plant that GM figured out how to implement the lean production system pioneered by Toyota. The plant is now the most efficient auto-manufacturing operation in Europe and the best within GM, with a productivity rate at least twice that of most North American assembly operations. Each of the new plants produces state-of-the-art vehicles for local consumption.

To realize scale economies, GM is also trying to design and build vehicles that share a common global platform. Engineering teams located in Germany, Detroit, South America, and Australia are designing these common vehicle platforms. Local plants are allowed to customize certain features of these vehicles to match the tastes and preferences of local customers. At the same time, adhering to a common global platform enables the company to spread its costs of designing a car over greater volume and to realize scale economies in the manufacture of shared components—both of which should help GM lower its overall cost structure. The first fruits of this effort include the 1998 Cadillac Seville, which was designed to be sold in more than 40 countries. GM's family of front-wheel-drive minivans was also designed around a common platform that allows the vehicles to be produced in multiple locations around the globe, as was the 1998 Opel Astra, which is GM's best-selling car in Europe. Ultimately, GM hopes the this coordinated global approach to designing cars will reduce the costs of developing a new vehicle by 15 to 25 percent. GM also hopes that sharing of common parts between GM cars will re-

duce by $3.5 billion its annual bill of $100 billion for component parts.

Despite its bold moves in the direction of greater global integration, numerous problems can still be seen on GM's horizon. Compared to Toyota, for example, GM still suffers from high costs, low perceived quality, and a profusion of brands. While its aggressive move into emerging markets may be based on the reasonable assumption that demand will grow strong in these areas, other automobile companies are also expanding their production facilities in the same markets, raising the specter of global excess capacity and price wars. Finally, and perhaps most significantly, there are those within GM who argue that the push toward "global cars" is misconceived. In particular, the German-based engineering staff at Opel's Russelsheim design facility, which takes the lead on design of many key global models, has voiced concerns that distinctively European engineering features they deem essential to a car's local success may be left by the wayside in a drive to devise what they see as blander "global" cars.

Source: R. Blumenstein, "GM Is Building Plants in Developing Nations to Woo New Markets," *Wall Street Journal*, August 4, 1997, p. A1; Haig Simonian, "GM Hopes to Turn Corner with New Astra," *Financial Times*, November 29, 1997, p. 15; D. Howes, "GM, Ford Play for Keeps Abroad," *Detroit News*, March 8, 1998, p. D1; "The Global Gambles of General Motors," *The Economist*, June 24, 2000, pp. 67–68; and J. Fahey, "Would You Buy a Chevy Saab?" *Forbes*, December 9, 2002, pp. 82–84.

Case Discussion Questions

1. How would you characterize the strategy pursued by GM in the (*a*) developing world and (*b*) Europe before 1997?

2. What do you think were the likely competitive effects of the pre-1997 strategy?

3. How would you characterize the strategy that GM has been pursuing since 1997? How should this strategy affect GM's ability to create value in the global automobile market?

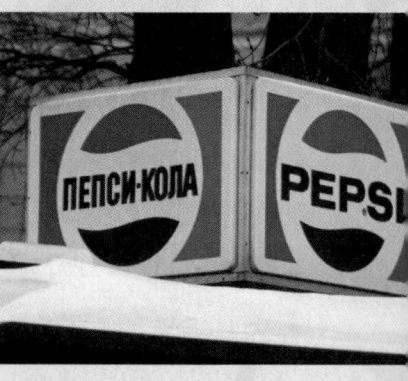

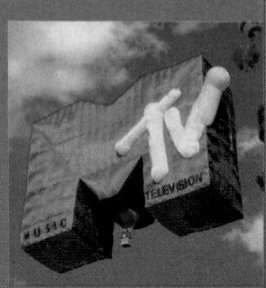

Chapter 13

The Organization of International Business

Introduction
Organizational Architecture
Organizational Structure
 Vertical Differentiation: Centralization
 and Decentralization
 Horizontal Differentiation: The Design
 of Structure
 Integrating Mechanisms
Control Systems and Incentives
 Types of Control Systems
 Incentive Systems
 Control Systems, Incentives, and
 Strategy in the International Business
Processes
Organizational Culture
 Creating and Maintaining
 Organizational Culture
 Organizational Culture and Performance
 in the International Business
Synthesis: Strategy and Architecture
 Multidomestic Firms
 International Firms
 Global Firms
 Transnational Firms
 Environment, Strategy, Architecture,
 and Performance
Organizational Change
 Organizational Inertia
 Implementing Organizational Change
Chapter Summary
Critical Discussion Questions
Closing Case: Organizational Change at
Royal Dutch/Shell

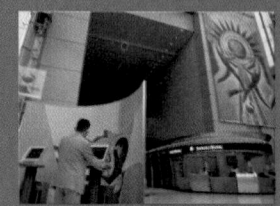

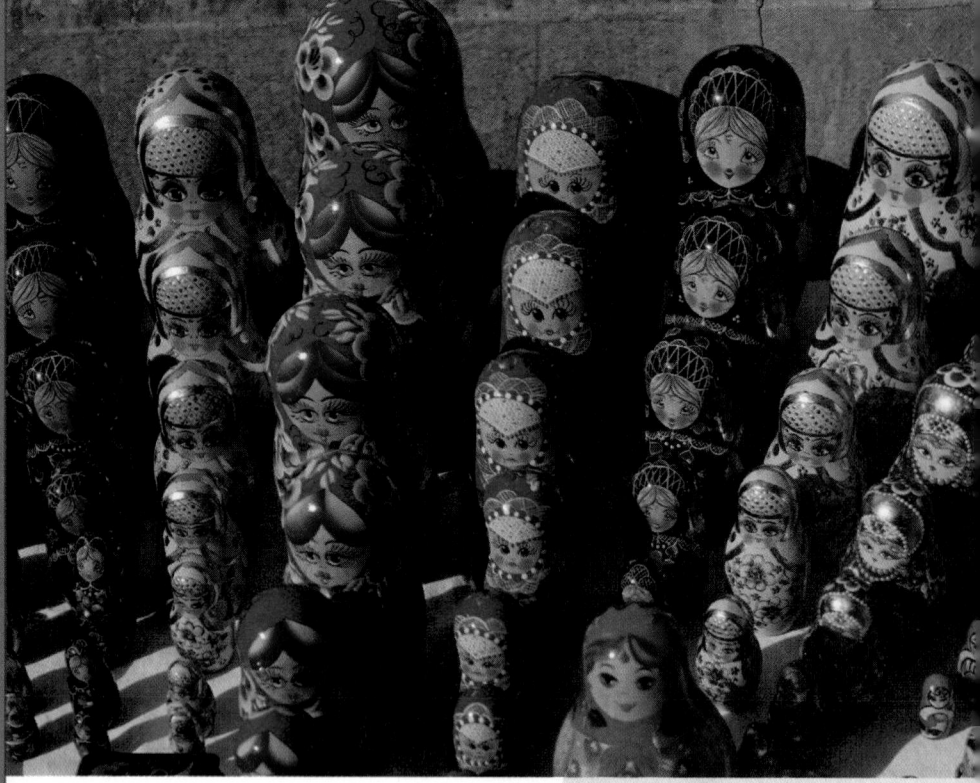

Organizational Change at Unilever

Unilever is one of the world's oldest multinational corporations with extensive product offerings in the food, detergent, and personal care businesses. It generates annual revenues in excess of $50 billion and sells more than 1,000 branded products in virtually every country. Detergents, which account for about 25 percent of corporate revenues, include well-known names such as Omo, which is sold in over 50 countries. Personal care products, which account for about 15 percent of sales, include Calvin Klein Cosmetics, Pepsodent toothpaste brands, Faberge hair care products, and Vaseline skin lotions. Food products account for the remaining 60 percent of sales and include strong offerings in margarine (where Unilever's market share in most countries exceeds 70 percent), tea, ice cream, frozen foods, and bakery products.

Historically, Unilever was organized on a decentralized basis. Subsidiary companies in each major national market were responsible for the production, marketing, sales, and distribution of products in that market. The company had 17 subsidiaries in Europe in the early 1990s, each focused on a different national market. Each was a profit center and each was held accountable for its own performance. This decentralization was viewed as a source of strength. The structure allowed local managers to match product offerings and marketing strategy to local tastes and preferences and to alter sales and distribution strategies to fit the prevailing retail systems. To drive the localization, Unilever recruited local managers to run local organizations; the U.S. subsidiary (Lever Brothers) was run by Americans, the Indian subsidiary by Indians, and so on.

To knit together the decentralized organization, Unilever worked to build a common organizational culture among its managers. For years, the company recruited people with similar backgrounds, values, and interests. The stated preference was for individuals with high levels of "sociability" who embrace the company's values, which emphasize cooperation and consensus building among managers. It is said that the company has been so successful at this that Unilever executives recognize one another at airports even when they have never met before. Unilever's senior management believes this corps of like-minded people is the reason its employees work so well together, despite their national diversity.

Unilever has also worked hard to periodically bring these managers together. Annual conferences on company strategy and executive education sessions at Unilever's management training center outside of London help establish connections between managers. The idea is to build an informal network of equals who know one another well and usually continue to meet and exchange experiences. Unilever also moves its young managers frequently, across borders, products, and divisions. This policy starts Unilever relationships early as well as increases know-how.

By the mid-1990s, the decentralized structure was increasingly out of step with a rapidly changing competitive environment. Unilever's global competitors, which include the Swiss firm Nestlé and Procter & Gamble from the United States, had been more successful than Unilever on several fronts—building global brands, reducing cost structure by consolidating manufacturing operations at a few choice locations, and executing simultaneous product launches in several national markets. Unilever's decentralized structure worked against efforts to build global or regional brands. It also meant lots of duplication, particularly in manufacturing, a lack of scale economies, and a high cost structure. Unilever also found that it was falling behind rivals in the race to bring new products to market. In Europe, for example, while Nestlé and Procter & Gamble moved toward pan-European product launches, it could take Unilever four to five years to "persuade" its 17 European operations to adopt a new product.

Unilever began to change all this in the mid-1990s. In 1996, it introduced a new structure based on regional business groups. Within each business group are a number of divisions, each focusing on a specific category of products. Thus, within the European Business Group is a division focusing on detergents, another on ice cream and frozen foods, and so on. These groups and divisions have been given the responsibility for coordinating the activities of national subsidiaries within their region to drive down operating costs and speed up the process of developing and introducing new products.

"Lever Europe" was established to consolidate the company's detergent operations. The 17 European companies now report directly to Lever Europe. Using its new-found organizational clout, Lever Europe consolidates the production of detergents in Europe in a few key locations to reduce costs and speed up new product introduction. Implicit in this new approach is a bargain: The 17 companies relinquished autonomy in their traditional markets in exchange for opportunities to help develop and execute a unified pan-European strategy. The number of European plants manufacturing soap has been cut from 10 to 2, and some new products will be manufactured at only one site. Product sizing and packaging are harmonized to cut purchasing costs and to accommodate unified pan-European advertising. By taking these steps, Unilever estimates it has saved as much as $400 million a year in its European detergent operations.

Lever Europe is also attempting to speed development of new products and to synchronize the launch of new products throughout Europe. Nonetheless, history still imposes constraints. While Procter & Gamble's leading laundry detergent carries the same brand name across Europe, Unilever sells its product under a variety of names. The company has no plans to change this. Having spent 100 years building these brand names, it believes it would be foolish to scrap them in the interest of pan-European standardization.

Sources: Guy de Jonquieres, "Unilever Adopts a Clean Sheet Approach," *Financial Times,* October 21, 1991, p. 13; C. A. Bartlett and S. Ghoshal, *Managing across Borders* (Boston: Harvard Business School Press, 1989); H. Connon, "Unilever's Got the Nineties Licked," *The Guardian,* May 24, 1998, p. 5; "Unilever: A Networked Organization," *Harvard Business Review,* November–December 1996, p. 138; C. Christensen and J. Zobel, "Unilever's Butter Beater: Innovation for Global Diversity," Harvard Business School Case #9-698-017, March 1998; and M. Mayer, A. Smith, and R. Whittington, "Restructuring Roulette," *Financial Times,* November 8, 2002, p. 8.

▌Introduction

This chapter identifies the organizational architecture that international businesses use to manage and direct their global operations. By **organizational architecture** we mean the totality of a firm's organization, including formal organization structure, control systems and incentives, processes, organizational culture, and people. The core argument outlined in this chapter is that superior enterprise profitability requires three conditions to be fulfilled. First, the different elements of a firm's organizational architecture must be internally consistent. For example, the control and incentive systems used in the firm must be consistent with the structure of the enterprise. Second, the organizational architecture must match or fit the strategy of the firm—strategy and architecture must be consistent. For example, if a firm is pursuing a global strategy but it has the wrong kind of architecture, it will likely be unable to execute that strategy effectively and poor performance may result. Third, the strategy and architecture of the firm must not only be consistent with each other, but they also must be consistent with competitive conditions prevailing in the firm's markets—strategy, architecture, and competitive environment must all be consistent. For example, a firm pursuing a multidomestic strategy might have the right kind of organizational architecture in place. However, if it competes in markets where cost pressures are intense and demands for local responsiveness are low, it will still have inferior performance because a global strategy is more appropriate in such an environment.

The opening case on Unilever touches on some of the important issues here. Historically, Unilever has competed in markets where local responsiveness has been very important. The production and marketing of food, detergent, and personal care products have traditionally been tailored to the tastes and preferences of consumers in different nations. Unilever satisfied this environmental demand for local responsiveness by pursuing a multidomestic strategy. Its organizational architecture reflected this strategy. Unilever operated with a decentralized structure that delegated responsibility for production, marketing, sales, and distribution decisions to autonomous national operating companies. This allowed local managers to configure product offerings, and marketing and sales activities, to the conditions prevailing in a particular nation. For a long time, this fit between strategy and architecture served Unilever well, helping it to become a dominant consumer products enterprise.

However, the competitive environment was changing by the early 1990s. Trade barriers between countries were falling, particularly in the European Union following the creation of a single market in 1992. This made it possible to manufacture certain items, such as detergents and margarine, at favorable central locations to realize the benefits associated with location and experience curve economies. Also, new products in areas such as frozen foods and margarine were gaining regional or even global acceptance. Unfortunately for Unilever, some of its global competitors moved more rapidly to exploit this change in the competitive environment. Unilever found itself disadvantaged by a high cost structure (caused by the duplication of manufacturing operations) and an inability to introduce new products in several national markets at once. In other words, the competitive environment changed, but Unilever did not change with it.

By the mid-1990s, Unilever had recognized its problems and changed both its strategy and its organizational architecture so that it better matched the new competitive realities. Unilever began to adopt a transnational strategic orientation, seeking to balance local responsiveness in marketing and sales with the centralization of manufacturing and product development activities to realize scale economies and execute pan-regional product launches. To implement this strategy, Unilever introduced a new organizational architecture based on regional business groups, each of which contained product divisions. These divisions were given the responsibility for centralizing manufacturing and product development activities, which implied a reduction in the autonomy traditionally granted to operating subsidiaries. To reestablish a fit between strategy, architecture, and environment, Unilever had to embrace the difficult process of strategic and organizational change.

To explore the issues illustrated by cases such as Unilever's, we open the current chapter by discussing in more detail the concepts of organizational architecture and fit. Next we turn to a more detailed exploration of various components of architecture—structure, control systems and incentives, organization culture, and processes—and explain how these components must be internally consistent. (We discuss the "people" component of architecture in Chapter 18, when we discuss human resource strategy in the multinational firm.) After reviewing the various components of architecture, we look at the ways in which architecture can be matched to strategy and the competitive environment to achieve high performance. The chapter closes with a discussion of organizational change, for as the Unilever case illustrates, periodically firms have to change their organization so that it matches new strategic and competitive realities.

Organizational Architecture ▮

As noted in the introduction, the term *organizational architecture* refers to the totality of a firm's organization, including formal organizational structure, control systems and incentives, organizational culture, processes, and people.[1] Figure 13.1 illustrates these different elements. By **organizational structure,** we mean three things: First, the formal division of the organization into subunits such as product divisions, national

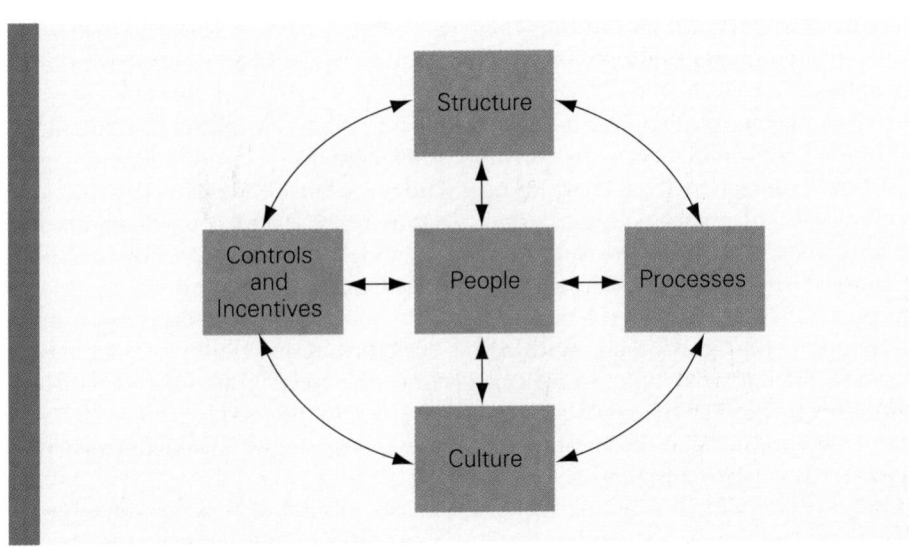

Figure 13.1

Organization Architecture

operations, and functions (most organizational charts display this aspect of structure); second, the location of decision-making responsibilities within that structure (e.g., centralized or decentralized); and third, the establishment of integrating mechanisms to coordinate the activities of subunits including cross-functional teams and or pan-regional committees.

Control systems are the metrics used to measure the performance of subunits and make judgments about how well managers are running those subunits. For example, Unilever historically measured the performance of national operating subsidiary companies according to profitability—profitability was the metric. **Incentives** are the devices used to reward appropriate managerial behavior. Incentives are very closely tied to performance metrics. For example, the incentives of a manager in charge of a national operating subsidiary might be linked to the performance of that company. Specifically, she might receive a bonus if her subsidiary exceeds its performance targets.

Processes are the manner in which decisions are made and work is performed within the organization. Examples are the processes for formulating strategy, for deciding how to allocate resources within a firm, or for evaluating the performance of managers and giving feedback. Processes are conceptually distinct from the location of decision-making responsibilities within an organization, although both involve decisions. While the CEO might have ultimate responsibility for deciding what the strategy of the firm should be (i.e., the decision-making responsibility is centralized), the process he or she uses to make that decision might include the solicitation of ideas and criticism from lower-level managers.

Organizational culture is the norms and value systems that are shared among the employees of an organization. Just as societies have cultures (see Chapter 3 for details), so do organizations. Organizations are societies of individuals who come together to perform collective tasks. They have their own distinctive patterns of culture and subculture.[2] As we shall see, organizational culture can have a profound impact on how a firm performs. Finally, by **people** we mean not just the employees of the organization, but also the strategy used to recruit, compensate, and retain those individuals and the type of people that they are in terms of their skills, values, and orientation (discussed in depth in Chapter 18).

As illustrated by the arrows in Figure 13.1, the various components of an organization's architecture are not independent of each other: Each component shapes, and is shaped by, other components of architecture. An obvious example is the strategy regarding people. This can be used proactively to hire individuals whose internal values are consistent with those that the firm wishes to emphasize in its organization culture. Thus, the people component of architecture can be used to reinforce (or not) the prevailing culture of the organization. This seems to have been the practice at Unilever, where an effort was made to hire individuals who were sociable and placed a high value on consensus and cooperation, values that the enterprise wished to emphasize in its own culture.

If a firm to going to maximize its profitability, it must pay close attention to achieving internal consistency between the various components of its architecture. Figure 13.2 shows an organizational chart for how Unilever's European operations might be structured (this chart is hypothetical). Note that there are several country subsidiaries, one for France, one for Germany, one for Spain, and so on, each reporting to the European Business Group. There are also several pan-European product divisions, one for detergents, one for frozen food, one for margarine, and so on, again each reporting to the European Business Group. Within this structure, responsibility for marketing, sales, and distribution decisions might be given to the country subsidiaries, while responsibility for product manufacturing might be given to the product divisions. As for control systems, imagine that profitability is the metric used to evaluate the performance of the country subsidiaries.

One problem with this arrangement is that the profitability of the country subsidiaries depends on manufacturing costs and new product development, and yet the

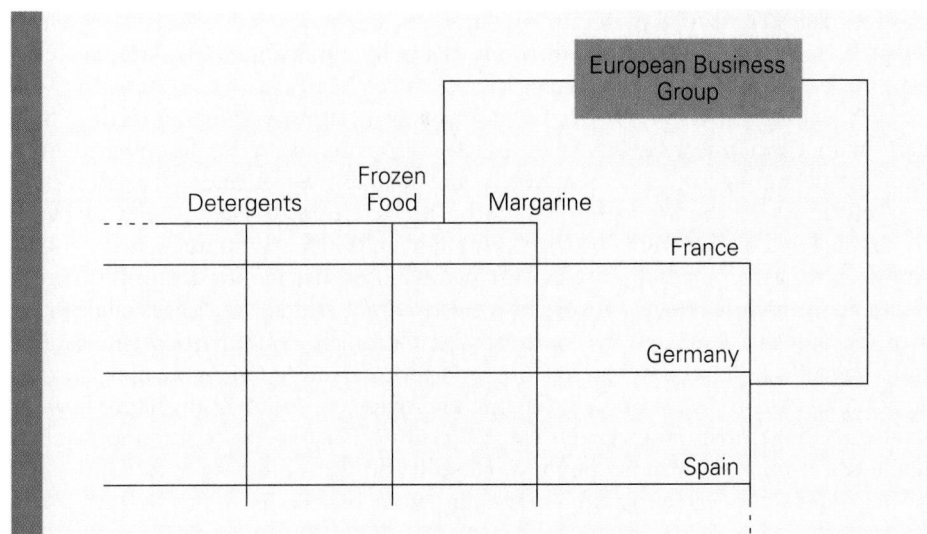

Figure 13.2

Fictional Organizational
Structure at Unilever

managers running the various country subsidiaries are not responsible for those important functions—responsibility resides in the product divisions! Thus, if the managers of the product divisions do not do their job properly, production costs may rise
and the profitability of the country subsidiaries might fall. In other words, the managers of the country subsidiaries are being evaluated according to a metric over which
they lack total control. If the performance of a subsidiary declines, they may argue that
this is not their fault; it was due to the inability of the managers in the pan-European
product divisions to drive down manufacturing costs. Thus, there is a potential conflict between structure and the control systems used; they are potentially inconsistent.

Some inconsistency is a fact of life in organizations. Perfection in the design of organization architecture is very difficult to achieve. Nevertheless, the inconsistency between different components of an organization's architecture can be minimized through
intelligent design. In the example just given, if the performance of each product division were assessed on the basis of manufacturing costs, it would give the managers of
the product division the incentive to optimize manufacturing efficiency. The problem
might be further alleviated if the heads of both the country subsidiaries and the European product divisions were rewarded according to the profitability of the *entire* European Business Group (for example, by having their bonus pay linked to the profitability
of the entire group). This would give the heads of the divisions a further reason to reduce manufacturing costs, and it would create an incentive for the heads of each subsidiary and division to share any best practices developed in their operation with
colleagues across Europe to the betterment of the entire European Business Group.

Internal consistency is a necessity but not a sufficient condition for high performance. Consistency between architecture and the strategy of the organization is also
required; architecture must fit strategy. When Unilever began to emphasize cost reduction as a major strategic goal, the firm had to change its architecture to match this
new strategic reality. It had to move away from a structure based primarily on stand-
alone operating subsidiaries in each country and toward one that looks more like the
structure depicted in Figure 13.2. Unilever had to create some entity, in this case the
product divisions, that could reduce the duplication of manufacturing operations
across country subsidiaries and consolidate manufacturing at a few choice locations.
Such change is easier said than done. It is relatively easy for senior managers to announce a radical change in strategy, but it is much harder to actually implement that
change. Doing so requires a change in architecture. Strategy is implemented through
architecture, and changing architecture is much more difficult than announcing a

change in strategy. We shall discuss why it is hard to change architecture later in this chapter. As we shall see, a prime reason is that organizations tend to be relatively inert; they are by nature difficult to change.

Even with internal consistency and a fit between strategy and architecture, high performance is not guaranteed. The firm must also ensure that the fusion between its strategy and architecture is consistent with the competitive demands of the market, or markets, in which the firm competes. In the 1980s, Unilever had a good fit between its strategy and architecture—it was pursuing a multidomestic strategy. A decentralized architecture composed of self-contained country subsidiaries was well suited to implementing this strategy. However, by the 1990s the strategy no longer made much sense because of a change in the competitive environment. Trade barriers between nations had fallen, and more efficient global competitors were emerging. Unilever's strategy no longer fit the environment in which it competed, so it had to change both its strategy and architecture to match the new reality. This type of organizational challenge is not unusual; markets rarely stand still, and firms often have to adjust their strategy and architecture to match new competitive realities.

Organizational Structure

Organizational structure means three things: (1) the formal division of the organization into subunits, which we shall refer to as horizontal differentiation; (2) the location of decision-making responsibilities within that structure, which we shall refer to as vertical differentiation; and (3) the establishment of integrating mechanisms. We begin by discussing vertical differentiation, then horizontal differentiation, and then integrating mechanisms.

Vertical Differentiation: Centralization and Decentralization

A firm's vertical differentiation determines where in its hierarchy the decision-making power is concentrated.[3] Are production and marketing decisions centralized in the offices of upper-level managers, or are they decentralized to lower-level managers? Where does the responsibility for R&D decisions lie? Are strategic and financial control responsibilities pushed down to operating units, or are they concentrated in the hands of top management? And so on. There are arguments for centralization and other arguments for decentralization.

Arguments for Centralization

Four main arguments support centralization. First, centralization can facilitate coordination. For example, consider a firm that has a component manufacturing operation in Taiwan and an assembly operation in Mexico. The activities of these two operations may need to be coordinated to ensure a smooth flow of products from the component operation to the assembly operation. This might be achieved by centralizing production scheduling at the firm's head office. Second, centralization can help ensure that decisions are consistent with organizational objectives. When decisions are decentralized to lower-level managers, those managers may make decisions at variance with top management's goals. Centralization of important decisions minimizes the chance of this occurring.

Third, by concentrating power and authority in one individual or a management team, centralization can give top-level managers the means to bring about needed major organizational changes. Fourth, centralization can avoid the duplication of activities that occurs when similar activities are conducted by various subunits within the organization. For example, many international firms centralize their R&D functions at one or two locations to ensure that R&D work is not duplicated. Production activities may be centralized at key locations for the same reason.

Arguments for Decentralization

There are five main arguments for decentralization. First, top management can become overburdened when decision-making authority is centralized, and this can result in poor decisions. Decentralization gives top management time to focus on critical issues by delegating more routine issues to lower-level managers. Second, motivational research favors decentralization. Behavioral scientists have long argued that people are willing to give more to their jobs when they have a greater degree of individual freedom and control over their work. Third, decentralization permits greater flexibility—more rapid response to environmental changes—because decisions do not have to be referred up the hierarchy unless they are exceptional in nature. Fourth, decentralization can result in better decisions. In a decentralized structure, decisions are made closer to the spot by individuals who (presumably) have better information than managers several levels up in a hierarchy. Fifth, decentralization can increase control. Decentralization can be used to establish relatively autonomous, self-contained subunits within an organization. Subunit managers can then be held accountable for subunit performance. The more responsibility subunit managers have for decisions that impact subunit performance, the fewer alibis they have for poor performance.

Strategy and Centralization in an International Business

The choice between centralization and decentralization is not absolute. Frequently it makes sense to centralize some decisions and to decentralize others, depending on the type of decision and the firm's strategy. Decisions regarding overall firm strategy, major financial expenditures, financial objectives, and the like are typically centralized at the firm's headquarters. However, operating decisions, such as those relating to production, marketing, R&D, and human resource management, may or may not be centralized depending on the firm's international strategy.

Consider firms pursuing a global strategy. They must decide how to disperse the various value creation activities around the globe so location and experience economies can be realized. The head office must make the decisions about where to locate R&D, production, marketing, and so on. In addition, the globally dispersed web of value creation activities that facilitates a global strategy must be coordinated. This creates pressures for centralizing some operating decisions.

In contrast, the emphasis on local responsiveness in multidomestic firms creates strong pressures for decentralizing operating decisions to foreign subsidiaries. In the classic multidomestic firm, foreign subsidiaries have autonomy in most production and marketing decisions. International firms tend to maintain centralized control over their core competency and to decentralize other decisions to foreign subsidiaries. This typically centralizes control over R&D and/or marketing in the home country and decentralizes operating decisions to the foreign subsidiaries. For example, Microsoft Corporation, which fits the international mode, centralizes its product development activities (where its core competencies lie) at its Redmond, Washington, headquarters and decentralizes marketing activity to various foreign subsidiaries. Thus, while products are developed at home, managers in the various foreign subsidiaries have significant latitude for formulating strategies to market those products in their particular settings.[4]

The situation in transnational firms is more complex. The need to realize location and experience curve economies requires some degree of centralized control over global production centers (as it does in global firms). However, the need for local responsiveness dictates the decentralization of many operating decisions, particularly for marketing, to foreign subsidiaries. Thus, in transnational firms, some operating decisions are relatively centralized, while others are relatively decentralized. In addition, global learning based on the multidirectional transfer of skills between subsidiaries, and between subsidiaries and the corporate center, is a central feature of a firm pursuing a transnational strategy. The concept of global learning is predicated on the notion that foreign subsidiaries within a multinational firm have significant freedom to

Figure 13.3

A Typical Functional Structure

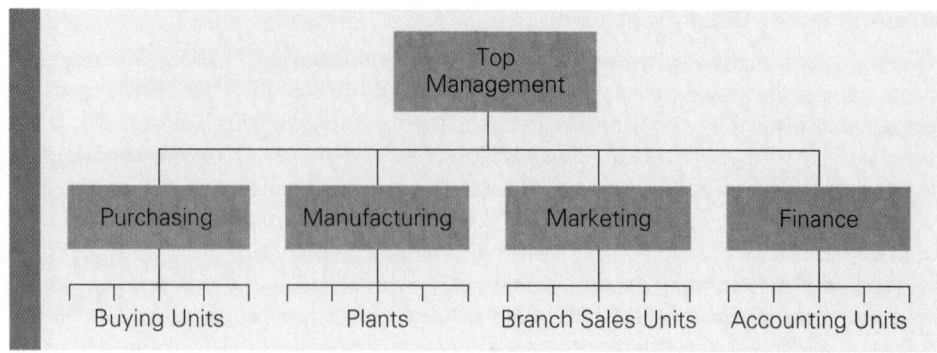

develop their own skills and competencies. Only then can these be leveraged to benefit other parts of the organization. A substantial degree of decentralization is required if subsidiaries are going to have the freedom to do this. For this reason too, the pursuit of a transnational strategy requires a high degree of decentralization.[5]

Horizontal Differentiation: The Design of Structure

Horizontal differentiation is concerned with how the firm decides to divide itself into subunits.[6] The decision is normally made on the basis of function, type of business, or geographical area. In many firms, just one of these predominates, but more complex solutions are adopted in others. This is particularly likely in the case of international firms, where the conflicting demands to organize the company around different products (to realize location and experience curve economies) and different national markets (to remain locally responsive) must be reconciled. One solution to this dilemma is to adopt a matrix structure that divides the organization on the basis of both products and national markets (as Unilever apparently did in Europe). In this section we look at different ways firms divide themselves into subunits.

The Structure of Domestic Firms

Most firms begin with no formal structure and are run by a single entrepreneur or a small team of individuals. As they grow, the demands of management become too great for one individual or a small team to handle. At this point the organization is split into functions reflecting the firm's value creation activities (e.g., production, marketing, R&D, sales). These functions are typically coordinated and controlled by top management (see Figure 13.3). Decision making in this functional structure tends to be centralized.

Further horizontal differentiation may be required if the firm significantly diversifies its product offering, which takes the firm into different business areas. For example, Dutch multinational Philips NV began as a lighting company, but diversification took the company into consumer electronics (e.g., visual and audio equipment), industrial electronics (integrated circuits and other electronic components), and medical systems (CT scanners and ultrasound systems). In such circumstances, a functional structure can be too clumsy. Problems of coordination and control arise when different business areas are managed within the framework of a functional structure.[7] For one thing, it becomes difficult to identify the profitability of each distinct business area. For another, it is difficult to run a functional department, such as production or marketing, if it is supervising the value creation activities of several business areas.

To solve the problems of coordination and control, at this stage most firms switch to a product divisional structure (see Figure 13.4). With a product divisional structure, each division is responsible for a distinct product line (business area). Thus, Philips created divisions for lighting, consumer electronics, industrial electronics, and medical systems. Each product division is set up as a self-contained, largely autonomous entity with its own functions. The responsibility for operating decisions is typically de-

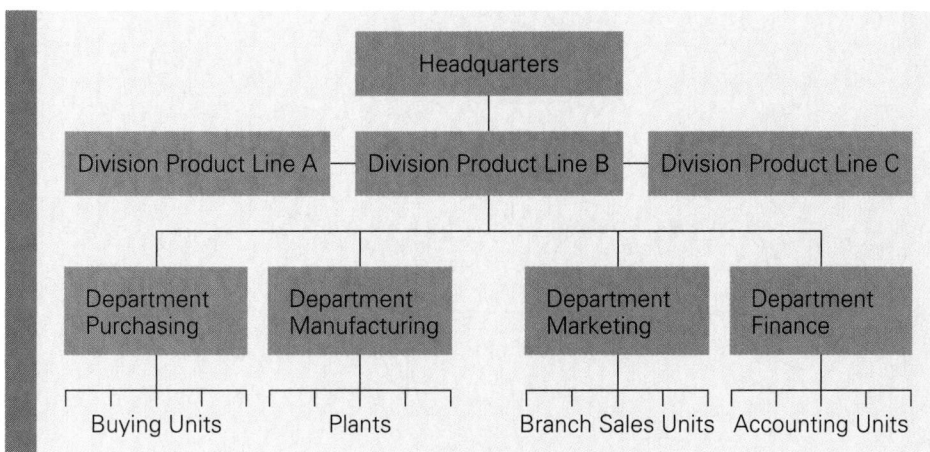

Figure 13.4

A Typical Product Divisional Structure

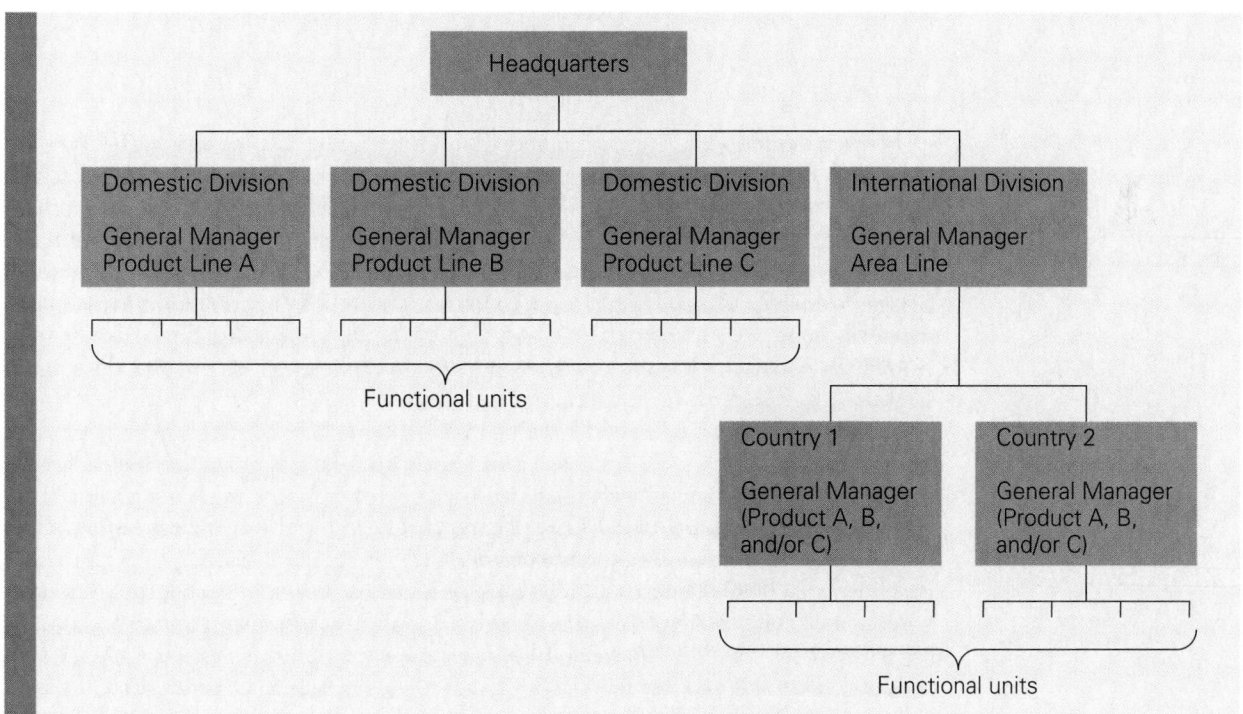

Figure 13.5

One Company's International Divisional Structure

centralized to product divisions, which are then held accountable for their performance. Headquarters is responsible for the overall strategic development of the firm and for the financial control of the various divisions.

The International Division

When firms initially expand abroad, they often group all their international activities into an international division. This has tended to be the case for firms organized on the basis of functions and for those organized on the basis of product divisions. Regardless of the firm's domestic structure, its international division tends to be organized on geography. Figure 13.5 illustrates this for a firm whose domestic organization is based on product divisions.

Figure 13.6

The International Structural
Stages Model

Source: Adapted from John M. Stopford and Louis T. Wells, *Strategy and Structure of the Multinational Enterprise* (New York: Basic Books, 1972).

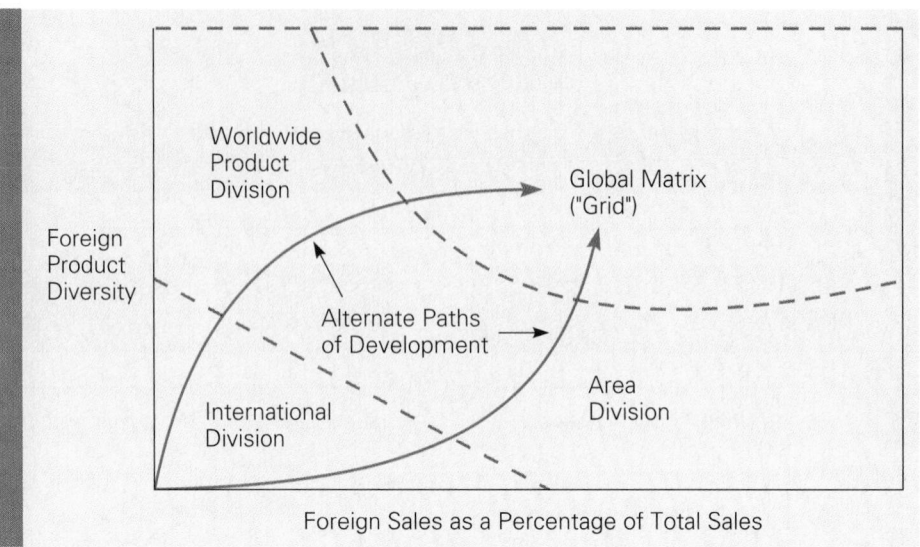

Many manufacturing firms expanded internationally by exporting the product manufactured at home to foreign subsidiaries to sell. Thus, in the firm illustrated in Figure 13.5, the subsidiaries in countries 1 and 2 would sell the products manufactured by divisions A, B, and C. In time, however, it might prove viable to manufacture the product in each country, and so production facilities would be added on a country-by-country basis. For firms with a functional structure at home, this might mean replicating the functional structure in every country in which the firm does business. For firms with a divisional structure, this might mean replicating the divisional structure in every country in which the firm does business.

This structure has been widely used; according to a Harvard study, 60 percent of all firms that have expanded internationally have initially adopted it. Nonetheless, it gives rise to problems.[8] The dual structure it creates contains inherent potential for conflict and coordination problems between domestic and foreign operations. One problem with the structure is that the heads of foreign subsidiaries are not given as much voice in the organization as the heads of domestic functions (in the case of functional firms) or divisions (in the case of divisional firms). Rather, the head of the international division is presumed to be able to represent the interests of all countries to headquarters. This effectively relegates each country's manager to the second tier of the firm's hierarchy, which is inconsistent with a strategy of trying to expand internationally and build a true multinational organization.

Another problem is the implied lack of coordination between domestic operations and foreign operations, which are isolated from each other in separate parts of the structural hierarchy. This can inhibit the worldwide introduction of new products, the transfer of core competencies between domestic and foreign operations, and the consolidation of global production at key locations so as to realize location and experience curve economies. These problems are illustrated in the Management Focus that looks at the experience of Abbott Laboratories with an international divisional structure.

As a result of such problems, most firms that continue to expand internationally abandon this structure and adopt one of the worldwide structures we discuss next. The two initial choices are a worldwide product divisional structure, which tends to be adopted by diversified firms that have domestic product divisions, and a worldwide area structure, which tends to be adopted by undiversified firms whose domestic structures are based on functions. These two alternative paths of development are illustrated in Figure 13.6. The model in the figure is referred to as the international structural stages model and was developed by John Stopford and Louis Wells.[9]

Management Focus

The International Division at Abbott Laboratories

With sales of about $18.8 billion in 2002, Abbott Laboratories is one of the world's largest health care companies. The company split itself into three divisions—pharmaceuticals, hospital products, and nutritional products—in the 1960s. This divisional structure still exists. Each division operates as a profit center, and each is relatively autonomous and self-contained, with its own R&D, manufacturing, and marketing functions. By the late 1960s, Abbott's foreign sales were growing rapidly; the company added an international division to handle the firm's non-U.S. operations on geographic rather than product lines.

Alongside these four divisions, however, a new business has grown up that is organized differently. Abbott's diagnostics business was established in the 1970s and became a world leader with global sales of $4 billion in 2002. Unlike the other divisions, the diagnostics business is organized on a global basis, operating in foreign countries through its own staff, rather than through the international division. Thus, Abbott handles global sales in two different ways—through an international division and through a global product division (the diagnostics business organization). The company is debating the best way of organizing international operations.

This debate is being informed by two changes occurring in Abbott's environment, changes that are pulling the company in different directions. One change is a shift toward global product development in the health care industry. To quickly recapture the costs of developing new products, which for pharmaceuticals can sometimes top $500 million, companies are trying to introduce new products as rapidly as possible

worldwide. Abbott has found that developing products first for the U.S. market and then modifying those products for foreign customers is slow and expensive. Instead, Abbott is trying to build global products that can be launched simultaneously around the world. This change is pulling Abbott toward adopting global product divisions for all its businesses. Some argue that only global product divisions would give Abbott the tight control over product development and product launch strategy that is deemed necessary.

On the other hand, bigger organizations with greater purchasing leverage, such as large hospital groups and health maintenance organizations, are coordinating their buying across a range of product lines in both the United States and elsewhere. These powerful customers prefer to have a single contact point at Abbott. Abbott develops stronger relations with key customers by having a single marketing organization in each country in which the company does businesses. This organization sells the products from each of Abbott's product divisions.

Executives at Abbott's international division support maintaining the geographic organization, while the heads of the product divisions favor a shift toward global product divisions. Top management seems to have decided there is no perfect solution to the company's organizational problems, and that imperfect as the current structure is, it works too well to contemplate a major change.

Sources: R. Walters, "Two's Company," *Financial Times*, July 7, 1995, p. 12; *Abbott Laboratories 2002 Annual Report;* and M. Santoli, "Patient Reviving," *Barron's*, February 28, 2000, pp. 24–26.

Worldwide Area Structure

A worldwide area structure tends to be favored by firms with a low degree of diversification and a domestic structure based on function (see Figure 13.7). Under this structure, the world is divided into geographic areas. An area may be a country (if the market is large enough) or a group of countries. Each area tends to be a self-contained, largely autonomous entity with its own set of value creation activities (e.g., its own production, marketing, R&D, human resources, and finance functions). Operations authority and strategic decisions relating to each of these activities are typically decentralized to each area, with headquarters retaining authority for the overall strategic direction of the firm and financial control.

This structure facilitates local responsiveness. Because decision-making responsibilities are decentralized, each area can customize product offerings, marketing strategy,

Figure 13.7

A Worldwide Area
Structure

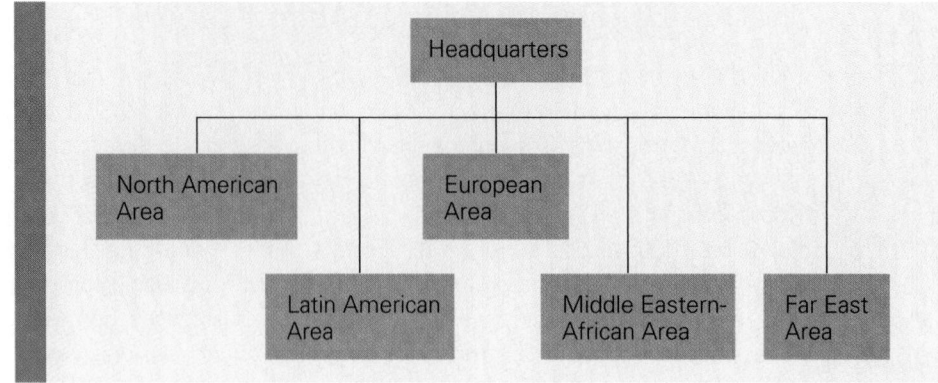

Figure 13.8

A Worldwide Product Divi-
sional Structure

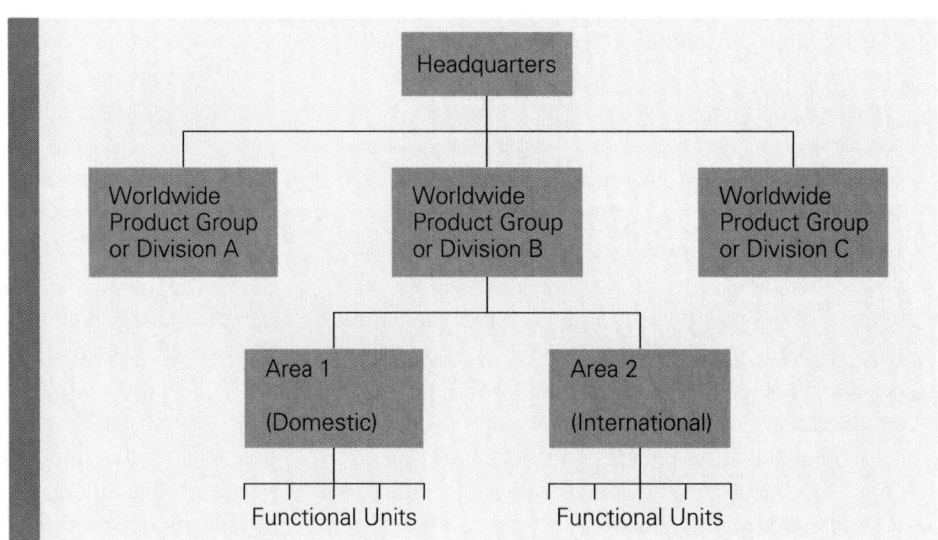

and business strategy to the local conditions. However, this structure encourages frag-
mentation of the organization into highly autonomous entities. This can make it difficult to transfer core competencies and skills between areas and to realize location and
experience curve economies. In other words, the structure is consistent with a multidomestic strategy but with little else. Firms structured on this basis may encounter significant problems if local responsiveness is less critical than reducing costs or
transferring core competencies for establishing a competitive advantage.

Worldwide Product Divisional Structure

A worldwide product division structure tends to be adopted by firms that are reasonably diversified and, accordingly, originally had domestic structures based on product
divisions. As with the domestic product divisional structure, each division is a self-
contained, largely autonomous entity with full responsibility for its own value creation
activities. The headquarters retains responsibility for the overall strategic development and financial control of the firm (see Figure 13.8).

Underpinning the organization is a belief that the value creation activities of
each product division should be coordinated by that division worldwide. Thus, the
worldwide product divisional structure is designed to help overcome the coordination problems that arise with the international division and worldwide area structures (see the Management Focus on Abbott Laboratories for a detailed example).
This structure provides an organizational context that enhances the consolidation

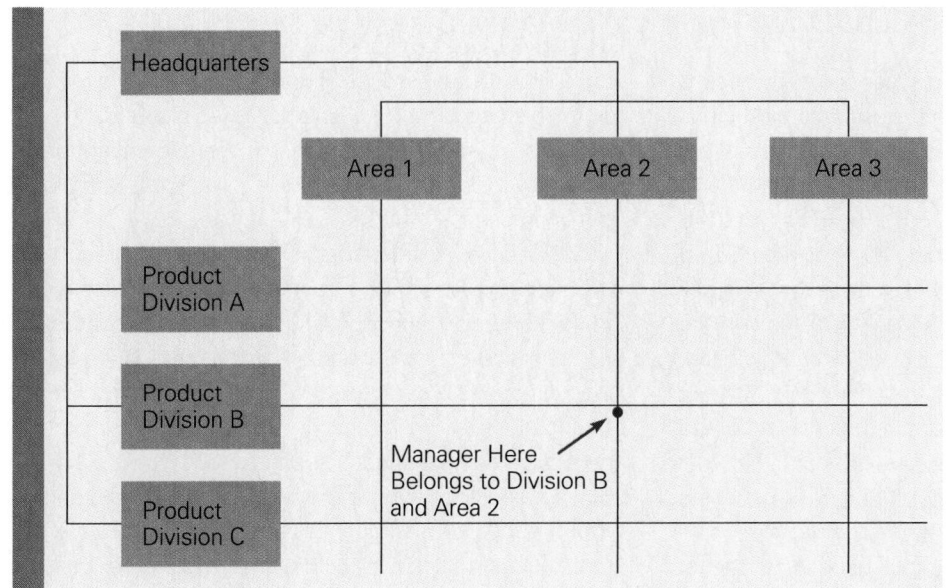

Figure 13.9

A Global Matrix Structure

of value creation activities at key locations necessary for realizing location and experience curve economies. It also facilitates the transfer of core competencies within a division's worldwide operations and the simultaneous worldwide introduction of new products. The main problem with the structure is the limited voice it gives to area or country managers, since they are seen as subservient to product division managers. The result can be a lack of local responsiveness, which, as we saw in Chapter 12, can be a fatal flaw.

Global Matrix Structure

Both the worldwide area structure and the worldwide product divisional structure have strengths and weaknesses. The worldwide area structure facilitates local responsiveness, but it can inhibit the realization of location and experience curve economies and the transfer of core competencies between areas. The worldwide product division structure provides a better framework for pursuing location and experience curve economies and for transferring core competencies, but it is weak in local responsiveness. Other things being equal, this suggests that a worldwide area structure is more appropriate if the firm's strategy is multidomestic, while a worldwide product divisional structure is more appropriate for firms pursuing global or international strategies. However, as we saw in Chapter 12, other things are not equal. As Bartlett and Ghoshal have argued, to survive in some industries, firms must adopt a transnational strategy. That is, they must focus simultaneously on realizing location and experience curve economies, on local responsiveness, and on the internal transfer of core competencies (worldwide learning).[10]

Many firms have attempted to cope with the conflicting demands of a transnational strategy by using a matrix structure (see Figure 13.2). In the classic global matrix structure, horizontal differentiation proceeds along two dimensions: product division and geographic area (see Figure 13.9). The philosophy is that responsibility for operating decisions pertaining to a particular product should be shared by the product division and the various areas of the firm. Thus, the nature of the product offering, the marketing strategy, and the business strategy to be pursued in area 1 for the products produced by division A are determined by conciliation between division A and area 1 management. It is believed that this dual decision-making responsibility should enable the firm to simultaneously achieve its particular objectives. In a classic matrix structure, giving product divisions and geographical areas equal status within the organization

The Rise and Fall of Dow Chemical's Matrix Structure

A handful of major players compete head to head around the world in the chemical industry. These companies are Dow Chemical and Du Pont of the United States, Great Britain's ICI, and the German trio of BASF, Hoechst AG, and Bayer. The barriers to the free flow of chemical products between nations largely disappeared in the 1970s. This along with the commodity nature of most bulk chemicals and a severe recession in the early 1980s ushered in a prolonged period of intense price competition. In such an environment, the company that wins the competitive race is the one with the lowest costs. Dow Chemical was long among the cost leaders.

For years, Dow's managers insisted that part of the credit should go to its matrix organization. Dow's organizational matrix had three interacting elements: functions (e.g., R&D, manufacturing, marketing), businesses (e.g., ethylene, plastics, pharmaceuticals), and geography (e.g., Spain, Germany, Brazil). Managers' job titles incorporated all three elements—for example, plastics marketing manager for Spain—and most managers reported to at least two bosses. The plastics marketing manager in Spain might report to both the head of the worldwide plastics business and the head of the Spanish operations. The intent of the matrix was to make Dow operations responsive to both local market needs and corporate objectives. Thus, the plastics business might be charged with minimizing Dow's global plastics production costs, while the Spanish operation might be charged with determining how best to sell plastics in the Spanish market.

When Dow introduced this structure, the results were less than promising; multiple reporting channels led to confusion and conflict. The large number of bosses made for an unwieldy bureaucracy. The overlapping responsibilities resulted in turf battles and a lack of accountability. Area managers disagreed with managers overseeing business sectors about which plants should be built and where. In short, the structure didn't work. Instead of abandoning the structure, however, Dow decided to see if it could be made more flexible.

Dow's decision to keep its matrix structure was prompted by its move into the pharmaceuticals industry. The company realized that the pharmaceutical business is very different from the bulk chemicals business. In bulk chemicals, the big returns come from achieving economies of scale in production. This dictates establishing large plants in key locations from which regional or global markets can be served. But in pharmaceuticals, regulatory and marketing requirements for drugs vary so much from country to country that local needs are far more important than reducing manufacturing costs through scale economies. A high

reinforces the idea of dual responsibility. Individual managers thus belong to two hierarchies (a divisional hierarchy and an area hierarchy) and have two bosses (a divisional boss and an area boss).

The reality of the global matrix structure is that it often does not work as well as the theory predicts. In practice, the matrix often is clumsy and bureaucratic. It can require so many meetings that it is difficult to get any work done. The need to get an area and a product division to reach a decision can slow decision making and produce an inflexible organization unable to respond quickly to market shifts or to innovate. The dual-hierarchy structure can lead to conflict and perpetual power struggles between the areas and the product divisions, catching many managers in the middle. To make matters worse, it can prove difficult to ascertain accountability in this structure. When all critical decisions are the product of negotiation between divisions and areas, one side can always blame the other when things go wrong. As a manager in one global matrix structure, reflecting on a failed product launch, said to the author, "Had we been able to do things our way, instead of having to accommodate those guys from the product division, this would never have happened." (A manager in the product division expressed similar sentiments.) The result of such finger-pointing can be that accountability is compromised, conflict is enhanced, and headquarters loses control over the organization (see the Management Focus on Dow Chemical).

In light of these problems, many transnational firms are now trying to build "flexible" matrix structures based more on firmwide networks and a shared culture and vi-degree of local responsiveness is essential. Dow realized its pharmaceutical business would never thrive if it were managed by the same priorities as its mainstream chemical operations.

Accordingly, instead of abandoning its matrix, Dow decided to make it more flexible so it could better accommodate the different businesses, each with its own priorities, within a single management system. A small team of senior executives at headquarters helped set the priorities for each type of business. After priorities were identified for each business sector, one of the three elements of the matrix—function, business, or geographic area—was given primary authority in decision making. The element with the lead varies according to the type of decision and the market or location in which the company was competing. Such flexibility required that all employees understand what was occurring in the rest of the matrix. Although this may seem confusing, for years Dow claimed this flexible system worked well and credited much of the company's success to the quality of the decisions the matrix system facilitated.

By the mid-1990s, however, Dow had refocused its business on the chemicals industry, divesting itself of its pharmaceutical activities where the company's performance had been unsatisfactory. Reflecting the change in corporate strategy, Dow in 1995 abandoned its matrix structure in favor of a more streamlined structure based on global business divisions. The change was also driven by realization that the matrix structure was just too complex and costly to manage in the intense competitive environment of the 1990s, particularly given the company's renewed focus on its commodity chemicals where competitive advantage often went to the low-cost producer. As Dow's then CEO put it in a 1999 interview, "We were an organization that was matrixed and depended on teamwork, but there was no one in charge. When things went well, we didn't know whom to reward; and when things went poorly, we didn't know whom to blame. So we created a global divisional structure, and cut out layers of management. There used to be 11 layers of management between me and the lowest level employees, now there are 5." In short, Dow ultimately found that a matrix structure was unsuited to a company that was competing in very cost-competitive global industries, and it had to abandon its matrix to drive down operating costs.

Sources: "Dow Draws Its Matrix Again, and Again, and Again," *The Economist*, August 5, 1989, pp. 55–56; "Dow Goes for Global Structure," *Chemical Marketing Reporter*, December 11, 1995, pp. 4–5; and R. M. Hodgetts, "Dow Chemical CEO William Stavropoulos on Structure and Decision Making," *Academy of Management Executive*, November 1999, pp. 29–35.

sion than on a rigid hierarchical arrangement. Within such companies, the informal structure plays a greater role than the formal structure. We discuss this issue when we consider informal integrating mechanisms in the next section.

Integrating Mechanisms

In the previous section, we explained that firms divide themselves into subunits. Now we need to examine some means of coordinating those subunits. One way of achieving coordination is through centralization. If the coordination task is complex, however, centralization may not be very effective. Higher level managers responsible for achieving coordination can soon become overwhelmed by the volume of work required to coordinate the activities of various subunits, particularly if the subunits are large, diverse, and/or geographically dispersed. When this is the case, firms look toward integrating mechanisms, both formal and informal, to help achieve coordination. In this section, we introduce the various integrating mechanisms that international businesses can use. Before doing so, however, let us explore the need for coordination in international firms and some impediments to coordination.

Strategy and Coordination in the International Business

The need for coordination between subunits varies with the strategy of the firm. The need for coordination is lowest in multidomestic companies, is higher in international companies, higher still in global companies, and highest of all in transnational companies. Multidomestic firms are primarily concerned with local responsiveness. Such firms are likely to operate with a worldwide area structure in which each area has considerable autonomy and its own set of value creation functions. Since each area is established as a stand-alone entity, the need for coordination between areas is minimized.

The need for coordination is greater in firms pursuing an international strategy and trying to profit from the transfer of core competencies and skills between units at home and abroad. Coordination is necessary to support the transfer of skills and product offerings between units. The need for coordination is also great in firms trying to profit from location and experience curve economies; that is, in firms pursuing global strategies. Achieving location and experience economies involves dispersing value creation activities to various locations around the globe. The resulting global web of activities must be coordinated to ensure the smooth flow of inputs into the value chain, the smooth flow of semifinished products through the value chain, and the smooth flow of finished products to markets around the world.

The need for coordination is greatest in transnational firms, which simultaneously pursue location and experience curve economies, local responsiveness, and the multidirectional transfer of core competencies and skills among all of the firm's subunits (referred to as global learning). As in global companies, coordination is required to ensure the smooth flow of products through the global value chain. As in international companies, coordination is required for ensuring the transfer of core competencies to subunits. However, the transnational goal of achieving multidirectional transfer of competencies requires much greater coordination than in international firms. In addition, transnationals require coordination between foreign subunits and the firm's globally dispersed value creation activities (e.g., production, R&D, marketing) to ensure that any product offering and marketing strategy is sufficiently customized to local conditions.

Impediments to Coordination

Managers of the various subunits have different orientations, partly because they have different tasks. For example, production managers are typically concerned with production issues such as capacity utilization, cost control, and quality control, whereas marketing managers are concerned with marketing issues such as pricing, promotions, distribution, and market share. These differences can inhibit communication between the managers. Quite simply, these managers often do not even "speak the same language." There may also be a lack of respect between subunits (e.g., marketing managers "looking down on" production managers, and vice versa), which further inhibits the communication required to achieve cooperation and coordination.

Differences in subunits' orientations also arise from their differing goals. For example, worldwide product divisions of a multinational firm may be committed to cost goals that require global production of a standardized product, whereas a foreign subsidiary may be committed to increasing its market share in its country, which will require a nonstandard product. These different goals can lead to conflict.

Such impediments to coordination are not unusual in any firm, but they can be particularly problematic in the multinational enterprise with its profusion of subunits at home and abroad. Differences in subunit orientation are often reinforced in multinationals by the separations of time zone, distance, and nationality between managers of the subunits.

For example, until recently the Dutch company Philips had an organization of worldwide product divisions and largely autonomous national organizations. The company has long had problems getting its product divisions and national organizations to cooperate on such things as new product introductions. When Philips developed a VCR format, the V2000 system, it could not get its North American subsidiary to introduce the product. Rather, the North American unit adopted the rival VHS format

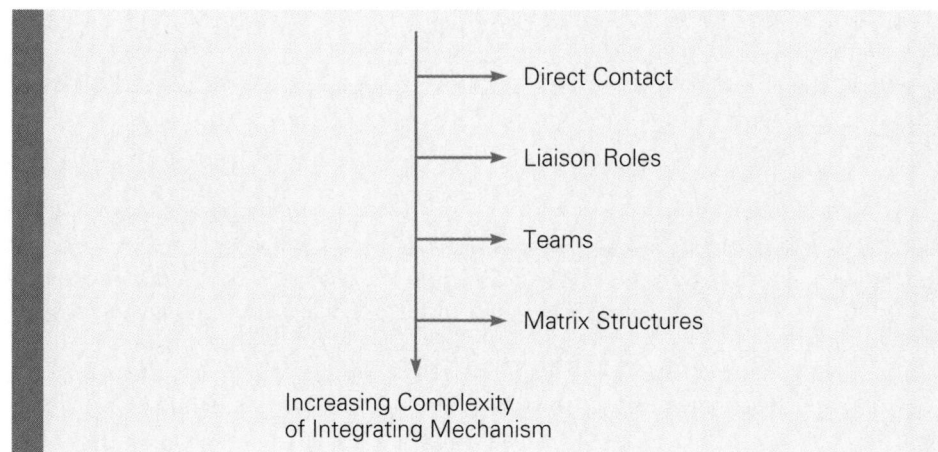

Figure 13.10

Formal Integrating
Mechanisms

produced by Philip's global competitor, Matsushita. Unilever experienced a similar problem in its detergents business. The need to resolve disputes between Unilever's many national organizations and its product divisions extended the time necessary for introducing a new product across Europe to several years. This denied Unilever the first-mover advantage crucial to building a strong market position.[11]

Formal Integrating Mechanisms

The formal mechanisms used to integrate subunits vary in complexity from simple direct contact and liaison roles, to teams, to a matrix structure (see Figure 13.10). In general, the greater the need for coordination, the more complex the formal integrating mechanisms need to be.[12]

Direct contact between subunit managers is the simplest integrating mechanism. Managers of the various subunits simply contact each other whenever they have a common concern. Direct contact may not be effective if the managers have differing orientations that act to impede coordination, as pointed out in the previous subsection.

Liaison roles are a bit more complex. When the volume of contacts between subunits increases, coordination can be improved by giving a person in each subunit responsibility for coordinating with another subunit on a regular basis. Through these roles, the people involved establish a permanent relationship. This helps attenuate the impediments to coordination discussed in the previous subsection.

When the need for coordination is greater still, firms tend to use temporary or permanent teams composed of individuals from the subunits that need to achieve coordination. They are typically used to coordinate product development and introduction, but they are useful when any aspect of operations or strategy requires the cooperation of two or more subunits. Product development and introduction teams are typically composed of personnel from R&D, production, and marketing. The resulting coordination aids the development of products that are tailored to consumer needs and that can be produced at a reasonable cost (design for manufacturing).

When the need for integration is very high, firms may institute a matrix structure, in which all roles are viewed as integrating roles. The structure is designed to facilitate maximum integration among subunits. The most common matrix in multinational firms is based on geographical areas and worldwide product divisions. This achieves a high level of integration between the product divisions and the areas so that, in theory, the firm can pay close attention to both local responsiveness and the pursuit of location and experience curve economies.

In some multinationals, the matrix is more complex still, structuring the firm into geographical areas, worldwide product divisions, and functions, all of which report directly to headquarters. Thus, within a company such as Dow Chemical before it

Figure 13.11

A Simple Management
Network

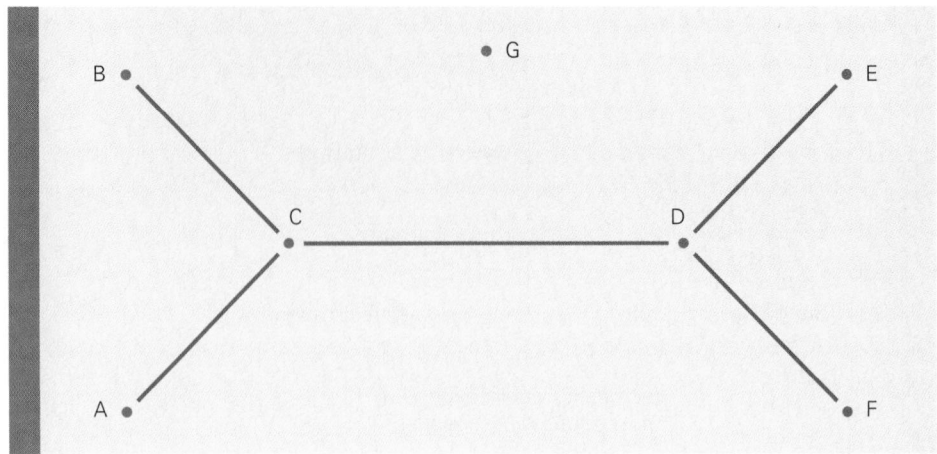

abandoned its matrix in the mid-1990s (see the Management Focus) each manager belongs to three hierarchies (e.g., a plastics marketing manager in Spain is a member of the Spanish subsidiary, the plastics product division, and the marketing function). In addition to facilitating local responsiveness and location and experience curve economies, such a matrix fosters the transfer of core competencies within the organization. This occurs because core competencies tend to reside in functions (e.g., R&D, marketing). A structure such as this in theory facilitates the transfer of competencies existing in functions from division to division and from area to area.

However, as discussed earlier, such matrix solutions to coordination problems in multinational enterprises can quickly become bogged down in a bureaucratic tangle that creates as many problems as it solves. Matrix structures tend to be bureaucratic, inflexible, and characterized by conflict rather than the hoped-for cooperation. For such a structure to work, it needs to be somewhat flexible and to be supported by informal integrating mechanisms.

Informal Integrating Mechanism: Management Networks

In attempting to alleviate or avoid the problems associated with formal integrating mechanisms in general, and matrix structures in particular, firms with a high need for integration have been experimenting with an informal integrating mechanism: management networks that are supported by an organization culture that values teamwork and cross-unit cooperation.[13] A **management network** is a system of informal contacts between managers within an enterprise.[14] The great strength of a network is that it can be used as a nonbureaucratic conduit for knowledge flows within a multinational enterprise.[15] For a network to exist, managers at different locations within the organization must be linked to each other at least indirectly. For example, Figure 13.11 shows the simple network relationships between seven managers within a multinational firm. Managers A, B, and C all know each other personally, as do managers D, E, and F. Although manager B does not know manager F personally, they are linked through common acquaintances (managers C and D). Thus, we can say that managers A through F are all part of the network, and also that manager G is not.

Imagine manager B is a marketing manager in Spain and needs to know the solution to a technical problem to better serve an important European customer. Manager F, an R&D manager in the United States, has the solution to manager B's problem. Manager B mentions her problem to all of her contacts, including manager C, and asks if they know of anyone who might be able to provide a solution. Manager C asks manager D, who tells manager F, who then calls manager B with the solution. In this way, coordination is achieved informally through the network, rather than by formal integrating mechanisms such as teams or a matrix structure.

For such a network to function effectively, however, it must embrace as many managers as possible. For example, if manager G had a problem similar to manager B's, he would not be able to utilize the informal network to find a solution; he would have to resort to more formal mechanisms. Establishing firmwide networks is difficult, and although network enthusiasts speak of networks as the glue that binds multinational companies together, it is far from clear how successful firms have been at building companywide networks. Two techniques being used to establish networks are information systems and management development policies.

Firms are using their computer and telecommunications networks to provide the physical foundation for informal information systems networks.[16] Electronic mail, videoconferencing, and high-speed data systems make it much easier for managers scattered over the globe to get to know each other. Without an existing network of personal contacts, however, worldwide information systems are unlikely to meet a firm's need for integration.

Firms are using their management development programs to build informal networks. Tactics include rotating managers through various subunits on a regular basis so they build their own informal network and using management education programs to bring managers of subunits together in a single location so they can become acquainted. Both of these tactics are used at Unilever to build its informal management network (see the opening case for details).

Management networks by themselves may not be sufficient to achieve coordination if subunit managers persist in pursuing subgoals that are at variance with firmwide goals. For a management network to function properly—and for a formal matrix structure to work, also—managers must share a strong commitment to the same goals. Consider again the case of manager B and manager F. As before, manager F hears about manager B's problem through the network. However, solving manager B's problem would require manager F to devote considerable time to the task. Insofar as this would divert manager F away from his own regular tasks—and the pursuit of subgoals that differ from those of manager B—he may be unwilling to do it. Thus, manager F may not call manager B, and the informal network would fail to provide a solution to manager B's problem.

To eliminate this flaw, an organization's managers must adhere to a common set of norms and values that override differing subunit orientations.[17] In other words, the firm must have a strong organizational culture that promotes teamwork and cooperation. When this is the case, a manager is willing and able to set aside the interests of his own subunit when doing so benefits the firm as a whole. If manager B and manager F are committed to the same organizational norms and value systems, and if these organizational norms and values place the interests of the firm as a whole above the interests of any individual subunit, manager F should be willing to cooperate with manager B on solving her subunit's problems.

Summary

Multinationals need integration—particularly if they are pursuing global, international, or transnational strategies—but it can be difficult to achieve because of the many impediments to coordination. Firms traditionally have tried to achieve coordination by adopting formal integrating mechanisms. These do not always work, however, since they tend to be bureaucratic and do not necessarily address the problems that arise from differing subunit orientations. This is particularly likely with a complex matrix structure, and yet a complex matrix structure is required for simultaneously achieving location and experience curve economies, local responsiveness, and the multidirectional transfer of core competencies within the organization. The solution to this dilemma seems twofold. First, the firm must try to establish an informal management network that can do much of the work previously undertaken by a formal matrix structure. Second, the firm must build a common culture. Neither of these partial solutions, however, is easy to achieve.[18]

Control Systems and Incentives

A major task of a firm's leadership is to control the various subunits of the firm—whether they be defined on the basis of function, product division, or geographic area—to ensure their actions are consistent with the firm's overall strategic and financial objectives. Firms achieve this with various control and incentive systems. In this section, we first review the various types of control systems firms use in their subunits. Then we briefly discuss incentive systems. We also look at how the appropriate control and incentive systems vary according to firms' international strategies.

Types of Control Systems

Four main types of control systems are used in multinational firms: personal controls, bureaucratic controls, output controls, and cultural controls. In most firms, all four are used, but their relative emphasis varies with the strategy of the firm.

Personal Controls

Personal control is control by personal contact with subordinates. This type of control tends to be most widely used in small firms, where it is seen in the direct supervision of subordinates' actions. However, it also structures the relationships between managers at different levels in multinational enterprises. For example, the CEO may use a great deal of personal control to influence the behavior of his or her immediate subordinates, such as the heads of worldwide product divisions or major geographic areas. In turn, these heads may use personal control to influence the behavior of their subordinates, and so on down through the organization. For example, Jack Welch, the longtime CEO of General Electric who retired in 2001, had regular one-on-one meetings with the heads of all of GE's major businesses (most of which are international).[19] He used these meetings to "probe" the managers about the strategy, structure, and financial performance of their operations. In doing so, he essentially exercised personal control over these managers and, undoubtedly, over the strategies that they favored.

Bureaucratic Controls

Bureaucratic control is control through a system of rules and procedures that directs the actions of subunits. The most important bureaucratic controls in subunits within multinational firms are budgets and capital spending rules. Budgets are essentially a set of rules for allocating a firm's financial resources. A subunit's budget specifies with some precision how much the subunit may spend. Headquarters uses budgets to influence the behavior of subunits. For example, the R&D budget normally specifies how much cash the R&D unit may spend on product development. R&D managers know that if they spend too much on one project, they will have less to spend on other projects, so they modify their behavior to stay within the budget. Most budgets are set by negotiation between headquarters management and subunit management. Headquarters management can encourage the growth of certain subunits and restrict the growth of others by manipulating their budgets.

Capital spending rules require headquarters management to approve any capital expenditure by a subunit that exceeds a certain amount (at GE, $50,000). A budget allows headquarters to specify the amount a subunit can spend in a given year, and capital spending rules give headquarters additional control over how the money is spent. Headquarters can be expected to deny approval for capital spending requests that are at variance with overall firm objectives and to approve those that are congruent with firm objectives.

Output Controls

Output controls involve setting goals for subunits to achieve and expressing those goals in terms of relatively objective performance metrics such as profitability, productivity, growth, market share, and quality. The performance of subunit managers is then judged by their ability to achieve the goals.[20] If goals are met or exceeded, subunit managers will be rewarded. If goals are not met, top management will normally intervene to find out why and take appropriate corrective action. Thus, control is achieved by comparing actual performance against targets and intervening selectively to take corrective action. Subunits' goals depend on their role in the firm. Self-contained product divisions or national subsidiaries are typically given goals for profitability, sales growth, and market share. Functions are more likely to be given goals related to their particular activity. Thus, R&D will be given product development goals, production will be given productivity and quality goals, marketing will be given market share goals, and so on.

As with budgets, goals are normally established through negotiation between subunits and headquarters. Generally, headquarters tries to set goals that are challenging but realistic, so subunit managers are forced to look for ways to improve their operations but are not so pressured that they will resort to dysfunctional activities to do so (such as short-run profit maximization). Output controls foster a system of "management by exception," in that so long as subunits meet their goals, they are left alone. If a subunit fails to attain its goals, however, headquarters managers are likely to ask some tough questions. If they don't get satisfactory answers, they are likely to intervene proactively in a subunit, replacing top management and looking for ways to improve efficiency.

Cultural Controls

Cultural controls exist when employees "buy into" the norms and value systems of the firm. When this occurs, employees tend to control their own behavior, which reduces the need for direct supervision. In a firm with a strong culture, self-control can reduce the need for other control systems. We shall discuss organizational culture later. McDonald's actively promotes organizational norms and values, referring to its franchisees and suppliers as partners and emphasizing its long-term commitment to them. This commitment is not just a public relations exercise; it is backed by actions, including a willingness to help suppliers and franchisees improve their operations by providing capital and/or management assistance when needed. In response, McDonald's franchisees and suppliers are integrated into the firm's culture and thus become committed to helping McDonald's succeed. One result is that McDonald's can devote less time than would otherwise be necessary to controlling its franchisees and suppliers.

Incentive Systems

Incentives refer to the devices used to reward appropriate employee behavior. Many employees receive incentives in the form of annual bonus pay. Incentives are usually closely tied to the performance metrics used for output controls. For example, setting targets linked to profitability might be used to measure the performance of a subunit, such as a global product division. To create positive incentives for employees to work hard to exceed those targets, they may be given a share of any profits above those targeted. If a subunit has set a goal of attaining a 15 percent return on investment and it actually reaches a 20 percent return, unit employees may be given a share in the profits generated in excess of the 15 percent target in the form of bonus pay. We shall return to the topic of incentive systems in Chapter 18 when we discuss human resource strategy in the multinational firm. For now, however, several important points need to be made.

First, the type of incentive used often varies depending on the employees and their tasks. Incentives for employees working on the factory floor may be very different from the incentives used for senior managers. The incentives must be matched to the type of work performed. The employees on the factory floor of a manufacturing plant may be broken into teams of 20 to 30 individuals, and they may have their bonus pay tied to the ability of their team to hit or exceed targets for output and product quality. In contrast, the senior managers of the plant may be rewarded according to metrics linked to the output of the entire operation. The basic principle is to make sure the incentive scheme for an individual employee is linked to an output target that he or she has some control over and can influence. The individual employees on the factory floor may not be able to exercise much influence over the performance of the entire operation, but they can influence the performance of their team, so incentive pay is tied to output at this level.

Second, the successful execution of strategy in the multinational firm often requires significant cooperation between managers in different subunits. For example, as noted earlier, some multinational firms operate with matrix structures where a country subsidiary might be responsible for marketing and sales in a nation, while a global product division might be responsible for manufacturing and product development. The managers of these different units need to cooperate closely with each other if the firm is to be successful. One way of encouraging the managers to cooperate is to link incentives to performance at a higher level in the organization. Thus, the senior managers of the country subsidiaries and global product divisions might be rewarded according to the profitability of the entire firm. The thinking here is that boosting the profitability of the entire firm requires managers in the country subsidiaries and product divisions to cooperate with each other on strategy implementation, and linking incentive systems to the next level up in the hierarchy encourages this. Most firms use a formula for incentives that links a portion of incentive pay to the performance of the subunit in which a manager or employee works and a portion to the performance of the entire firm, or some other higher level organizational unit. The goal is to encourage employees to improve the efficiency of their unit and to cooperate with other units in the organization.

Third, the incentive systems used within a multinational enterprise often have to be adjusted to account for national differences in institutions and culture. Incentive systems that work in the United States might not work, or even be allowed, in other countries. For example, Lincoln Electric, a leader in the manufacture of arc welding equipment, has used an incentive system for its employees based on piecework rates in its U.S. factories (under a piecework system, employees are paid according to the amount they produce). While this system has worked very well in the United States, Lincoln has found that the system is difficult to introduce in other countries. In some countries, such as Germany, piecework systems are illegal, while in others the prevailing national culture is antagonistic to a system where performance is so closely tied to individual effort. For further details, see the accompanying Management Focus.

Finally, it is important for managers to recognize that incentive systems can have unintended consequences. Managers need to carefully think through exactly what behavior certain incentives encourage. For example, if employees in a factory are rewarded solely on the basis of how many units of output they produce, with no attention paid to the quality of that output, they may produce as many units as possible to boost their incentive pay, but the quality of those units may be poor.

Control Systems, Incentives, and Strategy in the International Business

The key to understanding the relationship between international strategy, control systems, and incentive systems is the concept of performance ambiguity.

Performance Ambiguity

Performance ambiguity exists when the causes of a subunit's poor performance are not clear. This is not uncommon when a subunit's performance is partly dependent on the performance of other subunits; that is, when there is a high degree of interdependence between subunits within the organization. Consider the case of a French subsidiary of

Organizational Culture and Incentives at Lincoln Electric

Lincoln Electric is one of the leading companies in the global market for arc welding equipment. Lincoln's success has been based on extremely high levels of employee productivity. The company attributes its productivity to a strong organizational culture and an incentive scheme based on piecework. Lincoln's organizational culture dates back to James Lincoln, who in 1907 joined the company that his brother had established a few years earlier.

Lincoln had a strong respect for the ability of the individual and believed that, correctly motivated, ordinary people could achieve extraordinary performance. He emphasized that Lincoln should be a meritocracy where people were rewarded for their individual effort. Strongly egalitarian, Lincoln removed barriers to communication between "workers" and "managers," practicing an open-door policy. He made sure that all who worked for the company were treated equally; for example, everyone ate in the same cafeteria, there were no reserved parking places for "managers," and so on. Lincoln also believed that any gains in productivity should be shared with consumers in the form of lower prices, with employees in the form of higher pay, and with shareholders in the form of higher dividends.

The organizational culture that grew out of James Lincoln's beliefs was reinforced by the company's incentive system. Production workers receive no base salary but are paid according to the number of pieces they produce. The piecework rates at the company enable an employee working at a normal pace to earn an income equivalent to the average wage for manufacturing workers in the area where a factory is based. Workers have responsibility for the quality of their output and must repair any defects spotted by quality inspectors before the pieces are included in the piecework calculation. Since 1934, production workers have been awarded a semiannual bonus based on merit ratings. These ratings are based on objective criteria (such as an employee's level and quality of output) and subjective criteria (such as an employee's attitude toward cooperation and his or her dependability). These systems give Lincoln's employees an incentive to work hard and to generate innovations that boost productivity, for doing so influences their level of pay.

Lincoln's factory workers have been able to earn a base pay that often exceeds the average manufacturing wage in the area by more than 50 percent and receive a bonus on top of this that in good years could double their base pay. Despite high employee compensation, the workers are so productive that Lincoln has a lower cost structure than its competitors.

While this organizational culture and set of incentives works well in the United States, where it is compatible with the individualistic culture of the country, it did not translate easily into foreign operations. In the 1980s and early 1990s, Lincoln expanded aggressively into Europe and Latin America, acquiring a number of local arc welding manufacturers. Lincoln left local managers in place, believing that they knew local conditions better than Americans. However, the local managers had little working knowledge of Lincoln's strong organizational culture and were unable or unwilling to impose that culture on their units, which had their own long-established organizational cultures. Nevertheless, Lincoln told local managers to introduce the incentive systems in acquired companies. The company frequently ran into legal and cultural roadblocks. In many countries, piecework is viewed as an exploitive compensation system that forces employees to work ever harder. In Germany, where Lincoln made an acquisition, it is actually illegal. In Brazil, a bonus paid for more than two years becomes a legal entitlement! In many other countries, both managers and workers were opposed to the idea of piecework. Lincoln found that many European workers valued extra leisure more highly than extra income and were not prepared to work as hard as their U.S. counterparts. Many of the acquired companies were also unionized, and the local unions vigorously opposed the introduction of piecework. As a result, Lincoln was not able to replicate the high level of employee productivity that it had achieved in the United States, and its expansion pulled down the performance of the entire company.

Source: J. O'Connell, "Lincoln Electric: Venturing Abroad," Harvard Business School Case #9–398–095, April 1998, and www.lincolnelectric.com.

a U.S. firm that depends on another subsidiary, a manufacturer based in Italy, for the products it sells. The French subsidiary is failing to achieve its sales goals, and the U.S. management asks the managers to explain. They reply that they are receiving poor-quality goods from the Italian subsidiary. So the U.S. management asks the managers of the Italian operation what the problem is. They reply that their product quality is excellent—the best in the industry, in fact—and that the French simply don't know how to sell a good product. Who is right, the French or the Italians? Without more information, top management cannot tell. Because they are dependent on the Italians for their product, the French have an alibi for poor performance. U.S. management needs to have more information to determine who is correct. Collecting this information is expensive and time consuming and will divert attention away from other issues. In other words, performance ambiguity raises the costs of control.

Consider how different things would be if the French operation were self-contained, with its own manufacturing, marketing, and R&D facilities. The French operation would lack a convenient alibi for its poor performance; the French managers would stand or fall on their own merits. They could not blame the Italians for their poor sales. The level of performance ambiguity, therefore, is a function of the interdependence of subunits in an organization.

Strategy, Interdependence, and Ambiguity

Now let us consider the relationship among international strategy, interdependence, and performance ambiguity. In multidomestic firms, each national operation is a stand-alone entity and can be judged on its own merits. The level of performance ambiguity is low. In an international firm, the level of interdependence is somewhat higher. Integration is required to facilitate the transfer of core competencies and skills. Because the success of a foreign operation is partly dependent on the quality of the competency transferred from the home country, performance ambiguity can exist.

In global firms, the situation is still more complex. Recall that in a pure global firm the pursuit of location and experience curve economies leads to the development of a global web of value creation activities. Many of the activities in a global firm are interdependent. A French subsidiary's ability to sell a product depends on how well other operations in other countries perform their value creation activities. Thus, the levels of interdependence and performance ambiguity are high in global companies.

The level of performance ambiguity is highest of all in transnational firms. Transnational firms suffer from the same performance ambiguity problems that global firms do. In addition, because they emphasize the multidirectional transfer of core competencies, they also suffer from the problems characteristic of firms pursuing an international strategy. The extremely high level of integration within transnational firms implies a high degree of joint decision making, and the resulting interdependencies create plenty of alibis for poor performance. There is lots of room for finger-pointing in transnational firms.

Implications for Control and Incentives

The arguments of the previous section, along with the implications for the costs of control, are summarized in Table 13.1. The costs of control can be defined as the amount of time top management must devote to monitoring and evaluating subunits' performance. This is greater when the amount of performance ambiguity is greater. When performance ambiguity is low, management can use output controls and a system of management by exception; when it is high, managers have no such luxury. Output controls do not provide totally unambiguous signals of a subunit's efficiency when the performance of that subunit is dependent on the performance of another subunit within the organization. Thus, management must devote time to resolving the problems that arise from performance ambiguity, with a corresponding rise in the costs of control.

Table 13.1 reveals a paradox. We saw in Chapter 12 that a transnational strategy is desirable because it gives a firm more ways to profit from international expansion than

Strategy	Interdependence	Performance Ambiguity	Costs of Control
Multidomestic	Low	Low	Low
International	Moderate	Moderate	Moderate
Global	High	High	High
Transnational	Very high	Very high	Very high

Table 13.1

Interdependence, Performance Ambiguity, and the Costs of Control for the Four International Business Strategies

do multidomestic, international, and global strategies. But now we see that due to the high level of interdependence, the costs of controlling transnational firms are higher than the costs of controlling firms that pursue other strategies. Unless there is some way of reducing these costs, the higher profitability associated with a transnational strategy could be canceled out by the higher costs of control. The same point, although to a lesser extent, can be made with regard to global firms. Although firms pursuing a global strategy can reap the cost benefits of location and experience curve economies, they must cope with a higher level of performance ambiguity, and this raises the costs of control (in comparison with firms pursuing an international or multidomestic strategy).

This is where control systems and incentives come in. When we survey the systems that corporations use to control their subunits, we find that irrespective of their strategy, multinational firms all use output and bureaucratic controls. However, in firms pursuing either global or transnational strategies, the usefulness of output controls is limited by substantial performance ambiguities. As a result, these firms place greater emphasis on cultural controls. Cultural control—by encouraging managers to want to assume the organization's norms and value systems—gives managers of interdependent subunits an incentive to look for ways to work out problems that arise between them. The result is a reduction in finger-pointing and, accordingly, in the costs of control. The development of cultural controls may be a precondition for the successful pursuit of a transnational strategy and perhaps of a global strategy as well.[21] As for incentives, the material discussed earlier suggests that the conflict between different subunits can be reduced, and the potential for cooperation enhanced, if incentive systems are tied in some way to a higher level in the hierarchy. When performance ambiguity makes it difficult to judge the performance of subunits as stand-alone entities, linking the incentive pay of senior managers to the entity to which both subunits belong can reduce the resulting problems.

Processes ■

We defined processes as the manner in which decisions are made and work is performed within the organization.[22] Processes can be found at many different levels within an organization. There are processes for formulating strategy, processes for allocating resources, processes for evaluating new product ideas, processes for handling customer inquiries and complaints, processes for improving product quality, processes for evaluating employee performance, and so on. Often, the core competencies or valuable skills of a firm are embedded in its processes. Efficient and effective processes can lower the costs of value creation and add additional value to a product. For example, the global success of many Japanese manufacturing enterprises in the 1980s was based in part on their early adoption of processes for improving product quality and operating efficiency, including total quality management and just-in-time inventory systems. Today, the competitive success of General Electric can in part be attributed to a number of processes that have been widely promoted within the company. These include the company's six-sigma process for quality improvement, its process for "digitalization" of business (using corporate intranets and the Internet to automate activities and reduce operating costs), and its process for new idea generation, referred to within the company as "workouts," where managers and employees get together for intensive sessions over several days to identify and commit to ideas for improving productivity.

An organization's processes can be summarized by means of a flow chart, which illustrates the various steps and decision points involved in performing work. Many processes cut across functions, or divisions, and require cooperation between individuals in different subunits. For example, product development processes require employees from R&D, manufacturing, and marketing to work together in a cooperative manner to make sure new products are developed with market needs in mind and designed in such a way that they can be manufactured at a low cost. Because they cut across organizational boundaries, performing processes effectively often requires the establishment of formal integrating mechanisms and incentives for cross-unit cooperation (see above).

A detailed consideration of the nature of processes and strategies for process improvement and reengineering is beyond the scope of this book. However, it is important to make two basic remarks about managing processes, particularly in the context of an international business.[23] The first is that in a multinational enterprise, many processes cut not only across organizational boundaries, embracing several different subunits, but also across national boundaries. Designing a new product may require the cooperation of R&D personnel located in California, production people located in Taiwan, and marketing staff located in Europe, America, and Asia. The chances of pulling this off are greatly enhanced if the processes are embedded in an organizational culture that promotes cooperation between individuals from different subunits and nations, if the incentive systems of the organization explicitly reward such cooperation, and if formal and informal integrating mechanisms are used to facilitate coordination between subunits.

Second, it is particularly important for a multinational enterprise to recognize that valuable new processes that might lead to a competitive advantage can be developed anywhere within the organization's global network of operations.[24] New processes may be developed by a local operating subsidiary in response to conditions pertaining to its market. Those processes might then have value to other parts of the multinational enterprise. For example, in response to competition in Japan and a local obsession with product quality, Japanese firms were at the leading edge of developing processes for total quality management (TQM) in the 1970s. Because few U.S. firms had Japanese subsidiaries at the time, they were relatively ignorant of the trend until the 1980s when high-quality Japanese products began to make big inroads into the United States. An exception to this generalization was Hewlett-Packard, which had a very successful operating company in Japan, Yokogwa Hewlett-Packard (YHP). YHP was a pioneer of the total quality management process in Japan and won the prestigious Deming Prize for its achievements in improving product quality. Through YHP, Hewlett-Packard learned about the quality movement ahead of many of its U.S. peers and was one of the first Western companies to introduce TQM processes into its worldwide operations. Not only did Hewlett-Packard's Japanese operation give the company access to a valuable process, but the company also transferred this knowledge within its global network of operations, raising the performance of the entire company. The ability to create valuable processes matters, but it is also important to leverage those processes. This requires both formal and informal integrating mechanisms such as management networks.

Organizational Culture

Chapter 3 applied the concept of culture to nation-states. Culture is a social construct ascribed to societies, including organizations.[25] Thus, we can speak of organizational culture and organizational subculture. The basic definition of culture remains the same, whether we are applying it to a large society such as a nation-state or a small society such as an organization or one of its subunits. Culture refers to a system of values and norms that are shared among people. Values are abstract ideas about what a group believes to be good, right, and desirable. Norms mean the social rules and guidelines that prescribe appropriate behavior in particular situations. Values and norms express themselves as the behavior patterns or style of an organization that new employees are automatically encouraged to follow by their fellow employees. Although an organization's culture is rarely static, it tends to change relatively slowly.

Creating and Maintaining Organizational Culture

An organization's culture comes from several sources. First, there seems to be wide agreement that founders or important leaders can have a profound impact on an organization's culture, often imprinting their own values on the culture.[26] This was certainly the case with Lincoln Electric where the values of James Lincoln became the core values of Lincoln Electric (see the Management Focus). Another famous example of a strong founder effect concerns the founder of the Japanese firm Matsushita, Konosuke Matsushita, whose almost Zen-like personal business philosophy was codified in the "Seven Spiritual Values" of Matsushita that all new employees still learn today. These values are (1) national service through industry, (2) fairness, (3) harmony and cooperation, (4) struggle for betterment, (5) courtesy and humility, (6) adjustment and assimilation, and (7) gratitude. A leader does not have to be the founder to have a profound influence on organizational culture. Jack Welch is widely credited with having changed the culture of GE, primarily by emphasizing when he first became CEO a countercultural set of values, such as risk taking, entrepreneurship, stewardship, and boundaryless behavior. It is more difficult for a leader, however forceful, to change an established organizational culture than it is to create one from scratch in a new venture.

Another important influence on organizational culture is the broader social culture of the nation where the firm was founded. In the United States, for example, the competitive ethic of individualism looms large and there is enormous social stress on producing winners. Many U.S. firms find ways of rewarding and motivating individuals so that they see themselves as winners.[27] The values of U.S. firms often reflect the values of American culture. Similarly, the cooperative values found in many Japanese firms have been argued to reflect the values of traditional Japanese society, with its emphasis on group cooperation, reciprocal obligations, and harmony.[28] Thus, there may be something to the argument that national culture influences organizational culture.

A third influence on organizational culture is the history of the enterprise, which may shape the values of the organization. In the language of historians, organizational culture is the path-dependent product of where the organization has been through time. For example, Philips NV, the Dutch multinational, long operated with a culture that placed a high value on the independence of national operating companies. This culture was shaped by the history of the company. During World War II, Holland was occupied by the Germans. With the head office in occupied territories, power was devolved by default to various foreign operating companies, such as Philips subsidiaries in the United States and Great Britain. After the war ended, these subsidiaries continued to operate in a highly autonomous fashion. A belief that this was the right thing to do became a core value of the company.

Decisions that subsequently result in high performance tend to become institutionalized in the values of a firm. In the 1920s, 3M was primarily a manufacturer of sandpaper. Richard Drew, who was a young laboratory assistant at the time, came up with what he thought would be a great new product: a glue-covered strip of paper, which he called "sticky tape." Drew saw applications for the product in the automobile industry, where it could be used to mask parts of a vehicle during painting. He presented the idea to the company's president, William McKnight. An unimpressed

McKnight suggested that Drew drop the research. Drew didn't; instead he developed the "sticky tape" and then went out and got endorsements from potential customers in the auto industry. Armed with this information, he approached McKnight again. A chastened McKnight reversed his position and gave Drew the go-ahead to start developing what was to become one of 3M's main product lines—sticky tape—a business it dominates to this day.[29] From then on, McKnight emphasized the importance of giving 3M researchers free rein to explore their own ideas and experiment with product offerings. This soon became a core value at 3M and was enshrined in the company's famous "15 percent rule," which stated that researchers could spend 15 percent of their company time working on ideas of their own choosing. Today, new employees are often told the Drew story, which is used to illustrate the value of allowing individuals to explore their own ideas.

Culture is maintained by a variety of mechanisms. These include: (1) hiring and promotional practices of the organization, (2) reward strategies, (3) socialization processes, and (4) communication strategy. The goal is to recruit people whose values are consistent with those of the company. Lincoln Electric, for example, hires individuals who are very self-reliant, which is necessary in the company's individualistic culture. To further reinforce values, a company may promote individuals whose behavior is consistent with the core values of the organization. Merit review processes may also be linked to a company's values, which further reinforces cultural norms. Thus, at Lincoln Electric, the merit review process rewards people for behavior that is consistent with the attainment of high productivity.

Socialization can be formal, such as training programs that educate employees in the core values of the organization. Informal socialization may be friendly advice from peers or bosses or may be implicit in the actions of peers and superiors toward new employees. As for communication strategy, many companies with strong cultures devote a lot of attention to framing their key values in corporate mission statements, communicating them often to employees, and using them to guide difficult decisions. Stories and symbols are often used to reinforce important values (e.g., the Drew and McKnight story at 3M).

Organizational Culture and Performance in the International Business

Management authors often talk about "strong cultures."[30] In a strong culture, almost all managers share a relatively consistent set of values and norms that have a clear impact on the way work is performed. New employees adopt these values very quickly, and employees that do not fit in with the core values tend to leave. In such a culture, a new executive is just as likely to be corrected by his subordinates as by his superiors if he violates the values and norms of the organizational culture. Firms with a strong culture are normally seen by outsiders as having a certain style or way of doing things. Lincoln Electric, profiled in the Management Focus, is an example of a firm with a strong culture. Lincoln's organizational culture places a high value on individual achievements, meritocracy, and egalitarian behavior. Unilever, profiled in the opening case, is another example of a firm with a strong culture. Unilever places a high value on sociability, cooperation, and consensus-building behavior among its employees.

Strong does not necessarily mean good. A culture can be strong but bad. The culture of the Nazi Party in Germany was certainly strong, but it was most definitely not good. Nor does it follow that a strong culture leads to high performance. One study found that General Motors had a "strong culture," but it was a strong culture that discouraged lower level employees from demonstrating initiative and taking risks, which the authors argued was dysfunctional and led to low performance at GM.[31] Also, a strong culture might be beneficial at one point, leading to high performance, but inappropriate at another time. The appropriateness of the culture depends on the context. In the 1970s and early 1980s, when IBM was performing very well, several management authors sang the praises of its strong culture, which among other things placed a high value on consensus-based decision making.[32] These authors argued that such a decision-making process was appropriate given the substantial financial investments that IBM routinely made in new technology. However, this process turned out to be a weakness in the fast-moving computer industry of the late 1980s and 1990s. Consensus-based decision making was slow, bureaucratic, and not particularly conducive to corporate risk taking. While this was fine in the 1970s, IBM needed rapid decision making and entrepreneurial risk taking in the 1990s, but its culture discouraged such behavior. IBM found itself outflanked by then-small enterprises such as Microsoft.

One academic study concluded that firms that exhibited high performance over a prolonged period tended to have strong but "adaptive cultures." According to this study, in an adaptive culture, most managers care deeply about and value customers, stockholders, and employees. They also strongly value people and processes that create useful change in a firm.[33] While this is interesting, it reduces the issue to a very high level of abstraction; after all, no company would say it doesn't care deeply about customers, stockholders, and employees. A somewhat different perspective is to argue that the culture of the firm must match the rest of the architecture of the organization, the firm's strategy, and the demands of the competitive environment, for superior performance to be attained. All these elements must be consistent with each other. Lincoln Electric provides another useful example. Lincoln competes in a business that is very competitive, where cost minimization is a key source of competitive advantage. Both Lincoln's culture and incentive systems encourage employees to strive for high levels of productivity, which translates into the low costs that are critical for Lincoln's success.

The Lincoln example also demonstrates another important point for international businesses: A culture that leads to high performance in the firm's home nation may not be easy to impose on foreign subsidiaries! Lincoln's culture has clearly helped the firm to achieve superior performance in the U.S. market, but this same culture is very "American" in its form and difficult to implement in other countries. The managers and employees of several of Lincoln's European subsidiaries found the culture to be alien to their own values and were reluctant to adopt it. The result was that Lincoln found it very difficult to replicate in foreign markets the success it has had in the United States. Lincoln compounded the problem by acquiring established enterprises that already had their own organizational culture. Thus, in trying to impose its culture on foreign operating subsidiaries, Lincoln had to deal with two problems: how to change the established organizational culture of those units, and how to introduce an organizational culture whose key values might be alien to the values held by members of that society. These problems are not unique to Lincoln; many international businesses have to deal with exactly the same problems.

The solution Lincoln has adopted is to establish new subsidiaries, rather than acquiring and trying to transform an enterprise with its own culture. It is much easier to establish a set of values in a new enterprise than it is to change the values of an established enterprise. A second solution is to devote a lot of time and attention to transmitting the firm's organizational culture to its foreign operations. This was something Lincoln originally omitted. Other firms make this an important part of their strategy for internationalization. When MTV Networks opens an operation in a new country, it initially staffs that operation with several expatriates. These expatriates hire local employees whose values are consistent with the MTV culture and socialize those individuals into values and norms that underpin MTV's unique way of doing things. Once this has been achieved, the expatriates move on to their next assignment, and local employees run the operation. A third solution is to recognize that it may be necessary to change some aspects of a firm's culture so that it better fits the culture of the host nation. For example, many Japanese firms use symbolic behavior, such as company songs and morning group exercise sessions, to reinforce cooperative values and norms. However, such symbolic behavior does not go down well in Western cultures, where it is seen as odd, so many Japanese firms have not used such practices in Western subsidiaries.

The need for a common organizational culture that is the same across a multinational's global network of subsidiaries probably varies with the strategy of the firm. Shared norms and values can facilitate coordination and cooperation between individuals from different subunits.[34] A strong common culture may lead to goal congruence and can attenuate the problems that arise from interdependence, performance ambiguities, and conflict among managers from different subsidiaries. As noted earlier, a shared culture may help informal integrating mechanisms such as management networks to operate more effectively. As such, a common culture may be of greater value in a multinational that is pursuing a strategy that requires cooperation and coordination between globally dispersed subsidiaries. This suggests that it is more important to have a common culture in firms employing a transnational strategy than a multidomestic strategy, with global and international strategies falling between these two extremes.

Synthesis: Strategy and Architecture

In Chapter 12, we identified four international business strategies: multidomestic, international, global, and transnational. So far in this chapter we have looked at several aspects of organization architecture, and we have discussed the interrelationships between these dimensions and strategies. Now it is time to synthesize this material (see Table 13.2).

Multidomestic Firms

Firms pursuing a multidomestic strategy focus on local responsiveness. Table 13.2 shows that multidomestic firms tend to operate with worldwide area structures, within which operating decisions are decentralized to functionally self-contained country subsidiaries. The need for coordination between subunits (areas and country subsidiaries) is low. This suggests that multidomestic firms do not have a high need for integrating mechanisms, either formal or informal, to knit together different national operations. The lack of interdependence implies that the level of performance ambi-

Structure and Controls	Strategy			
	Multidomestic	**International**	**Global**	**Transnational**
Vertical differentiation	Decentralized	Core competency centralized; rest decentralized	Some centralized	Mixed centralized and decentralized
Horizontal differentiation	Worldwide area structure	Worldwide product division	Worldwide product division	Informal matrix
Need for coordination	Low	Moderate	High	Very high
Integrating mechanisms	None	Few	Many	Very many
Performance ambiguity	Low	Moderate	High	Very high
Need for cultural controls	Low	Moderate	High	Very high

Table 13.2

A Synthesis of Strategy, Structure, and Control Systems

guity in multidomestic concerns is low, as (by extension) are the costs of control. Thus, headquarters can manage foreign operations by relying primarily on output and bureaucratic controls and a policy of management by exception. Incentives can be linked to performance metrics at the level of country subsidiaries. Since the need for integration and coordination is low, the need for common processes and organization culture is also quite low. If these firms were unable to profit from the realization of location and experience curve economies, or from the transfer of core competencies, their organizational simplicity would make this an attractive strategy.

International Firms

Firms pursuing an international strategy attempt to create value by transferring core competencies from home to foreign subsidiaries. If they are diverse, as most of them are, these firms operate with a worldwide product division structure. Headquarters typically maintains centralized control over the source of the firm's core competency, which is most typically found in the R&D and/or marketing functions of the firm. All other operating decisions are decentralized within the firm to subsidiary operations in each country (which in diverse firms report to worldwide product divisions).

The need for coordination is moderate in such firms, reflecting the need to transfer core competencies. Thus, although such firms operate with some integrating mechanisms, they are not that extensive. The relatively low level of interdependence that results translates into a relatively low level of performance ambiguity. These firms can generally get by with output and bureaucratic controls and with incentives that are focused on performance metrics at the level of country subsidiaries. The need for a common organizational culture and common processes is not that great. An important exception to this is when the core skills or competencies of the firm are embedded in processes and culture, in which case the firm needs to pay close attention to transferring those processes and associated culture from the corporate center to country subsidiaries. Overall, although the organization of international firms is more complex than that of multidomestic firms, the increase in the level of complexity is not that great.

Global Firms

Firms pursuing a global strategy focus on the realization of location and experience curve economies. If they are diverse, as most of them are, these firms operate with a worldwide product division structure. To coordinate the firm's globally dispersed web of value creation activities, headquarters typically maintains ultimate control over most operating decisions. In general, global firms are more centralized than enterprises pursuing a multidomestic or international strategy. Reflecting the need for coordination of the various stages of the firms' globally dispersed value chains, the need for integration in these firms also is high. Thus, these firms tend to operate with an array of formal and informal integrating mechanisms. The resulting interdependencies can lead to significant performance ambiguities. As a result, in addition to output and bureaucratic controls, global firms tend to stress the need to build a strong organizational culture that can facilitate coordination and cooperation. They also tend to use incentive systems that are linked to performance metrics at the corporate level, giving the managers of different operations a strong incentive to cooperate with each other to increase the performance of the entire corporation. On average, the organization of global firms is more complex than that of multidomestic and international firms.

Transnational Firms

Firms pursuing a transnational strategy focus on the simultaneous attainment of location and experience curve economies, local responsiveness, and global learning (the multidirectional transfer of core competencies or skills). These firms may operate with matrix-type structures in which both product divisions and geographic areas have significant influence. The need to coordinate a globally dispersed value chain and to transfer core competencies creates pressures for centralizing some operating decisions (particularly production and R&D). At the same time, the need to be locally responsive creates pressures for decentralizing other operating decisions to national operations (particularly marketing). Consequently, these firms tend to mix relatively high degrees of centralization for some operating decisions with relative high degrees of decentralization for other operating decisions.

The need for coordination is particularly high in transnational firms. This is reflected in the use of an array of formal and informal integrating mechanisms, including formal matrix structures and informal management networks. The high level of interdependence of subunits implied by such integration can result in significant performance ambiguities, which raise the costs of control. To reduce these, in addition to output and bureaucratic controls, transnational firms need to cultivate a strong culture and to establish incentives that promote cooperation between subunits.

Environment, Strategy, Architecture, and Performance

Underlying the scheme outlined in Table 13.2 is the notion that a "fit" between strategy and architecture is necessary for a firm to achieve high performance. For a firm to succeed, two conditions must be fulfilled. First, the firm's strategy must be consistent with the environment in which the firm operates. We discussed this issue in Chapter 12 and noted that in some industries a global strategy is most viable, in others an international or transnational strategy may be most viable, and in still others a multidomestic strategy may be most viable (although the number of multidomestic industries is on the decline). Second, the firm's organization architecture must be consistent with its strategy.

If the strategy does not fit the environment, the firm is likely to experience significant performance problems. If the architecture does not fit the strategy, the firm is also likely to experience performance problems. Therefore, to survive, a firm must strive to achieve a fit of its environment, its strategy, and its organizational architecture. You will recall that we saw the importance of this concept in the opening case. Philips NV, the Dutch electronics firm, provides another illustration of the need for this fit. For reasons rooted in the history of the firm, Philips operated until recently with an organization typical of a multidomestic enterprise in which operating decisions were decentralized to largely autonomous foreign subsidiaries. Historically, electronics markets were segmented from each other by high trade barriers, so an organization consistent with a multidomestic strategy made sense. However, by the mid-1980s, the industry in which Philips competed had been revolutionized by declining trade barriers, technological change, and the emergence of low-cost Japanese competitors that utilized a global strategy. To survive, Philips needed to adopt a global strategy itself. The firm recognized this and tried to adopt a global posture, but it did little to change its organizational architecture. The firm nominally adopted a matrix structure based on worldwide product divisions and national areas. In reality, however, the national areas continued to dominate the organization, and the product divisions had little more than an advisory role. As a result, Philips' architecture did not fit the strategy, and by the early 1990s Philips was losing money. It was only after four years of wrenching change and large losses that Philips was finally able to tilt the balance of power in its matrix toward the product divisions. By the mid-1990s, the fruits of this effort to realign the company's strategy and architecture with the demands of its operating environment were beginning to appear in improved financial performance.[35]

Organizational Change

Multinational firms periodically have to alter their architecture so that it conforms to the changes in the environment in which they are competing and the strategy they are pursuing. To be profitable, Philips NV had to alter its strategy and architecture in the

1990s so that both matched the demands of the competitive environment in the electronics industry, which had shifted from a multidomestic to a global industry. While a detailed consideration of organizational change is beyond the scope of this book, a few comments are warranted regarding the sources of organization inertia and the strategies and tactics for implementing organizational change.

Organizational Inertia

Organizations are difficult to change. Within most organizations, there are strong inertia forces. These forces come from a number of sources. One source of inertia is the existing distribution of power and influence within an organization.[36] The power and influence enjoyed by individual managers are in part a function of their role in the organizational hierarchy, as defined by structural position. By definition, most substantive changes in an organization require a change in structure and, by extension, a change in the distribution of power and influence within the organization. Some individuals will see their power and influence increase as a result of organizational change, and some will see the converse. For example, in the 1990s, Philips NV increased the roles and responsibilities of its global product divisions and decreased the roles and responsibilities of its foreign subsidiary companies. This meant the managers running the global product divisions saw their power and influence increase, while the managers running the foreign subsidiary companies saw their power and influence decline. As might be expected, some managers of foreign subsidiary companies did not like this change and resisted it, which slowed the pace of change. Those whose power and influence are reduced as a consequence of organizational change can be expected to resist it, primarily by arguing that the change might not work. To the extent that they are successful, this constitutes a source of organizational inertia that might slow or stop change.

Another source of organizational inertia is the existing culture, as expressed in norms and value systems. Value systems reflect deeply held beliefs, and as such, they can be very hard to change. If the formal and informal socialization mechanisms within an organization have been emphasizing a consistent set of values for a prolonged period, and if hiring, promotion, and incentive systems have all reinforced these values, then suddenly announcing that those values are no longer appropriate and need to be changed can produce resistance and dissonance among employees. For example, Philips NV historically placed a very high value on local autonomy. The changes of the 1990s implied a reduction in the autonomy enjoyed by foreign subsidiaries, which was counter to the established values of the company and thus resisted.

Organizational inertia might also derive from senior managers' preconceptions about the appropriate business model or paradigm. When a given paradigm has worked well, managers might have trouble accepting that it is no longer appropriate. At Philips, granting considerable autonomy to foreign subsidiaries had worked very well in the past, allowing local managers to tailor product and business strategy to the conditions prevailing in a given country. Since this paradigm had worked so well, it was difficult for many managers to understand why it no longer applied. Consequently, they had difficulty accepting a new business model and tended to fall back on their established paradigm and ways of doing things. This made change difficult, for it required managers to let go of long-held assumptions about what worked and what didn't work, which was something many of them couldn't do.

Institutional constraints might also act as a source of inertia. National regulations including local content rules and policies pertaining to layoffs might make it difficult for a multinational to alter its global value chain. As with Unilever (see the opening case), a multinational might wish to take manufacturing control away from local subsidiaries, transfer that control to global product divisions, and consolidate manufacturing at a few choice locations. However, if local content rules (see Chapter 5) require some degree of local production and if regulations regarding layoffs make it difficult or expensive for a multinational to close operations in a country, a multinational may find that these constraints make it very difficult to adopt the most effective strategy and architecture.

Implementing Organizational Change

Although all organizations suffer from inertia, the complexity and global spread of many multinationals might make it particularly difficult for them to change their strategy and architecture to match new organizational realities. Yet at the same time, the trend toward globalization in many industries has made it more critical than ever that many multinationals do just that. In industry after industry, declining barriers to cross-border trade and investment have led to a change in the nature of the competitive environment. Cost pressures have increased, requiring multinationals to respond by streamlining their operations to realize economic benefits associated with location and experience curve economies and with the transfer of competencies and skills within the organization. At the same time, local responsiveness remains an important source of differentiation. To survive in this emerging competitive environment, multinationals must not only change their strategy, but they must also change their architecture so that it matches strategy in discriminating ways. The basic principles for successful organizational change can be summarized as follows: (1) unfreeze the organization through shock therapy, (2) move the organization to a new state through proactive change in the architecture, and (3) refreeze the organization in its new state.

Unfreezing the Organization

Because of inertia forces, incremental change is often no change. Those whose power is threatened by change can too easily resist incremental change. This leads to the big bang theory of change, which maintains that effective change requires taking bold action early to "unfreeze" the established culture of an organization and to change the distribution of power and influence. Shock therapy to unfreeze the organization might include the closure of plants deemed uneconomic or the announcement of a dramatic structural reorganization. It is also important to realize that change will not occur unless senior managers are committed to it. Senior managers must clearly articulate the need for change so employees understand both why it is being pursued and the benefits that will flow from successful change. Senior managers must also practice what they preach and take the necessary bold steps. If employees see senior managers preaching the need for change but not changing their own behavior or making substantive changes in the organization, they will soon lose faith in the change effort, which will flounder as a result.

Moving to the New State

Once an organization has been unfrozen, it must be moved to its new state. Movement requires taking action—closing operations; reorganizing the structure; reassigning responsibilities; changing control, incentive, and reward systems; redesigning processes; and letting people go who are seen as an impediment to change. In other words, movement requires a substantial change in the form of a multinational's organization architecture so that it matches the desired new strategic posture. For movement to be successful, it must be done with sufficient speed. Involving employees in the change effort is an excellent way to get them to appreciate and buy into the needs for change and to help with rapid movement. For example, a firm might delegate substantial responsibility for designing operating processes to lower-level employees. If enough of their recommendations are then acted on, the employees will see the consequences of their efforts and consequently buy into the notion that change is really occurring.

Refreezing the Organization

Refreezing the organization takes longer. It may require that a new culture be established, while the old one is being dismantled. Thus, refreezing requires that employees be socialized into the new way of doing things. Companies will often use management education programs to achieve this. At General Electric, where longtime CEO Jack Welch instituted a major change in the culture of the company, management education programs were used as a proactive tool to communicate new values to organization members. On their own, however, management education programs are not enough. Hiring policies must be changed to reflect the new realities, with an emphasis on hiring individuals whose own values are consistent with that of the new culture the firm is trying to build. Similarly, control and incentive systems must be consistent with the new realities of the organization, or change will never take. Senior management must recognize that changing culture takes a long time. Any letup in the pressure to change may allow the old culture to reemerge as employees fall back into familiar ways of doing things. The communication task facing senior managers, therefore, is a long-term endeavor that requires managers to be relentless and persistent in their pursuit of change. One striking feature of Jack Welch's two-decade tenure at GE, for example, is that he never stopped pushing his change agenda. It was a consistent theme of his tenure. He was always thinking up new programs and initiatives to keep pushing the culture of the organization along the desired trajectory.

ChapterSummary

This chapter identified the organizational architecture that can be used by multinational enterprises to manage and direct their global operations. A central theme of the chapter was that different strategies require different architectures; strategy is implemented through architecture. To succeed, a firm must match its architecture to its strategy in discriminating ways. Firms whose architecture does not fit their strategic requirements will experience performance problems. It is also necessary for the different components of architecture to be consistent with each other. The chapter made these major points:

1. Organizational architecture refers to the totality of a firm's organization, including formal organizational structure, control systems and incentives, processes, organizational culture, and people.

2. Superior enterprise profitability requires three conditions to be fulfilled: the different elements of a firm's organizational architecture must be internally consistent, the organizational architecture must fit the strategy of the firm, and the strategy and architecture of the firm must be consistent with competitive conditions prevailing in the firm's markets.

3. Organizational structure means three things: the formal division of the organization into subunits (horizontal differentiation), the location of decision-making responsibilities within that structure (vertical differentiation), and the establishment of integrating mechanisms.

4. Control systems are the metrics used to measure the performance of subunits and make judg-

ments about how well managers are running those subunits.

5. Incentives refer to the devices used to reward appropriate employee behavior. Many employees receive incentives in the form of annual bonus pay. Incentives are usually closely tied to the performance metrics used for output controls.

6. Processes refer to the manner in which decisions are made and work is performed within the organization. Processes can be found at many different levels within an organization. The core competencies or valuable skills of a firm are often embedded in its processes. Efficient and effective processes can help to lower the costs of value creation and to add additional value to a product.

7. Organizational culture refers to a system of values and norms that is shared among employees. Values and norms express themselves as the behavior patterns or style of an organization that new employees are automatically encouraged to follow by their fellow employees.

8. There are four main dimensions of organizational structure: vertical differentiation, horizontal differentiation, integration, and control systems.

9. Firms pursuing different strategies must adopt a different architecture to implement those strategies successfully. Firms pursuing multidomestic, global, international, and transnational strategies all must adopt an organizational architecture that matches their strategy.

10. While all organizations suffer from inertia, the complexity and global spread of many multinationals might make it particularly difficult for them to change their strategy and architecture to match new organizational realities. At the same time, the trend toward globalization in many industries has made it more critical than ever that many multinationals do just that.

Critical Discussion Questions

1. "The choice of strategy for a multinational firm must depend on a comparison of the benefits of that strategy (in terms of value creation) with the costs of implementing it (as defined by organizational architecture necessary for implementation). On this basis, it may be logical for some firms to pursue a multidomestic strategy, others a global or international strategy, and still others a transnational strategy." Is this statement correct?

2. Discuss this statement: "An understanding of the causes and consequences of performance ambiguity is central to the issue of organizational design in multinational firms."

3. Describe the organizational architecture a transnational firm might adopt to reduce the costs of control.

4. What is the most appropriate organizational architecture for a firm that is competing in an industry where a global strategy is most appropriate?

5. If a firm is changing its strategy from an international to a transnational strategy, what are the most important challenges it is likely to face in implementing this change? How can the firm overcome these challenges?

Research Task | globalEDGE™ globaledge.msu.edu

Use the globalEDGE™ site to complete the following exercises:

1. The *Financial Times* newspaper and the PricewaterhouseCoopers conduct an annual survey and publish the rankings of World's Most Respected Companies. Although the recent rankings are available on a subscription basis, past years' rankings are publicly available. Locate the most recent publicly available ranking and focus on the success factors highlighted by the *Financial Times*.

Prepare an executive summary of the strategic and organizational success factors of a company of your choice.

2. The globalEDGE™ presents selected articles from the business print media. Locate the selected articles section and find an article that provides insights about the three reasons for failure in the globalization process. Prepare a description of these three reasons and the solutions that the authors recommend.

Notes

1. D. Naidler, M. Gerstein, and R. Shaw, *Organization Architecture* (San Francisco: Jossey-Bass, 1992).

2. G. Morgan, *Images of Organization* (Beverly Hills, CA: Sage Publications, 1986).

3. The material in this section draws on John Child, *Organizations* (London: Harper & Row, 1984).

4. Allan Cane, "Microsoft Reorganizes to Meet Market Challenges," *Financial Times*, March 16, 1994, p. 1.

5. For research evidence that is related to this issue, see J. Birkinshaw, "Entrepreneurship in the Multinational Corporation: The Characteristics of Subsidiary Initiatives," *Strategic Management Journal* 18 (1997), pp. 207–29, and J. Birkinshaw, N. Hood, and S. Jonsson, "Building Firm Specific Advantages in Multinational Corporations: The Role of Subsidiary Initiatives," *Strategic Management Journal* 19 (1998), pp. 221–41.

6. For more detail, see S. M. Davis, "Managing and Organizing Multinational Corporations," in C. A. Bartlett and S. Ghoshal, *Transnational Management* (Homewood, IL: Richard D. Irwin, 1992).

7. A. D. Chandler, *Strategy and Structure: Chapters in the History of the Industrial Enterprise* (Cambridge, MA: MIT Press, 1962).

8. Davis, "Managing and Organizing Multinational Corporations."

9. J. M. Stopford and L. T. Wells, *Strategy and Structure of the Multinational Enterprise* (New York: Basic Books, 1972).

10. C. A. Bartlett and S. Ghoshal, *Managing across Borders* (Boston: Harvard Business School Press, 1989).

11. Guy de Jonquieres, "Unilever Adopts a Clean Sheet Approach," *Financial Times*, October 21, 1991, p. 13.

12. See J. R. Galbraith, *Designing Complex Organizations* (Reading, MA: Addison-Wesley, 1977).

13. See Bartlett and Ghoshal, *Managing across Borders*, and F. V. Guterl, "Goodbye, Old Matrix," *Business Month*, February 1989, pp. 32–38.

14. M. S. Granovetter, "The Strength of Weak Ties," *American Journal of Sociology* 78 (1973), pp. 1360–80.

15. A. K. Gupta, and V. J. Govindarajan, "Knowledge Flows within Multinational Corporations," *Strategic Management Journal* 21, no. 4 (2000), pp. 473–96; V. J. Govindarajan and A. K. Gupta, *The Quest for Global Dominance* (San Francisco: Jossey-Bass, 2001); and U. Andersson, M. Forsgren, and U. Holm, "The Strategic Impact of External Networks: Subsidiary Performance and Competence Development in the Multinational Corporation," *Strategic Management Journal* 23 (2002), pp. 979–96.

16. For examples, see W. H. Davidow and M. S. Malone, *The Virtual Corporation* (New York: Harper Collins, 1992).

17. W. G. Ouchi, "Markets, Bureaucracies, and Clans," *Administrative Science Quarterly* 25 (1980), pp. 129–44.

18. For some empirical work that addresses this issue, see T. P. Murtha, S. A. Lenway, and R. P. Bagozzi, "Global Mind Sets and Cognitive Shift in a Complex Multinational Corporation," *Strategic Management Journal* 19 (1998), pp. 97–114.

19. J. Welsh and J. Byrne, *Jack: Straight from the Gut* (Warner Books: New York, 2001).

20. C. W. L. Hill, M. E. Hitt, and R. E. Hoskisson, "Cooperative versus Competitive Structures in Related and Unrelated Diversified Firms," *Organization Science* 3 (1992), pp. 501–21.

21. Murtha, Lenway, and Bagozzi, "Global Mind Sets."

22. M. Hammer and J. Champy, *Reengineering the Corporation* (New York: Harper Business, 1993).

23. T. Kostova, "Transnational Transfer of Strategic Organizational Practices: A Contextual Perspective," *Academy of Management Review* 24, no. 2 (1999), pp. 308–24.

24. Andersson, Forsgren, and Holm, "The Strategic Impact of External Networks: Subsidiary Performance and Competence Development in the Multinational Corporation."

25. E. H. Schein, "What Is Culture?" in P. J. Frost et al., *Reframing Organizational Culture* (Newbury Park, CA: Sage, 1991).

26. E. H. Schein, *Organizational Culture and Leadership*, 2nd ed. (San Francisco: Jossey-Bass, 1992).

27. G. Morgan, *Images of Organization* (Beverly Hills, CA: Sage, 1986).

28. R. Dore, *British Factory, Japanese Factory* (London: Allen & Unwin, 1973).

29. M. Dickson, "Back to the Future," *Financial Times*, May 30, 1994, p. 7.

30. See J. P. Kotter and J. L. Heskett, *Corporate Culture and Performance* (New York: Free Press, 1992), and M. L. Tushman and C. A. O'Reilly, *Winning through Innovation* (Boston: Harvard Business School Press, 1997).

31. Kotter and Heskett, *Corporate Culture and Performance*.

32. The classic song of praise was produced by T. Peters and R. H. Waterman, *In Search of Excellence* (New York: Harper & Row, 1982). Ironically, IBM's decline began shortly after Peters and Waterman's book was published.

33. Kotter and Heskett, *Corporate Culture and Performance*.

34. Bartlett and Ghoshal, *Managing across Borders*.

35. See F. J. Auilar and M. Y. Yoshino, "The Philips Group: 1987," Howard Business School Case, 388–050, 1987; "Philips Fights Flab," *The Economist*, April 7, 1990, pp. 73–74; and R. Van de Krol, "Philips Wins Back Old Friends," *Financial Times*, July 14, 1995, p. 14.

36. J. Pfeffer, *Managing with Power: Politics and Influence within Organizations* (Boston: Harvard Business School Press, 1992).

Organizational Change at Royal Dutch/Shell

The Anglo-Dutch company Royal Dutch/Shell is the world's largest non-state-owned oil company with activities in more than 130 countries and 2002 revenues of $235 billion. From the 1950s until 1994, Shell operated with a matrix structure invented for it by McKinsey, a management consulting firm that specializes in organizational design. Under this matrix structure, the head of each operating company reported to two bosses. One boss was responsible for the geographical region or country in which the operating company was based, while the other was responsible for the business activity that the operating company was engaged in (Shell's business activities included oil exploration and production, oil products, chemicals, gas, and coal). Thus, for example, the head of the local Shell chemical company in Australia reported both to the head of Shell Australia and to the head of Shell's entire chemical division, who was based in London. Both bosses had equal influence and status within the organization.

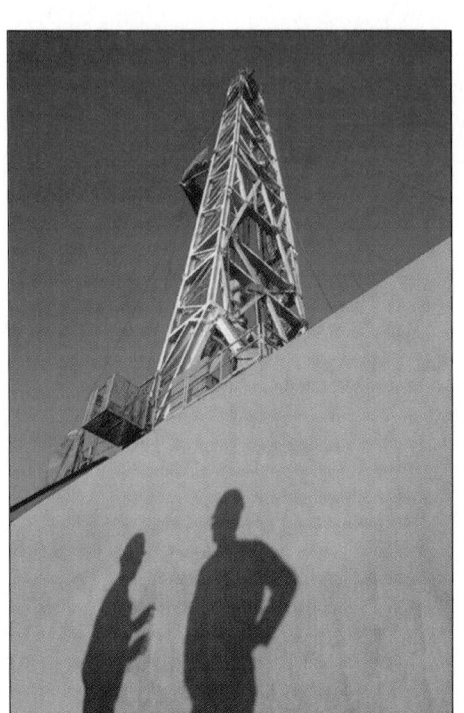

This matrix structure had two very visible consequences at Shell. First, because each operating company had two bosses to satisfy, decision making typically followed a pattern of consensus building, with differences of perspective between country (or regional) heads on the one hand and the heads of business divisions on the other being worked out through debate. Although this process could be slow and cumbersome, it was seen as a good thing in the oil industry where most big decisions are long-term ones that involve substantial capital expenditures and where informed debate between different viewpoints can clarify the pros and cons of issues, rather than hinder decision making. Second, because the decision-making process was slow, it was reserved for only the most important decisions (such as major new capital investments). The result was substantial decentralization by default to the heads of the individual operating companies, who were largely left alone to run their own operations. This decentralization helped Shell respond to local differences in government regulations, competitive conditions, and consumer tastes. Thus, for example, the head of Shell's Australian chemical company was given the freedom to determine pricing practices and marketing strategy in the Australian market. Only if Shell wished to undertake a major capital investment, such as building a new chemical plant, would the consensus-building decision-making system be invoked.

As desirable as this matrix structure seemed, in 1995 Shell announced a radical plan to dismantle it. The primary reason given by top management for the shift was continuing slack demand for oil and weak oil prices, which had put pressure on Shell's profit margins. Although Shell had traditionally been among the most profitable oil companies in the world, in the early 1990s its relative performance began to slip as other oil companies, such as Exxon, adapted more rapidly to a world of low oil prices by sharply cutting overhead costs and consolidating production in efficient facilities. Consolidating production at these companies often involved serving the world market from a smaller number of large-scale refining facilities and shutting down smaller facilities. In contrast, Shell still operated with a large head office, which was required to effect coordination within Shell's matrix structure, and substantial duplication of oil and chemical refining facilities across operating companies, each of which typically developed the facilities required to serve its own market.

In 1995, Shell's senior management realized that lowering operating costs required a sharp reduction in head office overhead and, where appropriate, the elimination of unnecessary duplication of facilities across countries. To achieve these goals, top executives decided to reorganize the company along divisional lines. Shell now operates with five main global product divisions—exploration and production, oil products, chemicals, gas, and coal. Each operating company reports to whichever global division is the most relevant. Thus, the head of the Australian chemical operation now reports directly to the head of the global chemical division. The thinking is that this will increase the power of the global chemical division and enable that division to eliminate any unnecessary duplication of facilities across countries. Eventually, production may be consolidated in larger facilities that serve an entire region, rather than a single country, thereby enabling Shell to reap greater scale economies.

The country (or regional) chiefs remain but their roles and responsibilities are reduced. Now their primary responsibility is coordination between operating companies within a country (or region) and relations with the local government. There is a solid line of reporting and responsibility between the heads of operating companies and the global divisions and only a dotted line between the heads of operating companies and country chiefs. Thus, for example, the ability of the head of Shell Australia to shape the major capital investment decisions of Shell's Australian chemical operation was substantially reduced as a result of these changes. Furthermore, the simplified reporting system reduced the need for a large head office bureaucracy, and Shell trimmed the workforce at its London head office by 1,170, driving down Shell's cost structure.

Sources: "Shell on the Rocks," *The Economist*, June 24, 1995, pp. 57–58; D. Lascelles, "Barons Swept out of Fiefdoms," *Financial Times*, March 30, 1995, p. 15; C. Lorenz, "End of a Corporate Era," *Financial Times*, March 30, 1995, p. 15; R. Corzine, "Shell Discovers Time and Tide Wait for No Man," *Financial Times*, March 10, 1998, p. 17; and R. Corzine, "Oiling the Group's Wheels of Change," *Financial Times*, April 1, 1998, p. 12.

Case Discussion Questions

1. What were the benefits of the matrix structure at Shell? What were the drawbacks? Did the matrix structure fit the environment of the global oil and chemical industries in the 1980s?

2. What shift occurred in Shell's operating environment in the 1990s? How did this shift affect the financial performance of the firm? What does this suggest about the fit between strategy and architecture?

3. What kind of structure did Shell adopt in 1995? In what ways did the architecture of Shell's organization after 1995 differ from that before 1995?

4. Comment on the fit between operating environment, strategy, and organizational architecture at Shell after the 1995 reorganization. Did the change lead to enhanced fit?

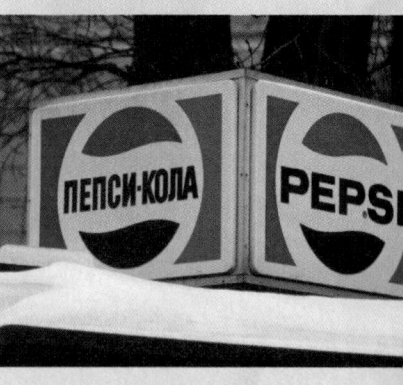

Chapter 14

Entry Strategy and Strategic Alliances

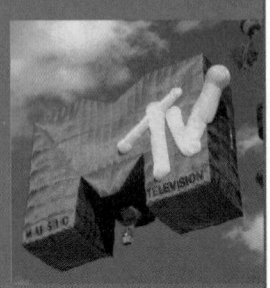

Introduction
Basic Entry Decisions
  Which Foreign Markets?
  Timing of Entry
  Scale of Entry and Strategic
  Commitments
  Summary
Entry Modes
  Exporting
  Turnkey Projects
  Licensing
  Franchising
  Joint Ventures
  Wholly Owned Subsidiaries
Selecting an Entry Mode
  Core Competencies and Entry Mode
  Pressures for Cost Reductions
  and Entry Mode
Establishing a Wholly Owned Subsidiary:
Green-Field Venture or Acquisition?
  Pros and Cons of Acquisitions
  Pros and Cons of Green-Field Ventures
  Green-Field Venture or Acquisition?
Strategic Alliances
  The Advantages of Strategic Alliances
  The Disadvantages of Strategic Alliances
Making Alliances Work
  Partner Selection
  Alliance Structure
  Managing the Alliance
Chapter Summary
Critical Discussion Questions
Closing Case: Merrill Lynch in Japan

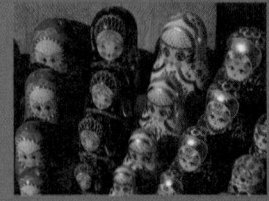

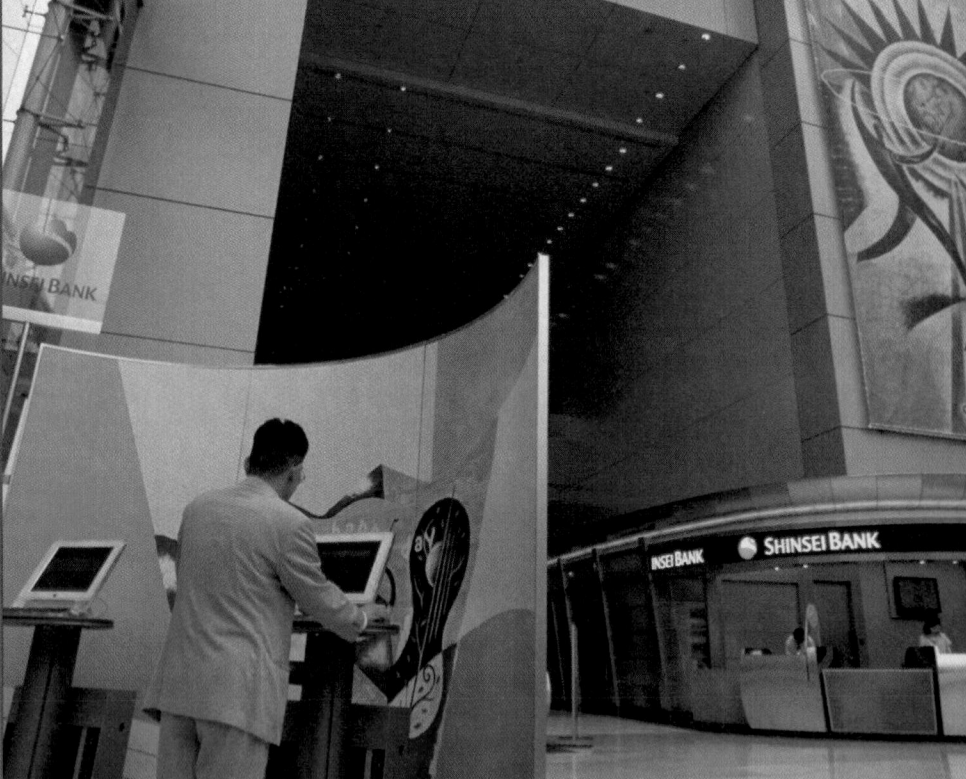

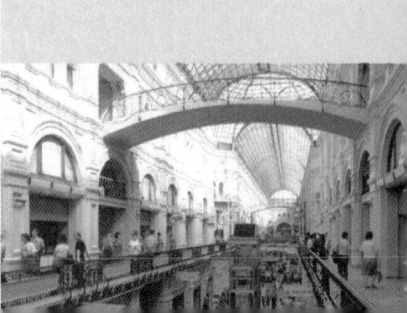

Diebold

For much of its 144-year history, Diebold Inc. did not worry much about international business. As a premier name in bank vaults and then automated teller machines (ATMs), the Ohio-based company found that it had its hands full focusing on U.S. financial institutions. The company first started to sell ATM machines in foreign markets in the 1980s. Wary of going it alone, Diebold forged a distribution agreement with the Dutch multinational electronics company Philips NV. Under the agreement, Diebold manufactured ATMs in the United States and exported them to foreign customers after Philips had made the sale.

In 1990, Diebold pulled out of the agreement with Philips and established a joint venture with IBM, Interbold, for the research, development, and distribution of ATM machines worldwide. Diebold, which owned a 70 percent stake in the joint venture, supplied the machines, while IBM supplied the global marketing, sales, and service functions. Diebold established a joint venture rather than setting up its own international distribution system because the company thought it lacked the resources to establish an international presence. In essence, Diebold was exporting its machines via IBM's distribution network.

By 1997, foreign sales had grown from the single digits to more than 20 percent of Diebold's total revenues, while sales in the United States were slowing due to a saturated domestic market. Looking forward, Diebold saw rapid growth in demand for ATMs in a wide range of developed and developing markets. Particularly enticing were countries such as China, India and Brazil, where an emerging middle class was starting to use the banking system in large numbers and demand for ATMs was expected to surge. It was at this point that Diebold decided to establish its own foreign distribution network.

As a first step, Diebold purchased IBM's 30 percent stake in the Interbold joint venture. In part, the acquisition was driven by Diebold's dissatisfaction with IBM's sales efforts, which often fell short of quota. Part of the problem was that for IBM's sales force, Diebold's ATMs were just part of their product portfolio, and not necessarily their top priority. Diebold believed it could attain a greater market share if it gained direct control over distribution.

The company also realized that in addition to local distribution, it would need a local manufacturing presence in a number of regions. Among the reasons for this were differences in the way ATMs are used, requiring cus-tomization of the product. In parts of Asia, for example, many customers pay their utility bills with cash via ATMs. To gain market share, Diebold had to design ATMs that both accept and count stacks of up to 100 currency notes, and weed out counterfeits. In other countries, ATMs perform multiple functions from filing tax returns to distributing theater tickets. Diebold believed that locating manufacturing close to key markets would help facilitate local customization.

To jump-start its international expansion, Diebold went on a foreign acquisition binge. In 1999 it acquired Brazil's Procomp Amazonia Industria Electronica, an electronics company with sales of $400 million and a big presence in ATMs. This was followed in quick succession by the acquisitions of the ATM units of France's Groupe Bull and Holland's Getronics, both major players in Europe for a combined $160 million. In China, where no substantial indigenous competitors were open to acquisition, Diebold established a manufacturing and distribution joint venture in which it took a majority ownership position. The result: by 2002 Diebold had a manufacturing presence in Asia, Europe, and Latin America as well as the United States and distribution operations in some 80 nations, the majority of which were wholly owned by Diebold. International sales accounted for some 37 percent of the company's $1.94 billion in revenues in 2002, and were forecast to grow at double-digit rates.

Interestingly, the acquisition of Brazil's Procomp also took Diebold into a new and potentially lucrative global business. In addition to its ATM business, Procomp had an electronic voting machine business. In 1999, Procomp won a $105 million contract, the largest in Diebold's history, to outfit Brazilian polling stations with electronic voting terminals. Diebold's management realized this might become a large global business. In 2001, Diebold expanded its presence in the electronic voting business by acquiring Global Election Systems Inc., a U.S. company that provides electronic voting technology for states and countries that want to upgrade from traditional voting technology.

Sources: H. S. Byrne, "Money Machine," *Barrons,* May 27, 2002, p. 24; M. Arndt, "Diebold," *Business Week,* August 27, 2001, p. 138; W. A. Lee, "After Slump, Diebold Pins Hopes on New ATM Market Features," *American Banker,* September 15, 2000, p. 1; and C. Keenan, "A Bigger Diebold, Phasing Out IBM Alliance, Will Market ATMs Itself," *American Banker,* July 3, 1997, p. 8.

Introduction

This chapter is concerned with three closely related topics: (1) the decision of which foreign markets to enter, when to enter them, and on what scale; (2) the choice of entry mode, and (3) the role of strategic alliances. Any firm contemplating foreign expansion must first struggle with the issue of which foreign markets to enter and the timing and scale of entry. The choice of which markets to enter should be driven by an assessment of relative long-run growth and profit potential. In the opening case, for example, we saw that in the late 1990s, Diebold decided to enter large developing markets such as China, India, and Brazil, primarily because of its assessment that long-term demand for automated teller machines (ATMs) in these markets would be high.

The choice of mode for entering a foreign market is another major issue with which international businesses must wrestle. The various modes for serving foreign markets are exporting, licensing or franchising to host-country firms, establishing joint ventures with a host-country firm, setting up a new wholly owned subsidiary in a host country to serve its market, or acquiring an established enterprise in the host nation to serve that market. Each of these options has advantages and disadvantages. The magnitude of the advantages and disadvantages associated with each entry mode is determined by a number of factors, including transport costs, trade barriers, political risks, economic risks, costs, and firm strategy. The optimal entry mode varies by situation, depending on these factors. Thus, whereas some firms may best serve a given market by exporting, other firms may better serve the market by setting up a new wholly owned subsidiary or by acquiring an established enterprise.

As we saw in the opening case, Diebold originally exported its ATMs to foreign countries. The company entered into distribution agreements with established multinationals such as Philips and IBM, which sold the machines for Diebold. By the mid-1990s, however, Diebold was becoming increasingly dissatisfied with this arrangement, and decided that if it was to expand its international presence, it needed to establish its own distribution system and set up manufacturing facilities in other countries. For Diebold, the issue was one of control—exporting through distributors did not give the company the control that it thought it needed to fully exploit international opportunities, so it decided to establish wholly or majority owned subsidiaries to manufacture and distribute its products internationally. To establish its presence quickly, Diebold acquired a number of foreign ATM companies, rather than building up operations by itself.

We touched on the topic of entry modes when we examined foreign direct investment (FDI) in Chapter 6. There we related economic theory to exporting, licensing, and foreign direct investment as means of entering foreign markets. Here we integrate that material with the material we discussed in Chapter 12 on firm strategy to present a comprehensive picture of the factors that determine the optimal entry mode. We consider a wider range of modes in this chapter as well as mixed entry modes. (For example, establishing joint ventures and wholly owned subsidiaries in another country are both FDI, but we did not make a distinction in Chapter 6.)

The final topic of this chapter is strategic alliances. Strategic alliances are cooperative agreements between actual or potential competitors. The term *strategic alliances* is often used to embrace a variety of arrangements between actual or potential competitors including cross-shareholding deals, licensing arrangements, formal joint ventures, and informal cooperative arrangements. The motives for entering strategic alliances are varied, but they often include market access; hence, the overlap with the topic of entry mode. Strategic alliances have advantages and disadvantages, and a firm must weigh these carefully before deciding whether to ally itself with an actual or potential competitor. Perhaps the biggest danger is that the firm will give away more to its ally than it receives. As we will see, firms can reduce this risk in the way they structure strategic alliances. We will also see how firms can build alliances that benefit both partners.

Basic Entry Decisions

In this section, we look at three basic decisions that a firm contemplating foreign expansion must make: which markets to enter, when to enter those markets, and on what scale.[1]

Which Foreign Markets?

There are more than 200 nation-states in the world. They do not all hold the same profit potential for a firm contemplating foreign expansion. Ultimately, the choice must be based on an assessment of a nation's long-run profit potential. This potential is a function of several factors, many of which we have studied in earlier chapters. In Chapter 2, we looked in detail at the economic and political factors that influence the potential attractiveness of a foreign market. There we noted that the attractiveness of a country as a potential market for an international business depends on balancing the benefits, costs, and risks associated with doing business in that country.

Chapter 2 also noted that the long-run economic benefits of doing business in a country are a function of factors such as the size of the market (in terms of demographics), the present wealth (purchasing power) of consumers in that market, and the likely future wealth of consumers. While some markets are very large when measured by number of consumers (e.g., China and India), low living standards may imply limited purchasing power and a relatively small market when measured in economic terms. We also argued that the costs and risks associated with doing business in a foreign country are typically lower in economically advanced and politically stable democratic nations, and they are greater in less developed and politically unstable nations.

This calculus is complicated by the fact that the potential long-run benefits bear little relationship to a nation's current stage of economic development or political stability. Long-run benefits depend on likely future economic growth rates, and economic growth appears to be a function of a free market system and a country's capacity for growth (which may be greater in less developed nations). This leads to the conclusion that, other things being equal, the benefit–cost–risk trade-off is likely to be most favorable in politically stable developed and developing nations that have free market systems, and where there is not a dramatic upsurge in either inflation rates or private-sector debt. The trade-off is likely to be least favorable in politically unstable developing nations that operate with a mixed or command economy or in developing nations where speculative financial bubbles have led to excess borrowing (see Chapter 2 for further details).

By applying the reasoning processes alluded to above and discussed in more detail in Chapter 2, a firm can rank countries in terms of their attractiveness and long-run profit potential. Preference is then given to entering markets that rank highly. In the case of Diebold, entering emerging markets such as Brazil and China made sense given the rapid growth of a middle class in these nations, their demand for banking service, and the low level of ATM penetration (see opening case).

One other fact we have not yet discussed is the value an international business can create in a foreign market. This depends on the suitability of its product offering to that market and the nature of indigenous competition.[2] If the international business can offer a product that has not been widely available in that market and that satisfies an unmet need, the value of that product to consumers is likely to be much greater than if the international business simply offers the same type of product that indigenous competitors and other foreign entrants are already offering. Greater value translates into an ability to charge higher prices and/or to build sales volume more rapidly.

Timing of Entry

Once attractive markets have been identified, it is important to consider the timing of entry. We say that entry is early when an international business enters a foreign market before other foreign firms and late when it enters after other international businesses have already established themselves. The advantages frequently associated with entering a market early are commonly known as first-mover advantages.[3] One first-mover advantage is the ability to preempt rivals and capture demand by establishing a strong brand name. A second advantage is the ability to build sales volume in that country and ride down the experience curve ahead of rivals, giving the early entrant a cost advantage over later entrants. This cost advantage may enable the early entrant to cut prices below that of later entrants, thereby driving them out of the market. A third advantage is the ability of early entrants to create switching costs that tie customers into their products or services. Such switching costs make it difficult for later entrants to win business.

There can also be disadvantages associated with entering a foreign market before other international businesses. These are often referred to as **first-mover disadvantages**.[4] These disadvantages may give rise to pioneering costs. **Pioneering costs** are costs that an early entrant has to bear that a later entrant can avoid. Pioneering costs arise when the business system in a foreign country is so different from that in a firm's home market that the enterprise has to devote considerable effort, time, and expense to learning the rules of the game. Pioneering costs include the costs of business failure if the firm, due to its ignorance of the foreign environment, makes some major mistakes. A certain liability is associated with being a foreigner, and this liability is greater for foreign firms that enter a national market early.[5] Research seems to confirm that the probability of survival increases if an international business enters a national market after several other foreign firms have already done so.[6] The late entrant may benefit by observing and learning from the mistakes made by early entrants.

Pioneering costs also include the costs of promoting and establishing a product offering, including the costs of educating customers. These costs can be significant when the product being promoted is unfamiliar to local consumers. In contrast, later entrants may be able to ride on an early entrant's investments in learning and customer education by watching how the early entrant proceeded in the market, by avoiding costly mistakes made by the early entrant, and by exploiting the market potential created by the early entrant's investments in customer education. For example, KFC introduced the Chinese to American-style fast food, but a later entrant, McDonald's, has capitalized on the market in China.

An early entrant may be put at a severe disadvantage, relative to a later entrant, if regulations change in a way that diminishes the value of an early entrant's investments. This is a serious risk in many developing nations where the rules that govern business practices are still evolving. Early entrants can find themselves at a disadvantage if a subsequent change in regulations invalidates prior assumptions about the best business model for operating in that country.

Scale of Entry and Strategic Commitments

Another issue that an international business needs to consider when contemplating market entry is the scale of entry. Entering a market on a large scale involves the commitment of significant resources. Entering a market on a large scale implies rapid entry. For an example, consider the entry of the Dutch insurance company ING into the U.S. insurance market in 1999 (described in detail in the accompanying Management Focus). ING had to spend several billion dollars to acquire its U.S. operations. Not all firms have the resources necessary to enter on a large scale, and even some large firms prefer to enter foreign markets on a small scale and then build slowly as they become more familiar with the market.

The consequences of entering on a significant scale—entering rapidly—are associated with the value of the resulting strategic commitments.[7] A strategic commitment has a long-term impact and is difficult to reverse. Deciding to enter a foreign market on a significant scale is a major strategic commitment. Strategic commitments, such as rapid large-scale market entry, can have an important influence on the nature of competition in a market. For example, by entering the U.S. financial services market on a significant scale, ING has signaled its commitment to the market (see Management Focus). This will have several effects. On the positive side, it will make it easier for the company to attract customers and distributors (such as insurance agents). The scale of entry gives both customers and distributors reasons for believing that ING will remain in the market for the long run. The scale of entry may also give other foreign institutions considering entry into the United States pause; now they will have to compete not only against indigenous institutions in the United States, but also against an aggressive and successful European institution. On the negative side, by committing itself heavily to the United States, ING may have fewer resources available to support expansion in other desirable markets, such as Japan. The commitment to the United States limits the company's strategic flexibility.

As suggested by the ING example, significant strategic commitments are neither unambiguously good nor bad. Rather, they tend to change the competitive playing field and unleash a number of changes, some of which may be desirable and some of which will not be. It is important for a firm to think through the implications of large-scale entry into a market and act accordingly. Of particular relevance is trying to identify how actual and potential competitors might react to large-scale entry into a market. Also, the large-scale entrant is more likely than the small-scale entrant to be able to capture first-mover advantages associated with demand preemption, scale economies, and switching costs.

The value of the commitments that flow from rapid large-scale entry into a foreign market must be balanced against the resulting risks and lack of flexibility associated with significant commitments. But strategic inflexibility can also have value. A famous example from military history illustrates the value of inflexibility. When Hernán Cortés landed in Mexico, he ordered his men to burn all but one of his ships. Cortés reasoned that by eliminating their only method of retreat, his men had no choice but to fight hard to win against the Aztecs—and ultimately they did.[8]

Balanced against the value and risks of the commitments associated with large-scale entry are the benefits of a small-scale entry. Small-scale entry allows a firm to learn about a foreign market while limiting the firm's exposure to that market. Small-scale entry is a way to gather information about a foreign market before deciding whether to enter on a significant scale and how best to enter. By giving the firm time to collect information, small-scale entry reduces the risks associated with a subsequent large-scale entry. But the lack of commitment associated with small-scale entry may make it more difficult for the small-scale entrant to build market share and to capture first- or early-mover advantages. The risk-averse firm that enters a foreign market on a small scale may limit its potential losses, but it may also miss the chance to capture first-mover advantages.

Summary

There are no "right" decisions here, just decisions that are associated with different levels of risk and reward. Entering a large developing nation such as China or India before most other international businesses in the firm's industry, and entering on a large scale, will be associated with high levels of risk. In such cases, the liability of being foreign is increased by the absence of prior foreign entrants whose experience can be a useful guide. At the same time, the potential long-term rewards associated with such a strategy are great. The early large-scale entrant into a major developing nation may be able to capture significant first-mover advantages that will bolster its long-run

International Expansion at ING Group

Management Focus

ING Group was formed in 1991 from the merger between the third largest bank in the Netherlands and the country's largest insurance company. Since then, the company has grown rapidly to become one of the top 10 financial services firms in the world, with operations in 65 countries and a wide range of products in banking, insurance, and asset management. ING's strategy has been to expand rapidly across national borders, primarily through a series of careful acquisitions. Its formula has been to pick a target that has good managers and a strong local presence, take a small stake in the company, win the trust of managers, and then propose a takeover. After the deal, the management and products of the acquired companies have been left largely intact, but ING has required them to sell ING products alongside their own. ING's big push has been the selling of insurance, banking, and investment products, something it has been doing in Holland since the original 1991 merger (in Holland, some 20 percent of ING's insurance products are sold through banks).

Two changes in the regulatory environment have helped ING pursue this strategy. One has been a trend to remove regulatory barriers that traditionally kept different parts of the financial services industry separate. In the United States, for example, a Depression-era law known as the Glass-Steagall Act forbad insurance companies, banks, and asset managers such as mutual fund companies from selling each other's products. The U.S. Congress repealed this act in 1999, opening the way for the consolidation of the U.S. financial services industry. Many other countries that had similar regulations removed them in the 1990s. ING's native Holland was one of the first countries to remove barriers between different areas of the financial services industry. ING took advantage of this to become a pioneer of banking and insurance combinations in Europe. Another significant regulatory development occurred in 1997 when the World Trade Organization struck a deal between its member nations that effectively removed barriers to cross-border investment in financial services. This made it much easier for a company such as ING to build a global financial services business.

ING's expansion was initially centered on Europe where its largest acquisitions have included banks in Germany and Belgium. However, in recent years the centerpiece of ING's strategy has been its aggressive moves into the United States. While ING's Dutch insurance predecessor, Nationale-Nederlanden, had owned several small, regional U.S. insurance companies since the 1970s, the big push into the United States began with the 1997 acquisition of Equitable Life Insurance Company of Iowa. This was followed by the acquisitions of Furman Selz, a New York investment bank, whose activities complement those of Barings, a British-based investment bank with significant U.S. activities that ING acquired in 1995. In 2000, ING acquired ReliaStar Financial Services and the nonhealth insurance units of Aetna Financial Services. These acquisitions combined to make ING one of the top 10 financial services companies in the United States.

ING was attracted to the United States by several factors. The United States is by far the world's largest financial services market, so any company aspiring to be a global player must have a significant presence there. Deregulation made ING's strategy of cross-selling financial service products feasible in the United

position in that market.[9] In contrast, entering developed nations such as Australia or Canada after other international businesses in the firm's industry, and entering on a small scale to first learn more about those markets, will be associated with much lower levels of risk. However, the potential long-term rewards are also likely to be lower because the firm is essentially forgoing the opportunity to capture first-mover advantages and because the lack of commitment signaled by small-scale entry may limit its future growth potential.

This section has been written largely from the perspective of a business based in a developing country considering entry into foreign markets. In a recent article, Christopher Bartlett and Sumantra Ghoshal pointed out the ability that businesses based in developing nations have to enter foreign markets and become global players.[10] Although such firms tend to be late entrants into foreign markets, and although their resources may be limited, Bartlett and Ghoshal argue that such late movers can

States. Despite some state-by-state regulation of insurance, ING says it is easier to do business in the United States than in the European Union, where the patchwork of languages and cultures makes it difficult to build a pan-European business with a single identity. Another lure is that with more and more Americans responsible for managing their own retirement with 401k plans and the like rather than traditional pensions, the personal investment business in the United States is booming, which has increased ING's appetite for U.S. financial services firms. In contrast, pensions are still primarily taken care of by national governments in Europe. Furthermore, in recent years U.S. insurance companies have traded at relatively low price–earnings ratios, making them seem like bargains compared to their European counterparts, which trade at higher valuations. Building a substantial U.S. presence also brings with it the benefits of geographic diversification, allowing ING to offset any revenue or profit shortfalls in one region with earnings elsewhere in the world.

Finally, ING has found it somewhat easier to make acquisitions in the United States than in Europe, where despite the rise of the European Union, national pride has made it difficult for ING to acquire local companies. ING's initial attempt to acquire a Belgium bank in 1992 was rebuffed, primarily due to nationalistic concerns, and it took ING until 1997 to make the acquisition. Similarly, a 1999 attempt to acquire a major French bank, Credit Commercial de France, in which it already held a 19 percent stake, was turned down. According to news reports, French regulators had expressed concerns over what would have been the first foreign acquisition of a French bank, and the board of CCF believed the acquisition should not proceed without the regulators' blessing

With ING's major U.S. presence established, its strategy now is to push forward with the cross-selling of its various insurance, banking, and asset management products. In mid-2000, the company announced the establishment of ING Direct, an online banking concept the company introduced in Canada, Australia, Spain, and France, where it has performed well. The online bank features a savings account paying above market interest rates, which ING Direct can afford due to its low cost structure. Although ING Direct does not offer checking accounts, which are money losers for traditional banks, it can electronically link an ING account to checking accounts that customers have at other banks, allowing them to easily transfer money. In addition to a savings account, ING Direct also offers consumer loans, mortgages, life insurance, and mutual funds. In an interesting move, instead of bank branches the company is setting up a scattering of cyber cafés where customers can drop in, buy a cup of coffee and a muffin, browse the Web, and access their online account. Despite initial skepticism, the concept seems to be doing well in the United States. As of early 2003, ING Direct has attracted more than a million new customers and $10 billion in assets.

Sources: J. Carreyrou, "Dutch Financial Giant Maps Its U.S. Invasion," *Wall Street Journal,* June 22, 2000, p. A17; J. B. Treaster, "ING Group Makes Its Move in Virtual Banking and Insurance," *New York Times,* August 26, 2000, p. C1; "The Lion's Friendly Approach," *The Economist,* December 18, 2000; and S. Kirsner, "Would You Like a Mortgage with Your Mocha?" *Fast Company,* March 2003, pp. 110–14.

still succeed against well-established global competitors by pursuing appropriate strategies. In particular, Bartlett and Ghoshal argue that companies based in developing nations should use the entry of foreign multinationals as an opportunity to learn from these competitors by benchmarking their operations and performance against them. Furthermore, they suggest that the local company may be able to find ways to differentiate itself from a foreign multinational, for example, by focusing on market niches that the multinational ignores or is unable to serve effectively if it has a standardized global product offering. Having improved its performance through learning and differentiated its product offering, the firm from a developing nation may then be able to pursue its own international expansion strategy. Even though the firm may be a late entrant into many countries, by benchmarking and then differentiating itself from early movers in global markets, the firm from the developing nation may still be able to build a strong international business presence. A good example of how this can

The Jollibee Phenomenon—A Philippine Multinational

Jollibee is one of the Philippines' phenomenal business success stories. Jollibee, which stands for "Jolly Bee," began operations in 1975 as a two-branch ice cream parlor. It later expanded its menu to include hot sandwiches and other meals. Encouraged by early success, Jollibee Foods Corporation was incorporated in 1978, with a network that had grown to seven outlets. In 1981, when Jollibee had 11 stores, McDonald's began to open stores in Manila, the capital city. Many observers thought Jollibee would have difficulty competing against McDonald's. However, Jollibee saw this as an opportunity to learn from a very successful global competitor. Jollibee benchmarked its performance against that of McDonald's and started to adopt operational systems similar to those used at McDonald's to control its quality, cost, and service at the store level. This helped Jollibee to improve its performance.

As it came to better understand McDonald's business model, Jollibee began to look for a weakness in McDonald's global strategy. Jollibee executives concluded that McDonald's fare was too standardized for many locals, and that the local firm could gain share by tailoring its menu to local tastes. Jollibee's hamburgers were set apart by a secret mix of spices blended into the ground beef to make the burgers sweeter than those produced by McDonald's, appealing more to Philippine tastes. It also offered local fare including various rice dishes, pineapple burgers, banana *langka* and peach mango pies for desserts. By pursuing this strategy, Jollibee maintained a leadership position over the global giant. By late 2002, Jollibee had 465 stores in the Philippines, a market share of more than 50 percent, and revenues of about $500 million. McDonald's, in contrast, had 237 stores.

In the mid-1980s, Jollibee had gained enough confidence to start expanding internationally. Its initial ventures were into neighboring Asian countries such as Indonesia, where it pursued the strategy of localizing the menu to better match local tastes, thereby differentiating itself from McDonald's. In 1987, Jollibee entered the Middle East, where a large contingent of expatriate Filipino workers provided a ready-made market for the company. The strategy of focusing on expatriates worked so well that in the late 1990s Jollibee decided to enter another foreign market where there was a large Filipino population—the United States. Between 1999 and 2002, Jollibee opened eight stores in the United States, all in California. Even though many believe the U.S. fast-food market is saturated, the stores have performed well. While the initial clientele was strongly biased toward the expatriate Filipino community, where Jollibee's brand awareness is high, non-Filipinos increasingly are coming to the restaurant. In the San Francisco store, which has been open the longest, more than half the customers are now non-Filipino. Today Jollibee has 28 international stores and a potentially bright future as a niche player in a market that has historically been dominated by U.S. multinationals.

Sources: Christopher Bartlett and Sumantra Ghoshal, "Going Global: Lessons from Late Movers," *Harvard Business Review*, March–April 2000, pp. 132–45; "Jollibee Battles Burger Giants in US Market," *Philippine Daily Inquirer*, July 13, 2000; www.jollibee.com.ph; and M. Ballon, "Jollibee Struggling to Expand in U.S.," *Los Angeles Times*, September 16, 2002, p. C1.

work is given in the accompanying Management Focus, which looks at how Jollibee, a Philippines-based fast-food chain, has started to build a global presence in a market dominated by U.S. multinationals such as McDonald's and KFC.

▪ Entry Modes

Once a firm decides to enter a foreign market, the question arises as to the best mode of entry. Firms can use six different modes to enter foreign markets: exporting, turnkey projects, licensing, franchising, establishing joint ventures with a host-country firm, or setting up a new wholly owned subsidiary in the host country. Each entry mode has advantages and disadvantages. Managers need to consider these carefully when deciding which to use.[11]

Exporting

Many manufacturing firms begin their global expansion as exporters and only later switch to another mode for serving a foreign market. This was the case with Diebold, for example, in the opening case. We take a close look at the mechanics of exporting in the next chapter. Here we focus on the advantages and disadvantages of exporting as an entry mode.

Advantages

Exporting has two distinct advantages. First, it avoids the often-substantial costs of establishing manufacturing operations in the host country. Second, exporting may help a firm achieve experience curve and location economies (see Chapter 12). By manufacturing the product in a centralized location and exporting it to other national markets, the firm may realize substantial scale economies from its global sales volume. This is how Sony came to dominate the global TV market, how Matsushita came to dominate the VCR market, how many Japanese automakers made inroads into the U.S. market, and how South Korean firms such as Samsung gained market share in computer memory chips.

Disadvantages

Exporting has a number of drawbacks. First, exporting from the firm's home base may not be appropriate if there are lower-cost locations for manufacturing the product abroad (i.e., if the firm can realize location economies by moving production elsewhere). Thus, particularly for firms pursuing global or transnational strategies, it may be preferable to manufacture where the mix of factor conditions is most favorable from a value creation perspective and to export to the rest of the world from that location. This is not so much an argument against exporting as an argument against exporting from the firm's home country. Many U.S. electronics firms have moved some of their manufacturing to the Far East because of the availability of low-cost, highly skilled labor there. They then export from that location to the rest of the world, including the United States.

A second drawback to exporting is that high transport costs can make exporting uneconomical, particularly for bulk products. One way of getting around this is to manufacture bulk products regionally. This strategy enables the firm to realize some economies from large-scale production and at the same time to limit its transport costs. For example, many multinational chemical firms manufacture their products regionally, serving several countries from one facility.

Another drawback is that tariff barriers can make exporting uneconomical. Similarly, the threat of tariff barriers by the host-country government can make it very risky. An implicit threat by the U.S. Congress to impose tariffs on imported Japanese autos led many Japanese auto firms to set up manufacturing plants in the United States. By 1990, almost 50 percent of all Japanese cars sold in the United States were manufactured locally—up from 0 percent in 1985.

A fourth drawback to exporting arises when a firm delegates its marketing, sales, and service in each country where it does business to another company. This is a common approach for manufacturing firms that are just beginning to expand internationally. The other company may be a local agent, or it may be another multinational with extensive international distribution operations (as was the case with Diebold, which exported its ATM machine through Philips and then IBM as detailed in the opening case). Local agents often carry the products of competing firms and so have divided loyalties. In such cases, the local agent may not do as good a job as the firm would if it managed its marketing itself. Similar problems can occur when another multinational takes on distribution. For example, in the opening case we saw how Diebold was dissatisfied with the way in which IBM distributed Diebold's products internationally. IBM's salespeople had a portfolio of products to sell and did not always give Diebold's products top priority.

The way around such problems is to set up wholly owned subsidiaries in foreign nations to handle local marketing, sales, and service. By doing this, the firm can exercise tight control over marketing and sales in the country while reaping the cost advantages of manufacturing the product in a single location, or a few choice locations. This was the strategy that Diebold ultimately pursued.

Turnkey Projects

Firms that specialize in the design, construction, and start-up of turnkey plants are common in some industries. In a **turnkey project,** the contractor agrees to handle every detail of the project for a foreign client, including the training of operating personnel. At completion of the contract, the foreign client is handed the "key" to a plant that is ready for full operation—hence, the term *turnkey*. This is a means of exporting process technology to other countries. Turnkey projects are most common in the chemical, pharmaceutical, petroleum refining, and metal refining industries, all of which use complex, expensive production technologies.

Advantages

The know-how required to assemble and run a technologically complex process, such as refining petroleum or steel, is a valuable asset. Turnkey projects are a way of earning great economic returns from that asset. The strategy is particularly useful where FDI is limited by host-government regulations. For example, the governments of many oil-rich countries have set out to build their own petroleum refining industries, so they restrict FDI in their oil and refining sectors. But because many of these countries lack petroleum-refining technology, they gain it by entering into turnkey projects with foreign firms that have the technology. Such deals are often attractive to the selling firm because without them, they would have no way to earn a return on their valuable know-how in that country. A turnkey strategy can also be less risky than conventional FDI. In a country with unstable political and economic environments, a longer-term investment might expose the firm to unacceptable political and/or economic risks (e.g., the risk of nationalization or of economic collapse).

Disadvantages

Three main drawbacks are associated with a turnkey strategy. First, the firm that enters into a turnkey deal will have no long-term interest in the foreign country. This can be a disadvantage if that country subsequently proves to be a major market for the output of the process that has been exported. One way around this is to take a minority equity interest in the operation. Second, the firm that enters into a turnkey project with a foreign enterprise may inadvertently create a competitor. For example, many of the Western firms that sold oil refining technology to firms in Saudi Arabia, Kuwait, and other Gulf states now find themselves competing with these firms in the world oil market. Third, if the firm's process technology is a source of competitive advantage, then selling this technology through a turnkey project is also selling competitive advantage to potential and/or actual competitors.

Licensing

A **licensing agreement** is an arrangement whereby a licensor grants the rights to intangible property to another entity (the licensee) for a specified period, and in return, the licensor receives a royalty fee from the licensee.[12] Intangible property includes patents, inventions, formulas, processes, designs, copyrights, and trademarks. For example, to enter the Japanese market, Xerox, inventor of the photocopier, established a joint venture with Fuji Photo that is known as Fuji-Xerox (for full details, see the accompanying Management Focus). Xerox then licensed its xerographic know-how to Fuji-Xerox. In return, Fuji-Xerox paid Xerox a royalty fee equal to 5 percent of the net sales revenue that Fuji-Xerox earned from the sales of photocopiers based on Xerox's patented know-how. In the Fuji-Xerox case, the license was originally granted for 10 years, and it has been renegotiated and extended several times since. The licensing agreement between Xerox and Fuji-Xerox also limited Fuji-Xerox's direct sales to the Asian Pacific region (although Fuji-Xerox does supply Xerox with photocopiers that are sold in North America under the Xerox label).[13]

Advantages

In the typical international licensing deal, the licensee puts up most of the capital necessary to get the overseas operation going. Thus, a primary advantage of licensing is that the firm does not have to bear the development costs and risks associated with opening a foreign market. Licensing is very attractive for firms lacking the capital to develop operations overseas. In addition, licensing can be attractive when a firm is unwilling to commit substantial financial resources to an unfamiliar or politically volatile foreign market. Licensing is also often used when a firm wishes to participate in a foreign market but is prohibited from doing so by barriers to investment. This was one of the original reasons for the formation of the Fuji-Xerox joint venture (see the Management Focus). Xerox wanted to participate in the Japanese market but was prohibited from setting up a wholly owned subsidiary by the Japanese government. So Xerox set up the joint venture with Fuji and then licensed its know-how to the joint venture.

Finally, licensing is frequently used when a firm possesses some intangible property that might have business applications, but it does not want to develop those applications itself. For example, Bell Laboratories at AT&T originally invented the transistor circuit in the 1950s, but AT&T decided it did not want to produce transistors, so it licensed the technology to a number of other companies, such as Texas Instruments. Similarly, Coca-Cola has licensed its famous trademark to clothing manufacturers, which have incorporated the design into their clothing.

Disadvantages

Licensing has three serious drawbacks. First, it does not give a firm the tight control over manufacturing, marketing, and strategy that is required for realizing experience curve and location economies (as global and transnational firms must do; see Chapter 12). Licensing typically involves each licensee setting up its own production operations. This severely limits the firm's ability to realize experience curve and location economies by producing its product in a centralized location. When these economies are important, licensing may not be the best way to expand overseas.

Second, competing in a global market may require a firm to coordinate strategic moves across countries by using profits earned in one country to support competitive attacks in another (see Chapter 12). By its very nature, licensing limits a firm's ability to do this. A licensee is unlikely to allow a multinational firm to use its profits (beyond those due in the form of royalty payments) to support a different licensee operating in another country.

A third problem with licensing is one that we encountered in Chapter 6 when we reviewed the economic theory of FDI. This is the risk associated with licensing technological know-how to foreign companies. Technological know-how constitutes the basis of many multinational firms' competitive advantage. Most firms wish to maintain control over how their know-how is used, and a firm can quickly lose control over its technology by licensing it. Many firms have made the mistake of thinking they could maintain control over their know-how within the framework of a licensing agreement. RCA Corporation, for example, once licensed its color TV technology to Japanese firms including Matsushita and Sony. The Japanese firms quickly assimilated the technology, improved on it, and used it to enter the U.S. market. Now the Japanese firms have a bigger share of the U.S. market than the RCA brand.

There are ways of reducing this risk. One way is by entering into a cross-licensing agreement with a foreign firm. Under a cross-licensing agreement, a firm might

The Evolution of the Fuji-Xerox Joint Venture

Fuji-Xerox is one of the most enduring and successful alliances between two companies from different countries. Established in 1962, today Fuji-Xerox is structured as a 25/75 joint venture between the Xerox Group, the U.S. maker of photocopiers, and Fuji Photo Film, Japan's largest manufacturer of film products (until 2001 Fuji Xerox was structured as a 50/50 joint venture). Fuji Xerox has revenues of about $8 billion, some 90 percent of which are generated in Japan.

The motivation to establish the joint venture was the Japanese government's refusal in the early 1960s to allow foreign companies to set up wholly owned subsidiaries in Japan. The joint venture was conceived as a marketing organization to sell xerographic products that would be manufactured by Fuji Photo under license from Xerox. However, when the Japanese government refused to approve the establishment of a joint venture intended solely as a sales company, the joint-venture agreement was revised to give Fuji-Xerox manufacturing rights. Management of the venture was placed in the hands of Japanese managers who were given autonomy to develop their own operations and strategy, subject to oversight by a board of directors that contained representatives from both Xerox and Fuji Photo.

Initially, Fuji-Xerox followed the lead of Xerox in manufacturing and selling the large high-volume copiers developed by Xerox in the United States. These machines were sold at a premium price to the high end of the market. However, Fuji-Xerox noticed that in the Japanese market, new competitors, such as Canon and Ricoh, were making significant inroads by building small, low-volume copiers and focusing on the mid- and low-priced segments of the market. This led to Fuji-Xerox's development of its first "homegrown" copier, the FX2200, which at the time was billed as the

world's smallest copier. Introduced in 1973, the FX2200 hit the market just in time to allow Fuji-Xerox to hold its own against a blizzard of new competition in Japan that followed the expiration of many of Xerox's key patents.

About the same time, Fuji-Xerox also embarked on a total quality control (TQC) program. The aims of the program were to speed up the development of new products, reduce waste, improve quality, and lower manufacturing costs. The first fruit of this program was the FX3500. Introduced in 1977, the FX3500 by 1979 had broken the Japanese record for the number of copiers sold in one year. Partly because of the success of the FX3500, in 1980 the company won Japan's prestigious Deming Prize. The success of the FX3500 was all the more notable because at the same time Xerox was canceling programs to develop low- to mid-level copiers and reaffirming its commitment to serving the high end of the market. Because of these cancellations, Tony Kobayashi, the CEO of Fuji-Xerox, was initially told to stop work on development of the FX3500. He refused, arguing that the FX3500 was crucial for the survival of Fuji-Xerox in the Japanese market. Given the arm's-length relationship between Xerox and Fuji-Xerox, Kobayashi was able to prevail.

By the 1980s, Fuji-Xerox was number two in the Japanese copier market with between 20 and 22 percent of the market, just behind that of market leader Canon. In contrast, Xerox was running into all sorts of problems in the United States. As Xerox's patents had expired, a number of companies, including Canon, Ricoh, Kodak, and IBM, began to take market share from Xerox. Canon and Ricoh were particularly successful by focusing on the low-end segment of the market, which Xerox had ignored. As a result, Xerox's market share in the Americas fell from 35 percent in 1975 to 25 percent in 1980, while its profitability slumped.

license some valuable intangible property to a foreign partner, but in addition to a royalty payment, the firm might also request that the foreign partner license some of its valuable know-how to the firm. Such agreements are believed to reduce the risks associated with licensing technological know-how, since the licensee realizes that if it violates the licensing contract (by using the knowledge obtained to compete directly with the licensor), the licensor can do the same to it. Cross-licensing agreements enable firms to hold each other hostage, which reduces the probability that they will behave opportunistically toward each other.[14] Such cross-licensing agreements are increasingly common in high-technology industries. For example, the U.S. biotechnology firm Amgen has licensed one of its key drugs, Nuprogene,

To recapture market share, Xerox began to sell Fuji-Xerox's FX3500 copier in the United States. Not only did the FX3500 help Xerox halt the rapid decline in its share of the U.S. market, but it also opened Xerox's eyes to the benefits of Fuji-Xerox's TQC program. Xerox found that the reject rate for Fuji-Xerox parts was only a fraction of the reject rate for American-produced parts. Visits to Fuji-Xerox revealed another important truth: quality in manufacturing does not increase real costs—it cuts costs by reducing defective products and service costs.

These developments forced Xerox to rethink the way it did business. From being the main provider of products, technology, and management know-how to Fuji-Xerox, Xerox in the 1980s became the willing pupil of Fuji-Xerox. In 1983, Xerox introduced its leadership through quality program, which was based on Fuji-Xerox's TQC program. As part of this effort, Xerox launched a quality training effort with its suppliers and was rewarded when the number of defective parts from suppliers subsequently fell from 25,000 per million in 1983 to 300 per million by 1992.

In 1985 and 1986, Xerox began to focus on its new product development process. One goal was to design products that, while customized to market conditions in different countries, also contained a large number of globally standardized parts. Another goal was to reduce the time it took to design new products and bring them to market. To achieve these goals, Xerox set up joint product development teams with Fuji-Xerox. Each team managed the design, component sources, manufacturing, distribution, and follow-up customer service on a worldwide basis. The use of design teams cut as much as one year from the overall product development cycle and saved millions of dollars.

One consequence of the new approach to product development was the 5100 copier. This was the first product designed jointly by Xerox and Fuji-Xerox for the worldwide market. The 5100 is manufactured in U.S. plants. It was launched in Japan in November 1990 and in the United States the following February. The 5100's global design reportedly reduced the overall time to market and saved the company more than $10 million in development costs.

As a result of the skills and products acquired from Fuji-Xerox, Xerox's position improved markedly during the 1980s and early 1990s. Due to its improved quality, lower costs, shorter product development time, and more appealing product range, Xerox was able to gain market share back from its competitors and to boost its profits and revenues. Xerox's share of the U.S. copier market increased from a low of 10 percent in 1985 to about 20 percent by 1995.

Unfortunately for Xerox, the connection with Fuji-Xerox was not enough to save the company from making a series of strategic mistakes during the second half of the 1990s, and by the early 2000s Xerox was once again a company in deep financial trouble with its market share under attack. To stave off possible bankruptcy, in 2001 Xerox sold half of its stake in Fuji-Xerox to Fuji Photo for $1.34 billion. In a testament to the importance of the joint venture, however, Xerox elected to maintain a 25 percent equity stake to be able to continue to access the technology and distribution clout of Fuji-Xerox.

Sources: R. Howard, "The CEO as Organizational Architect," Harvard Business Review, September–October 1992, pp. 106–23; D. Kearns, "Leadership through Quality," Academy of Management Executive 4 (1990), pp. 86–89; K. McQuade and B. Gomes-Casseres, "Xerox and Fuji-Xerox," Harvard Business School Case #9-391-156; E. Terazono and C. Lorenz, "An Angry Young Warrior," Financial Times, September 19, 1994, p. 11; and J. Bandler, "Xerox Will Sell Half of Its Interest in Fuji-Xerox," Wall Street Journal, March 7, 2001, p. B5.

to Kirin, the Japanese pharmaceutical company. The license gives Kirin the right to sell Nuprogene in Japan. In return, Amgen receives a royalty payment and, through a licensing agreement, gained the right to sell some of Kirin's products in the United States.

Another way of reducing the risk associated with licensing is to follow the Fuji-Xerox model and link an agreement to license know-how with the formation of a joint venture in which the licensor and licensee take important equity stakes. Such an approach aligns the interests of licensor and licensee, because both have a stake in ensuring that the venture is successful. Thus, the risk that Fuji Photo might appropriate Xerox's technological know-how, and then compete directly against Xerox in the global photocopier market, was reduced by the establishment of a joint venture in which both Xerox and Fuji Photo had an important stake.

Franchising

Franchising is similar to licensing, although franchising tends to involve longer-term commitments than licensing. **Franchising** is basically a specialized form of licensing in which the franchiser not only sells intangible property (normally a trademark) to the franchisee, but also insists that the franchisee agree to abide by strict rules as to how it does business. The franchiser will also often assist the franchisee to run the business on an ongoing basis. As with licensing, the franchiser typically receives a royalty payment, which amounts to some percentage of the franchisee's revenues. Whereas licensing is pursued primarily by manufacturing firms, franchising is employed primarily by service firms.[15] McDonald's is a good example of a firm that has grown by using a franchising strategy. McDonald's has strict rules as to how franchisees should operate a restaurant. These rules extend to control over the menu, cooking methods, staffing policies, and design and location of a restaurant. McDonald's also organizes the supply chain for its franchisees and provides management training and financial assistance.[16]

Advantages

The advantages of franchising as an entry mode are very similar to those of licensing. The firm is relieved of many of the costs and risks of opening a foreign market on its own. Instead, the franchisee typically assumes those costs and risks. This creates a good incentive for the franchisee to build a profitable operation as quickly as possible. Thus, using a franchising strategy, a service firm can build a global presence quickly and at a relatively low cost and risk, as McDonald's has.

Disadvantages

The disadvantages are less pronounced than in the case of licensing. Since franchising is often used by service companies, there is no reason to consider the need for coordination of manufacturing to achieve experience curve and location economies. But franchising may inhibit the firm's ability to take profits out of one country to support competitive attacks in another. A more significant disadvantage of franchising is quality control. The foundation of franchising arrangements is that the firm's brand name conveys a message to consumers about the quality of the firm's product. Thus, a business traveler checking in at a Hilton hotel in Hong Kong can reasonably expect the same quality of room, food, and service that she would receive in New York. The Hilton name is supposed to guarantee consistent product quality. This presents a problem in that foreign franchisees may not be as concerned about quality as they are supposed to be, and the result of poor quality can extend beyond lost sales in a particular foreign market to a decline in the firm's worldwide reputation. For example, if the business traveler has a bad experience at the Hilton in Hong Kong, she may never go to another Hilton hotel and may urge her colleagues to do likewise. The geographical distance of the firm from its foreign franchisees can make poor quality difficult to detect. In addition, the sheer numbers of franchisees—in the case of McDonald's, tens of thousands— can make quality control difficult. Due to these factors, quality problems may persist.

One way around this disadvantage is to set up a subsidiary in each country in which the firm expands. The subsidiary might be wholly owned by the company or a joint venture with a foreign company. The subsidiary assumes the rights and obligations to establish franchises throughout the particular country or region. McDonald's, for example, establishes a master franchisee in many countries. Typically, this master franchisee is a joint venture between McDonald's and a local firm. The proximity and the smaller number of franchises to oversee reduce the quality control challenge. In addition, because the subsidiary (or master franchisee) is at least partly owned by the firm, the firm can place its own managers in the subsidiary to help ensure that it is doing a good job of monitoring the franchises. This organizational arrangement has proven very satisfactory for McDonald's, KFC, Hilton Hotel Corp., and others.

Joint Ventures

A joint venture entails establishing a firm that is jointly owned by two or more otherwise independent firms. Fuji-Xerox, for example, was set up as a joint venture between Xerox and Fuji Photo (see Management Focus). Establishing a joint venture with a foreign firm has long been a popular mode for entering a new market. The most typical joint venture is a 50/50 venture, in which there are two parties, each of which holds a 50 percent ownership stake and contributes a team of managers to share operating control (this was the case with the Fuji-Xerox joint venture until 2001; it is now a 25/75 venture with Xerox holding 25 percent). Some firms, however, have sought joint ventures in which they have a majority share and thus tighter control.[17]

Advantages

Joint ventures have a number of advantages. First, a firm benefits from a local partner's knowledge of the host country's competitive conditions, culture, language, political systems, and business systems. Thus, for many U.S. firms, joint ventures have involved the U.S. company providing technological know-how and products and the local partner providing the marketing expertise and the local knowledge necessary for competing in that country. This was the case with the Fuji-Xerox joint venture. Second, when the development costs and/or risks of opening a foreign market are high, a firm might gain by sharing these costs andor risks with a local partner. Third, in many countries, political considerations make joint ventures the only feasible entry mode. Research suggests joint ventures with local partners face a low risk of being subject to nationalization or other forms of adverse government interference.[18] This appears to be because local equity partners, who may have some influence on host-government policy, have a vested interest in speaking out against nationalization or government interference.

Disadvantages

Despite these advantages, there are major disadvantages with joint ventures. First, as with licensing, a firm that enters into a joint venture risks giving control of its technology to its partner. Thus, a proposed joint venture in 2002 between Boeing and Mitsubishi Heavy Industries to build a new wide-body jet, raised fears that Boeing might unwittingly give away its commercial airline technology to the Japanese. However, joint-venture agreements can be constructed to minimize this risk. One option is to hold majority ownership in the venture. This allows the dominant partner to exercise greater control over its technology. The drawback with this is that it can be difficult to find a foreign partner who is willing to settle for minority ownership. Another option is to "wall off" from a partner technology that is central to the core competence of the firm, while sharing other technology.

A second disadvantage is that a joint venture does not give a firm the tight control over subsidiaries that it might need to realize experience curve or location economies. Nor does it give a firm the tight control over a foreign subsidiary that it might need for engaging in coordinated global attacks against its rivals. Consider the entry of Texas Instruments (TI) into the Japanese semiconductor market. When TI established semiconductor facilities in Japan, it did so for the dual purpose of checking Japanese manufacturers' market share and limiting their cash available for invading TI's global market. In other words, TI was engaging in global strategic coordination. To implement this strategy, TI's subsidiary in Japan had to be prepared to take instructions from corporate headquarters regarding competitive strategy. The strategy also required the Japanese subsidiary to run at a loss if necessary. Few if any potential joint-venture partners would have been willing to accept such conditions, since it would have necessitated a willingness to accept a negative return on investment. Indeed, many joint ventures establish a degree of autonomy that would make such direct control over strategic decisions all but impossible to establish.[19] Thus, to implement this strategy, TI set up a wholly owned subsidiary in Japan.

A third disadvantage with joint ventures is that the shared ownership arrangement can lead to conflicts and battles for control between the investing firms if their goals and objectives change or if they take different views as to what the strategy should be. This was apparently not a problem with the Fuji-Xerox joint venture. According to Tony Kobayashi, the former CEO of Fuji-Xerox, a primary reason is that both Xerox and Fuji Photo adopted an arm's-length relationship with Fuji-Xerox, giving the venture's management considerable freedom to determine its own strategy.[20] However, much research indicates that conflicts of interest over strategy and goals often arise in joint ventures. These conflicts tend to be greater when the venture is between firms of different nationalities, and they often end in the dissolution of the venture.[21] Such conflicts tend to be triggered by shifts in the relative bargaining power of venture partners. For example, in the case of ventures between a foreign firm and a local firm, as a foreign partner's knowledge about local market conditions increases, it depends less on the expertise of a local partner. This increases the bargaining power of the foreign partner and ultimately leads to conflicts over control of the venture's strategy and goals.[22]

❙Wholly Owned Subsidiaries

In a **wholly owned subsidiary,** the firm owns 100 percent of the stock. Establishing a wholly owned subsidiary in a foreign market can be done two ways. The firm either can set up a new operation in that country, often referred to as a green-field venture, or it can acquire an established firm in that host nation and use that firm to promote its products.[23] For example, as we saw in the Management Focus, ING's strategy for entering the U.S. market was to acquire established U.S. enterprises, rather than try to build an operation from the ground floor.

Advantages

There are three clear advantages of wholly owned subsidiaries. First, when a firm's competitive advantage is based on technological competence, a wholly owned subsidiary will often be the preferred entry mode, because it reduces the risk of losing control over that competence. (See Chapter 6 for more details.) Many high-tech firms prefer this entry mode for overseas expansion (e.g., firms in the semiconductor, electronics, and pharmaceutical industries). Second, a wholly owned subsidiary gives a firm tight control over operations in different countries. This is necessary for engaging in global strategic coordination (i.e., using profits from one country to support competitive attacks in another).

Third, a wholly owned subsidiary may be required if a firm is trying to realize location and experience curve economies (as firms pursuing global and transnational strategies try to do). As we saw in Chapter 12, when cost pressures are intense, it may pay a firm to configure its value chain in such a way that the value added at each stage is maximized. Thus, a national subsidiary may specialize in manufacturing only part of the product line or certain components of the end product, exchanging parts and products with other subsidiaries in the firm's global system. Establishing such a global production system requires a high degree of control over the operations of each affiliate. The various operations must be prepared to accept centrally determined decisions as to how they will produce, how much they will produce, and how their output will be priced for transfer to the next operation. Because licensees or joint-venture partners are unlikely to accept such a subservient role, establishing of wholly owned subsidiaries may be necessary.

Disadvantages

Establishing a wholly owned subsidiary is generally the most costly method of serving a foreign market from a capital investment standpoint. Firms doing this must bear the full capital costs and risks of setting up overseas operations. The risks associated with learning to do business in a new culture are less if the firm acquires an established host-country enterprise. However, acquisitions raise additional problems, including those associated with trying to marry divergent corporate cultures. These problems may more than offset any benefits derived by acquiring an established operation. Because the choice between green-field ventures and acquisitions is such an important one, we shall discuss it in more detail later in the chapter.

■ Selecting an Entry Mode

As the preceding discussion demonstrated, all the entry modes have advantages and disadvantages, as summarized in Table 14.1. Thus, trade-offs are inevitable when selecting an entry mode. For example, when considering entry into an unfamiliar country with a track record for nationalizing foreign-owned enterprises, a firm might favor a joint venture with a local enterprise. Its rationale might be that the local partner will help it establish operations in an unfamiliar environment and will speak out against nationalization should the possibility arise. However, if the firm's core competence is based on proprietary technology, entering a joint venture might risk losing control of that technology to the joint-venture partner, in which case the strategy may seem unattractive. Despite the existence of such trade-offs, it is possible to make some generalizations about the optimal choice of entry mode.[24]

Entry Mode	Advantages	Disadvantages
Exporting	Ability to realize location and experience curve economies	High transport costs Trade barriers Problems with local marketing agents
Turnkey contracts	Ability to earn returns from process technology skills in countries where FDI is restricted	Creating efficient competitors Lack of long-term market presence
Licensing	Low development costs and risks	Lack of control over technology Inability to realize location and experience curve economies Inability to engage in global strategic coordination
Franchising	Low development costs and risks	Lack of control over quality Inability to engage in global strategic coordination
Joint ventures	Access to local partner's knowledge Sharing development costs and risks Politically acceptable	Lack of control over technology Inability to engage in global strategic coordination Inability to realize location and experience economies
Wholly owned subsidiaries	Protection of technology Ability to engage in global strategic coordination Ability to realize location and experience economies	High costs and risks

Table 14.1

Advantages and Disadvantages of Entry Modes

Core Competencies and Entry Mode

We saw in Chapter 12 that firms often expand internationally to earn greater returns from their core competencies, transferring the skills and products derived from their core competencies to foreign markets where indigenous competitors lack those skills. We say that such firms are pursuing an international strategy. The optimal entry mode for these firms depends to some degree on the nature of their core competencies. A distinction can be drawn between firms whose core competency is in technological know-how and those whose core competency is in management know-how.

Technological Know-How

As was observed in Chapter 6, if a firm's competitive advantage (its core competence) is based on control over proprietary technological know-how, licensing and joint-venture arrangements should be avoided if possible to minimize the risk of losing control over that technology. Thus, if a high-tech firm sets up operations in a foreign country to profit from a core competency in technological know-how, it will probably do so through a wholly owned subsidiary. This rule should not be viewed as hard and fast, however. Sometimes a licensing or joint-venture arrangement can be structured to reduce the risk of licensees or joint-venture partners expropriating technological know-how. We will see how this might be achieved later in the chapter when we examine the structuring of strategic alliances. Another exception exists when a firm perceives its technological advantage to be only transitory, when it expects rapid imitation of its core technology by competitors. In such cases, the firm might want to license its technology as rapidly as possible to foreign firms to gain global acceptance for its technology before the imitation occurs.[25] Such a strategy has some advantages. By licensing its technology to competitors, the firm may deter them from developing their own, possibly superior, technology. Further, by licensing its technology, the firm may establish its technology as the dominant design in the industry (as Matsushita did with its VHS format for VCRs). This may ensure a steady stream of royalty payments. However, the attractions of licensing are frequently outweighed by the risks of losing control over technology and if this is a risk, licensing should be avoided.

Management Know-How

The competitive advantage of many service firms is based on management know-how (e.g., McDonald's). For such firms, the risk of losing control over the management skills to franchisees or joint-venture partners is not that great. These firms' valuable asset is their brand name, and brand names are generally well protected by international laws pertaining to trademarks. Given this, many of the issues arising in the case of technological know-how are of less concern here. As a result, many service firms favor a combination of franchising and subsidiaries to control the franchises within particular countries or regions. The subsidiaries may be wholly owned or joint ventures, but most service firms have found that joint ventures with local partners work best for the controlling subsidiaries. A joint venture is often politically more acceptable and brings a degree of local knowledge to the subsidiary.

Pressures for Cost Reductions and Entry Mode

The greater the pressures for cost reductions are, the more likely a firm will want to pursue some combination of exporting and wholly owned subsidiaries. By manufacturing in those locations where factor conditions are optimal and then exporting to the rest of the world, a firm may be able to realize substantial location and experience curve economies. The firm might then want to export the finished product to marketing subsidiaries based in various countries. These subsidiaries will typically be wholly owned and have the responsibility for overseeing distribution in their particular countries. Setting up wholly owned marketing subsidiaries is preferable to joint-venture arrangements and to using foreign marketing agents because it gives the firm tight control over marketing that might be required for coordinating a globally dispersed value chain. It also gives the firm the ability to use the profits generated in one market to improve its competitive position in another market. In other words, firms pursuing global or transnational strategies tend to prefer establishing wholly owned subsidiaries.

Establishing a Wholly Owned Subsidiary: Green-Field Venture or Acquisition? ■

A firm can establish a wholly owned subsidiary in a country by building a subsidiary from the ground up, the so-called green-field strategy, or by acquiring an enterprise in the target market. The volume of cross-border acquisitions has been growing at a rapid rate for two decades. Some 70 to 80 percent of all FDI inflows are in the form of mergers and acquisitions. In 2001, for example, mergers and acquisitions accounted for some 78 percent of all FDI inflows.[26]

❙Pros and Cons of Acquisitions

Acquisitions have three major points in their favor. First, they are quick to execute. By acquiring an established enterprise, a firm can rapidly build its presence in the target foreign market. Diebold's rapid rise in international revenues was primarily due to a number of acquisitions (see the opening case). When the German automobile company Daimler-Benz decided it needed a bigger presence in the U.S. automobile market, it did not increase that presence by building new factories to serve the United States, a process that would have taken years. Instead, it acquired the number three U.S. automobile company, Chrysler, and merged the two operations to form Daimler-Chrysler. When the Spanish telecommunications service provider Telefonica wanted to build a service presence in Latin America, it did so through a series of acquisitions, purchasing telecommunications companies in Brazil and Argentina. In all these cases, the firms made acquisitions because they knew that was the quickest way to establish a sizable presence in the target market.

Second, in many cases firms make acquisitions to preempt their competitors. The need for preemption is particularly great in markets that are rapidly globalizing, such as telecommunications, where a combination of deregulation within nations and liberalization of regulations governing cross-border foreign direct investment has made it much easier for enterprises to enter foreign markets through acquisitions. Such markets may see concentrated waves of acquisitions as firms race each other to attain global scale. In the telecommunications industry, for example, regulatory changes triggered what can be called a feeding frenzy, with firms entering each other's markets via acquisitions in order to establish a global presence. These included the $60 billion acquisition of Air Touch Communications in the United States by the British company Vodafone, which was the largest acquisition ever; the $13 billion acquisition of One 2 One in Britain by the German company Deutsche Telekom; and the $6.4 billion acquisition of Excel Communications in the United States by Teleglobe of Canada, all of which occurred in 1998 and 1999.[27] A similar wave of cross-border acquisitions occurred in the global automobile industry over the same time period, with Daimler acquiring Chrysler, Ford acquiring Volvo, and Renault acquiring Nissan.

Third, managers may believe acquisitions to be less risky than green-field ventures. When a firm makes an acquisition, it buys a set of assets that are producing a known revenue and profit stream. In contrast, the revenue and profit stream that a green-field venture might generate is uncertain because it does not yet exist. When a firm makes an acquisition in a foreign market, it not only acquires a set of tangible assets, such as factories, logistics systems, customer service systems, and so on, but it also acquires valuable intangible assets including a local brand name and managers' knowledge of the business environment in that nation. Such knowledge can reduce the risk of mistakes caused by ignorance of the national culture.

Despite the arguments for making acquisitions, acquisitions often produce disappointing results.[28] For example, a study by Mercer Management Consulting looked at 150 acquisitions worth more than $500 million each that were undertaken between January 1990 and July 1995.[29] The Mercer study concluded that 50 percent of these acquisitions ended up eroding, or substantially eroding, shareholder value, while another 33 percent created only marginal returns. Only 17 percent were judged to be successful. Similarly, a study by KPMG, an accounting and management consulting company, looked at 700 large acquisitions between 1996 and 1998. The study found that while some 30 percent of these actually created value for the acquiring company, 31 percent destroyed value, and the remainder had little impact.[30] In a major study of the postacquisition performance of acquired companies, David Ravenscraft and Mike Scherer concluded that many good companies were acquired during this period and, on average, their profits and market shares declined following acquisition.[31] They also noted that a smaller but substantial subset of those good companies experienced traumatic difficulties, which ultimately led to their being sold by the acquiring company. Ravenscraft and Scherer's evidence suggests that many acquisitions destroy rather than create value. While most of this research has looked at domestic acquisitions, the findings probably also apply to cross-border acquisitions.[32]

Why Do Acquisitions Fail?

Acquisitions fail for several reasons. First, the acquiring firms often overpay for the assets of the acquired firm. The price of the target firm can get bid up if more than one firm is interested in its purchase, as is often the case. In addition, the management of the acquiring firm is often too optimistic about the value that can be created via an acquisition and is thus willing to pay a significant premium over a target firm's market capitalization. This is called the "hubris hypothesis" of why acquisitions fail. The hubris hypothesis postulates that top managers typically overestimate their ability to create value from an acquisition, primarily because rising to the top of a corporation has given them an exaggerated sense of their own capabilities.[33] For example, Daimler acquired Chrysler in 1998 for $40 billion, a premium of 40 percent over the market value of Chrysler before the takeover bid. Daimler paid this much because it thought it could use Chrysler to help it grow market share in the United States. At the time, Daimler's management issued bold announcements about the "synergies" that would be created from combining the operations of the two companies. Executives believed they could attain greater scale economies from the global presence, take costs out of the German and U.S. operations, and boost the profitability of the combined entity. However, within a year of the acquisition, Daimler's German management was faced with a crisis at Chrysler, which was suddenly losing money due to weak sales in the United States. In retrospect, Daimler's management had been far too optimistic about the potential for future demand in the U.S. auto market and about the opportunities for creating value from "synergies." Daimler acquired Chrysler at the end of a multiyear boom in U.S. auto sales and paid a large premium over Chrysler's market value just before demand slumped.[34]

Second, many acquisitions fail because there is a clash between the cultures of the acquiring and acquired firm. After an acquisition, many acquired companies experience high management turnover, possibly because their employees do not like the acquiring company's way of doing things.[35] This happened at DaimlerChrysler; many senior managers left Chrysler in the first year after the merger. Apparently, Chrysler executives disliked the dominance in decision making by Daimler's German managers, while the Germans resented that Chrysler's American managers were paid two to three times as much as their German counterparts. These cultural differences created tensions, which ultimately exhibited themselves in high management turnover at

Chrysler.[36] The loss of management talent and expertise can materially harm the performance of the acquired unit.[37] This may be particularly problematic in an international business, where management of the acquired unit may have valuable local knowledge that can be difficult to replace.

Third, many acquisitions fail because attempts to realize synergies by integrating the operations of the acquired and acquiring entities often run into roadblocks and take much longer than forecast. Differences in management philosophy and company culture can slow the integration of operations. These problems are likely to be exacerbated by differences in national culture. Bureaucratic haggling between managers also complicates the process. Again, this reportedly occurred at DaimlerChrysler, where grand plans to integrate the operations of the two companies were bogged down by endless committee meetings and by simple logistical considerations such as the six-hour time difference between Detroit and Germany. By the time an integration plan had been worked out, Chrysler was losing money, and Daimler's German managers suddenly had a crisis on their hands.

Finally, many acquisitions fail due to inadequate preacquisition screening.[38] Many firms decide to acquire other firms without thoroughly analyzing the potential benefits and costs. They often move with undue haste to execute the acquisition, perhaps because they fear another competitor may preempt them. After the acquisition, however, many acquiring firms discover that instead of buying a well-run business, they have purchased a troubled organization. This may be a particular problem in cross-border acquisitions because the acquiring firm may not fully understand the target firm's national culture and business system.

Reducing the Risks of Failure

These problems can all be overcome if the firm is careful about its acquisition strategy.[39] Screening of the foreign enterprise to be acquired, including a detailed auditing of operations, financial position, and management culture, can help to make sure the firm (1) does not pay too much for the acquired unit, (2) does not uncover any nasty surprises after the acquisition, and (3) acquires a firm whose organization culture is not antagonistic to that of the acquiring enterprise. It is also important for the acquirer to allay any concerns that management in the acquired enterprise might have. The objective should be to reduce unwanted management attrition after the acquisition. Finally, managers must move rapidly after an acquisition to put an integration plan in place and to act on that plan. Some people in both the acquiring and acquired units will try to erect roadblocks to slow or stop any integration efforts, particularly when losses of employment or management power are involved, and managers should have a plan for dealing with such impediments before they arise.

Pros and Cons of Green-Field Ventures

The big advantage of establishing a green-field venture in a foreign country is that it gives the firm a much greater ability to build the kind of subsidiary company that it wants. For example, it is much easier to build an organization culture from scratch than it is to change the culture of an acquired unit. Similarly, it is much easier to establish a set of operating routines in a new subsidiary than it is to convert the operating routines of an acquired unit. This is a very important advantage for many international businesses, where transferring products, competencies, skills, and know-how from the established operations of the firm to the new subsidiary are principal ways of creating value. For example, when Lincoln Electric, the U.S. manufacturer of arc welding equipment, first ventured overseas in the mid-1980s, it did so by acquisitions, purchasing arc welding equipment companies in Europe. However, Lincoln's competitive advantage in the United States was based on a strong organizational culture and a unique set of incentives that encouraged its employees to do everything possible to increase productivity. Lincoln found through bitter experience that it was almost impossible to transfer its organizational culture and incentives to acquired firms, which had their own distinct organizational cultures and incentives. As a result, the firm switched its entry strategy in the mid-1990s and began to enter foreign countries by establishing green-field ventures, building operations from the ground up. While this strategy takes more time to execute, Lincoln has found that it yields greater long-run returns than the acquisition strategy.

Set against this significant advantage are the disadvantages of establishing a green-field venture. Green-field ventures are slower to establish. They are also risky. As with any new venture, a degree of uncertainty is associated with future revenue and profit prospects. However, if the firm has already been successful in other foreign markets and understands what it takes to do business in other countries, these risks may not be that great. For example, having already gained great knowledge about operating internationally, the risk to McDonald's of entering yet another country is probably not that great. Also, green-field ventures are less risky than acquisitions in the sense that there is less potential for unpleasant surprises. A final disadvantage is the possibility of being preempted by more aggressive global competitors who enter via acquisitions and build a big market presence that limits the market potential for the green-field venture.

Green-Field Venture or Acquisition?

The choice between acquisitions and green-field ventures is not an easy one to make. Both modes have their advantages and disadvantages. In general, the choice will depend on the circumstances confronting the firm. If the firm is seeking to enter a market where there are already well-established incumbent enterprises, and where global competitors are also interested in establishing a presence, it may pay the firm to enter via an acquisition. In such circumstances, a green-field venture may be too slow to establish a sizable presence. However, if the firm is going to make an acquisition, its management should be cognizant of the risks associated with acquisitions that were discussed earlier and consider these when determining which firms to purchase. It may be better to enter by the slower route of a green-field venture than to make a bad acquisition.

If the firm is considering entering a country where there are no incumbent competitors to be acquired, then a green-field venture may be the only mode. Even when incumbents exist, if the competitive advantage of the firm is based on the transfer of organizationally embedded competencies, skills, routines, and culture, it may still be preferable to enter via a green-field venture. Things such as skills and organizational culture, which are based on significant knowledge that is difficult to articulate and codify, are much easier to embed in a new venture than they are in an acquired entity, where the firm may have to overcome the established routines and culture of the acquired firm. Thus, as our earlier examples suggest, firms such as McDonald's and Lincoln Electric prefer to enter foreign markets by establishing green-field ventures.

Strategic Alliances

Strategic alliances refer to cooperative agreements between potential or actual competitors. In this section, we are concerned specifically with strategic alliances between firms from different countries. Strategic alliances run the range from formal joint ventures, in which two or more firms have equity stakes (e.g., Fuji-Xerox), to short-term contractual agreements, in which two companies agree to cooperate on a particular task (such as developing a new product). Collaboration between competitors is fashionable; recent decades have seen an explosion in the number of strategic alliances.

The Advantages of Strategic Alliances

Firms ally themselves with actual or potential competitors for various strategic purposes.[40] First, as noted earlier in the chapter, strategic alliances may facilitate entry into a foreign market. For example, Motorola initially found it very difficult to gain access to the Japanese cellular telephone market. In the mid-1980s, the firm complained loudly about formal and informal Japanese trade barriers. The turning point for Motorola came in 1987 when it allied itself with Toshiba to build microprocessors. As part of the deal, Toshiba provided Motorola with marketing help, including some of its best managers. This helped Motorola in the political game of securing government approval to enter the Japanese market and getting radio frequencies assigned for its mobile communications systems. Motorola no longer complains about Japan's trade barriers. Although privately the company admits they still exist, with Toshiba's help Motorola became skilled at getting around them.[41]

Strategic alliances also allow firms to share the fixed costs (and associated risks) of developing new products or processes. Motorola's alliance with Toshiba also was partly motivated by a desire to share the high fixed costs of setting up an operation to manufacture microprocessors. The microprocessor business is so capital intensive—Motorola and Toshiba each contributed close to $1 billion to set up their facility—that few firms can afford the costs and risks by themselves. Similarly, an alliance between Boeing and a number of Japanese companies to build the 767 was motivated by Boeing's desire to share the estimated $2 billion investment required to develop the aircraft.

Third, an alliance is a way to bring together complementary skills and assets that neither company could easily develop on its own.[42] In 2003, for example, Microsoft and Toshiba established an alliance aimed at developing embedded microprocessors (essentially tiny computers) that can perform a variety of entertainment functions in an automobile (e.g., run a back-seat DVD player or a wireless Internet connection). The processors will run a version of Microsoft's Windows CE operating system. Microsoft brings its software engineering skills to the alliance and Toshiba its skills in developing microprocessors.[43]

Fourth, it can make sense to form an alliance that will help the firm establish technological standards for the industry that will benefit the firm. For example, in 1999 Palm Computer, the leading maker of personal digital assistants (PDAs), entered into an alliance with Sony under which Sony agreed to license and use Palm's operating system in Sony PDAs. The motivation for the alliance was in part to help establish Palm's operating system as the industry standard for PDAs, as opposed to a rival Windows-based operating system from Microsoft.[44]

The Disadvantages of Strategic Alliances

The advantages we have discussed can be very significant. Despite this, some commentators have criticized strategic alliances on the grounds that they give competitors a low-cost route to new technology and markets.[45] Robert Reich and Eric Mankin have argued that many strategic alliances between U.S. and Japanese firms were part of an implicit Japanese strategy to keep higher-paying, higher-value-added jobs in Japan while gaining the project engineering and production process skills that underlie the competitive success of many U.S. companies.[46] They argued that Japanese success in the machine tool and semiconductor industries was built on U.S. technology acquired through strategic alliances. And they argued that U.S. managers were aiding the Japanese in achieving their goals by entering alliances that channel new inventions to Japan and provide a U.S. sales and distribution network for the resulting products. Although such deals may generate short-term profits, Reich and Mankin argue, in the long run the result is to "hollow out" U.S. firms, leaving them with no competitive advantage in the global marketplace.

Reich and Mankin have a point. Alliances have risks. Unless a firm is careful, it can give away more than it receives. But there are so many examples of apparently successful alliances between firms—including alliances between U.S. and Japanese firms—that their position seems extreme. It is difficult to see how the Motorola-Toshiba alliance or the Fuji-Xerox alliance fit Reich and Mankin's thesis. In these cases, both partners seem to have gained from the alliance. Why do some alliances benefit both firms while others benefit one firm and hurt the other? The next section provides an answer to this question.

Making Alliances Work

The failure rate for international strategic alliances seems to be high. One study of 49 international strategic alliances found that two-thirds run into serious managerial and financial troubles within two years of their formation, and that although many of these problems are solved, 33 percent are ultimately rated as failures by the parties involved.[47] The success of an alliance seems to be a function of three main factors: partner selection, alliance structure, and the manner in which the alliance is managed.

Partner Selection

One key to making a strategic alliance work is to select the right ally. A good ally, or partner, has three characteristics. First, a good partner helps the firm achieve its strategic goals, whether they are market access, sharing the costs and risks of product development, or gaining access to critical core competencies. The partner must have capabilities that the firm lacks and that it values. Second, a good partner shares the firm's vision for the purpose of the alliance. If two firms approach an alliance with radically different agendas, the chances are great that the relationship will not be harmonious, will not flourish, and will end in divorce. Third, a good partner is unlikely to try to opportunistically exploit the alliance for its own ends; that is, to expropriate the firm's technological know-how while giving away little in return. In this respect, firms with reputations for "fair play" to maintain probably make the best allies. For example, IBM is involved in so many strategic alliances that it would not pay the company to trample over individual alliance partners (in early 2003 IBM reportedly had more than 150 major strategic alliances).[48] This would tarnish IBM's reputation of being a good ally and would make it more difficult for IBM to attract alliance partners. Because IBM attaches great importance to its alliances, it is unlikely to engage in the kind of opportunistic behavior that Reich and Mankin highlight. Similarly, their reputations make it less likely (but by no means impossible) that such Japanese firms as Sony, Toshiba, and Fuji, which have histories of alliances with non-Japanese firms, would opportunistically exploit an alliance partner.

To select a partner with these three characteristics, a firm needs to conduct comprehensive research on potential alliance candidates. To increase the probability of selecting a good partner, the firm should:

1. Collect as much pertinent, publicly available information on potential allies as possible.
2. Collect data from informed third parties. These include firms that have had alliances with the potential partners, investment bankers who have had dealings with them, and former employees.
3. Get to know the potential partner as well as possible before committing to an alliance. This should include face-to-face meetings between senior managers (and perhaps middle-level managers) to ensure that the chemistry is right.

Alliance Structure

Having selected a partner, the alliance should be structured so that the firm's risks of giving too much away to the partner are reduced to an acceptable level. Figure 14.1 depicts four safeguards against opportunism by alliance partners. (Opportunism includes the theft of technology and/or markets that Reich and Mankin describe.) First, alliances can be designed to make it difficult (if not impossible) to transfer technology not meant to be transferred. The design, development, manufacture, and service of a

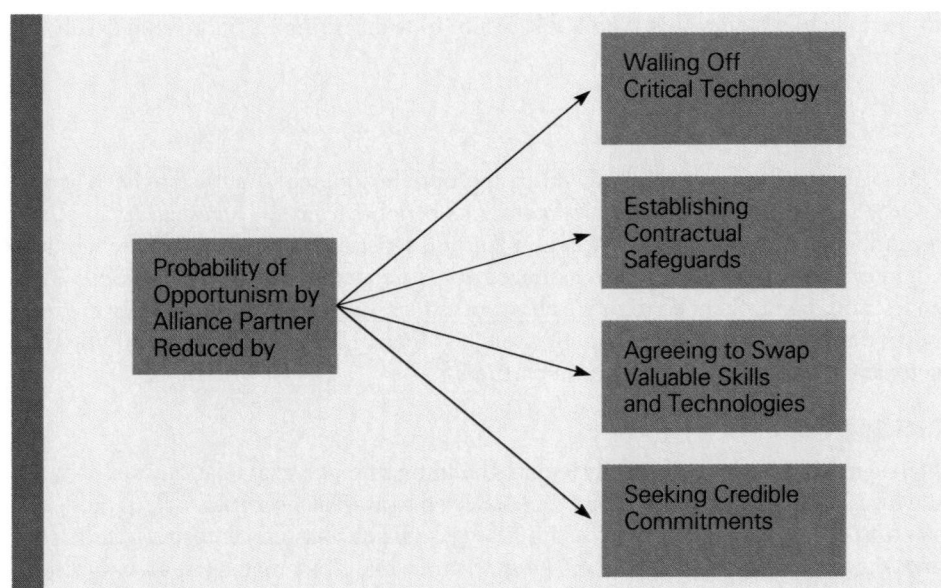

Figure 14.1

Structuring Alliances to
Reduce Opportunism

product manufactured by an alliance can be structured so as to wall off sensitive technologies to prevent their leakage to the other participant. In an alliance between General Electric and Snecma to build commercial aircraft engines, for example, GE reduced the risk of excess transfer by walling off certain sections of the production process. The modularization effectively cut off the transfer of what GE regarded as key competitive technology, while permitting Snecma access to final assembly. Similarly, in the alliance between Boeing and the Japanese to build the 767, Boeing walled off research, design, and marketing functions considered central to its competitive position, while allowing the Japanese to share in production technology. Boeing also walled off new technologies not required for 767 production.[49]

Second, contractual safeguards can be written into an alliance agreement to guard against the risk of opportunism by a partner. For example, TRW, Inc., has three strategic alliances with large Japanese auto component suppliers to produce seat belts, engine valves, and steering gears for sale to Japanese-owned auto assembly plants in the United States. TRW has clauses in each of its alliance contracts that bar the Japanese firms from competing with TRW to supply U.S.-owned auto companies with component parts. By doing this, TRW protects itself against the possibility that the Japanese companies are entering into the alliances merely to gain access to the North American market to compete with TRW in its home market.

Third, both parties to an alliance can agree in advance to swap skills and technologies that the other covets, thereby ensuring a chance for equitable gain. Cross-licensing agreements are one way to achieve this goal. For example, in the alliance between Motorola and Toshiba, Motorola has licensed some of its microprocessor technology to Toshiba, and in return, Toshiba has licensed some of its memory chip technology to Motorola.

Fourth, the risk of opportunism by an alliance partner can be reduced if the firm extracts a significant credible commitment from its partner in advance. The long-term alliance between Xerox and Fuji to build photocopiers for the Asian market perhaps best illustrates this. Rather than enter into an informal agreement or a licensing arrangement (which Fuji Photo initially wanted), Xerox insisted that Fuji invest in a 50/50 joint venture to serve Japan and East Asia. This venture constituted such a significant investment in people, equipment, and facilities that Fuji Photo was committed from the outset to making the alliance work in order to earn a return on its investment. By agreeing to the joint venture, Fuji essentially made a credible commitment to the alliance. Given this, Xerox felt secure in transferring its photocopier technology to Fuji.[50]

Managing the Alliance

Once a partner has been selected and an appropriate alliance structure has been agreed on, the task facing the firm is to maximize its benefits from the alliance. As in all international business deals, an important factor is sensitivity to cultural differences (see Chapter 3). Many differences in management style are attributable to cultural differences, and managers need to make allowances for these in dealing with their partner. Beyond this, maximizing the benefits from an alliance seems to involve building trust between partners and learning from partners.[51]

Building Trust

Managing an alliance successfully requires building interpersonal relationships between the firms' managers, or what is sometimes referred to as *relational capital*.[52] This is one lesson that can be drawn from a successful strategic alliance between Ford and Mazda. Ford and Mazda set up a framework of meetings within which their managers not only discuss matters pertaining to the alliance but also have time to get to know each other better. The belief is that the resulting friendships help build trust and facilitate harmonious relations between the two firms. Personal relationships also foster an informal management network between the firms. (Chapter 13 discusses informal management networks.) This network can then be used to help solve problems arising in more formal contexts (such as in joint committee meetings between personnel from the two firms).

Learning from Partners

Academics have argued that a major determinant of how much acquiring knowledge a company gains from an alliance is its ability to learn from its alliance partner.[53] For example, in a five-year study of 15 strategic alliances between major multinationals, Gary Hamel, Yves Doz, and C. K. Prahalad focused on a number of alliances between Japanese companies and Western (European or American) partners.[54] In every case in which a Japanese company emerged from an alliance stronger than its Western partner, the Japanese company had made a greater effort to learn. Few Western companies studied seemed to want to learn from their Japanese partners. They tended to regard the alliance purely as a cost-sharing or risk-sharing device, rather than as an opportunity to learn how a potential competitor does business.

Consider the alliance between General Motors and Toyota constituted in 1985 to build the Chevrolet Nova. This alliance was structured as a formal joint venture, called New United Motor Manufacturing, Inc., and each party had a 50 percent equity stake. The venture owned an auto plant in Fremont, California. According to one Japanese manager, Toyota quickly achieved most of its objectives from the alliance: "We learned about U.S. supply and transportation. And we got the confidence to manage U.S. workers."[55] All that knowledge was then transferred to Georgetown, Kentucky, where Toyota opened its own plant in 1988. On the other hand, possibly all GM got was a new product, the Chevrolet Nova. Some GM managers complained that the knowledge they gained through the alliance with Toyota has never been put to good use inside GM. They believe they should have been kept together as a team to educate GM's engineers and workers about the Japanese system. Instead, they were dispersed to various GM subsidiaries.

To maximize the learning benefits of an alliance, a firm must try to learn from its partner and then apply the knowledge within its own organization. It has been suggested that all operating employees should be well briefed on the partner's strengths and weaknesses and should understand how acquiring particular skills will bolster their firm's competitive position. Hamel, Doz, and Prahalad note that this is already standard practice among Japanese companies. They made this observation:

We accompanied a Japanese development engineer on a tour through a partner's factory. This engineer dutifully took notes on plant layout, the number of production stages, the rate at which the line was running, and the number of employees. He recorded all this despite the fact that he had no manufacturing responsibility in his own company, and that the alliance did not encompass joint manufacturing. Such dedication greatly enhances learning.[56]

For such learning to be of value, it must be diffused throughout the organization (as was seemingly not the case at GM after the GM-Toyota joint venture). To achieve this, the managers involved in the alliance should educate their colleagues about the skills of the alliance partner.

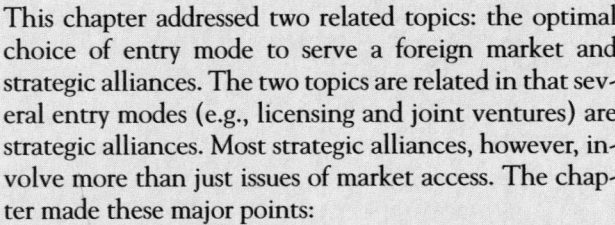

ChapterSummary

This chapter addressed two related topics: the optimal choice of entry mode to serve a foreign market and strategic alliances. The two topics are related in that several entry modes (e.g., licensing and joint ventures) are strategic alliances. Most strategic alliances, however, involve more than just issues of market access. The chapter made these major points:

1. Basic entry decisions include identifying which markets to enter, when to enter those markets, and on what scale.

2. The most attractive foreign markets tend to be found in politically stable developed and developing nations that have free market systems and where there is not a dramatic upsurge in either inflation rates or private-sector debt.

3. There are several advantages associated with entering a national market early, before other international businesses have established themselves. These advantages must be balanced against the pioneering costs that early entrants often have to bear, including the greater risk of business failure.

4. Large-scale entry into a national market constitutes a major strategic commitment that is likely to change the nature of competition in that market and limit the entrant's future strategic flexibility. The firm needs to think through the implications of such commitments before embarking on a large-scale entry. Although making major strategic commitments can yield many benefits, there are also risks associated with such a strategy.

5. There are six modes of entering a foreign market: exporting, creating turnkey projects, licensing, franchising, establishing joint ventures, and setting up a wholly owned subsidiary.

6. Exporting has the advantages of facilitating the realization of experience curve economies and of avoiding the costs of setting up manufacturing operations in another country. Disadvantages include high transport costs, trade barriers, and problems with local marketing agents. The latter can be overcome if the firm sets up a wholly owned marketing subsidiary in the host country.

7. Turnkey projects allow firms to export their process know-how to countries where FDI might be prohibited, thereby enabling the firm to earn a greater return from this asset. The disadvantage is that the firm may inadvertently create efficient global competitors in the process.

8. The main advantage of licensing is that the licensee bears the costs and risks of opening a foreign market. Disadvantages include the risk of losing technological know-how to the licensee and a lack of tight control over licensees.

9. The main advantage of franchising is that the franchisee bears the costs and risks of opening a foreign market. Disadvantages center on problems of quality control of distant franchisees.

10. Joint ventures have the advantages of sharing the costs and risks of opening a foreign market and of gaining local knowledge and political influence. Disadvantages include the risk of losing control over technology and a lack of tight control.

11. The advantages of wholly owned subsidiaries include tight control over technological know-how. The main disadvantage is that the firm must bear all the costs and risks of opening a foreign market.

12. The optimal choice of entry mode depends on the firm's strategy.

13. When technological know-how constitutes a firm's core competence, wholly owned

subsidiaries are preferred, since they best control technology.

14. When management know-how constitutes a firm's core competence, foreign franchises controlled by joint ventures seem to be optimal. This gives the firm the cost and risk benefits associated with franchising, while enabling it to monitor and control franchisee quality effectively.

15. When the firm is pursuing a global or transnational strategy, the need for tight control over operations to realize location and experience curve economies suggests wholly owned subsidiaries are the best entry mode.

16. When establishing a wholly owned subsidiary in a country, a firm must decide whether to do so by building a subsidiary from the ground up, the so-called green-field venture strategy, or by acquiring an established enterprise in the target market.

17. Relative to green-field ventures, acquisitions are quick to execute, may enable a firm to preempt its global competitors, and involve buying a known revenue and profit stream.

18. Acquisitions may fail when the acquiring firm overpays for the target, when the culture of the acquiring and acquired firms clash, when there is a high level of management attrition after the acquisition, and when there is a failure to integrate the operations of the acquiring and acquired firm.

19. The advantage of establishing a green-field venture in a foreign country is that it gives the firm a much greater ability to build the kind of subsidiary company that it wants. For example, it is much easier to build an organization culture from scratch than it is to change the culture of an acquired unit.

20. Strategic alliances are cooperative agreements between actual or potential competitors.

21. The advantage of alliances are that they facilitate entry into foreign markets, enable partners to share the fixed costs and risks associated with new products and processes, facilitate the transfer of complementary skills between companies, and help firms establish technical standards.

22. The disadvantage of a strategic alliance is that the firm risks giving away technological know-how and market access to its alliance partner in return for very little.

23. The disadvantages associated with alliances can be reduced if the firm selects partners carefully, paying close attention to the firm's reputation and the structure of the alliance so as to avoid unintended transfers of know-how.

24. Two keys to making alliances work seem to be building trust and informal communications networks between partners and taking proactive steps to learn from alliance partners.

Critical Discussion Questions

1. Review the Management Focus on ING. ING chose to enter the U.S. financial services market via acquisitions rather than green-field ventures. What do you think are the advantages to ING of doing this? What might the drawbacks be? Does this strategy make sense? Why?

2. Licensing proprietary technology to foreign competitors is the best way to give up a firm's competitive advantage. Discuss.

3. What kinds of companies stand to gain the most from entering into strategic alliances with potential competitors? Why?

4. Discuss how the need for control over foreign operations varies with firms' strategies and core competencies. What are the implications for the choice of entry mode?

5. A small Canadian firm that has developed some valuable new medical products using its unique biotechnology know-how is trying to decide how best to serve the European Community market. Its choices are:

   a. Manufacture the product at home and let foreign sales agents handle marketing.

   b. Manufacture the products at home and set up a wholly owned subsidiary in Europe to handle marketing.

   c. Enter into a strategic alliance with a large European pharmaceutical firm. The product would be manufactured in Europe by the 50/50 joint venture and marketed by the European firm.

The cost of investment in manufacturing facilities will be a major one for the Canadian firm, but it is not outside its reach. If these are the firm's only options, which one would you advise it to choose? Why?

Notes

1. For interesting empirical studies that deal with the issues of timing and resource commitments, see T. Isobe, S. Makino, and D. B. Montgomery, "Resource Commitment, Entry Timing, and Market Performance of Foreign Direct Investments in Emerging Economies," *Academy of Management Journal* 43, no. 3 (2000), pp. 468–84, and Y. Pan and P. S. K. Chi, "Financial Performance and Survival of Multinational Corporations in China," *Strategic Management Journal* 20, no. 4, (1999), pp. 359–74. A complementary theoretical perspective on this issue can be found in V. Govindarjan and A. K. Gupta, *The Quest for Global Dominance* (San Francisco: Jossey Bass, 2001). Also see F. Vermeulen and H. Barkeme, "Pace, Rhythm and Scope: Process Dependence in Building a Profitable Multinational Corporation," *Strategic Management Journal* 23 (2002), pp. 637–54.

2. This can be reconceptualized as the resource base of the entrant, relative to indigenous competitors. For work that focuses on this issue, see W. C. Bogenr, H. Thomas, and J. McGee, "A Longitudinal Study of the Competitive Positions and Entry Paths of European Firms in the U.S. Pharmaceutical Market," *Strategic Management Journal* 17 (1996), pp. 85–107; D. Collis, "A Resource-Based Analysis of Global Competition," *Strategic Management Journal* 12 (1991), pp. 49–68; and S. Tallman, "Strategic Management Models and Resource-Based Strategies among MNEs in a Host Market," *Strategic Management Journal* 12 (1991), pp. 69–82

3. For a discussion of first-mover advantages, see M. Liberman and D. Montgomery, "First-Mover Advantages," *Strategic Management Journal* 9 (Summer Special Issue, 1988), pp. 41–58.

4. J. M. Shaver, W. Mitchell, and B. Yeung, "The Effect of Own Firm and Other Firm Experience on Foreign Direct Investment Survival in the United States, 1987–92," *Strategic Management Journal* 18 (1997), pp. 811–24.

5. S. Zaheer and E. Mosakowski, "The Dynamics of the Liability of Foreignness: A Global Study of Survival in the Financial Services Industry," *Strategic Management Journal* 18 (1997), pp. 439–64.

6. Shaver, Mitchell, and Yeung, "The Effect of Own Firm and Other Firm Experience on Foreign Direct Investment Survival in the United States."

7. P. Ghemawat, *Commitment: The Dynamics of Strategy* (New York: Free Press, 1991).

8. R. Luecke, *Scuttle Your Ships before Advancing* (Oxford: Oxford University Press, 1994).

9. Isobe, Makino, and Montgomery, "Resource Commitment, Entry Timing, and Market Performance"; Pan and Chi, "Financial Performance and Survival of Multinational Corporations in China"; and Govindarjan and Gupta, *The Quest for Global Dominance*.

10. Christopher Bartlett and Sumantra Ghoshal, "Going Global: Lessons from Late Movers," *Harvard Business Review*, March–April 2000, pp. 132–45.

11. This section draws on several studies, including: C. W. L. Hill, P. Hwang, and W. C. Kim, "An Eclectic Theory of the Choice of International Entry Mode," *Strategic Management Journal* 11 (1990), pp. 117–28; C. W. L. Hill and W. C. Kim, "Searching for a Dynamic Theory of the Multinational Enterprise: A Transaction Cost Model," *Strategic Management Journal* 9 (Special Issue on Strategy Content, 1988), pp. 93–104; E. Anderson and H. Gatignon, "Modes of Foreign Entry: A Transaction Cost Analysis and Propositions," *Journal of International Business Studies* 17 (1986), pp. 1–26; F. R. Root, *Entry Strategies for International Markets* (Lexington, MA: D. C. Heath, 1980); A. Madhok, "Cost, Value and Foreign Market Entry: The Transaction and the Firm," *Strategic Management Journal* 18 (1997), pp. 39–61; and K. D. Brouthers and L. B. Brouthers, "Acquisition or Greenfield Start-up?" *Strategic Management Journal* 21, no. 1 (2000), pp. 89–97.

12. For a general discussion of licensing, see F. J. Contractor, "The Role of Licensing in International Strategy," *Columbia Journal of World Business*, Winter 1982, pp. 73–83.

13. See E. Terazono and C. Lorenz, "An Angry Young Warrior," *Financial Times*, September 19, 1994, p. 11, and K. McQuade and B. Gomes-Casseres, "Xerox and Fuji-Xerox," Harvard Business School Case #9-391-156.

14. O. E. Williamson, *The Economic Institutions of Capitalism*, (New York: Free Press, 1985).

15. J. H. Dunning and M. McQueen, "The Eclectic Theory of International Production: A Case Study of the International Hotel Industry," *Managerial and Decision Economics* 2 (1981), pp. 197–210.

16. Andrew E. Serwer, "McDonald's Conquers the World," *Fortune*, October 17, 1994, pp. 103–16.

17. For an excellent review of the basic theoretical literature of joint ventures, see B. Kogut, "Joint Ventures: Theoretical and Empirical Perspectives," *Strategic Management Journal* 9 (1988), pp. 319–32. More recent studies include T. Chi, "Option to Acquire or Divest a Joint Venture," *Strategic Management Journal* 21, no. 6 (2000), pp. 665–88; H. Merchant and D. Schendel, "How Do International Joint Ventures Create Shareholder Value?" *Strategic Management Journal* 21, no. 7, (2000), pp. 723–37; and H. K. Steensma and M. A. Lyles, "Explaining IJV Survival in a Transitional Economy though Social Exchange and Knowledge Based Perspectives," *Strategic Management Journal* 21, no. 8 (2000), pp. 831–51.

18. D. G. Bradley, "Managing against Expropriation," *Harvard Business Review*, July–August 1977, pp. 78–90.

19. J. A. Robins, S. Tallman, and K. Fladmoe-Lindquist, "Autonomy and Dependence of International Cooperative Ventures," *Strategic Management Journal* (October 2002), pp. 881–902.

20. Speech given by Tony Kobayashi at the University of Washington Business School, October 1992.

21. A. C. Inkpen and P. W. Beamish, "Knowledge, Bargaining Power, and the Instability of International Joint Ventures," *Academy of Management Review* 22 (1997), pp. 177–202, and S. H. Park and G. R. Ungson, "The Effect of National Culture, Organizational Complementarity, and Economic Motivation on Joint Venture Dissolution," *Academy of Management Journal* 40 (1997), pp. 279–307.

22. Inkpen and Beamish, "Knowledge, Bargaining Power, and the Instability of International Joint Ventures."

23. See Brouthers and Brouthers, "Acquisition or Greenfield Start-up?" and J. F. Hennart and Y. R. Park, "Greenfield versus Acquisition: The Strategy of Japanese Investors in the United States," *Management Science*, 1993, pp. 1054–70.

24. This section draws on Hill, Hwang, and Kim, "An Eclectic Theory of the Choice of International Entry Mode."

25. C. W. L. Hill, "Strategies for Exploiting Technological Innovations: When and When Not to License," *Organization Science* 3 (1992), pp. 428–41.

26. United Nations, *World Investment Report, 2002* (New York and Geneva: United Nations, 2002).

27. Ibid.

28. For evidence on acquisitions and performance, see R. E. Caves, "Mergers, Takeovers, and Economic Efficiency," *International Journal of Industrial Organization* 7 (1989), pp. 151–74; M. C. Jensen and R. S. Ruback, "The Market for Corporate Control: The Scientific Evidence," *Journal of Financial Economics* 11 (1983), pp. 5–50; R. Roll, "Empirical Evidence on Takeover Activity and Shareholder Wealth," in *Knights, Raiders and Targets*, ed. J. C. Coffee, L. Lowenstein, and S. Rose (Oxford: Oxford University Press, 1989); A. Schleifer and R. W. Vishny, "Takeovers in the 60s and 80s: Evidence and Implications," *Strategic Management Journal* 12 (Winter 1991 Special Issue), pp. 51–60; T. H. Brush, "Predicted Changes in Operational Synergy and Post Acquisition Performance of Acquired Businesses," *Strategic Management Journal* 17 (1996), pp. 1–24; and A. Seth, K. P. Song and R. R. Pettit, "Value Creation and Destruction in Cross Border Acquisitions," *Strategic Management Journal* 23 (October 2002), pp. 921–40.

29. J. Warner, J. Templeman, R. Horn, "The Case against Mergers," *Business Week*, October 30, 1995, pp. 122–34.

30. "Few Takeovers Pay Off for Big Buyers," *Investors Business Daily*, May 25, 2001, p. 1.

31. D. J. Ravenscraft and F. M. Scherer, *Mergers, Selloffs, and Economic Efficiency* (Washington, DC: Brookings Institution, 1987).

32. See P. Ghemawat and F. Ghadar, "The Dubious Logic of Global Mega-mergers," *Harvard Business Review*, July–August 2000, pp. 65–72.

33. R. Roll, "The Hubris Hypothesis of Corporate Takeovers," *Journal of Business* 59 (1986), pp. 197–216.

34. "Marital Problems," *The Economist*, October 14, 2000.

35. See J. P. Walsh, "Top Management Turnover Following Mergers and Acquisitions," *Strategic Management Journal* 9 (1988), pp. 173–83.

36. B. Vlasic and B. A. Stertz, *Taken for a Ride: How Daimler-Benz Drove Off with Chrysler* (New York: HarperCollins, 2000).

37. See A. A. Cannella and D. C. Hambrick, "Executive Departure and Acquisition Performance," *Strategic Management Journal* 14 (1993), pp. 137–52.

38. P. Haspeslagh and D. Jemison, *Managing Acquisitions* (New York: Free Press, 1991).

39. Ibid.

40. See K. Ohmae, "The Global Logic of Strategic Alliances," *Harvard Business Review*, March–April 1989, pp. 143–54; G. Hamel, Y. L. Doz, and

C. K. Prahalad, "Collaborate with Your Competitors and Win!" *Harvard Business Review*, January–February 1989, pp. 133–39; W. Burgers, C. W. L. Hill, and W. C. Kim, "Alliances in the Global Auto Industry," *Strategic Management Journal* 14 (1993), pp. 419–32; and P. Kale, H. Singh, H. Perlmutter, "Learning and Protection of Proprietary Assets in Strategic Alliances: Building Relational Capital," *Strategic Management Journal* 21 (2000), pp. 217–37.

41. "Asia Beckons," *The Economist*, May 30, 1992, pp. 63–64.

42. J. W. Spencer, "Firms' Knowledge Sharing Strategies in the Global Innovation System," *Strategic Management Journal* 24 (2003), pp. 217–33.

43. C. Souza, "Microsoft Teams with MIPS, Toshiba," *EBN*, February 10, 2003, p. 4.

44. M. Frankel, "Now Sony Is Giving Palm a Hand," *Business Week*, November 29, 2000, p. 50.

45. Kale, Singh, and Perlmutter, "Learning and Protection of Proprietary Assets."

46. R. B. Reich and E. D. Mankin, "Joint Ventures with Japan Give Away Our Future," *Harvard Business Review*, March–April 1986, pp. 78–90.

47. J. Bleeke and D. Ernst, "The Way to Win in Cross-Border Alliances," *Harvard Business Review*, November–December 1991, pp. 127–35.

48. E. Booker and C. Krol, "IBM Finds Strength in Alliances," *B to B*, February 10, 2003, pp. 3, 27.

49. W. Roehl and J. F. Truitt, "Stormy Open Marriages Are Better," *Columbia Journal of World Business*, Summer 1987, pp. 87–95.

50. McQuade and Gomes-Casseres, "Xerox and Fuji-Xerox."

51. See T. Khanna, R. Gulati, and N. Nohria, "The Dynamics of Learning Alliances: Competition, Cooperation, and Relative Scope," *Strategic Management Journal* 19 (1998), pp. 193–210, and Kale, Singh, and Perlmutter, "Learning and Protection of Proprietary Assets."

52. Kale, Singh, and Perlmutter, "Learning and Protection of Proprietary Assets."

53. Hamel, Doz, and Prahalad, "Collaborate with Competitors"; Khanna, Gulati, and Nohria, "The Dynamics of Learning Alliances: Competition, Cooperation, and Relative Scope"; and E. W. K. Tang, "Acquiring Knowledge by Foreign Partners from International Joint Ventures in a Transition Economy: Learning by Doing and Learning Myopia," *Strategic Management Journal*, 23, 2002, pp. 835–854.

54. Hamel, Doz, and Prahalad, "Collaborate with Competitors."

55. B. Wysocki, "Cross-Border Alliances Become Favorite Way to Crack New Markets," *Wall Street Journal*, March 4, 1990, p. A1.

56. Hamel, Doz, and Prahalad, "Collaborate with Competitors," p. 138.

Research Task | globalEDGE™   globaledge.msu.edu

Use the global EDGE™ site to complete the following exercises:

1. *The Entrepreneur* magazine annually publishes a list of its ranking of America's top 200 franchisors seeking international franchisees. Provide a list of the top 10 companies that pursue franchising as a mode of international expansion. Study one of these companies in detail and provide a description of its business model, its international expansion pattern, what qualifications it looks for in its franchisees, and what type of support and training it provides.

2. The U.S. Commercial Service prepares reports titled the "Country Commercial Guide" for each country of interest to U.S. Investors. Utilize the Country Commercial Guide for Brazil to gather information on this country. Considering that your company is producing laptop computers and is considering entering this country, select the most appropriate entry method, supporting your decision with the information collected from the commercial guide.

Merrill Lynch in Japan

Merrill Lynch is an investment banking titan. The U.S.-based financial services institution is the world's largest underwriter of debt and equity and the third largest mergers and acquisitions adviser behind Morgan Stanley and Goldman Sachs. Merrill Lynch's investment banking operations have long had a global reach. The company has a dominant presence in London and Tokyo. However, Merrill Lynch's international presence was limited to the investment banking side of its business until recently. In contrast, its private client business, which offers banking, financial advice, and stockbrokerage services to individuals, had historically been concentrated in the United States. This started to change in the mid-1990s. In 1995, Merrill Lynch purchased Smith New Court, the largest stockbrokerage in Great Britain. This was followed in 1997 by the acquisition of Mercury Asset Management, the United Kingdom's leading manager of mutual funds. Then in 1998, Merrill Lynch acquired Midland Walwyn, Canada's last major independent stockbrokerage. The company's boldest moves, however, have probably been in Japan.

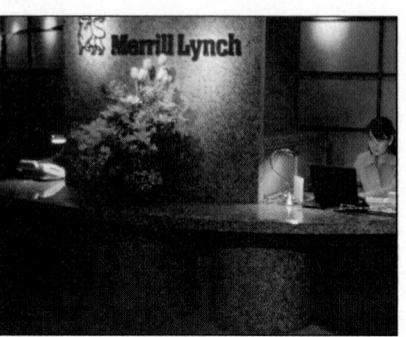

Merrill Lynch started a private client business in Japan in the 1980s but met with limited success. At the time, it was the first foreign firm to enter Japan's private client investment market. The company found it extremely difficult to attract employee talent and customers away from Japan's big four stockbrokerages, which traditionally had monopolized the Japanese market. Plus, restrictive regulations made it almost impossible for Merrill Lynch to offer its Japanese private clients the range of services it offered clients in the United States. For example, foreign exchange regulations meant it was very difficult to sell non-Japanese stocks, bonds, and mutual funds to Japanese investors. In 1993, Merrill Lynch admitted defeat, closed its six retail branches in Kobe and Kyoto, and withdrew from the private client market in Japan.

Over the next few years, however, things changed. In the mid-1990s, Japan embarked on a wide-ranging deregulation of its financial services industry. This led to the removal of many of the restrictions that had made it so difficult for Merrill Lynch to do business in Japan. For example, the relaxation of foreign exchange controls meant that by 1998, Japanese citizens could purchase foreign stocks, bonds, and mutual funds. Meanwhile,

Japan's big four stockbrokerages continued to struggle with serious financial problems that resulted from the 1991 crash of that country's stock market. In November 1997, in what was a shock to many Japanese, one of these firms, Yamaichi Securities, declared it was bankrupt due to $2.2 billion in accumulated "hidden losses" and that it would shut its doors. Recognizing the country's financial system was strained and in need of fresh capital, know-how, and the stimulus of greater competition, the Japanese government signaled that it would adopt a more relaxed attitude to foreign entry into its financial services industry. This attitude underlay Japan's wholehearted endorsement of a 1997 deal brokered by the World Trade Organization to liberalize global financial services. Among other things, the WTO deal made it much easier for foreign firms to sell financial service products to Japanese investors.

By 1997, it had become clear to Merrill Lynch that the climate in Japan had changed significantly. The big attraction of the market was still the same: the financial assets owned by Japanese households are huge, amounting to ¥1,220 trillion in late 1997, only 3 percent of which were then invested in mutual funds (most are invested in low-yielding bank accounts and government bonds). In mid-1997, Merrill Lynch started to consider reentering the Japanese private client market.

The company initially considered a joint venture with Sanwa Bank to sell Merrill Lynch's mutual fund products to Japanese consumers through Sanwa's 400 retail branches. The proposed alliance would have allowed Merrill Lynch to leverage Sanwa's existing distribution system, rather than having to build its own distribution system. However, the long-run disadvantage of such a strategy was that it would not have given Merrill Lynch the presence that it believed it needed to build a solid financial services business in Japan. Top executives reasoned that it was important for them to make a major commitment to the Japanese market to establish the company's brand name as a premier provider of investment products and financial advice to individuals. This would enable Merrill Lynch to entrench itself as a major player before other foreign institutions entered the market—and before Japan's own stockbrokerages rose to the challenge. At the same time, given their prior experience in Japan, Merrill Lynch executives were hesitant to go down this road because of the huge costs and risks involved.

The problem of how best to enter the Japanese market was solved by the bankruptcy of Yamaichi Securities. Suddenly Yamaichi's nationwide network of offices and 7,000 employees were up for grabs. In late December 1997, Merrill Lynch announced it would hire 2,000 of Yamaichi's employees and acquire 33 of Yamaichi's branch offices. The deal, which was enthusiastically endorsed by the Japanese government, significantly lowered Merrill Lynch's costs of establishing a retail network in Japan.

The company got off to a quick start. In February 1998, Merrill Lynch launched its first mutual fund in Japan and saw the value of its assets swell to $1 billion by April. By mid-2002, Merrill Lynch announced it had $12.9 billion under management in Japan. However, the collapse in global stock markets in 2001–02 hit Merrill's Japanese unit hard. After losing $500 million in Japan on its investment, in January 2002 the company fired 75 percent of its Japanese workforce and closed all but eight of its retail locations. Despite this costly downsizing, the company held onto almost all of the assets under management, continued to attract new accounts, and by mid-2002 was reportedly making a profit in Japan.

Sources: "Japan's Big Bang. Enter Merrill," *The Economist*, January 3, 1998, p. 72; J. P. Donlon, "Merrill Cinch," *Chief Executive*, March 1998, pp. 28–32; D. Holley, "Merrill Lynch to Open 31 Offices throughout Japan," *Los Angeles Times*, February 13, 1998, p. D1; A. Rowley, "Merrill Thunders into Japan," *The Banker*, March 1998, p. 6; J. Singer, "Merrill Reports Profits for Operation in Japan," *Wall Street Journal*, July 19, 2002, p. A9; and Merrill Lynch's website, www.ml.com.

Case Discussion Questions

1. Given the changes that have occurred in the international capital markets during the past decade, does Merrill Lynch's strategy of expanding internationally make sense? Why?

2. What factors make Japan a suitable market for Merrill Lynch to enter?

3. Review Merrill Lynch's 1997 reentry into the Japanese private client market. Pay close attention to the timing and scale of entry and the nature of the strategic commitments Merrill Lynch is making in Japan. What are the potential benefits associated with this strategy? What are the costs and risks? Do you think the trade-off between benefits and risks and costs makes sense? Why?

4. The collapse in stock market values in 2001–02 resulted in Merrill Lynch's Japanese unit incurring significant losses. In retrospect, was the Japanese expansion a costly blunder or did the company simply get hit by macroeconomic events that were difficult to predict and avoid?

5. Do you think Merrill Lynch should continue in Japan? Why?

Cases

BP: Creating a Global Brand   514

Restructuring Exide   514

Philips versus Matsushita:
A New Century, a New Round   517

BP: Creating a Global Brand 🎥

BP, formally British Petroleum, has long been one of the world's largest oil companies. Between 1999 and 2002, however, BP made a series of nine acquisitions in the United States and Europe that more than doubled the number of employees to 117,000. Most of the acquired companies were already international in scope. Many of the employees in this new company had no stake in the old British Petroleum. This created a problem for the company: How should it create an entity that operated as a unified global enterprise?

The company's solution to this problem was to articulate a set of common core values that are relevant around the world, and to rebrand the company around those values. The rebranding and values were both for external consumption—to project the new BP to stakeholders from customers to stockholders and various national governments—and for internal consumption—to give employees a common anchor.

The four key values that the company chose to emphasize came from extensive consultation with the employees of BP's various operating companies. The values are performance driven, innovative, progressive, and green. These core values are meant to affect how everyone at BP approaches the company. BP now refers to these core values as its corporate brand. This brand projects to both external and internal stakeholders what the company is all about.

BP believes that the core values transcend cultural differences in business environments across the globe. While ways of doing business may differ, BP asserts that the core values are things on which everyone can agree. As such, they form the basis for building a truly global company. Although delivery of the brand—the precise images used and communication messages employed—differs in small ways from nation to nation, the core values and overall brand image remain constant.

Case Discussion Questions

1. What are the strategic benefits to BP of emphasizing a common set of values and projecting a common corporate image worldwide?

2. What do you think are the internal impediments to building this kind of common corporate culture globally?

3. Do you think that the values BP has chosen transcend business and national culture?

4. What kind of company is BP trying to become through this process—multidomestic, international, global, or transnational?

Restructuring Exide

Introduction

In March 1999, Exide Corporation announced that Robert Lutz, the flamboyant, 67-year-old former Chrysler executive who helped turn that company around in the early 1990s, would become chairman, president, and chief executive office of Exide. Lutz, an outspoken former Marine known for his love of good cigars, fine wine, and flying jet fighters, would have his work cut out for him. Exide was a company in trouble. The world's largest manufacturer of lead acid batteries, the company had reportedly sacrificed profitability in its quest for market share leadership. For the financial year ending March 1999, Exide lost $9 million on global sales of $2.37 billion. A series of bank-financed acquisitions during the 1990s had left the company with a weak balance sheet, including $1.3 billion in debt that cost $100 million in annual interest payments to serve. Moreover, a price war in the lead battery industry was squeezing profit margins.

Exide's Business

Market Segments and Customers

Exide manufactures batteries for customers in two broad areas: industrial and automotive. The industrial area, which accounts for 37 percent of Exide's revenues, is broken into two segments. One, the motive power business, is engaged in the manufacture of batteries for electric vehicles including forklift trucks, golf carts, wheel chairs, and electric floor cleaning equipment. The other industrial segment, network power, makes standby batteries used for backup power applications, to ensure continuous power supply in case of main (primary) power failure or outage. The largest customers here are manufacturers of telecommunications equipment, which incorporate the batteries in their equipment to ensure that it continues to function in the case of a power outage (which is why you can still make phone calls, even if you do not have power at home). A second customer group is businesses that use standby batteries in computer installations so that the computer system stays up even if the power goes down.

In the industrial motive power business, most of Exide's batteries are sold through independent lift-truck dealers, or sold directly to large users of lift-trucks, such as Wal-Mart and Kroger. Exide's customers in the industrial network power business include manufacturers of telecommunications equipment, as well as telecommunications service providers. Customers include Lucent, Motorola, and Nokia, all major global producers of telecommunications equipment, and AT&T, British Telecom, China Telecom, Deutsche Telekom, GTE, Nippon Telephone and Telegraph, all service providers.

The automotive area of Exide's business, which accounts for 67 percent of global revenues, is comprised primarily of the manufacture and sale of lead acid batteries to automobile manufacturers and to aftermarket distributors. Principal original equipment manufacturer (OEM) customers include DaimlerChrysler, for whom Exide is the primary global battery supplier, Ford, Toyota, Mack Trucks, John Deere, Volvo, the Renault Group, Volkswagen, and BMW. Aftermarket batteries are sold principally though retail automotive parts chains and mass merchandisers. Customers in the United States include NAPA Distribution Centers, Wal-Mart, Kmart, and Les Schwab Tire. Customers in Europe include large national distributors such as Kwik Fit in the United Kingdom. In the United States, Exide batteries are sold in the aftermarket under the Exide and Champion brand names. In Europe, the brand names in the aftermarket vary from country to country and include Exide, Fulmen, DETA, Tudor, SONNAK, and Centra.

Competition

Exide is the global market share leader in both the motive power and network power segments of the industrial area. Major competitors include UK-based Invensys' Hawker battery group; C&D Technologies, another U.S. firm, and Yuasa of Japan. In the automotive area, Exide again leads with a 36 percent share of the global market for automobile batteries (both OEM and aftermarket). Exide's largest competitors in the United States automotive segment include Delphi Automotive and Johnson Controls. In Europe, Exide faces a number of strong local competitors including Varta, Fiamm, and Hoppeke. Price competition has long been intense in all markets, with major customers using their buying power to bargain down battery prices. Exide's financial troubles in the late 1990s, however, were due in part to an outbreak of extremely aggressive price competition in Europe.

Manufacturing, Employees, and Facilities

Lead is the principal material used in the manufacturing of batteries, accounting for about one-fifth of the cost of goods sold. Exide operates a number of lead recycling plants in both the United States and Europe. Exide reclaims lead from used batteries that end users return to distributors. Exide fulfills most of its lead requirements from its recycling plants. Other key raw materials include lead oxide and bulk chemicals.

Exide employs some 20,000 people, 8,500 in the United States and almost 11,000 in Europe. The company operates some 50 facilities, the bulk of which are in Europe and North America where most of the company's sales are concentrated. Exide has some 14 manufacturing facilities in North America, 16 in Western Europe, 2 in Australia, 1 in New Zealand, and 1 in Turkey. In Western Europe, there are manufacturing and lead recycling facilities in each major national market.

Lutz's Changes

Lutz moved rapidly to make a number of changes in Exide's business. One of his first decisions was to pull out of a supply agreement with Sears. Exide sold over 4.5 million batteries per year to Sears, but to get the agreement the company had to slash prices. The result was that Exide was making less from the Sears deal than it was from deals one-fifth of the size. Lutz also pushed the company to shift demand from low-price battery models to higher-price branded products, particularly in the automotive segment. Consistent with this theme, in June 1999, Exide introduced a new lead acid battery, the Select Orbital battery. While the battery cost $125, Exide claimed it was based on a radically new design and would retain its charge for over a year, substantially longer than for a conventional battery. Also, while a conventional battery has a life of 30 to 40 months, Exide claimed the Orbital would last five years and stand up to far more abuse.

Lutz also pushed the company to quickly solve its legal problems. The company was being sued in the United States for recycling old batteries and selling them as new through distributors such as Sears. Under Lutz direction, instead of fighting the lawsuits, Exide quickly settled them for a few million dollars and took a onetime charge against earnings.

Within some 15 months of his arrival, Lutz had replaced the entire board of directors and the majority of senior executives in both Europe and North America. Worldwide battery product capacity had been cut by some 20 percent through plant closures, the company's debt load had been substantially pared back by issuing additional stock and using the proceeds to pay down debt, and Exide had made a major acquisition, paying $368 million in stock and cash for GNB Technologies, a major supplier in the fast-growing market for standby batteries in telecommunications and computer equipment. Perhaps the most difficult change he initiated, however, was one in the organization structure of Exide's business.

Changing the Organization Structure: Product or Geography?

When he arrived at Exide, Lutz found a structure that was based on geography with 10 different country organizations. The genesis of this structure was rooted in history. Many of the country organizations had previously been independent businesses that Exide had acquired in its rush to gain global market share. After being acquired, the majority continued to function as self-contained operations with their own brands, manufacturing facilities, and distribution systems. Exide managed the different subsidiaries on an arm's-length basis, setting profit goals for each, and awarding local executives big bonuses if they exceeded those goals.

It soon became apparent to Lutz that this structure was causing problems for Exide, particularly in Europe. When Lutz arrived, Exide's European business was losing money. The various country managers in Europe blamed the losses on significant price discounting. After talking to competitors and customers, Lutz found that there indeed was significant price discounting in Europe, but in many cases, this was because different Exide subsidiaries were competing against each other for major customers. They were exporting into each other's territories, or competing aggressively for share in third countries. Thus, for example, the British subsidiary was gaining share in Australia from the Germany subsidiary by underselling the latter by 10 to 15 percent. Part of the blame for this competition could be laid at the feet of an incentive system that rewarded country managers for increasing the performance of their unit, irrespective of whether that was at the expense of another Exide unit.

Convinced that the structure had to change, Lutz held five management retreats between June 1999 and January 2000. "Where does our future lie?" Lutz asked the 30 senior executives assembled for the first meeting, "Does it lie in country management or in global business units?" Many of the country managers reacted with apprehension to the question. Several argued that their regions were in good shape, and that any problems that existed were due to weaknesses elsewhere or general industry conditions.

Between retreats, managers working in teams were assigned to grapple with the various dilemmas confronting the company, using existing and alternative models of the organization as solutions. In a typical assessment, one team looked at Exide's Asian expansion strategy. The members concluded that the geographic focus encouraged construction of manufacturing plants in each country Exide entered, even though it was not profitable to keep putting up plants like that. On the third retreat, the teams started to report their findings, and it quickly became apparent that many were concluding that only a product line structure could cure Exide's ills. After a vigorous debate, Lutz stood up and announced, "We don't have consensus yet . . . But I'm going to make a decision, and we are going to a global business unit structure."

Under the proposed structure that Lutz revealed at the next meeting, six global business units replaced the geographic organization. Each business unit was built around a distinct product line, such as network power, industrial motive power, and so on. It was the global business units that were now given responsibility for major strategic and operational decisions, such as what to produce where, how much to charge customers, and selling to major regional or global customers. Country managers were given a coordinating role and the responsibility for local sales efforts and distribution.

Although by now expected, the announcement was a blow for many country managers. Effectively, it meant a demotion. When one country manager frowned at the announcement, Lutz looked at him and asked, "Why don't you give this a try?" "No," the manager replied, "I'm out of here!" Another country manager told a consultant: "Being a country manager is my life. It's something I've worked for my entire life. I don't see how I'll have a role going forward." Subsequently, the manager was given the option of moving from Naples to Frankfurt, for less money, or leaving the company. He chose the former option, but his family refused to move and stayed in Naples. Other country managers came out of the process quite well. Albrecht Leuschner, the head of the German unit, found himself promoted to lead the global network power business unit, which was to be headquartered in Germany.

The Acquisition of GNB Technologies

Leuschner found himself in this position for just six weeks. In May 2000, Exide acquired GNB Technologies for its fast-growing network power business and industrial motive power businesses. The acquisition gave Lutz a problem; he feared that Mitchell Bregman, the well-regarded president of GNB's operation might leave once Exide folded his industrial battery business into its global network power and industrial motive power business units. Instead, Lutz approached Bregman and told him that after the acquisition, he would retain control over the North American industrial battery business. Effectively, after only six weeks, the global business unit structure was being amended. There was now a European business unit for network power headed by Leuschner, a European business unit for industrial motive power that was run out of the United Kingdom, and a North American industrial battery business headed by Bregman.

Initially, the decision gave rise to a turf battle between Leuschner and Bregman. The point of contention was over who should run China for Exide. Bregman wanted to form and direct a Chinese subsidiary, because China represented his unit's fastest growing market. Leuschner lobbied to form a joint venture in China that would be under his command. Bregman was finally persuaded to give in to Leuschner, but only after he had been given control over South American operations and had been guaranteed control over operations in Korea, Japan, and Taiwan.

Now all parties claim the structure is working well. The company still maintains separate industrial battery sales forces in North America and Europe, in what has become a de facto regional structure. However, teams from the European and North American units have begun making joint pitches to global customers such as Ford and Lucent.

Case Discussion Questions

1. What kind of industry environment does Exide operate in? Is it a global industry, a multidomestic industry, or something in between? What are the pressures for local responsiveness in this industry? What are the pressures for globalization?

2. How might a structure based on geography (country subsidiaries) result in inefficiencies at Exide?

3. What are the potential benefits to Exide of moving from a geographic structure based on country organizations to a product structure based on global business units? What are the potential drawbacks of such a structure?

4. Following the GNB acquisition, Lutz again changed the structure of Exide, at least on the industrial side of the organization. Why did he do this? Do you think this was a wise move, or might it create additional problems in the future?

Sources

1. Chappell, L. "Lutz Put Exide in Recovery." *Automotive News*, August 6, 2001, p. 49.

2. Exide 2000 and 2001 10K filed with Securities and Exchange Commission.

3. Lublin, J. S. "Place vs Product: It's Tough to Choose a Management Model." *Wall Street Journal*, June 27, 2001, pp. A1, A4.

4. Maynard, M. "Lutz Gets a Charge Out of a New Career. Excide CEO Achieves a Dream." *USA Today*, June 1, 1999, p. 12B.

5. Nauss, D. W. "Ex-Chrysler Exec Robert Lutz to Head Troubled Exide Corporation." *Los Angeles Times*, November 17, 1998, p. 3.

6. Puchalsky, A. "Exide Makes Tough Choices in Comeback." *Wall Street Journal*, March 26, 1999.

7. Sherefkin, R. "New One Two Punch at Exide." *Automotive News*, June 12, 2000, p. 22.

8. Taylor, A. "Getting Back in the Fast Lane." *Fortune*, March 6, 2000.

Philips versus Matsushita: A New Century, a New Round

Throughout their long histories, N. V. Philips (Netherlands) and Matsushita Electric (Japan) had followed very different strategies and emerged with very different organizational capabilities. Philips built its success on a worldwide portfolio of responsive national organizations while Matsushita based its global competitiveness on its centralized, highly efficient operations in Japan.

During the 1990s, both companies experienced major challenges to their historic competitive positions and organizational models, and at the end of the decade, both companies were struggling to reestablish their competitiveness. At the turn of the millennium, new CEOs at both companies were implementing yet another round of strategic initiatives and organizational restructurings. Observers wondered how the changes would affect their long-running competitive battle.

This case derives from an earlier case, "Philips versus Matsushita: Preparing for a New Round," HBS No. 399-102, prepared by Professor Christopher A. Bartlett, which was an updated version of an earlier case by Professor Bartlett and Research Associate Robert W. Lightfoot, "Philips and Matsushita: A Portrait of Two Evolving Companies," HBS Case No. 392-156. The section on Matsushita summarizes "Matsushita Electric Industrial (MEI) in 1987," HBS Case No. 388-144, by Sumantra Ghoshal (INSEAD) and Christopher A. Bartlett. Some early history on Philips draws from "Philips Group—1987," HBS Case No. 388-050, by Professors Frank Aguilar and Michael Y. Yoshino. This version was also prepared by Professor Bartlett.

Philips: Background

In 1892, Gerard Philips and his father opened a small lightbulb factory in Eindhoven, Holland. When their venture almost failed, they recruited Gerard's brother, Anton, an excellent salesman and manager. By 1900, Philips was the third largest lightbulb producer in Europe.

From its founding, Philips developed a tradition of caring for workers. In Eindhoven it built company houses, bolstered education, and paid its employees so well that other local employers complained. When Philips incorporated in 1912, it set aside 10 percent of profits for employees.

Technological Competence and Geographic Expansion

While larger electrical products companies were racing to diversify, Philips made only lightbulbs. This one-product focus and Gerard's technological prowess enabled the company to create significant innovations. Company policy was to scrap old plants and use new machines or factories whenever advances were made in new production technology. Anton wrote down assets rapidly and set aside substantial reserves for replacing outdated equipment. Philips also became a leader in industrial research, creating physics and chemistry labs to address production problems as well as more abstract scientific ones. The labs developed a tungsten metal filament bulb that was a great commercial success and gave Philips the financial strength to compete against its giant rivals.

Holland's small size soon forced Philips to look beyond its Dutch borders for enough volume to mass produce. In 1899, Anton hired the company's first export manager, and soon the company was selling into such diverse markets as Japan, Australia, Canada, Brazil, and Russia. In 1912, as the electric lamp industry began to show signs of overcapacity, Philips started building sales organizations in the United States, Canada, and France. All other functions remained highly centralized in Eindhoven. In many foreign countries Philips created local joint ventures to gain market acceptance.

In 1919, Philips entered into the Principal Agreement with General Electric, giving each company the use of the other's patents. The agreement also divided the world into "three spheres of influence": General Electric would control North America, Philips would control Holland; but both companies agreed to compete freely in the rest of the world. (General Electric also took a 20 percent stake in Philips.) After this time, Philips began evolving from a highly centralized company, whose sales were conducted through third parties, to a decentralized sales organization with autonomous marketing companies in 14 European countries, China, Brazil, and Australia.

During this period, the company also broadened its product line significantly. In 1918, it began producing electronic vacuum tubes; eight years later its first radios appeared, capturing a 20 percent world market share within a decade; and during the 1930s, Philips began producing X-ray tubes. The Great Depression brought with it trade barriers and high tariffs, and Philips was forced to build local production facilities to protect its foreign sales of these products.

Philips: Organizational Development

One of the earliest traditions at Philips was a shared but competitive leadership by the commercial and technical functions. Gerard, an engineer, and Anton, a businessman, began a subtle competition where Gerard would try to produce more than Anton could sell and vice versa. Nevertheless, the two agreed that strong research was vital to Philips' survival.

During the late 1930s, in anticipation of the impending war, Philips transferred its overseas assets to two trusts, British Philips and the North American Philips Corporation; it also moved most of its vital research laboratories to Redhill in Surrey, England, and its top management to the United States. Supported by the assets and resources transferred abroad, and isolated from their parent, the individual country organizations became more independent during the war.

Because waves of Allied and German bombing had pummeled most of Philips' industrial plant in the Netherlands, the management board decided to build the postwar organization on the strengths of the national organizations (NOs). Their greatly increased self-sufficiency during the war had allowed most to become adept at responding to country-specific market conditions—a capability that became a valuable asset in the postwar era. For example, when international wrangling precluded any agreement on three competing television transmission standards (PAL, SECAM, and NTSC), each nation decided which to adopt. Furthermore, consumer preferences and economic conditions varied: in some countries, rich, furniture-encased TV sets were the norm; in others, sleek, contemporary models dominated the market. In the United Kingdom, the only way to penetrate the market was to establish a rental business; in richer countries, a major marketing challenge was overcoming elitist prejudice against television. In this environment, the independent NOs had a great advantage in being able to sense and respond to the differences.

Eventually, responsiveness extended beyond adaptive marketing. As NOs built their own technical capabilities, product development often became a function of local market conditions. For example, Philips of Canada created the company's first color TV; Philips of Australia created the first stereo TV; and Philips of the United Kingdom created the first TVs with teletext.

While NOs took major responsibility for financial, legal, and administrative matters, 14 product divisions

(PDs), located in Eindhoven, were formally responsible for development, production, and global distribution. (In reality, the NOs' control of assets and the PDs' distance from the operations often undercut this formal role.) The research function remained independent and, with continued strong funding, set up eight separate laboratories in Europe and the United States.

While the formal corporate-level structure was represented as a type of geographic/product matrix, it was clear that NOs had the real power. NOs reported directly to the management board, which Philips enlarged from 4 members to 10 to ensure that top management remained in contact with and control of the highly autonomous NOs. Each NO also regularly sent envoys to Eindhoven to represent its interests. Top management, most of whom had careers that included multiple foreign tours of duty, made frequent overseas visits to the NOs. In 1954, the board established the International Concern Council to formalize regular meetings with the heads of all major NOs.

Within the NOs, the management structure mimicked the legendary joint technical and commercial leadership of the two Philips brothers. Most were led by a technical manager and a commercial manager. In some locations, a finance manager filled out the top management triad that typically reached key decisions collectively. This cross-functional coordination capability was reflected down through the NOs in front-line product teams, product-group-level management teams, and at the senior management committee of the NOs' top commercial, technical, and financial managers.

The overwhelming importance of foreign operations to Philips, the commensurate status of the NOs within the corporate hierarchy, and even the cosmopolitan appeal of many of the offshore subsidiaries' locations encouraged many Philips managers to take extended foreign tours of duty, working in a series of two- or three-year posts. This elite group of expatriate managers identified strongly with each other and with the NOs as a group and had no difficulty representing their strong, country-oriented views to corporate management.

Philips: Attempts at Reorganization

In the late 1960s, the creation of the Common Market eroded trade barriers within Europe and diluted the rationale for maintaining independent, country-level subsidiaries. New transistor- and printed circuit-based technologies demanded larger production runs than most national plants could justify, and many of Philips' competitors were moving production of electronics to new facilities in low-wage areas in East Asia and Central and South America. Despite its many technological innovations, Philips' ability to bring products to market began to falter. In the 1960s, the company invented the audiocassette but let its Japanese competitors capture the mass

market. A decade later, its R&D group developed the V2000 videocassette format—superior technically to Sony's Beta or Matsushita's VHS—but was forced to abandon it when North American Philips decided to outsource, brand, and sell a VHS product which it manufactured under license from Matsushita.

Over three decades, seven chairmen experimented with reorganizing the company to deal with its growing problems. Yet, entering the new millennium, Philips' financial performance remained poor and its global competitiveness was still in question. (See Exhibits 1 and 2.)

Van Reimsdijk and Rodenburg Reorganizations, 1970s

Concerned about what one magazine described as "continued profitless progress," newly appointed CEO Hendrick van Reimsdijk created an organization committee to prepare a policy paper on the division of responsibilities between the PDs and the NOs. Their report, dubbed the "Yellow Booklet," outlined the disadvantages of Philips' matrix organization in 1971:

> Without an agreement [defining the relationship between national organizations and product divisions], it is impossible to determine in any given situation which of the two parties is responsible . . . As operations become increasingly complex, an organizational form of this type will only lower the speed of reaction of an enterprise.

On the basis of this report, van Reimsdijk proposed rebalancing the managerial relationships between PDs and NOs—"tilting the matrix" in his words—to allow Philips to decrease the number of products marketed, build scale by concentrating production, and increase the flow of goods among national organizations. He proposed closing the least efficient local plants and converting the best into International Production Centers (IPCs), each supplying many NOs. In so doing, van Reimsdijk hoped that PD managers would gain control over manufacturing operations. Due to the political and organizational difficulty of closing local plants, however, implementation was slow.

In the late 1970s, his successor CEO, Dr. Rodenburg, continued this thrust. Several IPCs were established, but the NOs seemed as powerful and independent as ever. He furthered matrix simplification by replacing the dual commercial and technical leadership with single management at both the corporate and national organizational levels. Yet the power struggles continued.

Wisse Dekker Reorganization, 1982

Unsatisfied with the company's slow response and concerned by its slumping financial performance, upon becoming CEO in 1982, Wisse Dekker outlined a new initiative. Aware of the cost advantage of Philips' Japanese

Exhibit 1

Philips Group Summary Financial Data, 1970–2000 (millions of guilders unless otherwise stated)

	2000	1995	1990	1985	1980	1975	1970
Net sales	F83,437	F64,462	F55,764	F60,045	F36,536	F27,115	F15,070
Income from operations (excluding restructuring)	NA	4,090	2,260	3,075	1,577	1,201	1,280
Income from operations (including restructuring)	9,434	4,044	–2,389	N/A	N/A	N/A	N/A
As a percentage of net sales	11.3%	6.3%	–4.3%	5.1%	4.3%	4.5%	8.5%
Income after taxes	12,559	2,889	F–4,447	F1,025	F532	F341	F446
Net income from normal business operations	NA	2,684	–4,526	N/A	328	347	435
Stockholders' equity (common)	49,473	14,055	11,165	16,151	12,996	10,047	6,324
Return on stockholders' equity	42.8%	20.2%	–30.2%	5.6%	2.7%	3.6%	7.3%
Distribution per common share, par value F10 (in guilders)	F2.64	F1.60	F0.0	F2.00	F1.80	F1.40	F1.70
Total assets	86,114	54,683	51,595	52,883	39,647	30,040	19,088
Inventories as a percentage of net sales	13.9%	18.2%	20.7%	23.2%	32.8%	32.9%	35.2%
Outstanding trade receivables in month's sales	1.5	1.6	1.6	2.0	3.0	3.0	2.8
Current ratio	1.2	1.6	1.4	1.6	1.7	1.8	1.7
Employees at year-end (in thousands)	219	265	273	346	373	397	359
Wages, salaries and other related costs	N/A	N/A	F17,582	F21,491	F15,339	F11,212	F5,890
Exchange rate (period end; guilder$)	2.34	1.60	1.69	2.75	2.15	2.69	3.62
Selected data in millions of dollars:							
Sales	$35,253	$40,039	$33,018	$21,802	$16,993	$10,098	$4,163
Operating profit	3,986	2,512	1,247	988	734	464	NA
Pretax income	5,837	2,083	–2,380	658	364	256	NA
Net income	5,306	1,667	–2,510	334	153	95	120
Total assets	35,885	32,651	30,549	19,202	18,440	11,186	5,273
Shareholders' equity (common)	20,238	8,784	6,611	5,864	6,044	3,741	1,747

Note: Exchange rate December 31, 2000, was Euro/US$: 1.074

Source: Annual reports; Standard & Poor's *Compustat*; Moody's Industrial and International Manuals.

Exhibit 2

Philips Group, Sales by Product and Geographic Segment, 1985–2000 (millions of guilders)

	2000		1995		1990		1985	
Net Sales by Product Segment:								
Lighting	F11,133	13%	F 8,353	13%	F 7,026	13%	F 7,976	12%
Consumer electronics	32,357	39	22,027	34	25,400	46	16,906	26
Domestic appliances	4,643	6	—	—	—	—	6,644	10
Professional products/Systems	—	—	11,562	18	13,059	23	17,850	28
Components/Semiconductors	23,009	28	10,714	17	8,161	15	11,620	18
Software/Services	—	—	9,425	15	—	—	—	—
Medical systems	6,679	8	—	—	—	—	—	—
Origin	1,580	2	—	—	—	—	—	—
Miscellaneous	4,035	5	2,381	4	2,118	4	3,272	5
Total	83,437	100%	64,462	100%	F55,764	100%	F 64,266	100%
Operating Income by Sector:								
Lighting	1,472	16%	983	24%	419	18%	F 910	30%
Consumer electronics	824	9	167	4	1,499	66	34	1
Domestic appliances	632	7	—	—	—	—	397	13
Professional products/Systems	—	—	157	4	189	8	1,484	48
Components/Semiconductors	4,220	45	2,233	55	–43	–2	44	1
Software/Services	—	—	886	22	—	—	—	—
Medical systems	372	4	—	—	—	—	—	—
Origin	2,343	25	—	—	—	—	—	—
Miscellaneous	–249	–3	423	10	218	10	200	7
Increase not attributable to a sector	–181	–2	(805)	(20)	–22	–1	6	0
Total	9,434	100%	4,044	100%	2,260	100%	F 3,075	100%

Notes:

Conversion rate (December 31, 2000): 1 Euro: 2.20371 Dutch Guilders

Totals may not add due to rounding.

Product sector sales after 1988 are external sales only; therefore, no eliminations are made; sector sales before 1988 include sales to other sectors; therefore, eliminations are made.

Data are not comparable to consolidated financial summary due to restating.

Source: Annual reports

counterparts, he closed inefficient operations—particularly in Europe where 40 of the company's more than 200 plants were shut. He focused on core operations by selling some businesses (for example, welding, energy cables, and furniture) while acquiring an interest in Grundig and Westinghouse's North American lamp activities. Dekker also supported technology-sharing agreements and entered alliances in offshore manufacturing.

To deal with the slow-moving bureaucracy, he continued his predecessor's initiative to replace dual leadership with single general managers. He also continued to "tilt the matrix" by giving PDs formal product management responsibility, but leaving NOs responsible for local profits. And, he energized the management board by reducing its size, bringing on directors with strong operating experience, and creating subcommittees to deal with difficult issues. Finally, Dekker redefined the product planning process, incorporating input from the NOs, but giving global PDs the final decision on long-range direction. Still sales declined and profits stagnated.

Van der Klugt Reorganization, 1987

When Cor van der Klugt succeeded Dekker as chairman in 1987, Philips had lost its long-held consumer electronics leadership position to Matsushita, and was one of only two non-Japanese companies in the world's top 10. Its net profit margins of 1 percent to 2 percent not only lagged behind General Electric's 9 percent, but even its highly aggressive Japanese competitors' slim 4 percent. Van der Klugt set a profit objective of 3 percent to 4 percent and made beating the Japanese companies a top priority.

As van der Klugt reviewed Philips' strategy, he designated various businesses as core (those that shared related technologies, had strategic importance, or were technical leaders) and noncore (stand-alone businesses that were not targets for world leadership and could eventually be sold if required). Of the four businesses defined as core, three were strategically linked: components, consumer electronics, and telecommunications and data systems. The fourth, lighting, was regarded as strategically vital because its cash flow funded development. The noncore businesses included domestic appliances and medical systems, which van der Klugt spun off into joint ventures with Whirlpool and GE, respectively.

In continuing efforts to strengthen the PDs relative to the NOs, van der Klugt restructured Philips around the four core global divisions rather than the former 14 PDs. This allowed him to trim the management board, appointing the displaced board members to a new policy-making Group Management Committee. Consisting primarily of PD heads and functional chiefs this body replaced the old NO-dominated International Concern Council. Finally, he sharply reduced the 3,000-strong headquarters staff, reallocating many of them to the PDs.

To link PDs more directly to markets, van der Klugt dispatched many experienced product-line managers to Philips' most competitive markets. For example, management of the digital audio tape and electric-shaver product lines were relocated to Japan, while the medical technology and domestic appliances lines were moved to the United States.

Such moves, along with continued efforts at globalizing product development and production efforts, required that the parent company gain firmer control over NOs, especially the giant North American Philips Corp. (NAPC). Although Philips had obtained a majority equity interest after World War II, it was not always able to make the U.S. company respond to directives from the center, as the V2000 VCR incident showed. To prevent replays of such experiences, in 1987 van der Klugt repurchased publicly owned NAPC shares for $700 million.

Reflecting the growing sentiment among some managers that R&D was not market oriented enough, van der Klugt halved spending on basic research to about 10 percent of total R&D. To manage what he described as "R&D's tendency to ponder the fundamental laws of nature," he made R&D the direct responsibility of the businesses being supported by the research. This required that each research lab become focused on specific business areas (see Exhibit 3).

Finally, van der Klugt continued the effort to build efficient, specialized, multimarket production facilities by closing 75 of the company's 420 remaining plants worldwide. He also eliminated 38,000 of its 344,000 employees—21,000 through divesting businesses, shaking up the myth of lifetime employment at the company. He anticipated that all these restructurings would lead to a financial recovery by 1990. Unanticipated losses for that year, however—more than 4.5 billion Dutch guilders ($2.5 billion)—provoked a class-action lawsuit by angry American investors, who alleged that positive projections by the company had been misleading. In a surprise move, on May 14, 1990, van der Klugt and half of the management board were replaced.

Timmer Reorganization, 1990

The new president, Jan Timmer, had spent most of his 35-year Philips career turning around unprofitable businesses. With rumors of a takeover or a government bailout swirling, he met with his top 100 managers and distributed a hypothetical—but fact-based—press release announcing that Philips was bankrupt. "So what action can you take this weekend?" he challenged them.

Under "Operation Centurion," head count was reduced by 68,000 or 22 percent over the next 18 months, earning Timmer the nickname "The Butcher of Eindhoven." Because European laws required substantial compensation for layoffs—Eindhoven workers received 15 months' pay, for example—the first round of 10,000 lay-

Exhibit 3

Philips Research Labs by Location and Specialty, 1987

Location	Size (staff)	Specialty
Eindhoven, The Netherlands	2,000	Basic research, electronics, manufacturing technology
Redhill, Surrey, England	450	Microelectronics, television, defense
Hamburg, Germany	350	Communications, office equipment, medical imaging
Aachen, West Germany	250	Fiber optics, X-ray systems
Paris, France	350	Microprocessors, chip materials, design
Brussels	50	Artificial intelligence
Briarcliff Manor, New York	35	Optical systems, television, superconductivity, defense
Sunnyvale, California	150	Integrated circuits

Source: Philips, in *Business Week*, March 21, 1988, p. 156.

offs alone cost Philips $700 million. To spread the burden around the globe and to speed the process, Timmer asked his PD managers to negotiate cuts with NO managers. According to one report, however, country managers were "digging in their heels to save local jobs." But the cuts came—many from overseas operations. In addition to the job cuts, Timmer vowed to "change the way we work." He established new performance rules and asked hundreds of top managers to sign contracts that committed them to specific financial goals. Those who broke those contracts were replaced—often with outsiders.

To focus resources further, Timmer sold off various businesses including integrated circuits to Matsushita, minicomputers to Digital, defense electronics to Thomson, and the remaining 53 percent of appliances to Whirlpool. Yet profitability was still well below the modest 4 percent on sales he promised. In particular, consumer electronics lagged with slow growth in a price-competitive market. The core problem was identified by a 1994 McKinsey study that estimated that value added per hour in Japanese consumer electronic factories was still 68 percent above that of European plants. In this environment, most NO managers kept their heads down, using their distance from Eindhoven as their defense against the ongoing rationalization.

After three years of cost-cutting, in early 1994. Timmer finally presented a new growth strategy to the board. His plan was to expand software, services, and multimedia to become 40 percent of revenues by 2000. He was betting on Philips' legendary innovative capability to restart the growth engines. Earlier, he had recruited Frank Carrubba, Hewlett-Packard's director of research, and encouraged him to focus on developing 15 core technologies. The list, which included interactive compact disc (CD-i), digital compact cassettes (DCC), high definition television (HDTV), and multimedia software, was soon dubbed "the president's projects." But his earlier divestment of some of Philips' truly high-tech businesses and a 37 percent cut in R&D personnel left the company with few who understood the technology of the new priority businesses.

By 1996, it was clear that Philips' HDTV technology would not become industry standard, that its DCC gamble had lost out to Sony's Minidisc, and that CD-i was a marketing failure. While costs were lower, so too was morale, particularly among middle management. Critics claimed that the company's drive for cost-cutting and standardization had led it to ignore new worldwide market demands for more segmented products and higher consumer service.

Boonstra Reorganization, 1996

When Timmer stepped down in October 1996, the board replaced him with a radical choice for Philips—an outsider whose expertise was in marketing and Asia rather than technology and Europe. Cor Boonstra was a 58-year-old Dutchman whose years as CEO of Sara Lee, the U.S. consumer products firm, had earned him a reputation as a hard-driving marketing genius. Joining Philips in 1994, he headed the Asia Pacific region and the lighting division before being tapped as CEO.

Unencumbered by tradition, he immediately announced strategic sweeping changes designed to reach his target of increasing return on net assets from 17 percent to 24 percent by 1999. "There are no taboos, no sacred cows," he said. "The bleeders must be turned around, sold, or closed." Within three years, he had sold off 40 of Philips' 120 major businesses—including such well-known units as Polygram and Grundig. He also initiated a major worldwide restructuring, promising to transform a structure he described as "a plate of spaghetti" into "a neat row of asparagus." He said:

> How can we compete with the Koreans? They don't have 350 companies all over the world. Their factory in Ireland covers Europe and their manufacturing facility in Mexico serves North America. We need a more structured and simpler manufacturing and marketing organization to achieve a cost pattern in line with those who do not have our heritage. This is still one of the biggest issues facing Philips.

Within a year, 3,100 jobs were eliminated in North America and 3,000 employees were added in Asia Pacific, emphasizing Boonstra's determination to shift production to low-wage countries and his broader commitment to Asia. And after three years, he had closed 100 of the company's 356 factories worldwide. At the same time, he replaced the company's 21 PDs with seven divisions, but shifted day-to-day operating responsibility to 100 business units, each responsible for its profits worldwide. It was a move designed to finally eliminate the old PDNO matrix. Finally, in a move that shocked most employees, he announced that the 100-year-old Eindhoven headquarters would be relocated to Amsterdam with only 400 of the 3,000 corporate positions remaining.

By early 1998, he was ready to announce his new strategy. Despite early speculation that he might abandon consumer electronics, he proclaimed it as the center of Philips' future. Betting on the "digital revolution," he planned to focus on established technologies such as cellular phones (through a joint venture with Lucent), digital TV, digital videodisc, and web TV. Furthermore, he committed major resources to marketing, including a 40 percent increase in advertising to raise awareness and image of the Philips brand and de-emphasize most of the 150 other brands it supported worldwide—from Magnavox TVs to Norelco shavers to Marantz stereos.

While not everything succeeded (the Lucent cell phone joint venture collapsed after nine months, for example), overall performance improved significantly in the late 1990s. By 1999, Boonstra was able to announce that he had achieved his objective of a 24 percent return on net assets.

Kleisterlee Reorganization, 2001

In May 2001, Boonstra passed the CEO's mantle to Gerald Kleisterlee, a 54-year-old engineer (and career Philips man) whose turnaround of the components business had earned him a board seat only a year earlier. Believing that Philips had finally turned around, the board challenged Kleisterlee to grow sales by 10 percent annually and earnings 15 percent while increasing return on assets to 30 percent.

Despite its stock trading at a steep discount to its breakup value, Philips governance structure and Dutch legislation made a hostile raid all but impossible. Nonetheless, Kleisterlee described the difference as "a management discount" and vowed to eliminate it. The first sign of restructuring came within weeks, when mobile phone production was outsourced to CEC of China. Then, in August, Kleisterlee announced an agreement with Japan's Funai Electric to take over production of its VCRs, resulting in the immediate closure of the European production center in Austria and the loss of 1,000 jobs. The CEO then acknowledged that he was seeking partners to take over the manufacturing of some of its other mass-produced items such as television sets.

In mid-2001, a slowing economy resulted in the company's first quarterly loss since 1996 and a reversal of the prior year's strong positive cash flow. Many felt that these growing financial pressures—and shareholders' growing impatience—were finally leading Philips to recognize that its best hope of survival was to outsource even more of its basic manufacturing and become a technology developer and global marketer. They believed it was time to recognize that its 30-year quest to build efficiency into its global operations had failed.

Matsushita: Background

In 1918, Konosuke Matsushita (or "KM" as he was affectionately known), a 23-year-old inspector with the Osaka Electric Light Company, invested ¥100 to start production of double-ended sockets in his modest home. The company grew rapidly, expanding into battery-powered lamps, electric irons, and radios. On May 5, 1932, Matsushita's 14th anniversary, KM announced to his 162 employees a 250-year corporate plan broken into 25-year sections, each to be carried out by successive generations. His plan was codified in a company creed and in the "Seven Spirits of Matsushita" (see Exhibit 4), which, along with the company song, continued to be woven into morning assemblies worldwide and provided the basis of the "cultural and spiritual training" all new employees received during their first seven months with the company.

In the postwar boom, Matsushita introduced a flood of new products: TV sets in 1952; transistor radios in 1958; color TVs, dishwashers, and electric ovens in 1960. Capitalizing on its broad line of 5,000 products (Sony produced 80), the company opened 25,000 domestic retail outlets. With more than six times the outlets of rival Sony, the ubiquitous. "National Shops" represented 40 percent of appliance stores in Japan in the late 1960s. These not only provided assured sales volume, but also gave the company direct access to market trends and consumer reaction. When postwar growth slowed, however, Matsushita had to look beyond its

Exhibit 4

Matsushita Creed and Philosophy (Excerpts)

Creed
Through our industrial activities, we strive to foster progress, to promote the general welfare of society, and to devote ourselves to furthering the development of world culture.
Seven Spirits of Matsushita
Service through Industry Fairness Harmony and Cooperation Struggle for Progress Courtesy and Humility Adjustment and Assimilation Gratitude
KM's Business Philosophy (Selected Quotations)
"The purpose of an enterprise is to contribute to society by supplying goods of high quality at low prices in ample quantity."
"Profit comes in compensation for contribution to society . . . [It] is a result rather than a goal."
"The responsibility of the manufacturer cannot be relieved until its product is disposed of by the end user."
"Unsuccessful business employs a wrong management. You should not find its causes in bad fortune, unfavorable surroundings or wrong timing."
"Business appetite has no self-restraining mechanism . . . When you notice you have gone too far, you must have the courage to come back."

Source: "Matsushita Electric Industrial (MEI) in 1987," Harvard Business School Case No. 388-144.

expanding product line and excellent distribution system for growth. After trying many tactics to boost sales—even sending assembly line workers out as door-to-door salesmen—the company eventually focused on export markets.

The Organization's Foundation: Divisional Structure

Plagued by ill health, KM wished to delegate more authority than was typical in Japanese companies. In 1933, Matsushita became the first Japanese company to adopt the divisional structure, giving each division clearly defined profit responsibility for its product. In addition to creating a "small business" environment, the product division structure generated internal competition that spurred each business to drive growth by leveraging its technology to develop new products. After the innovating division had earned substantial profits on its new product, however, company policy was to spin it off as a new division to maintain the "hungry spirit."

Under the "one-product-one-division" system, corporate management provided each largely self-sufficient division with initial funds to establish its own development, production, and marketing capabil-

ities. Corporate treasury operated like a commercial bank, reviewing divisions' loan requests for which it charged slightly higher-than-market interest, and accepting deposits on their excess funds. Divisional profitability was determined after deductions for central services such as corporate R&D and interest on internal borrowings. Each division paid 60 percent of earnings to headquarters and financed all additional working capital and fixed asset requirements from the retained 40 percent. Transfer prices were based on the market and settled through the treasury on normal commercial terms. KM expected uniform performance across the company's 36 divisions, and division managers whose operating profits fell below 4 percent of sales for two successive years were replaced.

While basic technology was developed in a central research laboratory (CRL), product development and engineering occurred in each of the product divisions. Matsushita intentionally underfunded the CRL, forcing it to compete for additional funding from the divisions. Annually, the CRL publicized its major research projects to the product divisions, which then provided funding in exchange for technology for marketable applications. While it was rarely the innovator, Matsushita was usually very fast to market—earning it the nickname "Man-ishita," or copycat.

Matsushita: Internationalization

Although the establishment of overseas markets was a major thrust of the second 25 years in the 250-year plan, in an overseas trip in 1951 KM had been unable to find any American company willing to collaborate with Matsushita. The best he could do was a technology exchange and licensing agreement with Philips. Nonetheless, the push to internationalize continued.

Expanding through Color TV

In the 1950s and 1960s, trade liberalization and lower shipping rates made possible a healthy export business built on black-and-white TV sets. In 1953 the company opened its first overseas branch office—the Matsushita Electric Corporation of America (MECA). With neither a distribution network nor a strong brand, the company could not access traditional retailers, and had to resort to selling its products under their private brands through mass merchandisers and discounters.

During the 1960s, pressure from national governments in developing countries led Matsushita to open plants in several countries in Southeast Asia and Central and South America. As manufacturing costs in Japan rose, Matsushita shifted more basic production to these low-wage countries, but almost all high-value components and subassemblies were still made in its scale-intensive Japanese plants. By the 1970s, protectionist sentiments in the West forced the company to establish assembly operations in the Americas and Europe. In 1972, it opened a plant in Canada; in 1974, it bought Motorola's TV business and started manufacturing its Quasar brand in the United States; and in 1976, it built a plant in Cardiff, Wales, to supply the Common Market.

Building Global Leadership through VCRs

The birth of the videocassette recorder (VCR) propelled Matsushita into first place in the consumer electronics industry during the 1980s. Recognizing the potential mass-market appeal of the VCR—developed by Californian broadcasting company Ampex in 1956—engineers at Matsushita began developing VCR technology. After six years of development work, Matsushita launched its commercial broadcast video recorder in 1964 and introduced a consumer version two years later.

In 1975, Sony introduced the technically superior "Betamax" format, and the next year JVC launched a competing "VHS" format. Under pressure from MITI, the government's industrial planning ministry, Matsushita agreed to give up its own format and adopt the es-tablished VHS standard. During Matsushita's 20 years of VCR product development, various members of the VCR research team spent most of their careers working together, moving from central labs to the product divisions' development labs and eventually to the plant.

The company quickly built production to meet its own needs as well as those of OEM customers like GE, RCA, and Zenth, who decided to forgo self-manufacture and outsource to the low-cost Japanese. Between, 1977 and 1985, capacity increased 33-fold to 6.8 million units. (In parallel, the company aggressively licensed the VHS format to other manufacturers, including Hitachi, Sharp, Mitsubishi, and, eventually, Philips.) Increased volume enabled Matsushita to slash prices 50 percent within five years of product launch, while simultaneously improving quality. By the mid-1980s, VCRs accounted for 30 percent of total sales—over 40 percent of overseas revenues—and provided 45 percent of profits.

Changing Systems and Controls

In the mid-1980s, Matsushita's growing number of overseas companies reported to the parent in one of two ways: wholly owned, single-product global plants reported directly to the appropriate product division, while overseas sales and marketing subsidiaries and overseas companies producing a broad product line for local markets reported to Matsushita Electric Trading Company (METC), a separate legal entity. (See Exhibit 5 for METC's organization.)

Throughout the 1970s, the central product divisions maintained strong operating control over their offshore production units. Overseas operations used plant and equipment designed by the parent company, followed manufacturing procedures dictated by the center, and used materials from Matsushita's domestic plants. Growing trends toward local sourcing, however, gradually weakened the divisions' direct control. By the 1980s, instead of controlling inputs, they began to monitor measures of output (for example, quality, productivity, inventory levels).

About the same time, product divisions began receiving the globally consolidated return on sales reports that had previously been consolidated in METC statements. By the mid-1980s, as worldwide planning was introduced for the first time, corporate management required all its product divisions to prepare global product strategies.

Headquarters-Subsidiary Relations

Although METC and the product divisions set detailed sales and profits targets for their overseas subsidiaries, local managers were told they had autonomy on how to achieve the targets. "Mike" Matsuoko, president of the company's largest European production subsidiary in Cardiff, Wales, however, emphasized that failure to meet targets forfeited freedom. "Losses show bad health and invite many doctors from Japan who provide advice and support."

1985 Organization:

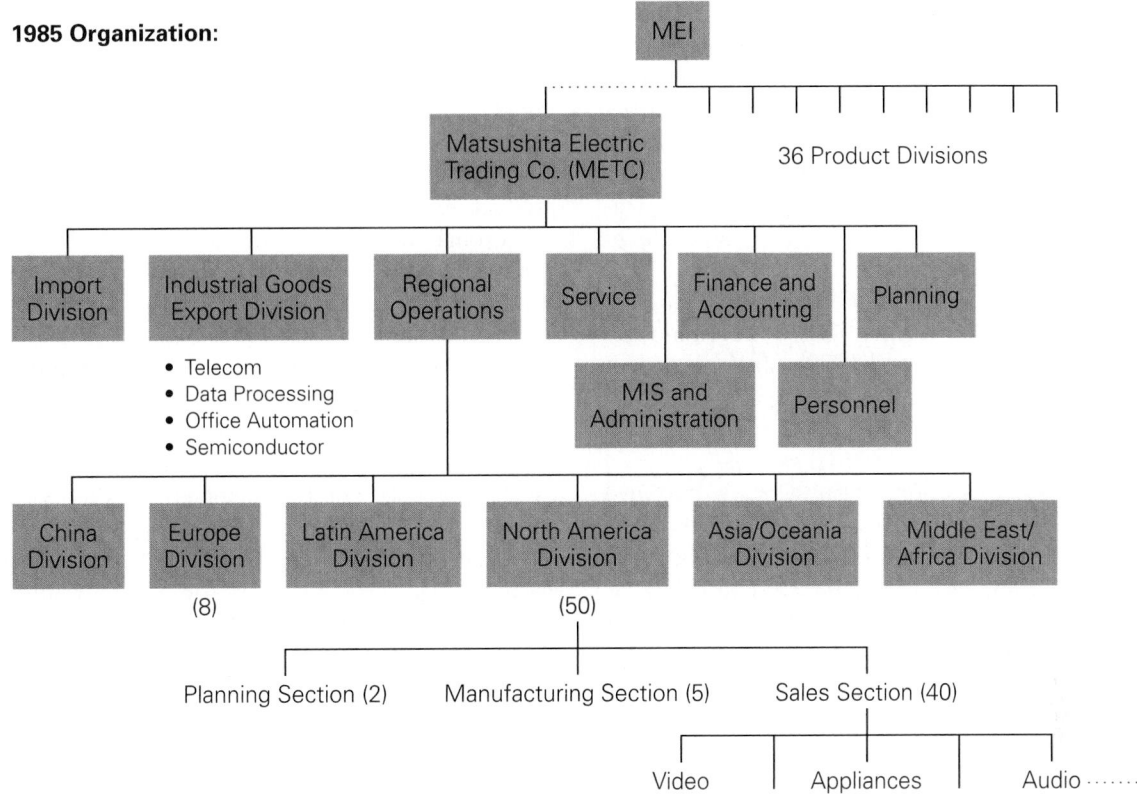

Exhibit 5

Organization of METC, 1985

Source: Harvard Business School Case No. 388-144.
Note: ( ) = number of people.

In the mid-1980s, Matsushita had over 700 expatriate Japanese managers and technicians on foreign assignment for four to eight years, but defended that high number by describing their pivotal role. "This vital communication role," said one manager, "almost always requires a manager from the parent company. Even if a local manager speaks Japanese, he would not have the long experience that is needed to build relationships and understand our management processes."

Expatriate managers were located throughout foreign subsidiaries, but there were a few positions that were almost always reserved for them. The most visible were subsidiary general managers whose main role was to translate Matsushita philosophy abroad. Expatriate accounting managers were expected to "mercilessly expose the truth" to corporate headquarters; and Japanese technical managers were sent to transfer product and process technologies and provide headquarters with local market information. These expatriates maintained relationships with senior colleagues at headquarters, who acted as career mentors, evaluated performance (with some input from local managers), and provided expatriates with information about parent company developments.

General managers of foreign subsidiaries visited Osaka headquarters at least two or three times each year—some as often as every month. Corporate managers reciprocated these visits, and, on average, major operations hosted at least one headquarters manager each day of the year. Face-to-face meetings were considered vital: "Figures are important," said one manager, "but the meetings are necessary to develop judgment." Daily faxes and nightly phone calls between headquarters and expatriate colleagues were a vital management link.

Yamashita's Operation Localization

Although international sales kept rising, as early as 1982 growing host country pressures caused concern about the company's highly centralized operations. In that year, newly appointed company President Toshihiko Yamashita launched "Operation Localization" to boost offshore production from less than 10 percent of value-added to 25 percent, or half of overseas sales, by 1990. To support the target, he set out a program of four localizations—personnel, technology, material, and capital.

Over the next few years, Matsushita increased the number of local nationals in key positions. In the United

States, for example, U.S. nationals became the presidents of three of the six local companies, while in Taiwan the majority of production divisions were replaced by Chinese managers. In each case, however, local national managers were still supported by senior Japanese advisors, who maintained a direct link with the parent company. To localize technology and materials, the company developed its national subsidiaries' expertise to source equipment locally, modify designs to meet local requirements, incorporate local components and adapt corporate processes and technologies to accommodate these changes. And by the mid-1980s, offshore production subsidiaries were free to buy minor parts from local vendors as long as quality could be assured, but still had to buy key components from internal sources.

One of the most successful innovations was to give overseas sales subsidiaries more choice over the products they sold. Each year the company held a two-week internal merchandising show and product planning meeting where product divisions exhibited the new lines. Here, overseas sales subsidiary managers described their local market needs and negotiated for change in features, quantities, and even prices of the products they wanted to buy. Product division managers, however, could overrule the sales subsidiary if they thought introduction of a particular product was of strategic importance.

President Yamashita's hope was that Operation Localization would help Matsushita's overseas companies develop the innovative capability and entrepreneurial initiatives that he had long admired in the national organizations of rival Philips. (Past efforts to develop such capabilities abroad had failed. For example, when Matsushita acquired Motorola's TV business in the United States, its highly innovative technology group atrophied as American engineers resigned in response to what they felt to be excessive control from Japan's highly centralized R&D operations.) Yet despite his four localizations, overseas companies continued to act primarily as the implementation arms of central product divisions. In an unusual act for a Japanese CEO, Yamashita publicly expressed his unhappiness with the lack of initiative at the TV plant in Cardiff. Despite the transfer of substantial resources and the delegation of many responsibilities, he felt that the plant remained too dependent on the center.

Tanii's Integration and Expansion

Yamashita's successor, Akio Tanii, expanded on his predecessor's initiatives. In 1986, feeling that Matsushita's product divisions were not giving sufficient attention to international development—in part because they received only 3 percent royalties for foreign production against at least 10 percent return on sales for exports from Japan—he brought all foreign subsidiaries under the control of METC. Tanii then merged METC into the parent company in an effort to fully integrate domestic

and overseas operations. Then, to shift operational control nearer to local markets, he relocated major regional headquarters functions from Japan to North America, Europe, and Southeast Asia. Yet still he was frustrated that the overseas subsidiary companies acted as little more than the implementing agents of the Osaka-based product divisions.

Through all these changes, however, Matsushita's worldwide growth continued generating huge reserves. With $17.5 billion in liquid financial assets at the end of 1989, the company was referred to as the "Matsushita Bank," and several top executives began proposing that if they could not develop innovative overseas companies, they should buy them. Flush with cash and international success, in early 1991 the company acquired MCA, the U.S. entertainment giant, for $6.1 billion with the objective of obtaining a media software source for its hardware. Within a year, however, Japan's bubble economy had burst, plunging the economy into recession. Almost overnight, Tanii had to shift the company's focus from expansion to cost containment. Despite his best efforts to cut costs, the problems ran too deep. With 1992 profits less than half their 1991 level, the board took the unusual move of forcing Tanii to resign in February 1993.

Morishita's Challenge and Response

At 56, Yoichi Morishita was the most junior of the company's executive vice presidents when he was tapped as the new president. Under the slogan "simple, small, speedy, and strategic," he committed to cutting headquarters staff and decentralizing responsibility. Over the next 18 months, he moved 6,000 staff to operating jobs. In a major strategic reversal, he also sold 80 percent of MCA to Seagram, booking a $1.2 billion loss on the transaction.

Yet the company continued to struggle. Japan's domestic market for consumer electronics collapsed—from $42 billion in 1989 to $21 billion in 1999. Excess capacity drove down prices and profits evaporated. And although offshore markets were growing, the rise of new competition—first from Korea, then China—created a global glut of consumer electronics, and prices collapsed.

With a strong yen making exports from Japan uncompetitive, Matsushita's product divisions rapidly shifted production offshore during the 1990s, mostly to low-cost Asian countries like China and Malaysia. By the end of the decade, its 160 factories outside Japan employed 140,000 people—about the same number of employees as in its 133 plants in Japan. Yet, despite the excess capacity and strong yen, management seemed unwilling to radically restructure its increasingly inefficient portfolio of production facilities.

In the closing years of the decade, Morishita began emphasizing the need to develop more of its technology and innovation offshore. Concerned that only 250 of the company's 3,000 R&D scientists and engineers were located outside Japan, he began investing in R&D partnerships and technical exchanges, particularly in fast emerging fields. For example, in 1998 he signed a joint R&D agreement with the Chinese Academy of Sciences, China's leading research organization. Later that year, he announced the establishment of the Panasonic Digital Concepts Center in California. Its mission was to act as a venture fund and an incubation center for the new ideas and technologies emerging in Silicon Valley. To some it was an indication that Matsushita had given up trying to generate new technology and business initiatives from its own overseas companies.

Nakamura's Initiatives

In April 2000, Morishita became chairman and Kunio Nakamura replaced him as president. Profitability was at 2.2 percent of sales, with consumer electronics at only 0.4 percent, including losses generated by onetime cash cows, the TV and VCR divisions. (Exhibits 6 and 7 provide the financial history for Matsushita and key product lines.) The new CEO vowed to raise this to 5 percent by 2004. Key to his plan was to move Matsushita beyond its roots as a "super manufacturer of products" and begin "to meet customer needs through systems and services." He planned to flatten the hierarchy and empower employees to respond to customer needs, and as part of the implementation, all key headquarters functions relating to international operations were transferred to overseas regional offices.

But the biggest shock came in November, when Nakamura announced a program of "destruction and creation," in which he disbanded the product division structure that KM had created as Matsushita's basic or-ganizational building block 67 years earlier. Plants, previously controlled by individual product divisions, would now be integrated into multiproduct production centers. In Japan alone 30 of the 133 factories were to be consolidated or closed. And marketing would shift to two corporate marketing entities, one for Panasonic brands (consumer electronics, information, and communications products) and one for National branded products (mostly home appliances).

They were radical moves, but in a company that even in Japan was being talked about as a takeover target, observers wondered if they were sufficient to restore its global competitiveness.

Case Discussion Questions

1. How did Philips become the most successful company in its business during a period when scores of electrical engineering companies were being formed (e.g., GE, RCA, EMI, Matsushita)? What did it do better than these others?

2. How was Matsushita able to overtake Philips in the consumer electronics industry? What distinctive strategic competencies gave it a competitive advantage? What organizational capabilities embedded them?

3. Why are both companies having such difficulties building the capabilities they both recognize as missing?

4. How effectively has Matsushita managed its change agenda of the 1980s and 1990s?

5. What advice would you have for the current CEO of Philips? What do you think of the company's outsourcing plans?

6. What advice would you have for the current CEO of Matsushita? Is the restructuring program at Matsushita attainable?

Exhibit 6

Matsushita, Summary Financial Data, 1970–2000*

	2000	1995	1990	1985	1980	1975	1970
In billions of yen and percent:							
Sales	¥7,299	¥6,948	¥6,003	¥5,291	¥2,916	¥1,385	¥932
Income before tax	219	232	572	723	324	83	147
As % of sales	3.0%	3.3%	9.5%	13.7%	11.1%	6.0%	15.8%
Net income	¥100	¥90	¥236	¥216	¥125	¥32	¥70
As % of sales	1.4%	1.3%	3.9%	4.1%	4.3%	2.3%	7.6%
Cash dividends (per share)	¥14.00	¥13.50	¥10.00	¥9.52	¥7.51	¥6.82	¥6.21
Total assets	7,955	8,202	7,851	5,076	2,479	1,274	735
Stockholders' equity	3,684	3,255	3,201	2,084	1,092	573	324
Capital investment	355	316	355	288	NA	NA	NA
Depreciation	343	296	238	227	65	28	23
R&D	526	378	346	248	102	51	NA
Employees (units)	290,448	265,397	198,299	175,828	107,057	82,869	78,924
Overseas employees	143,773	112,314	59,216	38,380	NA	NA	NA
As % of total employees	50%	42%	30%	22%	NA	NA	NA
Exchange rate {fiscal period end; ¥$}	103	89	159	213	213	303	360
In millions of dollars:							
Sales	$68,862	$78,069	$37,753	$24,890	$13,690	$4,572	$2,588
Operating income before depreciation	4,944	6,250	4,343	3,682	1,606	317	NA
Operating income after depreciation	1,501	2,609	2,847	2,764	1,301	224	NA
Pretax income	2,224	2,678	3,667	3,396	1,520	273	408
Net income	941	1,017	1,482	1,214	584	105	195
Total assets	77,233	92,159	49,379	21,499	11,636	4,206	2,042
Total equity	35,767	36,575	20,131	10,153	5,129	1,890	900

*Data prior to 1987 are for the fiscal year ending November 20; data 1988 and after are for the fiscal year ending March 31.

Source: Annual reports; Standard & Poor's *Compustat*; Moody's Industrial and International Manuals.

Exhibit 7

Matsushita, Sales by Product and Geographic Segment, 1985–2000 (billion yen)

	2000		1995		FY 1990		FY 1985	
By Product Segment:								
Video and audio equipment	¥1,706	23%	¥1,827	26%	¥2,159	36%	¥2,517	48%
Home appliances and household equipment	1,306	18	—	—	—	—	—	—
Home appliances	—	—	916	13	802	13	763	14
Communication and industrial equipment	—	—	1,797	26	1,375	23	849	16
Electronic components	—	—	893	13	781	13	573	11
Batteries and kitchen-related equipment	—	—	374	4	312	5	217	4
Information and communications equipment	2,175	28	—	—	—	—	—	—
Industrial equipment	817	11	—	—	—	—	—	—
Components	1,618	21	—	—	—	—	—	—
Others	—	—	530	8	573	10	372	7
Total	¥7,682	100%	¥6,948	100%	¥6,003	100%	¥5,291	100%
By Geographic Segment:								
Domestic	¥3,698	51%	¥3,455	50%	¥3,382	56%	¥2,659	50%
Overseas	3,601	49	3,493	50	2,621	44	2,632	50

Notes: Total may not add due to rounding.
Source: Annual reports

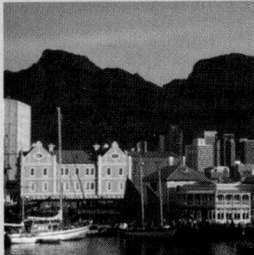

Part 6

Business
Operations

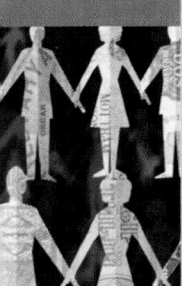

Chapter 15
Exporting, Importing, and Countertrade

Chapter 16
Global Manufacturing and Materials Management

Chapter 17
Global Marketing and R&D

Chapter 18
Global Human Resource Management

Chapter 19
Accounting in the International Business

Chapter 20
Financial Management in the International
Business

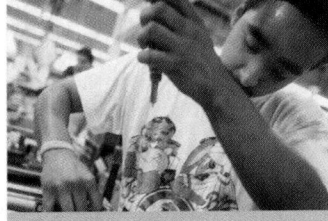

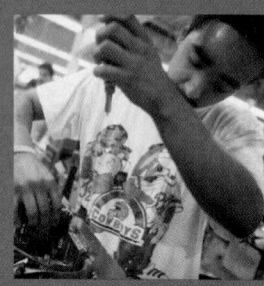

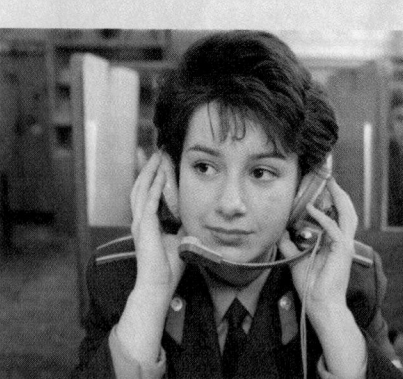

Chapter 15

Exporting,
Importing,
and
Countertrade

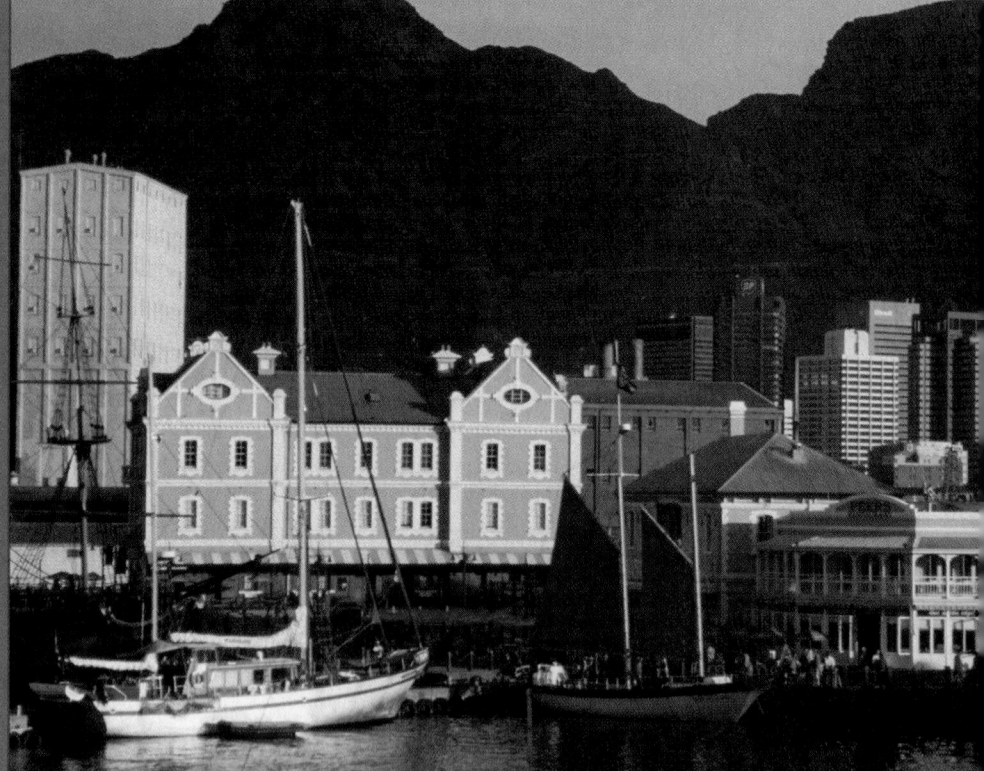

Introduction
The Promise and Pitfalls of Exporting
Improving Export Performance
  An International Comparison
  Information Sources
  Utilizing Export Management
  Companies
  Exporting Strategy
Export and Import Financing
  Lack of Trust
  Letter of Credit
  Draft
  Bill of Lading
  A Typical International Trade
  Transaction
Export Assistance
  Export–Import Bank
  Export Credit Insurance
Countertrade
  The Incidence of Countertrade
  Types of Countertrade
  The Pros and Cons of Countertrade
Chapter Summary
Critical Discussion Questions
Closing Case: Artais Weather Check

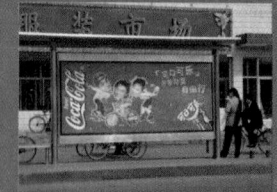

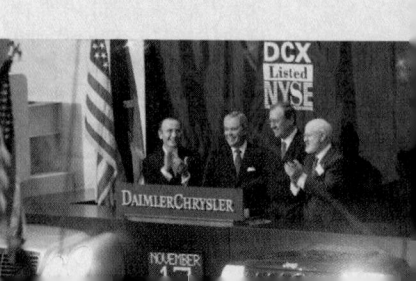

Megahertz Communications

Established in 1982, U.K.-based Megahertz Communications quickly established itself as one of Great Britain's leading independent broadcasting system builders. The company's core skill is in the design, manufacture, and installation of TV and radio broadcast systems, including broadcast and news-gathering vehicles with satellite links. In 1998, Megahertz's managing director, Ashley Coles, set up a subsidiary company, Megahertz International, to sell products to the Middle East, Africa, and Eastern Europe.

While the EU market for media and broadcasting is both mature and well served by large established companies, the Middle East, Africa, and Eastern Europe are growth markets with significant long-term potential for media and broadcasting. They also were not well served by other companies, and all three regions lacked an adequate supply of local broadcast engineers.

Megahertz International's export strategy was simple. The company aimed to provide a turnkey solution to emerging broadcast and media entities in Africa, the Middle East, and Eastern Europe, offering to custom design, manufacture, install, and test broadcasting systems. To gain access to customers, Megahertz hired salespeople with significant experience in these regions and opened a foreign sales office in Italy. Megahertz also exhibited at a number of exhibitions that focused on the targeted regions, sent mailings and e-mail messages to local broadcasters, and set up a Web page, which drew a number of international inquiries.

The response was swift. By early 2000, Megahertz had already been involved in projects in Namibia, Oman, Romania, Russia, Nigeria, Poland, South Africa, Iceland, and Ethiopia. The international operations had expanded to a staff of 75 and were generating £10 million annually. The average order size was about £250,000, and the largest £500,000. In recognition of the company's success, in January 2000 the British government picked Megahertz to receive a Small Business Export Award.

Despite the company's early success, however, it was not all smooth sailing. According to managing director Coles, preshipment financing became a major headache. Coles described his working life as a juggling act, with as much as 20 percent of his time spent chasing money. Due to financing problems, one week Megahertz could have next to nothing in the bank; the next it might have £300,000. The main problem was getting money to finance an order. Megahertz needed additional working capital to finance the purchase of component parts that go into the systems it builds for customers. The company found that banks were very cautious, particularly when they heard that the customers for the order were in Africa or Eastern Europe. The banks worried that Megahertz would not get paid on time, or at all, or that currency fluctuations would reduce the value of payments to Megahertz. Even when Megahertz had a letter of credit from the customer's bank and export insurance documentation, many lenders still saw the risks as too great and declined to lend bridging funds to Megahertz. As a partial solution, Megahertz turned to lending companies that specialize in financing international trade, but many of these companies charged interest rates significantly greater than those charged by banks, thereby squeezing Megahertz's profit margins.

Coles hoped these financing problems were temporary. Once Megahertz established a more sustained cash flow from its international operations, and once banks better appreciated the ability of Coles and his team to secure payment from foreign customers, he hoped that they would become more amenable to lending capital to Megahertz at rates that will help to protect the company's profit margins. By 2002, however, it was clear that the company's growth was too slow to achieve these goals anytime soon. As an alternative solution, in 2003 Coles agreed to sell Megahertz Communications to AZCAR of Canada. AZCAR acquired Megahertz to gain access to the expanding EU market and Megahertz's contacts in the Middle East. For Megahertz, the acquisition gave the company additional working capital that enabled it to take full advantage of export opportunities.

Sources: http://www.megahertz.co.uk; W. Smith, "Today Batley, Tomorrow the World?" *Director*, January 2000, pp. 42–49; and "AZCAR acquires 80% of Megahertz Broadcast Systems," Canadian Corporate Newswire, March 31, 2003.

Introduction

In the previous chapter, we reviewed exporting from a strategic perspective. We considered exporting as just one of a range of strategic options for profiting from international expansion. This chapter is more concerned with the "nuts and bolts" of exporting (and importing). Here we look at how to export.

Exporting is not just for large enterprises; many small firms such as Megahertz Communications have benefited significantly from the moneymaking opportunities of exporting. In the United States, for example, nearly 89 percent of firms that exported in 2001 were small businesses that employed less than 100 people. Their share of total U.S. exports grew steadily over the last decade to reach 21 percent by 2001.[1] Firms with less than 500 employees accounted for 97 percent of all U.S. exporters and almost 30 percent of all exports by value.[2] The situation is similar in several other nations. In Germany, for example, companies with less than 500 employees account for about 30 percent of that nation's exports.[3]

The volume of export activity in the world economy is increasing as exporting has become easier. The gradual decline in trade barriers under the umbrella of GATT and now the WTO (see Chapter 5) along with regional economic agreements such as the European Union and the North American Free Trade Agreement (see Chapter 8) have significantly increased export opportunities. At the same time, modern communication and transportation technologies have alleviated the logistical problems associated with exporting. Firms are increasingly using fax machines, the World Wide Web, toll-free 800 phone numbers, and international air express services to reduce the costs of exporting. Consequently, it is no longer unusual to find small companies such as Megahertz Communications that are thriving as exporters.

Nevertheless, as the opening case illustrates, exporting remains a challenge for many firms. Smaller enterprises can find the process intimidating. The firm wishing to export must identify foreign market opportunities, avoid a host of unanticipated problems that are often associated with doing business in a foreign market, familiarize itself with the mechanics of export and import financing (a problem that Megahertz Communications has had to grapple with), learn where it can get financing and export credit insurance, and learn how it should deal with foreign exchange risk. The process is made more problematic by currencies that are not freely convertible. As a result, there is the problem of arranging payment for exports to countries with weak currencies. This brings us to the complex topic of countertrade, by which payment for exports is received in goods and services rather than money. In this chapter, we will discuss all these issues with the exception of foreign exchange risk, which was covered in Chapter 9. We open the chapter by considering the promise and pitfalls of exporting.

The Promise and Pitfalls of Exporting

The great promise of exporting is that large revenue and profit opportunities are to be found in foreign markets for most firms in most industries. This was true for Megahertz Communications, profiled in the opening case. In another example, Landmark Systems of Vienna, Virginia, had virtually no domestic sales before it entered the European market. Landmark had developed a software program for IBM mainframe computers and located an independent distributor in Europe to represent its product. In its first year, 80 percent of sales were attributed to exporting. In the second year, sales jumped from $100,000 to $1.4 million—with 70 percent attributable to exports.[4] The international market is normally so much larger than the firm's domestic market that exporting is nearly always a way to increase the revenue and profit base of a company. By expanding the size of the market, exporting can enable a firm to achieve economies of scale, thereby lowering its unit costs. Firms that do not export often lose out on significant opportunities for growth and cost reduction.[5]

Studies have shown that while many large firms tend to be proactive about seeking opportunities for profitable exporting, systematically scanning foreign markets to see where the opportunities lie for leveraging their technology, products, and marketing skills in foreign countries, many medium-sized and small firms are very reactive.[6] Typically, such reactive firms do not even consider exporting until their domestic market is saturated and the emergence of excess productive capacity at home forces them to look for growth opportunities in foreign markets. Also, many small and medium-sized firms tend to wait for the world to come to them, rather than going out into the world to seek opportunities. Even when the world does come to them, they may not respond. An example is MMO Music Group, which makes sing-along tapes for karaoke machines. Foreign sales accounted for about 15 percent of MMO's revenues of $8 million in the mid-1990s, but the firm's CEO admits that this figure would probably have been much higher had he paid attention to building international sales during the 1980s and early 1990s. At that time, unanswered faxes and phone messages from Asia and Europe piled up while he was trying to manage the burgeoning domestic side of the business. By the time MMO did turn its attention to foreign markets, other competitors had stepped into the breach and MMO found it tough going to build export volume.[7]

MMO's experience is common, and it suggests a need for firms to become more proactive about seeking export opportunities. One reason more firms are not proactive is that they are unfamiliar with foreign market opportunities; they simply do not know how big the opportunities actually are or where they might lie. Simple ignorance of the potential opportunities is a huge barrier to exporting.[8] Also, many would-be exporters, particularly smaller firms, are often intimidated by the complexities and mechanics of exporting to countries where business practices, language, culture, legal systems, and currency are very different from the home market.[9] This combination of unfamiliarity and intimidation probably explains why exporters still account for only a tiny percentage of U.S. firms, less than 5 percent of firms with under 500 employees according to the Small Business Administration.[10]

To make matters worse, many neophyte exporters have run into significant problems when first trying to do business abroad and this has soured them on future exporting ventures. Common pitfalls include poor market analysis, a poor understanding of competitive conditions in the foreign market, a failure to customize the product offering to the needs of foreign customers, lack of an effective distribution program, a poorly executed promotional campaign in the foreign market, and problems securing financing (again, see the opening case on Megahertz Communications for an example).[11] Neophyte exporters tend to underestimate the time and expertise needed to cultivate business in foreign countries.[12] Few realize the amount of management resources that have to be dedicated to this activity. Many foreign customers require face-to-face negotiations on their home turf. An exporter may have to spend months learning about a country's trade regulations, business practices, and more before a deal can be closed.

Exporters often face voluminous paperwork, complex formalities, and many potential delays and errors. According to a UN report on trade and development, a typical international trade transaction may involve 30 parties, 60 original documents, and 360 document copies, all of which have to be checked, transmitted, reentered into various information systems, processed, and filed. The United Nations has calculated that the time involved in preparing documentation, along with the costs of common errors in paperwork, often amounts to 10 percent of the final value of goods exported.[13]

Improving Export Performance ■

Inexperienced exporters have a number of ways to gain information about foreign market opportunities and avoid common pitfalls that tend to discourage and frustrate novice exporters.[14] In this section, we look at information sources for exporters to increase their knowledge of foreign market opportunities, we consider the pros and cons of using export management companies (EMCs) to assist in the export process, and we review various exporting strategies that can increase the probability of successful exporting. We begin, however, with a look at how several nations try to help domestic firms in the export process.

An International Comparison

One big impediment to exporting is the simple lack of knowledge of the opportunities available. Often there are many markets for a firm's product, but because they are in countries separated from the firm's home base by culture, language, distance, and time, the firm does not know of them. Identifying export opportunities is made even more complex by the fact that more than 200 countries with widely differing cultures compose the world of potential opportunities. Faced with such complexity and diversity, it is not surprising that firms sometimes hesitate to seek export opportunities.

The way to overcome ignorance is to collect information. In Germany, one of the world's most successful exporting nations, trade associations, government agencies, and commercial banks gather information, helping small firms identify export opportunities. A similar function is provided by the Japanese Ministry of International Trade and Industry (MITI), which is always on the lookout for export opportunities. In addition, many Japanese firms are affiliated in some way with the *sogo shosha,* Japan's great trading houses. The sogo shosha have offices all over the world, and they proactively, continuously seek export opportunities for their affiliated companies large and small.[15]

German and Japanese firms can draw on the large reservoirs of experience, skills, information, and other resources of their respective export-oriented institutions. Unlike their German and Japanese competitors, many U.S. firms are relatively blind when they seek export opportunities; they are information disadvantaged. In part, this reflects historical differences. Both Germany and Japan have long made their living as trading nations, whereas until recently the United States has been a relatively self-contained continental economy in which international trade played a minor role. This is changing; both imports and exports now play a greater role in the U.S. economy than they did 20 years ago. However, the United States has not yet evolved an institutional structure for promoting exports similar to that of either Germany or Japan.

Information Sources

Despite institutional disadvantages, U.S. firms can increase their awareness of export opportunities. The most comprehensive source of information is the U.S. Department of Commerce and its district offices all over the country. Within that department are two organizations dedicated to providing businesses with intelligence and assistance for attacking foreign markets: the International Trade Administration and the United States and Foreign Commercial Service Agency.

These agencies provide the potential exporter with a "best prospects" list, which gives the names and addresses of potential distributors in foreign markets along with businesses they are in, the products they handle, and their contact person. In addition, the Department of Commerce has assembled a "comparison shopping service" for 14 countries that are major markets for U.S. exports. For a small fee, a firm can receive a customized market research survey on a product of its choice. This survey provides information on marketability, the competition, comparative prices, distribution channels, and names of potential sales representatives. Each study is conducted on-site by an officer of the Department of Commerce.

The Department of Commerce also organizes trade events that help potential exporters make foreign contacts and explore export opportunities. The department organizes exhibitions at international trade fairs, which are held regularly in major cities worldwide. The department also has a matchmaker program, in which department representatives accompany groups of U.S. businesspeople abroad to meet with qualified agents, distributors, and customers.

In addition to the Department of Commerce, nearly every state and many large cities maintain active trade commissions whose purpose is to promote exports. Most of these provide business counseling, information gathering, technical assistance, and financing. Unfortunately, many have fallen victim to budget cuts or to turf battles for political and financial support with other export agencies.

A number of private organizations are also beginning to gear up to provide more assistance to would-be exporters. Commercial banks and major accounting firms are more willing to assist small firms in starting export operations than they were a decade ago. In addition, large multinationals that have been successful in the global arena are typically willing to discuss opportunities overseas with the owners or managers of small firms.[16]

Utilizing Export Management Companies

One way for first-time exporters to identify the opportunities associated with exporting and to avoid many of the associated pitfalls is to hire an **export management company** (EMC). EMCs are export specialists who act as the export marketing department or international department for their client firms. EMCs normally accept two types of export assignments. They start exporting operations for a firm with the understanding that the firm will take over operations after they are well established. In another type, start-up services are performed with the understanding that the EMC will have continuing responsibility for selling the firm's products. Many EMCs specialize in serving firms in particular industries and in particular areas of the world. Thus, one EMC may specialize in selling agricultural products in the Asian market, while another may focus on exporting electronics products to Eastern Europe.

In theory, the advantage of EMCs is that they are experienced specialists who can help the neophyte exporter identify opportunities and avoid common pitfalls. A good EMC will have a network of contacts in potential markets, have multilingual employees, have a good knowledge of different business mores, and be fully conversant with the ins and outs of the exporting process and with local business regulations. However, the quality of EMCs varies.[17] While some perform their functions very well, others appear to add little value to the exporting company. Therefore, an exporter should review carefully a number of EMCs and check references from an EMC's past clients. One drawback of relying on EMCs is that the company can fail to develop its own exporting capabilities in-house.

Exporting Strategy

In addition to using EMCs, a firm can reduce the risks associated with exporting if it is careful about its choice of exporting strategy.[18] A few guidelines can help firms improve their odds of success. For example, one of the most successful exporting firms in the world, the Minnesota Mining and Manufacturing Co. (3M), has built its export success on three main principles—enter on a small scale to reduce risks, add additional product lines once the exporting operations start to become successful, and hire locals to promote the firm's products (3M's export strategy is profiled in the accompanying Management Focus). Another successful exporter, Red Spot Paint & Varnish, emphasizes the importance of cultivating personal relationships when trying to build an export business (see the Management Focus at the end of this section).

The probability of exporting successfully can be increased dramatically by taking a handful of simple strategic steps. First, particularly for the novice exporter, it helps to hire an EMC or at least an experienced export consultant to help identify opportunities and navigate the web of paperwork and regulations so often involved in exporting. Second, it often makes sense to initially focus on one market or a handful of markets. The idea is to learn about what is required to succeed in those markets, before moving on to other markets. The firm that enters many markets at once runs the risk of spreading its limited management resources too thin. The result of such a "shotgun approach" to exporting may be a failure to become established in any one market. Third, as with

Management Focus

Exporting Strategy at 3M

The Minnesota Mining and Manufacturing Co. (3M), which makes more than 40,000 products including tape, sandpaper, medical products, and the ever-present Post-it Notes, is one of the world's great multinational operations. In 2002, 55 percent of the firm's $16.3 billion in revenues was generated outside the United States. Although the bulk of these revenues came from foreign-based operations, 3M remains a major exporter with $1.5 billion in exports. The company often uses its exports to establish an initial presence in a foreign market, only building foreign production facilities once sales volume rises to a level that justifies local production.

The export strategy is built around simple principles. One is known as "FIDO," which stands for First In (to a new market) Defeats Others. The essence of FIDO is to gain an advantage over other exporters by getting into a market first and learning about that country and how to sell there before others do. A second principle is "make a little, sell a little," which is the idea of entering on a small scale with a very modest investment and pushing one basic product, such as reflective sheeting for traffic signs in Russia or scouring pads in Hungary. Once 3M believes it has learned enough about the market to reduce the risk of failure to reasonable levels, it adds additional products.

A third principle at 3M is to hire local employees to sell the firm's products. The company normally sets up a local sales subsidiary to handle its export activities in a country. It then staffs this subsidiary with local hires because it believes they are likely to have a much better idea of how to sell in their own country than American expatriates. Because of the implementation of this principle, just 160 of 3M's 39,500 foreign employees are U.S. expatriates.

Another common practice at 3M is to formulate global strategic plans for the export and eventual overseas production of its products. Within the context of these plans, 3M gives local managers considerable autonomy to find the best way to sell the product within their country. Thus, when 3M first exported its Post-it Notes in 1981 it planned to "sample the daylights" out of the product, but it also told local managers to find the best way of doing this. Local managers hired office cleaning crews to pass out samples in Great Britain and Germany; in Italy, office products distributors were used to pass out free samples; while in Malaysia, local managers employed young women to go from office to office handing out samples of the product. In typical 3M fashion, when the volume of Post-it Notes was sufficient to justify it, exports from the United States were replaced by local production. Thus, 3M found it worthwhile by 1984 to set up production facilities in France to produce Post-it Notes for the European market.

Sources: R. L. Rose, "Success Abroad," *Wall Street Journal*, March 29, 1991, p. A1; T. Eiben, "US Exporters Keep On Rolling," *Fortune*, June 14, 1994, pp. 128–31; and 3M's website at http://www.mmm.com.

3M, it often makes sense to enter a foreign market on a small scale to reduce the costs of any subsequent failure. Most importantly, entering on a small scale provides the time and opportunity to learn about the foreign country before making significant capital commitments to that market. Fourth, the exporter needs to recognize the time and managerial commitment involved in building export sales and should hire additional personnel to oversee this activity. Fifth, in many countries, it is important to devote a lot of attention to building strong and enduring relationships with local distributors and/or customers (see the Management Focus on Red Spot Paint for an example). Sixth, as 3M often does, it is important to hire local personnel to help the firm establish itself in a foreign market. Local people are likely to have a much greater sense of how to do business in a given country than a manager from an exporting firm who has previously never set foot in that country. Seventh, several studies have suggested the firm needs to be proactive about seeking export opportunities.[19] Armchair exporting does not work! The world will not normally beat a pathway to your door.

Finally, it is important for the exporter to keep the option of local production in mind. Once exports reach a sufficient volume to justify cost-efficient local production, the exporting firm should consider establishing production facilities in the foreign

Red Spot Paint & Varnish

Established in 1903 and based in Evansville, Indiana, Red Spot Paint & Varnish Company is in many ways typical of the companies that can be found in the small towns of America's heartland. The closely held company, whose CEO, Charles Storms, is the great-grandson of the founder, has 500 employees and annual sales of close to $90 million. The company's main product is paint for plastic components used in the automobile industry. Red Spot products are seen on automobile bumpers, wheel covers, grilles, headlights, instrument panels, door inserts, radio buttons, and other components. Unlike many other companies of a similar size and location, however, Red Spot has a thriving international business. International sales (which include exports and local production by licensees) now account for between 15 percent and 25 percent of revenue in any one year, and Red Spot does business in about 15 countries.

Red Spot has long had some international sales and won an export award in the early 1960s. To further its international business in the late 1980s, Red Spot hired a Central Michigan University professor, Bryan Williams. Williams, who was hired because of his foreign-language skills (he speaks German, Japanese, and some Chinese), was the first employee at Red Spot whose exclusive focus was international marketing and sales. His first challenge was the lack of staff skilled in the business of exporting. He found that it was difficult to build an international business without in-house expertise in the basic mechanics of exporting. According to Williams, Red Spot needed people who understood the nuts and bolts of exporting—letters of credit, payment terms, bills of lading, and so on. As might be expected for a business based in the heartland of America, there was not a ready supply of such individuals in the vicinity. It took Williams several years to solve this problem. Now Red Spot has a full-time staff of two who have been trained in the principles of exporting and international operations.

A second problem that Williams encountered was the clash between the quarter-to-quarter mentality that frequently pervades management practice in the United States and the long-term perspective that is often necessary to build a successful international business. Williams has found that building long-term personal relationships with potential foreign customers is often the key to getting business. When foreign customers visit Evansville, Williams often invites them home for dinner. His young children even started calling one visitor from Hong Kong "Uncle." Even with such efforts, however, the business may not come quickly. Meeting with potential foreign customers yields no direct business 90 percent of the time, although Williams points out that it often yields benefits in terms of competitive information and relationship building. He has found that perseverance pays. For example, Williams and Storms called on a major German automobile parts manufacturer for seven years before finally landing some business from the company.

Sources: R. L. Rose and C. Quintanilla, "More Small U.S. Firms Take Up Exporting with Much Success," *Wall Street Journal*, December 20, 1996, p. A1, A10; and interview with Bryan Williams of Red Spot Paint.

market. Such localization helps foster good relations with the foreign country and can lead to greater market acceptance. Exporting is often not an end in itself, but merely a step on the road toward establishment of foreign production (again, 3M provides an example of this philosophy).

Export and Import Financing ■

Mechanisms for financing exports and imports have evolved over the centuries in response to a problem that can be particularly acute in international trade: the lack of trust that exists when one must put faith in a stranger. In this section, we examine the financial devices that have evolved to cope with this problem in the context of international trade: the letter of credit, the draft (or bill of exchange), and the bill of lading. Then we will trace the 14 steps of a typical export–import transaction.

Figure 15.1

Preference of the U.S. Exporter

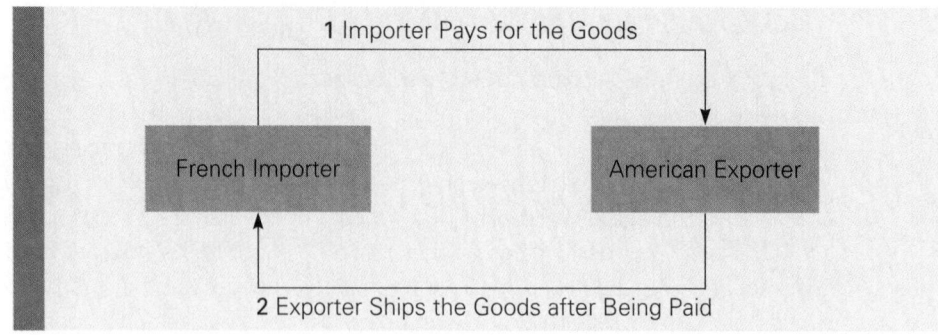

Figure 15.2

Preference of the French Importer

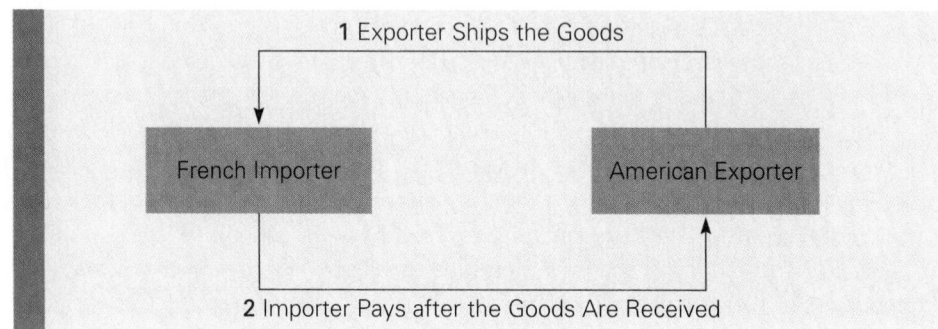

Lack of Trust

Firms engaged in international trade have to trust someone they may have never seen, who lives in a different country, who speaks a different language, who abides by (or does not abide by) a different legal system, and who could be very difficult to track down if he or she defaults on an obligation. Consider a U.S. firm exporting to a distributor in France. The U.S. businessman might be concerned that if he ships the products to France before he receives payment from the French businesswoman, she might take delivery of the products and not pay him. Conversely, the French importer might worry that if she pays for the products before they are shipped, the U.S. firm might keep the money and never ship the products or might ship defective products. Neither party to the exchange completely trusts the other. This lack of trust is exacerbated by the distance between the two parties—in space, language, and culture—and by the problems of using an underdeveloped international legal system to enforce contractual obligations.

Due to the (quite reasonable) lack of trust between the two parties, each has his or her own preferences as to how they would like the transaction to be configured. To make sure he is paid, the manager of the U.S. firm would prefer the French distributor to pay for the products before he ships them (see Figure 15.1). Alternatively, to ensure she receives the products, the French distributor would prefer not to pay for them until they arrive (see Figure 15.2). Thus, each party has a different set of preferences. Unless there is some way of establishing trust between the parties, the transaction might never occur.

The problem is solved by using a third party trusted by both—normally a reputable bank—to act as an intermediary. What happens can be summarized as follows (see Figure 15.3). First, the French importer obtains the bank's promise to pay on her behalf, knowing the U.S. exporter will trust the bank. This promise is known as a letter of credit. Having seen the letter of credit, the U.S. exporter now ships the products to France. Title to the products is given to the bank in the form of a document called a bill of lading. In return, the U.S. exporter tells the bank to pay for the products, which

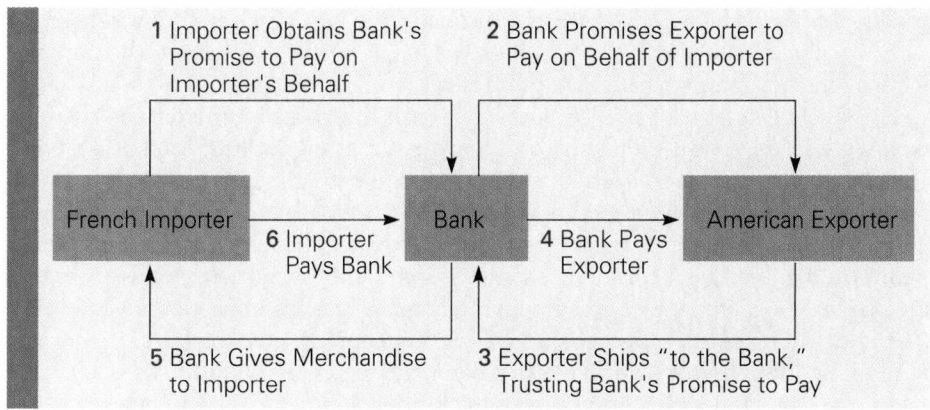

Figure 15.3

The Use of a Third Party

the bank does. The document for requesting this payment is referred to as a draft. The bank, having paid for the products, now passes the title on to the French importer, whom the bank trusts. At that time or later, depending on their agreement, the importer reimburses the bank. In the remainder of this section, we examine how this system works in more detail.

Letter of Credit

A letter of credit, abbreviated as L/C, stands at the center of international commercial transactions. Issued by a bank at the request of an importer, the **letter of credit** states that the bank will pay a specified sum of money to a beneficiary, normally the exporter, on presentation of particular, specified documents.

Consider again the example of the U.S. exporter and the French importer. The French importer applies to her local bank, say, the Bank of Paris, for the issuance of a letter of credit. The Bank of Paris then undertakes a credit check of the importer. If the Bank of Paris is satisfied with her creditworthiness, it will issue a letter of credit. However, the Bank of Paris might require a cash deposit or some other form of collateral from her first. In addition, the Bank of Paris will charge the importer a fee for this service. Typically this amounts to between 0.5 percent and 2 percent of the value of the letter of credit, depending on the importer's creditworthiness and the size of the transaction. (As a rule, the larger the transaction, the lower the percentage.)

Let us assume the Bank of Paris is satisfied with the French importer's creditworthiness and agrees to issue a letter of credit. The letter states that the Bank of Paris will pay the U.S. exporter for the merchandise as long as it is shipped in accordance with specified instructions and conditions. At this point, the letter of credit becomes a financial contract between the Bank of Paris and the U.S. exporter. The Bank of Paris then sends the letter of credit to the U.S. exporter's bank, say, the Bank of New York. The Bank of New York tells the exporter that it has received a letter of credit and that he can ship the merchandise. After the exporter has shipped the merchandise, he draws a draft against the Bank of Paris in accordance with the terms of the letter of credit, attaches the required documents, and presents the draft to his own bank, the Bank of New York, for payment. The Bank of New York then forwards the letter of credit and associated documents to the Bank of Paris. If all of the terms and conditions contained in the letter of credit have been complied with, the Bank of Paris will honor the draft and will send payment to the Bank of New York. When the Bank of New York receives the funds, it will pay the U.S. exporter.

As for the Bank of Paris, once it has transferred the funds to the Bank of New York, it will collect payment from the French importer. Alternatively, the Bank of Paris may allow the importer some time to resell the merchandise before requiring payment. This is not unusual, particularly when the importer is a distributor and not the final consumer of the merchandise, since it helps the importer's cash flow. The Bank of Paris will treat such an extension of the payment period as a loan to the importer and will charge an appropriate rate of interest.

The great advantage of this system is that both the French importer and the U.S. exporter are likely to trust reputable banks, even if they do not trust each other. Once the U.S. exporter has seen a letter of credit, he knows that he is guaranteed payment and will ship the merchandise. Also, an exporter may find that having a letter of credit will facilitate obtaining pre-export financing. For example, having seen the letter of credit, the Bank of New York might be willing to lend the exporter funds to process and prepare the merchandise for shipping to France. This loan may not have to be re-paid until the exporter has received his payment for the merchandise. As for the French importer, she does not have to pay for the merchandise until the documents have arrived and unless all conditions stated in the letter of credit have been satisfied. The drawback for the importer is the fee she must pay the Bank of Paris for the letter of credit. In addition, since the letter of credit is a financial liability against her, it may reduce her ability to borrow funds for other purposes.

Draft

A draft, sometimes referred to as a bill of exchange, is the instrument normally used in international commerce to effect payment. A **draft** is simply an order written by an ex-porter instructing an importer, or an importer's agent, to pay a specified amount of money at a specified time. In the example of the U.S. exporter and the French im-porter, the exporter writes a draft that instructs the Bank of Paris, the French im-porter's agent, to pay for the merchandise shipped to France. The person or business initiating the draft is known as the maker (in this case, the U.S. exporter). The party to whom the draft is presented is known as the drawee (in this case, the Bank of Paris).

International practice is to use drafts to settle trade transactions. This differs from domestic practice in which a seller usually ships merchandise on an open account, fol-lowed by a commercial invoice that specifies the amount due and the terms of pay-ment. In domestic transactions, the buyer can often obtain possession of the merchandise without signing a formal document acknowledging his or her obligation to pay. In contrast, due to the lack of trust in international transactions, payment or a formal promise to pay is required before the buyer can obtain the merchandise.

Drafts fall into two categories, sight drafts and time drafts. A **sight draft** is payable on presentation to the drawee. A **time draft** allows for a delay in payment—normally 30, 60, 90, or 120 days. It is presented to the drawee, who signifies acceptance of it by writing or stamping a notice of acceptance on its face. Once accepted, the time draft becomes a promise to pay by the accepting party. When a time draft is drawn on and accepted by a bank, it is called a banker's acceptance. When it is drawn on and ac-cepted by a business firm, it is called a trade acceptance.

Time drafts are negotiable instruments; that is, once the draft is stamped with an acceptance, the maker can sell the draft to an investor at a discount from its face value. Imagine the agreement between the U.S. exporter and the French importer calls for the exporter to present the Bank of Paris (through the Bank of New York) with a time draft requiring payment 120 days after presentation. The Bank of Paris stamps the time draft with an acceptance. Imagine further that the draft is for $100,000.

The exporter can either hold onto the accepted time draft and receive $100,000 in 120 days or he can sell it to an investor, say the Bank of New York, for a discount from the face value. If the prevailing discount rate is 7 percent, the exporter could receive $97,700 by selling it immediately (7 percent per annum discount rate for 120 days for $100,000 equals $2,300, and $100,000 − $2,300 = $97,700). The Bank of New York would then collect the full $100,000 from the Bank of Paris in 120 days. The exporter might sell the accepted time draft immediately if he needed the funds to finance mer-chandise in transit and/or to cover cash flow shortfalls.

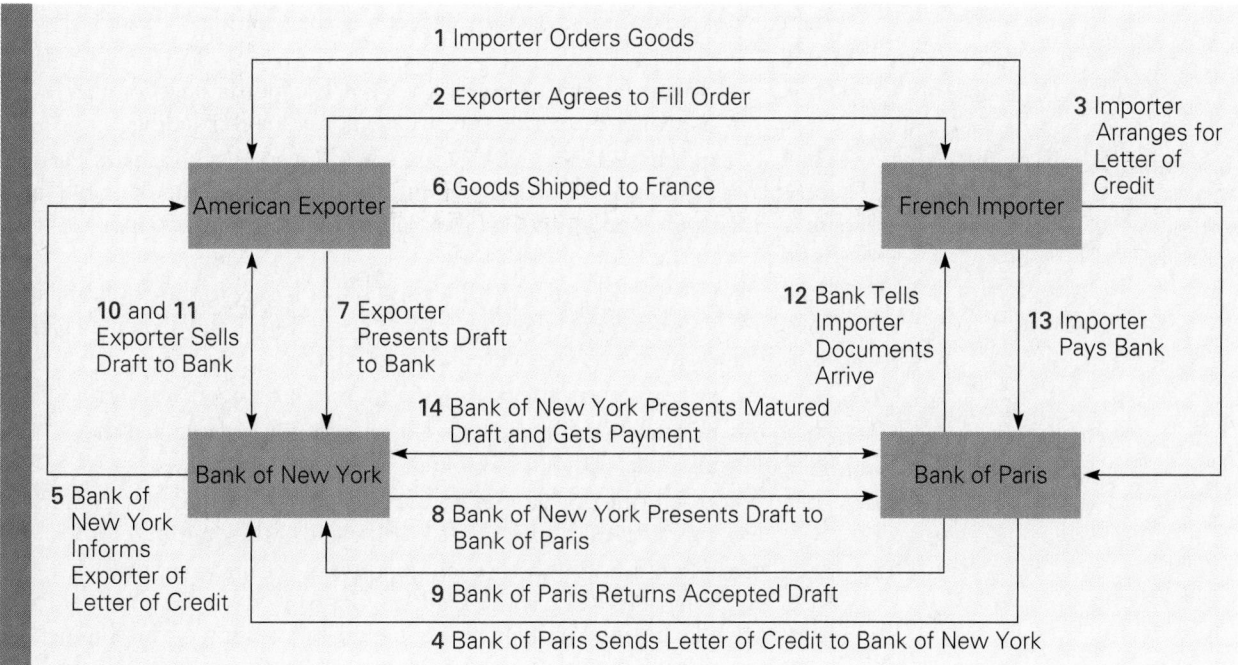

Figure 15.4

A Typical International Trade Transaction

Bill of Lading

The third key document for financing international trade is the bill of lading. The **bill of lading** is issued to the exporter by the common carrier transporting the merchandise. It serves three purposes: it is a receipt, a contract, and a document of title. As a receipt, the bill of lading indicates that the carrier has received the merchandise described on the face of the document. As a contract, it specifies that the carrier is obligated to provide a transportation service in return for a certain charge. As a document of title, it can be used to obtain payment or a written promise of payment before the merchandise is released to the importer. The bill of lading can also function as collateral against which funds may be advanced to the exporter by its local bank before or during shipment and before final payment by the importer.

A Typical International Trade Transaction

Now that we have reviewed the elements of an international trade transaction, let us see how the process works in a typical case, sticking with the example of the U.S. exporter and the French importer. The typical transaction involves 14 steps (see Figure 15.4).

1. The French importer places an order with the U.S. exporter and asks the American if he would be willing to ship under a letter of credit.
2. The U.S. exporter agrees to ship under a letter of credit and specifies relevant information such as prices and delivery terms.
3. The French importer applies to the Bank of Paris for a letter of credit to be issued in favor of the U.S. exporter for the merchandise the importer wishes to buy.
4. The Bank of Paris issues a letter of credit in the French importer's favor and sends it to the U.S. exporter's bank, the Bank of New York.

5. The Bank of New York advises the exporter of the opening of a letter of credit in his favor.

6. The U.S. exporter ships the goods to the French importer on a common carrier. An official of the carrier gives the exporter a bill of lading.

7. The U.S. exporter presents a 90-day time draft drawn on the Bank of Paris in accordance with its letter of credit and the bill of lading to the Bank of New York. The exporter endorses the bill of lading so title to the goods is transferred to the Bank of New York.

8. The Bank of New York sends the draft and bill of lading to the Bank of Paris. The Bank of Paris accepts the draft, taking possession of the documents and promising to pay the now-accepted draft in 90 days.

9. The Bank of Paris returns the accepted draft to the Bank of New York.

10. The Bank of New York tells the U.S. exporter that it has received the accepted bank draft, which is payable in 90 days.

11. The exporter sells the draft to the Bank of New York at a discount from its face value and receives the discounted cash value of the draft in return.

12. The Bank of Paris notifies the French importer of the arrival of the documents. She agrees to pay the Bank of Paris in 90 days. The Bank of Paris releases the documents so the importer can take possession of the shipment.

13. In 90 days, the Bank of Paris receives the importer's payment, so it has funds to pay the maturing draft.

14. In 90 days, the holder of the matured acceptance (in this case, the Bank of New York) presents it to the Bank of Paris for payment. The Bank of Paris pays.

■ Export Assistance

Prospective U.S. exporters can draw on two forms of government-backed assistance to help finance their export programs. They can get financing aid from the Export–Import Bank and export credit insurance from the Foreign Credit Insurance Association.

| Export–Import Bank

The Export–Import Bank, often referred to as Eximbank, is an independent agency of the U.S. government. Its mission is to provide financing aid that will facilitate exports, imports, and the exchange of commodities between the United States and other countries. Eximbank pursues this mission with various loan and loan-guarantee programs. The agency guarantees repayment of medium and long-term loans U.S. commercial banks make to foreign borrowers for purchasing U.S. exports. The Eximbank guarantee makes the commercial banks more willing to lend cash to foreign enterprises.

Eximbank also has a direct lending operation under which it lends dollars to foreign borrowers for use in purchasing U.S. exports. In some cases, it grants loans that commercial banks would not if it sees a potential benefit to the United States in doing so. The foreign borrowers use the loans to pay U.S. suppliers and repay the loan to Eximbank with interest.

| Export Credit Insurance

For reasons outlined earlier, exporters clearly prefer to get letters of credit from importers. However, sometimes an exporter who insists on a letter of credit will lose an order to one who does not require a letter of credit. Thus, when the importer is in a strong bargaining position and able to play competing suppliers against each other, an exporter may have to forgo a letter of credit.[20] The lack of a letter of credit exposes the exporter to the risk that the foreign importer will default on payment. The exporter can insure against this possibility by buying export credit insurance. If the customer defaults, the insurance firm will cover a major portion of the loss.

In the United States, export credit insurance is provided by the Foreign Credit Insurance Association (FCIA), an association of private commercial institutions operating under the guidance of the Export–Import Bank. The FCIA provides coverage against commercial risks and political risks. Losses due to commercial risk result from the buyer's insolvency or payment default. Political losses arise from actions of governments that are beyond the control of either buyer or seller.

Countertrade ∎

Countertrade is an alternative means of structuring an international sale when conventional means of payment are difficult, costly, or nonexistent. We first encountered countertrade in Chapter 9 in our discussion of currency convertibility. A government may restrict the convertibility of its currency to preserve its foreign exchange reserves so they can be used to service international debt commitments and purchase crucial imports.[21] This is problematic for exporters. Nonconvertibility implies that the exporter may not be able to be paid in his or her home currency; and few exporters would desire payment in a currency that is not convertible. Countertrade is a common solution.[22] **Countertrade** denotes a whole range of barterlike agreements; its principle is to trade goods and services for other goods and services when they cannot be traded for money. Some examples of countertrade are:

- An Italian company that manufactures power generating equipment, ABB SAE Sadelmi SpA, was awarded a 720 million baht ($17.7 million) contract by the Electricity Generating Authority of Thailand. The contract specified that the company had to accept 218 million baht ($5.4 million) of Thai farm products as part of the payment.
- Saudi Arabia agreed to buy 10 747 jets from Boeing with payment in crude oil, discounted at 10 percent below posted world oil prices.
- General Electric won a contract for a $150 million electric generator project in Romania by agreeing to market $150 million of Romanian products in markets to which Romania did not have access.
- The Venezuelan government negotiated a contract with Caterpillar under which Venezuela would trade 350,000 tons of iron ore for Caterpillar earthmoving equipment.
- Albania offered such items as spring water, tomato juice, and chrome ore in exchange for a $60 million fertilizer and methanol complex.
- Philip Morris ships cigarettes to Russia, for which it receives chemicals that can be used to make fertilizer. Philip Morris ships the chemicals to China, and in return, China ships glassware to North America for retail sale by Philip Morris.[23]

The Incidence of Countertrade

In the modern era, countertrade arose in the 1960s as a way for the Soviet Union and the Communist states of Eastern Europe, whose currencies were generally nonconvertible, to purchase imports. During the 1980s, the technique grew in popularity among many developing nations that lacked the foreign exchange reserves required to purchase necessary imports. Today, reflecting their own shortages of foreign exchange reserves, many of the successor states to the former Soviet Union and the Eastern European Communist nations are engaging in countertrade to purchase their imports. Consequently, according to some estimates, between 8 and 10 percent of world trade by value is now in the form of countertrade, up from only 2 percent in 1975.[24] There was a notable increase in the volume of countertrade after the Asian financial crisis of 1997. That crisis left many Asian nations with little hard currency to finance international trade. In the tight monetary regime that followed the crisis in 1997, many Asian firms found it very difficult to get access to export credits to finance their own international trade. Consequently, they turned to the only option available to them—countertrade.

Given the importance of countertrade as a means of financing world trade, prospective exporters will have to engage in this technique from time to time to gain access to international markets. The governments of developing nations sometimes insist on a certain amount of countertrade.[25] For example, all foreign companies contracted by Thai state agencies for work costing more than 500 million baht ($12.3 million) are required to accept at least 30 percent of their payment in Thai agricultural products. Between 1994 and mid-1998, foreign firms purchased 21 billion baht ($517 million) in Thai goods under countertrade deals.[26]

Types of Countertrade

With its roots in the simple trading of goods and services for other goods and services, countertrade has evolved into a diverse set of activities that can be categorized as five distinct types of trading arrangements: barter, counterpurchase, offset, switch trading, and compensation or buyback.[27] Many countertrade deals involve not just one arrangement, but elements of two or more.

Barter

Barter is the direct exchange of goods and/or services between two parties without a cash transaction. Although barter is the simplest arrangement, it is not common. Its problems are twofold. First, if goods are not exchanged simultaneously, one party ends up financing the other for a period. Second, firms engaged in barter run the risk of having to accept goods they do not want, cannot use, or have difficulty reselling at a reasonable price. For these reasons, barter is viewed as the most restrictive countertrade arrangement. It is primarily used for one-time-only deals in transactions with trading partners who are not creditworthy or trustworthy.

Counterpurchase

Counterpurchase is a reciprocal buying agreement. It occurs when a firm agrees to purchase a certain amount of materials back from a country to which a sale is made. Suppose a U.S. firm sells some products to China. China pays the U.S. firm in dollars, but in exchange, the U.S. firm agrees to spend some of its proceeds from the sale on textiles produced by China. Thus, although China must draw on its foreign exchange reserves to pay the U.S. firm, it knows it will receive some of those dollars back because of the counterpurchase agreement. In one counterpurchase agreement, Rolls-Royce sold jet parts to Finland. As part of the deal, Rolls-Royce agreed to use some of the proceeds from the sale to purchase Finnish-manufactured TV sets that it would then sell in Great Britain.

Offset

Offset is similar to counterpurchase insofar as one party agrees to purchase goods and services with a specified percentage of the proceeds from the original sale. The difference is that this party can fulfill the obligation with any firm in the country to which the sale is being made. From an exporter's perspective, this is more attractive than a straight counterpurchase agreement because it gives the exporter greater flexibility to choose the goods that it wishes to purchase.

Switch Trading

Switch trading refers to the use of a specialized third-party trading house in a countertrade arrangement. When a firm enters a counterpurchase or offset agreement with a country, it often ends up with what are called counterpurchase credits, which can be used to purchase goods from that country. Switch trading occurs when a third-party trading house buys the firm's counterpurchase credits and sells them to another firm that can better use them. For example, a U.S. firm concludes a counterpurchase agreement with Poland for which it receives some number of counterpurchase credits for purchasing Polish goods. The U.S. firm cannot use and does not want any Polish goods, however, so it sells the credits to a third-party trading house at a discount. The trading house finds a firm that can use the credits and sells them at a profit.

In one example of switch trading, Poland and Greece had a counterpurchase agreement that called for Poland to buy the same U.S.-dollar value of goods from Greece that it sold to Greece. However, Poland could not find enough Greek goods that it required, so it ended up with a dollar-denominated counterpurchase balance in Greece that it was unwilling to use. A switch trader bought the right to 250,000 counterpurchase dollars from Poland for $225,000 and sold them to a European sultana (grape) merchant for $235,000, who used them to purchase sultanas from Greece.

Compensation or Buybacks

A buyback occurs when a firm builds a plant in a country—or supplies technology, equipment, training, or other services to the country—and agrees to take a certain percentage of the plant's output as partial payment for the contract. For example, Occidental Petroleum negotiated a deal with Russia under which Occidental would build several ammonia plants in Russia and as partial payment receive ammonia over a 20-year period.

The Pros and Cons of Countertrade

Countertrade's main attraction is that it can give a firm a way to finance an export deal when other means are not available. Given the problems that many developing nations have in raising the foreign exchange necessary to pay for imports, countertrade may be the only option available when doing business in these countries. Even when countertrade is not the only option for structuring an export transaction, many countries prefer countertrade to cash deals. Thus, if a firm is unwilling to enter a countertrade agreement, it may lose an export opportunity to a competitor that is willing to make a countertrade agreement.

In addition, a countertrade agreement may be required by the government of a country to which a firm is exporting goods or services. Boeing often has to agree to counterpurchase agreements to capture orders for its commercial jet aircraft. For example, in exchange for gaining an order from Air India, Boeing may be required to purchase certain component parts, such as aircraft doors, from an Indian company. Taking this one step further, Boeing can use its willingness to enter into a counterpurchase agreement as a way of winning orders in the face of intense competition from its global rival, Airbus Industrie. Thus, for firms like Boeing, countertrade can become a strategic marketing weapon.

However, the drawbacks of countertrade agreements are substantial. Other things being equal, firms would normally prefer to be paid in hard currency. Countertrade contracts may involve the exchange of unusable or poor-quality goods that the firm cannot dispose of profitably. For example, a few years ago, one U.S. firm got burned when 50 percent of the television sets it received in a countertrade agreement with Hungary were defective and could not be sold. In addition, even if the goods it receives are of high quality, the firm still needs to dispose of them profitably. To do this, countertrade requires the firm to invest in an in-house trading department dedicated to arranging and managing countertrade deals. This can be expensive and time-consuming.

Given these drawbacks, countertrade is most attractive to large, diverse multinational enterprises that can use their worldwide network of contacts to dispose of goods acquired in countertrading. The masters of countertrade are Japan's giant trading firms, the *sogo shosha*, which use their vast networks of affiliated companies to profitably dispose of goods acquired through countertrade agreements. The trading firm of Mitsui & Company, for example, has about 120 affiliated companies in almost every sector of the manufacturing and service industries. If one of Mitsui's affiliates receives goods in a countertrade agreement that it cannot consume, Mitsui & Company will normally be able to find another affiliate that can profitably use them. Firms affiliated with one of Japan's *sogo shosha* often have a competitive advantage in countries where countertrade agreements are preferred.

Western firms that are large, diverse, and have a global reach (e.g., General Electric, Philip Morris, and 3M) have similar profit advantages from countertrade agreements. Indeed, 3M has established its own trading company—3M Global Trading, Inc.—to develop and manage the company's international countertrade programs. Unless there is no alternative, small and medium-sized exporters should probably try to avoid countertrade deals because they lack the worldwide network of operations that may be required to profitably utilize or dispose of goods acquired through them.[28]

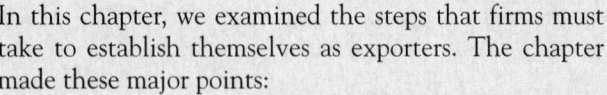

ChapterSummary

In this chapter, we examined the steps that firms must take to establish themselves as exporters. The chapter made these major points:

1. One big impediment to exporting is ignorance of foreign market opportunities.

2. Neophyte exporters often become discouraged or frustrated with the exporting process because they encounter many problems, delays, and pitfalls.

3. The way to overcome ignorance is to gather information. In the United States, a number of institutions, most important of which is the Department of Commerce, can help firms gather information in the matchmaking process. Export management companies can also help an exporter to identify export opportunities.

4. Many of the pitfalls associated with exporting can be avoided if a company hires an experienced export management company, or export consultant, and if it adopts the appropriate export strategy.

5. Firms engaged in international trade must do business with people they cannot trust and people who may be difficult to track down if they default on an obligation. Due to the lack of trust, each party to an international transaction has a different set of preferences regarding the configuration of the transaction.

6. The problems arising from lack of trust between exporters and importers can be solved by using a third party that is trusted by both, normally a reputable bank.

7. A letter of credit is issued by a bank at the request of an importer. It states that the bank promises to pay a beneficiary, normally the exporter, on presentation of documents specified in the letter.

8. A draft is the instrument normally used in international commerce to effect payment. It is an order written by an exporter instructing an importer, or an importer's agent, to pay a specified amount of money at a specified time.

9. Drafts are either sight drafts or time drafts. Time drafts are negotiable instruments.

10. A bill of lading is issued to the exporter by the common carrier transporting the merchandise. It serves as a receipt, a contract, and a document of title.

11. U.S. exporters can draw on two types of government-backed assistance to help finance their exports: loans from the Export–Import Bank and export credit insurance from the FCIA.

12. Countertrade includes a range of barterlike agreements. It is primarily used when a firm exports to a country whose currency is not freely convertible and may lack the foreign exchange reserves required to purchase the imports.

13. The main attraction of countertrade is that it gives a firm a way to finance an export deal when other means are not available. A firm that insists on being paid in hard currency may be at a competitive disadvantage vis-à-vis one that is willing to engage in countertrade.

14. The main disadvantage of countertrade is that the firm may receive unusable or poor-quality goods that cannot be disposed of profitably.

Critical Discussion Questions

1. A firm based in Washington state wants to export a shipload of finished lumber to the Philippines. The would-be importer cannot get sufficient credit from domestic sources to pay for the shipment but insists that the finished lumber can quickly be resold in the Philippines for a profit. Outline the steps the exporter should take to effect this export to the Philippines.

2. You are the assistant to the CEO of a small textile firm that manufactures quality, premium-priced, stylish clothing. The CEO has decided to see what the opportunities are for exporting and has asked you for advice as to the steps the company should take. What advice would you give the CEO?

3. An alternative to using a letter of credit is export credit insurance. What are the advantages and disadvantages of using export credit insurance rather than a letter of credit for exporting (a) a luxury yacht from California to Canada, and (b) machine tools from New York to the Ukraine?

4. How do you explain the popularity of countertrade? Under what scenarios might its popularity increase still further by the year 2010? Under what scenarios might its popularity decline by the year 2010?

5. How might a company make strategic use of countertrade schemes as a marketing weapon to generate export revenues? What are the risks associated with pursuing such a strategy?

Research Task | globalEDGE™ globaledge.msu.edu

Use the globalEDGE™ site to complete the following exercises:

1. The Internet is rich with resources that provide guidance to companies that wish to expand their markets through exporting; globalEDGE provides links to these "tutorial" websites. Identify five of these sources and provide a description of the services available for new exporters through each of these sources.

2. Utilize the globalEDGE™ Glossary of International Business Terms to identify the definitions of the following exporting terms: air waybill, certificate of inspection, certificate of product origin, wharfage charge, and export broker.

Notes

1. U.S. Department of Commerce, "A Profile of U.S. Exporting Companies, 2000–2001," February 2003. Report available at http://www.census.gov/foreign-trade/aip/index.html#profile.

2. Ibid.

3. W. J. Holstein, "Why Johann Can Export, but Johnny Can't," *Business Week*, November 4, 1991, pp. 64–65.

4. U.S. Small Business Administration, "Guide to Exporting," 2003. Report can be accessed at http://www.sba.gov/oit/info/Guide-To-Exporting/index.html.

5. R. A. Pope, "Why Small Firms Export: Another Look," *Journal of Small Business Management* 40 (2002), pp. 17–26.

6. S. T. Cavusgil, "Global Dimensions of Marketing," in *Marketing*, ed. P. E. Murphy and B. M. Enis (Glenview, IL: Scott, Foresman, 1985), pp. 577–99.

7. S. M. Mehta, "Enterprise: Small Companies Look to Cultivate Foreign Business," *Wall Street Journal*, July 7, 1994, p. B2.

8. W. Pavord and R. Bogart, "The Dynamics of the Decision to Export," *Akron Business and Economic Review*, 1975, pp. 6–11.

9. W. J. Burpitt and D. A. Rondinelli, "Small Firms' Motivations for Exporting: To Earn and Learn?" *Journal of Small Business Management*, October 2000, pp. 1–14.

10. Small Business Administration, "The State of Small Business 1999–2000: Report to the President," 2001. Can be accessed at http://www.sba.gov/advo/stats/stateofsb99_00.pdf.

11. A. O. Ogbuehi and T. A. Longfellow, "Perceptions of U.S. Manufacturing Companies concerning Exporting," *Journal of Small Business Management*, October 1994, pp. 37–59. U.S. Small Business Administration, "Guide to Exporting".

12. R. W. Haigh, "Thinking of Exporting?" *Columbia Journal of World Business* 29 (December 1994), pp. 66–86.

13. F. Williams, "The Quest for More Efficient Commerce," *Financial Times*, October 13, 1994, p. 7.

14. See Burpitt and Rondinelli, "Small Firms' Motivations for Exporting," and C. S. Katsikeas, L. C. Leonidou, and N. A. Morgan, "Firm Level Export Performance Assessment," *Academy of Marketing Science* 28 (2000), pp. 493–511.

15. M. Y. Yoshino and T. B. Lifson, *The Invisible Link* (Cambridge, MA: MIT Press, 1986).

16. L. W. Tuller, *Going Global* (Homewood, IL: Business One-Irwin, 1991).

17. Haigh, "Thinking of Exporting?"

18. M. A. Raymond, J. Kim, and A. T. Shao. "Export Strategy and Performance," *Journal of Global Marketing* 15 (2001), pp. 5–29, and P. S. Aulakh, M. Kotabe, and H. Teegen, "Export Strategies and Performance of Firms from Emerging Economies," *Academy of Management Journal* 43 (2000), pp. 342–61.

19. J. Francis and C. Collins-Dodd, "The Impact of Firms' Export Orientation on the Export Performance of High-Tech Small and Medium Sized Enterprises," *Journal of International Marketing* 8, no. 3 (2000), pp. 84–103.

20. For a review of the conditions under which a buyer has power over a supplier, see M. E. Porter, *Competitive Strategy* (New York: Free Press, 1980).

21. *Exchange Agreements and Exchange Restrictions* (Washington, DC: International Monetary Fund, 1989).

22. It's also sometimes argued that countertrade is a way of reducing the risks inherent in a traditional money-for-goods transaction, particularly with entities from emerging economies. See C. J. Choi, S. H. Lee, and J. B. Kim, "A Note of Countertrade: Contractual Uncertainty and Transactional Governance in Emerging Economies," *Journal of International Business Studies* 30, no. 1 (1999), pp. 189–202.

23. J. R. Carter and J. Gagne, "The Do's and Don'ts of International Countertrade," *Sloan Management Review*, Spring 1988, pp. 31–37, and W. Maneerungsee, "Countertrade: Farm Goods Swapped for Italian Electricity," *Bangkok Post*, July 23, 1998.

24. Estimate from the American Countertrade Association at http://freedonia.tpusa.com/infosrc/aca/. See also D. West, "Countertrade," *Business Credit* 104, no. 4 (2001), pp. 64–67, and B. Meyer, "The Original Meaning of Trade Meets the Future of Barter," *World Trade* 13 (January 2000), pp. 46–50.

25. Carter and Gagne, "The Do's and Dont's of International Countertrade."

26. Maneerungsee, "Countertrade: Farm Goods Swapped for Italian Electricity."

27. For details, see Carter and Gagne, "Do's and Dont's"; J. F. Hennart, "Some Empirical Dimensions of Countertrade," *Journal of International Business Studies*, 1990, pp. 240–60; and West, "Countertrade."

28. D. J. Lecraw, "The Management of Countertrade: Factors Influencing Success," *Journal of International Business Studies*, Spring 1989, pp. 41–59.

Artais Weather Check

Closing Case

Artais Weather Check, Inc., is a small Ohio-based company that manufactures an automated weather observation system, or AWOS, for small airports. Artais's AWOS system records runway conditions such as wind speed, direction, and temperature and converts the data into a voice message for pilots. Only three other companies besides Artais have been certified by the Federal Aviation Administration (FAA) to produce the equipment, and Artais dominates the market in the United States with a share of more than 80 percent.

Despite its dominant market share in the United States, Artais gets the majority of its $8 million in annual revenues from foreign markets. Within the United States, the market for automated weather observation systems is small. Although there are 18,000 public and private airports in the country, the largest have round-the-clock human weather watchers, while most of the smaller airports cannot afford the $45,000 to $60,000 required to install an AWOS. Thus, the prospects for growth in the United States seem to be limited to sales of about 75 systems per year nationwide.

To continue to grow the company's revenues, Artais has increasingly looked toward export sales. Initially, export sales were slow to develop, perhaps because Artais's management had very little international experience and spent several years simply trying to learn about foreign markets and the mechanics of exporting. However, exports have surged to account for close to two-thirds of the company's total revenues. But to get foreign orders, Artais has had to deal with frustrations it never encountered at home.

The first problem it came up against was one of name recognition. Although Artais is well-known within the United States, the company found that its name recognition was close to zero overseas. Another problem involves subsidized competition; according to Artais, its main competitors in some foreign markets are subsidized by their governments to protect jobs. Artais has also found that it needs to customize its products for foreign markets. To sell in Egypt, for example, its system had to be reprogrammed to relay weather information in Arabic as well as English. International customers also require that spare parts be located close by and that Artais employees install the equipment and provide on-site training, all of which raises the costs of doing business.

Political factors have also had a major impact on the outcome of some deals. For example, after working hard to secure a deal in Romania, Artais unexpectedly saw the deal fall through at the last moment. Instead, the deal went to a German competitor. According to some locals, the Romanian government, eager to improve trading relations with the European Union, gave the job to Artais's German competitor in an attempt to curry favor with the trading bloc's most powerful member. Artais has also lost several bids to competitors because it was unwilling to take payment in a foreign currency from an emerging market country, preferring instead to be paid in U.S. dollars.

Despite problems such as these, Artais has sold systems to airports in Taiwan, China, Ecuador, Saudi Arabia, and Egypt. Artais has found that such overseas contracts can be more lucrative than its domestic sales because of all the extras, such as spare parts, installation fees, and training. For the basic AWOS, the value of the foreign contracts has ranged from $200,000 to $2 million, compared with $45,000 to $60,000 in the United

States. Building on this success, Artais introduced a system designed to detect low-level wind shears. The system, which costs $350,000 per unit, was designed to be sold outside the United States. According to company representatives, Artais is disregarding the U.S. market because of the cost and time involved in meeting specifications established by the FAA. Systems built to FAA specifications can cost $1 million a unit, which is beyond the reach of many foreign buyers. The first two sales of the new system were to Saudi Arabia. The company believes that in time 20 percent of its annual sales will come from the wind-shear system, all of which will be generated overseas. In addition, the company believes that the bulk of revenues for its basic AWOS will continue to be generated overseas.

Source: S. N. Mehta, "Enterprise: Artais Finds That Smallness Isn't a Handicap in Global Market," *Wall Street Journal*, June 23, 1994, p. B2, and R. Carter, "Artais' New System to Help Airlines Harness the Wind," *Columbus Dispatch*, August 28, 1995, p. 8.

Case Discussion Questions

1. What is the motivation for Artais's shift toward a strategy of export-led growth? Why do you think the opportunities for growth might be greater in foreign markets? Do you think that developing countries are likely to be a major market opportunity for Artais? Why?

2. Could Artais have ramped up its foreign sales more rapidly? How?

3. What potential problems might Artais encounter selling its equipment to nations such as Egypt and Ecuador? How can the company deal with these problems?

4. Do you think that it is wise for the company to insist on being paid in dollars? What alternatives are open to the company? What are the risks associated with these alternatives? Should the company change its policy?

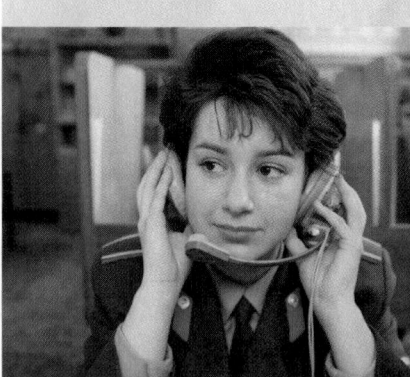

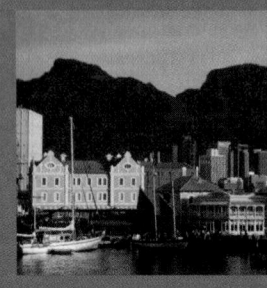

Chapter 16

Global Manufacturing and Materials Management

Introduction
Strategy, Manufacturing, and Logistics
Where to Manufacture
    Country Factors
    Technological Factors
    Product Factors
    Locating Manufacturing Facilities
The Strategic Role of Foreign Factories
Make-or-Buy Decisions
    The Advantages of Make
    The Advantages of Buy
    Trade-offs
    Strategic Alliances with Suppliers
Managing a Global Supply Chain
    The Role of Just-in-Time Inventory
    The Role of Organization
    The Role of Information Technology
    and the Internet
Chapter Summary
Critical Discussion Questions
Closing Case: Li & Fung

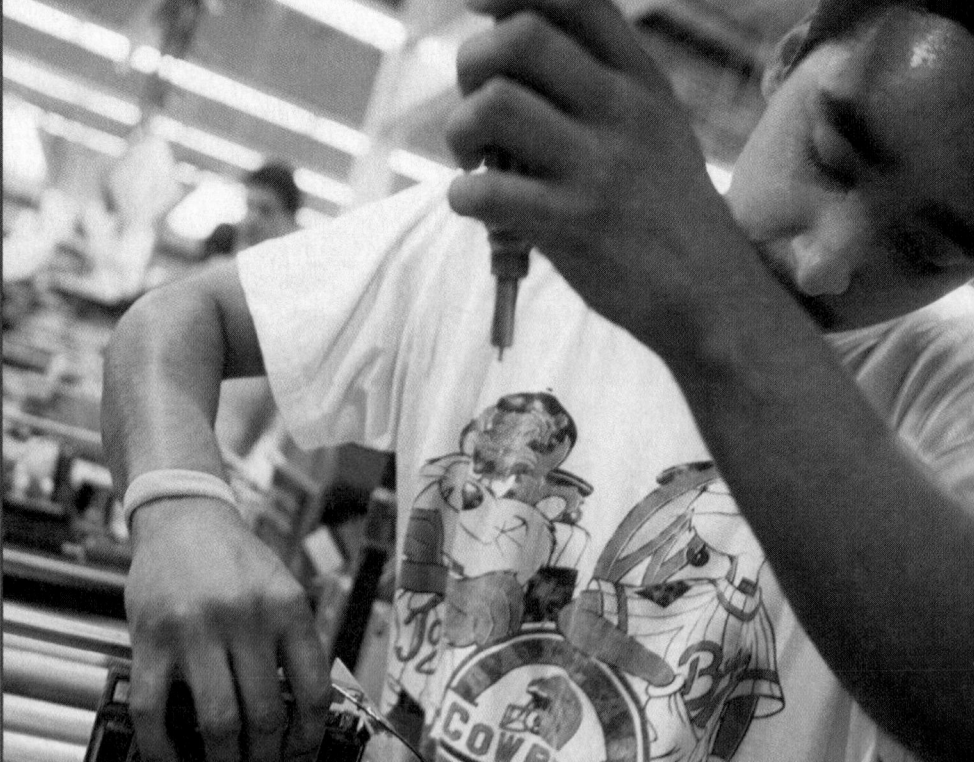

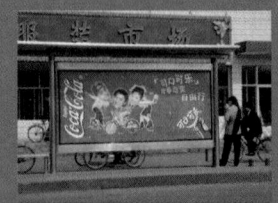

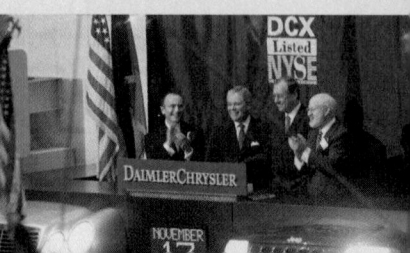

Competitive Advantage at Dell Computer

Michael Dell started Dell Computer Corporation in 1984 when he was an undergraduate student at the University of Texas. Two decades later, Dell has grown to become one of the world's great computer companies, with a leading share in the personal computer and server businesses. In fiscal 2003, a year in which most computer makers lost money due to slumping global demand for PCs, Dell saw its revenues jump by $5 billion to $36 billion, made $2.8 billion in operating profit, and gained 2.3 percent in global market share. Approximately one-third of Dell's sales were made outside the United States. Dell credits much of its strong performance in a tough environment to a cost structure that is the lowest in the industry. That cost structure is in part the result of Dell's global manufacturing and supply chain management strategy.

Dell has manufacturing sites in Brazil, Ireland, Malaysia, and China, in addition to the United States. The sites were chosen for low labor costs, the high productivity of the local workforce, and their proximity to important regional markets (wage rates in China for example, are 5 percent of those in the United States). Dell prefers to manufacture close to regional markets to reduce shipping costs and increase the speed of delivery to customers. In addition to manufacturing, much of Dell's customer support operations are also performed outside of the United States with a major center in Bangalore, India (U.S. customers calling Dell's customer support are likely to be connected to a service agent in India). India was chosen not just because of low wage rates, but also because of the availability of an educated and English-speaking workforce.

Dell's supply base is also global. Dell has some 200 suppliers, more than half of which are located outside the United States. Thirty suppliers account for about 75 percent of Dell's total purchases. Over 50 percent of its major suppliers are in Asia.

From inception, Dell's business model was based on direct selling to customers, cutting out wholesalers and retailers. The original thought was that by cutting out the middle of the distribution chain, Dell could offer consumers lower prices. Initially, direct selling was achieved through mailings and telephone contacts, but since the mid-1990s the majority of Dell's sales have been made over the Internet, and by 2003, some 85 percent of all sales were made through this medium. Internet selling has enabled Dell to offer its customers the ability to customize their orders, mixing and matching product features such as microprocessors, memory, monitors, internal hard drives, CD and DVD drives, keyboard and mouse format, and the like, to get the system that best suits their particular requirements.

While the ability to customize products, when combined with low prices, has made Dell attractive to customers, the real power of the business model is to be found in how Dell manages its global supply chain to minimize inventory while building PCs to individual customer orders within three days. Dell uses the Internet to feed real-time information about order flow to its suppliers. Dell's suppliers, wherever they are located, have up-to-the-minute information about demand trends for the components they produce, along with volume expectations for the next 4 to 12 weeks that are constantly updated as new information becomes available. Dell's suppliers use this information to adjust their own production schedules on a real-time basis, producing just enough components for Dell's needs and shipping them by the most appropriate mode, typically truck or air express so that they arrive just in time for production. This tight coordination is pushed far down the supply chain, with Dell sharing key data with its suppliers' principal suppliers. For example, Quanta of Taiwan makes notebook computers for Dell that incorporate digital signal processing chips from Texas Instruments. To better coordinate the supply chain, Dell passes information to Texas Instruments in addition to Quanta. This allows Texas Instruments to adjust its schedules to Quanta's needs, which in turn can adjust its schedule according to data from Dell.

Dell's ultimate goal is to drive all inventories out of the supply chain apart from those in transit between suppliers and Dell, effectively replacing inventory with information. Although Dell has not yet achieved this goal, the firm has reduced inventory to the lowest level in the industry. In 2003, Dell carried only three days of inventory, compared to 30, 45, or even 90 days' worth at competitors. This is a critical advantage in the computer inventory, where component costs account for 75 percent of revenues and typically fall by 1 percent per week due to rapid obsolescence. For example, when larger, faster hard drives are introduced, which occurs every three to six months, the value of previous-generation hard drives is significantly reduced. So if Dell holds one week of inventory, and a competitor holds four weeks, this translates immediately into 3 percent worth of component cost advantage to Dell, which can mean a 2 percent advantage on the bottom line. Driving inventory out of the system also dramatically reduces Dell's need for working capital and boosts the company's profitability.

Dell's Internet-based customer ordering and procurement systems have also allowed the company to synchronize demand and supply to an extent that few other companies can. For example, if Dell sees that it is running out of a particular component, say 17-inch monitors from Sony, it can manipulate demand by offering a 19-inch model at a lower price until Sony delivers more 17-inch monitors. By taking such steps to fine-tune the balance between demand and supply, Dell can meet customers' expectations. Also, balancing supply and demand allows the company to minimize excess and obsolete inventory. Dell writes off between 0.05 percent and 0.1 percent of total materials costs in excess or obsolete inventory. Its competitors write off between 2 percent and 3 percent, which again gives Dell a significant cost advantage.

Sources: D. Hunter, "How Dell Keeps from Stumbling," *Business Week,* May 14, 2001, pp. 38–40; "Enter the Eco-system: From Supply Chain to Network," *The Economist,* November 11, 2000; "Dell's Direct Initiative," *Country Monitor,* June 7, 2000, p. 5; B. Einhorn, "Quanta's Quantum Leap," *Business Week,* November 5, 2001, pp. 79–80; Dell Computer 10K statement for fiscal 2003, April 28, 2003; and J. E. Garten, "When Everything Is Made in China," *Business Week,* June 17, 2002, pp. 20–22.

■ Introduction

As trade barriers fall and global markets develop, many firms increasingly confront a set of interrelated issues. First, where in the world should manufacturing activities be located? Should they be concentrated in a single country, or should they be dispersed around the globe, matching the type of activity with country differences in factor costs, tariff barriers, political risks, and the like to minimize costs and maximize value added? Second, what should be the long-term strategic role of foreign production sites? Should the firm abandon a foreign site if factor costs change, moving production to another more favorable location, or is there value to maintaining an operation at a given location even if underlying economic conditions change? Third, should the firm own foreign manufacturing activities, or is it better to outsource those activities to independent vendors? Fourth, how should a globally dispersed supply chain be managed, and what is the role of Internet-based information technology in the management of global logistics? Fifth, should the firm manage global logistics itself, or should it outsource the management to enterprises that specialize in this activity?

In this chapter, we shall consider all these questions and discuss the various factors that influence decisions in this arena. The opening case provides a good example of how global manufacturing and logistic strategy can be used to establish a competitive advantage. Dell is the low-cost company in the computer industry. Its cost advantage comes in part from where it locates its global manufacturing and customer service functions, in part from its ability to tightly coordinate its global supply chain to remove inventory from the system, and in part from its direct selling model.

■ Strategy, Manufacturing, and Materials Management

In Chapter 12, we introduced the concept of the value chain and discussed a number of value creation activities, including production, marketing, materials management (logistics), R&D, human resources, and information systems. In this chapter, we will focus on two of these activities—production and materials management (logistics)—and attempt to clarify how they might be performed internationally to (1) lower the costs of value creation and (2) add value by better serving customer needs. We will discuss the contributions of information technology to these activities, which has become particularly important in the era of the Internet. In later chapters, we will look at other value creation activities in this international context (marketing, R&D, and human resource management).

In Chapter 12, we defined *production* as "the activities involved in creating a product." We used the term *production* to denote both service and manufacturing activities, since one can produce a service or produce a physical product. In this chapter, we focus more on manufacturing than on service activities, so we will use the term *manufacturing* rather than production. **Materials management** is the activity that controls

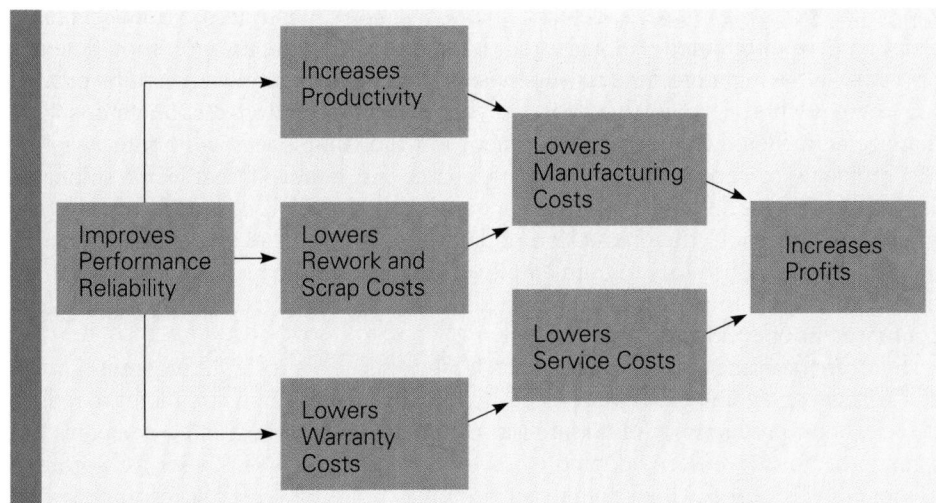

Figure 16.1

The Relationship between Quality and Costs

Source: Reprinted from "What Does Product Quality Really Mean?" by David A. Garvin, *Sloan Management Review 26* (Fall 1984), Figure 1, p. 37, by permission of the publisher. Copyright 1984 by Massachusetts Institute of Technology. All rights reserved.

the transmission of physical materials through the value chain, from procurement through production and into distribution. Materials management includes **logistics,** which refers to the procurement and physical transmission of material through the supply chain, from suppliers to customers. Manufacturing and materials management are closely linked, since a firm's ability to perform its manufacturing function efficiently depends on a continuous supply of high-quality material inputs, for which materials management is responsible.

The manufacturing and materials management functions of an international firm have a number of important strategic objectives.[1] One is to lower costs. Dispersing manufacturing activities to various locations around the globe where each activity can be performed most efficiently can lower costs. Costs can also be lowered by managing the global supply chain efficiently so as to better match supply and demand. Efficient supply chain management reduces the amount of inventory in the system and increases inventory turnover, which means the firm has to invest less working capital in inventory and is less likely to find excess inventory on hand that cannot be sold and has to be written off. A second strategic objective shared by manufacturing and materials management is to increase product quality by eliminating defective products from both the supply chain and the manufacturing process.[2] (In this context, *quality* means *reliability*, implying that the product has no defects and performs well.) The objectives of reducing costs and increasing quality are not independent of each other. As illustrated in Figure 16.1, the firm that improves its quality control will also reduce its costs of value creation. Improved quality control reduces costs in three ways:

- Increases productivity because time is not wasted manufacturing poor-quality products that cannot be sold, leading to a direct reduction in unit costs.
- Lowers rework and scrap costs associated with defective products.
- Lowers the warranty costs associated with fixing defective products.

The effect is to lower the costs of value creation by reducing both manufacturing and service costs.

The main management technique that companies utilize to boost their product quality is **total quality management** (TQM). TQM takes as its central focus the need to improve the quality of a company's products and services. The TQM philosophy was developed by a number of American consultants such as the late W. Edward Deming, Joseph Juran, and A. V. Feigenbaum.[3] Deming identified a number of steps that should be part of any TQM program. He argued that management should embrace the philosophy that mistakes, defects, and poor-quality materials are not acceptable and should be eliminated. He suggested that the quality of supervision should be improved by allowing more time for supervisors to work with employees and by providing them with the tools they need to do the job. Deming recommended that management should create an environment in which employees will not fear reporting problems or recommending improvements. He believed that work standards should not only be defined as numbers or quotas, but should also include some notion of quality to promote the production of defect-free output. He argued that management has the responsibility to train employees in new skills to keep pace with changes in the workplace. In addition, he believed that achieving better quality requires the commitment of everyone in the company.

In recent years many companies have adopted a successor to TQM programs known as a six sigma program. **Six sigma** is a statistically based philosophy that aims to reduce defects, boost productivity, eliminate waste, and cut costs throughout a company. Six sigma programs have been adopted by several major corporations, such as Motorola, General Electric, and Allied Signal. Sigma comes from the Greek letter that statisticians use to represent a standard deviation from a mean, the higher the number of "sigmas" the smaller the number of errors. At six sigma, a production process would be 99.99966 percent accurate, creating just 3.4 defects per million units. While it is almost impossible for a company to achieve such perfection, six sigma quality is a goal that several strive toward. Increasingly, companies are adopting six sigma programs to try to boost their product quality and productivity.[4]

The growth of international standards has also focused greater attention on the importance of product quality. In Europe, for example, the European Union requires that the quality of a firm's manufacturing processes and products be certified under a quality standard known as ISO 9000 before the firm is allowed access to the EU marketplace. Although the ISO 9000 certification process has proved to be somewhat bureaucratic and costly for many firms, it does focus management attention on the need to improve the quality of products and processes.[5]

In addition to lowering costs and improving quality, two other objectives have particular importance in international businesses. First, manufacturing and materials management must be able to accommodate demands for local responsiveness. As we saw in Chapter 12, demands for local responsiveness arise from national differences in consumer tastes and preferences, infrastructure, distribution channels, and host-government demands. Demands for local responsiveness create pressures to decentralize manufacturing activities to the major national or regional markets in which the firm does business or to implement flexible manufacturing processes that enable the firm to customize the product coming out of a factory according to the market in which it is to be sold.

Second, manufacturing and materials management must be able to respond quickly to shifts in customer demand. In recent years, time-based competition has grown more important.[6] When consumer demand is prone to large and unpredictable shifts, the firm that can adapt most quickly to these shifts will gain an advantage. As we shall see, both manufacturing and materials management play critical roles here. The opening case illustrated how Dell Computer uses real-time information about ordering patterns and inventory to bring demand and supply into close alignment, thereby quickly satisfying customer needs and taking excess inventory out of its supply chain.

Where to Manufacture

An essential decision facing an international firm is where to locate its manufacturing activities to achieve the goals of minimizing costs and improving product quality. For the firm contemplating international production, a number of factors must be considered. These factors can be grouped under three broad headings: country factors, technological factors, and product factors.[7]

Country Factors

We reviewed country-specific factors in some detail earlier in the book and we will not dwell on them here. Political economy, culture, and relative factor costs differ from country to country. In Chapter 4, we saw that due to differences in factor costs, certain countries have a comparative advantage for producing certain products. In Chapters 2 and 3, we saw how differences in political economy and national culture influence the benefits, costs, and risks of doing business in a country. Other things being equal, a firm should locate its various manufacturing activities where the economic, political, and cultural conditions, including relative factor costs, are conducive to the performance of those activities (for an example, see the next Management Focus feature, which looks at the Philips NV investment in China). In Chapter 12, we referred to the benefits derived from such a strategy as location economies. We argued that one result of the strategy is the creation of a global web of value creation activities.

Also important in some industries is the presence of global concentrations of activities at certain locations. In Chapter 6, we discussed the role of location externalities in influencing foreign direct investment decisions. Externalities include the presence of an appropriately skilled labor pool and supporting industries.[8] Such externalities can play an important role in deciding where to locate manufacturing activities. For example, because of a cluster of semiconductor manufacturing plants in Taiwan, a pool of labor with experience in the semiconductor business has developed. In addition, the plants have attracted a number of supporting industries, such as the manufacturers of semiconductor capital equipment and silicon, which have established facilities in Taiwan to be near their customers. This implies that there are real benefits to locating in Taiwan, as opposed to another location that lacks such externalities. Other things being equal, the externalities make Taiwan an attractive location for semiconductor manufacturing facilities.

Of course, other things are not equal. Differences in relative factor costs, political economy, culture, and location externalities are important, but other factors also loom large. Formal and informal trade barriers obviously influence location decisions (see Chapter 5), as do transportation costs and rules and regulations regarding foreign direct investment (see Chapter 7). For example, although relative factor costs may make a country look attractive as a location for performing a manufacturing activity, regulations prohibiting foreign direct investment may eliminate this option. Similarly, a consideration of factor costs might suggest that a firm should source production of a certain component from a particular country, but trade barriers could make this uneconomical.

Another country factor is expected future movements in its exchange rate (see Chapters 9 and 10). Adverse changes in exchange rates can quickly alter a country's attractiveness as a manufacturing base. Currency appreciation can transform a low-cost location into a high-cost location. Many Japanese corporations had to grapple with this problem during the 1990s and early 2000s. The relatively low value of the yen on foreign exchange markets between 1950 and 1980 helped strengthen Japan's position as a low-cost location for manufacturing. Between 1980 and the mid-1990s, however, the yen's steady appreciation against the dollar increased the dollar cost of products exported from Japan, making Japan less attractive as a manufacturing location. In response, many Japanese firms moved their manufacturing offshore to lower-cost locations in East Asia.

Technological Factors

This subsection is concerned with the technology that performs specific manufacturing activities. The type of technology a firm uses in its manufacturing can be pivotal in location decisions. For example, because of technological constraints, in some cases it is necessary to perform certain manufacturing activities in only one location and

Management Focus

Philips in China

The Dutch consumer electronics, lighting, semiconductor, and medical equipment conglomerate Philips NV has been operating factories in China since 1985 when the country first opened its markets to foreign investors. Then China was seen as the land of unlimited demand, and Philips, like many other Western companies, dreamed of Chinese consumers snapping up its products by the millions. But the company soon found out that one of the big reasons the company liked China—the low wage rates—also meant that few Chinese workers could afford to buy the products they were producing. Chinese wage rates are currently one-third of those in Mexico and Hungary, and 5 percent of those in the United States or Japan. So Philips hit on a new strategy; keep the factories in China but export most of the goods to the United States and elsewhere.

By 2002, Philips had invested some $2.5 billion in China. The company now operates 23 factories in China, 6 are wholly owned and 17 are joint ventures. Together they employ some 30,000 people. Philips exports nearly two-thirds of the $5 billion in products that the factories produce every year. Philips accelerated its Chinese investment in anticipation of China's entry into the World Trade Organization. The company also has plans to move even more production to China by 2005. In April 2003, Philips announced it would phase out production of electronic razors in the Netherlands, lay off 2,000 Dutch employees, and move production to China. A week earlier, Philips had stated that it would expand capacity at its semiconductor factories in China, while phasing out production in higher cost locations elsewhere.

The attractions of China to Philips include continuing low wage rates, an educated workforce, a robust Chinese economy, a stable exchange rate, a rapidly expanding industrial base that includes many other Western and Chinese companies that Philips uses as suppliers, and easier access to world markets given China's entry into the WTO. Philips has stated that ultimately its goal is to turn China into a global supply base from which the company's products will be exported around the world. In 2002, more than 20 percent of everything Philips made worldwide came from China, and executives say the figure is rising rapidly. Several products, such as CD and DVD players, are now made only in China. Moreover, Philips is also starting to give its Chinese factories a greater role in product development. In the TV business, for example, basic development used to occur in Holland and was moved to Singapore in the early 1990s. Now Philips is transferring TV development work to Suzhou near Shanghai. Similarly, basic product development work on LCD screens for cell phones was recently shifted to Shanghai.

Philips is hardly alone in this process. In 2002, more than half of all exports from China came from foreign manufacturers or their joint ventures in China. By 2002, China was the source of more than 50 percent of the cameras sold worldwide, 40 percent of all microwave ovens, 30 percent of the air conditioners, 25 percent of the washing machines, and 20 percent of all refrigerators.

Some observers worry however that Philips and companies pursuing a similar strategy might be overdoing it. Too much dependence on China could be dangerous if political, economic, or other problems disrupt production and the company's ability to supply global markets. Some observers believe that it might be better if the manufacturing facilities of companies like Philips were more geographically diverse as a hedge against problems in China. The fears of the critics were given some substance in early 2003 when an outbreak of the pneumonia-like SARS (severe acute respiratory syndrome) virus in China resulted in the temporary shutdown of several plants operated by foreign companies and disrupted their global supply chains. Although Philips was not directly affected, it did restrict travel by its managers and engineers to its Chinese plants.

Sources: B. Einhorn. "Philips' Expanding Asia Connections," *Business Week Online,* November 27, 2003; K. Leggett and P. Wonacott, "The World's Factory: A Surge in Exports from China Jolts the Global Industry," *Wall Street Journal,* October 10, 2002, p. A1; and "Philips NV: China Will Be Production Site for Electronic Razors," *Wall Street Journal,* April 8, 2003, p. B12.

serve the world market from there. In other cases, the technology may make it feasible to perform an activity in multiple locations. Three characteristics of a manufacturing technology are of interest here: the level of fixed costs, the minimum efficient scale, and the flexibility of the technology.

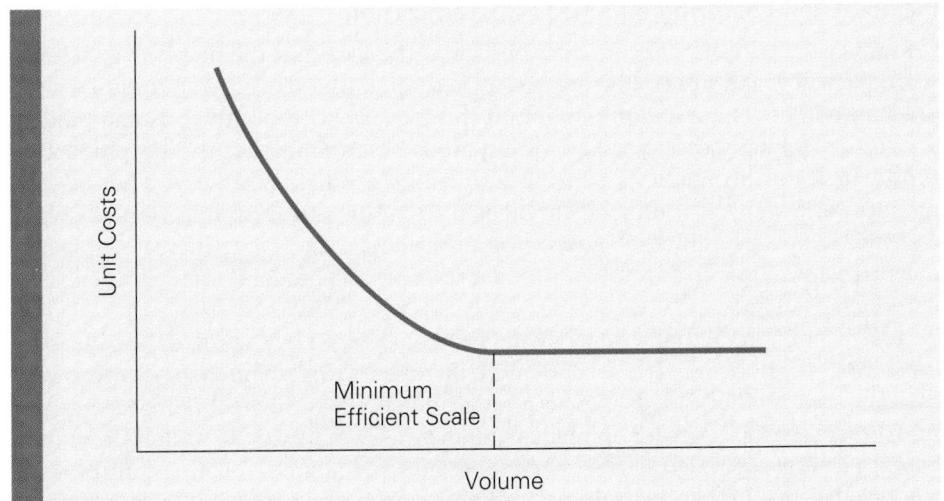

Figure 16.2

A Typical Unit Cost Curve

Fixed Costs

As we noted in Chapter 12, in some cases the fixed costs of setting up a manufacturing plant are so high that a firm must serve the world market from a single location or from a very few locations. For example, it now costs more than $1 billion to set up a state-of-the-art plant to manufacture semiconductor chips. Given this, other things being equal, serving the world market from a single plant sited at a single (optimal) location can makes sense.

Conversely, a relatively low level of fixed costs can make it economical to perform a particular activity in several locations at once. This allows the firm to better accommodate demands for local responsiveness. Manufacturing in multiple locations may also help the firm avoid becoming too dependent on one location. Being too dependent on one location is particularly risky in a world of floating exchange rates. Many firms disperse their manufacturing plants to different locations as a "real hedge" against potentially adverse moves in currencies.

Minimum Efficient Scale

The concept of economies of scale tells us that as plant output expands, unit costs decrease. The reasons include the greater utilization of capital equipment and the productivity gains that come with specialization of employees within the plant.[9] However, beyond a certain level of output, few additional scale economies are available. Thus, the "unit cost curve" declines with output until a certain output level is reached, at which point further increases in output realize little reduction in unit costs. The level of output at which most plant-level scale economies are exhausted is referred to as the **minimum efficient scale** of output. This is the scale of output a plant must operate at to realize all major plant-level scale economies (see Figure 16.2).

The implications of this concept are as follows: The larger the minimum efficient scale of a plant relative to total global demand, the greater the argument for centralizing production in a single location or a limited number of locations. Alternatively, when the minimum efficient scale of production is low relative to global demand, it may be economical to manufacture a product at several locations. For example, the minimum efficient scale for a plant to manufacture personal computers is about 250,000 units a year, while the total global demand exceeds 35 million units a year. The low level of minimum efficient scale in relation to total global demand makes it economically feasible for a company such as Dell to manufacture PCs in six locations (see opening case).

As in the case of low fixed costs, the advantages include allowing the firm to accommodate demands for local responsiveness or to hedge against currency risk by manufacturing the same product in several locations.

Flexible Manufacturing and Mass Customization

Central to the concept of economies of scale is the idea that the best way to achieve high efficiency, and hence low unit costs, is through the mass production of a standardized output. The trade-off implicit in this idea is between unit costs and product variety. Producing greater product variety from a factory implies shorter production runs, which in turn implies an inability to realize economies of scale. That is, wide product variety makes it difficult for a company to increase its production efficiency and thus reduce its unit costs. According to this logic, the way to increase efficiency and drive down unit costs is to limit product variety and produce a standardized product in large volumes.

This view of production efficiency has been challenged by the rise of flexible manufacturing technologies. The term **flexible manufacturing technology**—or **lean production,** as it is often called—covers a range of manufacturing technologies designed to (1) reduce setup times for complex equipment, (2) increase the utilization of individual machines through better scheduling, and (3) improve quality control at all stages of the manufacturing process.[10] Flexible manufacturing technologies allow the company to produce a wider variety of end products at a unit cost that at one time could be achieved only through the mass production of a standardized output. Research suggests the adoption of flexible manufacturing technologies may actually increase efficiency and lower unit costs relative to what can be achieved by the mass production of a standardized output, while at the same time enabling the company to customize its product offering to a much greater extent than was once thought possible. The term **mass customization** has been coined to describe the ability of companies to use flexible manufacturing technology to reconcile two goals that were once thought to be incompatible—low cost and product customization.[11] Flexible manufacturing technologies vary in their sophistication and complexity.

One of the most famous examples of a flexible manufacturing technology, Toyota's production system, is relatively unsophisticated, but it has been credited with making Toyota the most efficient auto company in the world. Toyota's flexible manufacturing system was developed by one of the company's engineers, Ohno Taiichi. After working at Toyota for five years and visiting Ford's U.S. plants, Ohno became convinced that the mass production philosophy for making cars was flawed. He saw numerous problems with mass production.

First, long production runs created massive inventories that had to be stored in large warehouses. This was expensive, both because of the cost of warehousing and because inventories tied up capital in unproductive uses. Second, if the initial machine settings were wrong, long production runs resulted in the production of a large number of defects (i.e., waste). Third, the mass production system was unable to accommodate consumer preferences for product diversity.

In response, Ohno looked for ways to make shorter production runs economical. He developed a number of techniques designed to reduce setup times for production equipment (a major source of fixed costs). By using a system of levers and pulleys, he reduced the time required to change dies on stamping equipment from a full day in 1950 to three minutes by 1971. This made small production runs economical, which allowed Toyota to respond better to consumer demands for product diversity. Small production runs also eliminated the need to hold large inventories, thereby reducing warehousing costs. Furthermore, small product runs and the lack of inventory meant that defective parts were produced only in small numbers and entered the assembly process immediately. This reduced waste and helped trace defects back to their source to fix the problem. In sum, these innovations enabled Toyota to produce a more diverse product range at a lower unit cost than was possible with conventional mass production.[12]

Flexible machine cells are another common flexible manufacturing technology. A flexible machine cell is a grouping of various types of machinery, a common materials handler, and a centralized cell controller (computer). Each cell normally contains four to six machines capable of performing a variety of operations. The typical cell is dedicated to the production of a family of parts or products. The settings on machines are computer controlled, which allows each cell to switch quickly between the production of different parts or products.

Improved capacity utilization and reductions in work-in-progress (that is, stockpiles of partly finished products) and in waste are major efficiency benefits of flexible machine cells. Improved capacity utilization arises from the reduction in setup times and from the computer-controlled coordination of production flow between machines, which eliminates bottlenecks. The tight coordination between machines also reduces work-in-progress inventory. Reductions in waste are due to the ability of computer-controlled machinery to identify ways to transform inputs into outputs while producing a minimum of unusable waste material. While freestanding machines might be in use 50 percent of the time, the same machines when grouped into a cell can be used more than 80 percent of the time and produce the same end product with half the waste. This increases efficiency and results in lower costs.

The efficiency benefits of installing flexible manufacturing technology can be dramatic. W. L. Gore, a privately owned company that manufactures a range of products from high-tech computer cables to its famous Gore-Tex fabric, has adopted flexible cells in several of its 46 factories. In its cable-making facilities, flexible cells have cut the time taken to make computer cables by 50 percent, reduced stock by 33 percent, and shrunk plant space by 25 percent. Similarly, Lexmark, a producer of computer printers, has also converted 80 percent of its 2,700-employee factory in Lexington, Kentucky, to flexible manufacturing cells, and it too has seen productivity increase by around 25 percent.[13]

Besides improving efficiency and lowering costs, flexible manufacturing technologies also enable companies to customize products to the unique demands of small consumer groups—at a cost that at one time could be achieved only by mass producing a standardized output. Thus, the technologies help a company achieve mass customization, which increases its customer responsiveness. Most important for international business, flexible manufacturing technologies can help a firm to customize products for different national markets. The importance of this advantage cannot be overstated. When flexible manufacturing technologies are available, a firm can manufacture products customized to various national markets at a single factory sited at the optimal location. And it can do this without absorbing a significant cost penalty. Thus, firms no longer need to establish manufacturing facilities in each major national market to provide products that satisfy specific consumer tastes and preferences, part of the rationale for a multidomestic strategy (Chapter 12).

Summary

A number of technological factors support the economic arguments for concentrating manufacturing facilities in a few choice locations or even in a single location. Other things being equal, when fixed costs are substantial, the minimum efficient scale of production is high, and/or flexible manufacturing technologies are available, the arguments for concentrating production at a few choice locations are strong. This is true even when substantial differences in consumer tastes and preferences exist between national markets, because flexible manufacturing technologies allow the firm to customize products to national differences at a single facility. Alternatively, when fixed costs are low, the minimum efficient scale of production is low, and flexible manufacturing technologies are not available, the arguments for concentrating production at one or a few locations are not as compelling. In such cases, it may make more sense to manufacture in each major market in which the firm is active if this helps the firm better respond to local demands. This holds only if the increased local responsiveness more than offsets the cost disadvantages of not concentrating manufacturing. With the advent of flexible manufacturing technologies and mass customization, such a strategy is becoming less attractive. In sum, technological factors are making it feasible, and necessary, for firms to concentrate manufacturing facilities at optimal locations. Trade barriers and transportation costs are major brakes on this trend.

Product Factors

Two product features affect location decisions. The first is the product's *value-to-weight* ratio because of its influence on transportation costs. Many electronic components and pharmaceuticals have high value-to-weight ratios; they are expensive and they do not weigh very much. Thus, even if they are shipped halfway around the world, their transportation costs account for a very small percentage of total costs. Given this, other things being equal, there is great pressure to manufacture these products in the optimal location and to serve the world market from there. The opposite holds for products with low value-to-weight ratios. Refined sugar, certain bulk chemicals, paint, and petroleum products all have low value-to-weight ratios; they are relatively inexpensive products that weigh a lot. Accordingly, when they are shipped long distances, transportation costs account for a large percentage of total costs. Thus, other things being equal, there is great pressure to manufacture these products in multiple locations close to major markets to reduce transportation costs.

The other product feature that can influence location decisions is whether the product serves universal needs, needs that are the same all over the world. Examples include many industrial products (e.g., industrial electronics, steel, bulk chemicals) and modern consumer products (e.g., handheld calculators and personal computers). Because there are few national differences in consumer taste and preference for such products, the need for local responsiveness is reduced. This increases the attractiveness of concentrating manufacturing at an optimal location.

Locating Manufacturing Facilities

There are two basic strategies for locating manufacturing facilities: concentrating them in a centralized location and serving the world market from there, or decentralizing them in various regional or national locations that are close to major markets. The appropriate strategic choice is determined by the various country-specific, technological, and product factors we have discussed in this section and are summarized in Table 16.1.

As can be seen, concentration of manufacturing makes most sense when:

- Differences between countries in factor costs, political economy, and culture have a substantial impact on the costs of manufacturing in various countries.
- Trade barriers are low.
- Externalities arising from the concentration of like enterprises favor certain locations.
- Important exchange rates are expected to remain relatively stable.
- The production technology has high fixed costs and high minimum efficient scale relative to global demand, or flexible manufacturing technology exists.
- The product's value-to-weight ratio is high.
- The product serves universal needs.

Alternatively, decentralization of manufacturing is appropriate when:

- Differences between countries in factor costs, political economy, and culture do not have a substantial impact on the costs of manufacturing in various countries.
- Trade barriers are high.
- Location externalities are not important.
- Volatility in important exchange rates is expected.

Country Factors	Concentrated Manufacturing Favored	Decentralized Manufacturing Favored	Table 16.1
Differences in political economy	Substantial	Few	Location Strategy and Manufacturing
Differences in culture	Substantial	Few	
Differences in factor costs	Substantial	Few	
Trade barriers	Substantial	Few	
Location externalities	Important in industry	Not important in industry	
Exchange rates	Stable	Volatile	
Technological Factors			
Fixed costs	High	Low	
Minimum efficient scale	High	Low	
Flexible manufacturing technology	Available	Not available	
Product Factors			
Value-to-weight ratio	High	Low	
Serves universal needs	Yes	No	

- The production technology has low fixed costs and low minimum efficient scale, and flexible manufacturing technology is not available.
- The product's value-to-weight ratio is low.
- The product does not serve universal needs (that is, significant differences in consumer tastes and preferences exist between nations).

In practice, location decisions are seldom clear cut. For example, it is not unusual for differences in factor costs, technological factors, and product factors to point toward concentrated manufacturing while a combination of trade barriers and volatile exchange rates points toward decentralized manufacturing. This seems to be the case in the world automobile industry. Although the availability of flexible manufacturing and cars' relatively high value-to-weight ratios suggest concentrated manufacturing, the combination of formal and informal trade barriers and the uncertainties of the world's current floating exchange rate regime (see Chapter 10) have inhibited firms' ability to pursue this strategy. For these reasons, several automobile companies have established "top-to-bottom" manufacturing operations in three major regional markets: Asia, North America, and Western Europe.

The Strategic Role of Foreign Factories

Whatever the rationale behind establishing a foreign manufacturing facility, the strategic role of foreign factories can evolve over time.[14] Initially, many foreign factories are established where labor costs are low. Their strategic role typically is to produce labor-intensive products at as low a cost as possible. For example, beginning in the 1970s, many U.S. firms in the computer and telecommunication equipment businesses established factories across Southeast Asia to manufacture electronic components, such as circuit boards and semiconductors, at the lowest possible cost. They located their factories in countries such as Malaysia, Thailand, and Singapore precisely because each of these countries offered an attractive combination of low labor costs, adequate infrastructure, and a favorable tax and trade regime. Initially, the components produced by these factories were designed elsewhere and the final product was assembled elsewhere. Over time, however, the strategic role of some of these factories has expanded; they have become important centers for the design and final assembly of products for the global marketplace. For example, Hewlett-Packard's operation in Singapore was established as a low-cost location for the production of circuit boards, but the facility has become the center for the design and final assembly of portable ink-jet printers for the global marketplace (see the accompanying Management Focus). A similar process seems to be occurring at some of the factories that Philips has established in China (see the Management Focus on Philips).

Such upward migration in the strategic role of foreign factories arises because many foreign factories upgrade their own capabilities.[15] This improvement comes from two sources. First, pressure from the center to improve a factory's cost structure and/or customize a product to the demands of consumers in a particular nation can start a chain of events that ultimately leads to development of additional capabilities at that factory. For example, to meet centrally mandated directions to drive down costs, engineers at HP's Singapore factory argued that they needed to redesign products so they could be manufactured at a lower cost. This led to the establishment of a design center in Singapore. As this design center proved its worth, HP executives realized the importance of co-locating design and manufacturing operations. They increasingly transferred more design responsibilities to the Singapore factory. In addition, the Singapore factory ultimately became the center for the design of products tailored to the needs of the Asian market. This too made good strategic sense because it meant products were being designed by engineers who were close to the Asian market and probably had a good understanding of the needs of that market, as opposed to engineers located in the United States.

A second source of improvement in the capabilities of a foreign factory can be the increasing abundance of advanced factors of production in the nation in which the factory is located. Many nations that were considered economic backwaters a generation ago have been experiencing rapid economic development during the past 20 years. Their communication and transportation infrastructures and the education level of the population have improved. While these countries once lacked the advanced infrastructure required to support sophisticated design, development, and manufacturing operations, this is often no longer the case. This has made it much easier for factories based in these nations to take on a greater strategic role.

Because of such developments, many international businesses are moving away from a system in which their foreign factories were viewed as nothing more than low-cost manufacturing facilities and toward one where foreign factories are viewed as globally dispersed centers of excellence.[16] In this new model, foreign factories take the lead role for the design and manufacture of products to serve important national or regional markets or even the global market. The development of such dispersed centers of excellence is consistent with the concept of a transnational strategy, which we introduced in Chapter 12. A major aspect of a transnational strategy is a belief in global learning—the idea that valuable knowledge does not reside just in a firm's domestic operations; it may also be found in its foreign subsidiaries. Foreign factories that upgrade their capabilities over time are creating valuable knowledge that might benefit the whole corporation.

Managers of international businesses need to remember that foreign factories can improve their capabilities over time, and this can be of immense strategic benefit to the firm. Rather than viewing foreign factories simply as sweatshops where unskilled labor churns out low-cost goods, managers need to view them as potential centers of excellence and to encourage and foster attempts by local managers to upgrade the capabilities of their factories and, thereby, enhance their strategic standing within the corporation.

Such a process does imply that once a foreign factory has been established and valuable skills have been accumulated, it may not be wise to switch production to

Hewlett-Packard in Singapore

In the late 1960s, Hewlett-Packard was looking around Asia for a low-cost location to produce electronic components that were to be manufactured using labor-intensive processes. The company looked at several Asian locations and eventually settled on Singapore, opening its first factory there in 1970. Although Singapore did not have the lowest labor costs in the region, costs were low relative to North America. Plus, the Singapore location had several important benefits that could not be found at many other locations in Asia. The education level of the local workforce was high. English was widely spoken. The government of Singapore seemed stable and committed to economic development, and the city-state had one of the better-developed infrastructures in the region, including good communication and transportation networks and a rapidly developing industrial and commercial base. HP also extracted favorable terms from the Singapore government with regard to taxes, tariffs, and subsidies.

To begin with, the plant manufactured only basic components. The combination of low labor costs and a favorable tax regime helped to make this plant profitable early. In 1973, HP transferred the manufacture of one of its basic handheld calculators from the United States to Singapore. The objective was to reduce manufacturing costs, which the Singapore factory was quickly able to do. Increasingly confident in the capability of the Singapore factory to handle entire products, as opposed to just components, HP's management transferred other products to Singapore over the next few years including keyboards, solid-state displays, and integrated circuits. However, all these products were still designed, developed, and initially produced in the United States.

The plant's status shifted in the early 1980s when HP embarked on a worldwide campaign to boost product quality and reduce costs. HP transferred the production of its HP41C handheld calculator to Singapore. The managers at the Singapore plant were given the goal of substantially reducing manufacturing costs. They argued that this could be achieved only if they were allowed to redesign the product so it could be manufactured at a lower overall cost. HP's central management agreed, and 20 engineers from the Singapore facility were transferred to the United States for one year to learn how to design application-specific integrated circuits. They then brought this expertise back to Singapore and set about redesigning the HP41C.

The results were a huge success. By redesigning the product, the Singapore engineers reduced manufacturing costs for the HP41C by 50 percent. Using this newly acquired capability for product design, the Singapore facility then set about redesigning other products it produced. HP's corporate managers were so impressed with the progress made at the factory that they transferred production of the entire calculator line to Singapore in 1983. This was followed by the partial transfer of ink-jet production to Singapore in 1984 and keyboard production in 1986. In all cases, the facility redesigned the products and often reduced unit manufacturing costs by more than 30 percent. The initial development and design of all these products, however, still occurred in the United States.

In the late 1980s and early 1990s, the Singapore plant started to take on added responsibilities, particularly in the ink-jet printer business. In 1990, the factory was given the job of redesigning an HP ink-jet printer for the Japanese market. Although the initial product redesign was a market failure, the managers at Singapore pushed to be allowed to try again, and in 1991 they were given the job of redesigning HP's DeskJet 505 printer for the Japanese market. This time the redesigned product was a success, garnering significant sales in Japan. Emboldened by this success, the plant has continued to take on additional design responsibilities. Today, it is viewed as a "lead plant" within HP's global network, with primary responsibility not just for manufacturing, but also for the development and design of a family of small ink-jet printers targeted at the Asian market.

Sources: K. Ferdows, "Making the Most of Foreign Factories," *Harvard Business Review,* March–April 1997, pp. 73–88, and "Hewlett-Packard: Singapore," Harvard Business School, case # 694–035.

another location simply because some underlying variable, such as wage rates, has changed.[17] HP has kept its facility in Singapore, rather than switching production to a location where wage rates are now much lower, such as Vietnam, because it recognizes that the Singapore factory has accumulated valuable skills that more than make up for the higher wage rates. Thus, when reviewing the location of production facilities, the international manager must bear in mind the valuable skills that may have been accumulated at various locations, and the impact of those skills on factors such as productivity and product design.

■ Make-or-Buy Decisions

International businesses frequently face **sourcing decisions,** decisions about whether they should make or buy the component parts that go into their final product. Should the firm vertically integrate to manufacture its own component parts or should it outsource them, or buy them from independent suppliers? Make-or-buy decisions are important factors of many firms' manufacturing strategies. In the automobile industry, for example, the typical car contains more than 10,000 components, so automobile firms constantly face make-or-buy decisions. Ford of Europe, for example, produces only about 45 percent of the value of the Fiesta in its own plants. The remaining 55 percent, mainly accounted for by component parts, comes from independent suppliers. In the athletic shoe industry, the make-or-buy issue has been taken to an extreme with companies such as Nike and Reebok having no involvement in manufacturing; all production has been outsourced, primarily to manufacturers based in low-wage countries.

Make-or-buy decisions pose plenty of problems for purely domestic businesses but even more problems for international businesses. These decisions in the international arena are complicated by the volatility of countries' political economies, exchange rate movements, changes in relative factor costs, and the like. In this section, we examine the arguments for making components and for buying them, and we consider the trade-offs involved in these decisions. Then we discuss strategic alliances as an alternative to manufacturing component parts within the company.

The Advantages of Make

The arguments that support making component parts in-house—vertical integration—are fourfold. Vertical integration may be associated with lower costs, facilitate investments in highly specialized assets, protect proprietary product technology, and facilitate the scheduling of adjacent processes.

Lower Costs

It may pay a firm to continue manufacturing a product or component part in-house if the firm is more efficient at that production activity than any other enterprise. Boeing, for example, has looked closely at its make-or-buy decisions with regard to commercial jet aircraft (for details see the accompanying Management Focus). It decided to outsource the production of some component parts but keep the design and final integration of aircraft. Boeing's rationale was that it has a core competence in large systems integration, and it is more efficient at this activity than any other comparable enterprise in the world. Therefore, it makes little sense for Boeing to outsource this particular activity.

Facilitating Specialized Investments

We first encountered the concept of specialized assets in Chapter 6 when we looked at the economic theory of vertical foreign direct investment. A variation of that concept explains why firms might want to make their own components rather than buy them.[18] When one firm must invest in specialized assets to supply another, mutual dependency is created. In such circumstances, each party fears the other will abuse the relationship by seeking more favorable terms.

Imagine Ford of Europe has developed a new, high-performance, high-quality, and uniquely designed fuel injection system. The increased fuel efficiency will help sell Ford cars. Ford must decide whether to make the system in-house or to contract out the manufacturing to an independent supplier. Manufacturing these uniquely designed systems requires investments in equipment that can be used only for this purpose; it cannot be used to make fuel injection systems for any other auto firm. Thus, investment in this equipment constitutes an investment in specialized assets.

Let us first examine this situation from the perspective of an independent supplier who has been asked by Ford to make this investment. The supplier might reason that once it has made the investment, it will become dependent on Ford for business since Ford is the only possible customer for the output of this equipment. The supplier perceives this as putting Ford in a strong bargaining position and worries that once the specialized investment has been made, Ford might use this to squeeze down prices for the systems. Given this risk, the supplier declines to make the investment in specialized equipment.

Now take the position of Ford. Ford might reason that if it contracts out production of these systems to an independent supplier, it might become too dependent on that supplier for a vital input. Because specialized equipment is required to produce the fuel injection systems, Ford cannot easily switch its orders to other suppliers who lack that equipment. (It would face high switching costs.) Ford perceives this as increasing the bargaining power of the supplier and worries that the supplier might use its bargaining strength to demand higher prices.

Thus, the mutual dependency that outsourcing would create makes Ford nervous and scares away potential suppliers. The problem here is lack of trust. Neither party completely trusts the other to play fair. Consequently, Ford might reason that the only safe way to get the new fuel injection systems is to manufacture them itself. It may be unable to persuade any independent supplier to manufacture them. Thus, Ford decides to make rather than buy.

In general, we can predict that when substantial investments in specialized assets are required to manufacture a component, the firm will prefer to make the component internally rather than contract it out to a supplier. Substantial empirical evidence supports this prediction.[19]

Proprietary Product Technology Protection

Proprietary product technology is technology unique to a firm. If it enables the firm to produce a product containing superior features, proprietary technology can give the firm a competitive advantage. The firm would not want competitors to get this technology. If the firm contracts out the manufacture of components containing proprietary technology, it runs the risk that those suppliers will expropriate the technology for their own use or that they will sell it to the firm's competitors. Thus, to maintain control over its technology, the firm might prefer to make such component parts in-house. An example of a firm that has made such decisions is given in the accompanying Management Focus, which looks at make-or-buy decisions at Boeing. While Boeing has decided to outsource a number of important components that go toward the production of an aircraft, it has explicitly decided not to outsource the manufacture of cockpits because it believes that doing so would give away key technology to potential competitors.

Improved Scheduling

The weakest argument for vertical integration is that production cost savings result from it because it makes planning, coordination, and scheduling of adjacent processes easier.[20] This is particularly important in firms with just-in-time inventory systems (which we discuss later in the chapter). In the 1920s, for example, Ford profited from tight coordination and scheduling made possible by backward vertical integration into steel foundries, iron ore shipping, and mining. Deliveries at Ford's foundries on the Great Lakes were coordinated so well that ore was turned into engine blocks within 24 hours. This substantially reduced Ford's production costs by eliminating the need to hold excessive ore inventories.

For international businesses that source worldwide, scheduling problems can be exacerbated by the time and distance between the firm and its suppliers. This is true whether the firms use their own subunits as suppliers or use independent suppliers. Ownership is

Management Focus

Make-or-Buy Decisions at the Boeing Company

The Boeing Company is one of the two premier manufacturers of commercial jet aircraft in the world with a 50 percent share of the global market for large commercial jet aircraft. Despite its large market share, in recent years Boeing has found it tough going. The company's problems are twofold. First, Boeing faces an aggressive competitor in Europe's Airbus Industrie. The dogfight between Boeing and Airbus for market share has enabled major airlines to play the two companies off against each other in an attempt to bargain down the price for commercial jet aircraft. Second, the airline business is quite cyclical and airlines sharply reduce orders for new aircraft when their own business is in a downturn. This occurred in the early 1990s and again after the events of September 11, 2001, hit the airline industry hard, and resulted in slumping orders for Boeing and Airbus.

During downturns, some of which can be extended, intense price competition often occurs between Airbus and Boeing as they struggle to maintain market share and order volume in the face of falling demand. Given these pricing pressures, the only way that Boeing can maintain its profitability is to reduce its own manufacturing costs. With this in mind, during the 1990s, Boeing launched a companywide review of its make-or-buy decisions. The objective was to identify activities that could be outsourced to subcontractors, both in the United States and abroad, to drive down production costs.

When making outsourcing decisions, Boeing applies a number of criteria. First, Boeing looks at the basic economics of the outsourcing decision. The central issue here is whether an activity could be performed more cost-effectively by an outside manufacturer or by Boeing. Second, Boeing considers the strategic risk associated with outsourcing an activity. Boeing decided it would not outsource any activity that it deemed to be part of its long-term competitive advantage, particularly design work and final integration and assembly. Third, Boeing looks at the operational risk associated with outsourcing an activity. The basic objective is to make sure Boeing does not become too dependent on a single outside supplier for critical components. Boeing's philosophy is to hedge operational risk by purchasing from two or more suppliers. Finally, Boeing considers whether it makes sense to outsource certain activities to a supplier in a given country to help secure orders for commercial jet aircraft from that country. This practice is known as offsetting, and it is common in many industries. For example, Boeing decided to outsource the production of certain components to China. This decision was influenced by forecasts suggesting that the Chinese will purchase more than $100 billion worth of commercial jets over the next 20 years. Boeing's hope is that pushing some subcontracting work China's way will help Boeing gain a larger share of this market than its global competitor, Airbus.

By 2002, Boeing was outsourcing some 64 percent of the work involved in building a commercial jet aircraft, up from 50 percent a decade earlier, with companies in Japan, Italy, and elsewhere shipping fuselage sections or even entire wings to Boeing. For its part, Boeing has decided to focus its efforts on design, final manufacturing integration and assembly, and marketing and sales. Every other activity can be potentially outsourced. Indeed, there are signs that Boeing will outsource substantially more work than ever before when making its latest jet, the 7E7, a "super-efficient" wide-body jet scheduled for market introduction in 2008.

Sources: D. Gates, "Boeing Buzzes about 'Source' of Work," *Seattle Times*, March 9, 2003, p. A1; S. Wilhelm, "Tough Contest Ahead over 7E7," *Puget Sound Business Journal*, April 11, 2002, p. 50; interviews between Charles Hill and senior management personnel at Boeing.

---

not the issue here. As we saw in the opening case, Dell Computer can achieve tight scheduling with its globally dispersed parts suppliers without vertical integration. Thus, although this argument for vertical integration is often made, it is not compelling.

The Advantages of Buy

The advantages of buying component parts from independent suppliers are that it gives the firm greater flexibility, it can help drive down the firm's cost structure, and it may help the firm to capture orders from international customers.

Strategic Flexibility

The great advantage of buying component parts from independent suppliers is that the firm can maintain its flexibility, switching orders between suppliers as circumstances dictate. This is particularly important internationally, where changes in exchange rates and trade barriers can alter the attractiveness of supply sources. One year Hong Kong might be the lowest-cost source for a particular component, and the next year, Mexico may be. Many firms source the same parts from suppliers based in two different countries, primarily as a hedge against adverse movements in factor costs, exchange rates, and the like.

Sourcing component parts from independent suppliers can also be advantageous when the optimal location for manufacturing a product is beset by political risks. Under such circumstances, foreign direct investment to establish a component manufacturing operation in that country would expose the firm to political risks. The firm can avoid many of these risks by buying from an independent supplier in that country, thereby maintaining the flexibility to switch sourcing to another country if a war, revolution, or other political change alters that country's attractiveness as a supply source.

However, maintaining strategic flexibility has its downside. If a supplier perceives the firm will change suppliers in response to changes in exchange rates, trade barriers, or general political circumstances, that supplier might not be willing to make specialized investments in plant and equipment that would ultimately benefit the firm.

Lower Costs

Although vertical integration is often undertaken to lower costs, it may have the opposite effect. When this is the case, outsourcing may lower the firm's cost structure. Vertical integration into the manufacture of component parts increases an organization's scope, and the resulting increase in organizational complexity can raise a firm's cost structure. There are three reasons for this.

First, the greater the number of subunits in an organization, the greater are the problems of coordinating and controlling those units. Coordinating and controlling subunits require top management to process large amounts of information about subunit activities. The greater the number of subunits, the more information top management must process and the harder it is to do well. Theoretically, when the firm becomes involved in too many activities, headquarters management will be unable to effectively control all of them, and the resulting inefficiencies will more than offset any advantages derived from vertical integration.[21] This can be particularly serious in an international business, where the problem of controlling subunits is exacerbated by distance and differences in time, language, and culture.

Second, the firm that vertically integrates into component part manufacture may find that because its internal suppliers have a captive customer in the firm, they lack an incentive to reduce costs. The fact that they do not have to compete for orders with other suppliers may result in high operating costs. The managers of the supply operation may be tempted to pass on cost increases to other parts of the firm in the form of higher transfer prices, rather than looking for ways to reduce those costs.

Third, vertically integrated firms have to determine appropriate prices for goods transferred to subunits within the firm. This is a challenge in any firm, but it is even more complex in international businesses. Different tax regimes, exchange rate movements, and headquarters' ignorance about local conditions all increase the complexity of transfer pricing decisions. This complexity enhances internal suppliers' ability to manipulate transfer prices to their advantage, passing cost increases downstream rather than looking for ways to reduce costs.

The firm that buys its components from independent suppliers can avoid all these problems and the associated costs. The firm that sources from independent suppliers has fewer subunits to control. The incentive problems that occur with internal suppliers do not arise when independent suppliers are used. Independent suppliers know they must continue to be efficient if they are to win business from the firm. Also, because independent suppliers' prices are set by market forces, the transfer pricing problem does not exist. In sum, the bureaucratic inefficiencies and resulting costs that can arise when firms vertically integrate backward and manufacture their own components are avoided by buying component parts from independent suppliers.

Offsets

Another reason for outsourcing some manufacturing to independent suppliers based in other countries is that it may help the firm capture more orders from that country. As noted in the Management Focus on Boeing, the practice of offsets is common in the commercial aerospace industry. For example, before Air India places a large order with Boeing, the Indian government might ask Boeing to push some subcontracting work toward Indian manufacturers. This kind of quid pro quo is not unusual in international business, and it affects far more than just the aerospace industry. Representatives of the U.S. government have repeatedly urged Japanese automobile companies to purchase more component parts from U.S. suppliers to partially offset the large volume of automobile exports from Japan to the United States.

Trade-offs

Clearly there are trade-offs in make-or-buy decisions. The benefits of manufacturing components in-house seem to be greatest when highly specialized assets are involved, when vertical integration is necessary for protecting proprietary technology, or when the firm is simply more efficient than external suppliers at performing a particular activity. When these conditions are not present, the risk of strategic inflexibility and organizational problems suggest it may be better to contract out component part manufacturing to independent suppliers. Because issues of strategic flexibility and organizational control loom even larger for international businesses than purely domestic ones, an international business should be particularly wary of vertical integration into component part manufacture. In addition, some outsourcing in the form of offsets may help a firm gain larger orders in the future.

Strategic Alliances with Suppliers

Several international businesses have tried to reap some benefits of vertical integration without the associated organizational problems by entering strategic alliances with essential suppliers. For example, there is an alliance between Kodak and Canon, under which Canon builds photocopiers for sale by Kodak, and an alliance between Apple and Sony, under which Sony builds laptop computers for Apple. By these alliances, Kodak and Apple have committed themselves to long-term relationships with these suppliers, which have encouraged the suppliers to undertake specialized investments. Strategic alliances build trust between the firm and its suppliers. Trust is built when a firm makes a credible commitment to continue purchasing from a supplier on reasonable terms. For example, the firm may invest money in a supplier—perhaps by taking a minority shareholding—to signal its intention to build a productive, mutually beneficial long-term relationship.

This kind of arrangement between the firm and its parts suppliers was pioneered in Japan by large auto companies such as Toyota. Many Japanese automakers have cooperative relationships with their suppliers that go back decades. In these relationships, the auto companies and their suppliers collaborate on ways to increase value added by, for example, implementing just-in-time inventory systems or cooperating in the design of component parts to improve quality and reduce assembly costs. These relationships have been formalized when the auto firms acquired minority shareholdings in many of their essential suppliers to symbolize their desire for long-term cooperative relationships with them. At the same time, the relationship between the firm and each essential supplier remains market mediated and terminable if the supplier fails to perform. By pursuing such a strategy, the Japanese automakers capture many of the benefits of vertical integration, particularly those arising from investments in specialized assets, without suffering the organizational problems that come with formal vertical integration. The parts suppliers also benefit from these relationships because they grow with the firm they supply and share in its success. Because of these strategies, Toyota manufactures only 27 percent of its component parts in-house, compared to 48 percent at Ford and 67 percent at GM. Of these three firms, Toyota appears to spend the least on component parts, suggesting it has captured many of the benefits that induced Ford and GM to vertically integrate.[22]

In general, the trends toward just-in-time inventory systems (JIT), computer-aided design (CAD), and computer-aided manufacturing (CAM) seem to have increased pressures for firms to establish long-term relationships with their suppliers. JIT, CAD, and CAM systems all rely on close links between firms and their suppliers supported by substantial specialized investment in equipment and information systems hardware. To get a supplier to agree to adopt such systems, a firm must make a credible commitment to an enduring relationship with the supplier—it must build trust with the supplier. It can do this within the framework of a strategic alliance.

Alliances are not all good. Like formal vertical integration, a firm that enters long-term alliances may limit its strategic flexibility by the commitments it makes to its alliance partners. As we saw in Chapter 14 when we considered alliances between competitors, a firm that allies itself with another firm risks giving away key technological know-how to a potential competitor.

Managing a Global Supply Chain ▮

Materials management, which encompasses logistics, embraces the activities necessary to get materials from suppliers to a manufacturing facility, through the manufacturing process, and out through a distribution system to the end user.[23] In the international business, the materials management function manages the global supply chain. The twin objectives of materials management are to manage a firm's global supply chain at the lowest possible cost and in a way that best serves customer needs, thereby lowering the costs of value creation and helping the firm establish a competitive advantage through superior customer service.

The potential for reducing costs through more efficient materials management is enormous. As we saw in the opening case, the competitive advantage of Dell Computer is based in part on the ability of the company to harness the power of the Internet to link orders from customers with its globally dispersed supply chain to match demand and supply, driving excess inventory out of its system and significantly reducing the company's cost structure. For the typical manufacturing enterprise, material costs account for between 50 and 70 percent of revenues, depending on the industry. Even a small reduction in these costs can have a substantial impact on profitability. According to one estimate, for a firm with revenues of $1 million, a return on investment rate of 5 percent, and materials costs that are 50 percent of sales revenues, a $15,000 increase in total profits could be achieved either by increasing sales revenues 30 percent or by reducing materials costs by 3 percent.[24] In a saturated market, it would be much easier to reduce materials costs by 3 percent than to increase sales revenues by 30 percent.

▮The Role of Just-in-Time Inventory

Pioneered by Japanese firms during the 1950s and 60s, just-in-time inventory systems now play a major role in most manufacturing firms. The basic philosophy behind just-in-time (JIT) systems is to economize on inventory holding costs by having materials arrive at a manufacturing plant just in time to enter the production process and not before. The major cost saving comes from speeding up inventory turnover. This reduces inventory holding costs, such as warehousing and storage costs. It means the company can reduce the amount of working capital it needs to finance inventory, freeing capital for other uses and/or lowering the total capital requirements of the enterprise. Other things being equal, this will boost the company's profitability as measured by return on capital invested. It also means the company is less likely to have excess unsold inventory that it has to write off against earnings or price low to sell.

In addition to the cost benefits, JIT systems can also help firms improve product quality. Under a JIT system, parts enter the manufacturing process immediately; they are not warehoused. This allows defective inputs to be spotted right away. The problem can then be traced to the supply source and fixed before more defective parts are produced. Under a more traditional system, warehousing parts for weeks before they are used allows many defective parts to be produced before a problem is recognized.

The drawback of a JIT system is that it leaves a firm without a buffer stock of inventory. Although buffer stocks are expensive to store, they can help a firm respond quickly to increases in demand and tide a firm over shortages brought about by disruption among suppliers. Such a disruption occurred after the September 11, 2001, attacks on the World Trade Center, when the subsequent shutdown of international air travel and shipping left many firms that relied upon globally dispersed suppliers and tightly managed "just-in-time" supply chains without a buffer stock of inventory. A less pronounced but similar situation occurred again in April 2003 when the outbreak of pneumonia-like SARS (severe acute respiratory syndrome) virus in China resulted in the temporary shutdown of several plants operated by foreign companies and disrupted their global supply chains.

There are ways of reducing the risks associated with a global supply chain that operates on just-in-time principles. To reduce the risks associated with depending on one supplier for an important input, some firms source these inputs from several suppliers located in different countries. While this does not help in the case of an event with global ramifications, such as September 11, 2001, it does help manage country-specific supply disruptions, which are more common. As for responding quickly to increases in consumer demand, the experience of Dell Computer shows that it is possible to do this while maintaining a JIT system by using real-time information to adjust product pricing, thereby bringing demand and supply into closer alignment (see the opening case).

The Role of Organization

As the number and dispersion of domestic and foreign markets and sources grow, the number and complexity of organizational linkages increase correspondingly. In a multinational enterprise, the challenge of managing the costs associated with purchases, currency exchange, inbound and outbound transportation, production, inventory, communication, expediting, tariffs and duties, and overall administration is massive. Figure 16.3 shows the linkages that might exist for a firm that sources, manufactures, and sells internationally. Each linkage represents a flow of materials, capital, information, decisions, and people. The firm must figure out the best organization to achieve tight coordination of the various stages of the value creation process.

A major requirement seems to be to separate out materials management as a function and give it equal weight, in organizational terms, with other more traditional functions such as manufacturing, marketing, and R&D. According to materials management specialists, purchasing, production, and distribution are not separate activities but three aspects of one basic task: controlling the flow of materials and products from sources of supply through manufacturing and distribution into the hands of customers.

Despite the apparent cost and quality control advantages of having a separate materials management function, all firms do not operate with such a function.[25] Those that do not include many firms in which purchasing costs, inventories, and customer service levels are important, interdependent aspects of establishing competitive advantage. Such firms typically operate with a traditional organizational structure simi-

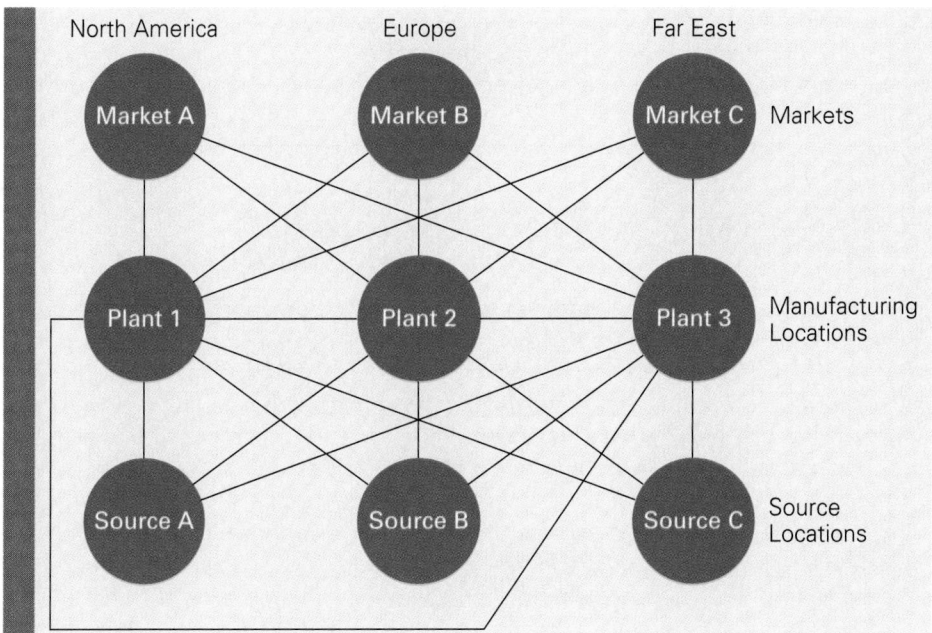

Figure 16.3

Potential Materials Management Linkages

lar to the one in Figure 16.4A. In such an organization, purchasing, production planning and control, and distribution are not integrated. Planning and control are part of the manufacturing function, while distribution is part of the marketing function. Such companies will be unable to establish materials management as a major strength and consequently may face higher costs. Figure 16.4B shows the structure of a typical organization in which materials management is a separate function. Purchasing, planning and control, and distribution are integrated within the materials management function. Such an arrangement allows the firm to transform materials management into an important strength.

With the legitimacy of materials management established, the next dilemma is determining the best structure in a multinational enterprise. In practice, authority is either centralized or decentralized.[26] Under a centralized solution, most materials management decisions are made at the corporate level, which can ensure efficiency and adherence to overall corporate objectives. This is the case at Dell Computer, for example. In large, complex organizations with many manufacturing plants, however, a centralized materials management function may become overloaded and unable to perform its task effectively. In such cases, a decentralized solution is needed.

A decentralized solution delegates most materials management decisions to the level of individual manufacturing plants within the firm, although corporate headquarters retains responsibility for overseeing the function. The great advantage of decentralizing is that it allows plant-level materials management groups to develop the knowledge and skills needed for interacting with foreign suppliers that are important to their particular plant. This can lead to better decision making. The disadvantage is that a lack of coordination between plants can result in less than optimal global sourcing. It can also lead to duplication of materials management efforts. These disadvantages can be attenuated, however, by information systems that enable headquarters to coordinate the various plant-level materials management groups.

The Role of Information Technology and the Internet

As we saw in the opening case on Dell Computer, Web-based information systems play a crucial role in modern materials management. By tracking component parts as they make their way across the globe toward an assembly plant, information systems enable a

Figure 16.4A

Traditional Organizational
Structure

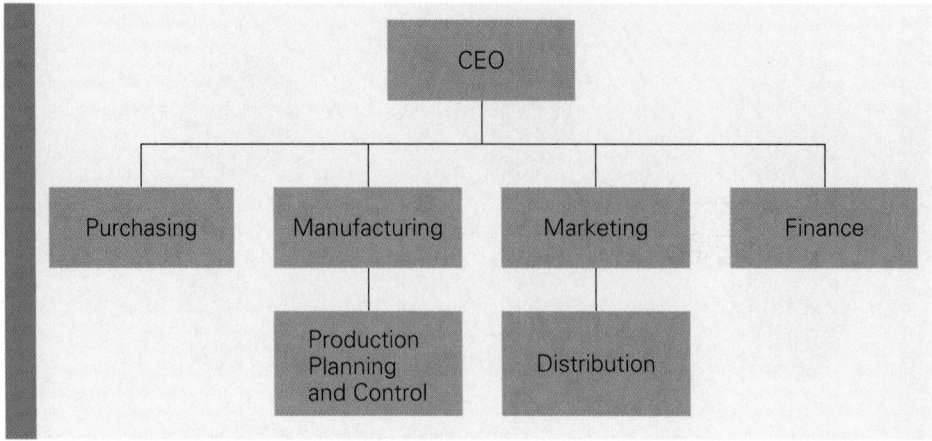

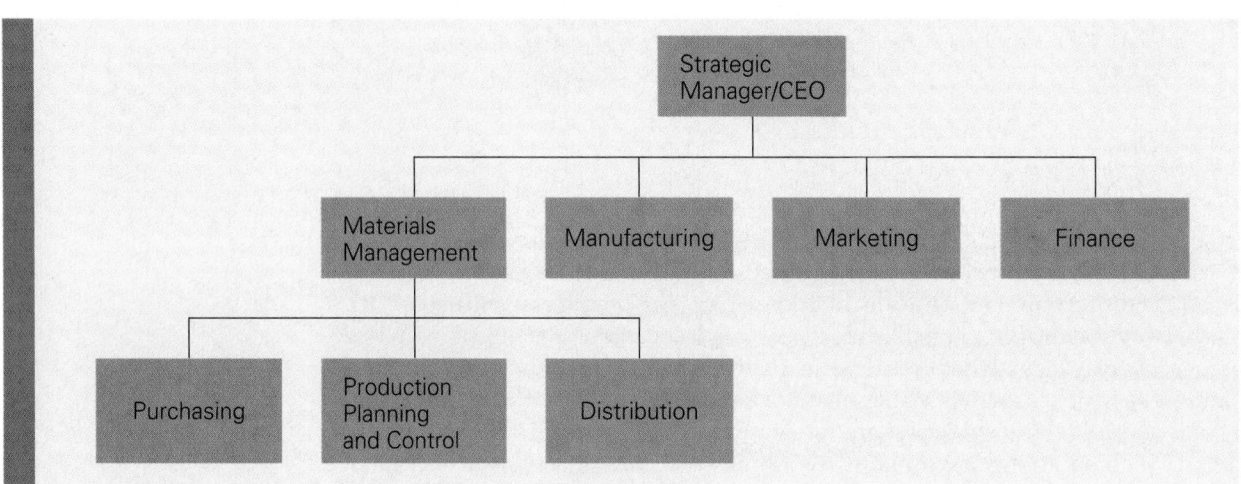

Figure 16.4B

Organizational Structure with Materials Management as Separate Function

firm to optimize its production scheduling according to when components are expected to arrive. By locating component parts in the supply chain precisely, good information systems allow the firm to accelerate production when needed by pulling key components out of the regular supply chain and having them flown to the manufacturing plant.

Firms increasingly use electronic data interchange (EDI) to coordinate the flow of materials into manufacturing, through manufacturing, and out to customers. As at Dell, the ultimate goal should be to replace inventory with information. EDI systems require computer links between a firm, its suppliers, and its shippers. Sometimes customers also are integrated into the system, as at Dell. These electronic links are then used to place orders with suppliers, to register parts leaving a supplier, to track them as they travel toward a manufacturing plant, and to register their arrival. Suppliers typically use an EDI link to send invoices to the purchasing firm. One consequence of an EDI system is that suppliers, shippers, and the purchasing firm can communicate with each other with no time delay, which increases the flexibility and responsiveness of the whole global supply system. A second consequence is that much of the paperwork between suppliers, shippers, and the purchasing firm is eliminated. Good EDI systems can help a firm decentralize materials management decisions to the plant level by giving corporate-level managers the information they need for coordinating and controlling decentralized materials management groups.

Before the emergence of the Internet as a major communication medium, firms and their suppliers normally had to purchase expensive proprietary software solutions to implement EDI systems. The ubiquity of the Internet and the availability of Web-based applications have made most of these proprietary solutions obsolete. Less expensive Web-based systems that are much easier to install and manage now dominate the market for global supply chain management software. These Web-based systems are rapidly transforming the management of globally dispersed supply chains, allowing even small firms to achieve a much better balance between supply and demand, thereby reducing the inventory in their systems and reaping the associated economic benefits. With increasing numbers of firms adopting these systems, those that don't may find themselves at a significant competitive disadvantage.

ChapterSummary

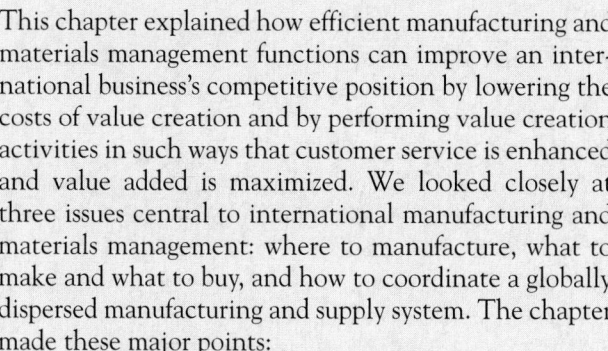

This chapter explained how efficient manufacturing and materials management functions can improve an international business's competitive position by lowering the costs of value creation and by performing value creation activities in such ways that customer service is enhanced and value added is maximized. We looked closely at three issues central to international manufacturing and materials management: where to manufacture, what to make and what to buy, and how to coordinate a globally dispersed manufacturing and supply system. The chapter made these major points:

1. The choice of an optimal manufacturing location must consider country factors, technological factors, and product factors.

2. Country factors include the influence of factor costs, political economy, and national culture on manufacturing costs, along with the presence of location externalities.

3. Technological factors include the fixed costs of setting up manufacturing facilities, the minimum efficient scale of production, and the availability of flexible manufacturing technologies that allow for mass customization.

4. Product factors include the value-to-weight ratio of the product and whether the product serves universal needs.

5. Location strategies either concentrate or decentralize manufacturing. The choice should be made in light of country, technological, and product factors. All location decisions involve trade-offs.

6. Foreign factories can improve their capabilities over time, and this can be of immense strategic benefit to the firm. Managers need to view foreign factories as potential centers of excellence and to encourage and foster attempts by local managers to upgrade factory capabilities.

7. An essential issue in many international businesses is determining which component parts should be manufactured in-house and which should be outsourced to independent suppliers.

8. Making components in-house facilitates investments in specialized assets and helps the firm protect its proprietary technology. It may improve scheduling between adjacent stages in the value chain, also. In-house production also makes sense if the firm is an efficient, low-cost producer of a technology.

9. Buying components from independent suppliers facilitates strategic flexibility and helps the firm avoid the organizational problems associated with extensive vertical integration. Outsourcing might also be employed as part of an "offset" policy, which is designed to win more orders for the firm from a country by pushing some subcontracting work to that country.

10. Several firms have tried to attain the benefits of vertical integration and avoid its associated organizational problems by entering long-term strategic alliances with essential suppliers.

11. Although alliances with suppliers can give a firm the benefits of vertical integration without dispensing entirely with the benefits of a market relationship, alliances have drawbacks. The firm that enters a strategic alliance may find its strategic flexibility limited by commitments to alliance partners.

12. Materials management encompasses all the activities that move materials to a manufacturing facility, through the manufacturing process, and out through a distribution system to the end user. The materials management function is complicated in an international business by distance, time, exchange rates, custom barriers, and other things.

13. Just-in-time systems generate major cost savings from reducing warehousing and inventory holding costs and from reducing the need to write off excess inventory. In addition, JIT systems help the firm spot defective parts and remove them from the manufacturing process quickly, thereby improving product quality.

14. For a firm to establish a good materials management function, it needs to legitimize materials management within the organization. It can do this by giving materials management equal footing with other functions.

15. Information technology, particularly Internet-based electronic data interchange, plays a major role in materials management. EDI facilitates the tracking of inputs, allows the firm to optimize its production schedule, lets the firm and its suppliers communicate in real time, and eliminates the flow of paperwork between a firm and its suppliers.

Critical Discussion Questions

1. An electronics firm is considering how best to supply the world market for microprocessors used in consumer and industrial electronic products. A manufacturing plant costs about $500 million to construct and requires a highly skilled workforce. The total value of the world market for this product over the next 10 years is estimated to be between $10 billion and $15 billion. The tariffs prevailing in this industry are currently low. Should the firm adopt a concentrated or decentralized manufacturing strategy? What kind of location(s) should the firm favor for its plant(s)?

2. A chemical firm is considering how best to supply the world market for sulfuric acid. A manufacturing plant costs about $20 million to construct and requires a moderately skilled workforce. The total value of the world market for this product over the next 10 years is estimated to be between $20 billion and $30 billion. The tariffs prevailing in this industry are moderate. Should the firm favor concentrated manufacturing or decentralized manufacturing? What kind of location(s) should the firm seek for its plant(s)?

3. A firm must decide whether to make a component part in-house or to contract it out to an independent supplier. Manufacturing the part requires a nonrecoverable investment in specialized assets. The most efficient suppliers are located in countries with currencies that many foreign exchange analysts expect to appreciate substantially over the next decade. What are the pros and cons of (a) manufacturing the component in-house and (b) outsource manufacturing to an independent supplier? Which option would you recommend? Why?

4. Explain how an efficient materials management function can help an international business compete more effectively in the global marketplace.

5. Read the opening case on Dell Computer.
   - What are the consequences for Dell's cost structure and profitability of replacing inventories with information?
   - Do you think that Dell's model can be imitated by other PC manufacturers and manufacturers in other industries?
   - What factors might make it difficult for other firms to adopt Dell's model?
   - What are the potential risks associated with Dell's supply chain strategy?

Research Task globalEDGE™ globaledge.msu.edu

Use the globalEDGE™ site to complete the following exercises:

1. The U.S. Department of Labor's Bureau of International Labor Affairs publishes a Chartbook of International Labor Comparisons. Locate the latest edition of this report and identify the hourly compensation costs for manufacturing workers in the United States, Japan, Korea, Taiwan, Germany, and the United Kingdom.

2. *IndustryWeek* magazine ranks the world's largest manufacturing companies by sales revenue. Identify the largest Chinese manufacturing companies as provided in the most recent ranking, paying special attention to the industries these companies operate in.

Notes

1. B. C. Arntzen, G. G. Brown, T. P. Harrison, and L. L. Trafton, "Global Supply Chain Management at Digital Equipment Corporation," *Interfaces* 25 (1995), pp. 69–93.

2. D. A. Garvin, "What Does Product Quality Really Mean," *Sloan Management Review* 26 (Fall 1984), pp. 25–44.

3. For general background information, see "How to Build Quality," *The Economist*, September 23, 1989, pp. 91–92; A. Gabor, *The Man Who Discovered Quality* (New York: Penguin, 1990); P. B. Crosby, *Quality Is Free* (New York: Mentor, 1980); M. Elliot et al., "A Quality World, a Quality Life," *Industrial Engineer*, January 2003, pp. 26–33.

4. G. T. Lucier and S. Seshadri, "GE Takes Six Sigma beyond the Bottom line," *Strategic Finance*, May 2001, pp. 40–46.

5. M. Saunders, "U.S. Firms Doing Business in Europe Have Options in Registering for ISO 9000 Quality Standards," *Business America*, June 14, 1993, p. 7.

6. G. Stalk and T. M. Hout, *Competing against Time* (New York: Free Press, 1990).

7. M. A. Cohen and H. L. Lee, "Resource Deployment Analysis of Global Manufacturing and Distribution Networks," *Journal of Manufacturing and Operations Management* 2 (1989), pp. 81–104.

8. P. Krugman, "Increasing Returns and Economic Geography," *Journal of Political Economy* 99, no. 3 (1991), pp. 483–99, and J. M. Shaver and F. Flyer, "Agglomeration Economies, Firm Heterogeneity, and Foreign Direct Investment in the United States," *Strategic Management Journal* 21 (2000), pp. 1175–93.

9. For a review of the technical arguments, see D. A. Hay and D. J. Morris, *Industrial Economics: Theory and Evidence* (Oxford: Oxford University Press, 1979). See also C. W. L. Hill and G. R. Jones, *Strategic Management: An Integrated Approach* (Boston: Houghton Mifflin, 2004).

10. See P. Nemetz and L. Fry, "Flexible Manufacturing Organizations: Implications for Strategy Formulation," *Academy of Management Review* 13 (1988), pp. 627–38; N. Greenwood, *Implementing Flexible Manufacturing Systems* (New York: Halstead Press, 1986); J. P. Womack, D. T. Jones, and D. Roos, *The Machine That Changed the World* (New York: Rawson Associates, 1990); and R. Parthasarthy and S. P. Seith, "The Impact of Flexible Automation on Business Strategy and Organizational Structure," *Academy of Management Review* 17 (1992), pp. 86–111.

11. B. J. Pine, *Mass Customization: The New Frontier in Business Competition* (Boston: Harvard Business School Press, 1993); S. Kotha, "Mass Customization: Implementing the Emerging Paradigm for Competitive Advantage," *Strategic Management Journal* 16 (1995), pp. 21–42; and J. H. Gilmore and B. J. Pine II, "The Four Faces of Mass Customization," *Harvard Business Review*, January–February 1997, pp. 91–101.

12. M. A. Cusumano, *The Japanese Automobile Industry* (Cambridge, MA: Harvard University Press, 1989); T. Ohno, *Toyota Production System* (Cambridge, MA: Productivity Press, 1990); and Womack, Jones, and Roos, *The Machine That Changed the World.*

13. "The Celling Out of America," *The Economist*, December 17, 1994, pp. 63–64.

14. K. Ferdows, "Making the Most of Foreign Factories," *Harvard Business Review*, March–April 1997, pp. 73–88.

15. This argument represents a simple extension of the dynamic capabilities research stream in the strategic management literature. See D. J. Teece, G. Pisano, and A. Shuen, "Dynamic Capabilities and Strategic Management," *Strategic Management Journal* 18 (1997), pp. 509–33.

16. T. S. Frost, J. M. Birkinshaw, and P. C. Ensign, "Centers of Excellence in Multinational Corporations," *Strategic Management Journal*, 23 (November 2002), pp. 997–1018.

17. C. W. L. Hill, "Globalization, the Myth of the Nomadic Multinational Enterprise, and the Advantages of Location Persistence," Working Paper, School of Business, University of Washington, 2001.

18. The material in this section is based primarily on the transaction cost literature of vertical integration; for example, O. E. Williamson, *The Economic Institutions of Capitalism* (New York: The Free Press, 1985).

19. For a review of the evidence, see Williamson, *The Economic Institutions of Capitalism*. See also L. Poppo and T. Zenger, "Testing Alternative Theories of the Firm: Transaction Cost, Knowledge Based, and Measurement Explanations for Make or Buy Decisions in Information Services," *Strategic Management Journal* 19 (1998), pp. 853–878.

20. A. D. Chandler, *The Visible Hand* (Cambridge, MA: Harvard University Press, 1977).

21. For a review of these arguments, see C. W. L. Hill and R. E. Hoskisson, "Strategy and Structure in the Multiproduct Firm," *Academy of Management Review* 12 (1987), pp. 331–41.

22. C. W. L. Hill, "Cooperation, Opportunism, and the Invisible Hand," *Academy of Management Review* 15 (1990), pp. 500–13.

23. See R. Narasimhan and J. R. Carter, "Organization, Communication and Coordination of International Sourcing," *International Marketing Review* 7 (1990), pp. 6–20, and Arntzen, Brown, Harrison, and Trafton, "Global Supply Chain Management at Digital Equipment Corporation."

24. H. F. Busch, "Integrated Materials Management," *IJPD & MM* 18 (1990), pp. 28–39.

25. J. G. Miller and P. Gilmour, "Materials Managers: Who Needs Them?" *Harvard Business Review*, July–August 1979, pp. 57–67.

26. Narasimhan and Carter, "Organization, Communication and Coordination of International Sourcing."

Li & Fung

Closing Case

Established in 1906, Hong Kong–based Li & Fung is now one of the largest multinational trading companies in the developing world, with annual sales of more than $4 billion in 2002. The company, which is still run by the grandson of the founder, Victor Fung, does not see itself as a traditional trading enterprise. Rather, it sees itself as an expert in supply chain management for its 350 or so major customers, providing the convenience of one-stop shopping for raw material sourcing, production planning and management, quality assurance, export documentation, and shipping consolidation. These customers are a diverse group and include clothing retailers and consumer electronics companies. Almost 75 percent of them are based in the United States. Li & Fung takes orders from customers and then sifts through its network of 7,000 independent suppliers located in 40 countries to find the right manufacturing enterprises to produce the product for customers at the most attractive combination of cost and quality. Attaining this goal frequently requires Li & Fung to break up the value chain and disperse different productive activities to manufacturers located in different countries depending on an assessment of factors such as labor costs, trade barriers, transportation costs, and so on. Li & Fung then coordinates the whole process, managing the logistics and arranging for the shipment of the finished product to the customer. Li & Fung has a policy of not owning any production facilities itself, preferring instead to shop around.

Typical of its customers is The Limited, Inc., a large U.S.-based chain of retail clothing stores. The Limited outsources much of its manufacturing and logistics func-

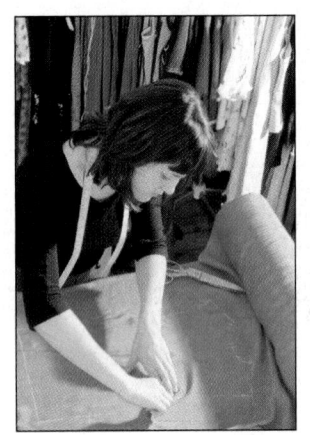

tions to Li & Fung. The process starts when The Limited comes to Li & Fung with designer sketches of clothes for the next fashion season. Li & Fung takes the basic product concepts and researches the market to find the right kind of yarn, dye, buttons, and so on, then assembles these into prototypes that The Limited can inspect. Once The Limited has settled on a prototype, it will give Li & Fung an order and ask for delivery within five weeks. The short time between an order and requested delivery is necessitated by the rapid rate of product obsolescence in the fashion clothing industry.

With order in hand, Li & Fung distributes the various aspects of the overall manufacturing process to different producers depending on their capabilities and costs. For example, Li & Fung might decide to purchase yarn from a Korean company but have it woven and dyed in Taiwan. So Li & Fung will arrange for the yarn to be picked up from Korea and shipped to Taiwan. The Japanese might have the best zippers and buttons, but they manufacture them mostly in China. So Li & Fung will go to YKK, a big Japanese zipper manufacturer, and order the right zippers from the Chinese plants. Then Li & Fung might decide that due to constraints imposed by export quotas and labor costs, the best place to make the final garments might be in Thailand. So everything will be shipped to Thailand. In addition, because The Limited, like many retail customers, needs quick delivery, Li & Fung might divide the order across five factories in Thailand. Five weeks after the order has been received, the garments will arrive on the shelves of The Limited, all looking like they came from one factory, with colors perfectly matched. The result is a product that may have a label that says "Made in Thailand," but it is a global product.

Li & Fung sees itself as a value added intermediary between the developed world and manufacturers in the developing world. Its core skill is the ability to coordinate a globally dispersed manufacturing process to get products quickly to customers at a low cost. When it comes to making attache cases, for example, Li & Fung buys leather in India, ships it to South Korea for tanning, and then sends it to China for final assembly with metal fittings made in Japan. Similarly, a talking toy assembled in China has a voice semiconductor made in Taiwan and sports clothes made in South Korea.

To better serve the needs of its customers, Li & Fung is divided into numerous small, customer-focused divisions. A theme store division serves a handful of customers such as Warner Brothers and Rainforest Café; there is a division for The Limited and another for Gymboree, a U.S.-based children's clothing store. Walk into one of these divisions, such as the Gymboree division, and you will see that all of the 40 or so people in the division are focused solely on meeting Gymboree's needs. On every desk is a computer with a direct software link to Gymboree. The staff is organized into specialized teams in areas such as design, technical support, merchandising, raw material purchasing, quality assurance, and shipping. These teams also have direct electronic links to dedicated staff in Li & Fung's branch offices in various countries where Gymboree buys in volume, such as China, Indonesia, and the Philippines.

Li & Fung was a leader in establishing real-time Internet-based links with its customers. At the same time, Li & Fung currently does not connect its Internet-based systems to the thousands of manufacturers who make its products, partly because communications systems aren't advanced enough in places like China, the Philippines, Bangladesh, and other Asian countries. Li & Fung relies on personal visits, phones, faxes, and couriers to keep in touch. The other reason manufacturers aren't linked to Li & Fung's system, however, is that it wants its own employees to make sure that materials have arrived, production has been scheduled, and shipping arrangements have been made. If it depended on manufacturers to directly enter that information, the quality of its data would be "like raw sewage," says Victor Fung. A manager in Pakistan could say, "Sure, we've started production; pay us," even if nothing was happening. Li & Fung personnel also have to be on the ground to make sure manufacturers comply with a customer's standards in terms of how they treat labor. For all these reasons, Victor Fung believes that it's unlikely the Internet will ever connect the complete supply chain.

Sources: J. Magretta, "Fast, Global, and Entrepreneurial: Supply Chain Management Hong Kong Style," *Harvard Business Review*, September–October 1998, p. 102–14; J. Ridding, "A Multinational Trading Group with Chinese Characteristics," *Financial Times*, November 7, 1997, p. 16; J. Ridding, "The Family in the Frame," *Financial Times*, October 28, 1996, p. 12; J. Lo, "Second Half Doubts Shadow Li & Fung Strength in Interims," *South China Morning Post*, August 27, 1998, p. 3; "Link in the Global Chain," *The Economist*, June 2, 2001, pp. 62–63; www.lifung.com; and W. J. Holstein, "Middleman Becomes Master," *Chief Executive*, October 2002, pp. 53–56.

Case Discussion Questions

1. At one time, many of Li & Fung's customers performed their own logistics and purchasing functions in-house. Now they outsource those functions to Li & Fung. Why? What is the value added that an intermediary such as Li & Fung delivers to its customers?

2. If Li & Fung is to execute on its promise to deliver value added to its customers, what skills and competencies must it have?

3. Why do you think that Li & Fung has a policy of not owning any production facilities?

4. Do you think Victor Fung is correct when he states that it is unlikely that the Internet will ever connect the complete supply chain? Why might he be correct? What might happen in the long run?

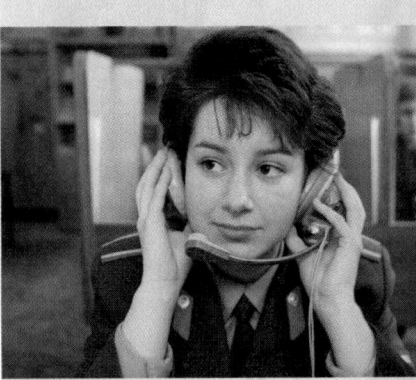

Chapter 17

Global Marketing and R&D

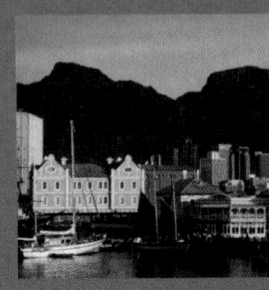

Introduction
The Globalization of Markets and Brands
Market Segmentation
Product Attributes
  Cultural Differences
  Economic Development
  Product and Technical Standards
Distribution Strategy
  Differences between Countries
  Choosing a Distribution Strategy
Communication Strategy
  Barriers to International
  Communication
  Push versus Pull Strategies
  Global Advertising
Pricing Strategy
  Price Discrimination
  Strategic Pricing
  Regulatory Influences on Prices
Configuring the Marketing Mix
New-Product Development
  The Location of R&D
  Integrating R&D, Marketing, and
  Production
  Cross-Functional Teams
Focus on Managerial Implications
Chapter Summary
Critical Discussion Questions
Closing Case: Procter & Gamble in Japan

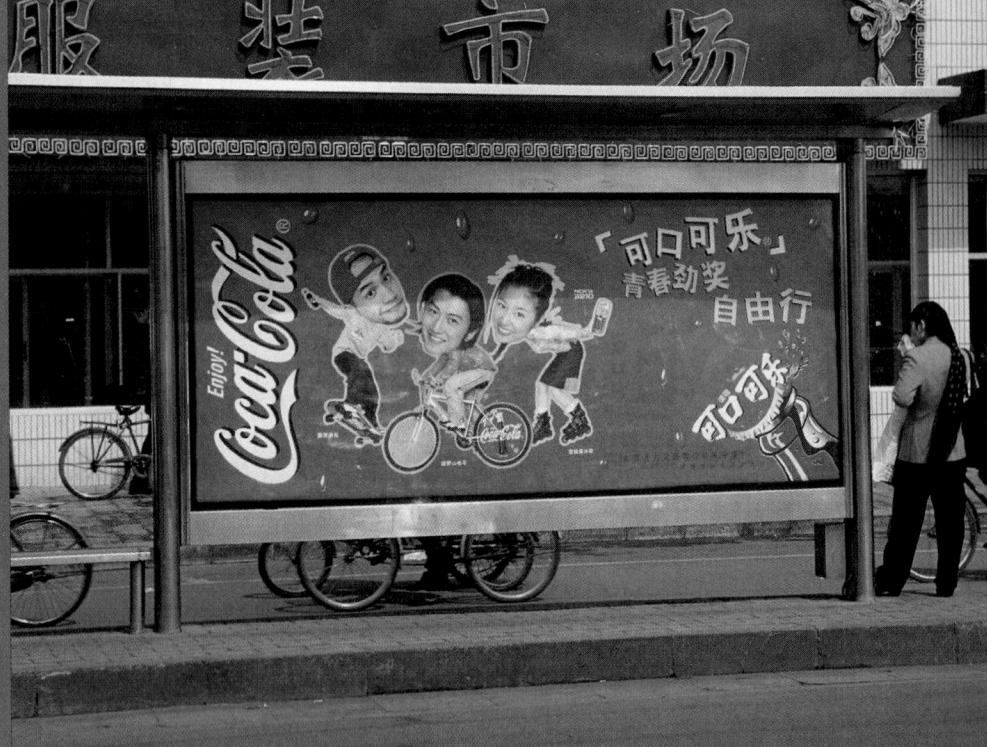

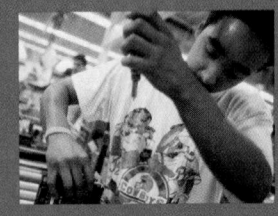

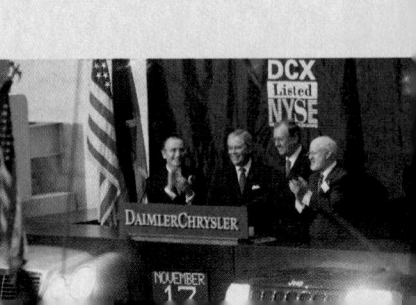

Marketing Coca-Cola in China

Since welcoming the company in 1975, China has grown to become a major market for Coca-Cola. The company now has 31 bottling plants and 30,000 employees in the country. China ended 2002 as the company's sixth largest market following a 14 percent year-on-year increase in consumption. Coca-Cola's goals call for China to become the company's largest overseas market within a decade, and quite possibly the largest market in the world, surpassing consumption in the United States. With a population four times the size of the United States, that goal seems attainable even if the Chinese do not consume as much on a per capita basis as Americans. Currently, the per capita consumption of Coke in the United States is 425 8-ounce servings per year, compared to around 9 servings per year in China.

To reach its goals for the Chinese market, Coca-Cola has embarked on an aggressive marketing campaign. The company has been aided by the Chinese acceptance of foreign brands. Whereas some 36 percent of consumers polled in India reject U.S. brands, and 19 percent in Indonesia, in China the figure is just 13 percent. Coca-Cola's biggest impediment to building sales volume is not brand acceptance or brand awareness, it is distribution. About half of China's 1.5 billion people do not have access to the product. Almost half of Coca-Cola's sales come from a handful of major cities and provincial capitals in China that account for just 8 percent of the population. For China to become the largest market for Coca-Cola, that must be changed.

Big cities dominate sales for a good reason. An explosion of major supermarket chains, including France's Carrefour and Wal-Mart, is creating the type of modern retail environment in which brands such as Coke thrive. In the rest of China, tiny shops and locally owned supermarkets prevail. Getting to these stores often requires hours of travel over rutted dirt roads, presenting a major logistical challenge, and those companies that are able to deliver products find that they are fighting for shelf space against local brands that are better entrenched in the rural hinterland of China than they are in major cities.

While Coke holds a 55 percent share of the cola market in China's big cities, in smaller cities and towns its share drops to 34 percent.

In the battle to grow volume, Coca-Cola's main weapon is market information. As recently as the mid-1990s, the company had little knowledge of who was drinking its product and where. Trucks would line up outside bottlers to collect products, but Coca-Cola didn't know where the products ended up. During the past few years, the company has been trying to map every supermarket, restaurant, small store, or market stall where a can of soda might be consumed. The company has 10,000 sales representatives that make regular visits to the myriad of small outlets, often on bicycle or foot, to ensure there is enough stock and to record what has been sold. All of the information is then put into a database, giving Coca-Cola perhaps the most accurate profile of consumer consumption in China. The data help refine point-of-sale and distribution strategies, thereby building sales volume. To help local distributors, Coca-Cola will buy the assets required to establish a distribution system—from the motorized tricycles used for deliveries to small refrigeration units—and then gradually let the distributors own the assets. It will then provide those distributors with the market information required to make sure that no outlet is ever short of product to sell.

In addition to distribution, another impediment to building volume has been pricing. High transportation costs have meant that Coke is most expensive in those parts of China where people are poorest. To bring the price down, Coca-Cola has started to open bottling plants closer to rural customers, and it is using recyclable bottles. Consistent with this strategy, in 2002 Coca-Cola opened two new bottling plants in China's hinterland.

Sources: G. Kahn, "Coke Works Harder at Being the Real Thing in the Hinterland," *Wall Street Journal*, December 26, 2002, pp. B1, B6; E. Louie, "In China, a New Signature for Soft Drink," *New York Times*, February 27, 2003, p. 3; N. Madden, "Brand Origin Not a Major Factor for Most Asians," *Advertising Age*, April 7, 2003, p. 33; "Coca-Cola Unwraps Logo for China," *China Daily*, February 19, 2003.

Introduction

In the previous chapter, we looked at the roles of global manufacturing and materials management in an international business. In this chapter, we continue our focus on specific business functions by examining the roles of marketing and research and development (R&D) in an international business. We focus on how marketing and R&D can be performed so they will reduce the costs of value creation and add value by better serving customer needs.

In Chapter 12, we spoke of the tension existing in most international businesses between the needs to reduce costs and at the same time to respond to local conditions, which tends to raise costs. This tension continues to be a persistent theme in this chapter. A global marketing strategy that views the world's consumers as similar in their tastes and preferences is consistent with the mass production of a standardized output. By mass-producing a standardized output, the firm can realize substantial unit cost reductions from experience curve and other scale economies. But ignoring country differences in consumer tastes and preferences can lead to failure. Thus, an international business's marketing function needs to determine when product standardization is appropriate and when it is not, and to adjust the marketing strategy accordingly. Similarly, the firm's R&D function needs to be able to develop globally standardized products when appropriate as well as products customized to local requirements.

We consider marketing and R&D within the same chapter because of their close relationship. A critical aspect of the marketing function is identifying gaps in the market so that new products can be developed to fill those gaps. Developing new products requires R&D; thus, the linkage between marketing and R&D. New products should be developed with market needs in mind, and only marketing can define those needs for R&D personnel. Also, only marketing can tell R&D whether to produce globally standardized or locally customized products. Research has long maintained that a major contributor to the success of new-product introductions is a close relationship between marketing and R&D.[1]

The opening case illustrates some issues we will be debating in this chapter. In trying to increase its sales volume in China, Coca-Cola has to battle with a distribution system that is very different from that in developed markets such as the United States. Rutted roads and small distributors present a barrier to getting the product close to people. Coca-Cola has been able to draw upon its extensive international experiences, however, to craft a distribution strategy that makes sense for China. In addition, the company uses more traditional glass bottles in China than in developed markets, so that recycling of containers can bring prices down and help grow consumption.

In this chapter, we begin by reviewing the debate on the globalization of markets. Then we discuss the issue of market segmentation. Next we look at four elements that constitute a firm's marketing mix: product attributes, distribution strategy, communication strategy, and pricing strategy. The **marketing mix** is the set of choices the firm offers to its targeted markets. Many firms vary their marketing mix from country to country depending on differences in national culture, economic development, product standards, distribution channels, and so on (as the opening case shows Coca-Cola has had to do in China). The chapter closes with a look at new-product development in an international business and at the implications of this for the organization of the firm's R&D function.

The Globalization of Markets and Brands

In a now-classic *Harvard Business Review* article, Theodore Levitt wrote lyrically about the globalization of world markets. Levitt's arguments have become something of a lightning rod in the debate about the extent of globalization. According to Levitt:

A powerful force drives the world toward a converging commonalty, and that force is technology. It has proletarianized communication, transport, and travel. The result is a new commercial reality—the emergence of global markets for standardized consumer products on a previously unimagined scale of magnitude.

Gone are accustomed differences in national or regional preferences . . . The globalization of markets is at hand. With that, the multinational commercial world nears its end, and so does the multinational corporation. The multinational corporation operates in a number of countries and adjusts its products and practices to each—at high relative costs. The global corporation operates with resolute consistency—at low relative cost—as if the entire world were a single entity; it sells the same thing in the same way everywhere.

Commercially, nothing confirms this as much as the success of McDonald's from the Champs Élysées to the Ginza, of Coca-Cola in Bahrain and Pepsi-Cola in Moscow, and of rock music, Greek salad, Hollywood movies, Revlon cosmetics, Sony television, and Levi's jeans everywhere.

Ancient differences in national tastes or modes of doing business disappear. The commonalty of preference leads inescapably to the standardization of products, manufacturing, and the institutions of trade and commerce.[2]

This is eloquent and evocative writing, but is Levitt correct? The rise of global media such as MTV and CNN, and the ability of such media to help shape a global culture, would seem to lend weight to Levitt's argument. If Levitt is correct, his argument has major implications for the marketing strategies pursued by international business. However, the consensus among academics is that Levitt overstates his case.[3] Although Levitt may have a point when it comes to many basic industrial products, such as steel, bulk chemicals, and semiconductor chips, globalization seems to be the exception rather than the rule in many consumer goods markets and industrial markets. Even a firm such as McDonald's, which Levitt holds up as the archetypal example of a consumer products firm that sells a standardized product worldwide, modifies its menu from country to country in light of local consumer preferences.[4]

Levitt is probably correct to assert that modern transportation and communications technologies, such as MTV, are facilitating a convergence of the tastes and preferences of consumers in the more advanced countries of the world. The popularity of sushi in Los Angeles, hamburgers in Tokyo, hip-hop music, and global media phenomena such as Pokémon, all support this. In the long run, such technological forces may lead to the evolution of a global culture. At present, however, the continuing persistence of cultural and economic differences between nations acts as a major brake on any trend toward global consumer tastes and preferences. In addition, trade barriers and differences in product and technical standards also constrain a firm's ability to sell a standardized product to a global market using a standardized marketing strategy. We discuss the sources of these differences in subsequent sections when we look at how products must be altered from country to country. Levitt's globally standardized markets seem a long way off in many industries.

Market Segmentation

Market segmentation refers to identifying distinct groups of consumers whose purchasing behavior differs from others in important ways. Markets can be segmented in numerous ways: by geography, demography (sex, age, income, race, education level, etc.), social-cultural factors (social class, values, religion, lifestyle choices), and psychological factors (personality). Because different segments exhibit different patterns of purchasing behavior, firms often adjust their marketing mix from segment to segment. Thus, the precise design of a product, the pricing strategy, the distribution channels used, and the choice of communication strategy may all be varied from segment to segment. The goal is to optimize the fit between the purchasing behavior of consumers in a given segment and the marketing mix, thereby maximizing sales to that

Marketing to Black Brazil

Brazil is home to the largest black population outside of Nigeria. Nearly half of the 160 million people in Brazil are of African or mixed-race origin. Despite this, until recently businesses have made little effort to target this numerically large segment. Part of the reason is rooted in economics. Black Brazilians have historically been poorer than Brazilians of European origin and thus have not received the same attention as whites. But after a decade of relatively strong economic performance in Brazil, an emerging black middle class is beginning to command the attention of consumer product companies. To take advantage of this, companies such as Unilever have recently introduced a range of skin care products and cosmetics aimed at black Brazilians, and Brazil's largest toy company recently introduced a black Barbie-like doll, Susi Olodum, sales of which quickly caught up with sales of a similar white doll.

But there is more to the issue than simple economics. Unlike the United States, where a protracted history of racial discrimination gave birth to the civil rights movement, fostered black awareness, and produced an identifiable subculture in U.S. society, the history of blacks in Brazil has been very different. Although Brazil did not abolish slavery until 1888, racism in Brazil has historically been much subtler than in the United States. Brazil has never excluded blacks from voting or had a tradition of segregating the races. Historically, too, the government encouraged intermarriage between whites and blacks in order to "bleach"

society. Partly due to this more benign history, Brazil has not had a black rights movement similar to that in the United States, and racial self-identification is much weaker. Surveys routinely find that African-Brazilian consumers decline to categorize themselves as either black or white, but instead choose one of dozens of skin tones and see themselves as being part of a culture that transcends race.

This subtler racial dynamic has important implications for market segmentation and tailoring the marketing mix in Brazil. Unilever had to face this issue when launching a Vaseline Intensive Care lotion for black consumers in Brazil. The company learned in focus groups that for the product to resonate with nonwhite women, its promotions had to feature women of different skin tones, excluding neither whites nor blacks. The campaign Unilever devised features three women with different skin shades at a fitness center. The bottle says the lotion is for "tan and black skin"—a description that could include many white women considering that much of the population lives near the beach. Unilever learned that the segment exists, but it is more difficult to define and requires more subtle marketing messages than the African-American segment in the United States or middle-class segments in Africa.

segment. Automobile companies, for example, use a different marketing mix to sell cars to different socioeconomic segments. Thus, Toyota uses its Lexus division to sell high-priced luxury cars to high-income consumers, while selling its entry-level models, such as the Toyota Corolla, to lower-income consumers. Similarly, personal computer manufacturers will offer different computer models, embodying different combinations of product attributes and price points, precisely to appeal to consumers from different market segments (e.g., business users and home users).

When managers in an international business consider market segmentation in foreign countries, they need to be cognizant of two main issues: the differences between countries in the structure of market segments and the existence of segments that transcend national borders. The structure of market segments may differ significantly from country to country. An important market segment in a foreign country may have no parallel in the firm's home country, and vice versa. The firm may have to develop a unique marketing mix to appeal to the purchasing behavior of a certain segment in a given country. An example of such a market segment is given in the accompanying Management Focus, which looks at the African-Brazilian market segment in Brazil, which as you will see is very different from the African-American segment in the

United States. In another example, a research project identified a segment of consumers in China in the 45-to-55 age range that has few parallels in other countries.[5] This group came of age during China's violent and repressive Cultural Revolution in the late 1960s and early 1970s. This group's values have been shaped by their experiences during the Cultural Revolution. They tend to be highly sensitive to price and respond negatively to new products and most forms of marketing. The existence of this group implies that firms doing business in China may need to customize their marketing mix to address the unique values and purchasing behavior of the group. The existence of such a segment constrains the ability of firms to standardize their global marketing strategy.

In contrast, the existence of market segments that transcend national borders clearly enhances the ability of an international business to view the global marketplace as a single entity and pursue a global strategy, selling a standardized product worldwide and using the same basic marketing mix to help position and sell that product in a variety of national markets. For a segment to transcend national borders, consumers in that segment must have some compelling similarities along important dimensions—such as age, values, lifestyle choices—and those similarities must translate into similar purchasing behavior. Although such segments exist in certain industrial markets, they are rare in consumer markets. However, one emerging global segment that is attracting the attention of international marketers of consumer goods is the so-called global youth segment. Global media are paving the way for a global youth segment. Evidence that such a segment exists comes from a study of the cultural attitudes and purchasing behavior of more than 6,500 teenagers in 26 countries.[6] The findings suggest that teens around the world are increasingly living parallel lives that share many common values. It follows that they are likely to purchase the same kind of consumer goods and for the same reasons. Even here though, marketing specialists argue that some customization in the marketing mix to account for differences across countries is required.

Product Attributes

A product can be viewed as a bundle of attributes.[7] For example, the attributes that make up a car include power, design, quality, performance, fuel consumption, and comfort; the attributes of a hamburger include taste, texture, and size; a hotel's attributes include atmosphere, quality, comfort, and service. Products sell well when their attributes match consumer needs (and when their prices are appropriate). BMW cars sell well to people who have high needs for luxury, quality, and performance, precisely because BMW builds those attributes into its cars. If consumer needs were the same the world over, a firm could simply sell the same product worldwide. However, consumer needs vary from country to country depending on culture and the level of economic development. A firm's ability to sell the same product worldwide is further constrained by countries' differing product standards. In this section, we review each of these issues and discuss how they influence product attributes.

Cultural Differences

We discussed countries' cultural differences in Chapter 3. Countries differ along a whole range of dimensions, including social structure, language, religion, and education. And as alluded to in Chapter 2, these differences have important implications for marketing strategy. For example, "hamburgers" do not sell well in Islamic countries, where the consumption of ham is forbidden by Islamic law. The most important aspect of cultural differences is probably the impact of tradition. Tradition is particularly important in foodstuffs and beverages. For example, reflecting differences in traditional eating habits, the Findus frozen food division of Nestlé, the Swiss food giant, markets fish cakes and fish fingers in Great Britain, but beef bourguignon and coq au vin in

France and vitéllo con funghi and braviola in Italy. In addition to its normal range of products, Coca-Cola in Japan markets Georgia, a cold coffee in a can, and Aquarius, a tonic drink, both of which appeal to traditional Japanese tastes.

For historical and idiosyncratic reasons, a range of other cultural differences exist between countries. For example, scent preferences differ from one country to another. S. C. Johnson Wax, a manufacturer of waxes and polishes, encountered resistance to its lemon-scented Pledge furniture polish among older consumers in Japan. Careful market research revealed that the polish smelled similar to a latrine disinfectant used widely in Japan in the 1940s. Sales rose sharply after the scent was adjusted.[8] In another example, Cheetos, the bright orange and cheesy-tasting snack from PepsiCo's Frito-Lay unit, do not have a cheese taste in China. Chinese consumers generally do not like the taste of cheese because it has never been part of traditional cuisine and because many Chinese are lactose-intolerant.[9]

There is some evidence of the trends Levitt talked about. Tastes and preferences are becoming more cosmopolitan. Coffee is gaining ground against tea in Japan and Great Britain, while American-style frozen dinners have become popular in Europe (with some fine-tuning to local tastes). Taking advantage of these trends, Nestlé has found that it can market its instant coffee, spaghetti bolognese, and Lean Cuisine frozen dinners in essentially the same manner in both North America and Western Europe. However, there is no market for Lean Cuisine dinners in most of the rest of the world, and there may not be for years or decades. Although some cultural convergence has occurred, particularly among the advanced industrial nations of North America and Western Europe, Levitt's global culture is still a long way off.

Economic Development

Just as important as differences in culture are differences in the level of economic development. We discussed the extent of country differences in economic development in Chapter 2. Consumer behavior is influenced by the level of economic development of a country. Firms based in highly developed countries such as the United States tend to build a lot of extra performance attributes into their products. These extra attributes are not usually demanded by consumers in less developed nations, where the preference is for more basic products. Thus, cars sold in less developed nations typically lack many of the features found in the West, such as air-conditioning, power steering, power windows, radios, and cassette players. For most consumer durables, product reliability may be a more important attribute in less developed nations, where such a purchase may account for a major proportion of a consumer's income, than it is in advanced nations.

Contrary to Levitt's suggestions, consumers in the most developed countries are often not willing to sacrifice their preferred attributes for lower prices. Consumers in the most advanced countries often shun globally standardized products that have been developed with the lowest common denominator in mind. They are willing to pay more for products that have additional features and attributes customized to their tastes and preferences. For example, demand for top-of-the-line four-wheel-drive sport utility vehicles, such as Chrysler's Jeep, Ford's Explorer, and Toyota's Land Cruiser, is almost totally restricted to the United States. This is due to a combination of factors, including the high-income level of U.S. consumers, the country's vast distances, the relatively low cost of gasoline, and the culturally grounded "outdoor" theme of American life.

Product and Technical Standards

Even with the forces that are creating some convergence of consumer tastes and preferences among advanced, industrialized nations, Levitt's vision of global markets may still be a long way off because of national differences in product and technological standards.

Differing government-mandated product standards can rule out mass production and marketing of a standardized product. Differences in technical standards also constrain the globalization of markets. Some of these differences result from idiosyncratic decisions made long ago, rather than from government actions, but their long-term effects are profound. For example, video equipment manufactured for sale in the United States will not play videotapes recorded on equipment manufactured for sale in Great Britain, Germany, and France (and vice versa). Different technical standards for television signal frequency emerged in the 1950s that require television and video equipment to be customized to prevailing standards. RCA stumbled in the 1970s when it failed to account for this in its marketing of TVs in Asia. Although several Asian countries adopted the U.S. standard, Singapore, Hong Kong, and Malaysia adopted the British standard. People who bought RCA TVs in those countries could receive a picture but no sound![10]

Distribution Strategy ■

A critical element of a firm's marketing mix is its distribution strategy: the means it chooses for delivering the product to the consumer. The way the product is delivered is determined by the firm's entry strategy, discussed in Chapter 14. In this section, we examine a typical distribution system, discuss how its structure varies between countries, and look at how appropriate distribution strategies vary from country to country.

Figure 17.1 illustrates a typical distribution system consisting of a channel that includes a wholesale distributor and a retailer. If the firm manufactures its product in the particular country, it can sell directly to the consumer, to the retailer, or to the wholesaler. The same options are available to a firm that manufactures outside the country. Plus, this firm may decide to sell to an import agent, which then deals with the wholesale distributor, the retailer, or the consumer. The factors that determine the firm's choice of channel are considered later in this section.

Differences between Countries

The three main differences between distribution systems are retail concentration, channel length, and channel exclusivity.

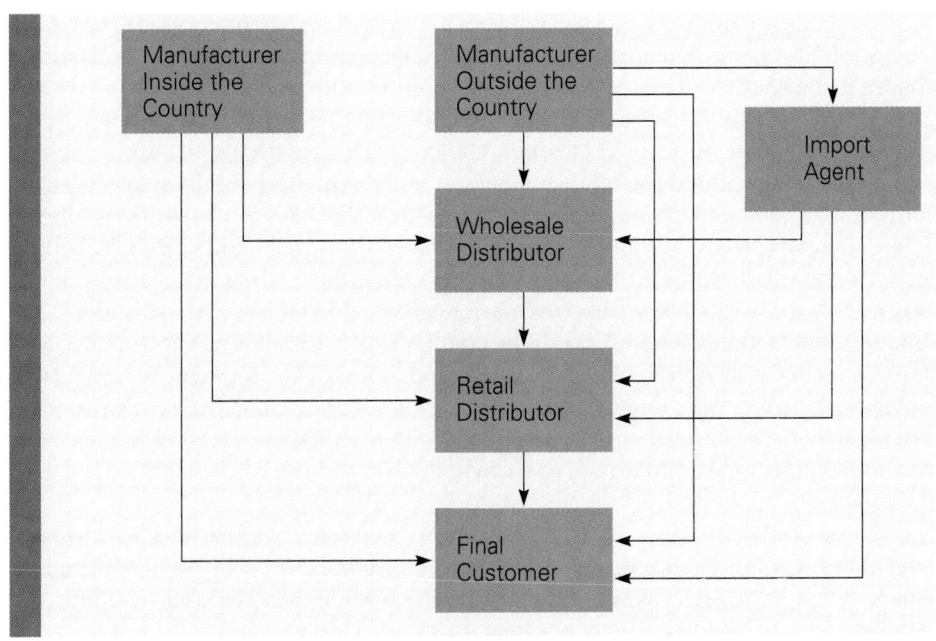

Figure 17.1

A Typical Distribution System

Retail Concentration

In some countries, the retail system is very concentrated, but it is fragmented in others. In a concentrated system, a few retailers supply most of the market. A fragmented system is one in which there are many retailers, no one of which has a major share of the market. Many of the differences in concentration are rooted in history and tradition. In the United States, the importance of the automobile and the relative youth of many urban areas have resulted in a retail system centered around large stores or shopping malls to which people can drive. This has facilitated system concentration. Japan's much greater population density together with the large number of urban centers that grew up before the automobile have yielded a more fragmented retail system of many small stores that serve local neighborhoods and to which people frequently walk. In addition, the Japanese legal system protects small retailers. Small retailers can block the establishment of a large retail outlet by petitioning their local government.

There is a tendency for greater retail concentration in developed countries. Three factors that contribute to this are the increases in car ownership, number of households with refrigerators and freezers, and number of two-income households. All these factors have changed shopping habits and facilitated the growth of large retail establishments sited away from traditional shopping areas. The last decade has seen consolidation in the global retail industry with companies such as Wal-Mart and Carrefour attempting to become global retailers by acquiring retailers in different countries. This has increased retail concentration.

In contrast, retail systems are very fragmented in many developing countries, which can make for interesting distribution challenges. In rural China, large areas of the country can be reached only by traveling rutted dirt roads (see the opening case). In India, Unilever has to sell to retailers in 600,000 rural villages, many of which cannot be accessed via paved roads, which means products can reach their destination only by bullock, bicycle, or cart (see the Management Focus on Unilever later in this chapter). In neighboring Nepal, the terrain is so rugged that even bicycles and carts are not practical, and businesses rely on yak trains and the human back to deliver products to thousands of small retailers.

Channel Length

Channel length refers to the number of intermediaries between the producer (or manufacturer) and the consumer. If the producer sells directly to the consumer, the channel is very short. If the producer sells through an import agent, a wholesaler, and a retailer, a long channel exists. The choice of a short or long channel is in part a strategic decision for the producing firm. However, some countries have longer distribution channels than others. The most important determinant of channel length is the degree to which the retail system is fragmented. Fragmented retail systems tend to promote the growth of wholesalers to serve retailers, which lengthens channels.

The more fragmented the retail system, the more expensive it is for a firm to make contact with each individual retailer. Imagine a firm that sells toothpaste in a country where there are over a million small retailers, as in rural India and China. To sell directly to the retailers, the firm would have to build a huge sales force. This would be very expensive, particularly since each sales call would yield a very small order. But suppose a few hundred wholesalers in the country supply retailers not only with toothpaste but also with all other personal care and household products. Because these wholesalers carry a wide range of products, they get bigger orders with each sales call, making it worthwhile for them to deal directly with the retailers. Accordingly, it makes economic sense for the firm to sell to the wholesalers and the wholesalers to deal with the retailers.

Because of such factors, countries with fragmented retail systems also tend to have long channels of distribution, sometimes with multiple layers. The classic example is Japan, where there are often two or three layers of wholesalers between the firm and retail outlets. In countries such as Great Britain, Germany, and the United States where the retail system is far more concentrated, channels are much shorter. When the retail sector is very concentrated, it makes sense for the firm to deal directly with retailers, cutting out wholesalers. A relatively small sales force is required to deal with a concentrated retail sector, and the orders generated from each sales call can be large. Such circumstances tend to prevail in the United States, where large food companies may sell directly to supermarkets rather than going through wholesale distributors.

The rapid development of the Internet in recent years has helped to shorten channel length. For example, the Seattle-based outdoor equipment retailer REI sells its products in Japan via a Japanese-language website, thereby eliminating the need for a retail presence on the ground in Japan, which obviously shortens the channel length between REI and its customers. However, there are obvious drawbacks with such a strategy. In the case of REI, consumers cannot receive the same level of advice over the Web as in physical retail stores, where salespeople can help customers choose the right gear for their needs. So although REI benefits from a short channel in Japan, it may lose significant sales due to the lack of point-of-sale service.

Channel Exclusivity

An exclusive distribution channel is one that is difficult for outsiders to access. For example, it is often difficult for a new firm to get access to shelf space in supermarkets. This occurs because retailers tend to prefer to carry the products of long-established manufacturers of foodstuffs with national reputations rather than gamble on the products of unknown firms. The exclusivity of a distribution system varies between countries. Japan's system is often held up as an example of a very exclusive system. In Japan, relationships between manufacturers, wholesalers, and retailers often go back decades. Many of these relationships are based on the understanding that distributors will not carry the products of competing firms. In return, the distributors are guaranteed an attractive markup by the manufacturer. As many U.S. and European manufacturers have learned, the close ties that result from this arrangement can make access to the Japanese market very difficult. However, it is possible to break into the Japanese market with a new consumer product. Procter & Gamble did during the 1990s with its Joy brand of dish soap. P&G was able to overcome a tradition of exclusivity for two reasons. First, after a decade of lackluster economic performance, Japan is changing. In their search for profits, retailers are far more willing than they have been historically to violate the old norms of exclusivity. Second, P&G has been in Japan long enough and has a broad enough portfolio of consumer products to give it considerable leverage with distributors, enabling it to push new products out through the distribution channel.

Choosing a Distribution Strategy

A choice of distribution strategy determines which channel the firm will use to reach potential consumers. Should the firm try to sell directly to the consumer or should it go through retailers; should it go through a wholesaler; should it use an import agent? The optimal strategy is determined by the relative costs and benefits of each alternative. The relative costs and benefits of each alternative vary from country to country, depending on the three factors we have just discussed: retail concentration, channel length, and channel exclusivity.

Because each intermediary in a channel adds its own markup to the products, there is generally a critical link between channel length, the final selling price, and the firm's profit margin. The longer a channel, the greater is the aggregate markup, and the higher the price that consumers are charged for the final product. To ensure that prices do not get too high due to markups by multiple intermediaries, a firm might be forced to operate with lower profit margins. Thus, if price is an important competitive weapon, and if the firm does not want to see its profit margins squeezed, other things being equal, the firm would prefer to use a shorter channel.

However, the benefits of using a longer channel often outweigh these drawbacks. As we have seen, one benefit of a longer channel is that it cuts selling costs when the retail sector is very fragmented. Thus, it makes sense for an international business to use longer channels in countries where the retail sector is fragmented and shorter channels in countries where the retail sector is concentrated. Another benefit of using a longer channel is market access—the ability to enter an exclusive channel. Import agents may have long-term relationships with wholesalers, retailers, and/or important consumers and thus be better able to win orders and get access to a distribution system. Similarly, wholesalers may have long-standing relationships with retailers and be better able to persuade them to carry the firm's product than the firm itself would.

Import agents are not limited to independent trading houses; any firm with a strong local reputation could serve as well. For example, to break down channel exclusivity and gain greater access to the Japanese market, Apple Computer signed distribution agreements with five large Japanese firms including business equipment giant Brother Industries, stationery leader Kokuyo, Mitsubishi, Sharp, and Minolta. These firms use their own long-established distribution relationships with consumers, retailers, and wholesalers to push Apple Macintosh computers through the Japanese distribution system. As a result, Apple's share of the Japanese market increased from less than 1 percent to 13 percent in the four years following the signing of the agreements.[11]

If such an arrangement is not possible, the firm might want to consider other, less traditional alternatives to gaining market access. Frustrated by channel exclusivity in Japan, some foreign manufacturers of consumer goods have attempted to sell directly to Japanese consumers using direct mail and catalogs. REI had trouble persuading Japanese wholesalers and retailers to carry its products, so it began a direct-mail campaign and then Web-based strategy to enter Japan that is proving very successful.

Communication Strategy

Another critical element in the marketing mix is communicating the attributes of the product to prospective customers. A number of communication channels are available to a firm, including direct selling, sales promotion, direct marketing, and advertising. A firm's communication strategy is partly defined by its choice of channel. Some firms rely primarily on direct selling, others on point-of-sale promotions or direct marketing, others on mass advertising; still others use several channels simultaneously to communicate their message to prospective customers. In this section, we will look first at the barriers to international communication. Then we will survey the various factors that determine which communication strategy is most appropriate in a particular country. After that we discuss global advertising.

Barriers to International Communication

International communication occurs whenever a firm uses a marketing message to sell its products in another country. The effectiveness of a firm's international communication can be jeopardized by three potentially critical variables: cultural barriers, source effects, and noise levels.

Cultural Barriers

Cultural barriers can make it difficult to communicate messages across cultures. We discussed some sources and consequences of cultural differences between nations in Chapter 3 and in the previous section of this chapter. Due to cultural differences, a message that means one thing in one country may mean something quite different in another. For example, when Procter & Gamble promoted its Camay soap in Japan in the 1980s it ran into unexpected trouble. In a TV commercial, a Japanese man walked into the bathroom while his wife was bathing. The woman began telling her husband all about her new soap, but the husband, stroking her shoulder, hinted that suds were not on his mind. This ad had been very popular in Europe, but it flopped in Japan because it is considered very bad manners there for a man to intrude on his wife.[12]

Benetton, the Italian clothing manufacturer and retailer, is another firm that has run into cultural problems with its advertising. The company launched a worldwide advertising campaign in 1989 with the theme "United Colors of Benetton" that had won awards in France. One of its ads featured a black woman breast-feeding a white baby, and another one showed a black man and a white man handcuffed together. Benetton was surprised when the ads were attacked by U.S. civil rights groups for promoting white racial domination. Benetton withdrew its ads and fired its advertising agency, Eldorado of France.

The best way for a firm to overcome cultural barriers is to develop cross-cultural literacy (see Chapter 3). In addition, it should use local input, such as a local advertising agency, in developing its marketing message. If the firm uses direct selling rather than advertising to communicate its message, it should develop a local sales force whenever possible. Cultural differences limit a firm's ability to use the same marketing message and selling approach worldwide. What works well in one country may be offensive in another. The accompanying Management Focus, which profiles Procter & Gamble's strategy for selling Tampax tampons internationally, demonstrates how cultural factors can influence the choice of communication strategy.

Source and Country of Origin Effects

Source effects occur when the receiver of the message (the potential consumer in this case) evaluates the message based on the status or image of the sender. Source effects can be damaging for an international business when potential consumers in a target country have a bias against foreign firms. For example, a wave of "Japan bashing" swept the United States in the early 1990s. Worried that U.S. consumers might view its products negatively, Honda responded by creating ads that emphasized the U.S. content of its cars to show how "American" the company had become. Many international businesses try to counter negative source effects by deemphasizing their foreign origins. When British Petroleum acquired Mobil Oil's extensive network of U.S. gas stations, it changed its name to BP, diverting attention away from the fact that one of the biggest operators of gas stations in the United States is a British firm.

A subset of source effects is referred to as *country of origin effects*. Country of origin effects refers to the extent to which the place of manufacturing influences product evaluations. Research suggests that country of origin is often used as a cue when evaluating a product, particularly if the consumer lacks more detailed knowledge of the product. For example, one study found that Japanese consumers tended to rate Japanese products more favorably than U.S. products across multiple dimensions, even when independent analysis showed that they were actually inferior.[13] When a negative country of origin effect exists, an international business may have to work hard to counteract this effect by, for example, using promotional messages that stress the positive performance attributes of their product. Thus, the South Korean automobile company Hyundai tried to overcome negative perceptions about the quality of its vehicle in the United States by running advertisements that favorably compare the company's cars to more prestigious brands.

Source effects and country of origin effects are not always negative. French wine, Italian clothes, and German luxury cars benefit from nearly universal positive source effects. In such cases, it may pay a firm to emphasize its foreign origins. In Japan, for example, there is strong demand for high-quality foreign goods, particularly those from Europe. It has become chic to carry a Gucci handbag, sport a Rolex watch, drink expensive French wine, and drive a BMW.

Overcoming Cultural Barriers to Selling Tampons

In 1997, Procter & Gamble purchased Tambrands, the manufacturer of Tampax tampons, for $1.87 billion. P&G's goal was to make Tampax a global brand. At the time of the acquisition, tampons were used by some 70 percent of women in North America and a significant majority in northwestern Europe. However, usage elsewhere was very low, ranging from single digits in countries such as Spain and Japan, to less than 2 percent throughout Latin America. P&G believed that it could use its global marketing skills and distribution networks to grow the product, particularly in underserved markets such as Latin America and Southern Europe. It has found it tough going.

A big part of the problem has been religious and cultural taboos. A persistent myth in many countries holds that if a girl uses a tampon, she might lose her virginity. This concern seems to crop up most often in countries that are predominantly Catholic. Although the Roman Catholic church states it has no official position on tampons, some priests have spoken out against the product, associating it with birth control and sexual activities that are prohibited by the church! Women must also understand their bodies to use a tampon. P&G is finding that in countries where school health education is limited, that understanding is difficult to foster.

After failed attempts to market the product in India and Brazil using conventional marketing strategies, such as print media advertising and retail distribution, P&G has decided to change to an approach based on direct selling and relationship marketing. It tested this model in Monterrey, Mexico. A centerpiece of the strategy has been the hiring of a sales force of counselors. The counselors are young women. They must first promise to become regular tampon users. Most have never tried a tampon. P&G trains each woman and observes her early classes. After passing a written test, the women are equipped with anatomy charts, a blue foam model of a woman's reproductive system, and a box of samples. In navy pantsuits or a doctor's white coat embroidered with the Tampax logo, the counselors are dispatched to speak in stores, schools, gyms, and anywhere women gather. The counselors talk to about 60 women a day, explaining how the product works with the aid of flip charts. About one-third end up buying a product.

The counselors also use these meetings as an opportunity to recruit young women to host gatherings in their homes. Modeled on Tupperware parties, about 20 women typically attend these "bonding sessions" where the counselor explains the product and how it is used, answers questions, and dispenses free samples. About 40 percent of women who attend these gatherings go on to host one.

P&G also found that about half of all doctors in Monterrey thought that tampons were bad for women. The company believes that this is based on ignorance; most of the doctors are men and they simply do not understand how the product works. To combat this, P&G used its sales force, which already called on doctors to sell products such as Pepto-Bismol and Metamucil, to give away tampons and explain how the product works. As a result, P&G believes it has reduced resistance among doctors to less than 10 percent.

Will this selling strategy work? The early signs were encouraging. In just a few months, sales of tampons grew from 2 percent to 4 percent of the total feminine hygiene market in Monterrey, and sales of the Tampax brand tripled. On the basis of these results, P&G decided to launch its first full campaign in Venezuela in early 2001, with several other Latin American countries following soon after.

Sources: E. Nelson and M. Jordan, "Seeking New Markets for Tampons, P&G Faces Cultural Barriers," *Wall Street Journal*, December 8, 2000, pp. A1, A8. Copyright 2000 by *Wall Street Journal*. Reproduced with permission of DOW JONES & COMPANY, INC., in the format textbook by the Copyright Clearance Center.

Noise Levels

Noise tends to reduce the probability of effective communication. Noise refers to the amount of other messages competing for a potential consumer's attention, and this too varies across countries. In highly developed countries such as the United States, noise is extremely high. Fewer firms vie for the attention of prospective customers in developing countries, and the noise level is lower.

Push versus Pull Strategies

The main decision with regard to communications strategy is the choice between a push strategy and a pull strategy. A **push strategy** emphasizes personal selling rather than mass media advertising in the promotional mix. Although very effective as a promotional tool, personal selling requires intensive use of a sales force and is relatively costly. A **pull strategy** depends more on mass media advertising to communicate the marketing message to potential consumers.

Although some firms employ only a pull strategy and others only a push strategy, still other firms combine direct selling with mass advertising to maximize communication effectiveness. Factors that determine the relative attractiveness of push and pull strategies include product type relative to consumer sophistication, channel length, and media availability.

Product Type and Consumer Sophistication

A pull strategy is generally favored by firms in consumer goods industries that are trying to sell to a large segment of the market. For such firms, mass communication has cost advantages, and direct selling is rarely used. An exception to this rule can be found in poorer nations with low literacy levels, where direct selling may be the only way to reach consumers (see the Management Focus on Unilever). A push strategy is favored by firms that sell industrial products or other complex products. Direct selling allows the firm to educate potential consumers about the features of the product. This may not be necessary in advanced nations where a complex product has been in use for some time, where the product's attributes are well understood, and where consumers are sophisticated. However, customer education may be very important when consumers have less sophistication toward the product, which can be the case in developing nations or in advanced nations when a complex product is being introduced.

Channel Length

The longer the distribution channel, the more intermediaries there are that must be persuaded to carry the product for it to reach the consumer. This can lead to inertia in the channel, which can make entry very difficult. Using direct selling to push a product through many layers of a distribution channel can be very expensive. In such circumstances, a firm may try to pull its product through the channels by using mass advertising to create consumer demand—once demand is created, intermediaries will feel obliged to carry the product.

In Japan, products often pass through two, three, or even four wholesalers before they reach the final retail outlet. This can make it difficult for foreign firms to break into the Japanese market. Not only must the foreigner persuade a Japanese retailer to carry her product, but she may also have to persuade every intermediary in the chain to carry the product. Mass advertising may be one way to break down channel resistance in such circumstances. However, in countries such as India, which has a very long distribution channel to serve its massive rural population, low literacy levels may imply that mass advertising may not work, in which case, the firm may need to fall back on direct selling, or rely on the good will of distributors (see the Management Focus on Unilever).

Media Availability

A pull strategy relies on access to advertising media. In the United States, a large number of media are available, including print media (newspapers and magazines), broadcasting media (television and radio), and the Internet. The rise of cable television in the United States has facilitated extremely focused advertising (e.g., MTV for teens and young adults, Lifetime for women, ESPN for sports enthusiasts). The same is true of the Internet where different websites attract different kinds of users. While this level of media sophistication is found in some other developed countries, it is not universal. Even

Unilever—Selling to India's Poor

One of the world's largest and oldest consumer products companies, Unilever has long had a substantial presence in many of the world's poorer nations, such as India. Outside of major urban areas, low income, unsophisticated consumers, illiteracy, fragmented retail distribution systems, and the lack of paved roads have made for difficult marketing challenges. Despite this, Unilever has built a significant presence among impoverished rural populations by adopting innovative selling strategies.

Take India as an example. The country's large rural population is dispersed among some 600,000 villages, more than 500,000 of which cannot be reached by a motor vehicle. Some 91 percent of the rural population lives in villages of fewer than 2,000 people, and of necessity, rural retail stores are very small and carry limited stock. The population is desperately poor, making perhaps a dollar a day, and two-thirds of that income is spent on food, leaving about 30 cents a day for other items. Literacy levels are low, and TVs are rare, making traditional media ineffective. Despite these drawbacks Hindustan Lever, Unilever's Indian subsidiary, has made a concerted effort to reach the rural poor. Although the revenues generated from rural sales are small, Unilever hopes that as the country develops and income levels rise, the population will continue to purchase the Unilever brands that they are familiar with, giving the company a long-term competitive advantage.

To contact rural consumers, Hindustan Lever tries to establish a physical presence wherever people frequently gather in numbers. This means ensuring that advertisements are seen in places where people congregate and make purchases, such as at village wells and weekly rural markets, and where they consume products, such as at riverbanks where people gather to wash their clothes using (the company hopes) Unilever soap. It is not uncommon to see the villages well plastered with advertisements for Unilever products. The company also takes part in weekly rural events, such as market day, where farm produce is sold and family provisions purchased. Hindustan Lever salesmen will visit these gatherings, display their products, explain how they work, give away some free samples, make a few sales, and seed the market for future demand.

The backbone of Hindustan Lever's selling effort, however, is a rural distribution network that encompasses 100 factories, 7,500 distributors, and an estimated 3 million retail stores, many of which are little more than a hole in a wall or a stall at a market. The total stock of Unilever products in these stores may be no more than a few sachets of shampoo and half a dozen bars of soap. A depot in each of India's states feeds products to major wholesalers, which then sell directly to retailers in thousands of small towns and villages that can be reached by motor vehicles. If access via motor vehicles is not possible, the major wholesalers sell to smaller second-tier wholesalers, which then handle distribution to India's 500,000 inaccessible rural villages, reaching them by bicycle, bullock, cart, or baskets carried on a human back.

Sources: K. Merchant, "Striving for Success—One Sachet at a Time," *Financial Times*, December 11, 2000, p. 14, and M. Turner, "Bicycle Brigade Takes Unilever to the People," *Financial Times*, August 17, 2000, p. 8.

many advanced nations have far fewer electronic media available for advertising than the United States. In Scandinavia, for example, until recently no commercial television or radio stations existed; all electronic media were state owned and carried no commercials, although this has now changed with the advent of satellite television deregulation. In many developing nations, the situation is even more restrictive because mass media of all types are typically more limited. A firm's ability to use a pull strategy is limited in some countries by media availability. In such circumstances, a push strategy is more attractive. For example, Unilever uses a push strategy to sell consumer products in rural India, where few mass media are available (see the Management Focus).

Media availability is limited by law in some cases. Few countries allow advertisements for tobacco and alcohol products on television and radio, though they are usually permitted in print media. When the leading Japanese whiskey distiller, Suntory, entered the U.S. market, it had to do so without television, its preferred medium. The firm spends about $50 million annually on television advertising in Japan.

The Push—Pull Mix

The optimal mix between push and pull strategies depends on product type and consumer sophistication, channel length, and media sophistication. Push strategies tend to be emphasized:

- For industrial products and/or complex new products.
- When distribution channels are short.
- When few print or electronic media are available.

Pull strategies tend to be emphasized:

- For consumer goods.
- When distribution channels are long.
- When sufficient print and electronic media are available to carry the marketing message.

Global Advertising

In recent years, largely inspired by the work of visionaries such as Theodore Levitt, there has been much discussion about the pros and cons of standardizing advertising worldwide.[14] One of the most successful standardized campaigns in history was Philip Morris's promotion of Marlboro cigarettes. The campaign was instituted in the 1950s, when the brand was repositioned, to assure smokers that the flavor would be unchanged by the addition of a filter. The campaign theme of "Come to where the flavor is. Come to Marlboro country" was a worldwide success. Marlboro built on this when it introduced "the Marlboro man," a rugged cowboy smoking his Marlboro while riding his horse through the great outdoors. This ad proved successful in almost every major market around the world, and it helped propel Marlboro to the top of the world market.

For Standardized Advertising

The support for global advertising is threefold. First, it has significant economic advantages. Standardized advertising lowers the costs of value creation by spreading the fixed costs of developing the advertisements over many countries. For example, Levi Strauss paid an advertising agency $550,000 to produce a series of TV commercials. By reusing this series in many countries, rather than developing a series for each country, the company enjoyed significant cost savings. Similarly, Coca-Cola's advertising agency, McCann-Erickson, claims to have saved Coca-Cola $90 million over 20 years by using certain elements of its campaigns globally.

Second, there is the concern that creative talent is scarce and so one large effort to develop a campaign will produce better results than 40 or 50 smaller efforts. A third justification for a standardized approach is that many brand names are global. With the substantial amount of international travel today and the considerable overlap in media across national borders, many international firms want to project a single brand image to avoid confusion caused by local campaigns. This is particularly important in regions such as Western Europe, where travel across borders is almost as common as travel across state lines in the United States.

Against Standardized Advertising

There are two main arguments against globally standardized advertising. First, as we have seen repeatedly in this chapter and in Chapter 3, cultural differences between nations are such that a message that works in one nation can fail miserably in another. Cultural diversity makes it extremely difficult to develop a single advertising theme that is effective worldwide. Messages directed at the culture of a given country may be more effective than global messages.

Second, advertising regulations may block implementation of standardized advertising. For example, Kellogg could not use a television commercial it produced in

Great Britain to promote its cornflakes in many other European countries. A reference to the iron and vitamin content of its cornflakes was not permissible in the Netherlands, where claims relating to health and medical benefits are outlawed. A child wearing a Kellogg T-shirt had to be edited out of the commercial before it could be used in France, because French law forbids the use of children in product endorsements. The key line, "Kellogg's makes their cornflakes the best they have ever been," was disallowed in Germany because of a prohibition against competitive claims.[15] Similarly, American Express ran afoul of regulatory authorities in Germany when it launched a promotional scheme that had proved very successful in other countries. The scheme advertised the offer of "bonus points" every time American Express cardholders used their cards. According to the advertisements, these "bonus points" could be used toward air travel with three airlines and hotel accommodations. American Express was charged with breaking Germany's competition law, which prevents an offer of free gifts in connection with the sale of goods, and the firm had to withdraw the advertisements at considerable cost.[16]

Dealing with Country Differences

Some firms are experimenting with capturing some benefits of global standardization while recognizing differences in countries' cultural and legal environments. A firm may select some features to include in all its advertising campaigns and localize other features. By doing so, it may be able to save on some costs and build international brand recognition and yet customize its advertisements to different cultures.

Pepsi-Cola used this kind of approach in a 1980s advertising campaign. The company wanted to use music to connect its products with local markets. Pepsi hired U.S. singer Tina Turner and rock stars from six countries to team up in singing and performing the Pepsi-Cola theme song in a big rock concert. The commercials were customized for each market by showing Turner with the rock stars from that country. Except for the footage of the local stars, all the commercials were identical. By shooting the commercials all at once, Pepsi saved on production costs. The campaign was extended to 30 countries, which relieved the local subsidiaries or bottlers of having to develop their own campaigns.[17]

■ Pricing Strategy

International pricing strategy is an important component of the overall international marketing mix.[18] In this section, we look at three aspects of international pricing strategy. First, we examine the case for pursuing price discrimination, charging different prices for the same product in different countries. Second, we look at what might be called strategic pricing. Third, we review some regulatory factors, such as government-mandated price controls and antidumping regulations, that limit a firm's ability to charge the prices it would prefer in a country.

▎Price Discrimination

Price discrimination exists whenever consumers in different countries are charged different prices for the same product.[19] Price discrimination involves charging whatever the market will bear; in a competitive market, prices may have to be lower than in a market where the firm has a monopoly. Price discrimination can help a company maximize its profits. It makes economic sense to charge different prices in different countries.

Two conditions are necessary for profitable price discrimination. First, the firm must be able to keep its national markets separate. If it cannot do this, individuals or businesses may undercut its attempt at price discrimination by engaging in arbitrage. Arbitrage occurs when an individual or business capitalizes on a price differential for a firm's product between two countries by purchasing the product in the country where prices

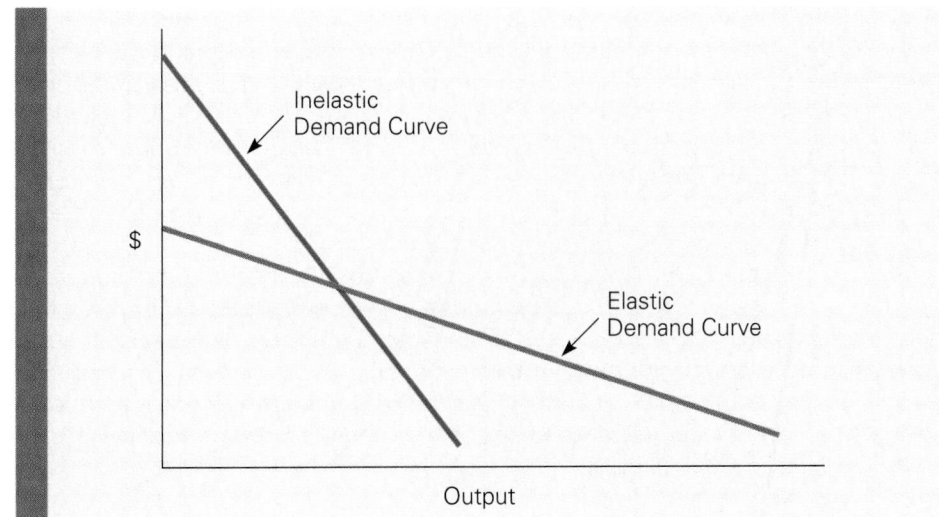

Figure 17.2

Elastic and Inelastic
Demand Curves

are lower and reselling it in the country where prices are higher. For example, many automobile firms have long practiced price discrimination in Europe. A Ford Escort once cost $2,000 more in Germany than it did in Belgium. This policy broke down when car dealers bought Escorts in Belgium and drove them to Germany, where they sold them at a profit for slightly less than Ford was selling Escorts in Germany. To protect the market share of its German auto dealers, Ford had to bring its German prices into line with those being charged in Belgium. Ford could not keep these markets separate.

However, Ford still practices price discrimination between Great Britain and Belgium. A Ford car can cost up to $3,000 more in Great Britain than in Belgium. In this case, arbitrage has not been able to equalize the price, because right-hand-drive cars are sold in Great Britain and left-hand-drive cars in the rest of Europe. Because there is no market for left-hand-drive cars in Great Britain, Ford has been able to keep the markets separate.

The second necessary condition for profitable price discrimination is different price elasticities of demand in different countries. The **price elasticity of demand** is a measure of the responsiveness of demand for a product to changes in price. Demand is said to be elastic when a small change in price produces a large change in demand; it is said to be inelastic when a large change in price produces only a small change in demand. Figure 17.2 illustrates elastic and inelastic demand curves. Generally, for reasons that will be explained shortly, a firm can charge a higher price in a country where demand is inelastic.

The Determinants of Demand Elasticity

The elasticity of demand for a product in a given country is determined by a number of factors, of which income level and competitive conditions are the two most important. Price elasticity tends to be greater in countries with low income levels. Consumers with limited incomes tend to be very price conscious; they have less to spend, so they look much more closely at price. Thus, price elasticities for products such as television sets are greater in countries such as India, where a television set is still a luxury item, than in the United States, where it is considered a necessity.

In general, the more competitors there are, the greater consumers' bargaining power will be and the more likely consumers will be to buy from the firm that charges the lowest price. Thus, many competitors cause high elasticity of demand. In such circumstances, if a firm raises its prices above those of its competitors, consumers will switch to the competitors' products. The opposite is true when a firm faces few competitors. When competitors are limited, consumers' bargaining power is weaker and

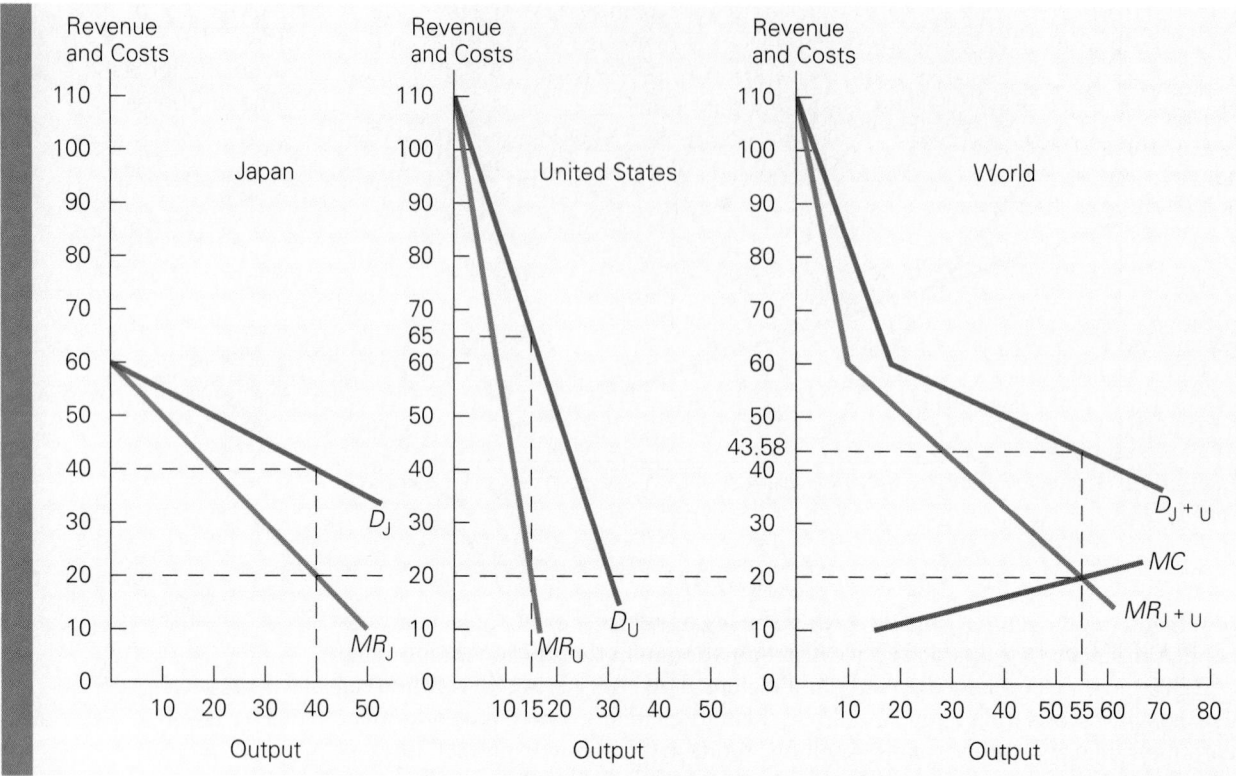

Figure 17.3

Price Discrimination

price is less important as a competitive weapon. Thus, a firm may charge a higher price for its product in a country where competition is limited than in a country where competition is intense.

Profit Maximizing under Price Discrimination

For those readers with some grasp of economic logic, we can offer a more formal presentation of the above argument. (Readers unfamiliar with basic economic terminology may want to skip this subsection.) Figure 17.3 shows the situation facing a firm that sells the same product in only two countries: Japan and the United States. The Japanese market is very competitive, so the firm faces an elastic demand curve (D_J) and marginal revenue curve (MR_J). The U.S. market is not competitive, so there the firm faces an inelastic demand curve (D_U) and marginal revenue curve (MR_U). Also shown in the figure are the firm's total demand curve (D_{J+U}), total marginal revenue curve (MR_{J+U}), and marginal cost curve (MC). The total demand curve is simply the summation of the demand facing the firm in Japan and the United States, as is the total marginal revenue curve.

To maximize profits, the firm must produce at the output where MR = MC. In Figure 17.3, this implies an output of 55 units. If the firm does not practice price discrimination, it will charge a price of $43.58 to sell an output of 55 units. Thus, without price discrimination, the firm's total revenues are $43.58 × 55 = $2,396.90. Look what happens when the firm decides to engage in price discrimination. It will still produce 55 units, since that is where MR = MC. However, the firm must now allocate this output between the two countries to take advantage of the difference in demand elasticity. Proper allocation of output between Japan and the United States can be determined graphically by drawing a line through their respective graphs at $20 to indicate that $20 is the marginal cost in each country (see Figure 17.3). To maximize profits, prices are now set in each country at that level where the marginal revenue for that country equals marginal costs. In Japan, this is a price of $40, and the firm sells 40 units. In the United States, the optimal price is $65, and it sells 15 units. Thus, reflecting the different competitive conditions, the price charged in the United States is more than 50 percent more than the price charged in Japan. Look at what happens to total revenues. With price discrimination, the firm earns revenues of

$$\$40 \times 40 \text{ units} = \$1,600$$

in Japan and

$$\$65 \times 15 \text{ units} = \$975$$

in the United States. By engaging in price discrimination, the firm can earn total revenues of

$$\$1,600 + \$975 = \$2,575,$$

which is $178.10 more than the $2,396.90 it earned before. Price discrimination pays!

Strategic Pricing

The concept of strategic pricing has three aspects, which we will refer to as predatory pricing, multipoint pricing, and experience curve pricing. Both predatory pricing and experience curve pricing may violate antidumping regulations. After we review predatory and experience curve pricing, we will look at antidumping rules and other regulatory policies.

Predatory Pricing

Predatory pricing is the use of price as a competitive weapon to drive weaker competitors out of a national market. Once the competitors have left the market, the firm can raise prices and enjoy high profits. For such a pricing strategy to work, the firm must normally have a profitable position in another national market, which it can use to subsidize aggressive pricing in the market it is trying to monopolize. Historically, many Japanese firms were accused of pursuing such a policy. The argument ran like this: Because the Japanese market was protected from foreign competition by high informal trade barriers, Japanese firms could charge high prices and earn high profits at home. They then used these profits to subsidize aggressive pricing overseas, with the goal of driving competitors out of those markets. Once this had occurred, so it is claimed, the Japanese firms then raised prices. Matsushita was accused of using this strategy to enter the U.S. TV market. As one of the major TV producers in Japan, Matsushita earned high profits at home. It then used these profits to subsidize the losses it made in the United States during its early years there, when it priced low to increase its market penetration. Ultimately, Matsushita became the world's largest manufacturer of TVs.[20]

Multipoint Pricing Strategy

Multipoint pricing becomes an issue when two or more international businesses compete against each other in two or more national markets. For example, multipoint pricing is an issue for Kodak and Fuji Photo because the companies compete against each other around the world. **Multipoint pricing** refers to the fact a firm's pricing strategy in one market may have an impact on its rivals' pricing strategy in another market. Aggressive pricing in one market may elicit a competitive response from a rival in another market. In the case of Kodak and Fuji, Fuji launched an aggressive competitive attack against

Kodak in the U.S. company's home market in January 1997, cutting prices on multiple-roll packs of 35mm film by as much as 50 percent.[21] This price cutting resulted in a 28 percent increase in shipments of Fuji color film during the first six months of 1997, while Kodak's shipments dropped by 11 percent. This attack created a dilemma for Kodak; the company did not want to start price discounting in its largest and most profitable market. Kodak's response was to aggressively cut prices in Fuji's largest market, Japan. This strategic response recognized the interdependence between Kodak and Fuji and the fact that they compete against each other in many different nations. Fuji responded to Kodak's counterattack by pulling back from its aggressive stance in the United States.

The Kodak story illustrates an important aspect of multipoint pricing—aggressive pricing in one market may elicit a response from rivals in another market. The firm needs to consider how its global rivals will respond to changes in its pricing strategy before making those changes. A second aspect of multipoint pricing arises when two or more global companies focus on particular national markets and launch vigorous price wars in those markets in an attempt to gain market dominance. In the Brazil market for disposable diapers, two U.S. companies, Kimberly-Clark Corp. and Procter & Gamble, entered a price war as each struggled to establish dominance in the market.[22] As a result, the cost of disposable diapers fell from $1 per diaper in 1994 to 33 cents per diaper in 1997, while several other competitors, including indigenous Brazilian firms, were driven out of the market. Kimberly-Clark and Procter & Gamble are engaged in a global struggle for market share and dominance, and Brazil is one of their battlegrounds. Both companies can afford to engage in this behavior, even though it reduces their profits in Brazil, because they have profitable operations elsewhere in the world that can subsidize these losses.

Pricing decisions around the world need to be centrally monitored. It is tempting to delegate full responsibility for pricing decisions to the managers of various national subsidiaries, thereby reaping the benefits of decentralization (see Chapter 13 for a discussion). However, because pricing strategy in one part of the world can elicit a competitive response in another part, central management needs to at least monitor and approve pricing decisions in a given national market, and local managers need to recognize that their actions can affect competitive conditions in other countries.

Experience Curve Pricing

We first encountered the experience curve in Chapter 12. As a firm builds its accumulated production volume over time, unit costs fall due to "experience effects." Learning effects and economies of scale underlie the experience curve. Price comes into the picture because aggressive pricing (along with aggressive promotion and advertising) can build accumulated sales volume rapidly and thus move production down the experience curve. Firms further down the experience curve have a cost advantage vis-à-vis firms further up the curve.

Many firms pursuing an **experience curve pricing** strategy on an international scale will price low worldwide in attempting to build global sales volume as rapidly as possible, even if this means taking large losses initially. Such a firm believes that in several years, when it has moved down the experience curve, it will be making substantial profits and have a cost advantage over its less-aggressive competitors.

| Regulatory Influences on Prices

The ability to engage in either price discrimination or strategic pricing may be limited by national or international regulations. Most important, a firm's freedom to set its own prices is constrained by antidumping regulations and competition policy.

Antidumping Regulations

Both predatory pricing and experience curve pricing can run afoul of antidumping regulations. Dumping occurs whenever a firm sells a product for a price that is less than the cost of producing it. Most regulations, however, define dumping more vaguely. For example, a country is allowed to bring antidumping actions against an importer under Article 6 of GATT as long as two criteria are met: sales at "less than fair value" and "material injury to a domestic industry." The problem with this terminology is that it does not indicate what is a fair value. The ambiguity has led some to argue that selling abroad at prices below those in the country of origin, as opposed to below cost, is dumping.

Such logic led the first Bush administration to place a 25 percent duty on imports of Japanese light trucks in 1988. The Japanese manufacturers protested that they were not selling below cost. Admitting that their prices were lower in the United States than in Japan, they argued that this simply reflected the intensely competitive nature of the U.S. market (i.e., different price elasticities). In a similar example, the European Commission found Japanese exporters of dot-matrix printers to be violating dumping regulations. To correct what they saw as dumping, the EU placed a 47 percent import duty on imports of dot-matrix printers from Japan and required that the import duty be passed on to European consumers as a price increase.[23]

Antidumping rules set a floor under export prices and limit firms' ability to pursue strategic pricing. The rather vague terminology used in most antidumping actions suggests that a firm's ability to engage in price discrimination also may be challenged under antidumping legislation.

Competition Policy

Most developed nations have regulations designed to promote competition and to restrict monopoly practices. These regulations can be used to limit the prices a firm can charge in a given country. For example, during the 1960s and 70s, the Swiss pharmaceutical manufacturer Hoffmann-LaRoche had a monopoly on the supply of Valium and Librium tranquilizers. The company was investigated in 1973 by the British Monopolies and Mergers Commission, which is responsible for promoting fair competition in Great Britain. The commission found that Hoffmann-LaRoche was overcharging for its tranquilizers and ordered the company to reduce its prices 35 to 40 percent. Hoffmann-LaRoche maintained unsuccessfully that it was merely engaging in price discrimination. Similar actions were later brought against Hoffmann-LaRoche by the German cartel office and by the Dutch and Danish governments.[24]

Configuring the Marketing Mix ■

A firm might vary aspects of its marketing mix from country to country to take into account local differences in culture, economic conditions, competitive conditions, product and technical standards, distribution systems, government regulations, and the like. Such differences may require variation in product attributes, distribution strategy, communications strategy, and pricing strategy. The cumulative effect of these factors makes it rare for a firm to adopt the same marketing mix worldwide.

For example, financial services is often thought of as an industry where global standardization of the marketing mix is the norm. However, while a financial services company such as American Express may sell the same basic charge card service worldwide, utilize the same basic fee structure for that product, and adopt the same basic global advertising message ("don't leave home without it"), differences in national regulations still mean that it has to vary aspects of its communications strategy from country to country (as pointed out earlier, the promotional strategy it had developed in the United States was illegal in Germany). Similarly, while McDonald's is often thought of as the quintessential example of a firm that sells the same basic standardized product worldwide, in reality it varies one important aspect of its marketing mix—its menu—from country to country. McDonald's also varies its distribution strategy. In Canada and the United States, most McDonald's are located in areas that are easily accessible by car, whereas in more densely populated and less automobile-reliant societies of the world,

Management Focus

Castrol Oil in Vietnam

Castrol is the lubricants division of the British chemical, oil, and gas concern Burmah Castrol. In Europe and in the United States, where Castrol has a 15 percent share of the do-it-yourself lubricants market, Castrol targets motorists who want to cosset their engine by paying a bit more for Castrol's high-margin GTX brand, rather than a standard lubricant. This differentiated positioning strategy is supported by sponsoring Formula 1 racing and the Indy car series in the United States and by heavy spending on television and in automobile magazines in both Europe and the United States.

Some of Castrol's most notable successes in recent years, however, have been in the developing nations of Asia where Castrol reaps only one-sixth of its sales, but more than one-quarter of its operating profits. In Vietnam, automobiles are still relatively rare, so Castrol has targeted motorcycle owners. Castrol's strategy is to target people who want to take care of their new motorcycles. The long-term goal is to build brand loyalty, so that when automobile ownership becomes common in Vietnam, as Castrol believes it will, former motorcycle owners will stick with Castrol when they trade up to cars. This strategy has already worked in Thailand. Castrol has held the leading share of the motorcycle market in Thailand since the early 1980s, and it now holds the leading share in that country's rapidly growing automobile market.

Unlike its practice in more developed countries, Castrol's communications strategy in Vietnam does not focus on television and glossy print media (there is relatively little of either in Vietnam). Rather, Castrol focuses on building consumer awareness through extensive use of billboards, car stickers, and some 4,000 signs at Vietnam's ubiquitous roadside garages and motorcycle cleaning shops. Castrol also developed a unique slogan that has a rhythmic quality in Vietnamese "Dau nhot tot nhat" (best quality lubricants) and sticks in consumers' minds. Castrol's researchers say the slogan is now recognized by a remarkable 99 percent of people in Ho Chi Minh City.

As elsewhere, Castrol has adopted a premium pricing strategy in Vietnam, which is consistent with the company's attempt to build a global brand image of high quality. Castrol oil costs about $1.5 per liter in Vietnam, about three times as much as the price of cheaper oil imported from Taiwan and Thailand. Despite the high price of its product, Castrol claims it is gaining share in Vietnam as its branding strategy wins converts.

Castrol has had to tailor its distribution strategy to Vietnam's unique conditions. In most countries where it operates, Castrol divides the country into regions and has a single distributor in each region. In Vietnam, however, Castrol will often have two distinct distributors in a region—one to deal with state-owned customers, of which there are still many in this nominally Communist country, and one to deal with private customers. Castrol acknowledges the system is costly but says it is the only way to operate in a country where there is still some tension between state and private entities.

Sources: V. Mallet, "Climbing the Slippery Slope," *Financial Times*, July 28, 1994, p. 7; A. Bolger, "Growth by Successful Targeting," *Financial Times*, June 21, 1994, p. 27; and "A Decade in Lubricants," *Vietnam Investment Review*, August 27, 2001.

such as Japan and Great Britain, location decisions are driven by the accessibility of a restaurant to pedestrian traffic. Because countries typically still differ along one or more of the dimensions discussed above, some customization of the marketing mix is normal.

However, there are often significant opportunities for standardization along one or more elements of the marketing mix.[25] Firms may find that it is possible and desirable to standardize their global advertising message and/or core product attributes to realize substantial cost economies. They may find it desirable to customize their distribution and pricing strategy to take advantage of local differences. In reality, the "customization versus standardization" debate is not an all or nothing issue; it frequently makes sense to standardize some aspects of the marketing mix and customize others, depending on conditions in various national marketplaces. An explicit example, that of Castrol Oil, is given in the accompanying Management Focus. Castrol sells a standardized product worldwide—lubricating oil—yet it varies other aspects of its marketing mix from country to country, depending on economic conditions, competitive conditions, and distribution systems. Decisions about what to customize and what to standardize should be driven by a detailed examination of the costs and benefits of doing so for each element in the marketing mix.

◾ New–Product Development

Firms that successfully develop and market new products can earn enormous returns. Examples include Du Pont, which has produced a steady stream of successful innovations such as cellophane, nylon, Freon, and Teflon (nonstick pans); Sony, whose successes include the Walkman, the compact disk, and the PlayStation; Pfizer, the drug company that during the 1990s produced several major new drugs including Viagra; 3M, which has applied its core competency in tapes and adhesives to developing a wide range of new products; Intel, which has consistently managed to lead in the development of innovative microprocessors to run personal computers; and Cisco Systems, which developed the routers that sit at the hubs of Internet connections, directing the flow of digital traffic.

In today's world, competition is as much about technological innovation as anything else. The pace of technological change has accelerated since the Industrial Revolution in the 18th century, and it continues to do so today. The result has been a dramatic shortening of product life cycles. Technological innovation is both creative and destructive.[26] An innovation can make established products obsolete overnight. But an innovation can also make a host of new products possible. Witness recent changes in the electronics industry. For 40 years before the early 1950s, vacuum valves were a major component in radios and then in record players and early computers. The advent of transistors destroyed the market for vacuum valves, but at the same time it created new opportunities connected with transistors. Transistors took up far less space than vacuum valves, creating a trend toward miniaturization that continues today. The transistor held its position as the major component in the electronics industry for just a decade. Microprocessors were developed in the 1970s and the market for transistors declined rapidly. The microprocessor created yet another set of new-product opportunities—handheld calculators (which destroyed the market for slide rules), compact disk players (which destroyed the market for analog record players), personal computers (which destroyed the market for typewriters), to name a few.

This "creative destruction" unleashed by technological change makes it critical that a firm stay on the leading edge of technology, lest it lose out to a competitor's innovations. As we explain in the next subsection, this not only creates a need for the firm to invest in R&D, but it also requires the firm to establish R&D activities at those locations where expertise is concentrated. As we shall see, leading-edge technology on its own is not enough to guarantee a firm's survival. The firm must also apply that technology to developing products that satisfy consumer needs, and it must design the product so that it can be manufactured in a cost-effective manner. To do that, the firm needs to build close links between R&D, marketing, and manufacturing. This is difficult enough for the domestic firm, but it is even more problematic for the international business competing in an industry where consumer tastes and preferences differ from country to country.[27] With all of this in mind, we move on to examine locating R&D activities and building links between R&D, marketing, and manufacturing.

▌The Location of R&D

Ideas for new products are stimulated by the interactions of scientific research, demand conditions, and competitive conditions. Other things being equal, the rate of new-product development seems to be greater in countries where:

- More money is spent on basic and applied research and development.
- Underlying demand is strong.
- Consumers are affluent.
- Competition is intense.[28]

Basic and applied research and development discovers new technologies and then commercializes them. Strong demand and affluent consumers create a potential market for new products. Intense competition between firms stimulates innovation as the firms try to beat their competitors and reap potentially enormous first-mover advantages that result from successful innovation.

For most of the post–World War II period, the country that ranked highest on these criteria was the United States. The United States devoted a greater proportion of its gross domestic product (GDP) to R&D than any other country did. Its scientific establishment was the largest and most active in the world. U.S. consumers were the most affluent, the market was large, and competition among U.S. firms was brisk. Due to these factors, the United States was the market where most new products were developed and introduced. Accordingly, it was the best location for R&D activities; it was where the action was.

Over the past 20 years, things have been changing quickly. The U.S. monopoly on new-product development has weakened considerably. Although U.S. firms are still at the leading edge of many new technologies, Asian and European firms are also strong players, with companies such as Sony, Sharp, Samsung, Ericsson, Nokia, and Philips NV driving product innovation in their respective industries. Both Japan and Germany are now devoting a greater proportion of their GDP to nondefense R&D than is the United States.[29] In addition, both Japan and the European Union are large, affluent markets, and the wealth gap between them and the United States is closing.

As a result, it is often no longer appropriate to consider the United States as the lead market. In video games, for example, Japan is often the lead market, with companies like Sony and Nintendo introducing their latest video game players in Japan some six months before they introduce them in the United States. In wireless telecommunications, Europe is generally reckoned to be ahead of the United States. Some of the most advanced applications of wireless telecommunications services are being pioneered not in the United States but in Finland, where more than 80 percent of the population has wireless telephones, compared to 40 percent of the U.S. population. However, it often is questionable whether any developed nation can be considered the lead market. To succeed in today's high-technology industries, it is usually necessary to simultaneously introduce new products in all major industrialized markets. When Intel introduces a new microprocessor, for example, it does not first introduce it in the United States and then roll it out in Europe a year later. It introduces it simultaneously around the world.

Because leading-edge research is now carried out in many locations around the world, the argument for centralizing R&D activity in the United States is now much weaker than it was two decades ago. (It used to be argued that centralized R&D eliminated duplication.) Much leading-edge research is now occurring in Japan and Europe. Dispersing R&D activities to those locations allows a firm to stay close to the center of leading-edge activity to gather scientific and competitive information and to draw on local scientific resources.[30] This may result in some duplication of R&D activities, but the cost disadvantages of duplication are outweighed by the advantages of dispersion.

For example, to expose themselves to the research and new-product development work being done in Japan, many U.S. firms have set up satellite R&D centers in Japan. Kodak's $65 million R&D center in Japan employs about 200 people. The company hired about 100 Japanese researchers and directed the lab to concentrate on electronic imaging technology. U.S. firms that have established R&D facilities in Japan include Corning, Texas Instruments, IBM, Digital Equipment, Procter & Gamble, Upjohn, Pfizer, Du Pont, Monsanto, and Microsoft.[31] The National Science Foundation (NSF) has documented a sharp increase in the proportion of total R&D spending by U.S. firms that is now done abroad.[32] For example, Motorola now has 14 dedicated R&D facilities located in seven countries, and Bristol-Myers Squibb has 12 facilities in six countries. At the same time, to internationalize their own research and gain access to U.S. talent, the NSF reports that many European and Japanese firms are investing in U.S.-based research facilities.

Integrating R&D, Marketing, and Production

Although a firm that is successful at developing new products may earn enormous returns, new-product development has a high failure rate. One study of product development in 16 companies in the chemical, drug, petroleum, and electronics industries suggested that only about 20 percent of R&D projects result in commercially successful products or processes.[33] Another in-depth case study of product development in three companies (one in chemicals and two in drugs) reported that about 60 percent of R&D projects reached technical completion, 30 percent were commercialized, and only 12 percent earned an economic profit that exceeded the company's cost of capital.[34] A study by the consulting division of Booz, Allen & Hamilton found that over one-third of 13,000 consumer and industrial products introduced over a five-year period failed to meet company-specific financial and strategic performance criteria.[35] Another study found that 45 percent of new products did not meet their profitability goals.[36] This evidence suggests that many R&D projects do not result in a commercial product, and that between 33 percent and 60 percent of all new products that do reach the marketplace fail to generate an adequate economic return. Two well-publicized product failures are Apple Computer's Newton, a personal digital assistant, and Sony's Betamax format in the video player and recorder market.

The reasons for such high failure rates are various and include development of a technology for which demand is limited, failure to adequately commercialize promising technology, and inability to manufacture a new product cost effectively. Firms can avoid such mistakes by insisting on tight cross-functional coordination and integration between three core functions involved in the development of new products: R&D, marketing, and production.[37] Tight cross-functional integration between R&D, production, and marketing can help a company to ensure that

1. Product development projects are driven by customer needs.
2. New products are designed for ease of manufacture.
3. Development costs are kept in check.
4. Time to market is minimized.

Close integration between R&D and marketing is required to ensure that product development projects are driven by the needs of customers. A company's customers can be a primary source of new-product ideas. Identification of customer needs, particularly unmet needs, can set the context within which successful product innovation occurs. As the point of contact with customers, the marketing function of a company can provide valuable information in this regard. Integration of R&D and marketing is crucial if a new product is to be properly commercialized. Without integration of R&D and marketing, a company runs the risk of developing products for which there is little or no demand.

Integration between R&D and production can help a company design products with manufacturing requirements in mind. Designing for manufacturing can lower costs and increase product quality. Integrating R&D and production can also help lower development costs and speed products to market. If a new product is not designed with manufacturing capabilities in mind, it may prove too difficult to build. Then the product will have to be redesigned, and both overall development costs and the time it takes to bring the product to market may increase significantly. Making design changes during product planning could increase overall development costs by 50 percent and add 25 percent to the time it takes to bring the product to market.[38] Many quantum product innovations require new processes to manufacture them, which makes it all the more important to achieve close integration between R&D and production. Minimizing time to market and development costs may require the simultaneous development of new products and new processes.[39]

Cross-Functional Teams

One way to achieve cross-functional integration is to establish cross-functional product development teams composed of representatives from R&D, marketing, and production. Because these functions may be located in different countries, the team will sometimes have a multinational membership. The objective of a team should be to take a product development project from the initial concept development to market introduction. A number of attributes seem to be important for a product development team to function effectively and meet all its development milestones.[40]

First, the team should be led by a "heavyweight" project manager who has high status within the organization and who has the power and authority required to get the financial and human resources the team needs to succeed. The "heavyweight" leader should be dedicated primarily, if not entirely, to the project. The leader should be someone who believes in the project (a champion) and who is skilled at integrating the perspectives of different functions and at helping personnel from different functions and countries work together for a common goal. The leader should also be able to act as an advocate of the team to senior management.

Second, the team should be composed of at least one member from each key function. The team members should have a number of attributes, including an ability to contribute functional expertise, high standing within their function, a willingness to share responsibility for team results, and an ability to put functional and national advocacy aside. It is generally preferable if core team members are 100 percent dedicated to the project for its duration. This assures their focus on the project, not on the ongoing work of their function.

Third, the team members should be physically co-located if possible to create a sense of camaraderie and to facilitate communication. This presents problems if the team members are drawn from facilities in different nations. One solution is to transfer key individuals to one location for the duration of a product development project. Fourth, the team should have a clear plan and clear goals, particularly with regard to critical development milestones and development budgets. The team should have incentives to attain those goals, such as receiving pay bonuses when major development milestones are hit. Fifth, each team needs to develop its own processes for communication and conflict resolution. For example, one product development team at Quantum Corporation, a California-based manufacturer of disk drives for personal computers, instituted a rule that all major decisions would be made and conflicts resolved at meetings that were held every Monday afternoon. This simple rule helped the team meet its development goals. In this case, it was also common for team members to fly in from Japan, where the product was to be manufactured, to the U.S. development center for the Monday morning meetings.[41]

Focus On Managerial Implications

The need to integrate R&D and marketing to adequately commercialize new technologies poses special problems in the international business because commercialization may require different versions of a new product to be produced for various countries.[42] To do this, the firm must build close links between its R&D centers and its various country operations. A similar argument applies to the need to integrate R&D and production, particularly in those international businesses that have dispersed production activities to different locations around the globe depending on a consideration of relative factor costs and the like.

Integrating R&D, marketing, and production in an international business may require R&D centers in North America, Asia, and Europe that are linked by formal and informal integrating mechanisms with marketing operations in each country in their regions and with the various manufacturing facilities. In addition, the international business may have to establish cross-functional teams whose members are dispersed around the globe. This complex endeavor requires the company to utilize the formal and informal integrating mechanisms that we discussed in Chapter 13 to knit its far-flung operations together so they can produce new products in an effective and timely manner.

While there is no one best model for allocating product development responsibilities to various centers, one solution adopted by many international businesses involves establishing a global network of R&D centers. Within this model, fundamental research is undertaken at basic research centers around the globe. These centers are normally located in regions or cities where valuable scientific knowledge is being created and where there is a pool of skilled research talent (e.g., Silicon Valley in the United States, Cambridge in England, Kobe in Japan, Singapore). These centers are the innovation engines of the firm. Their job is to develop the basic technologies that become new products.

These technologies are picked up by R&D units attached to global product divisions and are used to generate new products to serve the global marketplace. At this level, commercialization of the technology and design for manufacturing is emphasized. If further customization is needed so the product appeals to the tastes and preferences of consumers in individual markets, such redesign work will be done by an R&D group based in a subsidiary in that country or at a regional center that customizes products for several countries in the region.

Hewlett-Packard (HP) has four basic research centers located in Palo Alto, California; Bristol, England; Haifa, Israel; and Tokyo, Japan.[43] These labs are the seedbed for technologies that ultimately become new products and businesses. They are the company's innovation engines. The Palo Alto center, for example, pioneered HP's thermal ink-jet technology. The products are developed by R&D centers associated with HP's global product divisions. Thus, the Consumer Products Group, which has its worldwide headquarters in San Diego, California, designs, develops, and manufactures a range of imaging products using HP-pioneered thermal ink-jet technology. Subsidiaries might then customize the product so that it best matches the needs of important national markets. HP's subsidiary in Singapore, for example, is responsible for the design and production of thermal ink-jet printers for Japan and other Asian markets. This subsidiary takes products originally developed in San Diego and redesigns them for the Asian market. In addition, the Singapore subsidiary has taken the lead from San Diego in the design and development of certain portable thermal ink-jet printers. HP delegated this responsibility to Singapore because this subsidiary has acquired important competencies in the design and production of thermal ink-jet products, so it has become the best place in the world to undertake this activity.

Microsoft offers a similar example. The company has basic research sites in Redmond, Washington (its headquarters); Cambridge, England; Tokyo, Japan; and Silicon Valley, California. Staff at these research sites work on the fundamental problems that underlie the design of future products. For example, a group at Redmond is working on natural language recognition software, while another works on artificial intelligence. These research centers don't produce new products; rather, they produce the technology that is used to enhance existing products or help produce new products. The products are produced by dedicated product groups (e.g., desktop operating systems, applications). Customization of the products to match the needs of local markets is sometimes carried out at local subsidiaries. Thus, the Chinese subsidiary in Singapore will do some basic customization of programs such as Microsoft Office, adding Chinese characters and customizing the interface.

Chapter Summary

This chapter discussed the marketing and R&D functions in international business. A persistent theme of the chapter is the tension that exists between the need to reduce costs and the need to be responsive to local conditions, which raises costs. The chapter made these major points:

1. Theodore Levitt has argued that due to the advent of modern communications and transport technologies, consumer tastes and preferences are becoming global, which is creating global markets for standardized consumer products. However, this position is regarded as extreme by many commentators, who argue that substantial differences still exist between countries.

2. Market segmentation refers to the process of identifying distinct groups of consumers whose purchasing behavior differs from each other in important ways. Managers in an international business need to be aware of two main issues relating to segmentation: the extent to which there are differences between countries in the structure of market segments, and the existence of segments that transcend national borders.

3. A product can be viewed as a bundle of attributes. Product attributes need to be varied from country to country to satisfy different consumer tastes and preferences.

4. Country differences in consumer tastes and preferences are due to differences in culture and economic development. In addition, differences in product and technical standards may require the firm to customize product attributes from country to country.

5. A distribution strategy decision is an attempt to define the optimal channel for delivering a product to the consumer.

6. Significant country differences exist in distribution systems. In some countries, the retail system is concentrated; in others, it is fragmented. In some countries, channel length is short; in others, it is long. Access to distribution channels is difficult to achieve in some countries.

7. A critical element in the marketing mix is communication strategy, which defines the process the firm will use in communicating the attributes of its product to prospective customers.

8. Barriers to international communication include cultural differences, source effects, and noise levels.

9. A communication strategy is either a push strategy or a pull strategy. A push strategy emphasizes personal selling, and a pull strategy emphasizes mass media advertising. Whether a push strategy or a pull strategy is optimal depends on the type of product, consumer sophistication, channel length, and media availability.

10. A globally standardized advertising campaign, which uses the same marketing message all over the world, has economic advantages, but it fails to account for differences in culture and advertising regulations.

11. Price discrimination exists when consumers in different countries are charged different prices for the same product. Price discrimination can help a firm maximize its profits. For price discrimination to be effective, the national markets must be separate and their price elasticities of demand must differ.

12. Predatory pricing is the use of profit gained in one market to support aggressive pricing in another market to drive competitors out of that market.

13. Multipoint pricing refers to the fact that a firm's pricing strategy in one market may affect rivals' pricing strategies in another market. Aggressive pricing in one market may elicit a competitive response from a rival in another market that is important to the firm.

14. Experience curve pricing is the use of aggressive pricing to build accumulated volume as rapidly as possible to quickly move the firm down the experience curve.

15. New-product development is a high-risk, potentially high return activity. To build a competency in new-product development, an international business must do two things: disperse R&D activities to those countries where new products are being pioneered, and integrate R&D with marketing and manufacturing.

16. Achieving tight integration among R&D, marketing, and manufacturing requires the use of cross-functional teams.

Critical Discussion Questions

1. Imagine you are the marketing manager for a U.S. manufacturer of disposable diapers. Your firm is considering entering the Brazilian market. Your CEO believes the advertising message that has

been effective in the United States will suffice in Brazil. Outline some possible objections to this. Your CEO also believes that the pricing decisions in Brazil can be delegated to local managers. Why might she be wrong?

2. Within 20 years, we will have seen the emergence of enormous global markets for standardized consumer products. Do you agree with this statement? Justify your answer.

3. You are the marketing manager of a food products company that is considering entering the Indian market. The retail system in India tends to be very fragmented. Also, retailers and wholesalers tend to have long-term ties with Indian food companies, which makes access to distribution channels difficult. What distribution strategy would you advise the company to pursue? Why?

4. Price discrimination is indistinguishable from dumping. Discuss the accuracy of this statement.

5. You work for a company that designs and manufactures personal computers. Your company's R&D center is in North Dakota. The computers are manufactured under contract in Taiwan. Marketing strategy is delegated to the heads of three regional groups: a North American group (based in Chicago), a European group (based in Paris), and an Asian group (based in Singapore). Each regional group develops the marketing approach within its region. In order of importance, the largest markets for your products are North America, Germany, Great Britain, China, and Australia. Your company is experiencing problems in its product development and commercialization process. Products are late to market, the manufacturing quality is poor, costs are higher than projected, and market acceptance of new products is less than hoped for. What might be the source of these problems? How would you fix them?

Research Task | globalEDGE™   globaledge.msu.edu

Use the globalEDGE™ site to complete the following exercises:

1. Locate and retrieve the most current ranking of the global brands. Identify the criteria that are utilized in the ranking. Which country dominates the top 100 global brands list? Prepare a short report identifying the countries that possess global brands and the potential reasons for success.

2. Identify the twenty organizations with the highest advertising expenditure in the world. Prepare a short report regarding the country of origin of the companies with the most advertising spending, as well as the distribution of advertising expenditures by industry.

Notes

1. See R. W. Ruekert and O. C. Walker, "Interactions between Marketing and R&D Departments in Implementing Different Business-Level Strategies," *Strategic Management Journal* 8 (1987), pp. 233–48, and K. B. Clark and S. C. Wheelwright, *Managing New Product and Process Development* (New York: Free Press), 1993.

2. T. Levitt, "The Globalization of Markets," *Harvard Business Review*, May–June 1983, pp. 92–102. Reprinted by permission of *Harvard Business Review*, an excerpt from "The Globalization of Markets," by Theodore Levitt, May–June 1983. Copyright © 1983 by the President and Fellows of Harvard College. All rights reserved.

3. For example, see S. P. Douglas and Y. Wind, "The Myth of Globalization," *Columbia Journal of World Business*, Winter 1987, pp. 19–29; C. A. Bartlett and S. Ghoshal, *Managing across Borders: The Transnational Solution* (Boston: Harvard

Business School Press, 1989); V. J. Govindarajan and A. K. Gupta, *The Quest for Global Dominance* (San Francisco: Jossey Bass, 2001).

4. "Slow Food," *The Economist*, February 3, 1990, p. 64.

5. J. T. Landry, "Emerging Markets: Are Chinese Consumers Coming of Age?" *Harvard Business Review*, May–June 1998, pp. 17–20.

6. C. Miller, "Teens Seen as the First Truly Global Consumers," *Marketing News*, March 27, 1995, p. 9.

7. This approach was originally developed in K. Lancaster, "A New Approach to Demand Theory," *Journal of Political Economy* 74 (1965), pp. 132–57.

8. V. R. Alden, "Who Says You Can't Crack Japanese Markets?" *Harvard Business Review*, January–February 1987, pp. 52–56.

9.   T. Parker-Pope, "Custom Made," *Wall Street Journal*, September 26, 1996, p. 22.

10. "RCA's New Vista: The Bottom Line," *Business Week*, July 4, 1987, p. 44.

11. N. Gross and K. Rebello, "Apple? Japan Can't Say No," *Business Week*, June 29, 1992, pp. 32–33.

12. "After Early Stumbles P&G Is Making Inroads Overseas," *Wall Street Journal*, February 6, 1989, p. B1.

13. Z. Gurhan-Cvanli and D. Maheswaran, "Cultural Variation in Country of Origin Effects," *Journal of Marketing Research*, August 2000, pp. 309–17.

14. See M. Laroche, V. H. Kirpalani, F. Pons, and L. Zhou, "A Model of Advertising Standardization in Multinational Corporations," *Journal of International Business Studies*, 32 (2001), pp. 249–66, and D. A. Aaker and E. Joachimsthaler, "The Lure of Global Branding," *Harvard Business Review*, November–December 1999, pp. 137–44.

15. "Advertising in a Single Market," *The Economist*, March 24, 1990, p. 64.

16. D. Waller, "Charged Up over Competition Law," *Financial Times*, June 23, 1994, p. 14.

17. J. Lumbin, "Advertising: Tina Turner Helps Pepsi's Global Effort," *New York Times*, March 10, 1986, p. D13.

18. R. J. Dolan and H. Simon, *Power Pricing* (New York: Free Press, 1999).

19. B. Stottinger, "Strategic Export Pricing: A Long Winding Road," *Journal of International Marketing* 9 (2001), pp. 40–63, and S. Gil-Pareja "Export Process Discrimination in Europe and Exchange Rates," *Review of International Economics*, May 2002, pp. 299–312.

20. These allegations were made on a PBS "Frontline" documentary telecast in the United States in May 1992.

21. G. Smith and B. Wolverton, "A Dark Moment for Kodak," *Business Week*, August 4, 1997, pp. 30–31.

22. R. Narisette and J. Friedland, "Disposable Income: Diaper Wars of P&G and Kimberly-Clark Now Heat Up in Brazil," *Wall Street Journal*, June 4, 1997, p. A1.

23. "Printers Reflect Pattern of Trade Rows," *Financial Times*, December 20, 1988, p. 3.

24. J. F. Pickering, *Industrial Structure and Market Conduct* (London: Martin Robertson, 1974).

25. S. P. Douglas, C. Samuel Craig, and E. J. Nijissen, "Integrating Branding Strategy across Markets," *Journal of International Marketing* 9, no. 2 (2001), pp. 97–114

26. The phrase was first used by economist Joseph Schumpeter in *Capitalism, Socialism, and Democracy* (New York: Harper Brothers, 1942).

27. S. Kotabe, S. Srinivasan, and P. S. Aulakh. "Multinationality and Firm Performance: The Moderating Role of R&D and Marketing," *Journal of International Business Studies* 33 (2002), pp. 79–97.

28. See D. C. Mowery and N. Rosenberg, *Technology and the Pursuit of Economic Growth* (Cambridge, UK: Cambridge University Press, 1989), and M. E. Porter, *The Competitive Advantage of Nations* (New York: The Free Press, 1990).

29. C. Farrell, "Industrial Policy," *Business Week*, April 6, 1992, pp. 70–75.

30. W. Kuemmerle, "Building Effective R&D Capabilities Abroad," *Harvard Business Review*, March–April 1997, pp. 61–70, and C. Le Bas and C. Sierra, "Location versus Home Country Advantages in R&D Activities," *Research Policy* 31 (2002), pp. 589–609.

31. "When the Corporate Lab Goes to Japan," *New York Times*, April 28, 1991, sec. 3, p. 1.

32. D. Shapley, "Globalization Prompts Exodus," *Financial Times*, March 17, 1994, p. 10.

33. E. Mansfield. "How Economists See R&D," *Harvard Business Review*, November–December, 1981, pp. 98–106.

34. Ibid.

35. Booz, Allen, & Hamilton, "New Products Management for the 1980s," privately published research report, 1982.

36. A. L. Page, "PDMA's New Product Development Practices Survey: Performance and Best Practices," PDMA 15th Annual International Conference, Boston, October 16, 1991.

37. K. B. Clark and S. C. Wheelwright, *Managing New Product and Process Development* (New York: Free Press, 1993), and M. A. Shilling and C. W. L. Hill, "Managing the New Product Development Process," *Academy of Management Executive* 12, no. 3 (1998), pp. 67–81.

38. O. Port, "Moving Past the Assembly Line," *Business Week Special Issue: Reinventing America*, 1992, pp. 177–80.

39. K. B. Clark and T. Fujimoto, "The Power of Product Integrity," *Harvard Business Review*, November–December 1990, pp. 107–18; Clark and Wheelwright, *Managing New Product and Process Development*; S. L. Brown and K. M. Eisenhardt, "Product Development: Past Re-

search, Present Findings, and Future Directions," *Academy of Management Review* 20 (1995), pp. 348–78; and G. Stalk and T. M. Hout, *Competing against Time* (New York: Free Press, 1990).

40. Shilling and Hill, "Managing the New Product Development Process."

41. C. Christensen. "Quantum Corporation—Business and Product Teams," Harvard Business School Case # 9-692-023.

42. R. Nobel and J. Birkinshaw, "Innovation in Multinational Corporations: Control and Communication Patterns in International R&D Operations," *Strategic Management Journal* 19 (1998), pp. 479–96.

43. Information comes from the company's website, and from K. Ferdows, "Making the Most of Foreign Factories," *Harvard Business Review*, March–April 1997, pp. 73–88.

Procter & Gamble in Japan

Procter & Gamble (P&G), the large U.S. consumer products company, has a well-earned reputation as one of the world's best marketers. P&G manufactures and markets more than 200 products that it sells in 130 countries around the world, generating some $42 billion in revenues in 2002. Along with Unilever, P&G is a dominant global force in laundry detergents, cleaning products, personal care products and pet food products. P&G expanded abroad after World War II by exporting its products, brands, and marketing policies to Western Europe, initially with considerable success. Over the next 30 years, this policy of developing new products and marketing strategies in the United States and then transferring them to other countries became entrenched. Although some adaptation of marketing policies to accommodate country differences was pursued, it was minimal. In general, products were developed in the United States, manufactured locally, and sold using a marketing message created in Cincinnati.

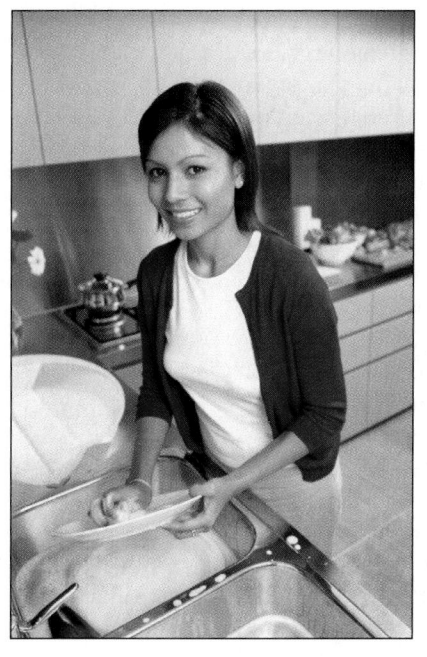

The first signs that this policy was no longer effective emerged in the 1970s, when P&G suffered a number of major setbacks in Japan. By 1985, after 13 years in Japan, P&G was still losing $40 million a year there. It had introduced disposable diapers in Japan and at one time had commanded an 80 percent share of the market, but by the early 1980s it held a miserable 8 percent. Three large Japanese consumer products companies were dominating the market. P&G's diapers, developed in the United States, were too bulky for the tastes of Japanese consumers. Kao, a Japanese company, had developed a line of trim-fit diapers that appealed more to Japanese tastes. Kao introduced its product with a marketing blitz and was quickly rewarded with a 30 percent share of the market. P&G realized it would have to modify its diapers if it were to compete in Japan. It did, and the company now has a 30 percent share of the Japanese market. Plus, P&G's trim-fit diapers have become a best-seller in the United States.

P&G had a similar experience in marketing education in the Japanese laundry detergent market. In the early 1980s, P&G introduced its Cheer laundry detergent in Japan. Developed in the United States, Cheer was promoted in Japan with the U.S. marketing message—Cheer works in all temperatures and produces lots of rich suds. But many Japanese consumers wash their clothes in cold water, which made the claim of working in all temperatures irrelevant. Also, many Japanese add fabric softeners to their water, which reduces detergents' sudsing action, so Cheer did not suds up as advertised. After a disastrous launch, P&G knew it had to adapt its marketing message. Cheer is now promoted as a product that works effectively in cold water with fabric softeners added, and it is one of P&G's best-selling products in Japan.

P&G's experience with disposable diapers and laundry detergents in Japan forced the company to rethink its product development and marketing philosophy. The company decided that its U.S.-centered way of doing business did not work. For the last decade, P&G has been delegating more responsibility for new-product development and marketing to its major subsidiaries in Japan and Europe. The company is more responsive to local differences in consumer tastes and preferences and more willing to admit that good new products can be developed outside the United States.

Evidence that this new approach is working can again be found in the company's activities in Japan. Until 1995, P&G did not sell dish soap in Japan. By 1998, it had Japan's best-selling brand, Joy, which now has a 20 percent share of Japan's $400 million market for dish soap. It made major inroads against the products of two domestic firms, Kao and Lion Corp., each of which marketed multiple brands and controlled nearly 40 percent of the market before P&G's entry. P&G's success with Joy was because of its ability to develop a product formula that was targeted at the unmet needs of Japanese consumers, to design a packaging format that appealed to retailers, and to create a compelling advertising campaign.

In researching the market in the early 1990s, P&G discovered an odd habit: Japanese homemakers squirted out excessive amounts of detergent onto dirty dishes, a clear sign of dissatisfaction with existing products. On further inspection, P&G found that this behavior resulted from the changing eating habits of Japanese consumers. The Japanese are consuming more fried food, and existing dish soaps did not effectively remove grease. Armed with this knowledge, P&G researchers in Japan went to work to create a highly concentrated soap formula based on a new technology developed by the company's scientists in Europe that was highly effective in removing grease. The company also designed a novel package for the product. The packaging of existing products had a clear weakness: the long-neck bottles wasted space on supermarket shelves. P&G's dish soap containers were compact cylinders that took less space in stores, warehouses, and delivery trucks. This improved the efficiency of distribution and allowed supermarkets to use their shelf space more effectively, which made them receptive to stocking Joy. P&G also devoted considerable attention to developing an advertising campaign for Joy. P&G's ad agency, Dentsu Inc., created commercials in which a famous comedian dropped in on homemakers unannounced with a camera crew to test Joy on the household's dirty dishes. The camera focused on a patch of oil in a pan full of water. After a drop of Joy, the oil dramatically disappeared.

With the product, packaging, and advertising strategy carefully worked out, P&G launched Joy throughout Japan in March 1996. The product almost immediately gained a 10 percent market share. Within three months the product's share had increased to 15 percent, and by year-end it was close to 18 percent. Because of strong demand, P&G was also able to raise prices as were the retailers that stocked the product, all of which translated into fatter margins for the retailers and helped consolidate Joy's position.

In the laundry detergent market too, P&G has been making inroads. Through market research, P&G found that Japanese consumers wanted detergents with stronger cleaning power, so the company developed and launched bleach-reinforced and antibacterial versions of its Ariel detergent in Japan. Both have been very successful, helping to take P&G's share of the Japanese laundry detergent market up to 20 percent by the early 2000s.

Sources: G. de Jonquieres and C. Bobinski, "Wash and Get into a Lather in Poland," *Financial Times*, May 28, 1992, p. 2; "Perestroika in Soapland," *The Economist*, June 10, 1989, pp. 69–71; "After Early Stumbles P&G Is Making Inroads Overseas," *Wall Street Journal*, February 6, 1989, p. B1; C. A. Bartlett and S. Ghoshal, *Managing across Borders: The Transnational Solution* (Boston: Harvard Business School Press, 1989); N. Shirouzu, "P&G's Joy Makes an Unlikely Splash in Japan," *Wall Street Journal*, December 10, 1997, p. B1; and A. Mollet, "Japan's Washaday Blues," *Chemical Week*, January 26, 2000, p. 26.

Case Discussion Questions

1. How would you characterize P&G's product development and marketing strategy toward Japan in the 1970s and 1980s. What were the advantages of this strategy? What were the drawbacks?

2. How would you characterize the strategy since the early 1990s? What are the advantages of this strategy? What are the potential drawbacks?

3. Which strategy has been more successful? Why?

4. What changes do you think P&G has had to make in its organization and company culture to implement this strategic shift?

5. What does P&G's experience teach us about the argument that consumer tastes and preferences across nations are converging and global markets are becoming more homogenous?

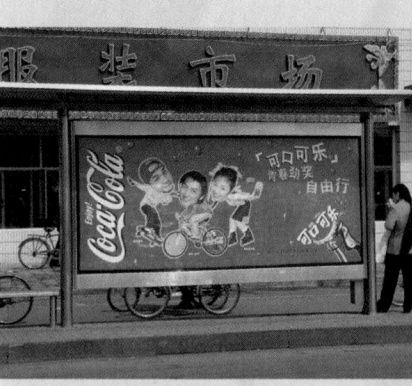

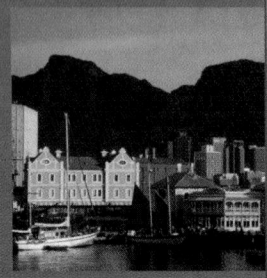

Chapter 18

Global Human Resource Management

Introduction
The Strategic Role of International HRM
Staffing Policy
  Types of Staffing Policy
  Expatriate Managers
Training and Management Development
  Training for Expatriate Managers
  Repatriation of Expatriates
  Management Development and
  Strategy
Performance Appraisal
  Performance Appraisal Problems
  Guidelines for Performance Appraisal
Compensation
  National Differences in Compensation
  Expatriate Pay
International Labor Relations
  The Concerns of Organized Labor
  The Strategy of Organized Labor
  Approaches to Labor Relations
Chapter Summary
Critical Discussion Questions
Closing Case: Degrussa: Strategy and
Human Resources in China

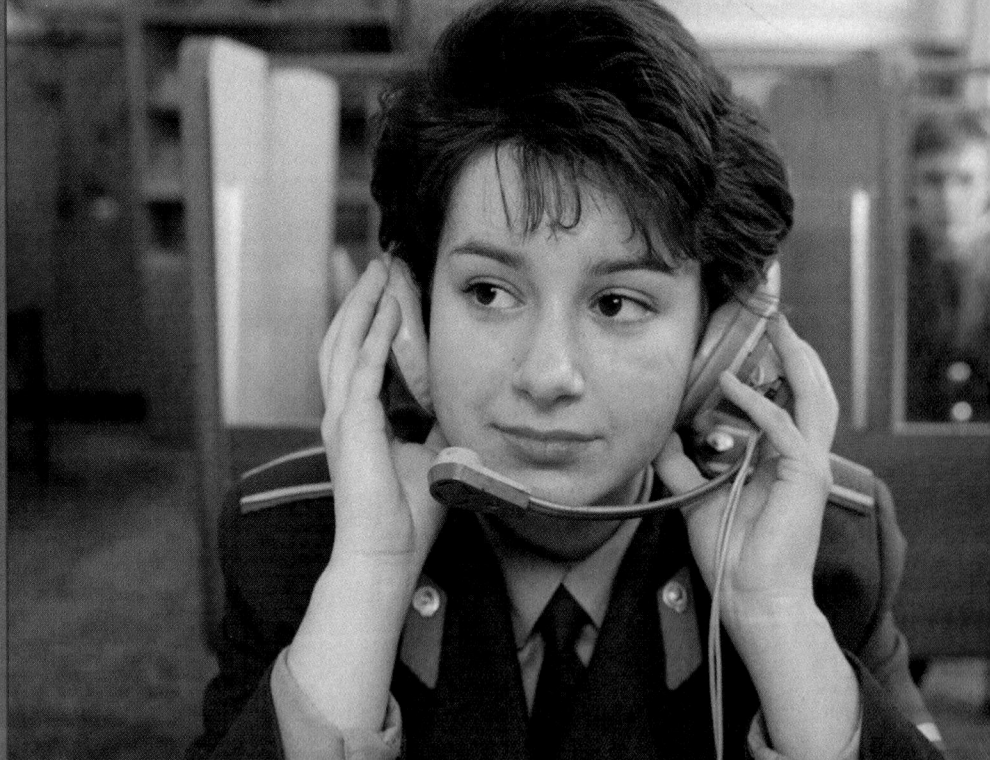

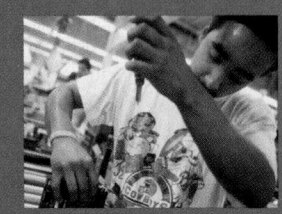

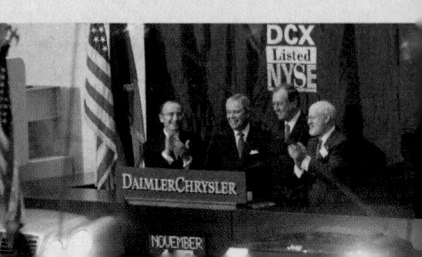

Molex

Molex, a 70-year-old manufacturer of electronic components based in Chicago, is the world's second largest manufacturer of electronic components. The company established an international division to coordinate exporting in 1967, opened its first overseas plant in Japan in 1970 and a second in Ireland in 1971. From that base, Molex has evolved into a global business that generated about 61 percent of its $1.76 billion in 2002 revenues outside of the United States. The company operates some 50 manufacturing plants in 21 countries and employs some 16,000 people worldwide, only one-third of whom are located in the United States. Molex's competitive advantage is based on a strategy that emphasizes a combination of low costs and excellent customer service. Manufacturing sites are located in countries where cost conditions are favorable and major customers are close. Since the 1970s, a key goal of Molex has been to build a truly global company that is at home wherever in the world it operates, and which proactively shares valuable knowledge across operations in different countries. The human resources function of Molex has always played a central role in meeting this goal.

As Molex grew rapidly overseas, the human resource management (HRM) function made sure that every new unit did the same basic things. Each new entity had to have an employee manual with policies and practices in writing, new employee orientation programs, salary administration with a consistent grading system, written job descriptions, written promotion and grievance procedures, standard performance appraisal systems that were written down, and so on. Beyond these things, however, Molex views HRM as the most localized of functions. Different legal systems, particularly with regard to employment law, different compensation norms, different cultural attitudes to work, different norms regarding vacation, and so on, all imply that policies and programs must be customized to the conditions prevailing in a country. To make sure this occurs, Molex's policy is to hire experienced HRM professionals from other companies in the same country in which it has operations. The idea is to hire people who know the language, have credibility, know the law, and know how to recruit in that country.

Molex's strategy for building a global company starts with its staffing policy for managers and engineers. The company frequently hires foreign nationals who are living in the United States, have just completed MBAs, and are willing to relocate if required. These individuals will typically work in the United States for a while, becoming familiar with the company's culture. Some of them will then be sent back to their home country to work there. Molex also carefully screens its American applicants, favoring those who are fluent in at least one other language. Molex is unusual for a U.S. company in this regard. However, with more than 15 languages spoken at its headquarters by native speakers, Molex is committed to multilingual competency. There is also significant hiring of managers and engineers at the local level. Here, too, a willingness to relocate internationally and foreign language competency are important, although this time English is the preferred foreign language. In a sign of how multinational Molex's management has become, it is not unusual to see foreign nationals holding senior positions at company headquarters. In addition to Americans, individuals of Greek, German, Austrian, Japanese, and British origin have all sat on the company's executive committee, its top decision-making body.

To help build a global company, Molex moves people around the world to give them experience in other countries and to help them learn from each other. It has five categories of expatriates: (1) regular expatriates who live in a country other than their home country for three-to-five-year assignments (there are approximately 50 of these at any one time), (2) "inpats" who come to the company's U.S. headquarters from other countries, (3) third-country nationals who move from one Molex entity to another (for example, Singapore to Taiwan), (4) short-term transfers who go to another Molex entity for 6 to 9 months to work on a specific project, and (5) medium terms who go to another entity for 12 to 24 months, again to work on a specific project.

Having a high level of intracompany movement is costly. For an employee making $75,000 in base salary, the total cost of an expatriate assignment can run as high as $250,000 when additional employee benefits are added in, such as the provision of schooling and housing, adjustments for higher costs of living, adjustments for higher tax rates, and so on. Molex also insists on treating all expatriates the same, whatever their country of origin, so a Singapore expatriate living in Taiwan is likely to be living in the same apartment building and sending his child to the same school as an American expatriate in Taiwan. This boosts the overall costs, but Molex believes that its extensive use of expatriates pays back dividends. It allows individuals to understand the challenges of doing business in different countries, it facilitates the sharing of useful knowledge across different business entities, and it helps to lay the foundation for a common company culture that is global in its outlook.

Molex also makes sure that expatriates know why they are being sent to a foreign country, both in terms of their own career development and Molex's corporate goals. To prevent expatriates from becoming disconnected from their home office, the HRM department touches base with them on a regular basis through telephone, e-mail, and direct visits. The company also encourages expatriates to make home office visits so that they do not become totally disconnected from their base and feel like a stranger when they return. Upon return, they are debriefed and their knowledge gained abroad is put to use by, for example, placing the expatriates on special task forces.

A final component of Molex's strategy for building a cadre of globally minded managers is the company's in-house management development programs. These are open to a wide range of managers who have worked at Molex for three years or more. Molex uses these programs not just to educate its managers in finance, operations, strategy, and the like, but also to bring together managers from different countries to build a network of individuals who know each other and can work together in a cooperative fashion to solve business problems that transcend borders.

Sources: J. Laabs, "Molex Makes Global HR Look Easy," *Workforce,* March 1999, pp. 42–46; C. M. Solomon; "Foreign Relations," *Workforce,* November 2000, pp. 50–56; C. M. Solomon, "Navigating Your Search for Global Talent," *Personnel Journal,* May 1995, pp. 94–100; A. C. Poe, "Welcome Back," *HR Magazine,* March 2000, pp. 94–105; and Molex SEC Form 10K, 2003.

▮ Introduction

Continuing our survey of specific functions within an international business, this chapter examines international human resource management (HRM). **Human resource management** refers to the activities an organization carries out to use its human resources effectively.[1] These activities include determining the firm's human resource strategy, staffing, performance evaluation, management development, compensation, and labor relations. None of these activities is performed in a vacuum; all are related to the strategy of the firm because, as we will see, HRM has an important strategic component.[2] Through its influence on the character, development, quality, and productivity of the firm's human resources, the HRM function can help the firm achieve its primary strategic goals of reducing the costs of value creation and adding value by better serving customer needs.

The strategic role of HRM is complex enough in a purely domestic firm, but it is more complex in an international business, where staffing, management development, performance evaluation, and compensation activities are complicated by profound differences between countries in labor markets, culture, legal systems, economic systems, and the like (see Chapters 2 and 3). For example,

- Compensation practices may vary from country to country depending on prevailing management customs.
- Labor laws may prohibit union organization in one country and mandate it in another.
- Equal employment legislation may be strongly pursued in one country and not in another.

If it is to build a cadre of managers capable of managing a multinational enterprise, the HRM function must deal with a host of issues. It must decide how to staff key management posts in the company, how to develop managers so that they are familiar with the nuances of doing business in different countries, and how to compensate people in different nations. HRM must also deal with a host of issues related to expatriate managers. (An **expatriate manager** is a citizen of one country who is working abroad in one of the firm's subsidiaries.) It must decide whom to send on expatriate postings, be clear about why they are doing it, compensate expatriates appropriately, and make sure that they are adequately debriefed and reoriented once they return home.

The opening case detailed how Molex deals with some of these issues. Molex is quite explicit about using the HRM function to help attain the strategic goal of building a global company that has a low cost structure, provides excellent customer service, and is comfortable doing business in many different countries and cultures. Molex uses its staffing policy to recruit managers who are fluent in more than one language and willing to relocate to other countries. It makes liberal use of expatriates. Foreign postings are seen as a way of developing managers and a means for transferring valuable know-how between country operations. The benefits package for expatriates is designed to make sure there is no bonus for being an American, which sends the message that all employees are viewed equally, regardless of national origin. Finally, Molex proactively uses its own in-house management development programs to help establish a network of managers from different countries who know each other, can share valuable information with each other, and can work together to solve business problems that transcend borders.

In this chapter, we will look closely at the role of HRM in an international business. We begin by briefly discussing the strategic role of HRM. Then we turn our attention to four major tasks of the HRM function: staffing policy, management training and development, performance appraisal, and compensation policy. We will point out the strategic implications of each of these tasks. The chapter closes with a look at international labor relations and the relationship between the firm's management of labor relations and its overall strategy.

The Strategic Role of International HRM ▪

A large and expanding body of academic research suggests a strong fit between human resources practices and strategy is required for high profitability.[3] Superior human resources can be a sustained source of high productivity and competitive advantage in the global economy. At the same time, research suggests that many international businesses have room for improving the effectiveness of their human resource function. In one study of competitiveness among 326 large multinationals, the authors found that human resources was one of the weakest capabilities in most firms, suggesting that improving the effectiveness of international human resource practices might have substantial performance benefits.[4]

In Chapter 12, we examined four strategies pursued by international businesses—the multidomestic, the international, the global, and the transnational. Multidomestic firms try to create value by emphasizing local responsiveness; international firms, by transferring core competencies overseas; global firms, by realizing experience curve and location economies; and transnational firms, by doing all these things simultaneously. In Chapter 13, we discussed the organizational requirements for implementing each of these strategies. Table 18.1, identical to Table 13.2, summarizes the relationships between international strategies, structures, and controls.

Structures or controls summarized in Table 18.1 don't mean much if the human resources that support them are not appropriate. Without the right kind of people in place, organizational structure is just a hollow shell. In Chapter 13, we explained that formal and informal structure and controls must be congruent with a firm's strategy for the firm to succeed. Success also requires HRM policies to be congruent with the firm's strategy and with its formal and informal structure and controls. For example, a transnational strategy imposes very different requirements for staffing, management development, and compensation practices than a multidomestic strategy does.

In many ways, Molex, which was profiled in the opening case, is pursuing a transnational strategy. Molex tries to drive down its cost structure by locating manufacturing plants in countries where cost conditions are favorable, but at the same time the firm devotes great attention to sharing valuable know-how among operations in different countries and uses management transfers (expatriates) and management development programs as a way of facilitating that. As indicated in Table 18.1, firms pursuing a transnational strategy need to build a strong corporate culture and

Structure and Controls	International Strategy			
	Multidomestic	**International**	**Global**	**Transnational**
Centralization of operating decisions	Decentralized	Core competency centralized Rest decentralized	Some centralized	Mixed centralized and decentralized Informal matrix
Horizontal differentiation	Worldwide area structure	Worldwide product division	Worldwide product division	Informal matrix
Need for coordination	Low	Moderate	High	Very high
Integrating mechanisms	None	Few	Many	Very many
Performance ambiguity	Low	Moderate	High	Very high
Need for cultural controls	Low	Moderate	High	Very high

Table 18.1

Strategy, Structure, and Control Systems

an informal management network for transmitting information within the organization. Through its employee selection, management development, performance appraisal, and compensation policies, the HRM function can help develop these things. For example, Molex's liberal use of expatriates, by creating a cadre of international managers with experience in various nations, should help to establish an informal management network. In addition, as at Molex, management development programs can build a corporate culture that supports strategic goals. In short, HRM has a critical role to play in implementing strategy. In each section that follows, we will review the strategic role of HRM in some detail.

Staffing Policy

Staffing policy is concerned with the selection of employees for particular jobs. At one level, this involves selecting individuals who have the skills required to do particular jobs. At another level, staffing policy can be a tool for developing and promoting corporate culture.[5] By corporate culture, we mean the organization's norms and value systems. We encountered the concept in Chapter 13 when we discussed the use of "cultural controls" in businesses, noting that strong cultural controls help the firm pursue its strategy. Firms pursuing transnational and global strategies have high needs for a strong unifying culture, and the need is somewhat lower for firms pursuing an international strategy and lowest of all for firms pursuing a multidomestic strategy (see Table 18.1).

In firms pursuing transnational and global strategies, we might expect the HRM function to pay significant attention to selecting individuals who not only have the skills required to perform particular jobs but who also "fit" the prevailing culture of the firm. General Electric, for example, which is positioned toward the transnational end of the strategic spectrum, is not just concerned with hiring people who have the skills required for performing particular jobs; it wants to hire individuals whose behavioral styles, beliefs, and value systems are consistent with those of GE. This is true whether an American is being hired, an Italian, a German, or an Australian and whether the hiring is for a U.S. operation or a foreign operation. The belief is that if employees are predisposed toward the organization's norms and value systems by their personality type, the firm, which has a significant need for integration, will experience fewer problems with performance ambiguity.

The need for integration is substantially lower in a multidomestic firm. There is less performance ambiguity and not the same need for cultural controls. In theory, this means the HRM function can pay less attention to building a unified corporate culture. In multidomestic firms, the culture can be allowed to vary from national operation to national operation. (Although, given the questionable viability of a multidomestic strategy in today's world, this might not be the best policy to pursue. Chapter 12 discusses the viability of this strategy.)

Types of Staffing Policy

Research has identified three types of staffing policies in international businesses: the ethnocentric approach, the polycentric approach, and the geocentric approach.[6] We will review each policy and link it to the strategy pursued by the firm. The most attractive staffing policy is probably the geocentric approach, although there are several impediments to adopting it.

The Ethnocentric Approach

An **ethnocentric staffing** policy is one in which all key management positions are filled by parent-country nationals. This practice was very widespread at one time. Firms such as Procter & Gamble, Philips NV, and Matsushita originally followed it. In the Dutch firm Philips, for example, all important positions in most foreign subsidiaries were at one time held by Dutch nationals who were referred to by their non-Dutch colleagues as the Dutch Mafia. In many Japanese and South Korean firms today, such as Toyota, Matsushita, and Samsung, key positions in international operations are still often held by home-country nationals. According to the Japanese Overseas Enterprise Association, in 1996 only 29 percent of foreign subsidiaries of Japanese companies had presidents who were not Japanese. In contrast, 66 percent of the Japanese subsidiaries of foreign companies had Japanese presidents.[7]

Firms pursue an ethnocentric staffing policy for three reasons. First, the firm may believe the host country lacks qualified individuals to fill senior management positions. This argument is heard most often when the firm has operations in less developed countries. Second, the firm may see an ethnocentric staffing policy as the best way to maintain a unified corporate culture. Many Japanese firms, for example, prefer their foreign operations to be headed by expatriate Japanese managers because these managers will have been socialized into the firm's culture while employed in Japan.[8] Procter & Gamble until recently preferred to staff important management positions in its foreign subsidiaries with U.S. nationals who had been socialized into P&G's corporate culture by years of employment in its U.S. operations. Such reasoning tends to predominate when a firm places a high value on its corporate culture.

Third, if the firm is trying to create value by transferring core competencies to a foreign operation, as firms pursuing an international strategy are, it may believe that the best way to do this is to transfer parent-country nationals who have knowledge of that competency to the foreign operation. Imagine what might occur if a firm tried to transfer a core competency in marketing to a foreign subsidiary without supporting the transfer with a corresponding transfer of home-country marketing management personnel. The transfer would probably fail to produce the anticipated benefits because the knowledge underlying a core competency cannot easily be articulated and written down. Such knowledge often has a significant tacit dimension; it is acquired through experience. Just like the great tennis player who cannot instruct others how to become great tennis players simply by writing a handbook, the firm that has a core competency in marketing—or anything else—cannot just write a handbook that tells a foreign subsidiary how to build the firm's core competency anew in a foreign setting. It must also transfer management personnel to the foreign operation to show foreign managers how to become good marketers, for example. The need to transfer managers overseas arises because the knowledge that underlies the firm's core competency resides in the heads of its domestic managers and was acquired through years of experience, not by reading a handbook. Thus, if a firm is to transfer a core competency to a foreign subsidiary, it must also transfer the appropriate managers.

Despite this rationale for pursuing an ethnocentric staffing policy, the policy is now on the wane in most international businesses for two reasons. First, an ethnocentric staffing policy limits advancement opportunities for host-country nationals. This can lead to resentment, lower productivity, and increased turnover among that group. Resentment can be greater still if, as often occurs, expatriate managers are paid significantly more than home-country nationals.

Second, an ethnocentric policy can lead to "cultural myopia," the firm's failure to understand host-country cultural differences that require different approaches to marketing and management. The adaptation of expatriate managers can take a long time, during which they may make major mistakes. For example, expatriate managers may fail to appreciate how product attributes, distribution strategy, communications strategy, and pricing strategy should be adapted to host-country conditions. The result may be costly blunders. They may also make decisions that are ethically suspect simply because they do not understand the culture in which they are managing.[9] In one highly publicized case in the United States, Mitsubishi Motors was sued by the federal Equal Employment Opportunity Commission for tolerating extensive and systematic sexual harassment in a plant in Illinois. The plant's top management, all Japanese expatriates, denied the charges. The Japanese managers may have failed to realize that behavior that would be viewed as acceptable in Japan was not acceptable in the United States.[10]

The Polycentric Approach

A **polycentric staffing** policy requires host-country nationals to be recruited to manage subsidiaries, while parent-country nationals occupy key positions at corporate headquarters. In many respects, a polycentric approach is a response to the shortcomings of an ethnocentric approach. One advantage of adopting a polycentric approach is that the firm is less likely to suffer from cultural myopia. Host-country managers are unlikely to make the mistakes arising from cultural misunderstandings to which expatriate managers are vulnerable. A second advantage is that a polycentric approach may be less expensive to implement, reducing the costs of value creation. Expatriate managers can be very expensive to maintain.

A polycentric approach also has its drawbacks. Host-country nationals have limited opportunities to gain experience outside their own country and thus cannot progress beyond senior positions in their own subsidiary. As in the case of an ethnocentric policy, this may cause resentment. Perhaps the major drawback with a polycentric approach, however, is the gap that can form between host-country managers and parent-country managers. Language barriers, national loyalties, and a range of cultural differences may isolate the corporate headquarters staff from the various foreign subsidiaries. The lack of management transfers from home to host countries, and vice versa, can exacerbate this isolation and lead to a lack of integration between corporate headquarters and foreign subsidiaries. The result can be a "federation" of largely independent national units with only nominal links to the corporate headquarters. Within such a federation, the coordination required to transfer core competencies or to pursue experience curve and location economies may be difficult to achieve. Thus, although a polycentric approach may be effective for firms pursuing a multidomestic strategy, it is inappropriate for other strategies.

The federation that may result from a polycentric approach can also be a force for inertia within the firm. After decades of pursing a polycentric staffing policy, food and detergents giant Unilever found that shifting from a multidomestic strategic posture to a transnational posture was very difficult. Unilever's foreign subsidiaries had evolved into quasi-autonomous operations, each with its own strong national identity. These "little kingdoms" objected strenuously to corporate headquarters' attempts to limit their autonomy and to rationalize global manufacturing.[11]

The Geocentric Approach

A **geocentric staffing** policy seeks the best people for key jobs throughout the organization, regardless of nationality. Molex is a good example of a company that has adopted a geocentric staffing policy (see the opening case). This policy has a number of advantages. First, it enables the firm to make the best use of its human resources. Second, and perhaps more important, a geocentric policy enables the firm to build a cadre of international executives who feel at home working in a number of cultures. Creation of such a cadre may be a critical first step toward building a strong unifying corporate culture and an informal management network, both of which are required for global and transnational strategies (see Table 18.1).[12] Firms pursuing a geocentric staffing policy may be better able to create value from the pursuit of experience curve and location economies and from the multidirectional transfer of core competencies than firms pursuing other staffing policies. In addition, the multinational composition of the management team that results from geocentric staffing tends to reduce cultural myopia and to enhance local responsiveness. Thus, other things being equal, a geocentric staffing policy seems the most attractive.

A number of problems limit the firm's ability to pursue a geocentric policy. Many countries want foreign subsidiaries to employ their citizens. To achieve this goal, they use immigration laws to require the employment of host-country nationals if they are available in adequate numbers and have the necessary skills. Most countries (including the United States) require firms to provide extensive documentation if they wish to hire a foreign national instead of a local national. This documentation can be time-consuming, expensive, and at times futile. A geocentric staffing policy also can be very expensive to implement. Training and relocation costs increase when transferring managers from country to country. The company may also need a compensation structure with a standardized international base pay level higher than national levels in many countries. In addition, the higher pay enjoyed by managers placed on an international "fast track" may be a source of resentment within a firm.

Summary

The advantages and disadvantages of the three approaches to staffing policy are summarized in Table 18.2. Broadly speaking, an ethnocentric approach is compatible with an international strategy, a polycentric approach is compatible with a multidomestic strategy, and a geocentric approach is compatible with both global and transnational strategies. (See Chapter 12 for details of the strategies.)

While the staffing policies described here are well known and widely used among both practitioners and scholars of international businesses, some critics have claimed that the typology is too simplistic and that it obscures the internal differentiation of management practices within international businesses. The critics claim that within some international businesses, staffing policies vary significantly from national subsidiary to national subsidiary; while some are managed on an ethnocentric basis, others are managed in a polycentric or geocentric manner.[13] Other critics note that the staffing policy adopted by a firm is primarily driven by its geographic scope, as opposed to its strategic orientation. Firms that have a very broad geographic scope are the most likely to have a geocentric mind-set.[14] Thus, Molex, which is involved in about 50 countries, is by this argument more likely to have a geocentric mind-set than a firm that is involved in only 3 countries.

Expatriate Managers

Two of the three staffing policies we have discussed—the ethnocentric and the geocentric—rely on extensive use of expatriate managers. As defined earlier, **expatriates** are citizens of one country who are working in another country. Sometimes the term *inpatriates* is used to identify a subset of expatriates who are citizens of a foreign country working in the home country of their multinational employer.[15] Thus, a citizen

Table 18.2

Comparison of Staffing
Approaches

Staffing Approach	Strategic Appropriateness	Advantages	Disadvantages
Ethnocentric	International	Overcomes lack of qualified managers in host nation Unified culture Helps transfer core competencies	Produces resentment in host country Can lead to cultural myopia
Polycentric	Multidomestic	Alleviates cultural myopia Inexpensive to implement	Limits career mobility Isolates headquarters from foreign subsidiaries
Geocentric	Global and transnational	Uses human resources efficiently Helps build strong culture and informal management network	National immigration policies may limit implementation Expensive

of Japan who moves to the United States to work at Molex would be classified as an inpatriate. With an ethnocentric policy, the expatriates are all home-country nationals who are transferred abroad. With a geocentric approach, the expatriates need not be home-country nationals; the firm does not base transfer decisions on nationality. A prominent issue in the international staffing literature is **expatriate failure**—the premature return of an expatriate manager to his or her home country.[16] Here we briefly review the evidence on expatriate failure before discussing a number of ways to minimize the expatriate failure rate.

Expatriate Failure Rates

Expatriate failure represents a failure of the firm's selection policies to identify individuals who will not thrive abroad.[17] The consequences include premature return from a foreign posting and high resignation rates, with expatriates leaving their company at about twice the rate of domestic managements.[18] Research suggests that between 16 and 40 percent of all American employees sent abroad to developed nations return from their assignments early, and almost 70 percent of employees sent to developing nations return home early.[19] Although detailed data are not available for other nationalities, one suspects that high expatriate failure is a universal problem. The costs of expatriate failure are high. One estimate is that the average cost per failure to the parent firm can be as high as three times the expatriate's annual domestic salary plus the cost of relocation (which is affected by currency exchange rates and location of assignment). Estimates of the costs of each failure run between $250,000 and $1 million.[20] In addition, approximately 30 to 50 percent of American expatriates, whose average annual compensation package runs to $250,000, stay at their international assignments but are considered ineffective or marginally effective by their firms.[21] In a seminal study, R. L. Tung surveyed a number of U.S., European, and Japanese multinationals.[22] Her results, summarized in Table 18.3, suggested that 76 percent of U.S. multinationals experienced expatriate failure rates of 10 percent or more, and 7 percent experienced a failure rate of more than 20 percent. Tung's work also suggests that U.S.-based multinationals experience a much higher expatriate failure rate than either European or Japanese multinationals.

Tung asked her sample of multinational managers to indicate reasons for expatriate failure. For U.S. multinationals, the reasons, in order of importance, were

1.   Inability of spouse to adjust.
2.   Manager's inability to adjust.

Recall Rate Percent	Percent of Companies
U.S. multinationals	
20–40%	7%
10–20	69
<10	24
European multinationals	
11–15%	3%
6–10	38
<5	59
Japanese multinationals	
11–19%	14%
6–10	10
<5	76

Table 18.3

Expatriate Failure Rates

Source: Data from R. L. Tung, "Selection and Training Procedures of U.S., European, and Japanese Multinationals," pp. 51–71. Copyright © by The Regents of the University of California. Reprinted from the *California Management Review*, Vol. 1.25, No. 1, by permission from The Regents.

3. Other family problems.
4. Manager's personal or emotional maturity.
5. Inability to cope with larger overseas responsibilities.

Managers of European firms gave only one reason consistently to explain expatriate failure: the inability of the manager's spouse to adjust to a new environment. For the Japanese firms, the reasons for failure were

1. Inability to cope with larger overseas responsibilities.
2. Difficulties with new environment.
3. Personal or emotional problems.
4. Lack of technical competence.
5. Inability of spouse to adjust.

The most striking difference between these lists is that "inability of spouse to adjust" was the top reason for expatriate failure among U.S. and European multinationals but only the number five reason among Japanese multinationals. Tung comments that this difference is not surprising, given the role and status to which Japanese society traditionally relegates the wife and the fact that most of the Japanese expatriate managers in the study were men.

Since Tung's study, a number of other studies have consistently confirmed that the inability of a spouse to adjust, the inability of the manager to adjust, or other family problems remain major reasons for continuing high levels of expatriate failure. One study by International Orientation Resources, an HRM consulting firm, found that 60 percent of expatriate failures occur due to these three reasons.[23] Another study found that the most common reason for assignment failure is lack of partner (spouse) satisfaction, which was listed by 27 percent of respondents.[24] The inability of expatriate managers to adjust to foreign postings seems to be caused by a lack of cultural skills on the part of the manager being transferred. According to one HRM management consulting firm, this is because the expatriate selection process at many firms is fundamentally flawed. "Expatriate assignments rarely fail because the person cannot accommodate to the technical demands of the job. Typically, the expatriate selections are made by line managers based on technical competence. They fail because of family and personal issues and lack of cultural skills that haven't been part of the selection process."[25]

Managing Expatriates at Royal Dutch/Shell

Royal Dutch/Shell is a global petroleum company with joint headquarters in both London and The Hague in the Netherlands. The company employs more than 100,000 people, approximately 5,500 of whom are at any one time living and working as expatriates. The expatriates at Shell are a very diverse group, made up of over 70 nationalities and located in more than 100 countries. Shell, as a global corporation, has long recognized that the international mobility of its workforce is essential to its success. By the early 1990s, however, Shell was finding it harder to recruit key personnel for foreign postings. To discover why, the company in 1993 interviewed more than 200 expatriate employees and their spouses to determine their biggest concerns. The data were then used to construct a survey that was sent to 17,000 current and former expatriate employees, expatriates' spouses, and employees who had declined international assignments.

The survey registered a phenomenal 70 percent response rate, clearly indicating that many employees thought this was an important issue. According to the survey, five issues had the greatest impact on the willingness of an employee to accept an international assignment. In order of importance, these were (1) separation from children during their secondary education (the children of British and Dutch expatriates were often sent to boarding schools in their home countries while their parents worked abroad), (2) harm done to a spouse's career and employment, (3) failure to recognize and involve a spouse in the relocation decision, (4) failure to provide adequate information and assistance regarding relocation, and (5) health issues. The underlying message was that the family is the basic unit of expatriation, not the individual, and Shell needed to do more to recognize this.

To deal with these issues, Shell implemented a number of programs designed to address some of these problems. To help with the education of children, Shell built elementary schools for Shell employees where there was a heavy concentration of expatriates. As for secondary school education, it worked with local schools, often providing grants, to help them upgrade their educational offerings. It also offered an education supplement to help expatriates send their children to private schools in the host country (before 1994, it would pay only for a child's boarding school education in its home country).

Helping spouses with their careers is a more vexing problem. According to the survey data, half of the spouses accompanying Shell staff on assignment were employed until the transfer. When expatriated, only 12 percent were able to secure employment, while a further 33 percent wished to be employed. Shell set up a spouse employment center to address the problem. The center provides career counseling and assistance in locating employment opportunities both during and immediately after an international assignment. The company also agreed to reimburse up to 80 percent of the costs of vocational training, further education, or reaccreditation, up to $4,400 per assignment.

Shell also set up a global information and advice network known as "The Outpost" to provide support for families contemplating a foreign posting. The Outpost has its headquarters in The Hague and now runs 40 information centers in more than 30 countries. The center recommends schools and medical facilities and provides housing advice and up-to-date information on employment, study, self-employment, and volunteer work.

Sources: E. Smockum, "Don't Forget the Trailing Spouse," *Financial Times,* May 6, 1998, p. 22; V. Frazee, "Tearing Down Roadblocks," *Workforce* 77, no. 2 (1998), pp. 50–54; C. Sievers, "Expatriate Management," *HR Focus* 75, no. 3 (1998), pp. 75–76; and J. Barbian, "Return to Sender," *Training,* January 2002, pp. 40–43.

The failure of spouses to adjust to a foreign posting seems to be related to a number of factors. Often spouses find themselves in a foreign country without the familiar network of family and friends. Language differences make it difficult for them to make new friends. While this may not be a problem for the manager, who can make friends at work, it can be difficult for the spouse who might feel trapped at home. The problem is often exacerbated by immigration regulations prohibiting the spouse from taking employment. With the recent rise of two-career families in many developed nations, this issue has become much more important. One recent survey found that 69 percent of expatriates are married, with spouses accompanying them 77 percent of the time. Of those spouses, 49 percent were employed before an assignment and only 11 percent were employed during an assignment.[26] Research suggests that a main reason managers now turn down international assignments is concern over the impact such an assignment might have on their spouse's career.[27] The accompanying Management Focus examines how one large multinational company, Royal Dutch/Shell, has tried to come to grips with this issue.

Expatriate Selection

One way to reduce expatriate failure rates is by improving selection procedures to screen out inappropriate candidates. In a review of the research on this issue, Mendenhall and Oddou state that a major problem in many firms is that HRM managers tend to equate domestic performance with overseas performance potential.[28] Domestic performance and overseas performance potential are not the same thing. An executive who performs well in a domestic setting may not be able to adapt to managing in a different cultural setting. From their review of the research, Mendenhall and Oddou identified four dimensions that seem to predict success in a foreign posting: self-orientation, others-orientation, perceptual ability, and cultural toughness.

1. *Self-orientation.* The attributes of this dimension strengthen the expatriate's self-esteem, self-confidence, and mental well-being. Expatriates with high self-esteem, self-confidence, and mental well-being were more likely to succeed in foreign postings. Mendenhall and Oddou concluded that such individuals were able to adapt their interests in food, sport, and music; had interests outside of work that could be pursued (e.g., hobbies); and were technically competent.

2. *Others-orientation.* The attributes of this dimension enhance the expatriate's ability to interact effectively with host-country nationals. The more effectively the expatriate interacts with host-country nationals, the more likely he or she is to succeed. Two factors seem to be particularly important here: relationship development and willingness to communicate. Relationship development refers to the ability to develop long-lasting friendships with host-country nationals. Willingness to communicate refers to the expatriate's willingness to use the host-country language. Although language fluency helps, an expatriate need not be fluent to show willingness to communicate. Making the effort to use the language is what is important. Such gestures tend to be rewarded with greater cooperation by host-country nationals.

3. *Perceptual ability.* This is the ability to understand why people of other countries behave the way they do; that is, the ability to empathize. This dimension seems critical for managing host-country nationals. Expatriate managers who lack this ability tend to treat foreign nationals as if they were home-country nationals. As a result, they may experience significant management problems and considerable frustration. As one expatriate executive from Hewlett-Packard observed, "It took me six months to accept the fact that my staff meetings would start 30 minutes late, and that it would bother no one but me." According to Mendenhall and Oddou, well-adjusted expatriates tend to be nonjudgmental and nonevaluative in interpreting the behavior of host-country nationals and willing to be flexible in their management style, adjusting it as cultural conditions warrant.

4. *Cultural toughness.* This dimension refers to the relationship between the country of assignment and how well an expatriate adjusts to a particular posting. Some countries are much tougher postings than others because their cultures are more unfamiliar and uncomfortable. For example, many Americans regard Great Britain as a relatively easy foreign posting, and for good reason—the two cultures have much in common. But many Americans find postings in non-Western cultures, such as India, Southeast Asia, and the Middle East, to

be much tougher.[29] The reasons are many, including poor health care and housing standards, inhospitable climate, lack of Western entertainment, and language difficulties. Also, many cultures are extremely male dominated and may be particularly difficult postings for female Western managers.

Mendenhall and Oddou note that standard psychological tests can be used to assess the first three of these dimensions, whereas a comparison of cultures can give managers a feeling for the fourth dimension. They contend that these four dimensions, in addition to domestic performance, should be considered when selecting a manager for foreign posting. However, current practice does not conform to Mendenhall and Oddou's recommendations. Tung's research, for example, showed that only 5 percent of the firms in her sample used formal procedures and psychological tests to assess the personality traits and relational abilities of potential expatriates.[30] Research by International Orientation Resources suggests that when selecting employees for foreign assignments, only 10 percent of the 50 Fortune 500 firms they surveyed tested for important psychological traits such as cultural sensitivity, interpersonal skills, adaptability, and flexibility. Instead, 90 percent of the time employees were selected on the basis of their technical expertise, not their cross-cultural fluency.[31]

Mendenhall and Oddou do not address the problem of expatriate failure due to a spouse's inability to adjust. According to a number of other researchers, a review of the family situation should be part of the expatriate selection process (see the Management Focus on Royal Dutch/Shell for an example).[32] A survey by Windam International, another international HRM management consulting firm, found that spouses were included in preselection interviews for foreign postings only 21 percent of the time, and that only half of them receive any cross-cultural training. The rise of dual-career families has added an additional and difficult dimension to this long-standing problem.[33] Increasingly, spouses wonder why they should have to sacrifice their own career to further that of their partner.[34]

Training and Management Development

Selection is just the first step in matching a manager with a job. The next step is training the manager to do the specific job. For example, an intensive training program might be used to give expatriate managers the skills required for success in a foreign posting. Management development is a much broader concept. It is intended to develop the manager's skills over his or her career with the firm. Thus, as part of a management development program, a manager might be sent on several foreign postings over a number of years to build her cross-cultural sensitivity and experience. At the same time, along with other managers in the firm, she might attend management education programs at regular intervals. The thinking behind job transfers is that broad international experience will enhance the management and leadership skills of executives. Recent research suggests this may be the case.[35]

Historically, most international businesses have been more concerned with training than with management development. Plus, they tended to focus their training efforts on preparing home-country nationals for foreign postings. Recently, however, the shift toward greater global competition and the rise of transnational firms have changed this. It is increasingly common for firms to provide general management development programs in addition to training for particular posts. In many international businesses, the explicit purpose of these management development programs is strategic. Management development is seen as a tool to help the firm achieve its strategic goals.

With this distinction between training and management development in mind, we first examine the types of training managers receive for foreign postings. Then we discuss the connection between management development and strategy in the international business.

Training for Expatriate Managers

Earlier in the chapter we saw that the two most common reasons for expatriate failure were the inability of a manager's spouse to adjust to a foreign environment and the manager's own inability to adjust to a foreign environment. Training can help the manager and spouse cope with both these problems. Cultural training, language training, and practical training all seem to reduce expatriate failure. We discuss each of these kinds of training here.[36] Despite the usefulness of these kinds of training, evidence suggests that many managers receive no training before they are sent on foreign postings. One study found that only about 30 percent of managers sent on one- to five-year expatriate assignments received training before their departure.[37]

Cultural Training

Cultural training seeks to foster an appreciation for the host country's culture. The belief is that understanding a host country's culture will help the manager empathize with the culture, which will enhance her effectiveness in dealing with host-country nationals. It has been suggested that expatriates should receive training in the host country's culture, history, politics, economy, religion, and social and business practices.[38] If possible, it is also advisable to arrange for a familiarization trip to the host country before the formal transfer, as this seems to ease culture shock. Given the problems related to spouse adaptation, it is important that the spouse, and perhaps the whole family, be included in cultural training programs.

Language Training

English is the language of world business; it is quite possible to conduct business all over the world using only English. For example, at ABB Group, a Swiss electrical equipment giant, the company's top 13 managers hold frequent meetings in different countries. Because they share no common first language, they speak only English, a foreign tongue to all but one.[39] Despite the prevalence of English, however, an exclusive reliance on English diminishes an expatriate manager's ability to interact with host-country nationals. As noted earlier, a willingness to communicate in the language of the host country, even if the expatriate is far from fluent, can help build rapport with local employees and improve the manager's effectiveness. Despite this, J. C. Baker's study of 74 executives of U.S. multinationals found that only 23 believed knowledge of foreign languages was necessary for conducting business abroad.[40] Those firms that did offer foreign language training for expatriates believed it improved their employees' effectiveness and enabled them to relate more easily to a foreign culture, which fostered a better image of the firm in the host country.

Practical Training

Practical training is aimed at helping the expatriate manager and family ease themselves into day-to-day life in the host country. The sooner a routine is established, the better are the prospects that the expatriate and her family will adapt successfully. One critical need is for a support network of friends for the expatriate. Where an expatriate community exists, firms often devote considerable effort to ensuring the new expatriate family is quickly integrated into that group. The expatriate community can be a useful source of support and information and can be invaluable in helping the family adapt to a foreign culture.

Repatriation of Expatriates

A largely overlooked but critically important issue in the training and development of expatriate managers is to prepare them for reentry into their home-country organization.[41] Repatriation should be seen as the final link in an integrated, circular process that connects good selection and cross-cultural training of expatriate managers with completion of their term abroad and reintegration into their national organization. However, instead of having employees come home to share their knowledge and encourage other high-performing managers to take the same international career track, expatriates too often face a different scenario.[42]

Often when they return home after a stint abroad—where they have typically been autonomous, well-compensated, and celebrated as a big fish in a little pond—they face an organization that doesn't know what they have done for the last few years, doesn't know how to use their new knowledge, and doesn't particularly care. In the worst cases, reentering employees have to scrounge for jobs, or firms will create standby positions that don't use the expatriate's skills and capabilities and fail to make the most of the business investment the firm has made in that individual.

Research illustrates the extent of this problem. According to one study of repatriated employees, 60 to 70 percent didn't know what their position would be when they returned home. Also, 60 percent said their organizations were vague about repatriation, about their new roles, and about their future career progression within the company, while 77 percent of those surveyed took jobs at a lower level in their home organization than in their international assignments.[43] Not surprisingly, 15 percent of returning expatriates leave their firms within a year of arriving home, while 40 percent leave within three years.[44]

The key to solving this problem is good human resource planning. Just as the HRM function needs to develop good selection and training programs for its expatriates, it also needs to develop good programs for reintegrating expatriates back into work life within their home-country organization, for preparing them for changes in their physical and professional landscape, and for utilizing the knowledge they acquired while abroad. For an example of the kind of program that might be used, see the accompanying Management Focus that looks at Monsanto's repatriation program.

Management Development and Strategy

Management development programs are designed to increase the overall skill levels of managers through a mix of ongoing management education and rotations of managers through a number of jobs within the firm to give them varied experiences. They are attempts to improve the overall productivity and quality of the firm's management resources.

International businesses increasingly are using management development as a strategic tool. This is particularly true in firms pursuing a transnational strategy, as increasing numbers are. Such firms need a strong unifying corporate culture and informal management networks to assist in coordination and control (see Table 18.2). In addition, transnational firm managers need to be able to detect pressures for local responsiveness, and that requires them to understand the culture of a host country.

Management development programs help build a unifying corporate culture by socializing new managers into the norms and value systems of the firm. In-house company training programs and intense interaction during off-site training can foster esprit de corps—shared experiences, informal networks, perhaps a company language or jargon—as well as develop technical competencies. These training events often include songs, picnics, and sporting events that promote feelings of togetherness. These rites of integration may include "initiation rites" wherein personal culture is stripped, company uniforms are donned (e.g., T-shirts bearing the company logo), and humiliation is inflicted (e.g., a pie in the face). All these activities aim to strengthen a manager's identification with the company.[45]

Bringing managers together in one location for extended periods and rotating them through different jobs in several countries help the firm build an informal management network. Such a network can then be used as a conduit for exchanging valuable performance-enhancing knowledge within the organization.[46] (Chapter 13 explained the importance of such networks in transnational firms.) Consider the Swedish telecommunications company L. M. Ericsson. Interunit cooperation is extremely im-

Management Focus

Monsanto's Repatriation Program

Monsanto is a global provider of agricultural products with revenues in excess of $4 billion and 10,000 employees. At any one time, the company will have 100 mid- and higher-level managers on extended postings abroad. Two-thirds of these are Americans who are being posted overseas, while the remainder are foreign nationals being employed in the United States. At Monsanto, managing expatriates and their repatriation begins with a rigorous selection process and intensive cross-cultural training, both for the managers and for their families. As at many other global companies, the idea is to build an internationally minded cadre of highly capable managers who will lead the organization in the future.

One of the strongest features of this program is that employees and their sending and receiving managers, or sponsors, develop an agreement about how this assignment will fit into the firm's business objectives. The focus is on why employees are going abroad to do the job, and what their contribution to Monsanto will be when they return. Sponsoring managers are expected to be explicit about the kind of job opportunities the expatriates will have once they return home.

Once they arrive back in their home country, expatriate managers meet with cross-cultural trainers during debriefing sessions. They are also given the opportunity to showcase their experiences to their peers, subordinates, and superiors in special information exchanges.

However, Monsanto's repatriation program focuses on more than just business; it also attends to the family's reentry. Monsanto has found that difficulties with repatriation often have more to do with personal and family-related issues than with work-related issues. But the personal matters obviously affect an employee's on-the-job performance, so it is important for the company to pay attention to such issues.

This is why Monsanto offers returning employees an opportunity to work through personal difficulties. About three months after they return home, expatriates meet for three hours at work with several colleagues of their choice. The debriefing session is a conversation aided by a trained facilitator who has an outline to help the expatriate cover all the important aspects of the repatriation. The debriefing allows the employee to share important experiences and to enlighten managers, colleagues, and friends about his or her expertise so others within the organization can use some of the global knowledge. According to one participant, "It sounds silly, but it's such a hectic time in the family's life, you don't have time to sit down and take stock of what's happening. You're going through the move, transitioning to a new job, a new house, the children may be going to a new school. This is a kind of oasis; a time to talk and put your feelings on the table." Apparently it works; since the program was introduced in the early 1990s, the attrition rate among returning expatriates has dropped sharply.

Sources: Excerpted from "Repatriation: Up, Down, or Out?" by C. M. Solomon, *Personnel Journal*, Copyright © January 1995, pp. 28–34. Used with permission of ACC Communications, Inc. *Personnel Journal* (now known as *Workforce*), Costa Mesa, CA. All rights reserved.

portant at Ericsson, particularly for transferring know-how and core competencies from the parent to foreign subsidiaries, from foreign subsidiaries to the parent, and between foreign subsidiaries. To facilitate cooperation, Ericsson transfers large numbers of people back and forth between headquarters and subsidiaries. Ericsson sends a team of 50 to 100 engineers and managers from one unit to another for a year or two. This establishes a network of interpersonal contacts. This policy is effective for both solidifying a common culture in the company and coordinating the company's globally dispersed operations.[47]

Performance Appraisal

A particularly thorny issue in many international businesses is how best to evaluate its expatriate managers' performance.[48] In this section, we look at this issue and consider some guidelines for appraising expatriate performance.

Performance Appraisal Problems

Unintentional bias makes it difficult to evaluate the performance of expatriate managers objectively. In most cases, two groups evaluate the performance of expatriate managers—host-nation managers and home-office managers—and both are subject to bias. The host-nation managers may be biased by their own cultural frame of reference and expectations. For example, Oddou and Mendenhall report the case of a U.S. manager who introduced participative decision making while working in an Indian subsidiary.[49] The manager subsequently received a negative evaluation from host-country managers because in India, the strong social stratification means managers are seen as experts who should not have to ask subordinates for help. The local employees apparently viewed the U.S. manager's attempt at participatory management as an indication that he was incompetent and did not know his job.

Home-country managers' appraisals may be biased by distance and by their own lack of experience working abroad. Home-office managers are often not aware of what is going on in a foreign operation. Accordingly, they tend to rely on hard data in evaluating an expatriate's performance, such as the subunit's productivity, profitability, or market share. Such criteria may reflect factors outside the expatriate manager's control (e.g., adverse changes in exchange rates, economic downturns). Also, hard data do not take into account many less-visible "soft" variables that are also important, such as an expatriate's ability to develop cross-cultural awareness and to work productively with local managers. Due to such biases, many expatriate managers believe that headquarters management evaluates them unfairly and does not fully appreciate the value of their skills and experience. This could be one reason many expatriates believe a foreign posting does not benefit their careers. In one study of personnel managers in U.S. multinationals, 56 percent of the managers surveyed stated that a foreign assignment is either detrimental or immaterial to one's career.[50]

Guidelines for Performance Appraisal

Several things can reduce bias in the performance appraisal process.[51] First, most expatriates appear to believe more weight should be given to an on-site manager's appraisal than to an off-site manager's appraisal. Due to proximity, an on-site manager is more likely to evaluate the soft variables that are important aspects of an expatriate's performance. The evaluation may be especially valid when the on-site manager is of the same nationality as the expatriate, since cultural bias should be alleviated. In practice, home-office managers often write performance evaluations after receiving input from on-site managers. When this is the case, most experts recommend that a former expatriate who served in the same location should be involved in the appraisal to help reduce bias. Finally, when the policy is for foreign on-site managers to write performance evaluations, home-office managers should be consulted before an on-site manager completes a formal termination evaluation. This gives the home-office manager the opportunity to balance what could be a very hostile evaluation based on a cultural misunderstanding.

▉ Compensation

Two issues are raised in every discussion of compensation practices in an international business. One is how compensation should be adjusted to reflect national differences in economic circumstances and compensation practices. The other issue is how expatriate managers should be paid.

National Differences in Compensation

Substantial differences exist in the compensation of executives at the same level in various countries. The results of a survey undertaken by Towers Perrin are summarized in Table 18.4. This survey looked at average compensation for four positions across

Table 18.4

Compensation for Four
Positions in 26 Countries

Source: Towers Perrin

	CEO	HR Director	Accountant	Mfg. Employee
Argentina	$860,704	$326,874	$63,948	$17,884
Australia	646,316	235,316	57,129	29,703
Belgium	655,390	286,222	63,883	34,336
Brazil	597,454	287,683	44,605	10,480
Canada	742,228	188,070	44,866	36,289
China (Shanghai)	93,393	58,278	14,552	3,021
France	540,260	224,112	69,554	34,741
Germany	421,622	189,785	61,375	36,934
Hong Kong SAR	635,186	211,321	56,711	16,691
Italy	567,685	254,138	59,388	29,469
Japan	545,233	235,536	59,107	51,997
Malaysia	350,558	130,771	24,522	7,453
Mexico	648,695	239,028	41,582	14,302
Netherlands	621,153	217,142	48,838	27,892
New Zealand	258,114	111,803	38,382	15,931
Singapore	621,871	239,376	51,733	16,912
South Africa	406,263	179,268	43,234	7,974
South Korea	194,421	109,637	41,365	17,904
Spain	399,423	196,305	56,332	22,746
Sweden	440,265	166,312	43,438	32,564
Switzerland	448,422	175,008	66,121	41,104
Taiwan	179,486	102,491	30,652	11,924
Thailand	145,173	98,120	19,175	6,293
United Kingdom	719,665	268,302	107,839	28,874
United States	1,403,899	306,181	66,377	44,680
Venezuela	609,097	272,212	41,192	11,221

26 countries in 2000.[52] The figures for CEOs and HR directors include both base compensation and performance-related pay bonuses, but do not include stock options. The figures for accountants and manufacturing employees refer just to base pay. As can be seen, wide variations exist across countries. The average compensation for a CEO in the United States was $1.4 million, compared to $545,260 in Japan and $179,486 in Taiwan. These figures underestimate the true differential because many U.S. executives earn considerable sums of money from stock option grants.[53] In 1996, stock option grants were used in only 10 of the 26 countries in the survey. By 2001, however, this figure had risen to 19 out of 26, suggesting that U.S.-style compensation packages that include stock option grants are becoming more frequent.[54]

Figure 18.1 summarizes additional data on CEO compensation from a subsequent Towers Perrin study of pay in midsize companies with annual revenues in the $500 million range. As can be seen, even among midsize firms, U.S. executives are paid significantly better than their peers in other nations. It should also be noted that this survey

Figure 18.1

National Differences in CEO Pay for Midsize Companies

Source: "Towers Perrin Study Finds Increasingly Similar Approaches to Corporate Pay in Different Global Markets," *Business Wire*, December 3, 2001.

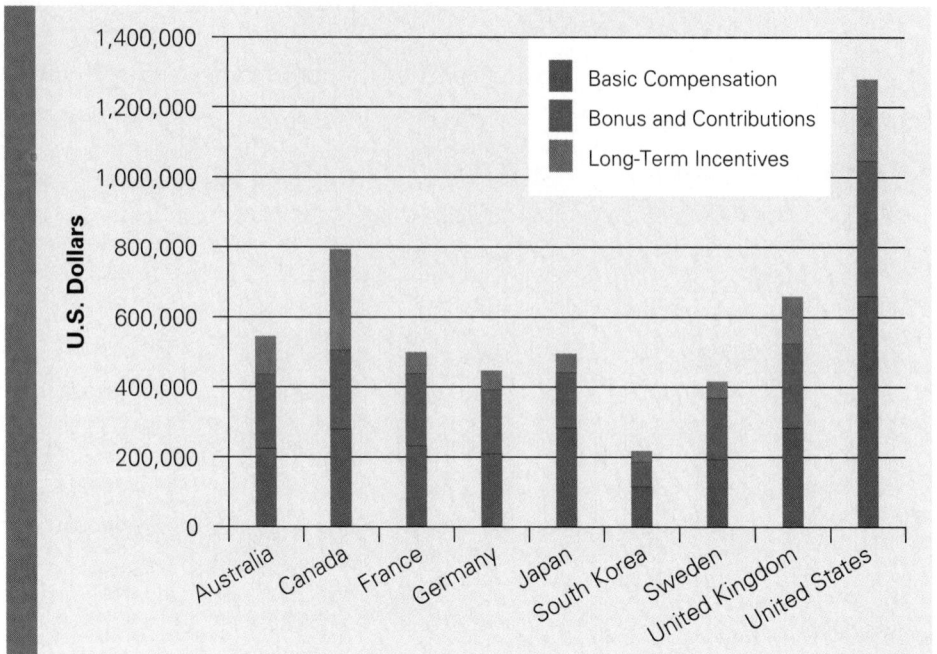

was undertaken in 2001, when long-term incentive pay in the United States fell due to a sluggish economy.

National differences in compensation raise a perplexing question for an international business: Should the firm pay executives in different countries according to the prevailing standards in each country, or should it equalize pay on a global basis? The problem does not arise in firms pursuing ethnocentric or polycentric staffing policies. In ethnocentric firms, the issue can be reduced to that of how much home-country expatriates should be paid (which we will consider later). As for polycentric firms, the lack of managers' mobility among national operations implies that pay can and should be kept country-specific. There would seem to be no point in paying executives in Great Britain the same as U.S. executives if they never work side by side.

However, this problem is very real in firms with geocentric staffing policies. A geocentric staffing policy is consistent with a transnational strategy. One aspect of this policy is the need for a cadre of international managers that may include many different nationalities. Should all members of such a cadre be paid the same salary and the same incentive pay? For a U.S.-based firm, this would mean raising the compensation of foreign nationals to U.S. levels, which could be very expensive. If the firm does not equalize pay, it could cause considerable resentment among foreign nationals who are members of the international cadre and work with U.S. nationals. If a firm is serious about building an international cadre, it may have to pay its international executives the same basic salary irrespective of their country of origin or assignment. The accompanying Management Focus contains several examples of how some international businesses have tried to deal with this problem.

Expatriate Pay

The most common approach to expatriate pay is the balance sheet approach. According to Organizational Resources Consulting, some 80 percent of the 781 companies it surveyed in 2002 use this approach.[55] This approach equalizes purchasing power across countries so employees can enjoy the same living standard in their foreign posting that they enjoyed at home. In addition, the approach provides financial incentives to offset qualitative differences between assignment locations.[56] Figure 18.2 shows a

Executive Pay Policies for Global Managers

A survey of human resource professionals in 45 large U.S. multinational companies undertaken by Organizational Resources Consulting, an international HRM consulting firm, found that all 45 companies viewed differing pay levels and perks as their biggest problem when trying to develop an international workforce. The root of the problem is cost; expatriate pay packages that are based on U.S. salaries and needs are increasingly seen as too expensive. To deal with this, many international businesses are trying to develop special pay schemes for their cadre of internationally mobile managers.

Hewlett-Packard transfers about 600 people a year across national borders. Although most of these transferees are on one- to two-year assignments, up to 25 percent are on indefinite assignments. HP ties the pay of short-term transferees to pay scales in their home country, but longer-term HP transferees are quickly switched to the pay scale of their host country and paid according to prevailing local standards. For employees moving from high-pay countries such as Germany to lower-pay countries, such as Spain, HP offers temporary bridging payments to ease the adjustment.

The Minnesota Mining and Manufacturing Co. (3M) has a completely different type of program for longer-term expatriates. The company developed the program because it drastically altered its international organization. In Europe, for example, 3M used to organize its operations on a country-by-country basis. However, 3M has established Europeanwide divisions, so many 3M executives who might have spent their career in one country are now being asked to move, perhaps permanently, to another country.

The 3M program compares net salaries in both the old and new country by subtracting the major costs, such as taxes and housing, from gross pay. The transferred executive then gets whichever pay packet is highest. Thus, when 3M transfers a German executive to France, the German remains on her home-country pay scale. But a British employee transferred to Germany, where salaries are higher, can expect to be switched to the German pay scale. Although the policy considers local housing costs, it doesn't compensate for higher housing costs through a special payment, as many traditional expatriate pay policies did. Any housing subsidy that resulted could last for the rest of an executive's career following a transfer and this would be very expensive.

The oil company Phillips Petroleum has adopted yet another policy. At Phillips, the policy used to be that when a third-country national, such as a British citizen, was transferred abroad (for example, from Britain to Kuwait), he would be paid in U.S. dollars and his salary would be raised to a level equivalent to that of someone in the United States doing a similar job. This was a very expensive policy given the generally high level of pay prevailing in the United States. Now Phillips has a "third-country nationals program." Under this program, the transferred employee is given generous housing allowances and educational assistance for his children. However, his salary is now pegged to the level prevailing in his home country.

Sources: Organizational Resource Counselors, *2002 Survey of International Assignment Policies and Practices,* March 2003; A. Bennett, "Executive Pay: What's an Expatriate?" *Wall Street Journal,* April 21, 1994, p. A5; and J. Flynn, "Continental Divide over Executive Pay," *Business Week,* July 3, 1995.

typical balance sheet. Note that home-country outlays for the employee are designated as income taxes, housing expenses, expenditures for goods and services (food, clothing, entertainment, etc.), and reserves (savings, pension contributions, etc.). The balance sheet approach attempts to provide expatriates with the same standard of living in their host countries as they enjoy at home plus a financial inducement (i.e., premium, incentive) for accepting an overseas assignment.

The components of the typical expatriate compensation package are a base salary, a foreign-service premium, allowances of various types, tax differentials, and benefits. We shall briefly review each of these components.[57] An expatriate's total compensation package may amount to three times what he or she would cost the firm in a home-country posting. Because of the high cost of expatriates, many firms have reduced their use of them in recent years. However, a firm's ability to reduce its use of

Figure 18.2

The Balance Sheet

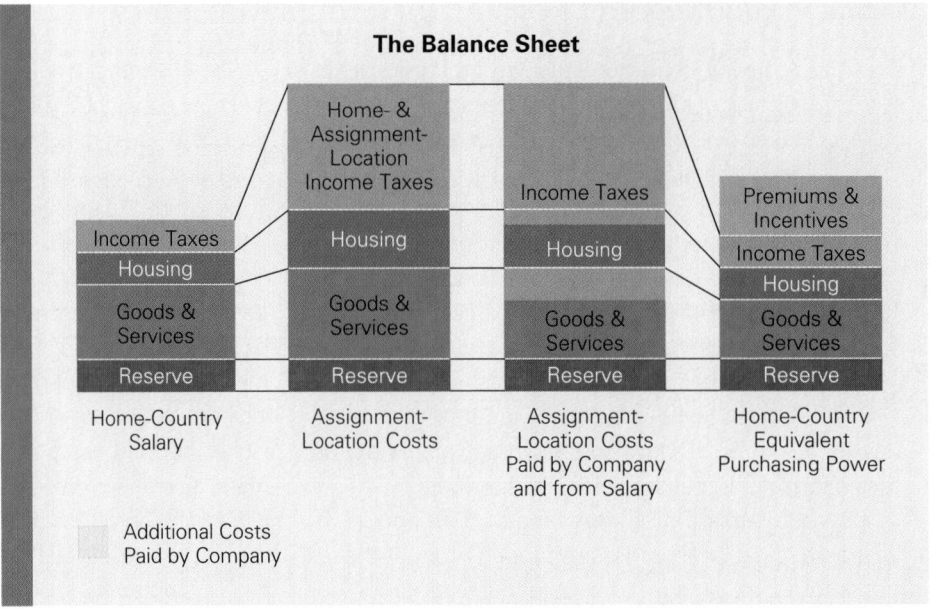

The Balance Sheet

expatriates may be limited, particularly if it is pursuing an ethnocentric or geocentric staffing policy.

Base Salary

An expatriate's base salary is normally in the same range as the base salary for a similar position in the home country. The base salary is normally paid in either the home-country currency or in the local currency.

Foreign Service Premium

A foreign service premium is extra pay the expatriate receives for working outside his or her country of origin. It is offered as an inducement to accept foreign postings. It compensates the expatriate for having to live in an unfamiliar country isolated from family and friends, having to deal with a new culture and language, and having to adapt to new work habits and practices. Many firms pay foreign service premiums as a percentage of base salary ranging from 10 to 30 percent after tax with 16 percent being the average premium.[58]

Allowances

Four types of allowances are often included in an expatriate's compensation package: hardship allowances, housing allowances, cost-of-living allowances, and education allowances. A hardship allowance is paid when the expatriate is being sent to a difficult location, usually defined as one where such basic amenities as health care, schools, and retail stores are grossly deficient by the standards of the expatriate's home country. A housing allowance is normally given to ensure that the expatriate can afford the same quality of housing in the foreign country as at home. In locations where housing is very expensive (e.g., London, Tokyo), this allowance can be substantial—as much as 10 to 30 percent of the expatriate's total compensation package. A cost-of-living allowance ensures that the expatriate will enjoy the same standard of living in the foreign posting as at home. An education allowance ensures that an expatriate's children receive adequate schooling (by home-country standards). Host-country public schools are sometimes not suitable for an expatriate's children, in which case they must attend a private school.

Taxation

Unless a host country has a reciprocal tax treaty with the expatriate's home country, the expatriate may have to pay income tax to both the home- and host-country governments. When a reciprocal tax treaty is not in force, the firm typically pays the expatriate's income tax in the host country. In addition, firms normally make up the difference when a higher income tax rate in a host country reduces an expatriate's take-home pay.

Benefits

Many firms also ensure that their expatriates receive the same level of medical and pension benefits abroad that they received at home. This can be very costly for the firm, since many benefits that are tax deductible for the firm in the home country (e.g., medical and pension benefits) may not be deductible out of the country.

International Labor Relations ▮

The HRM function of an international business is typically responsible for international labor relations. From a strategic perspective, the key issue in international labor relations is the degree to which organized labor can limit the choices of an international business. A firm's ability to integrate and consolidate its global operations to realize experience curve and location economies can be limited by organized labor, constraining the pursuit of a transnational or global strategy. Prahalad and Doz cite the example of General Motors, which gained peace with labor unions by agreeing not to integrate and consolidate operations in the most efficient manner.[59] General Motors made substantial investments in Germany—matching its new investments in Austria and Spain—at the demand of the German metalworkers' unions.

One task of the HRM function is to foster harmony and minimize conflict between the firm and organized labor. With this in mind, this section is divided into three parts. First, we review organized labor's concerns about multinational enterprises. Second, we look at how organized labor has tried to deal with these concerns. And third, we look at how international businesses manage their labor relations to minimize labor disputes.

The Concerns of Organized Labor

Labor unions generally try to get better pay, greater job security, and better working conditions for their members through collective bargaining with management. Unions' bargaining power is derived largely from their ability to threaten to disrupt production, either by a strike or some other form of work protest (e.g., refusing to work overtime). This threat is credible, however, only insofar as management has no alternative but to employ union labor.

A principal concern of domestic unions about multinational firms is that the company can counter its bargaining power with the power to move production to another country. Ford, for example, very clearly threatened British unions with a plan to move manufacturing to Continental Europe unless British workers abandoned work rules that limited productivity, showed restraint in negotiating for wage increases, and curtailed strikes and other work disruptions.[60]

Another concern of organized labor is that an international business will keep highly skilled tasks in its home country and farm out only low-skilled tasks to foreign plants. Such a practice makes it relatively easy for an international business to switch production from one location to another as economic conditions warrant. Consequently, the bargaining power of organized labor is once more reduced.

A final union concern arises when an international business attempts to import employment practices and contractual agreements from its home country. When these practices are alien to the host country, organized labor fears the change will reduce its influence and power. This concern has surfaced in response to Japanese multinationals that have been trying to export their style of labor relations to other countries. For example, much to the annoyance of the United Auto Workers (UAW), many Japanese auto plants in the United States are not unionized. As a result, union influence in the auto industry is declining.

The Strategy of Organized Labor

Organized labor has responded to the increased bargaining power of multinational corporations by taking three actions: (1) trying to establish international labor organizations, (2) lobbying for national legislation to restrict multinationals, and (3) trying to achieve international regulations on multinationals through such organizations as the United Nations. These efforts have not been very successful.

In the 1960s, organized labor began to establish international trade secretariats (ITSs) to provide worldwide links for national unions in particular industries. The long-term goal was to be able to bargain transnationally with multinational firms. Organized labor believed that by coordinating union action across countries through an ITS, it could counter the power of a multinational corporation by threatening to disrupt production on an international scale. For example, Ford's threat to move production from Great Britain to other European locations would not have been credible if the unions in various European countries had united to oppose it.

However, the ITSs have had virtually no real success. Although national unions may want to cooperate, they also compete with each other to attract investment from international businesses, and hence jobs for their members. For example, in attempting to gain new jobs for their members, national unions in the auto industry often court auto firms that are seeking locations for new plants. One reason Nissan chose to build its European production facilities in Great Britain rather than Spain was that the British unions agreed to greater concessions than the Spanish unions did. As a result of such competition between national unions, cooperation is difficult to establish.

A further impediment to cooperation has been the wide variation in union structure. Trade unions developed independently in each country. As a result, the structure and ideology of unions tend to vary significantly from country to country, as does the nature of collective bargaining. For example, in Great Britain, France, and Italy many unions are controlled by left-wing socialists, who view collective bargaining through the lens of "class conflict." In contrast, most union leaders in Germany, the Netherlands, Scandinavia, and Switzerland are far more moderate politically. The ideological gap between union leaders in different countries has made cooperation difficult. Divergent ideologies are reflected in radically different views about the role of a union in society and the stance unions should take toward multinationals.

Organized labor has also met with only limited success in its efforts to get national and international bodies to regulate multinationals. Such international organizations as the International Labor Organization (ILO) and the Organization for Economic Cooperation and Development (OECD) have adopted codes of conduct for multinational firms to follow in labor relations. However, these guidelines are not as far-reaching as many unions would like. They also do not provide any enforcement mechanisms. Many researchers report that such guidelines are of only limited effectiveness.[61]

Approaches to Labor Relations

International businesses differ markedly in their approaches to international labor relations. The main difference is the degree to which labor relations activities are centralized or decentralized. Historically, most international businesses have decentralized international labor relations activities to their foreign subsidiaries because labor laws, union power, and the nature of collective bargaining varied so much from country to country. It made sense to decentralize the labor relations function to local managers. The belief was that there was no way central management could effectively handle the complexity of simultaneously managing labor relations in a number of different environments.

Although this logic still holds, there is now a trend toward greater centralized control. This trend reflects international firms' attempts to rationalize their global operations. The general rise in competitive pressure in industry after industry has made it more important for firms to control their costs. Because labor costs account for such a large percentage of total costs, many firms are now using the threat to move production to another country in their negotiations with unions to change work rules and limit wage increases (as Ford did in Europe). Because such a move would involve major new investments and plant closures, this bargaining tactic requires the input of headquarters management. Thus, the level of centralized input into labor relations is increasing.

In addition, the realization is growing that the way work is organized within a plant can be a major source of competitive advantage. Much of the competitive advantage of Japanese automakers, for example, has been attributed to the use of self-managing teams, job rotation, cross-training, and the like in their Japanese plants.[62] To replicate their domestic performance in foreign plants, the Japanese firms have tried to replicate their work practices there. This often brings them into direct conflict with traditional work practices in those countries, as sanctioned by the local labor unions, so the Japanese firms have often made their foreign investments contingent on the local union accepting a radical change in work practices. To achieve this, the headquarters of many Japanese firms bargains directly with local unions to get union agreement to changes in work rules before committing to an investment. For example, before Nissan decided to invest in northern England, it got a commitment from British unions to agree to a change in traditional work practices. By its very nature, pursuing such a strategy requires centralized control over the labor relations function.

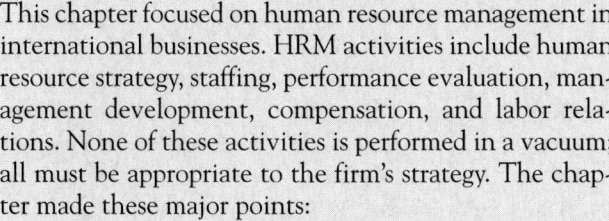

ChapterSummary

This chapter focused on human resource management in international businesses. HRM activities include human resource strategy, staffing, performance evaluation, management development, compensation, and labor relations. None of these activities is performed in a vacuum; all must be appropriate to the firm's strategy. The chapter made these major points:

1. Firm success requires HRM policies to be congruent with the firm's strategy and with its formal and informal structure and controls.

2. Staffing policy is concerned with selecting employees who have the skills required to perform particular jobs. Staffing policy can be a tool for developing and promoting a corporate culture.

3. An ethnocentric approach to staffing policy fills all key management positions in an international business with parent-country nationals. The policy is congruent with an international strategy. A drawback is that ethnocentric staffing can result in cultural myopia.

4. A polycentric staffing policy uses host-country nationals to manage foreign subsidiaries and

parent-country nationals for the key positions at corporate headquarters. This approach can minimize the dangers of cultural myopia, but it can create a gap between home- and host-country operations. The policy is best suited to a multidomestic strategy.

5. A geocentric staffing policy seeks the best people for key jobs throughout the organization, regardless of their nationality. This approach is consistent with building a strong unifying culture and informal management network and is well suited to both global and transnational strategies. Immigration policies of national governments may limit a firm's ability to pursue this policy.

6. A prominent issue in the international staffing literature is expatriate failure, defined as the premature return of an expatriate manager to his or her home country. The costs of expatriate failure can be substantial.

7. Expatriate failure can be reduced by selection procedures that screen out inappropriate candidates. The most successful expatriates seem to

be those who have high self-esteem and self-confidence, get along well with others, are willing to attempt to communicate in a foreign language, and can empathize with people of other cultures.

8. Training can lower the probability of expatriate failure. It should include cultural training, language training, and practical training, and it should be provided to both the expatriate manager and the spouse.

9. Management development programs attempt to increase the overall skill levels of managers through a mix of ongoing management education and rotation of managers through different jobs within the firm to give them varied experiences. Management development is often used as a strategic tool to build a strong unifying culture and informal management network, both of which support transnational and global strategies.

10. It can be difficult to evaluate the performance of expatriate managers objectively because of unintentional bias. A number of steps can be taken to reduce this bias.

11. Country differences in compensation practices raise a difficult question for an international business: Should the firm pay executives in different countries according to the standards in each country or equalize pay on a global basis?

12. The most common approach to expatriate pay is the balance sheet approach. This approach aims to equalize purchasing power so employees can enjoy the same living standard in their foreign posting that they had at home.

13. A key issue in international labor relations is the degree to which organized labor can limit the choices available to an international business. A firm's ability to pursue a transnational or global strategy can be significantly constrained by the actions of labor unions.

14. A principal concern of organized labor is that the multinational can counter union bargaining power with threats to move production to another country.

15. Organized labor has tried to counter the bargaining power of multinationals by forming international labor organizations. In general, these efforts have not been effective.

Critical Discussion Questions

1. What are the main advantages and disadvantages of the ethnocentric, polycentric, and geocentric approaches to staffing policy? When is each approach appropriate?

2. Research suggests that many expatriate employees encounter problems that limit both their effectiveness in a foreign posting and their contribution to the company when they return home. What are the main causes and consequences of these problems, and how might a firm reduce the occurrence of such problems?

3. What is the link between an international business's strategy and its human resource management policies, particularly with regard to the use of expatriate employees and their pay scale?

4. In what ways can organized labor constrain the strategic choices of an international business? How can an international business limit these constraints?

Research Task   globalEDGE™   globaledge.msu.edu

Use the globalEDGE™ to complete the following exercises:

1. The U.S. Department of State prepares quarterly reports for living costs abroad. Using the most current report identify the countries that are regarded as having a high cost of living and those that are perceived as risky. What are the living allowances and hardship differentials determined by the U.S. Department of State for those countries?

2. You work in the HR department at the headquarters of a multinational corporation. Your company is about to send several American managers overseas as expatriates. Utilize resources available on the globalEDGE website regarding expatriate life to compile a short checklist of concerns and steps for your company to go through before sending its managers overseas.

Notes

1. P. J. Dowling and R. S. Schuler, *International Dimensions of Human Resource Management* (Boston: PSW-Kent, 1990).

2. J. Millman, M. A. von Glinow, and M. Nathan, "Organizational Life Cycles and Strategic International Human Resource Management in Multinational Companies," *Academy of Management Review* 16 (1991), pp. 318–39.

3. See Peter Bamberger and Ilan Meshoulam, *Human Resource Strategy: Formulation, Implementation, and Impact* (Thousand Oaks, CA: Sage, 2000); P. M. Wright and S. Snell, "Towards a Unifying Framework for Exploring Fit and Flexibility in Human Resource Management; *Academy of Management Review* 23 (October 1998), pp. 756–72.

4. R. Colman, "HR Management Lags Behind at World Class Firms," CMA *Management*, July–August 2002, p. 9.

5. E. H. Schein, *Organizational Culture and Leadership* (San Francisco: Jossey-Bass, 1985).

6. H. V. Perlmutter, "The Tortuous Evolution of the Multinational Corporation," *Columbia Journal of World Business* 4 (1969), pp. 9–18; D. A. Heenan and H. V. Perlmutter, *Multinational Organizational Development* (Reading, MA: Addison-Wesley, 1979); D. A. Ondrack, "International Human Resources Management in European and North American Firms," *International Studies of Management and Organization* 15 (1985), pp. 6–32; and T. Jackson, "The Management of People across Cultures: Valuing People Differently," *Human Resource Management* 41 (2002), pp. 455–75.

7. V. Reitman and M. Schuman, "Men's Club: Japanese and Korean Companies Rarely Look Outside for People to Run Their Overseas Operations," *Wall Street Journal*, September 26, 1996, p. 17.

8. S. Beechler and J. Z. Yang, "The Transfer of Japanese Style Management to American Subsidiaries," *Journal of International Business Studies* 25 (1994), pp. 467–91. See also R. Konopaske, S. Warner, and K. E. Neupert, "Entry Mode Strategy and Performance: The Role of FDI Staffing," *Journal of Business Research*, September 2002, pp. 759–70.

9. M. Banai and L. M. Sama, "Ethical Dilemma in MNCs' International Staffing Policies," *Journal of Business Ethics*, June 2000, pp. 221–35.

10. Reitman and Schuman, "Men's Club: Japanese and Korean Companies Rarely Look Outside for People to Run Their Overseas Operations."

11. C. A. Bartlett and S. Ghoshal, *Managing across Borders: The Transnational Solution* (Boston: Harvard Business School Press, 1989).

12. S. J. Kobrin, "Geocentric Mindset and Multinational Strategy," *Journal of International Business Studies* 25 (1994), pp. 493–511.

13. P. M. Rosenzweig and N. Nohria, "Influences on Human Resource Management Practices in Multinational Corporations," *Journal of International Business Studies* 25 (1994), pp. 229–51.

14. Kobrin, "Geocentric Mindset and Multinational Strategy."

15. M. Harvey and H. Fung, "Inpatriate Managers: The Need for Realistic Relocation Reviews," *International Journal of Management* 17 (2000), pp. 151–59.

16. S. Black, M. Mendenhall, and G. Oddou, "Towards a Comprehensive Model of International Adjustment," *Academy of Management Review* 16 (1991), pp. 291–317, and J. Shay and T. J. Bruce, "Expatriate Managers," *Cornell Hotel & Restaurant Administration Quarterly*, February 1997, p. 30–40.

17. M. G. Harvey, "The Multinational Corporation's Expatriate Problem: An Application of Murphy's Law," *Business Horizons* 26 (1983), pp. 71–78.

18. J. Barbian, "Return to Sender," *Training*, January 2002, pp. 40–43.

19. Shay and Bruce, "Expatriate Managers." Also see J. S. Black and H. Gregersen, "The Right Way to Manage Expatriates," *Harvard Business Review*, March–April 1999, pp. 52–63.

20. Barbian, "Return to Sender."

21. Black, Mendenhall, and Oddou, "Towards a Comprehensive Model of International Adjustment."

22. R. L. Tung, "Selection and Training Procedures of U.S., European, and Japanese Multinationals," *California Management Review* 25 (1982), pp. 57–71.

23. C. M. Solomon, "Success Abroad Depends upon More Than Job Skills," *Personnel Journal*, April 1994, pp. 51–58.

24. C. M. Solomon, "Unhappy Trails," *Workforce*, August 2000, pp. 36–41.

25. Solomon, "Success Abroad Depends upon More Than Job Skills."

26. Solomon, "Unhappy Trails."

27. M. Harvey, "Addressing the Dual Career Expatriation Dilemma," *Human Resource Planning* 19, no. 4 (1996), pp. 18–32.

28. M. Mendenhall and G. Oddou, "The Dimensions of Expatriate Acculturation: A Review," *Academy of Management Review* 10 (1985), pp. 39–47.

29. I. Torbiorin, *Living Abroad: Personal Adjustment and Personnel Policy in the Overseas Setting* (New York: John Wiley & Sons, 1982).

30. R. L. Tung, "Selection and Training of Personnel for Overseas Assignments," *Columbia Journal of World Business* 16 (1981), pp. 68–78.

31. Solomon, "Success Abroad Depends upon More Than Job Skills."

32. S. Ronen, "Training and International Assignee," in *Training and Career Development*, ed. I. Goldstein (San Francisco: Jossey-Bass, 1985), and Tung, "Selection and Training of Personnel for Overseas Assignments."

33. Solomon, "Success Abroad Depends upon More Than Job Skills."

34. Harvey, "Addressing the Dual Career Expatriation Dilemma," and J. W. Hunt, "The Perils of Foreign Postings for Two," *Financial Times*, May 6, 1998, p. 22.

35. C. M. Daily, S. T. Certo, and D. R. Dalton, "International Experience in the Executive Suite: A Path to Prosperity?" *Strategic Management Journal* 21 (2000), pp. 515–23.

36. Dowling and Schuler, *International Dimensions of Human Resource Management*.

37. Ibid.

38. G. Baliga and J. C. Baker, "Multinational Corporate Policies for Expatriate Managers: Selection, Training, and Evaluation," *Advanced Management Journal*, Autumn 1985, pp. 31–38.

39. C. Rapoport, "A Tough Swede Invades the U.S.," *Fortune*, June 20, 1992, pp. 67–70.

40. J. C. Baker, "Foreign Language and Departure Training in U.S. Multinational Firms," *Personnel Administrator*, July 1984, pp. 68–70.

41. A 1997 study by the Conference Board looked at this in depth. For a summary, see L. Grant, "That Overseas Job Could Derail Your Career," *Fortune*, April 14, 1997, p. 166. Also see J. S. Black and H. Gregersen, "The Right Way to Manage Expatriates," *Harvard Business Review*, March–April 1999, pp. 52–63.

42. J. S. Black and M. E. Mendenhall, *Global Assignments: Successfully Expatriating and Repatriating International Managers* (San Francisco: Jossey-Bass, 1992), and K. Vermond, "Expatriates Come Home," *CMA Management*, October 2001, pp. 30–33.

43. Ibid.

44. Figures from the Conference Board study. For a summary, see Grant, "That Overseas Job Could Derail Your Career."

45. S. C. Schneider, "National v. Corporate Culture: Implications for Human Resource Management," *Human Resource Management* 27 (Summer 1988), pp. 231–46.

46. I. M. Manve and W. B. Stevenson, "Nationality, Cultural Distance and Expatriate Status," *Journal of International Business Studies* 32 (2001), pp. 285–303.

47. Bartlett and Ghoshal, *Managing across Borders*.

48. See G. Oddou and M. Mendenhall, "Expatriate Performance Appraisal: Problems and Solutions," in *International Human Resource Management*, ed. Mendenhall and Oddou (Boston: PWS-Kent, 1991); Dowling and Schuler, *International Dimensions*; R. S. Schuler and G. W. Florkowski, "International Human Resource Management," in *Handbook for International Management Research*, ed. B. J. Punnett and O. Shenkar (Oxford: Blackwell, 1996); and K. Roth and S. O'Donnell, "Foreign Subsidiary Compensation Strategy: An Agency Theory Perspective," *Academy of Management Journal* 39, no. 3 (1996), pp. 678–703.

49. Oddou and Mendenhall, "Expatriate Performance Appraisal."

50. "Expatriates Often See Little Benefit to Careers in Foreign Stints, Indifference at Home," *Wall Street Journal*, December 11, 1989, p. B1.

51. Oddou and Mendenhall, "Expatriate Performance Appraisal," and Schuler and Florkowski, "International Human Resource Management."

52. "Towers Perrin & Mercer Examine Pay Levels and Increases in 26 Countries," *Ioma's Report on Salary Surveys*, January 2001, pp. 2–4.

53. R. C. Longworth, "US Executives Sit on Top of the World," *Chicago Tribune*, May 31, 1998, p. C1.

54. "Towers Perrin Study Finds Increasingly Similar Approaches to Corporate Pay in Different Global Markets," *Business Wire*, December 3, 2001.

55. Organizational Resource Counselors, *2002 Survey of International Assignment Policies and Practices*, March 2003.

56. C. Reynolds, "Compensation of Overseas Personnel," in *Handbook of Human Resource Administration*, ed. J. J. Famularo (New York: McGraw-Hill, 1986).

57. M. Helms, "International Executive Compensation Practices," in *International Human Resource Management*, ed. M. Mendenhall and G. Oddou (Boston: PWS-Kent, 1991).

58. G. W. Latta, "Expatriate Incentives," *HR Focus* 75, no. 3 (March 1998), p. S3.

59. C. K. Prahalad and Y. L. Doz, *The Multinational Mission* (New York: The Free Press, 1987).

60. Ibid.

61. Schuler and Florkowski, "International Human Resource Management."

62. See J. P. Womack, D. T. Jones, and D. Roos, *The Machine That Changed the World* (New York: Rawson Associates, 1990).

Closing Case

Degrussa: Strategy and Human Resources in China

Germany's Degrussa AG is one of the largest chemical companies in the world with 2002 sales of euro 11.5 billion (approximately $11 billion). During the early 2000s, Degrussa underwent a major strategic transformation from a producer of low-margin commodity chemicals to high-margin specialty chemicals. Many of its products are customized to the unique needs of its customers and require significant investment in R&D and close collaboration with key customers.

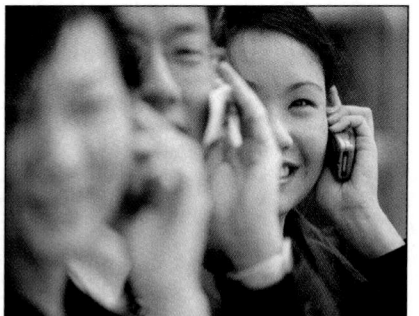

A major component of Degrussa's strategic shift, which involved numerous divestments and acquisitions, has been the establishment of significant operations in China. Degrussa sees China as the linchpin of its global strategy. By 2008, Degrussa anticipates that the Chinese specialty chemicals sector will leapfrog to a number two position, behind the European Union. Degrussa aims to be one of the major producers in specialty chemicals in China by that time period. In 2002, Degrussa generated euro 240 million from its Chinese operations, up from euro 210 million the previous year. The company has established 15 operating companies in China and an R&D center in Shanghai.

As part of its China strategy, Degrussa has established a goal of becoming one of China's most attractive employers. Degrussa believes that such a strategy is key if the company is going to achieve high productivity and profitability in China. One of the company's goals is to recruit as many exceptionally qualified young Chinese people as possible, many of whom will be slated to take on key management roles in China. To this end, Degrussa has established a "China Top Program." Emerging management personnel in the China region who display exceptional potential and outstanding performance are nominated for participation in this program by their business units. The nominees are then screened in a demanding assessment center set up by Degrussa for participation in the program. The first group to go through the program completed it in December 2002. This group will be assuming important management positions in Degrussa's Chinese companies in the near future. They will

also have the opportunity to aspire to leadership positions internationally within Degrussa's global network of operating companies. Already, the graduates of this program are working cooperatively across organizational boundaries, helping to establish the company's short- and midterm strategy for China.

More generally, Degrussa aspires to become the preferred employer in its industry in China. Among other things, this means a commitment to treating its Chinese employees on par with those in other locations around the world. As a practical matter, that means salary and benefit packages that are attractive relative to the local market. Degrussa's human resource policy is an extension of the company's corporate vision and its pledge to ensure the "fair treatment of our employees as well as deep respect for the diversity of different nationalities, cultures, and opinions." Also part of Degrussa's corporate vision is a commitment to include all members of Degrussa's staff in the process of defining the basic tenets and continually developing corporate culture. Emphasis is placed upon values that promote openness and fairness and upon flat hierarchies and team- or project-oriented work practices. The company also strives to foster innovation, encouraging every staff member, irrespective of nationality, to think like an entrepreneur.

Sources: "Like an Entrepreneur," *Asian Chemical News*, April 6, 2003, pp. 7–8; H. Tilton, "Executive Insight: Degrussa Is Poised to Explore New Markets," *Chemical Market Reporter*, April 21, 2003, p. 17; and "Successfully Different," *Asian Chemical News*, April 6, 2003, pp. 1–2.

Case Discussion Questions

1. How would you characterize Degrussa's staffing practices?

2. From a management development perspective, what is Degrussa trying to achieve through its China Top Program?

3. How does Degrussa's human resource strategy in China fit with the company's goals of attaining high productivity and profitability in China? How does it fit with the goals of fostering innovation and entrepreneurship?

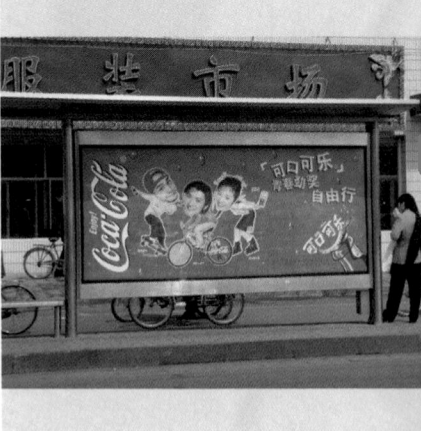

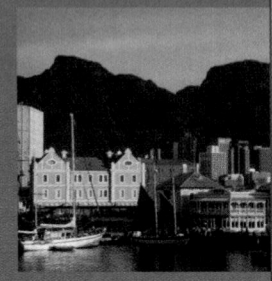

Chapter 19

Accounting in the International Business

Introduction
Country Differences in Accounting
Standards
  Relationship between Business and
  Providers of Capital
  Political and Economic Ties with Other
  Countries
  Inflation Accounting
  Level of Development
  Culture
  Accounting Clusters
National and International Standards
  Consequences of the Lack of
  Comparability
  International Standards
Multinational Consolidation and Currency
Translation
  Consolidated Financial Statements
  Currency Translation
  Current U.S. Practice
Accounting Aspects of Control Systems
  Exchange Rate Changes and Control
  Systems
  Transfer Pricing and Control Systems
  Separation of Subsidiary and Manager
  Performance
Chapter Summary
Critical Discussion Questions
Closing Case: China's Evolving
Accounting System

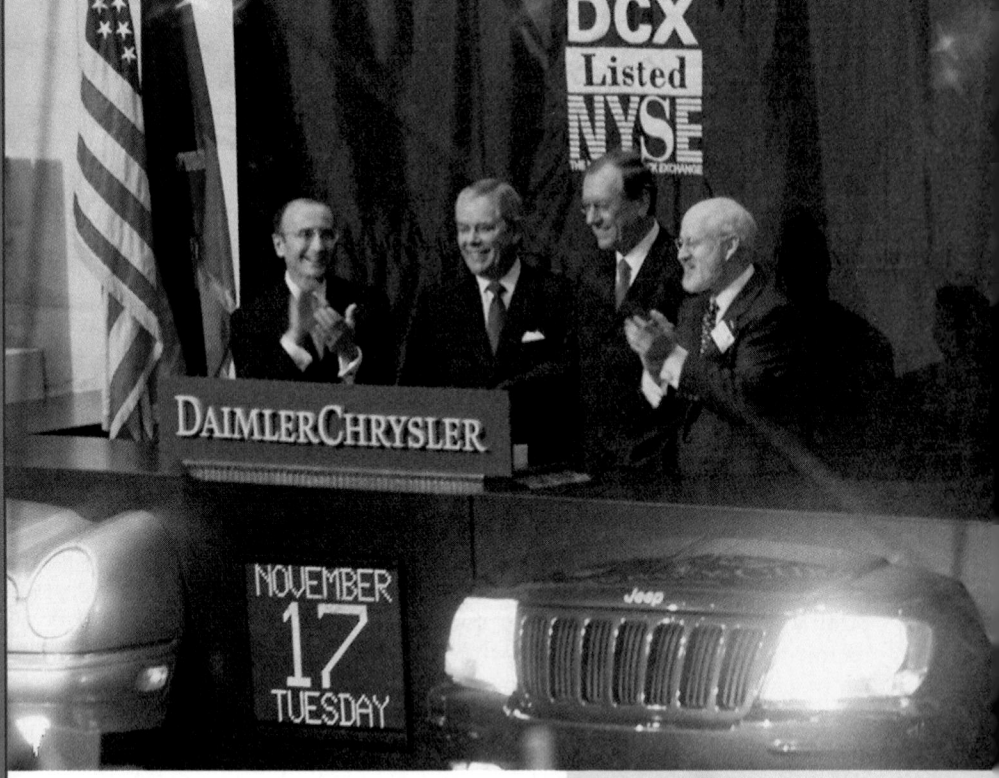

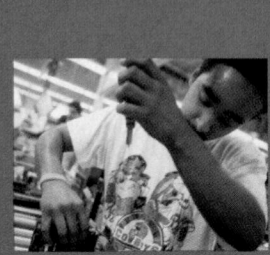

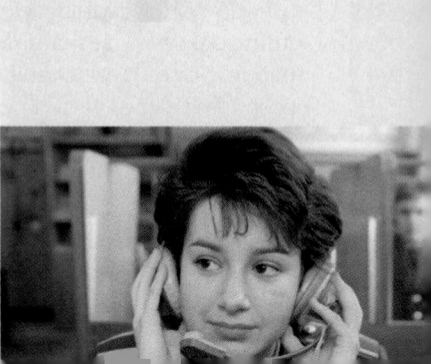

The Adoption of International Accounting Standards in Germany

A number of major German firms have begun to adopt international accounting standards that reveal far more about their financial performance than hitherto. This represents a major shift away from inscrutable German accounting standards that often hid as much about a company's financial performance as they revealed. The change has been driven by recognition that German capital markets are too narrow and illiquid to satisfy the future funding requirements of many major German companies. These corporations are realizing it is in their best interests to get a listing on the New York Stock Exchange (NYSE), the world's largest capital market, as a prelude to issuing equity and raising debt through the New York market.

Historically, German firms have almost never resorted to international capital markets to raise additional equity. Their view was that bank debt was adequate. However, the German market for debt has become expensive, while the possibility of raising additional equity in Germany has been limited by the relatively small and illiquid nature of the German equity market. The move among German firms to raise equity on international capital markets began in the early 1990s when a number of major German firms, including Daimler-Benz, Siemens, and Volkswagen, applied to the U.S. Securities and Exchange Commission (SEC) for a listing. The SEC, however, was not particularly responsive. In the SEC's view, German accounting standards were not comparable to those in the United States and did not provide sufficient information to investors. Among the SEC's objections was the German practice of not disclosing the size of a company's financial reserves and pension fund commitments, as well as the more liberal policy for writing down goodwill in Germany, which tended to overstate a firm's financial performance relative to that which would be reported under U.S. accounting rules.

However, Daimler-Benz announced in 1993 that it had reached an agreement with the SEC and would soon have a listing on the NYSE. To achieve this, Daimler-Benz had to issue two sets of accounts, one that adhered to German standards and another that adhered to U.S. generally accepted accounting principles (GAAP). When Daimler-Benz reported its 1994 financial results, the impact of using different accounting standards was readily apparent. Under German rules, Daimler-Benz reported a profit of more than $100 million, but under GAAP, the company reported a $1 billion loss!

Several other German firms announced they were willing to adopt international accounting standards. International accounting standards (IAS) are devised by the London-based International Accounting Standards Board (IASB). The IASB and its predecessor, the International Accounting Standards Committee (IASC), have been attempting to harmonize accounting rules that historically have varied significantly from country to country. The international standards are more forthcoming about financial performance than the German rules. However, they still fall short of the U.S. GAAP, primarily because they allow for a looser treatment of goodwill. In March 1995, the pharmaceutical company Schering AG became the first German firm to shift to international standards. It was followed by two other major German firms, Bayer AG and Hoechst AG. In 1997, Hoechst became the second German firm to list its shares on the NYSE. To support its listing, Hoechst issued two sets of accounts, one in accordance with IAS principles and one in accordance with GAAP. Under the IAS principles, Hoechst reported profits of $1.2 billion in 1995 and $1.4 billion in 1996. Under the more restrictive GAAP, it lost $40 million in 1995 and $708 million in 1996!

Even though adhering to GAAP apparently reduces the reported profit of German firms, others seem willing to follow these standards to gain access to the U.S. capital market. Allianz, a large German insurance company, adopted IAS principles as a prelude to seeking a listing on the NYSE. Allianz believes such a listing will help it finance acquisitions of other firms in the large U.S. insurance market. Under the IAS principles, Allianz became the first German insurance company to reveal the size of its "hidden reserves"—defined as the difference between the book value of its assets and their current market value. Because insurance companies generally invest the proceeds from insurance premiums in financial assets, such as stocks, and because the value of these assets tends to appreciate as the stock market rises, their market value can be substantial. However, their market value also fluctuates sharply with the value of the stock market, which is why German companies have preferred to keep them secret. In early 1998, the value of Allianz's hidden assets stood at $56.1 billion, but as the company pointed out, a sharp fall in the value of the stock market would cause a comparable fall in the assets. Nevertheless, because U.S. insurance companies always reveal the market value of such assets, Allianz must do so if it is to list its stock on the NYSE. The trend continued in 2001 when Deutsche Bank adopted U.S. GAAP principles as a prelude to its October 2001 listing on the NYSE. Also in 2001, Volkswagen, a company renowned for its opaque accounting practices, announced that as of 2002 it would issue two sets of accounts, one using German accounting standards and a second adhering to IAS rules. A taste of how this might change Volkswagen's reported results was given in the first six months of 2001 when Volkswagen announced that its pretax operating margin under German accounting rules rose to 3.4 percent from 3.2 percent a year earlier, but under IAS rules it fell from 5.6 percent to 4.8 percent.

Sources: P. Gumbel and G. Steinmetz, "German Firms Shift to More Open Accounting," *Wall Street Journal,* March 15, 1995, p. C1; "Daimler-Benz: A Capital Suggestion," *The Economist,* April 9, 1994, p. 69; L. Berton, "All Accountants May Soon Speak the Same Language," *Wall Street Journal,* August 29, 1995, p. A15; R. Atkins, "Allianz Plans to Seek New York Listing," *Financial Times,* May 29, 1998, p. 30; G. Meek, "Accountants Gather Round Different Standards," *Financial Times,* March 20, 1998, p. 12. D. I. Oyama, "World Watch," *Wall Street Journal,* June 30, 2001, p. A15; and R. Dzinkowski, "A View from Germany," *Financial Executive,* July–August 2002, pp. 20–23.

■ Introduction

Accounting has often been referred to as "the language of business."[1] This language finds expression in profit-and-loss statements, balance sheets, budgets, investment analysis, and tax analysis. Accounting information is the means by which firms communicate their financial position to the providers of capital investors, creditors, and government. It enables the providers of capital to assess the value of their investments or the security of their loans and to make decisions about future resource allocations (see Figure 19.1). Accounting information is also the means by which firms report their income to the government so the government can assess how much tax the firm owes. It is also the means by which the firm can evaluate its performance, control its internal expenditures, and plan for future expenditures and income. Thus, a good accounting function is critical to the smooth running of the firm.

International businesses face a number of accounting problems that do not confront purely domestic businesses. The opening case draws attention to one of these problems—the lack of consistency in the accounting standards of different countries. We begin this chapter by looking at the source of these country differences. Then we shift our attention to attempts to establish international accounting and auditing standards—the International Accounting Standards Board (IASB).

We will examine the problems arising when an international business with operations in more than one country must produce consolidated financial statements. As we will see, these firms face special problems because, for example, the accounts for their operations in Brazil will be in *real,* in Korea they will be in *won,* and in Japan they will be in *yen.* If the firm is based in the United States, it will have to decide what basis to use for translating all these accounts into U.S. dollars. The last issue we discuss is control in an international business. We touched on the issue of control in Chapter 13 in rather abstract terms. Here we look at control from an accounting perspective.

Figure 19.1

Accounting Information and Capital Flows

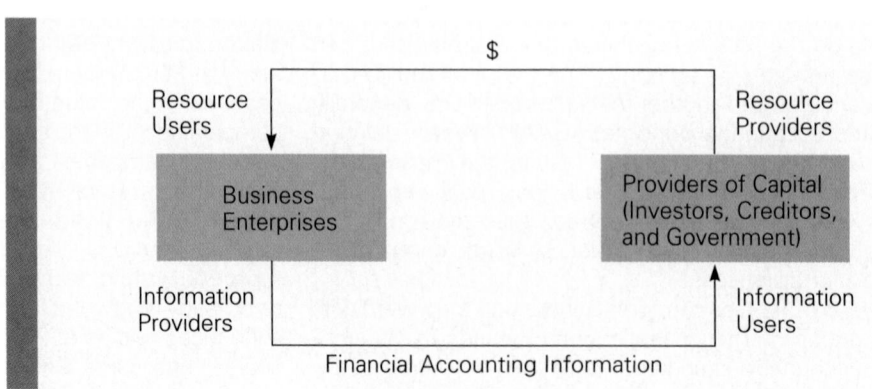

Country Differences in Accounting Standards ■

Accounting is shaped by the environment in which it operates. Just as different countries have different political systems, economic systems, and cultures, they also have different accounting systems.[2] In each country, the accounting system has evolved in response to the demands for accounting information.

An example of differences in accounting conventions concerns employee disclosures. In many European countries, government regulations require firms to publish detailed information about their training and employment policies, but there is no such requirement in the United States. Another difference is in the treatment of goodwill. A firm's goodwill is any advantage, such as a trademark or brand name (e.g., the Coca-Cola brand name), that enables a firm to earn higher profits than its competitors. When one company acquires another in a takeover, the value of the goodwill is calculated as the amount paid for a firm above its book value, which is often substantial. Under accounting rules prevailing in many countries, acquiring firms are allowed to deduct the value of goodwill from the amount of equity or net worth reported on their balance sheet. In the United States, goodwill has to be deducted from the profits of the acquiring firm over as much as 40 years (although firms typically write down goodwill much more rapidly). If two equally profitable firms, one German and one American, acquire comparable firms that have identical goodwill, the U.S. firm will report a much lower profit than the German firm, because of differences in accounting conventions regarding goodwill.[3]

Despite attempts to harmonize standards by developing internationally acceptable accounting conventions (more on this later), a myriad of differences between national accounting systems still remain. A study tried to quantify the extent of these differences by comparing various accounting measures and profitability ratios across 22 developed nations, including Australia, Britain, France, Germany, Hong Kong, Japan, Spain, and South Korea.[4] The study found that among the 22 countries, there were 76 differences in the way cost of goods sold was assessed, 65 differences in the assessment of return on assets, 54 differences in the measurement of research and development expenses as a percentage of sales, and 20 differences in the calculation of net profit margin. These differences make it very difficult to compare the financial performance of firms based in different nation-states.

Although many factors can influence the development of a country's accounting system, there appear to be five main variables:[5]

1. The relationship between business and the providers of capital.
2. Political and economic ties with other countries.
3. The level of inflation.
4. The level of a country's economic development.
5. The prevailing culture in a country.

Figure 19.2 illustrates these variables. We will review each in turn.

|Relationship between Business and Providers of Capital

The three main external sources of capital for business enterprises are individual investors, banks, and government. In most advanced countries, all three sources are important. In the United States, for example, business firms can raise capital by selling shares and bonds to individual investors through the stock market and the bond market. They can also borrow capital from banks and, in rather limited cases (particularly to support investments in defense-related R&D), from the government. The importance of each source of capital varies from country to country. In some countries, such

Figure 19.2

Determinants of National
Accounting Standards

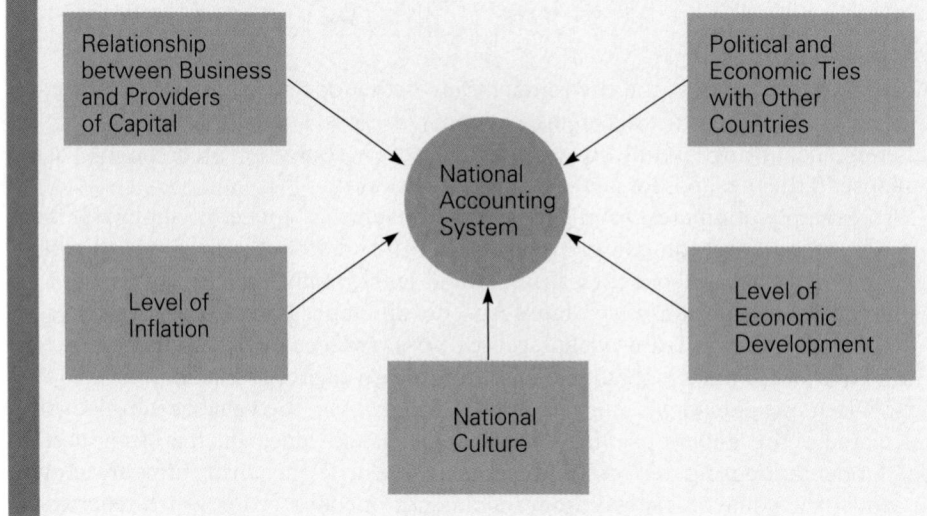

as the United States, individual investors are the major source of capital; in others, banks play a greater role; in still others, the government is the major provider of capital. A country's accounting system tends to reflect the relative importance of these three constituencies as providers of capital.

Consider the case of the United States and Great Britain. Both have well-developed stock and bond markets in which firms can raise capital by selling stocks and bonds to individual investors. Most individual investors purchase only a very small proportion of a firm's total outstanding stocks or bonds. As such, they have no desire to be involved in the day-to-day management of the firms in which they invest; they leave that task to professional managers. But because of their lack of contact with the management of the firms in which they invest, individual investors may not have the information required to assess how well the companies are performing. Because of their small stake in firms, individual investors generally lack the ability to get information on demand from management. The financial accounting system in both Great Britain and the United States evolved to cope with this problem. In both countries, the financial accounting system is oriented toward providing individual investors with the information they need to make decisions about purchasing or selling corporate stocks and bonds.

In countries such as Switzerland, Germany, and Japan, a few large banks satisfy most of the capital needs of business enterprises. Individual investors play a relatively minor role. In these countries, the role of the banks is so important that a bank's officers often have seats on the boards of firms to which it lends capital. In such circumstances, the information needs of the capital providers are satisfied in a relatively straightforward way—through personal contacts, direct visits, and information provided at board meetings. Consequently, although firms still prepare financial reports, because government regulations in these countries mandate some public disclosure of a firm's financial position, the reports tend to contain less information than those of British or U.S. firms. Because banks are the major providers of capital, financial accounting practices are oriented toward protecting a bank's investment. Thus, assets are valued conservatively and liabilities are overvalued (in contrast to U.S. practice) to provide a cushion for the bank in the event of default.

In still other countries, the national government has historically been an important provider of capital, and this has influenced accounting practices. This is the case in France and Sweden, where the national government has often stepped in to make loans or to invest in firms whose activities are deemed in the "national interest." In these countries, financial accounting practices tend to be oriented toward the needs of government planners.

Political and Economic Ties with Other Countries

Similarities in the accounting systems of countries are sometimes due to the countries' close political and/or economic ties. For example, the U.S. system has influenced accounting practices in Canada and Mexico, and since passage of NAFTA, the accounting systems in these three countries seem set to converge on a common set of norms. U.S.-style accounting systems are also used in the Philippines, which was once a U.S. protectorate. Another significant force in accounting worldwide has been the British system. The vast majority of former colonies of the British Empire have accounting practices modeled after Great Britain's. Similarly, the European Union has been attempting to harmonize accounting practices in its member countries. The accounting systems of EU members such as Great Britain, Germany, and France are quite different now, but if the EU has its way, they will converge on International Accounting Standards Board norms by 2005.

Inflation Accounting

In many countries, including Germany, Japan, and the United States, accounting is based on the **historic cost principle.** This principle assumes the currency unit used to report financial results is not losing its value due to inflation. Firms record sales, purchases, and the like at the original transaction price and make no adjustments in the amounts later. The historic cost principle affects accounting most significantly in the area of asset valuation. If inflation is high, the historic cost principle underestimates a firm's assets, so the depreciation charges based on these underestimates can be inadequate for replacing assets when they wear out or become obsolete.

The appropriateness of this principle varies inversely with the level of inflation in a country. The high level of price inflation in many industrialized countries during the 1970s and 1980s created a need for accounting methods that adjust for inflation. A number of industrialized countries adopted new practices. One of the most far-reaching approaches was adopted in Great Britain in 1980. Called **current cost accounting,** it adjusts all items in a financial statement—assets, liabilities, costs, and revenues—to factor out the effects of inflation. The method uses a general price index to convert historic figures into current values. The standard was not made compulsory, however, and once Great Britain's inflation rate fell in the 1980s, most firms stopped providing the data.

Level of Development

Developed nations tend to have large, complex organizations, whose accounting problems are far more difficult than those of small organizations. Developed nations also tend to have sophisticated capital markets in which business organizations raise funds from investors and banks. These providers of capital require that the organizations they invest in and lend to provide comprehensive reports of their financial activities. The work forces of developed nations tend to be highly educated and skilled and can perform complex accounting functions. For all these reasons, accounting in developed countries tends to be far more sophisticated than it is in less developed countries, where the accounting standards may be fairly primitive. In much of the developing world, the accounting system used was inherited from former colonial powers. Many African nations for example, have accounting practices based on either the British or French models, depending on which was the former colonial power. These models may not apply very well to small businesses in a poorly developed economy. Another problem in many of the world's poorer countries is a lack of trained accountants.[6]

Culture

A number of academic accountants have argued that the culture of a country has an important impact upon the nature of its accounting system.[7] Using the cultural typologies developed by Hofstede,[8] which we reviewed in Chapter 3, researchers have found that the extent to which a culture is characterized by uncertainty avoidance seems to have an impact on accounting systems.[9] **Uncertainty avoidance** refers to the extent to which cultures socialize their members to accept ambiguous situations and tolerate uncertainty. Members of high uncertainty avoidance cultures place a premium on job security, career patterns, retirement benefits, and so on. They also have a strong need for rules and regulations; the manager is expected to issue clear instructions, and subordinates' initiatives are tightly controlled. Lower uncertainty avoidance cultures are characterized by a greater readiness to take risks and less emotional resistance to change. According to Hofstede, countries such as Britain, the United States, and Sweden are characterized by low uncertainty avoidance, while countries such as Japan, Mexico, and Greece have higher uncertainty avoidance. Research suggests that countries with low uncertainty avoidance cultures tend to have strong independent auditing professions that audit a firm's accounts to make sure they comply with generally accepted accounting regulations.[10]

Accounting Clusters

Few countries have identical accounting systems. Notable similarities between nations do exist, however, and three groups of countries with similar standards are identified in Map 19.1.[11] One group might be called the British-American-Dutch group. Great Britain, the United States, and the Netherlands are the trendsetters in this group. All these countries have large, well-developed stock and bond markets where firms raise capital from investors. Thus, their accounting systems are tailored to providing information to individual investors. A second group might be called the Europe-Japan group. Firms in these countries have very close ties to banks, which supply a large proportion of their capital needs. Therefore, their accounting practices are geared to the needs of banks. A third group might be the South American group. The countries in this group have all experienced persistent and rapid inflation. Consequently, they have adopted inflation accounting principles.

National and International Standards

The diverse accounting practices discussed in the previous section have been enshrined in national accounting and auditing standards. **Accounting standards** are rules for preparing financial statements; they define what is useful accounting information. **Auditing standards** specify the rules for performing an audit—the technical process by which an independent person (the auditor) gathers evidence for determining if financial accounts conform to required accounting standards and if they are also reliable.

Lack of Comparability

An unfortunate result of national differences in accounting and auditing standards is the general lack of comparability of financial reports from one country to another. For example, consider the following:

- Dutch standards favor the use of current values for replacement assets; Japanese law generally prohibits revaluation and prescribes historic cost.
- Capitalization of financial leases is required practice in Great Britain, but it is not practiced in France.
- Research and development costs must be written off in the year they are incurred in the United States, but in Spain they may be deferred as an asset and need not be amortized as long as benefits that will cover them are expected to arise in the future.
- German accountants treat depreciation as a liability, whereas British companies deduct it from assets.

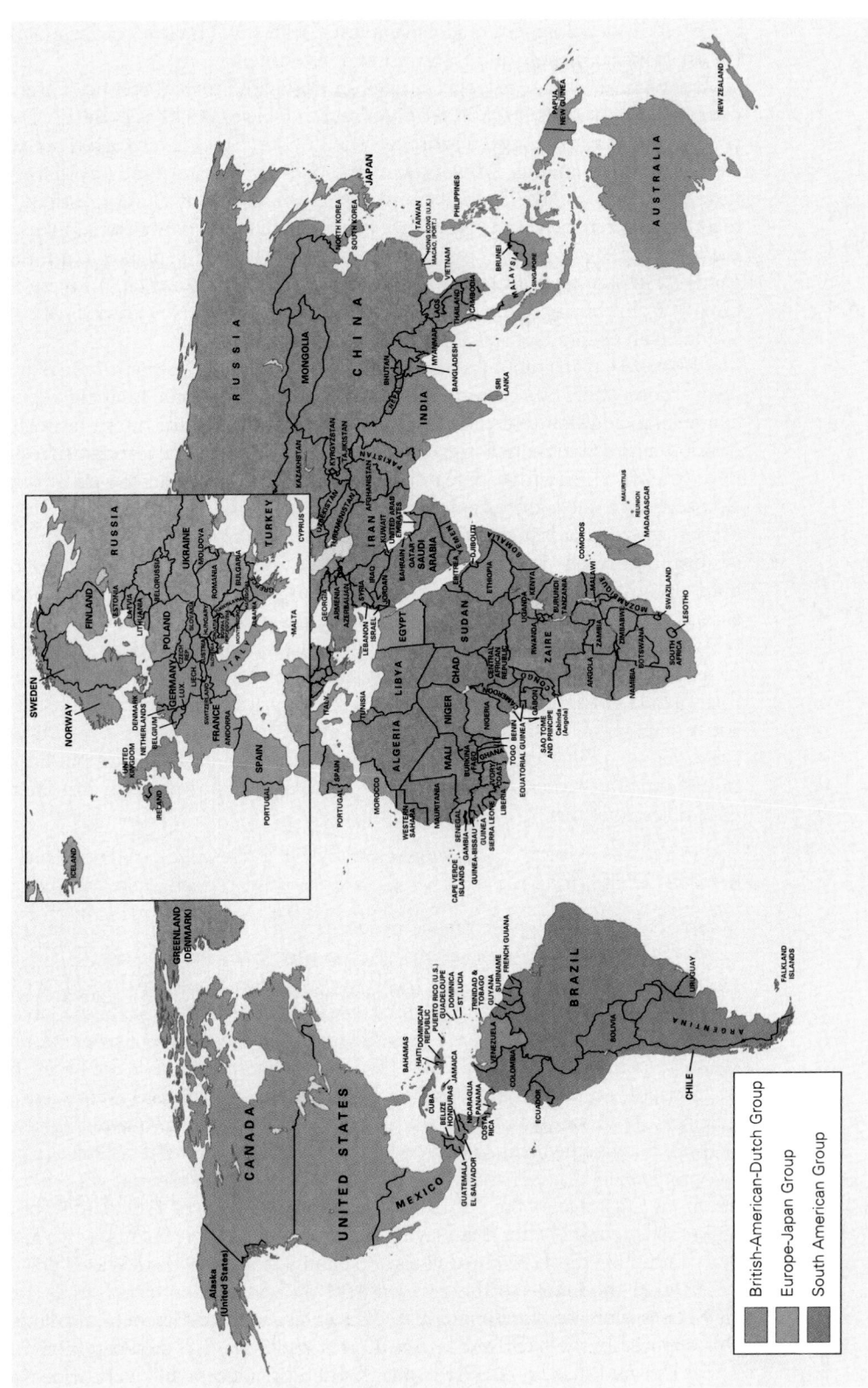

Map 19.1

Accounting Clusters

British-American-Dutch Group

Europe-Japan Group

South American Group

Such differences would not matter much if there was little need for a firm headquartered in one country to report its financial results to citizens of another country. However, as detailed in Chapter 11, one striking development of the past two decades has been the development of global capital markets. We have seen the growth of both transnational financing and transnational investment.

Transnational financing occurs when a firm based in one country enters another country's capital market to raise capital from the sale of stocks or bonds. A Danish firm raising capital by selling stock through the London Stock Exchange is an example of transnational financing. As we saw in the opening case, a number of large German firms are increasing their use of transnational financing by gaining listings, and ultimately issuing stock, on the New York Stock Exchange. Transnational investment occurs when an investor based in one country enters the capital market of another nation to invest in the stocks or bonds of a firm based in that country. An investor based in Great Britain buying General Motors stock through the New York Stock Exchange would be an example of transnational investment.

The rapid expansion of transnational financing and investment in recent years has been accompanied by a corresponding growth in transnational financial reporting. For example, in addition to its Danish financial reports, the Danish firm raising capital in London must issue financial reports that serve the needs of its British investors. Similarly, the U.S. firm with a large number of British investors might wish to issue reports that serve the needs of those investors. However, the lack of comparability between accounting standards in different nations can lead to confusion. For example, the Danish firm that issues two sets of financial reports, one set prepared under Danish standards and the other under British standards, may find that its financial position looks significantly different in the two reports, and its investors may have difficulty identifying the firm's true worth. Some examples of the confusion that can arise from this lack of comparability appear in the accompanying Management Focus.

In addition to the problems this lack of comparability gives investors, it can give the firm major headaches. The firm has to explain to its investors why its financial position looks so different in the two accountings. Also, an international business may find it difficult to assess the financial positions of important foreign customers, suppliers, and competitors.

International Standards

Substantial efforts have been made in recent years to harmonize accounting standards across countries.[12] The **International Accounting Standards Board** (IASB) is a major proponent of standardization. The IASB was formed in March 2001 to replace the International Accounting Standards Committee (IASC), which was established in 1973. The IASB has 14 members who are responsible for the formulation of new international financial reporting standards. By 2003, the IASB and its predecessor, the IASC, had issued 41 international accounting standards.[13] To issue a new standard, 75 percent of the 14 members of the board must agree. It can be difficult to get three-quarters agreement, particularly because members come from different cultures and legal systems. To get around this problem, most IASB statements provide two acceptable alternatives. As Arthur Wyatt, former chairman of the IASB, once said, "It's not much of a standard if you have two alternatives, but it's better than having six. If you can get agreement on two alternatives, you can capture the 11 required votes and eliminate some of the less used practices."[14]

Another hindrance to the development of international accounting standards is that compliance is voluntary; the IASB has no power to enforce its standards. Despite this, support for the IASB and recognition of its standards is growing. Increasingly, the IASB is regarded as an effective voice for defining acceptable worldwide accounting principles. Japan, for example, began requiring financial statements to be prepared on a consolidated basis after the IASB issued its initial standards on the topic. Russia and China have also stated their intention to adopt emerging international standards.

The Consequences of Different Accounting Standards

Management Focus

In 1999, the two major drug firms Zeneca and Astra merged to form AstraZeneca, based in the United Kingdom. In 2000 the profit of AstraZeneca was $865 million under U.S. accounting rules, but $3,318 million under British accounting rules. The largest difference between the two sets of accounts was the $1,756 million related to amortization and other acquisition-related costs. Under U.S. rules, the combination of Astra and Zeneca was treated as an acquisition, which required goodwill to be recognized with consequent amortization. Under British rules, any amortization was avoided as the combination was treated as a merger and so no goodwill arose.

U.S.-based SmithKline Beckman (SKB) merged with the British company Beecham Group in 1989. After the merger, SKB had quotations on both the London and New York stock exchanges, so it had to prepare financial reports in accordance with both U.S. and British standards. SKB's postmerger earnings, properly prepared in accordance with British accounting standards, were £130 million—quite a bit more than the £87 million reported in SKB's statement prepared in accordance with U.S. accounting standards. The difference resulted primarily from treating the merger as a pooling of assets for British purposes and as a purchase of assets for U.S. purposes. Even more confusing, the differences resulted in a shareholders' equity of £3.5 billion in the United States, but a negative £300 million in Great Britain! Not surprisingly, after these figures were released, SKB's stock was trading 17 percent lower on the London Stock Exchange than on the New York Stock Exchange.

In the mid-1980s, Telefonica, Spain's largest industrial company, was the first company in the world to float a multicountry stock offering simultaneously. In 1990, it reported net income under U.S. accounting standards of 176 billion pesetas, more than twice the 76 billion pesetas it reported under Spanish accounting standards. The difference was mainly due to an "add-back" of the incremental depreciation on assets carried at historic cost in the United States but reflecting more recent market value in the Spanish report. The effect of this difference on shareholders' equity was in the opposite direction; the equity reported in the U.S. accounts was 15 percent less than the equity reported in the Spanish accounts.

In 2000, British Airways reported a loss under British accounting rules of £21 million, but under U.S. rules, its loss was £412 million. Most of the difference could be attributed to adjustments for a number of relative small items such as depreciation and amortization, pensions, and deferred taxation. The largest adjustment was due to a reduction in revenue reported in the U.S. accounts of £136 million. This reduced revenue was related to frequent flyer miles, which under U.S. rules have to be deferred until the miles are redeemed. Apparently, this is not the case under British rules.

A final example is more hypothetical in nature, but just as revealing. Two college professors set up a computer model to evaluate the reported net profits of an imaginary company with gross operating profits of $1.5 million. This imaginary company operated in three different countries—the United States, Britain, and Australia. The professors found that holding all else equal (such as national differences in interest rates on the firm's debt), when different accounting standards were applied the firm made a net profit of $34,600 in the United States, $260,600 in Britain, and $240,600 in Australia.

Sources: S. F. O'Malley, "Accounting across Borders," *Financial Executive,* March–April 1992, pp. 28–31; L. Berton, "All Accountants May Soon Speak the Same Language," *Wall Street Journal,* August 29, 1995, p. A15; and "GAAP Reconciliations," *Company Reporting,* July 2001, pp. 3–6.

The impact of the IASB standards has probably been least noticeable in the United States because most of the standards issued by the IASB have been consistent with opinions already articulated by the U.S. **Financial Accounting Standards Board** **(FASB).** The FASB writes the generally accepted accounting principles by which the financial statements of U.S. firms must be prepared. In sharp contrast, some IASB standards have had a significant impact in many other countries because they eliminated a commonly used alternative.

Another body that promises to have substantial influence on the harmonization of accounting standards, at least within Europe, is the European Union (EU). In accordance with its plans for closer economic and political union, the EU is attempting to harmonize the accounting principles of its 15 member countries. The EU does this by issuing directives that the member states are obligated to incorporate into their own national laws. Because EU directives have the power of law, we might assume the EU has a better chance of achieving harmonization than the IASB does, but the EU is experiencing implementation difficulties. These difficulties arise from the wide variation in accounting practices among EU member countries. Accounting practices in Great Britain, for example, are closer to those of the United States than to those of France or Germany. Despite these difficulties, developments in the EU should be watched closely. If the EU achieves harmonization (in all probability, it eventually will), the accounting principles adopted in the EU could have a major influence on future IASB pronouncements. The current timeline calls for the EU to harmonize accounting standards among member states by 2005. Significantly, the EU is calling for harmonization under IASB standards. If implemented, the changes would be very significant. As of 2001, only one-fifth of the 300 leading companies in Europe employed IASB rules to compile their financial reports.[15]

Assuming that the EU is successful in achieving harmonization according to IASB standards, and that countries like Australia, Japan, China, and Russia follow suit as they have signaled that they will, by late in the decade, two major accounting bodies could have dominant influence on global reporting: FASB in the United States and IASB elsewhere. Under an agreement reached in 2002, these two bodies will increasingly work together to align their standards, suggesting that differences in accounting standards across countries may eventually disappear.

In a move that indicates the trend toward adoption of acceptable international accounting standards is accelerating, the IASB has developed accounting standards for firms seeking stock listings in global markets. Also, the FASB has joined forces with accounting standard setters in Canada, Mexico, and Chile to explore areas in which the four countries can harmonize their accounting standards (Canada, Mexico, and the United States are members of NAFTA, and Chile may join in the near future). The Securities and Exchange Commission has also dropped some of its objections to international standards, which could accelerate their adoption. In 1994, the SEC for the first time accepted three international accounting standards on cash flow data, the effects of hyperinflation, and business combinations for cross-border filings.[16] A taste of what is to come if increasing numbers of international firms adopt IASB principles can be found in the accompanying Management Focus, which details the impact of adopting these standards on Ciba, the Swiss pharmaceuticals and chemicals group.

Multinational Consolidation and Currency Translation

A consolidated financial statement combines the separate financial statements of two or more companies to yield a single set of financial statements as if the individual companies were really one. Most multinational firms are composed of a parent company and a number of subsidiary companies located in various other countries. Such firms typically issue consolidated financial statements, which merge the accounts of all the companies, rather than issuing individual financial statements for the parent company and each subsidiary. In this section, we examine the consolidated financial statements and then look at the related issue of foreign currency translation.

Consolidated Financial Statements

Many firms find it advantageous to organize as a set of separate legal entities (companies). For example, a firm may separately incorporate the various components of its business to limit its total legal liability or to take advantage of corporate tax regula-

Management Focus

Novartis Joins the International Accounting Club

Switzerland does not have a history of very detailed accounting rules. As a result, published financial statements by major Swiss firms such as Novartis, Roche Group, and Nestlé often obscured as much as they revealed. The standard set of accounts from a Swiss firm was viewed as being very unusual and difficult for international investors to understand and was described as being more like a statistical summary than the result of an integrated accounting system.

Swiss firms began to move toward adoption of IASC accounting principles in the early 1990s. The catalyst was increasing interest by foreign investors in the stock of major Swiss corporations. By the early 1990s, up to 40 percent of the stock of many of these firms was owned by foreign investors. As a group, these investors were demanding more detailed financial statements that were comparable to those issued by other multinational enterprises.

One of the first firms to respond to these pressures was Ciba, Switzerland's largest pharmaceuticals and chemicals firm and a major multinational enterprise with operations around the globe (Ciba subsequently became Novartis after it merged with another Swiss pharmaceutical company, Sandoz, in 1998). In 1993, the company announced that its 1994 financial statements would be in accordance with IASC guidelines. At the same time, it restated its 1992 results in line with IASC guidelines. The effect was to increase post-tax profits by 18 percent while raising inventories, cash, and marketable securities. Ciba's decision was motivated by a desire to appease foreign stockholders, who in 1994 held over one-third of Ciba's stock, and to position itself for the possibility of listings on the London and New York stock markets.

Ciba also decided to use the same international standards for internal financial reporting. Ciba set up a small international team to develop and implement its new system. While there were some preliminary problems in development of the system, including a

figure on the insurance value of fixed assets that was off by $690 million, the new system is now running smoothly and seems to have produced several major benefits.

Ciba discovered large savings as a result of the change, including tighter cash management, more efficient capital investment, a different approach to acquisitions, and more rigid asset management, which has reportedly reduced the value of inventories by 6 percent. The new system also enabled Ciba to benchmark its performance for the first time against its global competitors.

One big difference between the new and old systems was the move from the arguably more informative current cost accounting method, which Ciba had used for over 25 years and which regularly updates asset values to account for inflation, to historic cost accounting under international standards. However, Ciba's management admits this drawback is not serious given the low inflation rate in Switzerland and given the offsetting gains produced by the switch to a new system.

In 2000, Novartis, which was formed when Ciba merged with Sandoz in 1998, decided it needed to become more aggressive about attracting U.S. investors. Although Novartis already listed its shares as American Depositary Receipts (ADRs) on the American Stock Exchange, it decided to switch the listing to the more visible New York Stock Exchange and to double the amount of ADRs offered. Accompanying this shift, Novartis also decided that in addition to presenting its rules based on IASC principles, it needed to adopt full U.S. accounting principles. Novartis published its first complete set of U.S. accounts in 2002.

Sources: A. Jack, "Swiss Group Moves from Night to Day," *Financial Times,* March 30, 1994, p. 22; L. Berton, "All Accountants May Soon Speak the Same Language," *Wall Street Journal,* August 29, 1995, p. A15; and A. Beard, "Novartis Steps up the Pace of Its U.S. Charm Offensive," *Financial Times,* May 14, 2001, p. 23.

tions. Multinationals are often required by the countries in which they do business to set up a separate company. Thus, the typical multinational comprises a parent company and a number of subsidiary companies located in different countries, most of which are wholly owned by the parent. However, although the subsidiaries may be separate legal entities, they are not separate economic entities. Economically, all the companies in a corporate group are interdependent. For example, if the Brazilian subsidiary of a U.S. parent company experiences substantial financial losses that suck up corporate funds, the cash available for investment in that subsidiary, the U.S. parent company, and other subsidiary companies will be limited. Thus, the purpose of consolidated financial statements is to provide accounting information about a group of companies that recognizes their economic interdependence.

Transactions among the members of a corporate family are not included in consolidated financial statements; only assets, liabilities, revenues, and expenses with external third parties are shown. By law, however, separate legal entities are required to keep their own accounting records and to prepare their own financial statements. Thus, transactions with other members of a corporate group must be identified in the separate statements so they can be excluded when the consolidated statements are prepared. The process involves adding up the individual assets, liabilities, revenues, and expenses reported on the separate financial statements and then eliminating the intragroup ones. For example, consider these items selected from the individual financial statements of a parent company and one of its foreign subsidiaries:

	Parent	Foreign Subsidiary
Cash	$1,000	$ 250
Receivables	3,000*	900
Payables	300	500*
Revenues	7,000[†]	5,000
Expenses	2,000	3,000[†]

*Subsidiary owes parent $300.

[†]Subsidiary pays parent $1,000 in royalties for products licensed from parent.

The $300 receivable that the parent includes on its financial statements and the $300 payable that the subsidiary includes on its statements represent an intragroup item. These items cancel each other out and thus are not included in consolidated financial statements. Similarly, the $1,000 the subsidiary owes the parent in royalty payments is an intragroup item that will not appear in the consolidated accounts. The adjustments are as follows:

			Eliminations		
	Parent	Subsidiary	Debit	Credit	Consolidated
Cash	$1,000	$ 250			$ 1,250
Receivables	3,000*	900		$ 300	3,600
Payables	300	500*	$300		500
Revenues	7,000[†]	5,000		1,000	11,000
Expenses	2,000	3,000[†]	1,000		4,000

*Subsidiary owes parent $300.

[†]Subsidiary pays parent $1,000 in royalties for products licensed from parent.

Thus, while simply adding the two sets of accounts would suggest that the group of companies has revenues of $12,000 and receivables of $3,900, once intragroup transactions are removed from the picture, these figures drop to $11,000 and $3,600, respectively.

Preparing consolidated financial statements is becoming the norm for multinational firms. Investors realize that without consolidated financial statements, a multinational firm could conceal losses in an unconsolidated subsidiary, thereby hiding the economic status of the entire group. For example, the parent company in our illustration could increase its profit merely by charging the subsidiary company higher royalty fees. Since this has no effect on the group's overall profits, it amounts to little more than window dressing, making the parent company look good. If the parent does not issue a consolidated financial statement, however, the true economic status of the group is obscured by such a practice. With this in mind, the IASB has issued two standards requiring firms to prepare consolidated financial statements, and in most industrialized countries this is now required.

Currency Translation

Foreign subsidiaries of multinational firms normally keep their accounting records and prepare their financial statements in the currency of the country in which they are located. Thus, the Japanese subsidiary of a U.S. firm will prepare its accounts in yen, a Brazilian subsidiary in *real*, a Korean subsidiary in *won*, and so on. When a multinational prepares consolidated accounts, it must convert all these financial statements into the currency of its home country. As we saw in Chapter 9, however, exchange rates vary in response to changes in economic circumstances. Companies can use two main methods to determine what exchange rate should be used when translating financial statement currencies—the current rate method and the temporal method.

The Current Rate Method

Under the current rate method, the exchange rate at the balance sheet date is used to translate the financial statements of a foreign subsidiary into the home currency of the multinational firm. Although this may seem logical, it is incompatible with the historic cost principle, which, as we saw earlier, is a generally accepted accounting principle in many countries, including the United States. Consider the case of a U.S. firm that invests $100,000 in a Malaysian subsidiary. Assume the exchange rate at the time is $1 = 5 Malaysian ringgit. The subsidiary converts the $100,000 into ringgit, which gives it 500,000 ringgit. It then purchases land with this money. Subsequently, the dollar depreciates against the ringgit, so that by year-end, $1 = 4 ringgit. If this exchange rate is used to convert the value of the land back into U.S. dollars for preparing consolidated accounts, the land will be valued at $125,000. The piece of land would appear to have increased in value by $25,000, although in reality the increase would be simply a function of an exchange rate change. Thus, the consolidated accounts would present a somewhat misleading picture.

The Temporal Method

One way to avoid this problem is to use the temporal method to translate the accounts of a foreign subsidiary. The temporal method translates assets valued in a foreign currency into the home-country currency using the exchange rate that exists when the assets are purchased. Referring to our example, the exchange rate of $1 = 5 *ringgit*, the rate on the day the Malaysian subsidiary purchased the land, would be used to convert the value of the land back into U.S. dollars at year-end. However, although the temporal method will ensure the dollar value of the land does not fluctuate due to exchange rate changes, it has its own serious problem. Because the various assets of a foreign subsidiary will in all probability be acquired at different times and because exchange rates seldom remain stable for long, different exchange rates will probably have to be used to translate those foreign assets into the multinational's home currency. Consequently, the multinational's balance sheet may not balance!

Consider the case of a U.S. firm that on January 1, 2004, invests $100,000 in a new Japanese subsidiary. The exchange rate at that time is $1 = ¥100. The initial investment is therefore ¥10 million, and the Japanese subsidiary's balance sheet looks like this on January 1, 2004:

	Yen	Exchange Rate	U.S. Dollars
Cash	10,000,000	($1 = ¥100)	100,000
Owners' equity	10,000,000	($1 = ¥100)	100,000

Assume that on January 31, when the exchange rate is $1 = ¥95, the Japanese subsidiary invests ¥5 million in a factory (i.e., fixed assets). Then on February 15, when the exchange rate is $1 = ¥90, the subsidiary purchases ¥5 million of inventory. The balance sheet of the subsidiary will look like this on March 1, 2004:

	Yen	Exchange Rate	U.S. Dollars
Fixed assets	5,000,000	($1 = ¥95)	52,632
Inventory	5,000,000	($1 = ¥90)	55,556
Total	10,000,000		108,187
Owners' equity	10,000,000	($1 = ¥100)	100,000

Although the balance sheet balances in yen, it does not balance when the temporal method is used to translate the yen-denominated balance sheet figures back into dollars. In translation, the balance sheet debits exceed the credits by $8,187. The accounting profession has yet to adopt a satisfactory solution to the gap between debits and credits. The practice currently used in the United States is explained next.

Current U.S. Practice

U.S.-based multinational firms must follow the requirements of Statement 52, "Foreign Currency Translation," issued by the Financial Accounting Standards Board in 1981.[17] Under Statement 52, a foreign subsidiary is classified either as a self-sustaining, autonomous subsidiary or as integral to the activities of the parent company. (A link can be made here with the material on strategy discussed in Chapter 12. Firms pursuing multidomestic and international strategies are most likely to have self-sustaining subsidiaries, whereas firms pursuing global and transnational strategies are most likely to have integral subsidiaries.) According to Statement 52, the local currency of a self-sustaining foreign subsidiary is to be its functional currency. The balance sheet for such subsidiaries is translated into the home currency using the exchange rate in effect at the end of the firm's financial year, whereas the income statement is translated using the average exchange rate for the firm's financial year. But the functional currency of an integral subsidiary is to be U.S. dollars. The financial statements of such subsidiaries are translated at various historic rates using the temporal method (as we did in the example), and the dangling debit or credit increases or decreases consolidated earnings for the period.

Accounting Aspects of Control Systems

Corporate headquarters' role is to control subunits within the organization to ensure they achieve the best possible performance. In the typical firm, the control process is annual and involves three main steps:

1. Head office and subunit management jointly determine subunit goals for the coming year.
2. Throughout the year, the head office monitors subunit performance against the agreed goals.
3. If a subunit fails to achieve its goals, the head office intervenes in the subunit to learn why the shortfall occurred, taking corrective action when appropriate.

The accounting function plays a critical role in this process. Most of the goals for subunits are expressed in financial terms and are embodied in the subunit's budget for the coming year. The budget is the main instrument of financial control. The budget is typically prepared by the subunit, but it must be approved by headquarters management. During the approval process, headquarters and subunit managements debate the goals that should be incorporated in the budget. One function of headquarters management is to ensure a subunit's budget contains challenging but realistic performance goals. Once a budget is agreed to, accounting information systems are used to collect data throughout the year so a subunit's performance can be evaluated against the goals contained in its budget.

In most international businesses, many of the firm's subunits are foreign subsidiaries. The performance goals for the coming year are thus set by negotiation between corporate management and the managers of foreign subsidiaries. According to one survey of control practices within multinational enterprises, the most important criterion for evaluating the performance of a foreign subsidiary is the subsidiary's actual profits compared to budgeted profits.[18] This is closely followed by a subsidiary's actual sales compared to budgeted sales and its return on investment. The same criteria were also useful in evaluating the performance of the subsidiary managers. We will discuss this point later in this section. First, however, we will examine two factors that can complicate the control process in an international business: exchange rate changes and transfer pricing practices.

Exchange Rate Changes and Control Systems

Most international businesses require all budgets and performance data within the firm to be expressed in the "corporate currency," which is normally the home currency. Thus, the Malaysian subsidiary of a U.S. multinational would probably submit a budget prepared in U.S. dollars, rather than Malaysian ringgit, and performance data throughout the year would be reported to headquarters in U.S. dollars. This facilitates comparisons between subsidiaries in different countries, and it makes things easier for headquarters management. However, it also allows exchange rate changes during the year to introduce substantial distortions. For example, the Malaysian subsidiary may fail to achieve profit goals not because of any performance problems, but merely because of a decline in the value of the ringgit against the dollar. The opposite can occur, also, making a foreign subsidiary's performance look better than it actually is.

The Lessard–Lorange Model

According to research by Donald Lessard and Peter Lorange, a number of methods are available to international businesses for dealing with this problem.[19] Lessard and Lorange point out three exchange rates that can be used to translate foreign currencies into the corporate currency in setting budgets and in the subsequent tracking of performance:

- The **initial rate,** the spot exchange rate when the budget is adopted.
- The **projected rate,** the spot exchange rate forecast for the end of the budget period (i.e., the forward rate).
- The **ending rate,** the spot exchange rate when the budget and performance are being compared.

These three exchange rates imply nine possible combinations (see Figure 19.3). Lessard and Lorange ruled out four of the nine combinations as illogical and unreasonable; they are shaded in Figure 19.3. For example, it would make no sense to use the ending rate to translate the budget and the initial rate to translate actual performance data. Any of the remaining five combinations might be used for setting budgets and evaluating performance.

With three of these five combinations—II, PP, and EE—the same exchange rate is used for translating both budget figures and performance figures into the corporate

Figure 19.3

Possible Combinations of
Exchange Rates in the
Control Process

		Rate Used to Translate Actual Performance for Comparison with Budget		
		Initial (I)	Projected (P)	Ending (E)
Rate Used for Translating Budget	Initial (I)	(II) Budget at Initial Actual at Initial	Budget at Initial Actual at Projected	(IE) Budget at Initial Actual at Ending
	Projected (P)	Budget at Projected Actual at Initial	(PP) Budget at Projected Actual at Projected	(PE) Budget at Projected Actual at Ending
	Ending (E)	Budget at Ending Actual at Initial	Budget at Ending Actual at Projected	(EE) Budget at Ending Actual at Ending

currency. All three combinations have the advantage that a change in the exchange rate during the year does not distort the control process. This is not true for the other two combinations, IE and PE. In those cases, exchange rate changes can introduce distortions. The potential for distortion is greater with IE; the ending spot exchange rate used to evaluate performance against the budget may be quite different from the initial spot exchange rate used to translate the budget. The distortion is less serious in the case of PE because the projected exchange rate takes into account future exchange rate movements.

Of the five combinations, Lessard and Lorange recommend that firms use the projected spot exchange rate to translate both the budget and performance figures into the corporate currency, combination PP. The projected rate in such cases will typically be the forward exchange rate as determined by the foreign exchange market (see Chapter 9 for the definition of forward rate) or some company-generated forecast of future spot rates, which Lessard and Lorange refer to as the **internal forward rate.** The internal forward rate may differ from the forward rate quoted by the foreign exchange market if the firm wishes to bias its business in favor of, or against, the particular foreign currency.

Transfer Pricing and Control Systems

In Chapter 12 we reviewed the various strategies that international businesses pursue. Two of these strategies, the global strategy and the transnational strategy, give rise to a globally dispersed web of productive activities. Firms pursuing these strategies disperse each value creation activity to its optimal location in the world. Thus, a product might be designed in one country, some of its components manufactured in a second country, other components manufactured in a third country, all assembled in a fourth country, and then sold worldwide.

The volume of intrafirm transactions in such firms is very high. The firms are continually shipping component parts and finished goods between subsidiaries in different countries. This poses a very important question: How should goods and services transferred between subsidiary companies in a multinational firm be priced? The price at which such goods and services are transferred is referred to as the **transfer price.**

The choice of transfer price can critically affect the performance of two subsidiaries that exchange goods or services. Consider this example: A French manufacturing subsidiary of a U.S. multinational imports a major component from Brazil. It incorporates this part into a product that it sells in France for the equivalent of $230 per unit. The product costs $200 to manufacture, of which $100 goes to the Brazilian subsidiary to pay for the component part. The remaining $100 covers costs incurred in France. Thus, the French subsidiary earns $30 profit per unit.

	Before Change in Transfer Price	After 20 percent Increase in Transfer Price
Revenues per unit	$230	$230
Cost of component per unit	100	120
Other costs per unit	100	100
Profit per unit	30	10

Look at what happens if corporate headquarters decides to increase transfer prices by 20 percent ($20 per unit). The French subsidiary's profits will fall by two-thirds from $30 per unit to $10 per unit. Thus, the performance of the French subsidiary depends on the transfer price for the component part imported from Brazil, and the transfer price is controlled by corporate headquarters. When setting budgets and reviewing a subsidiary's performance, corporate headquarters must keep in mind the distorting effect of transfer prices.

How should transfer prices be determined? We discuss this issue in detail in the next chapter. International businesses often manipulate transfer prices to minimize their worldwide tax liability, minimize import duties, and avoid government restrictions on capital flows. For now, however, it is enough to note that the transfer price must be considered when setting budgets and evaluating a subsidiary's performance.

Separation of Subsidiary and Manager Performance

In many international businesses, the same quantitative criteria are used to assess the performance of both a foreign subsidiary and its managers. Many accountants, however, argue that although it is legitimate to compare subsidiaries against each other on the basis of return on investment (ROI) or other indicators of profitability, it may not be appropriate to use these for comparing and evaluating the managers of different subsidiaries. Foreign subsidiaries do not operate in uniform environments; their environments have widely different economic, political, and social conditions, all of which influence the costs of doing business in a country and hence the subsidiaries' profitability. Thus, the manager of a subsidiary in an adverse environment that has an ROI of 5 percent may be doing a better job than the manager of a subsidiary in a benign environment that has an ROI of 20 percent. Although the firm might want to pull out of a country where its ROI is only 5 percent, it may also want to recognize the manager's achievement.

Accordingly, it has been suggested that the evaluation of a subsidiary should be kept separate from the evaluation of its manager.[20] The manager's evaluation should consider how hostile or benign the country's environment is for that business. Further, managers should be evaluated in local currency terms after making allowances for those items over which they have no control (e.g., interest rates, tax rates, inflation rates, transfer prices, exchange rates).

ChapterSummary

This chapter focused on financial accounting within the multinational firm. We explained why accounting practices and standards differ from country to country and surveyed the efforts under way to harmonize accounting practices. We discussed the rationale behind consolidated accounts and looked at currency translation. We reviewed several issues related to the use of accounting-based control systems within international businesses. The chapter made these major points:

1. Accounting is the language of business: the means by which firms communicate their financial position to the providers of capital and to governments (for tax purposes). It is also the means by which firms evaluate their own performance, control their expenditures, and plan for the future.

2. Accounting is shaped by the environment in which it operates. Each country's accounting system has evolved in response to the local demands for accounting information.

3. Five main factors seem to influence the type of accounting system a country has: (*i*) the relationship between business and the providers of capital, (*ii*) political and economic ties with other countries, (*iii*) the level of inflation, (*iv*) the level of a country's development, and (*v*) the prevailing culture in a country.

4. National differences in accounting and auditing standards have resulted in a general lack of comparability in countries' financial reports.

5. This lack of comparability has become a problem as transnational financing and transnational investment have grown rapidly in recent decades (a consequence of the globalization of capital markets). Due to the lack of comparability, a firm may have to explain to investors why its financial position looks very different on financial reports that are based on different accounting practices.

6. The most significant push for harmonization of accounting standards across countries has come from the International Accounting Standards Committee (IASC) and its successor, the International Accounting Standards Board (IASB).

7. Consolidated financial statements provide financial accounting information about a group of companies that recognizes the companies' economic interdependence.

8. Transactions among the members of a corporate family are not included on consolidated financial statements; only assets, liabilities, revenues, and expenses generated with external third parties are shown.

9. Foreign subsidiaries of a multinational firm normally keep their accounting records and prepare their financial statements in the currency of the country in which they are located. When the multinational prepares its consolidated accounts, these financial statements must be translated into the currency of its home country.

10. Under the current rate translation method, the exchange rate at the balance sheet date is used to translate the financial statements of a foreign subsidiary into the home currency. This has the drawback of being incompatible with the historic cost principle.

11. Under the temporal method, assets valued in a foreign currency are translated into the home currency using the exchange rate that existed when the assets were purchased. A problem with this approach is that the multinational's balance sheet may not balance.

12. In most international businesses, the annual budget is the main instrument by which headquarters controls foreign subsidiaries. Throughout the year, headquarters compares a subsidiary's performance against the financial goals incorporated in its budget, intervening selectively in its operations when shortfalls occur.

13. Most international businesses require all budgets and performance data within the firm to be expressed in the corporate currency. This enhances comparability, but it distorts the control process if the relevant exchange rates change between the time a foreign subsidiary's budget is set and the time its performance is evaluated.

14. According to the Lessard–Lorange model, the best way to deal with this problem is to use a projected spot exchange rate to translate both budget figures and performance figures into the corporate currency.

15. Transfer prices also can introduce significant distortions into the control process and thus must be considered when setting budgets and evaluating a subsidiary's performance.

16. Foreign subsidiaries do not operate in uniform environments, and some environments are much tougher than others. Accordingly, it has been suggested that the evaluation of a subsidiary should be kept separate from the evaluation of the subsidiary manager.

Critical Discussion Questions

1. Why do the accounting systems of different countries differ? Why do these differences matter?

2. Why are transactions among members of a corporate family not included in consolidated financial statements?

3. At the right are selected amounts from the separate financial statements of a parent company (unconsolidated) and one of its subsidiaries. Given this,

    a. What is the parent's (unconsolidated) net income?

    b. What is the subsidiary's net income?

    c. What is the consolidated profit on the inventory that the parent originally sold to the subsidiary?

    d. What are the amounts of consolidated cash and receivables?

4. Why might an accounting-based control system provide headquarters management with biased information about the performance of a foreign subsidiary? How can these biases best be corrected?

	Parent	Subsidiary
Cash	$ 180	$ 80
Receivables	380	200
Accounts payable	245	110
Retained earnings	790	680
Revenues	4,980	3,520
Rent income	0	200
Dividend income	250	0
Expenses	4,160	2,960

Notes:

i. Parent owes subsidiary $70.

ii. Parent owns 100% of subsidiary. During the year, subsidiary paid parent a dividend of $250.

iii. Subsidiary owns the building that parent rents for $200.

iv. During the year, parent sold some inventory to subsidiary for $2,200. It had cost parent $1,500. Subsidiary, in turn, sold the inventory to an unrelated party for $3,200.

Research Task   globalEDGE™   globaledge.msu.edu

Use the globalEDGE™ site to complete the following exercises:

1. The globalEDGE™ site offers a country comparison tool that allows for comparing the countries based on statistical indicators. Utilize this tool to identify in which of the following countries the historic cost principle of accounting cannot provide accurate results: Argentina, Bulgaria, Ecuador, Indonesia, Latvia, Malaysia, Mexico, Romania, Russia, and Senegal. Utilize the "rank countries" tool to identify other countries in which the historic cost principle would not provide valid results.

2. Deloitte Touche Tohmatsu hosts an International Accounting Standards webpage that provides information and guidelines regarding the accounting procedures approved by IASC. Locate the website, the section on Standards, and prepare a short description of the international accounting standards of accounting for recording inventory levels.

Notes

1. G. G. Mueller, H. Gernon, and G. Meek, *Accounting: An International Perspective* (Burr Ridge, IL: Richard D. Irwin, 1991).

2. S. J. Gary, "Towards a Theory of Cultural Influence on the Development of Accounting Systems Internationally," *Abacus* 3 (1988), pp. 1–15, and R. S. Wallace, O. Gernon, and H. Gernon, "Frameworks for International Comparative Financial Accounting," *Journal of Accounting Literature* 10 (1991), pp. 209–64.

3. K. M. Dunne and G. A. Ndubizu, "International Acquisition Accounting Method and Corporate Multinationalism," *Journal of International Business Studies* 26 (1995), pp. 361–77.

4. W. A. Wallace and J. Walsh, "Apples to Apples: Profits Abroad," *Financial Executive,* May–June 1995, pp. 28–31.

5. Wallace, Gernon, and Gernon, "Frameworks for International Comparative Financial Accounting."

6. P. Walton, "Special Rules for a Special Case," *Financial Times*, September 18, 1997, p. 11.

7. Gary, "Towards a Theory of Cultural Influence on the Development of Accounting Systems Internationally," and S. B. Salter and F. Niswander, "Cultural Influences on the Development of Accounting Systems Internationally," *Journal of International Business Studies* 26 (1995), pp. 379–97.

8. G. Hofstede, *Culture's Consequences: International Differences in Work Related Values* (Beverly Hills, CA: Sage Publications, 1980).

9. Salter and Niswander, "Cultural Influences on the Development of Accounting Systems Internationally."

10. Ibid.

11. Mueller, Gernon, and Meek, *Accounting: An International Perspective*.

12. R. G. Barker, "Global Accounting Is Coming," *Harvard Business Review*, April 2003, pp. 2–3.

13. A current list can be accessed at www.iasb.org.uk. See also D. Tweedie, "Globalization, Here We Come," *Financial Times*, February 1, 2001, p. 2, and "Bean Counters, Unite!" *The Economist*, June 10, 1995, pp. 67–68.

14. P. D. Fleming, "The Growing Importance of International Accounting Standards," *Journal of Accountancy*, September 1991, pp. 100–06.

15. M. Peel, "Turbulence Forecast Worldwide," *Financial Times*, March 22, 2001, p. 2.

16. L. Berton, "All Accountants May Soon Speak the Same Language," *Wall Street Journal*, August 29, 1995, p. A15.

17. The statement can be accessed at http://www.fasb.org/st/summary/stsum52.shtml.

18. F. Choi and I. Czechowicz, "Assessing Foreign Subsidiary Performance: A Multinational Comparison," *Management International Review* 4 (1983), pp. 14–25.

19. D. Lessard and P. Lorange, "Currency Changes and Management Control: Resolving the Centralization/Decentralization Dilemma," *Accounting Review*, July 1977, pp. 628–37.

20. Mueller, Gernon, and Meek, *Accounting: An International Perspective*.

Closing Case

China's Evolving Accounting System

Attracted by its rapid transformation from a socialist planned economy into a market economy, economic annual growth rates of about 12 percent, and a population of nearly 1.3 billion, Western firms over the past 10 years have favored China as a site for foreign direct investment. Most see China as an emerging economic superpower with an economy that will be as large as that of Japan by 2005 and of the United States before 2010 if current growth projections hold true.

The Chinese government sees foreign direct investment as a primary engine of China's economic growth. To encourage such investment, the government has offered generous tax incentives to foreign firms that invest in China, either on their own or in a joint venture with a local enterprise. These tax incentives include a two-year exemption from corporate income tax following an investment, plus a further three years during which taxes are paid at only 50 percent of the standard tax rate. Such incentives when coupled with the promise of China's vast internal market have made the country a prime site for investment by Western firms. However, once established in China, many Western firms find themselves struggling to comply with the complex and often obtuse nature of China's rapidly evolving accounting system.

Accounting in China has traditionally been rooted in information gathering and compliance reporting designed to measure the government's production and tax goals. The Chinese system was based on the old Soviet system, which had little to do with profit or accounting systems created to report financial positions or the results of foreign operations. Although the system is changing rapidly, many problems associated with the old system still remain.

One problem for investors is a severe shortage of accountants, financial managers, and auditors in China, especially those experienced with market economy transactions and international accounting practices. As of 1995, there were only 25,000 accountants in China, far short of the hundreds of thousands that will be needed if China continues on its path toward becoming a market economy. Chinese enterprises, including equity and cooperative joint ventures with foreign firms, must be audited by Chinese accounting firms, which are regulated by the state. Traditionally, many experienced auditors have audited only state-owned enterprises, working through the local province or city authorities and the state audit bureau to report to the government entity overseeing the audited firm. In response to the shortage of accountants schooled in the principles of private-sector accounting, several large international auditing firms have established joint ventures with emerging Chinese accounting and auditing firms to bridge the growing need for international accounting, tax, and securities expertise.

A further problem concerns the somewhat halting evolution of China's emerging accounting standards. Current thinking is that China won't simply adopt the international accounting standards specified by the IASB, nor will it use the generally accepted accounting principles of any particular country as its model. Rather, accounting standards in China are expected to evolve in a rather piecemeal fashion, with the Chinese adopting a few standards as they are studied and deemed appropriate for Chinese circumstances.

In the meantime, current Chinese accounting principles present difficult problems for Western firms. For example, the former Chinese accounting system didn't need to accrue unrealized losses. In an economy where shortages were the norm, if a state-owned company didn't sell its inventory right away, it could store it and use it for some other purpose later. Similarly, accounting principles assumed the state always paid its debts—eventually. Thus, Chinese enterprises don't generally provide for lower-of-cost or market inventory adjustments or the creation of allowance for bad debts, both of which are standard practices in the West. Still, progress is being made. By January 2001, China's Ministry of Finance had issued some 15 accounting standards for business enterprises since it began doing so in the early 1990s. The majority of these conform with IASB standards, although there are some adaptations to accommodate China's "unique economy and society."

Sources: L. E. Graham and A. H. Carley, "When East Meets West," *Financial Executive*, July–August 1995, pp. 40–45; K. Theonnes and A. Yeung, "Playing Favorites," *Financial Executive*, July–August 1995, pp. 46–51; and P. Practer, "Emerging Trends," *Accountancy*, May 2001, p. 1293.

Case Discussion Questions

1. What factors have shaped the accounting system currently in use in China?

2. What problems does the accounting system currently in use in China present to foreign investors in joint ventures with Chinese companies?

3. If the evolving Chinese system does not adhere to IASB standards, but instead to standards that the Chinese government deems appropriate to China's "special situation," how might this affect foreign firms with operations in China?

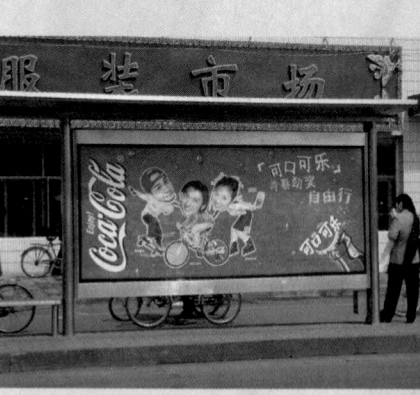

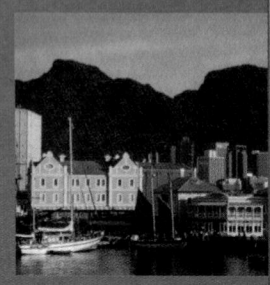

Chapter 20

Financial Management in the International Business

Introduction
Investment Decisions
  Capital Budgeting
  Project and Parent Cash Flows
  Adjusting for Political and Economic
  Risk
  Risk and Capital Budgeting
Financing Decisions
  Source of Financing
  Financial Structure
Global Money Management:
The Efficiency Objective
  Minimizing Cash Balances
  Reducing Transaction Costs
Global Money Management: The Tax
Objective
Moving Money across Borders: Attaining
Efficiencies and Reducing Taxes
  Dividend Remittances
  Royalty Payments and Fees
  Transfer Prices
  Fronting Loans
Techniques for Global Money
Management
  Centralized Depositories
  Multilateral Netting
Managing Foreign Exchange Risk
  Types of Foreign Exchange Exposure
  Tactics and Strategies for Reducing
  Foreign Exchange Exposure
  Developing Policies for Managing
  Foreign Exchange Exposure
Chapter Summary
Critical Discussion Questions
Closing Case Motorola's Global Cash
Management System

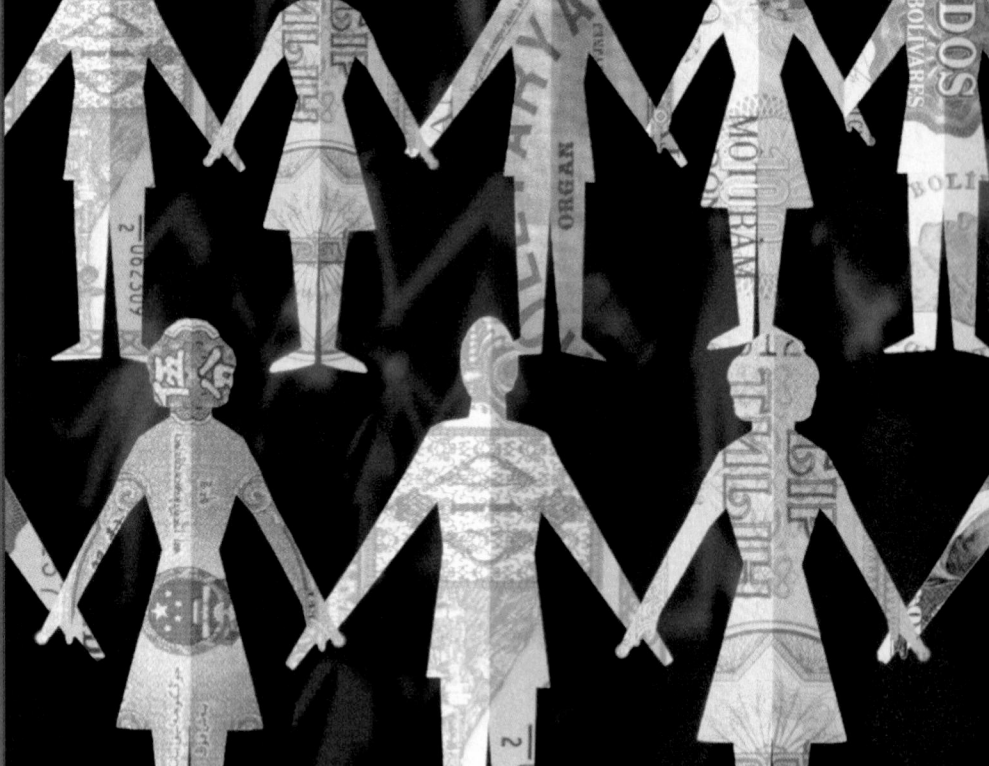

Global Treasury Management at Procter & Gamble

With more than 245 brands of paper, detergent, food, health, and cosmetics products sold in over 130 countries and over 60 percent of its $43 billion in 2002 revenues generated outside the United States, Procter & Gamble is the quintessential example of a global consumer products firm. Despite this global spread, P&G's treasury operations—which embrace investment, financing, money management, and foreign exchange decisions—were quite decentralized until the early 1990s. Essentially, each major international subsidiary managed its own investments, borrowings, and foreign exchange trades, subject only to outside borrowing limits imposed by the international treasury group at P&G's headquarters in Cincinnati.

Today P&G operates with a much more centralized system in which a global treasury management function at corporate headquarters exercises close oversight over the operations of different regional treasury centers around the world. This move was a response in part to the rise in the volume of P&G's international transactions and the resulting increase in foreign exchange exposures. Like many global firms, P&G has been trying to rationalize its global production system to realize cost economies by concentrating the production of certain products at specific locations, as opposed to producing those products in every major country in which it does business. As it has moved in this direction, the number and volume of raw materials and finished products that are being shipped across borders have been growing by leaps and bounds. This has led to a commensurate increase in the size of P&G's foreign exchange exposure, which now runs into billions of dollars. Also, more than one-third of P&G's foreign exchange exposure is now in nondollar exposures, such as transactions that involve the exchange of euros into won or sterling into yen.

P&G believes that centralizing the overall management of the resulting foreign exchange transactions can help the company realize a number of important gains. First, because its international subsidiaries often accumulate cash balances in the currency of the country where they are based, P&G now trades currencies between its subsidiaries. By cutting banks out of the process, P&G saves on transaction costs. Second, P&G has found that many of its subsidiaries purchase currencies in relatively small lots of, say, $100,000. By grouping these lots into larger purchases, P&G can generally get a better price from foreign trade dealers. Third, P&G is pooling foreign exchange risks and purchasing an "umbrella option" to cover the risks associated with various currency positions, which is cheaper than purchasing options to cover each position.

In addition to managing foreign exchange transactions, P&G's global treasury operation arranges for subsidiaries to invest their surplus funds in and to borrow money from other Procter & Gamble entities, instead of from local banks. Subsidiaries that have excess cash lend it to those that need cash, and the global treasury operation acts as a financial intermediary. P&G has cut the number of local banks that it does business with from 450 to about 200. Using intracompany loans instead of loans from local banks lowers the overall borrowing costs, which may result in annual savings on interest payments that run into tens if not hundreds of millions of dollars.

Sources: R. C. Stewart, "Balancing on the Global High Wire," *Financial Executive,* September–October 1995, pp. 35–39; S. Lipin, F. R. Bleakley, and B. D. Granito, "Portfolio Poker," *Wall Street Journal,* April 14, 1994, p. A1; and Procter & Gamble 10K report for 2000.

Introduction

As the opening case makes clear, this chapter focuses on financial management in the international business. Included within the scope of financial management are three sets of related decisions:

- *Investment decisions*, decisions about what activities to finance.
- *Financing decisions*, decisions about how to finance those activities.
- *Money management decisions*, decisions about how to manage the firm's financial resources most efficiently.

The opening case describes Procter & Gamble's approach toward these decisions. By managing investing, financing, and money management decisions centrally through its global treasury function, P&G has realized considerable cost economies. These economies help P&G compete more effectively in the global marketplace.

In an international business, investment, financing, and money management decisions are complicated by the fact that countries have different currencies, tax regimes, regulations concerning the flow of capital across their borders, norms regarding the financing of business activities, levels of economic and political risk, and so on. Financial managers must consider all these factors when deciding which activities to finance, how best to finance those activities, how best to manage the firm's financial resources, and how best to protect the firm from political and economic risks (including foreign exchange risk).

Good financial management can be an important source of competitive advantage. This is implicit in the opening case, where good financial management helps P&G attain cost economies and lower its overall cost structure. For another example, consider FMC, a Chicago-based producer of chemicals and farm equipment. FMC counts on overseas business for 40 percent of its sales. FMC attributes some of its success overseas to aggressive trading in the forward foreign exchange market. By trading in currency futures, FMC can provide overseas customers with stable long-term prices for three years or more, regardless of what happens to exchange rates. According to an FMC spokesman, "Some of our competitors change their prices on a relatively short-term basis depending on what is happening with their own exchange rate . . . We want to provide longer-term pricing as a customer service—they can plan their budgets knowing what the numbers will be—and we can hopefully maintain and build our customer base." FMC also offers its customers the option of paying in any of several currencies as a convenience to them and as an attempt to retain customers. If customers could pay only in dollars, they might give their business to a competitor that offered pricing in a variety of currencies. By adopting this policy, FMC deals with "the hassle of foreign exchange movements," says the spokesman, so its customers don't have to. By offering customers multicurrency pricing alternatives, FMC implicitly accepts the responsibility of managing foreign exchange risk for its business units that sell overseas. It has set up what amounts to an in-house bank to manage the operation, monitoring currency rates daily and managing its risks on a portfolio basis. This bank handles more than $1 billion in currency transactions annually, which means the company can often beat the currency prices quoted by commercial banks.[1]

Chapter 12 talked about the value chain and pointed out that creating a competitive advantage requires a firm to reduce its costs of value creation and/or add value by improving its customer service. P&G and FMC show how good financial management can help both reduce the costs of creating value and add value by improving customer service. By reducing the firm's cost of capital, eliminating foreign exchange losses, minimizing the firm's tax burden, minimizing the firm's exposure to unnecessarily risky activities, and managing the firm's cash flows and reserves in the most efficient manner, the finance function can reduce the costs of creating value. As the FMC example illustrates, good financial management can also enhance customer service, thus adding value.

We begin this chapter by looking at investment decisions in an international business. We will be most concerned with the issue of capital budgeting. Our objective is to identify the factors that can complicate capital budgeting decisions in an international business, as opposed to a purely domestic business. Most important, we will discuss how such factors as political and economic risk complicate capital budgeting decisions.

Then we look at financing decisions in an international business, focusing on the financial structure of foreign affiliates—the mix of equity and debt financing. Financial structure norms for firms vary widely from country to country. We will discuss the advantages and disadvantages of localizing the financial structure of a foreign affiliate to make it consistent with the norms of the country in which it is based.

Next we examine money management decisions in an international business. We will look at the objectives of global money management, the various ways businesses can move money across borders, and some techniques for managing the firm's financial resources efficiently.

The chapter closes with a section on managing foreign exchange risk. Foreign exchange risk was discussed in Chapter 9, but there our focus was on how the foreign exchange market works and the forces that determine exchange rate movements. In this chapter, we focus on the various tactics and strategies international businesses use to manage their foreign exchange risk.

Investment Decisions ■

A decision to invest in activities in a given country must consider many economic, political, cultural, and strategic variables. We have been discussing this issue throughout much of this book. We touched on it in Chapters 2 and 3 when we discussed how the political, economic, legal, and cultural environment of a country can influence the benefits, costs, and risks of doing business there and thus its attractiveness as an investment site. We returned to the issue in Chapter 6 with a discussion of the economic theory of foreign direct investment. We identified a number of factors that determine the economic attractiveness of a foreign investment opportunity. In Chapter 7, we looked at the political economy of foreign direct investment, and we considered the role that government intervention can play in foreign investment. In Chapter 12, we pulled much of this material together when we considered how a firm can reduce its costs of value creation and/or increase its value added by investing in productive activities in other countries. We returned to the issue again in Chapter 14 when we considered the various modes for entering foreign markets.

One role of the financial manager in an international business is to try to quantify the various benefits, costs, and risks that are likely to flow from an investment in a given location. This is done by using capital budgeting techniques.

▌Capital Budgeting

Capital budgeting quantifies the benefits, costs, and risks of an investment. This enables top managers to compare, in a reasonably objective fashion, different investment alternatives within and across countries so they can make informed choices about where the firm should invest its scarce financial resources. Capital budgeting for a foreign project uses the same theoretical framework that domestic capital budgeting uses; that is, the firm must first estimate the cash flows associated with the project over time. In most cases, the cash flows will be negative at first, because the firm will be investing heavily in production facilities. After some initial period, however, the cash flows will become positive as investment costs decline and revenues grow. Once the cash flows have been estimated, they must be discounted to determine their net present value using an appropriate discount rate. The most commonly used discount rate is either the firm's cost of capital or some other required rate of return. If the net present value of the discounted cash flows is greater than zero, the firm should go ahead with the project.[2]

Although this might sound quite straightforward, capital budgeting is a very complex and imperfect process. Among the factors complicating the process for an international business are these:

1. A distinction must be made between cash flows to the project and cash flows to the parent company.
2. Political and economic risks, including foreign exchange risk, can significantly change the value of a foreign investment.
3. The connection between cash flows to the parent and the source of financing must be recognized.

We look at the first two of these issues in this section. Discussion of the connection between cash flows and the source of financing is postponed until the next section, where we discuss the source of financing.

Project and Parent Cash Flows

A theoretical argument exists for analyzing any foreign project from the perspective of the parent company because cash flows to the project are not necessarily the same thing as cash flows to the parent company. The project may not be able to remit all its cash flows to the parent for a number of reasons. For example, cash flows may be blocked from repatriation by the host-country government, they may be taxed at an unfavorable rate, or the host government may require a certain percentage of the cash flows generated from the project be reinvested within the host nation. While these restrictions don't affect the net present value of the project itself, they do affect the net present value of the project to the parent company because they limit the cash flows that can be remitted to it from the project.

When evaluating a foreign investment opportunity, the parent should be interested in the cash flows it will receive—as opposed to those the project generates—because those are the basis for dividends to stockholders, investments elsewhere in the world, repayment of worldwide corporate debt, and so on. Stockholders will not perceive blocked earnings as contributing to the value of the firm, and creditors will not count them when calculating the parent's ability to service its debt.

But the problem of blocked earnings is not as serious as it once was. The worldwide move toward greater acceptance of free market economics (discussed in Chapter 2) has reduced the number of countries in which governments are likely to prohibit the affiliates of foreign multinationals from remitting cash flows to their parent companies. In addition, as we will see later in the chapter, firms have a number of options for circumventing host-government attempts to block the free flow of funds from an affiliate.

Adjusting for Political and Economic Risk

When analyzing a foreign investment opportunity, the company must consider the political and economic risks that stem from the foreign location.[3] We will discuss these before looking at how capital budgeting methods can be adjusted to consider risks.

Political Risk

We initially encountered the concept of political risk in Chapter 2. There we defined it as the likelihood that political forces will cause drastic changes in a country's business environment that hurt the profit and other goals of a business enterprise. Political risk tends to be greater in countries experiencing social unrest or disorder and countries where the underlying nature of the society makes the likelihood of social un-

Black Sea Energy Ltd.

In 1996, Black Sea Energy, Ltd., of Calgary, Canada, formed a 50-50 joint venture with the Tyumen Oil Company, then Russia's sixth largest integrated oil company. The objective of the venture, know as the Tura Petroleum Company, was to explore the Tura oil field in western Siberia. At the time, Tyumen was 90 percent owned by the Russian government; consequently Black Sea negotiated directly with representatives of the Russian government when establishing the joint venture. The agreement called for both parties to contribute more than $40 million to the formation of the venture, Black Sea in the form of cash, technology, and expertise, and Tyumen in the form of infrastructure and the licenses for oil exploration and production that it held in the region.

From an operational perspective, the venture proved to be a success. Following the injection of cash and technology from Black Sea Energy, production at the Tura field went from 4,000 barrels per day to nearly 12,000. However, Black Sea did not capture any of the economic profits flowing from this investment. In 1997, the Moscow-based Alfa Group, one of Russia's largest private companies, purchased a controlling stake in Tyumen from the Russian government. The new owners of Tyumen quickly concluded the Tura joint venture was not fair to them and they wanted it canceled. Their argument was that the value of the assets contributed by Tyumen to the joint venture was far in excess of $40 million, while the value of the technology and expertise contributed by Black Sea was significantly less than $40 million. The new owners also found some conflicting legislation that seemed to indicate the licenses held by Tura were owned by Tyumen, and that Black Sea therefore had no right to the resulting production. Tyumen took the issue to court in Russia and won, despite that fact that the original deal had been negotiated by the Russian government. Black Sea Energy had little choice but to walk away from the deal. According to Black Sea, by legal maneuvering, Tyumen was able to expropriate Black Sea's investment in the Tura venture. In contrast, the management of Tyumen claimed it had behaved in a perfectly legal manner.

Sources: D. J. Feils and F. M. Sabac, "The Impact of Political Risk on the Foreign Direct Investment Decision: A Capital Budgeting Analysis," *The Engineering Economist*, 45 (2000), pp. 129–34; Simon Kukes, "Letters to the Editor: Tura Joint Venture," *Wall Street Journal*, June 14, 1999, p. A21; and M. Whitehouse, "US Export-Import Bank Agrees to Give Russia's Tyumen Oil Loan Guarantee," *Wall Street Journal*, May 25, 1999, p. A21.

rest high. When political risk is high, there is a high probability that a change will occur in the country's political environment that will endanger foreign firms there.

In extreme cases, political change may result in the expropriation of foreign firms' assets. This occurred to U.S. firms after the Iranian revolution of 1979. In recent decades, outright expropriations have diminished substantially as a risk. However, a lack of consistent legislation and proper law enforcement, and no willingness on the part of the government to enforce contracts and protect private property rights can result in the de facto expropriation of the assets of a foreign multinational. The accompanying Management Focus provides an example of this that occurred in Russia during the late 1990s.

Political and social unrest may also result in economic collapse, which can render worthless a firm's assets. This occurred to many foreign companies' assets as a result of the bloody war following the breakup of the former Yugoslavia. In less extreme cases, political changes may result in increased tax rates, the imposition of exchange controls that limit or block a subsidiary's ability to remit earnings to its parent company, the imposition of price controls, and government interference in existing contracts. The likelihood of any of these events impairs the attractiveness of a foreign investment opportunity.

Many firms devote considerable attention to political risk analysis and to quantifying political risk. *Euromoney* magazine publishes an annual "country risk rating," which incorporates assessments of political and other risks and is widely used by businesses. The problem with all attempts to forecast political risk, however, is that they try to predict a future that can only be guessed at—and in many cases, the guesses are wrong. Few people foresaw the 1979 Iranian revolution, the collapse of communism in Eastern Europe, the dramatic breakup of the Soviet Union, the terrorist attack on the World Trade Center in September 2001; yet all these events have had a profound impact on the business environments of many countries. This is not to say that political risk assessment is without value, but it is more art than science.

Economic Risk

As with political risk, we first encountered the concept of economic risk in Chapter 2. There we defined it as the likelihood that economic mismanagement will cause drastic changes in a country's business environment that hurt the profit and other goals of a business enterprise. In practice, the biggest problem arising from economic mismanagement has been inflation. Historically, many governments have expanded their domestic money supply in misguided attempts to stimulate economic activity. The result has often been too much money chasing too few goods, resulting in price inflation. As we saw in Chapter 9, price inflation is reflected in a drop in the value of a country's currency on the foreign exchange market. This can be a serious problem for a foreign firm with assets in that country because the value of the cash flows it receives from those assets will fall as the country's currency depreciates on the foreign exchange market. The likelihood of this occurring decreases the attractiveness of foreign investment in that country.

There have been many attempts to quantify countries' economic risk and long-term movements in their exchange rates. (*Euromoney*'s annual country risk rating also incorporates an assessment of economic risk in its calculation of each country's overall level of risk.) As we saw in Chapter 9, there have been extensive empirical studies of the relationship between countries' inflation rates and their currencies' exchange rates. These studies show a long-run relationship between a country's relative inflation rates and changes in exchange rates. However, the relationship is not as close as theory would predict; it is not reliable in the short run and is not totally reliable in the long run. So, as with political risk, any attempts to quantify economic risk must be tempered with some healthy skepticism.

Risk and Capital Budgeting

In analyzing a foreign investment opportunity, the additional risk that stems from its location can be handled in at least two ways. The first method is to treat all risk as a single problem by increasing the discount rate applicable to foreign projects in countries where political and economic risks are perceived as high. Thus, for example, a firm might apply a 6 percent discount rate to potential investments in Great Britain, the United States, and Germany, reflecting those countries' economic and political stability, and it might use a 20 percent discount rate for potential investments in Russia, reflecting the political and economic turmoil in that country. The higher the discount rate, the higher the projected net cash flows must be for an investment to have a positive net present value.

Adjusting discount rates to reflect a location's riskiness seems to be fairly widely practiced. For example, a study of large U.S. multinationals found that 49 percent of them routinely added a premium percentage for risk to the discount rate they used in evaluating potential foreign investment projects.[4] However, critics of this method argue that it penalizes early cash flows too heavily and does not penalize distant cash flows enough.[5] They point out that if political or economic collapse were expected in the near future, the investment would not occur anyway. (This is borne out today in the case of Russia; Western companies are not investing there because they perceive the danger of political and economic collapse.) So for any investment decisions, the political and economic risk being assessed is not of immediate possibilities, but rather at some distance in the future. Accordingly, it can be argued that rather than using a higher discount rate to evaluate such risky projects, which penalizes early cash flows too heavily, it is better to revise future cash flows from the project downward to reflect the possibility of adverse political or economic changes sometime in the future. Surveys of actual practice within multinationals suggest that the practice of revising future cash flows downward is almost as popular as that of revising the discount rate upward.[6]

Financing Decisions

When considering its options for financing a foreign investment, an international business must consider two factors. The first is how the foreign investment will be financed. If external financing is required, the firm must decide whether to borrow from sources in the host country or elsewhere. The second factor is how the financial structure of the foreign affiliate should be configured.

Source of Financing

If the firm is going to seek external financing for a project, it will want to borrow funds from the lowest-cost source of capital available. As we saw in Chapter 11, firms increasingly are turning to the global capital market to finance their investments. The cost of capital is typically lower in the global capital market, by virtue of its size and liquidity, than in many domestic capital markets, particularly those that are small and relatively illiquid. Thus, for example, a U.S. firm making an investment in Denmark may finance the investment by borrowing through the London-based eurobond market rather than the Danish capital market.

However, host-country government restrictions may rule out this option. The governments of some countries require, or at least prefer, foreign multinationals to finance projects in their country by local debt financing or local sales of equity. In countries where liquidity is limited, this raises the cost of capital used to finance a project. Thus, in capital budgeting decisions, the discount rate must be adjusted upward to reflect this. However, this is not the only possibility. In Chapter 7, we saw that some governments court foreign investment by offering foreign firms low-interest loans, lowering the cost of capital. Accordingly, in capital budgeting decisions, the discount rate should be revised downward in such cases.

In addition to the impact of host-government policies on the cost of capital and financing decisions, the firm may wish to consider local debt financing for investments in countries where the local currency is expected to depreciate on the foreign exchange market. The amount of local currency required to meet interest payments and retire principal on local debt obligations is not affected when a country's currency depreciates. However, if foreign debt obligations must be served, the amount of local currency required to do this will increase as the currency depreciates, and this effectively raises the cost of capital. (We looked at this issue in Chapter 11 when we considered foreign exchange risk and the cost of capital.) Thus, although the initial cost of capital may be greater with local borrowing, it may be better to borrow locally if the local currency is expected to depreciate on the foreign exchange market.

Financial Structure

There is a difference in the financial structures of firms based in different countries. By financial structure we mean the mix of debt and equity used to finance a business. It is well known, for example, that Japanese firms rely far more on debt financing than do most U.S. firms. One study of firms in 23 countries found that debt-to-equity ratios varied from a low of 0.34 in Singapore to 0.76 in Italy. The average ratio in the United States was 0.55. It was also 0.55 in the United Kingdom, and 0.62 in Germany.[7] Another study of more than 4,000 firms in five countries found that the ratio of long-term debt to assets was 0.185 in the United States, 0.155 in Japan, 0.98 in the United Kingdom, 0.88 in Germany, and 0.145 in France, suggesting again that reliance on debt financing varies from country to country.[8]

It is not clear why the financial structure of firms should vary so much across countries. One possible explanation is that different tax regimes determine the relative attractiveness of debt and equity in a country. For example, if interest income were taxed at a high rate, a preference for debt financing over equity financing would be expected. However, according to empirical research, country differences in financial structure do not seem related in any systematic way to country differences in tax structure.[9] Another possibility is that these country differences may reflect cultural norms.[10] This explanation may be valid, although the mechanism by which culture influences capital structure has not yet been explained.

The interesting question for the international business is whether it should conform to local capital structure norms. Should a U.S. firm investing in Italy adopt the higher debt ratio typical of Italian firms for its Italian subsidiary, or should it stick with its more conservative practice? There are few good arguments for conforming to local norms. One advantage claimed for conforming to host-country debt norms is that management can more easily evaluate its return on equity relative to local competitors in the same industry. However, this seems a weak rationale for what is an important decision. Another point often made is that conforming to higher host-country debt norms can improve the image of foreign affiliates that have been operating with too little debt and thus appear insensitive to local monetary policy. Just how important this point is, however, has not been established. The best recommendation is that an international business should adopt a financial structure for each foreign affiliate that minimizes its cost of capital, irrespective of whether that structure is consistent with local practice.

Global Money Management: The Efficiency Objective

Money management decisions attempt to manage the firm's global cash resources—its working capital—most efficiently. This involves minimizing cash balances and reducing transaction costs.

Minimizing Cash Balances

For any given period, a firm must hold certain cash balances. This is necessary for serving any accounts and notes payable during that period and as a contingency against unexpected demands on cash. The firm does not sit on its cash reserves. It typically invests them in money market accounts so it can earn interest on them. However, it must be able to withdraw its money from those accounts freely. Such accounts typically offer a relatively low rate of interest. In contrast, the firm could earn a higher rate of interest if it could invest its cash resources in longer-term financial instruments (e.g., six-month certificates of deposit). The problem with longer-term instruments, however, is that the firm cannot withdraw its money before the instruments mature without suffering a financial penalty.

Thus, the firm faces a dilemma. If it invests its cash balances in money market accounts (or the equivalent), it will have unlimited liquidity but earn a relatively low interest rate. If it invests its cash in longer-term financial instruments (certificates of deposit, bonds, etc.), it will earn a higher rate of interest, but liquidity will be limited. In an ideal world, the firm would have minimal liquid cash balances. We will see later in the chapter that by managing its total global cash reserves through a centralized depository (as opposed to letting each affiliate manage its own cash reserves), an international business can reduce the amount of funds it must hold in liquid accounts and thereby increase its rate of return on its cash reserves.

|Reducing Transaction Costs

Transaction costs are the cost of exchange. Every time a firm changes cash from one currency into another currency it must bear a transaction cost—the commission fee it pays to foreign exchange dealers for performing the transaction. Most banks also charge a **transfer fee** for moving cash from one location to another; this is another transaction cost. The commission and transfer fees arising from intrafirm transactions can be substantial; according to the United Nations, 40 percent of international trade involves transactions between the different national subsidiaries of transnational corporations. As we will see later in the chapter, multilateral netting can reduce the number of transactions between the firm's subsidiaries, thereby reducing the total transactions costs arising from foreign exchange dealings and transfer fees.

Global Money Management: The Tax Objective ■

Different countries have different tax regimes. Table 20.1 illustrates top corporate income tax rates in 2003 for countries included in a survey by KPMG, an international accounting firm.[11] As can be seen, the top rates for corporate income tax varied from a high of 42 percent in Japan to a low of 12.5 percent in Ireland. However, the picture is much more complex than the one presented in Table 20.1. For example, in Germany and Japan, the tax rate is lower on income distributed to stockholders as dividends (36 and 35 percent, respectively), whereas in France the tax on profits distributed to stockholders is higher (42 percent). In the United States, the rate varies from state to state. The federal top rate is 35 percent, but states also tax corporate income, with state and local taxes ranging from 1 percent to 12 percent, hence the average effective rate of 40 percent.

Many nations follow the worldwide principle that they have the right to tax income earned outside their boundaries by entities based in their country.[12] Thus, the U.S. government can tax the earnings of the German subsidiary of an enterprise incorporated in the United States. Double taxation occurs when the income of a foreign subsidiary is taxed both by the host-country government and by the parent company's home government. However, double taxation is mitigated to some extent by tax credits, tax treaties, and the deferral principle.

A **tax credit** allows an entity to reduce the taxes paid to the home government by the amount of taxes paid to the foreign government. A **tax treaty** between two countries

Country	Top Corporate Income Tax Rate
Canada	36.6%
Chile	16.5
France	34.33
Germany	39.58
Hong Kong	17
Ireland	12.5
Japan	42
Mexico	34
Singapore	22
United Kingdom	30
United States	40

Table 20.1

Corporate Income Tax Rates, 2003

Source: KPMG Corporate Tax Survey, January 2003, www.kpmg.com.

is an agreement specifying what items of income will be taxed by the authorities of the country where the income is earned. For example, a tax treaty between the United States and Germany may specify that a U.S. firm need not pay tax in Germany on any earnings from its German subsidiary that are remitted to the United States in the form of dividends. A **deferral principle** specifies that parent companies are not taxed on foreign source income until they actually receive a dividend.

For the international business with activities in many countries, the various tax regimes and the tax treaties have important implications for how the firm should structure its internal payments system among the foreign subsidiaries and the parent company. As we will see in the next section, the firm can use transfer prices and fronting loans to minimize its global tax liability. In addition, the form in which income is remitted from a foreign subsidiary to the parent company (e.g., royalty payments versus dividend payments) can be structured to minimize the firm's global tax liability.

Some firms use **tax havens** such as the Bahamas and Bermuda to minimize their tax liability. A tax haven is a country with an exceptionally low, or even no, income tax. International businesses avoid or defer income taxes by establishing a wholly owned, nonoperating subsidiary in the tax haven. The tax haven subsidiary owns the common stock of the operating foreign subsidiaries. This allows all transfers of funds from foreign operating subsidiaries to the parent company to be funneled through the tax haven subsidiary. The tax levied on foreign source income by a firm's home government, which might normally be paid when a dividend is declared by a foreign subsidiary, can be deferred under the deferral principle until the tax haven subsidiary pays the dividend to the parent. This dividend payment can be postponed indefinitely if foreign operations continue to grow and require new internal financing from the tax haven affiliate. For U.S.-based enterprises, however, U.S. regulations tax U.S. shareholders on the firm's overseas income when it is earned, regardless of when the parent company in the United States receives it. This regulation eliminates U.S.-based firms' ability to use tax haven subsidiaries to avoid tax liabilities in the manner just described.

Moving Money across Borders: Attaining Efficiencies and Reducing Taxes

Pursuing the objectives of utilizing the firm's cash resources most efficiently and minimizing the firm's global tax liability requires the firm to be able to transfer funds from one location to another around the globe. International businesses use a number of techniques to transfer liquid funds across borders. These include dividend remittances, royalty payments and fees, transfer prices, and fronting loans. Some firms rely on more than one of these techniques to transfer funds across borders—a practice known as unbundling. By using a mix of techniques to transfer liquid funds from a foreign subsidiary to the parent company, unbundling allows an international business to recover funds from its foreign subsidiaries without piquing host-country sensitivities with large "dividend drains."

A firm's ability to select a particular policy is severely limited when a foreign subsidiary is owned partly either by a local joint-venture partner or by local stockholders. Serving the legitimate demands of the local co-owners of a foreign subsidiary may limit the firm's ability to impose the kind of dividend policy, royalty payment schedule, or transfer pricing policy that would be optimal for the parent company.

Dividend Remittances

Payment of dividends is probably the most common method by which firms transfer funds from foreign subsidiaries to the parent company. The dividend policy typically varies with each subsidiary depending on such factors as tax regulations, foreign exchange risk, the age of the subsidiary, and the extent of local equity participation. For example, the higher the rate of tax levied on dividends by the host-country government, the less attractive this option becomes relative to other options for transferring liquid funds. With regard to foreign exchange risk, firms sometimes require foreign subsidiaries based in "high-risk" countries to speed up the transfer of funds to the parent through accelerated dividend payments. This moves corporate funds out of a country whose currency is expected to depreciate significantly. The age of a foreign subsidiary influences dividend policy in that older subsidiaries tend to remit a higher proportion of their earnings in dividends to the parent, presumably because a subsidiary has fewer capital investment needs as it matures. Local equity participation is a factor because local co-owners' demands for dividends must be recognized.

Royalty Payments and Fees

Royalties represent the remuneration paid to the owners of technology, patents, or trade names for the use of that technology or the right to manufacture and/or sell products under those patents or trade names. It is common for a parent company to charge its foreign subsidiaries royalties for the technology, patents, or trade names it has transferred to them. Royalties may be levied as a fixed monetary amount per unit of the product the subsidiary sells or as a percentage of a subsidiary's gross revenues.

A fee is compensation for professional services or expertise supplied to a foreign subsidiary by the parent company or another subsidiary. Fees are sometimes differentiated into "management fees" for general expertise and advice and "technical assistance fees" for guidance in technical matters. Fees are usually levied as fixed charges for the particular services provided.

Royalties and fees have certain tax advantages over dividends, particularly when the corporate tax rate is higher in the host country than in the parent's home country. Royalties and fees are often tax-deductible locally (because they are viewed as an expense), so arranging for payment in royalties and fees will reduce the foreign subsidiary's tax liability. If the foreign subsidiary compensates the parent company by dividend payments, local income taxes must be paid before the dividend distribution, and withholding taxes must be paid on the dividend itself. Although the parent can often take a tax credit for the local withholding and income taxes it has paid, part of the benefit can be lost if the subsidiary's combined tax rate is higher than the parent's.

Transfer Prices

In any international business, there are normally a large number of transfers of goods and services between the parent company and foreign subsidiaries and between foreign subsidiaries. This is particularly likely in firms pursuing global and transnational strategies because these firms are likely to have dispersed their value creation activities to various optimal locations around the globe (see Chapter 12). As noted in Chapter 19, the price at which goods and services are transferred between entities within the firm is referred to as the **transfer price**.[13]

Transfer prices can be used to position funds within an international business. For example, funds can be moved out of a particular country by setting high transfer prices for goods and services supplied to a subsidiary in that country and by setting low transfer prices for the goods and services sourced from that subsidiary. Conversely, funds can be positioned in a country by the opposite policy: setting low transfer prices for goods and services supplied to a subsidiary in that country and setting high transfer prices for the goods and services sourced from that subsidiary. This movement of funds can be between the firm's subsidiaries or between the parent company and a subsidiary.

Benefits of Manipulating Transfer Prices

At least four gains can be derived by manipulating transfer prices.

1.   The firm can reduce its tax liabilities by using transfer prices to shift earnings from a high-tax country to a low-tax one.

2. The firm can use transfer prices to move funds out of a country where a significant currency devaluation is expected, thereby reducing its exposure to foreign exchange risk.

3. The firm can use transfer prices to move funds from a subsidiary to the parent company (or a tax haven) when financial transfers in the form of dividends are restricted or blocked by host-country government policies.

4. The firm can use transfer prices to reduce the import duties it must pay when an ad valorem tariff is in force—a tariff assessed as a percentage of value. In this case, low transfer prices on goods or services being imported into the country are required. Since this lowers the value of the goods or services, it lowers the tariff.

Problems with Transfer Pricing

Significant problems are associated with pursuing a transfer pricing policy.[14] Few governments like it.[15] When transfer prices are used to reduce a firm's tax liabilities or import duties, most governments believe they are being cheated of their legitimate income. Similarly, when transfer prices are manipulated to circumvent government restrictions on capital flows (e.g., dividend remittances), governments perceive this as breaking the spirit—if not the letter—of the law. Many governments now limit international businesses' ability to manipulate transfer prices in the manner described. The United States has strict regulations governing transfer pricing practices. According to Section 482 of the Internal Revenue Code, the Internal Revenue Service (IRS) can reallocate gross income, deductions, credits, or allowances between related corporations to prevent tax evasion or to reflect more clearly a proper allocation of income. Under the IRS guidelines and subsequent judicial interpretation, the burden of proof is on the taxpayer to show that the IRS has been arbitrary or unreasonable in reallocating income. The correct transfer price, according to the IRS guidelines, is an arm's-length price—the price that would prevail between unrelated firms in a market setting. Such a strict interpretation of what is a correct transfer price theoretically limits a firm's ability to manipulate transfer prices to achieve the benefits we have discussed. Many other countries have followed the U.S. lead in emphasizing that transfer prices should be set on an arm's-length basis.

Another problem associated with transfer pricing is related to management incentives and performance evaluation.[16] Transfer pricing is inconsistent with a policy of treating each subsidiary in the firm as a profit center. When transfer prices are manipulated by the firm and deviate significantly from the arm's-length price, the subsidiary's performance may depend as much on transfer prices as it does on other pertinent factors, such as management effort. A subsidiary told to charge a high transfer price for a good supplied to another subsidiary will appear to be doing better than it actually is, while the subsidiary purchasing the good will appear to be doing worse. Unless this is recognized when performance is being evaluated, serious distortions in management incentive systems can occur. For example, managers in the selling subsidiary may be able to use high transfer prices to mask inefficiencies, while managers in the purchasing subsidiary may become disheartened by the effect of high transfer prices on their subsidiary's profitability.

Despite these problems, research suggests that not all international businesses use arm's-length pricing but instead use some cost-based system for pricing transfers among their subunits (typically cost plus some standard markup). A survey of 164 U.S. multinational firms found that 35 percent of the firms used market-based prices, 15 percent used negotiated prices, and 65 percent used a cost-based pricing method. (The figures add up to more than 100 percent because some companies use more than one method.)[17] Only market and negotiated prices could reasonably be interpreted as arm's-length prices. The opportunity for price manipulation is much greater with cost-based transfer pricing. Other more sophisticated research has uncovered indirect evidence that many corporations do manipulate transfer prices to reduce global tax liabilities.[18]

Although a firm may be able to manipulate transfer prices to avoid tax liabilities or circumvent government restrictions on capital flows across borders, this does not mean the firm should do so. Since the practice often violates at least the spirit of the law in many countries, the ethics of engaging in transfer pricing are dubious at best. Also, tax authorities in many countries are increasing their scrutiny of this practice to stamp out abuses. A 2000 survey of some 600 multinationals undertaken by accountants Ernst & Young found that 75 percent of them believe that they will be the subject of a transfer pricing audit by tax authorities in the next two years.[19] Some 61 percent of the multinationals in the survey stated that transfer pricing was the top tax issue they faced.

Fronting Loans

A **fronting loan** is a loan between a parent and its subsidiary channeled through a financial intermediary, usually a large international bank. In a direct intrafirm loan, the parent company lends cash directly to the foreign subsidiary, and the subsidiary repays it later. In a fronting loan, the parent company deposits funds in an international bank, and the bank then lends the same amount to the foreign subsidiary. Thus, a U.S. firm might deposit $100,000 in a London bank. The London bank might then lend that $100,000 to an Indian subsidiary of the firm. From the bank's point of view, the loan is risk free because it has 100 percent collateral in the form of the parent's deposit. The bank "fronts" for the parent, hence the name. The bank makes a profit by paying the parent company a slightly lower interest rate on its deposit than it charges the foreign subsidiary on the borrowed funds.

Firms use fronting loans for two reasons. First, fronting loans can circumvent host-country restrictions on the remittance of funds from a foreign subsidiary to the parent company. A host government might restrict a foreign subsidiary from repaying a loan to its parent in order to preserve the country's foreign exchange reserves, but it is less likely to restrict a subsidiary's ability to repay a loan to a large international bank. To stop payment to an international bank would hurt the country's credit image, whereas halting payment to the parent company would probably have a minimal impact on its image. Consequently, international businesses sometimes use fronting loans when they want to lend funds to a subsidiary based in a country with a fairly high probability of political turmoil that might lead to restrictions on capital flows (i.e., where the level of political risk is high).

A fronting loan can also provide tax advantages. For example, a tax haven (Bermuda) subsidiary that is 100 percent owned by the parent company deposits $1 million in a London-based international bank at 8 percent interest. The bank lends the $1 million to a foreign operating subsidiary at 9 percent interest. The country where the foreign operating subsidiary is based taxes corporate income at 50 percent (see Figure 20.1).

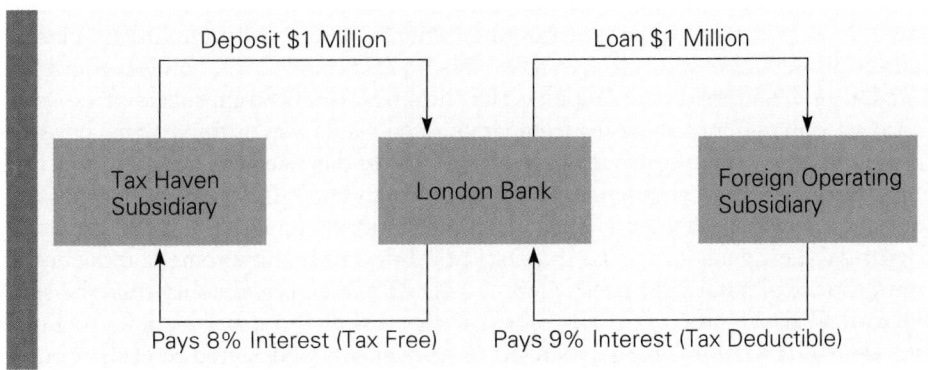

Figure 20.1

An Example of the Tax Aspects of a Fronting Loan

Under this arrangement, interest payments net of income tax will be as follows:

1. The foreign operating subsidiary pays $90,000 interest to the London bank. Deducting these interest payments from its taxable income results in a net after-tax cost of $45,000 to the foreign operating subsidiary.
2. The London bank receives the $90,000. It retains $10,000 for its services and pays $80,000 interest on the deposit to the Bermuda subsidiary.
3. The Bermuda subsidiary receives $80,000 interest on its deposit tax free.

The net result is that $80,000 in cash has been moved from the foreign operating subsidiary to the tax haven subsidiary. Because the foreign operating subsidiary's after-tax cost of borrowing is only $45,000, the parent company has moved an additional $35,000 out of the country by using this arrangement. If the tax haven subsidiary had made a direct loan to the foreign operating subsidiary, the host government may have disallowed the interest charge as a tax-deductible expense by ruling that it was a dividend to the parent disguised as an interest payment.

Techniques for Global Money Management

We now look at two money management techniques firms use in attempting to manage their global cash resources in the most efficient manner: centralized depositories and multilateral netting.

Centralized Depositories

Every business needs to hold some cash balances for servicing accounts that must be paid and for insuring against unanticipated negative variation from its projected cash flows. The critical issue for an international business is whether each foreign subsidiary should hold its own cash balances or whether cash balances should be held at a **centralized depository.** In general, firms prefer to hold cash balances at a centralized depository for three reasons.

First, by pooling cash reserves centrally, the firm can deposit larger amounts. Cash balances are typically deposited in liquid accounts, such as overnight money market accounts. Because interest rates on such deposits normally increase with the size of the deposit, by pooling cash centrally, the firm should be able to earn a higher interest rate than it would if each subsidiary managed its own cash balances.

Second, if the centralized depository is located in a major financial center (e.g., London, New York, or Tokyo), it should have access to information about good short-term investment opportunities that the typical foreign subsidiary would lack. Also, the financial experts at a centralized depository should be able to develop investment skills and know-how that managers in the typical foreign subsidiary would lack. Thus, the firm should make better investment decisions if it pools its cash reserves at a centralized depository.

Third, by pooling its cash reserves, the firm can reduce the total size of the cash pool it must hold in highly liquid accounts, which enables the firm to invest a larger amount of cash reserves in longer-term, less liquid financial instruments that earn a higher interest rate. For example, a U.S. firm has three foreign subsidiaries—one in Korea, one in China, and one in Japan. Each subsidiary maintains a cash balance that includes an amount for dealing with its day-to-day needs plus a precautionary amount for dealing with unanticipated cash demands. The firm's policy is that the total required cash balance is equal to three standard deviations of the expected day-to-day-needs amount. The three-standard-deviation requirement reflects the firm's estimate that, in practice, there is a 99.87 percent probability that the subsidiary will have sufficient cash to deal with both day-to-day and unanticipated cash demands. Cash needs are assumed to be normally distributed in each country and independent of each other (e.g., cash needs in Japan do not affect cash needs in China).

The individual subsidiaries' day-to-day cash needs and the precautionary cash balances they should hold are as follows (in millions of dollars):

	Day-to-Day Cash Needs (A)	One Standard Deviation (B)	Required Cash Balance (A + 3 × B)
Korea	$10	$1	$13
China	6	2	12
Japan	12	3	21
Total	$28	$6	$46

Thus, the Korean subsidiary estimates that it must hold $10 million to serve its day-to-day needs. The standard deviation of this is $1 million, so it is to hold an additional $3 million as a precautionary amount. This gives a total required cash balance of $13 million. The total of the required cash balances for all three subsidiaries is $46 million.

Now consider what might occur if the firm decided to maintain all three cash balances at a centralized depository in Tokyo. Because variances are additive when probability distributions are independent of each other, the standard deviation of the combined precautionary account would be:

$$\text{Square root of } (\$1,000,000^2 + 2,000,000^2 + 3,000,000^2)$$
$$= \text{Square root of } 14,000,000$$
$$= \$3,741,657$$

Therefore, if the firm used a centralized depository, it would need to hold $28 million for day-to-day needs plus (3 × $3,741,657) as a precautionary amount, or a total cash balance of $39,224,971. In other words, the firm's total required cash balance would be reduced from $46 million to $39,224,971, a saving of $6,775,029. This is cash that could be invested in less liquid, higher-interest accounts or in tangible assets. The saving arises simply due to the statistical effects of summing the three independent, normal probability distributions.

However, a firm's ability to establish a centralized depository that can serve short-term cash needs might be limited by government-imposed restrictions on capital flows across borders (e.g., controls put in place to protect a country's foreign exchange reserves). Also, the transaction costs of moving money into and out of different currencies can limit the advantages of such a system. Despite this, many firms hold at least their subsidiaries' precautionary cash reserves at a centralized depository, having each subsidiary hold its own day-to-day-needs cash balance. The globalization of the world capital market and the general removal of barriers to the free flow of cash across borders (particularly among advanced industrialized countries) are two trends likely to increase the use of centralized depositories.

Multilateral Netting

Multilateral netting allows a multinational firm to reduce the transaction costs that arise when many transactions occur between its subsidiaries. These transaction costs are the commissions paid to foreign exchange dealers for foreign exchange transactions and the fees charged by banks for transferring cash between locations. The volume of such transactions is likely to be particularly high in a firm that has a globally

Figure 20.2A

Cash Flows before
Multilateral Netting

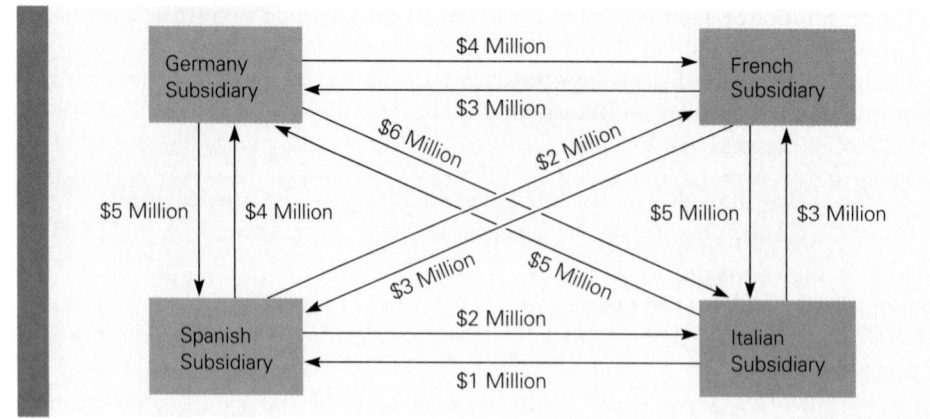

<table>
<tr><th></th><th colspan="6">Paying Subsidiary</th></tr>
<tr><th>Receiving
Subsidiary</th><th>Germany</th><th>France</th><th>Spain</th><th>Italy</th><th>Total
Receipts</th><th>Net Receipts
(payments)</th></tr>
<tr><td>Germany</td><td>—</td><td>$3</td><td>$4</td><td>$5</td><td>$12</td><td>($3)</td></tr>
<tr><td>France</td><td>$ 4</td><td>—</td><td>2</td><td>3</td><td>9</td><td>(2)</td></tr>
<tr><td>Spain</td><td>5</td><td>3</td><td>—</td><td>1</td><td>9</td><td>1</td></tr>
<tr><td>Italy</td><td>6</td><td>5</td><td>2</td><td>—</td><td>13</td><td>4</td></tr>
<tr><td>Total payments</td><td>$15</td><td>$11</td><td>$8</td><td>$9</td><td></td><td></td></tr>
</table>

Figure 20.2B

Calculation of Net Receipts (all amounts in millions)

Figure 20.2C

Cash Flows after Multilateral Netting

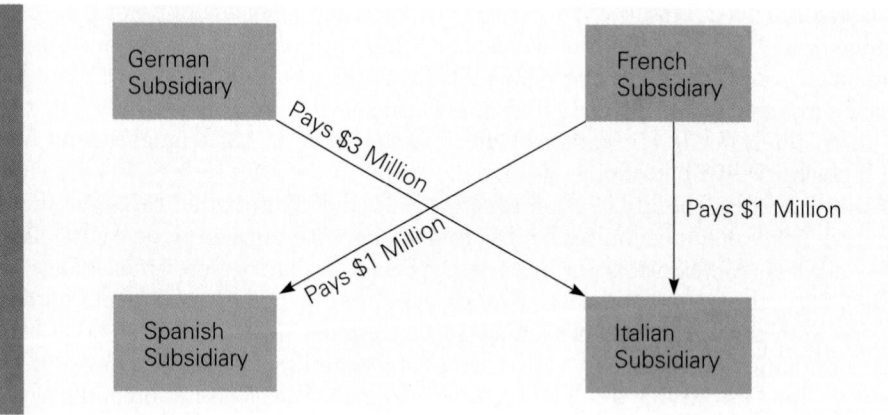

dispersed web of interdependent value creation activities. Netting reduces transaction costs by reducing the number of transactions.

Multilateral netting is an extension of **bilateral netting.** Under bilateral netting, if a French subsidiary owes a Mexican subsidiary $6 million and the Mexican subsidiary simultaneously owes the French subsidiary $4 million, a bilateral settlement will be made with a single payment of $2 million from the French subsidiary to the Mexican subsidiary, the remaining debt being canceled.

Under **multilateral netting,** this simple concept is extended to the transactions between multiple subsidiaries within an international business. Consider a firm that wants to establish multilateral netting among four European subsidiaries based in Germany, France, Spain, and Italy. These subsidiaries all trade with each other, so at the end of each month a large volume of cash transactions must be settled. Figure 20.2a shows how the payment schedule might look at the end of a given month. Figure 20.2b is a payment matrix that summarizes the obligations among the subsidiaries. Note that $43 million needs to flow among the subsidiaries. If the transaction costs (foreign exchange commissions plus transfer fees) amount to 1 percent of the total funds to be transferred, this will cost the parent firm $430,000. However, this amount can be reduced by multilateral netting. Using the payment matrix (Figure 20.2b), the firm can determine the payments that need to be made among its subsidiaries to settle these obligations. Figure 20.2c shows the results. By multilateral netting, the transactions depicted in Figure 20.2a are reduced to just three; the German subsidiary pays $3 million to the Italian subsidiary, and the French subsidiary pays $1 million to the Spanish subsidiary and $1 million to the Italian subsidiary. The total funds that flow among the subsidiaries are reduced from $43 million to just $5 million, and the transaction costs are reduced from $430,000 to $50,000, a savings of $380,000 achieved through multilateral netting.

Managing Foreign Exchange Risk

The nature of foreign exchange risk was discussed in Chapter 9. There we described how changes in exchange rates alter the profitability of trade and investment deals, how forward exchange rates and currency swaps enable firms to insure themselves to some degree against foreign exchange risk, and how relative inflation rates determine exchange rate movements. In this section, we focus on the various strategies international businesses use to manage foreign exchange risk. Buying forward, the strategy most discussed in Chapter 9, is just one of these. We will examine the types of foreign exchange exposure, the tactics and strategies firms adopt in attempting to minimize their exposure to foreign exchange risk, and things firms can do to develop policies for managing foreign exchange risk.

Types of Foreign Exchange Exposure

When we speak of **foreign exchange exposure,** we are referring to the risk that future changes in a country's exchange rate will hurt the firm. As we saw in Chapter 9, changes in foreign exchange values often affect the profitability of international trade and investment deals. Foreign exchange exposure is normally broken into three categories: transaction exposure, translation exposure, and economic exposure. Each is explained here.

Transaction Exposure

Transaction exposure is typically defined as the extent to which the income from individual transactions is affected by fluctuations in foreign exchange values. Such exposure includes obligations for the purchase or sale of goods and services at previously agreed prices and the borrowing or lending of funds in foreign currencies. Suppose a U.S. company has just contracted to import laptop computers from Japan. When the shipment arrives in 30 days, the company must pay the Japanese supplier ¥200,000 for each computer. The dollar/yen spot exchange rate today is $1 = ¥120. At this rate, each laptop computer would cost the importer $1,667 (i.e., 200,000/120 = 1,667). The importer knows it can sell each computer for $2,000 on the day the shipment arrives, so as the exchange rate stands, the U.S. company expects to make a gross profit of $333 on every computer it sells (2,000 − 1,667). If the dollar depreciates against the yen over the next 30 days, say, to $1 = ¥95, the U.S. company will still have to pay the Japanese company ¥200,000 per computer, but in dollar terms that would be $2,105 per laptop computer—more than the computers could be sold for. A depreciation in the value of the dollar against the yen from $1 = ¥120 to $1 = ¥95 would transform this profitable transaction into an unprofitable one. The transaction exposure per computer in this case is $2,105−$1,667 = $438, that being the amount of money per computer that has been lost due to an adverse movement in exchange rates between the time when the deal was signed and when the computers were paid for.

Translation Exposure

Translation exposure is the impact of currency exchange rate changes on the reported consolidated results and balance sheet of a company. This issue was discussed in Chapter 19 when we looked at currency translation practices. Translation exposure is basically concerned with the present measurement of past events. The resulting accounting gains or losses are said to be unrealized—they are "paper" gains and losses—but they are still important. Consider a U.S. firm with a subsidiary in Mexico. If the value of the Mexican peso depreciates significantly against the dollar this would substantially reduce the dollar value of the Mexican subsidiary's equity. In turn, this would reduce the total dollar value of the firm's equity reported in its consolidated balance sheet. This would raise the apparent leverage of the firm (its debt ratio), which could increase the firm's cost of borrowing and restrict its access to the capital market. Similarly, if a U.S. firm has a subsidiary in the European Union, and if the value of the euro depreciates rapidly against that of the dollar over a year, this will reduce the dollar value of the euro profit made by the European subsidiary, resulting in negative translation exposure. In fact, many U.S. firms suffered from significant translation exposure in Europe during 2000, precisely because the euro did depreciate rapidly against the dollar. Baxter International, a U.S. producer of medical products, was one of a host of U.S. companies that announced their financial results for late 2000 and probably much of 2001 would be lower than previously thought, due to negative translation exposure to the euro. On July 20, 2000, Baxter's CEO confidently predicted the company would hit its earnings and sales targets for all of 2000, and moreover, due to continuing strong global sales, would grow revenues and earnings by a figure in the mid-teens for 2001. Three months later, the CEO was less optimistic. While 2000 earnings and revenues were still on track, the company now expected much slower growth in 2001, which would reduce the projected increase in operating income by some $100 million. The CEO blamed the continuing weakness of the euro agains the U.S. dollar. At euro 1=$0.83 the euro had depreciated 10% since July, and 30% since early 1999. In 2003, by way of contrast, the euro rose in value against the dollar, boosting the profits of U.S. multinationals with significant operations in Europe.

Economic Exposure

Economic exposure is the extent to which a firm's future international earning power is affected by changes in exchange rates. Economic exposure is concerned with the long-run effect of changes in exchange rates on future prices, sales, and costs. This is distinct from transaction exposure, which is concerned with the effect of exchange rate changes on individual transactions, most of which are short-term affairs that will be executed within a few weeks or months. Consider the effect of the wide swings in the value of the dollar on many U.S. firms' international competitiveness during the 1980s. The rapid rise in the value of the dollar on the foreign exchange market in the early 1980s hurt the price competitiveness of many U.S. producers in world markets. U.S. manufacturers that relied heavily on exports (such as Caterpillar) saw their export volume and world market share plunge. The reverse phenomenon occurred in the following decade when the dollar declined against most major currencies. The fall in the value of the dollar between 1985 and 1995 increased the price competitiveness of U.S. manufacturers in world markets and helped produce an export boom in the United States.

Tactics and Strategies for Reducing Foreign Exchange Exposure

A number of strategies and tactics can help firms reduce their foreign exchange exposure. The tactics, which include buying forward and the use of leading and lagging strategies, are best suited to alleviating transaction exposure and translation exposure. The strategies addressing the configuration of a firm's assets across countries are best suited to reducing economic exposure.

Reducing Transaction and Translation Exposure

A number of tactics can help firms minimize their transaction and translation exposure. These tactics primarily protect short-term cash flows from adverse changes in exchange rates. We discussed two of these tactics in Chapter 9, buying forward and using currency swaps. They are important sources of insurance against the short-term effects of foreign exchange exposure. (For details, return to Chapter 9.)

In addition to buying forward and using swaps, firms can minimize their foreign exchange exposure through leading and lagging payables and receivables—that is, collecting and paying early or late depending on expected exchange rate movements. A **lead strategy** involves attempting to collect foreign currency receivables early when a foreign currency is expected to depreciate and paying foreign currency payables before they are due when a currency is expected to appreciate. A **lag strategy** involves delaying collection of foreign currency receivables if that currency is expected to appreciate and delaying payables if the currency is expected to depreciate. Leading and lagging involve accelerating payments from weak-currency to strong-currency countries and delaying inflows from strong-currency to weak-currency countries.

Lead and lag strategies can be difficult to implement, however. The firm must be in a position to exercise some control over payment terms. Firms do not always have this kind of bargaining power, particularly when they are dealing with important customers that are in a position to dictate payment terms. Also, because lead and lag strategies can put pressure on a weak currency, many governments limit leads and lags. For example, some countries set 180 days as a limit for receiving payments for exports or making payments for imports.

Several other tactics that can reduce transaction and translation exposure have already been discussed in this chapter. We have explained that:

- Transfer prices can be manipulated to move funds out of a country whose currency is expected to depreciate.
- Local debt financing can provide a hedge against foreign exchange risk.
- It may make sense to accelerate dividend payments from subsidiaries based in countries with weak currencies.
- Capital budgeting techniques can be adjusted to deflect the negative impact of adverse exchange rate movements on the current net value of a foreign investment.

Reducing Economic Exposure

Reducing economic exposure requires strategic choices that go beyond the realm of financial management. The key to reducing economic exposure is to distribute the firm's productive assets to various locations so the firm's long-term financial well-being is not severely affected by adverse changes in exchange rates. The post-1985 trend by Japanese automakers to establish productive capacity in North America and Western Europe can partly be seen as a strategy for reducing economic exposure (it is also a strategy for reducing trade tensions). Before 1985, most Japanese automobile companies concentrated their productive assets in Japan. However, the rise in the value of the yen on the foreign exchange market has transformed Japan from a low-cost to a high-cost manufacturing location. In response, Japanese auto firms have moved many of their productive assets overseas to ensure their car prices will not be unduly affected by further rises in the value of the yen. In general, reducing economic exposure necessitates that the firm ensure its assets are not too concentrated in countries where likely rises in currency values will lead to damaging increases in the foreign prices of the goods and services they produce.

Developing Policies for Managing Foreign Exchange Exposure

The firm needs to develop a mechanism for ensuring it maintains an appropriate mix of tactics and strategies for minimizing its foreign exchange exposure. Although there is no universal agreement as to the components of this mechanism, a number of common themes stand out.[20] First, central control of exposure is needed to protect resources efficiently and ensure that each subunit adopts the correct mix of tactics and strategies. Many companies have set up in-house foreign exchange centers. Although such centers may not be able to execute all foreign exchange deals—particularly in large, complex multinationals where myriad transactions may be pursued simultaneously—they should at least set guidelines for the firm's subsidiaries to follow.

Second, firms should distinguish between, on one hand, transaction and translation exposure and, on the other, economic exposure. Many companies seem to focus on reducing their transaction and translation exposure and pay scant attention to economic exposure, which may have more profound long-term implications.[21] Firms need to develop strategies for dealing with economic exposure. For example, Black & Decker, the maker of power tools, has a strategy for actively managing its economic risk. The key to Black & Decker's strategy is flexible sourcing. In response to foreign exchange movements, Black & Decker can move production from one location to another to offer the most competitive pricing. Black & Decker manufactures in more than a dozen locations around the world—in Europe, Australia, Brazil, Mexico, and Japan. More than 50 percent of the company's productive assets are based outside North America. Although each of Black & Decker's factories focuses on one or two products to achieve economies of scale, there is considerable overlap. On average, the company runs its factories at no more than 80 percent capacity, so most are able to switch rapidly from producing one product to producing another or to add a product. This allows a factory's production to be changed in response to foreign exchange movements. For example, as the dollar depreciated during the latter half of the 1980s, the amount of imports into the United States from overseas subsidiaries was reduced, and the amount of exports from U.S. subsidiaries to other locations was increased.[22]

Third, the need to forecast future exchange rate movements cannot be overstated, though, as we saw in Chapter 9, this is a tricky business. No model comes close to perfectly predicting future movements in foreign exchange rates. The best that can be said is that in the short run, forward exchange rates provide reasonable predictions of exchange rate movements, and in the long run, fundamental economic factors—particularly relative inflation rates—should be watched because they influence exchange rate movements. Some firms attempt to forecast exchange rate movements in-house; others rely on outside forecasters. However, all such forecasts are imperfect attempts to predict the future.

Fourth, firms need to establish good reporting systems so the central finance function (or in-house foreign exchange center) can regularly monitor the firm's exposure positions. Such reporting systems should enable the firm to identify any exposed accounts, the exposed position by currency of each account, and the time periods covered.

Finally, on the basis of the information it receives from exchange rate forecasts and its own regular reporting systems, the firm should produce monthly foreign exchange exposure reports. These reports should identify how cash flows and balance sheet elements might be affected by forecasted changes in exchange rates. The reports can then be used by management as a basis for adopting tactics and strategies to hedge against undue foreign exchange risks.

Surprisingly, some of the largest and most sophisticated firms don't take such precautionary steps, exposing themselves to very large foreign exchange risks. In 1990, the treasury department of the British food company Allied-Lyons apparently entered the forward foreign exchange market, not so much to hedge against future currency movements as to profit from placing large speculative bets that currencies would move one way or another. Unfortunately for Allied-Lyons, its treasury department made the incorrect speculative bets and it incurred losses of $240 million. Similarly, Showa Shell Sekiyu, the Royal Dutch/Shell group's Japanese affiliate, revealed in February 1993 that its treasury department had incurred some $1 billion in unrealized foreign exchange losses.[23]

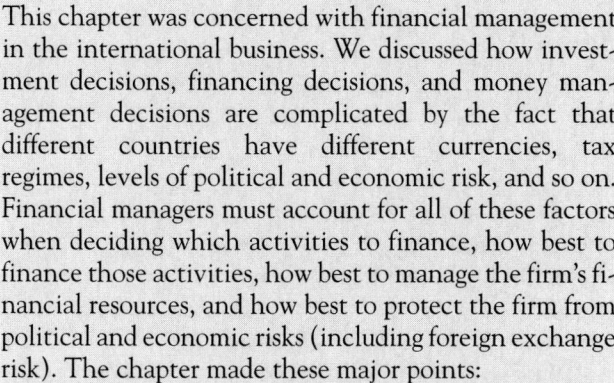

ChapterSummary

This chapter was concerned with financial management in the international business. We discussed how investment decisions, financing decisions, and money management decisions are complicated by the fact that different countries have different currencies, tax regimes, levels of political and economic risk, and so on. Financial managers must account for all of these factors when deciding which activities to finance, how best to finance those activities, how best to manage the firm's financial resources, and how best to protect the firm from political and economic risks (including foreign exchange risk). The chapter made these major points:

1. When using capital budgeting techniques to evaluate a potential foreign project, a distinction must be made between cash flows to the project and cash flows to the parent. The two will not be the same thing when a host-country government blocks the repatriation of cash flows from a foreign investment.

2. When using capital budgeting techniques to evaluate a potential foreign project, the firm needs to recognize the specific risks arising from its foreign location. These include political risks and economic risks (including foreign exchange risk).

3. Political and economic risks can be incorporated into the capital budgeting process either by using a higher discount rate to evaluate risky projects or by forecasting lower cash flows for such projects.

4. The cost of capital is typically lower in the global capital market than in domestic markets. Consequently, other things being equal, firms prefer to finance their investments by borrowing from the global capital market.

5. Borrowing from the global capital market may be restricted by host-government regulations or demands. In such cases, the discount rate used in capital budgeting must be revised upward to reflect this.

6. The firm may want to consider local debt financing for investments in countries where the local currency is expected to depreciate.

7. The principal objectives of global money management are to utilize the firm's cash resources in the most efficient manner and to minimize the firm's global tax liabilities.

8. Firms use a number of techniques to transfer funds across borders, including dividend remittances, royalty payments and fees, transfer prices, and fronting loans.

9. Dividend remittances are the most common method used for transferring funds across borders, but royalty payments and fees have certain tax advantages over dividend remittances.

10. The manipulation of transfer prices is sometimes used by firms to move funds out of a country to minimize tax liabilities, hedge against foreign exchange risk, circumvent government restrictions on capital flows, and reduce tariff payments.

11. Manipulating transfer prices in this manner runs counter to government regulations in many countries, it may distort incentive systems within the firm, and it has ethically dubious foundations.

12. Fronting loans involve channeling funds from a parent company to a foreign subsidiary through a third party, normally an international bank. Fronting loans can circumvent host-government restrictions on the remittance of funds and provide certain tax advantages.

13. By holding cash at a centralized depository, the firm may be able to invest its cash reserves more efficiently. It can reduce the total size of the cash pool that it needs to hold in highly liquid accounts, thereby freeing cash for investment in higher-interest-bearing (less liquid) accounts or in tangible assets.

14. Multilateral netting reduces the transaction costs arising when a large number of transactions

occur between a firm's subsidiaries in the normal course of business.

15. The three types of exposure to foreign exchange risk are transaction exposure, translation exposure, and economic exposure.

16. Tactics that insure against transaction and translation exposure include buying forward, using currency swaps, leading and lagging payables and receivables, manipulating transfer prices, using local debt financing, accelerating dividend payments, and adjusting capital budgeting to reflect foreign exchange exposure.

17. Reducing a firm's economic exposure requires strategic choices about how the firm's productive assets are distributed around the globe.

18. To manage foreign exchange exposure effectively, the firm must exercise centralized oversight over its foreign exchange hedging activities, recognize the difference between transaction exposure and economic exposure, forecast future exchange rate movements, establish good reporting systems within the firm to monitor exposure positions, and produce regular foreign exchange exposure reports that can be used as a basis for action.

Critical Discussion Questions

1. How can the finance function of an international business improve the firm's competitive position in the global marketplace?

2. What actions can a firm take to minimize its global tax liability? On ethical grounds, can such actions be justified?

3. You are the CFO of a U.S. firm whose wholly owned subsidiary in Mexico manufactures component parts for your U.S. assembly operations. The subsidiary has been financed by bank borrowings in the United States. One of your analysts told you that the Mexican peso is expected to depreciate by 30 percent against the dollar on the foreign exchange markets over the next year. What actions, if any, should you take?

4. You are the CFO of a Canadian firm that is considering building a $10 million factory in Russia to produce milk. The investment is expected to produce net cash flows of $3 million each year for the next 10 years, after which the investment will have to close because of technological obsolescence. Scrap values will be zero. The cost of capital will be 6 percent if financing is arranged through the eurobond market. However, you have an option to finance the project by borrowing funds from a Russian bank at 12 percent. Analysts tell you that due to high inflation in Russia, the Russian ruble is expected to depreciate against the Canadian dollar. Analysts also rate the probability of violent revolution occurring in Russia within the next 10 years as high. How would you incorporate these factors into your evaluation of the investment opportunity? What would you recommend the firm do?

Notes

1. L. Quinn, "Currency Futures Trading Helps Firms Sharpen Competitive Edge," *Crain's Chicago Business*, March 2, 1992, p. 20

2. For details of capital budgeting techniques, see R. A. Brealy and S. C. Myers, *Principles of Corporate Finance* (New York: McGraw-Hill, 1988).

3. D. J. Feils and F. M. Sabac, "The Impact of Political Risk on the Foreign Direct Investment Decision: A Capital Budgeting Analysis," *The Engineering Economist* 45 (2000), pp. 129–34.

4. J. C. Backer and L. J. Beardsley, "Multinational Companies' Use of Risk Evaluation and Profit Measurement for Capital Budgeting Decisions," *Journal of Business Finance*, Spring 1973, pp. 34–43.

5. For example, see D. K. Eiteman, A. I. Stonehill, and M. H. Moffett, *Multinational Business Finance* (Reading, MA: Addison-Wesley, 1992).

6. M. Stanley and S. Block, "An Empirical Study of Management and Financial Variables Influencing Capital Budgeting Decisions for Multinational Corporations in the 1980s," *Management International Review* 23 (1983), pp. 61–71.

7. W. S. Sekely and J. M. Collins, "Cultural Influences on International Capital Structure," *Journal of International Business Studies*, Spring 1988, pp. 87–100.

8. J. K. Wald, "How Firm Characteristics Affect Capital Structure: An International Comparison," *Journal of Financial Research* 22, no. 2, (1999), pp. 161–87.

9. J. Collins and W. S. Sekely, "The Relationship of Headquarters, Country, and Industry Classification to Financial Structure," *Financial Structure*, Autumn 1983, pp. 45–51; J. Rutterford, "An

International Perspective on the Capital Structure Puzzle," *Midland Corporate Finance Journal*, Fall 1985, p. 72; R. G. Rajan and L. Zingales, "What Do We Know about Capital Structure," *Journal of Finance* 50 (1995), pp. 1421–60; and Wald, "How Firm Characteristics Affect Capital Structure: An International Comparison."

10. Sekely and Collins, "Cultural Influences on International Capital Structure." See also A. C. W. Chui, A. E. Lloyd, and C. C. Y. Kwok, "The Determination of Capital Structure: Is National Culture the Missing Piece to the Puzzle?" *Journal of International Business Studies* 33 (2002), pp. 99–127.

11. KPMG, "KPMG Corporate Tax Rate Survey—January 2003," http://www.us.kpmg.com/microsite/Global_Tax/CTR_Survey/2003Corprorate TaxSurveyFINAL.pdf.

12. "Taxing Questions," *The Economist*, May 22, 1993, p. 73.

13. S. Crow and E. Sauls, "Setting the Right Transfer Price," *Management Accounting*, December 1994, pp. 41–47.

14. V. H. Miesel, H. H. Higinbotham, and C. W. Yi, "International Transfer Pricing: Practical Solutions for Inter-company Pricing," *International Tax Journal*, Fall 2002, pp. 1–22.

15. J. Kelly, "Administrators Prepare for a More Efficient Future," *Financial Times Survey: World Taxation*, February 24, 1995, p. 9.

16. Crow and Sauls, "Setting the Right Transfer Price."

17. M. F. Al-Eryani, P. Alam, and S. Akhter, "Transfer Pricing Determinants of U.S. Multinationals," *Journal of International Business Studies*, September 1990, pp. 409–25.

18. D. L. Swenson, "Tax Reforms and Evidence of Transfer Pricing," *National Tax Journal*, March 2001, pp. 7–25.

19. "Transfer Pricing Survey Shows Multinationals Face Greater Scrutiny," *The CPA Journal*, March 2000, p. 10.

20. For details on how various firms manage their foreign exchange exposure, see the articles contained in the special foreign exchange issue of *Business International Money Report*, December 18, 1989, pp. 401–12.

21. Ibid.

22. S. Arterian, "How Black & Decker Defines Exposure," *Business International Money Report*, December 18, 1989, pp. 404, 405, 409.

23. T. Corrigan, "Corporate Treasury Management," *Financial Times*, November 2, 1993, p. 31.

Research Task | globalEDGE™   globaledge.msu.edu

Use the globalEDGE™ site to complete the following exercises:

1. The top management of your company requested a report regarding the tax policies of the following countries: Argentina, Belgium, Bulgaria, China, Czech Republic, Denmark, Egypt, Germany, Italy, and United Kingdom. Prepare a table including the corporate and individual income tax rates and the value added tax rates (where applicable) for those countries.

2. One of the Marketing Potential Indicators for Emerging Markets is identified as the country risk. Utilizing the ranking provided by the globalEDGE™ site identify five emerging markets that exhibit the least risk for foreign investors.

Motorola's Global Cash Management System

Closing Case

A multinational corporation with operating companies in more than 80 countries and sales in excess of $23 billion, Motorola is one of the world's leading providers of wireless communications equipment, semiconductors, and advanced electronics systems and services. Separate Motorola companies act autonomously and trade with each other on an arm's-length basis, often across national borders. Historically, each operating company managed its own payments with other Motorola subsidiaries and with independent suppliers

and executed its own foreign exchange dealings. In the 1990s, however, Motorola built a global cash management system that managed transactions not only between Motorola operating companies, but also between Motorola companies and key suppliers.

The evolution of Motorola's global cash management system dates to 1976 when the company decided to develop a foreign currency netting system for transactions between Motorola companies. The objective of this system was to achieve cost savings by reducing both cash flows and the amount of foreign exchange deals required to execute cross-border payments. Under this system, all foreign currency transactions between Motorola companies are managed with a single payment or invoice from a London-based treasury management center to each Motorola company once every week. Figures C.1, C.2, and C.3 show how this system reduces organizational complexity, while the following table gives a numerical example using the exchange rates detailed in Figure C.3 between the dollar ($), pound (£), euro (E), and yen (¥).

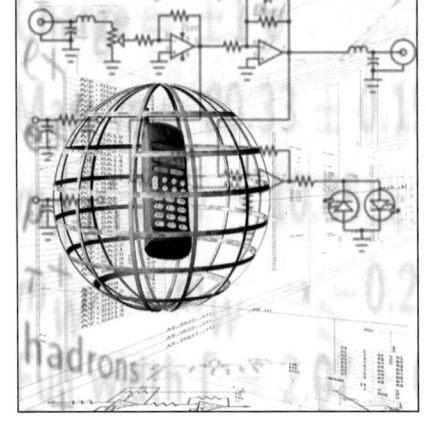

By use of the table, the net payments for each operating company can be easily calculated. Specifically,

Company A (£550 − £50 = £500).

Company B ($100 − $140 = −$40).

Company C (¥10,000 − ¥125,000 = −¥115,000).

Company D (E200 − E400 = −E200).

Before netting, the total amount of cash flows was the sum of all payments, which in dollar terms amounted to $1,320. The netted cash for each company is the sum of its payables less the sum of its receivables. In local currency, company A will receive £500, B will pay $40, C will pay ¥115,000, and D will pay E200. The netted cash flow in dollars is now $1,000. The center receives three different types of currencies, makes one payment to company A, and has a neutral cash position.

The benefits of this system are a reduction in cash flows and in the volume of foreign ex-

Figure C.1

Prenetting Information Flows

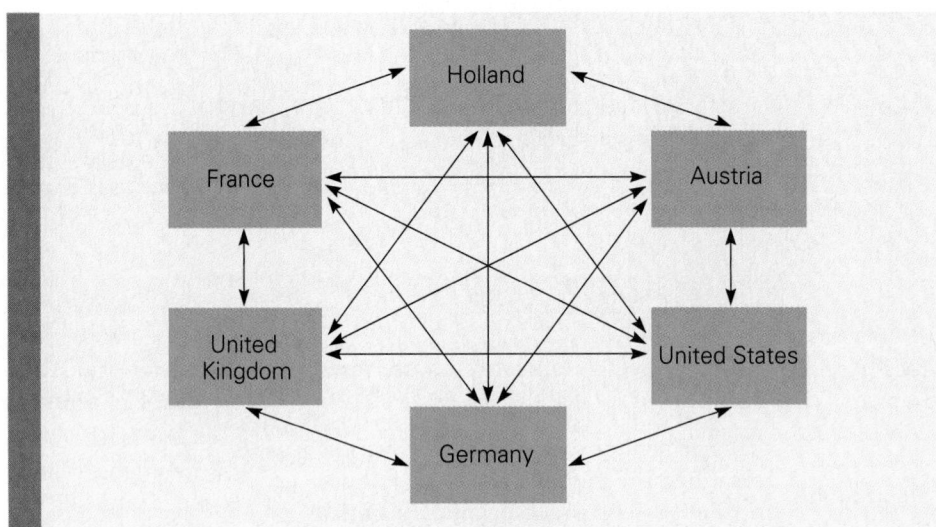

Figure C.2

Postnetting Information Flows

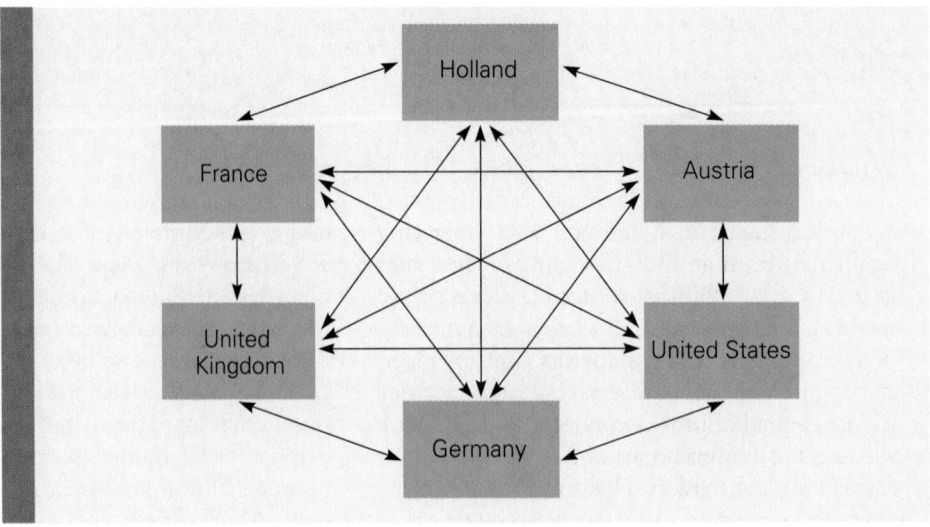

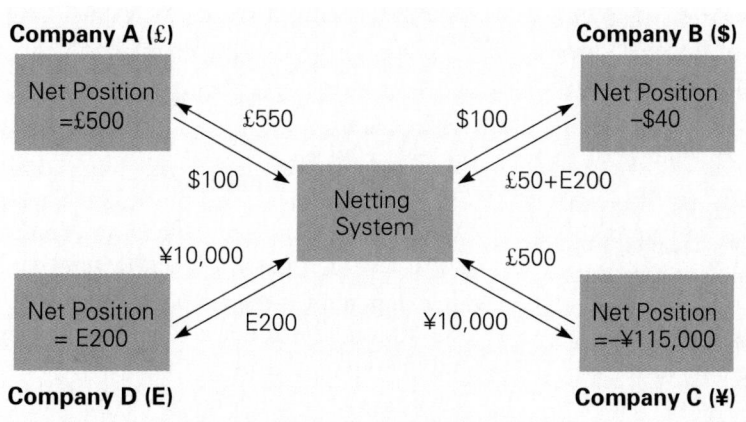

Figure C.3

Schematic Model of
Currency Netting

Accounts Payable	Accounts Receivable				Total Payable
	Company A (£)	Company B ($)	Company C (¥)	Company D (E)	
Company A	0	$100	0	0	
Company B	£50	0	0	E200	$140
Company C	£500	0	0	0	¥125,000
Company D	0	0	¥10,000	0	E400
Total receivable	£550	$100	¥10,000	E200	

change dealings. Moving from localized treasury management to one centralized system realized an estimated annual financial saving from lower transaction costs (bank fees and foreign exchange commissions) of about $6.5 million. However, this figure does not include administrative gains from more streamlined operations, which, while more difficult to quantify, are also probably quite substantial.

Motorola's success at implementing this system is attributed to a number of factors. First, senior management had the foresight to become committed to this initiative early. Management saw the system, and the information technology systems required to support it, as a source of strategic advantage. This was helpful in overcoming the normal resistance of operating managers to changes that take away some of their autonomy. Second, Motorola had already made substantial investments in building an information technology backbone to share manufacturing and logistics data between operating companies. Once this system was built, it could easily be extended to incorporate the data required for global treasury management. Third, Motorola took a gradual approach to implementing the system, which helped the company to perfect it before implementing it

organizationwide. A few sites were chosen as prototypes. After they had been integrated into the system and operating difficulties had been overcome, the inclusion of other sites proceeded smoothly. As a result, the number of participating Motorola entities rose from 38 in 1983 to 106 by the early 1990s.

Once the internal cash management system was working smoothly, Motorola extended the system to embrace key suppliers and customers. Extending the system was in principle relatively straightforward. Each week, the Motorola netting center collects data from each Motorola entity detailing payments that have to be made to suppliers. The global treasury function executes the required foreign exchange transactions, initiates payment orders, and advises Motorola companies of their net positions. After netting incoming payments with outgoing payments and combining common currencies, an approximate foreign exchange position is reached in which surplus currencies are sold and deficit currencies are purchased. The transaction value is about $100 million per week.

These payments are all handled by Citibank, which uses its own global information systems network to transfer funds between the various entities involved in the Motorola system, whether they are Motorola companies or independent vendors. Making this system work requires close electronic links between Motorola and Citibank, compatible information systems, a shared vision as to the purpose of the system, and ongoing cooperation between Motorola and Citibank to improve and manage the global flow of money.

As a result of this system, the net cash flow in 1991 between Motorola operating companies was $2.4 billion, a reduction of $2.38 billion from the value of payments settled in 1991. Without netting, Motorola would have had to engage in foreign exchange transactions valued at $4.3 billion. With netting, foreign exchange transactions were reduced to about $1.3 billion, which equates to annual direct savings in transaction costs of around $6.5 million.

Sources: C. P. Holland, G. Lockett, J. M. Richard, and I. Blackman, "The Evolution of a Global Cash Management System," *Sloan Management Review*, Fall 1994, pp. 37–47, and B. Ettorre, "How Motorola Closes Its Books in Two Days," *Management Review*, March 1995, pp. 84–89.

Case Discussion Questions

1. What are the strategic benefits to Motorola of the global cash management system described in this case?

2. How important is the relationship between Citibank and Motorola to the development, implementation, and smooth functioning of this system?

3. What factors helped Motorola to implement this system in a company where treasury operations had been decentralized to various national operations?

Cretors & Co.   694 🎥

Video Case: Cretors & Co. 🎥

Although it is a small business with annual sales of about $10 million, Cretors & Co. is the world's oldest and largest manufacturer of machines for popping and flavoring popcorn. It also makes machines for roasting and flavoring nuts, making cotton candy, and creating and serving other concession products. The company has been in business since 1885; it exported its first machine in 1897. Some 36 percent of the company's sales in 2002 were exports.

The bulk of Cretors' international sales are commercial machines for movie theaters. The company entered this market early and remains the dominant player. The company sells to a wide range of countries in Latin America and Europe. Almost all of the sales are made through distributors. Historically, many of these distributors have contacted Cretors and requested the opportunity to sell the company's equipment. However, Charlie Cretors, the great-grandson of the company's founder and its current CEO, notes that personal friendships have been very important in maintaining relationships with distributors and in growing the international market. To become a distributor for Cretors, the distributor also has to be able to provide after-sales service and support to end users.

Cretors has faced a number of problems when making international sales, including financing export sales, shipping products, and getting around import duties. Cretors insists on being paid in U.S. dollars, requires a 30 percent deposit on large orders, will ship large machines in containers and add other products that the distributor might want from the United States into that container, and is careful to classify equipment so that import duties are minimized.

Case Discussion Questions

1. How would you characterize Cretors' approach to building international sales? Do you think the company should change the way it builds international sales? Why?

2. Cretors makes extensive use of distributors to sell its products in foreign countries. What are the advantages of this approach? What are the potential disadvantages? Are there any circumstances where it might pay Cretors to sell directly with its own sales force?

3. What are the advantages to Cretors of requesting payment from foreign customers in U.S. dollars? What are the disadvantages?

4. What actions does Cretors take that make it an attractive company for foreign distributors to purchase products from?

Glossary

A

absolute advantage   A country has an absolute advantage in the production of a product when it is more efficient than any other country at producing it.

accounting standards   Rules for preparing financial statements.

ad valorem tariff   A tariff levied as a proportion of the value of an imported good.

administrative trade policies   Administrative policies, typically adopted by government bureaucracies, that can be used to restrict imports or boost exports.

Andean Pact   A 1969 agreement between Bolivia, Chile, Ecuador, Colombia, and Peru to establish a customs union.

antidumping policies   Designed to punish foreign firms that engage in dumping and thus protect domestic producers from unfair foreign competition.

antidumping regulations   Regulations designed to restrict the sale of goods for less than their fair market price.

arbitrage   The purchase of securities in one market for immediate resale in another to profit from a price discrepancy.

ASEAN (Association of South East Asian Nations) Formed in 1967, an attempt to establish a free trade area between Brunei, Indonesia, Malaysia, the Philippines, Singapore, and Thailand.

auditing standards   Rules for performing an audit.

B

backward vertical FDI   Investing in an industry abroad that provides inputs for a firm's domestic processes.

balance-of-payments accounts   National accounts that track both payments to and receipts from foreigners.

balance-of-trade equilibrium   Reached when the income a nation's residents earn from exports equals money paid for imports.

banking crisis   A loss of confidence in the banking system that leads to a run on banks, as individuals and companies withdraw their deposits.

barriers to entry   Factors that make it difficult or costly for firms to enter an industry or market.

barter   The direct exchange of goods or services between two parties without a cash transaction.

basic research centers   Centers for fundamental research located in regions where valuable scientific knowledge is being created; they develop the basic technologies that become new products.

bilateral netting   Settlement in which the amount one subsidiary owes another can be canceled by the debt the second subsidiary owes the first.

bill of exchange   An order written by an exporter instructing an importer, or an importer's agent, to pay a specified amount of money at a specified time.

bill of lading   A document issued to an exporter by a common carrier transporting merchandise. It serves as a receipt, a contract, and a document of title.

Bretton Woods   A 1944 conference in which representatives of 40 countries met to design a new international monetary system.

bureaucratic controls   Achieving control through establishment of a system of rules and procedures.

C

capital account   In the balance of payments, records transactions involving the purchase or sale of assets.

capital controls   Restrictions on cross-border capital flows that segment different stock markets; limit amount of a firm's stock a foreigner can own; and limit a citizen's ability to invest outside the country.

capital flight   Residents convert domestic currency into a foreign currency.

CARICOM   An association of English-speaking Caribbean states that are attempting to establish a customs union.

caste system   A system of social stratification in which social position is determined by the family into which a person is born, and change in that position is usually not possible during an individual's lifetime.

centralized depository   The practice of centralizing corporate cash balances in a single depository.

channel length   The number of intermediaries that a product has to go through before it reaches the final consumer.

civil law system   A system of law based on a very detailed set of written laws and codes.

class consciousness   A tendency for individuals to perceive themselves in terms of their class background.

class system   A system of social stratification in which social status is determined by the family into which a person is born and by subsequent socioeconomic achievements. Mobility between classes is possible.

collectivism   An emphasis on collective goals as opposed to individual goals.

COMECON   Now-defunct economic association of Eastern European Communist states headed by the former Soviet Union.

command economy   An economic system where the allocation of resources, including determination of what goods and services should be produced, and in what quantity, is planned by the government.

common law system   A system of law based on tradition, precedent, and custom. When law courts interpret common law, they do so with regard to these characteristics.

common market   A group of countries committed to (1) removing all barriers to the free flow of goods, services, and factors of production between each other and (2) the pursuit of a common external trade policy.

communist totalitarianism   A version of collectivism advocating that socialism can be achieved only through a totalitarian dictatorship.

communists   Those who believe socialism can be achieved only through revolution and totalitarian dictatorship.

comparative advantage   The theory that countries should specialize in the production of goods and services they can produce most efficiently. A country is said to have a comparative advantage in the production of such goods and services.

competition policy   Regulations designed to promote competition and restrict monopoly practices.

Confucian dynamism   Theory that Confucian teachings affect attitudes toward time, persistence, ordering by status, protection of face, respect for tradition, and reciprocation of gifts and favors.

constant returns to specialization   The units of resources required to produce a good are assumed to remain constant no matter where one is on a country's production possibility frontier.

contract   Document that specifies conditions of an exchange and details rights and obligations of involved parties.

contract law   Body of law that governs contract enforcement.

controlling interest   A firm has a controlling interest in another business entity when it owns more than 50 percent of that entity's voting stock.

control systems   Metrics used to measure performance of subunits.

copyright   Exclusive legal rights of authors, composers, playwrights, artists, and publishers to publish and dispose of their work as they see fit.

core competence   Firm skills that competitors cannot easily match or imitate.

cost of capital   Price of money.

Council of Ministers   Represents the interests of EU members and has authority to approve EU laws.

counterpurchase   A reciprocal buying agreement.

countertrade   The trade of goods and services for other goods and services.

countervailing duties   Antidumping duties.

Court of Justice   Supreme appeals court for EU law.

cross-cultural literacy   Understanding how the culture of a country affects the way business is practiced.

cross-licensing agreement   An arrangement in which a company licenses valuable intangible property to a foreign partner and receives a license for the partner's valuable knowledge; reduces risk of licensing.

cultural controls   Achieving control by persuading subordinates to identify with the norms and value systems of the organization (self-control).

culture   The complex whole that includes knowledge, belief, art, morals, law, custom, and other capabilities acquired by a person as a member of society.

currency board   Means of controlling a country's currency.

currency crisis   Occurs when a speculative attack on the exchange value of a currency results in a sharp depreciation in the value of the currency or forces authorities to expend large volumes of international currency reserves and sharply increase interest rates to defend the prevailing exchange rate.

currency speculation   Involves short-term movement of funds from one currency to another in hopes of profiting from shifts in exchange rates.

currency swap   Simultaneous purchase and sale of a given amount of foreign exchange for two different value dates.

currency translation   Converting the financial statements of foreign subsidiaries into the currency of the home country.

current account   In the balance of payments, records transactions involving the export or import of goods and services.

current account deficit   The current account of the balance of payments is in deficit when a country imports more goods and services than it exports.

current account surplus   The current account of the balance of payments is in surplus when a country exports more goods and services than it imports.

current cost accounting   Method that adjusts all items in a financial statement to factor out the effects of inflation.

current rate method   Using the exchange rate at the balance sheet date to translate the financial statements of a foreign subsidiary into the home currency.

customs union   A group of countries committed to (1) removing all barriers to the free flow of goods and services between each other and (2) the pursuit of a common external trade policy.

D

D'Amato Act   Act passed in 1996, similar to the Helms-Burton Act, aimed at Libya and Iran.

debt loan   Requires a corporation to repay loan at regular intervals.

deferral principle   Parent companies are not taxed on the income of a foreign subsidiary until they actually receive a dividend from that subsidiary.

democracy   Political system in which government is by the people, exercised either directly or through elected representatives.

deregulation   Removal of government restrictions concerning the conduct of a business.

diminishing returns to specialization   Applied to international trade theory, the more of a good that a country produces, the greater the units of resources required to produce each additional item.

dirty-float system   A system under which a country's currency is nominally allowed to float freely against other currencies, but in which the government will intervene, buying and selling currency, if it believes that the currency has deviated too far from its fair value.

draft   An order written by an exporter telling an importer what and when to pay.

drawee   The party to whom a bill of lading is presented.

dumping   Selling goods in a foreign market for less than their cost of production or below their "fair" market value.

E

eclectic paradigm   Argument that combining location-specific assets or resource endowments and the firm's own unique assets often requires FDI; it requires the firm to establish production facilities where those foreign assets or resource endowments are located.

e-commerce   Conducting business online through the Internet.

economic exposure   The extent to which a firm's future international earning power is affected by changes in exchange rates.

economic risk   The likelihood that events, including economic mismanagement, will cause drastic changes in a country's business environment that adversely affect the profit and other goals of a particular business enterprise.

economic union   A group of countries committed to (1) removing all barriers to the free flow of goods, services, and factors of production between each other, (2) the adoption of a common currency, (3) the harmonization of tax rates, and (4) the pursuit of a common external trade policy.

economies of scale   Cost advantages associated with large-scale production.

ecu   A basket of EU currencies that served as the unit of account for the EMS.

efficient market   A market where prices reflect all available information.

ending rate   The spot exchange rate when budget and performance are being compared.

equity loan   Occurs when a corporation sells stock to an investor.

ethical systems   Cultural beliefs about what is proper behavior and conduct.

ethnocentric behavior   Behavior that is based on the belief in the superiority of one's own ethnic group or culture; often shows disregard or contempt for the culture of other countries.

ethnocentric staffing   A staffing approach within the MNE in which all key management positions are filled by parent-country nationals.

ethnocentrism   Belief in the superiority of one's own ethnic group or culture.

eurobonds   A bond placed in countries other than the one in whose currency the bond is denominated.

eurocurrency   Any currency banked outside its country of origin.

eurodollar   Dollar banked outside the United States.

European Commission   Responsible for proposing EU legislation, implementing it, and monitoring compliance.

European Council   Consists of the heads of state of EU members and the president of the European Commission.

European Free Trade Association (EFTA)   A free trade association including Norway, Iceland, and Switzerland.

European Monetary System (EMS)   EU system designed to create a zone of monetary stability in Europe, control inflation, and coordinate exchange rate policies of EU countries.

European Parliament   Elected EU body that provides consultation on issues proposed by European Commission.

European Union (EU)   An economic group of 15 European nations: Austria, Belgium, Denmark, Finland, France, Germany, Great Britain, Greece, the Netherlands, Ireland, Italy, Luxembourg, Portugal, Spain, and Sweden. Established as a customs union, it is now moving toward economic union. (Formerly the European Community.)

exchange rate   The rate at which one currency is converted into another.

exchange rate mechanism (ERM)   Mechanism for aligning the exchange rates of EU currencies against each other.

exclusive channels   A distribution channel that outsiders find difficult to access.

expatriate   A citizen of one country working in another country.

expatriate failure   The premature return of an expatriate manager to the home country.

expatriate manager   A national of one country appointed to a management position in another country.

experience curve   Systematic production cost reductions that occur over the life of a product.

experience curve pricing   Aggressive pricing designed to increase volume and help the firm realize experience curve economies.

export management company   Export specialists who act as an export marketing department for client firms.

Export–Import Bank (Eximbank)   Agency of the U.S. government whose mission is to provide aid in financing and facilitate exports and imports.

exporting   Sale of products produced in one country to residents of another country.

externalities   Knowledge spillovers.

externally convertible currency   Nonresidents can convert their holdings of domestic currency into foreign currency, but the ability of residents to convert the currency is limited in some way.

F

factor endowments   A country's endowment with resources such as land, labor, and capital.

factors of production   Inputs into the productive process of a firm, including labor, management, land, capital, and technological know-how.

Financial Accounting Standards Board (FASB)   The body that writes the generally accepted accounting principles by which the financial statements of U.S. firms must be prepared.

financial structure   Mix of debt and equity used to finance a business.

first-mover advantages   Advantages accruing to the first to enter a market.

first-mover disadvantages   Disadvantages associated with entering a foreign market before other international businesses.

Fisher Effect   Nominal interest rates (i) in each country equal the required real rate of interest (r) and the expected rate of inflation over the period of time for which the funds are to be lent (I). That is, $i = r + I$.

fixed exchange rates   A system under which the exchange rate for converting one currency into another is fixed.

fixed-rate bond   Offers a fixed set of cash payoffs each year until maturity, when the investor also receives the face value of the bond in cash.

flexible machine cells   Flexible manufacturing technology in which a grouping of various machine types, a common materials handler, and a centralized cell controller produce a family of products.

flexible manufacturing technologies   Manufacturing technologies designed to improve job scheduling, reduce setup time, and improve quality control.

floating exchange rates   A system under which the exchange rate for converting one currency into another is continuously adjusted depending on the laws of supply and demand.

flow of foreign direct investment   The amount of foreign direct investment undertaken over a given time period (normally one year).

folkways   Routine conventions of everyday life.

foreign bonds   Bonds sold outside the borrower's country and denominated in the currency of the country in which they are issued.

Foreign Corrupt Practices Act   U.S. law regulating behavior regarding the conduct of international business in the taking of bribes and other unethical actions.

foreign debt crisis   Situation in which a country cannot service its foreign debt obligations, whether private-sector or government debt.

foreign direct investment (FDI)   Direct investment in business operations in a foreign country.

foreign exchange exposure   The risk that future changes in a country's exchange rate will hurt the firm.

foreign exchange market   A market for converting the currency of one country into that of another country.

foreign exchange risk   The risk that changes in exchange rates will hurt the profitability of a business deal.

foreign portfolio investment (FPI)   Investments by individuals, firms, or public bodies (e.g., national and local governments) in foreign financial instruments (e.g., government bonds, foreign stocks).

forward exchange   When two parties agree to exchange currency and execute a deal at some specific date in the future.

forward exchange rate   The exchange rates governing forward exchange transactions.

forward vertical FDI   Investing in an industry abroad that sells outputs of domestic processes.

franchising   A specialized form of licensing in which the franchiser sells intangible property to the franchisee and insists on rules to conduct the business.

free trade   The absence of barriers to the free flow of goods and services between countries.

free trade area   A group of countries committed to removing all barriers to the free flow of goods and services between each other, but pursuing independent external trade policies.

freely convertible currency   A country's currency is freely convertible when the government of that country allows both residents and nonresidents to purchase unlimited amounts of foreign currency with the domestic currency.

fronting loan   A loan between a parent company and a foreign subsidiary that is channeled through a financial intermediary.

fundamental analysis   Draws on economic theory to construct sophisticated econometric models for predicting exchange rate movements.

G

gains from trade   The economic gains to a country from engaging in international trade.

General Agreement on Tariffs and Trade (GATT) International treaty that committed signatories to lowering barriers to the free flow of goods across national borders and led to the WTO.

geocentric staffing   A staffing policy where the best people are sought for key jobs throughout an MNE, regardless of nationality.

global learning   The flow of skills and product offerings from foreign subsidiary to home country and from foreign subsidiary to foreign subsidiary.

global matrix structure   Horizontal differentiation proceeds along two dimensions: product divisions and areas.

global strategy   Strategy focusing on increasing profitability by reaping cost reductions from experience curve and location economies.

global web   When different stages of value chain are dispersed to those locations around the globe where value added is maximized or where costs of value creation are minimized.

globalization   Trend away from distinct national economic units and toward one huge global market.

globalization of markets   Moving away from an economic system in which national markets are distinct entities, isolated by trade barriers and barriers of distance, time, and culture, and toward a system in which national markets are merging into one global market.

globalization of production   Trend by individual firms to disperse parts of their productive processes to different locations around the globe to take advantage of differences in cost and quality of factors of production.

gold par value   The amount of currency needed to purchase one ounce of gold.

gold standard   The practice of pegging currencies to gold and guaranteeing convertibility.

green-field investment   Establishing a new operation in a foreign country.

gross domestic product (GDP)   The market value of a country's output attributable to factors of production located in the country's territory.

gross fixed capital formation   Summarizes the total amount of capital invested in factories, stores, office buildings, and the like.

gross national product (GNP)   The market value of all the final goods and services produced by a national economy.

group   An association of two or more individuals who have a shared sense of identity and who interact with each other in structured ways on the basis of a common set of expectations about each other's behavior.

H

Heckscher-Ohlin theory   Countries will export those goods that make intensive use of locally abundant factors of production and import goods that make intensive use of locally scarce factors of production.

hedge fund   Investment fund that not only buys financial assets (stocks, bonds, currencies) but also sells them short.

Helms-Burton Act   Act passed in 1996 that allowed Americans to sue foreign firms that use Cuban property confiscated from them after the 1959 revolution.

historic cost principle   Accounting principle founded on the assumption that the currency unit used to report financial results is not losing its value due to inflation.

home country   The source country for foreign direct investment.

horizontal differentiation   The division of the firm into subunits.

horizontal foreign direct investment   Foreign direct investment in the same industry abroad as a firm operates in at home.

host country   Recipient country of inward investment by a foreign firm.

Human Development Index   An attempt by the United Nations to assess the impact of a number of factors on the quality of human life in a country.

human resource management   Activities an organization conducts to use its human resources effectively.

I

import quota   A direct restriction on the quantity of a good that can be imported into a country.

incentives   Devices used to reward managerial behavior.

individualism   An emphasis on the importance of guaranteeing individual freedom and self-expression.

individualism versus collectivism   Theory focusing on the relationship between the individual and his or her fellows. In individualistic societies, the ties between individuals are loose and individual achievement is highly valued. In societies where collectivism is emphasized, ties between individuals are tight, people are born into collectives, such as extended families, and everyone is supposed to look after the interests of his or her collective.

inefficient market   One in which prices do not reflect all available information.

infant industry argument   New industries in developing countries must be temporarily protected from international competition to help them reach a position where they can compete on world markets with the firms of developed nations.

inflows of FDI   Flow of foreign direct investment into a country.

initial rate   The spot exchange rate when a budget is adopted.

innovation   Development of new products, processes, organizations, management practices, and strategies.

integrating mechanisms   Mechanisms for achieving coordination between subunits within an organization.

intellectual property   Products of the mind, ideas (e.g., books, music, computer software, designs, technological know-how). Intellectual property can be protected by patents, copyrights, and trademarks.

internal forward rate   A company-generated forecast of future spot rates.

internalization theory   Marketing imperfection approach to foreign direct investment.

International Accounting Standards Board (IASB)   Organization of representatives of professional accounting organizations from many countries that is attempting to harmonize accounting standards across countries.

international business   Any firm that engages in international trade or investment.

international division   Division responsible for a firm's international activities.

International Fisher Effect   For any two countries, the spot exchange rate should change in an equal amount but in the opposite direction to the difference in nominal interest rates between countries.

International Monetary Fund (IMF)   International institution set up to maintain order in the international monetary system.

international monetary system   Institutional arrangements countries adopt to govern exchange rates.

international strategy   Trying to create value by transferring core competencies to foreign markets where indigenous competitors lack those competencies.

international trade   Occurs when a firm exports goods or services to consumers in another country.

ISO 9000   Certification process that requires certain quality standards that must be met.

J

joint venture   A cooperative undertaking between two or more firms.

just-in-time (JIT)   Logistics systems designed to deliver parts to a production process as they are needed, not before.

L

lag strategy   Delaying the collection of foreign currency receivables if that currency is expected to appreciate, and delaying payables if that currency is expected to depreciate.

late-mover advantages   Benefits enjoyed by a company that is late to enter a new market, such as consumer familiarity with the product or knowledge gained about a market.

late-mover disadvantages   Handicap that late entrants to a market suffer.

law of one price   In competitive markets free of transportation costs and barriers to trade, identical products sold in different countries must sell for the same price when their price is expressed in the same currency.

lead market   Market where products are first introduced.

lead strategy   Collecting foreign currency receivables early when a foreign currency is expected to depreciate, and paying foreign currency payables before they are due when a currency is expected to appreciate.

lean production systems   Flexible manufacturing technologies pioneered at Toyota and now used in much of the automobile industry.

learning effects   Cost savings from learning by doing.

legal risk   The likelihood that a trading partner will opportunistically break a contract or expropriate intellectual property rights.

legal system   System of rules that regulate behavior and the processes by which the laws of a country are enforced and through which redress of grievances is obtained.

Leontief paradox   The empirical finding that, in contrast to the predictions of the Heckscher-Ohlin theory, U.S. exports are less capital intensive than U.S. imports.

letter of credit   Issued by a bank, indicating that the bank will make payments under specific circumstances.

licensing   Occurs when a firm (the licensor) licenses the right to produce its product, use its production processes, or use its brand name or trademark to another firm (the licensee). In return for giving the licensee these rights, the licensor collects a royalty fee on every unit the licensee sells.

local content requirement   A requirement that some specific fraction of a good be produced domestically.

location economies   Cost advantages from performing a value creation activity at the optimal location for that activity.

location-specific advantages   Advantages that arise from using resource endowments or assets that are tied to a particular foreign location and that a firm finds valuable to combine with its own unique assets (such as the firm's technological, marketing, or management know-how).

logistics   The procurement and physical transmission of material through the supply chain, from suppliers to customers.

M

Maastricht Treaty   Treaty agreed to in 1991, but not ratified until January 1, 1994, that committed the 12 member states of the European Community to a closer economic and political union.

maker   Person or business initiating a bill of lading (draft).

managed-float system   System under which some currencies are allowed to float freely, but the majority are either managed by government intervention or pegged to another currency.

management network   A network of informal contact between individual managers.

market economy   The allocation of resources is determined by the invisible hand of the price system.

market imperfections   Imperfections in the operation of the market mechanism.

market makers   Financial service companies that connect investors and borrowers, either directly or indirectly.

market power   Ability of a firm to exercise control over industry prices or output.

market segmentation   Identifying groups of consumers whose purchasing behavior differs from others in important ways.

marketing mix   Choices about product attributes, distribution strategy, communication strategy, and pricing strategy that a firm offers its targeted markets.

masculinity versus femininity   Theory of the relationship between gender and work roles. In masculine cultures, sex roles are sharply differentiated and traditional "masculine values" such as achievement and the effective exercise of power determine cultural ideals. In feminine cultures, sex roles are less sharply distinguished, and little differentiation is made between men and women in the same job.

mass customization   The production of a wide variety of end products at a unit cost that could once be achieved only through mass production of a standardized output.

materials management   The activity that controls the transmission of physical materials through the value chain, from procurement through production and into distribution.

mercantilism   An economic philosophy advocating that countries should simultaneously encourage exports and discourage imports.

MERCOSUR   Pact between Argentina, Brazil, Paraguay, and Uruguay to establish a free trade area.

minimum efficient scale   The level of output at which most plant-level scale economies are exhausted.

MITI   Japan's Ministry of International Trade and Industry.

mixed economy   Certain sectors of the economy are left to private ownership and free market mechanisms, while other sectors have significant government ownership and government planning.

money management   Managing a firm's global cash resources efficiently.

Moore's Law   The power of microprocessor technology doubles and its costs of production fall in half every 18 months.

moral hazard   Arises when people behave recklessly because they know they will be saved if things go wrong.

mores   Norms seen as central to the functioning of a society and to its social life.

multidomestic strategy   Emphasizing the need to be responsive to the unique conditions prevailing in different national markets.

Multilateral Agreement on Investment (MAI)   An agreement that would make it illegal for signatory states to discriminate against foreign investors; would have liberalized rules governing FDI between OECD states.

multilateral netting   A technique used to reduce the number of transactions between subsidiaries of the firm, thereby reducing the total transaction costs arising from foreign exchange dealings and transfer fees.

multinational enterprise (MNE)   A firm that owns business operations in more than one country.

multipoint competition   Arises when two or more enterprises encounter each other in different regional markets, national markets, or industries.

multipoint pricing   Occurs when a pricing strategy in one market may have an impact on a rival's pricing strategy in another market.

N

new trade theory   The observed pattern of trade in the world economy may be due in part to the ability of firms in a given market to capture first-mover advantages.

nonconvertible currency   A currency is not convertible when both residents and nonresidents are prohibited from converting their holdings of that currency into another currency.

norms   Social rules and guidelines that prescribe appropriate behavior in particular situations.

North American Free Trade Agreement (NAFTA)   Free trade area between Canada, Mexico, and the United States.

O

offshore production   FDI undertaken to serve the home market.

oligopoly   An industry composed of a limited number of large firms.

organizational architecture   Totality of a firm's organization.

organizational culture   Norms and values shared by employees.

organizational structure   Determined by the formal division into subunits, the location of decision making, and the coordination of activities of subunits.

Organization for Economic Cooperation and Development (OECD)   A Paris-based intergovernmental organization of "wealthy" nations whose purpose is to provide its 29 member states with a forum in which governments can compare their experiences, discuss the problems they share, and seek solutions that can then be applied within their own national contexts.

outflows of FDI   Flow of foreign direct investment out of a country.

output controls   Achieving control by setting goals for subordinates, expressing these goals in terms of objective criteria, and then judging performance by a subordinate's ability to meet these goals.

P

Paris Convention for the Protection of Industrial Property   International agreement to protect intellectual property; signed by 96 countries.

patent   Grants the inventor of a new product or process exclusive rights to the manufacture, use, or sale of that invention.

pegged exchange rate   Currency value is fixed relative to a reference currency.

people   Part of the organizational architecture that includes strategy used to recruit, compensate, and retain employees.

performance ambiguity   Occurs when the causes of good or bad performance are not clearly identifiable.

personal controls   Achieving control by personal contact with subordinates.

pioneering costs   Costs an early entrant bears that later entrants avoid, such as the time and effort in learning the rules, failure due to ignorance, and the liability of being a foreigner.

political economy   The study of how political factors influence the functioning of an economic system.

political risk   The likelihood that political forces will cause drastic changes in a country's business environment that will adversely affect the profit and other goals of a particular business enterprise.

political system   System of government in a nation.

political union   A central political apparatus coordinates economic, social, and foreign policy.

polycentric staffing   A staffing policy in an MNE in which host-country nationals are recruited to manage subsidiaries in their own country, while parent-country nationals occupy key positions at corporate headquarters.

positive-sum game   A situation in which all countries can benefit even if some benefit more than others.

power distance   Theory of how a society deals with the fact that people are unequal in physical and intellectual capabilities. High power distance cultures are found in countries that let inequalities grow over time into inequalities of power and wealth. Low power distance cultures are found in societies that try to play down such inequalities as much as possible.

predatory pricing   Reducing prices below fair market value as a competitive weapon to drive weaker competitors out of the market ("fair" being cost plus some reasonable profit margin).

price discrimination   The practice of charging different prices for the same product in different markets.

price elasticity of demand   A measure of how responsive demand for a product is to changes in price.

privatization   The sale of state-owned enterprises to private investors.

processes   Manner in which decisions are made and work is performed.

product liability   Involves holding a firm and its officers responsible when a product causes injury, death, or damage.

product life-cycle theory   The optimal location in the world to produce a product change as the market for the product matures.

product safety laws   Set certain safety standards to which a product must adhere.

production   Activities involved in creating a product.

profit   Difference between revenues and costs.

profitability   A rate of return concept.

projected rate   The spot exchange rate forecast for the end of the budget period.

property rights   Bundle of legal rights over the use to which a resource is put and over the use made of any income that may be derived from that resource.

pull strategy   A marketing strategy emphasizing mass media advertising as opposed to personal selling.

purchasing power parity (PPP)   An adjustment in gross domestic product per capita to reflect differences in the cost of living.

push strategy   A marketing strategy emphasizing personal selling rather than mass media advertising.

Q

quota rent   Extra profit producers make when supply is artificially limited by an import quota.

R

regional economic integration   Agreements among countries in a geographic region to reduce and ultimately remove tariff and nontariff barriers to the free flow of goods, services, and factors of production between each other.

relatively efficient market   One in which few impediments to international trade and investment exist.

religion   A system of shared beliefs and rituals concerned with the sacred.

representative democracy   A political system in which citizens periodically elect individuals to represent them in government.

right-wing totalitarianism   A political system in which political power is monopolized by a party, group, or individual that generally permits individual economic freedom but restricts individual political freedom, including free speech, often on the grounds that it would lead to the rise of communism.

royalties   Remuneration paid to the owners of technology, patents, or trade names for the use of same.

S

short selling   Occurs when an investor places a speculative bet that the value of a financial asset will decline, and profits from that decline.

sight draft   A draft payable on presentation to the drawee.

Single European Act   A 1997 act, adopted by members of the European Community, that committed member countries to establishing an economic union.

six sigma   Statistically based philosophy to reduce defects, boost productivity, eliminate waste, and cut costs.

Smoot-Hawley tariff   Enacted in 1930 by the U.S. Congress, this tariff erected a wall of barriers against imports into the United States.

social democrats   Those committed to achieving socialism by democratic means.

social mobility   The extent to which individuals can move out of the social strata into which they are born.

social strata   Hierarchical social categories.

social structure   The basic social organization of a society.

socialism   A political philosophy advocating substantial public involvement, through government ownership, in the means of production and distribution.

society   Group of people who share a common set of values and norms.

sogo shosha   Japanese trading companies; a key part of the *keiretsu*, the large Japanese industrial groups.

sourcing decisions   Whether a firm should make or buy component parts.

specialized asset   An asset designed to perform a specific task, whose value is significantly reduced in its next-best use.

specific tariff   Tariff levied as a fixed charge for each unit of good imported.

spot exchange rate   The exchange rate at which a foreign exchange dealer will convert one currency into another that particular day.

staffing policy   Strategy concerned with selecting employees for particular jobs.

state-directed economy   An economy in which the state plays a proactive role in influencing the direction and magnitude of private-sector investments.

stock of foreign direct investment   The total accumulated value of foreign-owned assets at a given time.

strategic alliances   Cooperative agreements between two or more firms.

strategic commitment   A decision that has a long-term impact and is difficult to reverse, such as entering a foreign market on a large scale.

strategic trade policy   Government policy aimed at improving the competitive position of a domestic industry and/or domestic firm in the world market.

strategy   Actions managers take to attain the firm's goals.

Structural Impediments Initiative   A 1990 agreement between the United States and Japan aimed at trying to decrease nontariff barriers restricting imports into Japan.

subsidy   Government financial assistance to a domestic producer.

swaps　The simultaneous purchase and sale of a given amount of foreign exchange for two different value dates.

systematic risk　Movements in a stock portfolio's value that are attributable to macroeconomic forces affecting all firms in an economy, rather than factors specific to an individual firm (unsystematic risk).

T

tariff　A tax levied on imports.

tax credit　Allows a firm to reduce the taxes paid to the home government by the amount of taxes paid to the foreign government.

tax haven　A country with exceptionally low, or even no, income taxes.

tax treaty　Agreement between two countries specifying what items of income will be taxed by the authorities of the country where the income is earned.

technical analysis　Uses price and volume data to determine past trends, which are expected to continue into the future.

temporal method　Translating assets valued in a foreign currency into the home currency using the exchange rate that existed when the assets were originally purchased.

theocratic law system　A system of law based on religious teachings.

theocratic totalitarianism　A political system in which political power is monopolized by a party, group, or individual that governs according to religious principles.

time draft　A promise to pay by the accepting party at some future date.

time-based competition　Competing on the basis of speed in responding to customer demands and developing new products.

timing of entry　Entry is early when a firm enters a foreign market before other foreign firms and late when a firm enters after other international businesses have established themselves.

total quality management　Management philosophy that takes as its central focus the need to improve the quality of a company's products and services.

totalitarianism　Form of government in which one person or political party exercises absolute control over all spheres of human life and opposing political parties are prohibited.

trade creation　Trade created due to regional economic integration; occurs when high-cost domestic producers are replaced by low-cost foreign producers in a free trade area.

trade deficit　See **current account deficit.**

trade diversion　Trade diverted due to regional economic integration; occurs when low-cost foreign suppliers outside a free trade area are replaced by higher-cost foreign suppliers in a free trade area.

trade surplus　See **current account surplus.**

Trade Related Aspects of Intellectual Property Rights　WTO agreement overseeing stricter intellectual property regulations.

trademark　Designs and names, often officially registered, by which merchants or manufacturers designate and differentiate their products.

transaction costs　The costs of exchange.

transaction exposure　The extent to which income from individual transactions is affected by fluctuations in foreign exchange values.

transfer fee　A bank charge for moving cash from one location to another.

transfer price　The price at which goods and services are transferred between subsidiary companies of a corporation.

translation exposure　The extent to which the reported consolidated results and balance sheets of a corporation are affected by fluctuations in foreign exchange values.

transnational corporation　A firm that tries to simultaneously realize gains from experience curve economies, location economies, and global learning, while remaining locally responsive.

transnational financial reporting　The need for a firm headquartered in one country to report its results to citizens of another country.

transnational strategy　Plan to exploit experience-based cost and location economies, transfer core competencies with the firm, and pay attention to local responsiveness.

Treaty of Rome　The 1957 treaty that established the European Community.

tribal totalitarianism　A political system in which a party, group, or individual that represents the interests of a particular tribe (ethnic group) monopolizes political power.

turnkey project　A project in which a firm agrees to set up an operating plant for a foreign client and hand over the "key" when the plant is fully operational.

U

unbundling　Relying on more than one financial technique to transfer funds across borders.

uncertainty avoidance　Extent to which cultures socialize members to accept ambiguous situations and to tolerate uncertainty.

United Nations　International institution with 191 member countries created to preserve peace.

United Nations Convention on Contracts for the International Sale of Goods　Agreement establishing a uniform set of rules governing contracts between businesses in different nations.

universal needs   Needs that are the same all over the world, such as steel, bulk chemicals, and industrial electronics.

V

value creation   Performing activities that increase the value of goods or services to consumers.

values   Abstract ideas about what a society believes to be good, right, and desirable.

vehicle currency   A currency that plays a central role in the foreign exchange market (e.g., the U.S. dollar and Japanese yen).

vertical differentiation   The centralization and decentralization of decision-making responsibilities.

vertical foreign direct investment   Foreign direct investment in an industry abroad that provides input into a firm's domestic operations, or foreign direct investment into an industry abroad that sells the outputs of a firm's domestic operations.

vertical integration   Extension of a firm's activities into adjacent stages of productions (i.e., those providing the firm's inputs or those that purchase the firm's outputs).

voluntary export restraint (VER)   A quota on trade imposed from the exporting country's side, instead of the importer's; usually imposed at the request of the importing country's government.

W

wholly owned subsidiary   A subsidiary in which the firm owns 100 percent of the stock.

World Bank   International institution set up to promote general economic development in the world's poorer nations.

World Trade Organization (WTO)   The organization that succeeded the General Agreement on Tariffs and Trade (GATT) as a result of the successful completion of the Uruguay round of GATT negotiations.

worldwide area structure   Business organizational structure under which the world is divided into areas.

worldwide product division structure   Business organizational structure based on product divisions that have worldwide responsibility.

Z

zero-sum game   A situation in which an economic gain by one country results in an economic loss by another.

Photo Credits

PO1.1	Piggy Banks	Royalty Free/Corbis
PO1.2	Palm Pilot	© Larry Williams/Corbis
PO1.3	Sun Sculpture	Royalty Free/Corbis
P1.1	German Wal-Mart	AFP/Corbis
P1.2	Piggy Banks	Royalty Free/Corbis
P1.3	Palm Pilot	© Larry Williams/Corbis
P1.4	Country Signs	© Torleif Svensson/Corbis
P1.5	Sun Sculpture	Royalty Free/ Corbis
C-1	Roses	© Owen Franken/Corbis
PO2.1	Dancers	© Lindsay Hebberd/Corbis
PO2.2	Varansi, India	© Fatima Martins/Corbis
PO2.3	Face of Buddha	© David Samuel Robbins/Corbis
P2.1	Regatta	© Frederic Haslin/Corbis
P2.2	Dancers	© Lindsay Hebberd/Corbis
P2.3	Varansi, India	© Fatima Martins/Corbis
P2.5	Face of Buddha	© David Samuel Robbins/Corbis
P2.6	Cranes	© Pawel Libera/Corbis
C-2	Girls playing game	© Reuters NewMedia Inc./Corbis
C-3	New Delhi McDonald's	© Baldev/Corbis SYGMA
PO3.1	Honda Employees	© China Features/Corbis SYGMA
PO3.2	EU Leaders	© Reuters NewMedia Inc./Corbis
PO3.3	Cotton Plants	© Richard Hamilton Smith/Corbis
P3.1	Computer College	© TUYAY EDWIN/CORBIS SYGMA
P3.2	Cows	© Joe Baraban/Corbis
P3.3	Starbucks	© Steve Raymer/Corbis
P3.4	Honda Employees	© China Features/Corbis SYGMA
P3.5	EU Leaders	© Reuters NewMedia Inc./Corbis
P3.6	Cotton Plants	© Richard Hamilton Smith/Corbis
C-4	Man Using Laptop	© Reuters NewMedia Inc./Corbis
C-5	Money Sign	Royalty Free/Corbis
C-6	Car Assembly Plant	© Bojan Brecelj/Corbis
C-7	Toyota Banner	© BISSON BERNARD/Corbis SYGMA
C-8	Deutsche Bank	© James Leynse/Corbis SABA
PO4.1	Exchange Rate	© AFP/Corbis
PO4.2	European Coins	Royalty Free/Corbis
PO4.3	Spices	© Dave Bartruff/Corbis
P4.1	Exchange Rate	© AFP/Corbis
P4.2	Grand Bazaar	© Wolfgang Kaehler/Corbis
P4.3	Online Sign	© AFP/Corbis
P4.4	Spices	© Dave Bartruff/Corbis
P4.5	European Coins	Royalty Free/Corbis
C-9	Thai Bhat	Royalty Free/Corbis
C-10	Man Carrying Bowl	© Ed Kashi/Corbis
C-11	Japanese City at Night	Royalty Free/Corbis
PO5.1	Dolls	© David Lawrence/Corbis
PO5.2	Pepsi Sign Moscow	© Peter Turnley/Corbis
PO5.3	Department Store	© Wolfgang Kaehler/Corbis
P5.1	MTV Balloon	© Jan Butchofsky-Houser/Corbis

P5.2	Dolls	© David Lawrence/Corbis
P5.3	ATM	© Tom Wagner/Corbis SABA
P5.4	Church	© David Ball/Corbis
P5.5	Pepsi Sign Moscow	© Peter Turnley/Corbis
P5.6	Department Store	© Wolfgang Kaehler/Corbis
C-12	Computer Screen	Royalty Free/Corbis
C-13	Oil Rig	Royalty Free/Corbis
C-14	Reception Desk	© Tom Wagner/Corbis SABA
PO6.1	Sailboats	© Nik Wheeler/Corbis
PO6.2	Paper Dolls	© David Lawrence/Corbis
PO6.3	Worker	© Ed Kashi/Corbis
P6.1	Sailboats	© Nik Wheeler/Corbis
P6.2	Worker	© Ed Kashi/Corbis
P6.3	Coca Cola Billboard	© Wolfgang Kaehler/Corbis
P6.4	Military Officer	© KEERLE GEORGES DE/Corbis SYGMA
P6.5	NYSE	© AFP/Corbis
P6.6	Paper Dolls	© David Lawrence/Corbis
C-15	Satellite Dishes	Royalty Free/Corbis
C-16	Seamstress	Royalty Free/Corbis
C-17	Washing Dishes	© Joyce Choo/Corbis
C-18	People Using Phones	© Randy Faris/Corbis
C-19	Chinese Currency	Royalty Free/Corbis
C-20	Phone in Globe	Royalty Free/Corbis

Index

Organization Index

ABB Group, 629
ABB SAE Sadelmi SpA, 547
Abbott Laboratories, 448, 449
Abercrombie and Fitch, 185
Accenture, 21, 143
Aetna Financial Services, 484
Ahold, 4
Air India, 549, 572
Air Touch Communications, 497
Airbus Industrie, 7, 163, 164, 192, 193, 549, 570
Alcan, 229
Alcoa, 229
Alfa Group, 671
Allianz, 645
Allied Signal, 558
Allied-Lyons, 687
American Express, 421, 598, 603
American Management Systems, 21
Amgen, 27, 490–491
Amstrad, 426
AOL, 277
Apple Computer, 170, 171, 228, 239, 321, 572, 592
Applied Materials, 328
Artais Weather Check, 552–553
AstraZeneca, 653
Atag Holdings NV, 293, 294
AT&T, 489, 515
AvtoVAZ, 237
AZCAR, 535

B&S Aircraft Alloys, 6
Bank of America, 143
Bank 24, 298–299
Barings, 484
BASF, 452
Baxter International, 684
Bayer AG, 452, 645
Bell Telephone Laboratories, 307
Benetton, 593
Bertelsmann, 277
Black & Decker, 686
Black Sea Energy Ltd., 671
BMW, 515, 587, 593
Boeing, 7, 11, 27, 147, 163, 164–165, 183, 192, 193, 211, 493, 501, 503, 549, 568, 569, 570, 572
Bombardier, 427
Bon Appetit Group, 214
Booz, Allen & Hamilton, 607
Bridgewater Pottery, 14, 22
Bristol-Myers Squibb, 239, 606
British Airways, 653
British Petroleum (BP), 4, 229, 230, 247, 514, 593
British Sky Broadcasting, 277
British Telecom (BT), 73, 515
Brooks Brothers, 185
Brother Industries, 592
Burlington Industries, 267
Burmah Castrol, 604

Canal Plus, 277
Canon, 160, 490, 572
Cardiac Science, 14, 22
Carrefour, 4, 5, 7, 243, 250, 583, 590
Castrol Oil, 604
Caterpillar, 7, 328, 335–336, 414, 430–431, 547, 684
Cato Institute, 304, 305
CBS, 128
CCF, 485
CEC, 524
Cemex, 20, 222–226, 232
Center for Marine Conservation, 201
Centra, 515
China Mobile Ltd., 134, 135, 379–382
China Telecommunications Corp., 133–134, 380, 515
China Unicom, 134–135
Chunghwa Telecom, 74
Ciba, 655
Cifera, 3
Cisco Systems, 27, 64, 605
Citicorp, 6, 103, 298, 381, 421, 691–692
Clear Vision, 415–418
Clinton Cards, 15
CNN, 16, 585
Coalition for Fair Lumber Imports (CFLI), 304–305
Coca-Cola, 6, 7, 57, 80, 409, 421, 426, 489, 583, 584, 585, 588, 597, 647
Coffee Partners, 213
Computer Associates, 175
Cone Mills, 272
Conservation International, 302
Consolidated Gold Field, 229
Corning, 606
Costco, 243, 250
Credit Commercial de France, 485
Cretors & Co., 694

DaimlerChrysler, 4, 230, 362, 371, 380, 497, 498–499, 515, 588, 645
Degrussa AG, 643
DeHavilland, 164–165
Dell Computer, 15–16, 64, 239, 317, 555–556, 558, 561, 570, 573–576
Delphi Automotive, 515
Dentsu Inc., 614
DETA, 515
Deutsche Bank, 298–299, 645
Deutsche Telekom, 4, 380, 382, 383, 399, 497, 515
Diebold, 479, 480, 481, 487–488, 497
Digital Equipment, 523, 606
Disney, 81, 115
Dixon Ticonderoga, 311–312
Dollops, 251
Dow Chemical, 393, 452–453, 455–456
Dresdner Bank, 298

E. I. du Pont, 273, 452, 605, 606
Eddie Bauer, 185
EDS, 21
Eli Lilly, 239
E-Mart, 243, 250

EMC, 239
EMI, 276, 277
Equitable Life Insurance Company, 484
Ericsson, 133, 134, 167, 169, 250, 426, 606, 630–631
Ernst & Young, 129, 175, 679
ESCO Korea Ltd., 213
ESPN, 595
Esquel Group, 184, 185
Excel Communications, 497
Exide Corporation, 514–517
Exxon, 22, 247, 476

Fair Labor Association, 129, 130, 131
Fair Trade Coffee, 302
Fairchild, 308
Federal Express, 186, 263
Fiamm, 515
Fiat, 267, 362
Finance One, 340
Flour Corp., 143
FMC, 668
Fokker, 164
Ford, 7, 22, 230, 236–237, 253, 267, 362, 414, 424, 425, 427, 497, 504, 515, 517, 568–569, 573, 588, 599, 638
Forrester Research, 13
Four Seasons, 413
Fox Broadcasting, 15
Freedom House, 67, 71
Friends of the Earth, 138
Fruit of the Loom Inc., 272
Fuji Film, 22, 225, 227, 502, 601–602
Fujitsu, 310
Fuji-Xerox, 160, 227, 488–494, 500, 501, 503–504
Fulmen, 515
Funai Electric, 524
Furman Selz, 484

G. W. Barth, 22
Gap, The, 81
Gateway, 239
Genentech, 189
General Electric, 3, 21, 211, 308, 335, 458, 463–464, 465, 473, 503, 518, 522, 526, 547, 550, 558, 620
General Motors, 22, 230, 237, 253, 263, 362, 417–418, 424, 425, 436–437, 466, 504, 573, 637
Getronics, 479
Global Election Systems, 479
Global Exchange, 128, 129, 131, 302
GNB Technologies, 516
Goldman Sachs, 379, 381, 510
Greenpeace, 138
Greenpoint Mortgage, 143
Groupe Bull, 479
Grundig, 522, 523
GTE, 515
Gucci, 593
Gymboree, 581

H. J. Heinz, 224, 421
Harwood Industries, 25

Hawker Siddely, 164–165
HBO, 16
Heritage Foundation, 71
Hewlett-Packard, 21, 422, 464, 566–568, 609, 627, 635
Hilton Hotels, 492, 493
Hindustan Lever Ltd., 251, 596
Hitachi, 115, 309, 310, 420, 430–431, 526
Hoechst AG, 452, 645
Hoffmann-LaRoche, 603
Home Depot, 21, 304
Honda, 227, 242, 260, 425, 427
Hoppeke, 515
Houghton Mifflin, 26
HSBC, 103
Hugo Boss, 185
Human Rights Watch, 80–81, 138
Hutchison Whampoa, 20
Hytech, 6
Hyundai, 186, 593

IBM, 21, 57, 80, 108, 111–112, 170, 171, 175, 239, 241, 242, 258–260, 263, 428, 466–467, 479, 480, 487, 490, 502, 536, 606
ICI, 452
IKEA, 428, 430–431
Infosys Technologies Ltd., 143
ING, 482–485, 494
Intel, 27, 187, 228, 308, 309, 420, 605
International Orientation Resources, 625
Invensys' Hawker, 515
Isuzu, 237, 253

John Deere, 515
Johnson & Johnson, 239
Johnson Controls, 515
Jollibee, 486
JVC, 11

Kao, 613, 614
Kellogg, 224, 421, 428, 597–598
KFC, 482, 486, 493
Kia Motors, 365
Kimberly-Clark Corp., 602
Kirin, 491
Kodak, 11, 22, 225, 227, 490, 572, 601–602, 606
Kokuyo, 592
Komatsu, 7, 328, 430–431
KPMG, 498, 675
Kroger, 515
Kwality, 251
Kwik Fit, 515

Landmark System, 536
Lands' End, 185
Lehman Brothers, 399
Les Schwab Tire, 515
Lever Brothers, 439–440
Levi Strauss, 115, 120, 130, 426, 585
Lexmark, 563
LG Semicon, 186
Li & Fung, 580–581
Lifetime, 595

Lik Sang, 87
Limited, The, 580, 581
Lincoln Electric, 460, 461, 465, 466, 467, 499–500
Lion Corp., 614
Lixi, Inc., 22
Lubricating Systems, Inc., 22
Lucent Technologies, 515, 517, 524

McCann-Erickson, 597
McDonald's, 6, 25, 26, 78, 89, 90, 115, 125, 233, 421, 422, 426, 427, 428, 459, 482, 486, 492, 493, 496, 500, 585, 603
Mack Trucks, 515
McKinsey, 476
Magnavox, 524
Magnet, 243
Marantz, 524
Marriott International, 413
Massachusetts General Hospital, 143
Matsushita, 11, 22, 114–115, 118, 225, 420, 426, 429, 455, 465, 487, 489, 496, 517–531, 601, 621
Maxblue, 298
Mazda, 253, 504
MCA, 528
Megahertz Communications, 535, 536, 537
Mercedes-Benz, 362, 371
Mercer Management Consulting, 498
Mercury Asset Management, 510
Merrill Lynch, 11, 298, 379, 381, 399, 421, 510–511
Micron Technology, 186, 308, 309
Microsoft, 27, 57, 64, 86–87, 115, 175, 176, 188, 239, 328, 329, 428, 445, 501, 606, 609
Midland Walwyn, 510
Milkfood, 251
Minolta, 592
Mitsubishi Heavy Industries, 164, 247, 310, 493, 526, 592, 622
Mitsui & Company, 550
MMO Music Group, 537
Mobil Oil, 593
Molex, 617–620, 623, 624
Monsanto, 188, 190, 606, 631
Morgan Stanley, 399
Motorola, 132, 134, 169, 170, 218, 250, 263, 309, 426, 500–501, 503, 515, 526, 528, 558, 689–692
MTV Networks, 16, 115, 409–410, 415, 421, 424, 426, 428, 432, 467, 585, 595

NAPA Distribution Centers, 515
National Association of Home Builders, 304
National Labor and Building Material Dealers Association, 304
Nationale-Nederlanden, 484
NEC Corporation, 309, 310
Nestlé, 439, 587–588, 655
New United Motor Manufacturing, 504
News Corporation, 15
Nike, 81, 128–131, 568
Nintendo, 7, 86–87, 606
Nippon Telephone and Telegraph (NTT), 383, 515
Nissan, 227, 242, 252, 362, 425, 497, 638, 639
Nokia, 4, 21, 133, 134, 167, 168–169, 218, 224, 225, 250, 426, 515, 606

Nordstrom, 185
Norelco, 524
Novartis, 655
Nucor Steel, 303

Occidental Petroleum, 549
Olivetti, 160
One 2 One, 497
Opel, 267
Oracle, 64, 175, 176
Organizational Resources Consulting, 634, 635
Oxfam, 179

Palm Computer, 501
Panasonic, 529
PeopleSoft, 176
PepsiCo, 7, 219, 585, 588, 598
Petroleos de Venezuela SA (PDVSA), 20, 247
Peugeot, 267
Pfizer, 414, 605, 606
Philip Morris, 547, 550, 597
Philips NV, 11, 420, 429, 446, 454–455, 465, 470–471, 479, 480, 487, 517–531, 559, 560, 606, 621
Phillips Petroleum, 635
Pokémon, 585
Polo Ralph Lauren, 185
Polygram Records, 277, 523
Posco, 399
PricewaterhouseCoopers (PwC), 130
Procomp Amazonia Industria Electronica, 479
Procter & Gamble, 3, 11, 22, 143, 224, 328, 421, 428, 439, 440, 591–594, 602, 606, 613–614, 621, 667, 668
Promodes, 243

Qualcomm, 4, 132–135
Quanta, 555
Quantum Group, 318–319, 608

Rainforest Café, 581
Rank-Xerox, 160, 227
RCA, 225, 489, 526, 589
Recreational Equipment Inc. (REI), 155, 591, 592
Reebok, 129, 130, 568
ReliaStar Financial Services, 484
Renault, 49, 497, 515
Revlon, 585
Ricoh, 490
Roche Group, 655
Rolex, 593
Rolls-Royce, 548
Royal Dutch/Shell, 136–139, 229, 230, 247, 476–477, 626, 627, 628, 687
RTZ, 229

S. C. Johnson Wax, 588
Samsung, 218, 243, 245, 246, 250, 251, 309, 487, 606, 621
Sandoz, 655
Sanwa Bank, 510
SAP, 176
Sazaby Inc., 213
Schering AG, 645
Seagram, 277
Sears, 515
Seattle Coffee, 213, 214, 215
Sega, 7
Sematech, 187

Severstal Steel, 237
Seyon, 130
Sharp, 526, 592, 606
Showa Shell Sekiyu, 687
Siemens, 250, 645
Sierra Club, 201
Silicon Graphics, 228
Smith New Court, 510
SmithKlein Beckman (SKB), 653
Snecma, 503
Softbank, 118
Somprasong Land, 339–340
SONNAK, 515
Sony, 6, 11, 21, 22, 86–87, 115, 118, 170, 225, 420, 426, 487, 489, 501, 502, 519, 523, 524, 526, 556, 572, 585, 605, 606, 607
Southland, 222
Sprint, 276
Standard & Poors, 333
Starbucks, 213–214, 215, 216, 225, 232, 302
Storage Technology, 21
Suntory, 596
Swan Optical, 7, 11, 22

Tata Oil Mills, 251
TCS, 175
Telebras Brazil, 75
Telefonica, 497, 653
Teleglobe, 497
Tesco, 4, 7, 243, 250
Texas Instruments, 143, 170, 242, 308, 309, 489, 493–494, 555, 606
Thaw, 155
3M Company, 293, 465–466, 539–541, 550, 605, 635
Time Warner, 276, 277
Tommy Hilfiger, 185
Toshiba, 170, 501, 502, 503
Total, 247
Towers Perrin, 632–633
Toyota, 7, 18, 214, 224, 226, 227, 242, 246, 248, 253, 255, 260, 263–264, 421, 424, 425, 427, 437, 504, 515, 562, 572, 573, 586, 588, 621
Toys "R" Us, 64, 254, 421, 428
Transparency International, 52
TRW, 503
Tudor, 515
Tura Petroleum Company, 671
Tyumen Oil Company, 671

Unilever, 3, 22, 251, 328, 432, 439–444, 455, 457, 466, 471, 586, 590, 596, 613, 622
U.S. Bancorp, 381
U.S. Department of Commerce, 305
Universal Pictures, 26, 277
Upjohn, 606

Varta, 515
Verizon, 132
Viacom, 409
Vivendi, 26, 277
Vodaphone, 497
Volkswagen, 229, 230, 237, 267, 293, 362, 515, 645–646
Volvo, 243, 245, 246, 250, 251, 252, 253, 497, 515

W. L. Gore, 563
Wal-Mart, 3–4, 5, 7, 81, 243, 250, 421, 428, 515, 583, 590

Warner Brothers, 581
Warner Music Group, 277
Westinghouse, 522
Weyerhaeuser, 21
Whirlpool, 522, 523
Windam International, 628
Wipro Ltd., 21, 143
World Economic Forum, 25
World Wildlife Fund (WWF), 200
WorldCom, 276

Xerox, 160, 227, 488–494, 503–504

Yamaichi Securities, 510, 511
YKK, 580
Yokogwa Hewlett-Packard (YHP), 464
Yuasa, 515

Zenith, 526

Name Index

Aaker, D. A., 611
Abacha, Sani, 54
Abbasi, S. M., 123
Ackerman, S. Rose, 54, 84
Adonis, A., 123
Agarwal, R., 174
Aggarwal, A., 201
Aguilar, Frank, 517
Aiyar, Shankar, 42
Akhter, S., 689
Alam, P., 689
Alchain, A. A., 174, 435
Alden, V. R., 611
Al-Eryani, M. F., 689
Allen, H. L., 338
Anand, J., 235
Anderson, J. E., 84, 507
Anderson, Kym, 209
Anderson, Lloyd, 155
Andersson, U., 435, 475
Andrews, E. L., 179, 189, 211
Annett, A., 123, 124
Aoki, M., 123, 124
Aris, B., 237
Aristotle, 44–45
Arndt, M., 479
Arndt, S., 338
Arntzen, B. C., 579
Arterian, S., 689
Ascarelli, S., 383
Atkins, R., 646
Auilar, F. J., 475
Aulakh, P. S., 612

Backer, J. C., 688
Bagozzi, R. P., 475
Baily, R., 189
Baker, G., 297, 333, 374
Baker, J. C., 629, 642
Balassa, B., 173
Baliga, G., 642
Ballon, M., 486
Bamberger, Peter, 641
Banai, M., 641
Bandler, J., 491
Barbian, J., 626, 641
Bardacke, T., 340
Bardhan, Pranab, 84, 86
Barkeme, H., 507
Barker, R. G., 664

Barney, J. B., 435
Bartlett, Christopher, 262, 426, 429, 432, 435, 440, 451, 474, 475, 484–485, 486, 507, 517, 611, 614, 641
Bartlett, D. L., 25, 35
Baskin, Roberta, 128
Batra, Ravi, 35
Baum, J., 74
Bazerman, M. H., 263
Beamish, P. W., 508
Beard, A., 655
Beardsley, L. J., 688
Beckett, P., 139
Beechler, S., 641
Behrman, J., 262, 263
Belman, D., 35
Ben-David, D., 35
Bennett, A., 635
Bennett, D., 214
Bernstein, A., 131, 143
Berton, L., 646, 653, 655, 664
Besanko, D., 434, 435
Bevan, D. L., 54
Bhagwati, J., 34, 209, 296
Biers, D., 135
Bigoness, W. J., 124
Birkinshaw, J. M., 435, 474, 579, 612
Black, J. S., 642
Black, S., 641
Blackman, I., 692
Blakely, G. L., 124
Bleakley, F. R., 667
Blecker, R. A., 35
Bleeke, J., 509
Block, R., 56
Block, S., 688
Block, Walter, 85
Bluestein, P., 344
Blumenstein, R., 437
Bobinski, C., 614
Bogart, R., 551
Bogenr, W. C., 507
Bokhari, F., 103
Bolger, A., 604
Bond, M. H., 124
Bongiorno, L., 431
Bono, 30
Booker, E., 509
Boonstra, Cor, 523–524
Borish, M. S., 85
Borrus, M., 310
Boulding, W., 174
Bounds, W., 131
Bove, Jose, 26
Bowen, H. P., 174
Bowman, L., 239
Brada, J. C., 85
Bradley, D. G., 508
Brander, J. A., 209
Branstetter, L. G., 262
Brealy, R. A., 688
Bregman, Mitchell, 516
Broder, John, 209
Brook, Stephen, 123
Brooks, G., 139
Brouthers, K. D., 236, 507, 508
Brouthers, L. B., 236, 507, 508
Brown, G. G., 579
Brown, S. L., 612
Bruce, T. J., 641
Bruno, Michael, 327, 338
Brush, T. H., 508
Buchan, D., 296
Buchanan, James, 45

Burgers, W., 509
Burns, J., 376
Burpitt, W. J., 551, 552
Burritt, C., 273
Burton, J., 333, 374
Busch, H. F.
Bush, George W., 145, 183, 302, 603
Byrne, H. S., 479
Byrne, J., 475

Caffrey, A., 306
Cane, Alan, 210, 474
Cannella, A. A., 508
Cardoso, Fernando Henrique, 404
Carley, A. H., 665
Carlton, Jim, 210
Carnegy, H., 431
Carns, A., 312
Carreyou, J., 485
Carroll, P., 373, 389
Carrubba, Frank, 523
Carter, J. R., 339, 552
Carter, Jimmy, 391
Carter, R., 553
Cavallo, Domingo, 358
Cavanagh, J., 297
Caves, R. E., 34, 235, 236, 508
Cavusgil, S. T., 551
Certo, S. T., 642
Chabrow, E., 155
Champy, J., 475
Chandler, A. D., 174, 475
Chandler, Alfred, 164
Chang, Shu-jung, 74, 235
Chao, J., 311
Chapman, T., 15
Chappell, L., 517
Chazan, G., 237, 344
Chen, Steve, 219
Chetty, S., 34
Chi, P. S. K., 507
Chi, T., 508
Chipello, C. J., 306, 435
Chirac, Jacques, 264
Choate, P., 35
Choi, C. J., 552
Choi, F., 664
Choudhury, R., 397
Christen, M., 174
Christensen, C., 440, 612
Chui, A. C. W., 689
Clark, K. B., 611, 612
Clinton, Bill, 80, 81, 138, 188, 191
Coffee, J. C., 508
Cohen, M. A., 579
Colchester, N., 296
Coleman, B., 374
Coles, Ashley, 535
Collier, P., 54
Collins, J. M., 688, 689
Collins, Susan M., 35
Collins-Dodd, C., 552
Colman, R., 641
Confucius, 104
Conner, H., 440
Conner, K. R., 435
Conners, L., 85
Contractor, F. J., 507
Coolidge, J., 54, 84
Cooper, H., 56
Copeland, T., 434
Corrigan, T., 689
Cortés, Hernán, 483
Corzine, R., 139, 477

Costa, I., 262
Craig, C. Samuel, 612
Crandall, R. W., 209
Cretors, Charlie, 694
Crosby, P. B., 579
Crow, S., 689
Cumby, R. E., 338
Cunningham, R., 87
Cushman, J. H., 201
Cusumano, M. A., 579
Czechowicz, I., 664

Daily, C. M., 642
Dalai Lama, 30
Dalton, D. R., 642
Dana, L., 90
Daniszewski, J., 237
Darlin, D., 311
Darling, J., 362
Davidow, W. H., 475
Davis, B., 311
Davis, D. R., 174
Davis, P., 297
Davis, S. M., 474, 475
Dean, J., 74
Deen, R., 131
DeGeorge, R. T., 124
de Jonquieres, Guy, 173, 189, 210, 262, 297, 435, 440, 475, 614
Dekker, Wisse, 519, 522
Dekmejian, R. H., 123
de la Torre, A., 296
Dell, Michael, 555
Delors, Jacques, 278
Deming, W. Edwards, 557–558
DePalma, A., 37
de Queiroz, R., 262
de Rocha, A., 4
Dertouzos, M. L., 122, 123, 124, 311
Devereux, M., 338
Dhillon, A., 125
Diamond, Jarad, 85
Diaz, Manuel, 26
Dib, L. A., 4
Dickens, P., 13, 397
Dickerson, M., 34
Dickson, M., 475
Dixit, A., 209, 263
Dobnik, V., 131
Dolan, R. J., 612
Dollar, D., 174
Domowitz, Ian, 397
Donaldson, Thomas, 121, 124
Donlon, J. P., 511
Dore, R., 122, 123, 475
Dornbusch, R., 173, 362, 389
Douglas, M., 122
Douglas, S. P., 611, 612
Dowds, C., 297
Dowling, P. J., 641, 642
Doz, Yves L., 435, 504–505, 508, 509, 637, 643
Draffen, C. M., 33
Dranove, D., 434, 435
Drew, Richard, 465–466
Drozdiak, W., 277
Duff, M., 431
Dunne, K. M., 663
Dunne, N., 146, 209, 311
Dunning, John, 228–229, 231, 235, 262, 507
Dzinokowski, R., 646

Easterly, William, 35

Edison, H. J., 338
Edison, J. R., 338
Edmondson, G., 169
Edwards, S., 373
Ehrlich, I., 86
Eiben, T., 540
Eichengreen, B., 373
Eigen-Zucchi, C., 297
Eilat, Y., 85
Einhorn, B., 135, 556, 560
Eisenhardt, K. M., 612
Eiteman, D. K., 688
Eliot, M., 579
Elliott, Kim A., 182
Elliott, Z. A., 209
Ellis, R., 122
Engardio, P., 21, 143
Engel, C., 338, 339
Enis, B. M., 551
Ensign, P. C., 579
Entous, A., 211
Erlanger, S., 373
Ernst, D., 509
Ettorre, B., 692

Fagerberg, J., 85
Fahey, J., 437
Fairlamb, D., 403
Fama, E., 338
Famularo, J. J., 642
Farnsworth, C. B., 306
Farrell, C., 612
Fayerweather, J., 263
Feigenbaum, A. V., 557
Feils, D. J., 671, 688
Feldstein, Martin, 297, 388–390, 397, 403
Ferdows, K., 435, 567, 579, 612
Fernald, J. G., 34
Finnigan, D., 15
Fischer, S., 173
Fisher, Irving, 329
Fisher, S., 85
Fladmoe-Lindquist, K., 508
Flagg, M., 4
Fleming, P. D., 664
Florkowski, G. W., 642, 643
Flyer, F., 235, 570
Flynn, J., 431
Forney, M., 135
Forsgren, M., 435, 475
Fossedal, G., 376
Francis, J., 552
Frankel, Jeffrey, 34, 157, 174
Frankel, M., 509
Frazee, V., 626
Freeland, C., 373
Freenstra, R. C., 262
Friberg, E. G., 297
Friedland, J., 612
Friedman, Milton, 45, 84, 338
Friedman, R., 84, 338
Friedman, T. L., 319
Frost, P. J., 475
Frost, T. S., 435, 579
Fry, L., 579
Fujimoto, T., 612
Fukuyama, Francis, 69, 70, 85
Fung, H., 641
Fung, Victor, 580, 581

Gagne, J., 297, 339, 552
Gagnon, J. E., 338
Galbraith, J. R., 475

Gandhi, Mahatma, 104
Garten, J. E., 556
Garvin, David A., 557, 579
Gary, S. J., 663, 664
Gates, D., 570
Gatignon, H., 507
Gay, G. D., 338
Gephardt, Richard, 309
Gerard, Leo, 302
Gernon, H., 663, 664
Gernon, O., 663
Gerstein, M., 474
Gerteis, J., 123
Ghadar, F., 508
Ghemawat, P., 507, 508
Ghosh, A. R., 373
Ghoshal, Sumantra, 262, 426, 429, 432, 435, 440, 451, 474, 475, 484–485, 486, 507, 517, 611, 614, 641
Gibbs, Donna, 128
Giddens, A., 84, 123
Giermanski, J. R., 273
Gilmore, J. H., 579
Gilmour, P.
Gil-Pareja, S., 612
Glassman, David, 415–416
Glen, Jack, 397
Goldsmith, E., 35
Goldsmith, James, 35
Goldstein, Alan, 209
Gomes-Casseres, B., 491, 507, 509
Goodman, N., 123
Goodwin, D., 124
Goodwin, J., 124
Gort, M., 174
Gottschalk, Peter, 35
Govindarajan, V. J., 435, 475, 507, 611
Graham, L. E., 665
Graham, R., 264
Granito, B. D., 667
Granovetter, M. S., 475
Grant, L., 642
Grant, M. E., 174
Greenfeld, V., 34
Greenhouse, S., 131
Gregersen, H., 642
Greider, William, 35
Groening, Matt, 15
Groombridge, M. A., 306
Gross, N., 611
Grosse, R. E., 262, 263
Grossman, G. M., 84, 174, 236
Guha, Krishna, 176
Gulati, R., 509
Gulde, A. M., 373
Gumble, P., 374, 646
Gunning, J. W., 54
Gupta, A. K., 435, 475, 507, 611
Gurhan-Cvanli, Z., 611
Guterl, F. V., 475
Gwartney, James, 85

Hagelstam, Jarl, 148, 173
Hagerty, J. R., 319
Haigh, R. W., 552
Hall, G., 435
Hall, K. G., 297
Hambrick, D. C., 508
Hamel, Gary, 504–505, 508, 509
Hamilton, Alexander, 191
Hamilton, C. A., 174
Hamilton, D., 311
Hamilton, H., 139
Hamilton, J. D., 339

Hamilton, M. N., 4
Hammer, M., 475
Hammonds, K. H., 21
Harding, Luke, 125
Hargreaves, D., 277
Harrison, T. P., 579
Harverson, P., 319
Harvey, M. G., 641, 642
Haspeslagh, P., 508
Haveman, H., 235
Hay, D. A., 579
Hayek, F. A., 85
Hayek, Friedrich von, 45
Hayes, F., 21
Heath, P. S., 123
Heckscher, Eli, 144–145, 147, 157–159, 166, 180
Heenan, D. A., 641
Helft, D., 223
Helms, M., 642
Helpman, E., 84, 174, 236
Henley, J., 26
Hennart, J. F., 236, 508, 552
Herbet, B., 131
Heskett, J. L., 475
Higinbotham, H. H., 689
Hill, C. W. L., 123, 235, 475, 507, 508, 509, 579, 612
Hill, Charles, 315, 570
Hirschman, A. O., 84, 85
Hitt, M. A., 434, 475
Hoagland, J., 139
Hodgetts, R. M., 453
Hoffman, K., 410
Hofheinz, P., 296
Hofstede, Geert, 91, 108, 111–112, 122, 123, 124, 650, 664
Holland, C. P., 692
Hollander, S., 173
Holley, D., 511
Hollman, K. W., 123
Holm, U., 435, 475
Holman, M., 376
Holmes, K. R., 85
Holstein, W. J., 33, 34, 551, 581
Holt, D. H., 124
Homes, S., 214
Hood, N., 20, 435, 474
Hood, S., 262
Horioka, Charles, 389
Horn, R., 508
Horwitz, T., 294
Hoskisson, R. E., 434, 475
Hout, T. M., 435, 579, 612
Howard, R., 491
Howell, S., 435
Howes, D., 437
Hudson, R., 139
Huertas, T. F., 397
Hufbauer, Gary, 182, 209, 303
Hume, David, 45, 148, 373
Hunt, J. W., 642
Hunter, D., 556
Huntington, Samuel, 69–70, 85, 93, 122
Hunya, G., 262
Huus, Kari, 210
Hwang, P., 507, 508
Hymer, S. H., 235

Ilbo, H., 243
Inglehart, R., 124
Inkpen, A. C., 508
Isobe, T., 507
Ito, K., 235

Ito, T., 338
Itoh, M., 262

Jack, A., 262, 264, 655
Jackson, J. O., 383
Jackson, T., 641
Jacobs, Irwin, 132, 134
Javetski, B. J., 319
Jefferson, Thomas, 146
Jemison, D., 508
Jennings, John, 138
Jensen, M. C., 508
Jeter, J., 56
Jiang Zemin, 135
Joachimsthaler, E., 611
John Paul II, Pope, 30
Johnson, Lyndon, 350
Johnson, M., 379
Johnston, C., 262
Jones, D. T., 123, 131, 435, 579, 643
Jones, G., 397
Jones, G. R., 579
Jones, Jim, 101
Jones, R. W., 174
Jonsson, S., 435, 474
Jordan, M., 586, 594
Jordan, Michael, 128
Jordan, Peter S., 209
Joseph, Joel, 128
Jospin, Lionel, 26
Juran, Joseph, 557

Kahn, G., 583
Kai-Cheng, Y., 124
Kale, P., 509
Kali, R., 124
Kalotay, K., 262
Kamm, T., 139
Kamprad, Ingvar, 430
Kapoor, A., 263
Katsikeas, C. S., 552
Kawai, H., 209
Kearns, D., 491
Keenan, C., 479
Kelly, J., 689
Kelly, K., 267
Kelly, M., 296
Kenel, P., 131
Kenen, P. B., 174
Khanna, T., 509
Kidron, M., 235
Kim, H., 434
Kim, J., 552
Kim, J. B., 552
Kim, W. C., 235, 507, 508, 509
Kim Young-Sam, 332, 364
King, N., 303
Kiriyenko, Sergei, 364
Kirkpatrick, M., 85
Kirpalani, V. H., 611
Kirsner, S., 485
Kivelidi, Ivan, 51
Kiyono, K., 262
Klebnikov, P., 84
Kleisterlee, Gerald, 524
Knickerbocker, F. T., 34, 226–227, 233, 235
Knight, Phil, 128–131
Kobayashi, Tony, 490, 494, 508
Kobrin, S. J., 641
Kogut, B., 174, 235, 508
Kold, R. W., 338
Koller, T., 434
Komiya, R., 262

Konopaske, R., 641
Koresh, David, 101
Kostova, T., 475
Kotabe, M., 552
Kotabe, S., 612
Kotha, S., 579
Kotter, J. P., 475
Kraay, A., 174
Kripalani, M., 21, 135, 143
Krol, C., 509
Krugman, Paul R., 35, 147, 173, 174, 193, 209, 235, 262, 310, 338, 373, 579
Kuemmerle, W., 612
Kukes, Simon, 671
Kuper, S., 262
Kuttner, R., 35
Kwok, C. C. Y., 689
Kynge, J., 374

Laabs, J., 618
Lambrecht, Bill, 209
Lancaster, K., 611
Landers, P., 115
Landry, J. T., 611
Laroche, M., 611
Lascelles, D., 477
Latta, G. W., 643
Lavine, A., 397
Lawrence, J. J., 124
Lawson, Robert, 85
Leamer, E. E., 174
Lecraw, D. J., 552
Lee, Charles S., 243
Lee, H. L., 579
Lee, L., 131
Lee, S. H., 552
Lee, T. M., 35
Lee, W. A., 479
Lee Kuan Yew, 65
Leggett, K., 560
Lenway, S. A., 475
Leonidou, L. C., 552
Leontief, Wassily, 158, 174
Lerman, Robert, 27, 35
Lessard, Donald, 659–660, 664
Lester, R. K., 122, 123, 124, 311
Leucke, R., 507
Leung, S., 435
Leuschner, Albrecht, 516–517
Levich, R. M., 338, 339
Levine, D. S., 339
Levitt, Theodore, 33, 425–426, 435, 584–585, 588, 597, 611
Lewis, K. K., 397
Li, J., 435
Li Ka-shing, 89
Liberman, M., 85, 507
Lichtenberg, F., 262
Lieberman, M. B., 174
Lifson, T. B., 552
Lightfoot, Robert W., 517
Limongi, F., 85
Lincoln, James, 461, 465
Lindquist, Diane, 223
Lindsey, B., 306
Lipin, S., 667
Lippman, T. W., 84, 123
Lipsey, R. E., 262
Listiev, Vladislav, 51
Lloyd, A. E., 689
Lockett, G., 692
Lomborg, B., 35
Longfellow, T. A., 551

Longworth, R. C., 642
Lorange, Peter, 659–660, 664
Lorenz, C., 477, 491, 507
Louie, E., 583
Loungani, P., 306
Lovett, S., 124
Lowenstein, L., 508
Lublin, J. S., 517
Luce, E., 247
Lucier, G. T., 579
Luck, C. G., 397
Lui, F., 86
Lukashenko, Alexander, 65, 69
Lula da Silva, Luiz Inacio, 404
Lumbin, J., 612
Luo, Y., 123
Lustog, N. C., 297
Lutz, Robert, 514–517
Lyles, M. A., 508
Lyons, R. K., 338

McAllister, I., 273
McCleery, R., 297
McGee, J., 507
McGinley, L., 56
McKinnon, Robert, 373
McKnight, William, 465–466
McLean, C., 214
McQuade, K., 491, 507, 509
McQueen, M., 507
Madden, N., 583
Madhavan, Ananth, 397
Madhok, A., 507
Magdoff, H., 262
Maggs, J., 201
Magnusson, P., 211, 262
Magretta, J., 581
Maheswaran, D., 611
Major, John, 138
Major, T., 299
Makino, S., 507
Mallet, V., 604
Malone, M. S., 475
Mandela, Nelson, 138
Mander, J., 35
Maneerungsee, W., 552
Mankin, Eric, 501, 502, 509
Mann, J., 247
Mansfield, E., 612
Manve, I. M., 642
Marcos, Ferdinand, 52
Marcouiller, D., 84
Marino, V., 37
Marsh, P., 435
Marx, Karl, 43
Maskus, K. E., 85, 174
Matsuoko, "Mike," 526
Matsushita, Konosuke, 465, 524–526, 529
Matthee, I., 34
Matthews, R. Guy, 303
Mauro, P., 86
Maynard, M., 517
Mead, R., 122, 123
Meek, G., 646, 663, 664
Mehta, S. N., 551, 553
Melick, W. R., 338
Mellow, C., 84
Mendenhall, M., 627–628, 632, 641, 642
Menem, Carlos, 358
Merchant, H., 508
Merchant, K., 596
Meshoulam, Ilan, 641
Meyer, B., 552
Meyer, M., 440

Miesel, V. H., 689
Miliband, R., 123
Mill, John Stuart, 45, 84
Miller, C., 611
Miller, M., 219
Miller, S., 122, 267
Millman, G. J., 397
Millman, J., 273, 641
Min, Sungwook, 174
Minder, L., 90
Ming Wang, Z., 124
Mitchell, W., 507
Mitra, P. K., 85
Mittee, Ledum, 138
Mitterand, François, 264
Mobutu Sese Seko, 374–376
Moden, K. M., 262
Moffett, M. H., 688
Mohamad, Mahathir bin, 319
Mollet, A., 614
Mondavi, Robert, 26
Montagu-Pollock, M., 74
Montgomery, D. B., 85, 174, 507
Monti, Mario, 277
Moody-Stuart, Mark, 138
Moore, Gordon, 34
Moore, P., 42
Moore, S., 139
Morales, Juan-Antino, 338
Morgan, E. J., 296
Morgan, G., 474, 475
Morgan, N. A., 552
Morishita, Yoichi, 528–529
Morris, D. J., 579
Mort, Jo-Ann, 86
Mosakowski, E., 507
Mosbacher, R. A., 34
Mowery, D. C., 612
Mueller, G. G., 663, 664
Mueller, S. L., 123
Mufson, S., 219
Mun, Thomas, 147
Murphy, K. M., 84, 85
Murphy, P. E., 551
Murrey, J. H., 123
Murrin, J., 434
Murtha, T. P., 475
Myers, S. C., 688
Myers, Steven L., 86

Nader, Ralph, 29, 35
Naidler, D., 474
Nakamoto, M., 310, 311
Nakamura, Kunio, 529
Nakane, C., 95, 123
Nalebuff, B., 209, 263
Namenwirth, J. Z., 122, 124
Namenwirth, Zvi, 91
Narain, S., 201
Narasimhan, R.
Narisette, R., 612
Narula, R., 235
Nathan, M., 641
Nauss, D. W., 362, 517
Ndubizu, G. A., 663
Neary, J. P., 174
Nellis, J., 85
Nelson, E., 594
Nelson, R. T., 155
Nemetz, P., 579
Neupert, K. E., 641
Newman, M., 169
Ng, Linda, 219
Nguyen, Thuyen, 129

Nijissen, E. J., 612
Niswander, F., 664
Nixon, Richard, 350
Nkrumah, Kwame, 306
Nobel, R., 612
Noel, M., 85
Nohria, N., 509, 641
Nonnemaker, L., 235
Nordstrom, H., 35
North, Douglass, 84, 85
Nurton, J., 56
Nydell, M. K., 123

Obstfeld, M., 209, 338, 373
Oddou, G., 627–628, 632, 641, 642
O'Donnell, S., 642
O'Driscoll, G. P., 85
Officer, L. H., 338
Ogbuehi, A. O., 551
O'Higgins, E. R. E., 239
Ohlin, Bertil, 144–145, 147, 157–159, 166, 174, 180
Ohmae, K., 508
Ohno, Taiichi, 562, 579
Ojeda, R. H., 297
Okuno, M., 262
Olson, M., 85
O'Malley, S. F., 653
Ondrack, D. A., 641
Ordonez, J., 214
O'Reilly, C. A., 475
O'Rourke, Dara, 130, 131
Ouchi, W. G., 475
Oyama, D. I., 646
Ozawa, T., 262
Ozretich, J., 155

Page, A. L., 612
Pan, Y., 507
Park, S. H., 508
Park, S. W., 243
Park, Y. R., 508
Parker-Pope, T., 611
Parthasarthy, R., 579
Passell, P., 146
Pauls, B. D., 373
Pavord, W., 551
Peel, M., 664
Peng, M. W., 90, 123
Perlmutter, H. V., 509, 641
Peters, T., 475
Peterson, M. F., 124
Pettigrew, Pierre, 303
Pettit, R. R., 235, 508
Pfeffer, J., 475
Pham, A., 87
Philips, Anton, 518, 519
Philips, Gerard, 518, 519
Philips, M., 297
Pickering, J. F., 612
Piggott, C., 223
Pine, B. J., II, 579
Pisano, G., 579
Plato, 43, 44
Platt, G., 397
Poe, A. C., 618
Pollard, S., 123
Pons, F., 611
Pope, H., 344
Pope, R. A., 551
Poppo, L., 579
Port, O., 612
Porter, Michael E., 108, 123, 147, 165–169, 174, 412–413, 434, 435, 552

Potterie, B., 262
Pottinger, M., 135
Powell, Colin, 70
Practer, P., 665
Prahalad, C. K., 435, 504–505, 509, 637, 643
Prestowitz, Clyde, 309
Pringle, D., 169
Pritchett, Lant, 35
Przeworski, A., 85
Puchalsy, A., 517
Pulley, B., 410
Punnett, B. J., 642
Putra, Hutomo Mandala, 365

Qiu, L. D., 262
Quinn, L., 688
Quintanilla, C., 541

Raddock, D. M., 262
Radrik, D., 35
Raghavan, A., 383
Rai, S., 176, 262
Raiffa, H., 263
Rajan, R. G., 689
Ralston, D. H., 124
Ram, R., 262
Ramamurti, R., 263
Rapach, R. D., 338
Rapoport, C., 642
Rather, Dan, 128
Ravenscraft, D. J., 235, 498, 508
Raymond, M. A., 552
Rebello, K., 611
Redstone, Sumner, M., 410
Reich, Robert, 7, 34, 252, 262, 394, 398, 417, 435, 501, 502, 509
Reitman, V., 641
Reynolds, C., 642
Rhoades, C., 122
Ricardo, David, 144–145, 147, 148, 150–158, 173, 180, 193, 194, 241
Richard, J. M., 692
Richardson, J., 338
Ricks, D. A., 123
Ridding, J., 374, 581
Riley, Alan, 296
Robins, J. A., 508
Robinson, S., 297
Robinson, W. T., 174
Robles, S., 262
Robock, S. H., 85
Rodriguez, Francisco, 174
Rodrik, Dani, 174
Roedy, William, 409
Roehl, W., 509
Rogoff, K., 174, 338, 339
Roll, R., 508
Romer, David, 157, 174
Romer, P. M., 84, 85, 262
Rondinelli, D. A., 551, 552
Ronen, S., 642
Roos, D., 123, 235, 435, 579, 643
Roosen, Gustavo, 247
Root, F. R., 507
Rose, E. L., 235
Rose, M., 139
Rose, R. L., 540, 541
Rose, S., 508
Rosenberg, N., 612
Rosenzweig, P. M., 641
Rotberg, R. I., 376
Roth, K., 642
Roulet, J., 397

Rowley, A., 511
Ruback, R. S., 508
Rudden, E., 435
Ruekert, R. W., 611
Ruggiero, Renato, 12
Rugman, A. M., 235
Runsten, D., 297
Rutterford, J., 688

Sabac, F. M., 671, 688
Sachs, Jeffrey, 30, 35, 66, 85, 157, 173, 174, 374, 375, 376, 405
Saggi, K., 262
Sahay, R., 85
St. George, Donna, 146
Salter, S. B., 664
Sama, L. M., 641
Samuelson, P., 173
Sapir, Edward, 123
Saro-Wiwa, Ken, 136–138
Sauls, E., 689
Saunders, M., 579
Savage, M., 123
Sazanami, Y., 209
Schein, E. H., 475, 641
Schendel, D., 508
Scherer, F. M., 235, 508
Scherer, Mike, 498
Schleifer, A., 508
Schlesinger, J., 311
Schneider, S. C., 642
Schuler, R. S., 641, 642, 643
Schultz, Howard, 213
Schuman, M., 243, 641
Schumpeter, Joseph, 612
Segal, R., 235
Seith, S. P., 579
Sekely, W. S., 688, 689
Seligman, S. D., 90
Selowsky, M., 85
Sen, Amartya, 62, 65, 66, 84
Serrat, A., 397
Serwer, Andrew E., 508
Seshadri, S., 579
Sesit, M. R., 383
Seth, A., 235, 508
Shan, W., 235
Shane, S. A., 123
Shanley, M., 434, 435
Shao, A. T., 552
Shapiro, C., 84
Shapley, D., 612
Shaver, J. M., 235, 507, 579
Shaw, R., 474
Shay, J., 641
Shelton, J., 373
Shenkar, O., 642
Shenon, P., 374
Sherefkin, R., 517
Shilling, M. A., 612
Shirouzu, N., 425, 614
Shleifer, A., 84, 85, 86
Shorrock, T. S., 374
Shuen, A., 579
Siddhartha Gautama, 104
Sierra, C., 612
Sievers, C., 626
Sikorski, R., 373
Simmons, L. C., 124
Simon, H., 612
Simonian, Haig, 264, 437
Singer, J., 399, 511
Singh, H., 509

Slater, Joanna, 42
Sly, L., 219
Smeeding, Timothy M., 35
Smith, Adam, 45, 60, 84, 119, 144, 148–149, 180, 193, 194, 241, 419, 440
Smith, G., 612
Smith, J. F., 223
Smith, P. B., 124
Smith, W., 535
Smockum, E., 626
Snell, S., 641
Solnik, Bruno, 384, 385, 397
Solomon, C. M., 618, 631, 641, 642
Solomon, R., 373
Solow, R. M., 122, 123, 124, 311
Son, Masayoshi, 118
Song, J., 235
Song, K. P., 235, 508
Soros, George, 318–319, 330
Southey, C., 189
Souza, C., 509
Spencer, J. W., 509
Spiegel, H. W., 84, 173
Srinivasan, S., 612
Stackhouse, Dale, 84
Stalk, G., 579, 612
Stanley, M., 688
Steele, J. B., 25, 35
Steensma, H. K., 508
Steinmetz, G., 646
Stern, R. M., 174
Stertz, B. A., 508
Stevenson, W. B., 642
Stewart, A., 34
Stewart, M., 34
Stewart, R. C., 667
Stiglitz, J. E., 35
Stonehill, A. I., 688
Stopford, John M., 448, 475
Storms, Charles, 541
Stottinger, B., 612
Stout, H., 131
Stuart, J., 37
Suharto, 52, 365, 367
Suzumura, K., 262
Sveikayskas, L., 174
Swann, D., 296
Sweeney, B., 297
Sweezy, P. M., 262
Swenson, D. L., 689

Tallman, S., 435, 507, 508
Tang, E. W. K., 509
Tanii, Akio, 528
Tanzer, A., 185, 209, 210, 410
Tao, Z., 262
Taylor, A., 517
Taylor, Edward, 91
Taylor, M. P., 338
Taylor, P., 176
Taylor, T., 174
Teece, D. J., 579
Teegen, H., 552
Templeman, J., 508
Terazono, E., 491, 507
Terpstra, R. H., 124
Thatcher, Margaret, 73
Theonnes, K., 665
Thevenot, B., 146
Thomas, A. S., 123
Thomas, H., 507
Thompson, E. P., 123

Thompson, G., 37
Thompson, M., 122
Thomsen, S., 235
Thorbecke, W., 297
Thornhill, J., 373, 374
Thurrow, R., 179
Tilton, H., 643
Timmer, Jan, 522–523
Tolchin, M., 262
Tolchin, S., 262
Torbiorin, I., 642
Torres, C., 373, 389
Trafton, L. L., 579
Trager, C. S., 34, 434
Treaster, J. B., 485
Trefler, D., 174
Trueheart, C., 26
Truitt, J. F., 509
Tuan, C., 219
Tuller, L. W., 552
Tung, R. L., 624, 625, 628, 641, 642
Turner, M., 297, 596
Turner, Tina, 598
Tushman, M. L., 475
Tweedie, D., 664
Tybout, J. R., 174
Tylor, E. B., 122
Tyson, L. A., 310

Ungar, Kenneth, 84
Ungson, G. R., 508
Urata, S., 209

Van de Krol, R., 475
van der Klught, Cor, 522
van Reimsdijk, Hendrick, 519
van Wolferen, K., 84
Varian, H. R., 84
Vaughan, S., 35
Vegh, C. A., 85
Vermeulen, F., 507
Vermond, K., 642
Vernon, Raymond, 147, 159–161, 174, 227
Vidal, J., 139
Vieth, W., 34, 210
Vishny, R. W., 84, 85, 86, 508
Vlasic, B., 508
von Glinow, M. A., 641

Wagstyle, S., 435
Wald, J. K., 688, 689
Walker, M., 299
Walker, O. C., 611
Wall, Howard J., 182
Wallace, R. S., 663
Wallace, W. A., 663
Wallach, Lori, 35
Waller, D., 397, 612
Walsh, J. P., 663
Walsh, P., 508
Walters, R., 449
Walton, P., 664
Warner, Andrew, 157, 173, 174
Warner, J., 508
Warner, S., 236, 641
Waterman, R. H., 475
Waters, R., 209
Weber, Max, 98, 100, 103–104, 105, 118–119, 123
Weber, R. B., 122, 124
Weber, Robert, 91

Weinstein, D. E., 174
Weiss, S., 262, 263
Weisweiller, R., 338
Wells, Louis T., 161, 174, 448, 475
Welsh, Jack, 458, 465, 473, 475
Wesson, R., 84
West, D., 552
Wha-Lee, J., 307
Wheelwright, S. C., 611, 612
Whitehouse, M., 671
Whittington, R., 440
Whorf, Benjamin Lee, 123
Wildavsky, A., 122
Wilhelm, S., 570
Wilhem, K., 135
Williams, Bryan, 541
Williams, F., 34, 189, 552
Williams, Frances, 210
Williamson, J., 338
Williamson, O. E., 236, 507, 579
Wilson, Rodney, 84
Wind, Y., 611
Winestock, G., 179, 211
Winters, A., 35
Wohar, M. E., 338
Wolf, Martin, 374
Wolff, C., 297
Wolff, G., 297
Wolverton, B., 612
Womack, J. P., 123, 235, 435, 579, 643
Wonacott, P., 560
Woods, Tiger, 128
Wright, P. M., 641
Wu Jichuan, 133–134
Wyatt, Arthur, 652
Wyploze, C., 296, 403
Wysocki, B., 509

Yamamura, K., 311
Yamashita, Toshihiko, 527, 528
Yeats, Alexander, 288–289, 297
Yeh, R. S., 124
Yeung, A., 665
Yeung, B., 507
Yi, C. W., 689
Yoon, S., 87
Yoshino, Michael Y., 475, 517, 552
Young, Andrew, 129
Young, J., 20
Young, S., 262

Zaheer, S., 507
Zahra, S., 85
Zang, J. Z., 641
Zang, K. H., 262
Zenger, T., 579
Zhan, X. J., 262
Zhou, L., 611
Zhu Rongi, 134
Zimmerman, R., 56
Zingales, L., 689
Zinnes, C., 85
Zobel, J., 440
Zysman, J., 310

Subject Index

Absolute advantage, 144, 148–150
Accounting, 644–665
  accounting clusters, 650, 651
  accounting information, 646
  adoption of international standards
    in Germany, 645–646
  in China, 664–665
  consolidated financial statements,
    654–657
  control systems and, *see* Control
    systems
  country differences in standards,
    647–654
  culture and, 649–650
  currency translation, 657–658
  inflation, 649
  introduction, 646
  lack of comparability, 650, 652
  level of development and, 649
  national and international
    standards, 650–654
  political and economic ties with
    other countries, 649
  relationship between business and
    providers of capital, 647–648
  uncertainty avoidance, 650
Accounting standards, 650–654
Acquisitions, 497–499, 500
Ad valorem tariffs, 181
Adaptive culture, 467
Administrative trade policies, 185–186
Advertising, 597–598
Aerospace industry, 163–165
Africa, 291–292
Agricultural subsidies, 179, 182–183
  WTO and, 203–204
AIDS, 56–57
Alliances; *see* Strategic alliances
Allowances, compensation, 636
American Depository Receipts (ADRs),
    379, 655
Andean Pact, 270, 287–288
Antidumping policies, 186, 602–603
Arbitrage, 322
Argentina's currency board, 358
Asia Pacific Economic Cooperation
    (APEC), 268, 290–291
Asian financial crisis of 1997–1998,
    23–24, 74, 79, 319, 330–333, 357,
    364–368, 548
  collapse of the Thai Baht, 339–341
  the crisis, 366–368
  debt bomb, 365
  excess capacity, 365
  expanding imports, 366
  investment boom, 364–365
Association of Southeast Asian Nations
    (ASEAN), 290
Attractiveness of a country as a market
    and/or an investment site, 77–80
  benefits, 77–78
  costs, 78–79
  economic risk, 79
  legal risk, 80
  overall attractiveness, 80
  political risk, 79
Auditing standards, 650, 652
Automobile industry, world, 424–425

Backward vertical foreign direct
    investment, 229

Balance-of-payments accounts,
    248–250, 252
Balance of trade, 147–148, 196
  adjustment to, 354, 355
  foreign direct investment and,
    248–250, 252
Balance-of-trade equilibrium, 347
Bandwagon effect, 319, 330
Banking crisis, 359
Bargaining power, 259–260
Barriers to trade and investment
  declining, 9–12
  firm strategy and, 205–206
  tariffs, *see* Tariffs
Barter, 548
"Big Mac Index," 324, 325
Bilateral netting, 682
Bill of lading, 545
Bolivia, 326–327
Brazil
  bailing out, 403–404
  marketing in, 586
Bretton Woods system, 345, 348–351
  collapse of, 346, 350–351
  IMF and, *see* International
    Monetary Fund (IMF)
  World Bank and, *see* World Bank
Bribery, 81–82, 121
Buddhism, 104
Bureaucratic controls, 458
Buy America Act, 184
Buybacks, 549

Canada
  NAFTA and, *see* North American
    Free Trade Agreement
    (NAFTA)
  softwood lumber dispute, 303–306
Capital, sources of, 647–648
Capital account, 248–249
Capital budgeting, 669–670
  risk and, 672–673
Capital flight, 335
Capital market; *see* Global capital
    market
Capitalism and the Protestant work
    ethic, 98, 100
Caribbean Community
    (CARICOM), 289
Cartagena Agreement, 287
Cases
  Artais Weather Check, 552–554
  bailing out Brazil, 403–404
  BP, 514
  collapse of the Thai Baht in 1997,
    339–341
  comparing Ghana and South Korea,
    306–307
  Cretors & Co., 694
  Degrussa: strategy and human
    resources in China, 643
  Deutsche Bank's pan-European
    retail banking strategy,
    298–299
  Dixon Ticonderoga, 311–312
  Ecuadorian Valentine roses, 36–37
  Ford and General Motors in Russia,
    236–237
  global strategy at General Motors,
    436–437
  International Monetary Fund,
    405–406
  Li & Fung, 580–581

  managed trade in the
    semiconductor industry,
    307–311
  McDonald's and Hindu culture, 125
  Merrill Lynch in Japan, 510–511
  money change, 402–403
  Motorola's global cash management
    system, 688–692
  Nike: the sweatshop debate,
    128–131
  organizational change at Royal
    Dutch/Shell, 476–477
  Philips *versus* Matsushita, 517–531
  piracy in the video game market,
    86–87
  politics of trade in steel, 302–303
  Procter & Gamble in Japan,
    613–614
  Qualcom's Chinese odyssey,
    132–135
  restructuring Exide, 514–517
  Royal Dutch/Shell: human rights in
    Nigeria, 136–139
  softwood lumber dispute, 303–306
  Starbucks video case, 302
  surging Samurai bond market,
    398–399
  tax breaks as export subsidies,
    210–211
  Toyota in France, 263–264
Cash balances, 674
Cash flows, 670
Centralization, 444
  decentralization *versus*, 445–446
Centralized depositories, 680–681
China
  accounting in, 664–665
  changing world order and, 22–23
  Degrussa: strategy and human
    resources in, 643
  foreign direct investment in,
    218–219
  guanxi in, 89–90, 105–106, 119,
    120
  marketing Coca-Cola in, 583, 584
  most favored nation status, 190–191
  Philips in, 560
  Qualcomm in, 132–135
  retaliatory trade policy and, 188
Christianity, 98
  economic implications of, 98, 100
Civil law system, 49–50
Class consciousness, 97
Class system, 91, 96–97
Collectivism, 43–44, 45
  individualism *versus*, 111, 112
Command economy, 48
Common law system, 49
Common market, 270
Communication strategy, 592–598
  channel length, 595
  country of origin effects, 593
  cultural barriers to, 592–593, 594
  global advertising, 597–598
  media availability, 595–596
  noise levels, 594
  product type and consumer
    sophistication, 595
  push *versus* pull strategies, 595–597
  source effects, 593
Communism, 44
  foreign direct investment and,
    240–241

Communist totalitarianism, 46
Comparative advantage, 144, 145,
    150–157
  basic message of, 153
  defined, 151
  diminishing returns, 154–156
  dynamic effects and economic
    growth, 156–157
  extensions of the Ricardian model,
    153–157
  gains from trade, 151–153
  immobile resources and, 154
  management focus, 155
  qualifications and assumptions, 153
  trade and growth, 157
Compensation, 632–637
  for expatriates, 634–637
  national differences in, 632–634
Competition
  foreign direct investment and,
    250–252
  pricing strategy and, 603
Competitive advantage
  culture and, 117–119
  at Dell Computer, 555–556
  national, *see* National competitive
    advantage
Confucian dynamism, 112–113
Confucianism, 89, 104–106
  economic implications of, 105–106
Congo, 374–376
Consolidated financial statements,
    654–657
Consumer protection, 188–190
Consumer tastes and preferences,
    424–426
Containerization, 14
Contract, 50
Contract law, 50–51
Control systems, 458–459, 658–661
  bureaucratic, 458
  cultural, 459
  defined, 442
  exchange rate changes and,
    659–660
  main steps of, 658
  output, 458–459
  performance ambiguity and,
    460–463
  personal, 458
  separation of subsidiary and
    manager performance, 661
  transfer pricing and, 660–661
Convention on Combating Bribery of
    Foreign Public Officials in
    International Business
    Transactions, 82
Copyrights, 53
Core competencies, 421
  entry strategy and, 496
Corruption, 52–53, 54
  ethics and, 81–82
Cost of capital, 381–382
  foreign exchange risk and, 394–395
Cost reduction, 422–424
  entry strategy and, 496–497
  make-or-buy decisions and, 568,
    571–572
Council of Ministers (EU), 270, 276
Counterpurchase, 548
Countertrade, 547–550
  barter, 548
  buybacks, 549

counterpurchase, 548
currency convertibility and,
      335–336
incidence of, 547–548
offset, 548
pros and cons of, 549–550
switch trading, 548–549
Countervailing duties, 186
Country of origin effects, 593
Crisis management by the IMF, 359–370
Argentina, 358
Asian, see Asian financial crisis of
      1997-1998
evaluating policy prescriptions,
      368–370
inappropriate policies, 368
lack of accountability, 369
Mexico, 360–361, 362
moral hazard, 369
observations, 369–370
in the post-Bretton Woods era,
      359–360
Russia, 361–364
Turkey, 343–344
types of crises, 359
Cross-cultural literacy, 90, 117
Cross-functional teams, 608
Cultural controls, 459
Cultural myopia, 622
Cultural toughness, 627–628
Cultural training, 629
Culture, 88–139
accounting system and, 649–650
as barrier to communication,
      592–593, 594
business ethics and, 119–121
changes in, 113–116
competitive advantage and, 117–119
cross-cultural literacy, 90, 117
defined, 91
determinants of, 93
education and, 107–108, 109
folkways and, 91–92
introduction, 90–91
managerial implications, 116–121
marketing and, 587–588, 598
mores and, 92
nation-state and, 92–93
norms and, 91–92
organizational, see Organizational
      culture
religions and, 98–106, see also
      specific religions
social structure, see Social structure
society and, 91, 92–93
spoken language and, 106–107
values and, 91–92
workplace and, 108, 111–113
Currency boards, 357
Argentinean, 358
Currency conversion, 317–318
Currency convertibility, 334–336
Currency crisis, 359
Currency management, 370
Currency speculation, 317–318
Currency swaps, 321
Currency translation, 657–658
Current account, 248–249
Current account deficit, 248
Current account surplus, 248
Current cost accounting, 649
Current rate method of currency
      translation, 657

Customs union, 270

D'Amato Act, 190
Debt loan, 381
Debt relief movement, 30
Decentralization, 445
centralization versus, 445–446
Deferred principle, 676
Demand conditions, 166–167
Demand elasticity, 599–600
Democracy, 46
economic progress and, 65–66
Demographics of globalization, 16–24
changing world order, 22–23
foreign direct investment, 18–19
global economy of the 21st century,
      23–24
multinational enterprises, 19–22
world output and world trade, 16–18
Department of Commerce, U.S.,
      538–539
Deregulation, 73
Dharma, 102
Differentiation strategy, 412
Diminishing returns, 154–156
Dirty float, 345
Distribution channels, 426–427
Distribution strategy, 589–592
channel exclusivity, 591
channel length, 590–591, 595
choosing a, 591–592
differences between countries,
      589–591
retail concentration, 590
typical distribution system, 589
Divided remittances, 676–677
Domestic rivalry, 167–168
Draft, 544
Dumping, 186
antidumping actions of the WTO,
      202–203
Dynamic effects of trade, 156–157

East African Community (EAC),
      291–292
Eclectic paradigm, 228–229
Economic development, 57–66
broader conceptions of, 62
democracy and, 65–66
differences in, 57–62
geography, education and, 66
innovation and entrepreneurship,
      62–65
market economy and, 64
marketing and, 588
political economy and, 62–66
required political system and, 65
strong property rights and, 64–65
Economic exposure, 684
reducing, 685–686
Economic independence, 252
Economic risk, 79, 672
Economic systems, 47–49
command economy, 48
costs of doing business and, 78
market economy, 47–48
mixed economy, 48–49
Economic union, 270
Economies of scale, 162
experience curve and, 419–420
Ecuador, 36–37
Education, 66
culture and, 107–108, 109

Efficient market, 324, 331
Elasticity of demand, 599–600
Electronic data interchange (EDI),
      576–577
Employment effects of foreign direct
      investment, 246–248
Ending spot exchange rate, 659–660
Entrepreneurship, 62–65
culture and, 94, 118, 119
Entry strategy, 478–500
acquisitions, 497–499, 500
basic decisions, 481–486
core competencies and, 496
cost reductions and, 496–497
Diebold and, 479
exporting, 487–488
franchising, 492–493
green-field ventures, 499–500
introduction, 480
joint ventures, 493–494
licensing agreements, 488–492
management know-how and, 496
scale of entry, 482–483
selecting a mode, 495–497
strategic alliances, see Strategic
      alliances
strategic commitments, 483
technological know-how and, 496
timing of entry, 482
turnkey projects, 488
which foreign markets?, 481
wholly owned subsidiaries, 494–495,
      497–500
Environmental issues, 27–29
GATT and, 199–202
Equal Employment Opportunity
      Commission, 622
Equity loan, 381
Ethical systems, 98
Ethics
corruption and, 81–82
culture and, 119–121
human rights and, 80–81
regulations and, 80–82
Ethnocentric staffing, 621–622
Ethnocentrism, 117
Euro, 279–282
benefits of, 280–281
costs of, 281–282
early experience, 282
transition to, 402–403
Eurobonds, 392–394
attraction of, 393–394
Eurocurrency market, 390–392
attractions of, 391–392
defined, 390
drawbacks of, 392
genesis and growth of, 390–391
European automobile market, 267,
      268–269
European Central Bank (ECB),
      281, 402
European Coal Steel Community, 274
European Commission, 267, 276
media industry mergers and, 277
European Community (EC), 271–272,
      274–275; see also European
      Union (EU)
European Council, 275–276
European Court of Justice, 278
European Parliament, 270, 278
European Union (EU), 144, 273,
      274–284, 293, 294–295

accounting standards and, 649, 654
agricultural subsidies in, 179,
      182–183
automobile industry in, 267,
      268–269
Common Agricultural Policy,
      182–183, 187, 193
enlargement of, 282–284
establishment of the Euro, 279–282
evolution of, 274–275
political structure of, 275–278
protecting consumers in, 188–190
Single European Act and, 278–279
steel industry in, 303
tax breaks and, 211
Exchange rates
arbitrage and, 322
bandwagon effect, 319, 330
control systems and, 659–660
currency boards and, 357–358
currency translation and, 657–658
defined, 316
economic theories and, 323–331
fixed, see Fixed exchange rates
floating, see Floating exchange rates
forecasting, see Forecasting
      exchange rates
forward, 320–321, 660
interest rates and, 329–330
investor psychology and, 330–331
law of one price and, 323–324
money supply and price inflation,
      326–328
pegged, 344–345, 356–357
in practice, 356–358
prices and, 323–329
purchasing power parity and,
      324–326, 328–329
spot, 318–320, 659–660
summary, 331
Expatriate managers, 623–628
compensation for, 634–637
defined, 618
failure rates, 624–627
repatriation of, 629–630
at Royal Dutch/Shell, 626
selection of, 627–628
training for, 629
Expatriates, 623
Experience curve pricing, 602
Experience curves, 418–420
economies of scale, 419–420
learning effects, 419
strategic significance, 420
Export management company
      (EMC), 539
Export-Import Bank, 546
Exporting, 534–553
assistance with, 546–547
countertrade, see Countertrade
credit insurance, 546–547
as entry strategy, 487–488, 495
export management companies, 539
Export-Import Bank, 546
financing, see Financing exports and
      imports
improving performance of, 537–541
information sources, 538–539
international comparison, 538
introduction, 536
Megahertz Communications, 535
promise and pitfalls of, 536–537
strategy of, 539–541

Externalities, 228
Externally convertible currency, 334–335

Factor endowments, 158, 166
Federal Aviation Administration (FAA), 552, 553
Fees, 677
Financial Accounting Standards Board (FASB), 653, 654
Financial management, 666–694
  financing decisions, 673–674
  foreign exchange risk, *see* Foreign exchange risk
  global treasury management, 667
  introduction, 668–669
  investment decisions, *see* Investment decisions
  money management, *see* Money management
  moving money across borders, *see* Moving money across borders
Financial services, 198–199
  deregulation of, 387–388
Financing decisions, 673–674
Financing exports and imports, 541–546
  bill of lading, 545
  draft, 544
  lack of trust and, 542–543
  letter of credit and, 543–544
  typical international trade transaction, 545–546
Firm strategy, structure and rivalry, 167–168
First-mover advantage, 78, 164, 170–171, 192
First-mover disadvantages, 482
Fisher Effect, 329–330
Fixed costs, 423, 561
Fixed exchange rates
  Bretton Woods system, 348–351
  case for, 354–355
  collapse of, 350–351
  defined, 345
  floating rates compared to, 355
  monetary discipline and, 354
  speculation and, 354–355
  trade balance adjustments and, 355
  uncertainty and, 355
Flexible machine cells, 562–563
Flexible manufacturing technology, 562
Floating exchange rates, 351–353
  case for, 353–354
  defined, 344
  fixed rates compared to, 355
  Jamaica agreement, 351
  monetary policy autonomy and, 354
  since 1973, 351–353
  trade balance adjustments and, 354
Flow of foreign direct investment, 215
Folkways, 91–92
Forecasting exchange rates, 331–334
  efficient market school, 331
  fundamental analysis, 333–334
  inefficient market school, 332
  technical analysis, 334
Foreign bonds, 392–393
Foreign Corrupt Practices Act, 53, 81–82
Foreign Credit Insurance Association (FCIA), 546–547
Foreign debt crisis, 359
Foreign direct investment (FDI), 212–237

  in China, 218–219
  defined, 9, 214
  direction of, 217–220
  flow of, 215
  green-field investment, 214, 221–223
  gross fixed capital formation and, 219–220
  horizontal, *see* Horizontal foreign direct investment
  inflows of, 215, 217–220
  introduction, 214–215
  managerial implications, 231–233
  mergers and acquisitions, 214, 221–223
  multinational enterprises and, 19–22, 214
  outflows of, 215, 220–221
  political economy of, *see* Political economy of foreign direct investment
  reducing barriers to, 10, 11
  regional economic integration and, 271
  slumping, 2001 and 2002, 217
  source of, 220–221
  by Starbucks, 213–214
  stock of, 215
  trends in, 18–19, 215–217
  vertical, *see* Vertical foreign direct investment
  in the world economy, 215–223
Foreign exchange exposure, 683–684
Foreign exchange market, 314–341
  arbitrage and, 322
  Axis hedges the Euro, 315
  currency conversion, 317–318
  currency convertibility, 334–336
  currency swaps, 321
  defined, 316
  efficient markets, 324
  exchange rates, *see* Exchange rates
  functions of, 316–321
  introduction, 316
  managerial implications, 336
  nature of, 322–323
  risks and, *see* Foreign exchange risk
Foreign exchange risk
  cost of capital and, 394–395
  currency swaps, 321
  defined, 316
  economic exposure, 684
  forward exchange rates and, 320–321
  managing, 683–687
  reducing, 685–686
  spot exchange rates and, 318–320
  transaction exposure, 684–685
  translation exposure, 684
Foreign policy objectives, 190
Foreign portfolio investment (FPI), 214
Foreign Sales Corporation (FSC), 210–211
Foreign service premium, 636
Forward exchange, 320–321
Forward exchange rates, 320–321
  internal, 660
Forward vertical foreign direct investment, 229
France
  protesting globalization in, 27
  Toyota in, 263–264
Franchising, 232–233

  as entry strategy, 492–493, 495
Free trade, 144, 180
  foreign direct investment and, 241–242, 244
  revised case for, 193
Free trade area, 269–270
Free Trade Area of the Americas (FTAA), 268, 289–290
Freely convertible currency, 334–335
Fronting loans, 679–680
Fundamental equilibrium, 349

Galápagos Declaration, 287–288
G8 meetings, 25
General Agreement on Tariffs and Trade (GATT), 8, 9, 10, 29, 55, 180, 268
  avoiding regulations, 196
  objective of, 195
  services and intellectual property, 197
  Uruguay Round, 196
Generally accepted accounting principles (GAAP), 645
Geocentric staffing, 623
Geography, 66
Germany, adoption of international accounting standards in, 645–646
Ghana, 306–307
Global capital market, 378–406
  accounting standards and, 652, *see also* Accounting
  attractions of, 381–386
  benefits of, 380–386
  bonds, 392–394
  cost of capital and, 381–382, 394–395
  deregulation and, 387–388
  equity, 394
  eurocurrency, *see* Eurocurrency market
  functions of, 380–381
  growth of, 386–390
  home bias puzzle and, 386
  information technology and, 386–387
  introduction, 380
  lower cost of capital and, 381–382
  managerial implications, 395–396
  Mexico and, 388–389
  portfolio diversification and, 382–386
  risks and, 388–390, 394–395
  Samurai bond market, 398–399
Global expansion, 416–422
  caveats concerning, 418
  core competencies and, 421
  creating a global web, 417–418
  economies of scale, 419–420
  experience effects, 418–420
  introduction, 416
  learning effects, 419
  location economies, 417–418
  strategic significance, 420
  subsidiary skills and, 421–422
Global learning, 430
Global matrix structure, 451–453
Global strategy, 429
  organizational architecture and, 468, 469
Global supply chain, 573–577
  information technology and the Internet, 575–577

  just-in-time inventory, 573–574
  organizations and, 574–575
Global web, 417–418
Globalization, 2–37
  debate over, 24–30
  declining trade and investment barriers, 9–12
  defined, 6
  demographics, *see* Demographics of globalization
  drivers of, 9–16
  emergence of global institutions, 8–9
  environment and, 27–29
  introduction, 4–6
  labor policies and, 27–29
  management and, 31–32
  of markets, 6–7, 584–585
  national sovereignty and, 29
  pencil industry and, 311–312
  poverty and, 29–30
  of production, 7–8
  protests against, 4–5, 24–25, 26
  technological change, *see* Technological change
Gold par value, 346
Gold standard, 346–348
  between 1918–1939, 347–348
  balance-of-trade equilibrium and, 347
  defined, 346
  mechanics of, 346
  strength of, 347
Government intervention, 186–193
  consumer protection, 188–190
  economic arguments for, 191–193
  in the foreign exchange market, 345, 371–372
  foreign policy objectives and, 190
  human rights protection, 190–191
  infant industries, 191–192
  job and industry protection, 187
  national security, 187
  political arguments for, 187–191
  retaliation for rules-breaking, 188
  strategic trade policy, 192–193
Government policy
  foreign direct investment and, 224, 254–257
  political economy and, *see* Political economy of international trade
  trade theory and, 147, 166, 168, 171–172
Great Britain, class divisions in, 91, 96–97
Great Depression, 194–195
Green-field investments/ventures, 214, 221–223, 499–500
Gross fixed capital formation, 219–220
Gross national income per capita (GNI), 57–59
Group of Five, 353
Groups, 94, 95
Guanxi, 89–90, 105–106, 119, 120, 218

Heckscher-Ohlin theory, 144, 145, 157–159, 166
  Leontief paradox and, 158–159
Hedge fund, 318
Helms-Burton Act, 190
Highly indebted poorer countries (HIPCs), 30
Hinduism, 102–104

economic implications of, 103–104
McDonald's and, 125
Historic cost principle, 649
Home countries and foreign direct
investments
benefits, 252, 253
costs, 252–253
government policies and, 254–255
international trade theory and,
253–254
Horizontal differentiation, 446–453
in an international division, 447–449
in domestic firms, 446–447
global matrix structure, 451–453
worldwide area structure, 449–450
worldwide product divisional
structure, 450–451
Horizontal foreign direct investment,
223–229
defined, 215
export impediments, 224
location-specific advantages and,
228–229
managerial implications, 231–233
market imperfections, 224–226
multipoint competition and, 227
oligopoly and, 226–227
product life cycle and, 227–228
sale of know-how, impediments to,
224–226
strategic behavior and, 226–227
transportation costs, 224
Hormone-treated beef, 188, 189
Host country benefits of foreign direct
investment, 244–251
balance-of-payments effects,
248–250
capital resources, 239, 245
competition and economic growth,
250–251
employment, 246–248
government policies and, 255–256
management, 246
resource-transfer effects, 244–246
technology, 245–246
Host country costs of foreign direct
investment, 251–252
balance of payments, 252
competition, 251–252
government policies and, 255–256
national sovereignty and
autonomy, 252
Host-government demands, 427
Human Development Index (HDI), 62
Human resources management (HRM),
616–643
compensation, 632–637
defined, 618
expatriates, see Expatriate managers
international labor relations,
637–639
introduction, 618–619
performance appraisal, 631–632
staffing policy, see Staffing policy
strategic role of international,
619–620
training and management
development, 628–631
Human rights, 80–81
government intervention and
protection of, 190–191
in Nigeria, 136–139
WTO and, 200–201
Hyperinflation, 326–327

Immobile resources, 154
Import quotas, 183–184
navigating around, 185
quota rent and, 184
Imports, financing; see Financing
exports and imports
Incentives, 459–460
defined, 442
performance ambiguity and,
460–463
India
changing political economy of,
41–42
Hinduism and, 102–104
selling to the poor in, 596
software industry in, 175–176
Individualism, 44–46
collectivism versus, 111, 112
Individuals, 94–95
Inefficient market, 332
Infant industries, 191–192
Inflation, 76, 672
accounting for, 649
interest rates and, 329–330
money supply and, 326–328
Inflows of foreign direct investment,
215, 217–220
Information sources, exporting, 538–593
Information technology, 386–387
global supply chain and, 575–577
Infrastructure and traditional
practices, 426
Initial spot exchange rates, 659–660
Innovation, 62–65
Inpatriates, 623–624
Integrating mechanisms, 453–457
formal, 455–456
impediments to coordination,
454–455
informal, 456–457
management networks, 456–457
strategy of the firm and
coordination, 453–454
summary, 457
Intellectual property, protection of,
53–57
GATT and, 197
threat of retaliation and, 188
WTO and, 204
Interest rates and exchange rates,
329–330
Internal forward rate of exchange, 660
Internalization theory, 224
International Accounting Standards
Board (IASB), 645, 646, 649,
652–654
International Accounting Standards
Committee (IASC), 645, 652, 655
International accounting standards
(IAS), 645–646; see also
Accounting
International Bank for Reconstruction
and Development (IBRD); see
World Bank
International Court of Arbitration for
the International Chamber of
Commerce, 51
International Development Agency
(IDA), 350
International Fisher Effect (IFE), 330
International institutions, 256–257; see
also specific institutions
International Labor Organization
(ILO), 638

International labor relations, 637–639
approaches to, 638–639
concerns of organized labor,
637–638
strategy of organized labor, 638
International Monetary Fund (IMF), 25,
243, 332
Brazil and, 403–404
case study, 405–406
crisis management by, see Crisis
management by the IMF
described, 8, 345–346
discipline and, 348–349
flexibility and, 349
role of, 348–349
Turkey's 18th program, 343–344
Zaire and, 375
International monetary system, 342–376
Argentina's currency board, 358
Bretton Woods system, see Bretton
Woods system
business strategy, 370–371
corporate-government relations,
371–372
currency management, 370
defined, 344
exchange rates and, see Exchange
rates
gold standard, see Gold standard
IMF, see International Monetary
Fund (IMF)
introduction, 344–346
management implications, 370–372
World Bank, see World Bank
International strategy, 428–429
organizational architecture and,
468, 469
International trade, 9
International trade secretariats (ITSs),
638
International trade theory, 142–176
absolute advantage, 144, 148–150
benefits of trade, 144–145
comparative advantage, see
Comparative advantage
economies of scale and, 162
first-mover advantage and, 164,
170–171
foreign direct investment and,
253–254
free trade, 144
government policy and, 147, 166,
168, 171–172
Heckscher-Ohlin theory, 144, 145,
157–159
introduction, 144
learning effects and, 163
Leontief paradox and, 158–159
location and, 169–170
management implications, 169–172
mercantilism, 144, 147–148
national competitive advantage, see
National competitive
advantage
new trade theory, 147, 162–165
overview of, 144–147
patterns of international trade, 145,
147
political economy and, see Political
economy of international trade
as a positive-sum game, 148–150,
153
product life-cycle theory, 145, 147,
159–161

U.S. knowledge-based economy,
143
Internet
globalization of, 12–14
information technology and,
575–577
Investment decisions, 669–673
capital budgeting, 669–670
discount rate, 672–673
economic risk, 672
political risk, 670–672
project and parent cash flows, 670
Investor psychology, 330–331
Irish miracle, 239
Islam, 100–102
banking in Pakistan, 103
division within, 92
economic implications of, 102
fundamentalism, 70, 101–102
resurgence of, 69–70
Islamic law, 50

Jamaica agreement, 351
Japan
administrative trade policies in, 186
competitive advantage in, 117–118
criminals in, 51
cultural change in, 113–115
distribution channels in, 591, 592
domestic rivalry in, 167–168
education in, 108
group membership in, 95
Procter & Gamble in, 613–614
Samurai bond market, 398–399
semiconductor industry, 307–311
Jobs and industries, protection of, 187
Joint ventures, 493–494, 495
evolution of the Fuji-Xerox,
490–491
Just-in-time (JIT) inventory, 573–574

Karma, 102
Know-how, impediments to sale of,
224–226, 230

Labor policies, 27–29
Lag strategy, 685
Language, 106–107
Language training, 629
Late-mover advantage, 78
Law of one price, 323–324
Lead strategy, 685
Lean production, 562
Learning effects, 163, 419
Legal risk, 80
Legal systems, 49–57
civil law, 49–50
common law, 49
contract law and, 50–51
costs of doing business and, 78–79
defined, 49
economic transformation and,
75–76
property rights, 51–53
theocratic law, 50
Leontief paradox, 158–159
Lessard-Lorange model, 659–660
Letter of credit, 543–544
Licensing, 215, 225–226, 231–233
as entry strategy, 488–492, 495
of technology, 245
Local content requirement, 184–185
Local responsiveness, 424–427

consumer tastes and preferences, 424–426
distribution channels, 426–427
host-government demands, 427
implications, 427
infrastructure and traditional practices, 426
"world cars," 424–425
Location economies, 417–418
Location of productive activities, 169–170
Location-specific advantages, 228–229
London Stock Exchange, 652
Long-term orientation, 112–113
Low cost strategy, 412
Lumber industry, 303–306

Maastricht Treaty, 279–281
Mafia, 51
Make-or-buy decisions, 568–573
advantages of buy, 570–572
advantages of make, 568–570
at Boeing, 570
strategic alliances, 572–573
tradeoffs, 572
Management development strategy, 630–631
Management focus
Atag Holdings NV, 294
Black Sea Energy Ltd., 671
Castrol Oil in Vietnam, 604
Comex's foreign acquisitions, 222–223
consequences of different accounting standards, 653
Deutsche Telekom taps the global capital market, 383
drug patents and the AIDS epidemic in South Africa, 56
European Commission and media industry mergers, 277
evolution of the Fuji-Xerox joint venture, 490–491
executive pay policies for global managers, 635
exporting strategy at 3M, 540
foreign direct investment by Volvo in South Korea, 243
free trade and REI, 155
George Soros-the man who moved currency markets, 318–319
Hewlett-Packard in Singapore, 567
Homer Simpson, 15
IKEA, 430–431
international division at Abbott Laboratories, 449
international expansion at ING Group, 484–485
Jollibee Phenomenon, 486
make-or-buy decisions at Boeing, 570
managing expatriates at Royal Dutch/Shell, 626
marketing to black Brazilians, 586
Matsushita and Japan's changing culture, 114–115
Mexican peso crisis and the automobile industry, 362
Monsanto's repatriation program, 631
navigating around import quotas, 185
Novartis joins the international accounting club, 655

organizational culture and incentives at Lincoln Electric, 461
overcoming cultural barriers to selling tampons, 594
Philips in China, 560
political economy, 77–82
Red Spot Paint & Varnish, 541
rise and fall of Dow Chemical's matrix structure, 452–453
rise of Finland's Nokia, 168–169
tailoring world cars to the U.S. market, 425
Unilever-selling to India's poor, 596
Wipro Ltd., 21
Management networks, 456–457
Management skills and foreign direct investment, 246
Manufacturing and materials management, 554–581
competitive advantage, 555–556
country factors, 559, 565
defined, 556–557
facilities location, 564–565
global supply chain, see Global supply chain
introduction, 556
make-or-buy, see Make-or-buy decisions
product factors, 564, 565
six sigma and, 558
strategic role of foreign factories, 565–568
strategy and, 556–558
technological factors, see Technological factors in locating manufacturing activities
total quality management and, 557–558
where to manufacture, 558–565
Maps
accounting clusters, 651
adult illiteracy rates, 110
APEC members, 291
economic freedom, 72
economic integration in the Americas, 284
European Union countries and applicants, 275
gross national income per capita, 58
growth in gross domestic product, 61
human development index, 63
percent of GNP spent on education, 109
political freedom, 68
purchasing power parity, 60
shape of the European Union after enlargement, 283
trade blocs in Africa, 292
world religions, 99
Market economy, 47–48
innovation, entrepreneurship and, 64
spread of, see States in transition
Market imperfections, 224–226, 230–231
Market makers, 381
Market segmentation, 585–587
Marketing, 582–614
advertising, 597–598
attributes of products and, 587–589
to black Brazilians, 586
Coca-Cola in China, 583, 584
communication strategy, see Communication strategy

cultural differences and, 587–588, 598
distribution strategy, see Distribution strategy
economic development and, 588
globalization of markets and brands, 584–585
introduction, 584
managerial implications, 608–609
new product development, 605–608
pricing strategy, see Pricing strategy
product and technical standards and, 588–589
segmentation of, 585–587
Unilever in India, 596
Marketing mix, 584
configuring the, 603–605
Markets, globalization of, 6–7
technological change and, 16
Masculinity versus femininity, 111, 112
Mass customization, 562
Materials management, 556–557; see also Manufacturing and materials management
Media availability, 595–596
Mercantilism, 144, 147–148
MERCOSUR, 268, 270, 288–289
Mergers and acquisitions, 214, 221–223
Mexico
currency crisis of 1995, 360–361, 362
global capital market and, 388–389
IBM's operations in, 241, 258–260
NAFTA, see North American Free Trade Agreement (NAFTA)
textile manufacturers in, 272–273
Microprocessors, 12
Minimum efficient scale, 561
Mixed economy, 48–49
Monetary discipline, 354
Monetary policy autonomy, 354
Money management, 674–676
centralized depositories, 680–681
defined, 674
minimizing cash balances, 674
multilateral netting, 681–683
reducing transaction costs, 675
taxes and, 675–676
transfer fee and, 675
Moral hazard, 369
Mores, 92
Morgan Guarantee Index, 352
Most favored nation (MFN) status, 190–191
Moving money across borders, 676–680
dividend remittances, 676–677
fronting loans, 679–680
royalty payments and fees, 677
transfer prices, 677–679
Mudarabah contract, 103
Multidomestic strategy, 429
organization architecture and, 468–469
Multilateral agreement on investment (MAI), 256–257
Multilateral netting, 681–683
Multinational enterprises (MNEs); see also Foreign direct investment (FDI)
defined, 214
demographics of, 19–22
mini-, 22
non-U.S., 20–21
political ideology and, 240–241

Multipoint competition, 227
Multipoint pricing, 601–602
Murabaha contract, 103

National competitive advantage, 147, 165–169
demand conditions and, 166–167
evaluation of theory, 168–169
factor endowments and, 165, 166
firm strategy, structure, and rivalry, 166, 167–168
related and supporting industries, 166, 167
National Science Foundation (NSF), 606–607
National security, 187
National sovereignty, 29
foreign direct investment and, 252
Nation-state, 92–93
Negotiations, 257–260
New-product development, 605–608
New trade theory, 147, 162–165
economies of scale and, 162
first-mover advantage and, 164
learning effects and, 163
New world order, 69–70
New York Stock Exchange (NYSE), 645, 652
Nigeria
corruption in, 54
human rights in, 136–139
Nirvana, 102–104
Noise levels, 594
Nonconvertible currency, 335
Nonverbal communications, 107
Norms, 91–92
North American Free Trade Agreement (NAFTA), 144, 155, 182, 257, 258, 268, 270, 285–287, 293, 294, 388
accounting standards and, 649, 654
case against, 285–286
case for, 285
contents of, 285
enlargement of, 287
first decade of, 286–287
labor and environmental issues and, 28
U.S. textile industry and, 272–273

Offsets, 548, 572
Ogoni people, 136–138
Oligopoly, 226–227
Organization for Economic Cooperation and Development (OECD), 27, 28, 82, 246, 247, 256, 638
Organization of International Business, 438–477
centralization, 444, 445–446
change and, see Organizational change
control systems and, see Control systems
culture and, see Organizational culture
decentralization, 445–446
environment, strategy, and performance, 470
global firms and, 468, 469
horizontal differentiation, see Horizontal differentiation
incentives and, see Incentives
integrating mechanisms, see Integrating mechanisms
international firms and, 468, 469

introduction, 440–441
multidomestic firms and, 468–469
organizational change at Unilever, 439–444
people and, 442
performance ambiguity and, 460–463
processes and, 442, 463–464
transnational firms and, 468, 469–470
vertical differentiation, 444–446
Organization of Petroleum Exporting Countries (OPEC), 54, 351–352, 390–391
Organizational architecture, 440–44
strategy and, 468–470
Organizational change, 470–473
implementing, 472–473
inertia, 471–472
moving to the new state, 472
refreezing, 472–473
at Royal Dutch/Shell, 476–477
unfreezing, 472
Organizational culture, 464–468
creating and maintaining, 465–466
defined, 442, 464–465
incentives and, 461
performance and, 466–468
"strong," 466–468
Organizational structure, 441–457
Organized labor; see International labor relations
Others-orientation, 627
Outflows of foreign direct investment, 215, 220–221
Output controls, 458–459
Outsourcing, 7

Pakistan, banking in, 103
Paris Convention for the Protection of Industrial Property, 54–55
Patents, 53–54
drug, 56
Pegged exchange rates, 344–345, 356–357
Pencil industry, 311–312
People, 442
Perceptual ability, 627
Performance ambiguity, 460–463
Personal controls, 458
Pioneering costs, 482
Plaza Accord, 353
Political economy, national differences in, 40–87
attractiveness of a country as a market and/or investment site, 77–80
command economy, 48
corruption and, 81–82
economic development and, see Economic development
economic systems, 47–49
ethics and, 80–82
human rights and, 80–81
India, 41–42
intellectual property, 53–57
introduction, 42–43
legal systems, see Legal systems
market economy, 47–48
mixed economy, 48–49
political systems, see Political systems
product liability, 57
product safety, 57
property rights, 51–53

regulations and, 81
states in transition, see States in transition
Political economy of foreign direct investment, 238–264
benefits to host countries, see Host country benefits of foreign direct investment
costs to host countries, 251–252
free market view of, 241–242, 244
government policy instruments and, 254–256
home countries and, see Home countries and foreign direct investments
ideology and, 240–244
international institutions and, 256–257
introduction, 240
Irish miracle, 239
managerial implications, 257–260
nature of negotiations, 257–260
pragmatic nationalism and, 242, 244
radical view of, 240–241, 244
Venezuela's petroleum industry, 247
Political economy of international trade, 178–211
agricultural subsidies and development, 179
development of the world trading system, see World trading systems
domestic politics and, 193
government intervention, see Government intervention
introduction, 180
managerial implications, 205–207
policy implications, 206–207
retaliation and trade war, 193
revised case for free trade, 193
trade barriers and firm strategy, 205–206
trade policy instruments, see Trade policy instruments
WTO and, see World Trade Organization (WTO)
Political risk, 79, 670–672
Political systems, 43–47
collectivism, 43–44
communism, 44
costs of doing business and, 78
defined, 43
democracy, 46
individualism, 44–46
social democracy, 44
socialism, 43–44
totalitarianism, 46–47
Political union, 270
Polycentric staffing, 622
Porter's diamond; see National competitive advantage
Portfolio's diversification, 382–386
Position-sum game, 148–150, 153
Poverty, 29–30
Power distance, 111, 112
Practical training, 629
Pragmatic nationalism, 242, 244
Predatory pricing, 601
Price discrimination, 598–599
profit maximizing under, 600–601
Price elasticity of demand, 599

determinants of, 599–600
Prices and exchange rates, 323–329
Pricing strategy, 598–603
antidumping regulations, 602–603
competition policy and, 603
determinants of demand elasticity, 599–600
discriminatory, 598–599
experience curve, 602
multipoint, 601–602
predatory, 601
profit maximizing, 600–601
strategic, 601–602
Private action, 51
Privatization, 44, 73–75
Processes, 442, 463–464
Product attributes, marketing of, 587–589
Product factors and location decisions, 564, 565
Product liability, 57
Product life-cycle theory, 145, 147, 159–161
foreign direct investment and, 227–228
Product safety, 57
Production, globalization of, 7–8
integrating R&D, marketing and, 607
technological change and, 15–16
Production possibility frontier (PPF), 149, 154, 156–157
Profit, 411
maximizing, under price discrimination, 600–601
Profitability, 411
Projected spot exchange rate, 659–660
Property rights, 51–53
corruption, 52–53, 54
defined, 51
Foreign Corrupt Practices Act, 53
innovation, entrepreneurship, and, 64–65
private action and, 51
public action and, 52
Protectionism
costs of, 182
pressures for greater, 195–196
WTO and, 203–204
Protestant work ethic, 98, 100
Public action, 52
Pull strategy, 595–597
Purchasing power parity (PPP), 59, 60, 324–326
empirical tests of, 328–329
Push strategy, 595–597

Quota rent, 184

Radical political ideology, 240–241, 244
Regional economic integration, 266–300
in Africa, 291–292
Andean Pact, 287–288
APEC, 290–291
ASEAN, 290
CARICOM, 289
case against, 273–274
Central American Common Market, 289
common market, 270
customs union, 270

defined, 268
economic case for, 271
economic union, 270
in Europe, see European Union (EU)
European automobile market, 267, 268–269
free trade area, 269–270
FTAA, 289–290
impediments to, 272–273
introduction, 268–269
levels of, 269–270
managerial implications, 292–295
MERCOSUR, 288–289
NAFTA, see North American Free Trade Agreement (NAFTA)
political case for, 271–272
political union, 270
trade creation and, 274
trade diversion and, 274
Regulations and ethics, 81
Related and supporting industries, 166, 167
Relational capital, 504
Religion, 98; see also specific religions
Repatriation of expatriates, 629–630, 631
Representative democracy, 46
Research and development (R&D), 605–608
cross-functional teams, 608
integrating marketing, production, and, 607, 608–609
introduction, 584, 605
location of, 605–607
Resource-transfer effects of foreign direct investment, 244–246
Retail concentration, 590
Retaliation
trade war and, 193
for trade-policy rules-breaking, 188
Right-wing totalitarianism, 47
Risks
capital budgeting and, 672–673
of doing business, 79–80
economic, 79, 672
foreign exchange, see Foreign exchange risk
global capital market, 388–390
political, 79, 670–672
systematic, 384
Royalties, 677
Russia
Black Sea Energy Ltd. in, 671
criminals in, 51
Ford and General Motors in, 236–237

Scheduling, 569–570
Sea turtles, 200–201
Securities and Exchange Commission (SEC), 645, 654
Self-orientation, 627
Semiconductor industry, 307–311
September 11, 10, 70, 217, 570, 574
Short selling, 318
Sight draft, 544
"Simpsons, The," 15
Singapore, 565–568
Single European Act, 267, 278–279
Six sigma, 558
Smoot-Hawley tariff, 195
Social democrats, 44
Social mobility, 96

Social structure, 93–98
class consciousness, 97
class system, 91, 96–97
groups and, 94, 95
individuals and, 94–95
mobility, 96–97
stratification, 96–98
Socialism, 43–44
Society, 91
nation-state and, 92–93
Softwood Lumber Agreement (SLA), 303–306
Source effects, 593
Sourcing decisions; *see* Make-or-buy decisions
South Africa, drug patents and AIDS in, 56–57
South Korea
collapse of the won, 332–333
foreign direct investment by Volvo in, 243
Ghana compared to, 306–307
Specific tariffs, 181
Speculation, currency, 354–355
Spoken language, 106–107
Spot exchange rates, 318–320
Lessard-Lorange model of, 659–660
Staffing policy, 620–628
ethnocentric, 621–622
expatriate managers, 623–628
geocentric, 623
introduction, 620–621
polycentric, 622
summary, 623
States in transition, 66–77
deregulation and, 73
implications of, 76–77
legal systems and, 75–76
nature of economic transformation, 73–76
new world order and global terrorism, 69–71
privatization and, 73–75
rocky road for, 76
spread of democracy, 67–69
spread of market-based systems, 71–73
Steel industry, 302–303
Stock of foreign direct investment, 215
Strategic alliances, 480, 500–505
advantages of, 500–501
building trust, 504
defined, 500
disadvantages of, 501–502
learning from partners, 504–505
make-or-buy decisions and, 572–573
managing, 504–505
partner selection, 502
structure of, 502–504
Strategic commitments, 483
Strategic pricing, 601–602
Strategic trade policy, 192–193; *see also* Trade policy instruments
Strategy of international business, 408–437
cost reduction and, 422–424
defined, 410–411
environment, architecture, and performance, 470
example of, 415–416
exporting, 539–541
firms and, 410–416

global expansion, *see* Global expansion
global strategy, 429, 468, 469
international strategy, 428–429, 468–469
introduction, 410
local responsiveness and, *see* Local responsiveness
at MTV Networks, 409–410
multidomestic strategy, 429, 468–469
profitability and, 411
strategic choices, 427–433
transnational strategy, 429–433, 468, 469–470
value chain and, 413–415
value creation and, 411–413
Strong culture, 466–467
Subsidiary skills, 421–422
Subsidies, 179, 181–183
as tax breaks, 210–211
Summit of the Americas, 289–290
Switch trading, 548–549
Systematic risk, 384

Taiwan, privatization in, 74
Tariffs, 9–10, 181
costs of, 182
Great Depression and, 195
lumber industry, 303–306
reduction of, 195
steel industry, 302–303
Tax breaks, 210–211
Tax credit, 675
Tax havens, 676
Tax treaty, 675–676
Taxes
expatriate compensation and, 637
fronting loans and, 679–680
global money management and, 675–676
transfer prices and, 677–679
Technical standards, 588–589
Technological change, 12–16
Internet/World Wide Web, 12–14
market globalization and, 16
microprocessors, 12
production globalization and, 15–16
telecommunications, 12
transportation, 13, 14
Technological factors in locating manufacturing activities, 559–564
fixed costs, 561
flexible machine cells, 562–563
flexible manufacturing, 562
mass customization, 562
minimum efficient scale, 561
other factors compared to, 565
summary, 563–564
Technology
benefits of, and foreign direct investment, 245–246
entry strategy and, 496
information, 386–387, 575–577
proprietary protection, 569
Telecommunications, 12, 198
Temporal method of currency translation, 657–658
Terrorism, 69–71
Thailand, 339–341
Theocratic law system, 50
Theocratic totalitarianism, 46–47

Time, 92
Time draft, 544
Total quality management (TQM), 557–558
Totalitarianism, 46–47
Trade creation, 274
Trade diversion, 274
Trade policy instruments, 180–186
administrative trade policies, 185–186
antidumping policies, 186
import quotas, 183–184
local content requirement, 184–185
subsidies, 181–183
tariffs, 181
voluntary export restraint, 183–184
Trade Related Aspects of Intellectual Property Rights (TRIPS), 55, 204
Trade war, 193
Trademarks, 53
Training and management development, 628–631
Transaction costs, 675
Transaction exposure, 683–684
reducing, 685
Transfer fee, 675
Transfer pricing
control systems and, 660–661
efficiencies, taxes and, 677–679
Translation exposure, 684
reducing, 685
Transnational financing, 652
Transnational investment, 652
Transnational strategy, 429–433
organizational architecture and, 468, 469–470
Transportation costs, 224
Transportation technology, 13, 14
Treaty of Rome, 274–275
Tribal totalitarianism, 47
Turkey and the IMF, 343–344
Turnkey projects, 488, 495

Uncertainty avoidance, 111, 112
accounting standards and, 650
United Auto Workers (UAW), 638
United Nations Convention on Contracts for the International Sale of Goods (CIGS), 51
United Nations (UN), 9, 179, 189, 235, 537
United States
costs of protectionism in, 182
decline in share of world output, 17
hollowing out of knowledge-based economy, 143
lumber industry, 303–306
semiconductor industry in, 307–311
steel industry, 302–303
textile industry, 272–273
United Steelworkers of America, 302
United Students Against Sweatshops (USAS), 130
Universal Declaration of Human Rights, 119–120, 138
Unspoken language, 107

Value chain, firm as, 413–415
Value creation, 411–413
Values, 91–92
changes in, 114–115, 116
Venezuela's petroleum industry, 247

Vertical differentiation, 444–446
Vertical foreign direct investment, 229–231
backward, 229
defined, 215
forward, 229
investment in specialized assets, 230–231
managerial implications, 231–233
market imperfections, 230–231
sale of know-how impediments, 230
strategic behavior, 229–230
Vietnam, 604
Voluntary export restraint (VER), 171, 183–184, 187, 196

Wealth of Nations, The (Smith), 45, 148–149
wholly owned subsidiary, 494–495
establishing, 497–500
Workers Rights Consortium (WRC), 130–131
Workplace culture, 108, 111–113
World Bank, 25, 76, 196, 307
described, 8
role of, 349–350
World Health Organization, 189
World order, changing, 22–23
World Trade Organization (WTO), 5, 144, 193, 218, 387, 510
agricultural protectionism, 203–204
antidumping actions, 202–203
China and, 134, 560
creation of, 197
described, 8, 180
Doha round, 204
expanding trade agreements, 198–199
experience to date, 197–202
foreign direct investment and, 256, 257
future of, 202–205
as global policeman, 197–198
intellectual property rights, 55–56, 204
lowering trade barriers, 9–10
lumber tariffs and, 304–305
national sovereignty issue and, 29
protests against, 24, 199–202
regional integration and, 268, 271, 274
in Seattle, 199–202
steel tariffs and, 303
tax breaks and, 210–211
trade in hormone-treated beef and, 189, 190
World trading systems, 194–205
disturbing trends, 195–196
GATT, 195–197
from Smith to the Great Depression, 194–195
WTO, *see* World Trade Organization (WTO)
World Values Survey, 114–115
World Wide Web, 12–14, 16
Worldwide area structure, 449–450
Worldwide product divisional structure, 450–451

Zaire, 374–376
Zero-sum game, 148

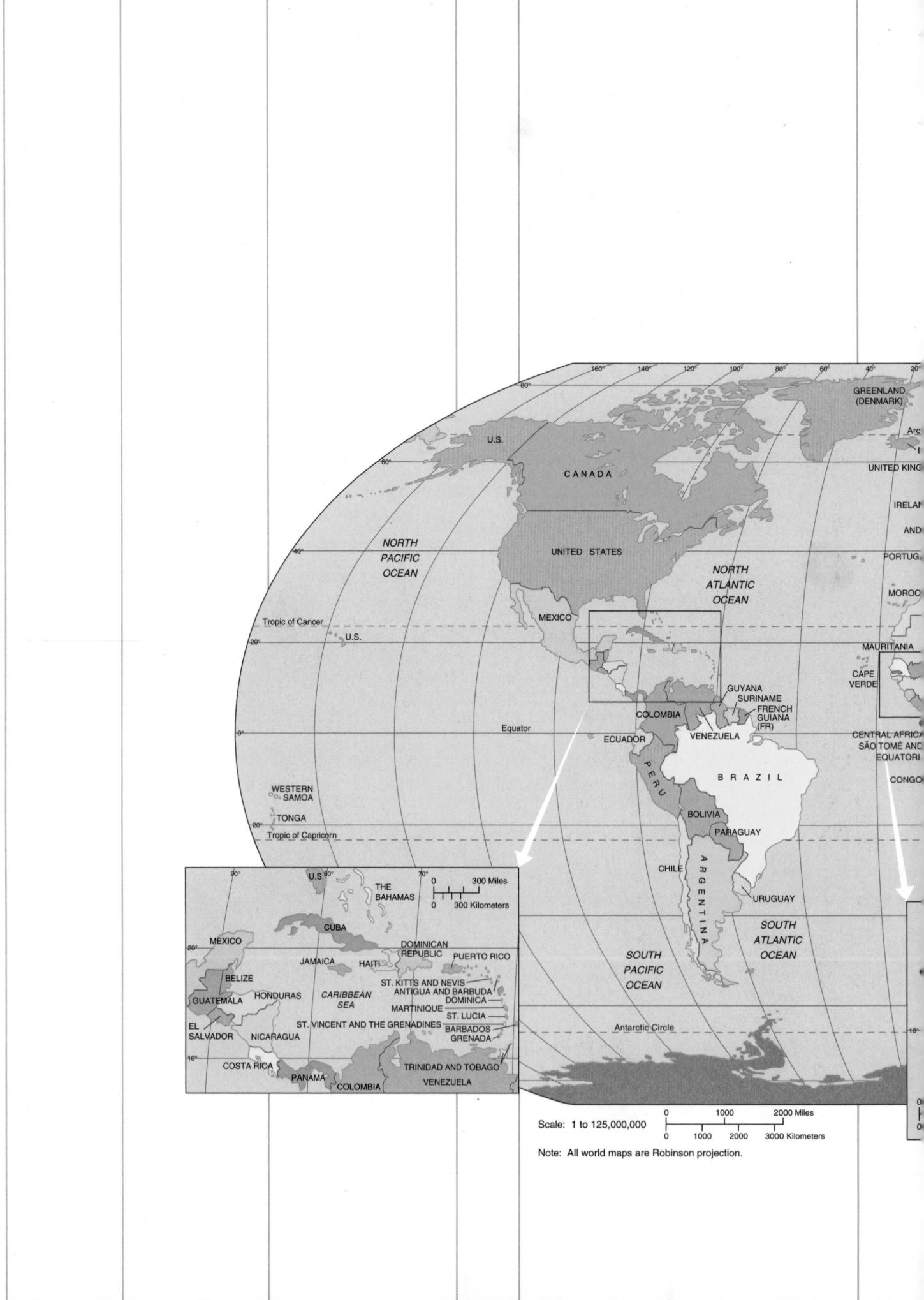

GREENLAND
(DENMARK)

Arc
I

UNITED KING

IRELAN

AND

PORTUG.

MOROC

U.S.

CANADA

NORTH
PACIFIC
OCEAN

UNITED STATES

NORTH
ATLANTIC
OCEAN

Tropic of Cancer

MEXICO

U.S.

MAURITANIA

CAPE
VERDE

GUYANA
SURINAME
FRENCH
GUIANA
(FR)

COLOMBIA

Equator

ECUADOR

VENEZUELA

CENTRAL AFRICA
SÃO TOMÉ AND
EQUATORI

BRAZIL

CONGO

PERU

WESTERN
SAMOA

TONGA

BOLIVIA

PARAGUAY

Tropic of Capricorn

CHILE

ARGENTINA

URUGUAY

SOUTH
ATLANTIC
OCEAN

SOUTH
PACIFIC
OCEAN

Antarctic Circle

U.S.

THE
BAHAMAS

0   300 Miles

0   300 Kilometers

CUBA

MEXICO

DOMINICAN
REPUBLIC

PUERTO RICO

JAMAICA

HAITI

BELIZE

GUATEMALA

HONDURAS

CARIBBEAN
SEA

ST. KITTS AND NEVIS
ANTIGUA AND BARBUDA
DOMINICA
MARTINIQUE
ST. LUCIA

EL
SALVADOR

NICARAGUA

ST. VINCENT AND THE GRENADINES

BARBADOS
GRENADA

COSTA RICA

PANAMA

COLOMBIA

TRINIDAD AND TOBAGO

VENEZUELA

Scale: 1 to 125,000,000

0   1000   2000 Miles

0   1000   2000   3000 Kilometers

Note: All world maps are Robinson projection.